Equine Internal Medicine

Equine Internal Medicine

Stephen M. Reed, DVM, Dip ACVIM
Professor, Department of Clinical Sciences
College of Veterinary Medicine
The Ohio State University
Columbus, Ohio

Warwick M. Bayly, BVSc, MS
Robert B. McEachern Distinguished
  Professor in Equine Medicine
College of Veterinary Medicine
Washington State University
Pullman, Washington

W.B. SAUNDERS COMPANY
A Division of Harcourt Brace & Company
Philadelphia   London   Toronto   Montreal   Sydney   Tokyo

W.B. SAUNDERS COMPANY
A Division of Harcourt Brace & Company

The Curtis Center
Independence Square West
Philadelphia, Pennsylvania 19106

Library of Congress Cataloging-in-Publication Data

Equine internal medicine / [edited by] Stephen M. Reed, Warwick M. Bayly.

p.   cm.

ISBN 0–7216–3524–5

1. Horses—Diseases.   2. Veterinary internal medicine.   I. Reed, Stephen M.
   II. Bayly, Warwick M.   [DNLM: 1. Horse Diseases.   SF 951 E638 1997]

SF951.E565 1998   636.1'0896—dc20

DNLM/DLC   95-48272

EQUINE INTERNAL MEDICINE   ISBN 0–7216–3524–5

Printed in the United States of America.

Last digit is the print number: 9   8   7   6   5   4   3   2   1

This book is dedicated to
Karen, Della, Abby, Nick,
Matthew, Daniel, Ben, and Caitlin.

Their continuing support and patience
has not gone unnoticed
and we are truly grateful for it.

Contributors

Dorothy M. Ainsworth, DVM, PhD
Associate Professor, Department of Clinical Sciences, New York State College of Veterinary Medicine, Cornell University, Ithaca, New York

Frank M. Andrews, DVM, MS, Dip ACVIM
Associate Professor and Section Chief, Department of Large Animal Clinical Sciences, College of Veterinary Medicine, University of Tennessee, Knoxville, Tennessee

Gordon J. Baker, BVSc, PhD, MRCVS, Dip ACVS
Professor and Chief, Equine Medicine and Surgery, and Chief of Staff, Large Animal Clinic, University of Illinois, College of Veterinary Medicine, Urbana, Illinois

Michelle Henry Barton, DVM, PhD, Dip ACVIM
Associate Professor, Department of Large Animal Medicine, College of Veterinary Medicine, University of Georgia, Athens, Georgia

Warwick M. Bayly, BVSc, MS
Robert B. McEachern Professor in Equine Medicine, College of Veterinary Medicine, Washington State University, Pullman, Washington

Laurie A. Beard, DVM, MS, Dip ACVIM
Assistant Professor, Department of Veterinary Clinical Science, College of Veterinary Medicine, The Ohio State University, Columbus, Ohio

Alicia L. Bertone, DVM, PhD
Professor, Department of Veterinary Clinical Sciences, College of Veterinary Medicine, The Ohio State University, Columbus, Ohio

Joseph J. Bertone, DVM, MS, Dip ACVIM
Monacacy Equine Veterinary Associates, Dickerson, Maryland

David S. Biller, DVM, MS
Associate Professor, Radiology Department, Kansas State University, Manhattan, Kansas

John D. Bonagura, DVM, MS, Dip ACVIM
Gilbreath-McLorn Professor of Veterinary Cardiology, Department of Veterinary Medicine and Surgery, University of Missouri—Columbia, Columbia, Missouri

Barbara A. Byrne, DVM, Dip ACVIM
Post DVM Research Assistant, Department of Veterinary Microbiology and Pathology, Washington State University, Pullman, Washington

E. Chirnside, PhD
Department of Infectious Diseases, Animal Health Trust, Newmarket, Suffolk, United Kingdom

Mark V. Crisman, DVM, MS, Dip ACVIM
Associate Professor, Large Animal Internal Medicine, Department of Large Animal Clinical Sciences, Virginia-Maryland Regional College of Veterinary Medicine, Blacksburg, Virginia

Douglas J. DeBoer, DVM
Associate Professor, Department of Medical Sciences, School of Veterinary Medicine, University of Wisconsin–Madison, Madison, Wisconsin

Wendy M. Duckett, DVM, MS, Dip ACVIM
Associate Professor, Department of Food Animal and Equine Medicine, North Carolina State College of Veterinary Medicine, Raleigh, North Carolina

Clara K. Fenger, DVM, PhD, Dip ACVIM
Equine Internal Medicine Consulting, Lexington, Kentucky

Jonathan H. Foreman, DVM, MS, Dip ACVIM
Associate Professor of Equine Medicine, Department of Equine Medicine and Surgery, University of Illinois, Urbana, Illinois

David E. Granstrom, DVM, PhD
Gluck Equine Research Center, Lexington, Kentucky

Bernard Hansen, DVM, Dip ACVIM
Department of Companion Animal Medicine, College of Veterinary Medicine, North Carolina State University, Raleigh, North Carolina

Patricia A. Harris, MRCVS, PhD
The Waltham Centre for Animal Nutrition, Waltham-on-the-Wolds, Leicestershire, England

Kenneth W. Hinchcliff, BVSc, MS, PhD, Dip ACVIM
Associate Professor, Department of Veterinary Clinical Sciences, College of Veterinary Medicine, The Ohio State University, Columbus, Ohio

David W. Horohov, PhD
Professor of Veterinary Immunology, School of Veterinary Medicine, Department of Veterinary Microbiology and Parasitology, Louisiana State University, Baton Rouge, Louisiana

John A. E. Hubbell, DVM, MS, Dip ACVA
Professor of Veterinary Clinical Sciences, The College of Veterinary Medicine, The Ohio State University, Columbus, Ohio

Heidi M. Immegart, DVM, MS, PhD, Dip ACT
Reproductive Diagnostics, Inc., Columbus, Ohio

Samuel L. Jones, MS, DVM
Division of Infectious Diseases, Washington University, St. Louis, Missouri

Thomas R. Klei, PhD
Boyd Professor, Parasitology and Veterinary Science, Department of Veterinary Microbiology and Parasitology, School of Veterinary Medicine, Louisiana State University, Baton Rouge, Louisiana

Catherine W. Kohn, DVM, Dip ACVIM
Professor, Department of Veterinary Clinical Sciences, College of Veterinary Medicine, The Ohio State University, Columbus, Ohio

Joseph J. Kowalski, DVM, PhD
Professor, The Ohio State University College of Veterinary Medicine, Columbus, Ohio

Bruce Kuesis, DVM, Dip ACVIM
Elgin Large Animal Medical Center, Elgin, Illinois

Hilary K. Matthews, DVM, PhD, Dip ACVIM
Postdoctoral Research Associate, Clinical Education and Family Practice, Department of Pediatrics, University of Tennessee Medical Center, Knoxville, Tennessee

Ian G. Mayhew, BSc, PhD
Royal DIK College of Veterinary Medicine, Edinburgh, Scotland

Jill J. McClure, DVM, MS, Dip ACVIM
Professor of Equine Medicine, School of Veterinary Medicine, Louisiana State University, Baton Rouge, Louisiana

Bonnie Rush Moore, DVM, MS, Dip ACVIM
Assistant Professor, College of Veterinary Medicine, Kansas State University, Manhattan, Kansas

Karen A. Moriello, DVM, Dip ACVIM
Clinical Associate Professor, Department of Medical Sciences, School of Veterinary Medicine, University of Wisconsin–Madison, Madison, Wisconsin

Debra Deem Morris, DVM, MS, Dip ACVIM
Owner and Veterinarian, North Jersey Animal Hospital, Wayne, New Jersey

William W. Muir III, DVM, PhD, Dip ACVA, Dip ACVECC
Professor of Veterinary Clinical Sciences, The College of Veterinary Medicine, The Ohio State University, Columbus, Ohio

Jennifer A. Mumford, PhD
Head, Department of Infectious Diseases, Animal Health Trust, Newmarket, Suffolk, United Kingdom

Edward D. Murphey, DVM, MS
Shriners of North America Fellow, Department of Surgery, Shriners Burn Institute, Department of Anesthesiology, University of Texas Medical Branch, Galveston, Texas

Michael J. Murray, DVM, MS
Associate Professor and Adelaide C. Riggs Chair in Equine Medicine, Marion duPont Scott Equine Medical Center, Virginia–Maryland Regional College of Veterinary Medicine, Virginia Tech University, Leesburg, Virginia

Nigel Perkins, BVSc, MS, Dip ACT
Senior Lecturer, Equine Theriogenology, Department of Veterinary Clinical Sciences, Massey University, Palmerston North, New Zealand

Stephen M. Reed, DVM, Dip ACVIM
Professor, Department of Clinical Sciences, College of Veterinary Medicine, The Ohio State University, Columbus, Ohio

Virginia B. Reef, DVM, Dip ACVIM
Associate Professor, University of Pennsylvania School of Veterinary Medicine, New Bolton Center, Kennett Square, Pennsylvania

Craig R. Reinemeyer, DVM, PhD
Professor, Department of Comparative Medicine, University of Tennessee, College of Veterinary Medicine, Knoxville, Tennessee

Yasuko Rikihisa, PhD
Professor, College of Veterinary Medicine, Department of Veterinary Biosciences, The Ohio State University, Columbus, Ohio

Luis Rivas, DVM, MS, Dip ACVIM
Private Equine Practitioner, Hillsboro, Ohio

Debra K. Rooney, PhD
Senior Clinical Research Associate, Ross Products Division, Abbott Laboratories, Columbus, Ohio

William J. Saville, DVM, Dip ACVIM
Department of Veterinary Preventive Medicine, The Ohio State University, College of Veterinary Medicine, Columbus, Ohio

David G. Schmitz, DVM, Dip ACVIM
Large Animal Clinic, College of Veterinary Medicine, Texas A&M University, College Station, Texas

Harold C. Schott, II, DVM, PhD, Dip ACVIM
Assistant Professor, Department of Large Animal Clinical Sciences, Michigan State University, East Lansing, Michigan

Susan D. Semrad, VMD, PhD
Associate Professor, Department of Medical Sciences, School of Veterinary Medicine, University of Wisconsin–Madison, Madison, Wisconsin

Robin Sinclair, PhD
Department of Infectious Diseases, Animal Health Trust, Newmarket, Suffolk, United Kingdom

Jack R. Snyder, DVM, PhD, Dip ACVS
Associate Professor, Department of Surgical and Radiological Sciences, School of Veterinary Medicine, University of California, and Chief of Equine Surgery, Veterinary Medical Teaching Hospital, Davis, California

Carla S. Sommardahl, DVM, Dip ACVIM
Postdoctoral Research Associate, University of Tennessee, College of Veterinary Medicine, Knoxville, Tennessee

Sharon J. Spier, DVM, PhD, Dip ACVIM
Associate Professor, Department of Medicine and Epidemiology, School of Veterinary Medicine, University of California, and Staff, Equine Field Service, Veterinary Medical Teaching Hospital, Davis, California

Randolph H. Stewart, DVM, MS
Veterinary Clinical Associate, Department of Veterinary Physiology and Pharmacology, College of Veterinary Medicine, Texas A&M University, College Station, Texas

Cyprianna E. Swiderski, DVM, Dip ACVIM
PhD Candidate in Immunology, Department of Veterinary Microbiology and Parasitology, School of Veterinary Medicine, Louisiana State University, Baton Rouge, Louisiana

Walter R. Threlfall, DVM, MS, PhD, Dip ACT
Professor and Head, Theriogenology, The Ohio State University, College of Veterinary Medicine, Columbus, Ohio

David A. Wilkie, DVM, MS, Dip ACVD
Associate Professor and Head, Ophthalmology, Department of Veterinary Clinical Sciences, The Ohio State University, Columbus, Ohio

W. David Wilson, BVMS, MS, Dip ACVIM
Professor, Department of Medicine and Epidemiology, and Director, California Center for Equine Health and Performance, School of Veterinary Medicine, University of California, Davis, California

Preface

The past 10 years have witnessed many exciting changes in the field of equine veterinary science. The greater availability of specialist training programs and the increased number of veterinarians taking advantage of postgraduate educational opportunities has resulted in a wealth of new knowledge, an increase in the number of veterinary specialists, and the maturing of an increasingly complex and challenging discipline—equine internal medicine. The delivery of superior health care and increased client expectations that have been associated with the growth of this discipline have led to the development of a specialist, the equine internist, and extremely well informed and astute equine general practitioners. Partly as a result of more training opportunities, the number of equine internists in practice is growing, and many veterinary teaching hospitals are now tertiary care facilities rather than secondary referral centers. More than ever before, equine internal medicine now stands as an autonomous specialty in our profession.

Much of the new knowledge that ushered in these advances is presented in this textbook. As a result of this information, veterinary students and practicing veterinarians can aspire to new levels of sophistication in the diagnosis and management of equine medical problems. In order for our profession to reach a higher level of understanding and to complete the task of managing the complex disease problems we observe today, it is essential to have an excellent understanding of the basic pathophysiologic mechanisms underlying the development of various equine diseases; hence, this textbook. It is devoted entirely to equine internal medicine and has been written for the veterinary student, practicing veterinarian, and discerning members of the horse-owning public. The aim of the book is to promote a clearer comprehension of medical disease processes in

order to better serve the horse and its owners. Consequently, the principles of disease or problem development are discussed in detail and then related to the clinical characteristics of each disease and its therapy and management.

While the bulk of the chapters address specific diseases along systems-based lines, we realize that the practitioner is initially confronted with a specific problem that may have its origin in one or more of the body's systems. The first section of the book is therefore devoted to an in-depth discussion of the basic mechanisms by which the problems may develop and the principles underlying the treatment to many of them. The reader can build on this foundation by reading about specific disorders in the second section of the book, which is divided into chapters dealing with problems of a particular body system or of a specific nature. Wherever possible, we have cross-referenced diseases listed as "rule outs" for a given problem in order to facilitate information retrieval by the reader.

We are proud of the expertise of the many different contributors to this text. It is their depth of knowledge that forms the backbone of the book and has resulted in the creation of a volume dedicated in its entirety to all aspects of equine internal medicine. As a result of their efforts, we hope *"Equine Internal Medicine"* will prove to be a book with universal appeal and application.

We would be remiss if we did not thank the many people at the W.B. Saunders Company for their persistence and educational efforts. David Kilmer, Ray Kersey, Linda Mills, and Stephanie Donley, in particular, are deserving of our gratitude. Our thanks also to our colleagues who so willingly contributed to the book and the many others who assisted in manuscript preparation, correspondence, and all the other tasks that must be accomplished to get a book like this into print.

STEPHEN M. REED, DVM
WARWICK M. BAYLY, BVSc, MS

Contents

DRUG NOTICE

Chapter 1

The Equine Immune System

1.1.

Contemporary Immunology

David W. Horohov, PhD

FROM "SOLUBLE FACTORS" TO CYTOKINES AND BEYOND

The field of immunology has witnessed an information explosion over the past several years. The phenomenological descriptions of antigens, receptors, and "soluble factors" have been replaced by DNA sequences, cloned genes, and recombinant proteins. These changes represent not only a simple adjustment in terminology but a logarithmic leap in our understanding of the processes of antigen recognition and immunoregulation. The application of this information has led to a better understanding of disease resistance, graft rejection, immunopathology, and immunodeficiencies, and to the development of novel therapeutics. The transfer of information and products from the laboratory to the clinic is occurring at an unprecedented rate. An example of this rapid transfer is the introduction of cytokines and monoclonal antibodies into the clinical setting.[1, 2]

As our understanding of various immune-mediated processes continues to expand, we may anticipate the transfer of additional products from the laboratory into the clinic. These products will be used for the treatment of neoplasia, infectious disease, immunodeficiencies, and autoimmunity. The effective use of these therapeutics will depend in part upon the clinician's understanding of the biology of the product and its role in regulating the immune response. While attempts to alter the function of the immune system are not new, these new products may permit the specific intervention in immune function that was not possible using earlier, broadly reactive immunostimulatory and immunosuppressive agents.

In this chapter we examine the state of contemporary immunology with specific emphasis on the issue of antigen specificity, recognition, and immunoregulation. Since a brief review of this kind cannot hope to cover in adequate depth all aspects of this rapidly growing field, the reader is referred to specific references that may provide additional information on the subject of interest. Additional information is also available from several recently published textbooks on immunology[3, 4] and veterinary immunology.[5] We begin first with a discussion of natural resistance and immunity.

NATURAL RESISTANCE AND IMMUNITY

Natural Resistance, or Innate Immunity

Every individual is under constant assault from a variety of microbes that share its living space. While most of these organisms are thought to be harmless, their disease-causing potential is evident when they occasionally cause *opportunistic infections.*[6] The host has evolved a variety of defensive measures to prevent such opportunistic infections from occurring. The first line of defense includes the physical barriers provided by the skin, the mucosa, and the digestive tract. In addition to providing a barrier to penetration, the surface of the skin contains various enzymes, fatty acids, and oils that inhibit the growth of bacteria, fungi, and viruses. Mucous membranes and mucosal secretions contain a variety of compounds that prevent colonization and penetration of these surfaces.[7] These include the bacteriolytic enzyme lysozyme, bactericidal basic polypeptides, mucopolysaccharides, and antibodies. Mucous also provides a physical barrier that entraps invading organisms and leads to their eventual disposal. Particles trapped in the mucous secretions of the respiratory tract, for example, are transported upward through the action of ciliary cells to the trachea, where they are either expectorated or swallowed. Once swallowed, the acidic secretions and digestive enzymes of the stomach destroy most organisms.

These physical barriers provide a formidable obstacle to most organisms. However, either as a result of injury or underlying disease, these barriers may be breached. Once breached, the host presents a variety of internal defense mechanisms to contain and eliminate the invaders. The plasma and interstitial fluids contain a variety of proteins that can inactivate foreign organisms. These include lysozyme,

Table 1–1. Acute Phase Proteins

C3, C4, and factor B	Ceruloplasmin
Ferritin	Kininogen
α_1-Acid glycoprotein	Haptoglobulin
Serum amyloid A (SAA)	Serum amyloid P (SAP)
α_1-Antichymotrypsin	C-reactive protein
α_2-Macroglobulin	Contrapsin
Cysteine protease inhibitor	Fibrinogen
Hemopexin	

interferons, lactoferrin, polyamines, antibodies, and various lytic proteins. Shortly after infection occurs, the concentration of some of these serum proteins, the *acute phase proteins* (Table 1–1), rapidly increases. Some of the acute phase proteins are part of the complement system, a major defense mechanism.

The complement system is composed of a number of different proteins that, when activated, serve as chemotactic factors, opsonins, and lytic agents. There are two pathways by which the complement system is activated (Fig. 1–1). The *classic pathway* involves the recognition and binding of C1 to antigen-antibody complexes. Bound C1 is a proteolytic enzyme and cleaves C4. Cleavage of C4 leads to the binding of C2 to C4b. C2 is in turn cleaved by C1 into C2a. The C4b,2a complex is referred to as the classic pathway C3 convertase since it is a protease capable of cleaving C3 into C3a and C3b. Another C3 convertase is generated via the *alternative pathway*. The activation of complement via the alternative pathway does not involve antibodies. Instead, certain microbial products (zymosan and lipopolysaccharide, LPS) stimulate the association of factor D, a proteolytic enzyme, with the complex of factor B and C3b, leading to the formation of the C3b,Bb complex, which is the alternative pathway C3 convertase. C3a, produced by the cleavage of C3 by the C3 convertases, can bind to mast cells, causing them to degranulate, and is thus referred to as an *anaphylatoxin*. C3b serves as an opsonin for C3b receptor-bearing phagocytic cells. C3b is also required for the formation of the *membrane attack complex* by the terminal complement components, C5 through C9. In this process C5 is cleaved

by either the C4b,2a,3b (classic pathway C5 convertase) or C3b,Bb and properidin (alternative pathway C5 convertase). C5 is cleaved into C5a and C5b. C5a is a chemotactic factor for neutrophils and monocytes. C5b forms a complex with C6, C7, and C8 on cell surfaces. This leads to the insertion and polymerization of C9, which forms a pore in the membrane leading to cell lysis. It is important to note that this process is regulated by a variety of regulatory proteins (C1 esterase inhibitor, C3b inactivator, etc.). Any alterations in the function of any of the complement proteins or its associated regulators results in clinical disease ranging from frequent bacterial infections to certain forms of anemia.

In addition to these humoral components, a cellular response is also elicited in response to the invading organism. The tissue-dwelling *macrophages* and their cousins, the granulocytes, constitute the first line of cellular defense. The phagocytic cells are derived from multipotent stem cells located chiefly in the bone marrow. Under the influence of a variety of signals provided from both within and outside the bone marrow, these stem cells become committed to developing into cells of the granulocyte-macrophage lineage. The critical signal is provided by a family of growth factors known as *colony-stimulating factors (CSFs)*.[8] The CSFs provide both proliferative as well as differentiative signals leading to the development of either monocytes or granulocytes. These cells leave the bone marrow and are carried by the blood to various sites in the body where the monocytes undergo further differentiation into macrophages. They provide the major line of defense by engulfing and destroying invading organisms. In addition, the macrophages secrete a variety of compounds that serve to stimulate the production of the acute phase proteins and attract other cells, including lymphocytes, into the area. Among those lymphoid cells attracted to the area are nonphagocytic cells, the *natural killer (NK)* cells, which are capable of lysing virus-infected and other abnormal cells. The production of interferon by macrophages and other infected cells enhances the cytolytic activity of the NK cells.[9] Other macrophages are also attracted to the site and they scavenge dead cells and debris, initiate wound healing, and participate in the induction of the adaptive immune response.[10]

The essential characteristic of the innate immune response is that the resistance mechanisms do not exhibit specificity for the invading organism. Thus the induction of the resis-

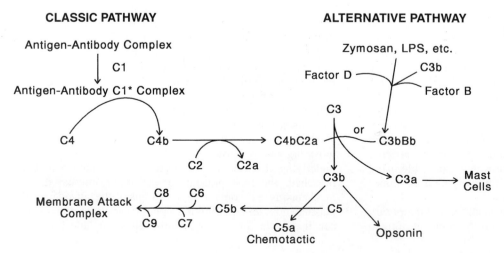

CLASSIC PATHWAY

Antigen-Antibody Complex

↓ C1

Antigen-Antibody C1* Complex

C4 → C4b → C4bC2a

C2 → C2a

C4b → C3b

C8 C6

Membrane Attack Complex ← C5b ← C5

C9 C7

C5a Chemotactic

ALTERNATIVE PATHWAY

Zymosan, LPS, etc.

Factor D — C3b

Factor B

C3

or C3bBb

C3b

C3a → Mast Cells

Opsonin

Figure 1–1. Classic and alternative pathways of complement activation. LPS, lipopolysaccharide.

tance mechanisms does not require prior exposure to the invading organism nor is it augmented by repeated exposure to the same organism. While resistance may be genetically controlled, the genes encoding resistance are not found within the gene complex that controls adaptive immune responses.[11] In most instances these mechanisms are adequate for eliminating casual invaders. However, pathogenic organisms have evolved various methods for avoiding elimination. In response to these organisms, the specialized cells and products of the adaptive immune response are mobilized.

Adaptive Immunity

The adaptive immune response is initiated in response to the encounter between lymphocytes and the foreign agent. In contrast to the nonspecific nature of the innate immune response, an important characteristic of the adaptive immune response is the specificity of this interaction. Thus exposure of the host to a particular microbe or parasite results in the induction of immune responses that are directed against that organism and do not affect unrelated organisms. The specificity of the adaptive immune response is the result of the interaction of specific molecules, or *antigens,* of the invader with antigen-specific receptors on lymphocytes. Each lymphocyte expresses its own unique antigen-specific receptor whose specificity is determined during the lymphocyte's development. An important facet of the immune response to a particular antigen is the clonal expansion of the antigen-specific lymphocytes. In addition to amplifying an ongoing immune response, clonal expansion also provides for the establishment of a population of *memory* lymphocytes. These memory cells are responsible for the rapid and enhanced immune response observed upon reexposure to the same antigen.

The adaptive immune response consists of both humoral and cellular effector mechanisms. The humoral component is mediated by *immunoglobulins,* or *antibodies,* which are found in plasma and tissue fluids. Antibodies are multimeric glycoproteins capable of binding to specific antigens. They are produced by differentiated B cells referred to as *plasma cells.* The activation, proliferation, and differentiation of B lymphocytes into plasma cells is dependent upon other cells, including T lymphocytes, which represent the cellular component of the adaptive immune response. The antigen-specificity of T lymphocytes is determined by the *T-cell receptor (TCR).* The TCR is analogous to, though distinct from, the immunoglobulin molecule of B cells. T lymphocytes have two major functions in the adaptive immune response: (1) as immune regulators and (2) as cytolytic effector cells. *Helper T lymphocytes* produce various cytokines necessary for the induction of both humoral and cellular immune responses. Other T cells inhibit or suppress the activity of other effector cells. Such *suppressor T cells* may play an important role in downregulating immune responses.[13] The other effector function of T cells is the cytolytic activity of *cytotoxic T lymphocytes (CTLs).* Antigen-specific CTLs play an important role in the destruction of virus-infected cells.[14] The induction of CTL activity is also regulated by helper and suppressor T cells.

The adaptive immune response thus differs from innate immunity in that it is antigen-driven and those cells that

mediate the adaptive immune responses express specific receptors for the antigen. Since the immune system will respond to the antigens of both live and killed pathogens, it is possible to stimulate immunity without causing infection. Indeed, this is the basis of vaccination. While this appears to be a rather obvious approach, it does not always yield the expected result. Why some vaccines work and others fail is a complex issue, a major component of which is the nature of antigen and the antigen-specific receptor of lymphocytes.

THE NATURE OF ANTIGEN AND ANTIGEN PROCESSING

Immunogens, Epitopes, and Haptens

All types of chemical structures can serve as antigens, but not all antigens can induce an immune response. *Immunogens,* antigens that can stimulate an immune response, are usually high-molecular-weight, chemically complex molecules. Proteins, nucleic acids, lipids, and polysaccharides can all serve as immunogens. Large immunogens, such as proteins, contain multiple *antigenic determinants,* or *epitopes,* which interact with lymphocytes via the antigen-specific receptor. *Haptens* consist of a single antigenic determinant and can effectively combine with the binding site of antibody molecules. However, haptens cannot stimulate an immune response unless they are physically attached to a larger molecule. This early observation led to the discovery that the induction of an antibody response required the interaction of B and T lymphocytes (see below) and to the realization that B and T cells recognized different epitopes.[15] Indeed, antigen recognition by B cells and T cells is fundamentally quite different. B cells and antibodies recognize antigens in solution or on cell surfaces in their native conformation. B-cell epitopes may be either linear or conformational. By contrast, T cells recognize only linear epitopes and are not capable of interacting with free antigen in its native conformation. Instead, T-cell epitopes must be partly degraded or *processed* and *presented* on the surface of *antigen-presenting cells.*

Antigen Processing[16]

Antigen processing refers to the partial degradation of complex antigens into T-cell epitopes within the phagolysosome of phagocytic cells, usually macrophages. Following phagocytosis, the phagosome containing the engulfed particle fuses with lysosomal vesicles to form the phagolysosome. In this environment of low pH and hydrolytic enzymes, the antigen is degraded. Portions of the degraded antigen may be expelled from the phagocyte through the process of exocytosis. Some of this degraded antigen remains associated with certain surface proteins of the phagocyte. This association of an epitope with particular cell surface proteins is referred to as *presentation.* This particular process has been recently referred to as the *exogenous* pathway of antigen processing since the antigen was initially acquired from outside the cell.[17] The *endogenous* pathway of antigen processing involves the partial degradation and transport to the surface of proteins synthesized within the cell itself, typically viral proteins.[17] The endogenously processed epitope is also presented in association with specific cell surface proteins.

However, antigens processed by the two pathways end up being associated with different, though related, cell surface proteins. The proteins the epitopes are associated with determine which T lymphocytes will recognize the presented epitope. Thus, helper T lymphocytes are typically induced by antigens processed via the exogenous pathway, whereas CTLs typically recognize antigens processed via the endogenous pathway.

The presentation of antigen to T lymphocytes has been shown to involve more than the expression of the processed antigen on the surface of the antigen-presenting cell. A second signal provided by the presenting cell is also required for activation of the T lymphocytes. This second signal appears to be mediated by soluble factors produced by the antigen-presenting cells. Thus paraformaldehyde-fixed antigen-presenting cells fail to stimulate T-cell responses unless supernatants from macrophage cultures are also added. The active component in these supernatants appears to be the cytokine *interleukin-1 (IL-1)*.[18] Besides serving as a second signal for lymphocyte activation, IL-1 affects a large number of physiologic processes in the body (Table 1–2).

In a complex immunogen, certain antigenic determinants are particularly effective at stimulating an antibody response. These *immunodominant* epitopes are often located at exposed areas of the antigen such as in polypeptide loops. These types of structures are often quite mobile and may allow for easier access to the antibody-binding site. T-cell epitopes have been shown to possess a particular structural characteristic in that they involve the formation of amphipathic helices.[19] However, structure alone does not determine the immunogenicity of a particular antigen. The ability of an immunogen to stimulate an immune response is genetically determined.[20] Studies of the immune responses of inbred strains of rodents to simple antigens led to the discovery that immunoresponsiveness was determined by those genes encoding the cell surface proteins that were involved in the presentation of antigens to T lymphocytes.[21] These genes were subsequently shown to be located on a single chromosome in a region that encoded the antigens of the *major histocompatibility complex (MHC),* a gene complex originally identified for its role in allograft rejection.[22]

THE MAJOR HISTOCOMPATIBILITY COMPLEX[23]

As mentioned above, the MHC was originally defined in terms of its role in allograft rejection. Following the rejection of a primary allograft, antibodies that reacted with the allograft could be found in the recipient's sera. These antibodies could be used to identify or type tissues in order to determine the suitability of a donor for transplantation. Using the sera from multiparous females, it was possible to identify a large number of these serologically defined transplantation antigens. Subsequent genetic analysis of the MHC region demonstrated that there were a number of closely linked genes encoding several different, though related antigens that were involved in allograft rejection. These closely related genes are collectively referred to as class I genes and their products as class I antigens.[24] In addition to the serologically defined class I antigens, another group of antigens was identified within the MHC. Antigens in this group were involved in the stimulation of mixed lymphocyte responses and the control of immunoresponsiveness. These class II antigens are structurally and functionally distinct from the class I antigens, except that both are involved in T-cell recognition of antigen. Class III genes encode proteins of the complement cascade and appear to be unrelated to the class I and class II genes.

Class I Antigens

Class I antigens are cell surface glycoproteins consisting of two noncovalently associated proteins, an MHC-encoded transmembrane protein of approximately 44 kD (α chain) and β_2-microglobulin, a 12-kD protein encoded outside the MHC. The structural organization of the class I antigen involves four disulfide-linked extracellular domains, three formed by the α chain (α_1, α_2, and α_3) and the fourth by β_2-microglobulin. X-ray crystallographic studies of a human class I antigen support this structural organization.[25] This structural organization is reminiscent of the immunoglobulin molecule and it has been proposed that the MHC antigens are a part of the *immunoglobulin superfamily*[26] (Fig. 1–2). In fact, class I α chains have been shown to exhibit over 30% sequence homology with immunoglobulin heavy chain constant regions. These data support the theory that immunoglobulins and MHC antigens are derived from a common ancestral gene.[27]

Class I antigens are expressed on the surface of most nucleated cells. The highest level of expression is on lymphoid cells with low-level expression on fibroblasts, muscle cells, and neural cells. Class I antigens are not detectable on early embryonal cells, placental cells, and some carcinomas. The level of expression of class I antigen can be modified by treatment with cytokines or infection with viruses. Treatment of cells with interferons (α, β, and γ) and tumor necrosis factor-alpha (TNF-α) augments class I antigen expression.[28] This augmented expression is the result of increased production of class I messenger RNA (mRNA). The regulatory region of the class I antigen genes has been shown to contain interferon- and TNF-α-responsive elements that control the transcriptional activity of these genes.

The MHC class I region of most animal species thus far studied, including the horse, contains a number of class I α-chain genes, some of which are pseudogenes and are not expressed.[24] Those genes that are expressed exhibit a great deal of polymorphism, including both isotypic and allelic

---

Table 1–2. Biological Activities of Interleukin-1

Activates T cells	Induces fever
Activates B cells	Cytotoxic for some tumor cells
Enhances natural killer cell killing	Cytostatic for other tumor cells
Fibroblast growth factor	Stimulates collagen production
Stimulates prostaglandin E synthesis	Stimulates keratinocyte growth
Stimulates bone resorption	Stimulates mesangial cell growth
Chemotactic for neutrophils	Activates neutrophils
Activates osteoclasts	Induces interleukin-6 production

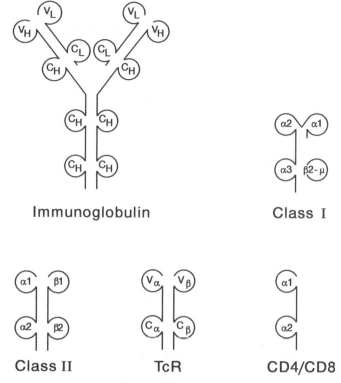

Immunoglobulin   **Class I**

Class II   **TcR**   **CD4/CD8**

Figure 1–2. The immunoglobulin superfamily. Immunoglobulin serves as the prototype model for the superfamily. Both the heavy and light chains of an immunoglobulin molecule can be divided into variable (V_H and V_L) and constant (C_H and C_L) domains. Analogous regions have been identified on a variety of other molecules involved in immune recognition, including class I and class II antigens, the T-cell antigen receptor (*TcR*), and the CD4 and CD8 antigens found on T cells (see text). Disulfide bonds forming the domains are not shown.

variations. Much of this polymorphism is localized in the α_1 and α_2 domains, the α_3 domain being more conserved. This high degree of polymorphism is attributed to recombination events between the different class I genes, including the pseudogenes. The polymorphism is probably related to the class I antigen's role in presenting antigen to T cells.

In addition to binding antibodies, the class I antigens also serve as the recognition structure for CTLs generated in response to the allograft.[29] However, the apparent physiologic role of class I antigens was defined when it was discovered that CTL lysis of virus-infected cells was restricted to target cells expressing the same MHC class I antigen as the CTLs.[30] This observation led to the realization that the CTLs, and T cells in general, recognized the combination of self-MHC and foreign antigen. The corollary of this is that non-self class I antigens (*alloantigens*) resemble the combination of self plus foreign antigen. The nature of the association between class I antigen and foreign antigen remained unclear until x-ray crystallographic studies of human class I antigen were performed.[25] In addition to revealing the structural organization of the domains of the class I antigen, the image also revealed a cleft that lay between the α_1 and α_2 domains. It was proposed that this cleft binds the

processed peptide epitopes for presentation to the TCR. Indeed, the cleft of the crystallized protein used for the x-ray diffraction studies was found to contain a contaminating peptide. Other experiments showed that the incubation of cells with purified viral peptides resulted in lysis of the cells by virus-specific, class I–restricted CTLs.[31] Together, these results support the notion that the endogenous processing of viral antigens leads to the association of the viral peptides with class I antigens on the surface of the infected cell and that this complex is recognized by the CTLs.

Class II Antigens

Class II antigens[32] are heterodimeric, transmembrane glycoproteins composed of an acidic α chain (25–35 kD) and a basic β chain (25–30 kD). A third chain, the invariant chain, has been shown to be associated with the class II antigen during assembly in the endoplasmic reticulum, but is not expressed on the cell surface. Both the α and β polypeptides are encoded within the MHC region. Both polypeptides possess two extracellular domains. The α chain has a single disulfide bond located in its membrane proximal (α_2) domain, while the β chain has a disulfide bond in both of its extracellular domains. Structurally, the class II antigens resemble class I antigens and are also members of the immunoglobulin superfamily (see Fig. 1–2).

The class II genes were originally defined as Ir genes because they determined the *immunor*esponsiveness of inbred strains of guinea pigs and mice to certain simple antigens.[20] The products of the Ir genes were referred to as Ia or *immune-a*ssociated antigens.[21] When the Ir genes were eventually mapped to the MHC region, they were designated class II genes, because they were functionally and structurally distinct from the class I genes. Unlike class I antigens, the class II antigens are restricted in their expression to certain cells of the immune system: B lymphocytes, dendritic cells, macrophages, and activated T lymphocytes of some species. Other cells may also express class II antigens after treatment with various cytokines. Interferon-γ, TNF-α, 1,25-dihydroxyvitamin D_3, and granulocyte-macrophage colony-stimulating factor can induce class II antigen expression on monocytes, macrophages, and other cells.[33] Interleukin-4 (IL-4), a T cell–produced cytokine, enhances class II antigen on B cells.[34] A number of agents have been shown to downregulate class II antigen expression, including glucocorticoids, prostaglandins, and alpha-fetoprotein.[33] Interferons-α and β have an antagonistic effect on interferon-γ induction of class II antigen expression. While it has been demonstrated that class II antigen expression is also regulated at the transcriptional level, no interferon or TNF-α response elements have been identified in the regulatory regions of class II genes. In fact, the regulatory regions of class I and class II genes are quite different[28] and are probably responsible for the differences in tissue distribution for these two MHC products.

Like the class I genes, the class II region contains genes for multiple class II antigens, some of which appear to be pseudogenes and are not expressed.[28] Those α and β chains that are expressed exhibit a high degree of allelic variability, though typically the β chain exhibits the most polymorphism. Unlike the class I genes, the variability in class

II genes is the result of point mutations. There is also correspondingly less polymorphism in the class II genes when compared with the class I genes. The MHC class II region of other species, including the horse, have been studied using human DNA probes, and extensive polymorphism involving several genes has been identified.

It is now known that antigen processed via the exogenous pathway is associated with class II antigens.[16] It has been proposed that the endocytosed antigen is partially degraded and associates with a class II molecule in a prelysosomal compartment of low pH and limited proteolytic activity. This association of the epitope with the class II molecule protects it from further degradation and leads to its subsequent presentation to the T cell. How this peptide associates with the class II antigen is not known. While class II antigens have not yet been analyzed by x-ray crystallography, analysis of the predicted amino acid sequences of α and β chains predicts the structure of class II antigens is similar to that of Class I antigens.[32] Thus the class II antigen probably contains a peptide-binding site at the junction of the α_1 and β_1 domains. Equilibrium dialysis binding studies of peptide–class II antigen associations support the notion that processed antigen binds to class II molecules.[35] These results are consistent with the model that antigen presentation to T cells, in particular helper T cells, in the context of class II antigens plays a central role in the induction of the immune response.

ANTIGEN-SPECIFIC RECEPTOR OF LYMPHOCYTES

It is now clear that class I and class II antigens function as peptide receptors for antigens processed via the two pathways. This peptide binding is nonspecific, whereas T-cell recognition of antigen in association with self-MHC is highly specific. Thus the specificity appears to be determined at the level of the T cell. However, the nature of the T-cell antigen-specific receptor remained elusive for a number of years. Recent advances in molecular biology techniques have begun to uncover some of its secrets. These advances resulted from studies of the immune system's other antigen-specific lymphocytes, the B cells.

B Cells

B lymphocytes are small lymphoid cells characterized by the cell surface expression of immunoglobulin molecules. B cells represent less than 15% of the circulating peripheral blood mononuclear cells, but are present in higher proportions in the lymph nodes and spleen. B cells are derived from the fetal liver and bone marrow of mammals and the bursa of Fabricius of birds. In the bone marrow, B cells are the products of a putative lymphoid stem cell derived from the pluripotent stem cell. Under the influence of various cytokines produced by bone marrow *stromal* cells, the B-cell precursor undergoes its 3-day development, which is characterized by the appearance of specific antigens on its surface.[36] During this process the genes encoding the immunoglobulin molecules are also rearranged. If these rearrangements are successful, the B cell, one of 10^{11} produced daily in humans, emerges from the bone marrow and enters the circulation.

In the circulation, B cells are mitotically inactive cells until stimulated with specific antigen. Following activation, distinctive changes in B-cell morphology and metabolic activity occur, including increases in cell size, RNA and DNA synthesis, rough endoplasmic reticulum cisternae, and expression of class II antigens.[37] These changes coincide with an increased turnover of phosphatidylinositol and the production of diacylglycerol and inositol triphosphate.[38] These second messengers lead to elevations of intracellular Ca^{2+} levels and the translocation of protein kinase C activity to the cytoplasmic membrane.[39] The resulting phosphorylation of cellular proteins leads to the proliferation and differentiation of the B cells. Most of the antigen-stimulated B cells will differentiate into antibody-secreting plasma cells. The remainder are thought to develop into the memory cell population, which will give rise to plasma cells upon reexposure to the antigen.[40] Each of the above processes appears to be controlled by cytokines produced by helper T cells.

General Structure of Antibody[41]

An antibody molecule is composed of two identical light chains and two identical heavy chains that form a disulfide-linked Y-shaped molecule (see Fig. 1–2). There are two forms of the light chain, denoted κ and λ, but a given B cell uses one form exclusively. Five different classes, or *isotypes,* of heavy chains have been identified, designated μ, δ, γ, α, and ε and corresponding to the five classes of immunoglobulin (Ig) molecules: IgD, IgM, IgG, IgA, and IgE. This association of light and heavy chains generates a bifunctional molecule. The antigen-binding region of an antibody molecule is formed by the association of the amino ends of a light and a heavy chain, while the immunologic function of an antibody is determined by its isotype (Table 1–3). Analysis of the heavy and light chains has identified distinct structural *domains,* which are conserved among different antibody molecules. Thus the light chain can be divided into two domains, a conserved carboxy-terminal domain and a highly variable amino-terminal domain. Analysis of various heavy chains revealed a similar domain structure, with the amino-terminal domain being highly variable and with several constant domains. The exact number of constant domains is dependent upon the isotype of the heavy chain; most have three domains while IgE has an extra domain. Some variation also exists in the distance between the first and second constant domains of the heavy chain. This *hinge* region plays an important role in antibody function, allowing the two antigen-binding sites (Fab) to move independently.

Membrane-bound IgM and IgD serve as the antigen-specific receptors for B lymphocytes. Each contains a membrane-spanning region near its carboxy end, which is inserted into the mRNA during differential splicing of the heavy chain exons.[42] Though rarely detectable in the circulation, IgD is present in large quantities on the surface of naive B lymphocytes. Following activation, the surface expression of IgD is lost, though the cell may continue to express the membrane form of IgM. Early on in an immune response, the B cell secretes large amounts of the pentameric form of IgM. As the immune response proceeds, the B cell will switch the isotype of its heavy chain. Isotype switching involves the substitution of one heavy chain constant region

Table 1–3. Immunoglobulin Isotypes

Isotype	Immunologic Function
IgD	Antigen receptor of naive B lymphocytes.
IgM	Surface IgM is found on naive, activated, and memory B cells.
	Secreted IgM is a pentamer and represents the major antibody produced during a primary response. IgM efficiently mediates agglutination, neutralization, opsonization, and complement activation.
IgG	The principle immunoglobulin found in plasma, representing up to 80% of the total immunoglobulin concentration. Various subclasses of IgG have been identified (see text). There are four IgG subclasses in the horse: IgGa, IgGb, IgGc, and IgG(B). The major functions of IgG include opsonization and neutralization reactions. IgG also fixes complement and participates in antibody-dependent cellular cytotoxicity (ADCC).
IgA	IgA, the most abundant antibody in secretions (tears, mucus, saliva, colostrum, etc.) is a dimer composed of 2 IgA molecules joined by a J chain. IgA in the plasma is predominantly monomeric. IgA antibodies can be neutralizing, but only activate complement via the alternative pathway.
IgE	Most IgE is found associated with the surface of mast cells and basophils and only very small amounts are present in the plasma. The cross-linking of two IgE molecules with specific antigen results in the degranulation of mast cells and basophils. Thus IgE is the primary antibody responsible for Type I hypersensitivity reactions and appears to play a central role in immunity to parasites.

in place of another.[44] The genes encoding the five different constant regions of the heavy chain are sequentially arranged on the chromosome (C_μ, C_δ, C_γ, C_ϵ, and C_α). Initially, the first two constant region genes encoding the μ and δ constant regions are used to form the heavy chain. The 5′ region of each constant region gene segment contains repetitive regions of DNA known as *switch sequences*.[43] The switch sequences appear to play a role in this rearrangement and may serve as the target for specific recombinases.[44] When switching occurs, a new constant region segment is selected and the intervening genes are removed either by splicing or looping out.[43, 44] Isotype switching affects only the heavy chain constant domains and has no effect on the antigen-specificity of the immunoglobulin molecule. The signal for B cells to undergo isotype switching is provided by T lymphocytes in the form of various cytokines.[45] IL-4 induces isotype switching to the IgE isotype, while interferon-γ blocks this induction and augments IgG production.[46] IgA is produced in response to the combination of IL-5 and transforming growth factor-β (TGF-β).[47]

Generation of Antibody Diversity[48]

The individual specificity of a particular antibody molecule and the B cell that produces it is determined by the light and heavy chain variable domains. The association of these two domains results in the formation of an antigen-binding groove, or pocket. This pocket contains regions of hypervariability, which appear to define the specificity of a particular antibody molecule. It has been estimated that over 10^8 different antibody-specificities are possible. The generation of this tremendous amount of diversity in antibody-specificity occurs during B-cell ontogeny in the bone marrow. Within a given B cell, the genes encoding the heavy and light chains of an antibody molecule are organized into specific gene segments. Thus the κ light chain is formed from variable (V_κ), joining (J_κ), and constant (C_κ) gene segments, which together form the variable and constant domains of the light chain.

In the germ line of an undifferentiated cell one finds several hundred different V_κ and several dozen J_κ gene segments (a somewhat different arrangement of λ light chain genes is observed, but the overall process is quite similar). Likewise, the heavy chain of a B lymphocyte is composed of V_H, diversity (D), and J_H segments, which form the variable domain, and these join to the constant region genes (C_μ, C_δ, C_γ, C_α, and C_ϵ) to form the complete heavy chain molecule. Similarly, in the germ line one finds a large number of V_H gene segments and a smaller number of D and J_H segments. During the differentiation of a B cell, there is subsequent selection and rearrangement of a V_L segment with a J_L segment and the accompanying deletion of intervening V_L and J_L segments. The subsequent rearranged VJC sequence is then transcribed into mRNA and translated into the light chain. A somewhat similar sequence follows for heavy chains, except that two rearrangements are necessary, a D to J_H rearrangement followed by a V_H to DJ_H rearrangement. Once completed, the VDJ segment is brought into proximity with the appropriate C_H segment and transcribed. Not all of the gene segment rearrangements produce functional genes. Since a B cell has two sets of heavy chain genes, one on each chromosome, and four sets of light chain genes, two each of κ and λ, it has several chances to form appropriate heavy and light chains. Once the heavy and light chain gene segments are successfully recombined, the genes on the sister chromosome neither recombine nor are they expressed. This process of *allelic exclusion* ensures that the B cell produces antibodies of a single specificity.[49]

While this random assortment of gene segments accounts for much of the diversity in antibody specificity, additional mechanisms are also involved, including *junctional diversity,* which results from the imprecise joining of gene segments and *somatic mutations*. Somatic mutations are point mutations in the hypervariable region of either the heavy or light chain that occur during proliferation of antigen-activated B lymphocytes. Such mutations appear to play a role in increasing antibody affinity for its antigen. Thus fewer than 1,000 genes can give rise to over 10^8 molecules of the various specificities needed to recognize the vast number of antigens the host may encounter.

T Cells

T lymphocytes are derived from a hemopoietic stem cell (prothymocyte) that enters the subcapsular region of the thymus from the bone marrow. Within the thymic environment the prothymocyte undergoes a developmental and se-lective process while emigrating through the cortex into the medullary region of the thymus.[50] Less than 3% of all the immature thymocytes found in the cortex survive to become peripheral T cells. This selection process involves both the acquisition of the T-cell antigen-specific receptor (TCR) through gene segment rearrangements and the subsequent selection for class I– or class II–restricted antigen recognition. It is this latter selection process that gives rise to the two populations of T lymphocytes, those that recognize antigen in association with, or restricted to, class I antigens and those that use class II antigens.[51]

T lymphocytes can be differentiated from B lymphocytes in that they do not express surface immunoglobulins but instead express the TCR. In addition to the TCR, all T cells also express another antigen called CD3 (The designation CD stands for *cluster designate* and is the result of an international workshop assembled to standardize the terminology used to describe leukocyte surface antigens recognized by monoclonal antibodies).[52] It turns out that TCR and CD3 form a multimeric complex on the T cell surface and that this complex is involved in antigen-specific recognition.

TCR and CD3 Complex[53, 54]

The TCR structure was first identified using anticlonotypic antibodies that recognized a surface antigen expressed on a cloned T lymphoma cell line.[55] This antibody recognized a disulfide-linked heterodimer composed of an acidic (α) and a basic (β) protein of 40 to 45 kD. Similar heterodimers were found on a variety of antigen-specific class I– and class II–restricted T-cell lines, but not on B cells. Peptide mapping studies of the α and β chains from many different T-cell lines demonstrated that they contained variable and constant domains reminiscent of immunoglobulin structure.[53] Using the procedure of subtractive hybridization, Hedrick and co-workers cloned the β chain of the TCR in 1984.[56] Analysis of the cloned gene demonstrated that it was related to, but distinct from, immunoglobulin genes. Further analysis indicated that, like immunoglobulin genes, the TCR β chain gene underwent gene rearrangements during T-cell development. Subsequently, three additional TCR genes were cloned, the α chain and two additional genes corresponding to the γ and δ chains of a second heterodimer. Thus two TCRs exist, an α/β heterodimer that constitutes the TCR on almost 90% of all T cells, and a γ/δ heterodimer present on approximately 10% of the T cells.[57] The significance of these two different TCR heterodimers has not yet been determined. It is clear that they represent functionally distinct populations of T cells, with the α/β cells representing typical cells, in that their antigen recognition function is restricted by class I and class II MHC antigens, whereas γ/δ cells may not be MHC-restricted in their recognition of antigen.[58] It has recently been proposed that γ/δ cells may constitute a primitive immunosurveillance mechanism because large numbers of them are found on mucosal surfaces.[59]

Analysis of the predicted amino acid sequences for the TCR proteins confirmed a structural similarity with antibody molecules placing these proteins in the immunoglobulin superfamily (see Fig. 1–2). One peculiarity in the structure of the TCR was observed from amino acid sequence analysis.

While both the α and β chains of the TCR contained a transmembrane region, both proteins had very short cytoplasmic tails. It therefore seemed unlikely that TCR itself could transmit any cytoplasmic signal in response to antigen binding. This led to the search for other proteins associated with the TCR. Solubilization of the T cell membranes with the triton-X100 revealed that five other proteins could be immunoprecipitated with the TCR.[59] Similar results were obtained when anti-CD3 antibodies were used. Thus the TCR heterodimer is noncovalently associated with the CD3 complex of proteins. The five components of the CD3 complex (γ, δ, ϵ and the ζ/η proteins), appear to be involved in signal transduction following TCR binding to antigen. Unlike the TCR α and β proteins, the CD3 proteins have large extracellular domains, some of which are phosphorylated in response to stimulation of the TCR.[54] In addition to providing a signaling mechanism for the TCR, the CD3 complex is also required for expression of the TCR heterodimer on the cell surface.[60]

Generation of TCR Diversity[61]

The generation of diversity in the TCR during T-cell ontogeny employs a mechanism that is quite similar to that used to generate immunoglobulin diversity. The TCR α and γ chains resemble immunoglobulin light chains in that they are composed of V, J, and C gene segments. The particular V, J, and C segments used are selected from a germ line configuration containing a few (C region) to several hundred (V region) gene segments. The selection and rearrangement of the gene segments are similar to those employed by the immunoglobulin light chain and appear to involve the same recombinase. Likewise, the β and δ chains resemble heavy chains, each being composed of V, D, J, and C gene segments, and their selection and rearrangement from germ line genes also parallel immunoglobulin heavy chain rearrangement. Thus the generation of diversity is the result of the combination of multiple gene segments and junctional diversity. However, unlike immunoglobulins, the TCR genes do not undergo somatic mutations.

CD4 and CD8 Antigens[62]

Mature thymocytes and T lymphocytes can be further divided into two distinct populations on the basis of their expression of either the CD4 or CD8 antigen. The expression of these antigens is directly correlated with the MHC specificity of the T cell. Thus, T cells expressing the CD8 antigen recognize antigen in association with class I antigens and CD4+ T cells recognize antigen in association with class II antigens. Furthermore, antibodies to CD4 and CD8 can block class II– and class I–restricted antigen recognition by T cells, respectively. These results indicate that there is a direct interaction between the MHC antigens of the antigen-presenting cell and the CD4 and CD8 antigens on the corresponding T cells. Thus, T cell recognition of antigen involves the engagement of a TCR-CD3-CD4 or TCR-CD3-CD8 complex with processed peptide in the cleft of a class II or class I molecule.

While it was originally proposed that the CD4-class II and CD8-class I interaction simply served to stabilize the

TCR-CD3-MHC complex, recent work has shown that the cytoplasmic domain of the CD4 and CD8 molecules is associated with a tyrosine kinase which is involved in the intracellular signaling process accompanying antigen stimulation of the T cell. Whatever their function, it is clear that the expression of CD4 and CD8 antigens determines the class of MHC antigen that a T cell recognizes during antigen presentation. Like the other members of this complex, the CD4 and CD8 molecules are members of the immunoglobulin superfamily (see Fig. 1–2). A number of other proteins are also associated with adhesion of T cells to antigen-presenting cells, including members of the *integrin* and *ICAM* (*i*ntracellular *a*dhesion *m*olecules) supergene families.[63] The interactions of these adhesions with their respective ligands may provide the initial interaction between T cells and antigen-presenting cells. Individuals with inherited deficiencies in the production of these molecules frequently present with immunodeficiency-like syndromes.[63]

While the T lymphocytes in the periphery express either CD4 or CD8 antigens, cortical thymocytes express both antigens.[50] During the process of thymic selection, these cells convert to either CD4+ or CD8+ cells or they are eliminated. It is at this stage of their development that T cells are said to "learn" to recognize antigen in the context of the appropriate MHC antigen.[51] It is also at this stage that autoreactive T cells are eliminated. While experimental studies have shown that both positive and negative selection of T cells is occurring,[50] the exact mechanism of these selective processes remains unknown. Interestingly, while T cells expressing the α/β heterodimer of the TCR can be either CD4+ or CD8+, γ/δ cells are either CD8+ or CD4−CD8−. These results suggest that the γ/δ cells undergo a different developmental process than the α/β cells.[57]

IMMUNOREGULATION

The generation of an immune response requires the interaction of multiple leukocyte subsets, including macrophages, B cells, and CD4+ and CD8+ T cells.[64] While the initial interactions of the B and T cells involves recognition of specific epitopes, which in the case of the T cell are presented in the context of MHC antigens, subsequent interactions are mediated by soluble factors, or *cytokines,* produced by the various cells. Macrophages, T cells, and even nonhematopoietic cells produce a variety of cytokines with immunoregulatory activity. However, it is the helper T cell that plays a central role in regulating immune responses.

Helper T Cells

The requirement for T cell help in the generation of an antibody response was discovered in experiments using haptens.[15] As was mentioned earlier, haptens are singular antigenic determinants that by themselves fail to elicit an immune response. When the hapten is attached to a larger antigen, referred to as a *carrier,* antihapten antibodies are stimulated and a memory B cell population is generated. Reexposure of the animal to the same hapten-carrier combination stimulates a memory response to the hapten. However, when the hapten is conjugated to a different carrier, no memory response is stimulated. This *carrier* effect is best explained by the model in which the B cell recognizes the hapten but fails to develop into memory or plasma cells unless T cells, which recognize antigenic determinants on the carrier, are also stimulated.[65] Subsequent work has shown that the help provided by the T cells was mediated by soluble proteins that serve as growth and differentiation factors for the B cells.[66] Much effort over the past decade has focused on the characterization of helper T cells and the soluble factors they produce.

While the definition of a helper T cell is primarily based on function, it was discovered that for many experimental models those T cells that mediated helper cell activity expressed the CD4 antigen.[67] This led to the classic division of T lymphocytes into helper (CD4+ class II antigen-restricted) and cytotoxic (CD8+ class I antigen-restricted) cells.[68] This division is quite artificial in terms of helper and cytotoxic function. CD4+ class II–restricted cytotoxic T cells have been identified and CD8+ class I–restricted T cells make some cytokines.[69, 70] Recently, it has been proposed that CD4+ helper cells may be further divided into distinct helper cell subsets based on the cytokines they produce.[71] Thus Th1 cells produce interferon-γ and IL-2, two cytokines involved in the induction of cell-mediated immune responses. Th2 cells, on the other hand, produce IL-4 and IL-5, two cytokines involved in the induction of antibody responses. The best evidence for separate helper T cell populations comes from the study of intracellular parasite infections in mice. Those strains of mice resistant to *Listeria donovani* infection develop a cell-mediated immune response characterized by activated macrophages and Th1 cells. By contrast, the susceptible BALB/c strain of mice generates a vigorous antibody response and Th2 cells.

It remains unclear as to what determines whether a helper cell will be a Th1 or Th2 cell. It has been proposed that the presentation of antigen to the T cell may determine its fate.[72] Thus, the presentation of soluble antigens by B cells may preferentially activate Th2 cells, which in turn produce those cytokines that drive B-cell responses. Antigen presentation by macrophages may preferentially activate Th1 cells that produce cytokines which stimulate cell-mediated responses, including macrophage activation and delayed-type hypersensitivity reactions. Additional work is needed to further define the function and role of helper cell subsets. This information would be very useful in designing vaccines that specifically stimulate desired immune responses.

Cytokines and Interleukins

Frequent mention has been made in this chapter of the role of cytokines regulating immune responses. Indeed, this particular area of immunology has seen the most growth over the past several years. This rapid acquisition of knowledge is the result of the application of modern molecular biology techniques to the identification and characterization of specific cytokines. To date, over 20 separate cytokines have now been cloned, sequenced, and synthesized in bacterial and eukaryotic expression systems. This has led to both a better understanding of cytokine function and to their application in a variety of clinical settings.

Initial studies of the role of soluble factors in the regulation of immune responses were often confounded by the heterogeneous nature of the culture supernatants used as the source of the cytokine activity.[73] Furthermore, the use of biological assays to identify specific cytokines resulted in the practice of assigning descriptive names to newly discovered cytokines (lymphocyte activating factor, T cell growth factor, etc.).[74] This quickly led to confusion since individual cytokines often exhibited multiple biological activities and the biological assays themselves were not specific for a particular cytokine. Once the genes for the cytokines had been cloned and the resulting proteins identified, it was possible to eliminate much of this confusion.[75] The adoption of the interleukin terminology for naming cloned cytokines has further clarified the biological function and role of particular cytokines.[76] Once a new cytokine's gene is identified and the biological activity of the purified protein characterized, it is assigned an interleukin designation. Table 1–4 contains a list of the 15 (as of this date) interleukins and their known biological activity. Not all cytokines have been given interleukin designation. Interferons, certain growth factors (platelet-derived growth factor, TGF-β), and TNF-α have retained their original names. It should also be emphasized that other cells besides T cells produce cytokines and interleukins. For example, monocytes and macrophages are the major source of IL-1, IL-6, and TNF-α. Thus the term *lymphokine,* which was originally used to describe immunoregulatory products of lymphocytes, has been replaced with *cytokine,* which denotes the more varied sources of immunoregulatory molecules.

The availability of cloned cytokines has permitted the subsequent identification and characterization of cytokine-specific receptors on T cells. The best characterized of these is the receptor for IL-2.[77] IL-2 is composed of three subunits: α, β, and γ. The β subunit is constitutively expressed on the T cell surface and has a low affinity for IL-2. The α chain is expressed upon activation of the T cell and was originally described as a T-cell activation antigen (Tac).[78] Alone, the α chain has higher affinity for IL-2, but it is the complex of α and β together that forms the high-affinity receptor for the cytokine. It appears that each of the different forms of the IL-2 receptor (α, β, and αβ) mediate different T-cell functions,[78] though the precise mechanism remains unknown. The answer may lie within the γ chain since it is thought to be involved in signal transduction once the IL-2 is attached to the receptor. It is clear that the binding of IL-2 to its high-affinity receptor drives the proliferation of the T cell. The expression of high-affinity IL-2 receptor and other cytokine receptors is transient. Over time the expression of the α chain diminishes and the T cell reverts to its quiescent state until it is restimulated with antigen. The receptors for other cytokines have also been identified, and in some cases cloned.[79] These receptors are typically multimeric structures and in some cases share common subunits. The isolation and characterization of cytokine receptors and the identification of their function remains an intensive area of investigation in immunologic research.

As was mentioned at the beginning of this chapter, the introduction of cloned cytokines into the clinical setting has proceeded at a rapid pace.[1] The first interleukin to be used in the clinical setting was IL-2.[80] Interest in the clinical use of IL-2 followed the discovery that high doses of IL-2 could induce cytotoxic cells, which could lyse a variety of freshly

Table 1–4. Interleukins

Interleukin	Biological Activities and Source
IL-1	*Lymphocyte activating factor.* Multiple biological activities affecting a variety of lymphoid and nonlymphoid cells (see Table 1–2); produced primarily by monocytes, though a variety of cell lines also produce IL-1-like activities
IL-2	*T-cell growth factor.* Provides proliferative signal for T cells; also affects B cells, macrophages, and natural killer (NK) cells; high concentrations of IL-2 stimulate cytolytic activity in NK cells and T cells; produced by activated Th1 and some CD8+ cells
IL-3	*Multi-colony-stimulating factor.* Promotes the growth of various hematopoietic cell precursors; produced by T cells and myelomonocytic cell lines
IL-4	*B-cell stimulatory factor 1.* Stimulates growth, maturation, and differentiation of B cells; growth and differentiation of some T cells; produced by Th2 cells
IL-5	*T-cell replacing factor.* Stimulates B-cell proliferation and immunoglobulin synthesis; stimulates T-cell proliferation and differentiation as well as eosinophil formation in bone marrow; produced by Th2 cells
IL-6	*B-cell differentiation factor.* Promotes maturation and immunoglobulin production by B cells; stimulates T-cell growth and IL-2 synthesis; induces production of acute phase proteins by hepatocytes; produced by macrophages, T cells, stromal cells, fibroblasts, and a variety of other cell lines
IL-7	*Pre-B-cell growth factor.* Stimulates proliferation and maturation of early B and T cells as well as mature T cells; produced by bone marrow–derived stromal cells
IL-8	Neutrophil chemotactic factor produced by monocytes and hepatocytes
IL-9	*P40.* Supports growth of certain T-cell clones; produced by CD4+ T cells
IL-10	*Cytokine synthesis inhibitory factor.* Inhibits production of IL-2 and interferon-γ; produced by Th2 cells
IL-11	An IL-6-like factor produced by stromal cells
IL-12	*Natural killer cell differentiation factor.* Augments NK cell function and stimulates generation of Th1 cells; produced by macrophages
IL-13	Produced by Th2 cells; downregulates cytokine production by macrophages and monocytes while activating B cells
IL-14	A high-molecular-weight B-cell growth factor produced by T cells and some B-cell lines
IL-15	A T-cell growth factor similar in function to IL-2

isolated tumor cells.[81] This *lymphokine-activated killer (LAK)* activity was subsequently shown to mediate tumor regression in vivo in mice and humans.[80] The initial success with IL-2 has prompted the introduction of other cytokines into the clinical setting. While none of these materials has moved beyond the experimental stage, one can anticipate their routine use in a variety of clinical settings, as immunomodulators and adjuvants. It is also clear, however, that before their full potential is realized, more basic information regarding their role in regulating immune responses is necessary.

A Model for the Role of Cytokines in Immunoregulation

The following model is proposed both as a general model for the induction of an immune response and as a means of summarizing the preceding information (Fig. 1–3). As in the case of all models, its design is heavily biased by the hand of the builder, though similar models have been proposed by others.[82] In this model the antigen, a virus, is phagocytosed by a macrophage (Mφ) and is processed via the exogenous pathway. The processed epitope is presented on the surface of the Mφ in the context of a class II antigen to a CD4+ T cell. Additionally the macrophage produces the cytokine IL-1, which, along with antigen presentation, activates the T cell. Meanwhile, CD8+ T cells encounter viral antigen on the surface of virus-infected cells. These epitopes have been processed via the endogenous pathway and are associated with the class I antigens on the surface of the infected cell. Once antigen-activated, the T cell begins to express the high-affinity form of the IL-2 receptor. The CD4+ Th1 cell produces IL-2 and IFN-γ. The interaction of IL-2 with its receptor drives the clonal proliferation of the activated CD8+ T cells. The IFN-γ then stimulates the CD8+ cell to differentiate into a cytotoxic effector cell. Meanwhile,

virus-specific B cells have also encountered antigen and present it to other CD4+ T cells, which produce the cytokine IL-5 that stimulates B-cell proliferation. IFN-γ can then cause some of these B cells to differentiate into IgG-secreting plasma cells, while IL-4 stimulates others to produce IgE.

Future Directions for Equine Immunology

The field of equine immunology continues to expand with the development of better reagents. Recent advances in gene-cloning technology have led to the cloning and expression of a number of equine cytokines. Thus the complementary DNA (cDNA) sequence for equine IL-2 was cloned using the polymerase chain reaction (PCR) and primers based on human and murine sequences.[83, 84] Similarly, the cDNA sequence for equine IL-4 was also amplified using PCR and sequenced.[85] One can anticipate additional equine cytokines being cloned and recombinant products produced for both experimental and clinical use.

Similar advances have been made in the characterization of cell surface antigens on equine B and T cells. Here the technique of monoclonal antibody production has been employed to develop specific antibodies that recognize various antigens on equine cells.[86] This has led to the initial characterization of equine MHC antigens and provided reagents for the preparation and analysis of equine lymphocyte subsets.

Perhaps the greatest advances in equine immunology will occur in the area of immunopathology. Horses experience a number of immunologically based hypersensitivities, many of which are resistant to therapeutic intervention or prevention. As more and more information becomes available implicating specific T-cell subsets in hypersensitivity reactions, intervention strategies may be developed. The recent implication of IgE in chronic obstructive pulmonary disease (COPD) points to one possible approach.[87, 88] IL-4 production by Th2 cells has been shown to play a critical role in IgE production in other species. Indeed, humans with asthma exhibit elevated levels of both IgE and IL-4 in bronchial secretions.[89] Inhibiting IL-4 production by Th2 cells could lead to reduced levels of IgE. Such an approach might employ anticytokine antibodies, soluble receptors, or other antagonistic cytokines (e.g., IL-12, IFN-γ). Such an approach would be limited only by the availability of such reagents.

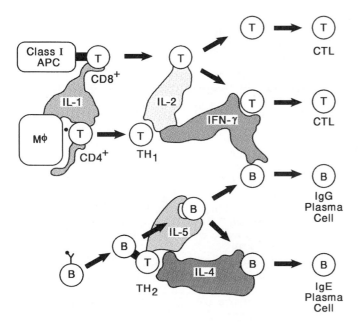

Figure 1–3. Cellular and cytokine interactions in the generation of humoral and cellular immunity. Developmental transitions of the cells (activation and differentiation) are indicated by the *horizontal arrows* and proliferation is indicated with *diagonal arrows*. See text for details. *APC,* antigen-presenting cell; *IL-2* and *IL-4,* interleukin-2 and -4; *CTL,* cytotoxic T lymphocyte; *IFN-γ,* interferon-gamma.

REFERENCES

1. Horohov DW, Siegel JP: Lymphokines: Progress and promise. *Drugs* 33:289, 1987.
2. Meeker TC, Lowder J, Maloney DG, et al: A clinical trial of anti-idiotype therapy for B cell malignancy. *Blood* 65:1349, 1985.
3. Paul WE: *Fundamental Immunology,* ed 2. New York, Raven Press. 1989, p 1123.
4. Roitt IM, Brostoff J, Male DK: *Immunology,* ed 2. New York, Harper & Row, 1989.
5. Halliwell REW, Gorman NT: *Veterinary Clinical Immunology.* Philadelphia, WB Saunders, 1989.

6. Prier JE, Friedman H: *Opportunistic Pathogens.* Baltimore, University Park Press, 1974.

7. Husband AJ: Perspectives in mucosal immunity: A ruminant model. *Vet Immunol Immunopathol* 17:357, 1987.

8. Stanley ER, Guilbert LJ: Methods for the purification, assay, characterization and target cell binding of a colony stimulating factor (CSF-1). *J Immunol Methods* 42:251, 1981.

9. Herberman RB, Ortaldo JR: Natural killer cells and their role in defenses against disease. *Science* 214:24, 1981.

10. Shevach EM: Macrophages and other accessory cells. In Paul WE, ed: *Fundamental Immunology.* New York, Raven Press, 1984, p 71.

11. Revel M: Host defense against infections and inflammations— Role of multifunctional IL-6/IFN-beta-2 cytokine. *Experientia* 45:549, 1989.

12. Mizel SB: The interleukins. *FASEB J* 3:2379, 1989.

13. Sy MS, Benacerraf B: Suppressor T cells, immunoglobulin and Igh restriction. *Immunol Rev* 101:132, 1988.

14. Rouse BT, Norley S, Martin S: Antiviral cytotoxic T lymphocyte induction and vaccination. *Rev Infect Dis* 10:16, 1988.

15. Benacerraf B, Unanue ER: *Textbook of Immunology.* Baltimore, Williams & Wilkins, 1979.

16. Braciale TJ, Morrison LA, Sweetser MT, et al: Antigen presentation pathways to class I and class II MHC-restricted T lymphocytes. *Immunol Rev* 98:95, 1987.

17. Townsend A, Bodmer H: Antigen recognition by class I–restricted T lymphocytes. *Annu Rev Immunol* 7:601, 1989.

18. Dinarello CA: Biology of interleukin 1. *FASEB J* 2:108, 1988.

19. Bastin J, Rothbard J, Davey J, et al: Use of synthetic peptides of influenza nucleoprotein to define epitopes recognized by class I–restricted cytotoxic T lymphocytes. *J Exp Med* 166:1508, 1987.

20. Paul WE: Immune response genes. In Paul WE, ed. *Fundamental Immunology.* New York, Raven Press, 1984, p 439.

21. Benacerraf B, Germain R: The immune response genes of the major histocompatibility complex. *Immunol Rev* 38:70, 1978.

22. Hood L, Steinmetz M, Malissen B: Genes of the major histocompatibility complex of the mouse. *Annu Rev Immunol* 1:529, 1983.

23. Sachs DH: The major histocompatibility complex. In Paul WE, ed. *Fundamental Immunology.* New York, Raven Press, 1984, p 303.

24. Nathenson SG, Geliebter J, Pfaffenbach GM, et al: Murine major histocompatibility complex class-I mutants: Molecular analysis and structure-function implications. *Annu Rev Immunol* 4:471, 1986.

25. Bjorkman PJ, Saper MA, Samraoui B, et al: The foreign antigen binding site and T cell recognition regions of class I histocompatibility antigens. *Nature* 329:512, 1987.

26. Hunkapiller T, Hood L: Diversity of the immunoglobulin gene superfamily. *Adv Immunol* 44:1, 1989.

27. Klein J, Figueroa F: Evolution of the major histocompatibility complex. *CRC Crit Rev Immunol* 6:295, 1985.

28. David-Watine B, Israel A, Kourilsky P: The regulation and expression of MHC class I genes. *Immunol Today* 11:286, 1990.

29. Townsend A, Bodmer H: Antigen recognition by class I–restricted T lymphocytes. *Annu Rev Immunol* 7:601, 1989.

30. Zinkernagel RM, Doherty PC: MHC-restricted cytotoxic T cells: Studies on the biological role of polymorphic major transplantation antigens determining T-cell restriction—specificity, function, and responsiveness. *Adv Immunol* 27:51, 1979.

31. Townsend ARM, Gotch FM, Davey J: Cytotoxic T cells recognize fragments of the influenza nucleoprotein. *Cell* 42:457, 1985.

32. Guillemot F, Auffray C, Orr HT, et al: MHC antigen genes. In Hames BD, Glover DM, eds. *Molecular Immunology.* Oxford, IRL Press, 1988, p 81.

33. Benoist C, Mathis D: Regulation of major histocompatibility complex class-II genes: X,Y and other letters of the alphabet. *Annu Rev Immunol* 8:681, 1990.

34. Paul WE: Interleukin 4/B cell stimulatory factor 1: One lymphokine, many functions. *FASEB J* 1:456, 1987.

35. Babbitt BP, Allen PM, Matsueda G, et al: Binding of immunogenic peptides to Ia histocompatibility molecules. *Nature* 317:359, 1985.

36. Lincade PW: Experimental models for understanding B lymphocyte formation. *Adv Immunol* 41:181, 1987.

37. Jelinek DF, Lipsky PE: Regulation of human B lymphocyte activation, proliferation, and differentiation. *Adv Immunol* 40:1, 1987.

38. Weigle WO: Factors and events in the activation, proliferation, and differentiation of B cells. *CRC Crit Rev Immunol* 7:285, 1987.

39. Altman A, Coggeshall KM, Mustelin T: Molecular events mediating T cell activation. *Adv Immunol* 48:227, 1990.

40. Kishimoto T, Hirano T: B lymphocyte activation, proliferation, and immunoglobulin secretion. In Paul WE, ed: *Fundamental Immunology.* New York, Raven Press, 1989, p 385.

41. Nezlin R: Internal movements in immunoglobulin molecules. *Adv Immunol* 48:1, 1990.

42. Singer PA, Singer HH, Williamson AR: Different species of messenger RNA encode receptor and secretory IgM mu chains differing at their carboxy termini. *Nature* 285:294, 1980.

43. Max EE: Immunoglobulins: molecular genetics. In Paul WE, ed. *Fundamental Immunology.* New York, Raven Press, 1989, p 235.

44. Cebra JJ, Komisar JL, Schweiter PA: CH Isotype "switching" during normal B-lymphocyte development. *Annu Rev Immunol* 2:493, 1984.

45. Finkelman FD, Holmes J, Katona IM, et al: Lymphokine control of in vivo immunoglobulin isotype selection. *Annu Rev Immunol* 8:303, 1990.

46. Coffman RL, Carty A: A T cell activity that enhances polyclonal IgE production and its inhibition by interferon-γ. *J Immunol* 136:949, 1986.

47. Coffman RL, Lebman DA, Shrader B: Transforming growth factor-beta specifically enhances IgA production by lipopolysaccharide-stimulated murine B lymphocytes. *J Exp Med* 170:1039, 1989.

48. Blackwell TK, Alt FW: Immunoglobulin genes. In Hames BD, Glover DM, eds: *Molecular Immunology,* Oxford, IRL Press, 1988, p 1.

49. Lai E, Wilson RK, Hood LE: Physical maps of the mouse and human immunoglobulin-like loci. *Adv Immunol* 46:1, 1989.

50. von Boehmer H: The developmental biology of T lymphocytes. *Annu Rev Immunol* 6:309, 1988.

51. Adkins B, Mueller C, Okada CY, et al: Early events in T-cell maturation. *Annu Rev Immunol* 5:325, 1987.

52. Reinherz EL, Haynes BF, Nadler LM, et al: *Leukocyte Typing,* vol 2. New York, Springer-Verlag, 1986, p 550.

53. Kronenberg M, Siu G, Hood LE, et al: The molecular genetics of the T-cell antigen receptor and T-cell recognition. *Annu Rev Immunol* 4:529, 1986.

54. Clevers H, Alarcon B, Wileman T, et al: The T cell receptor/CD3 complex: A dynamic protein ensemble. *Annu Rev Immunol* 6:629, 1988.

55. Allison JP, McIntyre BW, Bloch D: Tumor-specific antigen of murine T lymphoma defined with monoclonal antibody. *J Immunol* 129:2293, 1982.

56. Hedrick SM: T lymphocyte receptors. In Paul WE, ed: *Fundamental Immunology,* ed 2. New York, Raven Press, 1989, p 291.

57. Toyonaga B, Mak TW: Genes of the T-cell antigen receptor in normal and malignant T cells. *Annu Rev Immunol* 5:585, 1987.

58. Raulet DH: The structure, function, and molecular genetics of

the gamma/delta T cell receptor. *Annu Rev Immunol* 7:175, 1989.

59. Samelson LE, Harford HB, Klausner RD: Identification of the components of the murine T cell antigen receptor complex. *Cell* 43:223, 1985.

60. Fowlkes BJ, Pardoll DM: Molecular and cellular events of T cell development. *Adv Immunol* 44:207, 1989.

61. Terhorst C, Alarcon B, de Vries J, et al: T lymphocyte recognition and activation. In Hames BD, Glover DM, eds. *Molecular Immunology.* Oxford, IRL Press. 1988, p 145.

62. Parnes JR: Molecular biology and function of CD4 and CD8. *Adv Immunol* 44:265, 1989.

63. Kishimoto TK, Larson RS, Corbi AL: The leukocyte integrins. *Adv Immunol* 46:149, 1989.

64. Alm GV: Lymphokines in the regulation of immune responses. *Vet Immunol Immunopathol* 17:173, 1987.

65. Osborne DP, Katz DH: Antigen-induced deoxyribonucleic acid synthesis in mouse lymphocytes. I. The nature and specificity of lymphocyte activation by hemocyanin and dinitrophenyl carrier conjugates. *J Immunol* 111:1164, 1973.

66. Cantor H, Boyse EA: Regulation of cellular and humoral immunity by T cell subclasses. *Cold Spring Harbor Symp Quant Biol* 41:23, 1977.

67. Hodes RJ: T-cell-mediated regulation: Help and suppression. In Paul WE, ed. *Fundamental Immunology.* New York, Raven Press. 1989, p 587.

68. Cantor H, Boyse EA: Functional subclasses of T lymphocytes bearing different Ly antigens. II. Cooperation between subclasses of Ly+ cells in the generation of killer activity. *J Exp Med* 141:1390, 1975.

69. Hansen PW, Petersen CM, Povlsen JV, et al: Cytotoxic human HLA class II restricted purified protein derivative–reactive T-lymphocyte clones. IV. Analysis of HLA restriction pattern and mycobacterial antigen specificity. *Hum Immunol* 18:135, 1987.

70. Heeg K, Steeg C, Hardt C, et al: Identification of interleukin 2–producing T helper cells within murine Lyt-2+ T lymphocytes: Frequency, specificity and clonal segregation from Lyt-2+ precursors of cytotoxic T lymphocytes. *Eur J Immunol* 17:229, 1987.

71. Mosmann TR, Coffman RL: TH1 and TH2 cells: Different patterns of lymphokine secretion lead to different functional properties. *Annu Rev Immunol* 7:145, 1989.

72. Janeway CA, Carding S, Jones B, et al: CD4+ T cells: Specificity and function. *Immunol Rev* 101:39, 1989.

73. Rocklin RE, Benaltzen K, Greineder D: Mediators of immunity: Lymphokines and monokines. *Adv Immunol* 29:55, 1980.

74. Climens MJ, Morris AG, Gearing AJH: *Lymphokines and Interferons.* Oxford, IRL Press, 1987.

75. Devos R, Cheroutre H, Plaetinck G, et al: Identification and expression of cDNA plasmids corresponding to human interferon-gamma and interleukin 2. *Lymphokines* 13:21, 1987.

76. Mizel SB, Farrar JJ: Revised nomenclature for antigen-nonspecific T-cell proliferation and helper factors. *Cell Immunol* 48:433, 1979.

77. Smith KA: The interleukin 2 receptor. *Adv Immunol* 42:165, 1988.

78. Fung MR, Greene WC: The human interleukin 2 receptor: Insights into subunit structure and growth signal transduction. *Semin Immunol* 2:119, 1990.

79. Ohara J, Paul WE: Receptors for B-cell stimulatory factor-1 expressed on cells of haematopoietic lineage. *Nature* 325:537, 1987.

80. Rosenberg SA, Lotze MT: Cancer immunotherapy using interleukin-2 and interleukin-2–activated lymphocytes. *Annu Rev Immunol* 3:681, 1986.

81. Grimm EA, Mazumder A, Zhang HZ, et al: Lymphokine-activated killer cell phenomenon. Lysis of natural-resistant fresh solid tumor cells by interleukin 2–activated autologous human peripheral blood lymphocytes. *J Exp Med* 155:1823, 1982.

82. Miyajima A, Miyatake S, Schreurs J, et al: Coordinate regulation of immune and inflammatory response by T cell–derived lymphokines. *FASEB J* 2:2462, 1988.

83. Vandergrifft EV, Horohov DW: Molecular cloning and expression of equine interleukin 2. *Vet Immunol Immunopathol* 39:395, 1993.

84. Travenor AS, Allen WR, Butcher GW: cDNA cloning of equine interleukin-2 by polymerase chain reaction. *Equine Vet J* 25:242, 1993.

85. Vandergrifft EV, Swiderski CE, Horohov DW: Molecular cloning and expression of equine interleukin 4. *Vet Immunol Immunopathol* 40:379, 1994.

86. Antczak DF: Equine leucocyte antigen system: The future of clinical application. *Equine Vet J* 17:257, 1985.

87. Halliwell REW, McGorum BC, Irving P, et al: Local and systemic antibody production in horses affected with chronic obstructive pulmonary disease. *Vet Immunol Immunopathol* 38:201, 1993.

88. Dirscherl P, Grabner A, Buschmann H: Responsiveness of basophil granulocytes of horses suffering from chronic obstructive pulmonary disease to various allergens. *Vet Immunol Immunopathol* 38:217, 1993.

89. Romagnani S: Human TH1 and TH2 subsets: Regulation of differentiation and role in protection and immunopathology. *Int Arch Allergy Appl Immunol* 98:279, 1992.

1.2.

Immunogenetics

Jill J. McClure, DVM, MS

Immunogenetics is the branch of genetics concerned with the inheritance of antigenic and other characters related to the immune response. To an immunologist, the emphasis is placed on the "immuno-" portion of the word and generally refers to the two inherited systems involved in the immune system: the structural genetics of immunoglobulins, and the genes that constitute the major histocompatibility complex (MHC). However, the more broadly defined area of animal immunogenetics emphasizes "genetics" and includes study of the genetics of red blood cell antigens and even structural polymorphisms of proteins that have little connection to the immune system but are useful in blood typing.

The surfaces of cells are covered with molecules of various types and functions, the presence or absence of which is genetically determined. Alloantigens are molecules that differ among individuals of the same species and can be recognized as foreign by the immune system of animals of the same species *not* possessing them (e.g., by the production of antibody against them). A number of red and white blood cell surface molecules are alloantigens.

Red blood cell alloantigens form the basis for blood groups. There are seven different genetic systems or loci identified with the presence of red blood cell alloantigens in horses[1, 2] (Table 1–5). These seven systems comprise 34

Table 1–5. Blood Group Systems, Factors, and Alleles of the Horse Recognized by the International Society for Animal Genetics

System	Factors	Recognized Alleles
A	a*, b†, c, d, e, f, g	A^a, A^{adf}, A^{adg}, A^{abdf}, A^{abdg}, A^b, A^{bc}, A^{bce}, A^{be}, A^c, A^{ce}, A^e, A^-
C	a	C^a, C^-
D	a, b, c†, d, e, f, g, h, i, k, l, m, n, o, p, q, r	D^{adl}, D^{adlnr}, D^{adlr}, D^{bcmq}, D^{cefgmq}, $D^{cegimnq}$. D^{cfgkm}, D^{cfmqr}, D^{cmg}, D^{cdmp}, D^{cgmq}, D^{cgmqr}, D^{deklqr}, D^{delno}, D^{deloq}, D^{delq}, D^{dfkir}, D^{dghmp}, D^{dghmq}, D^{dghmqr}, D^{dki}, D^{dlnq}, D^{dlnqr}, D^{dlqr}, D^{dno}, D^{dq}, (D^-)
K	a	K^a, K^-
P	a†, b, c, d	P^a, P^{ac}, P^{acd}, P^{ad}, P^b, P^{bd}, P^d, P^-
Q	a*, b, c	Q^a, Q^{ub}, Q^{ube}, Q^{ac}, Q^b, Q^{bc}, Q^c, Q
U	a†	U^a, U^-

*Most common factors involved in neonatal isoerythrolysis.
†Previously reported to cause neonatal isoerythrolysis in at least one case.

serologically detectable factors internationally recognized as a result of interlaboratory comparison tests carried out under the auspices of the Society for Animal Genetics. Additional factors may be recognized by individual laboratories.[1, 2] Each factor is associated with only one locus or system. For example, seven of the factors are currently associated with the A system: A^a, A^b, A^c, A^d, A^e, A^f, and A^g. One factor each is associated with the C, K, and U systems, C^a, K^a, and U^a respectively. The D system has at least 17 factors associated with it.

The factors represent single antigenic sites (determinants) on the surface molecule and they are not synonymous with the whole gene product of the locus. The alleles are alternative forms of the gene that can occur at any given locus. Each allele controls the expression of a different singular molecule that may contain one or a combination of the detectable factors. A combination of factors inherited as a single unit (determined by a single allele) is known as a phenogroup[3] (see Table 1–5). For example, the A system has the following alleles made up of combinations of factors A^a through A^g; A^- (null, no factors detected), A^a (only A^a detected), A^{adf} (factors A^a, A^d, and A^f detected), A^{abdf}, A^{adg}, A^{abdg}, A^b, A^{bc}, A^{bce}, A^{be}, A^c, A^{ce}, and A^e. Not all "mathematically" possible combinations of factors or phenogroups occur. When multiple factors are present as one allele (e.g., A^{bc}) it probably represents more than one antigenic site on a single molecule determined by the gene; however, the presence of several molecules controlled by closely linked genes cannot be completely ruled out. It is sometimes possible to determine the genotype (e.g., which alleles are present) of an individual based on the phenotype, and sometimes not. For example, an individual in which blood factors A^a, A^c, and A^e are detected could be assumed to have inherited factor A^a from one parent and A^{ce} from the other (A^a/A^{ce}) whereas if only factors A^b and A^c were detected, it would not be possible to tell from blood typing whether the genotype of the individual was A^b/A^c or A^{bc}/A^{bc} or A^{bc}/A^b or A^{bc}/A^c. The frequencies of occurrence of each allele in the population vary among different breeds[1, 2] (Table 1–6).

There are three loci identified with the presence of leukocyte antigens in horses: ELA, ELY-1, and ELY-2.

The ELA locus is the major histocompatibility system of the horse.[4–9] The structure and function of these molecules is discussed in Chapter 1.1. There are several linked genes thus far identified in this system, including those coding for class I lymphocyte antigens (ELA-A, ELA-B), class II lymphocyte antigens, the fourth component of complement (C4), and steroid 21-hydroxylase.[10, 11] The A blood group system is also closely linked to the MHC.[12, 13]

The class I ELA-A locus has been best characterized as a result of a series of international workshops.[14–18] Thirteen serologic specificities (alleles) are well characterized and other specificities are known to exist. Class I antigens are found on virtually all nucleated cells in the body, although the amount of antigen per cell and the ease of detection varies. These antigens are conventionally assayed using peripheral blood mononuclear cells in a complement-mediated lymphocytotoxicity assay.

Another serologically defined class I ELA locus (ELA-B) has been described. Based on a series of recombinants between blood groups A, ELA-A, and ELA-B, the probable linear order of the genes on this segment of chromosomes is A,ELA-A,ELA-B.[10]

Horses and mice are unique in the expression of a soluble class I antigen called equine soluble class I (ESCI) in horses and Q10 in mice.[19, 20]

Three serologic specificities, W13, W22, and W23, appear to be alleles for another ELA-linked gene, which is separate from the ELA-A locus.[18] These alloantigens are believed to be class II genes (analogous to the D locus in humans) based on the molecular weights of the gene products.[18]

In most species class II antigens are found primarily on B cells and macrophages. Only about 20% of the peripheral blood mononuclear cells express the class II antigens, which makes serologic detection by cytotoxicity testing difficult. However, in horses, T lymphocytes also express class II antigens.[21] These antigens can be detected by serologic means (complement-mediated lymphocytotoxicity testing) or by mixed lymphocyte culture (MLC).[7, 22, 23] In MLC typing, the test animal's cells are cultured with a panel of lymphocytes from different individuals, each of which is known to be homozygous for a different class II antigen. The test animal's cells will not be stimulated by homozygous typing

Table 1–6. Gene Frequencies of Locus A Alleles for Seven Breeds of Horses in the United States*†

Locus	Allele	Breed						
		TB (n = 100)	AR (n = 100)	ST (n = 100)	MH (n = 84)	QH (n = 100)	PF (n = 108)	PP (n = 100)
A	adf	0.849	0.636	0.566	0.529	0.440	0.263	0.321
	adg	(0.001)‡	0.182	(0.001)	0.040	0.050	0.233	0.214
	a	0.000	0.000	0.000	0.000	0.000	0.000	0.000
	b	0.010	0.055	0.389	0.201	0.150	0.144	0.065
	c	0.007	0.007	0.000	0.037	0.010	0.042	0.004
	e	0.000	0.000	0.015	0.055	0.010	0.000	0.000
	bc	0.000	0.020	0.020	0.006	0.010	0.014	0.000
	be	0.000	0.000	(0.001)	0.000	0.000	0.000	0.000
	ce	0.000	0.000	0.000	0.010	0.000	0.000	0.000
	bce	0.000	0.000	0.000	(0.001)	0.000	0.000	0.000
	—	0.134	0.100	0.010	0.122	0.330	0.304	0.396

*Modified from Bowling AT, Clark RS: Blood group and protein polymorphism gene frequencies for seven breeds of horses in the United States. *Anim Blood Groups Biochem Genet* 16:93, 1985.

†Abbreviations: TB, Thoroughbreds; AR, Arabians; ST, standardbreds. MH, Morgans; QH, quarter horses; PF, Paso Fino; PP, Peruvian Pasos.

‡Specificity is present in the breed at frequency greater than or equal to 0.001, but was not found in the random sample under study.

cells with which they share a class II antigen, but they will be stimulated by cells with which they do not share a class II antigen.

ELY-1 and ELY-2 are each two-allele systems. ELY-1 has two alleles designated 1.1 and 1.2.[16, 24] ELY-2 has two alleles designated 2.1 and null (not detectable).[16, 25, 26] These systems are not linked to the MHC or to each other.[16, 25, 26] They are detected by serologic means using complement-mediated microlymphocytotoxicity testing. Their structure and function are not known.

Other types of genetic markers not directly relating to the immune system include polymorphic proteins and DNA polymorphisms (DNA "fingerprinting").

The genes controlling the structure of many plasma and cellular proteins have more than one allele, each of which produces a slightly structurally different molecule. The differences are generally minor and result in no difference in function of the molecule. However, the minor structural differences can result in differences in charge or size, or both, which can be detected using various types of electrophoresis. These structural differences serve as excellent genetic markers because they allow the genetic makeup to be directly inferred from the gene products detected by electrophoresis. If two different alleles are present in an individual, both molecular species are produced and can be detected, thus allowing the genotype to be inferred directly from the phenotype. A list of polymorphic proteins, many of which are used in equine blood typing, is shown in Table 1–7.

Attempts have been made to standardize the nomenclature relating to polymorphic protein systems. An abbreviation of the name of the genetic system (e.g., PI for protease inhibitor) is coupled with a letter indicating an allelic band pattern (e.g., PIF or PIN). The fastest allelic band pattern first described is called F and the slowest, S. This allows for the somewhat alphabetical assignment of additional alleles that might be discovered between or on either side of the F and S band patterns.[33] Most, but not all, allelic band terminology conforms to these guidelines. The variants (recognizable allelic band patterns) for the more commonly used protein polymorphisms in equine blood typing are listed in Table 1–8.

Table 1–7. Examples of Equine Polymorphic Proteins*

Abbreviation	Protein	Source
ALB	Albumin	Serum
TF	Transferrin	Serum
PI	Protease inhibitor	Serum
ES	Carboxylesterase	Serum
A1B	α1-β Glycoprotein	Serum
GC	Vitamin D–binding protein	Serum
PLG	Plasminogen	Serum
PEPA	Peptidase A	Serum
PGD	6-Phosphogluconate dehydrogenase	Red blood cells (RBC)
PGM	Phosphoglucomutase	RBC
GPI	Glucose phosphate isomerase	RBC
CAT	Catalase	RBC
CA	Carbonic anhydrase	RBC
HBA	Hemoglobin α	RBC
DIA	NAD diaphorase	RBC
AP	Acid phosphatase	RBC

*Data from references 2, 27–32.

Table 1–8. Variants of Commonly Used Protein Polymorphisms*

Marker†	Allelic Variants
ALB	A, I, B
TF	D, D2, E, F1, F2, F3, G, H1, H2, J, M, O, R
PI	E, F, G, H, I, J, K, L, L2, N, O, P, Q, R, R2, S, S3, T, U, V, W, X, Z
A1B	F, K, Q, S
ES	F, G, H, I, L, M, N, O, R, S
GC	F, S
PGD	D, F, I, S
CA	E, F, I, L, O, S
CAT	F, S
PGM	F, S, V
AP	F, S
HBA	A, AII, BI, BII, C, N, V
GPI	F, I, S
DIA	F, S
PEPA	F, S
PLG	1, 2

*Data from Bowling AT, Clark RS: Blood group and protein polymorphism gene frequencies for seven breeds of horses in the United States. *Anim Blood Groups Biochem Genet* 16:93, 1985.

†For abbreviations, see Table 1–7.

Technological advances have allowed detection of polymorphism at the level of DNA as well as at the level of gene products (e.g., proteins). The digestion of purified genomic DNA from nucleated cells with bacterial enzymes (called restriction enzymes) results in the DNA being "cut" wherever specific short sequences of base pairs (often only four to six bases in length), called restriction sites, occur. There are millions of digestion sites scattered somewhat randomly throughout the length of the DNA, and this enzymatic digestion results in production of a spectrum of fragments of DNA of various sizes, which can be separated by size using electrophoresis. A variation in DNA sequence that creates or eliminates a restriction site will alter the length of the resulting DNA fragment or fragments. The length variation in specific DNA fragments is referred to as DNA polymorphism, and the fragments are restriction fragment length polymorphisms (RFLPs).[34–37] The size distribution of the fragments produced by digestion is a function of the presence or absence of a given DNA restriction site and the length of the DNA between restriction sites, both of which depend upon the (inherited) DNA sequence.[36] Individual sites may be generated or abolished by mutations that change a single base pair or involve the insertion or deletion of DNA. The length of DNA between sites may vary depending upon which alleles of genes in that segment are present, as well as on the occurrence of deletions or insertions in that segment of the chromosome.[36, 37]

The RFLP is a potential genetic marker in that it is readily detectable and a number of distinguishable variants may exist in the population. Identification of a specific fragment from among the millions begins by sorting the fragments by size using electrophoresis. The fragment of interest is then located using a technique called Southern blotting, named after M.E. Southern, who developed it. This technique takes advantage of the fact that DNA can only pair according to set rules and so the sequence on one strand constitutes a unique match for the sequence on the other. To detect the presence of a specific sequence, a single-stranded copy of a DNA sequence can act as a probe to bind and detect the complementary sequence in the sample of DNA fragments that have been denatured to form single strands. The probe is a segment of DNA often chosen at random from a collection ("library") of cloned DNA fragments representing the whole genome. The probe is "labeled" (usually radioactively) and allowed to hybridize with the assortment of denatured DNA fragments. The labeled probe will find its complementary sequence among the fragments and "attach." The size fragment that contains the complementary sequence is identified by the presence of a radioactive band or bands on the electrophoresis blot. If the radioactive bands appear at different places on blots of DNA from different individuals, then the cloned DNA probe has detected a variable cutting pattern that results from DNA polymorphism. The probe and the RFLP it detects constitute a unique genetic marker system.

By digesting DNA with a variety of restriction enzymes that cut the DNA at different sites and generate different patterns of fragments and by looking with a variety of probes on each of these different digests, the number of permutations of possible combinations of genetic markers becomes very large and the likelihood of two individuals being identical becomes very remote, except in the case of identical twins. This forms the basis for a DNA fingerprint unique to an individual. Thus DNA polymorphisms are proving to be very powerful markers for animal identification.[35–37]

DNA polymorphisms also are powerful tools for the study of the genetic basis of disease. Sufficiently large numbers of RFLPs should provide genetic markers for each segment of chromosome. One can then look for the inheritance of the genetic marker (RFLP) in conjunction with some other character such as a disease.[35–38] Identification of an association between occurrence of disease and segregation of an RFLP suggests that (1) the RFLP may be a marker for the disease and (2) the gene(s) controlling the disease is located on that segment of DNA. This can form the basis for diagnostic testing and guide study of actual genetic mechanisms relating to the pathophysiology of the disease.

APPLICATION OF GENETIC MARKERS

Genetic markers in horses are used for identification, verification of parentage, and the study of the genetic basis of disease. The combined use of blood groups (red blood cell alloantigens) and other genetic markers is collectively called blood typing. The "blood type" is actually a composite result of many different tests used to detect the presence or absence of many different alleles at numerous loci.

The genetic markers commonly used in horse blood typing are autosomal but not all are independent of one another.[39] Several linkage groups have been identified wherein certain loci tend to be inherited together, which suggests that the genes controlling these markers are situated near one another on the chromosomes (Table 1–9).

Because an individual is (and in fact *must* be) a combina-

Table 1–9. Linkage Groups of Genetic Markers* [2, 11–13, 24, 26, 29, 30, 32, 40–42]

Linkage	Marker†
LG I	K, PGD
LG II	ALB, GC, ES
LG III	A, ELA
LG IV	GPI, A1b
LG V	U, Pi

*Data from references, 2, 11–13, 24, 26, 29, 30, 32, 40–42.
†Independent markers: C, D, P, Q, TF, PGM, CA, AP, HBA; undefined linkage: CAT, ELY-1, ELY-2, PLG. For abbreviations, see text and Table 1–7.

tion of the genetic material from its two parents, certain things are true. The individual will have no genes that are not present in one or both parents. The individual *must* have one of the two genes present at each locus from each parent. These facts form the basis for testing for parentage exclusions using genetic markers and blood typing.

A type I exclusion occurs when a foal possesses an antigen not present on either parent. Assuming that one of the parents is known for certain, usually the dam, then the other parent is excluded because it could not have contributed the antigen in question which the foal has. A type II exclusion occurs when the foal does not possess either antigen expressed by one stated parent (usually the sire). The foal must inherit one of the two antigens possessed by each parent. Both type I and II exclusions can be present simultaneously. The probabilities for making each type of exclusion can be calculated, with the theoretical maximum being 1.00 (100%). The combined probability of exclusions (CPE), calculated from the probability of making type I and type II exclusions for a particular locus, is the efficacy of the genetic system to exclude an incorrectly assigned sire. If neither type of exclusion is present, the parentage is not *proved* to be correct. It is only possible to exclude a parent with certainty.[43]

When evaluating pedigrees, each genetic marker system is treated as an independent unit. An exclusion in one system, even if all the other systems are "compatible," will allow exclusion of the stated parentage.

The effectiveness of blood typing in identifying animals and establishing parentage depends on the number of genetic systems tested, the number of different alleles for each system, and the distribution of the various alleles in the population. Some genetic marker systems are more "informative" than others. For example, if most horses have the same allele for a given locus, then that particular marker will not be very discriminating in distinguishing between two individuals because the likelihood will be that they will share the same type. Using a battery of 20 loci, including red blood cell typing and protein polymorphisms, blood typing is estimated to be 94% to 96% effective for recognizing incorrect paternity in Thoroughbreds, standardbreds, Arabians, quarter horses, Morgans, Paso Finos, and Peruvian Pasos.[2, 44] The same panel of markers is estimated to be 96% effective if both parents are incorrectly stated.[2] Using ELA

typing alone, approximately 67% of cases of questionable paternity can be resolved, and with a combination of ELA and other blood-typing markers, the percentage approaches 99%.[43] DNA fingerprinting will increase that probability even higher such that it will be essentially possible to "prove" biological parentage because the odds of incorrect inclusion will be negligible.

Another area of application of genetic markers is the study of the inherited basis of disease. A number of diseases have been "associated" with one or more genetic markers. An association means that the presence of the disease and the presence of the marker are positively correlated, that is, they tend to occur, to be inherited, together. This suggests that either some direct cause and effect exists (e.g., the marker is somehow directly associated with disease production) or that a possible linkage between the marker gene and the gene(s) that actually controls the disease trait exists (e.g., the genes are located on the same segment of chromosome). Several diseases have associations with the equine MHC (ELA antigens) including *Culicoides* hypersensitivity in Iceland ponies,[45] equine sarcoid,[46–48] and arytenoid chondritis.[49] The association of sarcoid is particularly strong but not absolute with W13, a class II antigen. Within families, sarcoid appears to be linked to particular class II alleles; however the particular allele varies among families, suggesting that some closely linked gene is responsible, not the class II antigen itself. RFLP analysis of DNA from horses with sarcoids using class II probes has not shown any constant fragment shared by all affected horses.[50]

A few other interesting associations have been noted such as the preponderance of a particular esterase (Es) variant in Swedish Trotters that never start a race.[51, 52] When attempts to identify the reason for this association were made, increased numbers of horses with leg problems and bad tempers were in the nonstarter group, but the association between these factors and Es was not statistically significant. The effect of Es on nonstarting appeared to decrease over time and it was suggested that any Es effect may have been overshadowed by changes in the environment of the horses (improvement in tracks and shoeing) made during the period of study. For the most part, however, current genetic markers have not been shown to be the gene products that are directly associated with disease occurrence and only a few have any confirmed disease association.

Theoretically, if the number of genetic markers were large enough and were sprinkled evenly throughout the chromosomes, eventually a marker for every genetically controlled disease could be found by comparing the inheritance of a disease trait with the inheritance of the genetic marker. The application of DNA polymorphisms promises to be a significant tool in this regard. By developing a set of probes which map all portions of the equine genome, it will be possible to study the linkage between genetic markers and disease traits (or any other genetic trait, for that matter). This will potentially allow detection of carriers of "defective" genes and allow for identification of the genes and their products involved in the pathogenesis of diseases.

REFERENCES

1. Bell K: The blood groups of domestic mammals. In Agar NS, Board PG, eds: *Red Blood Cells of Domestic Mammals.* Amsterdam, Elsevier Science, 1983.

2. Bowling AT, Clark RS: Blood group and protein polymorphism gene frequencies for seven breeds of horses in the United States. *Anim Blood Groups Biochem Genet* 16:93, 1985.

3. Stormont C: The language of phenogroups. *Haematologica* 6:73, 1972.

4. Antczak DF: Structure and function of the major histocompatibility complex in domestic animals. *J Am Vet Med Assoc* 181:1030, 1982.

5. Antczak DF, Bright SM, Remick LH, et al: Lymphocyte alloantigens of the horse. I. Serologic and genetic studies. *Tissue Antigens* 20:172, 1982.

6. Bailey E: Identification and genetics of horse lymphocyte alloantigens. *Immunogenetics* 11:499, 1980.

7. Lazary S, Bullen S, Muller J, et al: Equine leukocyte antigen system. II. Serological and mixed lymphocyte reactivity studies in families. *Transplantation* 30:210, 1980.

8. Lazary S, deWeck AL, Bullen S, Straub R, et al: Equine leukocyte antigen system. I. Serological studies. *Transplantation* 30:203, 1980.

9. Mottironi VD, Perryman LE, Pollara B, et al: x R, x P: Major histocompatibility locus in the Arabian horse. *Transplantation* 31:290, 1981.

10. Bernoco D, Byrns G, Bailey E, et al: Evidence of a second polymorphic ELA class I (ELA-B) locus and gene order for three loci of the equine major histocompatibility complex. *Anim Genet* 18:103, 1987.

11. Kay PH, Dawkins RL, Bowling AT, et al: Heterogeneity and linkage of equine C4 and steroid 21-hydroxylase genes. *J Immunogenet* 14:247, 1987.

12. Bailey E, Stormont C, Suzuki Y, et al: Linkage of loci controlling alloantigens of red blood cells and lymphocytes in the horse. *Science* 204:1317, 1979.

13. Guerin G, Varewyck H, Bertaud M, et al: Analysis of a horse family with a crossing-over between the ELA complex and the A blood group system. *Anim Genet* 19:1, 1988.

14. Antczak DF, Bailey E, Barger B, et al: Joint report of the Third International Workshop on Lymphocyte Alloantigens of the Horse, Kennett Square, Pennsylvania, 25–27 April 1984. *Anim Genet* 17:363, 1986.

15. Bailey E, Antczak DF, Bernoco D, et al: Joint report of the Second International Workshop on Lymphocyte Alloantigens of the Horse, held 3–8 October 1982. *Anim Blood Groups Biochem Genet* 15:123, 1984.

16. Bernoco D, Antczak DF, Bailey E, et al: Joint report of the Fourth International Workshop on Lymphocyte Alloantigens of the Horse, Lexington, Kentucky, 12–22 October 1985. *Anim Genet* 18:81, 1987.

17. Bull RW: Joint report of the First International Workshop of Lymphocyte Alloantigens of the Horse held 24–29 October 1981. *Anim Blood Groups Biochem Genet* 14:119, 1983.

18. Lazary S, Antczak DF, Bailey E, et al: Joint report of the Fifth International Workshop on Lymphocyte Alloantigens of the Horse, Baton Rouge, Louisiana, 31 October–1 November 1987. *Anim Genet* 19:447, 1988.

19. Lew AM, Bailey E, Valas RB, et al: The gene encoding the equine soluble class I molecule is linked to the horse MHC. *Immunogenetics* 24:128, 1986.

20. Lew AM, Valas RB, Maloy WL, et al: A soluble class I molecule analogous to mouse Q10 in the horse and related species. *Immunogenetics* 23:277, 1986.

21. Crepaldi T, Crump A, Newman M, et al: Equine T lymphocytes express MHC class II antigens. *J Immunogenet* 13:349, 1986.

22. Hesford F, Lazary S, Curty-Hanni K, et al: Biochemical evidence that equine leukocyte antigens W13,W22 and W23 are present on horse major histocompatibility complex class II molecules. *Anim Genet* 20:415, 1989.

23. McClure JJ, Muscoplat CC, Johnson DW, et al: Microculture method for mixed lymphocyte cultures in the horse. *Am J Vet Res* 39:337, 1978.

24. Lazary S, Gerber H, deWeck AL, et al: Equine leucocyte antigen system: III. Non-MHC linked alloantigenic system in horses. *J Immunogenet* 9:327, 1982.

25. Antczak DF: Lymphocyte alloantigens of the horse. III. ELY-2.1: A lymphocyte alloantigen not coded for by the MHC. *Anim Blood Groups Biochem Genet* 15:103, 1984.

26. Bailey E, Henny PJ: Comparison of ELY-2.1 with blood group and ELY-1 markers in the horse. *Anim Blood Groups Biochem Genet* 15:117, 1984.

27. Guttormsen SA, Weitkamp LR: Equine marker genes: Polymorphism for soluble erythrocyte malic enzyme. *Anim Blood Groups Biochem Genet* 12:53, 1981.

28. Kaminski M: *Distribution of Genetic Variants of Blood Proteins and Enzymes in Horses of Various Breeds.* Princeton, NJ, Veterinary Publications, 1978, p 243.

29. Kay PH, Dawkins RL, Bowling AT, et al: Electrophoretic polymorphism and molecular structure of equine C3. *Anim Genet* 17:209, 1986.

30. Kay PH, Dawkins RL, Bowling AT, et al: Polymorphism of the acetylcholine receptor in the horse. *Vet Rec* 120:363, 1987.

31. Rando A, Di Gregorio P, Masina P: Polymorphic restriction sites in the horse beta-globulin gene cluster. *Anim Genet* 17:245, 1986.

32. Weitkamp LR, Costello-Leary P, Guttormsen SA: Equine marker genes: Polymorphism for plasminogen. *Anim Blood Groups Biochem Genet* 14:219, 1983.

33. Braend M: Nomenclature of polymorphic protein systems. *Nature* 4988:1067, 1965.

34. Jones KW: New techniques in molecular genetics. *Equine Vet J* 21:241, 1989.

35. Summers KM: DNA polymorphisms in human population studies: A review. *Ann Hum Biol* 14:203, 1987.

36. Thein SL, Wainscoat JS: The clinical applications of DNA polymorphisms. *Dis Markers* 4:203, 1986.

37. White R, Lalouel J-M: Chromosome mapping with DNA markers. *Sci Am* 258(2):40, February, 1988.

38. Defesche JC, de Visser M, Bakker E, et al: DNA restriction fragment length polymorphisms in differential diagnosis of genetic disease: Application in neuromuscular diseases. *Hum Genet* 82:55, 1989.

39. Sandberg K, Andersson L: Genetic linkage in the horse. I. Linkage relationships among 15 blood marker loci. *Hereditas* 100:199, 1984.

40. Andersson L, Juneja RK, Sandberg K: Genetic linkage between the loci for phosphohexose isomerase (PHI) and a serum protein (Xk) in horses. *Anim Blood Groups Biochem Genet* 14:45, 1983.

41. Bowling AT: Genetic linkage between loci for a red cell alloantigen (U) and serum protease inhibitor (Pi) in the horse. *Anim Genet* 17:217, 1986.

42. Weitkamp LR, Guttormsen SA, Costello-Leary P: Equine gene mapping: Close linkage between the loci for soluble malic enzyme and Xk (Pa). *Anim Blood Groups Biochem Genet* 13:279, 1982.

43. Bailey E: Usefulness of lymphocyte typing to exclude incorrectly assigned paternity in horses. *Am J Vet Res* 45:1976, 1984.

44. Scott AM: Immunogenetic analysis as a means of identification in horses. In Bryans JT, Gerber H, eds: *Equine Infectious Diseases IV. Proceedings of the Fourth International Conference on Equine Infectious Diseases.* Princeton, NJ, Veterinary Publications, 1978, p 259.

45. Lazary S, Larsen HJ, Glatt A, et al: Distribution of ELA antigens in "sweet itch" of horses (abstract). Presented at 18th International Conference on Animal Blood Groups and

Biochemical Polymorphism, Ottawa, Canada, July 18–23, 1982, p 67.

46. Gerber H, Dubath M-L, Lazary S: Association between predisposition to equine sarcoid and MHC in multiple-case families. In Powell DG, ed: *Equine Infectious Diseases V: Proceedings of the Fifth International Conference.* 1988, p 272.

47. Lazary S, Gerber H, Glatt PA, et al: Equine leucocyte antigens in sarcoid-affected horses. *Equine Vet J* 17:283, 1985.

48. Meredith D, Elser AH, Wolf B, et al: Equine leukocyte antigens: Relationships with sarcoid tumors and laminitis in two pure breeds. *Immunogenetics* 23:221, 1986.

49. McClure JJ, Koch C, Powell M, et al: Association of arytenoid chondritis with equine lymphocyte antigens but no association with laryngeal hemiplegia, umbilical hernia and cryptorchidism. *Anim Genet* 19:427, 1988.

50. Bailey E, Woodward JG, Albright DG, et al: RFLP marker genes for physiologically and serologically identified traits of the equine MHC. In Warner CM, Rothschild MF, Lamont SJ, eds: *The Molecular Biology of the Major Histocompatibility Complex of Domestic Animal Species.* Ames, Iowa State University Press, 1988, p 135.

51. Andersson L, Arnason T, Sandberg K: Biochemical polymorphism in relation to performance in horses. *Theor Appl Genet* 73:419, 1987.

52. Andersson-Eklund L, Andersson L, Sandberg K: Association between serum esterase (Es) type and starting proportion in Swedish Trotters: Further observations. *Anim Genet* 20:93, 1989.

1.3.

Hypersensitivity Reactions

Cyprianna E. Swiderski, DVM

Hypersensitivity refers to an altered state of immunoreactivity resulting in self-injury.[1, 2] The term *allergy,* now used synonymously with hypersensitivity, originally denoted a differentiation of self from non-self that was specific and possessed immunologic memory.[2, 3] Thus, hypersensitivity is a more appropriate term for overexuberant immunologic reactions that may or may not be based on the differentiation of self from non-self.[2] Four types of hypersensitivity diseases were classified according to their pathogenesis by Gell and Coombs.[3] Deficits in this classification system have become apparent because it is based on pathogenesis and not etiology, and many diseases are characterized by more than one type of hypersensitivity reaction. This chapter utilizes a broader classification scheme which divides these reactions temporally into immediate and delayed-type hypersensitivity (DTH). Autoimmune diseases, in which inappropriate differentiation of self from non-self causes immune-mediated self-injury, also fit the definition of hypersensitivity and complicate classification systems. The pathogenesis of autoimmune disease as it applies to hypersensitivity is also addressed.

Relative to other, small domestic animal species, little is known with respect to the incidence, pathogenesis, and treatment of hypersensitivity reactions in the horse. The signs of hypersensitivity reactions may be so subtle and varied that the disease goes unnoticed or an alternative diagnosis is made. Study of equine hypersensitivity reactions is complicated by the inchoate state of our knowledge of equine immunology. T-cell subsets are not well characterized, cell markers are not readily available, and financial support for such studies is limited.

There are clinical similarities between human and equine hypersensitivity reactions.[4–9] For the sake of completeness this chapter reflects the current understanding of hypersensitivity reactions in human subjects. This picture may not always accurately reflect the pathogenesis of hypersensitivity reactions in the horse.

OVERVIEW (Fig. 1–4)

After dividing hypersensitivity reactions into immediate and DTH reactions, it becomes evident that the immediate-type reactions are initiated by antigen-antibody complexes, whereas delayed-type reactions require cellular immunity.[10, 11] All antibody-mediated reactions are immediate once antigen combines with antibody, but the exact time course varies with the antibody class mediating the reaction and the time required for antibody production.[2, 6] Immediate hypersensitivity can be divided into anaphylactic, or reaginic, hypersensitivity, and immune-complex reactions.[12, 13]

Anaphylactic hypersensitivity is triggered by the binding of antigen to antigen-specific *cell-bound* antibody.[12] Depending on the site of union of antigen and antibody, these reactions can manifest as severe systemic reactions or may occur locally, as seen with insect hypersensitivities.[10, 14–16] Nonreaginic immune-complex reactions are mediated by antigen-antibody combinations that initiate complement-mediated cytotoxicity or are cleared by the reticuloendothelial system.[2, 4, 10, 13] Antigens responsible for nonreaginic immune-complex reactions can be circulating as soluble agents or associated with cells that may be circulating or fixed at a particular tissue site. Therefore, as with anaphylactic reactions, immune-complex reactions can occur locally or systemically, as seen with drug eruptions and serum sickness, respectively.

DTH reactions are mediated by antigen-specific T cells that induce the formation of potent cytotoxic macrophage effector cells.[17] The reaction is termed *delayed* because of the protracted time from antigen exposure to clinical manifestation of the reaction. Allergic contact dermatitis is a DTH reaction.

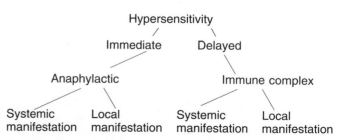

Figure 1–4. Schematic classification of hypersensitivity reactions.

IMMEDIATE-TYPE HYPERSENSITIVITY REACTIONS: ANAPHYLAXIS

Findings in other species suggest that the combination of antigen with antigen-specific cell-bound immunoglobulin contributes to the pathogenesis of many equine diseases, including adverse drug reactions,[2, 4, 6, 11, 16, 18–23] chronic obstructive pulmonary disease (COPD),[6, 11, 14, 15, 24–29] insect hypersensitivity,[2, 6, 11, 14–16, 20, 28, 30, 31] onchocerciasis,[16, 32] habronemiasis and other parasitic diseases,[6, 16, 33, 34] recurrent urticaria,[2, 16, 19, 20, 35, 36] angioedema,[2, 16, 20] food allergy,[2, 16, 18, 20, 28, 33, 37, 38] allergic rhinitis,[29, 39, 40] atopy,[2, 28, 35] and vasculitis.[2]

Pathogenesis

Anaphylactic hypersensitivity was once regarded as simply IgE-mediated histamine release. While the exact significance of histamine in equine anaphylactic hypersensitivity seems to vary with each disease entity, histamine cannot be considered the major mediator.[6, 11, 41, 42] Hypersensitivity is currently viewed as an inflammatory disease involving multiple cells and mediators. These mediators can either cause damage directly or serve as gatekeepers for recruitment of other cells that potentiate the inflammation with additional mediators. This causes a biphasic reaction with the first phase due to immediate release of preformed or newly synthesized mediators and a late phase due to mediators from secondarily recruited cells.[43–47] This biphasic reaction is reported in the horse.[31, 48]

Antigen, Antibody, and Cellular Characteristics

The antigen, antibody, and cells that bind the antibody are unique in anaphylactic hypersensitivity.[12, 43, 49–51] Only large antigens with molecular mass greater than 1,000 daltons are capable of cross-linking the Fab portions of surface-associated immunoglobulins that function as antigen receptors.[10, 43, 49] This cross-linking results in cellular activation and initiation of the hypersensitivity reaction.[5, 10, 12, 23, 43] Smaller antigens must combine with endogenous proteins to attain sufficient size to cross-link the cell's receptors.[4, 23, 49, 52]

Classically, anaphylactic hypersensitivity is associated with the production of IgE antibodies synthesized by B cells upon exposure to the appropriate antigen. IgE antibodies are sometimes called homocytotropic, indicating that the interaction between the immunoglobulin and cells it binds is species-specific.[1, 12, 53] IgE is the most significant homocytotropic antibody owing to high-affinity binding to the surface receptors of the mast cell and basophil via the Fc region of the antibody.[10, 12, 51, 54–56] This arrangement leaves the antigen-combining site (Fab portion) exposed (Fig. 1–5). Antigen cross-linking of the Fab portions of two or more IgE molecules stimulates cellular activation. Other antibody isotypes on mast cells and basophils are capable of inducing cellular activation when cross-linked by antigen but are less significant owing to their low-affinity binding to these cells.[12, 51, 54, 55, 57–61] The high-affinity binding of IgE to cell receptors accounts for the low serum concentration of IgE and the prolonged sensitivity to antigen after passive sensitization with small doses of antibody.[51, 62]

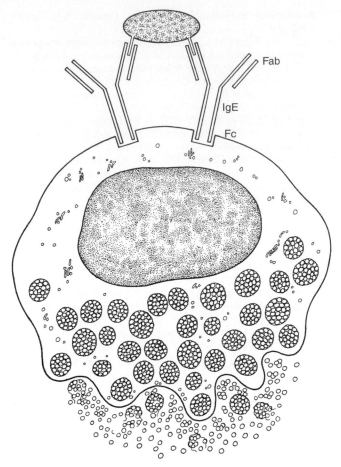

Mast cell degranulation with
release of mediators

Figure 1–5. Mast cell activation. Antigen cross-links the Fab portion of two or more IgE molecules, which are bound to the mast cell via high-affinity Fc surface receptors. Cross-linking triggers cell-associated enzyme cascades, leading to degranulation and the release of inflammatory mediators. (From Halliwell R, Gorman N: Mechanisms of immunological injury in hypersensitivity reactions. In Halliwell R, Gorman N, eds: *Veterinary Clinical Immunology.* Philadelphia, WB Saunders, 1989, p 213.)

IgE has demonstrated significance in the pathophysiology of equine hypersensitivity.[62a, 62b] Equine IgE exhibits physical characteristics of IgE from other species and is distinct from equine IgA, IgM, and all subclasses of equine IgG.[30, 31, 63, 64] In other non-equine species, certain subclasses of IgG are known to function as homocytotrophic antibody.[55, 57, 65] It is also possible that certain subclasses of equine IgG may mediate anaphylactic hypersensitivity reactions owing to the presence of low-affinity IgG receptors on the mast cell and basophil.[53, 66]

By virtue of their high-affinity IgE receptor, mast cells and basophils are the primary cell types that initiate anaphylactic hypersensitivity.[56] Macrophages, eosinophils, and platelets can also bind surface IgE but with much lower affinity, making them less significant in initiating the reaction.[17, 43, 56, 66, 67]

Mast cells and basophils are two distinct bone marrow–

derived cell types.[43, 55, 68] They have in common high histamine content, high-affinity IgE receptors, and triggering via receptor bridging, but differ structurally, morphologically, and functionally.[43, 55, 68] These cells appear to function not only in allergy but also in immunologic homeostasis.[43] Mast cells, because of their large number in connective tissue of mucosa, serosa, vessels, glands, ducts, nerves, and lymphoid tissue of humans and rats, appear to function in initial immunologic defense. Basophils seem to be more significant in mediating allergic and autoimmune disease, cutaneous hypersensitivity, and parasitic defense, and regulating DTH.

The anaphylactic reactions mediated by these cells may be severe systemic reactions characterized by cardiovascular and respiratory compromise, or may be localized, as with urticaria.[5, 10, 15, 16] Localized reactions are more common. Whether a local or systemic anaphylactic reaction develops depends on the challenge route, type, quantity, and site of mediator release, the response of the individual to the inflammatory mediators, and the activation requirements of the antigen.[69] The cellular and molecular events occurring in local and systemic anaphylaxis are identical.[10]

Altered Regulation of IgE Production

Antigen characteristics and the cytokines that are produced as a result of antigen interaction with T cells determine the immunoglobulin isotype that is synthesized during antigen challenge. In the majority of nonallergic humans, the production of IgE in response to a protein antigen is transient.[12] Subsequent interactions with the same antigen result in the production of IgG. However, atopic humans and certain strains of mice have an enhanced and persistent IgE response to low-dose antigen challenge, and despite chronic antigen stimulation do not complete the isotype switch to IgG production. This propensity for IgE production is genetic and affected individuals commonly develop immediate hypersensitivity reactions such as allergic rhinitis, bronchial asthma, atopic dermatitis, or food allergies to common environmental antigens. Atopy appears to be related to constitutive differences in cytokine production by the helper T cells of affected individuals.

Interleukin-4 (IL-4) and interferon-γ (IFN-γ) are cytokines of primary importance in IgE production.[12, 70–73] Activated T-helper 2 cells (Th2), as well as basophils and mast cells, are major sources of IL-4, whereas IFN-γ is derived from activated T-helper 1 cells (Th1), cytotoxic T-cells, and NK cells. IL-4 is required for the isotype switch of the B cell from surface IgM and IgD to IgE, and IFN-γ inhibits this switch to IgE.[70–73] In fact, disequilibrium between IL-4 and IFN-γ production may be responsible for increased IgE synthesis in allergic conditions such as atopy.[12, 70] Atopic humans are more likely to produce IL-4 secreting T-helper 2 cells (Th2) in response to environmental antigen challenge than non-atopic individuals who either fail to produce antigen-specific helper-T-cell clones or produce IFN-γ-secreting helper T-cell clones (Th1).[71, 73a, 73b] Glucocorticoids, which are frequently used to treat hypersensitivity disease, have been shown to induce helper T cell secretion of factors that augment the production of an IgE-suppressing factor.[74] Unfortunately, direct in vivo manipulation of IL-4 and IFN-γ using monoclonal antibodies to these cytokines in order to suppress IgE formation has not been successful.[12]

The persistent IgE response in genetically programmed individuals occurs only with low-dose antigen stimulation. Increasing the antigen dose creates a transient IgE response and an increase in IgG production.[12] This is the basis for using large antigen doses for desensitization.

In addition to differential cytokine production, alterations in calcium homeostasis, neutrophil respiratory burst, and accentuation of other inflammatory responses have been identified in allergic individuals.[70, 75, 76] An association between HLA class II antigens and allergen hyperresponsiveness has been determined in atopic individuals, indicating that allergen hyperresponsiveness is HLA class II–restricted.[77] Thus, in humans it appears that genetically controlled alterations in basophil and mast cell function, increased IgE synthesis, and hyperresponsiveness of the target organ are significant in the pathogenesis of allergic disease.[55]

Triggering of Mast Cells and Basophils

Mast cells and basophils may be triggered to release their inflammatory mediators either immunologically or nonimmunologically.[5, 10, 12, 43] Anaphylactic reactions that are immunologically triggered can occur in response to minute doses of antigen but require prior exposure to the antigen so that antigen-specific IgE can be synthesized. Immunologic triggering occurs when allergen cross-links two or more high-affinity IgE receptors on the mast cell surface. The Fc portion of the antigen-specific IgE molecule is bound to the mast cell or basophil high-affinity receptor leaving the Fab portion free to interact with antigen (see Fig. 1–5). Antigens capable of binding two or more Fab portions from different molecules produce a signal sufficient to alter cell membrane fluidity, which triggers a cell-associated enzyme cascade.

Nonimmunologic triggering occurs when mast cells and basophils are activated without direct antigen binding to surface IgE.[10, 43, 54] This reaction has been termed *anaphylactoid*.[52, 54, 69] Anaphylactoid reactions do not require prior exposure to the antigen and are clinically indistinguishable from immunologically triggered anaphylactic reactions. Complement products C3a and C5a, the anaphylatoxins, liberated via the alternative complement pathway, are capable of inducing nonimmunologic mast cell and basophil degranulation.[10, 54, 55, 78] Radiocontrast agents, certain complex polysaccharides, formyl methionine, gastrin, and substance P have been shown to directly stimulate the alternative pathway.[54] Many substances, including IL-3, hypertonic saline, nonsteroidal anti-inflammatory agents (NSAIDs), thiopental, codeine, opiates, neuromuscular blocking agents, mannitol, radiocontrast agents, polymyxin B, and vancomycin, are capable of inducing mast cell and basophil degranulation without C3a or C5a.[10, 43, 52, 54, 55, 69, 78] Because the same chemical mediators are produced during immunologically and nonimmunologically triggered reactions, the clinical signs and therapy of anaphylactic and anaphylactoid reactions are identical.[43, 69]

Immune complexes, which are capable of fixing complement, may trigger the release of mediators from mast cells and basophils by activating the classic pathway of complement, generating C3a and C5a.[10, 23, 78] Technically, this is nonimmunologic triggering because antigen does not bind to surface IgE, but this type of immediate hypersensitivity reaction does require prior antigen exposure for immunoglobulin synthesis.

Biochemical Events Induced by Receptor Bridging

IgE receptor bridging by antigen causes a local alteration in membrane fluidity, which activates membrane-associated enzymes. Though debated, it is likely that initial activation of tyrosine kinases, which phosphorylate and thereby activate phospholipase C (PLC), is the critical first step in mast cell signal transduction leading to degranulation. Other membrane-associated enzymes including serine proteases, methyltransferases, and adenylate cyclase, are subsequently activated in a cascade manner (Fig. 1–6).[12, 43, 68, 79] Activated PLC cleaves membrane phosphatidylinositol-1, 5-diphosphate (P2) to diacylglycerol (DAG) and inositol 1, 4, 5-triphosphate (IP$_3$). IP$_3$ triggers intracellular calcium mobilization. DAG is important in initiating the arachidonic acid cascade and forming membrane-active fusogens responsible for degranulation of the mast cell and basophil. In association with intracellular calcium, DAG activates phospholipase A$_2$ (PLA$_2$) and DAG lipase. PLA$_2$ cleaves arachidonic acid and lysophosphatidylcholine from membrane-derived phosphatidylcholine (PC). Once released, arachidonic acid reacts with cyclooxygenase and lipoxygenase to form the prostanoids and leukotrienes, respectively. DAG lipase activity results in the formation of fatty acids, monoacylglycerol (MAG), and lysophosphatidic acid (LPA). Lysophospholipids, DAG, MAG, and LPA are all membrane-active fusogens

that can cause degranulation. Adenylate cyclase activation and GTP-binding proteins both modulate this pathway. Thus, antigen binding to immunoglobulin on the basophil and mast cell surface results in release of inflammatory mediators from the cell's granules and stimulates prostanoid and leukotriene synthesis.

INFLAMMATORY MEDIATORS OF IMMEDIATE HYPERSENSITIVITY

The hypersensitivity reactions share common effector cells though the proportion of cell types varies. Accordingly, many mediators are common to the different types of hypersensitivity reactions, though their proportions may also vary. This accounts for the use of the same therapeutic agents in the treatment of many hypersensitivity diseases. For simplicity, the chemical mediators are discussed together. Three categories of inflammatory mediators of hypersensitivity exist: (1) those preformed within the secretory granule, (2) those synthesized upon cellular activation, and (3) those derived from recruited cells or from the actions of the preformed and newly generated mediators on tissue and plasma components.[43, 56, 80] Preformed mediators, also called primary mediators, include the biogenic amines histamine and serotonin; the proteoglycans heparin and chondroitin sulfate; and a plethora of enzymes including tryptase, chymase, acid hydrolases, kallikrein, and elastase. Newly generated mediators are those whose synthesis is stimulated by the perturbance of the basophil or mast cell membrane. These include the leukotrienes, prostanoids, kinins, and a

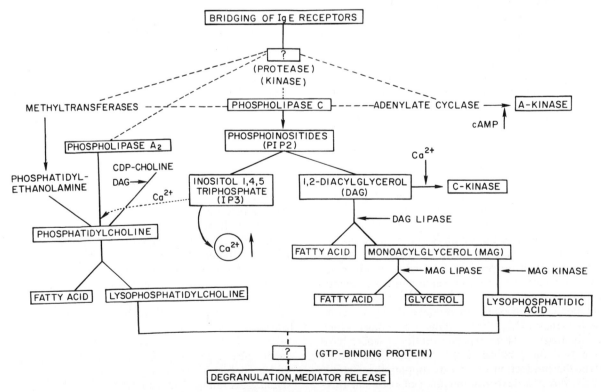

Figure 1–6. Enzyme cascade of IgE-dependent mediator release from mast cells and basophils. (From Ishizaka K, Ishizaka T: Allergy. In Paul W, ed: *Fundamental Immunology*. New York, Raven Press, 1989, p 876.)

variety of cytokines. The third set of mediators, called secondary mediators, includes mediators derived from cells other than mast cells and basophils which are attracted or activated by basophil- and mast cell–generated mediators. This group of mediators is extremely diverse and includes macrophage, neutrophil, eosinophil, and platelet products. Such mediators are especially significant in the late-phase reaction which occurs 2 to 4 hours after initial antigen exposure.[43] The multitude of mediators that are released or synthesized upon initiation of a hypersensitivity reaction explains the limited effects of therapeutic agents that act upon individual mediators, for example, antihistamines.[43] Few mediators of equine immediate hypersensitivity have been identified.

The mediators of immediate-type hypersensitivity reactions have multiple effects.[6, 10, 43, 51, 56, 67, 79, 81–88] Together, these mediators increase vascular permeability; constrict smooth muscle; dilate blood vessels; stimulate secretion of airway mucus, gastric acid, and adrenal catecholamines; alter platelet aggregation; activate chemoattractants of secondarily involved leukocytes; activate complement and coagulation cascades; and stimulate exocytosis of leukocyte lysozymes and granules. Clinically, human and equine immediate-type hypersensitivity reactions are similar.[4, 5, 88, 89] The clinical signs associated with mediator release vary with the quantity, site, and balance of mediator production, the anatomical distribution of target cells, and the sensitivity of target cells to stimulation.[4–6, 11, 23, 43, 69, 84, 90] Clinical signs in the horse include any combination of edema, urticaria, erythema, systemic hypotension, tachypnea, dyspnea, colic, tachycardia, and pruritus.*

Preformed Mediators

Histamine

Allergic reactions were once thought to be mediated simply by histamine.[43] Actually, histamine appears to be a minor mediator of equine immediate-type hypersensitivity reactions.[6, 11, 41, 42, 88] Though plasma histamine concentrations do increase significantly in equine experimental systemic anaphylaxis,[6, 89] antihistamines are relatively ineffective in the treatment of equine anaphylaxis, pruritus, and inflammatory dermatoses.[2, 11, 42, 88, 92] However, NSAIDs provide some benefit in the treatment of equine hypersensitivity reactions, suggesting that histamine and serotonin may be less significant than kinins, prostaglandins, and leukotrienes in mediating equine immediate hypersensitivity.[2, 41, 88]

The effects of histamine are mediated by stimulation of H_1, H_2, and H_3 receptors on a variety of cells.[93] H_1 receptor stimulation causes contraction of bronchial and gastrointestinal smooth muscle, neutrophil and eosinophil chemotaxis, and pain and pruritus.[43, 94] H_2 receptor activation stimulates airway mucous and gastric acid secretion.[43, 94, 95] H_2 receptor activation may also moderate the immune response by decreasing many immunologic events, including histamine release from basophils, neutrophil and eosinophil chemotaxis, cytokine release, T lymphocyte–mediated cytotoxicity, T lymphocyte mitogen response, and suppressor–T cell activity.[2, 16, 43, 54, 94–96] H_1 and H_2 receptor stimulation contributes

to vasodilation, increased vascular permeability, tachycardia, and pruritus, while stimulation of the sensory nerve endings of the vagus results in bronchoconstriction and cardiovascular depression.[6, 43, 56, 94]

A third category of histamine receptors termed H_3 was first detected on brain neurons.[97] More recent studies have detected H_3 receptors on lung mast cells, mesenteric perivascular nerve terminals, pig ileum, and human airway cholinergic and noncholinergic nonadrenergic nerves.[98–102] This receptor inhibits central nervous system (CNS) histamine synthesis and release, CNS serotonin release, peripheral histamine synthesis, and also peripheral norepinephrine, acetylcholine, and neuropeptide release.[97–105] The role of the H_3 receptor in hypersensitivity reactions is undetermined. It is postulated that H_3 receptor stimulation moderates these reactions.

Serotonin

Serotonin is released as an inflammatory mediator in the horse.[89, 106] Serotonin constricts smooth muscle and stimulates sensory nerves.[6, 28, 94] It has been detected in rodent mast cells[51, 80, 94, 107] but its significance in equine immediate hypersensitivity remains unclear.[41, 89] The serotonin antagonist methysergide did not protect against antigen-induced anaphylaxis in the horse.[88] Failure of methysergide does not rule out serotonin as a mediator of anaphylaxis. More likely, it simply reflects the multitude of mediators responsible for clinical signs.

Leukocyte Chemotactic Factors

Mast cell activation results in an influx of eosinophils, neutrophils, and macrophages. Early understanding of hypersensitivity attributed these activities to preformed proteins, the eosinophil and neutrophil chemotactic factors, which were released upon degranulation from the mast cell and basophil granule.[2, 11, 43, 51, 80] Growing understanding of the cytokine repertoire of the mast cell suggests that leukocyte chemotaxis and activation is the combined effort of a number of preformed and newly synthesized mast cell cytokines, synthesized mediators from the arachidonic acid cascade, as well as non-mast cell–derived cytokines.[108]

Studies in humans and rodents indicate that mast cells are capable of synthesizing IL-1, IL-3, IL-4, IL-5, and IL-6; tumor necrosis factor-alpha (TNF-α); granulocyte-macrophage colony-stimulating factor (GM-CSF); and IFN-γ.[108–111] TNF-α, IL-4, and possibly IL-6 exist as preformed mediators and TNF-α has been localized to the mast cell granule.[108, 110, 111] TNF-α attracts macrophages and neutrophils while IL-5 is chemotactic for eosinophils.[112, 113] Of these mast cell cytokines, IL-3, IL-5, GM-CSF, and TNF-α activate eosinophils; IFN-γ, TNF-α, and GM-CSF activate neutrophils; and IFN-γ, TNF-α, GM-CSF, IL-3, and IL-4 activate macrophages.

Tumor Necrosis Factor-Alpha

IgE-dependent activation of the mast cell results in release of preformed TNF-α as well as TNF-α synthesis.[108] TNF-α is a major initiator of leukocyte infiltration in IgE-dependent

---

*References 6, 10, 11, 43, 49, 56, 67, 69, 79, 81–85, 88, 89, 91.

reactions.[108, 111] Pretreatment with anti-TNF-α reduces leukocyte infiltration in IgE-dependent cutaneous inflammation of mice. TNF-α stimulates leukocyte adhesion and activation by increasing the expression of vascular adhesion molecules. TNF-α enhances neutrophil and macrophage phagocytosis, degranulation, and microbicidal activity, increases the expression of neutrophil complement receptors, and is chemotactic for neutrophils and macrophages.[112, 113] TNF-α also activates eosinophils, and stimulates the synthesis of the proinflammatory cytokines IL-1 and IL-6. TNF-α procoagulant activity promotes localized intravascular coagulation and capillary thrombosis. Systemic TNF-α causes shock and favors catabolic activity in most body tissues including adipose tissue, muscle, liver, and the gastrointestinal tract.[112, 113]

Proteoglycans

In humans and rodents, heparin and chondroitin E are bound to histamine within the granules of mast cells and basophils.[43, 56, 80] These two proteoglycans, which are liberated during degranulation, have been localized to distinct mast cell subsets in rodents and humans.[56] Heparin's net negative charge facilitates packaging of positively charged granule components such as the biogenic amines and calcium ions.[56, 80] Heparin is a potent anticoagulant with anti-inflammatory effects.[80, 114] Heparin is capable of inhibiting complement activation, activating kinin formation, blocking lymphocyte blastogenic responses, and stabilizing the mast cell enzyme tryptase.[43, 56, 80, 114–118] Chondroitin E, like heparin, chemically stabilizes granular histamine contents.[80] Chondroitin E inhibits the alternative complement pathway by attenuating formation of C3 convertase, inhibits the intrinsic coagulation cascade, and activates kinin formation.[80, 118]

Other Preformed Mediators

There appear to be a multitude of granule enzymes which may act directly to cause cellular damage, or may activate or inactivate other inflammatory mediators.[43, 51, 56, 68, 79, 119] These include chymase, tryptase, superoxide dismutase, peroxidase, elastase, cathepsin G, and the acid hydrolases arylsulfatase, β-hexosaminadase, and β-glucuronidase. Chymase, for example, in addition to converting angiotensin I to angiotensin II, also mediates the degradation of basement membranes and arteriolar vasoconstriction.[79, 120–123] Tryptase, a neutral fibrinolytic protease, catalyzes the conversion of C3 to C3a and C3b, complement mediators which enhance vasopermeability and can induce further mast cell and basophil degranulation.[56]

Newly Generated Mediators
Prostanoids

Prostanoids comprise the prostaglandins, thromboxanes, and prostacyclin (prostaglandin I_2, PGI_2).[79] These compounds are created by the action of cyclooxygenase on arachidonic acid (Fig. 1–7). The specific prostanoid formed depends on the site of inflammation. Various cells tend to produce certain of the metabolites.[43, 79] Prostanoids increase vascular permeability, are vasodilators, constrict smooth muscle, and alter platelet aggregation[43, 56] (Table 1–10). They are not chemotactic.[79, 82] PGE_2 is unique among the prostanoids in that

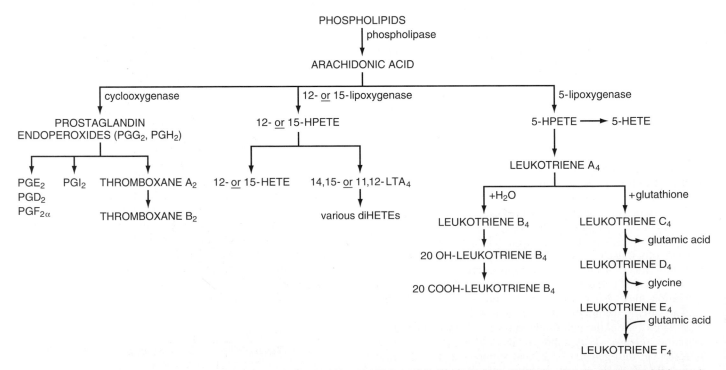

Figure 1–7. Cyclooxygenase and lipoxygenase products of arachidonic acid. (From Davies P, Bailey PJ, Goldenberg MM, et al: The role of arachidonic acid oxygenation products in pain and inflammation. *Annu Rev Immunol* 2:337, 1984. Reproduced with permission.)

Table 1–10. Physiologic Effects of Prostanoids*

Prostanoid	Action
PGE$_2$ (prostaglandin E$_2$)	Inhibits leukocyte chemotaxis; relaxes smooth muscle; inhibits mediator release
PGD$_2$	Constricts bronchial smooth muscle, dilates systemic vasculature, increases vascular permeability; inhibits platelet aggregation
PGF$_{2\alpha}$	Constricts smooth muscle
PGI$_2$ (prostacyclin)	Constricts smooth muscle; increases vascular permeability; inhibits platelet aggregation
TXA$_2$ (thromboxane A$_2$)	Constricts smooth muscle; aggregates platelets

*Data from references 43, 56, 79, 80, 84.

its activity inhibits the liberation of inflammatory mediators, leukocyte function, chemotaxis, and relaxes smooth muscle.[79]

Leukotrienes

Leukotrienes (LTs) are lipid mediators of immediate-type hypersensitivity reactions formed by the action of lipoxygenase on arachidonic acid[79] (see Fig. 1–7). The anaphylactic mediator, slow-reacting substance of anaphylaxis, is now known to be composed of LTC$_4$, LTD$_4$, and LTE$_4$.[84] Collectively, the leukotrienes increase vascular permeability, constrict bronchial smooth muscle, stimulate vasodilation, and are potent chemoattractants.[56, 79, 87] (Table 1–11). LTB$_4$ is the most potent neutrophil chemoattractant of the lipoxygenase products.[82, 85] The ability of LTC$_4$ to increase vascular perme-

Table 1–11. Physiologic Effects of Leukotrienes*

Leukotriene (LT)	Action
LTB$_4$	Chemoattractant of neutrophils; stimulates lysosome exocytosis; increases vascular permeability; constricts bronchial smooth muscle
LTC$_4$	Increases vascular permeability; constricts bronchial smooth muscle; increases bronchial mucous production; arteriolar constriction followed by vasodilation
LTD$_4$	Constricts bronchial smooth muscle; increases vascular permeability; arteriolar constriction followed by vasodilation
LTE$_4$	Constricts smooth muscle; vasodilation; increases vascular permeability

*Data from references 43, 56, 79, 82, 84, 85, 87, 194.

ability is 1,000 times that of histamine.[43] Leukotrienes are important mediators of allergic bronchoconstriction in humans,[79, 124] and there is evidence that leukotrienes are significant mediators of immediate-type hypersensitivities in the horse. Increased concentrations of LTB$_4$ have been detected in carrageenan-induced inflammation in ponies, and diethylcarbamazine, a leukotriene inhibitor, partially inhibited anaphylaxis in ponies.[88, 125]

Kinins

Kinins are potent vasoactive peptides that are enzymatically cleaved from α_2-globulins (kininogens) via enzymes called kininogenases.[10, 83] Kininogenases such as kallikrein are present in the mast cell and basophil granules of humans.[10] Kinins produce sustained smooth muscle contraction, mediate pain and itching, and in low doses stimulate vasodilation, increase capillary blood flow, and increase vascular permeability.[10] The vascular permeability effect of bradykinin is 100 times more potent than that of histamine.[83] Plasma kinin levels are increased in horses with experimental anaphylaxis.[89] Kinins are documented mediators of human allergic conditions.[126–131] Activation of the intrinsic coagulation cascade and kinin pathways is significant in the pathogenesis of the late-phase cutaneous reaction seen 2 to 4 hours after the initial immediate hypersensitivity.[44]

Secondary Mediators

In addition to the mast cells and basophils, secondary inflammatory cells, including neutrophils, macrophages, eosinophils, and platelets, are chemotactically recruited to participate in hypersensitivity reactions. These cells possess a repertoire of hundreds of mediators capable of inflammatory injury (Table 1–12). Though a discussion of these mediators is beyond the scope of this chapter, comprehension of the diversity of mediators from secondary cells is integral to developing a treatment protocol for hypersensitivity reactions.

Platelet Activating Factor

Platelet activating factor (PAF), actually two different molecules, is secreted by most leukocytes (including mast cells) and platelets.[10, 43, 56, 67, 80, 84] The effects of PAF are multiple. Infusion of PAF produces typical anaphylactic responses in rabbits, monkeys, and guinea pigs.[84] PAF activates platelets, neutrophils, eosinophils, and monocytes to aggregate and degranulate resulting in the generation of superoxide radicals.[43, 56, 84] PAF potently increases vascular permeability,[10] increases airway mucous secretion,[72] and constricts intestinal and bronchial smooth muscle.[10, 56, 67, 84, 91] PAF may produce vasoconstriction or vasodilation depending on the vascular site and existing vascular tone.[10, 67]

Cyclic Adenosine Monophosphate (cAMP) and Cyclic Guanosine Monophosphate (cGMP)

The cyclic nucleotides cAMP and cGMP act as intracellular effectors of inflammation. They are synthesized by many

Table 1–12. Secretory Products of Neutrophils, Eosinophils, and Macrophages*

Neutrophils

Lysozyme
Myeloperoxidase
Collagenase
Collagenolytic proteinase
Elastase
Cathepsin B, D, G (acid protcasc)
Leukokinins
N-acetyl-β-glucosaminadase
β-Glycerophosphatase
β-Glucuronidase
Acid lipase
Leukotrienes
Interleukin-1
Prostaglandins
Thromboxane
Basic proteins
Neutral protease
Fibrinolysin
Procoagulant factor
Mononuclear cell chemotactic factors
Oxidizing substances
  Superoxide ion
  Hydroxyl radicals
  Singlet oxygen
  Hypochlorous acid
  Perhydroxyl radical
  Hydrogen peroxide

Eosinophils

Acid phosphatase
Arylsulfatase
Major basic protein
Eosinophil peroxidase
Eosinophil cationic protein
Eosinophil-derived neurotoxin
Collagenase
Acetylcholinesterase
Acid glycerophosphatase
Platelet activating factor
Transforming growth factor-β
Transforming growth factor-α
Interleukin-1
β-Glucuronidase
Ribonuclease
Cathepsin
Acid phosphatase
Alkaline phosphatase
Histaminase

Eosinophils Continued

Phospholipase D
Leukotrienes
Adenosine biphosphatase
α-Mannosidase
Arylsulfatase
Catalase
Tumor necrosis factor-alpha

Macrophages

Interleukin-1
Interleukin-6
Interleukin-8
Tumor necrosis factor-alpha
Interferon-α, -β
Transforming growth factor-β
Platelet-derived growth factor
Epidermal growth factor
Fibroblast growth factor
Plasminogen activator
Angiotensin-converting enzyme
Tissue procoagulant
Coagulation factors V, VII, IX, X, prothrombin, prothrombinase
Complement proteins C2, C3, C4, C5; factors B, D, H, I
Apolipoprotein E
Platelet activating factor
Graulocyte colony-stimulating factor
Granulocyte-macrophage colony-stimulating factor
Elastase
Collagenase
Stromelysin
Lysozyme
Fibronectin
Oxygen metabolites
Nitrogen metabolites
Phosphatase
Arylsulfatase
Cholesteryl esterase
(Deoxy)ribonuclease
Triglyceride lipase
Glycosidase
Proteinases
Cathepsins B and D
Prostanoids
Leukotrienes

*Data from references 2, 13, 208, 209.

cells with mast cells being efficient producers.[56] These two nucleotides have opposing influences. Increases in cAMP or decreases in cGMP stabilize leukocytes and inhibit mediator release.[2, 12, 55] Conversely, decreases in cAMP or increases in cGMP favor the release of inflammatory mediators.[2] Many drugs used in the treatment of anaphylaxis alter cAMP and cGMP levels.[2, 55, 91, 132, 133] β-Adrenergic agents and methylxanthines tend to inhibit mediator release by increasing cAMP levels. Anticholinergic agents exert a similar effect by decreasing cGMP levels. Conversely, α-adrenergic agents, which decrease cAMP, as well as cholinergic agents, estrogen, and levamisole, which increase cGMP, favor mast cell degranulation. This is one justification for the use of β-adrenergic (epinephrine) and anticholinergic (atropine) agents in the treatment of anaphylaxis.

Complement Proteins

Complement proteins are significant mediators of immediate-type hypersensitivity reactions and are especially active in immune-complex disease.[6, 38] The critical activation step is the cleavage of C3 via the classic or alternative pathway (see discussion of immune-complex injury).[2, 38] C3a, C4a, and C5a, the anaphylatoxins, induce nonimmunologic triggering of mast cells, basophils, and platelets releasing granular mediators which stimulate smooth muscle contraction, increase capillary permeability, aggregate platelets, and stimulate intravascular coagulation.[2, 6, 10, 38] C5a attracts and activates neutrophils, precipitating enzymatic damage.[2, 38, 134, 135] C5b, another complement protein, is the initial step in assembling the membrane attack complex (Fig. 1–8) which lyses antigen-bearing cells by creating pores in the cell membrane.[134, 135] Through the formation of the membrane attack complex and the attraction of other inflammatory cells, the complement proteins assist in the destruction of many cells in the vicinity of the deposited immune complexes, resulting in tissue destruction, vasculitis, thrombosis, and hemorrhage.[6, 13]

NEUROIMMUNE INTERACTION

There appears to be a neurologic component in the pathogenesis of inflammation and immediate-type hypersensitivity reactions[136, 137] (Fig. 1–9). Direct stimulation of sensory nerves generates signs of immediate hypersensitivity reactions including vasodilation, and increased vascular permeability in the skin and lungs. If these sensory nerves are transected between the dorsal root ganglion and spinal cord, increased vascular permeability and vasodilation caused by direct sensory nerve stimulation are unchanged. Transection of the sensory nerves distal to the dorsal root ganglion eliminates the vasodilation associated with direct stimulation of these nerves. Local anesthesia of the nerve also eliminates vasodilation.

This indicates that an axonal reflex with an afferent limb mediated by stimulation of sensory nerves sending axons to the dorsal root ganglion, and an efferent limb mediated by nerves exiting the dorsal root ganglion and coursing to the site of inflammation, may contribute to the manifestation of certain hypersensitivity diseases. Currently it is believed that the sensory nerves are activated by polymodal nociceptors in the skin and that the inciting impulses spread retrograde along the axon of the sensory nerve toward the neuronal cell body (antidromic transmission). The axonal reflex is completed by efferent unmyelinated C fibers originating in the dorsal root ganglion.

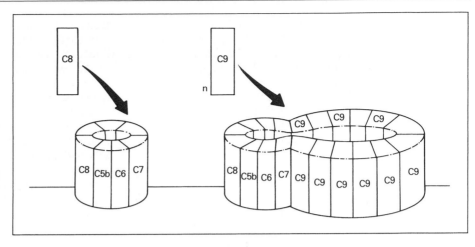

Figure 1–8. The membrane attack complex. Complement components C5b, C6, and C7 form a complex (C5b67) in the cell membrane. The C5b67 complex accepts complement protein C8, forming a channel across the lipid membrane. Osmotic lysis of the cell ensues. Complement component C9 may polymerize the C5b678 complex, forming a larger "hole" for more rapid lysis. (From Frank M.: The complement system. In Samter M, Talmage D, Frank M, et al, eds: *Immunological Diseases.* Boston, Little, Brown, 1988, p 222.)

C fibers appear to mediate vasodilation by releasing neuropeptides in the group tachykinins. Allergic mediators from mast cells, including histamine, and serotonin are capable of activating C fibers.[137] Substance P is by far the most significant tachykinin but neurokinin A, and calcitonin gene-related peptide are also active. Chemical depletion of substance P with capsaicin eliminates the flare response and attenuates inflammatory changes associated with sensory nerve stimulation. In fact, human patients with hyperactive rhinopathy have been treated successfully with capsaicin.[137]

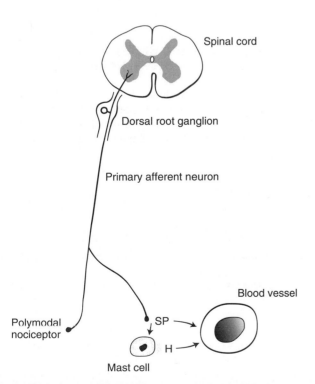

Figure 1–9. Axon-reflex model of neurogenic inflammation. *SP,* substance P; *H,* histamine. (From Foreman J: Neuropeptides and the pathogenesis of allergy. *Allergy* 42:2, 1987. Munksgaard International Publishers Ltd, Copenhagen, Denmark.)

THE LATE-PHASE REACTION

A late reexacerbation of signs is well characterized in certain human allergic conditions, including asthma, allergic rhinitis, and allergic cutaneous reactions.[44, 45, 51] This biphasic response has been noted in equine cutaneous reactions.[31, 48] The late-phase cutaneous reaction is characterized by erythema, edema, heat, and tenderness with or without pruritus, and may affect a larger area than that seen in the initial wheal and flare reaction.[45] Histologically, there is a predominance of neutrophils and mononuclear cells, with some eosinophils. Marked deposition of eosinophil and neutrophil granular protein (major basic protein, eosinophil-derived neurotoxin, and elastase) are noted by 1 to 3 hours.[45] Similar histologic changes have been noted in the horse.[48]

This reaction begins 3 to 4 hours after the initial antigen challenge, peaks by 6 to 12 hours, and usually resolves by 24 to 72 hours.[45] In humans, the reaction is antigen-induced and IgE-mediated. The exact mediators are not certain, but leukotrienes, kinins, and histamine are involved.[44] The reaction appears to be a cyclic reaction due to chemotactic recruitment of inflammatory cells by mediators released or synthesized in the acute phase of the reaction. These late-arriving cells release additional mediators which contribute to inflammation, recruit additional inflammatory cells, and degranulate additional mast cells or basophils.[43]

The late-phase response is most effectively treated with steroid therapy. It can be prevented by steroid pretreatment or by decreasing the initial mediator release in the immediate stage via antigen avoidance, treatment with cromolyn sodium, hyposensitization, or desensitization.[43]

IMMEDIATE-TYPE HYPERSENSITIVITY REACTIONS: IMMUNE-COMPLEX INJURY

Diseases mediated by the formation of immune complexes are categorized based on the site of antigen and antibody union and the relative ratio of antigen to antibody.[13] In the case of tissue antigens, antibody deposition and thus disease are fixed at the tissue site. This is an obvious overlap between immune-complex and autoimmune disease. In contrast, when soluble antigens react with antibody, the site of immune-complex deposition is dependent on the relative concentrations of antigen and antibody.[2, 6] In the classic Arthus-type reaction, antibody excess restricts immune-complex precipitation primarily to the site of antigen entry. In conditions of soluble antigen excess, systemic immune-complex formation occurs. Circulating immune complexes are removed by the reticuloendothelial system or are deposited in small capillaries of various tissues, resulting in the classic signs of serum sickness (vasculitis, lymphadenopathy, nephritis, vasculitis, arthritis, urticaria).[4, 6, 10, 38, 138] Cells that are injured in immune-complex reactions involving soluble antigen-antibody complex precipitation are truly "innocent bystanders" since they do not themselves bear foreign antigen.[6]

Immune-complex injury is mediated by both cellular and humoral factors.[13] The predominance of immune-complex injury is mediated by neutrophils recruited to the site of immune-complex deposition by complement components (Fig. 1–10). Monocytes and macrophages also act as cellular effectors of tissue injury. The role of complement proteins in immune-complex–mediated tissue injury is well characterized. When antibody isotypes capable of fixing complement combine via their Fab portion with antigen, the antibody undergoes a configurational change that exposes the C1 complex binding site within the antibody's constant region. The cascade of events that follows creates C3a, C3b, C4a, and C5a.[135] C3b, a potent opsonin, attaches to the antibody portion of the immune complex triggering the alternative pathway of complement. C5a potently attracts and activates neutrophils.[13, 134, 135] C3a, C4a, and C5a, the anaphylatoxins, induce nonimmunologic triggering of mast cells and basophils.[6, 10] C5b, the initial step in assembling the membrane attack complex (MAC), is also formed[134] (see Fig. 1–8). MAC lyses antigen-bearing cells independent of other leukocytes and may also lyse nearby cells that are not antigen-coated, creating pores in the cell membrane. Thus, a nonspecific inflammatory reaction is initiated at the site of the immune-complex deposition.[6]

Immune complexes precipitate in vessel walls and glomerular basement membranes as a result of electrostatic at-traction; the action of vasoactive amines, which increase permeability of the vessels to the complexes; and the filtering effect of these sites.[13] The mediators from cells responding to chemoattractants, and the MAC destroy many cells in the vicinity of the deposited immune complexes, resulting in tissue destruction, vasculitis, thrombosis, and hemorrhage[6] (see Fig. 1–10).

Though the triggering mechanism for immune-complex reactions is different from anaphylactic reactions, the mediators and secondarily recruited cells are similar. Clinical signs of immune-complex reactions occur days to weeks after exposure to the inciting agent.[23] Serum sickness, hemolytic anemia, neonatal isoerythrolysis, thrombocytopenia, immune synovitis, vasculitis, purpura hemorrhagica, angioedema, equine infectious anemia, systemic lupus erythematosus, hypersensitivity pneumonitis, neoplasia, bacterial and parasitic diseases, acute interstitial nephritis, acute glomerulonephritis, and some adverse drug reactions have immune-complex hypersensitivity reactions as part of their pathogenesis.[2, 11, 13, 23, 139]

DELAYED-TYPE HYPERSENSITIVITY REACTIONS

DTH reactions are classified as type IV reactions in the Gell and Coombs classification.[3] Unlike the immediate-type hypersensitivities described above, which can be passively transferred with serum, DTH reactions are cell-mediated and therefore cannot be passively transferred. DTH reactions are integral to defenses for graft rejection, infection, and neoplasia.[17, 140]

Pathogenesis of Delayed-Type Hypersensitivity Reactions

DTH reactions are characterized by an afferent phase in which antigen recognition occurs, and a response or efferent phase.[17, 140, 141] The afferent phase of the DTH reaction results in sensitization and requires a genetically restricted, antigen-

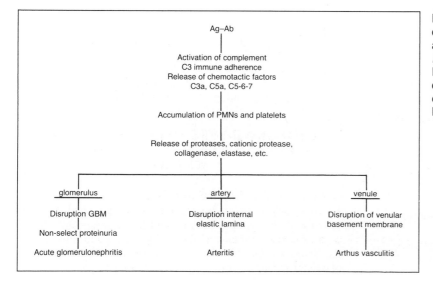

Figure 1–10. Immune injury of tissue by complement and neutrophils. *Ag-Ab,* antigen-antibody; *GBM,* glomerular basement membrane; *PMN,* polymorphonuclear leukocyte. (From Dixon F, Cochrane C, Theofilopoulos A: Immune complex injury. In Samter M, Talmage D, Frank M, et al, eds: *Immunological Diseases.* Boston, Little, Brown, 1988, p 246.)

specific interaction between antigen-specific helper T cells and an antigen-presenting cell (APC).[140] This interaction results in rapid division of, and cytokine production by, the antigen-sensitized T cells. Nonspecific accessory cells, predominately macrophages and fewer neutrophils, are activated by the helper T-cell cytokines including IFN-γ and act as nonspecific effectors of the response. That is, once activated by helper T cell cytokines, the macrophages and neutrophils display increased activity to many antigens, not simply the sensitizing antigen. Mast cells and basophils also participate in this reaction.

Specificity in the DTH is conferred via the antigen-specific receptor of the sensitized T cell.[142] However, neither macrophages nor the antigen-specific helper T cells alone are sufficient to carry out the reaction.[17] DTH reactions are regulated by a complex network of immune cells and cytokines which may either augment or suppress the actions of the antigen-specific helper T cell.[17, 142]

After exiting the vasculature, the antigen-specific T cell, via its secreted cytokines, interacts with mast cells and platelets.[142] Vasoactive mediators released from the mast cells and platelets further facilitate the entry of previously sensitized T cells into the tissues. Within the tissue, the antigen-specific helper T cell recognizes antigen on the surface of an APC in association with a major histocompatibility antigen (MHC). This interaction stimulates cytokine production by the helper T cell and the APC.[17, 141, 142] After presenting antigen to the antigen-specific helper T cell, the APC secretes IL-1, which activates T cells, causing proliferation and IL-2 synthesis.[141] IL-2 participates in a positive feedback loop with the T cell, further increasing IL-2 secretion and IL-2 receptor expression. IL-2 also induces IFN-γ production. Finally, IFN-γ enhances IL-1 and TNF production by monocytes.[141]

The effects of the cytokines are multiple (Table 1–13) and include leukocyte chemotaxis, activation, and mediator

release.[140] IFN-γ is a major cytokine responsible for immobilizing and activating leukocytes to increase phagocytic capabilities, increase receptor expression, and augment cytotoxic mechanisms.[17, 141, 142] Interaction of sensitized lymphocytes with macrophages throughout the body during sensitization also results in a nonspecific increase in resistance to pathogens unrelated to the sensitizing pathogen. This nonspecific increase in resistance is transient but can be reexpressed upon exposure to the original antigen.[17]

Allergic contact dermatitis is the best-characterized of the DTH diseases. In this disease, the sensitizing agents are usually simple chemicals (metals, soaps) that act as haptens and become complete antigens after binding with proteins on the surface of the APC, not skin proteins as previously believed.[20, 141]

The purpose of therapy in DTH reactions is to diminish cell-mediated immunity by regulating T-cell function and decreasing macrophage response to cytokines.[141, 142] Topical and systemic glucocorticoids are the mainstay of therapy in veterinary medicine. Glucocorticoids inhibit cell-mediated immunity at multiple points. Azathioprine, cyclophosphamide, and cyclosporine have been used to modify the DTH response in humans. Azathioprine modulates T-cell function, while cyclophosphamide has a primary effect on B cells and a minute effect on T cells. Cyclosporine moderates the DTH by interfering with IL-1 and IL-2 production. Downregulation of IL-1 and IL-2 limit macrophage and T-cell activation, respectively. Fortunately, allergic contact dermatitis, the most common DTH, generally responds to elimination of the antigen.

CLINICAL MANIFESTATIONS OF HYPERSENSITIVITY
(Tables 1–14 to 1–18)

The immune system is constantly challenged to differentiate self from non-self. During this process, sensitizing antigens are plentiful and may be in the form of altered self-antigens, molecules from bacteria, viruses, or other environmental antigens. Without proper checks and balances, these same humoral and cell-mediated immune reactions, which constantly defend the body from foreign antigens, have the potential to manifest as hypersensitivity reactions. A delicate network of immune cell interaction regulates these reactions.

Limited research leaves the role of hypersensitivity in equine disease processes poorly defined. Studies in human disease indicate that hypersensitivity reactions are significant in the pathogenesis of many diseases, including adverse drug reactions, glomerulonephritis, chronic active hepatitis, and demyelinating diseases such as the Guillian-Barré syndrome. These diseases have their equine counterparts. Tables 1–14 to 1–18 summarize what is known or *suspected* regarding the role of hypersensitivity reactions in equine diseases.

Adverse Drug Reactions

Adverse drug reactions may be nonimmunologically or immunologically mediated. Nonimmunologic reactions may be due to nonimmunologic triggering of effector pathways, drug overdose, cumulative toxicity, side effects, drug interactions, exacerbation of preexisting disease, and individual alter-

---

Table 1–13. Biological Activities of Selected Cytokines*

Growth factors
  Interleukin-1 (thymocytes, T lymphocytes)
  Interleukin-2 (T lymphocytes, natural killer cells)
  Interleukin-4 (B lymphocytes)
Differentiation factors
  Interleukin-1 (IL-2 production by T-cells)
  Interleukin-2 (IL-2 receptor expression on T-cells)
  Interleukin-3 (T-cell and mast cell maturation)
  Interferon-γ (multiple effects on lymphoid cells and other cells)
  Interleukins-4, -5, -6 (B-cell differentiation)
  Transfer factor (expression of specific delayed hypersensitivity)
Inflammatory factors
  Interleukin-1 (pyrogen)
  Chemotactic factors (IL-5, eosinophils; IL-8, neutrophils)
  Interferon-γ (activates macrophages)
  Tumor necrosis factor (solid tumors)

*This is a partial list of the major lymphokines and monokines. In parentheses are the principal targets or biological activities.

From Kirkpatrick C: Delayed hypersensitivity. In Samter M, Talmage D, Frank M, et al, eds: *Immunological Diseases*. Boston, Little, Brown, 1988, p 265.

Table 1–14. Diseases Associated with Systemic Anaphylactic Reactions

Disease	Antigens Implicated	Manifestation
Systemic anaphylaxis (immune-complex disease also implicated)[4, 6, 11, 16, 18, 23, 28, 138, 147, 156]	Sera, vaccines, antibiotics (penicillin, trimethroprim-sulfadiazine, neomycin, oxytetracycline, streptomycin), benzyl alcohol in vitamin B$_{12}$, vitamin E–selenium preparations, thiamine, phenothiazines, iron dextrans, *Hypoderma* larvae, anthelmintics, egg albumin	Acute death, urticaria, hypotension, respiratory distress due to laryngeal/ pharyngeal edema, bronchoconstriction, cardiac dysrhythmias, colic, gastrointestinal hypermotility, pulmonary emphysema, pulmonary edema, laminitis, purpura
Atopy-like dermatosis[2, 16, 35, 149]	Inhaled molds, pollens, dusts	Recurrent seasonal/nonseasonal dermatitis, ± pruritis

Table 1–15. Diseases Associated with Local Anaphylactic Reactions

Disease	Antigens Implicated	Manifestation
Angioedema (immune-complex disease also implicated)[16, 20, 36, 149]	Insect saliva, snake venoms, drug allergy, plant proteins, fishmeal	Sudden subcutaneous edema, predominantly affecting the head and feet
Urticaria (systemic anaphylaxis, immune complex, and DTH also implicated)[2, 11, 14, 16, 20–23, 28, 29, 35, 36, 92, 149]	Infectious agents *Streptococcus* spp., dermatophytes, *Trypanosoma equiperdum,* babesia, *Trypanosoma evansi*, horsepox virus Insect/arthropod venom *Culicoides* spp., *Onchocera cervicalis, Stomoxys calcitrans* Therapeutic agents Penicillin, phenylbutazone, aspirin, guaifenesin, phenothiazines, streptomycin, oxytetracycline, iron dextran, meperidine Biologicals *Streptococcus equi* vaccines, encephalomyelitis vaccines, *salmonella* bacterins, botulinum toxoid, tetanus toxoid Anesthetic agents Barbiturates, guaifenesin, halothane Inhaled allergens Pollens, mold Milk allergy Feed stuffs Oats, wheat, glucose, potatoes, beet pulp, buckwheat, clover, Saint Johnswort, tonics, barley, bran, chicory Snake bites Contactants; see Allergic contact dermatitis, Table 1–18 *Hypoderma* larvae Intestinal parasites	Multiple round, elevated plaques of pitting dermal edema
Insect hypersensitivity[2, 6, 11, 20, 29, 30]	Salivary antigens of: *Culicoides* spp., *Simulium* spp., *Stomoxys* spp., *Haematobia* spp.	Seasonal pruritus; papular crusting dermatitis, usually of the mane, tail, dorsum, and ventrum
Allergic rhinitis[29, 39, 40]	Inhaled allergens	Headshaking, sneezing, snorting, nasal discharge, coughing, excessive lacrimation

Table 1–16. Diseases Associated with Systemic Immune-Complex Reactions

Disease	Antigen Implicated	Manifestation
Serum sickness[4, 6, 16, 23]	In humans: serum, immunoglobulin products, penicillin, sulfonamides, streptomycin	Depression, lymphadenopathy, nephritis, vasculitis, neuropathy, arthritis, urticaria, fever, edema of head, pruritus, dyspnea, stiffness, cyanosis
Neonatal isoerythrolysis[8, 11]	Foal RBC antigens inherited from sire	Severe anemia, hemoglobinuria, jaundice, weakness, debilitation
Systemic lupus erythematosus[2, 13, 23, 210]	Altered native autologous antigen, generally nuclear antigen; also surface and cytoplasmic antigen of cells; in humans: isoniazid, griseofulvin, tetracycline, antimalarial drugs	Dependent lymphedema, panniculitis, alopecia, leukoderma, scaling, polyarthritis, thrombocytopenia, proteinuria, fever, depression, weight loss
Hemolytic anemia[4, 23]	Equine infectious anemia virus (EIA); drug metabolite or hapten on RBC; drug-induced RBC damage by penicillin, dipyrone, quinine, quinidine, stibophen, para-aminosalicylic acid, phenacetin, rifampin, methyldopa	Anemia, hepatomegaly, splenomegaly, hyperbilirubinemia, jaundice, bilirubinuria, weakness (hemoglobinemia, hemoglobinuria)
Immune-mediated thrombocytopenia[4, 23]	In humans: drug metabolite or hapten on platelet, drug-induced platelet damage; stibophen, sulfonamides, isoniazid, rifampin	Mucosal hemorrhages, coagulation defects
Transfusion reaction[6]	Self-antigens	Anemia, liver disease, bone marrow damage
Endocarditis[13]	Bacterial and viral antigens	Weight loss, intermittent depression, pyrexia
Agranulocytosis[4, 23]	In humans: phenylbutazone, amidopyrine, oxyphenbutazone, sulfonamides, cephalothins, β-lactam antibiotics, chloroamphenicol, para-aminosalicylic acid, phenothiazine, gold compounds, anticonvulsants, propylthiouracil, indomethacin, dipyrone, tolbutamide, barbiturates, antihistamines, arsenicals	Rare in horse

ations in drug metabolism.[143] Systemic and local anaphylaxis, immune-complex disease, and even DTH reactions are responsible for adverse reactions to various therapeutic agents.[11, 23, 52, 69]

Most drugs are too small for recognition by the immune system.[49, 52] Accordingly, immune recognition requires covalent bonding of the drug to endogenous proteins, polysaccharides, or nucleotides. This exogenous drug-hapten–endogenous protein-carrier relationship can result in immunologic recognition of endogenous proteins and resultant autoimmune disease.[52, 90] Generally parent drugs cannot form covalent bonds but the reactive metabolites of some parent compounds can bond covalently to endogenous proteins to initiate immunologic recognition.[23, 49, 52] For example, the penicilloyl moiety created by cleavage of the β-lactam ring is the primary reactive metabolite involved in human penicillin hypersensitivity reactions.[23] Because few parent drugs are capable of making such metabolites, anaphylactic reactions to therapeutic agents are not common.[23] The production of shared reactive metabolites explains cross-reactivity between related or seemingly unrelated drugs and explains why some drugs that do not make such metabolites are not associated with adverse reactions.[23, 49, 90] The sulfonamide antimicrobials, furosemide, thiazide diuretics, and sulfonylureas share a sulfamyl group which can act as a hapten, resulting in cross-reactivity.[23] The requirement for metabolic activation also explains organ-specific damage to the organ where the active metabolite is formed.[49, 90]

Host reactivity is also significant in the development of adverse drug reactions. In human medicine, females, persons with other allergies or severe illness, and persons with certain HLA types have an increased incidence of adverse drug reactions.[52]

Once an animal has been sensitized, the clinical signs manifested during hypersensitivity reactions depend on the quantity, persistence, distribution, and route of antigen challenge, the need for metabolic activation of the antigen, and the type, site, and quantity of mediators released.[23, 69, 80] In the case of anaphylaxis, the characteristic mast cell distribution and "shock organs" for the particular species also influence clinical signs.[4–6, 69] Inhalation of antigen is more likely to cause bronchoconstriction and conjunctivitis, topical exposure will likely cause urticaria, while oral and intravenous exposure may cause anaphylaxis, diarrhea, and angioedema.[23, 143] It is important to remember that producing antibody to a compound or metabolite does not equate with hypersensitivity. Most individuals treated with penicillin produce antibodies, but few have hypersensitivity reactions.[4, 144]

Systemic Anaphylaxis

In humans, the incidence of anaphylaxis is difficult to determine because minor reactions may go unreported and more severe reactions may be attributed to other disease processes.[69] This is most likely true also of equine anaphylaxis. The most severe clinical signs of systemic anaphylaxis in the horse are dyspnea and systemic hypotension resulting in collapse.[4, 11, 23]

Table 1–17. Diseases Associated with Local Immune-Complex Reactions

Disease	Antigens Implicated	Manifestation
Purpura haemorrhagica/cutaneous vasculitis/leukocytoclastic vasculitis (anaphylaxis and systemic immune-complex disease also implicated)[2, 6, 11, 20, 24, 25, 139, 150, 161, 211–213]	Bacteria, viruses: *Streptococcus equi, Streptococcus zooepidemicus, Rhodococcus, Ehrlichia,* equine viral arteritis, equine influenza virus, equine herpesvirus type 1; drugs; toxins; idiopathic	Generalized vasculitis; subcutaneous, and mucous membrane hemorrhages; infarction, necrosis, and exudation of skin; fever; depression; anorexia; renal disease; arthralgia
Chronic obstructive pulmonary disease (local anaphylaxis and DTH also implicated)[6, 11, 14, 24–27, 29]	Equine influenza virus, mold, dust, cold air, noxious gases	Respiratory distress, cough, wheezes, forced expiration, protrusion of costal arch
Pemphigus foliaceus[2, 16, 20, 157, 214]	Keratinocyte glycocalyx (autoantibody)	Annular thick crusts, erosions with epidermal collarettes, beginning on face and limbs; 50% have concurrent depression, fever, weight loss, anorexia
Uveitis[215, 216]	*Leptospira interrogans, Onchocerca, Toxoplasma gondii, Brucella* spp., *Streptococcus,* viral antigens, homologous ocular antigens	Blepharospasm, tearing, aqueous flare, hypopyon
Hypersensitivity pneumonitis[217]	Chicken feces	Respiratory distress; see Chronic obstructive pulmonary disease
Erythema multiforme[2, 16, 219]	In humans: infectious agents, pregnancy, therapeutic agents, tumor cells, contact irritants, idiopathic	Annular arciform areas which begin as maculopapular lesions, then undergo central clearing
Discoid lupus erythematosus[2]	Basement membrane protein	Patchy erythema; scaling; alopecia; face, neck, ear crusts; ± leukoderma and leukotrichia
Bullous pemphigoid[2, 16, 157, 214]	Basement membrane protein of skin and mucosa	Subepidermal vesicles, crusts and ulcers with epidermal collarettes, systemic disease
Glomerulonephritis (systemic immune-complex disease implicated)[13, 23, 216]	Equine infectious anemia virus, *Streptococcus* spp., in humans: *Onchocerca,* tumor cells, mercurials, gold, penicillamine, probenecid, lithium	Edema, weight loss, depression, anorexia, polyuria, polydipsia, proteinuria, hypoalbuminemia
Interstitial nephritis[23]	In humans, drug haptens or metabolites alter basement membrane: penicillin, sulfonamides, furosemide, thiazide diuretics, phenendion	
Hepatocellular injury[23]	In humans: halogenated anesthetics, acetaminophen, isoniazid, corticosteroids, anticonvulsants	Icterus, anorexia, increased γ-glutamyltransferase, hyperbilirubinemia, prolonged prothrombin time
Polyneuritis equi[218]	Myelin proteins, equine adenovirus type 1	Polyneuritis of sacral and coccygeal nerves ± cranial nerves (V, VII, VIII); paralysis of tail, rectum, anal sphincter, penis, bladder, urethral sphincter, ± rear limb ataxia, ± difficulty in mastication or swallowing

Table 1–18. Disease Associated with Delayed-Type Hypersensitivity Reactions

Diseases	Antigen Implicated	Manifestation
Allergic contact dermatitis (local anaphylaxis implicated)[6, 11, 16, 20, 92, 147]	Organophosphate insecticides, heavy metals, aniline dyes in tack, plants, bedding, soaps, blankets, neat's-foot oil, wool	Acute: urticaria, vesicles; chronic: hyperkeratosis, fibrosis, lichenification, variable pruritus; signs appear 5–21 days from initial contact; anamnestic response in 48 hr
Feedstuff hypersensitivity (anaphylactic and immune-complex hypersensitivity also implicated)[2, 11, 14, 16, 18, 19, 28, 33, 35–38, 149]	Concentrates, wheats, oats, barley, bran	Nonseasonal generalized pruritus ± urticaria; in humans: anaphylaxis, urticaria, abdominal pain, diarrhea

Table 1–19. Agents Implicated in Equine Urticaria*

Penicillin
Glucocorticoids
Iron dextran
Phenothiazines
Pethidine
Streptomycin
Oxytetracycline
Neomycin
Chloramphenicol
Sulfonamides
Phenylbutazone
Guaifenesin
Aspirin
Biologicals: antiserum, *Streptococcus equi* vaccines,
    tetanus toxoid, botulinum toxoid, encephalomyelitis
    vaccines
Foods: potatoes, distillers' waste, malt, beet pulp,
    buckwheat, clover, Saint Johns wort, wheat, oats,
    tonics, barley, bran, chicory
Organic iodides
Inhaled molds, pollens, feedstuffs
Infectious agents
Internal parasites

*Data from references 2, 6, 11, 16, 20, 23, 28, 35, 36, 92, 138, 149, 150, and George Martin, D.V.M., Baton Rouge, La.

clude hemoconcentration, increased hepatic and myocardial enzymes, and coagulation abnormalities consistent with disseminated intravascular coagulation.[69] Gastrointestinal hypermotility and colic occur as the result of smooth muscle effects of anaphylactic mediators and alterations in vascular permeability.[11]

Systemic anaphylactic or anaphylactic-like reactions have occurred after injections of sera, vaccines, vitamin E–selenium preparations, thiamine, iron dextrans, anthelmintics, phenothiazines, and antibiotics, including penicillin, neomycin, oxytetracycline, streptomycin, and trimethoprim-sulfadiazine[6, 11, 16, 18, 28, 138, 147, 148] (George Martin, D.V.M., Baton Rouge, La., personal communication). Rupture of *Hypoderma* larvae has also been reported to cause generalized allergic reactions in horses.[18] Urticaria is a reported complication with a variety of drugs in the horse[6, 16, 20, 21, 23, 28, 36, 92, 138, 147–150] (Table 1–19). Rare urticarial reactions have been reported with several anesthetic protocols. Though definitive identification of the inciting agent was not determined, thiamylal, guaifenesin, and halothane were implicated.[21, 22] Thiobarbiturate allergies are documented in humans.[52]

Hypersensitivity accounts for 6% to 10% of all human drug reactions.[4] Food, a host of therapeutic agents, and inhaled allergens are known causes of IgE-mediated anaphylaxis in humans[69, 151] (Table 1–20). It is likely that these and many other stimuli exist for the horse.[6, 11, 149] Anaphylactic

Clinical signs may vary from mild cardiovascular compromise to lethal shock.[4, 11, 23] Urticaria, the most common sign of anaphylaxis in humans, may be seen.[11, 23, 69] Death may occur from cardiac arrest, shock, or asphyxia.[6, 23] Signs usually occur within 30 minutes of exposure to the antigen, but may take several hours if the drug is not administered intravenously or if a metabolic byproduct is the sensitizing antigen.[23]

Hypersensitivity reactions can occur with any drug via any route at any time in the course of therapy. Such reactions are generally not dose-dependent.[4] There is a higher incidence of adverse drug reactions with parenteral dosing.[144] The lung and intestine are the reported "target organs" in equine experimental anaphylaxis.[6] Sudden severe edema of the skin, mucous membranes, and viscera (angioedema), purpura, erythema, urticaria, or even colic may occur in the acute phase.[11, 23] Vasodilation and increased capillary permeability caused by anaphylactic mediators result in hypotension, urticaria, angioedema, and systemic and pulmonary pooling of blood.[5] Laminitis may occur, presumably as a sequela of vascular changes in the hoof.[11] Respiratory distress and hypoxemia occur as a result of mediator-induced bronchospasm and pulmonary edema, or upper airway obstruction due to angioedema of the pharynx, glottis, and larynx, or any combination of these events may occur.[5, 23] Asphyxiation is a significant cause of death in human systemic anaphylaxis.[69, 145] Cardiac arrhythmias occur secondary to hypoxemia and hypotension-induced myocardial ischemia.[23] In humans, conduction abnormalities, atrial and ventricular arrhythmias, and hypoxic changes (ST segment depression, and tall T waves) are noted on the electrocardiogram (ECG).[69, 146] Biochemical abnormalities in humans in-

Table 1–20. Agents Causing Systemic Anaphylactic Reactions in Humans*

Antiserum	Thiamine
Tetanus toxoid	Folic acid
Relaxin	Penicillin
Insulin	Tetracycline
ACTH	Demethylchlortetracycline
Parathormone	Chlortetracycline
Methylprednisolone	Nitrofurantoin
Seminal plasma	Streptomycin
Chymotrypsin	Cephalosporins
Trypsin	Sulfasalazine
Penicillinase	Barbiturates
Chymopapain	Diazepam
Pollen	Phenytoin
Buckwheat	Isoniazid
Egg white	Succinylcholine
Cottonseed	Zomepirac
Pinto bean	Tripelennamine
Rice	2-Methyl-2-n-propyl-1,3-
Camomile tea	propanediol dicarbamate
Potato	Hymenoptera sting
Milk	Ethylene oxide
Nuts	Progesterone
Seafood	Procaine
Acacia	Organic mercurials
Glue	Organic iodides
Iron dextran	Fluorescein
Dextran	Congo red
Sulfobromophthalein (BSP)	Heparin
Sodium dehydrocholate	

Data from references 49, 69, 90, 151.

reactions reported in the horse may involve immunologic triggering via antigen-specific cell-associated antibody or complement-mediated triggering (via C3a and C5b) secondary to immune-complex formation. In the case of blood and serum product anaphylaxis, IgE from the donor can passively sensitize the recipient, resulting in anaphylaxis upon exposure to the antigen.[78]

Anaphylactoid reactions, which can occur without prior exposure to the stimulus, are clinically indistinguishable from immunologically mediated anaphylactic reactions.[5, 43, 69] Thiobarbiturates, opiates, NSAIDs, curare, highly charged antibiotics (polymyxin B), bromosulfophthalein, thiamine, dextran, neuromuscular blocking agents, and hyperosmolar solutions such as radiocontrast media, mannitol, and hypertonic saline are capable of inducing direct mast cell degranulation without binding of surface IgE.[10, 52, 69, 78, 143, 151–154]

Anaphylactic reactions should be differentiated from other adverse drug reactions, including accentuation of normal pharmacologic effects of the drug, drug interactions, and inappropriate route of administration.[23] Inadvertent intra-arterial injections can result in collapse, convulsions, coma, blindness, and death.[23] Intravenous administration of chloramphenicol, aminoglycosides, tetracyclines, polymyxin, drugs with limited water solubility, and propylene glycol can precipitate anaphylactic-like signs, including ataxia, shivering, dyspnea, and collapse.[4] In humans, the presence of eosinophils in the pulmonary capillaries and the spleen and liver sinusoids differentiate anaphylaxis from other causes of acute death.[151]

The inciting agent in anaphylaxis often remains uncertain. A meticulous historical review of environmental changes, including food, bedding, drugs, and exposure to pesticides, is critical. A complete blood count (CBC), serum biochemistry panel, and urinalysis are warranted to exclude any biochemical abnormalities, but can only be interpreted with an adequate history. Intradermal skin testing is useful if results are carefully scrutinized, but false-negative results can occur if the parent drug is not antigenic and the risk of precipitating an anaphylactic reaction should not be overlooked.[23] Experience in the treatment of human anaphylaxis indicates that lack of understanding of the early clinical signs results in therapy which is often too conservative and misdirected.[5]

Adverse Drug Reactions Mediated by Immune-Complex Formation

Therapeutic agents or their metabolites can function as the antigen in immune-complex reactions. These reactions manifest in three ways. A focal inflammatory reaction is seen if the soluble antigen meets an antibody excess.[6] Signs usually occur 6 hours after antigen exposure. This is the classic Arthus-type reaction. Localized vaccine reactions occurring in the face of high vaccinal titers may be an example of this type of reaction.

The second type of immune-complex disease occurs when circulating soluble antigen-antibody complexes precipitate on the surface of cells lining the vascular filters, especially of the kidney and joints.[90] Once coated by antigen-antibody complexes the cells are then destroyed either by antibody-dependent complement-mediated cytolysis or by antibody-dependent cellular cytotoxicity. This occurs in conditions of antigen excess and is mediated largely by IgG.[90] Signs usually occur 6 to 20 days into therapy but may occur in 2 to 3 days if the individual is previously sensitized.[4, 90] Any of the classic signs of serum sickness, fever, arthritis, nephritis, proteinuria, pruritus, lymphadenopathy, neuritis, edema, urticaria, and a papular rash ensue.[4, 23] Signs usually abate several days after therapy is discontinued. In humans, serum sickness has resulted from therapy with penicillin, sulfonamides, streptomycin, thiouracils, cholecystographic dyes, diphenylhydantoin, and serum products.[23, 90, 143]

The third type of immune-complex reaction is cytotoxic and may manifest as an autoimmune disease of one particular tissue or organ type (Table 1–21). This occurs in several ways.[90] The drug may react chemically with tissue epitopes rendering them antigenic, or the drug may precipitate on the cell surface, eliciting an antibody reaction.[4, 90, 143] Mistaken identity, in which the immune response to antigenic determinants of the drug cross-reacts with normal antigenic determinants of the body, can also occur.[4, 143, 155] In humans, hemolytic anemia associated with high-dose penicillin is mediated by haptenic drug metabolites on the red cell surface.[90] Occasionally, one particular organ may be affected due to formation of a toxic metabolite at this site. Such adverse drug reactions have been implicated in the development of skin eruptions, hemolytic anemia, thrombocytopenia, agranulocytosis, interstitial nephritis, hepatocellular injury, cholestasis, systemic lupus erythematosus, vasculitis, and polymyositis.[4, 23, 52, 90, 143]

Atopy-like Dermatosis

Atopy is a genetically programmed immediate-type hypersensitivity reaction to environmental allergens. The most common manifestation of atopy in small domestic animals is recurrent pruritic dermatitis. However, in humans, allergic rhinitis, bronchial asthma, and food allergies are also recognized atopic disorders. Certain pruritic dermatoses of the horse are likely atopic in origin although the role of reagenic antibody in these cases has not been documented.[11] Molds, pollens, and dusts are the primary allergens incriminated in the horse.[2, 35, 149] The condition may or not be seasonal and the distribution usually includes the face, ears, ventrum, and legs.[2]

Diagnosis of atopy can be frustrating and is often made by exclusion of other causes of pruritic dermatoses. Intradermal skin testing can be useful but false-positive reactions occur due to the presence of skin-sensitizing antibodies, excess antigen, dermatographism, physical trauma, and contaminants in solutions. False-negative reactions also occur.[2, 29] For these reasons, skin testing should be performed by an experienced person and interpreted in light of the patient's history.

Therapy is directed at avoiding the allergen if it can be identified. Hyposensitization has shown variable success, and is discontinued if not successful within 6 months.[2] If successful, however, booster injections are given as needed.[2] Systemic glucocorticoids (dexamethasone 0.05–0.2 mg/kg PO, IV, IM, s.i.d., or prednisolone 0.25–1.0 mg/kg PO s.i.d. for 5–7 days tapering to the lowest effective dose e.o.d.) are used in animals when hyposensitization fails or is not economically feasible.[2] Antihistamines, NSAIDs, diethylcar-

Table 1–21. Agents Causing Tissue-Specific Immune-Complex Reactions in Humans*

Skin eruptions	Aspirin, penicillin, blood products, sulfonamides, phenytoin, NSAIDs, allopurinol, thiazide diuretics, phenothiazines, quinidine
Hemolytic disorders	Methyldopa, penicillin, quinidine, tetracycline, sulfonamides, dipyrone, quinine, stibophen, para-aminosalicylic acid, phenacetin, rifampin, cephalothin
Thrombocytopenia	Sulfonamides, quinidine, quinine sulfonylureas, thiazides, gold, stibophen, isoniazid, rifampin, meprobamate, thiouracils, chloramphenicol
Agranulocytosis	Phenylbutazone, amidopyrine, oxyphenbutazone, dipyrone, sulfonamides, β-lactam antibiotics, chloramphenicol, phenothiazines, para-aminosalicylic acid, gold compounds, anticonvulsants, propylthiouracil, indomethacin, tolbutamide, barbiturates, antihistamines, arsenicals
Intersitial nephritis	High-dose penicillin, methicillin, hydantoin
Glomerulonephritis	Gold
Hepatocellular injury	Pyrazimide, rifampin, monoamine oxidase inhibitors, halothane, isoniazid, methyldopa, hydantoin, sulfonamides, indomethacin
Cholestasis	Phenothiazines, erythromycin estolate, nitrofurantoin, sulfonamides
Systemic lupus erythematosus	Isoniazid, hydralazine HCl, griseofulvin, tetracycline, procainamide, phenytoin, propylthiouracil
Pneumonitis	Nitrofurantoin, cromolyn sodium, sulfasalazine
Allergic rhinitis	Reserpine

*Data from references 4, 52, 143.

bamazine, and hydroxyzine have been used with little success.[2]

Urticaria and Angioedema

Urticarial reactions are fairly common in the horse.[2] These reactions are characterized by local or generalized pitting wheals of the head, neck, and trunk and occasionally the flanks and limbs. Pruritus, serum exudation, and hemorrhage are variable.[2, 16, 20] These reactions may be immunologically or nonimmunologically mediated.[2, 20] An immediate and a DTH reaction to salivary antigens of *Culicoides* and *Simulium* species are the most common causes of equine seasonal pruritic urticaria.[2, 20, 28] Urticarial reactions can also be seen with hepatitis; gastrointestinal parasitism; certain infectious diseases, including strangles, dermatophytosis, and babesiosis; a variety of drugs and biologicals; feedstuffs; inhaled allergens, including pollen and molds; insect bites and bee stings; and contact irritants such as saddle soap, leather conditioner, insecticides, and sneezeweed[2, 16, 20, 29, 150] (see Table 1–19).

Though many of these reactions have not been characterized, it is likely that they represent hypersensitivity reactions. Patch testing is considered useful in the diagnosis of contact hypersensitivity in humans. Intradermal skin testing, as with systemic anaphylaxis, may yield false-negative results if the parent antigen is not active.[23] Therapy is aimed at identification and avoidance of the provoking antigen, and palliative treatment with topical and systemic anti-inflammatory agents.[2] Avoidance alone is often the sole therapeutic measure required.[29, 35] In the case of drug-induced urticaria, therapeutic withdrawal of the offending agent should result in regression of the eruption in 10 to 14 days.[2] NSAIDs may be beneficial.[2, 88, 149, 156] As with most equine hypersensitivity reactions, antihistamine therapy alone is rarely beneficial.[2, 11, 35, 41, 42, 88, 92, 149] However, the finding that systemic histamine concentrations increase during equine immediate hypersensitivity provides some rationale for the use of antihistamines as one component of therapy for urticaria.[28] Systemic glucocorticoids (dexamethasone 0.05–0.2 mg/kg IV, IM, PO, or prednisone 0.25–1.0 mg/kg s.i.d. PO tapering to the lowest therapeutic dosage) may be warranted in refractory cases.[2, 35, 36, 149] Because urticaria may be a sign of systemic anaphylaxis, epinephrine (1:1,000, 5–10 mL/450 kg IM) is indicated if dyspnea or hypotension is present; a tracheostomy may also be necessary if dyspnea is severe.[2, 20, 29, 149]

Insect Hypersensitivity

An immediate and delayed-type hypersensitivity to the salivary antigens of *Culicoides* and *Simulium* species is the most common cause of pruritic skin disease of the horse.[2, 20, 28] The condition is seasonal in colder climates. Flies, including *Stomoxys* and *Haemotobia species,* are also implicated. Pruritic, papular crusting dermatitis with a dorsal (head, ears, neck, back, tailhead) or ventral distribution (legs, groin, axillae, ventral thorax, abdomen) is characteristic.[2, 20] There is evidence of a genetic tendency to develop *Culicoides* hypersensitivity.[2]

The primary goal of therapy is to control exposure to insect bites with the use of insecticides, both topically and within the horse's environment. Because *Culicoides* species feed primarily at dawn and dusk, the horses should be kept in stalls enclosed in fine-mesh netting during these hours. These insects are unable to fly in windy conditions and strategic placement of stall fans has been efficacious. Severe cases may require glucocorticoid therapy.

Parasite Hypersensitivity

Though not documented, hypersensitivity is thought to be significant in the pathogenesis of several parasitic diseases. A pruritic, seborrheic allergic dermatosis of foals has been associated with intestinal parasitism.[19] Cutaneous onchocerciasis and cutaneous habronemiasis may involve a hypersensitivity reaction to the microfilaria of *Onchocerca cervicalis* and the larvae of *Draschia* and *Habronema* species.[2, 20, 29, 157] Parasitic hypersensitivity was also suspected as the cause of chronic eosinophilic pancreatitis and ulcerative colitis in a 19-year-old mare with weight loss, coronary band alopecia, and buccal ulceration.[33]

It has been postulated that hypersensitivity plays a role in the development of clinical signs, intestinal lesions, and arterial lesions in *Strongylus vulgaris*–associated intestinal disease.[34] L3 larvae may produce factors that induce spasmodic colic.[158] However, hypersensitivity reactions to larvae killed by larvicidal anthelmintic therapy were not demonstrated in an experimental model.[159]

Therapy should be initially directed at eliminating the parasite with appropriate anthelmintic therapy. Concurrent glucocorticoid (dexamethasone 0.05–0.2 mg/kg IV, IM, PO, or prednisolone 0.25–1.0 mg/kg s.i.d. PO tapering to the lowest therapeutic dosage) therapy may be warranted if inflammation or pruritus is severe. Some authors recommend glucocorticoid therapy prior to anthelmintic treatment to minimize the possibility of an exacerbation of signs associated with parasite death.[20] Topical glucocorticoid therapy may be useful in some cases, for example, cutaneous habronemiasis.

Rhinitis

In humans, allergic rhinitis is considered an immediate-type hypersensitivity reaction to inhaled allergens.[40] A syndrome resembling allergic rhinitis of humans and dogs has been described in the horse.[29, 39, 40] Seasonal headshaking and tossing, rubbing of the muzzle, nasal irritation, sneezing and snorting, nasal discharge, and lacrimation were the presenting complaints. Many of these horses had concurrent COPD.

Vasculitis

Equine vasculitis is characterized by an acute onset of subcutaneous edema, necrosis, and ulceration of the extremities and oral mucosa which is not associated with local trauma or infection, hypoproteinemia, congestive heart failure, pleuritis, or peritonitis.[2, 139] Detection of immune complexes within vessel walls suggests that the vasculitis is the result of an immediate-type hypersensitivity reaction mediated by immune-complex injury.[2, 139, 160] Though the cause generally remains unknown, in the case of purpura hemorrhagica the vasculitis tends to occur 2 to 4 weeks after a respiratory infection.[20] In a study of 19 cases of equine vasculitis, only seven horses had a history of exposure to *Streptococcus equi*.[139] *Streptococcus equi, Streptococcus zooepidemicus,* influenza, equine herpesvirus type-1, and *Corynebacterium* have all been implicated.[2, 139] Drugs and toxins can also be the sensitizing antigen.[2, 28, 139, 160] Circulating immune complexes composed of IgA and *S. equi* M protein have been detected in horses with a history of purpura hemorrhagica.[161, 162]

Clinical signs include edema, erythema, crusts, and even necrosis and ulcers of the extremities.[2, 20, 139] Horses with purpura have profound edema of the limbs, head, and ventrum; petechiae of mucous membranes and skin; and show signs of systemic illness, including depression and stiffness.

Systemic immune-complex deposition can result in arthralgia and renal compromise.[139]

The differential diagnoses includes drug eruption, systemic lupus erythematosus, equine viral arteritis, equine infectious anemia, equine ehrlichiosis, and toxicoses.[2] With purpura hemorrhagica, the CBC may reveal a neutrophilia with or without a left shift, hyperglobulinemia, and hyperfibrinogenemia. The most common histologic finding in equine cutaneous vasculitis is leukocytoclastic vasculitis[139] but a mixed neutrophilic, eosinophilic, and lymphocytic infiltrate may be noted in edematous lesions.[2]

Therapy is aimed at reducing the edema, eliminating the antigenic stimulus, and inhibiting ongoing hypersensitivity reactions.[2] Hydrotherapy, counterpressure bandages, exercise, and diuretics may be useful in decreasing the edema. Penicillin (22,000–44,000 IU/kg b.i.d. to q.i.d. depending on the preparation, continued for 5 to 7 days after remission of clinical signs) is usually administered because streptococcal disease cannot be ruled out. Glucocorticoids (prednisolone 0.25–1.0 mg/kg PO, or dexamethasone 0.05–0.2 mg/kg IV or IM b.i.d. or s.i.d.) are continued until remission of clinical signs and then gradually tapered. The mean duration of glucocorticoid therapy in the 19 cases reported was 14 days.[139] NSAIDs are often administered. Tracheostomy may be required if edema of the head and neck is severe. Five of the 19 reported cases failed to respond to therapy.[139]

A photoactivated vasculitis affecting the white-skinned areas of the face and distal limbs during the summer is described. Therapy consists of systemic glucocorticoids for 30 days and avoiding exposure to the sun.[163]

Chronic Obstructive Pulmonary Disease

Although the pathogenesis of COPD is multifactorial, responses to provocative challenge exposure, cromolyn sodium, bronchodilators, immunotherapy, intradermal skin testing, and environmental manipulation indicate that immediate and DTH reactions are significant in the pathogenesis.[6, 11, 14, 24, 25, 27] Horses with COPD have greater concentrations of IgE in their bronchoalveolar lavage fluids than unaffected controls but show no difference in serum IgE concentrations.[62a] Horses with chronic pulmonary disease have a greater number of positive reactions to allergens on intradermal skin tests,[26] and basophils from COPD horses are more responsive to environmental allergen induced degranulation in vitro than unaffected controls.[62b] As previously described, many mediators are released during hypersensitivity reactions. In the lung these mediators have a variety of effects, including increased pulmonary resistance, decreased pulmonary compliance, bronchospasm, mucous secretion and plugging, decreased mucociliary clearance, and pulmonary edema.[6]

The significance of hypersensitivity in human asthma is well accepted.[164] A cycle of inhaled antigen challenge and associated leukocyte mediator release disrupts mucosal tight junctions, increasing mucosal permeability. This facilitates mediator and antigenic stimulation of submucosal mast cells, activating the immediate-type hypersensitivity pathways and a vicious circle of mediator release. Multiple infectious and environmental factors may be significant in initiating this cycle in the horse, including influenza viruses, molds, dust, cold air, and noxious gases[11, 26] (see Table 1–19).

Allergic Contact Dermatitis

Allergic contact dermatitis is a delayed hypersensitivity reaction to drugs or chemicals that associate with proteins on the APC.[141] APCs of the skin, the Langerhans' cells, are responsible for presenting the antigen to the antigen-specific T cell. Cytokines, including IL-1, IL-2, IFN-γ, and TNF, which are released from this cellular interaction, amplify the cellular infiltrate, which is predominately composed of macrophages. Initial signs appear after 5 to 21 days of sensitization.[92] Once sensitized, swelling and induration are seen at the site of antigen re-exposure within 24 hours. Contact allergic dermatitis has been incriminated in cutaneous reactions to insecticides, tack, metal within bits, dyes, bedding, soaps, blankets, neat's-foot oil, poison ivy, and wool.[11, 16, 20, 92, 149] Parabens, a preservative in topical medication, neomycin, and topical iodine solutions can cause allergic contact dermatitis in humans.[52]

Food Hypersensitivity

Food allergies in horses are poorly documented. Clover, Saint Johnswort, potatoes, distillers' waste, malt, beet pulp, buckwheat, glucose, chicory, and concentrates, including wheat, oats, barley, and bran, have been incriminated.[2, 16, 18, 19, 28, 36] The syndrome is characterized by nonseasonal pruritus or pruritic urticaria, but nonpruritic papules or plaques have been reported.[16, 28] Lesions may be found on the thorax, head, neck, and mucous membranes. Diagnosis is made using an elimination diet.[2] A hypoallergenic diet of oat hay for 3 to 4 weeks followed by alfalfa hay has been proposed. During this elimination trial, components of the original diet are reintroduced one at a time every week. Signs usually recur within 48 hours of reexposure to the offending allergen.

Therapy is avoidance of the offending feedstuff. The disease is reported to be poorly responsive to glucocorticoid therapy.[2] In humans, food allergy may be either an immediate or DTH reaction.[38] It has been postulated that the early substitution of artificial diets for mother's milk may enable uptake of and sensitization to dietary macromolecules.[38]

THERAPEUTIC MANAGEMENT OF IMMEDIATE HYPERSENSITIVITY REACTIONS

The diversity of chemical mediators that are released or synthesized by inflammatory cells during a hypersensitivity reaction explains the limited effect of therapeutic agents that act upon individual mediators.[43] Therapeutic agents used in the management of hypersensitivity reactions include α- and β-adrenergic agents, agents that increase cAMP, glucocorticoids, antihistamines, cromolyn sodium, oxygen, intravenous fluids, parasympatholytic agents, diethylcarbamazine, cyclooxygenase inhibitors, lipoxygenase inhibitors, phospholipase A$_2$ (PLA$_2$) inhibitors, PAF antagonists, calcium channel blockers, and calmodulin antagonists.[2, 14, 54, 55, 78, 164]

Sympathomimetic Agents

Multiple sympathomimetic agents are used to treat immediate hypersensitivity reactions.[5, 11, 165] The differing therapeutic effects of the sympathomimetic agents are due to their differing affinity for α- and β-adrenergic receptors and the tissue distribution of these receptors[165] (Table 1–22). Stimulation of α$_1$- and α$_2$-adrenergic receptors in vascular smooth muscle causes vasoconstriction. This decreases vascular permeability and peripheral blood flow with a resultant increase in blood pressure and decrease in vascular leakage, minimizing edema formation. Stimulation of β$_2$-adrenergic receptors relaxes bronchial and peripheral vascular smooth muscle (predominately in skeletal muscle) leading to bronchodilation and peripheral vasodilation. Stimulation of β$_1$-receptors located in the myocardium increases heart rate and stroke volume. This β$_1$-receptor stimulation has the beneficial effects of increasing cardiac output and blood pressure but can cause tachyarrhythmias and potentiate the myocardial ischemia that occurs during severe systemic anaphylactic reactions.[5]

Epinephrine

Epinephrine is the preferred initial treatment for anaphylactic and anaphylactoid reactions.[5, 11] By stimulating α- and β-adrenergic receptors, epinephrine counteracts the immediately life-threatening components of systemic anaphylactic reactions caused by inflammatory mediators.[5, 11, 42, 54, 145, 165] These are hypotension, which results from vasodilation and vascular leakage, and asphyxiation from upper airway angioedema and bronchoconstriction.[11] Stimulation of α-adrenergic receptors decreases vascular permeability, decreases edema formation, and increases blood pressure by constricting vascular smooth muscle.[11] β$_2$-Adrenergic receptor stimulation inhibits mediator release from mast cells and relaxes bronchial smooth muscle, causing bronchodilation.[5, 11] Use of epinephrine is not without drawbacks. While stimulation of cardiac β$_1$-adrenergic receptors increases cardiac output and blood pressure, this stimulation can cause tachyarrhythmias and potentiate the myocardial ischemia that occurs during systemic anaphylaxis.

The dose and route of epinephrine administration during an equine anaphylactic reaction is a matter of clinical judgment.[5, 23, 69] The potent sympathetic stimulation can cause excitement, especially if administered intravenously. Subcutaneous administration is not recommended because potent vasoconstriction can cause tissue necrosis, and absorption is unreliable with the cardiovascular collapse that occurs during anaphylaxis. Intramuscular administration is indicated if signs include mild respiratory difficulty or mild hypotension, as evidenced by poor peripheral pulse quality. Intravenous administration is indicated if significant airway obstruction or severe hypotension is present. Smaller doses should be administered intravenously. Epinephrine can be administered endotracheally if venous access cannot be achieved.

The half-life of epinephrine is short and dosages can be repeated every 15 to 20 minutes until a clinical response is noted.[5, 69] In the case of anaphylaxis associated with mild hypotension or dyspnea, the recommended intramuscular dosage is 0.01 to 0.02 mg/kg. This is equal to 5 to 10 mL of epinephrine 1:1,000 for a 450-kg horse. If dyspnea or hypotension is severe, intravenous epinephrine therapy is warranted. Administration of 0.003 to 0.005 mg/kg (1.5–2.25

Table 1–22. Catecholamines: Relative Potency and Tissue Distribution of Receptors*

Receptor Type	Tissue	Response	Potency of Agonists†
α	Blood vessels	Vasoconstriction	Epinephrine>norepinephrine>>>isoproterenol
β_1	Heart	Positive inotropic and chronotropic effects	Isoproterenol>epinephrine≥norepinephrine
β_2	Blood vessels	Vasodilation	Isoproterenol>epinephrine>>>norepinephrine

*From Adams R: Adrenergic and antiadrenergic drugs. In Booth N, McDonald L, eds: *Veterinary Pharmacology and Therapeutics.* Ames, Iowa State University Press, 1988, p 95.

†Symbols: >, greater than; ≥, greater than or equal; >>>, many times greater.

mL of a 1:1,000 dilution of epinephrine for a 450-kg horse) is recommended for the treatment of shock, but doses as high as 0.01 mg/kg (4.5 mL of a 1:1,000 dilution for a 450-kg horse) may be warranted.[166, 167] Intravenous epinephrine doses can be diluted tenfold prior to administration (i.e., 1 part 1:1,000 epinephrine to 9 parts normal saline). In human medicine, a constant slow infusion of diluted epinephrine is sometimes utilized with cardiac monitoring in cases refractory to repeated epinephrine boluses.[69]

Norepinephrine

Norepinephrine's primary therapeutic effect is increased blood pressure which is mediated by α-adrenergic constriction of vascular smooth muscle.[165] The vasoconstriction mediated by norepinephrine is not as potent as that of epinephrine. However, norepinephrine's primary advantage is that the myocardial stimulation is less potent than that of epinephrine[69, 165] (see Table 1–22). Norepinephrine, diluted in balanced polyionic fluid, is administered as a slow continuous IV infusion to human anaphylactic patients with refractory hypotension (0.1–0.2 μg/kg/min).[69] Its pressor effects last 1 to 2 minutes.[165] Norepinephrine should not be used alone in the treatment of hypersensitivity reactions if dyspnea is present. While norepinephrine can aid in reversing upper airway obstruction due to angioedema, limited β_2-adrenergic activity makes norepinephrine insufficient for reversal of bronchospasm.[165]

Pure β-Agonists

Agents that stimulate only β_1- and β_2-receptors, such as isoproterenol may be contraindicated in the treatment of hypersensitivity reactions characterized by hypotension.[69, 132, 165] In conditions of poor sympathetic tone, β_2-receptor stimulation of vascular smooth muscle causes vasodilation, which exacerbates hypotension. β-adrenergic receptor stimulation does improve cardiac output, and inhibits increases in vascular permeability, which improves blood pressure. However, the risk of vasodilation, decreased diastolic blood pressure, and myocardial hypoxia should be carefully considered with parenteral administration of β-agonists.[69, 165]

β₂-Agonists

Salbutamol, clenbuterol, and terbutaline are β_2-agonists which selectively cause bronchodilation, with minimal cardiac stimulation.[165] This effect is presumed to be mediated by an increase in cAMP associated with β-receptor stimulation.[55, 132] In a study of animal models, animals were more prone to anaphylaxis in conditions of high cGMP or low cAMP.[5] β-Adrenergic stimulation inhibits antibody-mediated granule release from mast cells and basophils and has been shown to decrease vascular permeability by decreasing the size of gaps formed between endothelial cells during mediator-induced contraction of these cells.[5, 54, 55, 133] β_2-Agonists may be useful in the treatment of horses experiencing dyspnea from mediator-induced bronchoconstriction. Owing to the vasodilator action of parenterally administered β_2-agonists, these agents should be administered via nebulization in the hypotensive horse. Terbutaline has been administered IV (3.3 μg/kg) and PO (66 μg/kg q.12.h.–130 μg/kg q.8.h.) to relieve bronchospasm (Ralph Beadle, D.V.M., Baton Rouge, La., personal communication, Feb. 1, 1991).[167]

Pure α-Agonists

Selective α-adrenergic stimulants, such as phenylephrine and metaraminol, have the beneficial effects of decreasing vascular permeability and edema formation by inducing vasoconstriction.[165] Unlike epinephrine, α-agonist-mediated vasoconstriction increases blood pressure with little cardiac stimulation. α-Agonists have been used to treat human anaphylaxis.[78] These agents can decrease respiratory distress due to upper airway and pulmonary edema but do not reverse bronchospasm.[11, 165] The recommended dosage of phenylephrine is 0.2 to 0.4 μg/kg/min. Phenylephrine bolus injections can cause reflex bradycardia, which is avoided by administering phenylephrine using constant infusion.[166, 167]

Phosphodiesterase Inhibitors

The phosphodiesterase inhibitors theophylline, aminophylline, and colforsin, indirectly increase cAMP by inhibiting its breakdown. These agents have been shown to decrease the release of inflammatory mediators from basophils and mast cells.[5, 23, 132] Phosphodiesterase inhibitors may be useful in cases of refractory bronchospasm, but side effects, including tachyarrhythmias, and exacerbation of hypotension limit their usefulness in the treatment of severe systemic anaphylaxis.[5] Phosphodiesterase inhibitors should not be used as first-line therapy for dyspnea associated with anaphylaxis owing to their negative side effects.

Glucocorticoids

Glucocorticoid therapy is the hallmark of treatment for hypersensitivity reactions. Glucocorticoids excel as therapeutic agents because they have potent effects on mediator release, accumulation, activation, and traffic of inflammatory cells.[164] The mechanisms of steroid effects are multiple. Glucocorticoids activate the transcription and translation of several proteins.[168-171] Lipocortin is probably the most significant. Lipocortin inhibits the action of PLA$_2$ in the cell membrane, inhibiting arachidonic acid liberation.[169, 170, 172] Without the arachidonic acid substrate, prostaglandin, leukotriene, and PAF formation are inhibited.[170, 171, 173, 174]

Glucocorticoids stabilize cellular and lysosomal membranes, and inhibit the synthesis and release of chemotactic inflammatory mediators from mast cells and basophils, including those that increase vascular permeability (LTC$_4$, LTD$_4$), and those causing vasodilation (PGD$_2$, PGE$_2$).[11, 164, 175] Glucocorticoids inhibit the production and release of multiple cytokines, including tumor necrosis factor alpha (TNFα), IFN-γ, granulocyte-macrophage colony-stimulating factor (GM-CSF), and interleukins 1, 2, 3, and 6.[175a] There is evidence that even after mediator release, glucocorticoids modify the effects of mediators at their target.[23] Glucocorticoids interfere with chemotaxis.[42] Glucocorticoids potentiate sympathetic tone, which exerts a direct effect on endothelial cells and vascular smooth muscle, inhibiting increased vascular permeability and vasodilation.[11, 42, 164, 175] The availability of circulating inflammatory cells is decreased by redistribution of eosinophils, monocytes, and T cells to the bone marrow and lymph nodes during glucocorticoid therapy.[42] There is also evidence that glucocorticoids facilitate bronchodilation by increasing the number of β_2-receptors on bronchial smooth muscle.[164]

Glucocorticoids do have a latent period before their inhibitory effects are noted. The best effect is achieved if they are given 8 hours prior to the stimulus-inciting hypersensitivity.[175] This is not clinically practical except in the rare instances where an expected exacerbation of signs can be foreseen. Despite the latent period, the potency of glucocorticoids and the diversity of their effects bring them to the forefront of hypersensitivity therapy. Hypersensitivity reactions are characterized by a vicious circle of mediator release, recruitment of secondary effector cells, and renewed mediator release. Glucocorticoid administration during the acute phase of hypersensitivity is rational.[23] Glucocorticoids limit the cyclic nature of hypersensitivity reactions and lessen the severity of ongoing inflammation. Glucocorticoids are the only therapeutic agents that prevent or lessen the severity of the late-phase reaction. Such therapy is especially indicated if bronchospasm and hypotension persist.[5] Parenteral prednisolone sodium succinate 0.25 to >10.0 mg/kg IV is most rapidly effective. Dexamethasone 0.05 to 0.2 mg/kg IV, IM, or PO or prednisolone 0.25 to 1.0 mg/kg PO) can be used for long-term therapy. The dosage should be tapered to the lowest effective dosage and administered every other day.

Antihistamines

Though antihistamines are considered part of the standard therapy for human anaphylaxis, they are relatively ineffec-

tive in the treatment of equine anaphylaxis and cutaneous hypersensitivity reactions.[2, 5, 11, 41, 42, 88] However, rationale for the use of antihistamines in treating anaphylaxis does exist because systemic levels of histamine increase during equine anaphylaxis.[89] Antihistamines should not be used alone in the treatment of equine anaphylactic reactions.

Antihistamines block H$_1$ receptors, but H$_1$-receptor stimulation mediates only a portion of the pathogenesis of hypersensitivity. Antihistamines do not address the plethora of other mediators, including leukotrienes and prostaglandins. Antihistamines cannot attenuate histamine's effects once it has combined with the H$_2$-receptor, and do not block some histamine-induced cascades.[23] Antihistamines cannot reverse the inflammatory process.[11] Antihistamines that have been used in the horse include pyrilamine maleate (1 mg/kg IV, IM, SQ), tripelenamine hydrochloride (1 mg/kg IM), diphenhydramine hydrochloride (0.66 mg/kg PO b.i.d.), chlorpheniramine, and hydroxyzine hydrochloride (1 mg/kg PO b.i.d.).[42, 88]

Cromolyn Sodium

Cromolyn sodium inhibits in vitro release of mediators from mast cells and possibly basophils.[11, 176] The mechanism by which cromolyn sodium inhibits mediator release is the subject of controversy. There is evidence that it inhibits activation of protein kinase C,[177] alters calcium channels in the plasma membrane,[178] inhibits phosphodiesterase,[179] and alters membrane proteins via phosphorylation.[180]

Cromolyn sodium is used prophylactically to prevent human asthma.[54] Its efficacy in the treatment of equine COPD is controversial. Nebulized doses of 80 mg for 4 consecutive days prevented clinical signs in horses with COPD for 3 weeks and single doses provide protection for 3 to 5 days.[181, 182] Other investigators have not detected an improvement in clinical signs with prechallenge cromolyn doses as high as 500 mg despite finding that cromolyn sodium treatment prior to antigen challenge maintains pulmonary resistance, transpulmonary pressure, and tidal volume at prechallenge levels.[183]

Parasympatholytic Agents

The parasympatholytic agents atropine (0.01 mg/kg IV or IM) and glycopyrrolate (0.005 mg/kg IV) are useful in treating reflex vagal bronchospasm and increased mucous secretion occurring during hypersensitivity reactions and acute respiratory distress associated with COPD.[5, 11, 184] These agents block muscarinic receptors, decreasing acetylcholine-mediated production of cGMP.[184] Decreased cGMP stabilizes granule and lysosomal membranes.[185-187] Because of the untoward side effects of the parasympatholytic agents, namely tachyarrhythmias and ileus, they should always bc uscd judiciously. Glycopyrrolate may be a more appropriate choice for the treatment of systemic anaphylaxis because the danger of tachyarrhythmias is lower than with atropine.[184]

Diethylcarbamazine

Diethylcarbamazine (DEC) has been shown to inhibit the release of prostaglandins, histamine, and leukotrienes in various species in vitro.[188–190] DEC caused a mild reduction in the severity of systemic hypotension and respiratory obstruction in experimental equine anaphylaxis.[41, 88] In the treatment of summer pasture–associated COPD, DEC has not resulted in significant improvement in clinical signs (Ralph Beadle, D.V.M., Baton Rouge, La., personal communication).

Nonsteroidal Anti-Inflammatory Agents

Cyclooxygenase Inhibitors

Cyclooxygenase inhibitors, including aspirin and meclofenamic acid, are reported to control the respiratory and cardiovascular manifestations of immediate systemic hypersensitivity in horses, which suggests that kinins and prostaglandins are more significant than bioamines in mediating equine hypersensitivity.[41, 42, 88] In addition to inhibiting prostaglandin formation, cyclooxygenase inhibitors antagonize vascular permeability and smooth muscle contraction induced by kinins and interfere with kinin formation by preventing kallikrein activation.[41, 42]

Twenty percent of humans with asthma experience an exacerbation of respiratory dyspnea after administration of cyclooxygenase inhibitors.[191] It has been postulated that by blocking the cyclooxygenase pathway with cyclooxygenase inhibitors, shunting of arachidonic acid metabolism to the lipoxygenase pathway increases histamine release from basophils, disturbing the balance between the unique anti-inflammatory effects of PGE_2 and the inflammatory effects of leukotrienes.[54, 192] Nonetheless, in vitro experiments indicate that cyclooxygenase inhibitors tend to enhance antigen-induced contraction of tracheal smooth muscle, but decrease bronchial smooth muscle contraction.[193] By inhibiting the formation of secondary mediators of anaphylaxis, the cyclooxygenase inhibitors may be a useful adjunct in the treatment of hypersensitivity, including hypersensitivity-induced dyspnea.

Lipoxygenase Inhibitors

Leukotrienes (LTs) are potent mediators of inflammation during hypersensitivity reactions. Pure inhibitors of the lipoxygenase pathway and dual inhibitors of the lipoxygenase and cyclooxygenase pathway, such as benoxaprofen and lonapalene, moderated LT-mediated inflammation in human subjects but were removed from the market due to liver toxicity.[194] Ketoprofen, a bradykinin antagonist, has demonstrated lipoxygenase inhibition in controlled in vitro systems.[194a, 194b] However, initial study of ketoprofen-treated horses has not demonstrated lipoxygenase inhibition.[194c] Lipoxygenase inhibitors have been shown to block antigen-induced immediate and late airway hypersensitivity responses, including bronchoconstriction, in allergic sheep and guinea pigs.[86, 193, 195] Newer lipoxygenase inhibitors including zileuton, piripost, and docebenone, and combined lipoxygenase/cyclooxygenase inhibitors such as tenidap have completed phase II human clinical trials and show great promise in the treatment of human inflammatory diseases.[195a, 195b] Though untested in equine patients, this class of NSAIDs is sure to be significant in future management of equine inflammatory disorders, including COPD.

Platelet Activating Factor Inhibitors

Platelet activating factor antagonists have shown little therapeutic promise in animal models of hypersensitivity.[196]

Phospholipase Inhibitors

Recognition that the anti-inflammatory action of glucocorticoids resulted from the production of a PLA_2-inhibiting protein, lipocortin, has created interest in other phospholipase inhibitors. Liberation of arachidonic acid by PLA_2 is an integral step in the cascade of mediators created by basophil and mast cell degranulation.[54] Basophil histamine release is inhibited by phospholipase inhibitors.[197] Phospholipase inhibitors are being studied experimentally in allergy,[198] human septic shock,[199] and myocardial disease.[200] These include vitamin E and plipastatins derived from bacterial products.[201, 202] Recombinant human lipocortin has been used in the treatment of certain human dermatoses, such as psoriasis.[203] The usefulness of phospholipase inhibitors in the treatment of equine hypersensitivity and inflammatory conditions has not been determined.

Calcium Channel Blockers

Calcium channel blockers include such drugs as nifedipine, verapamil, and dantrolene. The rationale for the use of calcium channel blockers in hypersensitivity reactions is that they interfere with the calcium-dependent steps in the formation and release of chemical mediators.[75] The calcium channel blockers nifedipine, and verapamil decrease leukotriene, thromboxane, and PAF synthesis and inhibit lysosome release.[75] Activation of PLA_2, 5-lipoxygenase, and calmodulin is calcium-dependent. Dantrolene, mepacrine, nifedipine, and nisoldipine appear to antagonize PLA_2 independent of their calcium channel blocking activity.[204, 205] To date, there is no literature on the use of calcium channel blockers in the treatment of equine hypersensitivity reactions. These agents have shown variable inhibitory effects on allergic and nonallergic histamine release in human subjects.[75] Because histamine is only a minor mediator of equine hypersensitivity, calcium channel blockers may provide some therapeutic benefit, but further research is needed in this area prior to clinical use.

Calmodulin Antagonists

Trifluoperazine and compound W7, both calmodulin antagonists, inhibit IgE-mediated histamine release and leukotriene synthesis in vivo.[206] They may also inhibit PLA_2.[207]

THERAPEUTIC APPROACH TO ACUTE SYSTEMIC ANAPHYLAXIS

The therapeutic goals in treating systemic anaphylaxis are to (1) prevent or reverse the complications caused by mediator release (2) maintain respiratory integrity, and (3) maintain cardiovascular stability.[5] Not all anaphylactic reactions require therapy. However, rapid recognition of those that do is critical to patient survival. Sudden dyspnea; hypotension, as evidenced by poor peripheral pulse character; rapid onset of urticaria; and collapse are significant cause for alarm.

Some horses respond to simply eliminating the allergen. The inciting antigen should be removed. Intravenous access via an indwelling intravenous catheter and airway patency should be instituted immediately because cardiovascular collapse and upper airway obstruction due to angioedema can occur rapidly.[5, 23, 69, 78] The conscious horse does not tolerate tracheal intubation so emergency tracheotomy may be required. Oxygen should be administered if available because bronchoconstriction and cardiovascular collapse result in hypoxemia.[5, 69, 151]

Cardiac monitoring by vigilant cardiac auscultation and electrocardiogram (ECG) is warranted. Many drugs used in the treatment of hypersensitivity reactions potentiate the effects of myocardial ischemia, and arrhythmias are common. The fluid requirement of horses in anaphylactic shock is not known but large volumes of balanced polyionic fluid should be administered rapidly to combat mediator-induced hypotension and cardiovascular collapse. Volumes of 400 mL/kg/24 hours may be used in the treatment of human anaphylaxis.[5, 69] Epinephrine is a potent sympathetic stimulant and its administration may cause excitement in the horse. Epinephrine is indicated and should be administered IM (10–20 μg/kg, equivalent to 5–10 mL of 1:1,000 dilution of epinephrine for a 450-kg horse) if dyspnea or hypotension are mild.[5] Epinephrine should not be administered subcutaneously because its potent vasoconstriction can lead to poor absorption and tissue necrosis.[5, 23] If dyspnea or hypotension is severe, epinephrine should be administered intravenously or endotracheally if there is no venous access (3–5 μg/kg or 1.5–2.25 mL of 1:1,000 dilution of epinephrine for a 450-kg horse).[5] Epinephrine doses can be repeated every 15 to 20 minutes until hypotension improves.[5, 69] The side effects of epinephrine therapy are tachyarrhythmias, and myocardial ischemia, which can in themselves be life-threatening. Alternatively, an epinephrine or norepinephrine drip can be instituted for cases of refractory hypotension.[5, 69]

Selective α-adrenergic receptor agonists, such as phenylephrine, which cause vasoconstriction, may be useful to improve blood pressure and decrease edema formation.[165, 167] Their limited β-adrenergic receptor stimulation makes α-agonists ineffective for reversing bronchospasm.[11, 165] Therefore, α-agonists should not be used alone in treating systemic hypersensitivity reactions.

Selective β1-adrenergic agonists such as isoproterenol are contraindicated in the treatment of anaphylactic reactions.[69] β-Agonists stimulate cardiac smooth muscle and relax peripheral vasculature, which potentiates vasodilation, hypotension, and myocardial hypoxia.

β2-Adrenergic agonists such as terbutaline may have a place in the treatment of systemic anaphylactic reactions with refractory bronchospasm.[145] Stimulation of β2-receptors selectively relaxes bronchial smooth muscle with less cardiac stimulation then epinephrine. Terbutaline can be administered IV to horses (3.3 μg/kg).[167] However, because parenterally administered β2-agonists cause some stimulation of cardiac muscle, vasodilation in skeletal muscle, and sweating, nebulization is the preferred route of administration of the β2-agonists during systemic anaphylaxis.[145, 167, 184] Parenteral administration of terbutaline should be restricted to normovolemic normotensive animals experiencing bronchospasm.

Antihistamines are considered part of the standard therapy for human anaphylaxis.[5] Their use as a sole therapeutic agent has shown little benefit in the treatment of equine anaphylaxis.[11, 41, 42, 88] However, because histamine concentration does increase during equine anaphylaxis, there is some rationale for their use.[89]

In humans, pressor agents such as dopamine or dobutamine are used to treat hypotension that is refractory to intravenous fluid and epinephrine therapy.[69] However, dopamine therapy is controversial because it may potentiate the release of hypersensitivity mediators through stimulation of dopaminergic receptors.[42] Dobutamine does not activate dopaminergic receptors. Dopamine has the advantage over dobutamine of preserving renal blood flow at low doses (1–10 μg/kg/min). Dopamine is administered very slowly as a diluted solution via an intravenous drip.[166, 167] Dopamine (200 mg) is diluted in 1 L of 5% dextrose and administered at a rate of 3 to 20 μg/kg/min (1–8 drops/sec/450 kg using a standard 10-drop/mL IV set). If dopamine is not available, dobutamine can also be used as a pressor agent. Dobutamine (50 mg) is diluted in 500 mL of 5% dextrose and administered at a rate of 1 to 5 μg/kg/min (1–4 drops/sec/450 kg). Pressor agents are administered until hypotension and pulse character improve. A maintenance drip may be necessary to maintain blood pressure. Pressor agents may reverse hypotension within seconds of initiating therapy. Overdosing occurs rapidly causing tachyarrhythmias and hypertension. For this reason the use of pressor agents should be limited to situations where hypotension is severe and potentially fatal. If hypotension is less severe, pressor agents should only be used if careful cardiac monitoring via an ECG is possible.

Though its effects may be delayed, glucocorticoid therapy is indicated to help reverse persistent bronchospasm, angioedema, and break the cycle of mediator-induced inflammation triggered during hypersensitivity reactions.[5, 69] Glucocorticoid therapy during the acute phase will aid in preventing the late-phase reaction.[78] Prednisolone sodium succinate 0.25 to 10.0 mg/kg, should be administered IV.

REFERENCES

1. *Dorland's Illustrated Medical Dictionary,* ed 26. Philadelphia, WB Saunders, 1985.
2. Scott DW: Immunologic diseases In Pederson D, ed: *Large Animal Dermatology.* Philadelphia, WB Saunders, 1988, pp 284–333.
3. Coombs RRA, Gell PGH: Classification of allergic reactions responsible for clinical hypersensitivity and disease. In Gell P, Coombs R, Lachmann P, eds. *Clinical Aspects of Immunology.* Oxford, Blackwell, 1975, pp 761–781.
4. Davis LE: Hypersensitivity reactions induced by antimicrobial drugs. *J Am Vet Med Assoc* 185:1131–1136, 1984.
5. Lucke WC, Thomas H: Anaphylaxis: Pathophysiology, clinical presentations and treatment. *J Emerg Med* 1:83–95, 1983.
6. Hanna CJ, Eyre P, Wells PW, et al: Equine immunology 2: Immunopharmacology—biochemical basis of hypersensitivity. *Equine Vet J* 14:16–24, 1982.
7. Tizard I: Type I hypersensitivity. In Tizard I, ed: *Veterinary Immunology: An Introduction.* Philadelphia, WB Saunders, 1992, pp 335–350.
8. Tizard I: Erythrocyte antigens and type II hypersensitivity. In Tizard I, ed: *Veterinary Immunology: An Introduction.* Philadelphia, WB Saunders, 1992, pp 351–360.

9. Tizard I: Type III hypersensitivity. In Tizard I, ed: *Veterinary Immunology: An Introduction.* Philadelphia, WB Saunders, 1992, pp 361–371.

10. Hamilton RG, Adkinson NF Jr: Mechanisms of acute allergic reactions. *Artif Organs* 8:311–317, 1984.

11. Eyre P, Hanna CJ: Equine allergies. *Equine Pract* 2:40–46, 1980.

12. Ishizaka K, Ishizaka T: Allergy. In Paul WE, ed: *Fundamental Immunology.* New York, Raven Press, 1989, pp 867–888.

13. Dixon FJ, Cochrane CC, Theofilopoulos AN: Immune complex injury. In Samter M, Talmage DW, Frank MM, et al, eds. *Immunological Diseases.* Boston, Little Brown, 1988, pp 233–260.

14. Schultz KT: Type I and type IV hypersensitivity in animals. *J Am Vet Med Assoc* 181:1083–1087, 1982.

15. Magro AM, Rudofsky UH, Schrader WP, et al: Characterization of IgE-mediated histamine release from equine basophils in vitro. *Equine Vet J* 20:352–356, 1988.

16. Mullowney PC: Dermatologic diseases of horses, V. Allergic, immune-mediated, and miscellaneous skin diseases. *Compendium Continuing Educ Pract Vet* 7:S217–S228, 1985.

17. Meltzer MS, Nacy CA: Delayed-type hypersensitivity and the induction of activated, cytotoxic macrophages. In Paul WE, ed: *Fundamental Immunology.* New York, Raven Press, 1989, pp 765–777.

18. Campbell SG: Diseases of allergy. In Catcott EJ, Smithcors JF, eds. *Equine Medicine and Surgery: A Text and Reference Work.* Wheaton, Ill, American Veterinary Publications, 1972, pp 227–237.

19. Kral F, Schwartzman RM: Allergic dermatoses. In *Veterinary and Comparative Dermatology.* Philadelphia, JB Lippincott, 1964, pp 110–121.

20. Manning T, Sweeney C: Immune-mediated equine skin diseases. *Compendium Continuing Educ Pract Vet* 8:979–987, 1986.

21. Klein L: Urticaria in the horse after anesthesia. *N Z Vet J* 31:206, 1983.

22. Goldberg GP, Short CE: Challenge in equine anesthesia: A suspected allergic reaction during acetylpromazine, guaifenesin, thiamylal, and halothane anesthesia. *Equine Pract* 10:5–10, 1988.

23. Davis LE: Adverse drug reactions in the horse. *Vet Clin North Am* 3:153–179, 1987.

24. Bryans JT, Gerber H, eds. *Equine Diseases III.* Basel, Karger, 1973, pp 448–457.

25. Gerber H: Chronic pulmonary disease in the horse. *Equine Vet J* 5:26–33, 1973.

26. Halliwell REW, Fleischman JB, Mackay-Smith M, et al: The role of allergy in chronic pulmonary disease of horses. *J Am Vet Med Assoc* 174:277–281, 1979.

27. McPherson EA, Thomson JR: Chronic obstructive pulmonary disease in the horse 1: Nature of the disease. *Equine Vet J* 15:203–206, 1983.

28. Walton GS: Allergic responses involving the skin of domestic animals. *Adv Vet Sci Comp Med* 15:201–240, 1971.

29. Beech J: Allergic diseases in the horse: Diagnosis and treatment. *Proc Am Assoc Equine Pract* 325–331, 1983.

30. Morrow AN, Quinn PJ, Baker KP: Some characteristics of the antibodies involved in allergic skin reactions of the horse to biting insects. *Br Vet J* 143:59–69, 1987.

31. Matthews AG, Imlah P, McPherson EA: Reagin-like antibody in horse serum. *Vet Res Commun* 6:13–23, 1983.

32. Scott DW: Parasitic diseases. In Pedersen D, ed: *Large Animal Dermatology.* Philadelphia, WB Saunders, 1988, pp 207–269.

33. Breider MA, Kiely RG, Edwards JF: Chronic eosinophilic pancreatitis and ulcerative colitis in a horse. *J Am Vet Med Assoc* 186:809–811, 1985.

34. Klei TR: Immunity and potential of vaccination. *Vet Clin North Am* 2:395–402, 1986.

35. Evans AG: Recurrent urticaria due to inhaled allergens. In Robinson NE, ed: *Current Therapy in Equine Medicine,* vol 2. Philadelphia, WB Saunders, 1987, pp 619–621.

36. Halliwell RE: Urticaria and angioedema. In Robinson NE, ed: *Current Therapy in Equine Medicine.* Philadelphia, WB Saunders, 1983, pp 535–536.

37. Atkins FM, Metcalfe DD: Food allergy in adults. In Lichtenstein LM, Fauci AS, eds: *Current Therapy in Allergy and Immunology.* Burlington, Ont, BC Decker, 1983, pp 39–45.

38. Van Dijk JE, Fledderus A, Mouwen JMVM, et al: Gastrointestinal food allergy and its role in large domestic animals. *Vet Res Commun* 12:47–59, 1988.

39. Francqueville M, Sabbah A: Allergic rhinitis in the horse: First case. *Allerg Immunol* (Paris) 22:56–60, 1990.

40. Lane JG, Mair TS: Observations on headshaking in the horse. *Equine Vet J* 19:331–335, 1987.

41. Chand N, Eyre P: Nonsteroidal anti-inflammatory drugs: A review. New applications in hypersensitivity reactions of cattle and horses. *Can J Comp Med* 41:233–240, 1977.

42. Eyre P, Hanna CJ, Wells PW, et al: Equine immunology 3: Immunopharmacology—anti-inflammatory, and antihypersensitivity drugs. *Equine Vet J* 14:277–281, 1982.

43. Smith TF: Allergy and pseudoallergy: An overview of basic mechanisms. *Prim Care* 14:421–434, 1987.

44. Atkins PC, Miragliotta G, Talbot SF, et al: Activation of plasma Hageman factor and kallikrein in ongoing allergic reactions in the skin. *J Immunol* 139:2744–2748, 1987.

45. Leiferman KM, Fujisawa T, Beulah H, et al: Extracellular deposition of eosinophil and neutrophil granule proteins in the IgE-mediated cutaneous late phase reaction. *Lab Invest* 62:579–589, 1990.

46. Dolovich J, Hargreave F, Chalmers R, et al: Late cutaneous allergic responses in isolated IgE dependent reactions. *J Allergy Clin Immunol* 52:38–46, 1973.

47. Solley G, Gleich G, Jordan R, et al: The late phase of the immediate wheal and flare skin reaction. Its dependence upon IgE antibodies. *J Clin Invest* 58:408–420, 1976.

48. Suter M, Tscharner C, Arnold P: Histologische und morphologische Charakterisierung von Pferde-Reagin (IgE) mittels Prausnitz-Küstner-technik. *Schweiz Arch Tierheilk* 123:647–654, 1981.

49. Uetrecht J: Mechanism of hypersensitivity reactions: Proposed involvement of reactive metabolites generated by activated leukocytes. *Trends Pharmacol Sci* 10:463–467, 1989.

50. Ishizaka K, Ishizaka T: Reversed type allergic skin reactions by anti-gamma E globulin antibodies in human and monkeys. *J Immunol* 100:554–562, 1968.

51. Leid RW: Chemical mediators of immediate hypersensitivity reactions. *Vet Clin North Am Large Anim Pract* 1:35–42, 1979.

52. Anderson JA, Adkinson NF: Allergic reactions to drugs and biologic agents. *J Am Vet Med Assoc* 258:2891–2899, 1987.

53. Wells PW, McBeath DG, Eyre P, et al: Equine immunology: An introductory review. *Equine Vet J* 13:218–222, 1981.

54. Marone G: The role of mast cell and basophil activation in human allergic reactions. *Eur Respir J* 2(suppl 6):446s–455s, 1989.

55. Marone G, Casolaro V, Cirillo R, et al: Pathophysiology of human basophils and mast cells in allergic disorders. *Clin Immunol Immunopathol* 50:s24–s40, 1989.

56. Schwartz LB: Mediators of human mast cells and human mast cell subsets. *Ann Allergy* 58:226–235, 1987.

57. Grant JA, Lichtenstein LM: Reversed in vitro anaphylaxis induced by anti-IgG: Specificity of the reaction and compari-

son with antigen-induced histamine release. *J Immunol* 109:20–25, 1972.

58. Fagan DL, Slaughter CA, Capra D, et al: Monoclonal antibodies to immunoglobulin G$_4$ induce histamine release from human basophils in vitro. *J Allergy Clin Immunol* 70:399–406, 1982.

59. Marone G, Tamburini M, Giudizi G, et al: Mechanism of activation of human basophils by *Staphylococcus aureus* Cowan 1. *Infect Immunol* 55:803–809, 1987.

60. Mueller GH, Kirk RW, Scott DW: Immunologic Diseases. In *Small Animal Dermatology*. Philadelphia, WB Saunders, 1983, 380–400.

61. Parish WD: A human heat-stable anaphylactic or anaphylactoid antibody which may participate in pulmonary disorders. In Austen KF, Lichtenstein LM, eds. *Asthma: Physiology, Immunopharmacology and Treatment*. New York, Academic Press, 1973, pp 71–89.

62. Burka JF, Briand H, Scott-Savage P, et al: Leukotriene D4 and platelet-activating factor—acether antagonists on allergic and arachidonic acid–induced reactions in guinea pig airways. *Can J Physiol Pharmacol* 67:483–490, 1989.

62a. Halliwell REW, McGorum BC, Irving P, et al: Local and systemic antibody production in horses affected with chronic obstructive pulmonary disease. *Vet Immunol Immunopathol* 38:201–215, 1993.

62b. Dirscherl P, Grabner A, Buschmann H: Responsiveness of basophil granulocytes of horses suffering from chronic obstructive pulmonary disease to various allergens. *Vet Immunol Immunopathol* 38:217–227, 1993.

63. Suter M, Fey H: Isolation and characterization of equine IgE. *Zentralbl Veterinarmed* [B] 28:414–420, 1981.

64. Suter M, Fey H: Further purification and characterization of horse IgE. *Vet Immunol Immunopathol* 4:545–553, 1983.

65. Stechschulte DJ, Orange RP, Austen KF: Two immunochemically distinct homologous antibodies capable of mediating immediate hypersensitivity reactions in the rat, mouse, and guinea pig. In Serafini U, ed. *Proceedings of the Seventh International Congress on Allergology-New Concepts in Allergy and Clinical Immunology*. Amsterdam, Excerpta Medica, 1971, pp 245–254.

66. Fridman WH, Bonnerot C, Daeron M, et al: Structural bases of Fcτ receptor functions. *Immunol Rev* 125:49–76, 1992.

67. Barnes PJ, Chung KF, Page CP: Platelet-activating factor as a mediator of allergic disease. *J Allergy Clin Immunol* 81:919–934, 1988.

68. Schulman ES, MacGlashan DW, Schleimer RP, et al: Purified human basophils and mast cells: Current concepts of mediator release. *Eur J Respir Dis* 64:53–61, 1983.

69. Bleeker ER, Lichtenstein LM: Systemic anaphylaxis. In Lichtenstein LM, Fauci AS eds: *Current Therapy in Allergy and Immunology*. Burlington, Ont, BC Decker, 1983, pp 78–83.

70. Ricci M: Immunoregulation in clinical diseases: An overview. *Clin Immunol Immunopathol* 50:S3–S12, 1989.

71. Romagnani S, Del Prete G, Maggi E, et al: Role of interleukins in induction and regulation of human IgE synthesis. *Clin Immunol Immunopathol* 50:S13–S23, 1989.

72. Herrod HG: Interleukins in immunologic and allergic diseases. *Ann Allergy* 63:269–272, 1989.

73. Del Prete G, Maggi E, Parronchi P, et al: IL-4 is essential factor for the IgE synthesis induced in vitro by human T cell clones and their supernatants. *J Immunol* 140:4193–4198, 1988.

73a. Kapsenberg ML, Wierenga EA, Bos JD, et al: Functional subsets of allergen-reactive human CD4$^+$ T-cells. *Immunol Today* 12:392–395, 1991.

73b. Romagnani S: Human TH1 and TH2 subsets: Doubt no more. *Immunol Today* 12:256–257, 1991.

74. Jardieu P, Akasaki M, Ishizaka K: Association of I-J determinants with lipomodulin/macrocortin. *Proc Natl Acad Sci U S A* 83:160–164, 1986.

75. Chand N, Perhach JL Jr, Diamantis W: Heterogeneity of calcium channels in mast cells and basophils and the possible relevance to pathophysiology of lung diseases: A review. *Agents Actions* 17:407–417, 1986.

76. Styrt B, Rocklin RE, Klempner MS: Characterization of the neutrophil respiratory burst in atopy. *J Allergy Clin Immunol* 81:20–26, 1988.

77. Marsh DG, Meyers DA, Freidhoff LR, et al: HLA-Dw2: A genetic marker for human immune response to short ragweed pollen allergen Ra5. *J Exp Med* 155:1452–1463, 1982.

78. Sheffer AL: Idiopathic anaphylaxis. In Lichtenstein LM, Fauci AS, eds. *Current Therapy in Allergy and Immunology*. Burlington, Ont, BC Decker, 1983, pp 84–87.

79. Bisgaard H: Leukotrienes and prostaglandins in asthma. *Allergy* 39:413–420, 1984.

80. Schwartz LB, Austen KF: The mast cell and mediators of immediate hypersensitivity. In Samter M, Talmage DW, Frank MM, et al, eds: *Immunological Diseases*. Boston, Little, Brown, 1988, pp 157–202.

81. Kaplan AP, Silverberg M, Ghebrehiwet B, et al: Pathways of kinin formation and role in allergic diseases. *Clin Immunol Immunopathol* 50:s41–s51, 1989.

82. Malmsten CL: Leukotrienes: Mediators of inflammation and immediate hypersensitivity reactions. *CRC Crit Rev Immunol* 4:307–334, 1985.

83. Proud D, Baumgarten CR, Naclerio RM, et al: The role of kinins in human allergic disease. *N Engl Reg Allergy Proc* 7:213–218, 1986.

84. O'Flaherty JT: Lipid mediators of inflammation and allergy. *Lab Invest* 47:314–329, 1982.

85. Goetzl EJ, Burrall BA, Baud L, et al: Generation and recognition of leukotriene mediators of hypersensitivity and inflammation. *Dig Dis Sci* 33:36s–40s, 1988.

86. Kreutner W, Sherwood J, Sehring S, et al: Antiallergy activity of Sch 37224, a new inhibitor of leukotriene formation. *J Pharmacol Exp Ther* 247:997–1003, 1988.

87. Higgins AJ: The biology, pathophysiology and control of eicosanoids in inflammation. *J Vet Pharmacol Ther* 8:1–18, 1985.

88. Eyre P: Preliminary studies of pharmacological antagonism of anaphylaxis in the horse. *Can J Comp Med* 40:149–152, 1976.

89. Eyre P, Lewis AJ: Acute systemic anaphylaxis in the horse. *Br J Pharmacol* 48:426–437, 1973.

90. Parker MD: Drug allergy. *N Engl J Med* 292:511–514, 1985.

91. Gronneberg R, Lagerholm B: Histopathological support of antagonism of allergen-induced mast cell mediator release in human skin by a beta(2)-agonist. *Allergy* 41:71–74, 1986.

92. Byars TD: Allergic skin disease in the horse. *Vet Clin North Am Large Anim Pract* 6:87–90, 1984.

93. Ash ASF, Schild HO: Receptors mediating some actions of histamine. *Br J Pharmacol Chemother* 27:427–439, 1966.

94. Douglas WW: Histamine and 5-hydroxytryptamine (serotonin) and their antagonists. In Gilman AG, Goodman LS, Rall TW, et al, eds: *The Pharmacological Basis of Therapeutics*. New York, Macmillan, 1985, pp 605–638.

95. Black JW, Duncan WA, Durant CJ, et al: Definition and antagonism of histamine H2-receptors. *Nature* 236:385–390, 1972.

96. Melmon KL, Rocklin RE, Rosenkranz RP: Autacoids as modulators of the inflammatory and immune response. *Am J Med* 71:100–106, 1981.

97. Arrang JM, Garbarg M, Schwartz JC: Auto-inhibition of brain histamine release mediated by a novel class (H3) of histamine receptor. *Nature* 302:832–837, 1983.

98. Arrang JM, Garbarg M, Lancelot JC, et al: Highly potent and

selective ligands for histamine H3-receptors. *Nature* 327:117–123, 1987.

99. Ishikawa S, Sperelakis N: A novel class (H3) of histamine receptors on perivascular nerve terminals. *Nature* 327:158–160, 1987.

100. Trzeciakowski JP: Inhibition of guinea pig ileum contractions mediated by a class of histamine receptor resembling the H3 subtype. *J Pharmacol Exp Ther* 243:874–880, 1987.

101. Ichinose M, Barnes PJ: Inhibitory histamine H3-receptors on cholinergic nerves in human airways. *Eur J Pharmacol* 163:383–386, 1989.

102. Ichinose M, Barnes PJ: Histamine H3-receptor mediated inhibition of non-adrenergic, non-cholinergic bronchoconstriction in guinea-pig in vivo (abstract). *Am Rev Respir Dis* 139:A236, 1989.

103. Van der Werf JF, Bast A, Bijloo GJ, et al: HA autoreceptor assay with superfused slices of rat brain cortex and electrical stimulation. *Eur J Pharmacol* 138:199–206, 1987.

104. Schlicker E, Betz R, Gothert M: Histamine H3 receptor–mediated inhibition of serotonin release in the rat brain cortex. *Arch Pharmacol* 337:588–590, 1988.

105. Tamura K, Palmer J, Wood J: Presynaptic inhibition produced by histamine at nicotinic synapses in enteric ganglia. *Neuroscience* 25:171–179, 1988.

106. Burka JF, Deline TF, Holroyde MC, et al: Chemical mediator of anaphylaxis (histamine, 5-HT, and SRS-A) released from horse lung and leukocytes in vitro. *Res Commun Chem Pathol Pharmacol* 13:379–388, 1976.

107. Ichikawa A, Kaneko H, Mori Y, et al: Release of serotonin from mast cells induced by N-(2-ethylhexyl)-3-hydroxybutyramide and catecholamine. *Biochem Pharmacol* 26:197–202, 1977.

108. Galli SJ, Gordon JR, Wershil BK: Cytokine production by mast cells and basophils. *Curr Opin Immunol* 3:865–873, 1991.

109. Plaut M, Pierce JH, Watson CJ, et al: Mast cell lines produce lymphokines in response to cross-linkage of FcΣRI or to calcium ionophores. *Nature* 339:64–67, 1989.

110. Arm JP, Lee TH: The pathobiology of bronchial asthma. *Adv Immunol* 51:323–382, 1992.

111. Galli SJ: New concepts about the mast cell. *N Engl J Med* 328:257–265, 1993.

112. Tizard I: Lymphokines and cytokines. In Tizard I, ed: *Veterinary Immunology: An Introduction.* Philadelphia, WB Saunders, 1992, pp 97–108.

113. Beutler B, Cerami A: The biology of cachectin/TNF—a primary mediator of the host response. *Annu Rev Immunol* 7:625–655, 1989.

114. Rosenberg RD, Lam L: Correlation between structure and function of heparin. *Proc Natl Acad Sci* U S A 76:1218–1222, 1979.

115. Kazatchkine MD, Fearon DT, Silbert JE, et al: Surface-associated heparin inhibits zymosan-induced activation of the human alternative complement pathway by augmenting the regulatory action of the control proteins on particlebound C3b. *J Exp Med* 150:1202–1215, 1979.

116. Hojima Y, Cochrane CG, Wiggins RC, et al: In vitro activation of the contact (Hageman Factor) system of plasma by heparin and chondroitin sulfate. *Blood* 63:1453–1459, 1984.

117. Schwartz LB, Bradford TM: Regulation of tryptase from human lung mast cells by heparin: Stabilization of the active tetramer. *J Biol Chem* 261:7372–7379, 1986.

118. Loos M, Volankis JE, Stroud RM: Mode of interaction of different polyanions with the first (C1), second (C2), and the fourth (C4) component of complement. III. Inhibition of C4 and C2 binding site(s) of C1s by polyanions. *Immunochemistry* 13:789–791, 1976.

119. Gorman NT, Halliwell REW: Mechanisms of immunological injury in hypersensitivity reactions. In Halliwell REW, Gorman NT, eds: *Veterinary Clinical Immunology.* Philadelphia, WB Saunders, 1989, pp 212–252.

120. Wintroub BU, Schechter NB, Lazarus GS: Angiotensin I conversion by human and rat chymotrypic proteinases. *J Invest Dermatol* 83:336–339, 1984.

121. Reilly CF, Tewksbury DA, Schechter NM, et al: Rapid conversion of angiotensin I to angiotensin II by neutrophil and mast cell proteinases. *J Biol Chem* 257:8619–8622, 1982.

122. Wintroub BU, Kaempfer CE, Schechter NM, et al: A human lung mast cell chymotrypsin-like proteinase: Identification and partial characterization. *J Clin Invest* 77:196–201, 1986.

123. Briggaman RA, Schechter NM, Fraki J, et al: Degradation of the epidermal-dermal junction by a proteolytic enzyme from human skin and human polymorphonuclear leukocytes. *J Exp Med* 160:1027–1042, 1984.

124. Creese BR, Temple DM: The mediators of allergic contraction of human airway smooth muscle: A comparison of bronchial and lung parenchymal strip preparations. *Clin Exp Pharmacol Physiol* 13:103–111, 1986.

125. Higgins A, Lees P: Detection of leukotriene B4 in equine inflammatory exudate. *Vet Rec* 115:275, 1984.

126. Newball HH, Meier HL, Kaplan AP, et al: Activation of Hageman factor by protease released during antigen challenge of human lung. *Trans Assoc Am Physicians* 94:126–133, 1981.

127. Meier HL, Kaplan AP, Lichtenstein LM, et al: Anaphylactic release of a prekallikrein activator from human lung in vitro. *J Clin Invest* 72:574–581, 1983.

128. Proud E, MacGlashan DW, Newball HH, et al: Immunoglobulin E mediated release of a kininogen from purified human lung mast cells. *Am Rev Respir Dis* 132:405–408, 1985.

129. Meier HL, Flowers B, Silverberg M, et al: The IgE dependent release of a Hageman factor cleaving factor from human lung. *Am J Pathol* 123:146–154, 1986.

130. Proud D, Togias A, Naclerio RM, et al: Kinins are generated in vivo following nasal airway challenge of allergic individuals with antigen. *J Clin Invest* 72:1678–1685, 1983.

131. Christiansen S, Bohn CB, Proud D, et al: Kininogenase activity in bronchoalveolar lavage (BAL) fluids in asthma (abstract). *J Allergy Clin Immunol* 75:177, 1985.

132. Inagaki N, Miura T, Daikoka M, et al: Inhibitory effects of beta-adrenergic stimulants on increased vascular permeability caused by passive cutaneous anaphylaxis, allergic mediators, and mediator releasers in rats. *Pharmacology* 39:19–27, 1989.

133. Ohuchi K, Hirasawa N, Takeda H, et al: Mechanism of antianaphylactic action of beta-agonists in allergic inflammation of air pouch type in rats. *Int Arch Allergy Appl Immunol* 82:26–32, 1987.

134. Widman FK: The complement system. In Widman FK ed: *An Introduction to Clinical Immunology.* Philadelphia, FA Davis, 1989, pp 123–145.

135. Frank M: The complement system. In Samter M, Talmage DW, Frank MM, et al, eds: *Immunological Diseases.* Boston: Little, Brown, 1988, pp 203–232.

136. Foreman JC: Neuropeptides and the pathogenesis of allergy. *Allergy* 42:1–11, 1987.

137. Saria A: Neuroimmune interactions in the airways: Implications for asthma, allergy, and other inflammatory airway diseases. *Brain Behav Immun* 2:318–321, 1988.

138. Keen P, Livingston A: Adverse reactions to drugs. *In Practice* 5:174–180, 1983.

139. Morris DD: Cutaneous vasculitis in horses: 19 cases (1978–1985). *J Am Vet Med Assoc* 191:460–464, 1987.

140. Kirkpatrick CH: Delayed hypersensitivity. In Samter M, Talmage DW, Frank MM, et al, eds: *Immunological Diseases.* Boston, Little, Brown, 1988, pp 261–278.

141. Belsito DV: The pathophysiology of allergic contact hypersensitivity. *Clin Rev Allergy* 7:347–379, 1989.

142. Askenase PW: Effector and regulatory mechanisms in delayed-type hypersensitivity. In Middleton E, Reed CE, Ellis EF, et al, eds: *Allergy Principles and Practice*. St Louis, Mosby–Year Book, 1988, pp 247–279.

143. Wintroub BU, Wasserman SI: Allergic reactions to drugs. In Samter M, Talmage DW, Frank MM, et al, eds. *Immunological Diseases*. Boston, Little, Brown, 1988, pp 699–714.

144. Adkinson NF Jr, Wheeler B: Risk factors for IgE-dependent reactions to penicillin. In Steffen C, Ludwig H, eds. *Clinical Immunology and Allergology: Proceedings of the Symposia at the XIth Congress of the European Academy of Allergology and Clinical Immunology*. New York, Elsevier-Holland Biomedical Press, 1981, pp 55–61.

145. Bochner BS, Lichtenstein LM: Anaphylaxis. *N Engl J Med* 324:1785–1790, 1991.

146. Haskins S: Monitoring the anesthetized patient. In Short CE, ed: *Principles and Practice of Veterinary Anesthesia*. Baltimore, Williams & Wilkins, 1987, pp 455–477.

147. Karns PA, Luther DG: A survey of adverse effects associated with ivermectin use in Louisiana horses. *J Am Vet Med Assoc* 185:782–783, 1984.

148. Allpress RG, Heathcote R: Adverse reactions in horses to intramuscular penicillin. *Vet Rec* 126:411–412, 1986.

149. Ackerman LJ: Allergic skin disorders. In Ackerman LJ, ed: *Practical Equine Dermatology*. Goleta, Calif, American Veterinary Publications, 1989, pp 85–110.

150. Greatorex JC: Urticaria, blue nose, and purpura haemorrhagica in horses. *Equine Vet J* 1:157–160, 1969.

151. Austen KF: The anaphylactic syndrome. In Samter M, Talmage DW, Frank MM, et al, eds. *Immunological Diseases*. Boston, Little, Brown, 1989, pp 1119–1134.

152. Findlay SR, Dvorak AM, Kagey-Sobotka A, et al: Hyperosmolar triggering of histamine release from human basophils. *J Clin Invest* 67:1604–1613, 1981.

153. Eggleston PA, Kagey-Sobotka A, Schleimer RP, et al: Interaction between hyperosmolar and IgE-mediated histamine release from basophils and mast cells. *Am Rev Respir Dis* 130:86–91, 1984.

154. Rockoff SD, Brasch R, Kuhn C, et al: Contrast media as histamine liberators. *Invest Radiol* 5:503–509, 1970.

155. Schwartz RS, Datta SK: Autoimmunity and autoimmune disease. In Paul WE, ed: *Fundamental Immunology*. New York, Raven Press, 1989, pp 819–866.

156. Eyre P, Burka JF: Hypersensitivity in cattle and sheep: A pharmacological review. *J Vet Pharmacol Ther* 1:97–109, 1978.

157. Scott DW: Autoimmune skin disease of large animals. *Vet Clin North Am Large Anim Pract* 6:79–86, 1984.

158. Berry CR, Merritt AM, Burrows CF, et al: Evaluation of the myoelectrical activity of the equine ileum infected with *Strongylus vulgaris* larvae. *Am J Vet Res* 47:27–30, 1986.

159. Turk MAM, Klei TR, Holmes RA, et al: Pathologic and immunologic responses of ponies to repeated infections of *Strongylus vulgaris* followed by sequential ivermectin treatments. *Proceedings of the Second Colic Seminar and Research Symposium*. Athens, GA, 1986, pp 18–20.

160. Fauci AS: The vasculitic syndromes. In Wyngaarden JB, Smith LH, eds: *Cecil Textbook of Medicine*, ed 17. Philadelphia, WB Saunders, 1985, pp 1937–1940.

161. Galan JE, Timoney JR: *Streptococcus equi* associated immune complexes in the sera of horses with purpura haemorrhagica (abstract). Presented at *Conference on Research Work in Animal Diseases*, November 12–13, 1984, 98.

162. Galan JE, Timoney JF: Immune complexes in purpura hemor-

rhagica of the horse contain IgA and M antigen of *Streptococcus equi*. J Immunol 135:3134–3137, 1985.

163. Stannard AA: Photoactivated vasculitis. In Robinson NE, ed: *Current Therapy in Equine Medicine*, vol 2. Philadelphia, WB Saunders, 1987, pp 646–647.

164. Norn S, Clementsen P: Bronchial asthma: Pathophysiology mechanisms and corticosteroids. *Allergy* 43:401–405, 1988.

165. Adams HR: Adrenergic and antiadrenergic drugs. In Booth NH, McDonald LE, eds: *Veterinary Pharmacology and Therapeutics*. Ames, Iowa State University Press, 1988, pp 91–136.

166. Muir W, Hubbell J: Cardiac emergency and shock. In *Handbook of Veterinary Anesthesia*. St. Louis, Mosby–Year Book, 1989, pp 285–308.

167. Plumb D: *Veterinary Drug Handbook*. White Bear Lake, Minn, PharmaVet Publishing, 1991.

168. Baxter JD, Forsham PH: Tissue effects of glucocorticoids. *Am J Med* 53:573–589, 1972.

169. Hanson JM, Morley J: Pharmacological aspects of glucocorticosteroids. In Hogg JC, Ellul-Micallef R, Brattsand R, eds: *Glucocorticosteroids, Inflammation and Bronchial Hyperreactivity*. Amsterdam, Excerpta Medica, 1985, pp 11–20.

170. Blackwell GJ, Carnuccio R, Rosa M, et al: Macrocortin: A polypeptide causing the anti-phospholipase effect of glucocorticoids. *Nature* 287:147–149, 1980.

171. Di Rosa M, Persico P: Mechanism of inhibition of prostaglandin biosynthesis by hydrocortisone in rat leukocytes. *Br J Pharmacol* 66:161–163, 1979.

172. Hirata F, Schiffmann E, Venkatasubramanian K, et al: A phospholipase A_2 inhibitory protein in rabbit neutrophils induced by glucocorticoids. *Proc Natl Acad Sci U S A* 77:2533–2536, 1980.

173. Bray MA, Gordon D: Prostaglandin production by macrophages and the effect of anti-inflammatory drugs. *Br J Pharmacol* 63:635–642, 1978.

174. Parente L, Rosa M, Flower RJ, et al: Relationship between the anti-phospholipase and anti-inflammatory effects of glucocorticoid-induced proteins. *Eur J Pharmacol* 99:233–239, 1984.

175. Inagaki N, Miura T, Nagai H, et al: Inhibition of vascular permeability increase in mice. *Int Arch Allergy Appl Immunol* 87:254–259, 1988.

175a. Schimmer BP, Parker KL: Adrenocorticotropic hormone; adrenocortical steroids and their synthetic analogs; inhibitors of the synthesis and actions of adrenocortical hormones. In Hardman JG, Limbird LE, eds. *The Pharmacological Basis of Therapeutics*, ed 9. New York, McGraw-Hill, 1996, pp 1459–1485.

176. Pelikan Z: The effects of disodium cromoglycate and beclomethasone dipropionate on the late nasal mucosa response to allergen challenge. *Ann Allergy* 132:986–992, 1982.

177. Lucas AM, Shuster S: Cromolyn inhibition of protein kinase C activity. *Biochem Pharmacol* 36:562–565, 1987.

178. Mazurek K, Schindler H, Schurholz T, et al: The cromolyn binding protein constitutes the Ca^{2+} channel of basophils opening upon immunological stimulus. *Proc Natl Acad Sci USA* 81:6841–6845, 1984.

179. Roy AC, Warren BT: Inhibition of cAMP phosphodiesterase by disodium cromoglycate. *Biochem Pharmacol* 23:917–920, 1974.

180. Theoharides TC, Sieghart W, Greengard P, et al: Anti-allergic drug cromolyn may inhibit histamine secretion by regulating phosphorylation of a mast cell protein. *Science* 207:80–82, 1980.

181. Murphy JR, McPherson EA, Lawson GHK: The effects of sodium cromoglycate on antigen inhalation challenge in two horses affected with chronic obstructive pulmonary disease (COPD). *Vet Immunol Immunopathol* 1:89–95, 1979.

182. Thomson JR, McPherson EA: Prophylactic effects of sodium cromoglycate on chronic obstructive pulmonary disease in the horse. *Equine Vet J* 13:243–246, 1981.

183. Soma CR, Beech J, Gerber NH Jr: Effects of cromolyn in horses with chronic obstructive pulmonary disease. *Vet Res Commun* 11:339–351, 1987.

184. Adams R: Cholinergic pharmacology: Autonomic drugs. In Booth NH, McDonald LE, eds. *Veterinary Pharmacology and Therapeutics.* Ames, Iowa State University Press, 1988, pp 117–136.

185. Kaliner M, Austen KF: A sequence of biochemical events in the antigen induced release of chemical mediators from sensitized human lung tissue. *J Exp Med* 138:1077–1094, 1973.

186. Kaliner M: IV immunologic mechanisms for release of chemical mediators of anaphylaxis from human lung tissue. *Can Med Assoc J* 110:431–435, 1974.

187. Advenier C, Mallard B, Santais MC, et al: The effects of atropine on anaphylactic shock in the guinea pig. *Agents Actions* 12:103–107, 1982.

188. Ishizaka T, Ishizaka K, Orange RP, et al: Pharmacologic inhibition of the antigen-induced release of histamine and slow-reacting substance of anaphylaxis (SRS-A) from monkey lung tissues mediated by human IgE. *J Immunol* 106:1267–1273, 1971.

189. Bakhle YS, Smith TW: Release of spasmogenic substances induced by vasoactive amines from isolated lungs. *Br J Pharmacol* 46:543–546, 1972.

190. Orange RP, Valentine MD, Austen KF: Inhibition of the release of slow-reacting substance of anaphylaxis in the rat with diethylcarbamazine. *Proc Soc Expl Biol Med* 127:127–132, 1968.

191. Samter M, Stevenson DD: Reactions to aspirin and aspirin-like drugs. In Samter M, Talmage DW, Frank MM, et al, eds. *Immunological Diseases.* Boston, Little, Brown, 1988, pp 1135–1148.

192. Marone G, Sobotka AK, Lichtenstein LM: Effects of arachidonic acid and its metabolites on antigen-induced histamine release from human basophils in vitro. *J Immunol* 123:1669–1677, 1979.

193. Hand JM, Schwalm SF, Lewis AJ: Antagonism of antigen-induced contraction of isolated guinea-pig trachea by 5-lipoxygenase inhibitors. *Int Arch Allergy Appl Immunol* 79:8–13, 1986.

194. Greaves MW: Pharmacology and significance of nonsteroidal anti-inflammatory drugs in the treatment of skin diseases. *J Am Acad Dermatol* 16:751–764, 1987.

194a. Walker JL: Interrelationship of SRS-A production and arachidonic acid metabolism in human lung tissue. In Samuelsson B, ed. *Advances in Prostaglandin and Thromboxane Research.* New York, Raven Press, 1980, pp 115–120.

194b. Dawson W, Boot JR, Harvey J, et al: The pharmacology of benoxaprofen with particular reference to effects on lipoxygenase product formation. *Eur J Rheumatol Inflamm* 5:61–68, 1982.

194c. Jackman BR, Moore JN, Barton MH, et al: Comparison of the effects of ketoprofen and flunixin meglumine on the in vitro response of equine peripheral blood monocytes to bacterial endotoxin. *Can J Vet Res* 58:138–143, 1994.

195. Abraham WM, Steveson JS, Garrido R: A leukotriene and thromboxane inhibitor (Sch 37224) blocks antigen-induced immediate and late responses and airway hyperresponsiveness in allergic sheep. *J Pharmacol Exp Ther* 247:1004–1011, 1988.

195a. Insel P: Analgesic-antipyretic and antiinflammatory agents and drugs employed in the treatment of gout. In Hardman JG, Limbird LE, eds. *The Pharmacological Basis of Therapeutics,* ed 9. New York, McGraw-Hill, 1996, pp 617–657.

195b. Cohn J: Zileuton (A-64077) A 5-lipoxygenase inhibitor. In Lewis AJ, Furst DE, eds. *Nonsteroidal Anti-Inflammatory Drugs—Mechanisms and Clinical Uses,* ed 2. New York, Marcel Decker, 1994, pp 367–390.

196. Pretolani M, Lefort J, Vargaftig BB: Limited interference of specific Paf antagonists with hyper-responsiveness to Paf itself of lungs from actively sensitized guinea-pigs. *Br J Pharmacol* 97:433–442, 1989.

197. Marone G, Kagey-Sobotka A, Lichtenstein LM: Possible role of phospholipase A$_2$ in triggering histamine secretion from human basophils *in vitro. Clin Immunol Immunopathol* 20:231–239, 1981.

198. Chand N, Pillar J, Diamantis W, et al: Inhibition of histamine secretion from rat peritoneal mast cells and rabbit leukocytes by p-bromophenacyl bromide a phospholipase A$_2$ inhibitor. *Res Commun Chem Pathol Pharmacol* 55:17–24, 1987.

199. Vadas P, Stefanski E, Pruzanski W: Potential therapeutic efficacy of inhibitors of human phospholipase A$_2$ in septic shock. *Agents Actions* 19:194–202, 1986.

200. Zalewski A, Goldberg S, Maroko PR: The effects of phospholipase A$_2$ inhibition on experimental infarct size, left ventricular hemodynamics, and regional myocardial blood flow. *Int J Cardiol* 21:247–257, 1988.

201. Douglas CE, Chan AC, Choy PC: Vitamin E inhibits platelet phospholipase A$_2$. *Biochim Biophys Acta* 876:639–645, 1986.

202. Nishikiori T, Naganawa H, Muraoka Y, et al: Plipastatins: New inhibitors of phospholipase a$_2$, produced by *Bacillus cereus* BMG302-fF67.III Structural elucidation of plipastatins. *J Antibiot (Tokyo)* 39:755–761, 1986.

203. Cartwright PH, Ilderton E, Sowden JM, et al: Inhibition of normal and psoriatic epidermal phospholipase A$_2$ by picomolar concentrations of recombinant human lipocortin I. *Br J Dermatol* 121:155–160, 1989.

204. Fletcher JE, Kistler P, Rosenberg H, et al: Dantrolene and mepacrine antagonize the hemolysis of human red blood cells by halothane and bee venom phospholipase A$_2$. *Toxicol Appl Pharmacol* 90:410–419, 1987.

205. Chang J, Blazek E, Carlson RP: Inhibition of phospholipase A$_2$ (PLA$_2$) activity by nifedipine and nisoldipine is independent of their calcium-channel-blocking activity. *Inflammation* 11:353–364, 1987.

206. Marone G, Columbo M, Poto S, et al: Possible role of calmodulin in the control of histamine release from human basophil leukocytes. *Life Sci* 39:911–922, 1986.

207. Watanabe T, Hashimoto Y, Teramoto T, et al: Calmodulin-independent inhibition of platelet phospholipase A$_2$ by calmodulin antagonists. *Arch Biochem Biophys* 246:699–709, 1986.

208. Meltzer MS, Nacy CA: Delayed-type hypersensitivity and the induction of activated, cytotoxic macrophages. In Paul WE, ed: *Fundamental Immunology.* New York, Raven Press, 1989, pp 765–780.

209. Samter M, Gleich GJ: The eosinophil. In Samter M, Talmage DW, Frank MM, et al, eds: *Immunological Diseases.* Boston, Little, Brown, 1988, pp 279–300.

210. Vrins A, Feldman BF: Lupus erythematosus-like syndrome in a horse. *Equine Pract* 5:18–25, 1983.

211. Biggers JD, Ingram PL: Studies on equine purpura haemorrhagica. Review of the literature. *Vet J* 104:214, 1948.

212. O'Dea JC: Comments on vaccination against strangles. *J Am Vet Med Assoc* 155:427, 1969.

213. Schalm OW, Carlson GP: The blood and blood-forming organs. In Mansmann RA, McAllister ES, Pratt PW, eds: *Equine Medicine and Surgery.* Santa Barbara, Calif, American Veterinary Publications, 1982, pp 377–413.

214. Manning TO, Scott DW, Rebhun WC, et al: Pemphigus-pemphigoid in a horse. *Equine Pract* 3:38–44, 1981.

215. Hines MT: Immunologically mediated ocular disease in the Horse. *Vet Clin North Am* 6:501–512, 1984.
216. Halliwell REW, Gorman NT: Miscellaneous immune-mediated diseases. In Halliwell REW, Gorman NT, eds: *Veterinary Clinical Immunology.* Philadelphia, WB Saunders, 1989, pp 378–421.
217. Mansmann RA, Osburn BI, Wheat JD, et al: Chicken hypersensitivity pneumonitis in horses. *J Am Vet Med Assoc* 166:673–677, 1975.
218. Kadlubowski M, Ingram PL: Circulating antibodies to the neuritogenic myelin protein, P2, in neuritis of the cauda equina of the horse. *Nature* 293:299–301, 1981.
219. Scott DW, Walton DK, Murray GB: Erythema multiforme in a horse. *Equine Pract* 6:26–30, 1984.

1.4.

Disorders of the Immune System

Debra Deem Morris, DVM, MS

IMMUNODEFICIENCY

Defects can occur in almost every aspect of the immune system. Immunodeficiency causes an increased susceptibility to infections, the consequences of which vary with the nature and degree of immune dysfunction. History and clinical signs that suggest the presence of immunodeficiency include (1) onset of infections during the first 6 weeks of life; (2) repeated infections that respond poorly to accepted therapy; (3) increased susceptibility to organisms with low pathogenicity; (4) infection with organisms that rarely occur in other animals; (5) illness following the administration of modified live virus vaccines; and (6) marked neutropenia or lymphopenia that persists for several days.[1]

Classification and Characterization

Immunodeficiencies can be classified by the system affected, or mechanistically as primary or secondary. Categorizing the disorder as involving the lymphoid system, phagocytic system, or complement system is useful because diagnostic testing is usually performed on this basis. A primary immunodeficiency is heritable. Secondary immunodeficiencies develop in animals that are capable of producing normal defense mechanisms, but have suffered another problem that precludes adequate immune function.

Clinical tests of B-cell function include serum immunoglobulin (Ig) quantitation and measurement of specific antibody responses. Serum immunoglobulin concentration can be crudely estimated by the total serum globulins derived by subtracting the albumin concentration from the total protein concentration. Because quantitation of albumin by the bromcresol green dye binding test may yield erroneous results, this method of globulin quantitation is not accurate.[2] Serum protein electrophoresis (based on the migration of serum proteins in an electric field) allows for more accurate quantitation of albumin and globulin concentrations. Serum protein electrophoresis is useful as an initial screen for assessing total immunoglobulin concentration. Hypogammaglobulinemia may occur with failure of passive transfer, primary immunodeficiency involving B cells, or diseases that cause protein loss via hemorrhage, exudation, enteropathy, or nephropathy.

The single radial immunodiffusion (SRID) test allows quantitation of species-specific, class-specific immunoglobulin based on the ability of antigen and antibody to precipitate at equivalence when combined in proportion in agar gel plates.[3] The serum being tested is added to punched-out wells in agar, impregnated with antibody to the specific immunoglobulin class being measured, and allowed to diffuse outward and bind with the anti-class-specific antisera. A precipitate forms when equivalence is reached and the area within the precipitate ring is directly proportional to the concentration of the patient's immunoglobulin class. The SRID test requires an 18- to 24-hour incubation period, which hampers its clinical utility.

A crude estimate of immunoglobulin concentration in the equine neonate can be obtained by the zinc sulfate turbidity test, glutaraldehyde coagulation test, latex agglutination, or by enzyme immunoassay.[4] Addition of serum to zinc sulfate solution causes precipitation of immunoglobulins, principally IgG. Although the degree of resultant turbidity is usually proportional to the IgG concentration, turbidity may be increased by hemolysis in the sample, poor operating conditions, and poor-quality reagents.[5, 6] In the glutaraldehyde coagulation test, glutaraldehyde forms insoluble complexes with basic proteins in the serum.[5] Gel formation in 10 minutes or less is equated with a serum IgG concentration of 800 mg/dL or greater, whereas a positive reaction in 60 minutes is indicative of at least 400 mg IgG/dL serum. Like the zinc sulfate turbidity test, hemolysis may falsely overestimate the IgG concentration. In the latex agglutination test (Foalcheck, Haver Mobay Corp., Shawnee, Kans.), the patient's serum is mixed with the anti-equine IgG absorbed to latex particles. Macroscopic agglutination is proportional to serum IgG. In the enzyme-linked immunosorbent assay (ELISA) test kit (Cite Test, AgriTech Systems, Inc., Portland, Me.), IgG present in the patient's serum is "captured" by anti-equine IgG antibody immobilized in a membrane filter. Enzyme-linked anti-equine IgG antibody is then added, followed by a chromogenic substrate. Subsequent color development is proportional to the concentration of IgG in the sample. The results of this assay technique are comparable to the SRID test.[7] B-cell function can also be measured by monitoring antibody production in response to immunization or disease. Serum antibody titers before and 4 weeks after immunization for influenza or rhinopneumonitis are readily available through most state diagnostic laboratories.

Because the majority of lymphocytes in the peripheral blood are T cells (80%), a reduction in the total peripheral lymphocyte count is indicative of T cell deficiency.[1] Lymph node biopsies may yield useful information in that B cells populate the cortical area, whereas T cells predominantly occupy the paracortical zone. Sparsity of lymphocytes in lymphoid organs is suggestive of immunodeficiency. Specific quantitation of T or B cells for precise classification of immunodeficiency is possible with immunofluorescence, enzyme labeling, or rosetting techniques.[1, 4, 8, 9] B cells are most commonly enumerated by direct immunofluorescence to detect the presence of surface immunoglobulin. B cells also bear surface receptors for complement and can be identified by erythrocyte-antigen-complement rosetting techniques. Equine T cells can be identified by their ability to spontaneously bind guinea pig red blood cells, forming rosettes.[10]

Lymphocyte function can be evaluated in vitro by the lymphocyte blastogenesis test.[9, 11] Mitogens added to isolated lymphocytes in culture cause proliferation that can be quantitated by tritiated thymidine uptake by the cells. Depending on the specific mitogen, either T-cell or B-cell blastogenesis can be assessed. Lipopolysaccharide is predominantly a B-cell stimulant, whereas phytohemagglutinin (PHA) and concanavalin A are T-cell mitogens. Reaction to intradermal PHA has been used as a specific indicator of T-cell function in vivo in horses.[12] A delayed-type hypersensitivity reaction to PHA develops in normal animals without prior sensitization. A 50-μg dose of PHA in 0.5 mL of phosphate-buffered saline is injected intradermally, while 0.5 mL of phosphate-buffered saline is administered intradermally at a distant site. At the PHA site, an increase in wheal size of 0.6 mm or less indicates a defect in cell-mediated immunity.

Other than determining absolute number, neutrophil functional defects are difficult to document clinically. A variety of assays for chemotaxis, phagocytosis, and killing function have been developed, but most are only available on a research basis. Tests of neutrophil chemotaxis determine the ability of isolated neutrophils to migrate through a semipermeable membrane toward a specific chemoattractant. Phagocytosis can be evaluated by observing ingestion of bacteria or particles, with or without opsonization. The respiratory burst that follows phagocytosis is commonly measured by chemiluminescence. Bactericidal activity is assessed by incubating a known number of bacteria with neutrophils and plotting killing over time. A crude estimate of the bactericidal ability of neutrophils can be made by their in vitro incubation with beads soaked with nitroblue tetrazolium dye. If beads are ingested and the dye is enzymatically reduced to generate a blue color, the bactericidal activity of the neutrophils is intact.

Defined Immunodeficiency Disorders

Failure of Passive Transfer

Failure of passive transfer is the most common immunodeficiency disorder of horses.[8, 9] It occurs in all breeds secondary to inadequate absorption of colostral antibodies. Failure of passive transfer is significantly correlated with increased susceptibility to infectious disease and death in neonatal foals.[13–16] The newborn foal is fully capable of mounting a normal immune response; however, it has had no prior antigenic exposure and thus has not yet accumulated immunoglobulins and other forms of adaptive immunity. During the first 1 to 2 months of life, foals are dependent upon passive immunity (immunity not dependent upon innate host defense mechanisms) for protection from infectious disease. Unlike in humans, immunoglobulin transfer to foals does not occur in utero because of the diffuse epitheliochorial nature of the equine placenta. Thus the foal is born essentially agammaglobulinemic and acquires passive immunity by the ingestion and absorption of colostrum from the dam.[17–19] Colostrum is a specialized form of milk containing immunoglobulins, that are produced during the last 2 weeks of gestation under hormonal influences.[18, 20] Colostrum contains primarily IgG and IgG(T), with small quantities of IgA and IgM, all of which have been concentrated into mammary secretions from the mare's blood.[20, 21] Colostrum is only produced one time each pregnancy and is replaced by milk that contains negligible immunoglobulins within 24 hours of the initiation of lactation.[18, 22] The absorptive capacity of the foal's gastrointestinal tract for immunoglobulins is greatest during the first 6 hours after birth, then steadily declines until immunoglobulins can no longer be absorbed when the foal is 24 hours old. This "closure" of the gut to absorption of large intact molecules is due to replacement of specialized enterocytes by more mature cells.[23] The incidence of failure of passive transfer is highly variable among groups of horses and seems to depend primarily on management factors that insure early colostral ingestion.[6] The reported prevalences of at least partial failure of passive transfer have ranged from 3% to 24%.[6, 9, 14]

Clinical Signs and Laboratory Findings. There are no clinical signs of failure of passive transfer, per se. Generalized or localized bacterial infections such as septicemia, pneumonia, enteritis, and arthritis that develop during the first 3 weeks of life are suggestive of failure of passive transfer. Exposure to highly pathogenic bacteria cannot be ruled out based solely on the time of onset and the specificity of colostral immunoglobulins may be inappropriate for infecting agents.

Routine laboratory findings may be suggestive of sepsis, but the presence of infection in the neonatal period is not pathognomonic for failure of passive transfer. Common abnormalities include neutropenia or neutrophilia, hypoglycemia, and hyperfibrinogenemia. The total plasma protein may be low, normal, or elevated in foals with failure of passive transfer due to the wide variation in normal presuckle total plasma protein and the confounding effects of dehydration secondary to sepsis.

Etiology and Pathogenesis. Causes for failure of passive transfer in foals include (1) failure of the foal to ingest an adequate volume of colostrum in the early postpartum period; (2) loss of colostrum via premature lactation; (3) inadequate immunoglobulin content of the colostrum; and (4) insufficient immunoglobulin absorption via the intestine.[8, 17, 18, 21, 24–26] There is a high negative correlation between foal serum IgG concentration and the incidence of severe infections[14]; however, the minimum amount of IgG necessary for protection of a foal from infection varies with the amount and virulence of environmental pathogens, concomitant stress factors, and colostral antibody titer against specific pathogens. Although a serum IgG concentration of at least 400 mg/dL has been considered evidence of adequate passive transfer, most normal foals attain values more than twice this high[6, 14] and serum IgG greater than 800 mg/dL may be required for adequate immunity.[16] Numerous other colostral factors may be important for the immune protection of foals. Colostrum regulates cell-mediated immunity,[27] activates granulocytes, promotes intestinal absorption of macromolecules,[28] decreases intestinal colonization by pathogens,[29] and contains constituents of innate immunity (e.g., complement) that have a local protective role in the neonatal digestive tract.[30]

Neonatal weakness or lack of maternal cooperation (common in maiden mares) are common reasons for the foal to ingest an inadequate volume of colostrum. If colostral ingestion is delayed beyond 6 hours, the absorption of immunoglobulins is significantly reduced. Lactation prior to parturition is another common reason for failure of passive transfer, since colostrum is only produced one time each gestation. The causative factors for premature lactation are unknown at this time, but foals from mares that "leak" milk hours to days prior to parturition are likely to suffer failure of passive transfer.

Subnormal colostral immunoglobulin content (<3,000 mg/dL) is rare in mares that do not prelactate,[6] but wide individual variation in colostral concentration of immunoglobulins does occur.[6, 22, 31] A genetic defect in the mare's ability to produce colostrum has been suggested[1, 32] and poorquality colostrum will undoubtedly cause failure of passive transfer. Colostral immunoglobulin content can be estimated by specific gravity (Lane Manufacturing, Denver, Colo.) or quantitated by SRID.[33]

Malabsorption is implicated as a cause of failure of passive transfer when foals are known to have ingested an adequate volume of good-quality colostrum within 12 hours of birth. Since glucocorticoids hasten the maturation of specialized enterocytes, stress-causing endogenous corticosteroid release has been suggested as a cause of reduced immunoglobulin absorption.[17, 24] Obvious stress factors are often not found in foals with apparent impaired ability to absorb IgG.[6]

Diagnosis. Subnormal serum IgG concentration 24 hours after birth is the basis for diagnosis of failure of passive transfer. Serum IgG of less than 200 mg/dL is indicative of complete failure of passive transfer, while 200 to 800 mg/dL should be considered partial failure of passive transfer. Many foals under good management conditions may remain healthy if the serum IgG is at least 400 mg/dL.[34] The most quantitatively accurate method to determine serum IgG is the SRID test (VMRD, Pullman, Wash.); however, this assay is time-consuming and expensive, thus inappropriate for the diagnosis of failure of passive transfer when timely therapeutic intervention is paramount.[3] Numerous field screening procedures for IgG have been evaluated.[5, 7, 35, 36] Criteria for selecting a screening test for equine failure of passive transfer must include overall accuracy, the time necessary to perform the test, ease of performance, and cost.[5] Although the zinc sulfate turbidity[35] and glutaraldehyde coagulation[5] tests are inexpensive and provide results within 1 hour, the ease and accuracy of latex agglutination[6] and enzyme immunoassay[7] procedures make them preferable in most practice situations. All screening tests are highly accurate in identifying foals with complete failure of passive transfer; however, there is variation in their ability to detect marginally deficient foals.

Treatment. If failure of passive transfer is anticipated because of premature lactation, neonatal weakness, dam death,

or low-specific-gravity colostrum, an alternative colostral source can be given orally. A minimum of 2 L of equine colostrum given in 500-mL increments during the first 8 hours after birth is optimal. Bovine colostrum may be safely substituted if equine colostrum is not available[37]; however, foals given bovine colostrum may also require plasma transfusion since bovine immunoglobulins have a very short halflife in foals and are not specifically directed against equine pathogens.

If the foal is more than 12 hours old when failure of passive transfer is suspected or diagnosed, an intravenous plasma transfusion is indicated. There are numerous commercial sources of equine plasma (Lake Immunogenetics, Ontario, N.Y.; Veterinary Dynamics Inc., Chino, Calif.; Ameri-Vet Labs, Addison, Ill.). Use of these products is convenient, saves time, and is safe since donors are free of alloantibodies and negative for infectious diseases. The only potential drawback to the use of commercial plasma is that antibodies specific for pathogens in the foal's environment may be lacking. Optimal plasma would be obtained from a local blood-typed donor, known to lack serum alloantibodies and alloantigens Aa and Qa (see Chapter 11). The volume of plasma necessary to bring serum IgG into an acceptable range cannot be accurately predicted because it is dependent on the severity of failure of passive transfer, the immunoglobulin content of the plasma, and on concomitant diseases, which may hasten immunoglobulin catabolism. Generally, 1 L of plasma will increase the serum IgG concentration of a 50-kg foal by 200 to 300 mg/dL,[38] thus 2 to 4 L may be necessary to achieve serum IgG greater than 800 mg/dL. A therapeutic dose of plasma should be administered, then foal serum IgG remeasured. If the desired concentration has not been attained, more plasma is necessary. Some foals with partial failure of passive transfer may do well without plasma therapy if there are no preexisting infections and exposure to pathogens is minimized. These foals should be monitored closely for the development of infections.

Client Education. The prognosis for foals with failure of passive transfer depends upon the degree of failure, the environment to which the foal is exposed, the foals's age at the time of diagnosis, and the presence and severity of secondary infections. Management factors that insure the ingestion of at least 2 L of high-quality colostrum within 6 hours of birth are paramount in failure of passive transfer prevention. Foalings should be witnessed so that any mispresentations can be corrected, and foals that do not readily nurse within 3 hours can be given colostrum via nasogastric tube. The evaluation of colostral specific gravity with a hydrometer (Lane Manufacturing, Denver, Colo.) may aid in prediction of failure of passive transfer.[33] A colostral specific gravity of 1.060 corresponds to approximately 3,000 mg/dL IgG, which is the minimum acceptable value. When dam colostral specific gravity is less than 1.060, some degree of failure of passive transfer should be suspected in the foal and corrected. Routine screening of foal serum IgG at 24 to 48 hours after birth allows necessary plasma therapy before the onset of infections.

Foals that are born prematurely, are weak, or from prelactating mares should be provided with an alternative colostral source within 6 hours of birth. A colostrum bank can be established by collecting and freezing (−20 °C) 250 mL of colostrum from mares that have not prelactated within 6 hours of foaling, once their own foals have suckled.[24] Ideally, banked colostrum should be screened for alloantibodies, although they are unlikely if the mare's own foal remains healthy. The immunoglobulins in banked frozen colostrum are stable for at least 1 year.

Combined Immunodeficiency

Combined immunodeficiency (CID) is a lethal primary immunodeficiency characterized by failure to produce functional B and T lymphocytes.[1, 39–41] The vast majority of affected foals are of the Arabian breed, in which the condition is inherited as an autosomal recessive trait.[42, 43] The incidence of combined immunodeficiency among foals of Arabian breeding is at least 2% to 3%,[42, 43] which suggests a carrier prevalence rate between 25% and 26%. There is currently no reliable method for detection of carriers except production of an affected foal. The disorder is rarely reported in other breeds.[44]

Clinical Signs and Laboratory Findings. Affected foals are clinically normal at birth, but develop signs of infection during the first 2 months of life. The age of onset of infection depends upon the adequacy of passive transfer and degree of environmental challenge. Bronchopneumonia is a prominent disease, often caused by adenovirus or *Pneumocystis carinii.*[39, 41] Enteritis, arthritis, and omphalophlebitis subsequent to a variety of mildly pathogenic agents are common. Signs include nasal discharge, coughing, dyspnea, diarrhea, fever, and weight loss. Although antibiotics, plasma, and supportive care prolong the course of disease, death invariably occurs before 5 months of age.[41]

A consistent hematologic finding is absolute lymphopenia ($<1,000/\mu L$). Depending upon the neutrophil response, the total white blood cell (WBC) count may be low, normal, or increased. Total serum globulins and serum IgG may be low, but the degree of passive transfer often makes these data impossible to interpret.

Etiology and Pathogenesis. Foals with combined immunodeficiency have a defect of lymphoid stem cells that may be attributable to altered purine metabolism.[45] Full immunologic reconstitution is possible by bone marrow transplants from a histocompatible donor, which suggests that the bone marrow and thymic microenvironments of foals with combined immunodeficiency are not altered.[46] Thymic hormones necessary for differentiation of stem cells are produced, but specific maturation pathways of cortical thymocytes are blocked.[47] There is a deficiency of interferon-γ.[48] Numbers, surface receptors, and the phagocytic capacity of neutrophils and macrophages are normal,[49] as is the complement system[40] supporting the theory that the hereditary defect affects only lymphocytes.[47, 50]

Although innate immunity is intact, the absence of adaptive immune function causes foals with combined immunodeficiency to be susceptible to even minor pathogens. Passively transferred immunoglobulins are rapidly catabolized during the first 4 weeks, with the half-life of maternally derived IgG between 20 and 23 days.[51] Endogenous immunoglobulin is detectable in normal foals by 2 weeks of age but does not reach adult concentrations until they are 4 to 6 months old.[32] Total immunoglobulin in the foal is lowest between 1 and 2 months and it is at this time that foals with combined immunodeficiency usually develop infections and first show signs. Owing to their inability to mount humoral or cell-mediated immunity, foals with combined immunodeficiency rapidly deteriorate after 2 months of age.

Research on serum uric acid concentrations (an end product of purine metabolism) suggested that there may be two autosomal recessive combined immunodeficiency diseases.[45] Some combined immunodeficiency carriers have extremely high serum concentrations of uric acid, whereas in others serum uric acid is normal. The genetic defect in offspring from the latter group of horses may affect another site or be unrelated to purine metabolism.

Diagnosis. Antemortem diagnosis of combined immunodeficiency is suggested by appropriate clinical signs in a foal of Arabian breeding with persistent marked lymphopenia (usually $<500/\mu L$) and the absence of serum IgM by SRID.[8, 9] The approximate half-life of equine IgM is 4 to 5 days and all derived from the colostrum should be depleted by 3 weeks after birth. If presuckle serum is unavailable for testing (which would be negative for IgM in foals with combined immunodeficiency), serum IgM cannot be used as a diagnostic aid until the foal is older than 3 weeks. Because the diagnosis of combined immunodeficiency implies that both the sire and dam are carriers of the trait, all suspected cases should be confirmed by necropsy. Criteria for definitive diagnosis are gross and histologic evidence of lymphoid hypoplasia in thymus, spleen, and lymph nodes.[1, 52]

Treatment. Supportive care may prolong the course of disease, but affected foals eventually die by 5 months. Immunologic reconstitution by transplantation of stem cells from bone marrow is possible[46]; however, histocompatibility must be exact lest fatal graft-versus-host disease develops.[53, 54] This option is not practical at the present time.

Client Education. Prevention of combined immunodeficiency requires identification of carriers and their removal from the breeding population. Heterozygosity for the lethal trait can only be confirmed by birth of an affected foal, which implicates both sire and dam. Approximately one in four foals that result from mating two carriers has combined immunodeficiency and two others are carriers. Mating of a carrier with a noncarrier produces no foals with combined immunodeficiency, but half the offspring would be carriers. All Arabian foals should be screened by an absolute lymphocyte count soon after birth. Foals with lymphopenia should be carefully monitored. The diagnosis of combined immunodeficiency should be pursued in any Arabian foal less than 5 months of age that has infectious disease.

Selective IgM Deficiency

Selective IgM deficiency is characterized by substantially reduced or absent serum IgM with normal or increased concentrations of other immunoglobulins and no other evidence of immunodeficiency.[9, 55] The syndrome has been most frequently described in Arabians and quarter horses, although the diagnosis has been made in other breeds.

Clinical Signs and Laboratory Findings. Three clinical syndromes have been described. Most affected horses develop severe pneumonia, arthritis, and enteritis with or without septicemia and die before 10 months of age. Gram-negative bacterial infections are common (especially with *Klebsiella* species) and age at onset of signs is generally older than in foals with combined immunodeficiency. The second category of affected foals generally have a history of repeated bacterial infections that respond temporarily to therapy but recur once antimicrobials are discontinued. These foals grow poorly and generally die within 2 years. The third presentation involves horses between 2 and 5 years of age, most of which have or ultimately develop lymphosarcoma. These individuals may have external or internal lymphadenopathy or both. Chronic weight loss, depression, and other nonspecific signs usually accompany lymphosarcoma.

Routine laboratory findings are not diagnostically specific. Hematologic abnormalities consistent with chronic inflammatory disease, such as anemia, neutrophilia, and hyperfibrinogenemia, are commonly present. The total plasma protein and serum globulins are usually normal. Serum biochemistry may reflect the involved organ systems.

Etiology and Pathogenesis. It is unknown whether serum IgM is decreased from insufficient production, excessive loss, or hypercatabolism. Although a genetic basis is suspected, the pathogenesis of selective IgM deficiency is unknown.[9, 55] Neoplastic lymphocytes in one horse with IgM deficiency were shown to have suppressor activity, which could downregulate B-cell function and IgM synthesis.[56] It seems likely that there are primary and secondary forms of this syndrome.

Diagnosis. Definitive diagnosis of selective IgM deficiency is made by quantitating the major serum immunoglobulins by SRID and determining the absolute lymphocyte count. Horses with selective IgM deficiency have serum IgM concentrations persistently less than 2 SD below that of age-matched controls (<15 mg/dL at 4–8 months; <25 mg/dL at >8 months) coupled with normal concentrations of IgG (≥400 mg/dL), and a normal lymphocyte count.[9, 50, 55] Since seriously ill foals may have transiently depressed serum IgM concentration, suspected cases should be tested at least twice to document that IgM concentrations remain low. All other immunoglobulin concentrations are normal.

Treatment. Other than supportive care and antimicrobial therapy, there is no effective treatment for selective IgM deficiency. Transfused plasma concentrations of IgM are low and the half-life is quite short, thus any benefit would be only temporary.

Client Education. The prognosis must be guarded; however, recovery has been reported.[9] Since primary immunodeficiency is likely in foals affected during the first year of life, it may be inadvisable to remate the sire and dam.

Transient Hypogammaglobulinemia

Transient hypogammaglobulinemia is a very rare immunodeficiency characterized by delayed onset of immunoglobulin synthesis.[34, 50] The only reported cases have involved Arabians[9, 14]; however, it is likely that this condition is more prevalent than reports suggest and may involve other breeds.[34] Affected foals manifest signs consistent with bacterial and viral infections when passively acquired immunoglobulins are catabolized to nonprotective concentrations. Hematologic studies may be suggestive of chronic infection, although total plasma protein is normal or reduced slightly.

For unknown reasons, the onset of autologous immunoglobulin production, which generally occurs at birth, is delayed until these foals are approximately 3 months of age. Because passively derived immunoglobulins are usually catabolized to nonprotective concentrations by 8 weeks post partum, foals with transient hypogammaglobulinemia are susceptible to infections until autologous immunoglobulin synthesis occurs.

Diagnosis is based on the presence of low serum IgG (<200 mg/dL) and IgG(T) (<20 mg/dL) at 2 to 4 months of age, with low-normal serum IgM (>15 mg/dL) and IgA (>20 mg/dL).[50, 57] Lymphocyte counts are normal. Antimicrobial therapy and plasma transfusions are necessary to minimize infections. Affected foals usually survive if they have not concomitantly suffered failure of passive transfer, and they receive appropriate support between 2 and 4 months of age.

Agammaglobulinemia

Agammaglobulinemia is a rare primary immunodeficiency of horses characterized by absence of B lymphocytes and failure to produce immunoglobulins, in the presence of normal cell-mediated immunity.[58] All documented cases have been colts of Thoroughbred, standardbred or quarter horse breeds.[58–61] Clinical signs commence between 2 and 6 months of age and include evidence of bacterial infections such as pneumonia, enteritis, and arthritis. Multisystemic infections that respond poorly to therapy are common and laboratory changes reflect chronic inflammatory disease. The total plasma protein is generally subnormal owing to the lack of immunoglobulins.

This syndrome has only been described in colts, which suggests an X-linked mode of inheritance, as occurs in a similar disease of humans.[62] A maturation defect from stem cells to B cells has been suggested. Affected foals have persistently subnormal serum concentrations of all immunoglobin classes and normal lymphocyte counts. Serum IgM and IgA are generally absent at the time of evaluation and maternally derived IgG and IgG(T) decline with time. At 2 months of age, IgG is less than 300 mg/dL, which declines to less than 100 mg/dL by 6 months. There is no serologic response to immunization, and B lymphocytes, as determined by immunofluorescence, are absent. Tests of cell-mediated immune function such as intradermal PHA and in vitro blastogenesis are normal. Plasma and antimicrobial therapy only result in transient improvement. Affected horses die from disseminated infection between 1 and 2 years of age.

Unclassified Immunodeficiencies

Unclassified immunodeficiencies, characterized by deficits in immune function that cannot be ascribed to the currently recognized categories, occur in horses. Numerous disease states or drugs can result in secondary immunodeficiency.

Nutritional deficiencies or excesses, certain microbial or parasitic infections, neoplasia, and corticosteroid or other hormonal therapy may be involved. Secondary unclassified immunodeficiency syndromes in horses include perinatal equine herpesvirus type 1 (EHV-1) infection, oral candidiasis and septicemia in foals, and adult acquired immunodeficiency.[34]

Foals that are infected late in gestation with EHV-1 are often born weak with interstitial pneumonia and develop a variety of bacterial diseases.[63] Affected foals have profound lymphopenia and generally die, despite therapy. The immunodeficiency is thought to be due to viral-induced lymphoid damage, since necropsy reveals marked necrosis of lymphoid tissue in the thymus, spleen, and lymph nodes. No treatment is effective and prevention is based on immunization of pregnant mares against EHV-1.

A group of foals with oral candidiasis and bacterial septicemia between 2 weeks and 4 months of age were found to have laboratory or histologic evidence of immunodeficiency that did not fulfill diagnostic criteria for any of the recognized primary immunodeficiencies.[64] Oral lesions ranged from focal white plaques on tongue margins to a generalized thick, white pseudomembrane covering the tongue and gingiva. Affected foals showed bruxism, ptyalism, fever, and depression in addition to pneumonia, arthritis, or diarrhea, singly or severally. The lymphocyte counts of the foals were usually normal. Several foals had IgM deficiency coupled with depressed blastogenesis, suggesting cellular immune dysfunction. Many of the foals had low or marginally reduced serum IgG in addition to IgM deficiency or reduced blastogenesis. It was not determined whether the immunologic defects were primary or secondary. All foals died despite extensive therapy with parenteral antimicrobials, topical antimycotics, and intravenous plasma.

Acquired immunodeficiency was identified in a 7-year-old appaloosa gelding that had no history of previous illness.[65] Clinical signs included lethargy, anorexia, and dyspnea. Pneumonia and septicemia due to *Rhodococcus equi* were confirmed by tracheal wash and blood culture, respectively. Immunologic evaluation revealed marked lymphopenia, subnormal serum IgG and IgA with marginally low IgG concentrations, failure to respond serologically to immunization, and reduced in vitro lymphocyte blastogenesis. Histologic examination of lymph nodes and spleen revealed lymphoid atrophy.

REFERENCES

1. Perryman LE: Primary and secondary immune deficiencies of domestic animals. *Adv Vet Sci Comp Med* 23:23, 1979.
2. Duncan JP, Prasse KW: Proteins, lipids, and carbohydrates. In Duncan JP, Prasse KW, eds: *Veterinary Laboratory Medicine,* ed 2. Ames, Iowa State University Press, 1986, p 105.
3. Rumbaugh GE, Ardans AA, Gino D, et al: Measurement of neonatal equine immunoglobulins for assessment of colostral immunoglobulin transfer: Comparison of single radial immunodiffusion with the zinc sulfate turbidity test, serum electrophoresis, refractometry for total serum protein and the sodium sulfite precipitation test. *J Am Vet Med Assoc* 172:321, 1978.
4. Henry MM: Techniques for evaluating the immune system. In Colahan P, Mayhew IG, Merritt AM, et al eds: *Equine Medicine and Surgery,* ed 4. Goleta, Calif., American Veterinary Publications, 1991, pp 1965–1971.
5. Clabough DL, Conboy HS, Roberts MC: Comparison of four screening techniques for the diagnosis of equine neonatal hypogammaglobulinemia. *J Am Vet Med Assoc* 194:1717, 1989.
6. Morris DD, Meirs DA, Merryman GS: Passive transfer failure in the horse: Incidence and causative factors on a breeding farm. *Am J Vet Res* 46:2294, 1985.
7. Bertone JJ, Jones RL, Curtis CR: Evaluation of a kit for determination of serum immunoglobulin G concentration in foals. *J Vet Intern Med* 2:181, 1988.
8. Morris DD: Immunologic disease of foals. *Compendium Continuing Educ Pract Vet* 8:S139, 1986.
9. Perryman LE, McGuire TC: Evaluation for immune system failures in horses and ponies. *J Am Vet Med Assoc* 176:1374, 1980.
10. Tarr MJ, Olsen RG, Karakowka S, et al: Erythrocyte rosette formation of equine peripheral blood lymphocytes. *Am J Vet Res* 38:1775, 1977.
11. Halliwell RW, Gorman NT: Disease associated with immunodeficiency. In Halliwell RW, Gorman NT, eds: *Veterinary Clinical Immunology.* Philadelphia, WB Saunders, 1989, p 449.
12. Hodgin EC, McGuire TC, Perryman LE, et al: Evaluation of delayed hypersensitivity responses in normal horses and immunodeficient foals. *Am J Vet Res* 39:1161, 1978.
13. McGuire TC, Poppie MJ, Banks KL: Hypogammaglobulinemia predisposing to infection in foals. *J Am Vet Med Assoc* 166:71, 1975.
14. McGuire TC, Crawford TB, Hallowell AL, et al: Failure of colostral immunoglobulin transfer as an explanation for most infections and deaths in neonatal foals. *Am J Vet Res* 170:1302, 1977.
15. Crawford TB, Perryman LE: Diagnosis and treatment of failure of passive transfer in the foal. *Equine Pract* 2:17, 1980.
16. Koterba AM, Brewer BD, Tarplee FA: Clinical and clinicopathological characteristics of the septicemic neonatal foal: Review of 38 cases. *Equine Vet J* 16:376, 1984.
17. Jeffcott LB: Passive immunity and its transfer with special reference to the horse. *Biol Rev* 47:439, 1972.
18. Jeffcott LB: Studies on passive immunity in the foal. I. Gammaglobulin and antibody variations associated with the maternal transfer of immunity and the onset of active immunity. *J Comp Pathol* 84:93, 1974.
19. Naylor JM: Colostral immunity in the calf and the foal. *Vet Clin North Am Large Anim Pract* 1:331, 1979.
20. Rouse BT, Ingram DG: The total protein and immunoglobulin profile of equine colostrum and milk. *Immunology* 19:901–907, 1970.
21. McGuire TC, Crawford TB: Passive immunity in the foal: Measurement of immunoglobulin classes and specific antibody. *Am J Vet Res* 34:1299, 1973.
22. Pearson RC, Hallowell AL, Bayly WM, et al: Times of appearance and disappearance of colostral IgG in the mare. *Am J Vet Res* 45:186, 1984.
23. Jeffcott LB: Duration of permeability of the intestine to macromolecules in the newly born foal. *Vet Rec* 88:340, 1971.
24. Jeffcott LB: Some practical aspects of the transfer of passive immunity to newborn foals. *Equine Vet J* 6:109, 1974.
25. Rumbaugh GE, Ardans AA, Gino D, et al: Identification and treatment of colostrum-deficient foals. *J Am Vet Med Assoc* 174:273, 1979.
26. DeShazo RD, Lopez M, Salevaggio JE: Use and interpretation of diagnostic immunologic laboratory tests. *J Am Med Assoc* 27:3011, 1987.
27. Radosevich JK, Scott GH, Olson GB: Delayed-type hypersensitivity responses induced by bovine colostral components. *Am J Vet Res* 46:875, 1985.
28. Jensen PT, Pedersen KB: The influence of sow colostrum trypsin inhibitor on immunoglobulin absorption in newborn piglets. *Acta Vet Scand* 23:161, 1982.
29. Francis GL, Read LC, Ballard FJ, et al: Purification and partial

sequence analysis of insulin-like growth factor-1 from bovine colostrum. *Biochem J* 233:207, 1986.

30. Reiter B: Review of nonspecific antimicrobial factors in colostrum. *Ann Rech Vet* 9:205, 1978.

31. Townsend HGG, Tabel H, Bristol FM: Induction of parturition in mares: Effect on passive transfer of immunity to foals. *J Am Vet Med Assoc* 182:255, 1983.

32. Perryman LE: Immunological management of young foals. *Conpendium Continuing Educ Pract Vet* 3:S223, 1981.

33. LeBlanc MM, McLaurin BI, Boswell R: Relationships among serum immunoglobulin concentration in foals, colostral specific gravity, and colostral immunoglobulin concentration. *J Am Vet Med Assoc* 189:57, 1986.

34. McClure JJ: Immunologic disorders. In Smith BP, ed: *Large Animal Internal Medicine*. St Louis, Mosby–Year Book, 1990, p 1598.

35. Le Blanc MM, Hurtgen JP, Lyle S: A modified zinc sulfate turbidity test for the detection of immune status in newly born foals. *Equine Vet Sci* 10:36, 1990.

36. Bauer JE, Brooks TB: Immunoturbidometric quantitation of serum immunoglobulin G concentration in foals. *Am J Vet Res* 51:1211, 1990.

37. Lavoie JP, Spenseley MS, Smith BP, et al: Absorption of bovine colostral immunoglobulins G and M in newborn foals. *Am J Vet Res* 50:1598, 1989.

38. Koterba AM, Brewer B, Drummond WH: Prevention and control of infection. *Vet Clin North Am Equine Pract* 1:41, 1985.

39. McGuire TC, Poppie MJ, Banks KL: Combined (B-and T-lymphocyte) immunodeficiency: A fatal genetic disease in Arabian foals. *J Am Vet Med Assoc* 164:70, 1974.

40. McGuire TC, Banks KL, Poppie MJ: Combined immunodeficiency in horses. Characterization of the lymphocyte defect. *Clin Immunol Immunopathol* 3:555, 1975.

41. Perryman LE, McGuire TC, Crawford TB: Maintenance of foals with combined immunodeficiency: Causes and control of secondary infections. *Am J Vet Res* 39:1043, 1978.

42. Perryman LE, Torbeck RL: Combined immunodeficiency of Arabian horses: Confirmation of autosomal recessive mode of inheritance. *J Am Vet Med Assoc* 176:1250, 1980.

43. Poppie MJ, McGuire TC: Combined immunodeficiency in foals of Arabian breeding: Evaluation of mode of inheritance and estimation of prevalence of affected foals and carrier mares and stallions. *J Am Vet Med Assoc* 170:31, 1977.

44. Perryman LE, Boreson CR, Conaway MW, et al: Combined immunodeficiency in an Appaloosa foal. *Vet Pathol* 21:547, 1984.

45. Kettler MK, Weil MR, Perryman LE: Serum uric acid concentrations in horses heterozygous for combined immunodeficiency. *Am J Vet Res* 50:2155, 1989.

46. Perryman LE, Bue CM, Magnuson NS, et al: Immunologic reconstitution of foals with combined immunodeficiency. *Vet Immunol Immunopathol* 17:495, 1987.

47. Splitter GA, Perryman LE, Magnuson NS, et al: Combined immunodeficiency of horses: A review. *Dev Comp Immunol* 4:21, 1980.

48. Yilma T, Perryman LE, McGuire TC: Deficiency of interferon-gamma but not interferon-beta in Arabian foals with severe CID. *J Immunol* 129:931, 1982.

49. Banks KL, McGuire TC: Surface receptors on neutrophils and monocytes from immunodeficient and normal horses. *Immunology* 28:581, 1975.

50. Riggs MW: Evaluation of foals for immune deficiency disorders. *Vet Clin North Am Equine Pract* 3:515, 1987.

51. MacDougall DF: Immunoglobulin metabolism in the neonatal foal. *J Reprod Fertil* 23:739, 1975.

52. McGuire TC, Banks KL, Davis WC: Alterations of the thymus and other lymphoid tissue in young horses with combined immunodeficiency. *Am J Pathol* 84:39, 1976.

53. Perryman LE, Liu IKM: Graft versus host reactions in foals with combined immunodeficiency. *Am J Vet Res* 41:187, 1980.

54. Ardans AA, Trommershausen-Smith A, Osburn BI, et al: Immunotherapy in two foals with combined immunodeficiency, resulting in graft versus host reaction. *J Am Vet Med Assoc* 170:167, 1977.

55. Perryman LE, McGuire TC, Hilbert BJ: Selective immunoglobulin M deficiency in foals. *J Am Vet Med Assoc* 170:212, 1977.

56. Perryman LE, Wyatt CR, Magnuson NS: Biochemical and functional characterization of lymphocytes from a horse with lymphosarcoma and IgM deficiency. *Comp Immunol Microbiol Infect Dis* 7:53, 1984.

57. Coignoul FL, Bertram TA, Roth JA, et al: Functional and ultrastructural evaluation of neutrophils from foals and lactating and nonlactating mares. *Am J Vet Res* 45:898–902, 1984.

58. Deem DA, Traver DS, Thacker HL: Agammaglobulinemia in a horse. *J Am Vet Med Assoc* 175:469, 1979.

59. Banks KL, McGuire TC, Jerrells TR: Absence of B-lymphocytes in a horse with primary agammaglobulinemia. *Clin Immunopathol* 5:282, 1976.

60. McGuire TC, Banks KL, Evans DR, et al: Agammaglobulinemia in a horse with evidence of functional T lymphocytes. *Am J Vet Res* 37:41, 1976.

61. Perryman LE, McGuire TC, Banks KL: Animal model of human disease—infantile X-linked agammaglobulinemia: Agammaglobulinemia in horses. *Am J Pathol* 111:125, 1983.

62. Rosen FS, Cooper MD, Wedgewood RJP: The primary immunodeficiencies. *N Engl J Med* 311:235, 1984.

63. Bryans JT, Swerczek TW, Darlington RW, et al: Neonatal foal disease associated with perinatal infection by equine herpesvirus 1. *J Equine Med Surg* 1:20, 1977.

64. McClure JJ, Addison JD, Miller RI: Immunodeficiency manifested by oral candidiasis and bacterial septicemia in foals. *J Am Vet Med Assoc* 186:1195, 1985.

65. Freestone JF, Hietala S, Moulton J, et al: Acquired immunodeficiency in a seven-year-old horse. *J Am Vet Med Assoc* 190:689, 1987.

1.5.

Immunomodulators

Jill J. McClure, DVM, MS

There are many ways by which the body defends itself. One of them is the immune response. It is recognized, however, that disease is not always the result of a virulent external force overpowering host defenses. In some cases, disease also results from either failure of the host to respond to even a modest challenge or from the host's production of an inappropriate or overexuberant immune response. It has been a goal of immunology to increase normal, restore deficient, and temper overexuberant host responses to more effectively resist disease. For these reasons, modulation of the immune system, which provides critical defense against many types of disease, has become an area of intense interest in clinical medicine. The therapeutic usefulness of immunomodulators includes a wide array of areas: as adjuvants to poorly immunogenic vaccines, boosting of anti-infectious defenses, immunotherapy of immunodeficiency syndromes and cancers, and correcting the immunosuppressive effects of chemotherapeutic agents.

An *immunomodulator* can be defined as a biological or nonbiological substance that directly influences a specific immune function or modifies one or more components of the immunoregulatory network to achieve an indirect effect on a specific immune function.[1] The term *biological response modifier* is sometimes used synonymously, although it is often used to refer to newer approaches to immunotherapy, including the use of highly purified molecules such as interleukins and interferons and monoclonal antibodies.[2, 3] Immunotherapy can be divided into two overlapping categories, active and passive. Active immunotherapy is involved with stimulation of the host response, whereas passive relies on the administration of biologically active agents.[2] Immunomodulators can also be considered specific or nonspecific with regard to their effect on an immune response.[3] Both immunostimulants and immunodepressants should be considered immunomodulators.[4] Immunomodulators can also be classified based on their origin: physiologic products (actual components of the immune response), microbial products, and chemically defined agents. Immunomodulation also includes bone marrow transplantation and irradiation.

While a scientific basis for the use of immunomodulators exists, a major limitation is clearly the complexity of the network to be modulated. We are faced with several major problems in the rational clinical application of immunomodulators. Our current diagnostic methods do not allow us to precisely identify the in vivo defects, deficiencies, or excesses of substances or regulators present within the network. Therefore, we have no way of knowing which substances are required to effect the most beneficial changes in total response. Every action initiated within the network prompts other actions, often opposing actions. The immune response is a complex network in which no single activity or compound can be modified in isolation without perturbing the entire system.[1, 4] It is important to realize that the same general result can be achieved through opposite mechanisms. That is, one may increase the functional capacity of the effector phase or one may depress the downregulatory mechanisms and produce the same net result. Stimulation of suppressor functions can result in net reduction of immunity, even following the administration of a bona fide immunostimulant.[4] Whether a particular substance or action produces a *net* stimulation or suppression often depends on the dose, the time course, and the status of other mediators. Immunomodulation is a two-edged sword and within the limits of our current knowledge, we have no practical, reliable way to predict the outcome of our intervention.

Much of the information on which we base our use of immunomodulators has come from controlled, experimental studies, some performed in vitro and others in vivo. In clinical patients, often expectations based on information extrapolated from these types of studies are not realized. One reason is that the temporal relationship between drug administration and the initiation of an immune response is critical.[4, 5] The same drug in the same dose given at different times after initiation may have opposing effects. In a controlled situation, when the initiation of challenge is known with regard to the timing of drug administration, some conclusions can be drawn with respect to effects. In a clinical patient we seldom have reference to the exact time frame of the immune response. Another reason why results may not be achieved is the fact that in the whole organism, a network of functions is activated, not an isolated part. The effect that will be manifested in vivo when activation occurs "in context" is not predictable from the response observed in vitro. An agent that "stimulates" some immune function in vitro may not have the same effect in vivo. It has also become apparent that it is the "coordination" of mediators and activities within the network that is critical and that the principle of simply applying more of a mediator is not an effective way to enhance a response.

Any single immunomodulator cannot be expected to work in all situations, just as penicillin might be appropriate for treating a streptococcal infection but would be inappropriate and ineffective in the treatment of a gram-negative infection. Whereas antimicrobial therapy can be guided by culture and antibiotic sensitivity testing, no such practically applicable methods to guide the selection of immunomodulators are available. Because of the complexity of the immune network, the rational use of immunomodulators is considerably more difficult than the use of antimicrobial agents.

It is sometimes difficult, if not impossible (and perhaps artificial), to separate the *immuno*modulatory functions from the *inflammatory* modulatory effects of various agents. Some of the clinical effects attributed to immunomodulators may in actuality be the result of effects on inflammation as opposed to effects on the specific immune responses.

Immunomodulators have been embraced by clinicians with great enthusiasm and the concept of their use remains very appealing, but in fact, because of the great difficulty in rationally applying them to patients, they have not currently realized their potential. We should look very critically at the immunomodulatory drugs on the market and make attempts to objectively evaluate the effects of therapy. Many agents that have been discarded for use in humans are being resurrected for veterinary use. Is it realistic to expect better results in veterinary patients?

Genetic engineering has allowed the production of many biological mediators on a large scale, making them available for research and clinical trials. As each mediator has become available, its clinical evaluation has proceeded with great hopes and expectations. While some results have been encouraging, in general these mediators have not lived up to expectations. Expectations for these biological products have been raised in an almost unprecedented fashion by the news media and investment brokers attempting to attract venture capital for research and development of these agents.

PHYSIOLOGIC PRODUCTS

Molecular cloning and hybridoma technology have allowed for the large-scale production of some forms of biological mediators such as interferon and interleukins and large numbers of monospecific antibodies. This has provided the opportunity to explore the use of some of these substances in clinical situations. Results have been poor to mixed. These compounds have not answered the problem of immunomodulation.

Immunoglobulins

Immunoglobulins (Ig) may be effector and regulatory mediators of the immune response. In the sense of effectors, the combination of antibody with antigen can activate complement, neutralize viruses, and promote opsonization by phagocytes. As regulators, antibodies against cell receptors or antigen-combining sites of other antibodies (anti-idiotype) can affect the way other mediators interact with receptors and can downregulate the immune response.

Most immunoglobulin products available for horses, with the exception of tetanus antitoxin, are normal plasma products as opposed to concentrated or purified gamma globulin preparations with high specific activity.

The major application of immunoglobulin administration is in treatment of failure of passive transfer, a situation in which antibodies are needed transiently to provide protection until the host levels of immunoglobulin reach protective levels.[6-9] While administration of immunoglobulins would be useful in the treatment of *any* antibody or immunoglobulin deficiency, in the case of primary deficiencies, repeated administration over the lifetime of the patient would be needed. Plasma is often used in the treatment of hypoproteinemia, but the effect in these cases is related to the protein content and effect on oncotic pressure, not to the specific immunoglobulin content of the plasma.

Monoclonal antibodies have been very useful for in vitro diagnosis, but in vivo applications have been limited. Theoretically, it is possible to couple monoclonal antibodies with isotopes, drugs, or toxins and deliver these substances to specific sites based on the antibody-specificity of the monoclonal antibody.[2] This is particularly significant in the treatment of cancer in which drugs, toxins, or isotopes are used to attack the tumor independent of immune effector functions. However, cross-reactivity between the target and "normal" tissue has made this problematic. Also, because the antibodies are of mouse origin, they may not function as well as host species-specific antibodies in immune effector functions and they are quickly metabolized and rapidly removed from the circulation. The potential for anaphylaxis initiated by introduction of a foreign protein and the development of an antiglobulin response characterized by production of anti-mouse immunoglobulin antibody, which can form immune complexes and result in damage, is also of concern.[2]

Monoclonal antibodies can conceivably be used to regulate immune functions if they are directed against the receptors for other mediators to either block or stimulate them. Monoclonal antibodies have been produced that combine with the receptors on T cells involved in acute allograft rejection.[1] This approach has also been taken in a limited sense in some forms of acquired immunodeficiency syndrome (AIDS) therapy wherein monoclonal antibodies are used to block the lymphocyte receptors to which the virus attaches, thereby preventing infection of the cell.[1]

Some peptide fragments of immunoglobulins (fragments from the Fc region) released by enzymatic degradation have immunomodulating properties. One such product, tuftsin, which has been chemically synthesized, has been shown to stimulate phagocytic functions, whereas other fragments exhibit inhibitory activity. Some neuropeptides compete with tuftsin for binding sites on phagocytic cells.[10]

Thymic Peptides and Hormones

A variety of substances produced by the epithelial cells of the thymus have immunomodulatory activity. Some of these peptides are available as thymic extracts, generally of bovine origin; others, which are chemically defined, have been either synthesized chemically or by genetic engineering. In general these peptides tend to induce specific T-cell markers on precursor immature lymphocytes and promote T-cell function. The most important use of these substances has been in the clinical management of thymus-dependent diseases such as in children with hypothymic function and in adults with secondary T-cell deficiencies associated with cancer and autoimmune disease. These compounds are virtually untested in horses, but clinical trials in immunodeficiencies of foals would seem to be justified.[10-12]

Peptides from Other Serum Proteins and Foodstuffs

Peptide segments (often only a few amino acids in length) from other serum proteins, including β_2-microglobulin, fibrin degradation products, prealbumins, C-reactive protein, alpha-fetoprotein, and components of the complement cascade, have been shown to have immunomodulating properties. Proteolysis of these compounds (e.g., by macrophage proteases) may represent the physiologic mechanism by which these substances are produced and elicit their immunoregulatory activity. Effects may be stimulatory, as in the case of enhancement of cytotoxicity with low doses of β_2-microglobulin fragments, or inhibitory, as in the case of suppression of lymphocyte proliferation by fragments from fibrin-fibrinogen.

Peptides isolated from ovine colostrum and human casein following enzymatic digestion have been shown to promote phagocytosis and to stimulate antibody production in a dose-dependent fashion. Presumably, similar peptides may exist in other species.[10]

Interferons

Interferon was first discovered by its ability to inhibit viral replication in vitro. Interferon is now known to encompass several families of molecules that exhibit a wide range of effects, including some modulation of the immune system, and are considered members of the class of intercellular messengers, cytokines.[13, 14]

There are various forms of antigenically distinct interferon produced by different cells in the body. Interferon-α (INF-α) is produced primarily by leukocytes, INF-β by fibroblasts, and INF-γ (immune interferon) by lymphocytes. IFN-γ differs considerably structurally from IFN-α and IFN-β. Numerous forms of IFN-α have been identified. The heterogeneity of IFN-β and IFN-γ appears limited.

Interferons are largely species-specific, although there are limited examples of species cross-reactivity. In general, interferon from one species is not effective in another. Interferons are glycoproteins. They are degraded by gastric acid in the stomach and thus systemic effects cannot be achieved by oral use.

It is difficult to generalize about the immunomodulatory functions of interferon because there is a diversity of effects depending upon the time of administration, the amount given, and so forth. Immune perturbations evoked by interferon include decreased immunoglobulin synthesis, increased expression of cell surface membrane antigens, suppression of hematopoiesis, enhanced cytotoxic responses of various types, increased graft rejection, decreased graft-versus-host disease, macrophage activation and transiently increased natural killer (NK) cell activity with decreased activity with continuous administration, variable but often decreased antibody-dependent cellular cytoxicity, decreased lymphoproliferative responses, and variable effects on monocyte activation.[13, 15, 16] The overall pattern of perturbation is arguably more immunosuppressive than immunostimulatory.

Interferons have in common the ability to inhibit the replication of most viruses and some malignant and normal cells.[2, 17] The antiviral and antitumor effects of interferon do not seem to be directly related to or mediated by the effects of interferon on the immune system but rather on their effects on cellular metabolic processes. Researchers have had little success in correlating the immunomodulatory effects of interferon with desired clinical endpoints, either in malignant or viral diseases.[1]

Because of its in vitro effect on virus replication, interferon held great promise as an antiviral agent in vivo. This expectation has not been realized. Systemic administration of interferon has not had great efficacy as therapy for disseminated viral disease. Interferon is largely ineffective after clinical signs have begun.[14, 16]

Interferon has been useful in the treatment of local viral infections such as papillomavirus infections, including recurrent laryngeal papillomatosis and condyloma acuminatum in humans.[1, 15] Interferon has local activity when applied to mucous membranes. It has not lived up to its potential as a cure or preventive for the common cold when used as a nasal spray because of failure of consistent results and a multitude of side effects.

Viral infections are accompanied by the production of significant amounts of endogenous interferon. A deficiency in this response appears to be rare. Therefore the value of increasing the dose is questionable. Deficient production of IFN-γ by neonates may contribute to compromised immune mechanisms along with lack of preformed antibody.[13]

The presence of interferon in viral infections is at least partially responsible for the clinical signs of headache, malaise, chills, myalgia, and so on that characterize viral infections. In fact, in clinical trials, the side effects observed with interferon have frequently been indistinguishable from the signs of viral infection.[1, 14]

Some forms of cancer are responsive to IFN-α, whereas others are nonresponsive. The response of IFN-β and IFN-γ has been less well studied, but seems to show a similar inconsistent pattern. The response of cancers to interferon seems to be unrelated to any measurable immune parameters and may not be immunologically mediated. A non-cross-resistance between interferon-γ and interferon-α has been documented.[1] Because one interferon does not work does not mean that another will not. Interferon, in doses sufficient to produce clinical effects on tumors, is significantly toxic. Signs include fever, malaise, and hematologic, hepatic, gastrointestinal, and central neurologic toxicities.[1]

Large doses of interferon are needed to effect a response in humans. In general, more interferon is needed to effect an immune response than to effect viral replication.[14] Extrapolation of doses to horses would suggest the need for a substantial amount of interferon to generate any effect.

A human IFN-α product extracted from lymphocytes is available for use in horses (Equiferon, Immunomodulators Laboratories, Stafford, Tex.) to prevent or alleviate the signs of viral respiratory disease. The recommended route of administration is oral with the solution distributed throughout the oral cavity. The recommended dose is 10 IU/lb (e.g., 10,000 IU for a 1,000-1 lb horse) which is minuscule compared doses as high as 14×10^6 units intranasally in humans in the treatment of respiratory viruses.[14]

Interleukins

Interleukins are cytokines (or lymphokines in the case of those produced by lymphocytes) produced by cells as a means to communicate with other cells. A series of interleukins have been identified that have varying effects on a variety of cell populations. (See Chapter 1.1.) Several are being produced in large quantities using genetic engineering and have undergone preliminary clinical trials.

Although perhaps originally identified as a result of their specific activity in vitro, in general the actions of interleukins are not selective on a single phase of the immune response. They interact in the network and produce a myriad of activities, not all of which may be congruent with a desired overall therapeutic effect. Initial studies have clearly shown that prediction of an in vivo effect from in vitro data is not reliable.

Interleukin-1 (IL-1, lymphocyte activating factor, LAF) is a monokine, and is primarily a product of macrophages, although nearly every antigen-presenting cell produces IL-1. It plays a pivotal role in the initiation of lymphocyte activation and development of increased host defense mechanisms (both immunologic and nonimmunologic) in the presence of antigen. It is probably the common denominator, the mediator, in the actions of many substances with adjuvant effects, including endotoxin, muramyl peptides, and staphylococcal exotoxins. IL-1 seems to enhance antibody production in vivo which correlates with the fact that adjuvants that increase antibody production are known to induce IL-1 production. The enhancement of antibody response by IL-1 is partially associated with hyperthermia (IL-1 is an endogenous pyrogen), which enhances the synthesis of immunoglobulins and other immune functions. IL-1 induces the production of IL-2, which promotes T-cell activation.[1, 13]

IL-1 is active in the inflammatory as well as the immune response. IL-1 induces systemic acute-phase changes, including neutrophilia, hypozincemia, hypoferremia, and increased hepatic synthesis of fibrinogen, haptoglobin, complement components, serum amyloid A protein, C-reactive protein, and α_2-macroglobulin. It also induces production of granulocyte-macrophage colony-stimulating factor and interferon and acts on the brain to initiate fever, adrenocorticotropic hormone release, and sleep. These changes augment host defense mechanisms, albeit not by an effect on the immune system.[1]

Purified IL-1, with its numerous biological activities in addition to production of lymphocyte activation, is too toxic for direct use as an adjuvant or immunotherapeutic agent although it bestows immunomodulatory properties on many other agents with recognized immunomodulatory properties[1] (Table 1–23).

Table 1–23. Water-Soluble Adjuvants That Induce Interleukin-1*

Direct	Indirect
Tumor necrosis factor	Interferon-γ
Lymphotoxin	Interferon-α
Colony-stimulating factors	Tuftsin
Interleukin-2	Isoprinosine
Endotoxin	
Peptidoglycans	
Muramyl peptides	
Muramyl dipeptides	
Klebsiella glycoprotein	
Staphylococcal exotoxins	
Streptococcal exotoxins	
Poly I: poly C12U	

*Data from Fauci AS, Rosenberg SA, Sherwin SA, et al: Immunomodulators in clinical medicine. Ann Intern Med 106:421, 1987.

The production of IL-1 has also been hypothesized to play a significant role in the pathogenesis of some diseases, including rheumatoid arthritis, by the recruitment of cells and overactivation of other mediators.[13]

IL-2 (T-cell growth factor) is produced by T cells. IL-2 causes proliferation of T cells, including both helper/inducer and suppressor/cytotoxic subsets. IL-2 also enhances the cytotoxicity of NK cells and stimulates the production of IFN-γ and tumor necrosis factor (TNF). It may also stimulate the production of lymphokines, which activate B lymphocytes.[13, 16, 18]

As with IL-1, the activity of IL-2 is essential for normal function of the immune response, but attempts to manipulate the immune response by exogenous administration have been unrewarding. In general, no consistent immunologic benefit has been found and significant side effects, often life-threatening, including fever, diarrhea, hypotension, fluid retention, anemia, and hepatic and renal dysfunction, have been reported with use of therapeutic doses. In most cases, the toxicity outweighs the therapeutic gain.[2, 16, 18]

Most clinical trials with IL-2 have involved treatment of cancer and AIDS. Adoptive transfer of in vitro IL-2–treated lymphokine-activated killer (LAK) cells has shown some success in treatment of some types of cancer.[1, 2]

Leukocyte Extracts

A number of products extracted from disrupted lymphocytes have been employed in immunotherapy.[19, 20] The chemical definition of the active substances and mechanisms of action is unknown. Dialyzable leukocyte extract (DLE) and transfer factor (TF) are two such preparations. Both nonspecific and specific transfer (with TF) of delayed hypersensitivity have been reported. Sporadic success in the treatment of patients with a variety of immunodeficiency syndromes, neoplasia, and viral, fungal, and mycobacterial diseases has been reported. Failures of this form of therapy have been attributed by some to the lack of use of the "correct" TF with the right specificity for the disease being treated. Some view

these substances as immunity inducers capable of transferring the immunologic memory of lymphocytes to another individual and consider this a potential mechanism for vaccination. The unpredictable outcomes associated with therapy have limited their clinical use.

BACTERIAL PRODUCTS

A variety of bacterial and fungal microorganisms or microbial products have been identified which have an immunomodulating effect on the immune system (Table 1–24). A common feature of many of these products is a nonspecific adjuvant effect, probably associated with the stimulation of IL-1 production by macrophages. This mechanism helps explain the similar effects of a diverse group of substances. Of the microbial products available, only cyclosporine, an immunosuppressive agent, has proved to be of significant clinical value in human medicine.

Mycobacterial Products

A whole range of mycobacterial fractions have been identified with immunomodulating ability. The minimal structure with immunologic (adjuvant) activity is muramyl dipeptide (MDP). Preparations commercially available for use in horses include BCG (bacille Callumet-Guérin), a modified live human tuberculosis vaccine, and protein-free mycobacterial cell wall extracts (Nomagen, Fort Dodge Laboratories, Inc., Fort Dodge, Ia.; Equimune I.V., Vetrepharm Inc., London, Ont.). While there is some variability in the effects of the various fractions, most act as adjuvants. Mycobacterial products are "active" agents which require a functional immune system for effect and as such are not effective in restoring immune responses in primary immunodeficiency patients. These products have a nonspecific stimulatory effect, particularly involving macrophage activation and cell-mediated immunity, and the responses are not specific for mycobacterial antigens. Their effect is believed to be mediated by release of IL-1 from macrophages.[3, 27, 28]

The application of mycobacterial fractions in the treatment of tumors was rationalized on the basis that macrophages are capable of killing many types of tumor cells in vitro. However, the ability of macrophages to regulate tumor growth or rejection in vivo is controversial and has not been proved by adoptive transfer of macrophages. Lymphocytes, not macrophages, may be more important in tumor rejection.[27]

Mycobacterial products are probably more useful at local sites (e.g., intralesionally in tumors) than as general systemic immunostimulators.[27] These agents have been effective in treatment of some animal models of viral and chemically induced cancers. However, naturally occurring tumors (e.g., not chemically or virally induced) tend to be less responsive to treatment, perhaps because they are less immunogenic and do not express tumor-specific antigens. Therefore, stimulation of the immune response is of little value since the tumors are not recognized by the immune system. Response in humans has been sporadic and side effects are common. Thus these compounds have been largely discarded in human medicine.[24]

Table 1–24. Selected Immunomodulatory Agents*

Physiologic Agents	Microbial Agents	Chemically Defined Compounds
Interferon	Mycobacterial organisms, fractions, and derivatives	Levamisole
Transfer factor	*Propionibacterium acnes (Corynebacterium parvum)*	Isoprinosine
Interleukins	derivatives	Thiabendazole
Thymic hormones	*Nocardia* derivatives	Poly I: poly C12U
Immunoglobulins	Staphylococcal cell wall products	Dimethylglycine
Hyperimmune sera	Streptococcal components	Nonsteroidal anti-inflammatory agents
Normal plasma	Endotoxin of gram-negative bacteria	Clotrimazole
Monoclonal antibodies	Cyclosporine	Tilorone
Corticosteroids	*Bordetella pertussis* components	Azimexon
Tuftsin	*Brucella abortus* components	Tuftsin
	Bacillus subtilis components (spores)	Azathioprine
	Klebsiella pneumoniae components	Methotrexate
	Statolon	Cyclophosphamide
	Bestatin	Griseofulvin
	Zymosan	Metronidazole
	Glucan	Amikacin
	Lentinan	Cefotaxime
		Piperacillin
		Mezlocillin
		Chloramphenicol
		Halothane
		Cyproheptadine

*Data from references 1–4, 11, 21–26.

In horses, the major application has been in the intralesional treatment of sarcoids, particularly periocular sarcoids.[29–34] Sarcoids are believed to be viral-induced (papillomavirus) tumors,[35] which suggests that success in horses parallels that seen in other systems.

Use of BCG has two potential hazards: infection of the host with the modified mycobacterial organism and anaphylaxis associated with the protein components of the vaccine. While infection is not a problem with the cell wall extract, anaphylaxis has been reported.[31, 36]

Propionibacterium acnes (Corynebacterium parvum) Products

Propionibacterium acnes is a gram-positive organism which exhibits adjuvant activity in heat-killed and formalin-treated suspensions. The effect of *P. acnes* on the immune system is complex. It appears to stimulate antibody production to some antigens with a variable effect on others. In some tumor models, tumor regression was observed; in others, potentiation of the tumor was noted. Suppressor cells can be induced, which may depress the overall response to immunization rather than potentiate it. The timing and route of administration with regard to administration of antigen has been shown to be crucial as to whether potentiation or suppression of responses occurs.[3] The fact that the stage of the immune response is critical presents obvious problems for use of the substance in a clinical setting where the stage is unknown.

Side effects, such as high fever, headache, vomiting, and hypertension, have been reported in humans.[3] *P. acnes* has been used in the treatment of several types of cancer in humans with variable success and significant side effects. The inconsistency of results and the frequency of adverse reactions have brought into question the usefulness of this preparation in humans.[24]

A *P. acnes* (*C. parvum*) preparation (EqStim, Immunovet, Inc., Tampa, Fla.) is marketed for use in treatment of viral respiratory disease in horses.

Endotoxin (Lipopolysaccharide, LPS)

Administration of endotoxin of gram-negative bacteria results in a myriad of effects, including the release of mediators such as IL-1 and TNF, lymphokines with demonstrable effects on the immune system. The immunomodulating effects of LPS are the result of lymphokine and cytokine production. LPS acts directly on lymphocytes in some species to produce polyclonal B-cell stimulation.[3, 28]

The major problem with the use of endotoxin as an adjuvant is its toxicity, even in small amounts. Chemical modifications of structure to decrease toxicity while preserving adjuvanticity have been attempted with some success. The efficacy of some gram-negative vaccines is probably in part related to the endotoxin present in the antigen preparations.[28]

Cyclosporine

Cyclosporine is a fungal derivative which selectively inhibits proliferation, cytotoxicity, and lymphokine production of T cells by blocking early activation events.[16] Of the microbial products that have immunomodulating activity, cyclosporine has emerged as a major immunosuppressive agent for allograft survival. This drug is widely used in organ transplantation to prevent graft rejection and is finding some application in the treatment of some immune-mediated (autoimmune) diseases. The drug is efficacious in suppressing specific immune responses with minimal nonspecific toxic effects on polymorphonuclear leukocytes, monocytes, and macrophages. Thus, immunosuppressed patients suffer fewer severe secondary infections.[37] The development of secondary malignancies has been reported with long-term drug use.[37]

The use of cyclosporine in horses has not been evaluated.

CHEMICALLY DEFINED AGENTS

A large number of drugs have been shown to have an effect on some phase of the immune response of the host, either in vitro or in vivo, including many drugs commonly used for other purposes including non-steroidal anti-inflammatory agents (NSAIDs), antibiotics, and anthelmintics.

Levamisole

Levamisole is an anthelmintic which was shown to reverse immunologic anergy in some cancer patients. This finding led to extensive research on the effects of the drug on the immune system.[38] Levamisole appears to have little effect on the normal immune system but it appears to stimulate a subnormal response and suppress hyperactive responses. The effects are dose-related and low doses seem to enhance, whereas higher doses seem to suppress, responses. Enhancement of inflammatory responses involving neutrophils may also be a feature of its action. Low efficacy and side effects have prompted a search for more effective agents in humans.[24]

Corticosteroids

Corticosteroids (which might also be considered under physiologic agents) are classic examples of immunosuppressive agents. Corticosteroids exhibit a myriad of effects. It is difficult to separate their immunosuppressive effects from their anti-inflammatory effects. Corticosteroids decrease the production of IL-1 by monocytes and IL-2 by lymphocytes. They have profound effects on cell traffic, including lymphocytes, allowing fewer lymphocytes to reach sites of chronic inflammation. The effect on antibody varies with the species, but in species where lympholysis is not a feature (humans and probably the horse), then antibody production is not significantly affected. Reduced phagocytosis of antibody-coated cells by the reticuloendothelial system (RES) rather than decreased antibody production is probably the mechanism whereby corticosteroids are efficacious, as in immune-mediated hemolytic anemia. Corticosteroids decrease the production of prostaglandins, which has an effect on the immune system as well as on inflammation.[24, 26, 39, 40]

Nonsteroidal Anti-inflammatory Agents

NSAIDs include such drugs as phenylbutazone, flunixin, aspirin, and indomethacin.

NSAIDs share common properties, including inhibition of prostaglandin synthesis by blocking the cyclooxygenase and lipoxygenase pathways. The role of prostaglandins in local pain and inflammation is well recognized; however, prostaglandins, particularly prostaglandins E_1 (PGE_1) and E_2 (PGE_2), have significant suppressive effects on a host of immune functions, as well as inflammatory activity. PGE_2 suppresses most in vitro manifestations of T-lymphocyte function, including lymphocyte proliferation, IL-2 production, and generation of cytotoxic cells. It also suppresses NK cell, antibody-dependent, and monocyte cytotoxicity activity. PGE also enhances antibody production, probably by inhibiting suppressor cells.[22]

Monocytes are stimulated to produce PGE_2 by the same stimuli that induce them to produce IL-1. Thus, the same stimuli that turn on or upregulate the immune response simultaneously turn on the system that downregulates or turns off the immune system. NSAIDs block the formation of PGE, thus blocking the downregulation of the immune response, theoretically effecting a net increase or stimulation of the immune response. However, NSAIDs by inhibiting PGE production, also "stimulate" the activity of suppressor cells, making the outcome less certain.[22, 26]

Certain groups of humans have been identified that have a decreased sensitivity to the suppressive effects of prostaglandins. That is, their responses are not shut down effectively. This may explain the propensity for development of autoimmune disorders in these persons. Physical exercise causes lymphocytes to become more sensitive to PGE and may explain depressed cellular immune function following physical stress.[22]

CONCLUSIONS

Inconsistent results and low efficacy plague many of the immunomodulating agents. In part, this probably reflects our inability to adequately identify situations in which specific drugs would be of most therapeutic value.

The quest for immunomodulators should not be abandoned. The search for practical testing of these agents, as well as the development of new drugs, is essential for the rational clinical use of these agents. At present, we cannot be certain that we are doing no harm when we use immunomodulators, even if we are doing no good. Until the tools become available for us to evaluate the need for, and the effects of, immunomodulation, we are administering blindly.

REFERENCES

1. Fauci AS, Rosenberg SA, Sherwin SA, et al: Immunomodulators in clinical medicine. *Ann Intern Med* 106:421, 1987.
2. Foon KA: Biological response modifiers: The new immunotherapy. *Cancer Res* 49:1621, 1989.
3. Gialdroni-Grassi G, Grassi C: Bacterial products as immunomodulating agents. *Int Arch Allergy Appl Immunol* 76:119, 1985.
4. Spreafico F: Problems and challenges in the use of immunomodulating agents. *Int Arch Allergy Appl Immunol* 76:108, 1985.
5. Hadden JW: The immunopharmacology of immunotherapy. *Springer Semin Immunopathol* 2:35, 1979.

6. Jeffcott LB: Some practical aspects of the transfer of passive immunity to newborn foals. *Equine Vet J* 6:109, 1974.

7. McGuire TC, Crawford TB, Hallowell AL, et al: Failure of colostral immunoglobulin transfer as an explanation for most infections and deaths of neonatal foals. *J Am Vet Med Assoc* 170:1302, 1977.

8. McGuire TC, Poppie MJ, Banks KL: Hypogammaglobulinemia predisposing to infection in foals. *J Am Vet Med Assoc* 166:71, 1975.

9. Rumbaugh GE, Ardans AA, Ginno D, et al: Identification and treatment of colostrum deficient foals. *J Am Vet Med Assoc* 174:273, 1979.

10. Werner GH: Natural and synthetic peptides (other than neuropeptides) endowed with immunomodulating activities. *Immunol Lett* 16:363, 1987.

11. Low TLK, Goldstein AL: Thymosin and other thymic hormones and their synthetic analogues. *Springer Semin Immunopathol* 2:169, 1979.

12. Naylor PH, Goldstein AL: Thymosin: Cyclic nucleotides and T cell differentiation. *Life Sci* 25:301, 1979.

13. Boumpas DT, Tsokos GC: Pathophysiologic aspects of lymphokines. *Clin Immunol Rev* 4:201, 1985.

14. Tyrrell DAJ: Interferons and their clinical value. *Rev Infect Dis* 9:243, 1987.

15. Balkwill FR: Interferons. *Lancet* 1:1060, 1989.

16. Fahey JL, Sarna G, Gale RP, et al: Immune interventions in disease. *Ann Intern Med* 106:257, 1987.

17. Bonnem EM, Spiegel RJ: Interferon-alpha: Current status and future promise. *J Biol Response Mod* 3:580, 1984.

18. Oliver RTD: The clinical potential of interleukin-2. *Br J Cancer* 58:405, 1988.

19. Fudenberg HH: "Transfer factor": An update. *Proc Soc Exp Biol Med* 178:327, 1985.

20. Tsang KY, Fudenberg HH: Transfer factor and other T cell products. *Springer Semin Immunopathol* 9:19, 1986.

21. Esber HJ, Ganfield D, Rosenkrantz H: Staphage lysate: An immunomodulator of the primary immune response in mice. *Immunopharmacology* 10:77, 1985.

22. Goodwin JS: Immunologic effects of nonsteroidal anti-inflammatory agents. *Med Clin North Am* 69:793, 1985.

23. Graber CD, Goust JM, Glassman AD, et al: Immunomodulating properties of dimethylglycine in humans. *J Infect Dis* 143:101, 1981.

24. Hadden JW: Immunomodulation and immunotherapy. *JAMA* 258:3005, 1987.

25. Roszkowski W, Ko HL, Roszkowski K, et al: Antibiotics and immunomodulation: Effects of cefotaxime, amikacin, mezlocillin, piperacillin and clindamycin. *Med Microbiol Immunol* 173:279, 1985.

26. Salaman JR, Miller JJ: Nonspecific chemical immunosuppression. *Transplant Proc* 11:845, 1979.

27. Baldwin RW, Byers VS: Immunoregulation by bacterial organisms and their role in the immunotherapy of cancer. *Springer Semin Immunopathol* 2:79–100, 1979.

28. Warren HS, Chedid LA: Future prospects for vaccine adjuvants. *CRC Crit Rev Immunol* 8:83, 1988.

29. Houlton JEF: Treatment of periocular equine sarcoids. In Barnett KC, Rossdale PD, Wade JF, eds. *Equine Ophthalmology.* London: British Equine Veterinary Association. *Equine Vet J* Suppl 2:117, 1983.

30. Lavach JD, Sullins KE, Roberts SM, et al: BCG treatment of periocular sarcoid. *Equine Vet J* 17:445, 1985.

31. Owen RaR, Jagger DW: Clinical observations of the use of BCG cell wall fraction for treatment of periocular and other equine sarcoids. *Vet Rec* 1200:548, 1987.

32. Schwartzman SM, Cantrell JL, Ribi E, et al: Immunotherapy of equine sarcoid with cell wall skeleton (CWS)–trehalose dimycolate (TDM) biologic. *Equine Pract* 6:13, 1984.

33. Vanselow BA, Abetz I, Jackson ARB: BCG emulsion immunotherapy of equine sarcoid. *Equine Vet J* 20:444, 1988.

34. Wyman M, Rings MD, Tarr MJ, et al: Immunotherapy in equine sarcoid: A report of two cases. *J Am Vet Med Assoc* 171:449, 1977.

35. Trenfield K, Spradbrow PB, Vanselow B: Sequences of papillomavirus DNA in equine sarcoids. *Equine Vet J* 17:449, 1985.

36. Landsheft WB, Anderson GF: Reaction of equine sarcoid therapy. *J Am Vet Med Assoc* 185:839, 1984.

37. Kahan BD: Pharmacokinetics and pharmacodynamics of cyclosporine. *Transplant Proc* 21:9, 1989.

38. Verhaegen H, de Cree J, de Beukelaar A, et al: The immunological evaluation of levamisole treatment in cancer patients. *Postgrad Med J* 54:799, 1978.

39. Claman HN: Anti-inflammatory effects of corticosteroids. *Clin Immunol Allergy* 4:317, 1984.

40. Dannenberg AM: The antiinflammatory effects of glucocorticoids: A brief review of the literature. *Inflammation* 3:329, 1979.

Chapter 2

Mechanisms of Infectious Disease

Bacterial and Mycotic Infections

Joseph J. Kowalski, DVM, PhD

The bacteria that cause infections in horses are in some cases relatively specific to a species such as *Streptococcus equi* subsp. *equi* or, as is the case with other organisms, such as *Salmonella*, they may have a broader animal host range.

The major bacteria in infections associated with horses are discussed with respect to organism characteristics, source of the organism, virulence factors of the organism, pathogenesis of infections, clinical significance, laboratory diagnosis, and, when applicable, prevention through immunization.

ACTINOBACILLUS

Organism Characteristics. Several different strains of *Actinobacillus* are associated with infections in the horse. One of these, *A. equuli*, is well documented as an equine pathogen. However, other strains of equine *Actinobacillus* are less well characterized, and there is some discrepancy with respect to their identification. Strains of actinobacilli isolated from horses that are nonhemolytic tend to be identified as *A. equuli*. In contrast, other strains are isolated that exhibit hemolysis of variable intensity on blood agar (BA) medium. Their biochemical characteristics closely resemble those of *A. suis* because of positive o-nitrophenyl-B-D-galactopyranoside and esculin reactions, and, depending on the number of biochemical tests performed, they may be identified as *A. suis*.[1] These organisms have been described as "*A. suis*-like" because of differing carbohydrate fermentation reactions.[1,2] Additional strains of actinobacilli have been isolated from horse specimens that cannot be characterized as *A. equuli* or *A. suis*-like.[2]

Following 24 hours of incubation on BA, equine actinobacilli are flat and gray with 1- to 3-mm colonies. A number of isolates have the characteristic of being somewhat "sticky." This property, which makes the isolate adhere to the surface of the plate and may be lost by subculture, is probably associated with surface antigens.[2] In the diagnostic laboratory, the ability of actinobacilli to grow on MacConkey (MAC) medium is variable. Some strains fail to grow on MAC, whereas others grow as well as they do on BA.

Biberstein indicates that he examined strains that routinely grew on MAC.[2] Other strains will grow, but in variable numbers that do not reflect those obtained on BA. When growth is apparent on MAC, colonies of *Actinobacillus* appear as 1-mm lactose-positive (magenta) colonies. Actinobacilli are gram-negative coccobacillary to rod-shaped organisms, which often exhibit a considerable pleomorphism.

Source of Organism. The habitat of equine actinobacilli is the mucous membranes of the alimentary tract. Thus, infections, especially those in adults, are often endogenous and likely follow fecal contamination or extension from oral mucous membranes. Some cases may be associated with larval migrations. Infections, which are particularly important in foals and often follow umbilical contamination, are likely derived from their mares after foaling or after environmental contamination. Fetal infection may occur following transplacental transmission, in which case infected foals are often born very weak, or dead, and foals that are born alive may require aggressive postnatal care. Despite intensive supportive care and the use of antimicrobial therapy, these animals often die with evidence of infection at other body sites, particularly the kidneys.

Virulence Factors. Toxins have not been demonstrated in actinobacilli associated with equine infections. The role of a capsule has not been clarified, but in other bacterial species capsules are generally thought to exhibit antiphagocytic properties.

Clinical Significance. Clinical signs in infected foals may be observed within 24 hours of birth. The most obvious clinical sign in foals is enteritis, and mortality may be quite high in neonates. Animals that survive the acute episode can exhibit lesions at several sites including the kidneys, joints, and respiratory tract. Further discussion of the clinical aspects as a result of infections with the actinobacilli may be obtained in Chapter 6. In adult animals, actinobacilli are isolated from a number of infectious processes including abscesses and tracheal washings and less frequently from conjunctival, urinary tract, joint, guttural pouch, and genital infections. Gay and associates *(Australian Veterinary Journal)* described *Actinobacillus* as a cause of peritonitis in adult horses. Excluding enteric infections associated with *Salmonella*, actinobacilli may be the most frequently encountered gram-negative organism in horses. Several of the isolates are identified as *A. suis*-like because of their similarity to *A. suis*, although differences in fermentation of carbohydrates is observed, especially with arabinose.[2]

Specimens. Actinobacilli may be isolated from aspirates or swabs, depending on the site of infection involved. Actinobacilli do not survive well when maintained in the laboratory, and the expectation is that recovery from clinical specimens could be very unrewarding if the time between collection and cultivation is prolonged. Specimens should be inoculated on an enriched medium, such as sheep or bovine BA, and a selective medium such as MAC, although as mentioned earlier, it is not unusual for actinobacilli not to grow on MAC agar. Growth of *Actinobacillus* is not always quantitative on MAC and may vary from no growth to growth comparable to BA, or somewhere in between. Laboratory identification is based on the use of biochemical tests that will speciate the various isolates of actinobacilli. Especially noteworthy is the isolation of β-hemolytic strains from equine specimens. Because of their similarity to *A. suis*, these strains are referred to as *A. suis*-like. Biberstein examined these isolates and concluded that separation of *A. suis*-like organisms from *A. suis* requires additional investigation.

STREPTOCOCCUS

Organism Characteristics. The streptococci are gram-positive cocci that occur singly, in pairs, and in chains of variable length. Chain length is much longer when streptococci are multiplying in fluid environments such as abscesses, milk, or broth culture media. It is common for streptococci to become decolorized as they age; therefore, it is not unusual for gram-positive and gram-negative staining cocci to occur in the same chain. This staining pattern may also be observed in stained smears prepared from clinical specimens.[3] The streptococci are catalase-negative and facultatively anaerobic, although these bacteria prefer microaerophilic environments for growth. The most important streptococcal pathogens of the horse produce a beta or clear type of hemolysis when cultivated on BA. The most frequent and important equine isolates of β-hemolytic streptococci are *Streptococcus equi* subsp. *zooepidemicus*; *S. equi* subsp. *equi*; and *S. dysgalactiae* subsp. *equisimilis*.

Although the nomenclature for these organisms has been recently changed, it is not uncommon for them to be referred to by their former designations (i.e., *S. equi*, *S. zooepidemicus*, and *S. equisimilis*). *S. equi* subsp. *zooepidemicus* is the beta streptococcus most frequently isolated from horses and may actually be the most frequent isolate compared with all bacteria isolated from horses. Following 18 to 24 hours of incubation, colonies on BA are 1 to 3 mm in diameter and watery (mucoid), because the organism produces a hyaluronic acid capsule. This capsule is often hydrolyzed during incubation by a hyaluronidase produced by the organism that results in a flat, transparent, matt-type colony. *S. equi* subsp. *equi* likewise produces a mucoid type of colony because of the elaboration of a hyaluronic acid capsule. Matt-type colonies may also be observed with *S. equi* subsp. *equi* colonies. These colonies may be related to lysogeny of the isolate by a bacteriophage, which is thought to induce the production of a hyaluronidase and result in hydrolysis of the capsule, thus producing the alternate colony type.[4, 5]

S. equi subsp. *equi* has been isolated from natural disease conditions only in horses and related animal species.[4] It is imperative that the laboratory distinguish between *S. equi*

subsp. *equi* and *S. equi* subsp. *zooepidemicus* in order to initiate appropriate management procedures prior to excessive transmission of *S. equi* subsp. *equi* within a herd.

The third beta streptococcus isolated from horse specimens, *S. dysgalactiae* subsp. *equisimilis*, is nonmucoid, resulting in colonies that are 1 to 2 mm in diameter and that have a dry, dewdrop shape. *S. dysgalactiae* subsp. *equisimilis* is isolated with less frequency from equines than either *S. equi* subsp. *zooepidemicus* or *S. equi* subsp. *equi*.

For all the major equine β-streptococci, the zone of beta hemolysis is relatively large in comparison with the colony size. Because they are gram-positive, these organisms do not grow on MAC. They are catalase negative, and all three are Lancefield Group C streptococci.

Source of Organism. The β-hemolytic streptococci are residents of the skin, upper respiratory, and lower genital tracts of horses, although *S. equi* subsp. *equi* is not commonly isolated from normal horses.[6, 7] Approximately 30% of apparently normal mares may be vaginal carriers of β-hemolytic streptococci, most notably *S. zooepidemicus*. Transmission of the organism is likely to occur by respiratory, genital, and alimentary routes after contact with infected horses, humans, and fomites, such as buckets and halters. Contact with pus from infected animals results in exposure to high numbers of organisms. Pharyngeal tissues are an important temporary habitat of *S. equi* subsp. *equi*.[6] Vectors, such as flies and other insects or humans may be implicated in transmission.[8] The carrier state, especially in an animal recovering from an infection, often plays a role in outbreaks that occur after the introduction of such an animal to a farm with a low disease prevalence.[4, 5, 9] Nasal shedding can last for up to 6 weeks in animals that have been infected with *S. equi* subsp. *equi*.[4, 9] In some animals several months of shedding have been detected, but this is not apparently a common occurrence.[4, 9]

Virulence Factors. Pathogenicity of the β-hemolytic streptococci may be related to the presence of surface virulence factors and to some extent to the elaboration of extracellular metabolites, although the role of metabolites has not been well documented. Two of the major surface factors that are associated with infection involve the presence of the hyaluronic acid capsule in the case of *S. equi* subsp. *equi* and *S. equi* subsp. *zooepidemicus*, which is in all likelihood antiphagocytic, as well as the presence of the surface antigen, M protein.[4, 6, 9, 10] There is one type of M protein in *S. equi* subsp. *equi* common to all strains as evidenced by the fact that there is a lack of immunologic variation in M proteins of *S. equi* subsp. *equi*. This homogeneity may be demonstrated by a variety of immunologic methods, including serum neutralization procedures, gel immunodiffusion, and immunoblot examinations.[4, 6] The identical relatedness of *S. equi* subsp. *equi* has also been demonstrated by DNA restriction analysis.[11]

M protein has been associated with resistance to phagocytosis in those streptococcal species that possess the proteins.[4, 6, 10, 12, 13] A number of vaccines for prevention of strangles utilize *S. equi* subsp. *equi* M protein as the primary immunogen. M proteins may function as superantigens, inducing deleterious host immune reactions because of their relatedness to mammalian tissue. Antibody cross-reactivity has been detected between M proteins and a number of mammalian tissues, including those in joints, heart, kidney, and skin. M proteins, at least in *S. pyogenes*, do not function in bacterial adhesion to host cell surfaces.

Following attachment to cells of the upper respiratory and alimentary tracts, especially to pharyngeal tissues and adjacent lymphoid tissue, *S. equi* subsp. *equi* migrate via the lymphatics to the lymph nodes of the head.[4, 10] Multiplication of the organism with chain formation is followed by an influx of polymorphonuclear cells, ultimately resulting in abscess formation. Many components of *S. equi* subsp. *equi* cell walls activate the host's leukocyte response. The latter response is mediated by the interaction of streptococcal cell wall peptidoglycan with the C3 component of complement.[4] Organisms multiply extracellularly as well as intracellularly, survival being associated with the release of bacterial toxins such as streptolysin O, a leukocidin and a hemolysin, which inhibits the action of leukocytes against the organism.[4, 14] The presence of the previously referred to surface antiphagocytic components, particularly M protein, is important to the survival of *S. equi* subsp. *equi*. Of particular importance is the binding of fibrinogen to M proteins. There are several mechanisms by which this is accomplished. In one scenario, M protein binds complement H control factor, which then binds C3b so that it is unavailable for complex formation with C3 convertase, keeping C3b at a depressed level and thus failing to activate the alternate complement pathway that ultimately results in diminished phagocytosis.[4] The presence of fibrinogen on the surface of *S. equi* subsp. *equi* also prevents the deposition of C3 on the bacterial cell surface, which not only inhibits phagocytosis but also enhances the survival of intracellular streptococci.[4, 14] Developing abscesses in the head and neck region may serve as a nidus of organisms at body sites distant to the primary infection, such as the brain and organs in the abdominal and thoracic cavities.

The pathogenesis of infections by *S. equi* subsp. *zooepidemicus* or *S. dysgalactiae* subsp. *equisimilis* have not been characterized to the same degree as those caused by *S. equi* subsp. *equi*. Infections associated with these organisms are, nonetheless, very important, especially those associated with *S. equi* subsp. *zooepidemicus*. In contrast with *S. equi* subsp. *equi*, the M proteins of *S. equi* subsp. *zooepidemicus* occur as several immunologic variants.[6, 10, 12] These M proteins induce bactericidal antibodies in mice, which are protective.[4, 10]

Clinical Significance. Of the important equine β-hemolytic streptococci, *S. equi* subsp. *zooepidemicus* is the most frequently encountered organism, but *S. equi* subsp. *equi* is the economically more important pathogen because of the high morbidity and significant mortality in susceptible herds. Clinical signs of *S. equi* subsp. *equi* infections can involve entire farms and may be related to the introduction of an infected or recovering carrier animal. The other beta streptococci cause infections in individual animals that can markedly affect performance, but they are not typically noted as highly communicable diseases.

S. equi subsp. *equi* infections, commonly referred to as "strangles," is characterized initially by a fever and nasal discharge that eventually lead to an abscess of the lymph nodes of the head and neck. Infections with *S. equi* subsp. *equi* are highly communicable and may be associated with significant economic losses, even though the mortality is not often excessively high.[5, 9] Infections occur most frequently in foals and immature adults, but animals of any age may become infected.[9] Infected animals may have elevated temperatures, pharyngitis, and a serous nasal discharge that later becomes mucopurulent. Abscessed lymph nodes eventually rupture, a feature that often signals recovery.[4, 9] Several complications may result from the abscess of some of the lymph nodes, especially the retropharyngeal nodes. Rupture of the retropharyngeal nodes may result in drainage into the guttural pouch or aspiration of some of the contents.[4] Rupture of the abscesses often coincides with clinical improvement and subsequent recovery of infected animals.[4, 9]

In some animals, the organisms following hematogenous metastasis are carried to lymph nodes in the thoracic and abdominal cavities or in some cases the brain and lungs.[3–5] This form of the disease, referred to as "bastard strangles," is associated with a mortality rate of 10%, which is somewhat higher than that associated with classical strangles.[3, 9] This aberrant form of *S. equi* subsp. *equi* infection may follow antimicrobial therapy in which modification of an organism's cellular components may diminish the animal's immune response.[3]

In an outbreak of strangles described in 1988, approximately 20% of the animals on the farm had various manifestations of atypical strangles.[5] Several animals involved in the outbreak exhibited signs of purpura hemorrhagica, a condition that may occur as a sequela to *S. equi* subsp. *equi* infections. Other atypical manifestations of *S. equi* subsp. *equi* infections include myocarditis related either to streptolysin O activity or perhaps an immune-mediated pathway in which antibodies to M protein cross-react with myosin.[4] In the course of infections with *S. equi* subsp. *equi*, a low percentage of animals exhibit an acute vasculitis, purpura hemorrhagica, which is observed several weeks (2 to 4 weeks) after the acute respiratory episode and is characterized by edema of the limbs, ventral abdomen, and head where evidence of this condition is initially observed because of involvement of the nostrils, which become edematous resulting in a narrowing of the nares. The pathogenesis of the vasculitis has been associated with high levels of antibody to M protein and other *S. equi* subsp. *equi* proteins, along with an elevation in C3 that results in the formation of immune complexes composed of IgG and IgA.[3, 4] The bacterial antigens associated with the immune complexes may be derived from the population of organisms found within abscesses.[4] It has been observed that horses that develop purpura hemorrhagica tend to engender greater antibody levels than are usually detected in animals in which this manifestation is not observed. Some cases of purpura hemorrhagica have been associated with recent exposure to vaccinal antigen.[3, 4]

S. equi subsp. *zooepidemicus* is the β-hemolytic streptococcus that is most frequently isolated from horses. The pathogenesis of equine *S. equi* subsp. *zooepidemicus* infections has not been characterized to the same degree as infections with *S. equi* subsp. *equi*. These organisms share antigens with *S. equi* subsp. *equi*, but these are not likely to be important in terms of cross-protection. The M proteins of *S. equi* subsp. *zooepidemicus* differ from those of *S. equi* subsp. *equi*. The organism should be considered in any equine pyogenic infection. Infections associated with this organism include respiratory infections that may be secondary to viral infections, wound infections, lymph node abscess, joint infections, eye infections, and genital infections. In many of these infections, *S. equi* subsp. *zooepidemicus* is the predominant organism, although simultaneous isolation of other organisms, such as actinobacilli, may be made. It is an opportunist that is present on normal respiratory and vaginal mucous membranes.

S. dysgalactiae subsp. *equisimilis* is isolated less frequently than *S. equi* subsp. *zooepidemicus* or *S. equi* subsp. *equi* but can be isolated from similar types of infections. Antigens are shared with *S. equi* subsp. *equi* and *S. equi* subsp. *zooepidemicus*, but details associated with their role in pathogenesis are not entirely known.

S. pneumoniae is isolated occasionally from transtracheal washings obtained from horses presented to the Ohio State University for diagnosis and treatment. This organism is an accepted human respiratory pathogen and should in all likelihood be considered significant when isolated from equine respiratory specimens, especially in the absence of bacteria usually isolated from equine specimens.

Specimens. Swabs and aspirates are suitable for isolation of β-hemolytic streptococci from clinical specimens. Gram-stained smears may provide useful information pending the results of cultures.

In specimens that are fluid, such as those from abscesses or transtracheal washings, streptococci generally form relatively long chains. Although streptococci are gram-positive, it is not unusual for some organisms to become decolorized because of age variability of organisms within a chain. Streptococci require enriched media for growth. On BA, colonies are surrounded by a zone of clear hemolysis, but *S. dysgalactiae* subsp. *equisimilis* is readily distinguishable from *S. equi* subsp. *equi* or *S. equi* subsp. *zooepidemicus*, because in contrast to the latter two bacteria it is not encapsulated and, therefore, does not have a mucoid colonial appearance.

These organisms do not grow on selective media, such as MAC, which are used to isolate gram-negative enteric bacteria. They are catalase negative. The three species are classified as Lancefield Group C streptococci on the basis of the presence of a common cell wall polysaccharide. Although grouping is not routinely performed, it may be important in some circumstances for epidemiologic studies. The differentiation of the three important β-hemolytic streptococci may be made by evaluating differences in their ability to ferment sugars, most notably sorbitol trehalose, mannitol, and lactose.[9]

S. pneumoniae can be recognized on BA plates because colonies are typically mucoid and are surrounded by a zone of alpha (green) hemolysis. Confirmatory tests for *S. pneumoniae* should include an optochin test, which is a procedure in which a 6-mm paper disk impregnated with optochin (ethyl hydrocuprein hydrochloride) is placed on a lawn of *S. pneumoniae* followed by overnight incubation at 37 °C, preferably in an elevated carbon dioxide environment. A positive test result is one in which the zone of inhibition around the disk is 14 mm or greater. An alternative screen for *S. pneumoniae* is a bile solubility test in which a suspension of organisms is mixed with bile (10% sodium taurocho-

late) and observed for clearing of the suspension because of autolysis of the organism.

Immunity. Following recovery from an outbreak of strangles, approximately 75% of infected animals will have an extended period of resistance to reinfection, although infections can occur in previously infected animals as early as 6 months after clinical disease.[3, 4] Animals that fail to develop immunity fail to produce mucosal IgA and IgG antibodies or circulating opsonic IgG antibodies, which appear later in the convalescent period.[4]

Mucosal antibodies to M protein, which requires topical stimulation, are detected earlier than are circulating antibodies and may prevent adherence of the organism to mucosal and pharyngeal tissue. Milk from mares contains IgG and IgA antibodies to M protein.[4] This is especially true in mares that have recovered from strangles. In all probability the level of antibody engendered following immunization would be dependent on the strength of the immune response of the mare.

There are a number of vaccines currently in use for the control of strangles. These include bacterins or M protein component vaccines. Immunity is obtained in no more than half of the immunized animals and then only when the components are incorporated in adjuvants or when multiple injections (preferably three) were given.[3, 4, 10, 15] While immunization does not lead to development of absolute resistance to infection, immunized animals respond with a more rapid and higher level of circulating antibody. In experimental challenges, vaccinates generally develop clinical signs that were less severe, although experimental infections tend to be more severe when intranasal challenge is utilized.[3, 10] Bacterin preparations are generally formulated with an adjuvant such as aluminum hydroxide (Equibac II, Fort Dodge). M protein vaccines are prepared by hot acid extraction organisms (Strepvax, Coopers Animal Health) or treatment of whole cells of *S. equi* subsp. *equi* with a cell wall hydrolyzing enzyme, a mutalysin (Bayer Corporation).

At least three injections of M protein vaccines are required for any meaningful resistance to develop, and horses that receive fewer than the recommended sequence could acquire an infection.[9, 15] Antibodies in serum may be detected following immunization or infection using several different methodologies, including serum-bactericidal antibodies, mouse protection tests, radioimmunoassay, *enzyme-linked immunosorbent assay* (ELISA), and agar gel immunodiffusion.[3] Which of these assays is reflective of resistance has not been determined. For example, horses, with detectable serum-bactericidal activity engendered by M protein vaccines or bacterin, exhibited clinical signs of strangles despite the presence of antibody just prior to the outbreak of disease. Animals brought onto a farm should be not be allowed to mingle with other horses but should be kept in designated areas or be placed in quarantine before their introduction to other animals on the farm. Consideration should be given to the collection of several nasal specimens for culture in an attempt to identify carrier animals.

RHODOCOCCUS

Organism Characteristics. The only important animal pathogen in this genus is *Rhodococcus equi*. This organism was previously known as *Corynebacterium equi*, but because of several characteristics including habitat, pigment production, cell wall composition antigenic analysis, and DNA homology it was assigned the generic name of *Rhodococcus*.[16–19, 20] Rhodococci contain cell wall lipids that are related to the mycolic acids of the acid-fast bacteria, the mycobacteria.[16, 19] The mycolic acids in the *Rhodococcus* cell wall may vary in chain length from C34 to C66 with *R. equi* mycolic acids falling in the C34 to C52 range. Another mycobacterial component identified in the genus is tuberculostearic acid.[19] Rhodococci are gram-positive coccoid to rod-shaped bacteria, although more coccoid forms predominate with continued laboratory cultivation. With few exceptions, such as nitrate reduction and urease and catalase production, *R. equi* is relatively biochemically inactive.[7, 19] *R. equi* is an aerobic organism, whose optimal temperature for growth is 30 °C, although multiplication does occur at temperatures above this, including incubator temperatures.[16, 19–21] The organism produces a polysaccharide capsule.[22, 23] *R. equi* may be shed in the feces of horses, thus contaminating the environment.[17, 19] The organism has also been detected in the feces of other herbivores, including sheep, goats, cattle, deer, wild birds, and pigs.[17, 19, 24] The presence of *R. equi* in the gut of adult horses apparently occurs in the absence of any multiplication, perhaps because of the aerobic metabolism of the organism and the inhibiting effect of the anaerobic flora. In contrast, intestinal multiplication occurs in foals up to 8 to 12 weeks of age.[19, 25, 26] Multiplication of the organisms begins once the stool is passed into the environment, where given suitable moisture, nutrients, and temperature, the organism's numbers may increase 10,000-fold over a period of 2 weeks.[16, 17, 20, 21, 25] The optimal temperature for growth is 30 °C (86 °F), but similar growth results at incubator temperatures (35 °C or 97 °F), temperature ranges that may be achieved in the spring and early summer in temperate climates. The organism does not multiply at temperatures below 10 °C.[19, 25] Isolation of the organism may be made from soil, where it is able to survive for prolonged periods, especially in feces-enriched environments. As a result, the soil, especially at the surface, on contaminated farms serves as a major source of organisms for susceptible foals especially on farms where infections are routinely diagnosed.[26]

R. equi has been isolated from farm soils on which there has been no history of horses on the premises.[17] In contrast with other related organisms, acidic soils do not appear to be inhibitory for *R. equi*, and the organism is able to survive in dry or wet soils. Soils that are sandy may be particularly suitable for the organism to survive.[16, 17] However, isolations of *R. equi* occur more readily from dry environments rather than from wet environments.[16, 17, 27] Not all environmental isolates of *R. equi* are virulent for foals or mice, which are the laboratory animals used for induction of experimental infections.[26]

Selective media have been developed that may be used to isolate *R. equi* from the environmental and fecal specimens, including such media as TANP and NANAT.[17, 27] These media are very similar, both containing potassium tellurite and cycloheximide. Individually, inhibitors incorporated into TANP include penicillin, whereas NANAT contains nalidixic acid and novobiocin in addition to tellurite and amphotericin B. Other selective media including M3 and modified Tins-dale medium have been used for the selective isolation of *R. equi*.

The portal of entry in most infections is the respiratory tract, following the inhalation of organism-laden dust. Elevated bacterial numbers may be detected in the air on windy, dry days. Other routes of infection include the alimentary tract following ingestion of contaminated soil or because of the coprophagic nature of foals or following the ingestion of expectorated exudates; transplacental and umbilical cord contamination have also been reported. Intestinal multiplication of *R. equi* does not occur in adult animals, although intestinal multiplication has been documented in foals up to 3 months of age, when multiplication ceases, perhaps when the anaerobic normal flora become fully established.[19, 21, 25, 27]

Source of Organism. *R. equi* may be shed in the feces of horses and other herbivores, thus, contaminating the environment. Wild birds have been implicated as mechanical vectors. The organism is found in soil, especially in soil enriched by organic acid found in the feces of herbivores.[17]

Pathogenesis. *R. equi* is a facultative intracellular pathogen. While *R. equi* virulence factors have not been definitively identified, a number of cell constituents and metabolites have been implicated in the infectious process. There are virulent and avirulent forms of *R. equi*.[27, 28] These forms may be differentiated because virulent strains are characterized by the presence of an 85 or 90 kb plasmid, which codes for 15- to 17-kDa surface proteins, which are present in virulent strains but absent in strains avirulent for mice.[19, 26, 28] Furthermore, analysis of 102 environmental isolates revealed that 25 of the strains had the plasmid and were virulent for mice, whereas the remaining strains were avirulent for mice and did not have the virulence plasmid.[26] Analysis of an additional 14 isolates from infected foals indicated that the plasmid was present in these strains as well.[26]

Other organism components for which a virulence role has been proposed, although not yet clarified, are the so-called "equi factors."[28] The several components thus classified are enzymes, cholesterol oxidase and phospholipase C (choline phosphorylase), which may be active as membranolytic exoenzymes and apparently act to allow penetration of the organism into cells resulting in abscess formation.[19, 28]

Another possible virulence factor is the presence of cell wall mycolic acid containing glycolipids, which in a mouse model induced more granulomas, and strains that possess them are more likely to be lethal.[19] The chain length of the mycolic acids is apparently critical, because increased virulence is attributed to *R. equi* that have mycolic acids with fatty acid chain lengths ranging from 34 to 66 carbons in length.[19]

Another possible virulence factor is the polysaccharide capsule associated with the organism, which probably inhibits phagocytosis by host cells, although in in vitro experiments, foal alveolar macrophages rapidly ingested opsonized *R. equi*.[19, 23, 28] The capsule of *R. equi* is serologically variable, and at least 27 capsular serotypes have been identified.[19] There is no apparent relationship between capsular serotype and virulence.[19, 21, 28]

It is apparent that ingested organisms can survive phagocytosis. Electron microscopic studies of macrophages revealed that the survival of an organism may be related to an inability of phagosome-lysosome fusion. In an in vitro model, opsonization enhances all aspects of the phagocytic process including ingestion, lysosome-phagosome fusion, and destruction by macrophages.[19–21] In other in vitro studies, neutrophils from either foals or adults exhibited bactericidal activity against opsonized *R. equi*.[21, 24] Degranulation of lysosomes may contribute to local tissue damage, eventually resulting in the characteristic suppurative lesion.[19]

Most infections with *R. equi* follow inhalation of dust in contaminated stables and paddocks. Grass-covered soils are less likely to be a source of infection because the organisms are not as readily aerosolized and are less likely to reach the respiratory tract. Environmental conditions that predispose foals to infections with *R. equi* include windy days and dry, dusty soil, which is enriched with herbivore feces; soil pH ranging from acidic soil with a pH as low as 4.8 or slightly alkaline ranges above 7; temperatures fluctuating in the range of 15 °C to 37 °C for a period of time; and a population of *R. equi* accumulating in soil on a farm is associated with horse production. The organisms are deposited in respiratory alveoli, where phagocytosis by macrophages occurs. In the absence of the antibody, organisms are able to survive intracellularly while continuing to multiply. A neutrophilic response eventually occurs that produces the characteristic suppurative response of *R. equi* infections.[19] Some of the lesions that occur may be the result of the lysosomal degranulation in macrophages with engulfed *R. equi*.[19] Organisms that are found in tracheal secretions may be coughed up, swallowed, and passed through the gut in the intestinal contents.[19] In some cases penetration and ulceration of the intestinal mucosa occur, resulting in enlargement of mesenteric lymph nodes and subsequent diarrhea.[19, 20]

Clinical Disease. The usual clinical disease associated with *R. equi* infections in foals is suppurative bronchopneumonia, which is characterized by the presence of large, coalescing abscesses throughout the lungs. The age of foals at the time of infection is usually between 2 and 3 months.[18, 19, 21, 24] Foals with lung abscesses may appear normal until some of the abscesses rupture, leading to the development of pleuritis. Enteritis and sometimes peritonitis may be observed in some animals. This form of *R. equi* infection occurs less frequently. Sometimes abortions may follow uterine infections. Less commonly, *R. equi* may be isolated from the joints of some animals, although some joint involvement is nonseptic and is suggestive of an immunologic component.[20, 21, 29]

Laboratory Diagnosis. In the living animal, transtracheal aspirates, joint aspirates, and uterine swabs are typical specimens that should be obtained for the diagnosis of *R. equi* infections. A Gram stain is a useful adjunctive procedure that could be done while waiting for culture results, especially from transtracheal and joint aspirates. A stained smear prepared from aspirates will reveal the presence of coccoid to short intracellular and extracellular gram-positive rods and neutrophils and macrophages.[23]

Specimens in which *R. equi* is suspected may be processed as routine specimens by inoculation on BA and MAC media. *R. equi* will grow only on BA medium and will appear after incubation overnight at 37 °C as colonies with a diameter of less than 1 mm and a water-like appearance because of capsule formation by the organism. After 48 hours of incubation, the mucoid colonies are about 2 mm in diameter. With continued incubation, the mucoid nature of the colonies becomes more apparent, as does the salmon pink color.[19, 21] The color does not become distinct until the third or fourth day of incubation, and at this time the colony size is approximately 3 to 4 mm. Other colonial variants have been described, but these occur infrequently.[19] Colonies suspected to be *R. equi* should have a Gram stain done to confirm a Gram reaction and morphology. A positive catalase reaction should be obtained. *R. equi* are catalase, urea positive and nitrate reduction positive, but they do not oxidize or ferment any of the usual sugars including dextrose, lactose, maltose, mannitol, or sucrose.[19] The organism does produce a CAMP-like reaction in sheep, bovine, or rabbit BA. This test is performed by streaking a culture of *Corynebacterium pseudotuberculosis*, which elaborates phospholipase D or β-toxin producing *Staphylococcus* along the equator of a BA plate, then streaking the *R. equi* suspect, which secretes the "equi factors" at right angles to it.[19] Strains that fail to produce "equi factors" have not been described.[19] A potentiation of hemolysis results in the vicinity where the two streaked colonies meet because of an interaction between the metabolites of the two cultures. Most respiratory specimens yield pure cultures of *R. equi*, although it is possible to isolate various environmental organisms in poor quality specimens, or, such pathogens as actinobacilli or β-hemolytic streptococci as co-pathogens.[21]

Immunity. The identity of antigens that elicit antibodies that can opsonize *R. equi* is unknown.[19] Antibody as evidence of exposure may be measured by various serologic tests, including ELISA, agar gel immunodiffusion, agglutination reactions, synergistic hemolysis inhibition, and complement fixation.[18] Immunoblotting has been used to identify important antigens for which their role as virulence factors has been proposed.[26, 28] Some studies suggest that passive immunity using plasma derived from horses immunized with live *R. equi* was protective in experimental *R. equi* infections, as demonstrated by the fact that foals receiving antibody containing plasma had clinical signs that were less severe than those found in animals receiving plasma from nonimmunized animals. There were discrepancies in this study in that at least one animal with a low level of antibody survived, and an animal with a high titer died.[19] The importance of antibody or other serum factors such as complement as mediators of phagocytosis has been well documented.[19]

Typical of most intracellular pathogens, cell-mediated immunity is likely to be very important although definitive research is needed. As has been demonstrated with antibody, alveolar macrophages obtained from foals experimentally infected with *R. equi* phagocytized and destroyed opsonized or nonopsonized *R. equi* with greater efficiency than did macrophages from non-challenged foals. This finding emphasizes the importance of antibody and activated macrophages in *R. equi* infections.[19] A key intermediary in cellular immunity is the CD4+ lymphocyte, which results in activation of macrophages through the lymphokine intermediary, interferon-γ.[19, 25] These cells also stimulate growth and differentiation of B cells to produce antibody.[24] Alternatively, macrophages, such as CD8$^+$ cells, may be activated by other secretory inflammatory constituents such as tumor necrosis factor (TNF).[19]

Bacterins have not proved to be useful because critical antigens may have been destroyed, or perhaps because immunity against many intracellular pathogens is best achieved by the use of living immunizing agents, or because antigen is not presented by an appropriate route.[20, 25] Antigenic stimulation of a foal's immune system in the intestinal tract may be important.[19] Infections are more likely in immunologically compromised animals that may have a predilection for becoming infected or in foals that fail to receive adequate colostrum and in animals exposed to increased numbers of organisms in contaminated environments.[16, 19, 25]

STAPHYLOCOCCUS

Organism Characteristics. The staphylococci are gram-positive cocci that occur singly, in pairs, in short chains, and in clusters. A reclassification has occurred among the staphylococci so that instead of two or three species, now about 29 species exist.[30]

Most of the new species are coagulase-negative species and are not usually associated with infection. The major equine pathogens from the genus are the coagulase-positive staphylococci that are now identified as *Staphylococcus aureus* or *S. intermedius* on the basis of their biochemical characteristics.

Source. Staphylococci are not common pathogens of the horse. It is likely that many of the infections that occur are derived from human nasal and skin carriers, and the infections would best be described as iatrogenic.[22, 31]

Virulence Factors. Staphylococci elaborate many toxins and enzymes, some of which may be implicated in infection. Coagulase is an enzyme that results in the clotting of plasma; however, equine plasma is not usually clotted, making its role in equine infections problematic. In addition, when a coagulase-positive staphylococcus was rendered coagulase negative, the altered organism retained its virulence for mice.[32] Nonetheless, this enzyme is a commonly used criterion for designation of staphylococci as being potentially pathogenic.

Alpha hemolysin lyses sheep and rabbit red blood cells by inducing pore formation in the cell membrane, causes dermonecrosis when injected intradermally in experimental animals, and is lethal following intravenous inoculation.[32] Other potential virulence factors include leukocidin, which affects the viability of leukocytes; whereas hyaluronidase lyses hyaluronic acid and is implicated as a spreading factor; and deoxyribonuclease, which hydrolyzes deoxyribonucleic acid. Lipases and proteases are also produced by staphylococci. Some of these metabolites have a role in certain situations, but their role in other types of infections is unknown. Lipase, for example, has been shown to degrade skin fatty acids that exhibit antimicrobial activity.[30] Whether this enzyme is essential to pathogenicity in other body sites is not known. Surface antigens may also contribute to the pathogenicity of staphylococci *S. aureus/intermedius* have a cell wall polysaccharide, ribitol teichoic acid, which covers the underlying mucopeptide and may protect from cell wall lysing enzymes such as lysozyme. In contrast, the coagulase-negative and usually nonpathogenic staphylococci have a glycerol teichoic acid that appears to be less protective of cell wall mucopeptide. Teichoic acids may be protective by diminishing the ability of the organism to be phagocytized. Another important cell wall component of *S. aureus* is protein A, a substance that binds the Fc portion of IgG and that fixes complement. Protein A may also be antiphagocytic.[30] Some strains possess an obvious capsule, but this is not a universal characteristic among staphylococci.[30]

Pathogenesis. Staphylococcal infections occur infrequently in horses and are commonly associated with sequestered sites, such as joints, spermatic cord, wound infections, or uterus.[22, 31, 33] Infections in other body areas are uncommon. Although skin infections caused by coagulase-positive staphylococci are diagnosed, they are not particularly common and are often secondary to other conditions that result in injury to the skin.[33, 34]

Introduction of organisms may follow procedures involving the ultimate site of infection, for example, joint taps.[22, 31] Once the organisms are introduced, the presence of ribitol teichoic acid and protein A may enable staphylococci to resist phagocytosis or to survive intracellular digestion once phagocytized.[30] Extracellular metabolites, including leukocidin and alpha hemolysin may exert an antileukocyte effect. Inasmuch as horse plasma is not clotted by staphylococcal coagulase, it may not play a role in staphylococcal infections of horses or for that matter in other species.[30]

Clinical Disease. Coagulase-positive staphylococci are uncommon equine pathogens. Infections caused by these organisms include joint infections and usually have a history of joint invasion following surgery or aspiration procedures; skin infections; metritis; and botryomycosis, the most common equine manifestation being an infection of the remnant of the spermatic cord following castration; and other wound infections.

Laboratory Diagnosis. Specimens include joint aspirates, skin biopsies, and uterine swabs using guarded swabs and exudates from draining lesions. Smears for cytologic staining by the Wright-Giemsa stain or especially by a Gram stain would provide preliminary evidence of the etiology. *S. aureus/intermedius* grows on BA but not on MAC. The pathogenic staphylococci isolated from animals usually produce a double zone of hemolysis on BA, which is characterized by the presence of a clear inner zone of hemolysis and a darker zone of incomplete hemolysis to the outside.

A Gram stain will reveal gram-positive cocci occurring singly, in pairs, in short chains, and in clumps. They are coagulase positive in that rabbit plasma inoculated with *S. aureus* or *intermedius* will result in clot formation. *S. aureus* and *S. intermedius* are also catalase positive and are quite similar biochemically. Differentiation may be accomplished by use of commercial test kits, although tests may be required that are not in the kits, such as polymyxin B susceptibility and an ortho-nitro-phenyl galactosidase test.

Prevention. Bacterins are not available and are probably not indicated in staphylococcal diseases of the horse. Enzymatic whole cell lysates are available but are not used in horses. Control is best accomplished by preventing contamination through the use of aseptic surgical and aspiration techniques, because in most cases a human source of the organism is involved.

SALMONELLA

Organism. Several schemes are utilized to classify salmonellae, leading to considerable confusion. Even a recent proposal to classify *Salmonella* in a single species, *S. enterica*, containing seven serogroups, has been modified to place organisms into two species, the second one being *S. bongori*.[35] Under this scheme one of the subgroups in the LeMinor proposal was accorded species status, thus reducing the number of subgroups to six. Thus, the two species of *Salmonella* in the scheme would be *S. enterica* and *S. bongori*, and the six subgroups of *S. enterica* would be *enterica*, *salamae*, *arizonae*, *diarizonae*, *indica*, and *houtenae*. While these proposals more accurately describe genetic relationships among the salmonellae, common usage continues to use the more simplified binomial nomenclature. Even though an isolate might be designated as a *S. enterica* subspecies *enterica* serovar *krefeld*, common usage would simply designate this isolate as *S. krefeld*.[36]

An important characteristic of salmonellae is their inability to ferment either lactose or sucrose or to utilize lactose slowly.[36] The slow fermentation of lactose is a characteristic of salmonellae that belong to subgroups *arizonae* and *diarizonae*, and these organisms are not common horse pathogens. The biochemical characteristics of salmonellae have been utilized in the development of media for isolation of salmonellae from mixed bacterial populations.[35, 37] On BA these organisms have typical colonies that are generally indistinguishable from many other enteric bacteria, including *E. coli*. They may be presumptively recognized on selective and differential media, such as MAC agar, where they appear as colorless, lactose-negative colonies or on brilliant green as lactose/sucrose negative, pink colonies. Suspect *Salmonella* colonies are often screened using a minimal number of laboratory tests, such as triple sugar iron (TSI) agar and lysine iron agar (LIA).[35] Definitive identification requires additional biochemical tests, either as tubed media or commercially available rapid identification schemes such as API 20E or Sensititre. Each of these latter procedures should generate a number code that is compatible with the genus *Salmonella*. In addition to being lactose and sucrose negative, salmonellae are gram-negative rods that are oxidase negative.[37]

Further identification of the more than 2,000 subspecies requires the use of serologic procedures by evaluating the O antigens of the cell wall and the H antigens of the flagella.[35, 37] Some serotypes, such as *S. typhimurium* and *S. dublin*, have bacteriophages that may be utilized in their identification. *Salmonella* are divided into serogroups on the basis of their O cell wall antigen profile and then into serotypes on the basis of their H flagellar antigens. *Salmonella* that have been commonly isolated from horses include *S. agona*, *S. ohio*, *S. krefeld*, *S. typhimurium*, and *S. newport*.[35, 38]

Source of Organism. *Salmonella* infections generally occur following some alteration associated with the gastrointestinal tract. Organisms may be derived from various sources, such as water and feed or the feces of rodents, birds, and other infected animals, including horses. Activation of the carrier state that may occur has reported to be about 3% to 30%.[35, 38] *Salmonella* infections frequently occur when horses are stressed as a result of poor sanitation; following transportation, surgery, or the use of broad-spectrum antimicrobial agents; or in the aftermath of some diagnostic procedures.

Pathogenesis. Although salmonellae may infect an animal at many body sites, infections are most likely to occur following oral uptake of the organisms, and subsequent survival at local environments such as gastric pH or the absence of a normal bacterial flora that could favor the establishment of salmonellae within the intestinal tract.[35, 39] Establishment of salmonellae within the intestine is dependent on a number of factors, including the animal's health and age, the serotype, and the number of bacteria ingested.[40] The presence of an intact normal microbial flora may preclude the establishment of salmonella by competing for nutrients and keeping the salmonella from making contact with the mucosal cells of the intestine.[35, 39] Salmonellae may remain in the intestinal lumen by attaching to cells through their organelles of attachment, the pili or fimbriae, an example of which are mannose-sensitive hemagglutinins, which are type 1 fimbriae and which may serve as a cellular charge attractant, or through some other cell surface intermediary, such as a mannose-resistant adhesion, which has been identified as a mediator of cell attachment in in vitro *Salmonella* models.[41] Type 1 fimbriae are not essential for adherence in all cases but probably enhance cell invasion.[41] In the case of some *Salmonella*, flagella may have a role in the initiation of infection by enabling the organism to come in contact with the intestinal mucosa.[42] The presence of organisms in the proximity of the intestinal mucosa results in transient enterocyte degeneration, permitting organisms to penetrate the intestinal cells by direct passage through the microvilli or at the intercellular junction, which is otherwise difficult to penetrate.[40–42] The organisms may then cause an enteritis and associated diarrhea by the production of enterotoxin. Enterotoxin causes a flow of fluid into the intestine by altering the flow of sodium, potassium, bicarbonate, and water out of the cell and into the lumen.[35]

Organisms may pass into the enterocyte by endocytosis, which is followed by direct passage to the underlying lamina propria where an inflammatory response consisting of neutrophils and macrophages is elicited.[35] Even though organisms are present within phagocytic cells, *Salmonella* are able to survive intracellularly by one of several mechanisms including tolerance of acid pH, resistance to super oxygen molecules, or by inhibiting phagosome-lysosome fusion, although multiplying *Salmonella* have been recognized within phagolysosomes.[41] *Salmonella* multiply within these cells and eventually destroy them, allowing for dissemination to other areas of the body.[35]

The mediators of tissue damage may include endotoxin, which is released following lysis of *Salmonella*. The absorption of endotoxin occurs even in normal animals in the course of the multiplication and death of organisms that comprise the normal flora.[39, 40] It is only when endotoxin is absorbed beyond the capabilities of fixed macrophages to filter additional endotoxin that resultant elevated quantities lead to the various clinical signs associated with endotoxin activity.[39, 40, 43] When endotoxin enters the circulation, binding to lipopolysaccharide-binding protein (LBP) occurs.[39, 44–46] This complex in turn reacts with receptors on macrophage surfaces to synthesize the inflammatory mediators involved in the pathophysiologic changes associated with endotoxin.[39] However, not all endotoxin binding to monocytes is LBP mediated.[44]

Endotoxin is a heat-stable cell wall component of gram-negative bacteria that is chemically a complex lipopolysaccharide.[40, 47] The polysaccharide portion consists of a conserved core portion that is common to many gram-negative bacteria.[39, 45, 48] This portion imparts to the organism the characteristic of "roughness" of gram-negative organisms whereby some or all of the variable portion of the polysaccharide portion is absent.[39] Strains of enteric bacteria, such as *E. coli* and J5, which contain the rough form of lipopolysaccharide, are being evaluated as a universal immunizing agent for various gram-negative infections.[39, 40, 43, 48] Attached to the core polysaccharide is the more diverse O-specific polysaccharide, which imparts to the various salmonella antigenic variation that results in their serogrouping and may lead to the induction of specific immunity.[39, 40, 47, 48]

The other component of endotoxin (lipopolysaccharide) is lipid A, the portion of endotoxin with which toxicity is generally associated.[39, 40, 48, 49] However, the molecule must occur as intact lipopolysaccharide for toxicity to result. Lipid A is essential for viability of gram-negative bacteria, because organisms that lack lipid A fail to survive.[45] Animals may readily cope with the release of small quantities of endotoxin that occur in the "normal" animal. When released in lesser amounts, the effects of endotoxin may not necessarily be life threatening and in fact may be beneficial. However, in the course of many gram-negative infections, including salmonellosis, intensification of endotoxic effects may result because of the release of greater, and therefore more stimulatory, quantities of toxin. When endotoxins are released at the time of cell lysis, their various pathophysiologic effects may be expressed. The toxic effects are similar regardless of the gram-negative bacterial source of the toxin. Fever results from the action of endotoxin by stimulating the release of various cytokines, such as TNF and interleukin (IL)-1, which are then carried by the bloodstream to act on the hypothalamic thermoregulatory center and act as endogenous pyrogens.[40, 48, 50] In addition to indirectly affecting the thermal regulatory center, endotoxin, through the release of internal cytokine mediators, may also result in the induction of various reactions by the host, some of which may be beneficial, notably T-cell activation, B-cell stimulation, and induction of nonspecific macrophage activity.[47] The reactions that may result, following stimulation by endotoxin, are mediated through the release of endogenous cytokine components, including IL-1, IL-6, and TNF.[44, 49] These cytokines induce a complex interaction of mediators and result in endothelial damage and marked hemodynamic and metabolic alterations.[48, 50, 51]

IL-1, which like other cytokines frequently acts as a cofactor in endotoxic reactions, is produced by mononuclear macrophages, endothelial cells, and blood mononuclear cells.[52] IL-1 has other properties in addition to its fever-inducing properties, including T-cell activation, enhanced nonspecific macrophage defense against infection, as well

as a variety of untoward acute endotoxin-induced effects, including the production of acute phase proteins, such as complement and various coagulation proteins along with the release of neutrophils, insulin, and the adrenal hormones corticotropin and cortisol.[39, 53, 54] IL-1 also mediates the stimulation of endothelial cells, contributing to a procoagulant state, prostaglandin release, and hypotension.[51, 53, 54] The procoagulant effect is associated with a surface monocyte thromboplastin-like component that results in the deposition of fibrin on the cell membrane, which induces the development of thrombi within small blood vessels.[53, 55] A more generalized thrombosis may occur when the procoagulant effect becomes more pronounced.

TNF is also produced by macrophages following exposure to endotoxin, often resulting in a series of complex reactions involving mediators that are produced following TNF release, including IL-1.[39, 46, 52, 54] The elevated levels of TNF in experimental and clinical endotoxemia coincide with the appearance of signs compatible with release of the various mediators.[39] TNF functions as an endogenous pyrogen in conjunction with IL-1. As a result of the action of TNF on endothelial cells, TNF is important in the developing hemostasis and intravascular coagulopathy and contraction of pulmonary smooth muscle.[48, 53, 54] The importance of TNF in endotoxic shock is corroborated by several findings, including increased TNF levels following injection of endotoxin.[54] In addition, signs that follow the injection of recombinant TNF mimic those obtained with endotoxin, and finally, the untoward TNF effects could be eliminated or mitigated by the use of monoclonal antibody.[39, 46, 48, 53, 54] TNF, which is in all likelihood the same as cachectin, is an inhibitor of lipoprotein lipase.[45, 50, 53, 54] Like IL-1, TNF is also associated with the release of prostaglandins and platelet activating factor (PAF) along with other mediators of shock, by increasing vasoactivity, including increased neutrophil adherence, and vascular permeability.[48, 54] As with IL-1, TNF in humans with sepsis, increases in proportion to hypotension and organ failure due to hypoperfusion.[54] Even though there are similarities in signs of TNF and IL-1 activity, the receptors for these two cytokines are different, supporting the fact that these are separate mediators.[50, 52] Nonetheless, TNF and IL-1 act together to stimulate the expression of inflammation, shock, and eventually death in animals in whom endotoxin is serving as a cytokine inducer.[39, 50] Following stimulation of macrophages, TNF is detected in the circulation very rapidly, but after distribution in tissues it is rapidly broken down.[53, 56]

IL-6, along with TNF, has been shown to be elevated in foals injected with endotoxin.[56] In one study, animals given 0.25 μg/kg of body weight of endotoxin, were divided into three groups, two of which were pretreated with polymyxin B or hyperimmune serum against an Re mutant of *S. typhimurium*, a strain deficient in a portion of its LPS polysaccharide.[57] Animals treated with polymyxin B had clinical signs of lesser intensity than did untreated controls. In contrast, in this study, animals treated with *S. typhimurium* antiserum had signs that were more severe than those found in the untreated controls. Explanations for antiserum failure include differences in core structure that limited cross-reaction and failure of the antibody to effectively block the toxic lipid A portion.[57] IL-6 stimulates the differentiation of B lymphocytes into antibody-producing cells as well as its involvement in stimulating the production of hepatic acute-phase proteins.[46, 54] The increase in IL-6 levels coincides with the increase in IL1 and TNF, and IL-6 levels are elevated to a greater degree when stimulation by both IL-1 and TNF occurs.[46, 54] There appears to be a correlation between mortality and elevated levels of IL-6.[46, 54]

Another effect of endotoxin is the activation of complement through the normal or alternative pathways resulting in vasodilation, smooth muscle contraction, and in the case of C5a, the chemotaxis of inflammatory cells.[52, 53] The classical pathway is activated by the binding of lipid A portion of endotoxin to C1 component of complement.[47, 53] On the other hand, activation of the alternate pathway may depend on determinants within the polysaccharide portion of endotoxin.[53]

The biologically active components within the complement cascade stimulate the release of leukotrienes, cyclooxygenase products, platelet agglutinating factor, and toxic oxygen radicals (metabolites), although many signs of endotoxic shock may be independent of complement.[52] As a result of interacting with the macrophage surface, a membrane-bound enzyme, phosphorylase A_2 is activated.[54] Phosphorylase A_2 generates the formation of arachidonic acid.[54, 58] The liberated arachidonic acid is metabolized by lipooxygenase or cyclooxygenase to yield active byproducts.[53, 54] In the case of cyclooxygenase, these end products are prostaglandins and thromboxane A_2.[40] Prostaglandin I_2 causes vasodilation and inhibits platelet aggregation with subsequent inadequate perfusion of tissues.[40, 49, 54] Thromboxane A_2 induces vasoconstriction, which also reduces platelet aggregation.[39, 40, 49, 54] Tissue hypertension mediated by thromboxane A_2 precedes the vasodilation induced by prostaglandin I_2.[39, 54] By increasing platelet aggregation, thromboxane A_2 contributes to the coagulopathy of endotoxin shock.

In the alternative arm of arachidonic acid metabolism, leukotrienes are generated by the action of lipooxygenase.[49, 53, 54] The leukotrienes are vasoactive and chemoattractant.[40, 54] They result in constriction of bronchioles and blood vessels.[40, 53] In addition, leukotriene B_4 is a chemoattractant for neutrophils in inflamed areas, including adherence of neutrophils to endothelial cells and obstruction of capillary blood flow.[40, 53]

With the continued activation effect of endotoxin, dissemination intravascular coagulopathy and organ failure result in the demise of the animal. Endotoxin acts on endothelial cells, but it also activates Hageman factor (factor XII), which results in vasodilation and increased vascular permeability.[54] Activated Hageman factor results in the formation of bradykinin, which is the byproduct of the coagulation system that is responsible for many vascular changes.[52, 54] Endotoxin also induces monocytes and macrophages to produce a number of clot-forming substances, among them coagulation factors VII, VIII, IX, IL1, platelet activating factor, and thromboplastin.[52, 53, 59] Thromboplastin is the procoagulant produced in the highest concentration and is the most active, although its action is dependent on factor VII for expression.[55, 60] PAF may play a particularly important role in endotoxin-associated death. PAF is released by a number of cells, including basophils, neutrophils, endothelial cells, and macrophages.[53, 54, 60] In addition to its role in aggregation of platelets, PAF induces aggregation of neutrophils, causes visceral smooth muscle contraction (e.g., bronchoconstriction) and is associated with cardiac abnormalities such as

arrhythmias.[54, 60] The increase in PAF is followed by a decrease in blood pressure and cardiac output.[53, 54, 60] Other manifestations of PAF include increased vascular permeability resulting in edema to hemoconcentration.[53, 54, 60] It should be noted that PAF antagonists may ameliorate the effects of PAF.[53, 54, 60]

Endotoxic shock in horses is characterized by an enhanced coagulable state that results in the formation of microthrombi, resulting in a decreased tissue perfusion with manifestation such as laminitis and generalized organ failure.[39, 60]

Disseminated intravascular coagulation is an important manifestation of systemic sepsis and is contributory to a fatal outcome of gram-negative infection in animals. It is characterized by thrombocytopenia-increased fibrin degradation products and prolonged prothrombin time.[55, 61] The most likely cause of death in most horses with endotoxic shock is cardiac failure.[54] A more detailed discussion of the pathogenesis of endotoxemia may be found in Chapter 12.

Specimens. In the live animal the usual specimen submitted for culture is feces. It may sometimes be difficult to isolate the organism from infected animals. Several steps may be taken to ensure isolation of salmonellae. These steps may include the collection of multiple fecal specimens over the course of several days, because the shedding of organisms may not occur on a persistent basis, or the use of larger quantities of the specimen or the use of rectal biopsies.[38] It is not unusual for salmonellae to be isolated from animals following necropsy when repeated attempts at isolation in the living animal were negative. In one study, salmonellae were isolated from 52% (34) rectal biopsies and 32% (21) of the concurrently obtained fecal specimens.[62] No complications were observed in the study.[62] In addition to the collection of multiple specimens, cultures must include the use of selective and enrichment media. A typical laboratory procedure would include the inoculation of BA, MAC, and brilliant green (BG) agar plates as well as an enrichment broth, such as selenite BG or tetrathionate broths. The quantity of feces inoculated into enrichment broths is critical, because larger quantities of specimen should improve the chances for the isolation of salmonellae. A pea- to lima bean-sized quantity of fecal material is inoculated into 10 mL of enrichment broth. The enrichment broth is subcultured to a fresh brilliant green agar plate after 12 to 16 hours of incubation at 37 °C to minimize eventual overgrowth by organisms initially inhibited by the components of the enrichment broth. Incubation beyond 16 hours diminishes the efficiency of enrichment broths. Colonies typical of salmonella are then identified using commercial kits or laboratory designed identification schemes. It may be useful to submit cultures identified as salmonella to a reference laboratory for serologic identification. In an animal that is bacteremic, a blood culture may be indicated. Culture with growth should be subcultured on BA and MAC agar plates for isolation, then definitive identification should be made.

In some circumstances, it may be desirable to determine the plasma levels of circulatory endotoxin. The most efficacious procedure used for this determination is a chromogenic *Limulus* amebocyte assay.[55]

NON-SALMONELLA ENTERIC BACTERIA

Organism Characteristics. The bacteria that are in this category and that are more frequently isolated would include: *Escherichia coli, Klebsiella, Enterobacter,* and *Proteus,* but other organisms in the family Enterobacteriaceae may be isolated from infections, especially from wounds and body cavity infections. The first three of the previously mentioned bacteria are collectively referred to as coliforms. These organisms are medium-sized gram-negative bacteria that rapidly utilize lactose. Thus, when cultivated on lactose containing selective media such as MAC, these organisms often yield reactions that are characteristic of rapid lactose fermenters. *Escherichia coli,* which may be mucoid or nonmucoid, and a species of *Klebsiella,* which is mucoid, are more consistent in their morphologic appearance on MAC, whereas *Enterobacter* exhibits more variability in that colonies may appear colorless, slightly pink, or magenta.

While preliminary identification of the coliforms may be suspected on the basis of colonial morphology on MAC, definitive identification is based on biochemical tests using either tubed media or commercially available kits. The other enteric organism commonly isolated from clinical specimens is *Proteus.* This organism is lactose negative on MAC agar, and its growth on BA results in swarming, a phenomenon in which the organism grows over the entire surface of the plate in characteristic waves. Whenever swarming is observed, consideration must always be given to the possible presence of other organisms in the specimen that could be masked by the *Proteus* owing to overgrowth, especially on BA. These organisms must then be isolated by subculture into media that inhibit the swarming of *Proteus,* such as phenylethyl alcohol BA medium if gram-positive bacteria are present, thus allowing the overgrown organisms to grow unimpeded. Swarming is usually not observed on MAC, allowing *Proteus* to be separated from other gram-negative enterics. In Gram stains, *Proteus* appear as medium-sized gram-negative rods, which makes them indistinguishable from many other related enteric bacteria. More infrequently, other enteric bacteria, such as *Citrobacter* or *Serratia,* may be associated with infections. Infections with these organisms often occur at sites where fecal or environmental contamination results.

Pathogenesis. All of the enteric organisms are characterized by the presence of endotoxin in their cell walls, which is released at the time of cell lysis. The signs of endotoxin effects are most apparent when elevated levels of toxin are released and absorbed. The effects of endotoxin have been summarized under *Salmonella* in this chapter and in Chapter 12. While not commonly reported in horses, multiplication of *E. coli* in the gastrointestinal tract of young animals may result in the release of enterotoxin, as LT or heat-labile toxin, or ST or heat-stable toxin, which exert their effects on mucosal cells resulting in water and electrolyte imbalances. An LT-like enterotoxin producing *E. coli* was isolated from the gut of foals, although its role in diarrhea is not well documented and requires additional investigation. In addition to the elaboration of enterotoxin, enterotoxigenic *E. coli* must also possess pilus or fimbrial antigen, which enables the organisms to bind to corresponding receptors on enterocytes. *E. coli* isolates from foals have been identified,

and these isolates possess fimbriae designated as K99 and F41. The adherence of organism to enterocytes places the organism in proximity to the cell where the level of enterotoxin would be elevated.

Clinical Disease. The non-salmonella enterics may be involved in a number of infections. Although not well documented, *E. coli* should always be considered as a possible enteropathogen in foals. *E. coli* is a common isolate from uterine specimens, but its importance may be difficult to establish. Any of the enterics may be isolated from body cavity and wound infections. *E. coli,* perhaps as a result of umbilical infections, is an important cause of septicemia in foals. Related manifestations in septicemic foals are joint infections and central nervous system infections.

Specimens. Infections involving enteric bacteria may be difficult to interpret because of the ubiquitous nature of the organisms. Proper specimen collection is therefore an important prerequisite in order to obtain good results. Of particular importance is the use of aseptic technique in the course of specimen collection. Wound infections must be cleansed with nonantiseptic soap and water prior to specimen collection. Uterine specimens should be collected using a guarded swab, such as a Teglund swab, in order to minimize contamination with vaginal or cervical flora. Aseptic technique should be used to obtain aspirates from body cavities and transtracheal washings.

Laboratory. Infections with many of the enteric bacteria are mixed infections and often contain anaerobic bacteria. A stained smear of specimens from wounds and body cavities should be made to obtain preliminary information regarding the variety and number of different bacterial types present. There could be some confusion between enteric bacteria and other gram-negative respiratory pathogens. Actinobacilli are more commonly isolated from equine respiratory specimens than are enteric bacteria. All specimens should be plated on BA and MAC agar plates, followed by incubation at 37 °C. Because wounds and body fluid specimens also have a high likelihood of containing anaerobic bacteria, some provision for anaerobic culture should be considered.

EHRLICHIA RISTICII

Organism Characteristics. *Ehrlichia risticii* is an equine intracellular rickettsial parasite of white blood cells, especially mononuclear leukocytes, although organisms are found in the enterocytes of the mucosal epithelium as well as macrophages and mast cells. The organism is the causative agent of equine monocytic ehrlichiosis (EME) or Potomac horse fever.[63] The reproductive type of the organism form of the organism is the elementary body, which can be detected intracellularly in monocytes in peripheral blood smears stained with Wright-Giemsa stain or specifically stained using fluorescent antibody techniques.[63] There is cross-reactivity between *E. risticii* and *E. sennetsu.*[63, 64]

Source of Organism. The disease occurs seasonally during the warm months of the year, usually May through September or October, although an occasional infection may be diagnosed during cold weather months.[62–64] The warm weather distribution of the majority of infections suggests that EME is a vector-mediated disease, although evidence indicates that ticks may not be involved in the transmission of EME.[63, 65] It is a noncontagious disease.[63] Accidental transmission may, however, occur through the use of non-sterile injection techniques inasmuch as experimental contamination of blood with tissue culture-derived organisms infected horses.[63] Animals may also become infected by the oral route.[65] Some of the clinical signs associated with EME include fever, listlessness, anorexia, depression, mild to severe colic, leukopenia, followed by leukocytosis and in its advanced stages, diarrhea.[63, 65, 66] The diarrhea that may occur in less than 60% of the cases may be hemorrhagic, and differential diagnosis would include other enteric infections including salmonellosis and giardiasis.[64] In some cases there is concurrent *Salmonella* infection.[64] Laminitis may be observed, but it occurs in fewer than a third of infected horses. There may be up to a 30% fatality rate.[63, 64] Clinical disease is at a relatively low level, less than 5%, except during epizootics when evidence of infection is greater (20% to 50%).[65]

Laboratory Diagnosis. Several different procedures may be used to diagnose *E. risticii* infections. Blood or buffy coat smears may be stained with Wright-Giemsa stain or with fluorescent-labeled antibody. Isolation of *E. risticii* from monocytes or intestinal mucosa may be attempted in cell culture using human histiocytes or canine monocytes and subsequent staining with fluorescein-labeled antibody. Because of the difficulty in culturing the organism in tissue culture systems, relatively few laboratories perform this procedure on a routine basis.[63, 64]

Perhaps the most practical means to identify infected animals is through the use of serology. The most practical method to accomplish this is through the use of indirect fluorescent antibody procedures using infected cell cultures or ELISA.[64, 66] Sera should be obtained as early in the course of disease as possible. Sera may be screened at a titer of 1:20, and sera with positive screening titers are then titrated using serial two-fold dilution to obtain an endpoint. Titers from animals that are ill with EME will be greater than or equal to 1:80.[65, 66] Paired serum samples, one obtained when signs are first observed and a second about 7 days later, should be tested.[65] Ideally, a four-fold increase in titer should be observed; however, if the acute specimen was obtained when the antibody was increasing such an increase may not be observed.[65] Less frequently utilized diagnostic procedures include ELISA, competitive ELISA, and gene probes. A more complete discussion of this disease and the procedures available for diagnosis are described elsewhere in this text.

Immunization. A killed vaccine (PHF-VAX, Schering-Plough, Inc.) is commercially available. In most situations an immunization protocol is recommended twice a year, especially in endemic areas, with the first dose of vaccine being administered in the spring.[65] While absolute protection does not result, immunized animals have clinical signs that are less severe or have a lower mortality rate. Infections do occur in immunized animals, perhaps reflecting the fact that critical protective antigens are lacking in the killed vaccine.[65] It may also be a reflection that CMI may be important. Vaccinal titers may be as high as 1:640, but these disappear over the course of 6 to 9 months.[65]

LEPTOSPIROSIS

Organism Characteristics. Leptospira are organisms that morphologically are spirochetes.[67] They are thin, spiral, or coiled organisms, which may be hooked at one or both ends and exhibit rotational motility associated with the pair of flagella that transverse the full length of the organism and are referred to as axial filaments. The genus *Leptospira* is divided into two complexes. One of these divisions encompasses nonpathogenic, but free-living leptospira that are designated as *Leptospira biflexa*.[67] The second complex, which includes organisms pathogenic for many domestic and wild animals and also humans is designated *L. interrogans*.[67] The pathogenic complex is further divided into several groups of serologically related leptospira that are called serogroups. Within the serogroup are leptospira that share cellular components but that also have unique antigenic constituents of their own. Because of this uniqueness, they are classified as serovars, a nomenclature similar to species designation in other organisms except that the identification was serologically rather than biochemically derived. Thus, as an example, a pathogenic serovar of leptospira would be designated as *L. interrogans* var. *autumnalis*. Restriction endonuclease analysis is a more accurate method used to identify leptospiral isolates. The leptospira, which are more important in horses, include *L. pomona, L. icterohemorrhagiae, L. bratlislava*, and *L. autumnalis*.[67–70, 71] Leptospira are aerobic organisms that utilize fatty acids as carbon and energy sources. Special media (e.g., EMJH, DIFCO Laboratories), are required for cultivation of leptospira.

Source of Organism. The ultimate source of leptospira is an infected animal, either one in which a serovar is maintained as a reservoir host or an animal species to which the leptospira has developed an adaptation, or an animal that is an accidental nonadapted host.[67, 70] Infection occurs following penetration of most mucous membranes or through an abrasion or cuts on skin surfaces. In the infected animal following a leptospiremic phase, organisms are present in the proximal convoluted tubules of the kidney and are shed in urine for varying periods depending on whether a host-adapted or non-host-adapted serovar is involved.[67, 70, 72]

Pathogenesis. After leptospira pass through intact mucous membranes or the damaged barrier of the skin, the organisms enter the circulation and spread hematogenously to various body sites. During the leptospiremic episode, organisms multiply in the liver, spleen, kidney, eye, brain, milk, and developing fetus in gravid animals. At such sites organisms release a variety of metabolites including a hemolysin and lipases, which may be complicated by immune-mediated damage leading to clinical signs associated with the disease.[70, 72] These signs, which may vary depending on the serovar involved, include hemolytic anemia, abortion, mastitis, hepatic abnormalities, and renal failure.[70] Infections with a host-adapted serovar tend to be less severe, and urinary shedding is more prolonged than in infection with non–host-adapted serovars. It appears that in the horse it is likely that serovar *bratislava* is a host-adapted leptospira, whereas other serovars such as *pomona* and *icterohemorrhagiae* are non–host-adapted serovars. With the appearance of antibody, leptospira are cleared from most body sites except those that are sequestered and inaccessible to the antibody. Such sites include the eye, brain, uterus, and proximal tubules of the kidney, the site from which organisms exit the body and contaminate the environment.[67, 70, 72] Clinical signs coincide with the level of host resistance, the virulence of the organism, including the type of toxic metabolites elaborated and the body site that is infected. In horses the observed forms of leptospirosis include systemic infection with kidney localization, which may include sporadic cases of abortion.[67, 69–71, 73]

One study, which examined equine abortions occurring during a 7-year period, revealed that abortions occurred from 140 days to full term of the gestation period.[73] Antibody was demonstrated in 96 of 104 fetuses and stillborn foals after 140 days of gestation and in 104 of 113 aborting mares. In addition, organisms were detected using a direct fluorescent antibody procedure in the placenta and tissues of 56 of 92 fetuses and foals and in the urine of 23 of 76 aborting mares. In all cases, isolates were identified as serovar *pomma* type *kennewicki* by restriction endonuclease analysis. Further documentation of leptospiral involvement was the documentation of organisms compatible with leptospira in kidney and fetal placenta when stained by Warthin-Starry technique.

Immunity. The immune response associated with leptospirosis can be difficult to interpret. The antibody response is serovar and is to some extent serogroup specific.[74] The agglutinating IgM antibody associated with exposure may not be a reflection of an animal's resistance to infection, because serovar-specific IgM retards the growth but does not kill leptospira. Immune lysis of leptospira is generally associated with an IgG class of antibody that appears several days later in infection and is less reliably detected by microscopic agglutination test (MAT).[70]

The immune response may be a reflection of T-cell hypersensitivity to leptospiral antigens, as observed in recurrent uveitis.[69] Alternatively clinical signs of recurrent uveitis may occur because of a cross-reaction between the leptospiral antigen and protein constituents of the cornea and lens.[67, 70] Exposure of the horse to the eliciting agent, in this case leptospiral antigens, leads to the manifestations of the clinical disease. Equine recurrent uveitis associated with leptospira may be difficult to document and is further complicated by the fact that a number of other infections, among which are brucellosis, salmonellosis, toxoplasmosis, and onchocerciasis, may cause uveitis. In several reported cases of equine recurrent uveitis, antibody titers to selected leptospiral serovars are higher in the aqueous humor than are corresponding titers in sera collected at the same time.[69]

Diagnosis. The diagnosis of leptospirosis is usually accomplished by use of a MAT by surveying for antibodies to leptospiral serovars endemic in a given geographic area. Titers in excess of 1:100 are an indication of exposure,

although an evaluation of the titers obtained from paired serum samples is more definitive.[67] Several important aspects of testing must be kept in mind when performing leptospiral serology. A number of clinically normal horses may harbor low serum leptospiral titers.[68, 75] In recurrent uveitis, a more definitive conclusion may be made by determining antibody levels in a carefully collected specimen obtained from the aqueous humor. Chronic recurrent uveitis was diagnosed in a horse in which serum titers to several leptospiral serovars were 1:50 to 1:100, whereas the titer in aqueous humor to *L. autumnalis* was 1:800, while leptospiral titers in the aqueous humor to other serovars were similar to titers obtained in serum. MAT titers in aborting mares may be quite high ranging from 1:1,600 to 3,276,800 in outbreaks where serovar *pomona* was implicated.[73] Other diagnostically useful procedures include culture, direct fluorescent antibody staining of urine sediment, and staining of tissue sections (e.g., kidney or placenta) with Warthin-Starry stain.[73]

Because leptospira require long-chain fatty acids, cultures require the use of special media such as BSA-Tween 80 (e.g., EMIH, Difco Laboratories) supplemented with 100 to 200 μg/mL of fluorouracil to control overgrowth of contaminants. Administration of furosemide enhances the likelihood of leptospiral isolation. The urine obtained from the second urination following administration of furosemide is submitted for culture.[67, 73]

For fluorescent antibody examination, urine is centrifuged, and the sediment is stained with leptospiral conjugate then examined at a magnification of $100\times$.[68, 73]

BORDETELLA

Organism Characteristics. The only species of *Bordetella* that is associated with equine respiratory infections is *B. bronchiseptica*. The organism is a small gram-negative rod to a coccobacillary organism that grows only under aerobic conditions.[72] While *B. bronchiseptica* infections are not as common in horses as other organisms, it should always be considered a possibility when pinpoint colonies are isolated from transtracheal aspirates on BA and MAC media.[72] Susceptibilities are indicated for this organism because antimicrobial susceptibility may be variable.

Pathogenesis. *Bordetella bronchiseptica* has been isolated from respiratory tract infections in horses with variable frequency.[72] The factors that are associated with equine infections have not been elucidated; however, in other animal species, *B. bronchiseptica* can adhere to respiratory epithelium through several intermediaries. These intermediaries include filamentous hemagglutinin (FHA) pertactin and fimbriae. These intermediaries enable bordetellae to adhere to respiratory cilia of infected animals and to resist the action of macrophages, while the production of extracellular metabolites such as tracheal cytotoxin and adenylcyclase toxin may contribute to the establishment of infection in the respiratory tract.[72] The latter toxins may function by inhibiting the action of phagocytic cells and by damaging respiratory epithelium, thus inhibiting the action of cilia. These mechanisms have been studied in other animal species, and presumably similar mechanisms are functional in the horse. Canine isolates of the organism also produce the extracellular enzyme, adenylcyclase, which can immobilize cilia and affect the organism's ability to survive phagocytosis. Other toxins are produced by *B. bronchiseptica*, some of which have been implicated in diseases of other animals, such as atrophic rhinitis in pigs.

Specimens. The specimen to obtain for diagnosis of respiratory infections associated with *B. bronchiseptica* is a transtracheal aspirate. A smear for cytology and for Gram stain may be prepared, but the organism probably cannot be differentiated from other gram-negative rods isolated from aspirates. In a Wright-Giemsa–stained cytologic smear, the organism appears as a blue staining small rod to coccobacillary organism, while in the gram-stained smear the organism will appear morphologically the same but will be pink or gram-negative. The aspirate should be plated on BA and MAC agar plates, followed by incubation at 37 °C for at least 48 hours. The organism grows very slowly on laboratory media. On BA medium, the organism is pinpoint following overnight incubation and reaches 1 to 2 mm in diameter following an additional 24 to 48 hours of incubation. The colonies are tan colored and somewhat dewdrop shaped, with no or weak hemolysis. Colonies also develop slowly on MAC agar. By 48 hours the colonies are about 1 mm in diameter and lactose negative.

Susceptibility tests should be completed on all *B. bronchiseptica* isolates because of the variability of their antimicrobial patterns. Commonly used antimicrobial agents for *Bordetella* infections are chloramphenicol, aminoglycosides, and amoxicillin/clavulanic acid. The susceptibility of the organism to cephalosporins is variable, and the antibiotic should be used only following documentation of susceptibility. The unresponsiveness of *B. bronchiseptica* infections is undoubtedly related to the presence of the organism in the lumen of the respiratory tree rather than in the lung parenchyma. In small animals, medication of this site is often accomplished by nebulization of an aminoglycoside, usually gentamicin.

PSEUDOMONAS AERUGINOSA

Organism Characteristics. There are many species of organism within the genus *Pseudomonas*, but the most important organism routinely encountered is *P. aeruginosa*. Less commonly *P. fluorescens*, and the reclassified organisms *Xanthomonas maltophilia* and *Shewanella putrefaciens* may be isolated from specimens. In some parts of the world *P. mallei* and *P. pseudomallei* are important pathogens of horses. The latter organism causes glanders, and the former organism is associated with pseudoglanders. Pseudomonads are medium-sized, gram-negative, nonfermentative, oxidase-positive bacteria.[76] In the laboratory, all of the organisms will grow only in the presence of oxygen; therefore, they do not undergo fermentative reactions and are thus considered aerobic organisms. However, under growth conditions in which nitrate is used as an electron acceptor, anaerobic growth may occur.[77] They exhibit motility by virtue of polar flagella, which may be a useful identifying characteristic, although staining of flagella may be a tedious and often unrewarding process.[76] The presence of polar flagella, an oxidase-positive reaction, and the inability to ferment carbohydrates differentiates pseudomonads from gram-negative bacteria in the family *Enterobacteriaceae*.

P. aeruginosa and *P. fluorescens*, and *P. putida* fluoresce because they produce a yellow, water-soluble pigment, fluorescein. Pyocyanin, a blue-green pigment, extractable with chloroform, is a metabolite produced only by *P. aeruginosa*.[76] A major concern with *P. aeruginosa* is its resistance to many antimicrobial agents.[76] This is often related to the presence of porins within the cell wall that can restrict the passage of many molecules into the cell, including antimicrobial agents. Of the antimicrobial agents commonly used in equine medicine, amikacin has the best antipseudomonal activity followed by gentamicin, although increased resistance is being observed with the latter antimicrobial agent. Use of ceftazidime has gained some acceptance in veterinary medicine for treatment of animal infections in which *P. aeruginosa* and other resistant gram-negative organisms are involved.

Source of Organism. Species in the genus *Pseudomonas* are widely distributed in nature and commonly occur in water and soil.[76] Pseudomonads are readily isolated from sinks and drains. In some cases, *P. aeruginosa* may be isolated from equine fecal specimens. This could lead to confusion with *Salmonella* in the early stages of laboratory identification, because they appear as lactose-negative organisms on selective media. Because of its ubiquitous nature, contamination of medical instruments with *P. aeruginosa* may occur and may be very difficult to eliminate if not properly disinfected, because *P. aeruginosa* is more resistant to the action of some disinfectants than other vegetative bacteria.[76] This could result in nosocomial infections or could at least yield laboratory results that may be difficult to interpret. *P. aeruginosa* is an opportunistic pathogen.

Virulence Factors. *P. aeruginosa* possess fimbriae that enable them to attach to body surfaces. Cells contain a surface protein fibronectin that inhibits bacterial adherence, and loss or disruption of the fibronectin coating encourages bacterial adhesion. Another adhesin associated with *P. aeruginosa* is exozyme S.[76] In addition, *P. aeruginosa* elaborate a number of potentially toxic substances, including endotoxins, exotoxins, and enzymes, some of which undoubtedly play a role in some animal infections. Enzymes elaborated by *P. aeruginosa* include phospholipases, hemolysins, elastases, fibrinolysin, and collagenase. As with other gram-negative bacteria, *P. aeruginosa* elaborates an endotoxin that can produce all of the systemic signs associated with endotoxin release in infections with other gram-negative bacteria. Exotoxin A is a pseudomonal toxin that is cidal for monocytes as well as bone marrow cells and is lethal for mice following experimental intravenous inoculation. Its toxic activity results from blockage of cell protein synthesis in eukaryotic cells.[76] Some of these enzymes may be associated with corneal damage in pseudomonal keratitis. Pili may also be involved in the adherence of *P. aeruginosa* to corneal tissue.

Clinical Significance. It may be difficult to determine the significance of *P. aeruginosa* in an infectious process. Specimens must be taken in an aseptic manner to minimize contamination; even so it may be necessary to obtain repeat specimens to ensure that the presence of the organism in the specimen is reproducible. In the equine corneal infections associated with *P. aeruginosa*, timely results are important because failure to adequately treat this organism may lead to keratomalacia, with eventual keratorhexis. The organism may be associated with wound infections, and infrequently, uterine infections, including abortions, but in both of these situations good quality specimens must be obtained to minimize the possibility of obtaining spurious results. Mixed microbial infections of the guttural pouch might include *P. aeruginosa*.

Geographically, infection with *P. pseudomallei*, which occurs as a soil organism in parts of Africa, the Far East, and Australia, is referred to as melioidosis.[76] Melioidosis is not a particularly contagious disease. The host range is fairly broad with infections being observed in ruminants, pigs, dogs, cats, and primates as well as horses. Infections follow ingestion, inhalation, or wound contamination and are characterized by abscess formation. The typical infections are chronic with abscesses in various organs and tissues following a septicemic episode. The mechanism of pathogenicity is unknown, except that *P. pseudomallei* elaborates an exotoxin that is similar in action to exotoxin A of *P. aeruginosa*.

P. mallei, a pathogen of the horse, dog, cat, and human, is the etiologic agent of glanders, a disease that occurs in horses and less frequently in carnivores, especially cats. The geographic distribution of this organism includes Eastern Europe, parts of Asia, and Africa. Horses become infected following inhalation of the organism, resulting in lesions in the respiratory tract. Tubercle-like granulomatous abscesses may develop in the nose and other locations, including the respiratory tract and skin. Dermatologic infections occur following contact of the organism with abraded skin. The skin form of glanders is often referred to as farcy. The disease is readily spread from one animal to another and can be fatal if untreated. The most common test to identify infected animals is the mallein test in which a heat extract of a culture is injected intrapalpebrally. Infected animals respond with a delayed hypersensitivity reaction of the eyelid.

Specimens. *P. aeruginosa* grows well on the usual laboratory media. On BA, the colonies will be flat, spreading, and gray, often with a rough surface and an irregular border. A narrow zone of beta (clear) hemolysis will be observed around most colonies. The hemolytic zone may initially be barely discernible but will become more apparent with continued incubation. A distinctive odor may be noted. On MAC, *P. aeruginosa* is lactose-negative, because of the elaboration of a bluish-green pigment that diffuses into the medium. Because *P. aeruginosa* is an aerobe, a biochemical test that is dependent on atmospheric growth should be evaluated. Commercial kits are available, such as API NFT (Bio Merieux Vitek, Inc., Hazelwood, MO 63042-2395).

Variant strains of *Pseudomonas* are isolated. Some of the variant characteristics include mucoid colonies and small (as opposed to the large colonies), flat, spreading colonies of typical isolates, and some may fail to produce pigment.

TAYLORELLA EQUIGENITALIS

Organism Characteristics. *Taylorella equigenitalis* is a gram-negative coccobacillary to rod-shaped organism that is nonmotile and may be encapsulated. The disease caused by this organism is known as contagious equine metritis (CEM).[78] The organism is facultatively anaerobic and requires a 5% to 10% environment of carbon dioxide. Enriched media such as eugon agar, chocolate blood agar, or chocolatized eugon agar prepared with horse blood are preferred.[78] Following 24 hours of incubation at 37 °C, colonies are quite small and rarely exceed 1 mm. *T. equigenitalis* is biochemically rather innocuous, being positive for catalase, oxidase, and phosphatase reactions.[78, 79]

Source. The organism is a parasite of the equine genital tract. Isolation of the organism may be made from the cervix, urethra, and especially the clitoral fossa of mares.[80] In the stallion, the prepuce and urethral fossa are the principal sources of the organism.[78, 79, 81] Stallions harbor the organism within preputial epithelial tissues but exhibit no clinical signs; however, stallions are a source of organisms that are venereally transmitted.[78, 79] In mares, the disease is characterized by a cervicitis and metritis that is characterized by thick, purulent discharge passed from the vagina and results in infertility. Early abortions occur, but these may or may not be observed. Precaution must be exercised to decontaminate any medical instruments used to examine the genital tract to preclude accidental transmission via fomites to other animals.

Virulence Factors. The mare is generally infected by a carrier stallion or organisms obtained following contact with fomites.[78] After multiplication in the distal genital tract, it is probable that infection progresses from an initial vaginitis and cervicitis to a metritis. Virulence factors such as pili or exotoxins have not been identified, nor has the role of the endotoxin been elucidated.

Clinical Signs. The infected male does not exhibit any obvious signs of infection, although the organism may be isolated from the urethral fossa and smegma.[78] In the infected female, the most obvious sign of infection with *T. equigenitalis* is the copious purulent fluid emanating from the vulva.[78] Organisms, some of which are engulfed by phagocytes, are contained in these fluids. The infection appears to be restricted to the mucous membranes of the genital tract.[78] A preferred site for isolation of the organism from mares is the clitoral fossa since the organism may be isolated for extended periods from this location. Swabs used for submission of specimens should be forwarded to the laboratory in Amies Transport Medium with charcoal, using a coolant.[79]

Laboratory Diagnosis. Serology and culture may have a place in the diagnosis of CEM in the mare. Serology is not as useful in the male because infected males do not serologically convert.[78] Carrier females may also be serologically negative. Serologic diagnosis of CEM is accomplished by the complement fixation test in which antibodies are detected somewhat later in the infection.[79] Infected animals have titers that are greater than 1:20. Alternative serologic tests include a passive hemagglutination test, which may be used to detect animals in the early stages of infection.[81]

Enriched media must be used to isolate the organism from clinical specimens. The medium of choice is eugon agar with chocolatized horse blood. Because the specimens from horses are likely to be contaminated with normal flora and environmental bacteria, selective media as well as nonselective media should be inoculated to improve the likelihood of isolation of *T. equigenitalis* from such specimens. Two types of selective media should be utilized. One of these media incorporates 200 µg/mL of streptomycin, while the second utilizes clindamycin at 5 µg/mL, trimethoprim at 1 µg/mL, and amphotericin B at 1 µg/mL in the previously mentioned chocolatized eugon agar. Isolates have been observed that are sensitive to streptomycin.[80] All plates for isolation of *T. equigenitalis* should be incubated at 37 °C in which the carbon dioxide level is 5% to 10%. *T. equigenitalis* isolates should be stained using a Gram stain to reveal gram-negative coccobacillary organisms that are positive when tested for oxidase, catalase, and phosphatase. The organism is otherwise biochemically inactive.

CORYNEBACTERIUM PSEUDOTUBERCULOSIS

Organism Characteristics. *Corynebacterium pseudotuberculosis* is a gram-positive pleomorphic rod-shaped organism, which in stained smears may be beaded and have swollen ends. Colonies of *C. pseudotuberculosis* grow in air at 37 °C. Following 24 hours of incubation, colonies are quite small and generally pinpoint in diameter, and they are surrounded by a weak zone of beta (clear) hemolysis, which is more apparent when the colony is moved. It will also be obvious, when touched with a microbiologic loop, that the colonies of *C. pseudotuberculosis* are not buttery, but rather hard, dry, and crumbly and can be pushed virtually intact on the surface of the plate. The organism is catalase, urea, and glucose positive, but fermentation of lactose, maltose, and sucrose is variable. *C. pseudotuberculosis* interacts with metabolites of *Rhodococcus equi* to produce a characteristic CAMP-like reaction when inoculated on BA medium. In this procedure, an *R. equi* is inoculated in a straight line at right angles to a single streaked line of *C. pseudotuberculosis*. Following overnight incubation, an enhanced zone of clear hemolysis is observed where metabolic byproducts from the two organisms co-mingle.

Source of Organism. *C. pseudotuberculosis* may be found on the skin and mucous membranes of animals. Most infections probably result from injury to the skin following trauma or the bite of an arthropod vector.[82] The organism is most commonly associated with infections in sheep and goats, but these isolates are different biotypes.[33, 83] In horses, *C. pseudotuberculosis* is associated with a form of ulcerative lymphangitis on the limbs or with abscesses of the pectoral and abdominal musculature.[33] In the latter case, internal abscesses may develop following hematogenous and lymphatic spread.[33, 82]

Pathogenesis. The organism is a facultative intracellular pathogen. *C. pseudotuberculosis* elaborates an exotoxin that has activity consistent with phospholipase D.[83, 84] This toxin has been shown to exhibit dermonecrotic activity and is lethal when injected intravenously, but this role may not be critical in natural infections. An alternative activity for this metabolite is as phosphorylase C, which increases capillary permeability.[82, 84] Animals with clinical disease, or animals that are from a locale in which infections occur, have antibody to the exotoxin.[82] The cell wall of *C. pseudotuberculosis* contains a lipid substance that enables the organism to resist phagocytic activity and contributes to reactions that result in abscess formation, a characteristic of infections with this organism, especially in sheep and goats.[84] The role of *C. pseudotuberculosis* metabolites has been implicated in disease in sheep and goats, but their role in the pathogenesis of equine infections has not been established.

Clinical Significance. There are three clinical entities associated with *C. pseudotuberculosis*. In some locations the agent has been isolated from cases of ulcerative lymphangitis. Penetration of the organisms in all likelihood results following traumatic injuries, especially on the limbs of horses.[82] The infection spreads centripetally along lymphatic vessels, and occasionally ulcerated nodules develop along the pathway of the vessels. In the western states of the United States, particularly California, the organism has been isolated from abscesses of the pectoral or abdominal muscles of horses and is commonly referred to as "pigeon fever."[33, 82–84] An arthropod vector has been implicated in transmission of the disease because of the seasonal nature of most of the cases, which occur in late summer or early fall.[83] *C. pseudotuberculosis* has also been isolated from cases of folliculitis in horses.[82] This infrequently recognized infection occurs in skin areas that have been traumatized or that have another underlying condition.[82, 83] Circumscribed nodular lesions that enlarge eventually result in alopecia and crusts. Upon removal of the crusts, purulent exudates may be observed.[82] The lesions may or may not be pruritic.[82] Similar follicular lesions have been diagnosed on horses from which unspeciated corynebacterium has been isolated. Lesions have a dermal distribution that coincides with the use of riding hardware. Trauma and other conditions of the skin may predispose the establishment of the infection.[82, 83]

Specimens. Specimens from horses with suspected ulcerative lymphangitis should have a biopsy obtained from the ulcerated nodule. The nodule is preferred to a swab specimen, because a deeper specimen can be obtained that improves the quality of the specimen and minimizes surface contamination. In addition, *Sporothrix schenckii* is an alternative etiologic agent for this type of lesion, and a biopsy would be a more suitable specimen for both of these organisms.[33] For corynebacterial abscesses, suppurative material from a previously cleansed lesion could be obtained by aspiration of an intact abscess or with a swab from a lesion that has already ruptured. Biopsies from old and maturing lesions should be submitted for culture and histopathology in corynebacterial folliculitis, although histologic examinations have not been found to be particularly fruitful.

The preferred medium for inoculation of specimens is a BA plate. Even though corynebacteria do not grow on selective media such as MAC, selective media should be inoculated in case a pathogen that does is involved. Swab specimens can be directly applied to one edge of the BA, but biopsy specimens should be cut in half or macerated prior to the material being applied to the plate. The BA plates should be incubated at 37 °C, and examined daily. At least 48 hours are required for colonies of *C. pseudotuberculosis* to reach a size adequate for a Gram stain, and biochemical tests could be performed. The key preliminary characteristics of *C. pseudotuberculosis* include weak beta (clear) hemolysis after 48 hours of incubation, a small, gram-positive pleomorphic rod, and a positive catalase reaction. If the specimen is obtained from a case of ulcerative lymphangitis, fungal media such as Brain Heart Infusion with cycloheximide and chloramphenicol (BHICC) should be inoculated with the consideration that *S. schenckii* is involved. In cases of folliculitis where crusty lesions may be observed, the possibility of *Dermatophilus congolensis* must be considered.[33, 82]

DERMATOPHILUS CONGOLENSIS

Organism Characteristics. *Dermatophilus congolensis* is an aerobic filamentous, branching gram-positive organism.[85, 86] Infections are referred to as dermatophilosis, streptotrichosis, or rain scald.[85] The organism forms characteristic filamentous structures that result from the longitudinal and horizontal division within the bacterial filament to form a zoospore.[85, 86] The microscopic arrangement of the zoospores into parallel rows is suggestive of a series of railroad ties, in which each tie consists of a series of coccoid zoospores lined up side by side. The individual zoospores are motile, a property that can be useful for isolation of the organism from clinical specimens when a culture is undertaken to isolate the organism from an infected animal.[85, 86] Even though it is a filamentous organism, *D. congolensis* is not a fungus but has a mucopeptide-containing cell wall that is similar to other bacteria.

Source. Since the organism survives in crust for several months, the major source of *D. congolensis* is an infected animal, which could be another horse, sheep, cattle, or goats or fomites that have been in contact with an infected animal. Flies that have come in contact with an infected area of skin may transfer the agent from one animal to another.[85] The organism may live in crusts for up to 3 to 4 months.[85]

Pathogenesis. Skin that is likely to become infected has usually been moistened or otherwise traumatized by riding gear or biting insects. The zoospores make contact with the surface of the skin, then germinate to form a filament that extends to the viable layers of the epidermis.[85] Infection does not extend to the dermis. An inflammatory reaction ensues, which contains inflammatory cells along with serous exudate.[85, 87] Eventually the thick crusts characteristic of dermatophilosis result. As opposed to remaining in the nonliving keratinized layers, which is characteristic of dermatophytes, infection with *D. congolensis* extends into living tissue. The infective zoospores are attracted to deeper layers of skin by the elevated levels of carbon dioxide found at this depth.[87]

Clinical Signs. The infection is confined to living epidermal tissue, thus restricting infections in horses to skin and hair.[87] The infectious zoospores migrate to the deeper layers of the epidermis where multiplication of the coccoid organism begins, resulting in the formation of the unique filament of *D. congolensis*. An inflammatory reaction develops into the characteristic crusty lesions associated with *Dermatophilus*.[85, 87] Dampness exacerbates the developing lesion.[85] Lesions occur primarily on the back and rump. The crusts may be easily removed as a scab revealing a moist, erythematous area underneath. The lesions, which can be several millimeters in diameter, are unsightly but are usually not pruritic or painful.[85] The lesion must be differentiated from staphylococcal dermatitis, corynebacterial folliculitis, and dermatophytosis.[82]

Laboratory Diagnosis. Crusts collected for diagnostic procedures should be transferred to the laboratory in a container that precludes the trapping of moisture, which would increase the growth of contaminating organisms present within the scab. Rapid diagnosis of dermatophilosis may be undertaken by maceration of the scabs to release organisms within the scab. The scabs should be placed into a suitable vessel, covered with a small quantity of water or saline, and macerated with a glass rod or a pipette. Following maceration, only 0.25 to 0.5 mL of turbid fluid should be present above the scab debris. Addition of too large a volume of fluid could dilute the specimen excessively, making it more difficult to locate small numbers of *Dermatophilus* organisms. The fluid is removed with a pipette. Several drops of macerated crusts are placed on a slide and then spread over an area approximating 1 cm × 3 cm. After air drying and fixation by gentle heat or alcohol, the slide is stained with Wright-Giemsa stain, Gram's stain, or Giemsa stain. After final washing, the stained smears are examined with an oil immersion objective for the characteristic branching and nonbranching filaments of *Dermatophilus*. The arrangement of the spores is such that the filament has the configuration of a series of railroad ties.

The organism will grow on BA under 5% to 10% carbon dioxide following 48 hours of incubation at 37 °C. The organisms are usually β-hemolytic. Smears are often preferred to cultures because of the frequency with which cultures are overgrown with contaminants. If cultures are desired, contamination can be diminished by placing the suspension of macerated scabs in a vessel with elevated carbon dioxide (e.g., a candle jar).[11] The suspension is first held at room temperature for several hours, then placed in the candle jar for about 15 minutes after which time some of the suspension is removed. The motile zoospores migrate to the surface of the fluid layer where they concentrate. The fluid may be drawn off with a pipette and cultured on BA in an elevated carbon dioxide environment. Colonies initially are small and shaped like a dewdrop, and they increase to 4 mm with continued incubation. The color of the colony changes from white to yellow or yellow-orange and is usually surrounded by a zone of beta (clear) hemolysis.

BORRELIA BURGDORFERI

Organism Characteristics. The disease associated with *Borrelia burgdorferi* is commonly referred to as Lyme disease or Lyme borreliosis.[58, 88, 89] *Borrelia* are spirochetes that measure 0.2 to 0.5 μm by 8 to 30 μm. Under a Gram stain the organisms appear gram-negative, but the organism stains very faintly. Other stains such as Giemsa stain or Wright's stain may be used, and these stains are generally preferred. Darkfield microscopy may be used to evaluate motility and loose spirals of viable organisms. *Borrelia* are motile by means of an axial filament, a flagellar-like appendage that traverses the full length of the organism and enables the organism to exhibit motility as the filament contracts and relaxes.[89]

Source. The horse is an incidental host for Lyme borreliosis. The usual infectious pathway involves an ixodid tick in the *Ixodes ricinus* group as the vector and the white-footed mouse (*Peromyscus leucopus*) as the usual intermediate host for the larval and nymph stage with deer (*Odocoileus virginianus*) as the typical final host for the adult in a life cycle that occurs once over a 2-year period.[88] Other animals, including horses, dogs, rabbits, birds, bats, and humans, may become infected when bitten by a stage of tick harboring the organism. Ixodid ticks that have been implicated are *Ixodes dammini, I. ricinus, I. pacificus, I. scapulosis,* and *Dermacentor variabilis,* although the last tick is not a particularly efficient vector.[88–90] *I. dammini* is found primarily in the eastern half of the United States in an area coinciding with the population of white-tailed deer.[88, 89] The ecologic habitat of the tick has slowly widened, perhaps related to the presence of *I. dammini* on birds.[88] *I. pacificus* is found primarily in the western half of the United States. The adult *I. dammini* feed primarily on deer, whereas the tick during the larval and nymphal stages feeds on the white-footed mouse and on other wild animals, including small rodents, birds, and squirrels, thus having a less restricted range.[88] Higher percentages of *I. dammini* (25% to 50%) than *I. pacificus* (1% to 6%) carry the spirochete.[88, 89] Ticks often become infected during the larval stage while feeding on the white-footed mouse.[88, 89] During the larval and nymphal stages, the feeding host's range broadens to include rabbits, birds, squirrels, and the domestic species.[88] The adults tend to feed on large animals including deer, horses, cows, and dogs. Ticks must feed for a sustained period of time (24 hours is adequate) for transfer of the organism to occur.[89] Transovarial transmission occurs but is not particularly important in transmission of the organism within the tick stages.[88, 89] Rather, infections are acquired and transmitted during the larval and nymphal stages of the life cycle.[88, 89]

Virulence Factors. The organism has a number of important detectable antigens, some that may be important determinants of virulence, in addition to being diagnostically useful. Among these antigens are outer surface proteins A and B (Osp A and Osp B).[88, 89] In addition to genes for Osp A and Osp B, other important genes that occur as plasmids have been detected.[88, 89] Several passages of *B. burgdorferi* in laboratory media coincide with the loss of plasmids and subsequent loss of virulence.[88, 89]

Pathogenesis and Clinical Signs. The organism multiplies at the site of the tick bite and eventually becomes bacteremic. Fever, lymphadenopathy, and joint involvement are the major systemic early signs of infection. The major clinical sign observed in horses is lameness due to joint disease, laminitis and cardiomyopathy, and neurologic and ocular manifestations are also observed, although Madigan found

no correlation between serum antibody to *B. burgdorferi* and uveitis in a small population (30) of horses.[58, 88, 89, 91] Since the organism is gram-negative, the release of endotoxin has been implicated as a mediator of clinical signs. Titers to *B. burgdorferi* have been detected in mares with early pregnancy failure, but the study did not establish a causal relation between the two.[91]

Specimens. Culture of the organism is not particularly rewarding; therefore, most diagnoses are based on serologic tests. Selective media are available for culture, and in one report isolation for *B. burgdorferi* from the brain of a horse with encephalitis was made.[90] The most commonly used diagnostic tests are enzyme immunoassay (e.g., ELISA) or indirect immunofluorescence procedures. A comparative study of these two methodologies revealed essentially no difference in the ability of the types of diagnostic procedures to identify infected and noninfected animals.[89, 92] Individual laboratories should be contacted for their interpretation of test results. Attempts at culture of specimens such as blood and cerebrospinal fluid involve the use of modified Kelly's medium, such as Barbour-Stoenner-Kelly medium, an enriched, selective medium.[88–90] The organism grows slowly in this medium, and cultures are often overgrown by contaminants that may be reduced by the addition of antimicrobial agents to the medium.[88] Cross-reactions with leptospira may be observed, but cross-reactive interference should not be considered a major problem.[58, 89, 93] Caution must be exercised when interpreting serologic titers. An elevated titer may simply be a reflection of exposure to the organism and may not be indicative of current disease.[88, 89]

ANAEROBIC INFECTIONS

Organisms. Anaerobic bacteria are widely distributed in the horse's environment. Some of these organisms (e.g., clostridia) may be found in soil and vegetation, in addition to comprising the normal flora of various body sites. The oral cavity, skin, and especially the intestinal tract are sites in which anaerobes comprise a significant portion of the normal flora.[94] The anaerobes that have been implicated in the majority of equine infections include various species of the following genera:[94]

1. *Clostridium*
2. *Propionibacterium*
3. *Fusobacterium*
4. *Bacteroides*
5. *Prevotella*
6. *Peptococcus*
7. *Peptostreptococcus*

Of the aforementioned anaerobic genera, *Clostridium* is a large gram-positive spore forming rod, while *Fusobacterium, Bacteroides,* and *Prevotella* are gram-negative small to filamentous rods. Some of the fusobacteria often contain granules and have pointed ends.[94] *Prevotella,* a newer genus, contains some organisms previously designated as *Bacteroides,* such as *B. melaninogenicus. Peptococcus* and *Peptostreptococcus* are gram-positive cocci.[94]

Source. Organisms may be derived by extension from normal flora sites to wounds, such as injection sites and other traumatic injuries, or following other clinical diseases (e.g., colic, dental injuries). In other cases, contamination by organisms found in soil or fecal material may lead to the establishment of exogenous organisms in wounds and injection sites.

Among the more important anaerobic equine pathogens are the clostridia, which may be found in various environments, including soil, although a number of clostridia may comprise a portion of the normal flora of some body sites including the intestinal tract and skin. The ability of the clostridia to form spores allows the organism to survive until germination and growth occur.

Virulence Factors. The clostridia elaborate some of the most potent exotoxins known. Some of these toxins are released continually during growth of the organism, whereas in other cases the toxin is released when lysis of the organism occurs during the normal growth cycle. The toxin may be released in the course of antimicrobial agent therapy, which leads to cell lysis.[95–98]

Under laboratory conditions of growth, maximal quantity of the *C. tetani* neurotoxin is released at the time of cell lysis, releasing its protoplasmic toxin.[95, 96] The toxin is released as a single peptide, which is cleaved or nicked by proteases into a heavy chain and a light chain, which are held together by disulfide bonds and noncovalent bond mechanisms.[96, 99] The toxin of *C. tetani* that is responsible for clinical signs of disease is a neurotoxin, tetanospasmin, which is produced at a localized lesion and is transported to its site of action in the central nervous system by one of two mechanisms.[95, 96] In the first case, exotoxin may be carried to remote sites through the vascular systems, eventually binding to ganglioside receptors of motor nerves.[96, 99] Movement of toxin may also proceed along peripheral and spinal nerve tracts.[96, 99] The toxin suppresses the release of synaptic inhibitors, resulting in continuous stimulation of muscles by neurotransmitters (e.g., gamma-aminobutyric acid or glycine). Clonic or tonic spasms of skeletal muscle occur, and the effects of the extensor muscles predominate.[95, 96, 99] This type of widespread toxin distribution is associated with more severe clinical signs because of extensive involvement of synapses throughout the body.

C. perfringens and *C. septicum* are associated with infections that may be termed gas gangrene or myonecrosis. Infections by these organisms are more extensive, as evidenced by the fact that larger masses of tissue are involved. The organisms elaborate a number of toxins and enzymes, which result in clinical signs that are similar for several clostridia associated with myonecrosis.[95, 100] *C. perfringens* is particularly active in this respect.

Some of the toxic substances produced by *C. perfringens* include collagenases, proteinases, hyaluronidases, and deoxyribonuclease.[94, 101] *C. perfringens* elaborates four major toxins (alpha, beta, epsilon, and iota) and an enterotoxin.[95, 99, 100] A number of minor toxins are also produced. Necrotizing or lethal properties have been associated with alpha, beta, epsilon, and iota toxins.[99] Epsilon toxin is elaborated as a protoxin that is converted to active toxin by proteolytic enzymes.[99] The four major toxins are used to classify *C.*

perfringens into five types, designated A through E.[95, 99, 100] For example *C. perfringens*, type A, elaborates primarily the alpha toxins, whereas type E *C. perfringens* elaborate alpha and iota toxins. Most animal infections are associated with a type A *C. perfringens*. *C. perfringens* also elaborates an enterotoxin that acts in the small intestine of some animals and results in an inflow of fluid into the intestinal lumen, resulting in diarrhea.[99, 101]

C. septicum produces similar substances that have lethal, necrotizing, and hemolytic exotoxic activities.[99, 100] The toxins of *C. septicum* are designated alpha, beta, gamma, and delta toxins.[99, 100] Infections involving skeletal muscle are referred to as "malignant edema," a form of gas gangrene or myonecrosis, which is characterized by expansive swelling of skeletal muscle following contamination of wounds, usually with spores. Open fractures that become contaminated with soil or feces may contain a number of bacteria, including *C. septicum*.

In addition to gas gangrene some clostridia, including *C. perfringens*, types B and C, *C. sordelli*, and *C. difficile*, have been implicated in hemorrhagic necrotizing enterocolitis.[94, 102] Clinical signs include colic, diarrhea, dehydration, depression, and weakness. Infections may involve portions of the small and large intestines. Organisms may be isolated from the gastric reflux.[94]

C. difficile elaborates an enterotoxin (toxin A) and a cytotoxin (toxin B).[95, 99, 102] The cytotoxin may be the more important toxin, being up to 1,000 times more active than toxin A.[95, 99, 102] Histotoxic damage with toxin B occurs following prior mucosal damage associated with toxin A or by some other mechanism.[102] In humans, *C. difficile* is important in antibiotic-associated gastrointestinal disease, especially following therapy with ampicillin or clindamycin.[95]

C. botulinum has been associated with cases of toxicoinfectious botulism, wound infections, and ingestion of preformed toxin in feeds.[103, 104] There are seven toxin types, A to G, elaborated by *C. botulinum*, all of which are pharmacologically similar but serologically distinct.[97] *C. botulinum* type B is common in the geographical area to the east of the Mississippi River, whereas type A *C. botulinum* is more common in the western United States.[104, 105] The organism has been isolated from necrotic foci such as the stomach, ulcers, wounds, and abscesses.[103, 104] A consistent site of stomach ulcers and erosions in cases of toxicoinfectious botulism was at the margo plicatus.[105] In these cases toxin is produced by *C. botulinum* within the lesion in the gastrointestinal tract. At these sites *C. botulinum* elaborates its toxin, which is then absorbed. The horse is exquisitely susceptible to this toxin.[104–106] The marked susceptibility of the horse to toxin can present a diagnostic dilemma, because the amount of exotoxin that will kill a horse may or may not have any effect on mice, the laboratory animal of choice to detect toxin when injected intraperitoneally. Low levels of toxin may therefore go undetected. Outbreaks of *C. botulinum* intoxication have been associated with bone meal.[104, 106] The types of *C. botulinum* are based on the various toxins elaborated by the organism. *C. botulinum* type B, has been implicated in most of the equine cases. The toxin of *C. botulinum* is also a protoplasmic toxin, which is released at the time of cell lysis at the site of infection or in contaminated feed.[95, 98, 103–105, 107] The released toxin is then absorbed and carried by the bloodstream to neurons, where it blocks passage of impulses to muscle by blocking release of acetylcholine, resulting in a flaccid paralysis. Because horses are very susceptible to the effects of the toxin, absorption of small quantities of toxin is required to initiate clinical signs. In some cases botulism can result from ingesting preformed toxin. In one report, an outbreak of botulism in eight horses was associated with the feeding of alfalfa hay to horses.[98] Organisms and toxin were detected in cecal and colonic contents of some of the horses as well as a sample of alfalfa hay. Death as a result of the toxin action is due to paralysis of the respiratory system and collapse of the circulatory system.[104]

The gram-negative anaerobes *Bacteroides* and *Fusobacterium* are commonly associated with animal infections.[94, 108] These organisms comprise a significant segment of the normal flora of animal intestinal tract, particularly the colon. Recently, some organisms in the genus *Bacteroides* were placed in the genus *Prevotella*. Enterotoxigenic strains of *B. fragilis* have been implicated in diarrhea in foals.[94, 108, 109] Of the most common species of *Fusobacterium*, *F. necrophorum* and *F. nucleatum* are the most frequently isolated from clinical specimens. *F. necrophorum* is probably the more important.[108] The organism elaborates a necrotizing endotoxin and a potent leukotoxin.[94, 108] Clinical specimens from which gram-negative anaerobes may be isolated include pleuritis, peritonitis, wounds, abscesses, and septic arthritis.[94]

Peptococcus and especially *Peptostreptococcus* are isolated from a variety of clinical specimens, including pleuropneumonia and other respiratory infections. Their role in infections has been not well characterized nor have their toxic metabolites been described in any detail. Frequently infections involving anaerobic bacteria also contain aerobic or facultative bacteria, thus treatment must be appropriately directed.

Clinical Signs. A prerequisite for establishment of anaerobic bacteria is a low oxidation-reduction potential that can result from the presence of necrotic tissue following mechanical or chemical injuries or decreased blood flow at the site of infection.[94] Infections involving anaerobic bacteria often occur with aerobic or facultatively anaerobic organisms that can multiply in the presence of oxygen.[94] In the course of an infection, these oxygen-utilizing organisms will preferentially metabolize oxygen, thus creating a more suitable environment for the multiplication of anaerobic bacteria.[94] In the course of microbial growth, metabolites will be released that result in additional tissue damage. The additive effect of these interactions creates a suitable environment for anaerobic infections. These infections are characterized by the presence of necrosis or suppurative exudates, including abscesses, which often have a disagreeable odor because of the elaboration of volatile fatty acids and amino acids by anaerobic bacteria.[94] The involvement of anaerobic bacteria should be considered in abscesses, wounds that sometimes are crepitant, and infections involving pleural and abdominal cavities and sinuses, especially if teeth are involved.[94]

In the case of anaerobic infections associated with the exotoxins of *C. tetani* or *C. botulinum*, the specific targets of the toxins result in a generally predictable set of clinical signs. In tetanus, these signs may include prolapse of the nictitating membrane, extension of the limbs, and convulsions. The lesions in which *C. tetani* multiply may be difficult to locate.[96] The clinical signs of tetanus are associated with the proteinaceous neurotoxin, tetanospasmin.[95, 96] Clinical signs of tetanus in horses include a sawhorse appearance, opisthotonos, and spasms of the larynx, diaphragm, and intercostal muscles resulting in respiratory failure.[96] As with *C. botulinum* toxin, tetanospasmin is a protoplasmic toxin that is released at the time of cell lysis.

Clinical signs of botulism occur in horses following contamination of wounds with *C. botulinum*, by ingestion of preformed *C. botulinum* toxin in feed, or after ingestion of *C. botulinum* organisms that multiply in gastrointestinal lesions (toxicoinfectious botulism) and elaborate toxin.[98, 104, 105, 107] The absorbed toxin blocks acetylcholine release from the neuromuscular junction, resulting in motor paralysis.[103] Signs of botulism include an initial stiffness of limbs, stilted gait, trembling when attempts are made to stand (shaker foal), and recumbency in which attempts to stand are increasingly infrequent.[98, 104, 107] Affected animals are dysphagic and have poor eyelid, tail, and tongue tone.[103, 107] Death results from respiratory collapse.[104, 107]

Several clostridia including *C. difficile*, *C. perfringens*, and types B and C and *C. sordelli* have been implicated in hemorrhagic necrotizing enteritis. Clinical signs include weakness, colic, and diarrhea. Animals that die have hemorrhagic enteritis.

Infections involving anaerobic bacteria, often combined with bacteria that grow under atmospheric conditions, should be considered in sinusitis; body cavity infections; and wound, joint, and bone infections. Attempts to isolate anaerobic bacteria from such body sites require that specimens be collected and submitted to the laboratory, minimizing exposure to atmospheric oxygen.

EQUINE FUNGAL INFECTIONS

General. Fungi are organisms that share general morphologic structure with mammalian cells in that they have a eukaryotic cell structure. In contrast to bacteria, which are prokaryotic, eukaryotic cells have a membrane-bound nucleus, possess cytoplasmic organelles such as mitochondria, have sterols in their cell membrane, and exhibit resistance to common antibacterial antimicrobial agents such as penicillin or gentamicin. While all eukaryotic cell membranes contain sterols, the sterol in mammalian cells is cholesterol, and importantly, the sterol in fungal cells is ergosterol. It is this difference in the sterol component that the selective toxicity of a number of antifungal agents is directed, including amphotericin B, miconazole, clotrimazole, ketoconazole, and itraconazole.

Fungi can occur as molds or yeasts. Fungi that are able to vary from one form to another are termed dimorphic. The basic unit of a mold is a hypha, a tubular structure, which grows by apical extension and branching into a fungal colony, the mycelium. Fungal hyphae are usually septate, but the hyphae of the *Phycomycetes*, such as *Mucor*, are aseptate. Fungal hyphae may differentiate into reproductive structures, including microconidia or macroconidia, or sometimes arthroconidia. Fungi may often be identified on the basis of their macroconidia or the characteristic microconidial-containing reproductive unit. With some molds, the hyphae may be pigmented, usually imparting a pigmented color (e.g., brown) to the fungal elements. Pigmented hyphae may sometimes be seen when microscopic examination is made from a biopsy sample from clinical specimens. These pigmented hyphae may be fungal elements of *Alternaria* if a skin scraping is examined, or, it may be evidence of a pathogen if the specimen is from a case of chromomycoses or maduromycoses. Yeasts are unicellular fungi, in which reproduction is characterized by formation of a bud or blastospore from the mother cell. Yeast cells may be 10 to 20 times larger than bacteria, and their colonies, unlike those of molds, have a buttery consistency like bacterial colonies.

Dermatophytes

Organism. Dermatophytes are mold fungi that infect body tissues that contain keratin (i.e., skin, hair, or hooves [nails]), causing infections commonly referred to as ringworm.[110] Three genera of dermatophytes can cause infections of these tissues, but animal infections are generally associated with only two of them—*Microsporum* and *Trichophyton*.[110, 111] *Epidermophyton* is a human pathogen and is infrequently isolated from animal specimens.

Equine infections are most commonly caused by *Trichophyton equinum* or *T. mentagrophytes*.[112] Less frequently, *Microsporum gypseum, M. canis,* or *T. verrucosum* may also be implicated in infections of the horse.[112]

It is important to understand the variations in fungal morphology that are observed in tissue in the course of infection compared with fungal structures found in culture. Septate hyphae are formed by dermatophytes in the body and in culture. In infected tissue, arthroconidia or arthrospores are formed by both *Microsporum* and *Trichophyton* following hyphal differentiation. Arthroconidia are not produced by dermatophytes in culture. In cultures, *Microsporum* form numerous characteristic macroconidia that may be used to speciate isolates. Species of *Trichophyton* cannot usually be readily differentiated morphologically. Numerous microconidia are usually formed in culture by isolates of *Trichophyton*, but macroconidia occur very infrequently. Furthermore, unlike *Microsporum*, which produce characteristic macroconidia, the macroconidia of *T. equinum* and *T. mentagrophytes* are generally indistinguishable. Some isolates may be recognized as *Trichophyton* because they produce specialized hyphal structures, such as coiled hyphae that bear a resemblance to springs, but coiled hyphae do not aid in speciation. Speciation of *Trichophyton* is usually based not on morphologic characteristics but on the nutritional requirement for specific growth factors, usually vitamins and amino acids.[113] *T. equinum* is able to grow only when the growth medium contains nicotinic acid.

Source. The ultimate source of the dermatophyte, which infects horses, is another infected animal following contact with fungal structures.[112] Indirect transmission results when fomites, including grooming supplies, blankets, and saddles (riding tack), become contaminated with fungal structures.[112] *M. gypseum* is an infrequent equine pathogen, and a possible source of this (geophilic) organism is soil.[110, 112] Infections with human pathogens are possible but are infrequently reported. Direct transmission from one animal to another may occur.[112]

Pathogenesis. Dermatophyte infections arise following direct or indirect contact of the animal with some fungal structure. The infecting structure might be a spore or part of a hypha that contacts nonliving dermal tissue and is able to become established by resisting mechanical removal.[110, 112] To further develop, the dermatophyte must compete with resident microbial flora and resist natural host defense mechanisms.[110, 114] The fungal element will begin to grow in the epidermis, eventually penetrating a hair follicle where hair within the follicle is attacked. Downward growth will continue until viable tissue is encountered.[111, 114] Infection of hair that is in the growth phase will occur, but the dermatophytes do not infect or multiply in hair in the resting stage.[115] Since fungal growth does not continue in resting hair, with time, infection within these follicles may be spontaneously resolved. Establishment of infection is also dependent on the virulence of the organism, the presence of tissue nutrients, and elaboration of fungal metabolites.[110]

Dermatophytes eleborate a keratin-hydrolyzing enzyme, keratinase, and it would be easy to propose a primary role for such an enzyme in pathogenesis.[110, 113, 114] However, some dermatophytes produce relatively small quantities of the enzyme, while other organisms such as *Streptomyces* actively hydrolyze keratin and are essentially non-pathogens. A surface emulsion containing fatty acids, inorganic salt, and protein may inhibit the superficial growth of pathogenic organisms, including the dermatophytes.[110, 114] Tissue iron has been implicated as an important growth factor for dermatophyte infections. The presence of unsaturated transferrin in the skin might lead to binding of iron, making the iron unavailable for the fungus.[110, 114] One of the characteristics of dermatophyte infections is their general aversion for growth in inflammatory lesions.[110, 115] This tends to occur when the dermatophytes elaborate soluble toxins or allergens and is characterized by erythema, scaling, and crusting.[112, 113] Lesions that are highly inflammatory will often resolve without therapy. The inflammation associated with some dermatophyte lesions may be related to immediate or delayed-type hypersensitivity reactions.[110, 114]

Abrasions and maceration of the dermis increase the likelihood of dermatophyte infection by providing a portal of entry.[110, 114] Dermatophyte lesions in horses, especially those associated with species of *Trichophyton*, are not typically inflamed but are generally crusty, though in some horses lesions may appear as vesicles.[112] Pruritus is observed in many cases.[112] Rapid presumptive diagnosis of dermatophyte infections in horses is based on the collection of skin and hair specimens and examining them microscopically following digestion with 10% to 20% potassium hydroxide for 15 to 20 minutes.[113] Other modifications of a microscopic examination of skin scrapings include the addition of dimethylsulfoxide to hasten clarification or the use of chlorphenolac as an alternative clarifying agent.[113, 116]

The specimen should be scanned for evidence of infection using the 10 or 20× objective. At this magnification, infected hair should be examined, beginning at the base end, while looking for loss of normal architecture, such as thickened hair and a darkening in and around the hair. Evidence of dermatophytes may be difficult to observe under low power, unless fungal structures are present in large quantities. Dermatophyte structures that are observed microscopically are hyphae and arthrospores. They are refractile and appear green in color when viewed microscopically. Reliable identification of hyphae and/or arthrospores requires examination of the digest at a magnification of 40×.[113]

Quite frequently, fungal hyphae and macroconidia of environmental fungi may be observed in KOH digests. These fungal elements are often pigmented a golden yellow. *Alternaria* is commonly observed in KOH preparations.

Isolation of the specific agent may be attempted using dermatophyte test medium (DTM) or Fungassay.[112–115] A positive presumptive reaction for a dermatophyte is the development of a red-colored medium within 10 to 14 days of inoculation.[113] Color changes after that time can often be attributable to the growth of environmental contaminants, especially *Alternaria*. Delayed color changes or lack of growth can occur with dermatophytes in cases where antifungal agents were begun prior to specimen collection for culture.[110, 115] Dermatophyte growth results in the development of a red color around fungal growth, which diffuses into the medium beginning as early as 4 to 5 days after inoculation of the medium.[114] With time, there is rapid intensification of this color. Red medium color as a result of growth with contaminants does not usually begin until 10 days after medium inoculation because the cycloheximide in the medium is inhibitory and not fungicidal for contaminant fungi, eventually allowing the contaminant to break through the inhibitory effects of the cycloheximide. The red color develops in DTM because dermatophytes preferentially utilize protein constituents of the medium, producing alkaline byproducts. Saprophytic fungi initially use the carbohydrates in the medium, but with their exhaustion, protein will be utilized, resulting in the development of delayed red color. In addition to delayed growth, dermatophyte growth often may be differentiated from contaminant growth by the color of the fungal colony. In addition to the development of a more rapid red color, dermatophytes are white to buff colored on the surface.[113, 115] The colonial growth of many contaminants is colored black, brown, gray, or green.[112] Contaminant overgrowth may be minimized by cleansing a lesion with alcohol or non-antiseptic soap prior to specimen collection to remove any loosely adhered organisms.

Care should be taken not to overinoculate DTM with skin and hair or to tighten the cap on the DTM because this can encourage contaminant overgrowth.[110] If there is a strong suspicion of a dermatophyte infection in the face of a negative DTM culture, it is possible that isolation of a dermatophyte did not occur because *Trichophyton equinum* has a nutritional requirement for niacin that, if absent from the medium, may preclude growth of the organism.

Identification of species of the genus *Microsporum* is based on the development of numerous characteristic macroconidia. Observations of fungal structures may be made by attaching some of the fungal growth to the adhesive side of clear cellophane tape and placing the tape on a drop of lactophenol cotton blue stain on a microscopic slide.[113, 114] A second drop of lactophenol cotton blue and a coverslip may be placed on the top of the tape.[113] The slide should be scanned with a 10× objective, switching to the 40× objective when more definitive structures such as macroconidiae and coiled hyphae are seen. On the other hand, identification of species of *Trichophyton* is more difficult. Generic characteristics include formation of numerous microconidia, and in some cases formation of specialized hyphal structures,

most notably coiled or spiral hyphae. Characteristic macrospores are not typically formed. Speciation of *Trichophyton* is often based on a determination of the nutritional requirements of the clinical isolates, especially vitamins and amino acids.

CRYPTOCOCCUS

Organism. The major pathogenic species of *Cryptococcus* that is associated with equine infections is *C. neoformans*. There are two varieties, *C. neoformans* var. *neoformans* and *C. neoformans* var. *gattii*.[117] There are four serotypes, A through D, within the species *C. neoformans*.[117] *C. neoformans* var. *neoformans* is a soil organism that is particularly numerous in areas enriched with nitrogenous compounds associated with bird droppings.[117] Birds themselves do not become infected but may distribute the organism in nature.[117] The second variety of *C. neoformans* var. *gattii* (serotype B) has a more restricted distribution, which includes Southern California, Australia, Africa, and Southeast Asia. This variety appears to have an environmental association with the flowery eucalyptus tree, though the growth factor supplied by the eucalyptus tree has not been identified.[117] This organism occurs as a round to ovoid yeast that is surrounded by a large polysaccharide capsule.[117] While in its soil environment, the capsule tends to be smaller, thus facilitating aerosolization of the organism.[117] Newly formed budding organisms are typically attached to the mother cell by a narrow base.

Source. *Cryptococcus* is found in many areas, but especially large numbers of organisms are found where there is environmental enrichment by the creatinine found in bird droppings. Infections usually result following inhalation of organisms, and it has been suggested that the yeast phase as well as the spores of the sexual mold phase may be involved.[117] The yeast cells have smaller capsules, which permits the organism to become airborne. Sinuses are initially infected, with extension to the eye and the central nervous system occurring as frequent secondary manifestations following extension from the primary sinus infection.

Virulence Factors. The virulence of *Cryptococcus* is in part related to the presence but not the size of the polysaccharide alpha-1-3 mannan capsule containing xylose and glucuronic acid side chains.[117] Noncapsulated strains are less virulent.[117] An important effect of the capsule is depression of inflammation and the inhibition of phagocytosis by masking the surface components of the organism.[117] Other effects include activation of the alternate complement pathway by capsular glucuronoxylomannan and inhibition of humoral and cellular immunity, with the latter effect resulting from an increase in the number of suppressor cells that inhibit multiplication of T and B cells. There is some evidence that the extracellular enzyme phenol oxidase may function as a virulence factor. This enzyme converts hydroxylbenzoic substrates (e.g., catecholamine) into brown and black pigments, and this may be correlated with the neurotropism of *C. neoformans* because of the abundance of these substrates in the central nervous system.[117] The presence of this enzyme may protect the organism from oxidative host defenses.[117] Because of the ubiquitous distribution of *C. neoformans* in the environment, it is likely that animals exposed to large numbers of organisms or those with a depressed immune system are more likely to become infected.[117] Successful resistance to cryptococcosis requires intact cellular-mediated immunity.[117]

Clinical Signs. This infrequently occurring infection is most often associated with sinus infections. However, there may be ocular and central nervous system involvement. The eye lesion observed is a chorioretinitis, which may lead to blindness.

Specimens. Diagnosis of cryptococcosis is generally based on recognition of typical organisms in smears following cytologic examination and cultural identification. Nasal discharges may be collected with a swab and then smeared on a slide using a roll smear technique. The smears should then be fixed with alcohol and stained using a staining procedure such as Wright-Giemsa. On smears cryptococci appear as spherical organisms 5 to 7 μm in diameter and have a capsule of varying thickness.[117] Less frequently buds are attached with a narrow base. Nasal exudates should be plated on media that will support the organism and permit its isolation from specimens that are likely to contain environmental organisms. Colonies of *Cryptococcus* may be seen after several days to a week of incubation on Sabouraud's agar plates containing either 50 μg/ml of chloramphenicol or 25 μg/ml of gentamicin and incubated at 37°C. Fungal media that contain cycloheximide should not be used to isolate *Cryptococcus* because this organism and most other fungi in the yeast phase are inhibited by the antibiotic. Blood agar will also support growth of the organism. Colonies are usually cream colored and may or may not be mucoid. On some media, and with prolonged incubation, *C. neoformans* may form colonies that are brown in color because of the production of melanin by phenol oxidase if the medium contains an appropriate substrate (e.g., caffeic acid). It should be noted that the nonpathogenic species of *Cryptococcus* do not grow at 37°C. Yeast colonies may be screened as possible *Cryptococcus* by positive reactions following inoculation of Christensen's urea agar. Definitive identification is based on evaluation of carbohydrate assimilation tests that are commercially available. Colonies suspected to be *Cryptococcus* may also be suspended in India ink to permit visualization of the capsule that surrounds the organism. The organism with its capsule will appear refractile against the dark background of India ink particles. Serologic tests can detect capsular material that becomes solubilized in body fluids. Latex particles coated with rabbit anti-*C. neoformans* antibody are mixed with the body fluid, and agglutination occurs if the capsular antigen is present. The reliability of this test for localized infections is unknown.

SPOROTHRIX SCHENCKII

Organism Characteristics. *Sporothrix schenckii* is a dimorphic fungus in which the yeast phase of the organism demonstrated in tissue is known as a "cigar body" because of its elongated appearance. In cultures incubated at 37 °C, ovoid-shaped organisms and pseudohyphae may be observed in addition to the cigar-shaped forms. The yeast form of the organism is found in specimens from tissue and in cultures incubated at 37 °C, although tissue forms are present in low numbers. The colonies formed by yeast-like colonies are initially cream colored but turn brown with continued incubation. Cultures that are incubated at room temperature will develop into the mold form of the colony, in which septate hyphae are formed, which develop characteristic reproductive structures commonly referred to as flowerettes because some of the microconidia are arranged in a petal-like fashion at the ends of reproductive hyphae, the conidiophores. On occasion, cultures incubated at room temperature may form yeast-like cream-colored colonies that may be somewhat media dependent.

Source. *S. schenckii* is found in soil and decaying vegetation (e.g., peat moss). Infection in animals usually occurs following a wound, most commonly on a limb. Of the domestic animals, horses are most susceptible. Infections are infrequent in dogs and cats, the other domesticated species in which infections have been reported.

Clinical Signs. The organism will multiply in the skin and subcutaneous tissue at the entry site, eventually developing an observable nodule 1 to 5 μm in diameter that often ulcerates. The infection spreads centripetally along a lymphatic vessel and coincides with the appearance of new nodules, some of which ulcerate. An enlargement of the lymphatic vessel may be apparent. Evidence of infection is usually observed on the inner or outer aspects of the limbs. Depending on the nature of the wound, lesions may be detected at other body sites. At the Ohio State University, a case of sporotrichosis was observed involving the perineal region in a mare following trauma incurred after service by a stallion. Histologically, the lesions are granulomatous in nature. Dissemination to other body sites may occur infrequently.

Virulence Factors. Virulence factors have not been identified, but proteases produced by the organism have been implicated in pathogenesis.

Specimens. The preferred specimen for diagnosis of sporotricosis is the removal of a nodule. The nodule should be cut in two, and several serial impression smears should be prepared for staining from the cut surface of one of the pieces. One of the slides should be stained with a Wright-Giemsa stain and examined for evidence of "cigar bodies." If available, a second slide could be stained with an anti-*Sporothrix* fluorescent antibody. Typically, examination of Wright-Giemsa–stained smears has not been particularly fruitful for demonstration of organisms. On the other hand, specifically labeled antibody has been shown to be more useful in this regard.

The cut surface of the other piece is used to inoculate a fungal media such as BHICC, in addition to a BA plate as well as a second fungal medium such as SABGM. The BHICC should be incubated at room temperature, a condition that leads to the isolation of the mold form of the organism. Microscopic examination of a slide prepared from a colony suspected to be *Sporothrix schenckii* should have the characteristic previously described flowerettes. This should be performed only in laboratories with an appropriate biological hood in order to preclude an accidental airborne laboratory infection. Culture media incubated at 37 °C will result in the development of the yeast phase of the fungus. The pasty yeast colony will initially be cream colored but will turn brown after continued incubation. A Gram stain from the colony will reveal the presence of budding yeasts, some of which may appear as pseudohyphae, which are elongated yeast forms that remain attached together.

ASPERGILLUS INFECTIONS

Organism Characteristics. The species of *Aspergillus* are molds that have septate hyphae and produce reproductive structures characteristic of the formation of an aerial hypha, which is swollen at the end and is designated the vesicle. The vesicle is covered by bowling pin-like structures from which are formed unicellular asexual spores—the microconidia or microaleurospores. Importantly, microconidia are not usually formed in vivo except at sites where growth is particularly luxuriant, such as the sinuses, lungs, and air sacs.

The genus is identified on the basis of the formation of the characteristic fruiting body and the color of the mycelial growth. Spore formation coincides with pigmentation of colonial growth on agar plates. Some colonies form green to blue-green colonies, whereas others are black.

Source. Aspergilli are widely distributed in the environment, being found in soil, dust, air, and feed. Infections may follow contamination after direct or airborne contact with fungal elements, including their spores.

Virulence Factors. Aspergilli produce a number of extracellular metabolites, including mycotoxins, for which there is no known role in equine disease. However, the elaboration of proteinases such as elastase may be associated with tissue damage attributable to the organism when ocular infections with this organism occur.

Clinical Signs. The major equine infections associated with species of *Aspergillus* are mycotic keratitis and guttural pouch infections, although other fungi may be associated with either condition.

In ocular infections, fungal airborne microconidia adhere to corneal tissue and form a localized ulcer. The cornea becomes opaque and vascularized. Untreated infections can lead to a deepening of the ulcer and lead eventually to complete penetration of the cornea. Many of the horses that develop corneal aspergillosis have been treated for prolonged periods with topical antibiotic/steroid formulations.

Aspergilli are among several fungi that have been associated with guttural pouch infections. Fungal growth can often be visualized endoscopically on the wall of the pouch. The elaboration of histolytic enzymes could lead to a breakdown of the wall of the guttural pouch as well as the wall of the carotid artery that is nearby, resulting in life-threatening hemorrhage.

Specimens. For a diagnosis of mycotic keratitis, a thin portion of cornea must be obtained using an instrument such as a Beaver scalpel. A specimen can also be obtained by carefully scraping the cornea. The specimen may be forwarded to the laboratory, where a portion of the cornea may be digested with 10% KOH and then examined for the presence of hyphae. Another portion of the cornea may be cultured on a fungal medium such as Sabouraud's agar, containing 25 μg/mL of gentamicin. The organism will also grow on BA. Cultures may be incubated at either room temperature or 37 °C. Colonies will appear in 2 to 3 days and may be microscopically identified by examining tape mounts for the characteristic reproductive structures.

EQUINE INFECTIONS BY BODY SITE

The organisms involved in equine body site infections constitute the isolates that are most commonly obtained and are listed in Figure 2–1. They are by no means the only pathogenic organisms that may be isolated from specimens. In many situations organisms other than those listed might be obtained. In some cases, the bacteria isolated from a clinical specimen may be insignificant and may be reflective of an improperly collected specimen or may be part of the normal flora. It must be emphasized that the quality of the laboratory result in many cases is only as good as the specimen that is presented to the laboratory.

Eye Infections

Many different types of bacteria and fungi may be isolated from eye specimens of normal animals, and these include *Bacillus*, *Corynebacterium*, *Staphylococcus*, *Streptococcus*, and *Moraxella*.[118] Fungi have also been isolated and include species of *Aspergillus*, *Fusarium*, and *Cladosporium* as well as the *Phycomycetes*, which include the genera *Mucor* and *Rhizopus*.[118]

Isolation of these organisms presents a problem in interpretation because many of these organisms are likely to be considered environmental contaminants and may be of little or no clinical significance, especially in the absence of clinical signs.

Several bacteria are commonly associated with conjunctivitis and keratitis. Even in infected eyes, corneal lesions may or may not exhibit ulcerations. β-Hemolytic streptococci, either *S. zooepidemicus* or *S. equisimilis*, are among the more common clinically significant gram-positive bacteria isolated from eyes with ocular disease. *Actinobacillus equuli* and *A. suis*-like organisms are among the more frequently isolated gram-negative bacteria. Neither the streptococci nor the actinobacilli should present any diagnostic or therapeutic problems, except that these organisms are fragile and require submission of specimens in a timely fashion using a moistened polyester swab/transport medium culture system.[118, 119] While most streptococci grow readily on BA, nutritionally variant streptococci, which require supplementation with pyridoxal, have been isolated from specimens obtained from horses with corneal ulcerations.[118, 119] Diagnosis of ocular infections involving *Pseudomonas aeruginosa* must be made with minimal delay because corneal lesions progress rapidly as a result of corneal digestion by pseudomonal enzymes.[118] Proper and prompt selection of an

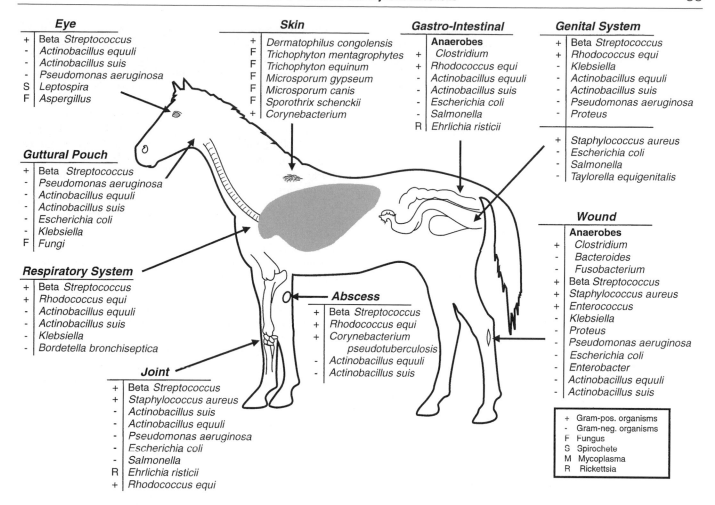

Eye

+	Beta *Streptococcus*
-	*Actinobacillus equuli*
-	*Actinobacillus suis*
-	*Pseudomonas aeruginosa*
S	*Leptospira*
F	*Aspergillus*

Guttural Pouch

+	Beta *Streptococcus*
-	*Pseudomonas aeruginosa*
-	*Actinobacillus equuli*
-	*Actinobacillus suis*
-	*Escherichia coli*
-	*Klebsiella*
F	*Fungi*

Respiratory System

+	Beta *Streptococcus*
+	*Rhodococcus equi*
-	*Actinobacillus equuli*
-	*Actinobacillus suis*
-	*Klebsiella*
-	*Bordetella bronchiseptica*

Joint

+	Beta *Streptococcus*
+	*Staphylococcus aureus*
-	*Actinobacillus suis*
-	*Actinobacillus equuli*
-	*Pseudomonas aeruginosa*
-	*Escherichia coli*
-	*Salmonella*
R	*Ehrlichia risticii*
+	*Rhodococcus equi*

Skin

+	*Dermatophilus congolensis*
F	*Trichophyton mentagrophytes*
F	*Trichophyton equinum*
F	*Microsporum gypseum*
F	*Microsporum canis*
F	*Sporothrix schenckii*
+	*Corynebacterium*

Abscess

+	Beta *Streptococcus*
+	*Rhodococcus equi*
+	*Corynebacterium pseudotuberculosis*
-	*Actinobacillus equuli*
-	*Actinobacillus suis*

Gastro-Intestinal

	Anaerobes
+	*Clostridium*
+	*Rhodococcus equi*
-	*Actinobacillus equuli*
-	*Actinobacillus suis*
-	*Escherichia coli*
-	*Salmonella*
R	*Ehrlichia risticii*

Genital System

+	Beta *Streptococcus*
+	*Rhodococcus equi*
-	*Klebsiella*
-	*Actinobacillus equuli*
-	*Actinobacillus suis*
-	*Pseudomonas aeruginosa*
-	*Proteus*

+	*Staphylococcus aureus*
-	*Escherichia coli*
-	*Salmonella*
-	*Taylorella equigenitalis*

Wound

	Anaerobes
+	*Clostridium*
-	*Bacteroides*
-	*Fusobacterium*
+	Beta *Streptococcus*
+	*Staphylococcus aureus*
+	*Enterococcus*
-	*Klebsiella*
-	*Proteus*
-	*Pseudomonas aeruginosa*
-	*Escherichia coli*
-	*Enterobacter*
-	*Actinobacillus equuli*
-	*Actinobacillus suis*

+	Gram-pos. organisms
-	Gram-neg. organisms
F	Fungus
S	Spirochete
M	Mycoplasma
R	Rickettsia

Figure 2–1. Equine body site infections. (© Kowalski-Vojt, the Ohio State University.)

antimicrobial agent may minimize the damage that can occur in infections with this organism. *P. aeruginosa* is usually susceptible to polymyxin B, with tobramycin, gentamicin, and ciprofloxacin providing other suitable topical antimicrobial choices.

Another organism that provides a diagnostic and therapeutic challenge as a common cause of keratitis is *Aspergillus*.[118, 120] Other fungi such as *Cladosporium* and the *Phycomycetes* (Mucor) may be isolated, but it is likely that in most cases these organisms are environmental contaminants. Occasional isolations of *Fusarium* have been made from clinically affected corneas. Fungal infections appear to occur in animals that have been treated for extended periods with antibiotic or steroid ophthalmic formulations.[120] Since fungi are resistant to the antibacterial antibiotics, fungal overgrowth may result. A laboratory diagnosis may be made by obtaining a portion of affected cornea using an instrument such as a Beaver blade or by carefully scraping the cornea with a scalpel following sedation. The specimen should be examined microscopically, using reduced light, following digestion with 10% KOH or following staining with a Wright-Giemsa stain.[118, 120] Fungal hyphae and arthrospores would be observed on microscopic examination. A part of the specimen should be inoculated onto a fungal medium such as Sabouraud's agar, which contains chloramphenicol

(50 μg/mL), or gentamicin (25 μg/mL) as antibacterial antibiotics in addition to culturing for routine bacterial pathogens. Fungal media containing cycloheximide should not be used, because the antibiotic could completely inhibit or delay the growth of most of the fungi associated with keratitis. Mycotic keratitis has been treated successfully with miconazole (Monistat IV) using subpalpebral lavage through a canula placed in the eyelid so that five or six treatments may be administered daily.[118]

Leptospirosis should be considered in horses that exhibit a loss of vision because of signs of equine recurrent uveitis (ERU, night blindness, periodic ophthalmia).[69] Signs of this condition, which alternate between periods of acute and quiescent disease, would include epiphora, ocular pain, blepharospasm, and a cloudy-appearing anterior chamber of the eye, although uveitis has been reported in the absence of overt clinical signs.[69]

The diagnosis of periodic ophthalmia is never ensured, but several approaches may be used to make a diagnosis, including the evaluation of any corneal lesions by the use of fluorescein dyes, to ensure that there is no corneal ulceration, leptospiral serology, and culture. In some cases leptospira have been isolated from fluids collected from the eye. Several leptospiral serovars have been isolated from cases of ERU, but the most common serovar is *pomona*.[71] Serology may be used for diagnostic purposes, but results may be equivocal. Serologic evaluation should be performed on serum and ocular fluid, and in several cases antibody titers in aqueous fluid were shown to be elevated.[69] Frequently, leptospiral titers in serum do not differ between normal horses and ERU suspects. In general, titers to the leptospiral serovar involved should be higher for the suspect serovar in ocular fluids than in serum. In one report the leptospiral titer was 16-fold higher in the aqueous humor than in serum for the suspect serovar.[71] Titers for other serovars were the same in serum and in aqueous humor. Other infectious agents including onchocercosis, toxoplasmosis, streptococci, and viral agents have been implicated in ERU.

Skin Infections

Dermatologic manifestations of infections in equine skin are most commonly associated with fungi or higher bacteria, although less frequently bacterial pathogens may be involved, including the coagulase-positive staphylococci (i.e., *S. aureus* or *S. intermedius*), streptococci, or corynebacteria. Corynebacteria cause a folliculitis that is manifested as encrusted areas of alopecia, which may be recognized initially as papules and pustules.[82] Specimens should be obtained from a follicle using a swab or a punch biopsy that is forwarded to the laboratory in appropriate transport media such as Stuart's medium.[82] Dermatologic manifestation of *C. pseudotuberculosis* infection may be seen with ulcerative lymphangitis and abscesses of the pectoral musculature and abdominal wall.[33, 82, 83]

Infections with higher bacteria are associated with *Dermatophilus congolensis*. Lesions may vary in size and are crusty with hair protruding through the crusts.[33, 34, 85] Specimens for laboratory examination can be obtained by grasping a tuft of the protruding hair in the involved area and removing the affected area as a crusty sheet, leaving a moist, reddened area beneath.[33, 34, 85] The simplest and most rapid way to obtain a diagnosis of dermatophilosis is to perform a microscopic examination of smears prepared from macerated crusts using various stains, including the Giemsa stain or Wright-Giemsa stains.[85] Smears may be prepared by placing portions of the crusts in a container, such as a test tube, then adding small increments of water and macerating the crusts with a glass rod or similar utensil until the small quantity of water above the moistened scab becomes turbid. The supernate is aspirated, and several drops of the fluid are placed on a glass slide and then spread over a 1 cm × 3 cm area. The slide is air dried the covered with alcohol or gently heated for fixation, followed by staining with a Giemsa or Wright-Giemsa stain for 10 to 15 minutes. After staining, the smears are gently rinsed with water, air dried, and scanned at high power, but definitive identification of *Dermatophilus* requires examination with an oil immersion objective.[85] A smear should be examined for at least 5 minutes before it is deemed negative for organisms resembling *Dermatophilus*. The organism appears as a blue-staining filament or branching filament with the appearance of a series of railroad ties. Cultures for *D. congolensis* are problematic because of the likelihood that the organisms will be overgrown by contaminants found within the scab. Special procedures to isolate motile zoospores may be attempted, but a procedure that is time consuming is generally not attempted.[33, 86]

While isolations of species of *Microsporum*, including *M. canis* or *M. gypseum* from horses may occur, the majority of equine dermatophyte infections are caused by species of *Trichophyton*.[34, 112] Most commonly two species of *Trichophyton*, *T. mentagrophytes* or *T. equinum* are involved, but occasionally isolations of *T. verrucosum* are made.[112] Species of *Trichophyton* do not fluoresce when exposed to a Wood lamp; therefore, a rapid presumptive diagnosis of a dermatophyte would be based on examination of KOH-digested skin scrapings or infected hair for the presence of hyphae or arthroconidia.[112, 121] Definitive identification of a dermatophyte etiology is dependent on the isolation of the organisms on a suitable medium such as Dermatophyte Test Medium (DTM) or Fungassay.[121] It is important to remember that *T. equinum* requires niacin as a growth supplement; therefore, failure to isolate the organism may be a reflection of the absence or inactivation of this essential nutrient.[122] Species identification is based on the nutritional requirement for growth factors by the different species of *Trichophyton*. *T. equinum* and *T. mentagrophytes* are essentially indistinguishable when cultural and microscopic characteristics are evaluated.

While species of *Microsporum* are less frequently associated with horse skin infections, they are more easily identified than are species of *Trichophyton*, because cultures generally yield numerous characteristic macroconidia. Almost 50% of *M. canis* fluoresce, thus this could be a useful though perhaps not practical diagnostic procedure in equine medicine.[112, 116, 122]

Infections with *Sporothrix schenckii*, a dimorphic fungus, generally occur on the limbs because the soil-borne organism can gain entrance most easily through wounds to the skin on the limbs.[112, 116, 122] Clinical signs are characterized by lymphangitis, with the presence of periodic, ulcerating and nonulcerating nodules along the lymphatic tract.[112] Diagnosis of infections with this organism is best accomplished by excision of a nodule followed by culture on BA medium or SABGM (25 μg/mL) incubated at 37 °C to obtain the yeast phase of the organism and a fungal medium such as BHICC incubated at room temperature to isolate the mold phase of the organism. Media containing cycloheximide should not be incubated at 37 °C for any fungus that has a yeast phase, because yeasts are inhibited by this antibiotic.

Examination of stained impression smears for the presence of *Sporothrix* is generally unrewarding, although some measure of success has been reported using specific fluorescent-labeled antibody.[112, 122] The fluorescent reagent is not, however, readily available.

Other fungal infections involving skin and dermal tissue include maduromycosis, which are mycotic granulomas that contain granules or microcolonies of organisms associated with several saprophytic fungi, such as *Helminthosporium spiciferum*, *Curvularia geniculuta*, and *Monosporium apiospermum*.[112]

Gastrointestinal Infections

Without question the single most important enteric pathogens of the horse are the various serotypes of *Salmonella*.[36, 112] Infections are characterized by fever, a range of consistency of stools, and leukopenia at some stages of infection in addition to the clinical signs mediated by the intermediaries such as IL-1 and TNF induced by endotoxin. Several characteristics must be kept in mind when salmonellosis is under consideration. Many animals are asymptomatic carriers of the organisms and may shed relatively low numbers of organisms. Second, even in an animal with clinical signs the shedding of organisms may be intermittent; thus, in either situation, salmonellae may not be detected unless multiple specimens are collected, or in some cases, a relatively large quantity of fecal contents cultured.[38, 123] Utilization of enrichment procedures such as selenite-brilliant green broth should always be included.

Intestinal actinobacillosis is of clinical importance primarily in foals, and alimentary tract carriage by adults may serve as a source of the organism for young animals.[1] Infections are most important in animals younger than 3 or 4 days of age. Signs of infection include diarrhea in 30% or more of infected foals in the first week of life. With the progression of infection, arthritis may be evident, and foals that die may have visceral abscesses, particularly involving the kidneys.[124]

An enteric form of *Rhodococcus equi* infection in foals is characterized by colonic invasion of the organism and the presence of mesenteric lymphadenopathy.[19, 21, 24] Lymph node involvement may result in interference of normal intestinal function and result in signs of diarrhea. In addition, foals may have a potbellied appearance because of weight loss and ascites. Involvement of the mesenteric lymph undoubtedly occurs following infection of the lungs and the development of a cough, whereby organisms are swallowed following expectoration, or perhaps following ingestion of soil-borne organisms.[21]

Clostridial infections usually involve the small or large intestine. Several species of *Clostridium* have been associated with enterocolitis especially *C. perfringens*, types A, B, C, and D, and *C. difficile*.[94, 102, 125] Most of these species may be isolated from fecal specimens in the absence of clinical disease. Infections are characterized by the development a hemorrhagic diarrhea.[102] Diagnosis requires the isolation of the suspect organism and where appropriate demonstration of the toxins as with *C. perfringens* and *C. difficile*. The demonstration of increased numbers of large gram-positive rods may be supportive of clostridial enterocolitis, but this finding should not be construed to be definitive especially in animals that have died because of the propensity for resident clostridia to multiply rapidly in tissues. Specimens for demonstration of toxins should be obtained as soon after death as possible because of the labile nature of some of the toxins.

Escherichia coli has not received significant notoriety as an enteric pathogen of horses or foals, and there are few reports implicating this organism.[126–129]

Infections with *Ehrlichia risticii* should be considered in horses that exhibit a diarrhea that may be bloody, especially during the summer when insect vectors are likely to be a problem. Signs include inappetence, fever, leukopenia, and in some animals laminitis.[64, 66] The diagnosis of EME or Potomac horse fever may be approached in several ways. Giemsa-stained blood smears may be examined in a laboratory with personnel experienced with identification of these organisms. For laboratories that have appropriate cell cultures, isolation of *E. risticii* from the buffy coats may be attempted. For routine purposes, serologic examination of serum using a fluorescent antibody procedure, preferably with paired sera, a practical, cost-effective procedure that is available at a number of laboratories.[64]

Since the clinical signs of salmonellosis and equine ehrlichiosis cannot be readily differentiated, treatment with tetracycline should be considered until serologic test results for equine erhlichiosis are available.

Peritonitis occurs as a secondary condition following any one of several intestinal diseases such as colic, intussusception, or intestinal perforation. There will be a mixed population of bacteria, including facultative organisms such as *E. coli*, *Klebsiella*, or *Proteus* and anaerobes such as *Fusobacterium*, *Bacteroides*, and *Clostridium*.

Enterotoxigenic *Bacteroides fragilis* has been isolated from foals with diarrhea.[109] The importance of this organism as a routine enteropathogen in horses remains undocumented.[109, 128, 129]

Genital System Infections

Genital infections in mares have a major economic consequence. The most convenient way to collect a uterine specimen is through the use of a guarded swab that diminishes contamination.

Viral agents, especially rotaviruses, may be an important cause of diarrhea in foals.[126, 129] Rapid diagnosis may be made using commercially available ELISA tests.[130] Bacteria have been isolated from the vagina, vestibule, clitoral fossa, and occasionally the uterus of normal animals.[130] The greatest variety and number of bacteria are isolated from the clitoral fossa, followed in decreasing order by the vestibule, vagina, and uterus.[130] Some of the organisms isolated from apparently normal animals, especially the clitoral fossa, are *S. zooepidemicus, E. coli*, and other coliforms, and alpha streptococcus as well as anaerobes.[130, 131] Some of these organisms, especially *S. zooepidemicus*, are thought to be among the more important pathogens isolated from the metritis, infertility, and abortion.[132, 133] If there is to be a delay in inoculation of laboratory culture media, the swab should be preserved with a transport medium such as Stuart's medium. Under these conditions, the more common genital pathogens may be isolated even when kept at room temperature for up to 72 hours.

Several bacteria are associated with infertility or abortion. Perhaps the most important of these are the β-hemolytic streptococci, most notably *S. zooepidemicus*, which is the most common isolated organism from equine genital specimens.[133] Less frequently, other β-streptococci, including *S. equisimilis* and occasionally *S. equi*, may be isolated.[132]

Gram-negative enteric-type bacteria such as *E. coli, Klebsiella*, and *Pseudomonas aeruginosa* are isolated from uterine specimens, including abortions.[132–134] No simple criteria are available to designate these organisms as pathogens when they are isolated, and their incrimination as pathogens is difficult to assess because all of the aforementioned organisms may be isolated from normal animals. Many of the organisms comprise the normal flora of the intestinal tract, and contamination of the perivulvular area is to be expected. The cultural reliability of uterine specimens is dependent on the quality of the specimen collected. The numbers of organisms isolated on primary culture and on follow-up cultures may provide useful information. Evidence of inflammation in a uterine biopsy may provide support for an ongoing infectious process.[135] Some serotypes of *Salmonella* such as *S. abortus-equi* have been implicated as genital-specific pathogens, although not in the United States. *Actinobacillus equuli* and *A. suis*-like organisms are potential pathogens because foals infected with actinobacilli often succumb to infections within 24 to 48 hours of birth, possibly following in utero infections.[133]

Coagulase-positive staphylococci (e.g., *S. aureus*) are frequently isolated from uterine specimens, but in most of the cases it is not usually considered significant.[133] However, staphylococci may be associated with important infections of the spermatic cord in stallions following castration.

Taylorella equigenitalis does not cause clinically apparent infections in the stallion. The male is important as a carrier and thus may be an important source of the organism for the mare. Detection of male carriers is best accomplished by culturing the urethral fossa. Infections in mares are associated with infertility and early abortion as a result of metritis, cervicitis, and vaginitis. Thick, white vulvular discharge may be observed. The mucus may be collected with a swab for shipment to the laboratory for culture. The preferred transport medium for *T. equigenitalis* is a charcoal-containing medium such as Amies Transport medium. Transport should not be prolonged beyond 48 hours. The organism will grow on chocolatized media, such as eugon agar in the presence of carbon dioxide. Fungi have been incriminated as causative agents of uterine infections and abortion in mares. Among the more frequently isolated organisms are *Aspergillus fumigatus, Mucor,* or species in the genus *Candida.*[131–134]

Wound Infections

Several important characteristics of wound infections must be considered to ensure that infections are being properly managed. Many of the lesions are mixed infections in which organisms with differing antimicrobial susceptibility patterns are involved. Thus, specimens often yield a diverse population of gram-positive and gram-negative bacteria, including aerobes, anaerobes, and facultative anaerobes, necessitating the use of compatible, but efficacious, antimicrobial combinations for therapy.[136] Satisfactory resolution of wound infections also requires improved local environments through drainage or debridement of infection sites.[136] Bacteria that contaminate wounds may come from a variety of sources including soil, feces, or use of contaminated supplies.[136] Thus, organisms such as *Clostridium, Bacteroides, Fusobacterium, Peptostreptococcus* and gram-negative enterics such as *E. coli,* are frequently found as fecal or environmental wound contaminants.[136]

Another important gram-negative organism associated with wound infections is *P. aeruginosa,* an organism susceptible to relatively few antimicrobial agents such as amikacin and gentamicin.[136] Enterococci and some other gram-positive bacteria are likely to be associated with fecal contamination. Beta streptococci, especially *S. zooepidemicus* are commonly isolated from wound infections.[136] Soil-borne wound infections associated with clostridial gas gangrene or myonecrosis are particularly important. A prominent sign of many clostridial wound infections is swelling and crepitation. Clostridia such as *C. perfringens, C. septicum,* and *C. sordelli* are among the more important anaerobic spore-forming organisms isolated from wound infections.[136] In contrast to the gaseous and gangrenous nature of most clostridial infections, sites contaminated with *C. tetani,* where toxin production plays a prominent role, may be small and difficult to locate. Clinical signs are associated with the elaboration of an exotoxin produced at the site of infection. There should be an awareness of the signs of *C. botulinum* intoxication because of the unique susceptibility of horses.[103, 137]

Abscesses

The most common organisms isolated from equine abscesses are β-hemolytic streptococci. The most important, although not the most frequently isolated beta streptococcus of the horses is *S. equi,* the causative agent of strangles. Organisms may be isolated from nasal discharges and transtracheal aspirates as well as abscesses. The beta streptococcus most frequently isolated from equine suppurative specimens is *S. zooepidemicus.* Biochemical differentiation of *S. equi* and *S. zooepidemicus* is critical because of the similarity in colonial morphology of the two organisms. *S. equisimilis* is isolated from abscesses with lesser frequency than *S. equi* or *S. zooepidemicus,* and unlike the latter two organisms *S. equisimilis* forms nonmucoid colonies when cultivated on BA media.

The formation of kidney and other parenchymal abscesses is common in foals infected with actinobacilli, especially following neonatal septicemia; however, *Actinobacillus equuli* and *A. suis*-like organisms may be isolated from abscesses in horses of all ages.[124]

Rhodococcus equi is an important cause of suppurative bronchopneumonia.[19, 21, 29] Involvement of *R. equi* should be considered in any foal up to the age of 6 months during the months of February to August.[18, 19, 23] In some animals the enteric form of *R. equi* infection may be observed and is characterized by enlargement and abscessation of mesenteric lymph nodes. These animals frequently exhibit signs of diarrhea.[21]

Abscess formation by *Corynebacterium pseudotuberculosis* takes one of two forms, ulcerative lymphangitis and "pigeon breast," a condition in which abscesses are present in the pectoral musculature and abdominal wall.[82, 83] The more commonly recognized infection, ulcerative lymphangitis, must be differentiated from sporotrichosis.[33] Clinical evidence of infection in both of the latter cases generally occurs on the limbs following a traumatic event. Differentiation of the two etiologies is based on culture of tissue biopsy obtained from a nodule and should include a histopathologic examination. Both organisms will grow on BA at 37 °C. *Sporothrix schenckii* may be isolated as a mold on a fungal medium such as BHICC incubated at room temperature and as a yeast on BA at 37 °C, while *C. pseudotuberculosis* will grow on BA. The second form of *C. pseudotuberculosis* is referred to as "pigeon breast" and is a disease that has been diagnosed principally in California and other western states.[33, 83] In this condition, abscesses are associated with the musculature of the chest and abdomen wall.[82, 83] Most of the cases occur during the late summer and may be associated with a currently unidentified insect or arthropod vector.[83]

Fistulous withers is a chronic infection involving the supraspinous bursa.[135, 138, 139] Organisms that have been historically associated with the infection are *Brucella abortus* and *Actinomyces bovis*, although other bacteria have been isolated from infected bursae, including *S. zooepidemicus, E. coli,* and *P. aeruginosa.*[139–141]

The diagnosis would include a routine culture, bearing in mind that *B. abortus* requires use of enriched media and incubation at 37 °C under increased carbon dioxide, whereas *A. bovis* requires anaerobic conditions with increased carbon dioxide. It appears that in recent years involvement of *B. abortis* has been less frequently isolated, and it is likely that *S. zooepidemicus* is the most important organism isolated from these specimens.[140] Serology may also be used to diagnose cases associated with *B. abortus,* although the significant titer for identification of an animal positive with *B. abortus* is inconclusive.[139, 141] Titers of *B. abortus* should be greater than 1:50 and preferably greater than 1:100 or 1:150.[139, 141] Seropositive horses are more likely to exhibit evidence of osteomyelitis on radiographic examination.[139]

Synovial Fluid Infections

Infections involving synovial fluid include the fluid found in joints and tendon sheaths. Joints may become infected by extension of a localized infection into a joint, following hematogenous spread or by direct penetration of the joint.[22, 31, 142] In foals, joint involvement often follows a bacteremic episode.[121] There is often a coexisting osteomyelitis or tenosynovitis.[32, 121, 142] Blood culture media may improve isolation of bacteria because of the neutralization of antibiotics and other antibacterial constituents of the aspirate by components of the medium.[143, 144]

β-Hemolytic streptococci, especially *S. zooepidemicus* and to a lesser extent *S. equisimilis,* are important causes of equine joint disease. *Actinobacillus equuli* and *A. suis*-like organisms are also frequently isolated from equine joints.[121, 142] In actinobacillosis-infected foals that survive the acute septicemic episode for more than 24 or 48 hours, joint involvement along with other manifestations of infection is common.[121] Joint infections with the coagulase-positive organisms, *S. aureus* or *S. intermedius,* while not common, should be considered iatrogenic infections.[22, 31] These infections are invariably associated with a procedure in which joint space was intentionally or accidentally entered. A similar scenario might be proposed for infections associated with enteric bacteria such as *E. coli, Klebsiella, Salmonella,* and *Pseudomonas aeruginosa,* among others, although a hematogenous spread is also an important consideration.[31, 121, 142] *E. coli* is especially important in septic foals.[121] Umbilical infections are an important nidus for the septicemia. All of the above-mentioned infections may be diagnosed by use of routine laboratory procedures, including cytology joint cultures and blood cultures when appropriate. A successful culture of synovial fluid should include the inoculation of broth media and could include the use of blood culture media.[143, 144]

Up to 25% of horses infected with *Ehrlichia risticii* may exhibit signs of laminitis.[63, 64, 66] Many of these animals may also exhibit signs of diarrhea, which is sometimes bloody. The diagnosis of infections may be made by submitting paired sera for fluorescent antibody procedures or, less commonly, isolation of the agent in monocyte tissue cultures.

Respiratory System Infections

Respiratory tract infections involve the lung parenchyma as evidenced by consolidation, atelectasis, and abscesses. In some cases a pleuropneumonia can result in which there is an accumulation of suppurative exudates and fibrin on the pleural surfaces.[145, 146] A variety of anaerobic and aerobic organisms may be isolated from respiratory specimens.

The genera that are associated with the majority of routine respiratory infections in horses are the streptococci and actinobacilli. The β-hemolytic *Streptococcus* that is involved in the majority of cases is *S. zooepidemicus.*[146, 147] Less frequently, *S. equisimilis* and seasonally *S. equi* may be isolated. Either *Actinobacillus equuli* or *A. suis*-like has been implicated in respiratory infections. On some occasions, infections of mixed etiology may be demonstrated.

Bronchopneumonia associated with *Rhodococcus equi* also exhibits a seasonal distribution, with most cases occurring between February and September in foals younger than 3 months of age but may involve animals up to 6 months of age.[147] Respiratory infections may occasionally be associated with other bacteria that can be cultivated under atmospheric conditions, including *P. aeruginosa, E. coli, Klebsiella pneumoniae,* and *Bordetella bronchiseptica.*[146, 148] Perhaps the two most consistently isolated of these organisms are *K. pneumoniae* and *B. bronchiseptica.*

All of the bacteria may be isolated from transtracheal aspirates or bronchoalveolar lavages using routine laboratory cultural procedures.[147]

Quite often Gram-stained smears of pleural fluid or transtracheal aspirates can provide useful information on which to base initial antimicrobial therapy until the results of culture and susceptibility tests are obtained.[147, 148] Gram-positive cocci, especially if chains are observed, would suggest the presence of *Streptococcus,* whereas the presence of gram-negative rods would suggest *Actinobacillus* or an enteric organism. Coagulase-positive staphylococci are occasionally implicated in equine respiratory disease.[146–149]

Demonstration of anaerobic organisms in transtracheal aspirate or bronchoalveolar lavages generally occurs in mixed infections with aerobic or facultative organisms.[145, 147] Species of *Bacteroides* are among the more common isolates, along with species of *Clostridium* and *Peptostreptococcus.*[145, 146, 148] With involvement of anaerobes, the breath of the affected animals or the aspirates may have a fetid odor.

In animals with pneumonia or lung abscesses, infections of parenchymal tissue may eventually involve the pleura and pleural cavity as a pleuritis or pyothorax. Bacteria that may be involved are *S. zooepidemicus, E. coli,* and anaerobes, including *Bacteroides, Fusobacterium,* and *Peptostreptococcus.*[145, 146, 148]

Guttural Pouch Infections

Guttural pouch infections are characterized by the fact that they occur as mixed infections. Often one of the components of the mixed microbial population isolated from guttural pouch specimens is a fungal component, such as *Alternaria* or *Aspergillus*. Clinical evidence of fungal involvement may be obtained by endoscopic examination of the guttural pouch, where a fungal plaque may be observed on the wall of the pouch. Bacteria involved are mixed and may include β-hemolytic streptococci, actinobacilli, *P. aeruginosa*, and the enterics such as *E. coli* or *Klebsiella*.

A washing obtained from the pouch may be examined cytologically for preliminary laboratory information and by culture for more definitive identification of the etiology. Attempts to isolate fungi are best accomplished by utilization of a selective fungal medium, such as SABGM. Guttural pouch infections may be considered life-threatening when fungi are involved, because fungal growth may encroach on the carotid artery and weaken the wall of the artery, which may eventually rupture.

REFERENCES

1. Jang SS, Biberstein EL, Hirsh DC: *Actinobacillus suis*-like organisms in horses. *Am J Vet Res* 48:1036, 1987.
2. Samitz EM, Biberstein EL: *Actinobacillus suis*-like organisms and evidence of hemolytic strains of *Actinobacillus lignieresii* in horses. *Am J Vet Res* 52:1245, 1991.
3. Sweeney CR, Benson CE, Whitlock RH, et al: *Streptococcus equi* infection in horses, Part II. *Compend Contin Educ Pract Vet* 9:845, 1987.
4. Timoney JF: Strangles. *Vet Clin North Am* 9:365, 1993.
5. Sweeney CR, Whitlock RH, Meirs DA, et al: Complications associated with *Streptococcus equi* infection on a horse farm. *J Am Vet Med Assoc* 191:1446, 1987.
6. Timoney JF, Mukhtar M, Galan J, et al: M proteins of the equine group C streptococci. In Dunny GM, Cleary PP, McKay LL, eds. *Genetics and Molecular Biology of Streptococci, Lactococci, and Enterococci*. Washington, DC, American Society for Microbiology, 1991, p 160.
7. Timoney JF: The role of *Streptococcus equi* subsp. *zooepidemicus* in lower respiratory tract infections of foals. *Equine Infect Dis VII*. Tokyo, Japan, 1994, p 319.
8. Poirier TP, Taylor RK, Kehoe MA, et al: Expression of group A streptococcal M protein in live oral vaccines. In Dunny GM, Cleary PP, McKay LL, eds. *Genetics and Molecular Biology of Streptococci, Lactococci, and Enterococci*. Washington, DC, American Society for Microbiology, 1991, p 165.
9. Sweeney CR, Benson CE, Whitlock RH, et al: *Streptococcus equi* infection in horses, Part I. *Compend Contin Educ Pract Vet* 9:689, 1987.
10. Timoney JF, Mukhtar MM: The protective M proteins of the equine group C streptococci. *Vet Microbiol* 37:389, 1993.
11. Galan JE, Timoney JF: Immunologic and genetic comparison of *Streptococcus equi* isolates from the United States and Europe. *J Clin Microbiol* 26:1142, 1988.
12. Causey RC, Todd WJ, Paccamonti DL: Evidence for M protein in *Streptococcus zooepidemicus* isolated from the equine uterus. Equine Infect Dis VII. Tokyo, Japan, 1994, p 360.
13. Timoney JF, Umbach A, Boschwitz JE, et al: *Streptococcus equi* subsp. *equi* expresses 2 M-like proteins including a homologue of the variable M-like protective protein of subsp. *zooepidemicus*. *Equine Infect Dis VII*. Tokyo, Japan, 1994, p 189.
14. Chanter N, Collin NC, Mumford JA: Resistance of *Streptococcus equi* in vitro to equine polymorphonuclear leukocytes. *Equine Infect Dis VII*. Tokyo, Japan, 1994, p 201.
15. Staempfli HR, Hoffman AM, Prescott JF, et al: *Clinical Evaluation of a Commercial M-protein Vaccine in Naturally Infected Foals*. San Francisco, Am Assoc Equine Pract, 1991.
16. Barton MD: The ecology and epidemiology of *Rhodococcus equi*. *Equine Infect Dis* 6:77–82, 1992.
17. Barton MD, Hughes KL: Ecology of *Rhodococcus equi*. *Vet Microbiol* 9:65, 1984.
18. Gaskin JM, King RR, Lane TJ, et al: Serological detection of *Rhodococcus equi* infections of foals. Proc. 8th ACVIM Forum. Washington, DC, 1990.
19. Prescott JF: *Rhodococcus equi*: An animal and human pathogen. *Clin Microbiol Rev* 4:20, 1991.
20. Prescott JF, Hoffman AM: *Rhodococcus equi*. *Vet Clin North Am* 9:375, 1993.
21. Vivrette S: The diagnosis, treatment, and prevention of *Rhodococcus equi* pneumonia in foals. *Vet Med* February, 89:144, 1992.
22. Madison JB, Sommer M, Spencer PA: Relations among synovial membrane histopathologic findings, synovial fluid cytologic findings, and bacterial culture results in horses with suspected infectious arthritis: 64 cases (1979–1987). *J Am Vet Med Assoc* 198:1655, 1991.
23. Zertuche JML, Hillidge CJ: Therapeutic considerations for *Rhodococcus equi* pneumonia in foals. *Compend Contin Educ Pract Vet* 9:965, 1987.
24. Maxwell VA: *Rhodococcus equi*: Pathogen of foals and humans. Proc. 11th ACVIM Forum, Washington, DC, 1993, p 177.
25. Prescott JF, Yager JA: The control of *Rhodococcus equi* pneumonia in foals. *Equine Infect Dis* 6:21–25, 1992.
26. Takai S, Ozawa T, Tsubaki S: Virulence-associated antigens of *Rhodococcus equi*. *Equine Infect Dis* 6:45–48, 1992.
27. Takai S, Takahagi J, Sato Y, et al: Molecular Epidemiology of Virulent *Rhodococcus equi* in Horses and Their Environment. *Equine Infect Dis VII*. Tokyo, Japan, 1994, p 183.
28. Takai S, Koike K, Ohbushi S, et al: Identification of 15- to 17-kilodalton antigens associated with virulent *Rhodococcus equi*. *J Clin Microbiol* 29:439, 1991.
29. Desjardins MR, Vachon AM: Surgical management of *Rhodococcus equi* metaphysitis in a foal. *J Am Vet Med Assoc* 197:608, 1990.
30. Jonsson P, Wadstrom T: *Staphylococcus*. In Gyles CL, Thoen CO, eds. *Pathogenesis of Bacterial Infections in Animals*. Ames, Iowa, Iowa State University Press, 1993.
31. Hanie EA: Antibiotic therapy for infections of skeletal and synovial structures, Part I. *Equine Pract* 11:50, 1989.
32. Hanie EA: Antibiotic therapy for infections of skeletal and synovial structures, Part II. *Equine Pract* 11:7, 1989.
33. Mullowney PC, Fadok VA: Dermatologic diseases of horses. Part II: Bacterial and viral skin diseases. *Compend Contin Educ Pract Vet* 6:s16, 1984.
34. Fadok VA: The Differential Diagnosis of Scaling and Crusting Dermatoses in Horses. Proc. 8th ACVIM Forum, Washington, DC, 1990.
35. Farmer III JJ, Kelly MT: *Enterobacteriaceae*. In Balows A, Hausler Jr WJ, Herrmann KL, et al, eds. *Manual of Clinical Microbiology*, ed 5. Washington, DC, American Society for Microbiology, 1991.
36. Spier SJ: *Salmonellosis*. *Vet Clin North Am* 9:385, 1993.
37. Hirsh DC: *Salmonella*. In Biberstein EL, Zee YC, eds. *Review of Veterinary Microbiology*. Boston, Blackwell Scientific Publications, 1990.
38. Walker RL, Madigan JE, Hird DW, et al: An outbreak of equine neonatal salmonellosis. *J Vet Diagn Invest* 3:223, 1991.
39. Moore JN, Morris DD: Endotoxemia and septicemia in horses: Experimental and clinical correlates. *J Am Vet Med Assoc* 200:1903, 1992.
40. Timmins LM: Management of equine endotoxaemia. *Aust Vet Pract* 21:90, 1991.

41. Finlay BB, Leung KY, Rosenshine I, et al: Salmonella interactions with the epithelial cell. *ASM News* 58:486, 1992.

42. Ginocchio CC: The initial bacterial and host cell events of *Salmonella* infections. *Clin Microbiol Up* 7:1, 1995.

43. Morris DD, Whitlock RH, Corbeil LB: Endotoxemia in horses: Protection provided by antiserum to core lipopolysaccharide. *Am J Vet Res* 47:544, 1986.

44. Prins JM, van Deventer SJH, Kuijper EJ, et al: Clinical relevance of antibiotic-induced endotoxin release. *Antimicrob Agents Chemother* 38:1211, 1994.

45. LeGrand EK: Endotoxin as an alarm signal of bacterial invasion: Current evidence and implications. *J Am Vet Med Assoc* 197:454, 1990.

46. Holbrook TC: Endotoxin tolerance in horses. Proc. 13th ACVIM Forum, Lake Buena Vista, Florida, 1995.

47. Lindberg AA, Karnell A, Weintraub A: The lipopolysaccharide of *Shigella* bacteria as a virulence factor. *Rev Infect Dis* 13:s279, 1991.

48. Bone RC: Gram-negative sepsis: a dilemma of modern medicine. *Clin Microbiol Rev* 6:57, 1993.

49. Cullor JS, Smith WL: Endotoxin and disease in food animals. *Compend Contin Educ Pract Vet* 18:s31, 1996.

50. White SL: Pathophysiology of fever. Proc. 7th ACVIM Forum. San Diego, 1989.

51. Breider MA: Endothelium and inflammation. *J Am Vet Med Assoc* 203:300, 1993.

52. Olson NC, Dodam JR, Kruse-Elliot KT: Endotoxemia and gram-negative bacteremia in swine: Chemical mediators and therapeutic considerations. *J Am Vet Med Assoc* 200:1884, 1992.

53. Morrison DC, Ryan JL: Endotoxins and disease mechanisms. *Annu Rev Med* 38:417, 1987.

54. Morris DD: Endotoxemia in horses. *J Vet Intern Med* 5:167, 1991.

55. Henry MM, Moore JN: Clinical relevance of monocyte procoagulant activity in horses with colic. *J Am Vet Med Assoc* 198:843, 1991.

56. Morris DD, Moore JN, Crowe N: Serum tumor necrosis factor activity in horses with colic attributable to gastrointestinal tract disease. *Am J Vet Res* 52:1565, 1991.

57. Durando MM, MacKay RJ, Linda S, et al: Effects of polymixin B and *Salmonella typhimurium* antiserum on horses given endotoxin intravenously. *Am J Vet Res* 55:921, 1994.

58. Magnarelli LA, Anderson JF, Shaw E, et al: Borreliosis in equids in northeastern United States. *Am J Vet Res* 49:359, 1988.

59. Henry MM, Moore JN: The clinical significance of procoagulant activity in equine colic. Proc. 8th ACVIM Forum, Washington, DC, 1990.

60. Carrick JB, Morris DD, Moore JN: Platelet activating factor: Another mediator of endotoxic shock. Proc. 7th ACVIM Forum, San Diego, 1989.

61. Morris DD, Beech J: Disseminated intravascular coagulation in six horses. *J Am Vet Med Assoc* 183:1067, 1983.

62. Palmer JE: Potomac horse fever: Epidemiology and treatment. Proceedings of the 4th annual veterinary medicine and forum, 1986, p 23.

63. Breider MA, Henton JE: Equine monocytic ehrlichiosis (Potomac horse fever). *Equine Pract* 9:20, 1987.

64. Goetz TE: Equine monocytic ehrlichiosis—EME (synonym: Potomac horse fever). Proceedings of the 4th annual veterinary medicine and forum, 1986, p 17.

65. Palmer JE: Potomac horse fever. *Vet Clin North Am* 9:399, 1993.

66. Rikihisa Y, Reed SM, Sams RA, et al: Serosurvey of horses with evidence of equine monocytic ehrlichiosis. *J Am Vet Med Assoc* 197:1327, 1990.

67. Bernard WV: Leptospirosis. *Vet Clin North Am* 9:435, 1993.

68. Bernard WV, Williams D, Tuttle PA, et al: Hematuria and leptospiruria in a foal. *J Am Vet Med Assoc* 203:276, 1993.

69. Abrams KL, Brooks DE: Equine recurrent uveitis: Current concepts in diagnosis and treatment. *Equine Pract* 12:27, 1990.

70. Heath SE, Johnson R: Leptospirosis. *J Am Vet Med Assoc* 205:1518, 1994.

71. Schwink K, Crisman M, Rigg D: Chronic recurrent uveitis in a horse with an elevated aqueous humor antibody titer to *Leptospira interrogans* serovar autumnalis. *Equine Pract* 11:41, 1989.

72. Bemis DA, Burns JEH: *Bordetella*. In Gyles CL, Thoen CO, eds. *Pathogenesis of Bacterial Infections in Animals*, ed 2. Ames, Iowa, Iowa State University Press, 1993.

73. Poonacha KB, Donahue JM, Smith BJ, et al: The role of *Leptospira interrogans* serovar pomona type *kennewicki* as a cause of abortion and stillbirth in mares. Equine Infect Dis VII. Tokyo, Japan, 1994, p 113.

74. Prescott JF, Zuerner RL: *Leptospira*. In Gyles CL, Thoen CO, eds. *Pathogenesis of Bacterial Infections in Animals*. Ames, Iowa, Iowa State University Press, 1993.

75. Bernard WV, Bolin C, Riddle T, et al: Leptospiral abortion and leptospiruria in horses from the same farm. *J Am Vet Med Assoc* 202:1285, 1993.

76. Gyles CL: *Pseudomonas* and *Moraxella*. In Gyles CL, Thoen CO, eds. *Pathogenesis of Bacterial Infections in Animals*. Ames, Iowa, Iowa State University Press, 1993.

77. Murray PR: *Pseudomonas* and related nonfermenters. In Murray PR, Kobayashi GS, Pfaller MA, et al, eds. *Medical Microbiology*, ed 2. St. Louis, CV, Mosby, 1994.

78. *Haemophilus* and *Taylorella*. In Carter GR, Chengappa MM, eds. *Essentials of Veterinary Bacteriology and Mycology*, ed 4. Philadelphia, Lea & Febiger, 1991.

79. *Taylorella equigenitalis*. In Quinn PJ, Carter ME, Markey B, et al, eds. *Clinical Veterinary Microbiology*. London, Wolfe Publishing, 1994.

80. Engvall A, Olsson E, Bleumink-Pluym N, et al: Epidemiology and control of contagious equine metritis in Sweden. *Equine Infect Dis* 6:89–93, 1992.

81. Eguchi M, Kamada M, Tsukuda S, et al: Use of the modified passive hemagglutination test for detection of *Taylorella equigenitalis* infected mares. *Equine Infect* VII:207, 1993.

82. Heffner KA, White SD, Frevert CW, et al: *Corynebacterium folliculitis* in a horse. *J Am Vet Med Assoc* 193:89, 1988.

83. Welsh RD: *Corynebacterium pseudotuberculosis* in the horse. *Equine Pract* 12:7, 1990.

84. Songer JG, Prescott JF: *Corynebacterium*. In Gyles CL, Thoen CO, eds. *Pathogenesis of Bacterial Infections in Animals*, ed 2. Ames, Iowa, Iowa State University Press, 1993.

85. Evans AG: Dermatophilosis: Diagnostic approach to nonpruritic, crusting dermatitis in horses. *Compend Contin Educ Pract Vet* 14:1618, 1992.

86. *Actinomyces, nocardia*, and *dermatophilus*. In Carter GR, Chengappa MM, eds. *Essentials of Veterinary Bacteriology and Mycology*, ed 4. Philadelphia, Lea & Febiger, 1991.

87. The skin as a microbial habitat: Bacterial skin infections. In Biberstein EL, Zee YC, eds. *Review of Veterinary Microbiology*. Boston, Blackwell Scientific Publications, 1990.

88. Patterson WH: Lyme spirochetosis in equine, bacteriologic, epidemiologic and clinical aspects of *Borrelia burgdoferi* infection in equine. Proc. 8th ACVIM Forum, Washington, DC, 1990, p 677.

89. Madigan JE: Lyme disease (Lyme borreliosis) in horses. *Vet Clin North Am* 9:429, 1993.

90. Burgess EC, Mattison M: Encephalitis associated with *Borrelia burgdorferi* infection in a horse. *J Am Vet Med Assoc* 191:1457, 1987.

91. Sorensen K, Neely DP, Grappell PM, et al: Lyme disease

antibodies in thoroughbred broodmares: Correlation to early pregnancy failure. *Equine Vet Sci* 10:166, 1990.

92. Magnarelli LA, Meegan JM, Anderson JF, et al: Comparison of an indirect fluorescent-antibody test with an enzyme-linked immunosorbent assay for serological studies of Lyme disease. *J Clin Microbiol* 20:181, 1984.

93. Greene RT, Walker RL, Nicholson WL, et al: Immunoblot analysis of immunoglobulin G response to the Lyme disease agent (*Borrelia burgdorferi*) in experimentally and naturally exposed dogs. *J Clin Microbiol* 26:648, 1988.

94. Moore RM: Pathogenesis of obligate anerobic bacterial infections in horses. *Compend Contin Educ Pract Vet* 15:278, 1993.

95. Allen SD, Baron EJ: *Clostridium.* In Balows A, Hauser JWJ, Herrman KL, et al, eds. *Manual of Clinical Microbiology*, ed 5. Washington, DC, American Society for Microbiology, 1991.

96. Bizzini B: *Clostridium tetani.* In Gyles CL, Thoen CO, eds. *Pathogenesis of Bacterial Infections in Animals*, ed 2. Ames, Iowa, Iowa State University Press, 1993.

97. Rocke TE: *Clostridium botulinum.* In Gyles CL, Thoen CO, eds. *Pathogenesis of Bacterial Infections in Animals.* Ames, Iowa, Iowa State University Press, 1993.

98. Wichtel JJ, Whitlock RH: Botulism associated with feeding alfalfa hay to horses. *J Am Vet Med Assoc* 199:471, 1991.

99. Hatheway CL: Toxigenic clostridia. *Clin Microbiol Rev* 3:66, 1990.

100. Gyles CL: Histotoxic clostridia. In Gyles CL, Thoen CO, eds. *Pathogenesis of Bacterial Infections in Animals.* Ames, Iowa, Iowa State University Press, 1993.

101. Niilo L: Enterotoxemic *Clostridium perfringens.* In Gyles CL, Thoen CO, eds. *Pathogenesis of Bacterial Infections in Animals.* Ames, Iowa, Iowa State University Press, 1993.

102. Jones RL, Adney WS, Alexander AF, et al: Hemorrhagic necrotizing enterocolitis associated with *Clostridium difficile* infection in four foals. *J Am Vet Med Assoc* 193:76, 1988.

103. Bernard W, Divers TJ, Whitlock RH, et al: Botulism as a sequel to open castration in a horse. *J Am Vet Med Assoc* 191:73, 1987.

104. Whitlock RH, Messick JB: Botulism in cattle and horses. Proc. 4th ACVIM Forum, Washington, DC, 1986.

105. Swerczek TW: Toxicoinfectious botulism in foals and adult horses. *J Am Vet Med Assoc* 176:217, 1980.

106. Swerczek TW: Experimentally induced toxicoinfectious botulism in horses and foals. *Am J Vet Res* 41:348, 1980.

107. Herbert KS: Botulism can kill. *The Blood-Horse* 23:2002, 1994.

108. Prescott JF: Gram-negative anaerobes. In Gyles CL, Thoen CO, eds. *Pathogenesis of Bacterial Infections in Animals.* Ames, Iowa, Iowa State University Press, 1993.

109. Myers LL, Shoop DS, Byars TD: Diarrhea associated with enterotoxigenic *Bacteroides fragilis* in foals. *Am J Vet Res* 48:1565, 1987.

110. Weitzman I, Summerbell RC: The dermatophytes. *Clin Microbiol Rev* 8:240, 1995.

111. DeBoer DJ, Moriello KA, Cairns R: Clinical update on feline dermatophytosis, Part II. *Compend Contin Educ Pract Vet* 17:1471, 1995.

112. Mullowney PC, Fadok VA: Dermatologic diseases of horses. Part III: Fungal skin diseases. *Compend Contin Educ Pract Vet* 6:s324, 1984.

113. DeBoer DJ, Moriello KA: Clinical update on feline dermatophytosis, Part I. *Compend Contin Educ Pract Vet* 17:1197, 1995.

114. Thomas MLE, Scheidt VJ, Walker RL: Inapparent carriage of *Microsporum canis* in cats. *Compend Contin Educ Pract Vet* 11:563, 1989.

115. Medleau L, Ristic Z: Diagnosing dermatophytosis in dogs and cats. *Vet Med* 87:1086, 1992.

116. Merchant SR: Zoonotic diseases with cutaneous manifestations, Part II. *Compend Contin Educ Pract Vet* 12:515, 1990.

117. Mitchell TG, Perfect JR: Cryptococcosis in the era of AIDS—100 years after the discovery of *Cryptococcus neoformans. Clin Microbiol Rev* 8:515, 1995.

118. McLaughlin SA, Gilger BC, Whitley RD: Infectious keratitis in horses: Evaluation and management. *Compend Contin Educ Pract Vet* 14:372, 1992.

119. da Silva Curiel JMA, Murphy CJ, Jang SS, et al: Nutritionally variant streptococci associated with corneal ulcers in horses: 35 cases (1982–1988). *J Am Vet Med Assoc* 197:624, 1990.

120. Coad CT, Robinson NM, Wilhelmus KR: Antifungal sensitivity testing for equine keratomycosis. *Am J Vet Res* 46:676, 1985.

121. Brewer BD, Koterba AM: Bacterial isolates and susceptibility patterns in a neonatal intensive care unit. *Compend Contin Educ Pract Vet* 12:1773, 1990.

122. Equine Dermatology. Proc. 8th ACVIM Forum, Washington, DC, 1990.

123. Palmer JE, Whitlock RH, Benson CE, et al: Comparison of rectal mucosal cultures and fecal cultures in detecting *Salmonella* infection in horses and cattle. *Am J Vet Res* 46:697, 1985.

124. Morris DD: Bacterial infections of the newborn foal. Part I: Clinical presentation, laboratory findings, and pathogenesis. *Compend Contin Educ Pract Vet* 6:s332, 1984.

125. Cudd TA, Pauly TH: Necrotizing enterocolitis in two equine neonates. *Compend Contin Educ Pract Vet* 9:88, 1987.

126. Holland RE, Sriranganathan N, DuPont L: Isolation of enterotoxigenic *Escherichia coli* from a foal with diarrhea. *J Am Vet Med Assoc* 194:389, 1989.

127. Ward ACS, Sriranganathan N, Evermann JF, et al: Isolation of piliated *Escherichia coli* from diarrheic foals. *Vet Microbiol* 12:221, 1986.

128. Holland RE, Schmidt A, Sriranganathan N, et al: Survey of infectious causes of diarrhoea in foals. *Equine Infect Dis* 6:55–60, 1992.

129. Traub-Dargatz JL, Gay CC, Evermann JF, et al: Epidemiologic survey of diarrhea in foals. *J Am Vet Med Assoc* 192:1553, 1988.

130. Hinrichs K, Cummings MR, Sertich PL, et al: Clinical significance of aerobic bacterial flora of the uterus, vagina, vestibule, and clitoral fossa of clinically normal mares. *J Am Vet Med Assoc* 193:72, 1988.

131. Liu IKM: Uterine infections in the mare. *Equine Pract* 11:26, 1989.

132. Swerczek TW: Identifying the bacterial causes of abortion in mares. *Vet Med* 86:1210, 1991.

133. Giles RC, Donahue JM, Hong CB, et al: Causes of abortion, stillbirth, and perinatal death in horses: 3,527 cases (1986–1991). *J Am Vet Med Assoc* 203:1170, 1993.

134. Acland HM: Abortion in mares: Diagnosis and prevention. *Compend Contin Educ Pract Vet* 9:318, 1987.

135. Jasko DJ: Endometritis and cervicitis in a mare. *Compend Contin Educ Pract Vet* 9:329, 1987.

136. Lundin CM: Antimicrobial therapy for soft tissue infections in the horse. *Equine Pract* 12:35, 1990.

137. Mitten LA, Hinchcliff KW, Holcombe SJ, et al: Mechanical ventilation and management of botulism secondary to an injection abscess in an adult horse. *Equine Vet J* 26:420, 1994.

138. Swerczek TW: Identifying the mycotic causes of abortion in mares. *Vet Med* 87:62, 1992.

139. Cohen ND, McMullan WC, Carter GK: Fistulous withers: The diagnosis and treatment of open and closed lesions. *Vet Med* 86:416, 1991.

140. Gaughan EM, Fubini SL, Dietze A: Fistulous withers in

horses: 14 cases (1978–1987). *J Am Vet Med Assoc* 193:964, 1988.

141. Rashmir-Raven A, Gaughan EM, Modransky P, et al: Fistulous withers. *Compend Contin Educ Pract Vet* 12:1633, 1990.

142. Martens RJ, Auer JA, Carter GK: Equine pediatrics: Septic arthritis and osteomyelitis. *J Am Vet Med Assoc* 188:582, 1986.

143. Montgomery RD, Long IR, Milton JL, et al: Comparison of aerobic culturette, synovial membrane biopsy, and blood culture medium in detection of canine bacterial arthritis. *Vet Surg* 18:300, 1989.

144. Honnas CM, Schumacher J, Cohen ND, et al: Septic tenosynovitis in horses: 25 cases (1983–1989). *J Am Vet Med Assoc* 199:1616, 1991.

145. Pipers FS: Pathophysiology of pleuropneumonia in the equine. Proc. 7th ACVIM Forum, San Diego, 1989.

146. Sweeney CR, Holcombe SJ, Barningham SC, et al: Aerobic and anaerobic bacterial isolates from horses with pneumonia or pleuropneumonia and antimicrobial susceptibility patterns of the aerobes. *J Am Vet Med Assoc* 198:839, 1991.

147. Spurlock SL: Antimicrobial use in equine respiratory disease. *Equine Pract* 11:6, 1989.

148. Chaffin MK, Carter GK, Byars TD: Equine bacterial pleuropneumonia. Part III: Treatment, sequelae, and prognosis. *Compend Contin Educ Pract Vet* 16:1585, 1994.

149. Spurlock SL, Spurlock GH, Donaldson LL: Consolidating pneumonia and pneumothorax in a horse. *J Am Vet Med Assoc* 192:1081, 1988.

2.2

Respiratory Viral Diseases

E. Chirnside, BSc, PhD
R. Sinclair, BSc, PhD
J.A. Mumford, BSc, PhD

VIRAL ARTERITIS

Although equine viral arteritis (EVA) has been known for almost 40 years, disease outbreaks are identified infrequently and field isolates of the causative agent, equine arteritis virus, are rare. The only reported host for EVA is the horse, in which clinical signs of infection vary widely, with the most severe form of infection causing abortion. Two important routes for transmission of viral arteritis are venereal infection, when a susceptible mare is served by a carrier stallion or inseminated with infected semen, and aerosol spread of EVA in respiratory secretions of an acutely infected horse. Carrier stallions, shedding virus in semen, act as a reservoir of the disease long after an outbreak has occurred. The prevention and control of outbreaks of EVA is largely dependent on continuous surveillance and detection of carrier stallions.

Etiologic Agent

EVA is a small, enveloped, positive-stranded RNA virus. The virion has a diameter of 50 to 70 nm and consists of an isometric nucleocapsid (35 nm) surrounded by an envelope that carries ring-like subunits with a diameter of 12 to 15 nm.[1-3] The nucleocapsid consists of an infectious, polyadenylated, single-stranded genomic RNA with a size of 12.7 kb and a 12 kD phosphorylated core protein (N).[1, 4-6] The envelope contains a 16-kDa non-glycosylated protein (M) and two further glycosylated proteins of 21 kD (G;) and 30 to 42 kD (G_l).

The virion is resistant to trypsin and survives freeze-drying and long storage at −70 °C. EVA is sensitive to ether; is inactivated by 1M magnesium chloride at 50 °C; and is reliably destroyed by a 1:32 dilution of a commercial sodium hypochlorite solution (Chloros).[7]

In contrast to alpha and rubiviruses, assembly of EVA occurs solely by intracellular budding.[8] During virus replication, a nested set of six subgenomic RNAs are synthesised in EVA-infected cells in addition to genomic RNA.[9] In view of these observations, EVA has been assigned to the novel genus arterivirus.[10] The nucleotide sequence of the genome of EVA contains eight overlapping open reading frames (ORFs).[4] The organization and expression of the EVA genome is remarkably similar to those of coronaviruses (infectious bursal disease virus, IBV; transmissible gastroenteritis virus, TGEV; feline infectious peritonitis virus, FIP; mouse hepatitis virus, MHV), and toroviruses (Berne virus, Breda virus) with a gene order 5′ replicase-envelope-nucleocapsid 3′. However, the virion architecture of EVA is fundamentally different from the coronaviruses and toroviruses and more closely resembles lactate dehydrogenase-elevating virus (LDV) and simian hemorrhagic fever virus (SHFV). Evidence is accumulating that the virus causing porcine reproductive and respiratory syndrome (PRRS) is also an arterivirus.

No nucleotide sequence information is available at present to ascertain if differences exist between isolates of EVA from different geographical areas. However, EVA isolates from the United States, Europe, New Zealand, and South Africa show differences in oligonucleotide fingerprint patterns.[11] This indicates that sequence differences are likely to exist between virus isolates. However, the biological significance of this genomic variability remains to be determined.

There is only one recognized serotype of EVA, although some evidence of antigenic variation among different isolates exists.[11, 12] Using a complement fixation test, it was demonstrated (in 1977) that there were minor antigenic differences between EVA isolates with homologous and heterologous equine antiserum.[12] There is also variation in the severity of clinical signs in disease caused by different EVA isolates. Reproducibly different tissue culture growth characteristics have also been demonstrated with respect to virus shed in the semen of different carrier stallions.[13]

Epizootiology

Infections with EVA occur in all types of horses due to the highly contagious nature of the disease and its transmission by both respiratory and venereal routes. The incidence of EVA infection based on serologic evidence is very low within the equine Thoroughbred population (0.5% to 6%), with variation between countries, and high in most other equine types studied; as many as 80% of Standardbred horses have serum antibodies to EVA. The Thoroughbred horse appears to suffer more overt clinical signs and deeper physical distress owing to EVA infection than do other horse breeds.

Equine arteritis virus is spread by direct contact with infected horses and their secretions. During the acute phase of infection virus is shed in all bodily secretions, including urine; and aerosol transmission is the most potent means of spreading the virus.

Until recently, the chief mode of virus transmission during EVA outbreaks was reported to be by direct contact via nasal droplet spray.[14, 15] In the Kentucky outbreak of 1984, a high percentage (36%) of stallions infected via the respiratory route continued to shed virus in their semen after recovery, resulting in transmission of EVA to susceptible mares to which they were bred.[16] Two carrier states exist in the stallion: a short-term state during convalescence (duration of 1 to 3 weeks) and a long-term chronic condition that may persist for years after clinical infection.[13, 16–18] In experimental infections of stallions, long-term carrier rates of 62.5% with persistence of EVA were achieved in the vas deferens, ampullae, seminal vesicles, prostate, and bulbourethral glands.[18] Increasing evidence suggests that the carrier stallion plays a pivotal epizootiologic role in the dissemination and perpetuation of EVA.

There are no reports of mares becoming EVA carriers or chronic shedders, nor of virus passage by the venereal route from a seropositive mare causing clinical disease or seroconversion in a stallion. Foals born to seropositive mares acquire maternal antibodies to EVA via colostrum.[19] These maternal antibodies decline to extinction within 2 to 6 months, resulting in the foal becoming seronegative unless subsequently infected with EVA. After clinical recovery from respiratory EVA infection, there is no significant decrease in the fertility of shedding stallions.[20, 21] Mares infected after service by a carrier stallion do not appear to have any related long-term fertility problems.

Pathogenesis

The pathogenicity of EVA strains appears to vary considerably, and the explanation for this remains unknown. EVA pathogenesis has been investigated by sequential studies on horses sacrificed at intervals following intranasal challenge with virulent virus. These studies established that EVA is a panvasculitis with viral replication occurring in most components of the cardiovascular system.

The initial virus replication occurs in bronchoalveolar macrophages in the lung, and by the second day of infection the virus has reached the bronchial lymph nodes. The virus then disseminates throughout the horse via the circulatory system, and by the third day the mesenteric lymph nodes, spleen, liver, kidney, nasopharynx, lung, serum, pleural fluid, abdominal fluid, and urine all contain EVA, the only exception being brain tissue. The main sites of viral replication are macrophages and endothelial tissue, with medial cells, mesothelium, and the epithelium of certain organs (adrenal) being identified as secondary sites. Vascular lesions develop

in the medial cells and endothelium. Infiltration of neutrophils into endothelial lesions causes damage to the internal elastic lamina of the small arteries. Lesions in the vascular and lymphatic systems subside by the 10th day of infection; however, arterial damage may persist for several weeks thereafter. The infectious virus persists in the kidney for up to 3 weeks after infection and can be isolated from urine during this time.

Abortion due to EVA is thought to be caused as a result of myometrial necrosis and edema leading to placental detachment and fetal death.[22] The occurrence of EVA-carrier stallions, with virus persisting in the genitourinary tract, indicates a viral tropism to specific cells. Carrier stallions persistently shed virus, even in the presence of high virus-neutralizing antibody. It has been demonstrated that persistence of the virus is mediated either directly or indirectly by testosterone and is consequently dependent on the presence of the testes.[23] Additional evidence that viral persistence is dependent on testosterone includes a failure of virus persistence to develop in prepubertal colts, a seasonal fluctuation in viral output coincident with fluctuations in serum testosterone levels, the apparent elimination of EVA from the reproductive tract following castration, and the absence of any carrier state in the mare.

Clinical Signs

Consequences of EVA infection range from subclinical disease, only recognized by seroconversion,[24] to acute illness causing abortigenic disease and deaths among foals. Studies of epizootics have shown that subclinical infections are up to six-fold more prevalent than are clinical infections.[25, 26]

The clinical signs observed in cases of EVA vary considerably in range and clinical severity. Typical cases present with the following: fever of 5 to 9 days' duration; limb edema, especially of the hind limbs; nasal and ocular discharges; rhinitis and conjunctivitis; periorbital or supraorbital edema; anorexia and depression; skin rash; edema of the scrotum and prepuce of the stallion; and abortion in the pregnant mare. Other clinical signs associated with arteritis include lameness, diarrhea, coughing, general weakness, and ataxia.[13, 26–29] Adult horses generally make an uneventful recovery after a viremic phase that may persist for up to 40 days after infection[18]; however, EVA infection may cause death among foals.[30–32] There has been one reported case of fatal, congenitally acquired EVA infection in a neonatal Thoroughbred.[33]

The major concern in clinical disease is abortion with an incidence in exposed mares of up to 50%. EVA may cause abortions in mares between 3 and 10 months of gestation.[25, 34] Abortion usually occurs concurrent with or shortly after infection.[17, 27, 29, 30]

Differential Diagnosis

Equine viral arteritis must be differentiated from other infections indicated by respiratory disease. These include equine influenza, equine herpesvirus (EHV) 1 and 4, equine rhinovirus, equine adenovirus, and equine infectious anemia virus. A complete diagnosis of arteriviral infection depends on information derived from an accurate history, a physical examination, and, most important, laboratory data. EVA can only be distinguished from the other prevalent equine respiratory viruses by discriminating laboratory-based tests. In abortion storms, EHV-1 is the most likely alternative infectious cause.

Laboratory Diagnosis
Sample Selection

In order to confirm the diagnosis of viral arteritis, the correct samples must be submitted for laboratory testing. In cases of respiratory disease whole and clotted blood, nasopharyngeal swabs stored in virus transport medium, and a urine sample should be taken, kept cool (4 °C), and submitted as quickly as possible to the diagnostic laboratory. The clinical history and recent transport history of the horse may also help in the selection of laboratory tests. Corticosteroids are cytotoxic to some cell types in tissue culture and interfere with EVA virus neutralization (VN) test, therefore any drugs already being prescribed should be noted.

In EVA abortion, both fetus and placenta are heavily contaminated with virus, and samples of these should be collected in a sterile manner and submitted for isolation of the virus. EVA virus can be isolated from the placenta, fetal spleen, lung, and kidney, and fetal and placental fluids.[34]

Samples of semen should be collected if a stallion is suspected of shedding virus. Samples should be taken from the sperm-rich fraction of full ejaculates (not dismount samples) and stored at 4 °C for rapid transport to the laboratory. In addition, serum samples from mares to which the stallion has been bred within the past 3 months are useful for providing test-mating confirmation of a positive virus isolation from semen.

Virus Isolation

Acute viral arteritis may be diagnosed by virus isolation from nasopharyngeal swabs or washings and from the buffy coat of EDTA-treated or citrated blood samples.[35] The diagnosis of abortion due to EVA is largely dependent on isolation of the virus from the placenta or fetal tissues.

EVA virus has been isolated directly by culture on equine kidney, rabbit kidney (RK-13), and Vero cells by serial blind passage of material from aborted fetuses and foals. In the latter cases, cytopathic effects were only recognizable after two to eight passages.[30, 36]

Isolation of EVA virus from field cases can prove difficult and has failed in some cases; nasopharyngeal swabs taken from febrile horses during an outbreak in Switzerland and from swabs and buffy coats during an outbreak in Kentucky produced no cytopathic effect in tissue culture inoculations.[28, 31] The latter workers were able to show virus transmission by inoculation of blood from febrile horses into susceptible animals followed by virus isolation from nasal swabs and blood of the experimentally infected horses.

The EVA carrier state was first demonstrated in naturally infected stallions by both test matings and virus isolation on RK-13 cells.[17] Virus culture from semen samples is currently the recognized method of identifying shedding stallions. Recently a new method independent of virus isolation in tissue culture has been used to demonstrate the presence of EVA virus in semen samples.[38] The methodology can detect 60 plaque-forming units/mL of semen and is equally sensitive as tissue culture isolation. The technique rapidly amplifies the quantity of viral genetic material in the sample. The advantages of this methodology over tissue culture are: (1) in the speed of virus detection (48 hours compared with 1 to 3 weeks), (2) in specificity (only EVA RNA is detected), (3) in its applicability to a wide range of clinical samples, and (4) it is not dependent on intact virus being present, only viral RNA. This methodology has been used to confirm tissue culture isolation results from Swedish semen shedders.[21]

Serology

Antibodies to EVA virus can be demonstrated by complement fixation (CF) and VN tests.[36, 39–41] The CF test is most useful for studying immunity to arteritis during the first 4 months after exposure, because the titer peaks 2 to 4 weeks after infection and decreases below detectable limits after 8 months.[12] CF tests have a role in diagnosing recent infection, because CF antibody titers decrease more rapidly than do VN antibody titers. VN antibody titers develop simultaneously to CF titers, are maximal 2 to 4 months after infection, and remain stable for several years.[28]

The laboratory diagnosis of seropositive horses is based on the complement-dependent virus neutralization test using the Bucyrus strain of EVA virus for tissue culture infection.[42] A titer of 1:4 in duplicate sera is deemed to be EVA seropositive. VN test procedures, although more expensive and laborious than CF tests, are more sensitive for the detection of antibody to EVA as a result of previous exposure to the virus. The VN test is unable to differentiate serum antibody elicited by vaccination from that caused by natural infection.

Enzyme-linked immunosorbent assay (ELISA) tests have been developed in Canada and England to detect EVA-specific antibody levels.[43, 44] These tests use purified EVA virus as the antigen in the ELISA, which is recognized by EVA-positive horse sera. The major problem encountered by EVA ELISAs are their failure to provide clear, sensitive results when the horse being tested has been previously vaccinated with any tissue culture-derived virus vaccine, such as those used to prevent EHV infection. In such cases the high background color development due to nonspecific binding of antibodies to tissue culture-derived antigen can mask the EVA ELISA result.

Disease Management
Treatment

Virtually all naturally infected horses recover from EVA, although some fatalities have been induced by experimental infections. Pyrexia in stallions can lead to sperm damage and temporary infertility, thus treatment with nonsteroidal anti-inflammatory preparations may be indicated to control pyrexia. Sexual rest following acute EVA infection is important to reduce the likelihood of a stallion becoming a chronic EVA carrier.[32]

Natural Immunity

Previously exposed horses are immune to experimental reinfection with virulent virus.[45] Natural immunity persists for up to 7 years and, although difficult to demonstrate,[28] is presumed to be lifelong. During recovery from EVA infection, high levels of serum neutralizing antibody are induced and have long duration. High levels of antibody correlate very well with protection from respiratory and venereal infection.[46]

Vaccination

Research work on EVA vaccines has concentrated on the safety and efficacy of a whole inactivated virus vaccine and an attenuated live virus vaccine.

Early studies demonstrated that virulent EVA could be attenuated by passage in tissue culture while retaining immunogenicity.[47] Serial passage through horse kidney, rabbit kidney, and equine dermis cells has served to attenuate virulent virus, resulting in a modified live vaccine (MLV).[46, 48–52] This type of vaccine was widely used during the EVA outbreak in Kentucky during 1984. Use of the MLV does not produce any side effects apart from a short-term abnormality of sperm morphology and a mild fever with no overt clinical signs.[52] The virus can be isolated sporadically from the nasopharynx and blood samples generally for up to 7 days and in a few cases for up to 32 days after vaccination.[52, 53] Vaccine virus has never been isolated from semen or urine after vaccination with MLV.[52, 53] VN antibody titers are induced within 5 to 8 days of vaccination and persist for at least 2 years.[51, 52]

Vaccination with MLV protects against clinical disease and reduces the amount of virus shed from the respiratory tract during challenge infection. Horses in contact and mares served by vaccinated stallions are not infected by EVA.[52, 54] Vaccinated mares challenged by artificial insemination were protected from clinical infection.[46] However, the latter worker (McCollum[46]) demonstrated the need for vaccinated animals, when challenged venereally, to be isolated, because one mare in contact with a vaccinated, venereally challenged mare became EVA seropositive.

The MLV was used to good effect in the containment of an outbreak of EVA on Kentucky stud farms in 1984. However, vaccination of horses precipitates shedding of virus from the nasopharynx after vaccination and does not prevent infection with EVA. To be universally accepted for use both on stud farms and within training stables as a preventive vaccine, these problems need to be addressed.

The use of a formalin-inactivated EVA vaccine has been pioneered.[55, 56] Secondary immunization 4 weeks after primary vaccination results in SN antibody titers of up to 1:5,120. The antibody titer decreases rapidly, but a third immunization after 2 months results in a VN titer of between 1:80 and 1:320, which persists for 6 months. The 50% protective dose was calculated as a VN antibody titer of 1:43. However, even though clinical disease was averted, not all horses with high antibody levels were protected from infection, because live virus was recovered from blood samples after challenge infection. The value of this type of vaccine in disease control within stables is unclear, because it is unknown if the vaccinated horses showed reduced levels of virus excretion from the nasopharynx. Recently, the inactivated vaccine has been shown to prevent stallions from becoming semen shedders after challenge infection.[57]

Outbreak Control

During an outbreak of EVA, the spread of infection should be controlled by movement restrictions, isolation of infected animals on stud farms followed by a quarantine period after recovery, allocation of personnel to deal solely with infected animals, diagnostic surveillance, and the implementation of a vaccination policy to immunize animals at risk of infection. The use of the MLV vaccine will result in a population of seropositive animals due to infection or live virus immunization, both groups having the potential to infect susceptible animals brought into close contact. As a result, a strict EVA control program must be conducted following the outbreak both within the control area and among animals resident within the area at the time of the outbreak, which have subsequently departed from it. This should involve annual vaccination of all noncarrier stallions and teasers prior to the breeding season and vaccination of seronegative mares served by carrier stallions. Following vaccination with the MLV, animals should be isolated for up to 21 days from nonvaccinated horses. Additionally, mares bred to seropositive stallions must be isolated for 14 days after service, shedding stallions housed and bred in separate facilities and any seropositive nonshedding stallion checked for two seasons by monitoring the serologic status of mares bred to that stallion. Stallions and mares that become clinically infected during the breeding season should not be used further during that season.

The use of an MLV as an integral part of an EVA control program is advocated in the state of New York and in New Zealand and remains an option in areas where either clinical disease or seropositive animals exist.[58, 59] However, the widespread vaccination of horses with a modified live EVA vaccine entails the risk that the vaccine virus could revert to virulence and that vaccinates could spread the attenuated strain out with the vaccination program either by virus shedding directly after vaccination or by inducing semen shedders. This does not appear to have occurred in Kentucky. However, in an equine population free of diseased and seropositive animals, import regulations excluding seropositive and clinically ill animals together with internal diagnostic surveillance is the safest and most effective method of disease prevention. In the event that a new outbreak occurs within a susceptible population, management procedures should follow those practiced in Kentucky, ideally with the substitution of a killed or subunit vaccine for the modified live vaccine.

EQUID HERPESVIRUS TYPE 1 AND EQUID HERPESVIRUS TYPE 4

The horse is the natural host of at least four different herpesviruses. Equid herpesvirus type 1 (EHV-1) and equid herpesvirus type 4 (EHV-4) are closely related viruses associated with a range of clinical syndromes including respiratory disease, perinatal foal disease, and abortion. EHV-1 can, in addition, cause neurologic disease.[60-62] EHV-2 is a relatively nonpathogenic virus. It is sometimes isolated from animals suffering mild respiratory disease, but it can also be isolated from animals that show no clinical signs of infection. EHV-3 infects the genital tract causing coital exanthema, which is characterized by pustular lesions on the external genitalia, lips, external nares, nasal mucosae, and conjunctiva.[63-65]

Etiologic Agent

EHV-1 and EHV-4 are large, enveloped viruses that contain a linear double-stranded DNA genome. In common with most enveloped viruses, they are sensitive to ether, high temperature, desiccation, and an acidic pH. The overall morphology of the virion closely resembles that described for a typical member of the Herpesviridae family.[66, 67] There are four main structural features: (1) the internal DNA core, (2) an icosahedral capsid, (3) the tegument, and (4) the outer envelope. The core is an electron-dense "toroid" structure with a less electron dense central cylinder around which the linear genome is wound. This is surrounded by 162 capsomers arranged to form an icosahedron that is approximately 100 nm in diameter.[65] Surrounding the capsid is an ill-defined tegument region, which is, in turn, surrounded by a triple-layered outer envelope containing glycoprotein, phosphoprotein, and lipid.[68, 69] The virion comprises at least 28 structural polypeptides. The most frequently used nomenclature is that described by Turtinen and Allen in which viral polypeptides are assigned the prefix VP and numbered from 1 to 28 in descending order of molecular weight.[70] Polypeptides incorporating glucosamine have been assigned the prefix gp instead of VP. The genes encoding six viral glycoproteins have been identified with DNA sequence homology to herpes simplex virus (HSV) envelope glycoproteins B, C, D, E, I, and H.[71-75] The polypeptides homologous to HSV gB, gC, and gD have been identified as gp14, gp13, and gp18a, respectively.[76] At least five minor glycoproteins with no apparent homologue in HSV have also been identified.

Electrophoretic analyses of the structural polypeptides of EHV-1 and EHV-4 have demonstrated a similar number of proteins in both virions, with an approximate molecular weight range of 13 to 300 kD. Despite gross similarities, the electrophoretic polypeptide profiles are sufficiently different to enable differentiation between EHV-1 and EHV-4. Intertypic mobility differences have been identified in gp 2, gp 13, gp 14, gp 18a, and gp 25 and also in VP 24a, 26a, and 26b.[60, 70]

Antigenic variation has been demonstrated among North American EHV-1 isolates using monoclonal antibodies directed against gp 13. From 72 different isolates tested with 42 monoclonal antibodies, 16 different isolate groups have been differentiated. However, no clinical or pathologic significance has been attributed to these variants to date.[77]

The genome of EHV-1 has been studied more widely than the genome of EHV-4 and will therefore be the focus of this section. It consists of a linear double-stranded molecule of DNA with an approximate molecular mass of 90 to 94 MDa and forms approximately 9% of the particle dry weight. It has a buoyant density of 1.1716 g/cm^3, a melting temperature of 51.4 °C, and a G + C content of 57 moles %.[65, 78, 79] Restriction endonuclease analysis and electron microscopy

have identified two segments, designated long (L) and short (S).[80-82] Both the L and the S are unique sequences (U_L and U_s) of 111 and 39 kb pairs respectively and S, but not L, is flanked by two inverted repeats (TR;/IR;). This allows the S component to invert relative to L thus giving rise to two possible arrangements of the genome. These are present in approximately equal proportions in a single population of DNA.[81] The complete nucleotide sequence of the British EHV-1 isolate designated AB4 has been sequenced and contains 80 potential open reading frames.[83] DNA-DNA hybridization studies with other alpha herpesviruses has demonstrated a high degree of colinearity of genes, particularly in the L segment of the genome.[81, 84-87]

Comparisons between the genome of EHV-1 and EHV-4 by restriction endonuclease analysis have demonstrated significant differences in their nucleotide sequences.[81, 88, 89] However, comparisons among isolates of the same type, recovered from disease outbreaks in North America and Australasia, show a high degree of genetic homogeneity.[90-92] From 300 North American isolates examined, using five different restriction enzymes, 16 variants with different DNA fingerprint patterns were identified. Two electropherotypes were associated with more than 90% of EHV-1 abortions among Kentucky mares and were designated 1P (prototype) and 1B.[60] The 1B variant was more frequently associated with multiple abortions among vaccinated herds. A greater degree of diversity was identified among EHV-4 isolates. Thirteen variants were identified from 21 isolates examined, although the biological significance of this variation remains to be determined. This contrasts with the high degree of genetic diversity reported for HSV, in which no two epidemiologically unrelated isolates exhibit the same restriction profiles.[93, 94]

Epizootiology

Serologic surveys suggest widespread distribution of EHV-1 and EHV-4 in the general horse population. However, the prevalence of these viruses is difficult to determine because of the subclinical nature of infections, particularly in older animals, and also the lack of a type-specific serologic diagnostic test. Horses acquire infection via the respiratory route, either directly in aerosols or indirectly via contaminated food, water, bedding, and other fomites. During the acute phase of disease, virus is shed into the environment via the respiratory tract. In young immunologically naive animals, virus can be recovered from the nasopharynx for up to 12 days postinfection, although in older animals with prior exposure to the virus, recovery may be possible for as little as 1 to 2 days. The virus can sometimes be recovered from the leukocyte fraction of blood for periods that can vary from 1 day to several months. This is most commonly detected with EHV-1 infections, although it can also occur with EHV-4. The rate of spread of the virus through the horse population varies considerably, depending on factors such as the proximity of individual animals, movement of animals between premises and within premises, sharing of common air space and drinking or feeding facilities, and the quality of general management procedures. Virus spread can be very rapid when animals are housed in close proximity, such as in American barns, whereas in horses at pasture it may take several weeks.[95]

In young animals, the most frequent outcome of infection is mild respiratory disease, although this can sometimes be severe following stressful situations such as weaning or transportation.[96] Sporadic outbreaks of respiratory disease or subclinical infections are not a significant threat to the general horse population; however, for Thoroughbreds in training, the consequences to an individual animal's performance can be severe.[97, 98] Of greater concern are outbreaks of EHV-1 abortion; these are usually sporadic and involve small numbers of mares but can sometimes occur in which the incidence of abortion is as high as 30% to 70% of infected animals.[95, 99] Outbreaks of EHV-1 neurologic disease can also be severe, resulting in up to 90% morbidity and 60% mortality.[100–102] During outbreaks of perinatal foal disease, which has been attributed to infection of the fetus late in gestation, foals are born alive but die during the first few hours or days of life, either from viral pneumonia or from secondary bacterial infection.[61, 62]

The ability of both viruses to exist in a latent carrier state has been demonstrated in experimental situations.[103, 104] Several months after infection, the virus can be reactivated by administration of high levels of corticosteroids.[103] The site of latency for both EHV-1 and EHV-4 is the lymphoid tissues, particularly those draining the respiratory tract, although EHV-1 is also found in peripheral lymphoid tissue.[105, 106] After reactivation of virus with corticosteroids, EHV-2 is frequently recovered from the nasopharynx and circulating lymphocytes prior to EHV-1.[103] This has led to speculation that EHV-2 may transactivate EHV-1 (or EHV-4) from its latent state, which is supported by data from cross-hybridization experiments that have demonstrated that the immediate early genes of EHV-1, EHV-2, and EHV-4 possess shared homology.[107]

The significance of latent infections in the epizootiology of EHV-1 and EHV-4 is difficult to quantify; however, early studies of closed herd populations have demonstrated its potential role in initiating outbreaks of disease.[97, 108] In these studies, virus was isolated from nasopharyngeal swabs and blood samples from several horses following stressful situations such as weaning, castration, and relocation. In a recent survey of abattoir horses, latent virus was identified in approximately 60% of animals by cocultivation of explanted tissue.[107] These findings are consistent with observations made during field outbreaks, in which the source of infection is frequently unidentified and is not associated with the introduction of new stock or contact with an infected animal.

Clinical Signs

The clinical signs of infection may vary from subclinical disease to acute illness leading to severe respiratory distress, abortion, paralysis, and neonatal foal death. Infection of young, immunologically naive horses with either EHV-1 and EHV-4 results in acute respiratory disease accompanied by serous nasal discharge, pyrexia with temperatures reaching 106 °F in severe cases, anorexia, and depression. Occasionally, replication of the virus in the lungs may result in the development of a viral bronchopneumonia. Secondary bacterial infection is a common sequel to respiratory infection, resulting in a mucopurulent nasal discharge and sometimes swelling of the local lymphoid tissue, which may lead to abscess formation. In older animals, clinical signs of respiratory infection are mild and are often not recognized. Because immunity to infection is short-lived, horses may suffer reinfections at frequent intervals (4 to 6 months) throughout their lives. The clinical signs of neurologic disease can vary from a mild ataxia, causing abnormalities in gait and general weakness, to complete hind limb paralysis and, in some cases, quadriplegia. Other clinical signs include ocular lesions, edema of the limbs and scrotum, and incontinence.[101, 109]

Pathogenesis

Both EHV-1 and EHV-4 are respiratory viruses, with primary replication occurring in the epithelial surfaces and local lymphoid tissues of the respiratory tract.[110, 111] Experimental infections in young foals have demonstrated that isolates of EHV-1 and EHV-4 have different pathogenic potential.[112] Thus, EHV-1 isolates from cases of neurologic disease demonstrate a tropism for vascular endothelial cells, particularly in the nasal mucosa, lungs, and central nervous system. EHV-1 is disseminated throughout the horse by a cell-associated viremia; the intracellular location of the virus providing an immunologically protected mechanism by which it can access secondary sites of virus replication, even in the presence of neutralizing antibody. The cell types implicated in viremia include mononuclear cells, macrophages, and lymphocytes.[107, 113, 114] In cases of neurologic disease caused by EHV-1, viral infection of endothelial cells in the brain and spinal cord causes local vasculitis and thrombosis, hypoxic degeneration of the local neurophil; the disease has therefore been called "equine stroke."[115] The characteristic vasculitis may represent a cell-mediated Arthus-type reaction to viral antigen; productive viral infection of neural tissue had not been demonstrated until recently.[116–118, 118a, 118b]

Recent experimental work indicates that endothelial infection may also be central to EHV-1 abortigenic disease.[119, 120] Productive infection of blood vessels in the uterus has been demonstrated in pregnant mares following intranasal EHV-1 challenge and may be associated with thrombosis and focal cotyledonary infarction, presenting a potential route for leakage of free virus or infected cells across the placenta to infect the fetus, which is subsequently aborted. Sites of viral replication and damage in fetal tissues have been well documented.[121] In early acute experimental infections where endometrial vasculitis is widespread, the associated cotyledonary infarction may be so severe as to cause detachment of the placenta and abortion before the fetus has become infected.[122] The field incidence of this phenomenon is not known.

Differential Diagnosis

The diagnosis is complicated because of the wide range of clinical symptoms that can be associated with EHV-1 and EHV-4 infection. It is important to differentiate between these and other respiratory viruses such as influenza subtypes 1 and 2, rhinovirus types 1 and 2, picornavirus, and arteritis virus. It is also important to differentiate EHV-1 from EHV-4 infection because of their differences in pathogenicity. The diagnosis can be aided by knowledge of the clinical details and vaccination history of the affected animals, although appropriate laboratory test results are essential for an unequivocal diagnosis.

Laboratory Diagnosis

An accurate laboratory diagnosis requires stringent selection of the appropriate clinical specimen, good technique in sample collection, and rapid transport to the diagnostic laboratory in suitable media. For unequivocal diagnosis, the virus must be isolated in culture and then identified using an appropriate test.

In suspected cases of EHV-1 or EHV-4 respiratory infection, nasopharyngeal swabs, heparinized blood, and whole clotted blood samples should be sent to the diagnostic laboratory. Virus can be isolated by inoculation of the nasal swab specimens directly onto susceptible cells; usually an equine cell line derived from fetal lung or kidney and also a nonequine cell line such as rabbit kidney (RK13). Inoculation onto these cell types may allow preliminary typing of isolates because EHV-1, but not EHV-4, causes a cytopathic effect in RK13 cells. Once identified, the virus can be typed using pools of monoclonal antibodies by immunofiltration or immunofluorescence test.[123, 124] With heparinized blood samples, the buffy coat fraction of blood containing leukocytes is harvested and used as the inoculum. Although isolation of virus is the definitive method of confirming diagnosis, the development of cytopathic effect can sometimes take 1 to 2 weeks, which is of limited value in disease management. More rapid diagnostic procedures include an antigen capture enzyme-immunoassay incorporating monoclonal and polyclonal antibodies and also the polymerase chain reaction that detects small quantities of virus specific DNA.[125, 126]

In cases of EHV-1 or EHV-4 abortion, the diagnosis is based on observation of typical histologic lesions in the fetal tissues and isolation of the virus in tissue culture or detection of viral DNA by the polymerase chain reaction.[121, 127] Suitable tissues for examination are fetal liver, lung, adrenal gland, thymus, and spleen collected into neutral buffered formalin and virus transport medium. For rapid screening purposes, or where only fixed tissues are available to the laboratory, immunofluorescence and immunoperoxidase techniques permit specific visualization of viral antigen in histologic sections.[128, 129]

The EHV-1 neurologic case presents a diagnostic challenge. Ideally, full postmortem examination and removal of the brain and spinal cord should be undertaken to ensure that the characteristic lesions of vasculitis are sampled to exclude other causes of paresis. Immunoperoxidase examination at sites of vasculitis has been shown to be of considerable value in confirming the diagnosis in adult horses in which high levels of neutralizing antibody may hinder attempts at virus isolation.[130] Appropriate tissues for histopathology and virus isolation where a full postmortem is not practical are specimens of medulla, spinal cord, turbinate, submandibular lymph node, lung, and spleen collected into neutral buffered formalin and virus transport medium.

A wide range of procedures has been developed for monitoring herpesvirus serum antibody levels, including immunofluorescence, neutralization, complement fixation, enzyme immunoassay, and single radial immunodiffusion.[128, 131–133]

The complement fixation test is the method of choice as a routine diagnostic test. Antibody levels can be compared in "acute" and "convalescent" phase serum samples and a four-fold rise in titer used to identify infected animals. Additionally, the short duration of CF antibody in sera (2 to 3 months) enables high levels of antibody in single samples to be used as a diagnostic indicator. The main drawback of the CF test is lack of differentiation between EHV-1 and EHV-4 because of the antigenic cross-reactivity between these viruses and a long assay time of 24 hours. The development of a 4-hour ELISA using recombinant viral antigen should improve the diagnosis of these viruses, although the development of a rapid type-specific serologic test remains an important goal for laboratory researchers.[134]

Disease Control

Immunity

Because of the high prevalence of EHV-1 and EHV-4 among the horse population, the majority of newborn foals are infected early in their lives. In some cases, passively derived maternal antibody may protect against respiratory infection; however, in other cases, it may only be sufficient to prevent clinical symptoms of disease but not viral replication and subsequent shedding of virus into the nasopharynx.[135] Immunity to reinfection of the respiratory tract is generally short-lived, although immunity to abortion appears to be of longer duration.[60] Repeated infection is thought to boost immunity such that respiratory infections in older animals become subclinical. The ability of one virus type to cross-protect against challenge with the heterologous type has been studied experimentally by Allen and Bryans.[60] Primary infection with one type was sufficient to protect against reinfection 4 weeks later with the homologous type; however, protection against the heterologous type required repeated exposure to the virus. This study contrasted with that by Edington and Bridges who were unable to demonstrate that successive infections with EHV-4 protected against infection by EHV-1, although repeat infection with EHV-1 protected against both homologous and heterologous virus.[136]

Both cellular and humoral immune responses contribute to host immunity. However, attempts to assess the immune status of individual animals using in vitro assays have been inconclusive. Experimental studies suggest that animals with high levels of serum neutralizing antibodies are less susceptible to respiratory infections; however, attempts to correlate neutralizing antibody levels with protection in field cases have been unsuccessful.[95] Conflicting results have been reported in studies of the cell-mediated immune response. In some cases, higher levels of immunity (assessed by lymphocyte proliferation) appeared to correlate with protection against abortion whereas, in other cases, no differences were detected between the levels of immunity in mares that aborted from those that foaled at full term.[137, 138] Recent observations suggest that EHV-1 infections can cause long-term nonspecific depression of the cell-mediated immune response, which is not related to the decreased numbers of circulating lymphocytes and neutrophils occurring in the acute stage of infection.[139] Cell-associated viremia frequently occurs in parallel with a decrease in white blood cell count, lymphocyte proliferation, and PHA stimulation[137] as reported for human influenza and herpesvirus infections.[140] Cell-mediated responses can also be depressed during pregnancy, with maximum suppression occurring during the last trimester, possibly accounting for the 95% incidence of EHV-1 abortions during this period.

Vaccination

Attempts to produce a vaccine to protect animals from infection and clinical disease have been of limited success. Early attempts to produce inactivated vaccines were hindered by the low immunogenicity of the preparations and the adverse local and systemic reactions to the antigens that were derived from the tissue of infected hamsters.[141] Both problems were overcome to a certain extent by administration of attenuated, live virus in a "planned infection" program.[142] The rationale was to vaccinate mares in the early stages of pregnancy, at which time most animals are relatively insusceptible to abortion, in order to mimic the short-lived immunity produced by natural infection. However, the program was later abandoned because of requirements for complicated herd management, a quarantine period for vaccinated horses, and reports of vaccine-related abortions. Attempts were made to improve the safety of live vaccines by further attenuation of virus strains.[143] The first attenuated vaccine licensed for use in the United States was derived from hamster-adapted virus that had been further attenuated by passage in equine cell culture.[141] It is still widely used in training stables in order to reduce the incidence of respiratory disease, although is not recommended for use in pregnant mares because of the potential risk of abortion.[144]

Attempts have been made to improve the efficacy of inactivated vaccines, and the problems associated with the use of crude hamster-derived antigen have been largely overcome. A commercial vaccine has been derived from formalin inactivated, cell-cultured virus antigen incorporated with adjuvant.[145] The vaccine appears to boost the horse's natural immunity, reducing the duration of virus excretion from the nasopharynx as well as providing a degree of short-term protection against abortion. However, cases of EHV-1 abortion in fully vaccinated mares are not infrequent, and it remains a major goal of vaccine researchers to produce an efficacious vaccine, ideally with longer lasting immunity than that provided by natural infections.

Good management procedures play a key role in minimizing the risk of virus spread in the event of an EHV-1 or EHV-4 outbreak. Infections tend to spread slowly through groups of horses by direct contact between animals, handlers, and contaminated surfaces. The spread of infection can be minimized by restricting movement of horses and by implementing isolation procedures for those that are infected. In the case of EHV-1, abortion, or neurologic disease, it is particularly important to restrict movement of animals from affected premises. When possible, animals should be divided into small groups or separated individually and screened at regular intervals until the end of the outbreak.

EQUINE INFLUENZA VIRUS

Equine influenza is a highly infectious respiratory disease that affects horses, donkeys, mules, and zebras. It is rarely fatal, but deaths have been reported during some epidemics, particularly in donkeys. Outbreaks of a disease resembling influenza have been reported as early as 1751; however, the etiologic agent was not isolated until 1956. The distribution of equine influenza is worldwide, with the exception of Australia and New Zealand.

Etiologic Agent

Equine influenza viruses belong to the orthomyxovirus family, which includes three types of virus, designated A, B, and C, distinguishable on the basis of the internal nucleoprotein (NP) and matrix (M) protein. All equine isolates are type A viruses. There are two subtypes of equine influenza; influenza A/equine/1 represented by the prototype virus Prague/56 and influenza A/equine/2 represented by the prototype Miami/63.[146, 147] These subtypes are classified on the basis of the antigenic character of their surface glycoproteins the hemagglutinin (HA) and the neuraminidase (NA) with A/equine/1 viruses carrying an H7HA and an N7NA and A/equine/2 viruses carrying an H3HA and an N8NA. In 1989, an H3N8 virus was isolated from horses in China that was not directly related to other equine H3N8 viruses and was believed to originate from an avian H3N8 virus. This virus does not appear to have persisted in the equine population.[148]

Equine influenza viruses are pleomorphic enveloped particles with an approximate diameter of 80 to 120 nm. The lipid envelope carries the two surface glycoproteins (HA, NA) of which the HA is most abundant representing 25% of the virus protein. Internally, the virus consists of an NP closely associated with the RNA segments and surrounded by M protein.[149] Influenza viruses are single-stranded RNA viruses with a segmented genome. The eight segments code for the structural proteins (HA, NA, NP, and M) and the nonstructural proteins (NS1, P1, P2, and P3) involved in virus replication.

An important characteristic of influenza viruses is their ability to undergo antigenic drift, whereby mutations occur in the genes coding for the HA and NA particularly, resulting in amino acid substitutions and change in the antigenic character of the surface glycoproteins. These changes allow the virus to avoid neutralization by antibody present in the equine population and thus infect seropositive animals. Occasionally antigenic shift occurs when surface glycoproteins change as a result of recombinational events with influenza viruses of other species. Antigenic shift gives rise to the viruses that result in pandemics in susceptible populations, which occurred with the appearance of the subtype 2 influenza virus in 1963.

Within H7N7 (subtype 1) viruses, minor antigenic drift has been identified,[150] whereas among H3N8 (subtype 2) viruses more extensive antigenic drift has been detected, such that variants have been identified represented by the prototypes A/Kentucky/81 and A/Fontainebleau/79.[151]

Epizootiology

Equine influenza has been reported in North and South America, Europe, the former Soviet Union, the Middle East, India, Singapore, Japan, China, and South Africa. The only large equine populations that have not yet been affected are those of Australia and New Zealand. In some countries the infection appears to be enzootic, and outbreaks occur annually,[152, 153] whereas in other countries that have experienced major epidemics, such as South Africa[154] and India,[155] the infection appears to have been eliminated from the population.

The intrinsic ability of influenza viruses to change has an important impact on the epizootiology, which is also influenced by the pathogenesis of the disease and the immune response of the horse to infection and vaccination. Additionally, the structure and activities of the equine industry have had a profound influence on the spread of influenza in recent years. Equine influenza is a highly infectious disease and is characterized by rapid spread in susceptible populations. Morbidity rates are consequently high.[156, 157]

Infection of the epithelial lining of the respiratory tract results in a frequent and explosive cough that effectively disseminates an aerosol of virus over distances of 32 meters or more.[158] Additionally, there is good evidence that the virus can be transmitted by personnel and by contact with contaminated vehicles and housing.[159] Nevertheless, the virus is susceptible to sunlight and disinfectants and does not persist in the environment for long periods, unless protected by proteinaceous solutions (e.g., dirty water).

There is no evidence that variation in the prevalence of equine influenza is influenced by climatic conditions, although it is noteworthy that the infection is not endemic in persistently hot climates. Outbreaks of disease are more frequently related to movement of horses and introduction of young stock into endemic areas.

Many outbreaks in recent years have occurred as a result of horses with subclinical infections traveling long distances by air and being introduced into susceptible populations without adequate quarantining. In some areas of the world, horses move freely for racing and breeding purposes and are thus a potent source for new outbreaks. The partial immunity often conferred by vaccination suppresses clinical signs but may still allow the virus to shed.[160, 161] Such animals are not recognizable as a source of infection but are likely to play an important role in the maintenance and spread of the disease. Immunity stimulated by vaccination and infection is short-lived. Vaccinated animals are susceptible to infection 2 to 3 months after vaccination, while natural immunity may persist for a year.[162] It is not entirely clear how much this phenomenon relates to the immune system of the horse and how much antigenic drift in equine influenza viruses may play a role. While it has been recognized that antigenic variants exist among A/equine/2 viruses, their relevance to vaccine efficacy has not yet been clearly defined. Nevertheless, the widespread epidemics caused by variants of the H3N8 subtype in the United States and Europe in 1979 and 1980[151] and in Europe in 1989[163] raises the possibility that antigenic drift plays a major role in the epizootiology of equine influenza.

Pathogenesis

Influenza virus infects the epithelial cells of the upper and lower airways. The hemagglutinin spike is a key component of the virus and is the means by which the virus particle attaches to epithelium and gains entry to the cells. Infection of ciliated epithelium results in the loss of cilia within 3 to 4 days of infection and thus compromises the mucociliary clearance mechanism. The degree of damage and severity of clinical signs is affected by the dose of virus to which the horse is exposed.[164]

In the upper airways, laryngitis and tracheitis are observed and in the lower airways, bronchitis and bronchiolitis are accompanied by interstitial pneumonia, congestion, edema, and neutrophil infiltration.[157] In uncomplicated cases, the pathology has resolved within 2 to 3 weeks. However, damage to the ciliated epithelium often results in the establishment of secondary bacterial infections. Although local antibody is thought to be important for immunity to respiratory infections, there is a rapid inflammatory response resulting in leakage of serum antibody into the respiratory tract early in infection. Thus, humoral antibody is likely to be predominant in the first few weeks following infection and is instrumental in neutralizing the virus.[165]

Clinical Signs

In unprimed animals, the clinical signs of equine influenza are highly characteristic. A high temperature develops within 1 to 3 days of infection and may persist for 7 to 10 days. The onset of pyrexia is followed by a harsh, dry cough that may persist for 2 to 3 weeks. Animals suffer inappetance and depression. A seronasal discharge becomes mucopurulent, particularly if secondary bacterial infection occurs.

One of the most notable features in an outbreak of influenza is the rapid spread of disease within a group. In general, subtype 2 infections produce more severe clinical disease than do subtype 1 infections.[166] However, the latter virus has not been isolated in the last decade. The duration of pyrexia and coughing may relate not only to the subtype involved but also to the exposure dose.[164]

Mortality rates are usually very low in uncomplicated cases, with the exception of young foals that lack maternal antibody and develop pneumonia.[158] Mortality in donkeys has been reported to be associated with secondary bacterial infection.[167] Unusual clinical signs, including enteritis and high mortality, were reported in an outbreak of influenza in China in 1989. However, this virus was of avian origin and has not persisted in the equine population.[148]

Secondary complications and sequelae to equine influenza are common in stressed or neglected animals. Bacterial infections, particularly *Streptococcus zooepidemicus*, *S. equi*, *S. pneumoniae*, *Actinobacillus equuli*, and *Bordetella bronchiseptica* result in purulent nasal discharge, conjunctivitis and, in some cases, pneumonia. Long-term coughing in horses with asthmoid bronchitis following influenza has been attributed to inadequate rest and early resumption of hard work, poor environmental conditions, and inadequate antibacterial therapy. Other signs sometimes encountered are dyspnea and myalgia and, in severe cases, icterus. Cardiac damage has been encountered in animals worked during the acute phase of the disease.

In animals that have been previously infected or are vaccinated, the clinical signs are modified such that it is not possible to distinguish between influenza and other respiratory pathogens, with individuals developing no more than a transient mild pyrexia or occasional cough. In these cases, laboratory tests are required to confirm a diagnosis.

Diagnosis

Traditionally, influenza viruses have been isolated from nasopharyngeal exudates by inoculation of embryonated hens' eggs or tissue cultures such as Madin-Darby canine kidney cells. In partially immune animals, only low levels of virus are excreted for a short (1 to 2 days) period of time. Thus, it is often necessary to repeatedly take nasopharyngeal samples in culture before the virus is detected. A more rapid diagnosis can be obtained using an antigen capture ELISA test in which virus nucleoprotein (a highly abundant protein produced during infection) is captured using a specific monoclonal antibody. This test can provide a diagnosis within a matter of hours but does not differentiate between the two subtypes.[168] Other group specific methods such as immunofluorescent staining of infected respiratory epithelial cells have also been used.[169] Although detection of virus antigen in ELISA tests is quicker and usually more sensitive than isolation of the virus, it is important that attempts are always made to obtain isolates of the virus. New viruses can then be compared with those used on vaccines to determine whether major antigenic changes have occurred that could affect vaccine efficacy. A retrospective diagnosis may also be achieved by measuring antibody in acute and convalescent sera using hemagglutination inhibition or single radial hemolysis tests. This approach provides information about the subtype of the infecting viruses.

Prevention and Control

Prevention and control of equine influenza relies on two approaches: (1) rapid diagnosis and restriction of movement of horses, and (2) vaccination. Although equine influenza is a highly infectious disease, its spread can be minimized or even halted by restricting transport of horses from infected areas. Additionally, within premises or yards the impact of the disease on groups of horses can be lessened by reducing infection pressure and stress. Immediate isolation of affected animals reduces the level of virus in the environment, and reduction in work programs can reduce the severity of clinical disease that develops. It has been clearly demonstrated that both the duration of virus excretion and clinical signs are dependent on the infecting dose.[164] To further reduce risk of infections, housing and transport vehicles should be thoroughly disinfected before reuse by uninfected animals, and personnel should not move between infected and uninfected premises.

Vaccination against equine influenza can markedly reduce the severity of disease and decrease the spread of infection. However, at the present time, vaccines rarely prevent infection. All current vaccines contain inactivated antigens of both A/equine/1 and A/equine/2 viruses, and most products contain two A/equine/2 viruses—the original prototype virus Miami/63 and a representative of the 1979 to 1981 variants.

Both whole virus and subunit vaccines are available. Whole virus vaccines in an aqueous form or with adjuvants, such as oil, aluminum hydroxide or a polymer, and subunit vaccines containing micelles or immune-stimulating complexes (ISCOMs) have been developed.[163]

The efficacy of influenza vaccines is determined largely by the HA content of the vaccine and the potency of the adjuvant or antigen presentation system. The protection against infection and disease provided by inactivated vaccines relates directly to the level of antibody stimulated to HA.[170] Thus, all vaccination programs should aim to sustain high levels of antibody to HA between booster doses of vaccine. In young animals receiving their primary course of three doses, it is particularly difficult to sustain high levels of HA antibody for more than a few weeks after vaccination, and this group of animals is at particular risk. Vaccine manufacturers recommend a primary course of two doses of vaccine 4 to 6 weeks apart followed by a booster dose at 6 months. Vaccination can begin at 3 to 6 months of age or when maternal antibody has waned. In foals with no maternal immunity, successful vaccination can be initiated in much younger animals. Antibody to inactivated vaccines is short-lived, and animals often become susceptible within 6 to 8 weeks of their second dose of vaccine; thus, it may be beneficial in high-risk situations to give the third dose of vaccine before 6 months.

A significant observation in a vaccinated population is the occurrence of individuals who fail to develop antibody. The immunologic basis for this is not understood, but the presence of "poor responders" in a population is important in the epizootiology of the disease. As vaccine-induced immunity relates directly to antibody to HA, these individuals are highly susceptible to infection and may play a key role in the introduction of infection into new populations. Identification and repeated vaccination of poor responders will contribute to herd immunity.

Vaccines were first introduced in the late 1960s, and original products contained the A/equine/1 isolate, Prague/56 and the A/equine/2 isolate, and Miami/63. Following the identification of antigenic variants among H3N8 viruses represented by Fontainebleau/79 and Kentucky/81,[151] some vaccine manufacturers included the recent isolates in their vaccines. However, relatively little emphasis has been placed on the need to update vaccine strains to combat antigenic drift, probably as a result of the observation that postvaccination horse sera were highly cross-reactive in HI tests with a wide range of A/equine/2 isolates.[171] It has thus been assumed that immunity conferred by such vaccines would be similarly cross-reactive. This conclusion was challenged during the 1989 epidemic of influenza in Great Britain, when horses experienced clinical influenza despite high levels of vaccine-induced antibody that nevertheless reacted with the outbreak strain.

Analysis of the nucleotide sequence of the HA gene of a 1989 isolate revealed nucleotide changes resulting in amino acid substitution in all four antigenic sites on the HA compared with previous isolates such as Fontainebleau/79.[172] These changes resulted in antigenic differences between vaccine and outbreak strains that could be detected using postinfection horse sera in reciprocal HI but not with sera from repeatedly vaccinated animals.[163] The significance of the observed antigenic drift in relation to vaccine efficacy has now been demonstrated in the target species. Vaccine prepared from the recent isolate almost eliminated viral shedding following challenge with the homologous strain, whereas vaccines composed of earlier viruses allowed shedding of the virus for several days.[173] These observations suggest that the significance of antigenic drift in H3N8 viruses in relation to vaccine efficacy, particularly the ability to prevent spread within a group, may have been underrated.

Thus, more regular updating of vaccine virus may significantly improve control by vaccination.

REFERENCES

1. Hyllseth B: Structural proteins of equine arteritis virus. *Arch ges Virusforsch* 40:177, 1973.
2. Murphy FA: Togavirus morphology and morphogenesis. In Schlesinger RW, ed. *The Togaviruses: Biology Structure and Replication.* New York, Academic Press, 1980, p. 241.
3. Horzinek MC: *Non-arthropod Borne Togaviruses.* New York, Academic Press, 1981.
4. Den Boon JA, et al: Equine arteritis virus is not a togavirus but belongs to the coronavirus-like "superfamily." *J Virol* 65:2910, 1991.
5. Zeegers JJW, et al: The structural proteins of equine arteritis virus. *Virology* 73:200, 1976.
6. De Vries AAF, et al: All subgenomic RNAs of equine arteritis virus contain a common leader sequence. *Nucleic Acids Res* 18:3241, 1990.
7. Burki F: The virology of equine arteritis virus. In Proceedings of the Second International Conference of Equine Infectious Diseases, Paris. Basel, Karger, 1970, p 125.
8. Magnusson P, et al: Morphological studies on equine arteritis virus. *Arch ges Virusforsch* 30:105, 1970.
9. Van Berlo MF, et al: Equine arteritis virus-infected cells contain six polyadenylated virus-specific RNAs. *Virology* 118:345, 1982.
10. Westaway FG, et al: Togaviridae. *Intervirology* 24:125, 1985.
11. Murphy TW, et al: Genomic variability among globally distributed isolates of equine arteritis virus. *Vet Microbiol* 32:101, 1992.
12. Fukunaga Y, McCollum WH: Complement fixation reactions in equine viral arteritis. *Am J Vet Res* 38:2043, 1977.
13. Timoney PJ, et al: The carrier state in equine arteritis virus infection in the stallion with specific emphasis on the venereal mode of transmission. *J Reprod Fertil Suppl* 35:95, 1987a.
14. McCollum WH, et al: The recovery of virus from horses with experimental cases of equine arteritis using monolayer cell cultures of equine kidney. *Am J Vet Res* 23:465, 1961a.
15. McCollum WH, et al: Propagation of equine arteritis virus in monolayer cultures of equine kidney. *Am J Vet Res* 22:731, 1961b.
16. Timoney PJ: Clinical, virological and epidemiological features of the 1984 outbreak of equine viral arteritis in the Thoroughbred population in Kentucky, USA. In Proceedings of the Grayson Foundation International Conference of Thoroughbred Breeders Organizations, Dromoland Castle, Ireland, 1985, p 24.
17. Timoney PJ, et al: Demonstration of the carrier state in naturally acquired equine arteritis virus infection in the stallion. *Res Vet Sci* 41:279, 1986.
18. Neu SM, et al: Persistent infection of the reproductive tract in stallions persistently infected with equine arteritis virus. In Powell DG, ed. Proceedings of the Fifth International Conference on Equine Infectious Disease. Lexington, Kentucky University Press, 1988, p 149.
19. McCollum WH: Studies of passive immunity in foals to equine viral arteritis. *Vet Microbiol* 1:45, 1976.
20. Timoney PJ, et al: Status of EAV in Kentucky 1985. *J Am Vet Med Assoc* 191:36, 1987c.
21. Klingeborn B, et al: Prevalence of antibodies to equine arteritis virus in Sweden, shedding of the virus in semen from Swedish breeding stallions and evaluation of its possible influence on fertility. In Plowright W, Rossdale PD, Wade JF, eds. Proceedings of the Sixth International Conference on Equine Infectious Diseases, Cambridge, 1991. Newmarket, R & W Publications, 1992, p 319.
22. Coignoul FL, Cheville NF: Pathology of the maternal genital tract, placenta and foetus in equine viral arteritis. *Vet Pathol* 21:333, 1984.
23. Little TV, et al: Output of equine arteritis virus from persistently infected stallions is testosterone-dependent. In Plowright W, Rossdale PD, Wade JF, eds. Proceedings of the Sixth International Conference on Equine Infectious Diseases, Cambridge, 1991. Newmarket, R & W Publications, 1992, p 225.
24. McCollum WH, Bryans JT: Serological identification of infection by equine arteritis virus in horses of several countries. In Proceedings of the Third International Conference on Equine Infectious Diseases, Paris 1972. Basel, Karger, 1973, p 256.
25. Timoney PJ, McCollum, WH: The epidemiology of equine arteritis virus. *Proc Am Assoc Equine Pract* 31:545, 1985.
26. Collins JK, et al: Equine viral arteritis in a veterinary teaching hospital. *Prev Vet Med* 4:389, 1987.
27. Doll ER, et al: An outbreak of abortion caused by the equine arteritis virus. *Cornell Vet* 47:69, 1957.
28. Gerber H, et al: Serological investigations on equine viral arteritis. In Proceedings of the Fourth International Conference on Equine Infectious Diseases, Lyons, 1976. Veterinary Publications Inc, 1978, p 461.
29. Clayton H: The 1986 outbreak of EVA in Alberta, Canada. *J Equine Vet Sci* 7:101, 1987.
30. Golnik W, et al: Natural viral arteritis in foals. *Schweiz Arch Tierheilkd* 123:523, 1981.
31. Carman S: Equine arteritis virus isolated from a standardbred foal with pneumonia. *Can Vet J* 29:937, 1988.
32. Timoney PJ, McCollum, WH: Equine viral arteritis—epidemiology and control. *J Equine Vet Sci* 8:54, 1988.
33. Vaala WE, et al: Fatal, congenitally acquired infection with equine arteritis virus in a neonatal Thoroughbred. *Equine Vet J* 24:155, 1992.
34. Cole JR, et al: Transmissibility and abortigenic effect of equine viral arteritis in mares. *J Am Vet Med Assoc* 189:769, 1986.
35. Geering WA, Forman AJ: Exotic diseases; Australian Bureau of Animal Health/Australian Government Publishing Service, Canberra. *Anim Health Australia* 9:104, 1987.
36. Burki F: Eigenschaften des virus der Equinen Arteritis. *Pathologia Microbiol* 28:939, 1965.
37. McCollum WH, Swerczek TW: Studies of an epizootic of equine viral arteritis in racehorses. *Equine Vet J* 2:293, 1978.
38. Chirnside ED, Spaan WJM: Reverse transcription and cDNA amplification by the polymerase chain reaction of equine arteritis virus (EAV). *J Virol Methods* 30:133, 1990.
39. Matumoto M, et al: Constat anticorps contre le virus de l'arterite equine dans le serum de juments indienne. *C R Soc Biol* 159:1262, 1965.
40. Burki F, Gerber H: Ein virologisch gesicherter Groszausbruch von Equiner Arteritis. *Berl Munch Tierarztl Wochenschr* 79:391, 1966.
41. Hyllseth B, Petersson U: Neutralisation of equine arteritis virus; enhancing effect of guinea pig serum. *Arch ges Virusforsch* 37:337, 1970.
42. Senne DA, et al: Equine viral arteritis: A standard procedure for the virus neutralisation test and comparison of results of a proficiency test performed at five laboratories. In Proceedings of the 89th Annual Meeting of the United States Animal Health Association, Milwaukee, Wisconsin, 1985, p 29.
43. Lang G, Mitchell WR: A serosurvey by ELISA for antibodies to EAV in Ontario racehorses. *J Equine Vet Sci* 4:153, 1984.
44. Cook RF, et al: The effects of vaccination with tissue culture-derived viral vaccines on detection of antibodies to equine

arteritis virus by enzyme-linked immunosorbent assay (ELISA). *Vet Microbiol* 20:181, 1989.

45. McCollum WH: Vaccination for equine arteritis virus. In Proceedings of the Second International Conference on Equine Infectious Diseases, Paris. Basel, Karger, 1970, p 143.

46. McCollum WH, et al: Responses of vaccinated and non-vaccinated mares to artificial insemination with semen from stallions persistently infected with equine arteritis virus. In Powell D, ed. Proceedings of the Fifth International Conference on Equine Infectious Diseases, Lexington, 1991. Lexington, University Press of Kentucky, 1988, p 13.

47. Doll ER, et al: Immunisation against equine viral arteritis using modified live virus propagated in cell cultures of rabbit kidney. *Cornell Vet* 58:497, 1968.

48. McCollum WH: Development of a modified virus strain and vaccine for equine viral arteritis. *J Am Vet Med Assoc* 155:318, 1969.

49. McCollum WH: Pathological features of horses given avirulent virus intramuscularly. *Am J Vet Res* 42:1218, 1981.

50. Harry TO, McCollum WH: Stability of viability and immunising potency of lyophilised, modified equine arteritis live virus vaccine. *Am J Vet Res* 42:1501, 1981.

51. McCollum WH: Responses of horses vaccinated with avirulent modified-live equine arteritis virus propagated in E. derm (NBL-6) cell line to nasal inoculations with virulent virus. *Am J Vet Res* 47:1931, 1986.

52. Timoney PJ, et al: Safety evaluation of a commercial modified live equine arteritis virus vaccine for use in stallions. In Powell D, ed. Proceedings of the Fifth International Conference on Equine Infectious Diseases, Lexington 1987. Lexington, University Press of Kentucky, 1988, p 19.

53. Fukunaga Y, et al: Effect of the modified *Bucyrus* strain of equine arteritis virus experimentally inoculated into horses. *Bull Equine Res Inst* 19:97, 1982.

54. McKinnon AO, et al: Vaccination of stallions with a modified live equine arteritis virus vaccine. *J Equine Vet Sci* 6:66, 1986.

55. Fukunaga Y, et al: Tentative preparation of an inactivated virus vaccine for equine viral arteritis. *Bull Equine Res Inst* 21:56, 1984.

56. Fukunaga Y, et al: Induction of immune response and protection from equine viral arteritis (EVA) by formalin inactivated-virus vaccine for EVA in horses. *J Vet Med* 37:135, 1990.

57. Fukunaga Y, et al: An attempt to protect persistent infection of equine viral arteritis in the reproductive tract of stallions using formalin inactivated virus vaccine. In Plowright W, Rossdale PD, Wade JF, eds. Proceedings of the Sixth International Conference on Equine Infectious Diseases, Cambridge, 1991. Newmarket, R & W Publications, 1992, p 239.

58. McKenzie J: Equine viral arteritis and trade in horses from the USA. *Surveillance* 15:6, 1988.

59. McKenzie J: Survey of stallions for equine viral arteritis. *Surveillance* 16:17, 1990.

60. Allen GP, Bryans, JT: Molecular epizootiology, pathogenesis, and prophylaxis of equine herpesvirus-1 infections. In Pandy R, Karger S, eds. *Progress in Veterinary Microbiology and Immunology*, vol 1. Basel, Karger, 1986, p 78.

61. Bryans JT, et al: Neonatal foal disease associated with perinatal infection by equine herpesvirus 1. *J Equine Med Surg* 1:20, 1977.

62. Hartley WJ, Dixon RJ: An outbreak of foal perinatal mortality due to equid herpesvirus type-1: Pathological observations. *Equine Vet J* 11:215, 1979.

63. Krosgrud J, Onstad O: Equine coital exanthema: Isolation of virus and transmission experiments. *Acta Vet Scand* 12:1, 1971.

64. Studdert MJ: Comparative aspects of equine herpesviruses. *Cornell Vet* 64:94, 1974.

65. O'Callaghan DJ, et al: The equine herpesvirus. In *The Viruses*, vol. 2. New York, Plenum Press, 1983, p 215.

66. Plummer G, Waterson AP: Equine herpesviruses. *Virology* 19:412, 1963.

67. O'Callaghan DJ, Randall CC: Molecular anatomy of herpesviruses: Recent studies. *Prog Med Virol* 22:152, 1976.

68. O'Callaghan DJ, et al: Structure and replication of equine herpesvirus. In: Powell D (ed): Proceedings of the 4th International Conference on Equine Infectious Diseases. Princeton, NJ, Veterinary Publications, 1978, p 1.

69. Spear PG, Roizman B: Proteins specified by herpes simplex virus. V: Purification of structural proteins of the herpes virion. *J Virol* 9:143, 1980.

70. Turtinen LW, Allen GP: Identification of the envelope surface glycoproteins of equine herpesvirus type-1. *J Gen Virol* 63:481, 1982.

71. Allen GP, Coogle LD: Characterization of an equine herpesvirus type 1 gene (gp13) encoding a glycoprotein with homology to herpes simplex virus glycoprotein C. *J Virol* 62:2850, 1988.

72. Whalley JM, et al: Identification and nucleotide sequence of a gene in equine herpesvirus 1 analogous to the herpes simplex virus gene encoding the major envelope glycoprotein gB. *J Gen Virol* 70:383, 1989.

73. Audonnet JC, et al: Equine herpesvirus type 1 unique short fragment encodes glycoproteins with homology to herpes simplex virus type 1 gD, gI and gE. *J Gen Virol* 71:2969, 1990.

74. Elton DM, et al: Location of open reading frames coding for equine herpesvirus type 1 glycoproteins with homology to gE and gI of herpes simplex virus. *Am J Vet Res* 52:1252, 1991.

75. Robertson GR, et al: Sequence characteristics of a gene in equine herpesvirus 1 homologous to glycoprotein H of herpes simplex virus. *DNA Seq* 1:241, 1991.

76. Allen GP, et al: Molecular dissection of two major equine herpesvirus-1 glycoprotein antigens (gB and gC) that elicit humoral immune responses in the horse. In Plowright W, Rossdale PD, Wade JF, eds. Proceedings of the 6th International Conference on Equine Infectious Diseases, Cambridge, 1991. 1992, p 181.

77. Allen GP, et al: Equid herpesvirus-1 glycoprotein 13 (gp13): epitope analysis, gene structure, and expression in *E. coli*. In Powell D, ed. Proceedings of the 5th International Conference on Equine Infectious Diseases. Lexington, Kentucky, 1988, p 103.

78. Darlington RW, Randall, CC: The nucleic acid content of equine abortion virus. *Virology* 19:322, 1963.

79. Soehner RL, et al: Some physiochemical properties of equine abortion virus nucleic acid. *Virology* 26:394, 1965.

80. Henry BE, et al: Structure of the genome of equine herpesvirus type-1. *Virology* 115:97, 1981.

81. Whalley JM, et al: Analysis of equine herpesvirus type-1: Arrangement of cleavage sites for restriction endonucleases *Eco*RI, *Bgl*II and *Bam*HI. *J Gen Virol* 57:307, 1981.

82. Ruyechan WT, et al: Electron microscopic study of equine herpesvirus type-1 DNA. *J Virol* 42:297, 1982.

83. Telford EA, et al: The DNA sequence of equine herpesvirus-1. *Virology* 189:304, 1992.

84. Fitzpatrick DR, et al: Nucleotide sequence of bovine herpesvirus type-1 glycoprotein gIII, a structural model for gIII as a new member of the immunoglobulin superfamily, and implications for the homologous glycoprotein of other herpesviruses. *Virology* 173:46, 1989.

85. Davison AJ, Wilkie NM: Location and orientation of homologous sequences in the genomes of five herpesviruses. *J Lab Clin Med* 63:5, 1983.

86. Ben-Porat T, et al: Localization of the regions of homology

between the genomes of herpes simplex virus types 1 and pseudorabies virus. *Virology* 127:194, 1983.

87. Cullinane AA, et al: Characterization of the genome of equine herpesvirus-1 subtype-2. *J Gen Virol* 69:1570, 1988.

88. Sabine M, et al: Differentiation of subtypes of equine herpesvirus 1 by restriction endonuclease analysis. *Aust Vet J* 57:148, 1981.

89. Turtinen LW, et al: Serological and molecular comparisons of several equine herpesvirus type-1 strains. *Am J Vet Res* 42:2099, 1983.

90. Allen GP, et al: Molecular epizootiological studies of equine herpesvirus-1 infections by restriction endonuclease fingerprinting viral DNA. *Am J Vet Res* 44:263, 1983.

91. Allen GP, et al: A new field strain of equine abortion virus (equine herpesvirus-1) among Kentucky horses. *Am J Vet Res* 46:138, 1985.

92. Studdert MJ, et al: The molecular epidemiology of equine herpesvirus 1 in Australasia. *Aust Vet J* 69:104, 1992.

93. Buchman TG, et al: Restriction endonuclease fingerprinting of herpes simplex DNA: A new epidemiological tool applied to a nosocomial outbreak. *J Infect Dis* 138:488, 1978.

94. Lonsdale DM, et al: Variations in herpes simplex virus isolated from human ganglia and a study of herpes simplex virus isolated from human ganglia and a study of clonal variation in HSV-1. *Ann N Y Acad Sci* 354:291, 1980.

95. Mumford JA, et al: Serological and virological investigation of an equid herpesvirus 1 (EHV-1) abortion storm on a stud farm in 1985. *J Reprod Fertil Suppl* 35:509, 1987.

96. Bryans JT: Herpesviral disease affecting reproduction in the horse. *Vet Clin North Am Large Animal Pract* 2:303, 1980.

97. Burrows R, Goodridge D: Observations of picornavirus, adenovirus and equine herpesvirus infections in the Pirbright pony herd. In Proceedings of the 4th International Conference on Equine Infectious Diseases, Lyon, 1976. Princeton, NJ, Veterinary Publications, 1978, p 155.

98. Mumford JA, Rossdale PD: Virus and its relationship to the "poor performance" syndrome. *Equine Vet J* 12:3, 1980.

99. Doll ER, Bryans JT: Epizootiology of equine viral rhinopneumonitis. *J Am Vet Med Assoc* 142:31, 1963.

100. Saxgaard F: Isolation and identification of equine rhinopneumonitis virus from cases of abortion and paralysis. *Nord Vet* 18:504, 1966.

101. Greenwood RES, Simpson ARB: Clinical report of a paralytic syndrome affecting stallions, mares and foals on a thoroughbred stud farm. *Equine Vet J* 12:112, 1980.

102. Chowdhury SI, et al: Equine herpesvirus type-1 induced abortions and paralysis in a Lipizzaner stud: A contribution to the classification of equine herpesvirus. *Arch Virol* 90:273, 1986.

103. Edington N, et al: Experimental reactivation of equid herpesvirus 1 following the administration of corticosteroids. *Equine Vet J* 17:769, 1985.

104. Browning GF, et al: Latency of equine herpesvirus type 4. *Vet Rec* 123:518, 1988.

105. Welch HM, et al: Latent equid herpesvirus 1 and 4: Detection and distinction using the polymerase chain reaction and co-cultivation from lymphoid tissues. *J Gen Virol* 73:261, 1992.

106. Edington N, Welch HM, Griffith L: The prevalence of latent equine herpesviruses in the tissues of 40 abbatoir horses. *Equine Vet J* 26:140, 1994.

107. Edington N: Latency of equine herpesviruses. In Plowright W, Rossdale PD, Wade JF, eds. Proceedings of the 6th International Conference on Equine Infectious Diseases, Cambridge, 1991. 1992, p 195.

108. Burrows R, Goodridge D: Studies of persistent and latent equid herpesvirus 1 and herpesvirus 3 infections in the Pirbright pony herd. In *Latent Herpesvirus Infections in Veterinary Medicine*. Boston, Nijhoff, 1984, p 307.

109. Crowhurst FA, et al: An outbreak of paresis in mares and

110. Prickett ME: The pathology of the disease caused by equine herpesvirus 1. In Bryans JT, Gerber H, eds. Proceedings of the 2nd International Conference on Equine Infectious Diseases, Paris, 1969. 1970, p 24.

111. Campbell TM, Studdert MJ: Equine herpesvirus type-1. *Vet Bull* 53:135, 1983.

112. Patel JR, et al: Variation in cellular tropism between isolates of equine herpesvirus-1 in foals. *Arch Virol* 74:41, 1982.

113. Dutta SK, et al: Lymphocyte responses to virus and mitogen in ponies during experimental infection with equine herpesvirus 1. *Am J Vet Res* 41:2066, 1980.

114. Scott JC, et al: In vivo harboring of equine herpesvirus-1 in leukocyte populations and sub-populations and their quantitation from experimentally infected ponies. *Am J Vet Res* 44:1344, 1983.

115. Edington N, et al: Endothelial cell infection and thrombosis in paralysis caused by equid herpesvirus-1: Equine stroke. *Arch Virol* 90:111, 1986.

116. Platt H, et al: Pathological observations on an outbreak of paralysis in broodmares. *Equine Vet J* 12:118, 1980.

117. Thorsen J, Little PB: Isolation of equine herpesvirus 1 from a horse with an acute paralytic disease. *Can J Comp Med* 39:358, 1975.

118. Whitwell KE, Blunden AS: Pathological findings in horses dying during an outbreak of the paralytic form of equid herpesvirus type-1 infection. *Equine Vet J* 24:2, 1992.

118a. Slater JD, Borchers K, Thackray AM, Field HJ: The trigeminal ganglion is a location for equine herpesvirus 1 latency and reactivation in the horse. *J GH Vir* 75:2007, 1995.

118b. Bari MK, Efstathion S, Lawrence G, et al: The detection of latency associated transcripts of equine herpesvirus 1 in ganglionic neurons. *J GH Vir* 76:3113, 1995.

119. Edington N, et al: The role of endothelial cell infection in the endometrium, placenta and foetus of equid herpesvirus 1 abortions. *J Comp Pathol* 104:379, 1991.

120. Smith K, et al: An immunohistological study of the uterus of mares following experimental infection with EHV-1. *Equine Vet J* 20:36, 1993.

121. Westerfield C, Dimock WW: The pathology of equine abortion. *J Am Vet Med Assoc* 109:101, 1946.

122. Smith K, et al: Abortion of virologically negative foetuses following experimental challenge of pregnant mares with equid herpesvirus 1. *Equine Vet J* 24:256, 1992.

123. Yeargan MR, et al: Rapid subtyping of equine herpesvirus 1 with monoclonal antibodies. *J Clin Microbiol* 21:694, 1985.

124. Sinclair R: Equid herpesvirus type-1: Antigenic analysis and diagnosis of infection using monoclonal antibodies. PhD Thesis, CNAA, London, 1991.

125. Sinclair R, Mumford JA: Rapid detection of equine herpesvirus type-1 antigens in nasal swab specimens using an antigen capture enzyme-linked immunosorbent assay. *J Virol Methods* 39:299, 1992.

126. Sharma PC, et al: Diagnosis of equid herpesvirus 1 and 4 polymerase chain reaction. *Equine Vet J* 24:20, 1992.

127. Ballagi-Pordany A, et al: Equine herpesvirus type 1: Detection of viral DNA sequences in aborted fetuses with the polymerase chain reaction. *Vet Microbiol* 22:373, 1990.

128. Smith IM, et al: The fluorescent antibody technique in the diagnosis of equine rhinopneumonitis virus abortion. *Can J Com Med* 36:303, 1972.

129. Whitwell KE, et al: An immunoperoxidase method applied to the diagnosis of equine herpesvirus abortion, using conventional and rapid microwave techniques. *Equine Vet J* 24:10, 1992.

130. Blunden AS, et al: An outbreak of paralysis associated with

geldings associated with equid herpesvirus 1. *Vet Rec* 109:527, 1981.

equid herpesvirus type-1 infection in a livery stable. *Prog Vet Neurol* 3:95, 1992.

131. Thomson GR, et al: Serological detection of equid herpesvirus 1 infections in the respiratory tract. *Equine Vet J* 8:58, 1976.

132. Dutta SK, et al: Detection of equine herpesvirus 1 antigen and the specific antibody by enzyme-linked immunosorbent assay. *Am J Vet Res* 36:445, 1983.

133. Gradil C, Joo HS: A radial immunodiffusion enzyme immunoassay for detection of antibody to equine rhinopneumonitis virus in horse serum. *Vet Microbiol* 17:315, 1988.

134. Sinclair R, Binns MM, Chirnside ED, Mumford JA: Detection of antibodies against equid herpesvirus type 1 and type 4 using recombinant antigen derived from an immunodominant region of glycoprotein B. *J Clin Microbiol* 31:265, 1993.

135. Kendrick JW, Stevenson W: Immunity to equine herpesvirus-1 infection in foals during the first year of life. *J Reprod Fertil Suppl* 27:615, 1979.

136. Edington N, Bridges CG: One way protection between equid herpesvirus 1 and 4 *in vivo*. *Res Vet Sci* 48:235, 1990.

137. Pachciarz JA, Bryans JT: Cellular immunity to equine rhinopneumonitis virus in pregnant mares. In Powell D, ed. Proceedings of the 4th International Conference of Equine Infectious Diseases, Lyon, 1976. 1978, p 115.

138. Dutta SK, Campbell DL: Cell mediated immunity in equine herpesvirus type-1 infection. 1: *In vitro* lymphocyte blastogenesis and serum neutralization antibody in normal parturient and aborting mares. *Can J Comp Med* 41:404, 1977.

139. Hannant DH, et al: Evidence for non-specific immunosuppression during the development of immune responses to equid herpesvirus-1. *Equine Vet J Suppl* 12:41, 1991.

140. Cambridge G, et al: Cell mediated immune response to influenza virus infections in mice. *Infect Immun* 13:36, 1976.

141. Doll ER: Immunization against viral rhinopneumonitis of horses with live virus propagated in hamsters. *J Am Vet Med Assoc* 139:1324, 1961.

142. Doll ER, Bryans JT: A planned infection program for immunizing mares against viral rhinopneumonitis. *Cornell Vet* 53:249, 1963.

143. Dutta SK, Shipley WD: Immunity and the level of neutralization antibodies in foals and mares vaccinated with a modified live-virus rhinopneumonitis vaccine. *Am J Vet Res* 36:445, 1975.

144. Burrows R, Goodridge D: Equid herpesvirus 1: Some observations on the epizootiology of infections and on the innocuity testing of live virus vaccines. In Proceedings of the 24th Annual Conference of the American Association of Equine Practitioners, St. Louis, 1978. 1979, p 17.

145. Bryans JT: Immunization of pregnant mares with an inactivated equine herpesvirus 1 vaccine. In Powell D, ed. Proceedings of the 4th International Conference on Equine Infectious Diseases, Lyon, 1976. 1978, p 83.

146. Sovinova O, et al: Isolation of a virus causing respiratory disease in horses. *Acta Virol* 2:52, 1958.

147. Wadell GH, et al: A new influenza virus associated with equine respiratory disease. *J Am Vet Med Assoc* 143:587, 1963.

148. Guo, YJ, et al: Equine influenza epidemic again in North-East China. *Virus Information Exchange Newsletter for South-East Asia and the Western Pacific* 7:146, 1990.

149. Hay AH, Skehel JJ: The structure and replication of influenza virus. In Beare AS, ed. *Basic and Applied Influenza Research.* Florida, CRC Press, 1982.

150. Gibson CA, et al: Haemagglutinin gene sequencing studies of equine-1 influenza A virus. In Powell DG, ed. Proceedings of the 5th International Conference on Equine Infectious Diseases. Kentucky University Press, 1988, p 51.

151. Hinshaw VS, et al: Analysis of antigenic variation in equine 2 influenza A viruses. *Bull World Health Organ* 61:153, 1983.

152. Higgins WP, et al: Surveys of equine influenza outbreaks during 1983 and 1984. *J Equine Vet Sci* 6:15, 1986.

153. Berg M, et al: Genetic drift of equine 2 influenza A virus (H3N8), (1963–1988). Analysis by oligonucleotide mapping. *Vet Microbiol* 22:225, 1990.

154. Kawaoka Y, et al: Origin of the A/equine/Johannesburg/86 (H3N8) virus: Antigenic and genetic analysis of equine-2 influenza A hemagglutinins. In Powell DG, ed. Equine infectious Diseases V. Lexington, Kentucky University Press, 1988, p 47.

155. Uppal PK, Yadav MP: Isolation of A/equi-2 virus during 1987 equine influenza epidemic in India. *Equine Vet J* 21:364, 1989.

156. Mumford JA, et al: Experimental infection of ponies with equine influenza (H3N8) viruses by intranasal inoculation or exposure to aerosols. *Equine Vet J* 22:93, 1990.

157. Gerber H: Clinical features, sequelae and epidemiology of equine influenza. In *Equine Infectious Diseases.* New York, Phiebig, 1970, p 63.

158. Miller WMC: Equine influenza: Further observations on the coughing outbreak 1965. *Vet Rec* 77:455, 1965.

159. Erasmus BJ: Veterinary Research Institute, Ondestepoort, South Africa, 1986, unpublished data.

160. Mumford JA, et al: Studies with inactivated equine influenza vaccine 2. Protection against experimental infection with influenza virus A/equine/Newmarket/79 (H3N8). *J Hyg Camb* 90:385, 1983.

161. Mumford JA, et al: Protection against experimental infection with influenza virus A/equine/Miami/63 (H3N8) provided by inactivated whole virus vaccines containing homologous virus. *Epidemiol Infect* 100:501, 1988.

162. Hannant D, et al: Duration of circulating antibody and immunity following infection with equine influenza virus. *Vet Rec* 122:125, 1988.

163. Mumford JA: Progress in the control of equine influenza. In Plowright W, Rossdale PD, Wade JF, eds. *Equine Infectious Diseases VI.* Newmarket, R & W Publications, 1991, p 207.

164. Mumford JA, et al: Experimental infection of ponies with equine influenza (H3N8) viruses by intranasal inoculation or exposure to aerosols. *Equine Vet J* 22:93, 1990.

165. Hannant D, et al: Antibody isotype responses in the serum and respiratory tract to primary and secondary infections with equine influenza virus (H3N8). *Vet Microbiol* 19:293, 1989.

166. Lucam F, et al: La Grippe Equine. Caracters de la maladie expérimentale et de l'immunité post-vaccinal. *Rev Med Vét* 125:1273, 1974.

167. Rose MA, et al: Influenza in horses and donkeys in Britain, 1969. *Vet Rec* 86:768, 1970.

168. Cook RF, et al: Detection of influenza nucleoprotein antigen in nasal secretions from horses infected with A/equine influenza (H3N8) viruses. *J Virol Methods* 20:1, 1988.

169. Anestad G, Maagaard O: Rapid diagnosis of equine influenza. *Vet Rec* 126:550, 1990.

170. Mumford JA, Wood J: Establishing an acceptability threshold for equine influenza vaccines. Symposium on an International Harmonization of Veterinary Biologicals. In Developments in Biological Standardization, 79, 1992, p 137.

171. Burrows R, Denyer M: Antigenic properties of some equine influenza viruses. *Arch Virol* 73:15, 1982.

172. Binns MM, et al: Genetic and antigenic analysis of an equine influenza isolate from the 1989 epidemic. *Arch Virol* 1992.

173. Mumford JA, et al: The effect of antigenic drift on the efficacy of equine influenza vaccines. In Options for the control of influenza II. (Abstract) 1992b.

2.3

Internal Parasite Infections

Thomas R. Klei, PhD

Horses serve as hosts for numerous parasites, which induce a wide range of pathologic and immunologic responses.[1] Many of the latter are of a hypersensitive nature and also result in disease conditions. Immune responses leading to protective resistance against reinfection occur, but the level of this resistance is most often incomplete. Mechanisms associated with these responses have not been investigated extensively in the horse, but information is available from other host-parasite systems that is relevant to the equine. The purpose of this section is to acquaint the reader with contemporary thoughts on host-parasite interactions. Because of their prevalence, major importance to the equine and information available, coverage is limited to helminth parasites that occur in most developed and nontropical countries.

PARASITE-INDUCED LESIONS

Infection with most metazoan parasites results in inflammation and structural and functional changes of the organs invaded. The outcome of these changes is an alteration of the host's physiologic state. The degree of alteration is dependent on the existing physiologic condition of the animal, which is dictated to a great degree by its age, nutritional status, and previous immunologic experience with the parasite. The numbers of parasites introduced and the specific parasite also affect the degree of physiologic change that occurs. When these factors favor major alterations, the results are readily identifiable clinical signs of infection. Subclinical infections, although less apparent, are potentially important to the general health of the animal and continued transmission of the agent. The pathophysiologic effects of infection by ectoparasites, helminths, and microorganisms is in many cases similar.[2] Abnormalities in weight gain, skeletal growth, reproduction, and lactation may result from infections with any of these agents. These changes are often directly related to parasite-induced anorexia, disruption of metabolic processes, and anemia. An understanding of the morphologic and biochemical lesions produced by specific parasites clarifies the role of these agents in clinical and subclinical conditions associated with the infections. A majority of detailed studies on the pathophysiology of parasitic infections have been conducted in laboratory animal models and domestic animal species other than the horse.[2] However, the classical pathology of parasitic infections of the horse has been reviewed.[3, 4] The following discussion outlines some recent observations on host-parasite interactions that may be of significance to equine medicine. Examples of host-parasite interactions responsible for alterations in host homeostasis are presented as they relate to the gastrointestinal tract, lungs, and skin.

Gastrointestinal Tract

Internal parasites are most important to equine health as mediators of gastrointestinal symptoms such as colic and diarrhea. Although almost all internal parasites have been inferentially implicated as causative agents of colic at some time, large strongyles, principally *Strongylus vulgaris* and to a lesser extent *Parascaris equorum*, have classically been considered major pathogens in this regard. Details of the pathogenesis of colic associated with migration of *S. vulgaris* through the mesenteric arteries and the resultant thrombosis infarctions and necrosis of the intestine have been described in detail elsewhere.[3, 4] Although this condition has been well described, some points are particularly noteworthy. Histologic studies of experimentally infected parasite-free pony foals during the initial stages of the infection indicate that the severity of the lesions produced in the intestine cannot be attributed solely to mechanical disruption caused by larval migrations and that these larval stages induce some biological amplification system within the mucosa, which results in the degree of inflammation observed.[5] Although the mechanisms involved in this response have not been investigated, the histologic nature of the lesion is characteristic of an Arthus reaction suggesting an involvement of the immune response. Other experimental studies using the parasite-free pony–*S. vulgaris* system have implicated a role for the immune response in the mediation and regulation of the arterial lesions produced by this parasite. Passive transfer of immune serum but not normal serum reduced the severity of arteritis seen and clinical signs associated with experimental infections without reducing the numbers of parasites that develop in these ponies. However, treatment with immune serum also induced an anamnestic eosinophilia and marked perivascular infiltration of eosinophils in the cecum. The reduction in intravascular lesions may have been associated with an inactivation of parasite-secreted inflammatory factors either by antibody or serum enzymes. This serum may also have contained nonspecific host-derived anti-inflammatory substances. The exacerbation of the eosinophil response may have been associated with the formation of immune complexes. Although the mechanisms are unknown, the results suggest that the immune response may simultaneously modulate and potentiate inflammation. It has been postulated that larvacidal treatment of *S. vulgaris*-infected horses and killing of intravascular larvae may release a bolus of antigenic factors from these larvae within the mesenteric vasculature, resulting in an exacerbation of arterial and intestinal lesions and colic. Experimental testing of this hypothesis indicates that this phenomenon does not occur and further that viable larvae are necessary to maintain the arteritis and eosinophilia seen.[6, 7]

Parascaris equorum-associated colic in foals has been related to intestinal impaction and rupture and is not considered to be of major significance in adult horses.[8] However, ascarid nematodes are particularly potent sources of allergens, and it is not inconceivable that the hypersensitized mature horse may respond to low-level infections with this parasite. Observations made in the author's laboratory are noteworthy in this regard. Two mature *Parascaris*-free adult horses were inoculated intradermally with less than 90 μg of saline-soluble somatic extract of adult *P. equorum* in order to test for immediate hypersensitivity to this antigen. Both

in their apparent normal host, as has been described for *D. arnfieldi.*

Age resistance to *P. equorum* and *S. vulgaris* has been described to occur in horses by comparing susceptibility of young and old ponies reared under parasite-free conditions. It is apparent that the reaction of the lung to migrating *P. equorum* larvae is more marked in mature horses and suggests that an immune response occurs in this site.[9, 10] Initial reports on age-acquired resistance to *S. vulgaris* infection have not been substantiated by further experimentation, and these results remain equivocal.[22]

The occurrence of acquired resistance to equine parasites can be inferred from the observation that older chronically exposed horses generally have lower burdens of parasites than do similarly exposed young horses. Using these criteria, acquired resistance is apparent to infections of *S. westeri, P. equorum, Strongylus* sp., and cyathostome sp. Extensive experiments are limited, however, to those on *S. vulgaris.*

The level of resistance that is acquired in most cases is partial and of a concomitant type; that is, some stages of the parasite, such as arterial larvae of *S. vulgaris*, may reside within the horse in the face of an active acquired resistance against newly acquired infective stages. Resistance to infection with *S. westeri* adult parasites is inferred by the short duration of their life cycle within the small intestine and the failure of subsequent exposures to establish patent infections. Mares, however, remain infected with arrested third-stage larvae, which subsequent to foaling are transmitted to the foals in milk 4 days postpartum. Although not studied in horses, similar phenomena occur in swine strongyloidosis. In these infections, there is an apparent protective resistance against the migrating L_3, which is effective in preventing re-establishment of the intestinal infection but is ineffective against L_3, which are sequestered in the abdominal fat of the sow.[23] Similar epidemiologic phenomena occur in *S. westeri* infection of horses, and it may be implied that similar immunologic mechanisms are also active.

Immunologic mechanisms associated with protective resistance are presented primarily as they relate to parasites that inhabit the lumen of the gastrointestinal tract and secondly as those that undergo extensive extra-intestinal tissue migration.

Gastrointestinal Parasites

Immune responses directed toward gastrointestinal nematodes have been demonstrated to vary significantly among hosts and against different parasite species within a given host.[24] However, some generalities may be stated that may serve as a background for understanding these responses in the horse. A phenomenon termed "self-cure" has been described in sheep, in which the ingestion of significant numbers of infective larvae induces the expulsion of existing adult parasites. This expulsion is initiated by a species-specific immediate-type hypersensitivity response that may cause the nonspecific expulsion of other nematode species. Although this phenomenon has not been examined in the equine, experimental infections of naturally parasitized ponies with large numbers of *S. vulgaris* L_3 induced a dramatic decrease in preexisting strongyle fecal egg counts, suggesting that a self-cure–like reaction may occur under some conditions.

More typically, establishment of primary infections results at some time in spontaneous expulsions of these worms due either to senility or, as demonstrated in laboratory animal model systems, to active acquired immune responses. This phenomenon occurs experimentally in the absence of re-infection and is thus separate from the self-cure phenomenon. A confusing number of immune effectors have been identified with this phenomenon in various model systems, and it is likely that some if not all are at some time active in the equine intestine. The mechanisms involved are T-cell dependent. Antibodies may be involved but are not sufficient in themselves to induce expulsion. T-cell–mediated mastocytosis, eosinophilia, and goblet cell hyperplasia have all been demonstrated to be related to expression of expulsion in some systems. These accessory cells are involved in the nonspecific efferent arm of this response. Mediators of inflammation, such as vasoactive amines, prostaglandins, and increased mucus production, have been linked to immune elimination of primary infections in some but not all model systems. It is likely that a number of specific immunologic events initiate several nonspecific effector mechanisms, resulting in this expulsion. These mechanisms vary with the species of parasite involved. The elimination of adult *S. westeri* and *P. equorum* from maturing horses and the hypothetical seasonal turnover in *Strongylus* spp. and cyathostome spp. may be mediated by such responses.

In addition to immune responses that occur during tissue migrations, protective resistance to reinfection by gastrointestinal nematodes occurs at the surface of the epithelium. This reaction, termed rapid expulsion or immune exclusion, is separate from self-cure or immune expulsion of primary infection. Infective larvae are expelled from the intestine in a matter of hours. Again mechanisms of expulsion described vary between parasite and host species. However, anaphylactic reactions and mucus entrapment have been observed. Some experiments using the *T. spiralis*-rat system suggest that alterations in the epithelial cells in immune animals are directly involved in the exclusion of these parasites. Although immune-mediated damage of intestinal helminths such as decreased fecundity, reduced size, and morphologic alterations have been noted, infective larvae expelled by rapid expulsion mechanisms remain viable and undamaged. It may be speculated that reactions of this nature are responsible, in part, for resistance to reinfection of equines with cyathostomes.

Tissue-Migrating Parasites

A number of intestinal helminths as well as others migrate through extraintestinal tissues as part of their life cycle. These include parasites such as *P. equorum, S. westeri,* and *Strongylus* spp., all of which stimulate an acquired immune response in the horse. During this migration these larvae are vulnerable to attack by immune effectors that may either encapsulate them in an immune-mediated inflammatory response, disrupt their migrations by interfering with important metabolic or invasive processes, or inhibit molting from the L_3 to L_4 stages. The most studied phenomenon in this regard is antibody-mediated adherence of inflammatory cells, which may result in killing of the larvae. This phenomenon has been demonstrated to involve many different cell types and immunoglobulin isotypes in different host-parasite systems. In vitro studies of this nature have been conducted using *S. vulgaris* third-stage larvae and equine immune effectors in the author's laboratory. In these experiments, an antibody-dependent adherence of cells was demonstrated and shown to be parasite species-specific. In vitro killing was mediated by eosinophils and not by neutrophils or monocytes. Activated eosinophils were necessary to mediate this response, and *S. vulgaris* infections have been demonstrated to activate eosinophils and neutrophils in vivo.[25] Although it is not certain that eosinophils are essential in this protective immune response, an anamnestic eosinophilia is characteristic in immune ponies but not nonimmune ponies following experimental *S. vulgaris* challenge. Due to its prominence, compelling in vitro and correlative in vivo data, the eosinophil has been considered to be a major effector in immune-mediated helminth killing. However, recent studies in murine parasite model systems in which eosinophilia was blocked by anti-IL₅ treatment suggest that this type of cell is not essential for protective resistance in some systems.[26] It is possible, in vivo, that a number of cells function as effectors and may overcome the absence of sufficient eosinophils under some circumstances. Antibody reactivity with parasite-secreted enzymes and molting fluids, factors important in parasite homeostasis, have been demonstrated in vitro; and similar reactions may be important in vivo.

T-cell responses are essential for the induction of protective resistance to tissue-migrating helminths in most systems studied, including the experimental *S. vulgaris* pony model. This dependency is likely due to the T-cell dependency of the antibody response and to the mediation of secondary effector cell responses. It is likely that antigenic substances secreted or excreted (ES) by migrating nematodes are important in the induction of these responses. It is probable that a combination of immune responses elicited by a combination of specific parasite antigens, including surface antigens and ES products, is necessary to induce an immune response sufficient to provide protective resistance.

PARASITE EVASION OF IMMUNE EFFECTORS

Some parasites that live for long periods within a host have been shown to modulate the host response in both a specific and a nonspecific fashion, as described previously for filarial infections. It is inferred that this modulation inhibits immune responses associated with protective resistance. In addition, blocking antibodies have been demonstrated that inhibit antibody-dependent eosinophil killing of schistosome larvae in both rodent models and in sera from infected patients. The role of these types of antibodies in other infections is unclear.

A number of parasite-driven mechanisms have been described that promote parasite survival within hosts possessing strong immune responses directed toward their antigenic components.[27] Others mask themselves to avoid recognition or directly inactivate immune effectors. Host molecules shown to be attached to the surface of parasites include glycolipids of blood group antigens, glycoproteins, serum proteins, and class I and class II MHC molecules. In some instances, host-like molecules have been demonstrated to be encoded in parasitic helminth genomes and expressed on their surfaces. This phenomenon, termed molecular mimicry, has been postulated to be a mechanism evolved by the parasite mask itself from the host immune surveillance systems.

Some parasites, notably tapeworm larvae, have been demonstrated to produce factors that activate complement and thus may produce a state of localized complement depletion in vivo. Other factors from tapeworm larvae have been shown to disrupt the coagulation cascade and others to have anti-inflammatory activity.[28] Filarial nematodes synthesize prostaglandins from host arachidonic acid and release these in vitro and potentially in vivo.[29] It has been suggested that these molecules may be responsible for local modulation of inflammatory cell function and play a role in the survival of parasites.

These types of mechanisms have been identified in most host-parasite systems examined and are likely active in the horse. These intriguing phenomena, however, have yet to be investigated in equine parasite infections.

REFERENCES

1. Jacobs DE: *A Colour Atlas of Equine Parasites.* Philadelphia, Lea & Febiger, 1986.
2. Symons LEA: *Pathophysiology of Endoparasitic Infection Compared with Ectoparasitic Infestation and Microbial Infection.* San Diego, Academic Press, 1989.
3. Slocombe JOD: Pathogenesis of helminths in equines. *Vet Parasitol* 18:139, 1985.
4. Herd RP: *The Veterinary Clinics of North America Equine Practice.* Vol. 2: *Parasitology.* Philadelphia, WB Saunders, 1986.
5. McCraw BM, Slocombe JOD: Early development of *Strongylus vulgaris* in pony foals (abstr). *Proc Am Assoc Vet Parasitol* 57, 1990.
6. Klei TR, Turk MAM, McClure JR, et al: Effects of repeated experimental *Strongylus vulgaris* infections and subsequent ivermectin treatment on mesenteric arterial pathology in pony foals. *Am J Vet Res* 51:54, 1990.
7. Holmes RA, Klei TR, McClure JR, et al: Sequential mesenteric arteriography in pony foals during a course of repeated experimental *Strongylus vulgaris* infections and ivermectin treatments. *Am J Vet Res* 51:661, 1990.
8. Clayton HM: Ascarids: Recent advances In Herd RP, ed. *The Veterinary Clinics of North America Equine Practice Parasitology.* Philadelphia, WB Saunders, 1986 p 313.
9. Beroza GA, Barclay WP, Phillips TN, et al: Cecal perforation and peritonitis associated with *Anoplocephala perfoliata* infection in three horses. *J Am Vet Med Assoc* 183:804, 1983.
10. Barclay WP, Phillips TN, Foerner JJ: Intussusception associated with *Anoplocephala perfoliata.* *Vet Rec* 124:34, 1989.
11. Owen RR, Jagger DW, Quan-Taylor R: Cecal intussusceptions in horses and the significance of *Anoplocephala perfoliata.* *Vet Rec* 124:34, 1989.
11a. Proudman CJ, Edwards GB, Gareth B: Are tapeworms associated with equine colic? A case control study. *Equine Vet J* 25:224, 1993.
12. Uhlinger CA: Effects of three anthelmintic schedules on the incidence of colic. *Equine Vet J* 22:251, 1991.
13. Uhlinger CA: Equine small strongyles: Epidemiology, pathology and control. *Compend Contin Educ Pract Vet* 13:863, 1991.
14. Castro GA: Immunophysiology of enteric parasitism. *Parasitol Today* 5:11, 1989.

15. Bueno L, Ruckenbusch Y, Dorchies PH: Disturbances of digestive motility in horses associated with strongyle infection. *Vet Parasitol* 5:253, 1979.
16. Lester GD, Bolton JR, Cambridge H, et al: The effect of *Strongylus vulgaris* larvae on the equine intestinal myoelectrical activity. *Equine Vet J Suppl* 7:8, 1989.
17. Berry CR, Merrit AM, Burrows CF, et al: Evaluation of the myoelectrical activity of the equine ileum infected with *Strongylus vulgaris* larvae. *Am J Vet Res* 87:27, 1986.
18. Kaiser L, Tithof PK, Williams JF: Depression of endothelium-dependent relaxation of filarial parasite products. *Am J Physiol* 254:H648, 1990.
19. McKenzie CD: *Immune responses in onchocerciasis and* dracunculiasis. In Soulsby EJL, ed. *Immune Responses in Parasitic Infections: Immunology, Immunopathology and Immunoprophylaxis*. Vol. I. *Nematodes*. Boca Raton, CRC Press, 1987.
20. King CL, Nutman TB: Regulation of immune responses in lymphatic filariasis and onchocerciasis. *Immunol Today* 3:A54, 1991.
21. Foil LD, Klei TR, Miller RI, et al: Seasonal changes in density and tissue distribution of *Onchocerca cervicalis* microfilariae in ponies and related changes in *Culicoides varnipennis* populations in Louisiana. *J Parasitol* 73:320, 1987.
22. Ogbourne CP, Duncan JR: *Strongylus vulgaris in the Horse: Its Biology and Veterinary Importance*, ed 2. Misc. Pub. No. 9. St. Albans, U.K., Commonwealth Institute of Parasitology.
23. Murrell KD: Induction of protective immunity to *Strongyloides ransomi* in pigs. *Am J Vet Res* 42:1915, 1981.
24. Loyd S, Soulsby EJL: Immunobiology of gastrointestinal nematodes of ruminants. In Soulsby EJL, ed. *Immune Responses in Parasitic Infections: Immunology, Immunopathology and Immunoprophylaxis*. Vol I: *Nematodes*. Boca Raton, CRC Press, 1987, p 1.
25. Dennis VA, Klei TR, Chapman MR, et al: *In vivo* activation of equine eosinophils and neutrophils by experimental *Strongylus vulgaris* infections. *Vet Immunol Immunopathol* 20:61, 1988.
26. Finkelman FD, Pearce EJ, Urban JF, et al: Regulation and biological function of helminth-induced cytokine responses. *Immunol Today* 12:A62, 1991.
27. Sher A, Colley DG: Immunoparasitology. In Paul WE, ed. *Fundamental Immunology*, ed 2. New York, Raven Press, 1989, p 957.
28. Loyd S: Cysticercoses. In Soulsby EJL, ed. *Immune Responses in Parasitic Infections: Immunology, Immunopathology and Immunoprophylaxis*. Vol II: *Trematodes and Cestodes*. Boca Raton, CRC Press, 1987, p 183.
29. Liu, LX, Weller PF: Arachidonic acid metabolism in filarial parasites. *Exp Parasitol* 71:496, 1990.

2.4

Rickettsial Diseases

Yasuko Rikihisa, PhD

Potomac horse fever and equine ehrlichiosis are two rickettsial diseases known to affect horses. Diagnosis of these diseases requires an awareness of the typical pattern of clinical signs, hematologic values, seasonal pattern, and prevalence of the disease in the area. Because of the frequent international and domestic transport of horses, knowledge of the previous location of the horse may also aid in the diagnosis. Equine ehrlichiosis is most likely transmitted by the tick. Potomac horse fever is not contagious and is considered to be vector-borne.

For Potomac horse fever, serologic testing by indirect fluorescent antibody (IFA) and for equine ehrlichiosis, direct observation of blood buffy coat smears is the primary method of laboratory diagnosis. Polymerase chain reaction (PCR) methods have been gaining acceptance for detection of both *Ehrlichia* spp. When correctly diagnosed at acute stages of infection and treated properly, the prognosis of equine ehrlichiosis is excellent and that of Potomac horse fever is excellent to good in uncomplicated cases.

POTOMAC HORSE FEVER
Geographical Distribution

Potomac horse fever (equine monocytic ehrlichiosis, equine ehrlichial colitis, acute equine diarrhea syndrome), a rickettsial disease of equidae, was originally recognized in 1979 along the Potomac River in Montgomery County, Maryland.[1] The disease may have also existed in Northern California since the 1970s.[1a] It is now known to occur serologically in 43 of the United States, two provinces (Ontario and Saskatchewan) in Canada, France, Italy, Venezuela, India, and Australia.* However, confirmation by isolation of the etiologic agent has been made only in the United States. The disease is caused by a rickettsial organism named *Ehrlichia risticii*, which is serologically distinguishable from other pathogenic species infecting horses.

Etiology

In 1983, it was shown that the disease can be transmitted between horses by whole blood transfusion.[1] This finding made laboratory experiments under controlled conditions possible. In 1984, serologic cross-reactivity of sera of infected horses with *Ehrlichia sennetsu*, a human *Sennetsu fever* agent in Japan, was noted.[2] In the same year, the presence of ehrlichial organisms in macrophages and glandular epithelial cells of the intestinal wall of affected horses was demonstrated by transmission electron microscopy.[3] The etiologic agent was independently isolated in three different laboratories using human histiocytic lymphoma U-937 cells,[4, 5] canine primary monocytes,[2] and murine $P388D_1$ cells.[6] The agent was confirmed to reproduce the disease in horses and was re-isolated from horses with experimentally induced disease.

The causative agent of Potomac horse fever was later named *Ehrlichia risticii*.[7] *E. risticii* is currently classified among eight *Ehrlichia* spp. that cause diseases in various species of animals, including humans. The genus *Ehrlichia* belongs to the tribe Ehrlichieae, which contains obligate intracellular bacteria with a tropism for leukocytes. None of the tribe Ehrlichieae has been cultured outside of eukaryotic cells or in yolk sac. Success in culturing *E. risticii* in macrophage cell lines made it possible to obtain the quantities of

*Personal communication 7/2/93, Dr. Cynthia Holland, Protatek Reference Laboratory, Chandler, Arizona.

organisms needed for basic research at the molecular and cellular levels and for vaccine development.

The tribe Ehrlichieae is included in the family Rickettsiaceae along with the tribes Rickettsieae and Wolbachieae.[8] 16S rRNA gene sequence comparison is currently considered to be the most reliable method to determine phylogenetic relatedness among bacteria. Recent studies have shown relatedness (81.7%) in the sequences of the 16S rRNA gene in *E. risticii* and *Rickettsia prowazekii*, which is the etiologic agent of epidemic typhus, a well-known rickettsial disease responsible for the deaths of millions of people during wartime and natural disasters. Both microorganisms belong to the α subdivision of the purple bacteria.[9] The percentage of 16S rRNA gene sequence homology between *E. risticii* and *E. sennetsu* was 98.9%, and surprisingly the next related bacterium was *Neorickettsia helminthoeca* (94.8% 16S rRNA gene sequence homology).[10] *N. helminthoeca* belongs to the tribe Ehrlichieae and is the etiologic agent of salmon poisoning disease of the dog. *N. helminthoeca* is antigenically cross-reactive with *E. risticii* and biologically and morphologically resembles *E. risticii*.[11] Furthermore, the 16S rRNA gene of the fluke *Stellantchasmus falcatus* isolate (SF agent) is 99.1% homologous to that of *E. risticii*.[11a] Since vector hosts and their parasites tend to co-evolve, *E. risticii* and *E. sennetsu* may infect the helminth as *N. helminthoeca* and the SF agent do. Within 11 *E. risticii* strains, a maximum of 10 nucleotides are different (0.7% divergence).[12]

Although they are currently classified in the same genus, *E. risticii* is divergent from *E. equi* and *E. canis*, which is the type species of the genus *Ehrlichia* by 16S rRNA gene sequence comparison, homology being 83.3% and 82.4%, respectively.

E. risticii is a tiny gram-negative coccus and stains dark blue to purple with Romanowsky staining (Fig. 2–2). *E. risticii* tend to occupy one side of the cytoplasm rather than being symmetrically or evenly distributed. *E. risticii* are

generally round but are sometimes pleomorphic and may be elongated, especially in tissue culture. They divide by binary fission. The organisms are found in membrane-lined vacuoles within the cytoplasm of infected eukaryotic host cells, primarily macrophages and glandular epithelial cells in the intestine of the horse. *E. risticii* is seen in at least two different forms: multiple dark, small organisms (0.2 to 0.4 μm) enveloped by the host membrane (called morulae) and relatively light, large forms (0.8 to 1.5 μm) individually tightly wrapped with host membrane.[13, 14] Morulae appear to interchange with individually enveloped forms, since an intermediate stage appearing as moderately dense *Ehrlichia* cells tightly enveloped with the host membrane, which is continuous with the membrane surrounding a morula, has been seen.[15] *E. risticii* in T-84, P388D₁, and U-937 cells, in primary equine monocyte culture, and in infected equine tissues are primarily seen as individual forms, especially in intestinal epithelial cells.[14, 16] However, several of recent *E. risticii* isolates make inclusions as large and as tightly packed as *E. canis* inclusion.[16a, 62] Vacuoles containing *E. risticii* have been shown not to fuse with lysosomes.[17] The inhibition of lysosomal fusion is not a generalized process but rather is restricted to vesicles that contain *E. risticii*.[17]

Transmission electron microscopy showed that *E. risticii* have distinct ribosomes and DNA strands.[15] Clumps of ribosomes are homogenously distributed in the cytoplasm rather than marginated beneath the cytoplasmic membrane. Compared with those of the rickettsiae or ordinary bacteria, the DNA and ribosomes in *E. risticii* are more loosely packed in the cytoplasm except for the small, dense form. Thus, the electron density of ehrlichial organisms is similar to that of the host cell cytoplasmic background, and this low contrast makes it difficult to find *E. risticii* in infected tissue at low magnification under the electron microscope. *E. risticii* are surrounded by thin, bileaflet outer and inner membranes (Fig. 2–3). Unlike the rickettsiae, ehrlichial organisms show no thickening of either leaflet of the outer membrane.[14, 15] Morphologically, *E. risticii* does not appear to contain significant amounts of peptidoglycan.[15] Peptidoglycan is counterproductive when considering their intracellular life, because it requires the provision of an effective diffusion rather than mechanical protection by peptidoglycan.

No plasmid or phage has been detected by agarose gel electrophoresis of DNA fractions from *E. risticii* cultured in vitro. A weak endotoxin activity is detectable by Limulus amebocyte lysate assay, but a significant level of lipid A was detected in the phenol phase extracted by host phenol method by immunoblot analysis using a monoclonal antibody against lipid A.[20] No endospore-like structure has been reported, although minicell-like structures resulting from uneven binary fission and apparent outer membrane vesicles of various sizes have been seen in *E. risticii*.[14]

E. risticii appears to perform aerobic and asaccharolytic catabolism. The metabolic activities of *E. risticii* have been investigated. *E. risticii* can utilize glutamine and glutamate and generate ATP as rickettsiae do[19, 21]; however, unlike rickettsiae, *E. risticii* prefers to use glutamine rather than glutamate, because it is enveloped by the host membrane and glutamine penetrates phagosomes better than glutamate. Unlike members of the genera *Chlamydia* and *Wolbachia*, but like those of the genus *Rickettsia*, *E. risticii* cannot utilize glucose-6-phosphate or glucose.[19] In this sense, *E.*

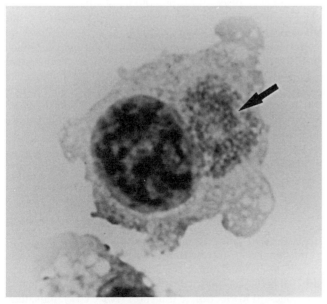

Figure 2–2. *Ehrlichia risticii* in the cytoplasm of P388D₁ cells. Organisms are stained dark purple by Diff-Quik staining (*arrow*). Magnification, ×4,000.

risticii is similar to the genus *Rickettsia*, but the rate of adenosine triphosphate (ATP) synthesis per milligram of protein in vitro is one fifth that of *Rickettsia typhi* when Percoll density gradient–purified *E. risticii* is tested.[21] The greatest metabolic activity of *E. risticii* is observed at a pH of 7.2 to 8.0 and declines drastically at a pH below 7.[19] This finding suggests that *E. risticii* has an ability to prevent both acidification and lysosomal fusion of the vacuole where it resides.

Epizootiology

There is no sex, age, or breed predilection in terms of seropositive rate based on serotesting results in Ohio.[22] The disease is seen mainly during the summer and is most common from June through September. The mode of transmission of Potomac horse fever is unknown. The seasonal nature, sporadic existence,[1] presence of *E. risticii* in horse blood monocytes, and experimental transmission by the intradermal route suggest a blood-sucking arthropod as the vector.[23] *Dermacentor variabilis*, black flies, eye gnats, biting midges, and mosquitoes have been found to be negative for *E. risticii* transmission.[24] Experimental oral transmission of the disease has been demonstrated,[25] although epizootiologic study rejects the feco-oral route of transmission.[26] Genetic relatedness of *E. risticii* to *N. helminthoeca*[10] and SF agent[11a] suggests that *E. risticii* is also transmitted by the fluke.

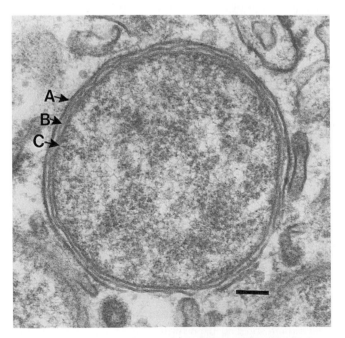

Figure 2–3. Transmission electron micrograph of *Ehrlichia risticii* in the cytoplasm of a macrophage in the large colon of a horse. *E. risticii* is tightly enveloped by the host membrane (A) and has its own outer (B) and inner (C) membranes. Magnification, ×105,000. Bar = 0.1μm. (Reproduced with permission of Yasuko R: Ultrastructure of rickettsiae with special emphasis on ehrlichiae. In Williams JE, Kakoma I, eds. Ehrlichiosis. Dordrecht, The Netherlands, Kluwer Academic Press, 1990. Reprinted by permission of Kluwer Academic Publishers.)

Experimental injection of cell cultured *E. risticii* or infected horse blood and re-isolation of the organism have revealed that dogs, cats, mice, and non-human primates can be infected, although only mice and cats developed significant clinical signs.[27–30] Potomac horse fever may have a zoonotic potential, because *E. risticii* can cause mild clinical signs in primates.[30]

Seroepizootiologic studies showed that cats, dogs, foxes, pigs, and goats in an endemic area of Maryland had antibodies to *E. risticii*.[31, 32] Since *E. risticii* has not been isolated from these species of animals in these studies, it is not known whether they harbor *E. risticii* and can serve as reservoirs. Recently, clinical cases of canine ehrlichiosis with a seropositive reaction to *E. risticii* but not to *E. canis* and isolation of *Ehrlichia* spp. whose 16S rRNA base sequence is identical to *E. risticii* were reported, suggesting that a strain of *E. risticii* may infect and cause disease in dogs.[33] However, whether the canine isolate can infect horses and cause Potomac horse fever was not investigated.

Owners and veterinarians should be aware of the sporadic nature of the disease. On some farms and racetracks, the disease recurs several summers in a row, or the disease may show up suddenly in isolated areas where no previous Potomac horse fever cases have been reported. Usually, if clinical cases are serologically confirmed on a farm, racetrack, or horseshow, there are several additional seropositive horses that show no clinical signs.

Pathogenesis/Immune Responses
Establishment of Infection

E. risticii can establish infection in mice and horses with or without causing apparent clinical illness. Based on a murine model for Potomac horse fever, the disease is apparently dose dependent; that is, with a lower dosage of *E. risticii*, innate defense mechanisms appear to contain *Ehrlichia* cells below threshold level.[34] Only at higher dosages can the organism cause disease and pathologic changes.

E. risticii can be consistently re-isolated from the peripheral blood monocytes from day 1 to day 28 postinfection, which is 8 days after spontaneous resolution of clinical signs.[35] *E. risticii* may persist much longer in the intestinal walls of clinically recovered horses, since the homogenate of intestinal tissues recovered from two ponies at 2 months post infection contained *E. risticii* antigens.[36] Furthermore, in a pregnant mare-fetus system, *E. risticii* infection persists up to 4 months, since *E. risticii* was isolated from the spleen, bone marrow, and mesenteric and colonic lymph nodes of a 7-month-old fetus of a mare that was infected experimentally during the third month of gestation.[37]

Mechanism of Diarrhea

E. risticii infects blood monocytes and has a predilection for the intestinal wall, especially that of the large colon where it infects tissue macrophages,[3, 14] intestinal glandular (crypt) epithelial cells, and mast cells.[13, 14] Watery diarrhea is caused by a reduction in electrolyte transport (Na^+, Cl^-); thus, there is a lack of water resorption, mainly in the large and small colons.[38] Infected intestinal epithelial cells lose microvilli,[16, 38] which may contribute to the reduced electrolyte transport and water resorption. An increase in intracellular cyclic adenosine monophosphate (AMP) is found in infected mouse macrophages and infected mouse and horse intestinal tissues.[38-40] This change in cyclic AMP content may also contribute to the reduced luminal absorption of Na^+ and Cl^- in the colon and thus to the lack of water absorption and diarrhea.

Cellular Damage and Cytokines

In contrast with cells infected with virulent strains of the genus *Rickettsia*, host cells infected with *E. risticii* show little cytolysis in vivo or in vitro until the cytoplasm is completely filled with infecting organisms and the cells burst. Plaque formation in a monolayer of monocytes-macrophages rarely occurs; rather frequently, infected macrophages dissociate from the bottom of the culture flask and float. This, too, is different from the situation with the genus *Rickettsia*. Ehrlichial release appears to occur not only by cell lysis but also through exocytosis by fusion of the inclusion membrane with the plasma membrane. In the case of intestinal epithelial cells, which make a monolayer tightly connected by circumferential zones of intercellular junctions, ehrlichial organisms appear to be transmitted between adjacent cells in vitro by a coupled exocytosis in one cell and endocytosis in an adjacent cell.[16]

Dissimilar to ordinary gram-negative bacteria, *E. risticii* do not fully activate macrophages in vitro,[39] *E. risticii* induces only low levels of tumor necrosis factor (TNF) and prostaglandin E_2 production in macrophages.[39] This may be caused by a lack of typical lipopolysaccharide in *E. risticii*. *E. risticii* in general does not induce a severe inflammatory reaction in equine tissues.[14, 38] In part this may be due to the low TNF-α production. In contrast, infected macrophages produce large amounts of interleukin-1 (IL-1), and this may be related to the pathogenesis of the disease.[39]

Mechanism of Infection of Macrophages

Since *E. risticii* are obligate intracellular bacteria, it is essential for *E. risticii* to bind to the proper receptor, to induce internalization, and to maintain an intracellular environment adequate for survival and proliferation. In vitro, professional phagocytes-monocytes and macrophages of host animal species have no intrinsic resistance to infection with *E. risticii*. In addition, intestinal epithelial cells and mast cells, which are normally not very phagocytic, are induced to take up *E. risticii*. *E. risticii* binds to equine macrophage but not polymorphonuclear leukocytes (PMNs).[41] Both host cell receptor and *E. risticii* ligand appear to be proteins.[41] It was found that ehrlichial internalization, proliferation, and intercellular spreading, but not binding, were highly dependent on host clathrin, microfilament, or microtubule systems,[42] as well as Ca^{2+}-calmodulin[43] and protein tyrosine kinase.[43a]

E. risticii entry into P388D$_1$ cells is blocked by monodansylcadaverine, an inhibitor of clathrin assembly, suggesting that *E. risticii* enters by receptor-mediated endocytosis.[41] *E. risticii* can be readily taken up by equine PMNs but is rapidly destroyed in them.[41] Polyclonal equine antiserum to *E. risticii* does not inhibit binding or internalization of *E. risticii* to P388D$_1$ macrophages, but internalized antibody-

coated *E. risticii* fails to survive.[44] Since the Fab fragment of the equine anti-*E. risticii* IgG blocks the binding of *E. risticii* to P388D$_1$ macrophages, antibody-coated *E. risticii* most likely enters macrophages via the Fc receptor. The mechanisms of destruction of antibody-coated *E. risticii* in macrophages are presently unknown. Fc-receptor–mediated uptake may deliver *E. risticii* to the intracellular compartment susceptible to lysosomal fusion. Alternatively, since ^{14}C-L-glutamine metabolism by purified host cell-free *E. risticii* was blocked by polyclonal antibody, direct metabolic inhibition may make *E. risticii* unable to survive in the macrophage.[44]

Immune Response

It has been reported that recovered horses are immune to reinfection for at least 20 months.[45] Both humoral and cell-mediated immune responses appear to have significant roles in this protection. *E. risticii* induces a specific antibody response in the natural host or in experimental animals, regardless of the presence of clinical signs. The presence of the antibody, however, does not always correlate with the clearance of the *Ehrlichia* spp. and the presence of protective immunity. An immunoglobulin M (IgM) response occurs a few days after the initial infection and lasts for less than 2 months.[46] A challenge injection did not elicit an IgM response.[46] Several days after *E. risticii* infection of the horse, tests for IgG antibody became significantly positive.[46]

Development of neutralizing antibodies in infected horses was also demonstrated using a cell culture system[35, 47] and a murine model for Potomac horse fever.[35, 49] Three mechanisms of antibody neutralization have been shown. In the first mechanism, antibody blocks ehrlichial binding to its specific receptor, instead making it bind through the Fc receptor. In the second mechanism, the antibody directly inhibits ehrlichial metabolism as demonstrated by reduced ^{14}C-CO_2 production from ^{14}C-L-glutamine in host-cell free *E. risticii* in the presence of the antibody.[44] The third mechanism is antibody dependent cell-mediated cytotoxicity. Macrophages infected with *E. risticii* present ehrlichial antigens on their surface similar to virus-infected cells and are found to be lysed when incubated with anti-ehrlichial antibody and normal equine peripheral blood monocytes.[49] Five to seven major antigens were identified on the surface exposed.[48] These antigens are considered to be the target in antibody-mediated neutralization.

IFN-γ has the ability to activate both uninfected and infected macrophages and transform them into effector cells.[50] Using murine peritoneal macrophages, the ehrlichiacidal mechanism exhibited by interferon-γ (IFN-γ) was investigated. *E. risticii* was found to be very sensitive to nitric oxide, which was generated by macrophage cytoplasmic nitric oxide synthase induced by IFN-γ.[50] Ehrlichial killing by IFN-γ was blocked by a competitive inhibitor of nitric oxide synthase, N, N^G-monomethyl L-arginine.[50] Activities of T cells that generate(s) IFN-γ are, however, found generally severely depressed in infected mice in a time- and dose-related manner.[34] One cause for depressed T-cell response was found in macrophages. Class II histocompatibility antigen (Ia antigen) induction on the surface of *E. risticii*-infected macrophages (antigen-presenting cells) is suppressed in vitro,[51] suggesting inhibition of antigen-specific T-cell activation in *E. risticii* infection. Thus, an understanding of the immunodepression mechanism and identification of neutralizable ehrlichial antigens is the key toward developing an improved, more effective vaccine for Potomac horse fever.

Clinical Findings

The incubation period for *E. risticii* infection is approximately 1 to 3 weeks. Clinical signs are an acute onset of fever up to 107 °F, depression, anorexia, decreased borborygmi in all abdominal quadrants, subcutaneous edema of the legs and ventral abdomen, dehydration, and diarrhea.[52] Laminitis and severe abdominal pain occur in 15% to 25% and 5% to 10% of cases, respectively, which are the major reasons for euthanasia.[52] Laminitis may progress, despite resolution of the rest of the clinical signs. Diarrhea may be mild to severe "pipestream" and occurs in 10% to 30% of cases. In some horses the diarrhea may be transient; in others cases it persists for several days; and still other horses may have no diarrhea. Owners and veterinarians should be aware of the variable nature of the clinical signs. The case fatality rate varies from 5% to 30%. Transplacental transmission of *E. risticii* is reported[37] and the organism may induce abortion or resorption of the fetus or produce maladjusted foals, which require extensive neonatal care. Recurrence of diarrhea and on and off prolonged illness in antibiotic-treated horses has been observed.[53] Leukopenia (white blood cell [WBC] count <5,000/μL) with a left shift and rebound leukocytosis (WBC >14,000/μL) are prominent hematologic changes.[54] Anemia, plasma protein concentration, increase in packed cell volume, and thrombocytopenia may be also observed.[54]

Diagnosis

In contrast with *E. equi* infection, visual observation of blood smears of suspected horses after Romanowsky staining is useless for diagnosis of *E. risticii* infection, because only a few blood monocytes are infected with very few organisms even at the acute stage of infection.

Serologic Diagnosis

All ehrlichial agents induce specific humoral immune responses. These responses are the basis for serologic diagnosis of ehrlichial diseases. However, since serologic response occurs in every animal exposed to *E. risticii* regardless of whether infection is established or disease is present, serologic testing alone, with no supporting information, provides limited information for the diagnosis of disease. Serologic diagnosis of ehrlichial infections can be accomplished either by IFA[46, 55] or by enzyme-linked immunosorbent assay (ELISA).[46] The cut-off titer for positive serology may vary with the laboratory. In the author's laboratory, IgG IFA titers of 20 or higher represent a positive serology. For serologic testing for *E. risticii* infection, the higher the titer, the greater is the correlation with Potomac horse fever clinical disease.[22] The chance of healthy horses having a titer of 40 or less is similar to that of ill horses (early and late stages, and low levels of infection with *E. risticii* or possible cross-reaction with other microorganisms). Thus, at a titer of 40 or less, although the horse is seropositive, the current disease is not likely to be caused by *E. risticii*. The chance of having a titer of 80 or less and 640 or less is approximately four times higher in ill horses than in healthy horses, and the chance of having titers higher than 1,280 is 12 to 26 times higher in ill horses.[22] All experimentally infected horses had an IFA titer of 80 or higher at the onset of clinical disease.

E. risticii have been adapted to grow in a continuous murine monocyte-macrophage cell line and other cell lines; thus, the antigen slides are relatively easy to prepare.[46, 56] An enzyme-linked immunosorbent assay has been developed using purified *E. risticii* as the antigen. The IgM titer rises earlier during the course of infection than the IgG titer. A rise in IgM titer occurs only at the time of initial infection, and the titer becomes negative in 1 to 2 months.[46] Thus, an IgM ELISA is not useful for detecting chronic or multiple infections but is useful for early diagnosis of a primary infection.

Of horses at two racetracks in Ohio, 13% (138 of 840) to 20% (116 of 574) were exposed to *E. risticii*, according to the results of a serosurvey conducted in the summer of 1986.[22] Of the seropositive horses, 80% to 90% did not show clinical signs of infection.

IFA testing may produce false-positive results in equine sera when they bind nonspecifically to the infected cells. There are several means of solving this problem: First, *E. risticii* organisms should be seen clearly in the cytoplasm of the host cells by IFA staining at 1000× magnification. If staining is blurred, morphologically different from the positive control staining or Giemsa-stained infected cells, or extracellular objects are stained, it should not be judged positive. The person who reads slides should be trained to have a clear visual concept of the appearance of IFA-positive *E. risticii* on each batch of antigen slides prepared. Second, positive and negative control equine sera must be tested to ensure the quality of the entire IFA procedure each time, including the quality of the antigen slides used and FITC anti-horse IgG. Third, to reduce non-specific binding, our laboratory uses 0.02% Tween-20 in the phosphate buffered saline washes. Usually serial dilution of the serum takes care of the problem of nonspecific binding if the titer of the sera is sufficiently high. If none of these procedures work, the author pre-absorbs the equine sera with uninfected macrophages cultured and prepared under the same condition as the *E. risticii*-infected macrophage antigen. Several other serologic tests such as latex agglutination[57] and monoclonal antibody based competitive ELISA have been reported.[58] However, to date a rapid and reliable field serodiagnostic test is not yet available.

There is no serologic cross-reactivity between the tribe Ehrlichieae and the tribes Rickettsieae and Chlamydieae by the IFA test.[2, 7, 59] *E. risticii* has only minor heat-sensitive antigenic determinants, unlike the genus *Rickettsia*. By Western blot (immunoblot) analysis,[18] however, 55 kDa heat-shock protein 60 homolog crossreacts with those of other *Ehrlichia* spp. and *Rickettsia* spp.[59a]

Several ehrlichial species antigenically cross-react within the genus when tested by IFA or Western blot analysis.[11] Within the genus *Ehrlichia*, *E. risticii* and *E. sennetsu* have the strongest common antigenicity. *E. sennetsu* is non-pathogenic to horses but it protects them from *E. risticii* infection.[60]

Immunologic cross-reactivity among members of the tribe Ehrlichieae does not create a serious problem in serologic diagnosis because of the host animal specificity of *Ehrlichia* spp. in nature, and different clinical signs. However, since homologous spp. antigen provides the most sensitive serodiagnosis, it is still important to identify the species. Even misdiagnosed with other species, tetracycline series of antibiotics are effective for all of the ehrlichial diseases, especially at early stages of infection.

Recently, our laboratory found that one of six *E. risticii* Ohio isolates and three Kentucky isolates are quite divergent from *E. risticii*, Illinois isolate (ATCC VR-986) in their antigen profiles by Western immunoblot analysis and by IFA using two panels of monoclonal antibodies.[16a, 62] They are also different in the base sequence of 16S rRNA and in the growth morphology in the cell.[62] An isolate that has less difference in antigenic profile than our four isolates was described.[61] Thus, it is likely that there are multiple strains or subspecies of *E. risticii*, or *Ehrlichia* spp. in the field, which can be distinguished by Western immunoblotting or monoclonal antibody labeling of antigens but not by IFA or ELISA serologic testing of infected horse sera. The existence of divergent antigenic variants should be taken into consideration in improving the serodiagnosis and efficacy of vaccines for Potomac horse fever in the field.

In summary, recommendations for the serologic confirmation of Potomac horse fever include demonstration of seroconversion, a four-fold rise or fall in titer, or the presence of IgM antibody specific to *E. risticii*. It should be emphasized, however, that the initial diagnosis and treatment of Potomac horse fever should be made on clinical signs, negative test results for other pathogens such as salmonella, for which the use of tetracyclines may be contraindicated, and initial IFA test results if available within 1 to 2 days. Treatment should not be delayed until laboratory confirmation is obtained from a second IFA test. It is important to point out that in the field Potomac horse fever and salmonellosis can occur concurrently.[56] Weak seropositive or seronegative results of vaccinated horses when they develop clinical signs compatible with Potomac horse fever are useful for ruling out the possibility of this infection. Seropositive results in vaccinated horses are useless unless a four-fold rise in titer is seen.

Isolation of E. risticii *and Polymerase Chain Reaction*

The isolation of *E. risticii*[35] is accomplished by inoculating buffy coat or mononuclear cell fractions of peripheral blood of affected animals into cell culture.[62] Murine monocyte-macrophage P388D$_1$ cells, human histiocytic lymphoma U-937 cells, or canine primary monocytes are used for isolating *E. risticii*. The procedure is more sensitive than is direct observation. Even if a single organism cannot be seen in the original buffy coat smear, the organisms can be isolated by this procedure.[35]

Isolation procedures for diagnosing infection, however, are impractical for clinical laboratories because they take too long (3 days to 1 month) relative to the rapid course of Potomac horse fever and require a reasonable tissue culture technique and facility. Although positive isolation provides a definitive diagnosis, negative results do not necessarily indicate the absence of infection.

A polymerase chain reaction (PCR) that detects 16S rRNA gene or an uncharacterized *E. risticii* gene in peripheral blood monocytes and feces of experimentally infected animals has been developed.[63, 64, 64a] Applicability of this test in field cases has been tested.[63] Although cell culture isolation gives superior sensitivity to PCR procedure for field specimens, PCR procedure will be used more often in the future because of its convenience.[63]

Postmortem Identification of Ehrlichial Organisms

E. risticii can be demonstrated in intestinal epithelial cells and macrophages in paraffin-embedded tissue specimens with a silver stain or an immunoperoxidase procedure using a specific antibody to *E. risticii*.[65] Immunoperoxide staining detects fewer *E. risticii* than does silver staining, presumably due to partial inactivation of antigens owing to fixation and paraffin embedding. However, silver staining produces background reactions in some specimens and thus is less specific than immunoperoxidase staining.[65] These procedures have not been adapted for routine diagnosis.

Pathologic Findings

The most obvious postmortem findings are the grossly distended large colon and cecum filled with watery contents (Fig. 2–4). There are few other consistent gross pathologic changes in horses with Potomac horse fever except for patchy hyperemia along the wall of the large intestine.[38] There is no destruction, foul odor, or significant inflammatory infiltration such as in enterocolitis caused by salmonella, which may cause similar clinical signs or may co-infect with *E. risticii* in nature.[38] However, remarkable goblet cell mucus depletion and reduced height and increased basophilia of mucosal epithelial cells, dilatation of intestinal glands, and entrapment of cellular debris in the glandular lumens are

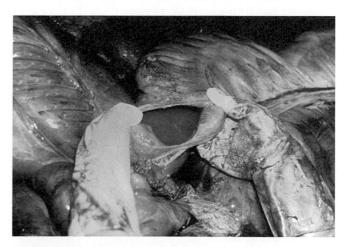

Figure 2–4. Fluid-filled large colon of a horse with Potomac horse fever.

seen in experimental *E. risticii* infection.[38, 60, 66] Mesenteric lymph nodes are relatively small and consist of prominent sheets of histiocytes, macrophages, occasional giant cells, and severely depleted inactive lymphoid cells.[60] Lack of severe lesions and absence of neutrophil infiltration are thus important in the differential diagnosis of Potomac horse fever.

Therapy

In vitro *E. risticii* is susceptible to doxycycline, demeclocycline, and oxytetracycline but is resistant to erythromycin and nalidixic acid.[67] As with other rickettsiae, *E. risticii* is resistant to aminoglycosides because they penetrate host cells poorly. Although oxytetracycline alone is bacteriostatic, it was found to induce lysosomal fusion with ehrlichia-containing vacuoles in P388D$_1$ cells,[17] thus becoming bactericidal. Oxytetracycline and doxycycline frequently correct the pyrexia and other clinical signs within 24 to 48 hours, which by itself is diagnostic.[53] Although doxycycline is more effective than is oxytetracycline in vitro and is highly effective in mice inoculated with *E. risticii*,[67, 68] oxytetracycline is preferred for the equine species because intravenous administration of doxycycline has an acute toxic effect.[69] Intravenous oxytetracycline at 6.6 mg/kg of body weight twice a day for 7 days was effective in 71% (five of seven) of cases of experimentally infected ponies when the ponies were treated after the development of severe clinical signs.[53] Oxytetracycline is also reported to be effective when given immediately after the development of fever but before the development of diarrhea.[70] In the murine model for Potomac horse fever, doxycycline, given on the fifth day, has the best effect on the immune response. When doxycycline is given on the third or seventh day after infection, immunodepression due to *E. risticii* infection is more severe.[68] Although erythromycin or rifampin alone has a poor effect in controlling *E. risticii* infection in vitro or in infected mice,[67, 68] the use of the oral combination of erythromycin and rifampin has been efficacious in the treatment of experimentally infected horses.[71]

Other supportive therapy is frequently required for acutely ill horses if they are to show clinical improvement. Dehydration is corrected by the oral or intravenous administration of polyionic isotonic fluids. Brief therapy (2 to 7 days) with nonsteroidal anti-inflammatory agents (e.g., phenylbutazone, flunixin, meglumine, aspirin) for horses may be valuable early in the course of treatment to help in the management of clinical signs of Potomac horse fever.[66]

Prevention

Vector transmission is probably the only means of spread under natural circumstances, because susceptible animals housed for several months adjacent to infected animals do not have a higher incidence of the disease than those kept far from infected animals.[26] However, since a blood-sucking arthropod does not seem to be the vector, treatment with insecticide is unlikely to be helpful. Research toward finding vectors should be continued.

Since infection-induced immunity is excellent[45] and a vaccine made of β-propiolacton–inactivated host cell-free *E.*

risticii protects mice from homologous challenge based on clinical, pathologic, and immunologic criteria,[72] vaccination is expected to be very effective in controlling Potomac horse fever. Vaccines prepared from inactivated cell-cultured *E. risticii* are available for Potomac horse fever from three commercial sources. Formalin-inactivated whole organism vaccine with aluminum hydroxide adjuvant has been reviewed.[73] Studies published in 1987 reported 78% prevention of all clinical signs except fever.[74] Protection conferred by this vaccine appears to be much shorter in duration when compared with infection-induced protection.[73] IFA titers measured after vaccination are also lower and drop rapidly in contrast to what occurs in natural infection.[73] Therefore, improvement of vaccine for Potomac horse fever is desired.

Vaccination is not necessary for up to 2 years in the horse that has recovered from illness or has a high IFA titer due to natural exposure or subclinical infection, because infection-induced immunity provides better protection than do the vaccines.

For nonexposed animals, considering the time required to develop immunity after vaccination, the short-lasting immunity to even the homologous strain of *E. risticii*, and the existence of antigenic variants in the field, it is unknown how much benefit the vaccine will provide in the field challenge.

The vaccine is reported to cause no ill effects in horses except for swelling at the injection site in 10% of the animals.[73] Recombinant clones that produce several *E. risticii* antigenic proteins have been produced in the author's and other laboratories. Using the murine model for Potomac horse fever, a combination of two recombinant clones that express 44-kDa and 70-kDa antigens was shown to confer protection against *E. risticii* challenge.[75] The protection was slightly less effective than the protection given by whole *E. risticii* antigen. The efficacy of recombinant antigens for the protection of horses from Potomac horse fever has not been reported.

EQUINE EHRLICHIOSIS
Geographical Distribution

Equine ehrlichiosis and *E. equi* in the cytoplasm of blood neutrophils and eosinophils in affected horses were initially reported in 1969.[76] The disease has been observed chiefly in California. In addition, sporadic cases have been reported in Colorado, Illinois, Florida, Washington, and New Jersey and also in Germany,[77] Switzerland,[78] Sweden,[79] and Israel.[80] In the United States, the disease occurs much less frequently than does Potomac horse fever.

Etiology

E. equi is classified along with *E. risticii* in the genus *Ehrlichia* in the tribe Ehrlichieae. Recent 16S rRNA gene sequence analysis revealed that only up to three bases are different among *E. equi*, *E. phagocytophila*, which infects ruminants, primarily sheep and goats in Europe, and recently discovered human granulocytic ehrlichiosis (HGE) agent.[81, 90] As a matter of fact, recently equine granulocytic ehrlichiosis caused by an agent that has 16S rDNA sequence identical to that of HGE agent was reported in Connecticut[81a] and

Sweden.[81b] Intravenous inoculation of infected human blood produces a disease indistinguishable from that caused by *E. equi*,[81c] indicating equine ehrlichiosis is caused by at least two strains of organisms.

By 16S rRNA gene sequence comparison, relatedness between *E. risticii* and *E. equi* is low—83.3%.[12] Interestingly, *E. equi* is closely related (96.6% homology) to *Anaplasma marginale* in 16S rRNA base sequence. *A. marginale* causes infectious anemia in cattle. By IFA, *E. equi* was reported to strongly cross-react with *Cowdria ruminantium* but not with *E. risticii*.[82, 83] *C. ruminantium* infects endothelial cells and neutrophils in ruminants and causes heartwater in Africa. Recent 16S rRNA gene sequence analysis revealed 92.1% relatedness between *E. equi* and *C. ruminantium*.[12] In contrast, relatedness between *E. risticii* and *C. ruminantium* is 83%.[12] Clearly, *E. equi* and *E. risticii* are very different organisms. *E. equi* has been cultured in vitro using the tick-embryo cell line IDE8 and a human promyelocytic leukemia cell line HL60.[83a] Contrary to previous speculation by some researchers, *E. equi* is a distinct species different from *E. ewingii*, another granulocytic ehrlichia that infects dogs in the United States, as 16S rRNA gene sequence homology is 92.4%.[12, 59]

E. equi appears as round, dark purple, small dots or loose aggregates that appear as "mulberries" (morulae) in the cytoplasm of blood granulocytes, primarily in neutrophils and eosinophils by Romanowsky staining.[76] By electron microscopy, several loosely packed ovoid, round, or rod-shaped *E. equi* organisms are seen in several membrane-lined vacuoles of equine neutrophils and eosinophils.[84] The size of vacuoles ranges from 1.5 to 5 μm in diameter.[85]

Epizootiology

In contrast to Potomac horse fever, the disease is found during late fall, winter, and spring. Like Potomac horse fever, in some areas equine ehrlichiosis is endemic and in others the disease is absent. In one seroepidemiologic survey, horses residing in the foothills of northern California have greater exposure to *E. equi* than did those residing in the Sacramento Valley.[86] Since most of the seropositive horses in this study are healthy, subclinical infection with *E. equi* seems to occur as Potomac horse fever. Recent findings indicate that the western black-legged tick, *Ixodes pacificus*, is able to transmit *E. equi* and may act as a competent vector in the field.[86a] *E. equi* can cause parasitemia in dogs, cats, goats, sheep, and nonhuman primates, with mild to no clinical signs.[76, 88, 91] Cattle, rats, mice, guinea pigs, hamsters, or rabbits were not susceptible to infection.[88, 89] Gribble suggested that the horse may be an accidental host, based on the low incidence of the disease.[76] Whether other species of animals can serve as a reservoir for equine ehrlichiosis is unknown, although white-footed mice were recently shown to serve as an enzootic reservoir of HGE agent.[92]

Pathogenesis/Immune Response

Infected animals develop antibody detectable by IFA, and leukocytes from infected animals show inhibition of migration when mixed with *E. equi* antigen.[91] Since *E. equi* has not been propagated in vitro in sufficient quantity, an antigen prepared from the buffy coat cells of an experimentally infected horse is used as the antigen for immunologic studies.[91] Spontaneously recovered animals are immune to reinfection from 2.5 to 20 months.[76] Maternal antibody protects foals from the disease for up to 2 months but not from establishment of infection.[76] When challenged, small numbers of infected neutrophils were seen in a 15-day-old foal born to an immune mare.[76] Oxytetracycline treatment eliminates *E. equi* from horses, but rechallenge induces minimal clinical signs, suggesting the development of protective immunity in the recovered horse.[91] Although the blood of recovered horses is reported not to be infectious,[87] blood collected from ponies at 81 or 114 days after primary infection with *E. equi* induced mild clinical signs (fever, mild thrombocytopenia) in susceptible recipient ponies but did not protect the recipient animals against a second challenge 100 days later.[91] It thus appears that *E. equi* may persist in small numbers despite the concomitant presence of antibodies and the demonstrable inhibition of leukocyte migration.[91]

Clinical Findings

With experimental transmission using fresh blood from an infected horse, the incubation period is 1 to 9 days.[76] Clinical signs of the disease are fever lasting 1 to 9 days, depression, partial anorexia, limb edema, petechiation, icterus, ataxia, and reluctance to move.[89] In contrast to *E. risticii* infection, laminitis does not develop in equine ehrlichiosis.[87] Experimental inoculation of seven pregnant mares caused clinical signs of various severity, but none of the mares aborted.[76] Hematologic changes observed are thrombocytopenia, elevated plasma icterus index, decreased packed-cell volume, and marked leukopenia, first involving lymphocytes and then granulocytes. The disease is inapparent to mild and is usually not fatal except for injury resulting from ataxia or secondary infection. *E. equi* morulae are found in the cytoplasm of neutrophils and eosinophils only during the acute phase of the disease. The infection rate of peripheral blood neutrophils varies from 0.5% to 73%.[76] Chronic cases have not been reported.

Diagnosis

Direct microscopic examination of Romanowsky (the author prefers Giemsa or Diff-Quik) -stained peripheral blood buffy coat smears is simple and inexpensive and provides a permanent record. *E. equi* can be seen in granulocytes of buffy coat smears during the acute phase of the disease at 1,000× magnification. When more than three ehrlichial inclusion bodies (morulae) are seen, it is considered at definitive diagnosis.[87] A reliable isolation method for *E. equi* from the blood has not been developed. An IFA test using the buffy coat cells of the infected horse as the antigen has been developed and has been useful in detecting and titrating antibody in recovered horses.[91] Infected ponies become positive in the *E. equi* IFA test by 21 days after inoculation, and antibody titers as high as 1:1,280 were recorded at day 75 after inoculation. Nested PCR has been developed for detection of *E. equi* 16S rRNA in horse blood and ticks.[93] None of these methods distinguishes *E. equi* from HGE agent infection. DNA sequencing including three base regions that

Table 2–1. Comparison of Biological Features of *Ehrlichia risticii* and *E. equi*

	E. risticii	*E. equi*
Distribution	United States, Canada, Europe	United States, Europe
Natural host	Horse	Horse
Experimental host	Mouse, nonhuman primate, cat, dog	Cat, dog, sheep, goat, nonhuman primate but not mouse, rat, guinea pig, rabbit, cow
Host cell	Monocyte/macrophage intestinal epithelial cells, mast cells	Neutrophils, eosinophils
Appearance of inclusion	Individually tightly enveloped by host membrane or densely packed morulae (some of recent Ohio and Kentucky isolates)	Loosely packed small morulae

are different between these two organisms is required to distinguish them.

Pathologic Findings

The characteristic gross lesions are petechial hemorrhages and edema accompanied by proliferative and necrotizing vasculitis of small arteries and veins in the legs. In mature males, orchitis may also be seen.[76]

Therapy

Intravenous oxytetracycline at a dosage of 7 mg/kg of body weight is reported to be effective in treatment of *E. equi* infection.[87] After the initial 48 hours of treatment with oxytetracycline, defervescence is seen in all horses treated. After treatment with oxytetracycline at 7 mg/kg every 24 hours

intravenously for 3 to 7 days, oxytetracycline at 22 mg/kg orally every 12 hours for 7 days can be given additionally to prevent recurrence of the disease. However, such prophylactic measures must be considered carefully because oral oxytetracycline therapy has been incriminated in the onset of diarrhea in some horses.

Prevention

Since *E. equi* is most likely transmitted by *Ixodes* sp. ticks, tick repellent and insecticide are therefore expected to be effective for prevention. A vaccine has not been developed for this disease.

SUMMARY

Tables 2–1 and 2–2 summarize the biological and clinical features of Potomac horse fever and equine ehrlichiosis.

Table 2–2. Comparison of Clinical Features of Potomac Horse Fever and Equine Ehrlichiosis

	Potomac Horse Fever	Equine Ehrlichiosis
Mortality	Low to high	None
Acute disease	Yes	Yes
Chronic disease	No	No
Severity	Mild to severe	Mild to moderate
Leukopenia	Yes	Yes
Thrombocytopenia	Yes/no	Yes
Anemia	Yes/no	Yes
Pyrexia; anorexia; depression	Yes	Yes
Laminitis	Yes/no	No
Diarrhea	Yes/no	No
Abortion	Yes/no	No
Ehrlichia	Rarely seen in the blood	Blood granulocytes
Differential diagnosis	Colitis X	Encephalitis
	Salmonellosis	Liver disease
	Endotoxic shock	Purpura hemorrhagica
	Antibiotic-associated diarrhea	Equine infectious anemia
	Dietary changes	Equine viral arteritis
	Intoxications	

In recent years, because of outbreaks of Potomac horse fever in the United States, and discovery of HGE agent, which is closely related to *E. equi*, there has been an increased awareness of the importance of rickettsial diseases in horses. With rickettsial diseases, wild animals and vector arthropods or helminths are usually reservoirs of rickettsiae, and domestic animals and humans are accidental deadend hosts. Because environmental exposure of horses to vectors and reservoirs is relatively high, it is important to improve diagnostic, therapeutic, and vaccine procedures.

REFERENCES

1. Knowles RC, Anderson CW, Shipley WD, et al: Acute equine diarrhea syndrome (AEDS): A preliminary report. *Proc Annu Meet Am Assoc Equine Pract* 29:353, 1983.
1a. Madigan JE, Barlough JE, Rikihisa Y, et al: Identification of the "Shasta River Crud" syndrome as Potomac horse fever (Equine monocytic ehrlichiosis). *J Eq Vet Sci*, submitted for publication.
2. Holland CJ, Ristic M, Cole AI, et al: Isolation, experimental transmission and characterization of causative agent of Potomac horse fever. *Science* 227:522, 1985.
3. Rikihisa Y, Perry BD, Cordes DO: Rickettsial link with acute equine diarrhea. *Vet Rec* 115:390, 1984.
4. Rikihisa, Perry BD: Causative agent of Potomac horse fever. *Vet Rec* 115:554, 1984.
5. Rikihisa Y, Perry BD: Causative ehrlichial organisms in Potomac horse fever. *Infect Immun* 49:513, 1985.
6. Dutta SK, Myrup AC, Rice RM, et al: Experimental reproduction of Potomac horse fever in horses with a newly isolated *Ehrlichia* organism. *J Clin Microbiol* 22:256, 1985.
7. Holland CJ, Weiss E, Burgdorfer W, et al: *Ehrlichia risticii* sp. nov.: Etiological agent of equine monocytic ehrlichiosis (synonym, Potomac horse fever). *Int J System Bacteriol* 35:524, 1985.
8. Ristic M, Huxsoll D: Tribe II. *Ehrlichiae. In* Krieg NR, Holt JG, eds. *Bergey's Manual of Systematic Bacteriology*, vol. 1. Baltimore, Williams & Wilkins, 1984, p 704.
9. Weisburg WG, Dobson ME, Samuel JE, et al: Phylogenetic diversity of the rickettsiae. *J Bacteriol* 171:4202, 1989.
10. Pretzman C, Ralph D, Stotherd D, et al: 16SrRNA sequence relatedness of *Neorickettsia helminthoeca* to *Ehrlichia risticii* and *Ehrlichia sennetsu. Int J Syst Bacteriol* 45:207, 1995.
11. Rikihisa Y: Cross-reacting antigens between *Neorickettsia helminthoeca* and *Ehrlichia* spp. shown by immunofluorescence and Western immunoblotting. *J Clin Microbiol* 29:2024, 1991.
11a. Wen B, Rikihisa Y, Yamamoto S, et al: Characterization of SF agent, an *Ehrlichia* sp. isolated from *Stellantchasmus falcatus* fluke, by 16S rRNA base sequence, serological, and morphological analysis. *Int J Syst Bacteriol* 46:149, 1996.
12. Wen B, Rikihisa Y, Fuerst PA, et al: Analysis of 16S rRNA genes of ehrlichial organisms isolated from horses with clinical signs of Potomac horse fever. *Int J Syst Bacteriol* 45:315, 1995.
13. Rikihisa Y: Ultrastructural studies of ehrlichial organisms in the organs of ponies with equine monocytic ehrlichiosis (synonym, Potomac horse fever). In Winkler H, Ristic M, eds. *Microbiology.* Washington, DC, American Society of Microbiology, 1986, p 200.
14. Rikihisa Y, Perry BD, Cordes DO: Ultrastructural study of rickettsial organisms in the large colon of ponies experimentally infected with Potomac horse fever. *Infect Immun* 49:505, 1985.
15. Rikihisa Y: Ultrastructure of rickettsiae with special emphasis on ehrlichia. In Williams JC, Kakoma I, eds. *Ehrlichiosis: A*

Vector-Borne Disease of Animals and Humans. Boston, Kluwer Academic Publishers, 1990, p. 22.
16. Rikihisa Y: Growth of *Ehrlichia risticii* in human colonic epithelial cells. In Hechemy K, Paretsky D, Walker DH, et al, eds. Rickettsiology: Current issues and perspectives. *Ann N Y Acad Sci* 590:104, 1990.
16a. Chaichanasiriwithaya W, Rikihisa Y, Yamamoto S, et al: Antigenic, morphologic, and molecular characterization of 9 new *Ehrlichia risticii* isolates. *J Clin Microbiol* 38:3026, 1994.
17. Wells MY, Rikihisa Y: Lack of lysosomal fusion with phagosomes containing *Ehrlichia risticii* in P388D1 cells: Abrogation of inhibition with oxytetracycline. *Infect Immun* 56:3209, 1988.
18. Dasch GA, Weiss E, Williams JC: Antigenic properties of the ehrlichiae and other rickettsiaceae. In Williams JC, Kakoma I, eds. *Ehrlichiosis: A Vector-Borne Disease of Animals and Humans.* Boston, Kluwer Academic Publishers, 1990, p 32.
19. Weiss E, Dasch GA, Kang Y-H, et al: Substrate utilization by *Ehrlichia sennetsu* and *Ehrlichia risticii* separated from host constituents by renografin gradient centrifugation. *J Bacteriol* 170:5012, 1988.
20. Chaichanasiriwithaya W, Rikihisa Y, Quareshi N: *Ehrlichia risticii* has lipid A but cosignal activity for nitric oxide production in response to interferon-γ residues in carbohydrate residue. *Infect Immun*, submitted for publication.
21. Weiss E, Williams JC, Dasch GA, et al: Energy metabolism of monocytic *Ehrlichia. Proc Natl Acad Sci USA* 86:1674, 1989.
22. Rikihisa Y, Reed SM, Sams RA, et al: Serosurvey of horses with evidence of equine monocytic ehrlichiosis (Potomac horse fever). *J Am Vet Med Assoc* 197:1327, 1990.
23. Perry BD, Rikihisa Y, Saunders G: Transmission of Potomac horse fever by intradermal route. *Vet Rec* 116:246, 1985.
24. Schmidtmann ET, Rice RM, Roble MG, et al: Search for an arthropod vector of *Ehrlichia risticii*. In Proceedings of the Symposium on Potomac Horse Fever, Lawrenceville, NJ, Veterinary Learning Systems, 1988, p 9.
25. Palmer JE, Benson CE: Oral transmission of *Ehrlichia risticii* resulting in Potomac horse fever. Vet Rec 112:635, 1988.
26. Perry BD, Palmer JE, Troutt HF, et al: A case control study of Potomac horse fever. *Prev Vet Med* 4:69, 1986.
27. Dawson JE, Holland CJ, Ristic M: Susceptibility of cats to infection with *E. risticii*, causative agent of equine monocytic ehrlichiosis (Potomac horse fever). *Am J Vet Res* 49:1497, 1988.
28. Ristic M, Dawson J, Holland CJ, et al: Susceptibility of dogs to infection with *Ehrlichia risticii*, causative agent of equine monocytic ehrlichiosis (Potomac horse fever). *Am J Vet Res* 49:1497, 1988.
29. Jenkins SJ, Jones NK, Jenny AL: Potomac horse fever agent in mice. *Vet Rec* 117:556, 1985.
30. Stephenson EH: Experimental ehrlichiosis in nonhuman primates. In Williams JC, Kakoma I, eds. *Ehrlichiosis: A Vector-Borne Disease of Animals and Humans.* Boston, Kluwer Academic Publishers, 1990, p 93.
31. Dawson JE, Holland CJ, Ristic M: Susceptibility of dogs and cats to infection with *Ehrlichia risticii* causative agent of Potomac horse fever (Abstract). In Proceedings, 67th Annual Meeting and Conference of Research Workers in Animal Disease, 1986, p 349.
32. Perry BD, Schmidtmann ET, Rice RM, et al: Epidemiology of Potomac horse fever: An investigation into the possible role of non-equine mammals. *Vet Rec* 125:83, 1989.
33. Kakoma I, Hansen RD, Anderson BE, et al: Cultural, molecular, and immunological characterization of the etiologic agent for atypical canine ehrlichiosis. *J Clin Microbiol* 32:170, 1994.
34. Rikihisa Y, Johnson GJ, Burger CJ: Reduced immune responsiveness and lymphoid depletion in mice infected with *Ehrlichia risticii. Infect Immun* 55:2215, 1987.

35. Rikihisa Y, Wada R, Reed SM, et al: Development of neutralizing antibodies in horses infected with *Ehrlichia risticii*. *Vet Microbiol* 36:139, 1993.

36. Messick JB, Rikihisa Y, Reed SM: Unpublished observation, 1990.

37. Dawson JE, Ristic M, Holland CJ, et al: Isolation of *Ehrlichia risticii*, the causative agent of Potomac horse fever, from the fetus of an experimentally infected mare. *Vet Rec* 121:232, 1987.

38. Rikihisa Y, Johnson GJ, Wang Y-Z, et al: Loss of adsorptive capacity for sodium chloride as a cause of diarrhea in Potomac horse fever. *Res Vet Sci* 52:353, 1992.

39. van Heeckeren A, Rikihisa Y, Park J, et al: Tumor necrosis factor-α, interleukin-1α and prostaglandin E_2 production in murine peritoneal macrophages infected with *Ehrlichia risticii*. *Infect Immun* 61:4333, 1993.

40. Rikihisa Y, Perry BD, Lin YC: Increase in intestinal cyclic AMP in mouse model for Potomac horse fever. Abstract 1353, Annual Meeting of the American Society of Cell Biology, Atlanta, 1985, p 357a.

41. Messick JB, Rikihisa Y: Characterization of *Ehrlichia risticii* binding, internalization, and growth in host cells by flow cytometry. *Infect Immun* 61:3803, 1993.

42. Rikihisa Y, Zhang Y, Park J: Role of clathrin, microfilament, and microtubule on infection of mouse peritoneal macrophages with *Ehrlichia risticii*. *Infect Immun* 62:5126, 1994.

43. Rikihisa Y, Zhang Y, Park J: Role of CA^{2+} and calmodulin on ehrlichial survival in macrophages. *Infect Immun* 63:2310, 1996.

43a. Zhang Y, Rikihisa Y: Tyrosine phosphorylation is required for ehrlichial internalization and replication in P388D cells. *Infect Immun*, submitted for publication. 1996.

44. Messick JB, Rikihisa Y: Inhibition of binding, entry or survival of *Ehrlichia risticii* in P388$_1$ cells by anti-*E. risticii* IgG and Fab fragments. *Infect Immun* 62:3156, 1994.

45. Palmer JE, Benson CE, Whitlock RH: Equine ehrlichial colitis: Resistance to rechallenge in experimental horses and ponies. *Am J Vet Res* 51:763, 1990.

46. Pretzman CT, Rikihisa Y, Ralph D, et al: Enzyme-linked immunosorbent assay for detecting Potomac horse fever disease. *J Clin Microbiol* 25:31, 1987.

47. Williams NM, Timoney PJ: In vitro killing of *Ehrlichia risticii* by activated and immune mouse peritoneal macrophages. *Infect Immun* 61:861, 1993.

48. Kaylor SP, Crawford TB, McElwain TF, et al: Passive transfer of antibody to *Ehrlichia risticii* protects mice from ehrlichiosis. *Infect Immun* 60:3079, 1992.

49. Messick JB, Rikihisa Y: Presence of parasite antigens on the surface of P388D$_1$ cells infected with *Ehrlichia risticii*. *Infect Immun* 60:3079, 1992.

50. Park J, Rikihisa Y: L-arginine-dependent killing of intracellular *Ehrlichia risticii* by macrophages treated with interferon-gamma. *Infect Immun* 60:3504, 1992.

51. Messick JB, Rikihisa Y: Suppression of I-A^d on P388D$_1$ cells by *Ehrlichia risticii* infection in response to gamma interferon. *Vet Immunol Immunopathol* 32:225, 1992.

52. Whitlock RH, Palmer JE, Benson CE, et al: Potomac horse fever clinical characteristics and diagnostic features. American Association of Veterinary Laboratory Diagnosticians, 27th Annual Proceedings 103, 1984.

53. Jernigan A, Rikihisa Y, Hinchcliff KW: Pharmacokinetics of oxytetra-cycline in ponies with Potomac horse fever. In Proceedings of the 70th Annual Meeting and Conference of Research Workers in Animal Disease, Chicago, 1989, p 35.

54. Zimmer LE, Whitlock RH, Palmer JE, et al: Clinical and hematologic variables in ponies with experimentally induced equine ehrlichial colitis (Potomac horse fever). *Am J Vet Res* 48:63, 1987.

55. Ristic M, Holland CJ, Dawson JE, et al: Diagnosis of equine monocytic ehrlichiosis (Potomac horse fever) by indirect immunofluorescence. *J Am Vet Med Assoc* 189:39, 1986.

56. Rikihisa Y, Reed SM, Sams RA, et al: A serological survey and the clinical management of horses with Potomac horse fever. In Proceedings of a Symposium on Potomac Horse Fever. Lawrenceville, NJ, Veterinary Learning Systems, 1988, p 41.

57. Holland CJ, Ristic M, Dawson J, et al: Comparative evaluation of the PLAT and IFA test for diagnosis of Potomac horse fever. In Proceedings of a Symposium on Potomac Horse Fever. Lawrenceville, NJ, Veterinary Learning Systems, 1988, p 101.

58. Shankarappa B, Dutta S, Sanusi J, et al: Monoclonal antibody mediated, immunodiagnostic competitive enzyme-linked immunosorbent assay for equine monocytic ehrlichiosis. *J Clin Microbiol* 27:24, 1989.

59. Rikihisa Y: The tribe Ehrlichieae and ehrlichial diseases. *Clin Microbiol Rev* 4:286, 1991.

59a. Zhang Y, Ohashi N, Lee EH, et al: Cloning, sequencing, expression of heat shock-protein 60 homolog of *Ehrlichia sennetsu* and its antigenic comparison with those of other rickettsiae. *FEMS Immunol Med Microbiol*, submitted for publication.

60. Rikihisa Y, Pretzman CI, Johnson GC, et al: Clinical and immunological responses of ponies to *Ehrlichia sennetsu* and subsequent *Ehrlichia risticii* challenge. *Infect Immun* 56:2960, 1988.

61. Vemulapalli R, Biswas B, Dutta SK: Pathogenic, immunologic, and molecular differences between two *Ehrlichia risticii* strains. *J Clin Microbiol* 33:2987, 1995.

62. Rikihisa Y, Chaichanasiriwithaya W, Reed SM, et al: Distinct antigenic differences of new *Ehrlichia risticii* isolates. In Proceedings of the 7th International Conference on Equine Infectious Diseases, Tokyo, June 8–11, 1994. R&W Publishing, Newmarket, UK, 1994, p. 211.

63. Mott J, Rikihisa Y, Zhang Y, et al: Comparison of PCR and culture isolation to indirect fluorescence antibody test for diagnosis of Potomac horse fever. *J Clin Microbiol*, in press, 1996.

64. Biswas B, Mukherjee D, Mattingly-Napier B, et al: Diagnostic application of polymerase chain reaction for detection of *Ehrlichia risticii* in equine monocytic ehrlichiosis (Potomac horse fever). *J Clin Microbiol* 29:2228, 1991.

64a. Barlough JE, Rikihisa Y, Madigan JE: Nested polymerase chain reaction for detection of *Ehrlichia risticii* genomic DNA in infected horses. *Vet Parasitol*, in press, 1996.

65. Steele K, Rikihisa Y, Walton A: Demonstration of *Ehrlichia* in Potomac horse fever using a silver stain. *Vet Pathol* 23:531, 1986.

66. Rikihisa Y, Johnson GC, Reed SM: Immune responses and intestinal pathology of ponies experimentally infected with Potomac horse fever. In Proceedings of the Symposium on Potomac Horse Fever. Lawrenceville, NJ, Veterinary Learning Systems, 1988, p 27.

67. Rikihisa Y, Jiang BM: In vitro susceptibility of *Ehrlichia risticii* to eight antibiotics. *Antimicrob Agents Chemother* 32:986, 1988.

68. Rikihisa Y, Jiang BM: Effect of antibiotics on clinical, gross pathologic, and immunologic responses of mice infected with *Ehrlichia risticii*: Protective effects of doxycycline. *Vet Microbiol* 19:253, 1989.

69. Riond J-L, Riviere JE, Duckett WM, et al: Cardiovascular effects and fatalities associated with intravenous administration of doxycycline to horses. *Equine Vet J* 24:41, 1992.

70. Palmer JE, Whitlock RH, Benson CE: Clinical signs and treatment of equine ehrlichial colitis. In Proceedings of a Symposium on Potomac horse fever. Lawrenceville, NJ, Veterinary Learning Systems, 1988, p 49.

71. Palmer J, Benson C: Effect of treatment with erythromycin

and rifampin during the acute stages of experimentally induced equine ehrlichial colitis in ponies. *Am J Vet Res* 53:2071, 1992.

72. Rikihisa Y: Protection against murine Potomac horse fever by an inactivated *Ehrlichia risticii* vaccine. *Vet Microbiol* 28:339, 1991.
73. Palmer JE: Prevention of Potomac horse fever (Editorial). *Cornell Vet* 79:201, 1989.
74. Ristic M, Holland CJ, Goetz TE: Evaluation of a vaccine for equine monocytic ehrlichiosis. In Proceedings of a Symposium on Potomac Horse Fever. Lawrenceville, NJ, Veterinary Learning Systems, 1987, p 89.
75. Shankarappa B, Dutta SK, Mattingly-Napier B: Identification of the protective 44-kilodalton recombinant antigen of *Ehrlichia risticii*. *Infect Immun* 60:612, 1992.
76. Gribble DH: Equine ehrlichiosis. *J Am Vet Med Assoc* 155:462, 1969.
77. Buscher G, Gandras R, Apel G, et al: Der erste Fall von Ehrlichiosis beim Pferd in Deutschland (Kurzmitteilung). *Dtsch Tieraerztl Wochenschr* 91:408, 1984.
78. Hermann M, Baumann D, Lutz H, et al: Erster diagnostizierter Fall von equine Ehrlichiose in der Schweiz. *Pferdeheilkunde* 1:247, 1985.
79. Björsdorff A, Christensson D, Johnson A, et al: Granulocytic ehrlichiosis in the horse—The first verified cases in Sweden. In Proceedings of IVth International Symposium on Rickettsiae Rickettsial Disease. Piešťány Spa, Czech and Slovak Federal Republich, 1990, p 69.
80. Gunders AE, Gottlieb D: Intra-granulocytic inclusion bodies of *Psammomys obesus* naturally transmitted by *Ornithodoros erraticus* (small race). *Refuah Vet* 34:5, 1977.
81. Anderson BE, Dawson JE, Jones DC, et al: *Ehrlichia chaffeensis*, a new species associated with human ehrlichiosis. *J Clin Microbiol* 29:2838, 1991.
81a. Madigan JE, Barlough JE, Dumler JS, et al: Equine granulocytic ehrlichiosis in Connecticut caused by an agent resembling the human granulocytotropic ehrlichia. *J Clin Microbiol* 34:434, 1996.
81b. Johansson K-E, Pettersson B, Uhlén M, et al: Identification of the causative agent of granulocytic ehrlichiosis in Swedish dogs and horses by direct solid phase sequencing of PCR products from the 16S rRNA gene. *Res Vet Sci* 58:109, 1995.
81c. Madigan JE, Richter PJ, Kimsey RB, et al: Transmission and passage in horses of the agent of human granulocytic ehrlichiosis. *J Infect Dis* 172:1141, 1995.

82. Logan LL, Holland CJ, Mebus CA, et al: Serological relationship between *Cowdria ruminantium* and certain ehrlichia. *Vet Rec* 119:458, 1986.
83. Holland CJ, Logan LL, Mebus CA, et al: The serological relationship between *Cowdria ruminantium* and certain members of the genus *Ehrlichia*. *Onderstepoort J Vet Res* 54:331, 1987.
83a. Goodman JL, Nelson C, Vitale B, et al: Direct cultivation of causative agent of human granulocytic ehrlichiosis. *N Engl J Med* 334:209, 1996.
84. Sells DM, Hildebrandt PK, Lewis GE, et al: Ultrastructural observations on *Ehrlichia equi* organisms in equine granulocytes. *Infect Immun* 13:273, 1976.
85. Lewis GE: Equine ehrlichiosis: A comparison between *E. equi* and other pathogenic species of *Ehrlichia*. *Vet Parasitol* 2:61, 1976.
86. Madigan JE, Hietala S, Chalmers S, et al: Seroepidemiologic survey of antibodies to *Ehrlichia equi* in horses of northern California. *J Am Vet Med Assoc* 196:1962, 1990.
86a. Richter PJ, Kimsey RB, Madigan JE, et al: *Ixodes pacificus* as a vector of *Ehrlichia equi*. *J Med Entomol* 33:1, 1995.
87. Madigan JE, Gribble D: Equine ehrlichiosis in northern California: 49 cases (1968–1981). *J Am Vet Med Assoc* 190:445, 1987.
88. Lewis GE, Huxsoll DL, Ristic M, et al: Experimentally induced infection of dogs, cats, and nonhuman primates with *Ehrlichia equi*, etiologic agent of equine ehrlichiosis. *Am J Vet Res* 36:85, 1975.
89. Stannard AA, Gribble DH, Smith RS: Equine ehrlichiosis: A disease with similarities to tick-borne fever and bovine petechial fever. *Vet Rec* 84:149, 1969.
90. Chen S-M, Dumler JS, Bakken JS, et al: Identification of a granulocytotropic *Ehrlichia* species as the etiologic agent of a human disease. *J Clin Microbiol* 32:589, 1994.
91. Nyindo MCA, Ristic M, Lewis GE Jr, et al: Immune responses of ponies to experimental infection with *Ehrlichia equi*. *Am J Vet Res* 39:15, 1978.
92. Telford III SR, Dawson JE, Katarolos P, et al: Perpetuation of the agent of human granulocytic ehrlichiosis in a deer tick–rodent cycle. *Proc Natl Acad Sci USA* 93:6209, 1996.
93. Barlough JE, Ma JE, DeRock E, et al: Nested polymerase chain reaction for detection of *Ehrlichia equi* genomic DNA in horses and ticks (*Ixodes pacificus*). *Vet Parasitol* 63:319, 1996.

Chapter 3

Clinical Approach to Commonly Encountered Problems

3.1

Syncope and Weakness

Mark V. Crisman, DVM, MS

Syncope is a clinical syndrome consisting of a generalized weakness, sudden collapse, and a transient cessation of consciousness. Syncopal episodes are uncommon in horses, and generally there is little or no premonitory warning or presyncopal (faintness) signs evident to the rider or handler. The subsequent loss of consciousness and collapse may potentially be harmful or dangerous to both the horse and the rider. Despite the infrequent reports of true syncopal episodes in horses, the clinical signs are sufficiently dramatic to cause great concern on the part of the owner. Syncope in horses has been virtually unstudied. Consequently, most of the following information has been drawn from studies of people and other animal species.

Although presyncopal signs have been well described in humans (i.e., dizziness, yawning, confusion, spots before the eyes), these signs are generally not evident in horses. Horses may stumble initially and go down or collapse completely. The depth and duration of unconsciousness may vary, but generally unconsciousness lasts for a few minutes. Horses may be slightly unsteady or struggle during recovery. After a syncopal attack, the horse will completely recover and appear "normal."

PATHOPHYSIOLOGY

Syncope results from a relatively sudden reduction in cerebral blood flow and subsequent cerebral ischemia. Cerebral blood flow is maintained primarily by arterial blood pressure and cerebrovascular resistance. In response to either falling or rising systemic blood pressure, the cerebral blood flow autoregulatory mechanism automatically regulates cerebral vessels to constrict or dilate. This control phenomenon maintains a relatively constant cerebral blood flow despite fluctuations in arterial blood pressure, whether or not these fluctuations are physiologic or pathologic in origin. If perfusion pressure in humans falls below 60 mm Hg, the cerebral blood flow autoregulatory mechanism may fail. Mean resting arterial pressure measured at the carotid artery in horses has been reported to be 97 $\pm$ 12 mm Hg at a heart rate of 42 $\pm$ 10 beats/min.[1] Systolic pressure in horses experiencing syncope has not been determined.

Disturbances in oxygen supply to the brain generally result from three primary causes: (1) anoxia, (2) anemia, and (3) ischemia. Although a variety of conditions or diseases may cause these disturbances, all three potentially deprive the brain of its critical oxygen supply.[2] Anoxia is generally described as insufficient oxygen reaching the blood so that both arterial oxygen content and tension are low. This results from either an inability of oxygen to cross the alveolar membrane (e.g., pulmonary disease) or low oxygen tension in the environment (e.g., high altitude). In situations of mild hypoxia, the cerebral blood flow autoregulatory mechanism maintains oxygen delivery to the brain. When the hypoxia is severe or the compensatory mechanism fails, cerebral hypoxia occurs and syncope may result.

Anemia is functionally defined as a decreased oxygen-carrying capacity of the blood. This may be characterized by several mechanisms, including a reduction in the amount of hemoglobin available to bind and transport oxygen or changes in hemoglobin that interfere with oxygen binding (e.g., methemoglobin). If the anemia is severe, the oxygen concentration drops below the brain's metabolic requirements despite increased cerebral blood flow.

Finally, cerebral ischemia results when cerebral blood flow is insufficient to supply cerebral tissue. Any disease that greatly reduces cardiac output, such as myocardial infarction or an arrhythmia, may ultimately result in cerebral ischemia. If any of these aforementioned conditions occurs and cerebral blood flow is interrupted or stops with resultant cerebral underperfusion, consciousness is lost. If tissue oxygenation is restored immediately, consciousness generally returns quickly without sequelae.

Areas of the brain that maintain or control consciousness have been the subject of much debate and research. Generally, the level of activity of the brain (alertness) is maintained through sensory input to the ascending reticular activating system in the rostral brain stem, thalamus, and cerebral cortex. More specifically, the bulboreticular facilitatory area within the reticular substance of the middle and lateral pons and mesencephalon are considered to be the central driving component of the excitatory area of the brain. Recent studies have identified the role of the midbrain reticular formation and the thalamic intralaminar nuclei in maintaining consciousness and arousal in animals and humans.[3] Syncope may result if regional cerebral blood flow to this area is disrupted for any reason.

In horses, syncope may be either cardiogenic or extracardiac (neurocardiogenic) in origin. The primary cause of syncope in horses is generally cardiovascular disease. Cardiogenic syncope may result from: (1) myocardial disease, (2) cardiac dysrhythmias (i.e., atrial fibrillation, third-degree heart block), (3) congenital heart disease, (4) pulmonary hypertension or stenosis, and (5) pericardial disease. Although many of these conditions are uncommon in horses, atrial fibrillation has been associated with several reports of syncope.[4]

Cardiovascular disease, resulting either in an inability to regulate heart rate or in stroke volume, will ultimately decrease cardiac output. Atrial fibrillation can lead to heart rates greater than 240 beats/min with submaximal exercise. The lack of effective atrial contraction prevents complete ventricular filling at the end of diastole, thus causing a marked reduction in effective cardiac output. Complete heart block may be persistent or intermittent and has also been associated with syncopal episodes in horses. When the block is complete and the pacemaker below the block fails to function, syncope occurs. This has been reported in both humans and horses as Stokes-Adams-Morgagni syndrome. This syndrome is the most frequent arrhythmic cause of syncope in humans.[5] Stokes-Adams-Morgagni attacks result from an advanced atrioventricular block and usually involve a momentary sense of weakness followed by an abrupt loss of consciousness. After cardiac standstill or prolonged periods of asystole, unconsciousness results from cerebral ischemia. These "cardiac faints" have been reported to occur several times a day in humans. Additional less common causes of cardiogenic syncope usually involve the distal conduction system (His-Purkinje system) and may be persistent or episodic. Heart block involving the atrioventricular node or proximal conduction system may be congenital or drug induced (e.g., digitalis) in origin. Sick sinus syndrome, a condition described in elderly humans, involves impaired sinoatrial impulse formation or conduction and has been associated with cerebral anoxia. With any of these conditions, cardiac output will not sufficiently increase during skeletal muscle exercise to meet peripheral oxygen demands. Blood will preferentially flow to exercising muscle, resulting in systemic arterial hypotension. This results in cerebral ischemia leading to weakness or syncope.

Extracardiac causes of syncope may indirectly involve the cardiovascular system and were previously referred to as vasovagal or vasodepressor syncope. The term "neurocardiogenic syncope" more accurately describes this phenomenon. This is the most common type of syncope reported in humans and is often precipitated by stress or pain.[6] Although not specifically described in horses, it is likely that a similar mechanism of collapse may exist. The critical cardiovascular features include hypotension and paradoxical sinus bradycardia, heart block, or sinus arrest after sympathetic excitation. Additionally, cardiac asystole may occur as an extreme manifestation of neurocardiogenic syncope. The mediating mechanisms of neurocardiogenic syncope are not well understood; however, several theories have been proposed. Hypercontractile states may cause excessive stimulation of the myocardial mechanoreceptors (C fibers) located in the left ventricle. The result is an exaggerated parasympathetic afferent signal carried by the vagus and glossopharyngeal nerves with a subsequent decrease in sympathetic tone. Inhibition of sympathetic vasoconstrictor activity results in vasodilation, which may be especially evident during periods of vigorous activity and increased heart rates and blood pressure. The excess vagal activity produces bradycardia and a decrease in cardiac output. This combination, along with a decrease in peripheral vascular resistance, ultimately leads to syncope.

Regardless of the specific cause, syncope results from a relatively sudden fall in cerebral blood flow. The loss of consciousness is caused by a reduction of oxygenation to the parts of the brain that maintain consciousness. In horses, syncope is usually caused by a fall in systemic blood pressure resulting from a decrease in cardiac output.

Additional less common causes of syncope in horses may include neurologic disease from space-occupying lesions or increased intracranial pressure. Syncopal episodes have been reported in foals with severe respiratory or congenital heart disease.[7] After minimal exercise or restraint in these foals, hypoxia and subsequently reduced cerebral blood flow may result in syncope. Certain drugs, specifically phenothiazine tranquilizers (acepromazine), have been reported to cause syncope in horses. These tranquilizers will produce antiadrenergic effects primarily through α_1-blockade with resultant vasodilation and hypotension. If phenothiazine tranquilizers are administered to severely hypovolemic horses or to horses that have hemorrhaged, severe hypotension and syncope may result.

Several disorders are often confused with syncope and should be carefully differentiated with an accurate history and thorough physical examination. These disorders include: (1) epilepsy, (2) hypoglycemia, (3) narcolepsy and cataplexy, (4) cerebrovascular disease, and (5) hyperkalemic periodic paralysis.

Epileptic seizures generally differ from syncope in that they have immediate onset and involve loss of consciousness, tonic and clonic convulsive activity with opistothotonus, and changes in visceral function (urination and defecation). Seizures commonly last for several minutes and are often followed by a postictal phase in which the horse may pace, appear blind, and not recognize its surroundings.

Metabolic disturbances such as hypoglycemia are frequently observed in neonatal foals and may be associated with weakness or syncopal-like episodes. Typically, foals are premature or are subject to perinatal stress with subsequent increased glucose utilization secondary to hypoxia or sepsis. Serum glucose determination is necessary to evaluate hypoglycemia.

Narcolepsy, an abnormal sleep tendency, and cataplexy may occasionally be difficult to distinguish from syncope as a cause of unconsciousness. Attacks of narcolepsy or cataplexy may be preceded by signs of weakness (buckling at the knees) followed by total collapse and areflexia. Rapid eye movements may occur with an absence of spinal reflexes. No other neurologic abnormalities are observed between attacks, although animals may appear sleepy between episodes. Provocative testing with physostigmine (0.05 mg/kg) may induce narcoleptic attacks and might be helpful in differentiating syncope from narcolepsy or cataplexy.

Cerebrovascular disease associated with head trauma and subarachnoid hemorrhage may cause temporary unconsciousness in horses. Clinical signs resulting from brain trauma are generally associated with focal cerebral dysfunction and, therefore, are readily distinguishable from syncope.

Hyperkalemic periodic paralysis causes weakness and collapse without alterations in consciousness. This autosomal dominant disorder has been reported in certain lines of registered Quarter Horses, Paints, and Appaloosas. A reliable DNA-based test is available to diagnose hyperkalemic periodic paralysis in horses.

EVALUATION OF SYNCOPE

1. *History*: Emphasis should be placed on obtaining a detailed history. Both the onset and the duration of the problem along with performance history should be determined.

2. *Physical Examination*: After a thorough physical examination and determination of vital signs, a detailed cardiovascular and neurologic examination should be performed. In addition to heart rate at rest and pulse characteristics, a thorough cardiac auscultation should be performed in a quiet room to identify any murmurs or cardiac dysrhythmias. An electrocardiogram and echocardiogram will also provide valuable information. A neurologic examination should carefully evaluate reflexes and sensory and motor function to identify any central or peripheral neuropathies.

3. *Complete Blood Count and Biochemical Profile*: To rule out other potential causes of syncope-like episodes (e.g., hypoglycemia, sepsis), a complete blood count and biochemical profile should be performed. Additionally, serum lactate dehydrogenase (isoenzymes 1 and 2) and creatine kinase (CK-2) concentration determinations may be helpful in identifying cardiac dysfunction.

4. *Exercise/Stress Test*: A thorough cardiac evaluation should be performed following strenuous exercise, including auscultation and an electrocardiogram. If available, a high-speed treadmill may be helpful in this phase of the evaluation. If any cardiac abnormalities are detected on physical examination, exercise testing on a treadmill will allow a more thorough evaluation of the cardiovascular system, although care must be taken to ensure that such testing does not exacerbate the horse's condition.

Diagnosis of the cause of syncope in horses is not always easy, because it should be considered a "symptom complex" rather than a primary disease. In addition to the infrequent reports of syncope, the history is often vague and the neurologic and cardiovascular examinations may not lead to a specific etiology. Even in the absence of apparently overt cardiovascular disease (e.g., atrial fibrillation), cardiac dysrhythmias cannot be excluded as the possible cause of syncope.

TREATMENT OF SYNCOPE

Options in the treatment of syncope in horses are very limited. Both the frequency of the syncopal attacks and the underlying cause (i.e., cardiogenic, neurocardiogenic) may determine if a course of treatment should be undertaken. Generally, treatment of syncope should be directed toward preventing or correcting the cause of the decreased cerebral perfusion. An accurate pathophysiologic diagnosis is essential for treating cardiogenic syncope. A few reports in the literature indicate successful treatment of syncope in horses associated with atrial fibrillation.[4] A horse with a complete heart block returned to work after implantation of a transvenous cardiac pacing system.[8]

REFERENCES

1. Physick-Shepard PW: Cardiovascular response to exercise and training in the horse. *Vet Clin North Am Equine Pract* 1:383, 1985.
2. Plum F, Posner JB: Multifocal, diffuse, and metabolic brain disease causing stupor or coma. In Plum F, Posner JB, eds. *The Diagnosis of Stupor and Coma*, ed 3. Philadelphia, FA Davis, 1986, pp 208–213.
3. Kinomura S, Larsson J, Gulyas B, et al: Activation by attention of the human reticular formation and thalamic intralaminar nuclei. *Science* 271:512–515, 1996.
4. Deegen E, Buntenkotter S: Behavior of the heart rate of horses with auricular fibrillation during exercise and after treatment. *Equine Vet J* 8:26–29, 1976.
5. O'Rourke RA, Walsh RA, Easton JD: Faintness and syncope. In Stein JH, ed. *Internal Medicine*, ed 4. St. Louis, CV Mosby, 1994, pp 1020–1025.
6. Sra JS, Jazayeri MR, Avitall B, et al: Comparison of cardiac pacing with drug therapy in the treatment of neurocardiogenic (vasovagal) syncope with bradycardia or systole. *N Engl J Med* 328:1085–1090, 1993.
7. Vitamus A, Bayly WM: Pulmonary atresia with dextroposition of the aorta and ventricular septal defect in three Arabian foals. *Vet Pathol* 19:160–168, 1982.
8. Reef VB, Clark ES, Oliver JA, et al: Implantation of a permanent transvenous pacing catheter in a horse with a complete heart block and syncope. *J Am Vet Med Assoc* 189:449–452, 1986.

3.2

Polyuria and Polydipsia

Catherine W. Kohn, DVM
Bernard Hansen, DVM

The complaint of excessive urination and drinking may be encountered with some frequency in equine practice. Before pursuing a lengthy diagnostic work-up, it is important to verify that 24-hour urine production and voluntary water consumption exceed reference ranges. Urine production in adult horses may range from 15 to 30 mL/kg/day, and values as high as 48 mL/kg/day have been reported.[1–4] Daily urine volume is affected by diet; more water is lost in the urine in horses fed pelleted diets and legume hays than in horses fed grass hay. The latter excrete more water in feces.[5, 6] Generally, any component of the diet that increases renal solute load will increase urine volume (e.g., high salt content in the diet).[7] Voluntary water intake is also affected by the ambient temperature (Table 3–1). When temperatures are high and evaporative water losses increase to cool the horse, voluntary water intake also increases. Diet and climatic conditions must therefore be considered when interpreting water consumption and urine production data. Water requirements are proportional to metabolic body size rather than to body weight. Thus, larger horses, particularly draft breeds, require less water per kilogram than do smaller horses, ponies, or miniature horses. In addition, fat is low in water content compared with lean body tissue, and fat animals require proportionately less water than do lean animals.[7]

Some owners may misinterpret polyalkiuria (frequent urination, usually small volume) as polyuria (PU). Quantitative collection of urine for a 24-hour period may be required to verify excessive urine production. Several relatively simple collection apparatuses have been described.[8, 9]

MAINTENANCE OF WATER BALANCE IN HEALTH

Maintenance of water homeostasis depends on establishing a balance between intake and excretion such that plasma osmolality remains constant (within approximately 2% of normal).[10] The primary determinant of renal water excretion is antidiuretic hormone (ADH).[11] ADH is a polypeptide synthesized in three nuclei in the hypothalamus (suprachiasmatic, paraventricular, and supraoptic nuclei)[12] and transported from the latter two nuclei in secretory granules down axons of the supraopticohypophyseal tract into the posterior lobe of the pituitary where ADH is stored.[11] Some ADH enters the cerebrospinal fluid or portal capillaries of the median eminence from the paraventricular nucleus.[11] In addition, neurons from the suprachiasmatic nucleus deposit ADH in other areas in the central nervous system.[12] In humans, lesions of the posterior pituitary or supraopticohypophyseal tract below the median eminence do not usually lead to permanent central diabetes insipidus because ADH still has access to systemic circulation in these cases.[11] The clinical importance of these anatomic relationships in horses is not known.

ADH increases renal water reabsorption and urine osmolality by augmenting water permeability of luminal membranes of cortical and medullary collecting tubules.[11] ADH

augments urea, and in some species NaCl, accumulation in the interstitium, therefore promoting medullary hypertonicity. The primary stimuli for ADH release are plasma hyperosmolality and depletion of the effective circulating blood volume. Osmoreceptors in the hypothalamus detect changes in plasma osmolality of as little as 1%.[11] Although the threshold for ADH release in the horse is not known, 24-hour water deprivation in healthy ponies resulted in approximately an 8 mOsm/kg increase in plasma osmolality (about 3%), from 287 ± 3 mOsm/kg to 295 ± 4 mOsm/kg, which was associated with an increase in plasma ADH concentration from 1.53 ± 0.36 pg/mL to 4.32 ± 1.12 pg/mL.[13] In another study of ponies, water deprivation for 19 hours resulted in an increase in plasma osmolality from 297 ± 1 mOsm/L to 306 ± 2 mOsm/L.[14] In humans, plasma osmolalities of 280 to 290 mOsm/L stimulate ADH release.[11] The organs that sense changes in effective circulating blood volume include arterial and left atrial baroreceptors. These stretch receptors function indirectly as volume sensors by responding to the reductions in intraluminal pressure that typically accompany loss of plasma volume. Reduced activation of these receptors by hypovolemia or heart failure is a potent cause of ADH release, even in the absence of increased plasma osmolality. ADH secretion may also be stimulated by stress (pain), nausea, hypoglycemia, and certain drugs including morphine and lithium.[11]

When the need for water in body fluids cannot be met by conservation via the renal/ADH axis, thirst is stimulated. Thirst is regulated primarily by plasma tonicity; however, in humans the threshold for stimulation of thirst is approximately 2 to 5 mOsm/kg greater than that for stimulation of ADH release.[11] Thirst is controlled by osmosensitive neurons in close proximity in the hypothalamus to osmoreceptors that mediate ADH secretion.[12] Thirst is sensed peripherally by oropharyngeal mechanoreceptors as dryness of the mouth. Thirst may also be stimulated by volume depletion through an incompletely understood mechanism. Experimental ponies drank when their plasma osmolalities increased by 3% after water deprivation, when plasma Na concentrations increased by approximately 5%, and after induction of a plasma volume deficit of 6%.[14]

MECHANISM OF URINE CONCENTRATION[15, 16]

In order for the kidney to make concentrated urine, ADH must be produced, the renal collecting tubules must respond to ADH, and the renal medullary interstitium must be hypertonic. Generation of medullary hypertonicity is initiated in the thick ascending limb of the loop of Henle by active transport of sodium chloride (NaCl) out of the lumen. As the thick ascending limb is impermeable to water, active resorption of NaCl results in hypotonicity of the fluid entering the distal tubule in the renal cortex (Fig. 3–1A). The distal tubules and cortical portions of the collecting ducts are permeable to water (Fig. 3–1B), which is reabsorbed down its concentration gradient into the interstitium. Reabsorbed water is rapidly transported out of the interstitium by the extensive cortical capillary network, and interstitial hypertonicity is preserved. Urea remains in the lumen of the distal tubule and cortical collecting duct and is further

Table 3–1. Voluntary Water Consumption in Healthy Horses

Ambient Temperature	mL/kg/day	L/450 kg
5–16 °C (41–61 °F)	44–61	19.8–27.5
25 °C (77 °F)	70	31.5

Data from Tasker JB: Fluid and electrolyte studies in the horse. III: Intake and output of water, sodium and potassium in normal horses. *Cornell Vet* 57:649–657, 1967; Rose BD: Clinical Physiology of Acid-Base and Electrolyte Disorders. New York, McGraw-Hill Information Services, 1989, pp 153–208, 609; and Groenedyk S, English PB, Abetz I: External balance of water and electrolytes in the horse. *Equine Vet J* 20:189–193, 1988.

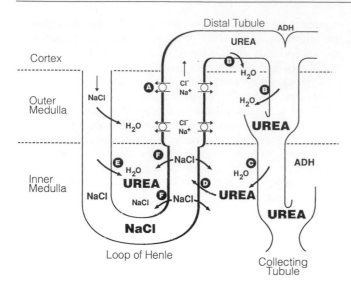

Figure 3–1. The countercurrent hypothesis identifies the roles of sodium chloride and urea transport in the generation of concentrated urine. (From Hansen B: Polyuria and polydipsia. In Fenner WR: Quick Reference to Veterinary Medicine, ed 2. Philadelphia, JB Lippincott, 1991. Adapted from Jamison RL, Maffly RH: The urinary concentration mechanism. N Engl J Med 295:1059–1067, 1976.)

concentrated. Luminal fluid flows into the medullary collecting duct, which is permeable to both water and urea when under the influence of ADH (Fig. 3–1C). Water is reabsorbed down its progressively steeper concentration gradient as luminal fluid moves through the medullary collecting ducts. Some urea is also reabsorbed into the interstitium. Reabsorbed water is efficiently removed by the vasa recta in the renal medulla. Since these blood vessels are also arranged in a hairpin loop configuration, minimal loss of medullary interstitial solute occurs with water removal. Some reabsorbed urea enters the loop of Henle (Fig. 3–1D) and is thus recycled, helping to maintain medullary hypertonicity. In the absence of ADH, the collecting ducts are relatively impermeable to water and urea, resulting in water and urea loss in urine and reduction of medullary solute. Prolonged diuresis of any cause may result in the loss of medullary hypertonicity (medullary washout) with subsequent impairment of renal concentrating ability. Water is reabsorbed down its concentration gradient from the thin descending limb of the loop of Henle (Fig. 3–1E) as a consequence of medullary hypertonicity. This segment of the nephron is impermeable to NaCl and urea, thus the osmolality of luminal fluid in the most distal portion of the loop approaches that of the interstitium. The thin ascending limb of the loop of Henle is permeable to NaCl. NaCl diffuses down its concentration gradient into the interstitium (Fig. 3–1F). As previously mentioned, this segment is also permeable to urea, and some interstitial urea enters the tubule lumen by diffusion down its concentration gradient. Luminal fluid entering the thick ascending limb of the loop of Henle is thus hypotonic to the interstitium.

When luminal fluid reaches the thick ascending limb of the loop of Henle, approximately 80% of the glomerular filtrate has been reabsorbed. Therefore, only 20% of the

glomerular filtrate is available for reabsorption via the action of ADH.

PRIMARY POLYDIPSIA

Excessive water intake may result in water diuresis. Primary polydipsia has been described in horses residing in the southern United States during months when ambient temperature and humidity are high.[8] Apparent psychogenic polydipsia may result from boredom, especially in stalled, young horses.[8] Psychogenic polydipsia has also been anecdotally reported in horses with chronic liver disease and central nervous system signs that had been treated with intravenous fluids.[17] Primary disorders of thirst are poorly understood in horses.

CAUSES OF POLYURIA WITH SECONDARY POLYDIPSIA (Table 3–2)

Increased urine flow may be induced by solute or water diuresis. Solute diuresis results in increased urine flow because of excessive renal excretion of a non-reabsorbed solute such as glucose or sodium. During solute diuresis, the urine osmolality is equal to or higher than the plasma osmolality. Primary renal insufficiency or failure (33% or fewer intact nephrons) result in solute diuresis, because each functional nephron must filter an increased amount of solute in order to maintain daily obligatory solute excretion. Fractional clearances of solutes such as sodium (Na), potassium (K), and chloride (Cl) will therefore appropriately increase. Solute diuresis due to glucosuria occurs in hyperglycemic horses when the maximal renal reabsorptive capacity for glucose is exceeded (180 to 200 mg/dL).[18] Solute diuresis due to glucosuria has been reported in horses with pituitary adenoma and in a hyperglycemic horse with bilateral granulosa cell tumors.[19, 20] Primary diabetes mellitus, a common cause of hyperglycemia and glucosuria in other species, is uncommon in the horse, although type II diabetes mellitus was diagnosed in a 15-year-old Quarter Horse mare.[21] Primary renal tubular glucosuria due to a defect in proximal tubular glucose reabsorption (as is seen in Basenji dogs with Fanconi-like syndrome)[15] has not been reported in horses. Psychogenic salt consumption has also been reported to cause solute diuresis in a horse.[22] Postobstructive solute diuresis is diagnosed uncommonly in horses because nephrolithiasis and ureterolithiasis are uncommon; when they occur the condition is often bilateral and associated with chronic renal failure, and treatment is usually unsuccessful.[23, 24]

Decreased water resorption in the collecting tubules or inappropriately large voluntary water intake causes water diuresis. The osmolality of the urine during water diuresis is less than that of plasma. Water diuresis may be caused by insufficient ADH secretion, insensitivity of the receptors of the distal collecting duct and collecting tubules to the action of ADH, renal medullary solute washout, or apparent psychogenic polydipsia. Insufficient secretion of ADH (central diabetes insipidus) may be associated with adenoma of the pars intermedia of horses but has never been documented,[25] and with head trauma, and potassium depletion in other species. A case of idiopathic central diabetes insipidus was

Table 3–2. Causes of Polyuria and Polydipsia

Solute Diuresis

Primary renal insufficiency or failure
Glucosuria (adenoma of the pars intermedia of the pituitary)
Psychogenic salt consumption
Diabetes mellitus
Postobstructive diuresis

Water Diuresis

Insufficient antidiuretic hormone (central diabetes insipidus)
    Adenoma of the pars intermedia of the pituitary
    Head trauma
    (Potassium depletion)
Insufficient response of collecting ducts to antidiuretic hormone
Acquired nephrogenic diabetes insipidus
    Hyperadrenocorticism (glucocorticoid excess with adenoma of
        the pars intermedia of the pituitary)
    Endotoxemia
    (Drugs: gentamicin, lithium, methoxyfluorane, amphotericin B,
        propoxyphene, etc)
(Congenital nephrogenic diabetes insipidus)
Renal medullary solute washout
    Chronic diuresis of any cause
    Inappropriate renal tubular sodium handling
Apparent psychogenic polydipsia
(Chronic liver disease)
(Polycythemia)
(Pyometra)
(Hypercalcemia)
(Potassium depletion)

Iatrogenic

Intravenous fluid therapy
Excess dietary salt
Drugs:
    Diuretics
    Glucocorticoids
    (Drugs causing acquired diabetes insipidus)

( ), not reported in horses.
Adapted from Hansen B: Polyuria and polydipsia. In Fenner WR: Quick Reference to Veterinary Medicine, ed 2. Philadelphia, JB Lippincott, 1991, pp 103–114.

reported in a Welsh pony.[26] Insensitivity of collecting duct receptors to ADH may occur during endotoxemia and hyperadrenocorticism (glucocorticoid excess associated with tumors of the pars intermedia). In other species, potassium depletion, hypercalcemia, and the administration of certain drugs (including gentamicin) have been reported to cause insensitivity of the collecting duct receptors to ADH.[15] Congenital diabetes insipidus has also been reported in other species.[26] True nephrogenic diabetes insipidus implies isolated dysfunction of response to ADH by collecting tubules that are not associated with other structural or metabolic lesions of the kidney. The occurrence of nephrogenic diabetes insipidus in two sibling Thoroughbred colts has suggested that the condition might be heritable in some horses.[27] Renal medullary washout (loss of medullary Na, Cl, and urea) leading to water diuresis may result from chronic diuresis of any cause. Diuresis is associated with increased tubular flow

rates and inability to adequately resorb sodium and urea from the tubular lumen.[15] Enhanced medullary blood flow may further deplete medullary solute.[15] Water diuresis has also been reported in association with pyometra, hypoadrenocorticism (chronic renal sodium loss), chronic liver disease (increased aldosterone concentration promotes sodium retention, smaller daily load of urea for excretion due to decreased conversion of ammonia to urea), primary polycythemia, hypercalcemia, and potassium depletion in other species.[15]

APPROACH TO THE HORSE WITH POLYURIA AND POLYDIPSIA (see Fig. 3–2)

Iatrogenic causes of polyuria and polydipsia (PUPD) (see Table 3–2) should be ruled out by careful assessment of the history and by documentation of return to normal urine volume and water intake after withdrawal of intravenous fluids, excess dietary salt, or drugs implicated in causing PUPD. Verification of 24-hour urine volume and water intake should be undertaken for horses suspected of having PUPD that do not display obvious PU (frequent large volume urination, stall very wet) and PD (water bucket always empty, overt thirst). Hemogram, serum biochemistries, and urinalysis should be assessed for all horses with PUPD. A hallmark finding in horses with PUPD is a decreased urine specific gravity (USG). Identification of other abnormalities on laboratory tests (e.g., increased blood urea nitrogen or creatinine (Cr) concentrations, hyperglycemia, hypokalemia) necessitates ruling out the presence of underlying diseases (such as renal insufficiency, adenoma of the pars intermedia of the pituitary) utilizing specialized laboratory tests.

The hydration status of horses should next be carefully assessed. Those horses that are dehydrated should be judiciously rehydrated with intravenous fluids, taking care not to overhydrate horses with renal insufficiency. After rehydration, when possible, creatinine clearance should be determined by utilizing a urine collection apparatus to allow 24-hour volumetric urine collection. A creatinine clearance value below the reference range (1.46 to 3.68 mL/min/kg)[28] suggests that renal insufficiency with decreased GFR and solute diuresis are likely present. A creatinine clearance within the reference range indicates that central diabetes insipidus (CDI), nephrogenic diabetes insipidus (NDI), or apparent psychogenic polydipsia (APP) is present. To distinguish among these differential diagnoses, an exogenous ADH challenge test should be performed (see later).

Horses with PUPD that are well hydrated and healthy based on physical examination and results of hemogram and serum biochemistry determinations should be subjected to a water deprivation test to assess renal ability to conserve water.[2, 29, 30] Water deprivation testing is contraindicated in a dehydrated horse with a low USG. Such horses have already undergone an endogenous water deprivation test (clinical dehydration is present) and have responded with an inappropriately low USG. The following guidelines for interpretation of water deprivation test results are based on practical experience and the limited data available. A positive response to water deprivation (USG >1.030) indicates that the horse has APP, whereas a negative response (USG <1.008) after 24 hours of water deprivation or greater than 5% weight loss[31] is consistent with a diagnosis of CDI, true NDI,

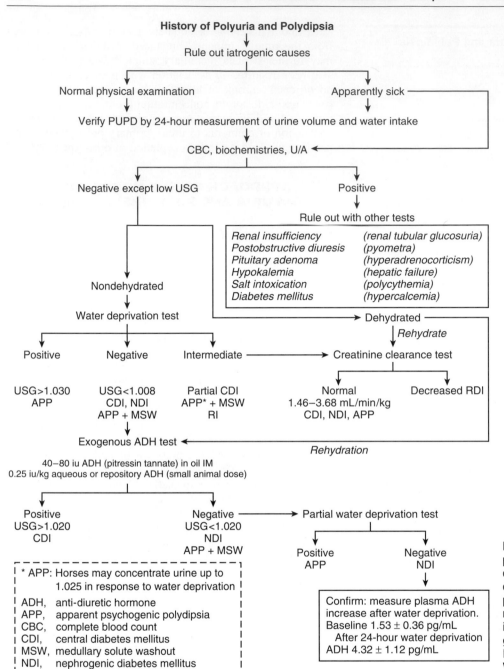

Figure 3–2. Approach to the polyuric patient. CDI, central diabetes mellitus; NDI, nephrogenic diabetes mellitus; APP, apparent psychogenic polydipsia; MSW, medullary solute washout; RI, renal insufficiency; USG, urine specific gravity. (Modified from Hansen B: Polyuria and polydipsia. In Fenner WF: Quick Reference to Veterinary Medicine, ed. 2. Philadelphia, JB Lippincott, 1991, p 110.)

insensitivity of collecting duct receptors to ADH, or apparent psychogenic polydipsia and medullary solute washout (APP plus MSW). Horses with a negative response to water deprivation testing should undergo an exogenous ADH challenge. Some horses may have an intermediate response to water deprivation. An intermediate response is consistent with partial CDI or APP plus MSW or RI, and assessment of creatinine clearance is indicated. Consult Chapter 16 for a more detailed discussion of water deprivation testing.

An evaluation of a response to the administration of exogenous ADH is indicated for horses that do not adequately concentrate their urine during water deprivation testing, for horses that required rehydration and subsequently demonstrated creatinine clearance values within reference ranges, and for rehydrated horses for which creatinine clearance determinations are impractical. Two regimens for exogenous ADH administration have been reported 40 to 80 IU ADH as pitressin tannate in oil IM[32] or 0.25 IU/kg aqueous or repository ADH IM.[31] There are few reports of responses of horses to exogenous ADH administration, and the following recommendations are based on clinical experience. A positive response to exogenous ADH (USG >1.020) confirms the diagnosis of CDI. A negative response (USG <1.020) implies that NDI or APP plus MSW is present.[31]

Medullary solute washout may result in a decreased USG despite the presence of adequate ADH. A partial water deprivation test should result in an increase in USG in horses with APP plus MSW but should have no effect on horses with true NDI or insensitivity of collecting duct receptors to ADH. The horse is allowed to consume its normal diet and water ad libitum. Voluntary water consumption is monitored closely for 3 to 4 days to establish a baseline. Water available to the horse is then decreased by 5% to 10% of the baseline voluntary intake. Water should be offered in aliquots several times a day to prevent the horse from consuming most of the water in a short time. Water intake should never be restricted below maintenance requirements (about 40 mL/kg/day). During water restriction, the horse is allowed to eat its regular diet. The horse should be weighed daily if possible and should be carefully observed for signs of dehydration (prolonged capillary refill time, increasing heart rate, prolonged skin tenting, hypernatremia). Moderate water restriction in the face of continued intake of dietary solutes facilitates reestablishment of the corticomedullary osmotic gradient.[15] Results of partial water deprivation tests in horses have been infrequently reported.

The diagnosis of true NDI or insensitivity of collecting duct receptors to ADH may be confirmed by measuring plasma ADH concentrations before and after partial water deprivation. ADH concentrations have been reported to increase from baseline values of 1.53 ± 0.36 pg/mL to 4.32 ± 1.12 pg/mL after 24 hours of water deprivation in ponies.[13]

Because DDI, NDI, and APP are relatively uncommon in horses, the presenting complaint of PUPD usually signifies other underlying disease. The most likely underlying disease is renal insufficiency. Pituitary adenoma should be considered in horses with compatible clinical signs (hirsutism, weight loss, laminitis) and supporting laboratory data (hyperglycemia, failure of suppression of cortisol production by dexamethasone).[33] Medullary washout may be a more common complication of primary diseases and their therapy in horses than has been reported to date. Potential causes of diuresis compatible with the case history and clinical signs should be investigated, and a partial water deprivation test should be considered when horses exhibit PUPD.

REFERENCES

1. Tasker JB: Fluid and electrolyte studies in the horses. III: Intake and output of water, sodium and potassium in normal horses. *Cornell Vet* 57:649–657, 1967.
2. Rumbaugh GE, Carlson GP, Harrold D: Urinary production in the healthy horse and in horses deprived of feed and water. *Am J Vet Res* 43:735–737, 1982.
3. Morris DD, Divers TJ, Whitlock RH: Renal clearance and fractional excretion of electrolytes over a 24-hour period in horses. *Am J Vet Res* 45:2431–2435, 1984.
4. Kohn CW, Strasser SL: 24-hour renal clearance and excretion of endogenous substances in the mare. *Am J Vet Res* 47:1332–1337, 1986.
5. Cymbaluk NF: Water balance of horses fed various diets. *Equine Pract* 11:19–24, 1989.
6. Rose RJ: Electrolytes: Clinical application. *Vet Clin North Am Equine Pract* 6:281–294, 1990.
7. Kohn CW, DiBartola SP: Composition and distribution of body

8. Roussel AJ, Carter GK: Polyuria and polydipsia. In *Problems in Equine Medicine*. Philadelphia, Lea & Febiger, 1989, pp 150–160.
9. Harris P: Collection of urine. *Equine Vet J* 20:86–88, 1988.
10. Humes HD: Disorders of water metabolism. In *Fluids and Electrolytes*. Philadelphia, WB Saunders, 1986, pp 118–149.
11. Rose BD: *Clinical Physiology of Acid-Base and Electrolyte Disorders*. New York, McGraw-Hill Information Services, 1989, pp 153–208, 609.
12. Zerbe RL, Robertson GL: Osmotic and nonosmotic regulation of thirst and vasopressin secretion. In *Maxwell and Kleeman's Clinical Disorders of Fluid and Electrolyte Metabolism*. New York, McGraw-Hill, 1994, pp 81–82.
13. Houpt KA, Thornton SN, Allen WR: Vasopressin in dehydrated and rehydrated ponies. *Physiol Behav* 45:659–661, 1989.
14. Suffit E, Houpt KA, Sweeting M: Physiological stimuli of thirst and drinking patterns in ponies. *Equine Vet J* 17:12–16, 1985.
15. Hansen B: Polyuria and polydipsia. In *Quick Reference to Veterinary Medicine*, ed 2. Philadelphia, JB Lippincott, 1991, pp 103–114.
16. Jamison RL, Maffly RH: The urinary concentrating mechanism. *N Engl J Med* 295:1059–1067, 1976.
17. Carlson GP: Discussion: Practical clinical chemistry. *Proc 23rd AAEP Convention*. Golden, CO, American Association of Equine Practitioners, 1977, pp 168–169.
18. Stewart J, Holman HH: The "blood picture" of the horse. *Vet Rec* 52:157–165, 1940.
19. Corke MJ: Diabetes mellitus: The tip of the iceberg. *Equine Vet J* 18:87–88, 1986.
20. McCoy DJ: Diabetes mellitus associated with bilateral granulosa cell tumors in a mare. *J Am Vet Med Assoc* 188:733–734, 1986.
21. Ruoff WW, Baker DC, Morgan SJ: Type II diabetes mellitus in a horse. *Equine Vet J* 18:143–144, 1986.
22. Buntain BJ, Coffman JR: Polyuria and polydipsia in a horse induced by psychogenic salt consumption. *Equine Vet J* 13:266–268, 1981.
23. Laverty S, Pascoe JR, Ling GV, et al: Urolithiasis in 68 horses. *Vet Surg* 21:56, 1992.
24. Ehnen SJ, Divers TJ, Gillette D, et al: Obstructive nephrolithiasis and ureterolithiasis associated with chronic renal failure in horses: Eight cases (1981–1987). *J Am Vet Med Assoc* 197:249, 1990.
25. Baker JR, Ritchie HE: Diabetes mellitus in the horse: A case report and review of the literature. *Equine Vet J* 6:7–11, 1974.
26. Breukink HJ, Van Wegen P, Schotman AJH: Idiopathic diabetes insipidus in a Welsh pony. *Equine Vet J* 15:284–287, 1983.
27. Schott HC, Bayly WM, Reed SM, et al: Nephrogenic diabetes insipidus in sibling colts. *J Vet Intern Med* 7:68–72, 1993.
28. Kohn CW, Chew DJ: Laboratory diagnosis and characterization of renal disease in horses. *Vet Clin North Am Equine Pract* 3:585–615, 1987.
29. Brobst DF, Bayly WM: Responses of horses to a water deprivation test. *J Equine Vet Sci* 2:51–56, 1982.
30. Genetzky RM, Loparco FV, Ledet AE: Clinical pathologic alterations in horses during a water deprivation test. *Am J Vet Res* 48:1007–1011, 1987.
31. Ziemer EL: Water deprivation test and vasopressin challenge. In *Equine Medicine and Surgery*. Goleta, CA, American Veterinary Publications, 1991, p 1544.
32. Whitlock RH: Polyuria. In Robinson NE, ed. *Current Therapy in Equine Medicine 3*. Philadelphia, WB Saunders, 1992, pp 620–622.
33. Madigan JE, Dybdal NO: Endocrine and metabolic diseases.

In *Large Animal Internal Medicine*. St Louis, CV Mosby, 1990, pp 1296–1300.
34. Groenedyk S, English PB, Abetz I: External balance of water and electrolytes in the horse. *Equine Vet J* 20:189–193, 1988.

3.3

Edema

Kenneth W. Hinchcliff, BVSc, MS, PhD

Edema is the excessive and abnormal accumulation of fluid in the interstitium. Interstitial fluid accumulates because of imbalances in the rates with which fluid enters and exits the interstitium. Factors that increase the rate of fluid flux from the capillary or impair lymph drainage sufficiently to overwhelm normal compensatory mechanisms result in accumulation of fluid and the development of edema.

PHYSIOLOGY

The volume of interstitial fluid and lymph fluid in the normal horse is 8% to 10% of body weight,[1] or 36 to 45 L in a 450-kg horse. Interstitial fluid consists of water, protein, and electrolytes. Compared with plasma, interstitial fluid has a slightly lower concentration of cationic electrolytes, a slightly higher concentration of chloride, and a much lower concentration of protein (1.2 versus 0.2 mOsmol/L of water).[2] The amount and function of plasma proteins within the interstitial space are not inconsequential. There is a constant circulation of plasma proteins between the vascular and interstitial spaces with about half of the protein circulating every 24 hours in humans. More than half of the plasma protein content of the body is contained within the interstitial space at any one time.[3] Plasma proteins within the interstitial space are important in the transport of water-insoluble substances from the vascular space and in resistance to infection.[3]

Interstitial fluid is contained within the interstitium, the intercellular connective tissues that lie between the cellular elements of the vascular and cellular compartments of the body. The extracellular tissue of the interstitium, except in the case of bone, consists of a three-dimensional collagen fiber network embedded in a proteoglycan gel matrix.[4] Interstitial water exists as both free water and as water within the proteoglycan gel. Normally, only a small proportion of interstitial fluid exists as free water, most of the water being contained in the interstitial gel. However, in edematous states, the proportion of fluid as free water within the interstitium increases.[2]

The source of interstitial fluid is the intravascular space. The volume of interstitial fluid is determined by the functional relationships of three major anatomic structures: the capillary; the interstitial space; and the lymphatics.[5] Functionally, the volume of fluid that accumulates in the intersti-

tium is determined by the rate of ingress of fluid from the vascular space, the compliance of the interstitium, and the rate at which fluid is evacuated from the interstitium. The net rate of ingress of fluid from capillaries into the interstitium is determined by a number of factors acting across the capillary membrane, the effects of which are related by the Starling equation:

$$J = Kf[(P_c - P_t) - \sigma(\pi_p - \pi_t)]$$

in which: J = volume flow across the capillary wall; Kf = filtration coefficient of the capillary wall (volume flow per unit time per 100 g of tissue per unit pressure); P_c = capillary hydrostatic pressure; P_t = interstitial fluid hydrostatic pressure; σ = osmotic reflection coefficient; π_p = colloid osmotic (oncotic) pressure of the plasma; π_t = colloid osmotic (oncotic) pressure of the interstitial fluid.[6] Although all these factors act in concert to determine the rate of net fluid efflux from the capillary, it is conceptually easier to consider them individually.

Filtration (Kf) and Reflection (σ) Coefficients

Together, the filtration and reflection coefficients describe the properties of the capillary membrane that determine the ease with which water, protein, and other plasma constituents move from the vascular space to the interstitium. The filtration coefficient, which is the product of the hydraulic permeability and surface area of the capillary, is a measure of the ease with which water crosses the capillary membrane. The reflection coefficient is an indicator of the degree to which the capillary membrane resists the passage of a substance, such as protein. A reflection coefficient can be defined for each substance; a reflection coefficient of 0 indicates that the molecule crosses the membrane as readily as does water, whereas a value of 1 indicates that the membrane is completely impermeable to the substance. The reflection coefficient for a substance may vary with the anatomic site of the capillary:[7, 8] Capillaries in the liver are quite permeable to albumin, whereas capillaries in muscle are much less permeable, and cerebral capillaries are among the least permeable to albumin.

The movement of fluid and protein across the vascular membrane is assumed to be passive, with plasma water and protein exiting the vascular space through pores in the capillary membrane. However, the rate with which various plasma constituents cross the capillary membrane varies considerably depending on the constituent and the tissue. For example, muscle capillary pores are very permeable to water molecules (reflection coefficient of 0) but very much less permeable to albumin (reflection coefficient of approximately 0.9).[2] Movement of solutes across the endothelium is not fully understood, being complex, but is affected by the concentration of the solutes on either side to the membrane, solute charge and interaction with other solutes, and capillary pore configuration.[9]

Together the filtration and reflection coefficients partially determine the rate of fluid flux across the capillary wall, and the composition of the fluid. For a given hydrostatic and oncotic pressure difference, tissues with higher filtration coefficients (whether due to a larger capillary surface area or more porous capillaries) will have a greater fluid flux. Conversely, under the same circumstance, increases in the reflection coefficient of the capillary wall reduce fluid flux. The differential permeability of the capillary membrane to water and protein has important consequences in the maintenance of the oncotic pressure difference between plasma and interstitial fluid.

Hydrostatic and Colloid Osmotic Pressures

Transcapillary fluid flow is the result of an imbalance between the hydraulic forces favoring movement of water from the capillary into the interstitium and the forces favoring movement of water in the reverse direction. The forces contributing to fluid movement out of the capillary are the intracapillary hydrostatic pressure and the interstitial colloid osmotic pressure, whereas those forces favoring movement of fluid from the interstitium to the capillary are the interstitial hydrostatic pressure (if it is positive) and the plasma colloid osmotic pressure.[10]

The principal force favoring fluid efflux from the capillary is the hydrostatic pressure within the capillary. Capillary hydrostatic pressure varies among different tissues and decreases along the length of the capillary. Hydrostatic pressure within a capillary is determined by the arterial and venous pressures and by the precapillary and postcapillary resistances.[11] Specifically, capillary pressure is determined by the ratio of the postcapillary resistance (R_a) to the precapillary resistance (R_v), and the arterial (P_a) and venous (P_v) pressures:

$$P_c = \{(R_v/R_a)P_a + P_v\}/\{1 + (R_v/R_a)\}$$

Thus, a small increase in venous pressure has a much more marked effect on capillary pressure than does an increase in arterial pressure. For this reason the hydrostatic pressure is greater in capillaries below the heart (e.g., legs) than in those above the heart (e.g., head).

The colloid osmotic pressure of the plasma is the principal force minimizing fluid efflux from the capillary. The colloid osmotic pressure is generated because the plasma and interstitial fluid are separated by a semipermeable membrane—the endothelium—and vary slightly, but significantly, in composition. As noted previously, the interstitial fluid has a lower protein concentration than does plasma but has essentially identical electrolyte concentrations. The difference in protein concentration across the semipermeable endothelium generates an osmotic force that tends to draw water from the interstitium into the plasma.

In addition to the capillary hydrostatic pressure, the colloid osmotic pressure and negative hydrostatic pressure of the interstitial fluid favor fluid movement out of the capillary. Fluid flux across the capillary is the result of the summation of these forces (Table 3–3). It should be recognized that these figures represent the forces at the midpoint of an idealized capillary and that the forces are dynamic, changing between tissues and even along the length of the capillary. In fact, there is a large net flux of fluid from the capillary at its arteriolar end, where capillary hydrostatic forces are

Table 3–3. Mean Forces (mm Hg) Influencing Fluid Movement Into or Out of the Capillary

Hydrostatic Pressures

Mean capillary pressure	17.0
Interstitial pressure	−5.3
Total hydrostatic pressure favoring filtration	22.3

Colloid Oncotic Pressures

Plasma oncotic pressure	28.0
Interstitial oncotic pressure	6.0
Total oncotic pressure opposing filtration	22.0

Total Pressure Favoring Filtration	**0.3**

Data from Guyton AC: Textbook of Medical Physiology, ed 8. Philadelphia, WB Saunders, 1986.

greatest and plasma oncotic forces are least, and a net flux of fluid into the capillary toward its venous end, where capillary hydrostatic forces are least and plasma oncotic pressure is greatest.

The small imbalance in filtration forces results in a net efflux of fluid from the capillary into the interstitial tissue. This fluid does not accumulate in the interstitium—it is removed by the lymphatics.

Lymphatics

The lymphatics drain the interstitium of fluid and substances, notably proteins, that are not absorbed by the capillaries. The lymphatics represent the only means by which interstitial protein is returned to the circulation. Interstitial fluid, and with it protein, moves down a pressure gradient into lymphatic capillaries through clefts between the lymphatic endothelial cells. Lymphatic endothelial cells are supported, and the lymphatic capillaries maintained patent, by anchoring filaments that attach the endothelial cells to surrounding connective tissue. Lymphatic fluid progresses centripetally through progressively larger vessels before draining into the great veins of the chest. Lymphatic valves prevent the retrograde flow of fluid from the lymphatics. Lymph is propelled by factors extrinsic to the lymphatics, including muscle activity, active and passive motion, posture, respiration, and blood vessel pulsation.[12] Exercise causes a significant increase in lymph flow, at least in part because of the increase in tissue pressure that is associated with muscle contraction, although passive motion also increases lymph flow.[12] Standing results in marked diminution or cessation of lymph flow from, and the prompt accumulation of interstitial fluid in, the lower extremities of humans.[12] In addition to the extrinsic factors affecting lymph flow, coordinated contractions of lymphatic vessels contribute substantially to the centripetal flow of lymph.[12]

MECHANISMS OF EDEMA FORMATION

Simply stated, accumulation of excessive fluid in the interstitial spaces—edema—results from an imbalance of the rates

Table 3–4. Pathogenesis of Edema

Increased Capillary Hydrostatic Pressure

Venous obstruction
   Thrombophlebitis
   Compression (mass, tourniquet)
Venous congestion
   Posture (dependent limbs)
   Congestive heart failure
Arteriolar dilation
   Inflammation
Increased body water

Decreased Plasma Oncotic Pressure

Panhypoproteinemia
Hypoalbuminemia

Increased Interstitial Oncotic Pressure

Increased capillary permeability

Decreased Lymph Flow

Lymphatic obstruction

---

of fluid filtration from the capillaries and drainage by the lymphatics. Perturbations of one or more of the forces that affect filtration across the capillary alter the rate at which fluid enters the interstitium. Increases in capillary hydrostatic pressure, decreases in plasma oncotic pressure, and increases in interstitial oncotic pressure all favor increased fluid filtration. Conversely, increased interstitial hydrostatic pressure and decreased interstitial oncotic pressure act to inhibit fluid filtration.

The fundamental mechanisms of accumulation of excessive interstitial fluid are listed in Table 3–4. Increases in capillary hydrostatic pressure, which occur with venous obstruction or arteriolar dilation, such as that associated with inflammation, increase net fluid efflux. The edema that occurs with congestive heart failure likely has an increase in capillary hydrostatic pressure as one of its causes, although the mechanism is complex.[13] Posture also affects capillary hydrostatic pressure; capillaries below the level of the heart have higher hydrostatic pressures than do capillaries above the level of the heart.

A decrease in the oncotic gradient across the capillary endothelium, which occurs with a decreased plasma oncotic pressure or an increased interstitial oncotic pressure, results in an increase in efflux of fluid from the capillary. A decrease in plasma oncotic pressure decreases the oncotic gradient that favors movement of fluid into the capillary. Consequently, the capillary hydrostatic pressure, which favors filtration, predominates and fluid accumulates in the interstitium. Plasma oncotic pressure decreases when plasma protein concentration declines. Albumin is the plasma protein that exerts the preponderance of the oncotic force;[8] therefore, clinically, edema is often associated with hypoalbuminemia. An increase in the permeability of the capillary membrane markedly increases both fluid and protein transport into the interstitium and decreases the ability of the

membrane to maintain a difference in oncotic pressure between the plasma and the interstitium.[5] Capillary permeability increases when the endothelium is damaged, such as by vasculitis or inflammatory reactions.

Lymphatic obstruction prevents the removal of interstitial fluid and protein. Filtration of fluid and passage of small amounts of protein into the interstitial space continues in the presence of lymphatic obstruction. The interstitial fluid is reabsorbed by the capillaries; however, the protein is not. Consequently, the protein content of the interstitial fluid gradually increases, with a resultant increase in interstitial oncotic pressure that favors filtration of fluid. The increased interstitial oncotic pressure causes fluid to accumulate in the interstitium, thus exacerbating the edema.[2]

Alterations in the magnitude of one or more of Starling's forces may be offset by compensatory changes in lymph flow and other of Starling's forces. In concert, Starling's forces and lymph flow act as "edema safety factors" to

---

Table 3–5. Common Causes of Peripheral or Ventral Edema in Horses

Congestive Heart Failure
   Valvular disease
   Myocarditis
   Monensin toxicosis
Vasculitis
   Equine viral arteritis
   Equine ehrlichiosis
   Purpura hemorrhagica
   Equine infectious anemia
Venous Obstruction and Congestion
   Catheter-related thrombophlebitis
   Disseminated intravascular coagulation
   Tight bandages
   Tumors
   Immobility
Cellulitis
   Staphylococcal
   Clostridial
   Counterirritant application
Lymphatic Obstruction
   Ulcerative lymphangitis
   Lymphadenitis (Streptococcus equi,
     Corynebacterium pseudotuberculosis)
   Lymphosarcoma
   Tumors
Hypoalbuminemia
   Parasitism
   Pleural and peritoneal effusions
   Protein loss (gastrointestinal, renal, wounds)
   Inadequate production (starvation)
   Hemodilution (subsequent to hemorrhage)
Shock
   Hemorrhagic
   Endotoxic
Pleuritis
Late-term pregnancy
Prepubic tendon rupture
Starvation
   Inadequate intake
   Malabsorption

prevent the excess accumulation of interstitial fluid and development of frank edema.[6] For example, lymph flow increases with the increased filtration associated with increased capillary hydrostatic pressure. Thus a larger volume of fluid enters and is removed from the interstitial space. The interstitial protein concentration decreases as increased fluid flow washes protein out of the interstitial space. Reduced interstitial space protein concentration increases the oncotic gradient, inhibiting fluid efflux from the capillary, and decreases the rate of movement of fluid from the capillary to the interstitial space.[6]

DIAGNOSTIC APPROACH TO THE PATIENT WITH EDEMA

Edema is not, of itself, a disease; rather, it is a sign of a disease process. Therefore, the diagnostic approach to the patient with edema is based on an understanding of the pathogenesis of edema and a knowledge of the diseases likely to be involved (Table 3–5). The diagnostic approach to an animal with edema should not be any different than for any other sign of disease. A clinical examination, including history and physical examination, will permit the development of a list of potential diagnoses and dictate the appropriate subsequent steps in confirming the diagnosis. The reader is referred to those sections of the text that deal with specific diseases for a description of the appropriate diagnostic aids.

When taking the history of a horse that presents with edema, one should focus on acquiring those facts that have the greatest diagnostic utility in differentiating among those diseases that have edema as a sign. Housing and season and geographical region should be considered. Vaccine and parasiticide administration should be determined. Exposure to other horses and diseases present within the herd should be ascertained. The duration of the edema, its distribution, and the presence of any other clinical signs should be questioned. The remainder of the history should be investigated depending on the responses to initial questions.

The physical examination should begin with a visual evaluation of the horse's attitude and physical condition. The temperature, pulse, and respiration should be recorded. While the physical examination should be complete, particular attention should be paid to those body systems that the preliminary examination indicated may be involved in the disease process. The physical examination will reveal the distribution and severity of edema. Edema that is localized to one extremity or is not bilaterally symmetric is more likely to be caused by local factors (e.g., lymphangitis or venous obstruction) than by systemic disease. Conversely, edema that involves several areas of the body and has a symmetric distribution is likely to be associated with systemic disease (e.g., the ventral edema of congestive heart failure).

Subsequent to the initial clinical examination, the clinician will have developed an ordered list of potential diagnoses. Confirmation, or elimination, of these diagnoses is dependent on subsequent diagnostic procedures, including the response to therapy. Refer to the sections of this text dealing with the specific disease processes for appropriate diagnostic procedures.

REFERENCES

1. Carlson GP: Blood chemistry, body fluids, and hematology. In Gillespie JR, Robinson NE, eds. *Equine Exercise Physiology 2.* Davis, CA, ICEEP Publications, 1987, p 393.
2. Guyton AC: The body fluid compartments: Extracellular and intracellular fluids; interstitial fluid and edema. In Guyton AC: *Textbook of Medical Physiology*, ed 8. Philadelphia, WB Saunders, 1986, p 274.
3. Renkin EM: Some consequences of capillary permeability to macromolecules: Starling's hypothesis revisited. *Am J Physiol* 250:H706–H710, 1986.
4. Comper WD: Interstitium. In Staub NC, Taylor AE, eds. *Edema.* New York, Raven Press, 1984, p 299.
5. Demling RH: Effect of plasma and interstitial protein content on tissue edema formation. *Curr Stud Hematol Blood Trans* 53:36–52, 1986.
6. Taylor AE: Capillary fluid filtration. Starling forces and lymph flow. *Circ Res* 49:557–575, 1981.
7. Taylor AE, Granger DN: Exchange of macromolecules across the microcirculation. In Renkin EM, Hoffman JF, Fanestil DD, et al, eds. *Handbook of Physiology*, Section 2, IV: 467–520, 1984.
8. Raj JU, Anderson J: Regional differences in interstitial fluid albumin concentration in edematous lamb lungs. J Appl Physiol 72:699–705, 1992.
9. Berne RM, Levy MN: The microcirculation and lymphatics. In Berne RM, Levy MN, eds. *Physiology*, ed 2. St. Louis, CV Mosby, 1986, p 500.
10. Michel CC: Microvascular permeability, venous stasis and oedema. *Inter Angiol* 8:9–13, 1984.
11. Green JF: *Fundamental Cardiovascular and Pulmonary Physiology.* Philadelphia, Lea & Febiger, 1987, p 128.
12. Gnepp DR: Lymphatics. In Staub NC, Taylor AE, eds. *Edema.* New York, Raven Press, 1984, p 263.
13. Weaver LJ, Carrico CJ: Congestive heart failure and edema. In Staub NC, Taylor AE, eds. *Edema.* New York, Raven Press, 1984, p 543.

3.4

Changes in Body Weight

Jonathan H. Foreman, DVM, MS, Diplomate ACVIM

An unwelcome or unexpected change in a horse's body weight is a commonly encountered problem in equine practice. Although obesity may be a more common problem, weight loss often represents a more serious situation, with potentially severe consequences. Normal or acceptable body weight is also in the eye of the beholder, because a horse with a given body weight might look overweight as an endurance horse, appropriate as a Thoroughbred racehorse, or too thin as a show hunter.

Whether dealing with a problem of weight loss or weight gain, the veterinarian should always investigate the feeding practices of the horse. It is not uncommon to have the owner report that the horse is receiving 3 lb of grain twice daily when the actual measuring device (usually the everyday coffee can) differs in net grain weight once the volume of the measuring device and grain density are taken into account. It may be necessary to observe firsthand the feeding practices of the stable in order to document that the horse is actually getting the reported amount of grain two or three times daily. Hay should be examined for type, quality (color, texture, leafiness, steminess), mold, weeds, and potentially toxic plants. The horse in question should be observed eating both hay and grain to ensure that it really does consume the amounts reported by the owner or feeder.

Nursing foals should also be observed by the veterinarian when suckling. The mare's udder should be examined before and after nursing to ensure that the mare is actually producing sufficient milk and that the foal is actually nursing the mare completely until her udder is empty. The milk itself should be examined from both halves of the udder to see that it appears grossly normal (no evidence of mastitis). The foal's nostrils should be examined after nursing to determine the presence of milk reflux due to dysphagia, esophageal obstruction, or gastric reflux associated with gastrointestinal ulcers.

DECREASED BODY WEIGHT

Losses in body weight are usually insidious and chronic in nature but may be surprisingly rapid in the face of acute overwhelming systemic infections (Table 3–6). Causes have been variously classified as gastrointestinal, nutritional, infectious, or hypoproteinemic.[1, 2] Differential mechanisms include decreased feed intake, decreased absorption of nutrients, decreased nutrient utilization, and increased loss of energy or protein leading to a catabolic "sink."[1–3]

Decreased feed intake may be caused by management factors, poor dentition, dysphagia, or esophageal obstruction. Management factors leading to weight loss may be multifactorial and include inadequate amounts of feed, inadequate quality of feed, or inability of the horse to eat the proper amounts of the feed given. A horse with severe lameness (e.g., chronic laminitis) may not be able to ambulate to the feed source. A horse low on the pecking order in a pasture hierarchy may be unable to eat because it cannot approach the feed without the other horses bullying it and fending it away. The feed must be palatable and digestible. Appropriate amounts and types of concentrates must be fed considering the horse's work schedule or pregnancy status. Proper investigation of stable feeding practices is described earlier.

Poor dentition may cause the horse to fail to eat some or all of its grain or hay. Parrot-mouthed horses, or aged horses with receding incisor teeth (more than 25 years old), may have difficulty in tearing off grass when grazing. A horse with one or more oral sores from a poorly fitting bit or from sharp cheek teeth may exhibit partial or complete inappetance due to pain associated with chewing. Sharp cheek teeth, wavemouth, or stepmouth may lead to poor digestion and incomplete absorption of nutrients due to inadequate mastication of hay leading to poor fiber utilization during the hindgut (cecum) fermentation process.

Dysphagia has many causes, including abnormal prehension, chewing, or swallowing.[4] Abnormal prehension can be

Table 3–6. Mechanisms and Differential Diagnoses for Decreased Body Weight

Decreased Dietary Intake
    Inadequate diet
    Lameness
    Pecking order
    Poor dentition
    Dysphagia
    Esophageal obstruction

Maldigestion/Malabsorption
    Lactose intolerance
    Gastrointestinal ulceration
    Parasitism
    Diarrhea
    Inflammatory intestinal disease
        Granulomatous enterocolitis
        Eosinophilic enterocolitis
        Lymphocytic/plasmacytic enterocolitis
    Gastrointestinal neoplasia

Inappropriate Hepatic Utilization

Inadequate Circulation/Respiration
    Heart failure
    Chronic obstructive pulmonary disease

Increased Rate of Protein/Energy Loss
    Infection
        Pneumonia
        Pleuritis
        Peritonitis
        Equine infectious anemia
    Protein-losing enteropathy
        Diarrhea
        Gastrointestinal ulceration
        Parasitism
        Inflammatory intestinal disease
        Gastrointestinal neoplasia
    Renal disease (glomerular)
    Increased metabolic energy utilization
        Chronic pain
        Secondary hyperadrenocorticism

due to tongue lacerations; dental, mandibular, or maxillary fractures; damage to nerves supplying the tongue or facial musculature (local trauma, equine protozoal myelitis [EPM], polyneuritis equi); or central neurologic disease (EPM). Basal ganglia lesions due to poisoning by ingestion of yellow star thistle or Russian knapweed prevent normal prehension in the pharynx.[5] Swallowing abnormalities may be due to neurologic (EPM, viral encephalitis, guttural pouch infection), muscular, or physical obstructions such as strangles, abscesses, or guttural pouch distention.[4] Muscular causes include hyperkalemic periodic paralysis in Quarter Horse foals, vitamin E or selenium deficiency in neonates, botulism in neonates and adults, and local trauma subsequent to laryngeal surgery (laryngoplasty).

Esophageal obstruction usually presents acutely because an apparently dysphagic horse regurgitates food from its nostrils while attempting to eat or drink. Chronic choke, or anorexia related to painful swallowing due to partial esophageal obstruction, may lead to weight loss without the owner realizing that the horse is not eating adequately. Esophageal endoscopy is usually diagnostic, but positive contrast radiography may be helpful and is sometimes necessary to establish an accurate diagnosis.

If the horse with weight loss has been observed to fully ingest adequate amounts of good-quality hay and grain, then decreased feed absorption must be considered to be a reason for weight loss. Maldigestion and malabsorption are not easily confirmed diagnoses, but tests based on luminal absorption of simple sugars (xylose or glucose tolerance tests) have been used to document malabsorption syndromes.[3, 6, 7] These tests are described in greater detail in this text in the section on small intestinal diseases (see Chapter 12.3). Malabsorption may be caused by parasitism, diarrhea, and inflammatory or neoplastic intestinal disease.

Gastrointestinal parasitism results in weight loss due to several mechanisms.[2] Parasites may compete directly for nutrients within the lumen of the bowel. Malabsorption may result from a lack of mucosal integrity, a decrease in intestinal villi size and number (and subsequent decrease in mucosal absorptive surface area), and a decrease in digestive enzymes that originate in the mucosa. Competition of parasites for protein sources may result in decreased availability of amino acids for production of digestive enzymes or mucosal transport proteins. Increased mucosal permeability due to leakiness in mucosal intercellular bridges may result in mucosal edema and increased transudation of intercellular fluid and its associated electrolytes, amino acids, and sugars into the lumen of the intestine.

Chronic diarrhea results in partial or complete anorexia, which contributes directly to weight loss. More rapid (decreased) gastrointestinal transit time results in increased losses of incompletely digested dietary feedstuffs. Malabsorption may result from decreased transit time and from villus blunting due to specific pathogens, such as in viral diarrhea (see the malabsorption section in small intestinal diseases). Bacterial pathogens may be in direct competition for luminal nutrients. Mucosal invasion by both viral and bacterial pathogens may cause mild-to-severe degrees of mucosal sloughing (ulcers), which result in maldigestion, malabsorption, and increased mucosal losses of intercellular fluid (e.g., in parasitism).

Given that the horse has adequate feed intake and absorption, inappropriate hepatic utilization of amino acids and sugars must be considered as a differential for weight loss. Chronic liver disease may result in weight loss due to inappetance, maldigestion (due to inadequate bile acid production), and inadequate or improper processing of amino acids into normal plasma proteins in the liver. These abnormalities may result in lowered concentrations of serum albumin, liver-dependent clotting factors (factors II, VII, IX, and X), and total plasma or serum protein. Lowered circulating proteins (especially albumin) may result in decreased plasma colloid osmotic pressure and thus may manifest as peripheral dependent edema in the distal limbs, pectoral region, and ventral midline. This peripheral edema may mask further weight loss by making the horse's torso appear to be heavier than it actually is. Decreases in clotting factors may result in bleeding diatheses. Hyperlipemia, hyperlipidemia, fatty liver syndrome, and ketosis may be seen in poorly fed ponies and in miniature horses with acute anorexia or overwhelming energy demands, such as pregnancy or lactation.[8]

Increased loss of protein or energy is a common cause of decreased body weight in horses. Luminal losses of fluid, electrolytes, and nutrients were described earlier for intestinal parasitism and diarrhea. Acute inflammatory protein losses may occur into major body cavities in overwhelming infections such as pleuritis or peritonitis. Chronic abscessing pneumonia, pleuritis, and peritonitis often result in increased, rather than acutely decreased, serum total protein due to increased γ-globulin production in response to chronic antigenic stimulation from the chronic infection. These chronic infections also usually have weight loss as an additional clinical sign due to the continuing catabolic processes associated with the infection itself. Equine infectious anemia (EIA) is a type of persistent systemic infection which, in its symptomatic form, may result in chronic weight loss and varying levels of anemia.[9] Asymptomatic EIA carriers may have no weight loss or other obvious clinical signs but can infect pasture mates via vector transmission.

Protein-losing enteropathy (PLE) is not a definitive diagnosis but is rather a group of diseases, each of which results in luminal losses of fluid, electrolytes, plasma proteins, and nutrients. Mechanisms of protein and fluid loss were described earlier for intestinal parasitism and diarrhea. Gastrointestinal ulcers have been reported to result in lowered serum total protein and weight loss.[10] One of the early indications of nonsteroidal anti-inflammatory drug toxicity is the detection of a lowered serum total protein. Such horses may also manifest varying degrees of inappetance and colic, especially associated with the immediate postprandial period. Intestinal neoplasia (usually lymphosarcoma) often manifests as a PLE with weight loss.[11]

Acute or chronic renal diseases, especially involving glomerulonephritis, can result in urinary protein loss and subsequent body weight loss.[12] Such horses may have polyuria and polydipsia as associated clinical signs. Polyuria is often reported by owners or handlers as increased wetness in stall bedding. Owners should be questioned thoroughly regarding the horse's water intake. The veterinarian may need to observe stable watering habits, often including actually measuring the volume of the subject's water buckets in order to definitively establish the presence of polydipsia. It may be necessary to turn off automatic waterers in the subject's stall or pasture and to offer the horse measured volumes of water from additional buckets in order to establish a diagnosis of polydipsia. Urine puddles in stalls, or collected urine samples, may foam excessively due to increased protein concentrations. Increased urinary protein concentrations can be quickly diagnosed on the farm with the proper interpretation of urine dipstick protein indicators.

Neoplasia or abscesses within the thorax or abdomen serve as catabolic energy and protein "sinks," resulting in chronic weight loss.[11, 13] Chronic pain, such as that associated with severe, unresponsive laminitis, results in increased catabolism and weight loss, probably as a result of chronically elevated systemic catecholamine levels. Increased circulating epinephrine and norepinephrine levels result in a whole-body catabolic state with increased breakdown of stored energy sources and ultimately result in chronic weight loss. Similar weight loss due to systemic catabolism can be the result of chronically elevated serum cortisol associated with pituitary adenoma and secondary hyperadrenocorticism.

Heart murmurs and resultant heart failure can cause

weight loss due to inefficiency of circulation of nutrients and oxygen to peripheral tissues. Chronic obstructive pulmonary disease (COPD) or heaves may result in weight loss due to an increase in the work of breathing and due to poor oxygenation of peripheral tissues. While ventral abdominal musculature may hypertrophy and result in a "heave line," weight loss will be manifested by increased depth between the ribs and decreased muscular thickness and definition along the dorsal midline. Suckling foals with severe pneumonia may manifest weight loss if they become inappetant due to decreased suckling related to their severe dyspnea.

Approach to the Horse with Decreased Body Weight

An appropriately taken history should document the type, amount, and quality of feed and hay being provided daily. Documentation of deworming products used and intervals of administration is critical. The history may also document the presence of anorexia, depression, polyuria, polydipsia, diarrhea, or other important historical signs that may point more quickly toward a specific cause of the weight loss.

The physical examination should reveal the presence of weight loss, a cardiac murmur, pneumonia or pleuropneumonia (increased lung sounds), COPD (increased abnormal expiratory lung sounds), dental abnormalities, peripheral edema, urine staining on the hindlimbs, diarrhea, icterus, nasal discharge (dysphagia, pneumonia), fever, or hirsutism (secondary hyperadrenocorticism). The rectal examination may document the presence of intra-abdominal masses (abscess, neoplasia), enlarged left kidney, thickened intestinal or rectal wall, colonic displacement, gritty peritoneal surfaces (peritonitis), gritty feces (sand impaction), or diarrhea.

Fecal flotation may serve as an adequate screening tool to determine whether there is any evidence of parasitism. In the event of a positive fecal flotation, Baermann's sedimentation may be necessary to quantitatively determine the severity of the patent parasitic load in the horse with weight loss. Fecal occult blood may be positive with gastrointestinal ulceration or neoplasia, but parasites or a recent rectal examination may also result in positive results.

Routine hematology (complete blood count, fibrinogen) should assist in diagnosing infectious conditions such as pleuritis or peritonitis. Decreased serum or plasma total protein and albumin concentrations are evidence of hypoproteinemia and make the following conditions more likely: severe malnutrition, PLE (diarrhea, parasitism, ulceration, intestinal neoplasia, inflammatory intestinal disease), glomerular disease, acute pleuritis or peritonitis, or chronic liver disease. Increased total protein concentrations, especially γ-globulins, make chronic closed cavity infections such as abscesses, peritonitis, or pleuritis more likely. Increased β-globulin fractions suggest the presence of parasitism.

Routine serum biochemistries should aid in diagnosing renal (renal azotemia, electrolyte abnormalities) and liver disease (increased gamma-glutamyltransferase, aspartate aminotransferase, serum alkaline phosphatase, lactate dehydrogenase). Urinalysis should reveal increased protein levels on dipstick or quantitative analysis in the event of glomerular protein losses. Metabolic alkalosis may be evident in the aftermath of salivary bicarbonate losses due to dysphagia or esophageal obstruction.

Endoscopy may aid in the diagnosis of causes of dysphagia or esophageal obstruction. Lengthy endoscopes are necessary for examination of large adult horses for suspected gastrointestinal ulcers, but shorter endoscopes may suffice for foals or shorter-necked adults (e.g., Arabians, ponies).

Peritoneal fluid analysis will document the presence of a transudate (equivocal infection) or exudate (probable infection).[14, 15] Both aerobic and anaerobic peritoneal fluid cultures should be performed if intra-abdominal infection is suspected. Exfoliative cytology may rarely document the presence of neoplastic cells due to intra-abdominal neoplasia.[11, 16]

Non-routine tests should be performed only as indicated and include oral absorption tests (see the section on small intestinal diseases) (Chapter 12.5) and biopsies of the liver, kidney, or intestinal wall. Abdominal or thoracic ultrasonography should help to rule in or out abnormalities of the liver or kidneys and may document the presence of abnormal fluid (peritonitis, pleuritis) or masses (abscesses, neoplasia). Cardiac ultrasound should be definitive in the event of a murmur and suspected heart failure. Radiography may also be helpful to document the presence of thoracic masses or COPD, but increased pleural fluid will obscure visualization of other intrathoracic structures.

INCREASED BODY WEIGHT

Overfeeding may be the most common cause of obesity in horses and may also be the easiest to correct. The stable's feeding practices and feed and hay sources should be investigated thoroughly. It is not uncommon for novice horse owners, single horse owners, and pony owners to overfeed their animals.

Ponies seem to be particularly susceptible to obesity, perhaps because their size renders them to be more easily overfed. However, at least one author has proposed that this tendency toward obesity in ponies receiving modern confinement diets may be due to their having evolved in the inhospitable ice age climates of northern Europe.[17] In that era, the lack of readily available grazing feedstuffs might have placed greater selection pressure on survival of ponies with more efficient dentition and better nutrient and fluid absorption from the gastrointestinal tract. It is argued that those ponies that had greater feed conversion efficiency would have been stronger, had longer lives, and been more available for breeding. Current illustrations of this theory may lie in the Welsh and Connemara pony breeds that still thrive and flourish in the wild in the relatively inhospitable north Atlantic climates of the western coasts of Wales and Ireland, respectively.

Pregnancy in mares is a normal physiologic event that leads to increased body weight. Surprisingly, many new owners of mares may not know that their new purchase is pregnant. It is not uncommon for an earlier negative pregnancy diagnosis to have been in error. Any mare that is gaining weight in an unexpected manner should be examined rectally, and ultrasonographically if necessary, for a possible pregnancy.

Hypothyroidism has been reported to be associated with weight gain and failure to become pregnant in broodmares.[18] Evidence for both hypothyroid-associated weight gain and infertility was lacking in surgically created hypothyroid pony[19] and quarter horse[20] subjects. There is, however, an abundance of field experience to infer a relationship between obesity, hypothyroidism, and infertility in mares.[17] Documentation of hypothyroidism must be by performance of a thyroid-stimulating hormone or thyroid-releasing hormone stimulation test,[21, 22] since resting thyroid levels vary diurnally[23] and are not truly reflective of thyroid function. It must also be remembered that only 5 days of normal phenylbutazone (PBZ) therapy results in abnormally low resting serum thyroid levels due to direct competition of PBZ with thyroid hormone for serum protein-binding sites.[21] The diagnosis and treatment of hypothyroidism is described in greater detail elsewhere in this text.

Approach to the Horse with Increased Body Weight

Differential diagnoses for increased body weight include overfeeding, pregnancy, hypothyroidism, and other conditions that result in abdominal distention, such as bloat, ascites, uroperitoneum, fetal hydrops, and rupture of the prepubic tendon or abdominal wall musculature. The latter conditions are described in greater detail in the following section titled Abdominal Distention.

Feeding practices should be investigated and observed firsthand if necessary. A positive pregnancy status should be an easy historical and rectal diagnosis. Most hematologic and biochemical tests will be normal in the pregnant or simply overweight horse. Thyroid status should be assessed appropriately, not by simple resting thyroid hormone concentrations, but by thyroid-stimulating hormone or thyroid-releasing hormone stimulation tests that have been described previously and that are presented elsewhere in this text.[21, 22]

Education of the client is important with regard to feeding practices, especially if it is determined that the overweight horse has simply been overfed by a novice owner. Dangerous consequences, including colic and laminitis, should be explained to the client.

REFERENCES

1. Ettinger SJ: Body weight. In Ettinger SJ, ed. *Textbook of Veterinary Internal Medicine*, ed 2. Philadelphia, WB Saunders, 1983, p 100.
2. Maas J: Alterations in body weight or size. In Smith BP, ed. *Large Animal Internal Medicine*. St. Louis, CV Mosby, 1990, p 171.
3. Brown CM: Chronic weight loss. In Brown CM, ed. *Problems in Equine Medicine*. Philadelphia, Lea & Febiger, 1989, p 6.
4. Brown CM: Dysphagia. In Robinson NE, ed. *Current Therapy in Equine Medicine 3*. Philadelphia, WB Saunders, 1992, p 171.
5. Oehme FW: Plant toxicities. In Robinson NE, ed. *Current Therapy in Equine Medicine 2*. Philadelphia, WB Saunders, 1987, p 672.
6. Roberts MC: Malabsorption syndromes in the horse. *Compend Contin Educ Pract Vet* 7:S637, 1985.
7. Jacobs KA, Bolton JR: Effect of diet on the oral D-xylose absorption test in the horse. *Am J Vet Res* 43:1856, 1982.
8. Moore BR, Abood AS, Hinchcliff KW: Hyperlipemia in 9 miniature horses and miniature donkeys. *J Vet Intern Med* 8:376, 1994.
9. Clabough DL: Equine infectious anemia: The clinical signs, transmission, and diagnostic procedures. *Vet Med* 85:1007, 1990.
10. Snow DH, Douglas TA, Thompson H, et al: Phenylbutazone toxicosis in Equidae: A biochemical and pathophysiologic study. *Am J Vet Res* 42:1754, 1981.
11. Traub JL, Bayly WM, Reed SM, et al: Intra-abdominal neoplasia as a cause of chronic weight loss in the horse. *Compend Contin Educ Pract Vet* 5:S526, 1983.
12. Divers TJ: Equine renal system. In Smith BP, ed. *Large Animal Internal Medicine*. St. Louis, CV Mosby, 1990, p 872.
13. Rumbaugh GE, Smith BP, Carlson GP: Internal abdominal abscesses in the horse: A study of 25 cases. *J Am Vet Med Assoc* 172:304, 1978.
14. Nelson AW: Analysis of equine peritoneal fluid. *Vet Clin North Am Large Anim Pract* 1:267, 1979.
15. Duncan JR, Prasse KW: Cytology. In Duncan JR, Prasse KW, eds. *Veterinary Laboratory Medicine*, ed 2. Ames, IA, Iowa State University Press, 1986, p 201.
16. Foreman JH, Weidner JP, Parry BA, et al: Pleural effusion secondary to thoracic metastatic mammary adenocarcinoma in a mare. *J Am Vet Med Assoc* 197:1193, 1990.
17. Schafer M: *An Eye for a Horse*. London, JA Allen, 1980, p 26.
18. Nachreiner RF, Hyland JH: Reproductive endocrine function testing in mares. In McKinnon AO, Voss JL, eds. *Equine Reproduction*. Philadelphia, Lea & Febiger, 1993, p 303.
19. Lowe JE, Kallfelz FA: Thyroidectomy and the T4 test to assess thyroid dysfunction in the horse and pony. *Proc Am Assoc Equine Pract* 16:135, 1970.
20. Vischer CM: Hypothyroidism and exercise intolerance in the horse. M. S. Thesis, University of Illinois, in preparation, 1996.
21. Morris DD, Garcia M: Thyroid-stimulating hormone response test in healthy horses, and effect of phenylbutazone on equine thyroid hormones. *Am J Vet Res* 44:503, 1983.
22. Foreman JH: Hematological and endocrine assessment of the performance horse. In Robinson NE, ed. *Current Therapy in Equine Medicine 3*. Philadelphia, WB Saunders, 1992, p 807.
23. Duckett WM, Manning JP, Weston PG: Thyroid hormone periodicity in healthy adult geldings. *Equine Vet J* 21:125, 1989.

3.5

Abdominal Distention

Jonathan H. Foreman, DVM, MS, Diplomate ACVIM

Increases in body weight due to overeating or pregnancy must be distinguished from increases in body girth due to bloat, ascites, uroperitoneum, fetal hydrops, or ruptured prepubic tendon. In each of these conditions, body weight may actually be increased due to fetal growth or fluid accumulation. More important, however, there is a perceptible change to the shape of the abdomen of the horse.

Bloat is usually associated with colic signs in horses and is due to gaseous intestinal distention secondary to ileus or simple obstruction of the large, or rarely small, intestine.

Ileus secondary to diarrhea, peritonitis, colic surgery, or parasympatholytic agents (e.g., atropine) can result in sufficient accumulation of intraluminal gas to be manifested as tympany, bloat, and mild-to-severe abdominal pain.[1] If optic topical atropine application is overly aggressive, secondary ileus and bloat may result. Rapid and severe gas production may follow grain overload; cecal and colonic fermentation of readily available carbohydrate sources results in rapid-onset colonic tympany and abdominal distention.[2] Exhaustion in endurance horses has also been associated with intestinal shutdown and subsequent abdominal distention.[3] In any of these bloat conditions, abdominal auscultation in the flank area reveals decreased or absent intestinal motility sounds (borborygmi) and perhaps increased gascous distention sounds ("pinging"). Decreased borborygmi in the right flank are specific for cecal ileus.

Simple colonic obstruction also results in tympany and bloat. Strangulating obstruction results in greater pain than is usually manifested in simple obstruction and bloat. Colonic displacements are more common in older postpartum mares.[4] They often present initially with mild colic signs and progressively develop more dramatic pain and abdominal distention. Miniature horses with simple obstructions due to fecoliths often have bloat as the initial clinical sign.[5] Such cases have the additional complication that rectal examination may be impossible for differentiation of the source of the bloat. Even in full-sized horses, rectal examination may reveal that the abdomen is so filled with distended colon that the examiner can push his or her arm into the rectum no farther than wrist-deep. Colonic or cecal bloat can be relieved by trocharization through the flank, but relief is merely palliative and is usually temporary because the cause of the obstruction has still not been resolved.

Ascites does not commonly occur in horses. It is usually secondary to peritonitis or abdominal neoplasia. Peritonitis is caused by septicemia, laparotomy, intestinal leakage, internal abscess, or a penetrating external wound resulting in inflammation and usually infection of the peritoneal lining of the abdomen. Such inflammation results in increased fluid production by the squamous abdominal epithelium. Initially, this increased abdominal fluid may be characterized as a transudate (low cell count, low total protein). If inflammation with infection persists, the character of the fluid may change to that of an exudate (increased cell count >5,000 nucleated cells/μL, increased neutrophil count, increased degenerate neutrophils, microscopically visible bacteria, and increased total protein).[6, 7] These increases in abdominal fluid volume can be substantive and can result in abdominal distention that eventually becomes clinically apparent. Fluid ballottement in the cquine abdomen is not an easily performed diagnostic technique but may be easier in foals, ponies, or miniature horses than in full-sized horses.

Ascites may also result from abdominal neoplasia. Tumors reported to cause ascites and weight loss in horses include lymphosarcoma, squamous cell carcinoma, mammary adenocarcinoma, and mesothelioma.[8, 9] Although rare, mesothelioma may cause the most fluid production, because it is a tumor of the fluid-producing cells of the peritoneal lining. Mesothelioma may result in the production of large volumes of fluid (several liters) in a short time (24 hours) after a similarly large volume was drained from the same horse via abdominal catheterization or trocharization.

Ascites may also result from any condition that produces lowered serum total protein and albumin. With lowered intravascular colloid osmotic pressure, fluid diffuses or moves from the vasculature and results in dependent peripheral edema. Fluid may also accumulate within the major body cavities (i.e., the thorax and the abdomen).[7] The mechanisms for such low-protein conditions include poor protein intake, malabsorption, poor hepatic utilization, and increased rate of protein loss such as in glomerular renal disease, peritonitis/pleuritis, or gastrointestinal transudation (diarrhea or ulceration). Causes of peripheral edema are described elsewhere in this text.

Increased preload due to right-sided heart failure can also result in a transudate fluid accumulation within the abdomen.[7] A horse in right-sided heart failure usually has tricuspid insufficiency and manifests other signs of right-sided heart failure, such as a murmur, exercise intolerance, jugular pulse, and edema of the ventral abdomen, pectoral muscles, and distal limbs. Severe mitral insufficiency can also result in right-sided heart failure, but only after the development of left-sided failure and its associated pulmonary edema, which is manifested by exercise intolerance, coughing, epistaxis, and increased respiratory effort.

Uroperitoneum results from leakage of urine from some part of the urinary tract into the abdomen. It is most commonly associated with a ruptured bladder in neonatal foals (usually male).[10–12] It may also result from a necrotic bladder secondary to neonatal sepsis and urachal abscesses. Such foals often present with pendulous, bloated abdomens that ballotte more easily than do the abdomens of adult horses with accumulation of fluid. Abdominal fluid may actually smell like urine, and peritoneal fluid creatinine concentrations will be high—often more than twice those of peripheral blood.[10–12] Since most classically described neonatal urinary bladder tears are dorsal near the trigone, the foal may still be able to produce a stream of urine despite having a leaking bladder. A ruptured urinary bladder abscess should be suspected in a septic foal that initially responded to therapy for sepsis and then, several days later, had acute onset depression, anorexia, ileus, and abdominal distention. Adults rarely have uroperitoneum; however, uroperitoneum has been associated with ruptured urinary bladders during stressful parturition in mares that manifest mild postpartum abdominal pain and abdominal distention.[12, 13]

Fetal hydrops results from an accumulation of excessive amounts of fluid within the amnion (hydrops amnion) or chorioallantois (hydrops allantois).[14] Hydrops results in a bilaterally pendulous abdomen in a late-term pregnant mare. A rapid accumulation of fluid over 10 to 14 days may make it difficult for the mare to walk or perhaps even breathe. A diagnosis may be made after taking history and performing a rectal examination, although it is usually difficult to palpate the fetus because the excess fluid causes the uterus to descend out of reach of the examiner. If necessary, a percutaneous ultrasonographic examination may be used to confirm the diagnosis by documenting the presence of increased intrauterine fluid within the fetal membranes.

A ruptured prepubic tendon results in a unilateral lowering of the abdominal margin and apparent distention of the abdomen only on the affected side. It is routinely associated with later term pregnancy in mares and is thought to occur simply due to the increased weight of the pregnant uterus pressing downward on the abdominal wall. Rupture of the rectus, transverse, or oblique abdominal muscles can also result in ventral dropping or herniation of the abdomen late in gestation.[14] Ruptures may be more common in older or more sedentary mares, probably due to decreased abdominal wall strength and tone. Other than a focal abdominal wall hernia, a unilateral prepubic tendon rupture results in the only form of prominent unilateral abdominal distention in horses. Mares with ruptured prepubic tendons may have elicitable pain in the local abdominal wall and may demonstrate a reluctance to walk. They may need assistance during parturition, because they may have difficulty performing an effective abdominal press to aid in fetal expulsion.

APPROACH TO THE HORSE WITH ABDOMINAL DISTENTION

Pregnancy, diarrhea, colic signs, colic surgery, and the use of parasympatholytic agents should be evident from the history. The rate of onset of abdominal distention may help to distinguish more acute conditions (e.g., gastrointestinal bloat from grain overload) from more chronic conditions (e.g., ascites due to heart or liver failure). Signalment and history may assist in indicating specific conditions. A depressed, 48- to 72-hour-old male foal with fluid abdominal distention may be a likely candidate to have a ruptured urinary bladder and uroperitoneum. Miniature horses with bloat and colic signs frequently have simple obstructions owing to fecoliths or enteroliths.

A complete physical examination will reveal the presence of a murmur that may be associated with heart failure and ascites. Other signs of heart failure may also be evident on physical examination. An actual defect in the integrity of the abdominal wall may be palpable upon external examination of the abdomen in a mare with a ruptured prepubic tendon or ruptured abdominal wall musculature.[14] Ballottement should be attempted to discern the presence of increased free abdominal fluid in suspected ascites or uroperitoneum. Fever may indicate the presence of an infectious peritonitis or umbilical abscess.

A rectal examination is a critical part of the examination of a horse with bloat or colic but may be difficult to accomplish if colonic distention is dramatic or if the patient is small (i.e., foal, pony, or miniature horse). A rectal examination may further document advanced pregnancy, resulting in mild bilateral abdominal distention (normal pregnancy), abnormal or severe bilateral distention (hydrops or bilateral ruptured prepubic tendon), or unilateral distention (unilateral ruptured prepubic tendon or focal abdominal wall hernia). A rectal examination may also reveal abnormalities of the urinary tract (enlarged kidney or ureter, abscess, or neoplasia), which may result in uroperitoneum in adults.

An ultrasonographic examination may be helpful and is sometimes necessary to examine the distended abdomen and fetus in a pregnant mare. Such an examination must be performed percutaneously in late gestation. Ultrasonography can determine the location of increased abdominal fluid (intrauterine or extrauterine) and the health status of the fetus. Percutaneous placement of base-apex electrocardiographic leads across the mare's abdomen may help to document that the fetus is still viable if an ultrasound examination does not produce definitive evidence (heart movement, gross fetal movement).[15]

Cardiac ultrasonography may help to document the presence of a cardiac valvular defect that can be the cause of ascites in a horse with heart failure. Abdominal radiography may assist in the diagnosis of abdominal distention due to intestinal obstruction in a foal or miniature horse. Percutaneous ultrasound examination may also assist in documenting the source of abdominal distention (e.g., intussusception) in smaller horses or foals[16, 17] and in characterizing umbilical and urachal abnormalities.[17]

Complete blood counts and plasma fibrinogen concentrations will assist in the diagnosis of inflammatory conditions such as infectious peritonitis. Urachal or urinary bladder abscesses may also be associated with inflammatory leukograms. Blood or peritoneal fluid cultures may assist in documenting the offending bacterial agent(s). Foals or adults with uroperitoneum will have elevated serum urea nitrogen, creatinine, and potassium and decreased serum sodium, chloride, and bicarbonate concentrations.[10, 11]

Abdominocentesis should be attempted to distinguish the cause of ascites. Care must be taken, however, to obtain peritoneal fluid from late-term pregnant mares in order to avoid penetrating directly into the distended uterus. Analysis of peritoneal fluid will reveal abdominal fluid to be a transudate (equivocal infection) or exudate (probable infection).[6, 7] Fluid should be cultured both aerobically and anaerobically when infectious peritonitis is suspected. Exfoliative cytology may rarely document the presence of neoplastic cells.[8, 9] Peritoneal fluid creatinine concentration will approach or often exceed (more than twice) that of serum if uroperitoneum is present.[10, 11] Serum and peritoneal urea nitrogen concentrations are less reliable for such a diagnosis because the peritoneal membrane does not differentially sequester urea nitrogen (but does creatinine) within the abdominal cavity.

REFERENCES

1. Ducharme NG, Fubini SL: Gastrointestinal complications associated with the use of atropine in horses. *J Am Vet Med Assoc* 182:229, 1983.
2. Huskamp B: Diseases of the stomach and intestine. In Dietz O, Wiesner F, eds. *Diseases of the Horse.* New York, Karger, 1984, p 186.
3. Swanson TD: The veterinarian's responsibilities at trail rides. In Robinson NE, ed. *Current Therapy in Equine Medicine 3.* Philadelphia, WB Saunders, 1992, p 80.
4. Sullins KE: Diseases of the large colon. In White NA, ed. *The Equine Acute Abdomen.* Philadelphia, Lea & Febiger, 1990, p 375.
5. Ragle CA, Snyder JR, Meagher DM, et al: Surgical treatment of colic in American miniature horses: 15 cases (1980–1987). *J Am Vet Med Assoc* 201:329, 1992.
6. Nelson AW: Analysis of equine peritoneal fluid. *Vet Clin North Am Large Anim Pract* 1:267, 1979.
7. Duncan JR, Prasse KW: Cytology. In Duncan JR, Prasse KW, eds. *Veterinary Laboratory Medicine,* ed 2. Ames, IA, Iowa State University Press, 1986, p 201.
8. Traub JL, Bayly WM, Reed SM, et al: Intra-abdominal neoplasia as a cause of chronic weight loss in the horse. *Compend Contin Educ Pract Vet* 5:S526, 1983.

9. Foreman JH, Weidner JP, Parry BA, et al: Pleural effusion secondary to thoracic metastatic mammary adenocarcinoma in a mare. *J Am Vet Med Assoc* 197:1193, 1990.
10. Behr MJ, Hackett RP, Bentinck-Smith J, et al: Metabolic abnormalities associated with rupture of the urinary bladder in neonatal foals. *J Am Vet Med Assoc* 178:263, 1981.
11. Richardson DW, Kohn CW: Uroperitoneum in the foal. *J Am Vet Med Assoc* 182:267, 1983.
12. Divers TJ: Equine renal system. In Smith BP, ed. *Large Animal Internal Medicine.* St Louis, CV Mosby, 1990, p 872.
13. Nyrop KA, DeBowes RM, Cox JH, et al: Rupture of the urinary bladder in two post-partum mares. *Compend Contin Educ Pract Vet* 6:S510, 1984.
14. Lofstedt RM: Miscellaneous diseases of pregnancy and parturition. In McKinnon AO, Voss JL, eds. *Equine Reproduction.* Philadelphia, Lea & Febiger, 1993, p 596.
15. Colles CM, Parkes RD, May CJ: Foetal electrocardiography in the mare. *Equine Vet J* 10:32, 1978.
16. Bernard WV, Reef VB, Reimer JM, et al: Ultrasonographic diagnosis of small intestinal intussusception in three foals. *J Am Vet Med Assoc* 194:395, 1989.
17. Reef VB: Ultrasonographic evaluation and diagnosis of foal diseases. In Robinson NE, ed. *Current Therapy in Equine Medicine 3.* Philadelphia, WB Saunders, 1992, p 417.

3.6

Dysphagia

Laurie A. Beard, DVM, MS

NORMAL EATING

Normal eating is complex and requires normal anatomic structures and neurologic function. The process of eating can be divided into prehension (uptake of food into the oral cavity) and deglutition (transport of food from the oral cavity to the stomach). Prehension requires the lips to grasp and the incisors to tear the food.[1] Motor innervation to the tongue, lips, and muscles of mastication is provided by the hypoglossal, facial, and trigeminal nerves. Sensory input is important for successful prehension and requires intact olfactory, optic, and trigeminal nerves, providing smell, sight, and sensation of the rostral oral mucosa and lips. Normal prehension depends on the central nervous system to coordinate movements of the tongue and lips.

Deglutition involves mastication, swallowing, and transport of food through the esophagus to the stomach. Mastication or chewing of food initiates mechanical digestion and insalivation. Mastication is specifically a function of the molars to grind feed and the tongue and buccal muscles to position the food. The facial nerve provides motor and sensory fibers to the tongue and pharynx. The glossopharyngeal nerve provides sensory fibers to the caudal third of the tongue. The trigeminal nerve is sensory to the teeth and provides the important parasympathetic fibers to the parotid salivary gland. Function of this gland is critical to help liquefy food and provides a small amount of digestive enzymes.

Swallowing is complex and is performed in a series of steps. Initially, food must be moved to the base of the tongue and formed into a bolus. This action requires coordinated movements of the tongue and pharynx. Second, the bolus is forced caudally. As this action takes place, the oropharynx relaxes and the soft palate elevates to seal the palatopharyngeal arch and nasopharynx.[1] Next, the bolus enters the oropharynx and the hyoid apparatus swings rostrodorsally, which draws the larynx and the common pharynx forward.[1, 2] The epiglottis is tipped caudally and prevents the bolus from entering the larynx.[1] Finally, the bolus is moved into the common pharynx with pharyngeal muscle contractions and enters the open cranial esophageal sphincter. The sphincter closes to prevent esophagopharyngeal reflux and aerophagia.[1] Herbivores are unique, because breathing continues uninterrupted during swallowing, unlike other animals.[1] The glossopharyngeal, vagus, and spinal accessory nerves provide both sensory and motor fibers to the pharynx, larynx, and soft palate.

The esophageal phase of eating involves the transport of the food bolus to the stomach, with primary peristaltic waves. The primary peristaltic waves are generated by continuous contraction of the pharyngeal peristalsis.[1] The bolus is transported to the caudal esophageal sphincter, which relaxes to allow the bolus to enter the stomach and then contracts to prevent gastroesophageal reflux. If reflux does occur, esophageal clearance is achieved by secondary peristaltic waves. Antiperistalsis is normal in ruminants during eructation and regurgitation but is not normal in horses.[1]

DYSPHAGIA

Dysphagia is defined as difficulty in swallowing but is often used to describe problems with eating.[2] Problems with eating may include problems with prehension, mastication, swallowing, and esophageal transport. In this section, the term dysphagia will be used in the broader sense to describe "problems with eating." Dysphagia can result from a number of disorders affecting any part of the upper gastrointestinal system (oral cavity, pharynx, and esophagus). Clinical signs of dysphagia vary depending on the cause and the location of the problem but may include ptyalism (excessive salivation), gagging, dropping food, nasal discharge, and coughing. Dysphagia can result from either morphologic or functional disorders. The causes of these diseases may be acquired or congenital. Morphologic causes of dysphagia include abnormal anatomy, obstruction of the upper gastrointestinal tract, inflammation, and pain. Examples of anatomic abnormalities include a cleft palate and subepiglottic cysts.[3, 4] Obstruction of the upper gastrointestinal tract most commonly includes feed impactions of the esophagus but can also include pharyngeal obstructions secondary to retropharyngeal lymph node masses or severe guttural pouch tympany.[5-10] Inflammatory conditions resulting in pain and dysphagia include periodontal diseases, foreign bodies, pharyngitis, epiglottitis, and mandibular or maxillary fractures.[3, 6]

Functional disorders resulting in dysphagia include neurologic, neuromuscular, and muscular diseases. Functional disorders frequently result in problems with swallowing, but less commonly involve mastication and prehension, and rarely occur with esophageal transport. Neurologic diseases resulting in dysphagia may be peripheral or central. Peripheral neurologic problems frequently result from abnormalities of the guttural pouch but can also include toxic peripheral neuropathies, such as lead toxicity. Problems of the guttural pouch include infection (tympany, empyema or mycosis), iatrogenic problems (infusion of caustic substances), and trauma (rupture of the longus capitis muscle from the basisphenoid bone and hemorrhage into the guttural pouch).[2, 11, 12] Central neurologic diseases may result in problems in prehension, mastication, or swallowing. Specific examples include equine protozoal myelitis (EPM), viral encephalitis (rabies, eastern and western encephalitis), toxic neuropathies (leukoencephalomalacia and nigropallidal encephalomalacia), and cerebral trauma.[1, 2, 7, 13–15] Neuromuscular problems resulting in dysphagia generally present as a systemic disease and include diseases such as botulism and organophosphate toxicity.[1, 2, 16, 17] Muscular diseases resulting in dysphagia are rare but include nutritional muscular dystrophy (white muscle disease) in foals.[18]

Basic Approach to Dysphagia

The initial evaluation of dysphagia is focused on determination of whether morphologic or functional abnormalities exist. In order to best answer these questions, a thorough history, physical examination (including observation of the horse eating), and additional tests (e.g., endoscopic examination and radiographs) are required. A history of an acute onset of dysphagia is often consistent with trauma, whereas a slow progressive onset of clinical signs is more consistent with a neurologic problem such as guttural pouch mycosis, EPM, or toxicities. Exposure to toxic substances or plants (lead or yellow star thistle) should be assessed. A history of treatment prior to the onset of dysphagia suggests trauma or injury to the pharynx. Use of a balling gun or flushing of guttural pouches may result in iatrogenic injury to the pharynx, esophagus, and guttural pouches. Concurrent problems in other horses (e.g., strangles or other bacterial infections of the submandibular lymph nodes) should be determined.

A physical examination should be performed, and careful attention should be paid to the head and neck. Because rabies is a potential cause of dysphagia, protective measures should be taken while performing a careful and thorough physical examination. Ideally, all clinicians working on horses should have an adequate rabies antibody titer. An examination of the oral cavity is best accomplished with a mouth speculum, good light, and, if necessary, the administration of sedation. The teeth should be examined carefully for retained deciduous caps, sharp points or hooks, wave mouth or stepmouth, dental fractures, or patent infundibula.[3] Foreign bodies may become wedged between the molars or under the tongue. The tongue should be examined for lacerations, foreign bodies, and evidence of neoplasia. The throat latch area and neck should be examined for heat or swelling, which might occur secondary to a ruptured esophagus. The lungs should be carefully auscultated to determine if the horse shows evidence of aspiration pneumonia secondary to dysphagia.

A valuable activity is to watch the horse eat. An important distinction between dysphagia and anorexia should be made. Dysphagic horses are usually hungry and will attempt to eat. Problems with prehension generally suggest a primary neurologic problem. It may be necessary to watch the horse try to graze and eat hay or grain. Ingestion of yellow star thistle or Russian knapweed results in basal ganglia lesions (nigropallidal encephalomalacia).[14] These horses are unable to prehend food (with lack of coordination of the lips and tongue), but they can swallow.[14] Their ability to drink water should be carefully evaluated, because some horses continue to drink despite having difficulty in swallowing. Horses that expel food while chewing may have problems with mastication. Coughing and nasal discharge indicate aspiration of food into the trachea. Aspiration may be caused by problems with swallowing or regurgitation. Esophageal obstruction results in regurgitation of food through the nares. Regurgitation is often observed during feeding but may occur shortly after or even hours after feeding. Ptyalism, without dysphagia, may result from ingestion of legume plants (especially second-cutting red clover) contaminated with *Rhizoctonia leguminicola*.[19] This fungus produces a mycotoxin called slaframine, which has parasympathomimetic properties.[19] This excess salivation disappears once the animal stops feeding on the plant.

Morphologic Abnormalities

Morphologic abnormalities that cause dysphagia are easier to diagnose than are functional disorders. Morphologic problems of the oral cavity generally result in problems of prehension or mastication. An oral examination (as outlined earlier) is particularly useful. The passing of a nasogastric tube, endoscopic examination, and radiographs (if necessary) are further diagnostic tests that may help to identify the anatomic localization and cause of dysphagia. Complete obstruction of the esophagus can be excluded if a nasogastric tube is passed successfully into the stomach. Feed impactions of the esophagus are common in horses. Esophageal impactions of feed may occur because of poor mastication or due to esophageal strictures or diverticulum.[5–7] The most common sites for obstructions occur in the cranial esophagus, at the thoracic inlet, and at the base of the heart.[7] Other esophageal abnormalities include rupture, fistula, cyst, megaesophagus, and neoplasia.[5, 20] An endoscopic examination allows visualization of the nasal passageways, nasopharynx, guttural pouches, pharynx, larynx, and esophagus. Inflammation of the pharynx, larynx, or esophagus is best assessed by endoscopic examination. Partial obstructions of the pharynx often result in dyspnea, especially during exercise, and can sometimes cause dysphagia. Retropharyngeal masses, guttural pouch tympany, and rarely neoplasia may result in pharyngeal obstruction and collapse.[2, 9, 10] Depending on the length of the endoscope available, all or part of the esophagus can be evaluated for inflammation or obstruction.

Radiographs can provide additional information in horses with morphologic causes of dysphagia; however, they are not required in all situations. Radiographs of the skull can help demonstrate the presence of periodontal disease, fractures of the mandible or maxilla, lesions of the temporomandibular joint, or radio-opaque foreign bodies.[3] Radiographs of the larynx or pharynx are indicated in cases of pharyngeal obstruction and are especially useful to evaluate retropharyngeal masses, neoplasia, or trauma.[8-10] Radiographs of esophageal perforations reveal subcutaneous air, which shows up as extraluminal radiolucencies.[6] Contrast studies of the esophagus, with the use of barium sulfate, may help differentiate cases of esophageal strictures, dilatation, or diverticulum.[5] Radiographs of the thorax are indicated in horses with nasal discharge and abnormal thoracic auscultation because of the concerns of aspiration pneumonia.

Functional Abnormalities

Functional disorders that cause dysphagia are more difficult to diagnose and should be pursued after morphologic causes are not identified. A functional abnormality should also be considered if the initial physical examination provides strong evidence of a neurologic, neuromuscular, or muscular problem. The initial step to evaluate functional causes of dysphagia is to perform a neurologic examination. The neurologic examination will help to establish a neuroanatomic localization by: (1) assessment of brain, brain stem, and spinal cord functions, (2) determining if the problem is focal, multifocal, or diffuse, and (3) determining if it is a peripheral or central problem.

Cerebral disease is usually manifested by seizures, head pressing, wandering, depression, and changes in mentation. Brain stem function can be assessed by cranial nerve examination. Evaluation of an abnormal response of the cranial nerves should establish the location of the problem within the brain stem. For example, the optic nerve can be assessed by the menace response (requiring the facial nerve) and by the pupillary light reflex (requiring the oculomotor nerve). Abnormalities of the oculomotor, trochlear, and abducens nerves are manifested by strabismus or by lack of a pupillary light reflex. Facial nerve paralysis (ear, eyelid, and muzzle droop) and vestibular disease (circling, nystagmus, and head tilt) often occur together because of the close proximity of these nerves as they exit the brain stem.[21] Endoscopic examination is a valuable tool to determine if pharyngeal or laryngeal paralysis is present. These problems may be caused either by peripheral or by central diseases. The dorsolateral wall of the medial compartment of the guttural pouch contains a plexus of nerves, including the glossopharyngeal nerve; branches of the vagus, spinal accessory, and hypoglossal nerves; and the cranial cervical ganglion. Mycotic plaques, empyema, and trauma (hematoma) of the guttural pouch can result in pharyngeal paralysis, dorsal displacement of the soft palate, laryngeal hemiplegia, and occasionally Horner's syndrome.[1, 2, 11, 12, 21] Skull radiographs should be obtained in many horses with dysphagia but are especially helpful when traumatic injuries are suspected. Rupture of the longus capitis muscle results in ventral deviation of the dorsal pharynx and narrowing of the nasopharynx.[12] Bony fragments may be evident ventral to the basisphenoid bones in these horses.[12] Otitis media and pathologic fracture of the petrous temporal bone frequently result in vestibular disease and facial nerve paralysis and occasionally in glossopharyngeal and vagus nerve involvement.[21] An endoscopic examination of the guttural pouches is helpful with this problem, because the distal stylohyoid bone is thickened and irregular. Ventrodorsal, lateral, and rostrolateral oblique radiographs may also reveal osseous changes of the stylohyoid bone, tympanic bulla, or petrous temporal bone.[21]

The clinical examination should include an evaluation of gait. Signs of ataxia, generalized weakness, and hypermetria along with cranial nerve signs may be observed with brain stem involvement. The horse should be evaluated at the walk, trot, down an incline, over a step, and backing and turning in tight circles. The clinician may wish to place the horse's feet in abnormal positions and determine if the horse can correctly reposition the leg in a reasonable time. Generalized weakness (without ataxia) may manifest with a decrease in tail, eyelid, and tongue tone and muscle fasciculations. Weakness generally suggests a neuromuscular (botulism, organophosphate poisoning) or muscular problem.[16-18] Equine lower motor neuron disease results in generalized weakness and weight loss; however, horses are not dysphagic and do not exhibit cranial nerve abnormalities.[22] Ataxia or hypermetria along with dysphagia suggest a diffuse or multifocal disease that affects the spinal cord and brain stem. Examples of such diseases include EPM, rabies, equine herpes myeloencephalopathy, polyneuritis equi, and a migrating parasite.[12, 23, 24] Further diagnostic tests are indicated in these cases, such as an evaluation of spinal fluid for cytology and chemistry and Western blot analysis for antibodies to *Sarcocystis neurona*.[25] Grass sickness, a disease found in Great Britain and in other northern European countries, results in ileus and colic.[26] Grass sickness can result in dysphagia, with problems in swallowing or esophageal transport.[26] Grass sickness is regarded as a fatal disease, resulting in ileus of the gastrointestinal tract, dysphagia, and weight loss, which is most likely caused by an unidentified neurotoxin. Grass sickness can be defined as a dysautonomia characterized by pathologic lesions in autonomic ganglia, enteric plexi, and specific nuclei in the central nervous system.[27] Additional information about the specific causes of dysphagia are covered elsewhere in this text.

REFERENCES

1. Watrous BJ: Dysphagia and regurgitation. In Anderson NY, ed. *Veterinary Gastroenterology,* ed 2. Malvern, PA, Lea & Febiger, 1992, pp 137–157.
2. Brown CM: Dysphagia. In Robinson NE, ed. *Current Therapy in Equine Medicine,* ed 3. Philadelphia, WB Saunders, 1992, pp 174–175.
3. Baum KH, Modransky PD, Halpern NE, et al: Dysphagia in horses: The differential diagnosis, Part I. *Compend Contin Educ Pract Vet* 10:1301–1307, 1988.
4. Stick JA, Boles C: Subepiglottic cyst in three foals. *J Am Vet Med Assoc* 177:62, 1980.
5. Stick JA: Esophageal disease. In Robinson NE, ed. *Current Therapy in Equine Medicine,* ed 2. Philadelphia, WB Saunders, 1987, pp 12–15.
6. Merrit AM: Dysphagia in horses. In Anderson NY, ed. *Veterinary Gastroenterology,* ed 2. Malvern, PA, Lea & Febiger, 1992, pp 597–602.
7. Baum GH, Halpern NE, Banish LD, et al: Dysphagia in horses: The differential diagnosis, Part II. *Compend Contin Educ Pract Vet* 10:1405–1408, 1988.
8. McCue PM, Freeman DE, Donawick WJ: Guttural pouch tympany: 15 cases (1977–1986). *J Am Vet Med Assoc* 12:1761–1763, 1989.
9. Sweeny CR, Benson CE, Whitlock RH, et al: *Streptococcus equi* infection in horses, Part I. *Compend Contin Educ Pract Vet* 9:689–693, 1987.

10. Todhunter RJ, Brown CM, Stickle R: Retropharyngeal infections in five horses. *J Vet Med Assoc* 187:600–604, 1985.
11. Greet TRC: Outcome of treatment in 35 cases of guttural pouch mycosis. *Equine Vet J* 19:483–487, 1987.
12. Sweeny CR, Freeman DE, Sweeny RW, et al: Hemorrhage into the guttural pouch (auditory tube diverticulum) associated with rupture of the longus capitis muscle in three horses. *J Am Vet Med Assoc* 202:1129–1131, 1993.
13. MacKay RJ, Davis SW, Dubey JP: Equine protozoal myeloencephalitis. *Compend Contin Educ Pract Vet* 14:1359–1367, 1992.
14. Oehme FW: Plant toxicities. In Robinson NE, ed. *Current Therapy in Equine Medicine,* ed 2. Philadelphia, WB Saunders, 1987, p 675.
15. Uhlinger C: Clinical and epidemiologic features of an epizootic of equine leukoencephalomalacia. *J Am Vet Med Assoc* 198:126–128, 1991.
16. Swerczek TW: Toxicoinfectious botulism in foals and adult horses. *J Am Vet Med Assoc* 176:217–220, 1980.
17. Oehme FW: Insecticides. In Robinson NE, ed. *Current Therapy in Equine Medicine,* ed 2. Philadelphia, WB Saunders, 1987, pp 656–660.
18. Moore RM, Kohn CW: Nutritional muscular dystrophy in foals. *Compend Contin Educ Pract Vet* 13:476–490, 1991.
19. Bowman KF: Salivary gland disease. In Robinson ED, ed. *Current Therapy in Equine Medicine,* ed 2. Philadelphia, WB Saunders, 1987, pp 2–5.
20. Green S, Green EM, Arson E: Squamous cell carcinoma: An unusual cause of choke in the horse. *Mod Vet Pract* December:870–875, 1986.
21. Power HT, Watrous BJ, de Lahunta A: Facial and vestibulocochlear nerve disease in six horses. *Am J Vet Med Assoc* 183:1076–1080, 1983.
22. Divers TJ, Mohammed HO, Cummings JR, et al: Equine lower motor neuron disease: Findings in 28 horses and proposal of a pathophysiological mechanism. *Equine Vet J* 26:409–415, 1994.
23. Kohn CW, Fenner WR: Equine herpes myeloencephalopathy. *Vet Clin North Am* 3:405–419, 1987.
24. Yvorchuk-St. Jean: Neuritis of the cauda equina. *Vet Clin North Am* 3:421–426, 1987.
25. Granstrom DE, Dubey JP, Davis SW, et al: Equine protozoal myeloencephalitis: Antigen analysis of cultured *Sarcocystis neurona* merozoites. *J Vet Diagn Invest* 5:88–90, 1993.
26. Doxey DL, Milne EM, Gilmour JS, et al: Clinical and biochemical features of grass sickness (equine dysautonomia). *Equine Vet J* 23:360–364, 1991.
27. Griffiths IR, Kydriakides E, Smith S, et al: Immunocytochemical and lectin histochemical study of neuronal lesions in autonomic ganglia of horses with grass sickness. *Equine Vet J* 25:446–452, 1993.

3.7

Respiratory Distress

Bonnie Rush Moore, DVM, MS

Respiratory distress is defined as labored breathing and is characterized by an inappropriate degree of effort to breathe on the basis of rate, rhythm, and subjective evaluation of respiratory effort.[1] Dyspnea is the sensation of arduous, uncomfortable, or difficult breathing that occurs when the demand for ventilation is in excess of the patient's ability to respond.[2] Dyspnea describes a symptom rather than a clinical sign, and although the term is often used, it is not technically applicable in veterinary medicine.[1] The clinical signs of respiratory distress vary with the severity and origin of impaired gas exchange. Clinical signs commonly observed in horses with respiratory distress include flared nostrils, exercise intolerance, inactivity, exaggerated abdominal effort, abnormal respiratory noise (stridor), anxious expression, extended head and neck, cyanosis, and synchronous pumping of the anus with the respiratory cycle.[1] Horses with chronic respiratory distress may develop a heave line resulting from hypertrophy of the cutaneous trunci and abdominal muscles, which assist during forced expiration.[3] Respiratory distress usually results from inefficient exchange of oxygen and carbon dioxide due to primary pulmonary disease, airway obstruction, or impairment of the muscles and supporting structures necessary for ventilation. In some cases, ventilation is increased in the absence of impaired gas exchange in response to pain, metabolic acidosis, or high environmental temperature.[3, 4] Familiarity with the mechanics of breathing and control of ventilation in healthy and diseased lungs will facilitate the diagnosis and treatment of respiratory distress.[3, 4]

CONTROL OF VENTILATION

The partial pressure of oxygen (PaO_2) and carbon dioxide ($PaCO_2$) in arterial blood are maintained within a narrow range through rigid control of gas exchange.[2] The center controller of respiration in the medulla alters the rate and depth of respiration via efferent signals to the muscles of respiration in response to afferent signals from chemoreceptors in the peripheral vasculature and central nervous system and mechanoreceptors in the upper and lower respiratory tract, diaphragm, and thoracic wall. The central controller, therefore, adjusts alveolar ventilation to the metabolic rate of the individual.[4]

Sensors

The chemoreceptors identify changes in metabolism and oxygen requirements and provide feedback to the central controller, thus allowing for modification of ventilation. Central chemoreceptors respond predominantly to hypercapnia, whereas peripheral chemoreceptors respond to both hypoxia and hypercapnia.[2] Central chemoreceptors, located in the ventral medulla, monitor alterations in the pH of intracerebral interstitial fluid and cerebrospinal fluid. The blood-brain barrier is impermeable to bicarbonate and hydrogen ions but is freely permeable to carbon dioxide (CO_2). Therefore, acidification of the intracerebral interstitial fluid and stimulation of the central chemoreceptors occur predominantly in response to hypercapnia. The severity of acidosis in the intracerebral interstitial fluid due to hypercapnia is amplified by two features of the central nervous system: (1) hypercapnia produces cerebral vasodilation, increasing the delivery of CO_2 to the central nervous system, and (2) cerebrospinal fluid has poor buffering capacity due to low total protein concentrations.[2]

Peripheral chemoreceptors are located in the arterial circulation and respond to acidemia, hypercapnia, and hypoxemia.[2] The carotid bodies are situated at the bifurcation of the common carotid artery, and the aortic bodies are located near the aortic arch. These receptors relay information to the central controller regarding arterial gas tensions via the glossopharyngeal and vagus nerves. Their responsiveness to alterations in $PaCO_2$ is less consequential than the central chemoreceptors; however, the peripheral chemoreceptors are solely responsible for the hypoxic ventilatory drive. The peripheral chemoreceptors demonstrate a nonlinear response to low arterial oxygen tension. They are insensitive to alterations in PaO_2 above 100 mm Hg, exhibit moderate response to arterial O_2 tensions between 50 and 100 mm Hg, and demonstrate a dramatic increase in responsiveness when the partial pressure of oxygen falls below 50 mm Hg in the arterial circulation.[2] The respiratory pattern elicited by hypoxia differs from that stimulated by hypercapnia.[5, 6] Hypoxia evokes an increase in respiratory frequency, whereas hypercapnia triggers an elevation in tidal volume. In addition, hypoxia stimulates recruitment of the inspiratory muscles, whereas hypercapnia potentiates the activity of both inspiratory and expiratory muscles.

The sensitivity of peripheral chemoreceptors should be considered in the treatment of patients with complex acid-base and blood-gas abnormalities.[4] A patient suffering from impaired gas exchange due to both pulmonary disease and metabolic acidosis secondary to shock will manifest respiratory distress in response to hypoxemia, hypercapnia, and acidosis. Oxygen supplementation will likely improve the patient's arterial oxygen tension. Such treatment, however, may abolish the hypoxic ventilatory drive and consequently slow the ventilatory rate. This decreased ventilation could exacerbate respiratory acidosis and may result in decompensation of the patient.[4] To avoid life-threatening acidemia, treatment of metabolic acidosis in addition to oxygen supplementation is indicated.

Receptors, located in the upper and lower respiratory tract, respond to both mechanical and chemical stimuli, and relay afferent information to the central controller of respiration via the vagus nerve.[1, 2] Vagal blockade abolishes tachypnea in horses with pulmonary disease; therefore, these receptors are likely to play an important role in development of respiratory distress associated with primary pulmonary disease.[7-9] Pulmonary stretch receptors, also called slow-adapting stretch receptors, are located within smooth muscle fibers in the walls of the trachea and bronchi.[1, 2, 4] These receptors are stimulated by pulmonary inflation and inhibit further inflation of the lung (Hering-Breuer reflex). Conversely, at end-expiration, they stimulate inspiratory activity. These receptors are considered to be partially responsible for controlling the depth and rate of respiration.

Irritant receptors (rapid adjusting stretch receptors) are believed to be located between epithelial cells of the conducting airways.[2] It is unlikely that they function in regulation of breathing in a normal resting horse.[4] Stimulation of these receptors by noxious stimuli triggers bronchoconstriction, cough, tachypnea, mucus production, and release of inflammatory mediators.[1, 2] Irritant receptors can be triggered by exogenous stimuli (smoke, irritant gases, dust) or by endogenously produced inflammatory mediators including histamine and prostaglandins. Production of histamine, pros-

taglandins, and other inflammatory mediators is increased in horses with chronic obstructive pulmonary disease.[10-12] Stimulation of irritant receptors by these inflammatory mediators may, in part, be responsible for bronchoconstriction, mucus production, and tachypnea observed in horses with allergic airway disease. In addition to their role as chemoreceptors, irritant receptors also function as mechanoreceptors.[1] An abrupt change in end-expiratory lung volume, such as occurs with pneumothorax or pleural effusion, produces a tachypneic breathing pattern attributed to stimulation of irritant receptors. Juxtacapillary receptors (J receptors) are believed to be located within the wall of the alveolus. Stimulation by increased interstitial fluid volume triggers the sensation of difficult breathing.[2] Nonmyelinated C fibers are located in the pulmonary parenchyma, conducting airways, and blood vessels. These receptors respond to pulmonary edema, congestion, and inflammatory mediators, and stimulation activates a tachypneic breathing pattern.[1] In addition, C-fiber receptors may stimulate the release of pulmonary neuropeptides, which produce bronchoconstriction, vasodilation, protein extravasation, and cytokine production.[1] Mechanoreceptors of the larynx are stimulated by increased negative pressure (upper airway obstruction) within the airway and produce prolongation of inspiratory time and activation of upper airway dilator muscles.[13]

Central Control of Respiration

The central controller consists of a group of motor neurons in the pons and medulla, which receive input from the peripheral and central receptors and initiate phasic activity of diaphragmatic, intercostal, and abdominal respiratory muscles.[2] The medullary respiratory center, which is located in the reticular formation, controls the rhythmic pattern of respiration. The dorsal respiratory group coordinates inspiratory activity by assimilating afferent information from the glossopharyngeal and vagus nerves and transmits efferent signals to the muscles of inspiration and neurons in the ventral respiratory group. The ventral respiratory group consists of both inspiratory and expiratory motor neurons. This nucleus is relatively inactive at rest and has a more dominant role during exercise.[2] The apneustic center, located in the pons, provides stimulatory input to inspiratory motor neurons. Damage to the apneustic center, due to trauma or neonatal maladjustment syndrome, results in prolonged inspiratory gasps, interrupted by transient expiratory efforts.[4] The pneumotaxic center, also located in the pons, is inhibitory to the inspiratory centers and regulates the volume and rate of respiration. The pneumotaxic center is not required to maintain a normal respiratory rhythm; instead, this center functions to "fine tune" the respiratory rhythm,[2] receiving afferent input from the vagus nerve regarding PaO_2, $PaCO_2$, and pulmonary inflation.

Effectors of Respiration

The muscles required for ventilation include the diaphragm, the external and internal intercostal muscles, and the abdominal muscles. The single most important muscle required for the inspiratory phase of the respiratory cycle is the diaphragm.[14] Contraction of the diaphragm forces the abdominal contents back, increasing the length of the thoracic cavity, and pulls the ribs abaxially, increasing the width of the abdominal cavity. In addition, the external intercostal muscles participate in inspiration by pulling the ribs abaxially to increase the width of the thoracic cavity. The net effect is an increase in the size of the thoracic cavity, producing subatmospheric intrathoracic pressure, to drive inspiration and pulmonary inflation. Expiration at rest is a passive process in most species and relies on elastic recoil of the lung to create positive intrathoracic pressure.[14] In horses, the first portion of expiration relies on elastic recoil of the lung to the point of relaxation volume, whereby the tendency for pulmonary collapse equals the tendency for expansion by the thoracic wall. However, horses further decrease lung volume by active compression of the chest wall, through contraction of the internal intercostal muscles and muscles of the abdominal wall.[15] Conversely, the first part of inhalation is passive until the relaxation volume is reached, at which point the diaphragm and external intercostal muscles complete the inspiratory phase. Mechanical (abdominal distention, trauma to the thoracic wall) and neuromuscular (botulism, phrenic nerve damage, nutritional muscular dystrophy) dysfunction of the diaphragm and intercostal muscles will prevent expansion of the thoracic wall and produce hypoventilation, hypoxemia, and respiratory distress.[4] Horses with torsion of the large colon develop marked abdominal distention and respiratory distress. Respiratory failure due to impaired diaphragmatic function plays an important role in the pathophysiology and mortality associated with this intestinal accident.

The diameter of the conducting airways is an important determinant of the degree of pulmonary resistance and work of breathing and is under the control of the autonomic nervous system. Vagal-mediated parasympathetic stimulation causes airway narrowing and is one mechanism of bronchoconstriction associated with allergic airway disease. Administration of atropine results in rapid relief of bronchoconstriction in some horses with chronic obstructive pulmonary disease, demonstrating the important role of parasympathetic bronchoconstriction in the pathogenesis of this disease.[16, 17] β_2-Receptor stimulation produces smooth muscle relaxation and bronchodilation. β_2-Adrenergic receptors are abundant throughout the lung; however, sympathetic innervation is sparse and beta receptors within the lung must rely on circulating catecholamines for stimulation.[4] Airways must be constricted for β_2-stimulation or atropine blockade to produce increased airway caliber.[18, 19] α-Adrenergic receptors are less abundant than β_2-receptors and play no important role in the regulation of airway diameter. However, alpha receptors appear to be up-regulated in horses with chronic obstructive pulmonary disease and contribute to bronchoconstriction associated with this disease.[20]

Nonadrenergic-noncholinergic (NANC) innervation also contributes to large airway diameter. Smooth muscles of the trachea and bronchi relax in response to activation of the inhibitory NANC system. In COPD-affected horses with clinical signs of airway obstruction, inhibitory NANC function is absent.[20a] Failure of the inhibitory NANC system may result from the inflammatory response during acute COPD or may be an inherent autonomic dysfunction of the conducting airways of COPD-affected horses.

HYPOXEMIA

Respiratory distress most often originates from inadequate pulmonary gas exchange to meet the metabolic demands of the individual resulting in hypoxia and hypercapnia. Hypoxia results from one or more of five basic pathophysiologic mechanisms: hypoventilation, ventilation-perfusion mismatch, right to left shunting of blood, diffusion impairment, and reduced inspired oxygen concentration.[21] The degree of hypercapnia and response to oxygen supplementation will vary, depending on the mechanism of impaired gas exchange. Determination of these two parameters is useful in identifying the pathophysiologic process predominantly responsible for the development of hypoxia.[21]

Hypoventilation

The hallmark of hypoventilation is hypercapnia.[21] The elevation in Pa_{CO_2} is inversely proportional to the reduction in alveolar ventilation; halving alveolar ventilation will double Pa_{CO_2}.[2] The reduction in arterial oxygen tension is almost directly proportional to the increase in CO_2. For instance, if Pa_{CO_2} increases from 40 to 80 mm Hg, then the Pa_{O_2} would decrease from 100 to 60 mm Hg.[21] Therefore, hypoxemia resulting from hypoventilation is rarely life-threatening. In addition, oxygen supplementation easily abolishes hypoxemia due to pure hypoventilation. Acidosis due to hypercapnia is the most clinically significant feature of hypoventilation and may threaten the life of the patient.[21] Metabolic alkalosis or central nervous system depression (head trauma, encephalitis, narcotic drugs) can produce hypoventilation; however, horses with these disorders may not demonstrate clinical signs of respiratory distress. The following disorders can cause alveolar hypoventilation, and affected patients usually demonstrate clinical signs of respiratory distress: mechanical (abdominal distention, trauma to the thoracic wall) and neuromuscular (botulism, phrenic nerve damage, nutritional muscular dystrophy) dysfunction of the diaphragm and intercostal muscles, restrictive pulmonary disease (silicosis, pulmonary fibrosis, pneumothorax, pleural effusion), and upper airway obstruction.[4]

Ventilation-Perfusion Mismatch

Ventilation-perfusion (V-Q) mismatch is the most common cause of hypoxemia and is characterized by unequal distribution of alveolar ventilation and blood flow.[4] Pulmonary regions that are overperfused in relation to ventilation (low V-Q ratio) contribute disproportionate amounts of blood with low arterial oxygen content to the systemic circulation.[2, 21] Respiratory diseases characterized by low V-Q ratios include chronic obstructive pulmonary disease, pulmonary atelectasis, and consolidation.[4] If ventilation exceeds perfusion (high V-Q ratio), the ventilated pulmonary units are inefficient for elimination of CO_2 and O_2 uptake. Ventilation of poorly or nonperfused units is wasted ventilation, termed alveolar dead space.[2, 21] Conditions associated with high V-Q ratios include pulmonary thromboembolism and shock (low pulmonary artery pressure). Patients with V-Q mismatch often have a normal arterial P_{CO_2}. The ventilatory drive to maintain normal Pa_{CO_2} is powerful. Because the CO_2 dissociation curve is basically a straight line (direct relationship), increased ventilation efficiently decreases $PaCO_2$ at both high and low V-Q ratios.[21] Due to the nearly flat shape of the O_2 dissociation curve, increasing ventilation is inefficient for proportionally increasing the arterial PO_2. Only pulmonary units with moderate to low V-Q ratios will benefit from increased ventilation. Therefore, the increased ventilatory effort to maintain normal $PaCO_2$ is wasted and unnecessarily increases the work of breathing. Oxygen supplementation will increase $PaCO_2$ in patients with a V-Q mismatch. However, elevation in arterial O_2 is delayed compared with hypoventilation and in some cases may be incomplete.[21] Compensatory mechanisms are present to minimize unequal distribution of ventilation and perfusion in diseased lungs to prevent the development of hypoxemia until pulmonary pathology is severe.[22] Reflex pulmonary arterial constriction (hypoxic vasoconstriction) prevents perfusion of unventilated alveolar units and attempts to redirect blood flow to alveoli that are adequately ventilated. Airway hypocapnia causes bronchoconstriction of airways that conduct to unperfused alveolar units, redirecting air flow to better perfused alveoli.

Shunt

Shunt is defined as blood that is not exposed to ventilated areas of the lung and is added to the arteries of the systemic circulation.[21] Shunting can occur as an extreme form of V-Q mismatch or with direct addition of unoxygenated blood to the arterial system. Physiologic shunting is defined as perfusion of nonventilated or collapsed regions of the lung and occurs with pulmonary consolidation, atelectasis, and edema. Congenital heart disease, such as tetralogy of Fallot and some cardiac septal defects, is an example of a direct right to left shunt wherein unoxygenated blood from the right side of the heart is added to oxygenated blood from the left heart. In these conditions, hypoxemia cannot be abolished by increasing the oxygen content of inspired air. The shunted blood is never exposed to the higher concentration of inspired oxygen in the alveolus, and the addition of a small amount of shunted blood with its low O_2 content greatly reduces the PO_2 of arterial blood.[22] When compared with that seen while breathing room air, the decrement in PO_2 is much greater at PO_2 levels associated with the inhalation of O_2-enriched air because the O_2 dissociation curve is so flat at high PO_2 levels. Only hypoxemia due to right-to-left shunting behaves in this manner when the patient is permitted to inspire high percentages of oxygen (70% to 100%). Shunts do not usually cause hypercapnia.[22] Excess arterial CO_2 is detected by chemoreceptors, and ventilation is increased to reduce the content of CO_2 in unshunted blood until arterial PCO_2 reaches the normal range. In some cases of shunt, the arterial PCO_2 is below normal due to hyperventilation stimulated by the hypoxemic ventilatory drive.

Diffusion Impairment

Gas exchange between the alveolus and the capillary occurs by passive diffusion, which is driven by the property of molecules to randomly move from an area of high concentration to one of low concentration.[22] Factors that determine the rate of gas exchange include the concentration gradient between the alveolus and capillary blood, solubility of the gas, surface area available for diffusion, and the width of the air-blood barrier. Diseases characterized by pure diffusion impairment are rare in veterinary medicine.[4] Diffusion impairment can occur with pulmonary fibrosis, interstitial pneumonia, silicosis, or edema due to increased width of the barrier or decreased surface area available for gas exchange.[22] The clinician should recognize that the major component of hypoxemia for these conditions is a V-Q mismatch; however, diffusion impairment can contribute the severity of hypoxemia. Supplemental oxygen therapy is effective in the treatment of hypoxemia due to diffusion impairment, because it creates a more favorable concentration gradient and increases the driving pressure of oxygen to move from the alveolus into the blood. Transport of CO_2 is less affected by diseases of diffusion impairment because of its greater solubility compared with O_2.[22]

Reduction of Inspired Oxygen

Hypoxemia due to decreased inspired oxygen content is uncommon and occurs only under special circumstances. High altitude and iatrogenic ventilation with a low oxygen concentration are the most common circumstances in which hypoxemia is attributed to reduction of inspired oxygen content.[21]

Most pulmonary diseases in horses incorporate more than one of these pathophysiologic mechanisms for the development of hypoxemia. Horses with pleuropneumonia, for example, may develop hypoxemia due to hypoventilation (extrapulmonary restriction by pleural effusion), V-Q mismatch (accumulation of exudate and edema within alveoli and conducting airways), and diffusion impairment (exudate and edema within the interstitial spaces).

OBSTRUCTIVE DISEASE

The location (intrathoracic or extrathoracic) and nature (fixed or dynamic) of airway obstruction will determine if impedance to air flow will occur during inspiration, expiration, or both.[3] The phase of the respiration cycle affected by air flow obstruction will be prolonged and may be associated with a respiratory noise (stridor or wheeze).[23, 24]

The horse is an obligate nasal breather and can only breathe efficiently through the nares.[4] Therefore, upper airway obstruction within the nasal passages cannot be bypassed by mouth breathing. In addition, approximately 80% of the total airway resistance to air flow is located in the upper airway.[24] A 50% decrease in the radius of an airway increases its resistance by 16-fold (Poiseuille's law).[14] Therefore, small changes in the upper airway diameter dramatically affect the overall resistance to air flow and work of breathing for the horse.[3] Extrathoracic airway pressures are subatmospheric during inspiration; therefore, poorly supported structures in the upper airway narrow or collapse during inspiration (dynamic collapse). The most common cause of non-fixed upper airway obstruction in horses is laryngeal hemiplegia, which produces inspiratory stridor during exercise.[3] Intraluminal masses and arytenoid chondritis cause fixed upper airway obstruction and produce inspiratory and expiratory respiratory distress.[3]

Twenty percent of the total airway resistance is attributable to the small airways.[24] Although the radius of individual bronchioles is small, there are many of them and the sum or "collective" radius is large, with the result that their overall contribution to pulmonary resistance is very low.[23] Because the resistance of the bronchioles is low, advanced disease must be present for routine measurements of airway resistance to detect an abnormality, and obstruction of these airways must be extensive before a horse would suffer from respiratory distress. During pulmonary inflation, intrathoracic pressures are subatmospheric. Small airways are pulled open by negative intrathoracic pressure and stretched parenchymal attachments at high lung volumes. Thus, resistance to air flow in small airways is low during the inspiratory phase of respiration.[23] During exhalation, intrathoracic pressure is positive and the diameter of small airways is decreased, and bronchioles may even close at low lung volumes. Therefore, resistance to air flow in small airways is greatest during the expiratory phase. In horses with chronic obstructive pulmonary disease, the airway diameter is reduced by inflammatory exudate, edema, and bronchoconstriction.[16, 17] As lung volume decreases during expiration, the narrowed bronchioles are compressed shut (dynamic airway collapse) and trap air distal to the site of closure.[4] This is an example of severe flow limitation, which may lead ultimately to the development of emphysema. Flow limitation forces horses with chronic obstructive pulmonary disease to breathe at higher lung volumes and maintain a higher functional residual capacity in order to reduce or avoid dynamic airway collapse. Affected horses attempt to reduce the end-expiratory lung volume by recruitment of abdominal muscles to increase the intrathoracic pressures during expiration. However, the greater the end-expiratory pressure, the greater will be the likelihood of small airway compression and collapse. Hypertrophy of the cutaneous trunci and expiratory abdominal muscles, especially the external abdominal oblique, produces the characteristic heave line associated with chronic obstructive pulmonary disease.[4] Because dynamic airway narrowing and collapse occurs during exhalation, wheezes are loudest at end-expiration in horses with chronic obstructive pulmonary disease.[16, 17]

RESTRICTIVE DISEASE

Restrictive disease is less common than is obstructive pulmonary disease in horses.[4] By definition, restrictive disease inhibits pulmonary expansion and leads to inspiratory respiratory distress.[25] The vital capacity and compliance (pulmonary or chest wall) are reduced, expiratory flow rates and elastic recoil are increased, and airway resistance is normal. The characteristic respiratory pattern in horses with restrictive pulmonary disease is rapid, shallow respiration at low lung volumes.[4] This strategy takes advantage of high pulmonary compliance at low lung volumes and decreases the work of breathing. This respiratory pattern has the disadvantage of increased ventilation of anatomic dead space.[25] Restrictive diseases may be classified as intrapulmonary (pulmonary fibrosis, silicosis,[26] interstitial pneumonia[27, 28]) and extrapulmonary (pleural effusion, pneumothorax, mediastinal mass,

botulism, nutritional muscular dystrophy).[4] Hypoxemia observed in horses with intrapulmonary restrictive disease is attributed to V-Q mismatch and diffusion impairment. Stimulation of J receptors may contribute to respiratory distress observed in these patients.[25] The pathophysiologic mechanism for hypoxemia in horses with extrapulmonary restriction is hypoventilation.[4] In cases of pleural effusion and pneumothorax, respiratory distress is likely to be exacerbated by thoracic pain.

NONPULMONARY RESPIRATORY DISTRESS

Respiratory distress does not always originate from dysfunction of the pulmonary system and its supporting structures. Nonpulmonary respiratory distress can occur due to inadequate oxygen-carrying capacity of the blood, compensation for metabolic acidosis, pain, and hyperthermia.

Impaired oxygen-carrying capacity of the blood may occur due to anemia (blood loss, hemolytic, aplastic) or dysfunction of red blood cells (methemoglobinemia, carbon monoxide toxicity). In these cases, the arterial Po_2 tension is normal; however, the oxygen content of the blood is greatly reduced.[2] Tachypnea and respiratory distress occur in response to impaired oxygen delivery and tissue hypoxia.[3]

The respiratory system can compensate for metabolic acidosis by increasing ventilation to lower $Paco_2$ and attenuate acidemia.[2] The ventilatory drive is increased in response to stimulation by peripheral chemoreceptors by circulating hydrogen ions. Hypocarbic compensation for mild to moderate metabolic acidosis is effective in returning blood pH to normal until renal compensatory mechanisms can be established.[2]

Pain and anxiety are physiologic causes of tachypnea and hyperpnea. Horses with musculoskeletal pain are unlikely to demonstrate marked respiratory distress; however, rhabdomyolysis and laminitis are painful musculoskeletal conditions that may produce tachypnea.[3] Marked respiratory distress is frequently observed in horses with abdominal pain; however, the respiratory distress is not solely due to pain and is exacerbated by abdominal distention, shock, acidosis, and endotoxemia.

Hyperthermia due to fever, high environmental temperature, exercise, and heat stress can produce respiratory distress in horses. Tachypnea and elevation in body temperature are the most prominent clinical signs in horses with anhidrosis.[29] Hyperpnea is an effective mechanism for heat dissipation in humans, dogs, and ruminants.[3] Unfortunately, increased ventilation is an inefficient mechanism for heat dissipation in horses and appears to be wasted effort.[3, 4]

CLINICAL EVALUATION OF RESPIRATORY DISTRESS

A thorough physical examination is essential to determine the origin of respiratory distress, identify concurrent disease, and direct further diagnostic testing. Prolonged inspiration is consistent with restrictive or extrathoracic, nonfixed, obstructive disease, whereas expiratory difficulty is exhibited by horses with intrathoracic airway obstruction.[3, 23] Respiratory distress associated with both inspiration and expiration may indicate an extrathoracic fixed obstruction. Stridor is an abnormal respiratory noise that is usually generated by obstruction of the upper airway and is most often heard during inspiration.[3] Horses with nonpulmonary respiratory distress demonstrate increased rate and depth of respiration, without producing abnormal respiratory noise.

Thoracic auscultation is performed to identify abnormal respiratory sounds (crackles and wheezes) or regions of decreased breath sounds due to pleural effusion, pneumothorax, or pulmonary consolidation. Percussion of the thoracic wall generates a resonant and hollow sound when performed over regions of normal lung. Pleural effusion and pulmonary consolidation sound dull and flat during thoracic percussion, whereas pneumothorax produces a hyperresonant sound.[30]

Normal air flow occurs in laminar flow, therefore, normal horses at rest do not generate easily audible sounds.[4] Respiratory sounds are generated from vibration in tissue and sudden changes in pressure of gas moving within the airway lumen. Airway narrowing and exudate generate audible sounds by creating disturbances in laminar flow, turbulence, and sudden changes in pressure of moving gas.[14] Crackles are intermittent or explosive sounds, generated by bubbling of air through secretions or by equilibration of airway pressures after sudden opening of collapsed small airways. The generation of crackles requires an air-fluid interface, and these abnormal lung sounds are observed in horses with pneumonia, interstitial fibrosis, chronic obstructive pulmonary disease, pulmonary edema, and atelectasis.[4] Wheezes are continuous, musical sounds that originate from oscillation of small airway walls before complete closing (expiratory wheeze) or opening (inspiratory wheeze).[14] Expiratory wheezes are the hallmark of obstructive pulmonary disease.[23]

Arterial blood-gas determination provides a quantitative evaluation of pulmonary function, alveolar ventilation, and acid-base status and may identify the origin of respiratory distress (hypercapnia, hypoxemia, acidemia).[21] The pathophysiologic mechanism of hypoxemia may be determined by examining the Pa_{CO_2} level and by investigating the response of Pa_{O_2} to supplemental oxygen therapy. In addition, response to bronchodilator, parasympathomimetic, or antiinflammatory therapy can be monitored by serial blood gas determination.

Additional diagnostic tests that may be indicated in horses with respiratory distress include thoracic radiography, thoracic ultrasonography, endoscopic examination of the upper airway, and atropine challenge. The findings during thoracic auscultation and percussion are valuable in determining indication for ultrasonography versus radiography.[31] Pulmonary consolidation, abscessation, fibrosis, interstitial pneumonia, peribronchial infiltration, and mediastinal mass are readily differentiated and diagnosed via thoracic radiography. Thoracic ultrasonography is superior to radiography in detection and characterization of pleural fluid and peripheral pulmonary abscessation and consolidation in horses. The ultrasound beam is reflected by air; therefore, deep pulmonary lesions will not be imaged by ultrasonography if the overlying lung is aerated.[31] An endoscopic examination of the upper airway is indicated in horses with inspiratory stridor and suspected upper airway obstruction.[32] Horses with extreme respiratory distress may resent endoscopic examination, and forced examination may precipitate a respiratory

crisis. Atropine administration in horses with chronic obstructive pulmonary disease may provide rapid relief of respiratory distress, if the major component of airway obstruction is reversible bronchoconstriction. Horses that respond to an atropine challenge will likely respond favorably to bronchodilator therapy. Incomplete response to atropine in horses with chronic obstructive pulmonary disease indicates that exudate or fibrosis is contributing to airway obstruction, and limited response to bronchodilator therapy is anticipated.[16, 17]

REFERENCES

1. Ainsworth DM, Davidow E: Respiratory distress in large animals. *12th ACVIM Forum* 589–591, 1994.
2. West JB: Control of Ventilation. In West JB, ed. *Respiratory Physiology—The Essentials.* Baltimore, Williams & Wilkins, 1990, pp 115–130.
3. Wilson WD, Lofstedt J: Alterations in respiratory function. In Smith BP, ed. *Large Animal Internal Medicine.* St Louis, CV Mosby, 1990, pp 47–100.
4. Derksen FJ: Applied respiratory physiology. In Beech J, ed. *Equine Respiratory Disorders.* Philadelphia, Lea & Febiger, 1991, pp 1–29.
5. Ainsworth DM, Ducharme NG, Hackett RP: Regulation of equine respiratory muscles during acute hypoxia and hypercapnia. *Am Rev Respir Dis* 147:A700, 1993.
6. Muir WW, Moore CA, Hamlin RL: Ventilatory alterations in normal horses in response to changes in inspired oxygen and carbon dioxide. *Am J Vet Res* 36:155–161, 1975.
7. Derksen FJ, Robinson NE, Slocombe RF: Ovalbumin induced allergic lung disease in the pony: Role of vagal mechanisms. *J Appl Physiol* 53:719–724, 1982.
8. Derksen F, Robinson N, Slocombe R: 3-Methylindole-induced pulmonary toxicosis in ponies. *Am J Vet Res* 43:603–607, 1982.
9. Derksen FJ, Robinson NE, Stick JA: Technique for reversible vagal blockade in the standing conscious pony. *Am J Vet Res* 42:523–531, 1981.
10. McGorum BC: Quantification of histamine in plasma and pulmonary fluids from horses with chronic obstructive pulmonary disease, before and after "natural (hay and straw) challenges." *Vet Immunol Immunopathol* 36:223–237, 1993.
11. Watson E, Sweeney C, Steensma K: Arachidonate metabolites in bronchoalveolar lavage fluid from horses with and without COPD. *Equine Vet J* 24:379–381, 1992.
12. Grunig G, Hermann M, Winder C, et al: Procoagulant activity in respiratory tract secretions from horses with chronic pulmonary disease. *Am J Vet Res* 49:705–709, 1988.
13. Sant'Ambrogio G, Mathew OP, Fisher JT: Laryngeal receptors responding to transmural pressure, airflow, and local muscle activity. *J Appl Physiol* 65:317–330, 1983.
14. West JB: Mechanics of breathing. In West JB, ed. *Respiratory Physiology—The Essentials.* Baltimore, Williams & Wilkins, 1990, pp 87–115.
15. Koterba AM, Kosch PC, Beech J: The breathing strategy of the adult horse (*Equus caballus*) at rest. *J Appl Physiol* 64:337–343, 1988.
16. Derksen FJ: Chronic obstructive pulmonary disease. In Beech J, ed. *Equine Respiratory Disorders.* Philadelphia, Lea & Febiger, 1991, pp 223–235.
17. Beech J: Chronic obstructive pulmonary disease. In Smith BP, ed. *Large Animal Internal Medicine.* St Louis, CV Mosby, 1990, pp 533–537.
18. Derksen FJ, Scott JS, Slocombe RF, et al: Effect of clenbuterol

on histamine-induced airway obstruction in ponies. *Am J Vet Res* 48:423–429, 1987.

19. Scott J, Broadstone R, Derksen F, et al: Beta adrenergic blockade in ponies with recurrent obstructive pulmonary disease. *J Appl Physiol* 64:2324–2328, 1988.

20. Scott JS, Garon HE, Broadstone RV, et al: Alpha 1 adrenergic induced airway obstruction in ponies with recurrent pulmonary disease. *J Appl Physiol* 65:686–791, 1988.

20a. Robinson NE, Derksen FJ, Olszewski MA, Buechner-Maxwell VA: The pathogenesis of chronic obstructive pulmonary disease of horses. *BVJ* 152:283–306, 1996.

21. West JB: Gas exchange. In West JB, ed. *Pulmonary Pathophysiology–The Essentials.* Philadelphia, Williams & Wilkins, 1990, pp 18–40.

22. West JB: Ventilation-perfusion relationships. In West JB, ed. *Respiratory Physiology—The Essentials.* Philadelphia, Williams & Wilkins, 1990, pp 51–68.

23. West JB: Obstructive diseases. In West JB, ed. *Pulmonary Pathophysiology—The Essentials.* Baltimore, Williams & Wilkins, 1990, pp 57–88.

24. Macklem PT, Mead J: Resistance of central and peripheral airways measured by retrograde catheter. *J Appl Physiol* 22:395–402, 1967.

25. West JB: Restrictive diseases. In West JB, ed. *Pulmonary Pathophysiology—The Essentials.* Baltimore, Williams & Wilkins, 1990, pp 89–107.

26. Berry CR, O'Brien TR, Madigan JE, et al: Thoracic radiographic features of silicosis in 19 horses. *J Vet Intern Med* 5:248–256, 1991.

27. Buergelt CD, Hines SA, Cantor G, et al: A retrospective study of proliferative interstitial lung disease of horses in Florida. *Vet Pathol* 23:750–756, 1986.

28. Lakritz J, Wilson WD, Berry CR, et al: Bronchointerstitial pneumonia and respiratory distress in young horses: Clinical, clinicopathologic, radiographic, and pathological findings in 23 cases (1984–1989). *J Vet Intern Med* 7:277–288, 1993.

29. Mayhew IG, Ferguson HO: Clinical, clinicopathologic, and epidemiologic features of anhidrosis in central Florida Thoroughbred horses. *J Vet Intern Med* 1:136–141, 1987.

30. Beech J: Examination of the respiratory tract. In Beech J, ed. *Equine Respiratory Disorders.* Philadelphia, Lea & Febiger, 1991, pp 27–40.

31. Reimer JM: Diagnostic ultrasonography of the equine thorax. *Compend Contin Educ Pract Vet* 12:1321–1327, 1990.

32. Robertson JT: Pharynx and larynx. In Beech J, ed. *Equine Respiratory Disorders.* Philadelphia, Lea & Febiger, 1991, pp 331–388.

3.8

Cough

Catherine W. Kohn, DVM

Cough, a sudden explosive expulsion of air through the glottis, is both a common sign of respiratory disease and a reflex pulmonary defense mechanism. Coughing facilitates the removal of noxious substances and excessive secretions from the airways by creating maximum expiratory air flow. A high velocity of air flow generates the shear forces required to separate mucus from the airway walls, enabling expulsion of exudate and debris from the airway.[1] An understanding of the cough reflex provides insight into the pathophysiology of diseases characterized by cough.

The cough reflex has been infrequently studied in horses. Descriptions of the cough cycle and the neural basis of cough presented here are based on data from other species. We infer that similar events occur in horses. Because there are differences among species regarding the cough reflex,[2] studies on horses will be required to define the physiologic events of the cough reflex in this species.

COUGH CYCLE

There are four phases of the cough cycle: inspiration, compression, expression, and relaxation.[1] Deep *inspiration,* which immediately precedes cough, increases lung volume. As lung volume increases, the ability to generate maximum expiratory air flow increases due to the greater force of contraction achieved by the muscles of respiration when their precontraction length is increased and due to the greater elastic recoil pressure of the lung at high lung value.[3] The velocity of expiratory airflow is thus maximized by pre-cough expansion of lung volume. Achievement of maximum expiratory air flow rates requires a "relatively gentle" expiratory effort, and air flow maxima are therefore independent of effort.[2]

After deep inspiration, the glottis closes. While the glottis remains closed, *compression* of the chest cavity is achieved by contraction of the thoracic and abdominal musculature during an active expiratory effort. Compression of the chest results in an increase in pleural pressure from 50 to 100 mm Hg.[2] This increase in pleural pressure is transmitted to pressure in the intrathoracic airways and trachea. Intra-alveolar pressures actually exceed intrapleural pressures by an amount equal to the elastic recoil pressure of the lung.[4]

Expression occurs when the glottis opens abruptly, thus producing a gradient in airway pressure (atmospheric at the pharynx and high in the alveoli), and air is forcefully expired. The velocity of air flow toward the mouth is maximized in larger airways by the occurrence of dynamic airway compression (Fig. 3–3). The intra-airway pressures vary in the respiratory system according to the instantaneous transpulmonary pressure.[3] At the "equal pressure point," the airway pressure is equal to the pleural pressure. Toward the mouth from the equal pressure point (downstream), the pleural pressure is greater than intrathoracic airway pressure, and the intrathoracic airways therefore are dynamically compressed.[4] Partial collapse of the airways downstream of the equal pressure point maximizes air flow velocities in these airways by decreasing their diameter. At high lung volumes, it is likely that the equal pressure point is in the larger airways and, therefore, only the intrathoracic trachea may be subject to dynamic compression and maximal air flow velocity.[4] Maximum air flow velocity produces high shearing forces that dislodge mucus and debris from airway walls, thus facilitating expectoration. Cough is therefore most effective as a defense mechanism for clearing the larger airways in healthy animals. Removal of noxious substances from the smaller peripheral airways is dependent on the presence of mucus in the airways, and irritants that stimulate cough may also stimulate mucus production.[5]

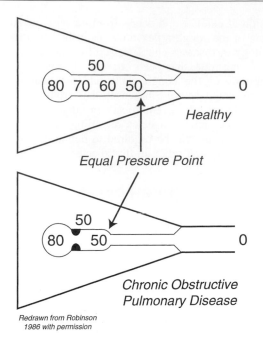

Figure 3–3. Dynamic airway compression during cough or maximum expiratory air flow. Lungs are represented at total lung capacity. When chronic obstructive pulmonary disease (COPD) is present, the equal pressure point moves toward the alveoli. This peripheral migration of the equal pressure point results in dynamic compression in more peripheral airways during cough than would be found in a healthy individual. (Redrawn from Robinson NE: Pathophysiology of Coughing. Proceedings of the 32nd Convention of the AAEP, 1986, pp 291–297.)

In diseases characterized by increased resistance in small peripheral airways due to partial obstruction (e.g., chronic obstructive pulmonary disease [COPD]), maximal expiratory flow rates are reduced. When small airways are partially obstructed, the equal pressure point moves toward the periphery of the lung during coughing because pressures in airways downstream of the partial obstruction are lower than are pressures in those airways in healthy lungs (see Fig. 3–3). This shift in the equal pressure point subjects more peripheral airways to dynamic compression. Coughing is likely to be less effective as a clearance mechanism when obstructive diseases of the small airways are present. Bronchodilator therapy may increase the effectiveness of cough in such patients by increasing expiratory air flow rates.[4]

The sound of cough is generated by vibration of laryngeal and pharyngeal structures caused by the rapid expulsion of air immediately after opening of the glottis,[3] by narrowing and deformation of airways and by vibration of surrounding lung tissue. Variations in the sound of cough are most likely related to the quantity and quality of mucus in the airway.[6]

At the end of cough, *relaxation* occurs. Intrapleural pressure falls, and the muscles of expiration relax. Transient bronchodilation occurs.[1]

NEURAL BASIS OF THE COUGH REFLEX

The afferent input for the cough reflex is carried predominantly in the vagus nerves, and the cough reflex is uniquely dependent on vagal afferents in the species studied.[5, 7, 8] Sensory myelinated nerves in the larynx respond to mechanical and chemical irritation and mediate both cough and changes in airway diameter.[7] There is still debate about the identity of receptors that initiate cough in the lower airways; however, all the receptors described here likely contribute to the cough response.[8] *Rapidly adapting receptors* are located in the airway mucosa in the region of the carina. These receptors are stimulated primarily by mechanical deformation produced, for example, by inhaled particles, mucus, or cellular debris accumulating near the carina. Chemical irritants (e.g., ammonia fumes, ozone, inflammatory mediators) evoke cough by stimulation of receptors located in the peripheral airways. *Pulmonary C fibers* may mediate a chemically evoked cough, although this issue is still debated. Chemical mediators known to stimulate pulmonary C fibers and cough when inhaled as aerosols by humans include bronchodilator prostaglandins, bradykinin, and capsaicin.[8] Forced expiration during coughing may be facilitated by the modulating effects of information from these receptors on central respiratory neurons.

Bronchoconstriction is a constant component of cough,[3, 6] and stimuli of cough may also cause bronchoconstriction; however, cough and bronchoconstriction are separate airway reflexes. Inhalation of dust and irritant gases causes reflex bronchoconstriction in the species studied.[9] Reflex bronchoconstriction has a relatively slow onset and is long lasting compared with the cough reflex.[9] Bronchoconstriction may increase the efficiency of cough by decreasing airway diameter and therefore increasing air flow velocity.[6] In some cases, bronchodilating drugs may suppress the cough reflex by desensitizing airway receptors that elicit cough.[6]

Sensory nerves mediating both bronchoconstriction and cough are distributed unevenly along the airways.[7] Laryngeal receptors and sensory nerves in the extrapulmonary airways may be more sensitive to mechanical stimuli, whereas intrapulmonary receptors may respond preferentially to chemical mediators and irritants.

Little is known about the brain stem neuronal pathways of the cough reflex. In the cat, the cough center is reported to be in the medulla at the level of the obex, alongside the solitary nucleus of the vagus and close to the expiratory neurons of the respiratory center.[3] On the motor side of the cough reflex, the vagal, phrenic, intercostal, and lumbar nerves and motor portions of the trigeminal, facial, hypoglossal, and accessory nerves are distributed to the striated and smooth muscles of respiration, the vocal fold abductors and adductors, and glands of the respiratory tract.[3]

STIMULI OF COUGH

Cough may be stimulated by airway smooth muscle contraction (bronchoconstriction), excessive mucus production, presence of inhaled particles in the airways, release of inflammatory mediators (infectious diseases), exposure to cold or hot air, intramural or extramural pressure or tension on the airways (tumor, granuloma, abscess, or decreased pulmonary compliance due to restrictive disease such as interstitial fibrosis or pleuritis), sloughing of airway epithelial cells, and enhanced epithelial permeability (pulmonary edema).[5] Epithelial sloughing and enhanced epithelial permeability theoretically increase the accessibility of cough receptors to the mechanical or chemical agents that stimulate them. Loss of the integrity of the epithelial lining of the respiratory tract is a common feature in many respiratory diseases associated with cough (infectious diseases); however, a cause and effect relationship between alterations in respiratory epithelium and cough has not been established.[5]

Diseases of the respiratory tract may alter the sensitivity of the cough reflex.[5] For example, viral diseases may increase the responsiveness of cough receptors to stimuli.

DELETERIOUS CONSEQUENCES OF COUGH

Although cough is an important defense mechanism of the respiratory system that promotes expectoration of inhaled noxious substances and voluminous airway secretions, cough may lose its original defensive function and may contribute to the morbidity and discomfort associated with bronchopulmonary disease.[8] This is especially true when the effort to cough is intense and when multiple coughs occur sequentially.[3] Chronic coughing is exhausting and, especially in foals, may decrease food intake. Paroxysmal or persistent cough may impair respiration.[3] Coughing may have profound effects on the cardiovascular system. During the deep inspiratory phase of cough, the rise in intra-abdominal pressure due to contraction of the diaphragm and the fall in intrathoracic pressure combine to aspirate blood from the vena cava to abruptly fill the right atrium and ventricle.[3] Because the pleural pressure is decreased, the pulmonary artery pressure is also decreased. During the expiratory phase of cough, there is an initial increase in systemic arterial blood pressure and a simultaneous and commensurate increase in cerebral venous and cerebrospinal fluid pressures. However, venous return to the heart soon decreases and within a few heartbeats, filling of the heart and stroke volume decrease.[2, 3] Hypotension ensues. Falling arterial blood pressure in the face of high cerebral venous pressures reduces the effective perfusion pressure of the brain. Cerebral hypoperfusion and anoxia may occur. Cough-induced syncope has been reported in humans[2] and in dogs.[10]

In chronic cough, bronchial muscular hypertrophy may develop. Chronic cough may be accompanied by bronchial mucosal edema or emphysema. During cough inspiration, inflammatory debris may be aspirated into previously uncontaminated areas of the lung. Cough in dogs has been associated with pneumothorax (from rupture of pre-existing pulmonary bullae) and lung lobe torsion.[11] Rib and vertebral fractures have been reported in humans with powerful coughs but have not been reported in horses.[2, 3]

CLINICAL APPROACH TO THE COUGHING HORSE (Fig. 3–4)

Cough is a common sign of respiratory disease in horses. The presence of cough is an indication of mechanical or irritant stimulation of cough receptors for which the potential causes are diverse. There are many clinical approaches to anatomic localization of the origin of the cough stimulus in respiratory disease and to discovery of its etiology. All methods have in common a systematic and thorough evaluation of the history and physical examination of the patient. To aid the clinician in formulating a rational approach to diagnosis, diseases associated with cough may be grouped according to those characterized by fever (current or historical) and those characterized by lack of an elevated body temperature. The clinician should keep in mind that there are always exceptions to generalizations concerning disease processes, and the following discussion is therefore meant to serve only as a guide to develop a logical approach to differentiation of diseases characterized by cough.

COUGH WITH FEVER

Horses with cough and fever should have a thorough physical examination (see Chapter 6 for a complete description of a physical examination for horses with respiratory disease). A minimum laboratory database for the coughing horse with fever should include the results of a hemogram and a fibrinogen determination. Careful auscultation of the thorax should be conducted in a quiet room with the horse breathing quietly. If the horse is not dyspneic or hypoxemic, auscultation during forced breathing should also be undertaken. A plastic bag loosely held over the horse's nostrils forces the horse to increase tidal volume and respiratory rate. This maneuver will cause many horses with exudate in the airways to cough, and deep breathing may be frankly painful for some horses with pleuropneumonia. Auscultation during forced breathing is not necessary in horses with obviously abnormal lung sounds during quiet breathing, nor is it advisable in horses with pneumonia (especially aspiration pneumonia) or in horses with foreign material in the trachea. Crackles and wheezes heard repeatedly during the inspiratory and early expiratory phases of breathing suggest that pulmonary parenchymal disease is present. Accentuated normal bronchovesicular sounds are sometimes present in horses with pulmonary consolidation, because of referral of sounds from the aerated lung. Absence of lung sounds in dependent portions of the thorax indicates that pulmonary consolidation, atelectasis, or fluid in the pleural cavity may be present. Thoracic percussion and sonographic evaluation are particularly helpful in documenting the presence of fluid in the pleural cavity. Ultrasonography may also show pleural irregularities and superficial parenchymal abscessation, atelectasis, or consolidation. Thoracic radiographs are especially helpful in demonstrating deeper parenchymal disease. Many equine practitioners will not have access to thoracic radiography but will be able to perform thoracic ultrasonography.

Abnormal lung sounds, percussion irregularities, and sonographic evidence of fluid or consolidation are indications for performing transtracheal aspiration (TTA) and bronchoalveolar lavage (BAL). When both procedures are to be performed on the same patient, TTA should be performed first so that a sample for culture is obtained before the airway is contaminated by the BAL tube. Many practitioners prefer to obtain TTA samples transendoscopically in order to avoid percutaneous aspiration. Despite the development of guarded culture swabs for transendoscopic use, this technique does not always prevent contamination of lower airway fluid samples.[12] One study demonstrated that *Pseudomonas* spp. and anaerobic bacteria in cultures of tracheal fluid obtained

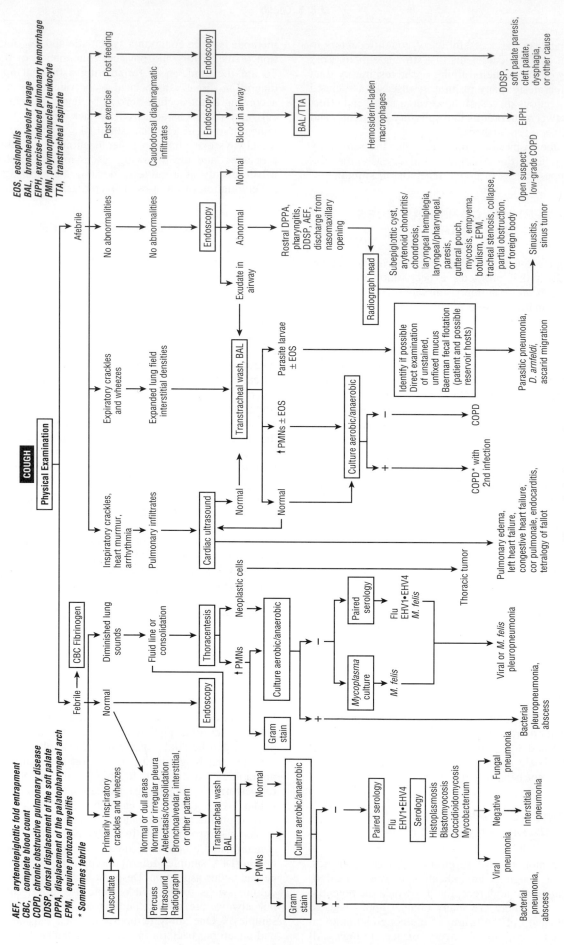

Figure 3–4. Approach to cough.

AEF, arytenoiepiglottic fold entrapment
CBC, complete blood count
COPD, chronic obstructive pulmonary disease
DDSP, dorsal displacement of the soft palate
DPPA, displacement of the palatopharyngeal arch
EPM, equine protozoal myelitis

* Sometimes febrile

EOS, eosinophils
BAL, broncheoalveolar lavage
EIPH, exercise-induced pulmonary hemorrhage
PMN, polymorphonuclear leukocyte
TTA, transtracheal aspirate

154

transendoscopically should be viewed as potential contaminants.[12]

Cytologic evaluation of the TTA/BAL, indicating an increase in polymorphonuclear leukocytes (PMNs), is consistent with parenchymal disease. Some PMNs may be degenerate. Although some clinicians feel that PMNs may be seen in the tracheal aspirates of normal horses, few PMNs are found in bronchoalveolar lavage fluids from healthy horses (4.4 ± 3.3 cells to 8.9 ± 1.2 cells/μL).[13] How well the environment of the lower airways is represented by results of cytologic evaluation of BAL fluids is a matter of some debate. Bronchoalveolar lavage fluids are harvested from a focal area of the lung. If parenchymal disease is not generalized, bronchoalveolar lavage may miss the diseased region. Results of BAL fluid analysis were normal in some horses with pneumonia and pleuropneumonia.[14] Transtracheal wash fluid consists of secretions from both lungs, and TTA cytology was abnormal in all horses with pneumonia and pleuropneumonia in one study.[14] The prevalence of PMNs in TTA fluid from horses without lower respiratory tract disease has not been determined.

The presence of degenerate PMNs, and extracellular or intracellular bacteria in TTA/BAL fluid is consistent with the diagnosis of a septic process. A Gram stain should be evaluated to guide the initial choice of antimicrobial agents while awaiting results of culture and sensitivity determinations. Growth of aerobic or anaerobic bacteria in a culture of TTA fluid confirms the presence of bacterial pneumonia if clinical and radiographic findings are also consistent with this disease process. Contamination of cultures of airway secretions obtained via TTA may occasionally occur. Lack of growth of bacterial pathogens from TTA fluid suggests that viral, interstitial, or fungal pneumonia might be present. These possibilities should be investigated by evaluating paired serum samples taken 10 to 14 days apart for influenza virus, EHV-1, EHV-4, rhinovirus, and equine viral arteritis. Serology for histoplasmosis, blastomycosis, coccidioidomycosis (southwestern United States especially), and possibly mycobacteria should be evaluated. Fungal cultures of tracheal fluid should be evaluated when other more common causes of pneumonia have been ruled out and if the clinical signs of the patient are consistent with this diagnosis. Negative results on serologic tests and fungal cultures in patients with a marked interstitial pattern on thoracic radiographs should prompt consideration of the diagnosis of interstitial pneumonia, a condition for which the inciting cause has not been established and for which the prognosis is grave.

Percussion, radiographic, or ultrasonic evidence of increased intrapleural fluid is an indication for thoracocentesis. Many horses with bacterial pleuropneumonia have elevated pleural fluid PMN concentrations, and PMNs may be degenerate. Intracellular or extracellular bacteria may be seen on cytologic evaluation. Occasionally, frankly neoplastic cells may be identified in thoracic fluid (usually squamous cells or lymphocytes). Many cytologists are uncomfortable diagnosing thoracic neoplasia based solely on an evaluation of pleural fluid. Thoracic fluid should be cultured aerobically and anaerobically. A positive culture identifies the cause of bacterial pleuritis; however, often pleural fluid cultures may be negative. Cultures of TTA fluid are more likely to be positive in horses with pleuropneumonia, and TTA cultures should be performed routinely for these patients. Primary

viral pleuritis, although rare in my experience, has been reported in horses, and paired serology for influenza virus and EHV-1/EHV-4 may be helpful when cultures are negative. One case of pleuritis due to *Mycoplasma felis* has been reported.[15] Culture of pleural fluid and paired serology for this organism should be performed in patients for whom other tests have not proved diagnostic.

Intrathoracic neoplasia may cause cough with or without accompanying fever. Confirmation of the presence of a thoracic tumor may require an ultrasound-guided biopsy or an exploratory thoracotomy and a biopsy. Secondary bacterial pleuritis may complicate thoracic neoplasia, and aerobic and anaerobic cultures of thoracic fluid from patients suspected of having thoracic neoplasia should be performed.

Some febrile coughing horses have no abnormalities on auscultation, percussion, thoracic radiography, or ultrasound. In such patients, occult pulmonary disease may be present and TTA/BAL and culture of TTA fluid are indicated. Alternatively, such horses may have upper airway disease (sinusitis, sinus tumor, guttural pouch empyema), and an endoscopic evaluation is also indicated.

COUGH WITHOUT FEVER

When auscultation of the thorax demonstrates primarily expiratory crackles and wheezes, thoracic percussion often reveals a caudoventral expansion of the lung borders. These findings suggest that COPD may be present. Thoracic radiographs usually show increased interstitial densities; radiographs are useful to rule out occult underlying pulmonary disease (such as a well walled off abscess) but are not required for diagnosis in most cases. TTA and BAL are indicated. Horses with COPD usually have an increase in well-preserved PMNs, and sometimes eosinophils, in TTA and BAL fluids. Growth of pathogens in aerobic or anaerobic culture of TTA fluid identifies secondary bacterial infection. No growth in cultures of TTA fluid is also consistent with the diagnosis of COPD. Occasionally, TTA/BAL fluids may contain parasite larvae or many eosinophils. If horses have historically been housed with donkeys or mules, *Dictyocaulus arnfeldi* infestation should be suspected. Coughing horses younger than 18 months of age with eosinophilic TTA fluid may be experiencing an aberrant migration of *Parascaris equorum* larvae. An attempt should be made to identify the larvae, although this may be difficult. A direct cytologic evaluation of unfixed, unstained, or iodine-stained mucus may be helpful to identify larvae of *D. arnfeldi*.[16] A Baermann flotation should be performed on feces from the patient and potential reservoir hosts but may not demonstrate ascarid larvae, because pulmonary migration may occur early in the prepatent period.[16] The diagnosis of pulmonary ascarid migration is based on ruling out other causes of pneumonia.

When TTA/BAL fluids have no abnormal cells, cultures should still be assessed. Afebrile coughing horses with thoracic auscultation findings of inspiratory crackles and wheezes and cardiac murmur or arrhythmia should have thoracic radiographs. The presence of diffuse pulmonary infiltrates in a bronchoalveolar pattern suggests that pulmonary edema may be present. A complete ultrasonic evaluation of the heart is indicated.

Some coughing, afebrile horses have no abnormalities on

auscultation or percussion, and endoscopy of the upper airway and trachea is indicated. Some horses will have endoscopic evidence of exudate in the trachea and likely have low-grade COPD. These horses should have thoracic radiographs if possible, and TTA/BAL should be performed followed by culture of TTA fluid. A transtracheal aspirate should not be obtained immediately after tracheoscopy because bacteria on the endoscope may contaminate airway cultures.

In other patients, cough may be a symptom of upper airway obstructive disease (dorsal displacement of the soft palate, rostral displacement of the palatopharyngeal arch, arytenoepiglottic fold entrapment, subepiglottic cyst, arytenoid chondritis/chondrosis, laryngeal hemiplegia, or tracheal stenosis, collapse, or partial obstruction) or maxillary or frontal sinusitis with discharge into the nasal passages via the nasomaxillary opening or laryngeal/pharyngeal paresis. The latter may be a symptom of guttural pouch mycosis, empyema, or systemic disease (e.g., botulism or equine protozoal myelitis). Cough may also be a symptom of the presence of a tracheal foreign body (e.g., a twig or TTA catheter). Horses with cough but no abnormalities on endoscopy should be suspected of having low-grade COPD.

Cough after exercise or feeding should also prompt an endoscopic evaluation. Evidence of hemorrhage in the trachea after exercise indicates that exercise-induced pulmonary hemorrhage is likely. This diagnosis can be confirmed by finding hemosiderin-laden macrophages in BAL or TTA fluid. Thoracic radiographs may show interstitial densities and pleural thickening in the caudodorsal lung field. Postprandial cough may be associated with soft palate paresis, dorsal displacement of the soft palate, cleft palate (neonates and foals), or dysphagia of any cause.

A detailed description of diagnostic and therapeutic strategies for diseases of the respiratory system can be found in Chapter 6.

REFERENCES

1. Fuller RE: Cough. In Crystal RG, West JB, eds. *The Lung: Scientific Foundation.* New York, Raven Press, 1991, pp 1861–1867.

2. Leith DE: Cough. In Brain JD, Proctor DF, Reid LM, eds. Respiratory Defense Mechanisms, Part II. In Lenfant C, ed. *Lung Biology in Health and Disease,* Vol. 5. New York, Marcel Dekker, 1977, pp 545–592.

3. Korpas J, Tomori Z: Cough and other respiratory reflexes. *Prog Respir Res* 12:15–148, 1979.

4. Robinson NE: *Pathophysiology of Coughing.* Proceedings of the 32nd Convention of the AAEP, 1986, pp 291–297.

5. Karlsson J-A, Sant'Ambrogio G, Widdicombe J: Afferent neuronal pathways in cough and reflex bronchoconstriction. *J Appl Physiol* 65:1007–1023, 1988.

6. Korpas J, Widdicombe JG: Aspects of the cough reflex. *Respir Med* 85 (Suppl A):3–5, 1991.

7. Karlsson J-A, Hansson L, Wollmer P, Dahlback M: Regional sensitivity of the respiratory tract to stimuli causing cough and reflex bronchoconstriction. *Respir Med* 85 (Suppl A):47–50, 1991.

8. Coleridge HM, Coleridge JCG: Pulmonary reflexes: Neural mechanisms of pulmonary defense. *Annu Rev Physiol* 56:69–91, 1994.

9. Widdicombe JG: Respiratory reflexes and defense. In Brain JD, Proctor DF, Reid LM, eds. Respiratory Defense Mechanisms, Part II. In Lenfant C, ed. *Lung Biology in Health and Disease,* Vol. 5. New York, Marcel Dekker, 1997, pp 593–630.

10. Ware WA: Disorders of the cardiovascular system. In Nelson RW, Couto CG, eds. *Essentials of Small Animal Internal Medicine.* St. Louis, Mosby-Year Book, 1992, pp 4–5.

11. Sherding R: Personal communication. The Ohio State University, June 1995.

12. Sweeney CR, Sweeney RW, Benson CE: Comparison of bacteria isolated from specimens obtained by use of endoscopic guarded tracheal swabbing and percutaneous tracheal aspiration in horses. *J Am Vet Med Assoc* 195:1225–1229, 1989.

13. Moore BR, Dradowka S, Robertson JT, et al: Cytologic evaluation of bronchoalveolar lavage fluid obtained from Standardbred racehorses with inflammatory airway disease. *Am J Vet Res* 56:562–567, 1995.

14. Rossier Y, Sweeney CR, Ziemer EL: Bronchoalveolar lavage fluid cytologic findings in horses with pneumonia or pleuropneumonia. *J Am Vet Med Assoc* 198:1001–1004, 1991.

15. Ogilvie TH, Rosendal S, Blackwell TE, et al: *Mycoplasma felis* as a cause of pleuritis in horses. *J Am Vet Med Assoc* 192:1374–1376, 1983.

16. Beech J: *Parascaris equorum* infection and *Dictyocaulus arnfeldi* infection. In Colahan PT, Mayhew IG, Merritt AM, Moore JN, eds. *Equine Medicine and Surgery.* Goleta, CA, American Veterinary Publications, 1991, pp 442–443.

Chapter 4

Pharmacologic Principles

4.1

Principles of Antimicrobial Therapy

Laurie A. Beard, DVM, MS

Clinical manifestations of infections are the result of interactions between the infecting organism and the host. Therapy for infectious diseases introduces a drug(s) into that relationship, producing a triad of elements that interact in multiple ways. Discussions of therapy for infectious diseases can legitimately encompass disinfectants, passive and active immunomodulatory drugs, anti-inflammatory drugs, and medications used for supportive measures as well as antimicrobial drugs. All except the last of these groups are mentioned here to remind the reader to keep antimicrobial drugs in their proper context while formulating rational therapeutic approaches. Antimicrobial therapy is more than "killing germs." The brevity of the following presentation of the principles of antimicrobial therapy is a reflection of the available space rather than the amount of information that is known to be relevant or believed to be relevant to the subject.

Principle 1: For antimicrobial therapy to be effective, an infectious organism must be the cause of the disease. If microbes are not the cause of the disease, antimicrobial drugs have no role in therapy against the disease. If antimicrobial drugs are used to treat non-infectious diseases, it is as if to say that animal is suffering from "antibiotic deficiency." The mere presence of microbes does not equate with infectious disease; the microbes should be participants in disease if they are to deserve therapeutic attention. Antimicrobial drugs may act properly but still not interfere with the development of the disease, because the microbes may be of minor importance in the development of the disease.

Principle 2: Antimicrobial medication is necessary to rid the host of the disease. An appropriate succession to principle 1 is that the host with a disease caused by an infectious agent requires the assistance of an antimicrobial drug to eliminate the disease or that the drug will enhance the host's ability to destroy the organism. Support for this requirement is not always readily apparent and may be a judgmental decision made by the attending veterinarian. Principles 3 and 4 help when making this decision.

Principle 3: The identity of the organism is known or is reasonably suspected. Some microbes produce lesions that are grossly discernible, and ancillary diagnostic assistance is not necessary. Other microbes have physical characteristics that allow them to be easily identified by light microscopy in samples of tissue or material from the site of the infection. Some microbes, however, cannot be identified without biochemical tests or specialized procedures that are only available at microbiological laboratories. Attempts should be made to identify the infecting organism before antimicrobial drugs are administered. Isolation of the organism is important and, for most infectious conditions, should be attempted. Light microscopic evaluation and a Gram's stain of a portion of the sample taken when it is submitted allows a preliminary identification, or at least a differential identification, of the organism.

Principle 4: The infecting organism is susceptible to the drug selected. The susceptibility of an infecting organism is not always confirmed when therapy is initiated. Initial treatment must be selected on the basis of the suspected causative agent and previously known antibiograms of the microbe or predictability of the microbe's susceptibility. An accumulation of antibiograms provides the veterinarian with reference about the antimicrobial susceptibilities of microbes encountered in his or her practice.

Tests to determine the susceptibility of bacteria to antimicrobial drugs in vitro have greatly aided the selection of drugs for appropriate treatment of infectious diseases. Tests have limitations, however, that must be recognized and considered when results of tests are used to formulate therapeutic strategies. Tests of susceptibility are better for determination of drugs not to select than they are for determination of drugs to select. If conditions in the animal and those in the laboratory are identical, it is reasonable to expect a similar response in the animal as in the laboratory. If different conditions exist, however, different responses by the animal are possible. It is appropriate to accept the clinical response over the laboratory results when the observed response is not supported by the results of the test in vitro.

Two explanations for disparity of results of susceptibility that are often overlooked are the microenvironment at the site of infection and the cause-effect relationship. Isolated pathogens do not necessarily cause the observed condition. If the patient is recovering and the antibiogram suggests that the choice of medication will not be successful, the isolated organism may not be the culprit. The microenvironment at the site of infection influences the activity of antimicrobial drugs and may differ considerably from that of the microenvironment in vitro. That microenvironment includes pH, partial pressures of oxygen and carbon dioxide, osmolality, concentrations of ions, and temperature. The microenvironment may enhance or inhibit activity of antimicrobial drugs and can be altered by ancillary treatments.

Principle 5: The host's defenses must contribute to the patient's recovery. Many infectious conditions can be resolved with specific antimicrobial support because the host's defenses are responsive and are "assisted" by the medication. If, however, the condition persists longer than is expected or readily recurs or is unresponsive, although all indications suggest that it should be resolving, inadequacy of the host's defenses should be suspected. The host's defenses, which include natural physical and physiologic barriers, such as the skin, mucosa, the blood-brain barrier, and the blood-testicular barrier, as well as the cellular and humoral defenses, should be evaluated. If the host's defenses are found to be inadequate for recovery, attempts should be made to improve them, if possible. The nature of the inadequacy dictates whether passive immune supplementation or active immune stimulation or a combination of the two is appropriate.

Host defenses can contribute adversely to the development of clinical signs. Modification of the host's response, therefore, becomes an important addendum to therapy. Because improvement or resolution of signs of inflammation is an indication of adequate antimicrobial therapy, abatement of the same signs subsequent to anti-inflammatory treatment may confuse the assessment of the antimicrobial treatment. Concurrent use of antimicrobial and anti-inflammatory drugs is a judgment to be made by the attending veterinarian and should be based on more than just the presence of inflammation, which can be expected with any infectious condition.

Because some pathogens incite reasonably consistent responses in the host, the type of inflammatory response can assist the veterinarian who is trying to make an initial diagnosis on which to base therapy. For instance, streptococcal and staphylococcal organisms incite pyogenic inflammatory reactions. *Pasteurella* species classically cause fibrinous reactions; *Rhodococcus equi* causes pyogranulomatous reactions; and clostridial organisms cause necrotizing or hemorrhagic inflammation. It is important, therefore, that the veterinarian assess the inflammatory cells in a sample of tissue or fluid that is representative of the site of the infection. This assessment can help in the formulation of a list of organisms that may be associated with the condition and expedite the selection and initiation of antimicrobial therapy.

Principle 6: Therapeutic concentrations of the drug are achieved at the site of infection, and the microenvironment at the site of infection is compatible with the activity of the drug. Whether the concentration of the drug at the site of infection is "therapeutic" is usually judged by the clinical response and is a function of activity of the host's defenses and the drug. The effect of the drug is usually concentration-dependent; however, in all conditions, concentrations that are bactericidal are not uniquely superior to those that are bacteriostatic. Concentrations of drugs at different sites are variable and influenced by host-related factors (dynamic biological processes) and drug-related factors that affect absorption, distribution, biotransformation, or elimination of the drug. The host-related factors may be altered considerably by disease. Biological variation among animals and within the same animal affect the results of studies of the distribution of drugs in animals. Diseases impose changes in those already variable processes that may restrict the clinical application of data that was derived from studies on healthy animals. Host-related factors include circulation of blood at the site of infection and the site of administration of the drug, the inflammatory response, the duration of the disease, the age concurrent disease, and the factors inherent to certain species that primarily influence absorption, biotransformation, or elimination of the drug. Drug-related factors include the drug's chemical nature, solubility, concentration, and concurrent medication.

To extrapolate the results of antimicrobial tests in vitro to therapeutics requires, among other things, the assumption that the microenvironment at the site of infection is comparable with that of the system used in vitro. Because the microenvironment at sites of infection is seldom evaluated clinically, the aforementioned assumption may not always be appropriate. Contents of abscesses in people are hyperosmotic, hyperionic, acidic, hypoxic, and hypercarbic and contain larger concentrations of potassium, magnesium, phosphate, and lactate and smaller concentrations of glucose than does plasma. Septic pleural fluid from horses is similar. These findings serve to remind the veterinarian of the benefit of ancillary treatment that alters the microenvironment to improve the activity of the drug. These findings also explain, in part, the lack of efficacy of some drugs in the treatment of certain conditions.

Principle 7: Concurrent use of more than one antimicrobial drug is appropriate in limited situations. Concurrent use of more than one antimicrobial drug is advantageous when one or more of the following criteria are met: the drugs are synergistic in vivo against the causative microbe; concurrent use prevents emergence of resistance; and the spectrum of antimicrobial activity is extended to include all microbes causing disease. Compatibility of the drugs is essential.

Synergy occurs when the antimicrobial effect of two drugs in combination is greater than that of the expected sum of the effects of the two drugs, individually. Units of synergy can be inhibitory or lethal concentrations of the drugs or the time of exposure required to kill or inhibit specific microbes. As with antimicrobial susceptibility, synergy is determined in vitro within specific, controlled conditions. Confusion arises when clinical significance is applied to the meaning of synergy. *Nowhere in the definition of synergy are there clinical implications.* Clinical importance can only be determined by appropriately performed clinical investigations. Studies may find a lack of clinical superiority of the combination relative to the individual drugs (i.e., equal response) and a greater synergistic response than that predicted from results in vitro or from clinical responses opposite from the in vitro response. Despite data from studies in vitro, convincing evidence that drugs used concurrently are therapeutically superior to the use of individual drugs is scarce at best or is arguably absent.

With very few exceptions, bacteria develop resistance to antimicrobial drugs. Although resistance develops by several mechanisms and at various rates, it is an important clinical concern. Resistance can develop simultaneously to multiple drugs (usually plasmid mediated). Resistance to individual drugs usually occurs independently and at different frequencies for the different drugs. Therefore, the probability of mutation to resistance to two drugs simultaneously is inversely related to the product of the frequencies of the individual drugs' mutation to resistance. The rationale for concurrent administration of more than one antimicrobial drug rests in these probability statistics, and it is most applicable when treating infections caused by one organism that readily develops resistance. A prime example of this is the treatment of tuberculosis in humans. Factual similarities with equine pathogens are not readily apparent; however, attempts have been made to prevent the emergence of resistant strains of *Pseudomonas aeruginosa* by applying this principle and by concurrently administering carbenicillin or ticarcillin with gentamicin or amikacin.

Bacteria may readily develop resistance to some drugs. Those drugs should not be administered as the sole antimicrobial drug. Rifampin is an example of such an agent. It should always be administered concurrently with another drug to which the microbe is also susceptible. In mixed infections, one microbe may actually protect other organisms from the effects of drugs to which they are susceptible in vitro, with the result that no response is observed clinically. This is exemplified by mixtures of penicillinase-producing bacteria (e.g., *Staphylococcus aureus* or *Escherichia coli*) and penicillin-susceptible bacteria (e.g., *Streptococcus* spp.) The streptococci may be susceptible to penicillin in vitro because they are tested as pure isolates; however, the staphylococci or the *E. coli* produce enough penicillinase in vivo in the microenvironment at the site of infection that the penicillin used to treat the streptococci is destroyed before it can affect the streptococci. This symbiotic relationship in infections is seldom considered and may be more common than is recognized.

The third indication for concurrent use of more than one antimicrobial drug is to extend the spectrum of activity of therapy. This is particularly appropriate for the initial treatment of a life-threatening disease. The decision to do so should be based on the presumption that nearly all, if not all, potential pathogens will be effectively opposed and that withholding or delaying that form of treatment will result in the patient's death. It is, therefore, obvious that the microbes must be identified initially and that historical susceptibilities of those microbes is predictable.

Care should be taken when applying this rationale, because it can be abused by substituting it for adequate collection of diagnostic data or by using it to appease urgent demands of clients. Risk of adverse reactions increases as the number of drugs administered increases. If adversity develops, it is not always clear if an element of therapy or the disease is responsible. As a result, therapeutic decisions to avoid deleterious consequences are more complicated. In most cases, single-drug regimens can provide adequate therapy, and the potential for adverse effects is minimized.

Probably the most common indication for concurrent administration of more than one antimicrobial drug is mixed bacterial infections. In these instances, the action of the drugs is usually directed toward different microbes and is assumed to be independent of the other drugs on the other microbes. The drugs should be chemicophysically compatible. Their activity (synergistic, additive, independent, or antagonistic) against one etiologic microbe may be quite different from their activity against another microbe. This may necessitate the recruitment of all one's cognitive and judgmental skills to make therapeutic adjustments. For example, a 3-month-old foal is found to have pneumonia caused by *Streptococcus zooepidemicus*, *Rhodococcus equi*, *Escherichia coli*, and bacteremia caused by *S. zooepidemicus*

and *E. coli*. Erythromycin may be used against the *S. zooepidemicus* and *R. equi*, whereas gentamicin is selected for treatment against the *E. coli*. This may not be an "ideal" combination of drugs because erythromycin and gentamicin are antagonistic (the minimum inhibitory concentration of erythromycin is increased by more than a factor of 10) against *R. equi* in vitro. The coliform bacteremia is judged more likely to be life-threatening than is the pneumonia; however, and alternative choices are not available. At this point, erythromycin may be temporarily excluded from the regimen until the bacteremia is controlled and the foal is stable. Alternatively, the regimen may be continued with recognition that, even though limited, the activity of the erythromycin against the *R. equi* is acceptable under the circumstances, and therapeutic concentrations can be attained by accumulation of the drug during the treatment schedule. The latter choice would allow the therapeutic protocol to concentrate primarily on the bacteremia, but not at the expense of the pneumonia.

SPECIFIC ANTIMICROBIAL AGENTS

β-Lactams: Penicillins and Cephalosporins

The β-lactam antibiotics are named for their structure, which contains a β-lactam ring and includes the penicillins and cephalosporins. The basic structure of the penicillins involves a β-lactam ring fused with a thiazoline ring. The basic structure of the cephalosporins include the same β-lactam ring fused with a 7-aminocephalosporanic acid nucleus. β-Lactams are commonly used antimicrobial agents in equine medicine, due to their effectiveness against a wide range of equine pathogens including a number of gram-positive organisms, some gram-negative organisms, and obligate anaerobes. These drugs are effective against *Streptococcus zooepidemicus* and *S. equi*, common equine pathogens resulting in respiratory tract infections.

Mechanism of Action

β-Lactam antibiotics inhibit cell wall synthesis and are bactericidal. The peptidoglycan component is essential for the integrity of the bacterial cell wall and consists of alternating units of *N*-acetylglucosamine and *N*-acetylmuramic acid cross-linked by short strands of peptides. Peptidoglycan synthesis is a complex process and involves several enzymes but can be divided into three stages. In stage 1, a peptidoglycan precursor is formed in the bacterial cytoplasm. Stage 2 involves the production of a peptidoglycan polymer. The final stage involves cross-linking of the peptidoglycan polymer by peptide bonds.[1] Penetration of the outer membrane of the bacteria through channels or porins is essential for the β-lactam to be effective. Once the antibiotic has penetrated the outer membrane, it must bind a target protein (penicillin-binding proteins [PBP]) located on the inner cellular membrane. The PBPs are enzymes involved in the various stages of cell wall synthesis and include transpeptidases, carboxypeptidases, and transglycosidases.[1] The number of PBPs and the affinity of the β-lactam for the PBP vary with bacterial species. The primary action of the β-lactam antibiotics is to inhibit the cross-linking of peptidoglycan by binding to a set of PBP responsible for transpeptidation.[1] In addition, some of the β-lactam antibiotics may cause de-inhibition of a number of endogenous bacterial enzymes, resulting in "autolysis."[1, 2]

Resistance to β-Lactams

Resistance to β-lactams started very early after the introduction of these drugs and continues despite the introduction of new and better compounds.[3] Resistance may be chromosomally or plasmid mediated. There are three important mechanisms by which bacteria may be resistant to β-lactams: (1) reduction of β-lactam permeability into the cell; (2) modification of the affinity of PBPs for β-lactams; and (3) inactivation of the drug by bacterially produced enzymes (β-lactamases).[1–3] Reduction of permeability of the β-lactams into a bacterial cell is the primary reason that gram-negative bacteria are resistant to β-lactams.[1, 2] The lipopolysaccharide and lipoprotein outer membranes of gram-negative bacteria make entry by β-lactam antibiotics to the outer-wall porins difficult to accomplish.[4] The activity of β-lactam antibiotics against gram-negative bacteria also relates to the rate at which the antibiotic can penetrate the outer membrane.[5] Ampicillin has a greater rate of penetration into gram-negative bacteria than does penicillin G, which improves ampicillin's activity against gram-negative bacteria.[4] Cephalosporins, in contrast to most penicillins, have the ability to penetrate the porins in the outer membrane of gram-negative bacteria.[1] Alterations of PBPs may result in decreased affinity of β-lactams to PBPs; however, this form of resistance is not very common.[1, 4, 7]

Production of bacterially produced β-lactamases is the most important and common mechanism of bacterial resistance. β-Lactamases cleave the β-lactam ring to produce inactive penicillin and cephalosporin derivatives.[8] β-Lactamases can be very specific for either cephalosporins (cephalosporinases) or penicillins (penicillinases) or may be generic and act on any β-lactam antibiotic.[1, 5] β-Lactamases can be induced by the presence of penicillin.[9] Gram-positive bacteria produce large quantities of extracellular β-lactamases (primarily penicillinases), which are usually plasmid-mediated. Gram-negative β-lactamases are retained in the periplasmic space, which increases the efficacy of the enzyme by increasing its proximity to the antibiotic site of action.[5] Five classes of gram-negative β-lactamases have been identified,[10] which may be chromosomally or extrachromosomally mediated.[1]

β-Lactamase Inhibitors

Overcoming bacterial resistance caused by β-lactamase production is possible by either modifying the β-lactam ring to produce an antibiotic that is resistant to the effects of β-lactamase (e.g., cloxacillin) or by producing a substance that can inactivate the β-lactamase enzymes.[8] β-Lactamase inhibitors are substrate analogs that prevent the β-lactamases from destroying penicillins or cephalosporins.[8] The combination of a β-lactam and a β-lactamase inhibitor significantly increases the spectrum of activity. Clavulanic acid is a widely used β-lactamase inhibitor in human and veterinary

medicine and is used in combination with the β-lactam ticarcillin (Timentin) in horses.[11]

Pharmacokinetics of β-Lactamases

Most β-lactamases are not suitable for oral administration, because horses do not adequately absorb them.[1, 12–15] Amoxicillin (oral bioavailability of 5.3% to 10.4%),[12, 13] penicillin V (1.65%),[14] and penicillin G (2.87%)[14] and cefadroxil[15] have low bioavailabilities following oral administration and are therefore not suitable as oral antimicrobial agents. Oral administration of penicillin G and V is associated with the development of colic and diarrhea.[14] However, oral administration of privampicillin, a prodrug of ampicillin, results in a bioavailability of 35.9% in adult horses.[12] Furthermore, the bioavailability of various β-lactams is affected by age, with amoxicillin and cephadril having bioavailabilities of 36% to 43% and 64%, respectively, in week-old foals.[14, 16] Oral administration of ampicillin trihydrate in 2- to 3-day-old foals resulted in detectable concentrations of ampicillin 1 hour after treatment.[17] β-Lactams are excreted by glomerular filtration or by renal secretion, and probenecid greatly decreases tubular secretion of β-lactams.[3] Cephalosporins, in contrast to penicillins, undergo significant hepatic biotransformation to active metabolites.[1, 18, 19] β-Lactamases have excellent distribution into most tissues (including across the placenta) and fluids (including synovial, pericardial, pleural, and peritoneal) with the exceptions of non-inflamed central nervous tissues and the eye.[18, 20–23]

Toxicity and Adverse Reactions

The β-lactams have minimal toxic effects. The most common adverse reactions include hypersensitivity reactions, which range from hives and skin eruptions to anaphylaxis.[1] There may also be cross-reactivity to other β-lactam antibiotics.[1] Procaine penicillin is the most commonly used antibiotic in equine medicine. Adverse reactions and occasionally deaths have been reported after intramuscular use and are believed to be caused by anaphylaxis to penicillin or procaine toxicity, with procaine toxicity being more likely the cause.[24] Veterinary procaine penicillin products may have a higher concentration of soluble procaine than do the human preparations.[24] Heating results in a further increase in the soluble procaine concentration, thus increasing the likelihood of procaine toxicity.[24] Other forms of penicillin toxicity reported in humans include seizures, platelet dysfunction, immune-mediated hemolytic anemia, liver damage, acute interstitial nephritis, and drug fever. Penicillin-induced immune mediated anemia, although uncommon, is reported in horses and results in extravascular and intravascular hemolysis and detection of antipenicillin antibodies in the serum.[26–28] Intramuscular administration of ceftiofur is associated with muscle soreness in horses.[29] Anecdotal reports have been made about diarrhea being induced by ceftiofur, with intravenous administration being the most incriminated cause.

TYPE OF β-LACTAMS
Penicillins

The natural penicillins include penicillin G (benzyl penicillin) and penicillin V (phenoxypenicillin), which have similar spectrums of activity. However, penicillin G remains the drug of choice for use in veterinary medicine. Penicillin G is active against most gram-positive and gram-negative aerobic cocci and some aerobic and anaerobic gram-positive bacilli (*Bacillus, Clostridium, Actinomyces,* and *Fusobacterium* spp).[2] However, it is not effective against β-lactamase–producing bacteria.[2] Sodium or potassium salts of penicillin G are chosen when rapid effects and high concentrations of the drug are needed. The potassium salts are the most frequently used, due to the high costs of the sodium salts. Each million units of potassium penicillin contains 1.7 mEq of potassium, and slow intravenous administration is recommended.

The procaine ester of penicillin G slows the absorption of the drug from intramuscular sites of administration. Intravenous injection results in adverse central nervous system reactions attributable to the procaine; therefore, procaine penicillin should not be administered intravenously.[24, 25] Benzathine penicillin G is absorbed slower from intramuscular sites and results in lower circulating concentrations than procaine penicillin G. Concentrations of penicillins at the site of infection and the response of systemic infections to penicillins are related to circulating concentrations of the drug. Therefore, the procaine and benzathine esters may not be as clinically effective as are the sodium or potassium salts. Cloxacillin, dicloxacillin, oxacillin, naficillin, and methicillin are natural penicillins, but they are resistant to penicillinase-producing bacteria. These drugs have a relatively narrow spectrum of activity and should be reserved for treatment of infections caused by penicillinase-producing microbes (e.g., *Staphylococcus aureus*).

Modification of the penicillin molecule has resulted in a group of extended-spectrum penicillins, although they are susceptible to penicillinases. These antibiotics have increased activity against many strains of gram-negative aerobes but have less activity against gram-positive organisms compared with penicillin G. Ampicillin is available in two preparations: sodium ampicillin and ampicillin trihydrate. Administration of sodium ampicillin (intravenous or intramuscular) results in higher plasma concentrations than the trihydrate form (intramuscular only). The absorption of ampicillin trihydrate is erratic and greatly influenced by the concentration of the formulation, the volume injected, and the site of injection.[30] The trihydrate salt, therefore, has limited value in the treatment of systemic infections.[30]

The anti-pseudomonal penicillins, which include carbenicillin, tricarcillin, piperacillin, azocillin, and mezlocillin, are all susceptible to penicillinases. Azlocillin, mezocillin, and piperacillin are semisynthetic derivatives of ampicillin. Adequate studies of these drugs in equine medicine are lacking. Therefore, their clinical use may be best delayed until sufficient data are available. The extended-spectrum penicillins have a similar spectrum to the aminopenicillins with greater activity against many Enterobacteriaceae, including strains of *Pseudomonas aeruginosa*. Ticarcillin and carbenicillin are similar in structure. Ticarcillin is available in a fixed combination with clavulanic acid, which greatly broadens its spectrum and increases its usefulness in equine medicine.[11]

Cephalosporins

Cephalosporins are resistant to penicillinase and are effective against *Staphylococcus aureus*, which is a known penicil-linase producer. Cephalosporins are effective against anaerobic bacteria, with the exception of *Bacteroides fragilis.* Cephalosporins can induce bacterial production of penicillinase; therefore, concurrent administration of a penicillin and a cephalosporin is not recommended. Cephalosporins are classified as first-, second-, or third-generation based on the chronology of their development and on general features of antimicrobial activity. First-generation cephalosporins are effective against many gram-positive bacteria and are moderately effective against gram-negative bacteria. They have been advocated for use following human and equine orthopedic procedures.[18] The pharmacokinetics for several first-generation cephalosporins are established in horses and include cephalothin, cefazolin, and cephapirin.[18, 20, 22, 23] Second- and third-generation agents have greater activity against gram-negative bacteria than do the first-generation cephalosporins but tend to lose their gram-positive spectrum.[21] Cefoxitin is a second-generation cephalosporin that has been evaluated in a limited number of horses.[21]

Ceftiofur is a β-lactamase-resistant, third-generation cephalosporin and is commonly used to treat respiratory infections in horses.[31, 32] Detectable concentrations of ceftiofur are reported in synovial fluid, peritoneal fluid, urine, and pleural fluid.[31, 32] However, in contrast with other third-generation cephalosporins, it attains poor concentration in cerebrospinal fluid (CSF). Cefotaxime and ceftazidime are third-generation cephalosporins that are recommended for treatment of neonatal pneumonia and sepsis.[33] Cefotaxime and ceftazidime provide high efficacy against gram-negative microbes and penetrate cerebrospinal fluid well.[33] Their use is limited due to the high costs of these drugs.

AMINOGLYCOSIDES

Aminoglycosides are polycationic, bactericidal antimicrobial agents that have an important place in equine medicine for treatment of gram-negative and staphylococcal infections. Aminoglycosides are active against aerobic gram-negative bacilli, many staphylococci, and certain mycobacteria. Their action against gram-positive bacteria is limited, although the uptake of aminoglycosides into gram-positive organisms is facilitated by the presence of inhibitors of synthesis of bacterial cell walls (e.g., β-lactam antimicrobial agents).[34] Aminoglycosides are not effective against anaerobic bacteria.[34] Gentamicin is the most commonly used aminoglycoside in equine medicine and is often used in combination with a β-lactam, resulting in broad-spectrum antimicrobial coverage. Amikacin is synthesized from kanamycin and is reserved for treatment of gram-negative infections that are not sensitive to cheaper antibiotics. This drug is generally more effective than is gentamicin.[35] The use of kanamycin has declined over the years as the spectrum of activity is limited. Neomycin is only available in the oral or topical forms and is not used systemically. Neomycin is the most potent in terms of nephrotoxicity. It is used topically for eye ointments or for sterilization of the gastrointestinal tract.

Mechanism of Action

Aminoglycosides are bactericidal agents that bind irreversibly to the 30S bacterial ribosome and interfere with the translation of messenger RNA, distort the codon-anticodon interaction, and impede translocation.[34] The initiation and elongation reactions of protein synthesis are also inhibited. The precise mechanism for their bactericidal effect remains unknown, because tetracycline and chloramphenicol also inhibit protein synthesis in a similar manner and are bacteriostatic. The aminoglycosides diffuse through aqueous channels formed by porin proteins in the outer membrane of gram-negative bacteria. The penetration of the aminoglycosides across the cytoplasmic (inner) cellular membrane is dependent on an oxygen-requiring process and passive diffusion.[34] The oxygen-dependent process involves an electron transport system, which causes the bacterial cytoplasm to become negatively charged. The positively charged aminoglycosides are thus attracted to the negative bacterial cytoplasm. Anaerobic bacteria are consequently resistant to aminoglycosides, because they do not utilize oxygen. The electron transport system is also present in the lysosomes and mitochondria and is a factor in aminoglycoside accumulation into these structures.[36]

There is an increase in resistance to aminoglycosides reported for human and equine isolates. *Klebsiella* and *Proteus* spp. are reported to have higher rates of resistance to gentamicin when compared with *E. coli, Enterobacter,* and *Pseudomonas* spp.[34, 35] There are three reported mechanisms of resistance, including ribosomal mediation, ineffective transport into the bacteria, and plasmid-mediated aminoglycoside-modifying enzymes.[34] The last represent the most important and common mechanism for bacterial resistance to aminoglycosides. Cross-resistance has been reported, although it is rarely reported for amikacin.[34, 35] Amikacin is less vulnerable to the inactivating enzymes because of protective molecular side chains.[34, 35]

Pharmacokinetics

Aminoglycosides are poorly absorbed from the gastrointestinal tract and must be administered by intravenous, intramuscular, or subcutaneous injection to attain adequate absorption.[36] After intramuscular or subcutaneous injection, absorption is almost complete in 30 to 60 minutes.[36–39] The volume of distribution approximates the extracellular fluid space; however, because of the polycationic nature of aminoglycosides, the penetration across membranes is limited.[36] Reasonable aminoglycoside concentrations are achieved in bone, synovial fluid, and peritoneal fluid in horses.[37] Peak synovial and peritoneal fluid amikacin concentrations are achieved 2 and 3 hours, respectively, after intramuscular administration.[37] CSF amikacin concentrations were only 0.97 μg/mL in a mare with meningitis, with no detectable CSF concentrations in normal horses.[37, 40] Very low gentamicin concentrations occur in aqueous humor and bronchial secretions in horses even with very high doses.[40, 41] Aminoglycosides are filtered primarily by the glomerulus and are not metabolized.

The pharmacokinetics of aminoglycosides in neonatal foals has been investigated in a number of studies because of the frequent use of these drugs for treatment of neonatal septicemia. It has been suggested that these subjects may be more susceptible to the nephrotoxic effects of aminoglycosides than are adult horses.[42] However, the process of glomerular filtration is more mature in foals than in neonates of other species.[38, 43, 44] Glomerular filtration rate in 2-day-old foals is not significantly different from that of their dams.[45] Aminoglycosides are distributed in the extracellular fluid space, and neonatal foals have larger total body water and extracellular fluid volumes compared with adult horses,[46] which result in a larger volume of distribution for aminoglycosides. The larger volume of distribution of aminoglycosides results in a lower plasma concentration than for the same dose given to an adult horse.[43, 46, 47] The extracellular fluid volume is also affected by the physiologic status of the patient, particularly the patient's hydration status.[44, 48, 49] The reduction in extracellular fluid volume resulting from dehydration can be reversed by treatment with intravenous fluids.[43]

Aminoglycosides have a low therapeutic index; thus, monitoring of patient serum aminoglycoside concentrations is recommended.[50–52] Serum creatinine concentrations are correlated with aminoglycoside clearance. The determination of aminoglycoside clearance from serum creatinine concentration is less than optimal, because serum creatinine concentration accounts for only 40.9% of the variability in the clearance of gentamicin in horses with sepsis.[51] Direct monitoring of circulating concentrations of aminoglycosides will prevent an accumulation of nephrotoxic concentrations and ensure that the peak therapeutic concentration is achieved. Therapeutic success with gentamicin and amikacin is associated with peak serum concentrations of more than 10 μg/mL and 25 μg/mL, respectively. To avoid nephrotoxicity, trough concentrations of gentamicin and amikacin should be less than 1 μg/mL and 5 μg/mL, respectively.[50, 51]

Toxicity and Adverse Reactions

Nephrotoxicity is the most important toxic effect associated with aminoglycoside use and is potentially reversible.[36, 50, 53] Reports of aminoglycoside nephrotoxicity in humans range from 8% to 26% of patients receiving aminoglycoside therapy.[53] The toxicity is a result of an accumulation of the drug in the proximal tubular cells. Because of their cationic nature, the aminoglycosides are attracted to anionic moieties and accumulate in acidic environments. At an acid pH, these drugs are maximally protonated. The drug is filtered by the glomerulus and is then taken up into the phospholipid bilayer of the brush border and basolateral membranes of the proximal tubular cells. The aminoglycosides bind to the acidic phospholipids phosphatidylinositol and phosphatidylserine.[53] The two tissues in which aminoglycosides accumulate (renal cortex and cochlear tissue) have disproportionately high amounts of phosphatidylinositol in their membranes compared with other tissue membranes.[36, 53] The aminoglycosides become submerged in the lipid bilayer and cause membrane aggregation around the positively charged drug. The interaction of the aminoglycoside-phospholipid interaction results in a number of alterations, including altered membrane permeability, altered membrane fluidity, phospholipiduria, lysosomal myeloid body formation, and inhibition of lysosomal phospholipases. The lysosomes become distended, leak, and then rupture resulting in cellular death.[36, 53] As the disease progresses, defects in renal concentrating ability, mild proteinuria, appearance of granular or hyaline casts, and a reduction in glomerular filtration rate (with an increase in serum creatinine concentration) are noted. Several factors influence nephrotoxicity including: (1) continuous administration resulting in aminoglycoside accumulation versus multiple or single dosing; (2) the specific aminoglycoside used, with neomycin concentrating in the renal cortex the most and streptomycin the least; (3) administration of concurrent drugs (amphotericin B, furosemide), and (4) other concurrent medical problems (e.g., hypovolemia, sepsis, endotoxemia).[36, 53] The administration of single versus multiple administration of aminoglycosides is elaborated on in the following sections.

Ototoxicity has not been reported in horses; however, vestibular and auditory dysfunction are described in humans. Ototoxicity is irreversible and, in contrast with nephrotoxicity, is correlated with peak serum concentrations of aminoglycosides. Neuromuscular blockade is a rare complication of aminoglycoside therapy, with neomycin being the most offending aminoglycoside. Studies indicate that aminoglycosides may inhibit prejunctional release of acetylcholine, with calcium overcoming the neurotoxic effect.[54] Neuromuscular blockade has not been recognized in horses; however, gentamicin does augment the neuromuscular blockade of atracurium in anesthetized horses.[54]

Once-a-Day Dosing

Currently there is a controversy with regard to what dosage regimens are the most effective and least toxic. A larger dose given at infrequent intervals should be more efficacious and least nephrotoxic. This dose estimate is based on a number of pharmacodynamic properties: (1) mechanisms of bactericidal activity; (2) first-exposure adaptive resistance; (3) post antibiotic effect, and (4) mechanism of aminoglycoside-induced nephrotoxicity.[41, 55, 56] The mechanism of bactericidal activity of the aminoglycosides is dependent on the extracellular concentration of the drug, with the higher serum concentration resulting in a greater uptake of drug into the bacteria.[55] First-exposure adaptive resistance is based on the chance of bacteria being resistant to the effects of subsequent drug administration, until the bacteria have been exposed to a drug-free environment for a period of time. Post-antibiotic effect is a term used to describe the persistent suppression of bacterial growth that follows exposure to an antimicrobial agent. Bacterial growth may be delayed for hours after drug levels have decreased below minimum inhibitory concentrations. The duration and dosage regimen are the two most important factors in the development of nephrotoxicity.[36, 55] Multiple and continuous infusion is associated with the development of aminoglycoside nephrotoxicity. Extended periods below trough concentrations will significantly decrease the risk of nephrotoxicity, as will short durations of aminoglycoside therapy.[55] Single daily dosing of gentamicin is reported in horses at a dose of 6.6 mg/kg and 8.8 mg/kg every 24 hours.[40, 41, 57] Gentamicin administered at 6.6 mg/kg every 24 hours for 10 days did not result in nephrotoxicosis (as assessed by urinalysis, blood urea nitrogen, and serum creatinine concentrations, and urine-glutamyltransferase:urine-creatinine ratios) in adult horses.[41] However, this dosage regime has not been studied extensively, and the use of daily aminoglycosides in neutropenic patients may be less than optimal due to a shortened post-antibiotic effect time.[58]

TETRACYCLINE

The tetracycline group includes several antimicrobials isolated from various species of *Streptomyces*, which includes tetracycline, chlortetracycline, oxytetracycline, doxycycline, and minocycline. However, oxytetracycline is the most commonly used tetracycline in veterinary medicine. Gram-positive and gram-negative bacteria, rickettsia, mycoplasma, and ehrlichia are usually susceptible to tetracycline. In the past, tetracycline was commonly used for anaerobic infections; however, recent studies indicate a 33% resistance to tetracyclines of the β-lactamase–producing *Bacteroides* species.[59] Oxytetracycline is the treatment of choice for ehrlichia infections in horses including *Ehrlichia equi* and *E. risticii*. In addition to the antimicrobial effects, oxytetracycline has been used to treat flexural deformities in young foals.[60, 61] Intravenous administration of oxytetracycline (44 mg/kg) resulted in significant, but transient, changes in metacarpophalangeal joint angles in normal foals.[60, 61]

Mechanism of Action

Tetracyclines are broad-spectrum, bacteriostatic antimicrobials that inhibit protein synthesis by binding to the 30S ribosomal subunit, prevent binding of aminoacyl tRNA to the messenger RNA molecule/ribosome complex, and prevent bacterial protein synthesis. Bacterial intracellular concentrations of tetracycline are a result of active and passive transport. Eukaryotic cells lack the active transport mechanism, but sufficient amounts of the drug enter the host's cells to be effective against obligate intracellular parasites. Bacterial resistance to tetracycline is primarily plasmid-mediated, resulting in decreased active transport of the drug and increased active transport of the drug out of the bacterial cytoplasm.

Pharmacokinetics

Routes of administration of tetracyclines include intravenous, intramuscular, and oral means. However, oral oxytetracycline has a poor bioavailability of 0.72% in horses,[62] and intramuscular administration is associated with cellulitis. Therefore, the recommended route of administration of tetracycline in horses is the intravenous route. Tetracyclines are widely distributed to many tissues (e.g., heart, kidney, lungs, muscle, pleural fluid, saliva, synovial fluid, and peritoneal fluid), which is a function of their high lipid solubility.[63] Tetracyclines cross the placenta and are found in high concentrations in milk, but penetration into CSF is poor. The elimination half-life of oxytetracycline is long, ranging from 12.9 to 14.9 hours, following intravenous administration at a dose of 10 mg/kg to horses and ponies.[64] The elimination half-life of oxytetracycline is apparently shorter in donkeys (6.5 hours) when administered intravenously at the same dose.[64] Tetracyclines are not metabolized to a significant extent and are eliminated by glomerular filtration and biliary routes. Enterohepatic circulation does occur. The primary route of elimination of doxycycline, however, is biliary.

Toxicity and Adverse Reactions

The adverse consequences of tetracycline administration in horses include diarrhea, nephrotoxicosis, and cardiovascular collapse and death. Severe and potentially fatal diarrhea have been associated with the use of oxytetracycline in horses.[65] The biliary route of excretion of tetracyclines may alter bacterial flora and lead to subsequent gastrointestinal superinfections.[65, 66] The use of oral tetracyclines is discouraged in horses because of potential gastrointestinal side effects. Oral administration of oxytetracycline is associated with an increase in fecal bacterial counts of coliforms, *Bacteroides* and *Streptococcus* spp., and the appearance of *Clostridium perfringens* type A in horses.[66] The nephrotoxic potential of tetracyclines has been reported in a number of species, including horses.[67] Intravenous administration of oxytetracycline (70 mg/kg or 3 g) to a newborn foal for treatment of flexor tendon contracture resulted in acute renal failure.[67] However, administration of oxytetracycline at 44 mg/kg to normal, newborn foals did not result in any significant changes in serum creatinine concentrations, but more sensitive assessments of renal function were not determined.[60] Tetracycline-induced nephrotoxicosis may be more likely in foals with concurrent sepsis, hypovolemia, or other disease processes.[60]

Cardiovascular collapse is associated with rapid intravenous administration of tetracycline in horses and is manifested by arrhythmias, muscle fasciculations, clinical signs of discomfort, and collapse and death.[68] Intravenous use of doxycycline in horses results in such severe cardiovascular side effects that it should not be used in horses.[68] Tetracycline-induced cardiovascular effects have been attributed to chelation of free calcium and result in impairment of myocardial muscle function.[68] Ionized calcium concentrations decrease in sheep after rapid administration of oxytetracycline but not in horses administered intravenous doxycycline.[68, 69] Neuromuscular blockade may also result from chelation of calcium in the central and peripheral nervous system but is likely not as clinically important as the cardiovascular side effects of the drug.[68, 70] Oxytetracycline may result in muscle relaxation due to calcium chelation, which explains the transient, but significant, changes in fetlock joint angle in foals.[60, 61] The cardiovascular effects of tetracyclines have also been associated with the different vehicles used for injection, with propylene glycol being incriminated in causing increased pulmonary artery pressures, and a decrease in cardiac output, stroke volume, and heart rates in calves.[71] It is recommended that slow administration of dilute oxytetracycline will help to prevent adverse reactions. The drug should be diluted 4- to 10-fold in isotonic saline, 5% dextrose solution, or sterile water.

SULFONAMIDE AND PYRIMIDINES
Sulfonamides

Sulfonamides are bacteriostatic, weak organic acids that have similar mechanisms of action. Agents in this group used in equine medicine include sulfamethoxazole, sulfadimidine, sulfamethazine, sulfadoxine, and sulfadiazine. Sulfonamides are one of the oldest antimicrobial agents still in use today, but widespread resistance has developed against them. Therefore, use of sulfonamides in equine medicine has been replaced with sulfonamide-pyrimidine combinations (potentiated sulfonamides). Sulfonamides interfere with folate synthesis. Sulfonamides are analogs and competitive antago-

nists of para-aminobenzoic acid (PABA) and inhibit synthesis of purines required for DNA synthesis.[72] Sulfonamides compete with PABA as the substrate for dihydropteroic synthetase, which is the enzyme responsible for incorporation of PABA into dihydropterorate acid, the immediate precursor to folic acid. This bacteriostatic mechanism is therefore inhibited by an excess of PABA. Sensitive bacteria are those that must synthesize their own folic acid; bacteria and mammalian cells that use pre-formed folic acid are not affected.

Pyrimidines

Pyrimidines include trimethoprim, pyrimethamine, ormethoprim, aditoprim, and bacquiloprim. Trimethoprim and pyrimethamine are diaminopyrimidines, whereas ormethoprim and aditoprim are diaminobenzylpyrimidines. Aditoprim and bacquiloprim are newer compounds. Ormethoprim is registered for use in dogs but not in horses. Pyrimidines are bacteriostatic antimicrobials that also inhibit folate synthesis. They inhibit the enzyme dihydrofolate reductase and prevent the synthesis of tetrahydrofolic acid from dihydrofolic acid.[72] Dihydrofolate reductase is also present in mammalian and bacterial cells; however, bacterial enzymes are inhibited by a much lower concentration of the drug than are mammalian cells. Pyrimidines interfere with the de novo synthesis of folates and also inhibit their recycling.[73] Trimethoprim has a greater affinity for bacterial enzymes, whereas pyrimethamine has a greater affinity for protozoal enzymes.

Potentiated Sulfonamides

The combination of a pyrimidine and a sulfonamide result in a synergistic effect, with the combined drugs having bactericidal activity, and these drugs are called "potentiated sulfonamides." Potentiated sulfonamides result in the minimum inhibitory concentration of each antimicrobial being lower, the antimicrobial spectrum being broader, and resistance being developed more slowly.[72] Potentiated sulfonamides are effective against a number of gram-positive and gram-negative and protozoal organisms and are effective in vitro against some obligate anaerobes. The in vivo activity of potentiated sulfonamides against anaerobic bacteria is generally not very effective.[59] Culture media used for sensitivity testing of potentiated sulfonamides should not contain thymidine or PABA, because these agents may reduce the in vitro activity. The most commonly used potentiated sulfonamides include a combination of a sulfonamide with trimethoprim. However, pharmacologic studies using a combination of sulfadimethoxine and ormethoprim have been performed in horses and foals.[74–78] Potentiated sulfonamides are prepared with a fixed 1:5 ratio and are designed to reach a 1:20 ratio in human plasma. The optimum concentration ratio in vitro and in vivo for most susceptible organisms is approximately 1:20; however, significant synergism may occur with a wide range of drug ratios.[72]

Resistance

Resistance to sulfonamides is common, associated with cross-resistance to other sulfonamides, and may be chromosomal or plasmid mediated.[2, 72] Chromosomal-mediated resistance is achieved by increased bacterial production of PABA or by reducing the affinity of the enzyme dihydropterase synthetase for the sulfonamide.[2, 72] An excess of PABA in necrotic tissue or abscesses may decrease the effectiveness of the sulfonamides.[73] The plasmid-mediated form of resistance is also achieved by production of the enzyme with reduced affinity for the sulfonamide.[2, 72] The major cause of resistance to trimethoprim is plasmid-mediated and results in the production of the enzyme dihydrofolate reductase, which lacks the capacity to bind trimethoprim. Resistance to trimethoprim may also be achieved chromosomally, resulting in the overproduction of dihydrofolate reductase.[2, 72]

Pharmacokinetics

The sulfonamides differ in their pharmacokinetic properties.[72] Absorption depends on the pK_a of the drug (the pH at which half of the drug is ionized and half is not), because the non-ionized form diffuses rapidly through cell membranes. At a physiologic pH, most sulfonamides are non-ionized and are rapidly absorbed from the gastrointestinal tract and distributed to all tissues and body fluids (including CSF and synovial fluid).[74-79] Concentrations of the sulfonamides are higher in plasma than tissues, whereas the tissue concentrations of trimethoprim may be higher than those of plasma concentrations.[72] The amount of protein binding is variable and is affected by species, drug, and concentration. Only the free, unbound drug is biologically active. Elimination of the sulfonamide and pyrimidine occur by renal excretion and liver metabolism.[72, 73, 80, 81] The bioavailability of pyrimethamine is reported to be 56% in adult horses.[82] Pyrimethamine concentrations in CSF of horses are 25% to 50% of the corresponding plasma concentrations, which exceeds the minimum inhibitory concentrations for many common equine pathogens, including *Sarcocystis neurona*, the etiologic agent of equine protozoal myelitis.[82-84] Dimethylsulfoxide is often used to treat neurologic disease in horses, and may increase delivery of substances across the blood-brain barrier. However, intravenous administration of dimethyl sulfoxide (DMSO) at 1 g/kg did not alter CSF concentrations of either trimethoprim or sulfamethizole in horses.[84]

Toxicity and Adverse Reactions

Toxicity and adverse reactions associated with potentiated sulfonamides in horses include nephrotoxicity, blood dyscrasias, cardiovascular collapse and death, and diarrhea. Nephrotoxicity is reported to occur with sulfonamide use, particularly the older sulfonamides that are not as soluble as the newer ones.[72] Crystalluria, hematuria, and obstruction of renal tubules may occur when water intake and urine pH are low.[72, 73]

Hematopoietic disorders, including hemolytic anemia, agranulocytosis, aplastic anemia, and thrombocytopenia, have been reported in humans.[73] Agranulocytosis and aplastic anemia may be a result of decreased folate availability. A decrease in the neutrophil count has been observed in horses receiving pyrimethamine (1 mg/kg orally every 24 hours for 10 days), although the counts were still within normal limits.[83] Although anemia has not been reported in

horses treated with potentiated sulfonamides, anecdotal reports have been made. Folinic acid supplementation to prevent anemia is sometimes recommended for horses that are treated with potentiated sulfonamides for a long time. Simultaneous administration of folinic acid or thymidine did not interfere with antibacterial activity of sulfamethoxazole-trimethoprim in experimentally infected mice.[85] Thrombocytopenia is most likely to be an immune-mediated event.[86] Severe postoperative hemorrhage is described in horses being treated with potentiated sulfonamides.[86]

The intravenous administration of a potentiated sulfonamide in horses can be associated with potentially fatal complications, including central nervous system signs (excitation and muscle fasciculations) and cardiovascular collapse.[78] The use of detomidine and a potentiated sulfonamide has been reported to be responsible for the death of several horses, and a combination of these drugs should be avoided.[87-89]

Diarrhea can be associated with the use of potentiated sulfonamides in horses; however, there are conflicting reports.[72, 90] Treatment with potentiated sulfonamides was not associated with diarrhea in horses at a veterinary teaching hospital.[90] Oral administration of potentiated sulfonamides did not result in significant changes in fecal bacterial counts.[66] Anorexic horses, however, may be more at risk for developing antibiotic-induced colitis.[72]

MACROLIDES

The macrolide antimicrobials are fermentation products of *Streptomyces* spp. and are characterized by a large lactone ring containing between 12 and 16 atoms. The macrolide antimicrobial family includes erythromycin, tylosin, roxithromyxin, erythromycylamine, tilmicosin, dirithromycin, and flurithromycin. However only erythromycin, tylosin, and tilmicosin are used in veterinary medicine, with erythromycin being the only macrolide used in equine medicine. Erythromycin, in combination with rifampin, is the treatment of choice for *Rhodococcus equi* infections in foals and has been demonstrated to be effective against *Ehrlichia risticii*, the etiologic agent of Potomac horse fever.[91-94] However, development of resistance to erythromycin and rifampin has been reported in a foal with *R. equi* pneumonia.[95]

Mechanism of Action

The mechanism of action of macrolides is still unclear, but all macrolides inhibit bacterial protein synthesis to varying extents.[96] Erythromycin is bacteriostatic at therapeutic concentrations and accumulates to a greater extent in gram-positive bacteria than in gram-negative ones.[96, 97] However, it may become bactericidal at higher concentrations.[96] The macrolides bind to the 50S ribosomal subunit with a specific target in the 23S ribosomal RNA molecule and to various ribosomal proteins.[96] Macrolides do not bind to mammalian ribosomes. Resistance to erythromycin may occur due to ribosomal alterations, mutations, and plasmid-mediated methods. Alteration of the bacterial ribosome results from methylation of the 50S drug receptor site on the ribosome, which prevents erythromycin from binding. Decreased permeability of the bacterial cytoplasm and hydrolysis of erythromycin also account for different mechanisms of bacterial resistance.[97, 98]

Pharmacokinetics

Erythromycin is a lipid-soluble antibiotic, which is rapidly inactivated in an acidic environment (e.g., the stomach). Enteric coatings and chemical modifications, including the formation of esters or salts from the bases, allow for better absorption from the small intestine.[99] There are several formulations of erythromycin for oral administration that include erythromycin estolate, ethylsuccinate, and erythromycin stearate. Erythromycin ethylsuccinate and estolate arc absorbed as inactive esters and are then hydrolyzed to the active form of the drug.[99] In contrast, erythromycin stearate and phosphate dissociate in the proximal small intestine and are absorbed as the free base.[99] Erythromycin estolate is recommended at a dose of 25 mg/kg orally four times a day (q.i.d.) for the treatment of *Rhodococcus equi* pneumonia in foals.[100, 101] However, recent studies indicate that erythromycin phosphate or stearate may be substituted for estolate in treatment of *R. equi* pneumonia at a dose of 37.5 mg/kg orally twice a day (b.i.d.),[99] which is less expensive and may result in better owner compliance. Erythromycin is distributed widely into intracellular and extracellular spaces but does not cross the blood-brain barrier. The drug achieves very high tissue concentrations compared with serum concentrations.[98] In addition, the drug accumulates rapidly intracellularly and demonstrates intrahepatic antimicrobial activity.[98] Elimination of erythromycin occurs predominantly through hepatic metabolism and biliary excretion.[97, 98]

Toxicity and Adverse Reactions

Adverse effects of erythromycin include gastrointestinal disturbances (diarrhea and altered motility) and interactions with other drugs.[97, 98] Diarrhea is thought to be the result of enterohepatic cycling, resulting in alterations of intestinal flora.[98] Anecdotal reports have been made that erythromycin-induced diarrhea is more severe in adult horses than in foals. Erythromycin should only be used in adult horses in reserved cases. There is evidence that erythromycin may increase intestinal motility by binding motilin receptors, and erythromycin has been used to treat postoperative ileus in horses. Interactions of erythromycin with other drugs may occur, including impairment of the clearance of theophylline, increasing the likelihood of theophylline toxicity. A combination of erythromycin and chloramphenicol is contraindicated due to competitive binding at the bacterial ribosome. A combination of gentamicin and erythromycin gave antagonistic interactions in horses.[101] Tilmicosin and tylosin should not be used in horses, because they may result in severe and potentially fatal enterocolitis. The linconsaides, including lincomycin and clindamycin, are similar to the macrolides in their mechanism of action and spectrum. However, the usefulness of these compounds is limited in horses due to gastrointestinal side effects and they should not be used in horses.[97]

RIFAMPIN

Rifampin is a semisynthetic, macrocyclic, bactericidal antibiotic, with excellent ability to penetrate tissues. Rifampin has a wide range of antibacterial spectrum and is effective at low tissue concentrations against some gram-negative and most gram-positive microorganisms, including *Mycobacterium tuberculosis*.[101, 102] Rifampin is also effective against many strains of obligate anaerobic bacteria.[101] Rifampin is lipid soluble and is capable of attaining high intracellular concentrations in phagocytic cells and abscesses. Therefore, it is efficacious against intracellular organisms, such as *R. equi*, *M. tuberculosis*, and *E. risticii*, which survive intracellularly in macrophages.[90, 91, 93] Rifampin should be used in combination with other antimicrobial agents to prevent the development of resistant bacteria. Rifampin in combination with erythromycin is the treatment of choice for foals with *R. equi* pneumonia.[90, 91, 93]

Mechanism of Action

Rifampin inhibits protein synthesis by binding to the b subunit of the bacterial DNA-dependent RNA polymerase and suppresses the initiation of the synthesis of the messenger RNA.[101] Inhibition of mammalian RNA polymerase by rifampin only occurs at very high drug concentrations.[101] The minimum inhibitory concentration of rifampin for gram-negative bacteria is highcr than for gram-positive ones and is attributed to the drug penetrating the outer membrane of gram-positive bacteria more readily than do gram-negative ones.[101, 103] Development of bacterial resistance to rifampin is very common and occurs quickly if rifampin is used alone. Resistance occurs by a single mutation of the amino acid sequence of the b-subunit of the RNA polymerase enzymes. Thus, the bacterial RNA polymerase binds rifampin with less affinity. An increase in the dose of rifampin may overcome bacterial resistance in vitro, and development of bacterial resistance is decreased if rifampin is used in combination with another antimicrobial agent.[101, 104] Therefore, it is important to use rifampin in combination with another drug, such as penicillin or erythromycin.[101] Rifampin is synergistic with trimethoprim and erythromycin and has an additive effect with penicillin G and ampicillin.[100]

Pharmacokinetics

Rifampin is rapidly absorbed from the gastrointestinal tract of adult and foals.[102, 103, 105–107] It is distributed widely in the extracellular and intracellular compartments and is highly lipid soluble. Antimicrobial concentrations are approached in all tissue compartments, including milk, bone, CSF, and exudates. Rifampin undergoes hepatic deacetylation with production of 25-desacetylrifampin, which is a bioactive metabolite. Rifampin and desacetylrifampin are eliminated in the bile and urine.[101] Rifampin may result in red-orange colored urine, sweat, feces, saliva, and tears. It also results in autoinduction of hepatic enzymes. This leads to an increase in the rate of elimination of rifampin in foals treated for 10 days with the drug.[107] Rifampin also increases metabolism of many substances including digitalis, warfarin, and corticosteroids.[101] Administration of rifampin results in a significant increase in the rate of elimination of phenylbutazone.[108] Rifampin is recommended at a dose of 5 to 10 mg/kg orally in adult horses and foals.[91, 92, 100] The rate of elimination of rifampin is slower in foals than adult horses, with rifampin having a longer half-life in foals.[105, 107] Therefore, a lower dose of 5 mg/kg may be sufficient to treat foals with susceptible gram-positive infections.[105, 107]

Toxicity and Adverse Effects

The most frequent side effect associated with rifampin in humans includes hypersensitivity reactions, mild pruritus, and gastrointestinal tract alterations, with immunosuppression and hepatotoxicosis reported in longer term use (> 3 months) in humans.[101] Adverse effects associated with rifampin therapy in horses are apparently rare, and, when reported, are associated with administration of the intravenous preparation of rifampin (which is not currently available). An acute anaphylactic reaction and death are reported in a foal receiving intravenous rifampin.[107] Intravenous administration of rifampin is reported to result in moderate sweating for approximately 8 hours after administration.[106] Treatment of foals with erythromycin and rifampin combinations is associated with diarrhea.[92, 96, 99] However, the erythromycin is believed to be the most likely source of diarrhea.[90, 92, 96, 101]

CHLORAMPHENICOL

Chloramphenicol is a broad-spectrum antibiotic, which historically has been used extensively in human and veterinary medicine. However, in view of the adverse reactions reported in humans, restrictions on its use have been imposed in veterinary medicine. These restrictions prohibit its administration to food animals in the United States of America. Its use is also prohibited in horses in Australia.[109] Chloramphenicol has a wide spectrum of activity that includes many gram-negative and gram-positive bacteria, including obligate anaerobes, and rickettsia. Chloramphenicol readily penetrates bacterial cells via facilitated diffusion and is effective against intracellular organisms. Chloramphenicol has three structural groups that determine its antimicrobial and toxic activities: (1) the *p*-nitrophenol group, (2) the dichloroacetyl group, and (3) an alcohol group.[110] Thiamphenicol, which has different biologic activity than does chloramphenicol, is produced when the *p*-nitrophenol group is replaced with a methylsulfyl group.[110]

Mechanism of Action

Chloramphenicol is a bacteriostatic antibiotic that inhibits protein synthesis in bacterial cells and to lesser extent in mammalian cells. Chloramphenicol binds to the 50S ribosomal subunit and interferes with the insertion of aminoacyl-tRNA, thus inhibiting the function of peptidyl transferase and protein synthesis. Several mechanisms of resistance are described for chloramphenicol, including the production of a chloramphenicol acetyltransferase enzyme that inactivates chloramphenicol, decreased bacterial cell wall permeability, altered binding capabilities at the 50S ribosome subunit, and inactivation of chloramphenicol by nitroreductase.[110]

Pharmacokinetics

The pharmacokinetics of chloramphenicol have been investigated in the horse in conjunction with oral and intravenous administration.[111–117] Chloramphenicol is highly lipid-soluble, and the oral bioavailability is good. However, the bioavailability and peak serum concentration decrease with repeated doses in adult horses.[112] There is also evidence that chloramphenicol damages the small intestinal mucosa in young calves.[118] The elimination half-life (approximately 1 hour) and maximum serum concentrations of chloramphenicol are lower in horses compared with other species.[112, 113, 115, 117, 119] Therefore, a relatively high and frequent dose is recommended in horses (50 mg/kg by mouth every 4 to 6 hours).[111, 112, 115, 117] Age influences the pharmacokinetics of chloramphenicol in horses.[107, 111, 114] Foals have a longer elimination half-life of chloramphenicol than do adult horses; however, differences disappear when foals are approximately 7 days of age.[107, 111] Chloramphenicol is well distributed in body fluids and readily reaches therapeutic concentrations in the CSF. Tissue concentrations may be higher than are those of serum.[119] The major route of elimination of chloramphenicol is via hepatic metabolism and production of glucuronide, which is then excreted into the urine by filtration and secretion.

Toxicity and Adverse Effects

Despite the adverse effects attributed to chloramphenicol in humans, few problems have been reported in horses.[119] The adverse reactions of chloramphenicol in humans include blood dyscrasias, including a dose-dependent suppression of the bone marrow precursor erythroid series and a fatal, dose-independent, idiosyncratic induction of aplastic anemia.[119] The dose-dependent suppression of bone marrow is the most common type of blood dyscrasia in humans and is reversible. The suppression usually occurs when plasma chloramphenicol levels are greater than 25 μg/mL.[119] The prevalence rate of the fatal, dose-independent, aplastic anemia is estimated to be 1:6,000 to 1:41,000 in humans.[119] There is evidence that the *p*-nitrophenol group of the chloramphenicol molecule is responsible for the toxic effects, as it undergoes reduction, leading to the production of toxic intermediates and resulting in stem cell damage in humans.[110] Elimination of the *p*-nitrophenol group (e.g., the case with the antimicrobial agent thiamphenicol) may prevent development of the chloramphenicol-associated aplastic anemia.[110]

The use of oral chloramphenicol in horses should be discouraged because of the high likelihood for human exposure when preparing and administering the drug to horses. No reports have been made of blood dyscrasias occurring subsequent to administration of chloramphenicol in horses, which may be due to the rapid clearance and difficulty in maintaining significant blood levels.[119] Chloramphenicol has inhibitory effects on the cytochrome P-450 system, which may affect the metabolism of other drugs. Potential interactions among chloramphenicol and other drugs (including acetylpromazine, phenylbutazone, and thiamylal) have been evaluated in horses.[108, 120]

METRONIDAZOLE

Metronidazole is a synthetic, bactericidal antimicrobial agent with antibacterial and antiprotozoal properties. Metronidazole's antimicrobial spectrum includes obligate anaerobic bacteria, which are common equine pathogens such as *Bacteroides* spp., and *Clostridium* spp.[121] Metronidazole is also effective against various protozoal organisms including *Entamoeba histolytica*, *Trichomonas*, *Giardia*, and *Balantidium coli*. Metronidazole, in combination with other antimicrobial agents (e.g., a β-lactam and an aminoglycoside), is frequently chosen as the antimicrobial therapy in horses with mixed aerobic and anaerobic infections that commonly occur with pleuritis, lung and abdominal abscesses, and soft tissue infections.[121]

Mechanism of Action

Metronidazole is effective against only obligate anaerobic bacteria but not against facultative anaerobic or aerobic bacteria.[59] Once metronidazole enters the bacteria, it functions as an electron sink for oxidation-reduction reactions.[122] The reduced metronidazole is responsible for the drug's antimicrobial activity. Apparently facultative anaerobic bacteria are incapable of reducing metronidazole to the active reduced form of the drug; thus, metronidazole is ineffective against them. Once metronidazole is reduced, the intracellular concentration of the drug decreases, and more drug accumulates within the bacteria.[122] The reduced compound is believed to interfere with DNA and nucleic acid synthesis.[122]

Pharmacokinetics

The pharmacokinetics of metronidazole is reported in horses in several studies.[123–126] The bioavailability of metronidazole administered orally or intragastrically ranges from 57% to 111%.[123–125] Rectal administration of metronidazole results in mean peak serum concentrations of 4.5 μg/mL, which is less than that reported for oral or intragastric administration (ranging from 9.1 to 13.1 μg/mL),[125, 126] suggesting that metronidazole administered per rectum is not as well absorbed as by oral administration. However, the mean peak serum concentration following rectal administration of metronidazole is greater than the minimum inhibitory concentration that is effective against 90% of *Bacteriodes* spp. and *Clostridium* spp. of animal origin.[126] Once absorbed, metronidazole is widely distributed throughout the body, and clinically significant concentrations are detected in synovial fluid, peritoneal fluid, CSF, and urine in horses.[125] However, endometrial concentrations of metronidazole are poor and below the minimum inhibitory concentration of many equine anaerobic pathogens.[125] Metronidazole is metabolized by the liver by several pathways. The metabolites and parent compound are eliminated by renal and hepatic excretion. Recommended doses include 15 to 25 mg/kg by mouth every 6 to 12 hours.[123, 124] However, adequate peak serum and fluid (synovial fluid, peritoneal fluid, and CSF) concentrations were obtained in horses that were administered oral and intragastric metronidazole with a loading dose of 15 mg/kg, followed by 7.5 mg/kg every 6 hours.[125]

Toxicity and Adverse Effects

Toxicity and adverse effects associated with metronidazole are apparently uncommon in horses. Adverse effects associated with metronidazole in humans include gastrointestinal disturbances (nausea and vomiting), dark urine, and skin reactions.[122] Anorexia is reported to occur in horses treated with metronidazole (4 of 200 horses), but resolves with discontinuation of the drug.[121] Central nervous system disorders including convulsions and peripheral neuropathy are reported in humans who are treated with high doses or long durations of metronidazole.[122] There is a report of postanesthetic hindlimb paralysis occurring in two horses that were treated with intraperitoneal metronidazole; however, the paralysis may have been associated with anesthesia and recumbency.[127]

FLUOROQUINOLONES

Fluoroquinolones, or quinolones, are a relatively new class of antimicrobial agents that are used in human and veterinary medicine. The quinolones in use in human medicine include norfloxan, ciprofloxacin, ofloxacin, enoxacin, and pefloxacin. Enrofloxacin is the only quinolone approved for veterinary use in the United States. Quinolones possess a broad spectrum of activity, including aerobic gram-negative and many gram-positive bacteria, mycoplasmas, and chlamydiae.[128] Activity against Enterobacteriaceae, including *Pseudomonas*, is excellent.[128] Gastrointestinal pathogens are also sensitive to quinolones, which include *Escherichia coli*, *Vibrio cholera*, *Aeromonas*, *Campylobacter*, *Yersinia*, and *Salmonella*.[128, 129] Bacteria that produce β-lactamases, including *Staphylococcus aureus*, are sensitive to quinolones; however, Streptococci spp. are not as sensitive, thus limiting the usefulness of quinolones in the treatment of respiratory tract infections.[128, 129] Quinolones are not effective against obligate anaerobes.[128, 130, 131] Enrofloxacin is not approved for use in horses, and recently its use in food animals has been prohibited. Enrofloxacin is not currently recommended for use in horses due to toxicity problems associated with cartilage and bone development.[130, 132] However, its use in the treatment of equine osteomyelitis has been increasing.

Mechanism of Action

The quinolones' mechanism of action is unique among antimicrobial agents. The specific target for all quinolones is the bacterial DNA gyrase (bacterial type II topoisomerase).[130, 131, 133] DNA gyrase plays a crucial role in the unwinding, cutting, and consecutive resealing of DNA.[130, 131] Inhibition of DNA gyrase by quinolones results in serious disruption of the spatial arrangement of bacterial DNA.[131] Quinolones are bactericidal even when bacteria are in a stationary growth phase, which is in contrast to other bactericidal antibiotics including β-lactams and aminoglycosides. Quinolones can potentially inhibit mammalian DNA gyrase, but significantly higher concentrations of the drug are necessary.[130, 131] Resistance to quinolones is uncommon but can occur by chromosomal mutations that either alter DNA gyrase or decrease permeability of the bacterial cell wall to quinolones. Plasmid-mediated resistance has not yet been described.[131]

Pharmacokinetics

Oral administration of quinolones is rapidly and substantially absorbed in monogastric species, including horses, with an 80% bioavailability being reported.[130] However, the oral bioavailability of ciprofloxacin is poor in ponies (6%).[134] The time to peak serum concentrations following oral administration of enrofloxacin in horses is 0.5 hours.[130] The bioavailability of the drug is decreased with administration of magnesium- and aluminum-containing compounds.[130, 131, 133] Quinolones have a very large volume of distribution and low protein binding (ranging from 14% to 25% for most quinolones).[128, 130, 131] Tissue concentrations of quinolones may sometimes exceed serum concentrations.[128] High concentrations of quinolones occur in the liver, genitourinary system, sputum, lung, and bone and are concentrated in phagocytic cells.[128, 130, 131] However, quinolones do not achieve very high CSF concentrations.[131] Elimination is achieved primarily by the kidneys and secondarily by the liver. Renal elimination of quinolones occurs via glomerular filtration and probenecid-sensitive tubular secretion.[130] Urinary drug concentrations can be 100 to 300 times greater than serum concentrations.[128]

Toxicity and Adverse Effects

Use of quinolones in human medicine is believed to be well tolerated and associated with few side effects.[131] However, administration of quinolones to juvenile animals is associated with lesions of weight-bearing cartilage, which is the most important adverse effect in veterinary medicine. Quinolones are associated with lesions of weight-bearing cartilage in beagle puppies that are administered very high doses of 30 to 60 mg/kg for 2 weeks.[128, 130] There are reports of cartilage lesions resulting from use of enrofloxacin in young horses, although this has not been well substantiated.[130, 132] For this reason, enrofloxacin is not currently recommended for use in horses.[132] Among other adverse effects of quinolones in human medicine are gastrointestinal problems including nausea, vomiting, and colitis.[131] Central nervous system symptoms associated with quinolone therapy include headaches and dizziness, and seizures are rarely reported. Urinary tract problems may result from the formation of crystals of the drug in the urinary tract, associated with high urinary concentrations of the agent, and decreased solubility in an acid pH. Several drug interactions are noted for quinolones. Quinolones decrease the clearance of theophylline, potentially resulting in theophylline toxicity.[131] A combination of quinolones and chloramphenicol is contraindicated and may decrease the effectiveness of the quinolone.[131]

ANTIFUNGAL AGENTS

Fungal infections, in contrast to bacterial agents, are relatively uncommon in horses. Fungal infections may be superficial and systemic or regional. Superficial infections include dermatophytosis (ringworm), guttural pouch mycosis, fungal keratitis, and endometrial fungal infections. Systemic or regional fungal infections include systemic candidiasis in neonatal foals, coccidioidomycosis, phycomycosis, and fungal pneumonia in horses. Treatment of superficial fungal infections is often achieved with topical antifungal therapy, whereas systemic or regional fungal infections must be treated systemically. The clinical outcome of antifungal therapy is dependent on a number of factors, including the efficacy of the specific antifungal agent, the ability of the drug to reach the organism (pharmacokinetics), and the toxicity of the drug. Polyene antifungal agents, including amphotericin B, nystatin, and natamycin, have a similar mechanism of action and bind the primary sterol (ergosterol) of the fungal cell wall. Polyene antifungals are not absorbed well after oral administration and are therefore administered intravenously or topically. Azole antifungal agents include clotrimazole, ketoconazole, miconazole, itraconazole, enilconazole, and fluconazole, and these agents exert their antifungal effects by inhibiting the synthesis of ergosterol. Clotrimazole and miconazole are restricted to topical administration, whereas ketoconazole and itraconazole may be used orally. Griseofulvin is an antifungal agent that inhibits fungal mitosis and is only effective against dermatophytes. Flucytosine is an antifungal agent that is converted to 5-fluorouracil and impairs DNA synthesis. Flucytosine use has not been described in equine medicine.

Amphotericin B

Amphotericin B is a polyene antifungal agent that is produced from *Streptomyces nodosus*. Amphotericin B possesses fungistatic properties but may be fungicidal at higher doses. The spectrum of antifungal activity is broad for amphotericin B and includes *Histoplasma capsulatum, Cryptococcus neoformans, Coccidioides immitis, Candida* spp., and many strains of *Aspergillus*. It has been used for the treatment of sporotrichosis and phycomycosis.[135] The systemic use of amphotericin B is limited in horses due to its pharmacokinetic properties and potential toxicity. Topical administration of amphotericin B in horses is reported for fungal keratitis[136] and fungal endometritis.[137] Amphotericin B has been used systemically to treat fungal pneumonia,[138, 139] systemic candidiasis,[140] fungal meningitis,[141] coccidioidomycosis,[142] and phycomycosis[143] in horses. Nystatin and natamycin are antifungal agents similar to amphotericin B. These agents cannot be used systemically, but they have been used topically for treatment of fungal keratitis[136] and guttural pouch mycosis in horses.[144, 145]

Mechanism of Action

Amphotericin B binds to the ergosterol in the fungal plasma membrane and changes the membrane fluidity and increases cellular permeability. Leakage of fungal cellular constituents results in the loss of electrolytes and eventual cell death. Amphotericin is also thought to possess some immunomodulatory effects, resulting in the stimulation or suppression of cell-mediated and humoral immunity.[146] Amphotericin B does not bind mammalian membranes to the same degree as it does fungal membranes, with the major cell sterol of mammalian membranes being cholesterol and not ergosterol.[147]

Pharmacokinetics

Pharmacokinetics of amphotericin B are unknown in horses and must be extrapolated from humans. It is poorly absorbed from the gastrointestinal tract, requiring that it be administered intravenously to achieve systemic absorption. It is recommended that for intravenous administration that the drug should be diluted in 5% dextrose (not in saline of lactated Ringer's solution) and be administered by slow intravenous injection over 1 hour.[135, 138] The initial dose of amphotericin should be low and increased slowly over the next few days.[138] Once absorbed, amphotericin is highly protein bound, and the agent is detected in pleural, peritoneal, and synovial fluid. CSF concentrations of amphotericin B are poor. Amphotericin is excreted slowly in the urine in humans.

Toxicity and Adverse Reactions

The most significant and common adverse effect associated with amphotericin B therapy in humans and companion animals is nephrotoxicity.[135] Although amphotericin B has not been reported to result in nephrotoxicity in horses, polyuria and polydypsia have been reported in a horse 4 weeks after the onset of amphotericin B therapy.[139] Other adverse reactions associated with amphotericin B in humans include chills, headaches, fever, phlebitis, anemia, hypokalemia due to renal tubular acidosis, and anaphylaxis-like reactions.[135] Transient fever, lethargy, and tachycardia are reported in horses and foals receiving intravenous amphotericin B for treatment of fungal pneumonia and systemic candidiasis.[139, 140] Frequent evaluation of serum creatinine and urinalysis to try to prevent renal failure is recommended when amphotericin B is administered to horses.[139, 140]

AZOLE ANTIFUNGAL AGENTS

Theazole derivatives include imidazole and triazoles and are broad-spectrum fungistatic agents that include clotrimazole, miconazole, ketoconazole, itraconazole, and enilconazole. Clotrimazole and miconazole were the first discovered but are unsuitable for oral use. Clotrimazole and miconazole have a smaller spectrum of activity compared with ketoconazole and are effective against *Candida* spp. and dermatophytes. Dermatophytosis, guttural pouch mycosis, and fungal keratitis have been treated with topical administration of both drugs.

Ketoconazole was the first orally active imidazole approved for use in 1979 in the United States. Ketoconazole is an imidazole antifungal derivative and is effective against a wide range of fungi, including *Candida* spp., *C. immitis*, and *H. capsulatum*. It is less effective against *C. neoformans*, *Sporotrichosis schenckii*, and *Aspergillus* spp. Ketoconazole has been used to treat coccidioidomycosis,[142] phycomycosis,[148] and guttural pouch mycosis in horses.[144, 145] However, treatment of coccidioidomycosis with ketoconazole is generally not effective.[142]

Itraconazole and enilconazole are two new antifungal agents. Itraconazole was approved for use in 1992 in the United States, but enilconazole is currently not available. Itraconazole has 5 to 100 times better in vitro and in vivo potency than does ketoconazole and has good activity against *Aspergillus* spp. Itraconazole is used to treat meningeal cryptococcosis and sporotrichosis in humans.[149] Use of itraconazole in equine medicine is relatively new. Successful treatment of coccidioidomycosis osteomyelitis is reported in a horse with systemic itraconazole, which is in contrast to ketoconazole.[142, 150] Systemic itraconazole and topical enilconazole therapy are reported to be successful in the treatment of guttural pouch mycosis in a horse that had dysphagia, which was not responding to topical miconazole therapy.[151] Eniloconazole is used for the treatment of dermatomycosis in large animals in the United Kingdom.

Mechanism of Action

Azole derivatives are fungistatic antifungal agents that inhibit the production of the primary sterol of the fungal cell wall, ergosterol.[152] Azoles inhibit the P-450–dependent lanosterol C_{14}-demethylase enzyme, which results in the depletion of ergosterol and an accumulation of C_{14}-methyl sterols in the cytoplasmic membrane. Absence of ergosterol leads to a lack of the fungal cell wall integrity, causing increased cellular permeability and cell death.[152] Azole derivatives affect cholesterol synthesis, the primary sterol in mammalian membranes, but to a lesser degree than they do fungal membranes.[152] Itraconazole appears to affect mammalian membranes to a lesser degree than does ketoconazole.[149]

Pharmacokinetics

Neither clotrimazole or miconazole is suitable for oral use, because clotrimazole results in autoinduction of hepatic enzymes causing undetectable plasma concentrations after several days and miconazole is poorly absorbed from the gastrointestinal tract. Ketoconazole was the first imidazole antifungal agent that was reported to result in good absorption following oral administration in humans and companion animals. However, the oral bioavailability in horses is poor (23%).[153] It may be necessary to dissolve the ketoconazole in 0.2N HCl and to administer the drug via a nasogastric tube to result in detectable serum concentrations.[153] The use of ketoconazole is limited in horses due to the low absorption from the gastrointestinal tract, the apparent need to administer the drug intragastrically, the cost, and the high likelihood that therapy will take a long time (several weeks to months).[153] The failure of treatment of coccidioidomycosis in horses with ketoconazole is likely due to the poor absorption following oral administration.[142, 153]

Toxicity and Adverse Reactions

Azole derivatives have fewer side effects compared with amphotericin B. The most common adverse effects in humans include nausea, anorexia, and vomiting. Ketoconazole is reported to result in altered testosterone, cortisol, and androgen synthesis due to inhibition of mammalian P-450. Adverse effects of azole derivative therapy have not been reported for horses.

GRISEOFULVIN

Griseofulvin is a fungistatic agent that is produced by *Penicillium griseofulvin dierckx*. Griseofulvin is primarily used to treat dermatophyte infections and is not effective against any other fungi, yeast, or bacteria. Griseofulvin works by disrupting the mitotic spindle of the fungi by interacting with the polymerized microtubules and inhibits fungal mitosis. The selective toxicity of the drug depends on energy-dependent uptake into susceptible fungi, which occurs preferentially to uptake in mammalian cells.

Pharmacokinetics

Absorption of griseofulvin is variable and dependent on the particle size of the drug. Microsized preparations are 25% to 75% absorbed, whereas the ultra-microsized preparations are 100% absorbed. Following absorption, griseofulvin can be detected in 48 to 72 hours within the stratum corneum. The drug is tightly bound to new keratinocytes, as the older fungal-infected keratin is shed. Treatment is usually of long duration until all the older keratin is shed.

Toxicity and Adverse Effects

Adverse effects of griseofulvin are associated with long-term treatment and results in mild and transient central nervous system and gastrointestinal problems. Griseofulvin is teratogenic in cats, and it is recommended that the drug not be given to pregnant animals. However, administration of griseofulvin to a pregnant mare had no apparent adverse effects.[154]

FLUCYTOSINE

Flucytosine is an antimetabolite from the fluoropyrimidine series that was originally designed as an anticancer agent. Flucytosine has a limited spectrum of activity but is effective against *C. neoformans* and several strains of *Candida*. It is not effective against *Aspergillius* spp., *S. schenckii*, *H. capsulatum*, and *C. immitis*. Flucytosine must first gain entry inside fungal cells and then be converted to 5-fluorouracil by fungal cytosine deaminase. 5-Fluorouracil is either incorporated into RNA or converted to a related compound that inhibits DNA synthesis. Mammalian cells lack cytosine deaminase and therefore are resistant to the effects of flucytosine.[135] Flucytosine is well absorbed in humans after oral administration and is distributed widely in the body, with significant concentrations being detected within CSF.[135] Use of flucytosine has not been reported in horses.

NON-STEROIDAL ANTI-INFLAMMATORY DRUGS

Non-steroidal anti-inflammatory drugs (NSAIDs) are commonly used in equine medicine. These agents exert their anti-inflammatory properties by inhibiting the cyclooxygenase enzyme, which converts arachidonic acid into mediators of inflammation, prostaglandins and thromboxane.[155, 156]

Commonly used NSAIDs in horses include phenylbutazone, flunixin meglumine, dipyrone, ketoprofen, meclofenamic acid, and naproxen. Chemically the NSAIDs are classified as either carboxylic or enolic acids, with subgroups classified by their structural differences. Phenylbutazone, oxyphenbutazone, and dipyrone are enolic acids and classified in a subgroup as pyrazolones.[156, 157] Carboxylic acid subgroups include the salicylates (sodium salicylate, acetyl salicylic acid), propionic acids (naproxen, ibuprofen), anthranilic acids (meclofenamic acid), aminonicotinic acids (flunixin meglumine), and indolines (indomethacin).[156] NSAIDs have other beneficial effects besides anti-inflammatory properties, which include analgesic, anti-endotoxic, anti-pyretic, and anti-platelet properties.

Anti-Inflammatory Properties

Mediators of the inflammatory process, including histamine, bradykinin, 5-hydroxytryptamine, leukotrienes, platelet activating factor, prostaglandins, and thromboxane, are produced when tissue damage occurs. Arachidonic acid is converted by cyclooxygenase to prostaglandins and thromboxane A_2 (TXA_2).[158] NSAIDs, such as phenylbutazone and flunixin meglumine, prevent the formation of prostaglandins (e.g., prostaglandin E_2 [PGE_2] and prostacyclin), which produce erythema and edema via vasodilation.[155-157, 159, 160] Plasma and urinary concentrations of NSAIDs do not always correlate with plasma prostaglandin and thromboxane concentrations or clinical effects. This may be due to increased concentrations of NSAIDs in inflammatory exudate or in synovial fluid of inflamed joints.[161, 162]

Analgesic Properties

NSAIDs reduce pain by reducing local prostaglandin production associated with inflammation. Prostaglandins produce pain in inflamed tissues and potentiate the pain response to chemical and mechanical stimuli by lowering the threshold of polymodal nociceptors of C fibers.[158] Therefore, an NSAID does not exhibit its analgesic properties until prostaglandins formed prior to its administration have dissipated. There is evidence that prostaglandins in the spinal cord play an important role in processing of pain information, and NSAIDs may have a central action by inhibiting the formation of prostaglandins within the spinal cord.[163, 164] For example, it is speculated that flunixin meglumine may have some central effect that accounts for its superior analgesic property in horses with colic. Flunixin meglumine (1 mg/kg) had a longer duration of analgesia in horses with postoperative pain, when compared with phenylbutazone (4 mg/kg) and carprofen (0.7 mg/kg).[165] However, phenylbutazone is usually preferred as an analgesic for musculoskeletal problems resulting in lameness (i.e., degenerative joint disease or laminitis).[156, 157]

Anti-Endotoxic Properties

Endotoxemia in horses is a serious disorder, and NSAIDs are frequently administered to horses with endotoxemia to alleviate the clinical signs associated with this problem. Flunixin meglumine is reported to be the most effective

NSAID in the treatment of experimental endotoxemia, compared with phenylbutazone and selective thromboxane inhibitors.[166–168] Pre-treatment with flunixin meglumine prevents endotoxin-induced increases in blood lactate and plasma prostaglandin concentrations and improves clinical signs of horses given endotoxin.[166, 168]

However, there is no difference between treatment with flunixin (1 mg/kg intravenously) or ketoprofen (2.2 mg/kg intravenously) on plasma prostaglandin, tumor necrosis factor, and leukotriene concentrations in horses given endotoxin.[169] Use of a low dose of flunixin meglumine (0.25 mg/kg intravenously), which is unlikely to mask clinical parameters necessary for further patient evaluation, significantly decreased plasma thromboxane concentrations and alleviated abdominal pain in ponies when administered prior to the endotoxin.[166]

Anti-pyretic Properties

Infection and inflammation lead to the formation of interleukin-1 and tumor necrosis factor, resulting in the increased production of PGE_2 in the vascular organs in the preoptic hypothalamic areas of the central nervous system.[158] PGE_2, mediated by cyclic adenosine monophosphate (AMP), acts locally within the hypothalamus to elevate the hypothalamic set point, the temperature about which body temperature is maintained. The anti-pyretic properties of NSAIDs have attributed to prevent the formation of PGE_2 and promote return of the body temperature's set point to normal. The NSAIDs do not influence body temperature when it is elevated by exercise or increased by ambient temperature. Phenylbutazone, flunixin meglumine, and dipyrone are frequently used as anti-pyretic agents, but dipyrone has poor analgesic and anti-inflammatory properties.

Anti-platelet Properties

TXA_2 is the principal eicosanoid synthesized by platelets and potent agonist of platelet aggregation and vasoconstriction.[158] NSAIDs possess anti-platelet properties by inhibiting platelet production of TXA_2 and preventing platelet aggregation.[170, 171] Phenylbutazone, flunixin meglumine, and aspirin decrease the production of TXA_2 in horses.[159, 172–174] However, aspirin results in a much longer duration of inhibition of TXA_2 synthesis in horses compared with phenylbutazone and flunixin meglumine.[159] Serum TXB_2 (the stable metabolite of TXA_2) synthesis is inhibited 100% by aspirin, 50% by phenylbutazone, and 63% by flunixin meglumine 24 hours after administration of the drugs.[159] Phenylbutazone, flunixin meglumine, and aspirin decrease platelet aggregation in horses; however, aspirin is the most potent and longest lasting drug and is the only one to increase template bleeding times in horses.[174, 175] Aspirin irreversibly inhibits cyclooxygenase, whereas phenylbutazone and other commonly used NSAIDs reversibly inhibit the enzyme (see the mechanism of action section).[159, 175] Platelets do not have the DNA material necessary to synthesize protein; therefore, irreversible inhibition of cyclooxygenase results in platelets being incapable of synthesizing TXA_2.[171] The anti-platelet actions of aspirin, therefore, last the life span of the platelet, which ranges from 8 to 10 days. Aspirin is effective when

administered every 48 hours, even though it has a shorter half-life than do other NSAIDs. Low aspirin doses and a long dosing interval minimize the risk of the toxic effects of NSAID therapy. In addition, low doses of aspirin will not affect the synthesis of prostacyclin, the principal prostaglandin synthesized by endothelial cells, a vasodilator and inhibitor of platelet aggregation. Administration of aspirin on alternate days may be valuable in the treatment of diseases associated with thrombus formation, including endotoxemia, thromboembolic colic, and thrombophlebitis.

Mechanism of Action

All NSAIDs inhibit the formation of prostaglandins and thromboxane through inhibition of the cyclooxygenase enzyme. Prostaglandins and thromboxane are a group of related lipid molecules that are derived from phospholipid portions of cellular membranes. Phospholipase A_2 releases arachidonic acid from phospholipids (phosphatidylcholine, phosphatidylethanolamine, and phosphatidylinositol).[176] Arachidonic acid is then metabolized by either lipooxygenase (resulting in leukotrienes) or cyclooxygenase (resulting in prostaglandins and thromboxane) pathways.[158] Cyclooxygenase, also known as prostaglandin G/H synthetase has both cyclooxygenase and peroxidase activities and catalyzes two reactions.[177] The first reaction is the cyclooxygenase reaction, in which arachidonic acid is converted to prostaglandin G_2 (PGG_2). The second reaction is a peroxidase reaction, reducing PGG_2 to prostaglandin H_2 (PGH_2).[176] NSAIDs only block the cyclooxygenase activity without affecting the peroxidase activity. There are actually two cyclooxygenase isoenzymes (COX-1 and COX-2).[176] COX-1 is expressed in many tissues and is involved in maintaining physiologic cellular functions, such as interaction between vascular endothelium and platelets. COX-2 is expressed only after cellular activation in response to various stimuli, including trauma and the presence of various cytokines.[176] Adverse effects of NSAIDs occur with inhibition of COX-1, whereas the beneficial anti-inflammatory effects are observed with inhibition of COX-2. The effect of different NSAIDs on either COX-1 or COX-2 may vary, but this variation is not recognized to be of clinical significance.[176] The exact mode of inhibition and magnitude of inhibition of COX varies and is complex. Aspirin irreversibly inhibits cyclooxygenase by acetylating a serine residue, whereas phenylbutazone, flunixin meglumine, and indomethacin inhibit cyclooxygenase reversibly.[177] Flunixin meglumine is the most potent NSAID used in equine medicine, with meclofenamic acid and phenylbutazone being moderate, and dipyrone and aspirin being the least potent.[159]

Pharmacokinetics

The bioavailability of phenylbutazone after oral administration is variable and is affected by type of feed and the product used (paste or powder) and may also be dependent on the time of day of administration.[159, 178] The volume of distribution is small for NSAIDs, owing to the high protein binding of the drugs.[156, 157] The majority of NSAIDs are metabolized to inactive metabolites, with the exception of phenylbutazone and dipyrone.[158, 179, 180] The main metabolites of phenylbutazone are oxyphenbutazone and gammahydroxyphenbutazone.[157, 178] Oxyphenbutazone is an active metabolite; however, it has less pharmacologic activity than does phenylbutazone.[157, 178]

Toxicity and Adverse Effects

The toxic and adverse effects of NSAIDs include gastrointestinal, renal, hematologic, and hepatic disease in humans and other species.[180, 181] Gastrointestinal and renal disease may result from excessively high doses and prolonged administration of NSAIDs to horses and foals.[182–189] Gastrointestinal disease resulting from use of NSAIDs frequently results in a protein-losing enteropathy with gastrointestinal ulcers predominantly occurring in the large colon.[182, 189] NSAIDs may result in renal papillary necrosis in horses, but pre-existing factors such as hypovolemia must usually be present.[183, 185] Gastrointestinal and renal toxicity induced by NSAID use can occur at the same time.[183]

Gastrointestinal Toxicity

Gastrointestinal disease caused by NSAIDs results in ulcers throughout the gastrointestinal tract and is due to loss of protective prostaglandins.[180] Prostaglandins have a physiologic role in protection and growth of the gastrointestinal tract. Prostaglandins (particularly PGE_2) increase mucosal blood flow and mucus secretion, decrease gastric acid and pepsin secretion, accelerate cell proliferation, and stabilize cell membranes.[180] Loss of these important prostaglandins caused by use of NSAIDs results in gastrointestinal ulcers occurring in the large colon (especially right dorsal) and cecum, small intestines, and oral mucosa.[180, 183, 186, 187] Absorption of phenylbutazone to the fibrous and cellulose components of hay and roughage and release of the drug on fermentation may account for the presence of lower gastrointestinal ulcers.[187] Ulcers range from shallow to deep and perforating, and bacterial invasion is common.[187] The large ulcers demonstrate marked vasculitis and thrombosis of submucosal vessels. The distribution of gastrointestinal ulcers caused by NSAIDs may differ between foals and adult horses, with gastric ulcers being more frequently reported in foals.[188]

The clinical signs of gastrointestinal disease induced by NSAIDs are usually nonspecific but include colic, fever, bruxism, and ventral edema.[183, 184, 187, 189] Diarrhea may or may not be present. Similar clinical signs are often present in horses with colitis (i.e., salmonellosis, Potomac horse fever), for which NSAIDs are indicated. The first hematologic and clinical chemistry abnormalities noticed are often hypoproteinemia and hypoalbuminemia.[182, 184, 186, 189] Serum albumin concentration is a very sensitive indicator of NSAID toxicity, and hypoalbuminemia is reported in horses receiving the recommended dose of phenylbutazone without any gross evidence of colonic ulcers at necropsy.[182] Neutropenia with a left shift and electrolyte abnormalities are frequently reported.[183, 184, 186]

Several factors influence the gastrointestinal toxicity of NSAIDs, including signalment, the specific NSAID, formulation of the NSAID (i.e., paste or powder), and the route of administration (parental or oral).[184] However, the dose and duration of administration of the drug used are the most important factors influencing gastrointestinal toxicity.[182, 184] Most reports of gastrointestinal toxicity due to NSAIDs involve phenylbutazone, with toxic doses including 8 to 14 mg/kg PO by mouth every 24 hours for 7 to 14 days, although toxicity may occur at lower dose rates.[182, 184, 186] Phenylbutazone is suggested to be the most likely to result in toxicity, with flunixin meglumine being moderately likely and ketoprofen being the least likely.[184] Both oral and systemic administration of NSAIDs may result in toxicity.[184, 186]

Renal Toxicity

The pathophysiology of renal disease induced by NSAIDs is due to the loss of protective prostaglandins in the kidney. Prostaglandins play an important role in modulating renal blood flow, glomerular filtration rate, renin release, concentrating mechanisms, and sodium and potassium hemostasis during hypovolemic crises.[181] PGE_2 exerts a marked protective role by functioning as a local vasodilator to maintain renal blood flow and glomerular filtration rate in the face of adverse circumstances (i.e., dehydration, hypotension).[181] Prostaglandins may accentuate renin release in response to β-adrenergic stimulation due to hemorrhage or dehydration. Prostaglandins also play a role in the regulation of sodium and chloride and influence water metabolism by antagonizing the effects of anti-diuretic hormone and medullary blood flow.[181]

Renal papillary necrosis, acute renal insufficiency, nephrotic syndrome, interstitial nephritis, sodium and fluid retention, and hyperkalemia can occur in humans who receive NSAIDs.[181] However, the only form of NSAID-induced nephrotoxicity recognized in horses is renal papillary necrosis.[185] In normal horses, the combination of NSAIDs and dehydration is necessary to induce renal papillary necrosis.[185] Papillary necrosis is thought to be secondary to medullary ischemia.[185]

The clinical signs in horses associated with renal disease associated with use of NSAIDs are also non-specific but include polyuria, polydypsia, weight loss, and depression. Hematologic and chemistry abnormalities include, but are not limited to, azotemia, hyponatremia, and hypochloremia. Urinalysis reveals isosthenuric urine in the face of an elevated serum creatinine concentration. Proteinuria and granular casts may also be detected on urinalysis.

Cellulitis

Cellulitis and thrombophlebitis are reported to occur with intramuscular, intravenous, or perivascular injections of various NSAIDs due to the acidic nature of the drug and concentration of the drug in solution. Flunixin meglumine is recommended for intravenous and intramuscular administration. However, intramuscular administration of flunixin meglumine has been associated with rare cases of clostridial myositis and cellulitis (including botulism) which is usually fatal. Phenylbutazone is recommended only for intravenous or oral administration. Perivascular injections result in extravascular inflammation and may cause sloughing of surrounding tissues and thrombophlebitis.

Other Adverse Effects

NSAIDs are associated with blood dyscrasias, hepatotoxicities (Reye's syndrome), premature closure of the ductus arteriosus, bronchoconstriction in asthmatic patients, and antagonization of the effects of anti-hypertensive drugs in humans. Blood dyscrasias are described in horses receiving phenylbutazone, but this syndrome is not well documented. Transient elevations in liver enzymes occur in horses given toxic doses of phenylbutazone, but values return to normal when the dose of phenylbutazone is decreased. Administration of NSAIDs to pregnant women may result in premature closure of the ductus arteriosus, leading to fetal pulmonary hypertension. This has not been reported to be a problem in foals, even with frequent administration of NSAIDs to pregnant mares. However, phenylbutazone does cross the placenta in horses, resulting in the potential for accumulation of NSAIDs in the fetus.[190] Aspirin is documented to potentate bronchoconstriction in asthmatic human patients. However, administration of NSAIDs to horses with chronic obstructive pulmonary disease does not change resistance or dynamic compliance.[191]

GLUCOCORTICOIDS

Corticosteroids are a group of drugs that are naturally and synthetically produced. The natural corticosteroids are synthesized from the adrenal cortex and are characterized as glucocorticoids (cortisol), mineralocorticoids (aldosterone), and adrenal sex hormones (testosterone and estrogen). Natural glucocorticoids affect protein, fat, and carbohydrate metabolism and possess some anti-inflammatory properties. Synthetic glucocorticoids possess predominantly anti-inflammatory properties and minimal metabolic effects compared with cortisol. Commonly used synthetic glucocorticoids in equine medicine include betamethasone, dexamethasone, prednisolone, prednisone, and triamcinolone and are largely used due to their potent anti-inflammatory effects.

In addition to their anti-inflammatory effects, glucocorticoids have a wide spectrum of activity including immunosuppressive, metabolic, and endocrine activities, some of which are beneficial, but many of which are detrimental. The exact mechanism of action of glucocorticoids remains unknown. However, all glucocorticoids are highly bound to proteins, including corticosteroid-binding globulin and albumin. Glucocorticoids then pass through the cell wall of the effector cell and bind an intracellular protein receptor. The receptor-glucocorticoid complex travels to the nucleus, binds DNA, and initiates transcription and synthesis of new proteins. The subsequent actions of the newly synthesized proteins leads to the wide spectrum of effects of glucocorticoids.

Anti-Inflammatory Properties

Glucocorticoids are potent anti-inflammatory agents. Their anti-inflammatory effects include stabilization of cellular membranes, decreased vascular permeability, inhibition of leukocyte migration and adherence,[192] inhibition of platelet aggregation, and reduction of the inflammatory processes that results in fibrosis.[193] The exact mechanism of the anti-inflammatory effects of glucocorticoids is still debated but is generally attributed to decreased production of eicosanoids (including prostaglandins, thromboxane, and leukotrienes), platelet activating factor, and tumor necrosis factor).[192] Tissue damage results in the release of arachidonic acid from actions of phospholipase A_2 (which is present in multiple forms) on cellular phospholipids.[194] Arachidonic acid is metabolized by cyclooxygenase (resulting in prostaglandins and thromboxane), lipooxygenase (resulting in production of leukotrienes), or platelet activating factor.[195] The ability of glucocorticoids to decrease production of eicosanoids is believed to be due to inhibition of phospholipase A_2.[196, 197] Glucocorticoids stimulate production of lipomodulin, which inactivates phospholipase A_2.[196, 197] Additional effects of glucocorticoids include synthesis of other proteins resulting in reduced cytokine formation, inhibition of histamine release, and inhibition of the induction of nitric oxide synthetase (the enzyme responsible for synthesis of nitric oxide).[198] However, not all studies support the hypothesis that glucocorticoids exert their anti-inflammatory effects by inhibition of eicosanoid production.[199–201] Dexamethasone (0.06 mg/kg) and betamethasone (0.08 mg/kg) resulted in clinical evidence of reduced inflammation, but eicosanoid concentrations of fluid exudates were not reduced in horses.[200, 201]

The intra-articular administration of glucocorticoids has been used for many years in equine medicine for treatment of various joint diseases. Triamcinolone acetonide, isoflupredone acetate, betamethasone acetate, betamethasone sodium phosphate, methylprednisolone acetate, and flumethasone are approved for intra-articular administration in the horse.[202] When injected intra-articularly, these drugs exhibit potent local anti-inflammatory and analgesic effects and inhibit catabolic and anabolic processes. Intra-articular glucocorticoids reduce the inflammatory vasodilation mediated through prostaglandin E_2 and prostacyclin and diminish the production of superoxide radicals and interleukin-1 (which stimulates chondrocyte production of catabolic enzymes).[203] Glucocorticoids also possess anti-anabolic effects, and the detrimental effects of intra-articular glucocorticoid therapy are covered later.

Immunosuppressive Properties

Glucocorticoids suppress the immune system by several mechanisms; however, a complete understanding of glucocorticoid-induced suppression is lacking. Species are characterized as being steroid-sensitive (mouse, rat, and rabbit) or steroid-resistant (humans, dogs, cattle, pigs, goats, and horses).[192, 204] The classification of steroid-sensitive and steroid-resistant is based on the ease and degree of induction of lymphopenia with exogenous glucocorticoids.[192, 204] The effects of glucocorticoids in steroid-sensitive species include severe lymphopenia due to cellular lysis.[192]

Glucocorticoids result in a change in leukocyte kinetics, phagocytic activity of macrophages, and cell-mediated immunity. These agents result in a peripheral mature neutrophilia, slight lymphopenia, and eosinopenia in horses and is called a "stress leukogram."[192, 205] The increase in neutrophil count is due to an increase in release of mature neutrophils from the bone marrow, their decreased margination and decreased vascular adherence, and decreased diapedesis of neutrophils out of the blood vessels. Redistribution of lymphocytes to nonvascular lymphatic compartments such as lymph nodes, bone marrow, and spleen results in lymphopenia and eosinopenia. Macrophages are more sensitive to the immunosuppressive effects of corticosteroids than are neutrophils,[206] and macrophage killing of ingested organisms is decreased.[207] The mechanism by which glucocorticoids effect macrophage phagocytosis is unknown; however, glucocorticoid-induced production of lipomodulin and inhibition of phospholipase A_2 is not responsible.[207] Cell-mediated immunity is decreased, documented by a decrease in lymphocyte blastogenesis response to T-cell mitogens and decreased production of a number of interleukins and cytokines. In contrast to cell-mediated immunity, humoral immunity (measured by immunoglobulin concentration) does not appear to be significantly affected by glucocorticoids.[192] Exogenous glucocorticoids increase serum iron concentration in horses and may allow for an increase in available iron for bacterial growth.[208]

Glucocorticoids are often used to treat conditions such as autoimmune diseases and hypersensitivity problems because of their immunosuppressive effects. Autoimmune disease in horses include hemolytic anemia, idiopathic thrombocytopenia, and pemphigus foliaceus. Although these agents are not effective at decreasing immunoglobulin synthesis, they are effective in treatment of autoimmune diseases because they decrease cellular interactions between T cells and B cells.[192] Hypersensitivity reactions in horses are frequently treated with glucocorticoids. Diseases believed to arise from hypersensitivity reactions include chronic obstructive pulmonary disease, immune-mediated vasculitis due to type III hypersensitivity (which includes purpura hemorrhagica and equine herpes virus I myeloencephalitis), and various pruritic problems (e.g., hives), resulting from a type I hypersensitivity reaction.

The immunosuppressive effects of glucocorticoids are related to the steroid potency, dose, and dose interval.[192] Immunosuppression is often associated with higher doses and more potent glucocorticoids. Administration of 1 mg/kg of dexamethasone to ponies once daily for 9 days resulted in a rapid but transient decrease in circulating lymphocytes, with the greatest decrease occurring in the T-lymphocyte population.[204] The lymphocyte count returned to baseline 24 hours after the last injection of dexamethasone.[204] A disseminated mycotic infection has been reported in an adult Quarter Horse receiving 600 mg of prednisolone, followed by 100 mg/day of dexamethasone for 15 days.[209] Even administration of a small dose of glucocorticoids may result in immunosuppression in a local area. In one study, bacteria were detected in 60% of joints in horses injected with *S. aureus* and 200 mg of methylprednisolone acetate compared with 40% of the joints injected with *S. aureus* alone.[210]

Metabolic Effects

Endogenous and exogenous glucocorticoids result in hyperglycemia, hyperlipidemia, and hyperinsulinemia in horses.[211–213] Glucocorticoids stimulate gluconeogenesis by mobilization of fat and protein for production of glucose, decrease peripheral utilization of glucose, and increase liver stores of glycogen. Adrenocorticotropic hormone (ACTH)

and cortisol stimulate hormone-sensitive lipase, increase the mobilization of free fatty acids from adipose cells, and increase plasma triglyceride concentrations. Glucocorticoids also antagonize the effects of insulin by inhibiting the cellular response to insulin at the receptor or at the post-receptor level.[213] Amino acids are mobilized from muscle and travel to the liver where they are synthesized into glucose and glycogen. The catabolic effects of these agents result in reduced muscle mass, thinning of the skin, loss of hair, and a negative nitrogen balance. Glucocorticoids may also decrease wound healing due to their catabolic effects. Glucocorticoids also inhibit the later stages of inflammation, including proliferation of capillaries and fibroblasts, deposition of collagen, and scar formation. Pituitary adenomas, which are common in older horses, produce ACTH and subsequently cortisol and cause hyperglycemia, glucosuria, and insulin resistance (documented by an increase insulin concentration in the face of hyperglycemia).[212] Hyperlipidemia associated with pituitary adenomas has been reported in horses.[211, 212]

Endocrine Effects

Glucocorticoids have pronounced effects on the endocrine system. Cortisol is produced in the body by the adrenal cortex, which is under control of ACTH released by the pars distalis of the anterior pituitary. Administration of ACTH (or increases in endogenous release) results in an increase in plasma cortisol concentrations. The rate of pituitary release of ACTH is under neuroendocrine control from the hypothalamus mediated via corticotropic-releasing hormone (CRH) and negative feedback inhibition by plasma cortisol concentrations. Exogenous glucocorticoids also result in negative feedback inhibition of ACTH and CRH release. Iatrogenic adrenal cortical insufficiency may result from sudden withdrawal of glucocorticoids in horses, especially with excessive and prolonged use and is discussed in a later section.[214–218]

Pharmacokinetics

Various glucocorticoids are available for use in equine medicine and in several different formulations and different routes of administration. The basic glucocorticoid molecule consists of a four-ring structure, and modification of this structure results in increased anti-inflammatory effects and decreased mineralocorticoid effects. Prednisone, prednisolone, methylprednisolone, and triamcinolone possess moderate anti-inflammatory effects and decreased mineralocorticoid effects. Dexamethasone and flumethasone are potent anti-inflammatory glucocorticoids, with minimal mineralocorticoid activities. Certain glucocorticoids, such as cortisone and prednisone, must first be metabolized by the liver to the active metabolite (cortisol and prednisolone). Addition of a double bond between C_1 and C_2 (such as with prednisolone) improves glucocorticoid activity. The addition of a methyl group at C_6 (such as with methylprednisolone) further improves the glucocorticoid effects. Further substitution of the 17-ester position results in a group of steroids with potent anti-inflammatory effects (betamethasone). The natural glucocorticoids (cortisol and hydrocortisone) possess mild anti-inflammatory effects. The formulation of the glucocorticoid alters the duration of action. Water-soluble (sodium phosphate, sodium succinate) and alcohol-soluble (the drug itself, e.g., dexamethasone) glucocorticoids result in a rapid absorption and effect from either intravenous or intramuscular injection. Water-insoluble ester formulations include acetate, diacetate, acetonide, valerate, and isonicotinatc and are generally long-acting due to the slow absorption of the drug when administered systemically. Intramuscular administration of prednisone acetate to horses resulted in a slow absorption, with prednisone detected in the plasma for 7 days.[218] A common misconception is that water-insoluble esters are long-acting when administered intra-articularly.[203, 219] The duration of action is based on the rate of hydrolysis of the ester within the joint.[203] Therefore, water-insoluble esters (e.g., methylprednisolone acetate, which is hydrolyzable in plasma) will be rapid-acting when administered intra-articularly (as opposed to being long-acting when administered intramuscularly). Water-soluble esters (e.g., methylprednisolone sodium succinate, which is not hydrolyzable in plasma) are unlikely to be efficacious intra-articularly.[220] Intra-articular administration of methylprednisolone acetate in horses resulted in detection of methylprednisolone acetate for only 2 to 6 days following injection, but methylprednisolone was detected up to 39 days after injection.[220] Triamcinolone acetonide has been shown to be a relatively short-acting steroid in horses when injected intra-articularly, and the drug is cleared from the joints in 4 days.[221] It has been assumed that with local administration the systemic side effects of the drug are avoided.[219] However, intra-articular administration of glucocorticoids results in systemic absorption and transient adrenal suppression. Intra-articular triamcinolone entered the blood only 1 hour after intra-articular administration in horses, and concentrations were detectable only for 48 hours after injection.[221]

Toxicity and Adverse Effects

Complications associated with intra-articular use of glucocorticoids are well recognized and include post-injection flare, osseous metaplasia, increased risk of septic arthritis, and steroid arthropathy.[202, 222] Post-injection flare is an inflammatory response that occurs 24 hours after intra-articular injection of glucocorticoids and is characterized by heat, swelling, and pain. The incidence is approximately 2% and varies with the glucocorticoid used. The reaction is most likely to be a sterile inflammatory response to the microcrystalline suspension of the ester formulations. The reaction is usually mild, transient, and self-limiting.[202, 222, 223] Septic arthritis is an adverse sequela of intra-articular glucocorticoid therapy.[209, 222] Glucocorticoids may result in decreased resistance to infectious organisms introduced either during injection or from hematogenous origin.[222] Glucocorticoids may have a masking effect on detection of infectious arthritis.[209] Lameness and increases in synovial fluid neutrophil counts may be delayed in horses with infectious arthritis following glucocorticoid injection.[209] Osseous metaplasia may result from injection of long-acting glucocorticoids in peri-articular soft tissue structures. This may be due to a reaction of the vehicle.[202, 222] Ossification may not occur for several months after injection.[222]

The intra-articular use of glucocorticoids is controversial. It is well documented that, in addition to possessing beneficial anti-catabolic effects, glucocorticoids suppress collagen synthesis by chondrocytes, glycosaminoglycan, decreased viscosity, and hyaluronic acid content of the synovial fluid.[224–226] Intra-articular injection of 120 mg/joint of methylprednisolone acetate for 8 weeks in horses' carpal joints resulted in chondrocyte necrosis and hypocellularity, loss of proteoglycan content, and decreased collagen synthesis.[226] The effects of intra-articular glucocorticoids in horses are long lived, and in one study the effects were present 16 weeks after a single injection.[226] Steroid arthropathy is characterized by an accelerated rate of joint destruction and degenerative joint disease.[202, 222] The development of steroid arthropathy is dependent on pre-existing degenerative joint disease and on continued exercise.[203, 224] Therefore, it is recommended that intra-articular glucocorticoids be used in horses with minimal or no radiographic changes before the injection and that horses are rested after the injection.[203] Use of a smaller dose of glucocorticoids may provide beneficial anti-inflammatory effects, without significant deleterious effects on chondrocyte metabolism.[203, 227] Injection of normal middle carpal joints in horses of 100 mg/joint of methylprednisolone acetate three times in 14-day intervals did not result in degenerative changes in articular cartilage.[227]

Adrenal insufficiency caused by sudden withdrawal of exogenous glucocorticoid therapy has been well documented in the horse.[214–218, 228, 229] Clinical signs of adrenal insufficiency in horses include anorexia, depression, hypoglycemia, muscle weakness, and a dull, dry hair coat.[215, 217] Electrolyte abnormalities associated with glucocorticoid-induced adrenal insufficiency are variable in horses, but hyperkalemia may occur.[217] Horses with adrenal insufficiency secondary to excessive doses of glucocorticoids usually have a decreased response to exogenous ACTH administration, owing to suppression of endogenous ACTH secretion and secondary adrenocortical atrophy.[214, 215] Iatrogenic adrenal insufficiency is also reported to occur due to excessive use of anabolic steroids and administration of ACTH in horses.[215]

The duration of adrenal suppression is dependent several factors including: (1) the potency of the corticosteroid; (2) the route of administration; (3) the formulation of the corticosteroid; and (4) the dose administered. In horses, triamcinolone suppresses plasma cortisol concentrations for a longer time than does dexamethasone.[217] Plasma cortisol concentrations were detectable for 192 hours (8 days) and were suppressed for 336 hours (48 days) in horses treated with 20 mg of intramuscular triamcinolone.[217] Plasma cortisol concentrations were decreased for 5 to 7 days after administration of dexamethasone to horses.[216, 217] The route of administration also changes the duration of adrenal suppression. Intramuscular administration of dexamethasone and prednisolone resulted in a longer duration of adrenal suppression than when the drugs were given intravenously.[217, 218] Intra-articular administration of triamcinolone resulted in adrenal suppression for 5 days after the injection.[221] The formulation of the corticosteroid also influences the duration of suppression, and administration of prednisolone acetate resulted in a significantly longer duration of adrenal suppression than did prednisolone sodium succinate.[218] Finally, the larger the dose of the drug, the longer will be the duration of adrenal suppression. Dexamethasone (0.044 mg/kg and 0.088 mg/

kg) resulted in suppression of plasma cortisol for 4 days after injection, with suppression being slightly longer for the higher dose in horses.[216] The adrenal suppression induced by dexamethasone appears to be transient and results in permanent detrimental effects on the adrenal cortex, documented by a normal ACTH response 8 days after six dexamethasone (0.088 mg/kg) injections were given at 5-day intervals.[218]

To prevent adrenal suppression associated with glucocorticoid administration, it is recommended that horses be tapered off the drug. A decrease in the frequency of administration (from once a day to alternate days) and a reduction of dosages of the corticosteroid may help to prevent induction of adrenal insufficiency. Rest and avoidance of stress are often sufficient treatment for horses with iatrogenic adrenal suppression. Exogenous glucocorticoid replacement may sometimes be necessary in certain cases, with slow withdrawal of the drug.[215]

Other serious adverse effects of glucocorticoid use in horses include immunosuppression and laminitis. Detrimental side effects associated with the immunosuppressive effects of glucocorticoids include the development of opportunistic fungal and bacterial infections. Fungal pneumonia, systemic fungal infections, and mycotic keratitis are reported to occur in horses receiving systemic corticosteroids and ophthalmic corticosteroid treatment.[210] Glucocorticoid-induced laminitis is a serious sequela reported in horses.[214, 216, 230] The mechanism by which glucocorticoids induce laminitis may be due to potentiation of vasoconstriction caused by catecholamines.[230] Triamcinolone has been more frequently associated with laminitis than other glucocorticoids.

THERAPEUTIC AGENTS FOR LOWER RESPIRATORY DISEASE

Diseases of the respiratory system are common in horses, and chronic obstructive pulmonary disease (COPD, or heaves) is one of the most common lower airway diseases. COPD is characterized by airway obstruction due to accumulation of mucus and exudate, edema in the airway wall, and bronchospasm induced by an allergen or irritant.[231, 232] The airway obstruction, which is frequently attributed to a hypersensitivity reaction from exposure to molds and poorly cured hay, results in the release of various inflammatory mediators including histamine, eicosanoids, platelet activating factor, and complement-derived mediators.[232] Treatment is directed primarily at removing the inciting allergen by modifying the environment. Additional therapeutic methods include suppressing the immune/inflammatory system with glucocorticoids and NSAIDs and bronchodilators to relieve lower airway obstruction.

The parasympathetic nervous system is the primary source of excitatory innervation of the airways.[231, 233] Afferent parasympathetic receptors become activated by several substances (e.g., histamine, allergens, and irritants).[231, 233] Activation of the post-ganglionic parasympathetic fibers results in the release of acetylcholine, which binds muscarinic M_3 receptors on bronchial smooth muscle. Activation of M_3 receptors increases the activity of phospholipase C, which subsequently hydrolyzes phosphoinositide to inositol triphosphate (IP_3) and diacylglycerol (DAG). Activation of M_3 receptors may also increase cyclic guanosine-5'-monophos-

phate concentration leading to bronchoconstriction.[231] IP_3 releases intracellular stores of calcium and causes bronchial smooth muscle contraction. Muscarinic M_2 receptors, located on the presynaptic nerve terminal of the parasympathetic neuromuscular junction, are inhibitory and decrease the release of acetylcholine.[234] M_2 receptors may become inactivated by some viruses and in an allergic response.[231] Bronchoconstriction is also produced by activation of adenosine receptors (A-1). Adenosine is an autocoid (a compound that exerts its effects in the same location in which it was produced) that has multiple effects in many different organ systems. Activation of adenosine receptors in the respiratory tract inhibits adenylate cyclase and reduces the rate of formation of cyclic AMP, resulting in bronchoconstriction.

There are two inhibitory nervous systems in equine airways, which include the sympathetic and the non-adrenergic, non-cholinergic (NANC) nervous systems. Activation of the adrenergic receptors in the respiratory tract causes bronchodilation and stabilization of mast cells. Catecholamines bind to β_2-adrenergic receptors located on bronchial smooth muscle, which causes activation of adenyl cyclase, increases cyclic AMP concentrations, and subsequent decreases in intracellular calcium concentration. The NANC system predominates in the lower airway and is mediated by neuropeptides.

ANTICHOLINERGIC AGENTS

Anticholinergic agents include atropine, glycopyrrolate, and ipratropium and prevent vagally induced bronchoconstriction. Atropine (administered as an aerosol) did not alter lung function in normal ponies or in ponies with COPD in remission.[235] However, it decreased pulmonary resistance in ponies having acute attack of airway obstruction.[235] Systemic administration of atropine at a dose of 0.015 mg/kg can be used to induce bronchodilation in horses with acute bronchoconstriction.

Mechanism of Action

Anticholinergic agents prevent the binding of acetylcholine to the M_3 receptor on bronchial smooth muscle. Therefore, these drugs will only be effective when the bronchospasm is mediated via the parasympathetic nervous system.[231] Bronchoconstriction in horses with COPD is usually mediated by parasympathetic innervation, and therefore these drugs are usually effective.[231] Atropine, glycopyrrolate, and ipratropium are nonspecific muscarinic antagonists. Therefore, they bind both the M_3 receptor and the prejunctional inhibitory M_2 receptor. There, these drugs may increase the release of acetylcholine while blocking the effect of acetylcholine at the muscle.[231] Specific M_3 receptor antagonists are not currently available.

Pharmacokinetics

The duration of action of atropine is short in horses, and adverse side effects are associated with its use. However, administration of atropine may be useful in horses with COPD to determine if the lower airway obstruction is reversible. An "atropine challenge test" includes the administration of atropine at a dose of 0.015 mg/kg to horses with clinical signs of lower airway obstruction. Horses in which clinical signs improve after the administration of atropine will respond more favorably to other bronchodilators.[236] Glycopyrrolate has also been used to manage COPD in horses at a dose rate of 0.004 mg/kg intramuscularly every 12 hours.[236] Glycopyrrolate, when administered as an aerosol, is twice as potent as atropine in causing bronchodilation. Ipratropium bromide is a quaternary ammonium anticholinergic drug. Ipratropium does not cross the blood-brain barrier and is not absorbed after inhalation. Aerosolized ipratropium bromide (1 to 3 μg/kg) decreased the maximum change in pleural pressures and pulmonary resistance and increased the dynamic compliance in horses with an acute episode of COPD for 4 to 6 hours.[237]

Toxicity and Adverse Effects

Atropine has been associated with several adverse effects in horses, including tachycardia and gastrointestinal dysfunction and therefore is not routinely used in equine medicine.[238] Administration of atropine sulfate (0.044 and 0.176 mg/kg) to clinically normal ponies resulted in decreased borborygmus and colic in 3 of 10 of the ponies.[238] Aerosolized ipratropium is believed not to be absorbed systemically and, therefore, does not have the adverse effects of tachycardia and colic.[237] The increase in heart rate produced by anticholinergics is due to the parasympathetic control of the heart in resting horses.[239, 240] Despite the increase in heart rate, cardiac output is not significantly increased in resting horses.[241]

ADRENERGIC AGONISTS

Adrenergic agonists include catecholamines (epinephrine, norepinephrine), isoproterenol, clenbuterol, terbutaline, albuterol, and salbutamol. These adrenergic agonists produce bronchodilation, increase heart rate and force of cardiac contraction, alter vasomotor tone, and alter carbohydrate and fat metabolism.[242] The physiologic effects of the adrenergic agonist vary according to the adrenergic receptor (α_1, α_2, β_1, and β_2) that is activated. Epinephrine, norepinephrine, and isoproterenol activate both α and β receptors and have multiple cardiovascular effects. Epinephrine is the drug of choice for anaphylaxis but is unsuitable for routine clinical use owing to its lack of specificity. Epinephrine and norepinephrine are associated with tachycardia and arrhythmias when administered to horses due to stimulation of β_1-receptors.[243, 244] Isoproterenol is a nonselective α and β agonist but possess stronger β_1 than β_2 effects, which results in unavoidable tachycardia.[245] Clenbuterol, terbutaline, albuterol, salbutamol, and pirbuterol are selective β_2-agonists and are therefore useful bronchodilators with minimal extrapulmonary effects. Of these only clenbuterol (which is not available in the United States) has been studied extensively in the horse.

Clenbuterol

Clenbuterol hydrochloride is an effective β_2-agonist with pronounced cardiopulmonary effects in horses.[246] Intrave-

nous administration of clenbuterol to eight healthy horses reduced pulmonary resistance by 33.6%.[246] This lasted for 3 hours.[246] Transient increases in heart rate and reductions in mean arterial pressure were also recorded.[246] Administration of clenbuterol to horses with COPD decreased the maximal change in pleural pressure during respiration.[247] Clenbuterol also increased the rate of mucociliary clearance in horses with COPD.[248] Not all studies have documented that clenbuterol (0.8 μg/kg by mouth b.i.d.) is effective in the treatment of horses with COPD.[249] This may depend on the dose used.[250] In a clinical trial, clenbuterol has been demonstrated to improve clinical signs in 75% of horses with reversible bronchoconstriction.[250] However, only 25% of horses responded to an oral dose of 0.8 μg/mL b.i.d.[250] Cumulatively, 50% of horses responded to a dose of 1.6% μg/kg or less and 75% responded to a 3.2 μg/kg dose or less.[250] In vitro studies have found equine airways to have a variable response to the relaxant effect of clenbuterol. Therefore, it may be necessary to administer clenbuterol to effect.[250] Administration of clenbuterol to normal horses does not markedly affect the cardiorespiratory responses of horses to exercise.[251–253] However, the effects of clenbuterol on responses to exercise has not been evaluated in horses with COPD.

Mechanism of Action

Adrenergic agonists produce bronchodilation by binding to β_2-receptors in bronchial smooth muscle. Activation of β_2-receptors results in activation of adenylate cyclase, with a resultant increase in the intracellular concentration of cyclic AMP, which lowers the intracellular concentration of calcium and causes smooth muscle relaxation. Stimulation of β_2-receptors on mast cells also increases cyclic AMP concentrations, stabilizes cell membranes, and prevents mast cell degranulation. Activation of α_2-receptors (which are present on the prejunctional nerve terminal of the parasympathetic neuromuscular junction) may inhibit release of acetylcholine and prevent bronchoconstriction.[234] This may account for the mechanism by which xylazine provides some relief for horses with COPD.

Pharmacokinetics

The β_2-agonists are resistant to enzymatic degradation, can be administered orally, and have a prolonged duration of action (5 to 8 hours). Intravenous administration may be associated with hypotension, tachycardia, and sweating. Administration as an inhalant aerosol may diminish some of the side effects.[231] The elimination half-life of clenbuterol is approximately 10 hours. The oral dose of clenbuterol to horses currently recommended is 0.8 μg/kg b.i.d.; however, this dose is only effective in 25% of horses with COPD.[250] Higher doses may be necessary for a beneficial effect. To avoid side effects, it is recommended that the dose must be increased slowly (from 0.8 μg/mL) over several days.[250]

Toxicity and Adverse Effects

The adverse effects of adrenergic agonist include β_1 stimulation (tachycardia, arrhythmias), and β_2 effects (sweating, nervousness, muscle tremor, colic tocolytic actions, and worsening of ventilation-perfusion abnormalities). Oral administration of clenbuterol resulted in mild sweating, muscle tremors, and nervousness in less than 7% of horses.[250] β_2-Agonists should be used with caution in horses near parturition because the tocolytic actions of the drugs may delay parturition. Bronchodilation may exacerbate ventilation-perfusion mismatches and decrease arterial blood oxygen tensions in some human patients; however, this has not been well documented in horses.

METHYLXANTHINES

The methylxanthines include theophylline, theobromine, and caffeine and are structurally related and have similar pharmacologic effects.[254] Aminophylline (theophylline ethylenediamine) is a soluble salt of theophylline. These drugs have been used for over a century to treat asthma in humans. In addition to their bronchodilator effects, the methylxanthines stimulate the central nervous and cardiovascular systems, induce diuresis, increase basal metabolic rate, and plasma concentrations of free fatty acids.[254] The clinical effects and pharmacokinetics of theophylline have been studied extensively in horses.

Theophylline has been recommended and used for treatment of COPD in horses. In vitro, theophylline causes relaxation of equine tracheal smooth muscle.[255] Administration of intravenous aminophylline to ponies with COPD decreased pulmonary resistance and increased pulmonary compliance, but the degree of bronchodilation was variable.[256] The effect of theophylline in the lung appears to be related to its plasma concentration.[257] Therefore, the variation in degree of bronchodilation may be related to plasma theophylline concentrations in treated horses.[256] Theophylline also induced a dose-dependent increase in heart rate, sweating, sensitivity to external stimuli, urine flow, and muscle tremors.[258] Theophylline has a narrow therapeutic index, and the pharmacokinetics and toxicity are discussed further.

Mechanism of Action

The precise mechanism by which methylxanthines induce bronchodilation is unknown. However, three mechanisms have been suggested, including: (1) decreases in cytoplasmic concentrations of calcium; (2) inhibition of phosphodiesterase (the enzyme responsible for breakdown of cyclic AMP) and therefore, subsequent accumulation of cyclic AMP; and (3) blockade of adenosine receptors (a bronchoconstrictor). Inhibition of phosphodiesterase is often cited to explain the mechanism of action of methylxanthines, but therapeutic concentrations of theophylline produced minimal inhibition of the hydrolysis of cyclic AMP.[254] Methylxanthines are, however, competitive of adenosine receptors at therapeutic concentrations.

Pharmacokinetics

Methylxanthines are well absorbed after oral administration in horses.[259–262] Theophylline has a long elimination half-life in horses of ranging from 12 to 17 hours.[257–259, 263] Protein binding of theophylline in horses (12%) is lower than that

reported in humans (36%).[260] Theophylline is available in oral or parenteral formulations. Oral preparations are available as a sustained-release formulation (Theo-Dur).[264, 265] Sustained-release theophylline formulations may provide relatively stable therapeutic plasma concentrations of theophylline with less fluctuation in peak and trough concentrations and require less frequent administration.[264] The slow-release preparation resulted in a lower peak blood concentration, but a sustained duration.[264] However, the slow-release formulation did not exhibit any advantage in prolonging the elimination half-life of theophylline in the horse.[265]

Theophylline possesses a low therapeutic index. Therapeutic concentrations of theophylline in humans range between 10 and 20 µg/mL, and concentrations greater than 20 µg/mL are associated with adverse clinical signs.[254, 266] However, horses appear to be more sensitive to the effects of theophylline and adverse effects (tachycardia, muscle tremors, sweating, and hypersensitivity) occurred when plasma theophylline concentrations approached 15 µg/mL.[258] Suggested therapeutic plasma concentrations of theophylline are 8 to 15 µg/mL in horses.[256] Close monitoring of clinical signs and plasma theophylline concentrations is recommended in horses treated with theophylline due to the individual variation of the drug's pharmacokinetics. Elimination of theophylline is primarily by hepatic metabolism, and clearance of theophylline is increased by phenytoin, barbiturates, and rifampin,[254] but erythromycin and cimetidine decreased clearance of theophylline (thus increasing the likelihood of theophylline toxicity).

Toxicity and Adverse Effects

Adverse effects associated with theophylline in humans includes sudden death, cardiac arrhythmias, tachycardia, dizziness, nausea, hypotension, restlessness, and agitation. Sudden death and cardiac arrhythmias may be associated with rapid intravascular injection. Therefore, intravenous preparations may be diluted in 5% dextrose or normal saline and administered slowly. Adverse effects of theophylline in horses includes central nervous system stimulation (nervousness and hypersensitivity to external stimuli), muscle tremors, sweating, and tachycardia.[236, 256, 258] The intravenous administration of theophylline is more likely to result in adverse effects than oral administration in horses.[236, 258] Clinical signs of theophylline toxicity was noted in horses administered intravenous theophylline at 5, 10, and 15 mg/kg.[258] A loading dose of 15 mg/kg followed by a maintenance dose of 5 mg/kg every 12 hours has been recommended.[262] Intragastric administration of theophylline at 5 mg/kg at 12-hour intervals is predicted to produce and maintain an average steady-state plasma theophylline concentration of 10 µg/mL in horses.[261] Adverse effects of oral theophylline administration are reported in horses receiving 10 mg/kg. Therefore, adverse effects of theophylline may be avoided if the dose is gradually increased over a period of time.[260]

CROMOLYN SODIUM

Cromolyn sodium (Intal) is not a bronchodilator but is a prophylactic agent in the treatment of bronchial asthma.[254]

Cromolyn inhibits the immediate and late asthmatic responses to antigenic stimulation or to exercise.[254] It is an inhibitor of mast cell degranulation and histamine release in humans.[254] However, in order to be effective, the drug must be administered prior to exposure to the antigen or irritant. There is conflicting evidence of the efficacy regarding the drug in the treatment of lower airway disease in horses.[267–270] Administration of cromolyn to horses with recurrent COPD increased the duration of protection against an antigen challenge for 4 to 5 days.[268] Treatment of 56 horses with cromolyn delayed the onset of clinical signs of COPD.[267] However, cromolyn treatment in horses with COPD did not improve clinical signs, although it did decrease pulmonary resistance and intrapleural pressures in treated horses.[269] Cromolyn has been reported to improve clinical signs and bronchoalveolar lavage metachromatic cell histamine content in young racehorses with lower airway disease.[270]

Mechanism of Action

The exact mechanism by which cromolyn stabilizes mast cell membranes is unknown. Cromolyn may reduce the accumulation of intracellular calcium induced by antigens in sensitized mast cells.[254] However, concentrations required to observe such effects are significantly higher than are therapeutic concentrations.[254] Cromolyn sodium may be a tachykinin antagonist and may have effects on reflex bronchoconstriction via interference with neurotransmitters.[271]

Pharmacokinetics

Cromolyn sodium is not absorbed after oral administration, and the therapeutic effects are only achieved by local administration; therefore, cromolyn sodium must be given by inhalation, either as a solution (delivered by aerosol spray or nebulization) or as a powdered drug (delivered by a turbo inhaler). Cromolyn sodium is usually administered to horses by nebulization. The variation in clinical response to cromolyn is likely dependent on the type of nebulizer system.[270] There may be a wide disparity between nebulizer systems with regard to the amount of aerosol reaching the distal airways.[270] Cromolyn is excreted unchanged in the urine and bile.[256] The drug can be detected in equine urine by the enzyme-linked immunoassay for 6 hours after an 80-mg dose given by nebulizer and for 17 hours after intratracheal administration.[272] There are several recommended doses for cromolyn sodium in horses. Eighty to 200 mg has been shown to be prophylactically effective to improve clinical signs in horses with lower airway disease.[270] However, a dose of 520 mg was ineffective in improving clinical signs of COPD in horses.[269]

Toxicity and Adverse Reactions

Adverse side effects or toxicity has not been reported in horses treated with cromolyn sodium. Adverse reactions in humans are minor and include bronchospasm, coughing, laryngeal edema, headache, rash, and nausea.[256] Very rare cases of anaphylaxis have been reported. ▪

LOOP DIURETICS

Furosemide, bumetanide, and ethacrynic acid are potent diuretics, and furosemide is used extensively in racehorses prior to racing. Furosemide has been shown to have beneficial effects in the lung independent of its diuretic activity.[273–275] Furosemide has been shown to be a bronchodilator in a number of species, including horses.[273–275] Inhaled furosemide prevents bronchoconstriction produced by irritants or allergens.[276–280] Intravenous and nebulized furosemide increases the dynamic compliance and decreases pulmonary resistance in ponies with COPD but does not affect PaO_2 and PCO_2.[281] However, administration of furosemide to normal ponies did not affect pulmonary dynamic compliance and resistance.[281] Furosemide also results in improvement in pulmonary gas exchange in dogs and humans with pulmonary edema.[282, 283] The mechanism by which furosemide decreases pulmonary edema may be due to increases in vascular compliance and capacitance, redistribution of blood away from edematous portions of the lungs, and reduction of the rate of lymph production.[243, 282] Furosemide is also used to reduce the incidence or severity of exercise-induced pulmonary hemorrhage in horses, but the efficacy is unclear.[284–286]

Mechanism of Action

The mechanism by which furosemide produces its diuretic effect is due to its direct action on renal tubular function.[243] Furosemide inhibits the reabsorption of sodium and chloride in the thick ascending loop of Henle by inhibiting the Na^+-K^+-Cl^- co-transporter at the luminal membrane.[287] Inhibition of this transporter prevents concentration or dilution of the tubular fluid, which increases the delivery of sodium and chloride to the distal tubule and results in the production of large volumes of isotonic urine.[243, 288]

The mechanism of action of furosemide on the airways and blood vessels is unknown but may be independent of its diuretic action.[275, 289, 290] Furosemide increased venous compliance[289] and decreased pulmonary wedge pressure[290] in animals with ligated ureters. It also decreased pulmonary artery and right atrial pressure in horses during exercise.[288, 291] There is evidence that prostaglandins may play a role in the extra-renal effects of furosemide.[273–275, 288] Flunixin meglumine blocked the furosemide-induced bronchodilation in horses with COPD but did not prevent diuresis.[275] Administration of furosemide and flunixin meglumine attenuated the furosemide-induced decreases in pulmonary artery and right atrial pressures in horses during exercise.[288] However, in a similar study, treatment with flunixin meglumine did not alter the effect of furosemide on pulmonary artery and pulmonary artery wedge pressure in horses during exercise.[291]

Pharmacokinetics

Furosemide may be administered by intravenous, intramuscular, and oral means or by inhalation. However the pharmacokinetics of furosemide after oral administration is unknown in horses, and it is most frequently administered as an intravenous or intramuscular injection. Furosemide is rapidly eliminated in the horse. The majority of the drug is eliminated unchanged in the urine within 4 hours.[243]

REFERENCES

1. Caprile KA: The cephalosporin antimicrobial agents: A comprehensive review. *J Vet Pharmacol Ther* 11:1, 1988.
2. Nathwani D, Woods MJ: Penicillins: A current review of their clinical pharmacology and therapeutic use. *Drugs* 45:866, 1993.
3. Dever LA, Dermody TS: Mechanisms of bacterial resistance to antibiotics. *Arch Intern Med* 151:886, 1991.
4. Wischart DF: Recent advances in antimicrobial drugs: The penicillins. *J Am Vet Med Assoc* 185:1106, 1984.
5. Neu MH: Beta-lactams: A perspective on the contribution of these enzymes to bacterial resistance. *Prostaglandin Med* 1:7, 1984.
6. Stratton CW, Gelfand MS, Gerdberg JL, et al: Characterization of mechanisms of resistance to β-lactam antibiotics and methicillin resistant strains of *Staphylococcus saprophyticus*. *Antimicrob Agents Chemother* 34:1780, 1990.
7. Kilgore WR, Simmons RD, Jackson JW: β-Lactamase inhibition: A new approach in overcoming bacterial resistance. *Compend Contin Educ Pract* 8:325, 1986.
8. Phillips I, Shannon K: Importance of β-lactamase induction. *Eur J Clin Microbiol Infect Dis* 12(Suppl):S19, 1993.
9. Rolinson GN: Evolution of beta-lactamase inhibitors. *Surg Gynecol Obstet* 172(Suppl):11, 1991.
10. Sparks SE, Jones RL, Kilgore WR: In vitro susceptibility of bacteria to a ticarcillin-clavulanic acid combination. *Am J Vet Res* 49:2038, 1988.
11. Ensink JM, Klein WR, Mevius DJ, et al: Bioavailability of oral penicillins in the horse: A comparison of pivampicillin and amoxicillin. *J Vet Pharmacol Ther* 15:221, 1992.
12. Wilson WD, Spensley MS, Baggot JD, et al: Pharmacokinetics and estimated bioavailability of amoxicillin in mares after intravenous, intramuscular, and oral administration. *Am J Vet Res* 49:1688, 1988.
13. Wilson WD, Baggot JD, Adamson PJW, et al: Cefadroxil in the horse: Pharmacokinetics and *in vitro* antibacterial activity. *J Vet Pharmacol Ther* 8:246, 1985.
14. Baggot JD, Love DN, Love RJ, et al: Oral dosage of penicillin V in adult horses and foals. *Equine Vet J* 22:290, 1990.
15. Horspool LJI, McKellar QA: Disposition of penicillin G sodium following intravenous and oral administration to Equidae. *Br Vet J* 151:1, 1995.
16. Henry MM, Morris DD, Lakritz J, et al: Pharmacokinetics of cephradine in neonatal foals after single oral dosing. *Equine Vet J* 24:242, 1992.
17. Brown MP, Gronwall R, Kroll WR, et al: Ampicillin trihydrate in foals: Serum concentrations and clearance after a single oral dose. *Equine Vet J* 16:371, 1982.
18. Ruoff WW, Sams RA: Pharmacokinetics and bioavailability of cephalothin in horse mares. *Am J Vet Res* 46:2085, 1985.
19. Thompson TD, Quay JF, Webber JA: Cephalosporin group of antimicrobial drugs. *J Am Vet Med Assoc* 185:1109, 1984.
20. Brown MP, Gronwall RR, Houston AE: Pharmacokinetics and body fluid and endometrial concentrations of cepharpirin in mares. *Am J Vet Res* 47:784, 1986.
21. Brown MP, Gronwall RR, Houston AE: Pharmacokinetics and body fluid and endometrial concentrations of cefoxitin in mares. *Am J Vet Res* 47:1743, 1986.
22. Brown MP, Gronwall R, Gossman TB: Pharmacokinetics and serum concentrations of cepharin in neonatal foals. *Am J Vet Res* 48:805, 1987.
23. Sams RA, Ruoff WW: Pharmacokinetics and bioavailability of cefazolin in horses. *Am J Vet Res* 46:348, 1985.
24. Chapman CB, Couage P, Nielsen IL: The role of procaine in adverse reactions to procaine penicillin in horses. *Aust Vet J* 69:129, 1992.
25. Neilsen IL, Jacobs KA, Hunington PJ, et al: Adverse reaction to procaine penicillin G in horses. *Aust Vet J* 65:181, 1988.
26. Blue JT, Dinsomore RP, Anderson KL: Immune-mediated hemolytic anemia induced by penicillin in horses. *Cornell Vet* 77:263, 1987.
27. McConnico RS, Roberts MC, Tompkins M: Penicillin-induced immune-mediated hemolytic anemia in a horse. *J Am Vet Med Assoc* 201:1402, 1992.
28. Robbins RL, Wallace SS, Brunner CJ, et al: Immune-mediated haemolytic disease after penicillin therapy in a horse. *Equine Vet J* 25:462, 1993.
29. Mahrt CR: Safety of ceftiofur sodium administered intramuscularly in horses. *Am J Vet Res* 53:2201, 1992.
30. Brown MP, Stover SM, Kelly RH, et al: Body fluid concentrations of ampicillin trihydrate in 6 horses after a single intramuscular dose. *Equine Vet J* 14:83, 1982.
31. Folz SD, Hanson AK, Griffin LL, et al: Treatment of respiratory infections in horses with ceftiofur sodium. *Equine Vet J* 24:300, 1992.
32. Yancey RJ, Kinney ML, Roberts BJ, et al: Ceftiofur sodium, a broad-spectrum cephalosporin: Evaluation *in vitro* and *in vivo* in mice. *Am J Vet Res* 48:1050, 1987.
33. Morris DD, Rutowski D: Therapy in two cases of neonatal foals and septicemia and meningitis with cefotaxime sodium. *Equine Vet J* 19:151, 1987.
34. Edson RS, Terrel CL: The aminoglycosides. *Mayo Clin Proc* 66:1158, 1991.
35. Orsini JA, Benson CE, Spencer PA, et al: Resistance to gentamicin and amikacin or gram-negative organisms isolated from horses. *Am J Vet Res* 50:923, 1989.
36. Brown SA, Riviere JE: Comparative pharmacokinetics of aminoglycoside antibiotics. *J Vet Pharmacol Ther* 14:1, 1991.
37. Brown MP, Embertson RM, Gronwall RR, et al: Amikacin sulfate in mares: Pharmacokinetics and body fluid and endometrial concentrations after repeated intramuscular administration. *Am J Vet Res* 45:1610, 1984.
38. Baggot JD, Love DN, Stewart J, et al: Gentamicin dosage in foals aged one month and three months. *Equine Vet J* 18:113, 1986.
39. Orsini JA, Soma LR, Rourke JE, et al: Pharmacokinetics of amikacin in the horse following intravenous or intramuscular administration. *J Vet Pharmacol Ther* 8:194, 1985.
40. Dohery TJ, Novotny MJ, Desjardins MR, et al: Gentamicin concentrations in body fluids of adult horses following high-dose administration. In AAEP 40th Annual Convention Proceedings, 1994, p 113.
41. Godber LM, Walker RD, Stein GE, et al: Pharmacokinetics, nephrotoxicosis, and *in vitro* antibacterial activity associated with single versus multiple (three times) daily gentamicin treatments in horses. *Am J Vet Res* 56:613, 1995.
42. Riviere JE, Cooper GL, Hinsman EJ, et al: Species dependent gentamicin pharmacokinetics and nephrotoxicity in the young horse. *Fund Appl Toxicol* 3:448, 1983.
43. Adland-Davenport P, Brown MR, Robinson JD, et al: Pharmacokinetics of amikacin in critically ill neonatal foals treated for presumed or confirmed sepsis. *Equine Vet J* 22:18, 1990.
44. Green SL, Conlon PD, Mama K, et al: Effects of hypoxaemia and azotemia on the pharmacokinetics of amikacin in neonatal foals. *Equine Vet J* 24:475, 1992.
45. Brewer BD, Clemmet SF, Lotz WS, et al: A comparison of insulin, para-aminohippuric acid, and endogenous creatinine clearance as measures of renal function in neonatal foals. *J Vet Intern Med* 4:30, 1990.

46. Golenz MR, Wilson WD, Carlson GP, et al: Effect of route of administration and age on the pharmacokinetics of amikacin administered by the intravenous and intraosseous routes to 3- and 5-day-old foals. *Equine Vet J* 26:367, 1994.

47. Cummings LE, Guthrie AJ, Harkins JD, et al: Pharmacokinetics of gentamicin in newborn to 30-day-old foals. *Am J Vet Res* 51:1988, 1990.

48. Green SL, Conlon PD: The pharmacokinetics of amikacin in hypoxic premature foals *Equine Vet J* 25:276, 1993.

49. Wichtel MG, Breuhaus BA, Aucoin D: Relationship between pharmacokinetics of amikacin sulfate and sepsis score in clinically normal and hospitalized neonatal foals. *J Am Vet Med Assoc* 200:1339, 1992.

50. Sweeney RW, MacDonald M, Hall J, et al: Kinetics of gentamicin elimination in two horses with acute renal failure. *Equine Vet J* 18:113, 1988.

51. Sweeney RW, Divers TJ, Rossier Y: Disposition of gentamicin administered intravenously to a horse with sepsis. *J Am Vet Med Assoc* 200:503, 1992.

52. Sojka JE, Brown SA: Pharmacokinetic adjustments of gentamicin dosing in horses with sepsis. *J Am Vet Med Assoc* 189:784, 1986.

53. Kaloyanides GL: Drug-phospholipid interactions: Role in aminoglycoside nephrotoxicity. *Ren Fail* 14:351, 1992.

54. Hildebenbrand SV, Hill III T: Interactions of gentamycin and atracurium in anaesthetised horses. *Equine Vet J* 26:209, 1994.

55. Marik PE, Lipman J, Kopilski S, et al: A prospective randomized study comparing once versus twice-daily amikacin in critically ill adults and pediatric patients. *J Antimicrob Chem* 28:753, 1991.

56. Zhanel GG, Ariano RE: Once daily aminoglycoside dosing: Maintained efficacy and reduced nephrotoxicosis? *Ren Fail* 14:1, 1992.

57. Magdesian KG, Hogan PM, Brumbaugh G, et al: Pharmacokinetics of gentamicin administered once daily by the intravenous and intramuscular routes in horses. In AAEP 40th Annual Convention Proceedings 1994, p 115.

58. Gilbert DN: Once-daily aminoglycoside therapy. *Antimicrob Agents Chemother* 35:399, 1991.

59. Moore RM: Diagnosis and treatment of obligate anaerobic bacterial infections in horses. *Compend Contin Educ Pract Vet* 15:989, 1993.

60. Madison JB, Garber JL, Rice B, et al: Effects of oxytetracycline on metacarpophalangeal and distal interphalangeal joint angles in newborn foals. *J Am Vet Med Assoc* 204:246, 1994.

61. Kasper CA, Clayton HM, Wright AK, et al: Effects of high doses of oxytetracycline on metacarpophalangeal joint kinematics in neonatal foals. *J Am Vet Med Assoc* 207:71, 1995.

62. McKellar QA, Horspool JI: Stability of penicillin G, ampicillin, amikacin, and oxytetracycline and their interactions with food in vitro simulated equine gastrointestinal contents. *Res Vet Sci* 58:227, 1995.

63. Brown MP, Stover SM, Kelly RH, et al: Oxytetracycline hydrochloride in the horse: Serum, synovial, peritoneal, and urine concentrations after single dose intravenous administration. *J Vet Pharmacol Ther* 4:7, 1981.

64. Horspool LJI, McKellar QA: Disposition of oxytetracycline in horses, ponies, and donkeys after intravenous administration. *Equine Vet J* 22:284, 1990.

65. Cook WR: Diarrhoea in the horse associated with stress and tetracycline therapy. *Vet Rec* 93:15, 1973.

66. White G, Prior SD: Comparative effects of oral administration of trimethoprim/sulphadiazine or oxytetracycline on the faecal flora of horses. *Vet Rec* 111:316, 1982.

67. Vivrette S, Cowgill LD, Pascoe J: Hemodialysis for treatment of oxytetracycline-induced acute renal failure in a neonatal foal. *J Am Vet Med Assoc* 203:105, 1993.

68. Roind JL, Riviere JE, Duckett WM, et al: Cardiovascular effects and fatalities associated with intravenous administration of doxycycline to horses and ponies. *Equine Vet J* 24:41, 1992.

69. Button C, Mulders MSG: Effects of oxytetracycline in propylene glycol, oxytetracycline in saline solution, and propylene glycol alone on blood ionized calcium and plasma total calcium in sheep. *Am J Vet Res* 45:1658, 1969.

70. Bowen JM, McMullan WC: Influence of induced hypermagnesemia and hypocalcemia on neuromuscular blocking property of oxytetracycline in the horse. *Am J Vet Res* 36:1025, 1975.

71. Gross DR, Kitzman JV, Adams HR: Cardiovascular effects of intravenous administration of propylene glycol in calves. *Am J Vet Res* 40:783, 1979.

72. Van Duijkeren EV, Vulto AG, Van Miert AS: Trimethoprim/sulfonamide combinations in the horse: A review. *J Vet Pharmacol Ther* 17:64, 1994.

73. Mandel GL, Sande MA: Antimicrobial agents: Sulfonamide, trimethoprim-sulfamethoxazole, quinolones and agents for urinary tract infections. In Gilman AG, Rall TW, Nies AS, et al, eds. *The Pharmacological Basis of Therapeutics,* ed 8. New York, Pergamon Press, 1990, p 1047.

74. Brown MP, Gronwall R, Castro I: Pharmacokinetics and body fluid endometrial concentrations of trimethoprim-sulfamethoxazole in mares. *Am J Vet Res* 49:918, 1988.

75. Brown MP, Gronwall RR, Cook LK, et al: Serum concentrations of ormetoprim/sulfadimethoxine in 1–3-day-old foals after a single dose of oral paste combination. *Equine Vet J* 25:73, 1993.

76. Brown MP, Gronwall RR, Houston AE: Pharmacokinetics and body fluid and endometrial concentrations of ormetoprim-sulfadimethoxine in mares. *Can J Vet Res* 53:12, 1989.

77. Brown MP, Kelly RH, Stover SM, et al: Trimethoprim-sulfadiazine in the horse: Serum, peritoneal, and urine concentrations after single-dose intravenous administration. *Am J Vet Res* 44:540, 1983.

78. Wilson RC, Hammond LS, Clark CH, et al: Bioavailability and pharmacokinetics of sulfamethazine in the pony. *J Vet Pharmacol Ther* 12:99, 1989.

79. Brown MP, McCartney JH, Gronwall R, et al: Pharmacokinetics of trimethoprim-sulphamethoxazole in two-day-old foals after a single intravenous injection. *Equine Vet J* 22:51, 1990.

80. Nouws JFM, Firth EC, Vree JB, et al: Pharmacokinetics and renal clearance of sulfamethazine, sulfamerazine, and sulfadiazine and their N4-acetyl and hydroxy metabolites in horses. *Am J Vet Res* 48:392, 1987.

81. Nouws JFM, Vree JB, Backman M, et al: Disposition of sulfadimidine and its N4-acetyl and hydroxy metabolites in horse plasma. *J Vet Pharmacol Ther* 81:303, 1985.

82. Clarke CR, Burrows GE, McAllister CG, et al: Pharmacokinetics of intravenously and orally administered pyrimethamine in horses. *Am J Vet Res* 53:2292, 1992.

83. Clarke CR, MacAllister CG, Burrows GE, et al: Pharmacokinetics, penetration into cerebrospinal fluid, and hematologic effects after multiple oral administration of pyrimethamine to horses. *Am J Vet Res* 53:2296, 1992.

84. Green SL, Mayhew IG, Brown MP, et al: Concentrations of trimethoprim and sulfamethoxazole in cerebrospinal fluid and serum in mares with and without a dimethyl sulfoxide pretreatment. *Can J Vet Res* 54:215, 1990.

85. Grunberg E: The effect of trimethoprim on the activity of sulfonamide and antibiotic in experimental infections. *J Infect Dis* 12:S478, 1973.

86. Dodd WJ: Sulfonamide and blood dyscrasias. *J Am Vet Med Assoc* 196:886, 1990.

87. Taylor PM, Rest RJ, Duckham TN, et al: Possible potentiated sulphonamide and detomidine interactions. *Vet Rec* 122:143, 1988.

88. Dick IGG, White SK: Possible potentiated sulfonamide-associated fatality in an anaesthetised horse. *Vet Rec* 121:288, 1987.

89. Wilson DA, MacFadden KE, Green EM, et al: Is the administration of trimethoprim-potentiated sulfonamides associated with the subsequent development of diarrhea in horses and ponies. In AAEP 41st Annual Convention Proceedings, 1995, p 189.

90. Prescott JF, Sweeny CR: Treatment of *Cornyebacterium equi* pneumonia in foals: A review. *J Am Vet Med Assoc* 187:725, 1985.

91. Sweeney CR, Sweeney RW, Divers TJ: *Rhodococcus equi* pneumonia in 48 foals: Response to antimicrobial therapy. *Vet Microbiol* 14:329, 1987.

92. Hillidge CJ: Use of erythromycin-rifampin combination in treatment of *Rhodococcus equi* pneumonia. *Vet Microbiol* 14:337, 1987.

93. Palmer JE, Benson CE: Effect of erythromycin and rifampin during the acute stages of experimentally induced equine ehrlichial colitis in ponies. Am J Vet Res 53;2071, 1992.

94. Kenney DG, Robbins SC, Prescott JF, et al: Development of reactive arthritis and resistance to erythromycin and rifampin in a foal during treatment for *Rhodococcus equi* pneumonia. *Equine Vet J* 25:246, 1994.

95. Maxxei T, Mini E, Novelli A, et al: Chemistry and mode of action of macrolides. *J Antimicrob Chemother* 31(Suppl C):1, 1993.

96. Burrows GE: Pharmacokinetics of macrolides, lincomycins, and spectinomycin. *J Am Vet Med Assoc* 176:1072, 1980.

97. Williams JD, Sefton AM: Comparison of macrolide antibiotics. *J Antimicrob Chemother* 31(Suppl C):11, 1993.

98. Ewing PJ, Burrows G, MacAllister CG, et al: Comparison of oral erythromycin formulations in the horse using pharmacokinetic profiles. *J Vet Pharmacol Ther* 17:17, 1994.

99. Prescott JF, Hoover DJ, Dohoo IR: Pharmacokinetics of erythromycin in foals and adult horses. *J Vet Pharmacol Ther* 6:67, 1983.

100. Prescott JF, Nicholson VM: The effects of combinations of selected antibiotics on the growth of *Corynebacterium equi*. *J Vet Pharmacol Ther* 7:61, 1984.

101. Frank LA: Clinical pharmacology of rifampin. *J Am Vet Med Assoc* 197:114, 1990.

102. Wilson WD, Spensley MS, Baggot JD, et al: Pharmacokinetics, bioavailability, and in vitro antibacterial activity of rifampin in the horse. *Am J Vet Res* 49:2041, 1988.

103. Kohn CW, Sams R, Kowalaski JJ, et al: Pharmacokinetics of single intravenous and single and multiple dose oral administration of rifampin in mares. *J Vet Pharmacol Ther* 16:119, 1993.

104. Wehril W: Rifampin: Mechanisms of action and resistance. *Rev Infect Dis* 5:S407, 1983.

105. Castro LA, Brown MP, Gronwall R, et al: Pharmacokinetics of rifampin given as a single oral dose in foals. *Am J Vet Res* 47:2584, 1986.

106. Burrows GE, MacAllister CG, Beckstom DA, et al: Rifampin in the horse: Comparison of intravenous, intramuscular, and oral administration. *Am J Vet Res* 46:442, 1985.

107. Burrows GE, MacAllister CG, Ewing P, et al: Rifampin disposition in the horse: Effects of age and method of oral administration. *J Vet Pharmacol Ther* 15:124, 1992.

108. Burrows GE, MacAllister CG, Ewing P, et al: Rifampin disposition in the horse: Effect of repeated dosage of rifampin or phenylbutazone. *J Vet Pharmacol Ther* 15:305, 1992.

109. Page SW: Chloramphenicol 1: Hazards of use and current regulatory environment. *Aust Vet J* 68:1, 1991.

110. Yunnis AA: Chloramphenicol: Relation of structure to activity and toxicity. *Ann Rev Pharmacol Toxicol* 28:83, 1988.

111. Adamson PJW, Wilson WD, Baggot JD, et al: Influence of age on the disposition kinetics of chloramphenicol in equine neonates. *Am J Vet Res* 52:426, 1991.

112. Gronwall RR, Brown MP, Merritt AM, et al: Body fluid concentrations and pharmacokinetics of chloramphenicol given to mares intravenously or by repeated gavage. *Am J Vet Res* 47:2591, 1986.

113. Brown MP, Kelly RH, Gronwall RR, et al: Chloramphenicol sodium succinate in the horse: Serum, synovial, peritoneal, and urine concentrations after single-dose intravenous administration. *Am J Vet Res* 45:578, 1984.

114. Brumbaugh GW, Martens RJ, Knight HD, et al: Pharmacokinetics of chloramphenicol in the neonatal horse. *J Vet Pharmacol Ther* 6:219, 1983.

115. Buonpane NA, Brown MP, Gronwall R, et al: Serum concentrations and pharmacokinetics of chloramphenicol in foals after a single oral dose. *Equine Vet J* 20:59, 1988.

116. Burrows CE, MacAllister CG, Tripp P, et al: Interactions between chloramphenicol, acepromazine, phenylbutazone, rifampin and thiamylal in the horse. *Equine Vet J* 21:34, 1989.

117. Varma KJ, Powers TE, Powers JD: Single- and repeat-dose pharmacokinetic studies of chloramphenicol in horses: Values and limitations of pharmacokinetics studies in predicting dosage regimens. *Am J Vet Res* 48:403, 1987.

118. Rollin RE, Mero KN, Kozisek RP, et al: Diarrhea and malabsorptive changes in calves associated with therapeutic doses of antibiotics: Absorption and clinical changes. *Am J Vet Res* 47:987, 1986.

119. Page SW: Chloramphenicol 3: Clinical pharmacology of systemic use in the horse. *Aust Vet J* 68:5, 1991.

120. Burrows GE, MacAllister CG, Tripp P, et al: Interactions between chloramphenicol, acepromazine, phenylbutazone, rifampin and thiamylal in the horse. *Equine Vet J* 21:34, 1989.

121. Sweeney RW, Sweeney CR, Weiher J: Clinical uses of metronidazole in horses: 200 cases (1984–1989). *J Am Vet Med Assoc* 198:1045, 1991.

122. Scully B: Metronidazole. *Med Clin North Am* 72:613, 1988.

123. Sweeney RW, Sweeney CR, Soma LR, et al: Pharmacokinetics of metronidazole given to horses by intravenous and oral routes. *Am J Vet Res* 47:1726, 1986.

124. Baggot JD, Wilson WD, Hietala S: Clinical pharmacokinetics of metronidazole in horses. *J Vet Pharmacol Ther* 11:417, 1988.

125. Specht TE, Brown MP, Gronwall RR, et al: Pharmacokinetics and body fluid and endometrial concentrations of metronidazole in horses. *Am J Vet Res* 53:1807, 1992.

126. Garber JL, Brown MP, Gronwall RR, et al: Pharmacokinetics of metronidazole after rectal administration in horses. *Am J Vet Res* 54:2060, 1993.

127. Owen RH, Ap Rh, Jagger DW, et al: Possible adverse reaction to metronidazole in the horse. *Vet Rec* 117:534, 1985.

128. Orsini JA, Perkons S: The fluoroquinolones: Clinical applications in veterinary medicine. *Compend Contin Educ Pract Vet* 6:1491, 1992.

129. Prescott JF, Yielding KM: In vitro susceptibility of selected veterinary bacterial pathogens to ciprofloxacin, endofloxacin, and norfloxacin. *Can J Vet Res* 54:195, 1990.

130. Hooper DC, Wolfson JS: Fluoroquinolone antimicrobial agents. *N Engl J Med* 324:384, 1991.

131. Berg J: Clinical indications for enrofloxacin in domestic animals and poultry. In Quinolones: A new class of antimicrobial agents for use in veterinary medicine. Proceedings of the West Veterinary Conference, Las Vegas, Nevada. Shawnee, KS, Mobay Corporation Animal Health Division, 1988, p 254.

132. Neer TM: Clinical pharmacologic features of fluoroquinolone antimicrobial drugs. *J Am Vet Med Assoc* 193:577, 1988.

133. Dowling PM: New developments of antimicrobial therapy for

large animals: Fluoroquinolones and florfenicol. In Proceedings of the 12th Annual ACVIM Forum, 1994, p 567.

134. Vancustem PM, Babish JG, Schwark WS: The fluoroquinolone antimicrobials: Structure, antimicrobial activity, pharmacokinetics, clinical use in domestic animals and toxicity. *Cornell Vet* 80:173, 1990.

135. Droughet E, Dupont B: Evolution of antifungal agents: Past, present, and future. *Rev Infect Dis* 9(Suppl 1):S4, 1987.

136. Beech J, Sweeney CCR, Irby N: Keratomycoses in 11 horses. *Equine Vet Suppl* 2:6, 1990.

137. Pugh DG, Bowen JM, Kloppe LH, et al: Fungal endometritis in mares. *Compend Contin Educ Vet Pract* 8:S173, 1986.

138. Ruoff WW: Fungal pneumonia in horses. In AAEP 34th Annual Convention Proceedings 988, 423.

139. Cornick JL: Diagnosis and treatment of pulmonary histoplasmosis in a horse. *Cornell Vet* 80:97, 1990.

140. Reilly LK, Palmer JE: Systemic candidiasis in four foals. *J Am Vet Med Assoc* 205:464, 1994.

141. Steckel RR, Adams SB, Long GG, et al: Antemortem diagnosis and treatment of cryptococcal meningitis in a horse. *J Am Vet Med Assoc* 180:1085, 1982.

142. Ziemer EL, Pappagianis D, Madigan JE, et al: Coccidioidomycosis in horses: 15 cases (1975–1984). *J Am Vet Med Assoc* 201:910, 1992.

143. McMullan WC, Joyce JR, Hanselka DV, et al: Amphotericin B for the treatment of localized subcutaneous phycomycosis in the horse. *J Am Vet Med Assoc* 170:1293, 1977.

144. Church S, Wyn-Jones G, Parks AH, et al: Treatment of guttural pouch mycosis. *Equine Vet J* 18:362, 1986.

145. Greet TRC: Outcome of treatment in 35 cases of guttural pouch mycosis. *Equine Vet J* 19:483, 1987.

146. Hauser WE, Remington JS: The effect of antibiotics on the humoral and cell-mediated immune responses. In Sabath LD, ed. *Action of Antibiotics in Patients.* Bern, Huber, 1982, p 127.

147. Bajtburg J, Powderly WG, Kobayashi GS, et al: Amphotericin B: Current understanding of mechanisms of action. *Antimicrob Agents Chemother* 34:183, 1990.

148. Eaton SA: Osseous involvement by *Pythium insidiosum*. *Compend Contin Educ Vet Pract* 2:485, 1993.

149. Van Cauteren H, Heykants J, De Coster R, et al: Itraconazole: Pharmacologic studies in animals and humans. *Rev Infect Dis* 9(Suppl 1):S43, 1987.

150. Foley JP, Legendre AM: Treatment of coccidioidomycosis osteomyelitis with itraconazole in a horse. *J Vet Intern Med* 6:333, 1992.

151. Davis EW, Legendre AM: Successful treatment of guttural pouch mycosis with itraconazole and topical enilconazole in a horse. *J Vet Intern Med* 8:304, 1994.

152. Moriello KA: Ketoconazole: Clinical pharmacology and therapeutic recommendations. *J Am Vet Med Assoc* 188:303, 1986.

153. Prades M, Brown MP, Gronwall R, et al: Body fluid and endometrial concentrations of ketoconazole in mares after intravenous injection or repeated gavage. *Equine Vet J* 21:211, 1989.

154. Hiddleston WA: The use of griseofulvin mycelium in equine animals (Letter). *Vet Rec* 87:119, 1970.

155. Higgins AJ, Lees P, Taylor JB: Influence of phenylbutazone on eicosanoid levels in equine acute inflammatory exudate. *Cornell Vet* 74:198, 1984.

156. Lees P, Higgins AJ: Clinical pharmacology and therapeutic uses of non-steroidal anti-inflammatory drugs in the horse. *Equine Vet J* 17:83, 1985.

157. Tobin T, Chay S, Kamerling S, et al: Phenylbutazone in the horse: A review. *J Vet Pharmacol Ther* 9:1, 1986.

158. Oates JA, Fitzgerald GA, Branch RA, et al: Clinical implications of prostaglandins and thromboxane A_2 formation. *N Engl J Med* 319:689, 1988.

159. Lees P, Ewins CP, Taylor JBO: Serum thromboxane in the horse and its inhibition by aspirin, phenylbutazone and flunixin. *Br Vet J* 143:462, 1987.

160. Lees P, Higgins AJ: Flunixin inhibits prostaglandin E_2 production in equine inflammation. *Res Vet Sci* 37:347, 1984.

161. Soma LR, Uboh CE, Rudy J, et al: Plasma concentration of flunixin in the horse: Its relationship to thromboxane B_2 production. *J Vet Pharmacol Ther* 15:292, 1992.

162. Owens JG, Kamerling SG, Barker SA: Pharmacokinetics of ketoprofen in healthy horses and horses with acute inflammation. *J Vet Pharmacol Ther* 18:187, 1995.

163. Malmber AB, Yaksh TL: Hyperalgesia mediated by spinal glutamate or substance P receptor blocked by spinal cyclooxygenase inhibition. *Science* 257:1276, 1992.

164. Cunningham FM, Lees P: Advances in anti-inflammatory therapy. *Br Vet J* 150:115, 1994.

165. Johnson GB, Taylor PM, Young SS, et al: Post-operative analgesia using phenylbutazone, flunixin or carprofen in horses. *Vet Rec* 133:336, 1993.

166. Semrad SD, Hardee GE, Hardee MM, et al: Low dose flunixin meglumine: Effects on eicosanoid production and clinical signs induced by experimental endotoxaemia in horses. *Equine Vet J* 19:201, 1987.

167. Semrad SD, Hardee GE, Hardee MM, et al: Flunixin meglumine given in small doses: Pharmacokinetics and prostaglandin inhibition in healthy horses. *Am J Vet Res* 46:2474, 1985.

168. Moore JN, Hardee MM, Hardee GE: Modulation of arachidonic acid metabolism in endotoxic horses: Comparison of flunixin meglumine, phenylbutazone, and a selective thromboxane synthetase inhibitor. *Am J Vet Res* 47:110, 1986.

169. Jackman BR, Moore JN, Barton MH, et al: Comparison of the effect of ketoprofen and flunixin meglumine on the *in vitro* response of equine peripheral blood monocytes to bacterial endotoxin. *Can J Vet Res* 58:138, 1994.

170. Meyers KM, Linder C, Katz J, et al: Phenylbutazone inhibition of equine platelet function. *Am J Vet Res* 40:265, 1979.

171. Patrono C: Aspirin as an antiplatelet drug. *N Engl J Med* 330:18, 1994.

172. Baxter GM, Moore JN: Effect of aspirin on ex vivo generation of thromboxane in healthy horses. *Am J Vet Res* 48:13, 1987.

173. Cambridge H, Lees P, Hooke RE, et al: Antithrombotic actions of aspirin in the horse. *Equine Vet J* 23:123, 1991.

174. Kopp KJ, Moore JN, Byars TD, et al: Template bleeding time and thromboxane generation in the horse: Effects of three non-steroidal anti-inflammatory drugs. *Equine Vet J* 17:322, 1985.

175. Trujillo O, Rois A, Maldonado R, et al: Effect of oral administration of acetylsalicylic acid on haemostasis in the horse. *Equine Vet J* 13:205, 1981.

176. Smith WL: Prostanoid biosynthesis and mechanisms of action. *Am J Physiol* 263:F181, 1992.

177. Brooks PM, Day RO: Nonsteroidal antiinflammatory drugs—differences and similarities. *N Engl J Med* 324:1716, 1991.

178. Gerring EL, Lees P, Taylor JB: Pharmacokinetics of phenylbutazone and its metabolites in the horse. *Equine Vet J* 13:152, 1981.

179. Sams R, Gerken DF, Ashcraft SM: Pharmacokinetics of ketoprofen after multiple intravenous doses to mares. *J Vet Pharmacol Ther* 18:108, 1995.

180. Cryer B, Feldman M: Effect of nonsteroidal anti-inflammatory drugs on endogenous gastrointestinal prostaglandins and therapeutic strategies for prevention and treatment of nonsteroidal anti-inflammatory drug-induced damage. *Arch Intern Med* 152:1145, 1992.

181. Clive DM, Stoff JS: Renal syndromes associated with nonsteroidal antiinflammatory drugs. *N Engl J Med* 310:563, 1984.

182. Snow DH, Douglas TA, Thompson H, et al: Phenylbutazone toxicosis in Equidae: A biochemical and pathophysiologic study. *Am J Vet Res* 42:1754, 1981.

183. MacKay RJ, French TW, Nguyen HT, et al: Effects of large doses of phenylbutazone administration to horses. *Am J Vet Res* 44:774, 1983.

184. MacAllister CG, Morgan SJ, Borne AT, et al: Comparison of adverse effects of phenylbutazone, flunixin meglumine, and ketoprofen in horses. *J Am Vet Med Assoc* 202:71, 1993.

185. Gunson DE: Renal papillary necrosis in horses. *J Am Vet Med Assoc* 182:263, 1983.

186. Collins LG, Tyler DE: Phenylbutazone toxicosis in the horse: A clinical study. *J Vet Med Assoc* 184:699, 1984.

187. Cohen ND, Carter GK, Mealy RH, et al: Medical management of right dorsal colitis in 5 horses: A retrospective study (1987–1993). *J Vet Intern Med* 9:272, 1995.

188. Carrick DM, Papich MG, Middleton DM, et al: Clinical and pathologic effects of flunixin meglumine administration to neonatal foals. *Can J Vet Res* 53:195, 1989.

189. Karcher LF, Dill SG, Anderson AI, et al: Right dorsal colitis. *J Vet Intern Med* 4:247, 1990.

190. Crisman MV, Wicke JR, Sams RA, et al: Concentration of phenylbutazone and oxyphenbutazone in post-parturient mares and their neonatal foals. *J Vet Pharmacol Ther* 14:330, 1991.

191. Gray PR, Derksen FE, Robinson NE, et al: The role of cyclooxygenase products in the acute airway obstruction and airway hyperreactivity of ponies with heaves. *Am Rev Respir Dis* 140:154, 1989.

192. Cohn LA: The influence of corticosteroids on host defense mechanisms. *J Vet Intern Med* 5:95, 1991.

193. Auer JA, Fackleman GE: Treatment of degenerative joint disease in the horse: A review and commentary. *Vet Surg* 10:80, 1981.

194. Smith WL: Prostanoid biosynthesis and mechanisms of action. *Am J Physiol* 263:F181, 1992.

195. Breider MA: Endothelium and inflammation. *J Am Vet Med Assoc* 203:300, 1993.

196. Flower RJ: Lipocortin and the mechanism of action of the glucocorticoids. *Br J Pharmacol* 94:987, 1988.

197. Duncan GS, Peers SH, Carey F, et al: The local anti-inflammatory action of dexamethasone in the rat carrageenan oedema model is reversed by an antiserum to lipocortin 1. *Br J Pharmacol* 108:62, 1993.

198. Moncada S, Palmer RM: Inhibition of the induction of nitric oxide synthase by glucocorticoids: Yet another explanation for their anti-inflammatory effects? *Trends Pharmacol Sci* 12:130, 1991.

199. Davidson FF, Dennis EA: Biological relevance of lipocortins and related proteins as inhibitors of phospholipase A_2. *Biochem Pharmacol* 38:3645, 1989.

200. Lane PJ, Lees P, Fink-Gremmels J: Action of dexamethasone in an equine model of acute non-immune inflammation. *Res Vet Sci* 48:87, 1990.

201. Lees P, Higgins AJ, Sedgwick AD, et al: Actions of betamethasone in models of acute non-immune inflammation. *Br Vet J* 143:143, 1987.

202. Harkins JD, Carney JM, Tobin T: Clinical use and characteristics of the corticosteroids. *Vet Clin North Am Equine Pract* 9:543, 1993.

203. Nixon AJ: Intra-articular medication. In Robinson NE, ed. *Current Veterinary Therapy in Equine Medicine 3.* Philadelphia, WB Saunders, 1992, p 127.

204. Magnuson NS, McGuire TC, Banks KL: In vitro and in vivo effects of corticosteroids on peripheral blood lymphocytes from ponies. *Am J Vet Res* 39:393, 1978.

205. Burgurez PN, Ousey J, Cash RSG, et al: Changes in blood neutrophil and lymphocyte counts following administration of cortisol to horses and foals. *Equine Vet J* 15:58, 1983.

206. Cupp TR, Fauci AS: Corticosteroid-mediated immunoregulation in man. *Immunol Rev* 65:133, 1982.

207. Schaffner A, Schaffner T: Glucocorticoid-induced impairment of macrophage antimicrobial activity: Mechanisms and dependence of the state of activation. *Rev Infect Dis* 9:S620, 1987.

208. Smith JE, DeBowes RM, Cipriano JE: Exogenous corticosteroids increase serum iron concentrations in mature horses and ponies. *J Am Vet Med Assoc* 188:1296, 1986.

209. Tulamo RM, Bramlage LR, Gabel AA: The influence of corticosteroids on sequential clinical and synovial fluid parameters in joints with acute infectious arthritis in the horse. *Equine Vet J* 21:332, 1989.

210. Smith DA, Maxie MG, Wilcock BP: Disseminated mycosis: A danger with systemic corticosteroid therapy. *Can Vet J* 22:276, 1981.

211. Naylor J, Kronfeld D, Acland H: Hyperlipemia in horses: Effects of undernutrition and disease. *Am J Vet Res* 41:899, 1980.

212. Moore BR, Abood SK, Hinchcliff KW: Hyperlipemia in miniature horses and miniature donkeys. *J Vet Intern Med* 5:356, 1994.

213. Freestone JF, Wolfsheimer KJ, Ford RB, et al: Triglyceride, insulin, and cortisol responses of ponies to fasting and dexamethasone administration. *J Vet Intern Med* 5:15, 1991.

214. Cohen ND, Carter GK: Steroid hepatopathy in a horse with glucocorticoid-induced hyperadrenocorticism. *J Am Vet Med Assoc* 200:1682, 1992.

215. Dowling PM, Williams HA, Clark TP: Adrenal insufficiency associated with long-term anabolic steroid administration in a horse. *J Am Vet Med Assoc* 203:1166, 1993.

216. MacHarg MA, Bottoms GD, Carter GK, et al: Effects of multiple intramuscular injections and doses of dexamethasone on plasma cortisol concentrations and adrenal responses to ACTH in horses. *Am J Vet Res* 46:2285, 1985.

217. Slone DE, Purohit RC, Ganjam VK, et al: Sodium retention and cortisol (hydrocortisone) suppression caused by dexamethasone and triamcinolone in equids. *Am J Vet Res* 44:280, 1983.

218. Toutain PL, Brandon RA, Pomyers H, et al: Dexamethasone and prednisone in the horse: Pharmacokinetics and actions on the adrenal gland. *Am J Vet Res* 45:1750, 1984.

219. Short CR, Beadle RE: Pharmacology of anti-arthritic drugs. *Vet Clin North Am* 8:401, 1978.

220. Autefage A, Alvinerie M, Toutain L: Synovial fluid and plasma kinetics of methylprednisolone and methylprednisolone acetate in horses following intra-articular administration of methylprednisolone acetate. *Equine Vet J* 18:193, 1986.

221. Chen CL, Sailor JA, Collier J, et al: Synovial and serum levels of triamcinolone following intra-articular administration of triamcinolone acetonide in the horse. *J Vet Pharmacol Ther* 15:240, 1992.

222. Hackett RP: Intra-articular use of corticosteroids in the horse. *J Am Vet Med Assoc* 181:292, 1982.

223. Nizolek DJH, White KK: Corticosteroids and hyaluronic acid treatments in equine degenerative joint disease: A review. *Cornell Vet* 71:355, 1981.

224. Owen RR, Marsh JA, Hallet FR, et al: Intra-articular corticosteroid- and exercise-induced arthropathy in a horse. *J Am Vet Med Assoc* 184:302, 1984.

225. Owen RR: Intra-articular corticosteroid therapy in the horse. *J Am Vet Med Assoc* 177:710, 1980.

226. Chunekamari S, Krook LP, Lust G, et al: Changes in articular cartilage after intra-articular injections of methylprednisolone acetate in horses. *Am J Vet Res* 50:1733, 1989.

227. Trotter GW, McIlwraith CW, Yovich JV, et al: Effects of

intra-articular administration of methylprednisolone acetate on normal equine articular cartilage. *Am J Vet Res* 52:83, 1991.

228. Hoffis GF, Murdick PW, Tharp VL, et al: Plasma concentrations of cortisol and corticosterone in the normal horse. *Am J Vet Res* 31:1379, 1970.

229. O'Conner JT: The untoward effects of corticosteroids in equine practice. *J Am Vet Med Assoc* 153:1614, 1968.

230. Eyre P, Elmes PJ, Strickland S: Corticosteroid-potentiated vascular responses of the equine digit: A possible pharmacologic basis for laminitis. *Am J Vet Res* 40:135, 1979.

231. Robinson NE: Bronchodilators in equine medicine. In Proceedings of the 10th Annual American College of Veterinary Internal Medicine Forum, 1992, p 287.

232. Derksen FJ, Robinson NE, Armstrong PJ, et al: Airway reactivity in ponies with recurrent airway obstruction (heaves). *J Appl Physiol* 58:598, 1985.

233. Buechner-Maxwell V: Airway hyperresponsiveness. *Compend Contin Educ Vet Pract* 5:1379, 1993.

234. Yu M, Wang Z, Robinson NE: Prejunctional α_2-adrenoreceptors inhibit acetylcholine release from cholinergic nerves in equine airways. *Am J Physiol* 265:L565, 1993.

235. Broadstone RV, Scott JS, Derksen FJ, et al: Effect of atropine in ponies with recurrent airway obstruction. *J Appl Physiol* 65:2720, 1988.

236. Pearson EG, Riebold TW: Comparison of bronchodilators in alleviating clinical signs in horses with chronic obstructive pulmonary disease. *J Am Vet Med Assoc* 194:1287, 1989.

237. Robinson NE, Derksen FJ, Berney C, et al: The airway response of horses with recurrent airway obstruction (heaves) to aerosol administration of ipratropium bromide. *Equine Vet J* 25:299, 1993.

238. Durcharme NG, Fubini SL: Gastrointestinal complications associated with the use of atropine in horses. *J Am Vet Med Assoc* 82:229, 1983.

239. Hamlin RL, Klepinger WL, Gilpin KW, et al: Autonomic control of heart rate in the horse. *Am J Physiol* 22:978, 1972.

240. Slinker BK, Campbell KB, Alexander JE, et al: Arterial baroreflex control of heart rate in the horse, pig, and calf. *Am J Vet Res* 43:1926, 1982.

241. Hinchcliff KW, McKeever KH, Muir WW: Hemodynamic effects of atropine, dobutamine, nitroprusside, phenylephrine, and propanolol in conscious horses. *J Vet Intern Med* 5:80, 1991.

242. Hoffman BB, Lefkowitz RJ: Catecholamines and sympathetic drugs. In Gilman AG, Rall TW, Nies AS, et al, eds. *The Pharmacologic Basis of Therapeutics,* ed 8. New York, McGraw-Hill, 1990, p 187.

243. Anderson MG, Aitken MM: Biochemical and physiologic effect of catecholamine administration in the horse. *Res Vet Sci* 22:357, 1977.

244. Snow DH: Metabolic and physiologic effects of adrenoreceptor agonist and antagonists in the horse. *Res Vet Sci* 27:372, 1979.

245. Adams HR: New perspectives in cardiopulmonary therapeutics: Receptor-selective adrenergic drugs. *J Am Vet Med Assoc* 185:966, 1984.

246. Shapland JE, Garner HE, Hatfield DG: Cardiopulmonary effects of clenbuterol in the horse. *J Vet Pharmacol Ther* 4:43, 1981.

247. Sasse HHL: Clinical aspects of current beta-agonist use in veterinary medicine. In Hanrahan JP, ed. *Beta-Agonists and Their Effects on Animal Growth and Carcass Quality.* Essex, Elsevier Applied Publishing, 1987, p 60.

248. Turgut K, Sasse HHL: Influence of clenbuterol on mucociliary transport in healthy horses and horses with chronic obstructive pulmonary disease. *Vet Rec* 125:526, 1989.

249. Traub-Dargatz JL, McKinnon AO, Thrall MA, et al: Evalua-

tion of clinical signs of disease, bronchoalveolar lavage and tracheal wash analysis, and arterial blood gas tensions in 13 horses with chronic obstructive pulmonary disease treated with prednisone, methyl sulfonmethane, and clenbuterol hydrochloride. *Am J Vet Res* 53:1908, 1992.

250. Erichsen DF, Aviad AD, Schultz RH, et al: Clinical efficacy and safety of clenbuterol HCl when administered to effect in horses with chronic obstructive pulmonary disease (COPD). *Equine Vet J* 26:331, 1994.

251. Rose RJ, Allen JR, Brock KA: Effects of clenbuterol hydrochloride on certain respiratory and cardiovascular parameters in horses performing treadmill exercises. *Res Vet Sci* 35:301, 1983.

252. Rose RJ, Evans DL: Cardiorespiratory effects of clenbuterol in fit Thoroughbred horses during a maximal exercise test. In Gillespie JR, Robinson NE, eds. *Equine Exercise Physiology 3.* Davis, CA, ICEEP Publications, 1987, p 117.

253. Slocombe RF, Covelli G, Bayly WM: Respiratory mechanics of horses during stepwise treadmill exercise tests, and the effect of clenbuterol pretreatment on them. *Aust Vet J* 69:221, 1992.

254. Rall TW: Drugs used in the treatment of asthma. In Gilman AG, Nies AS, Taylor P, eds. *The Pharmacological Basis of Therapeutics,* ed 8. New York, McGraw-Hill, 1990, p 618.

255. Ingvast-Larsson C: Relaxant effects of theophylline and clenbuterol on tracheal smooth muscle from horse and rat *in vitro*. *J Vet Pharmacol Ther* 14:310, 1991.

256. McKiernan BC, Kortiz GD, Scott JS, et al: Plasma theophylline concentration and lung function in ponies with recurrent obstructive lung disease. *Equine Vet J* 122:194, 1990.

257. Ingvast-Larsson C, Appelgren LE, Nyman G: Distribution studies of theophylline: Microdialysis in rat and horse and whole body autoradiography in rats. *J Vet Pharmacol Ther* 15:386, 1992.

258. Errecalde JO, Button C, Mulders MSG: Some dynamic and toxic effects of theophylline in horses. *J Vet Pharmacol Ther* 8:320, 1985.

259. Ingvast-Larsson C, Paalzow G, Paalzow L, et al: Pharmacokinetic studies of theophylline in horses. *J Vet Pharmacol Ther* 8:76, 1985.

260. Ingvast-Larsson C, Kallings P, Persson S, et al: Pharmacokinetics and cardiorespiratory effects of oral theophylline in exercised horses. *J Vet Pharmacol Ther* 12:189, 1989.

261. Erracelade JO, Button C, Baggot JD, et al: Pharmacokinetics and bioavailability of theophylline in horses. *J Vet Pharmacol Ther* 7:255, 1984.

262. Button C, Errecalde JO, Mulders MSG: Loading and maintenance dosage regimens for theophylline in horses. *J Vet Pharmacol Ther* 8:328, 1985.

263. Kowalczyk DF, Beech J, Littlejohn D: Pharmacokinetics of theophylline in horses after intravenous administration. *Am J Vet Res* 45:2272, 1984.

264. Goetz TE, Munsiff IJ, McKiernan BC: Pharmacokinetic disposition of an immediate release aminophylline and sustained-release theophylline formulation in the horse. *J Vet Pharmacol Ther* 12:369, 1989.

265. Errecalde JO, Landoni MF: The pharmacokinetics of a slow-release theophylline preparation in horses after intravenous and oral administration. *Vet Res Commun* 16:131, 1992.

266. Ayers JW, Pearson EG, Riebold TW, et al: Theophylline and dyphylline pharmacokinetics in the horse. *Am J Vet Res* 46:2500, 1985.

267. Thomson JL, McPherson EA: Prophylactic effects of sodium cromoglycate on chronic obstructive pulmonary disease in the horse. *Equine Vet J* 13:243, 1981.

268. Murphy JR, McPherson EA, Lawson GHK: The effects of sodium cromoglycate on antigen inhalation challenge in two

horses affected with chronic obstructive pulmonary disease (COPD). *Vet Immunol Immunopathol* 1:89, 1979.

269. Soma LR, Beech J, Gerber NH: Effect of cromolyn in horses with chronic obstructive pulmonary disease. *Vet Res Comm* 11:339, 1987.

270. Hare JE, Viel L, O'Byrne PM, et al: Effect of sodium cromoglycolate on light racehorses with elevated metachromatic cell numbers on bronchoalveolar lavage and reduced exercise tolerance. *J Vet Pharmacol Ther* 17:237, 1994.

271. Crossman DC, Dashwood MR, Taylor GW, et al: Sodium cromoglycate: Evidence of tachykinin antagonist activity in the human skin. *J Appl Physiol* 75:167, 1993.

272. Leavitt R, Farmer W, Paterson R, et al: Development and evaluation of an enzyme immunoassay for detection of sodium cromoglycate in equine urine. In Proceedings of the 9th International Conference of Racing Analysts and Veterinarians, 1992, p 203.

273. Hinchcliff KW, Muir WW: Pharmacology of furosemide in the horse: A review. *J Vet Intern Med* 5:211, 1991.

274. Hinchcliff KW, Mitten LA: Furosemide, bumetanide, and ethacrynic acid. *Vet Clin North Am Equine Pract* 3:511, 1993.

275. Rubie S, Robinson NW, Stoll M, et al: Flunixin meglumine blocks furosemide-induced bronchodilation in horses with chronic obstructive pulmonary disease. *Equine Vet J* 25:138, 1993.

276. Bianco S, Vahgi A, Robushi M, et al: Prevention of exercise-induced bronchoconstriction by inhaled furosemide. *Lancet* 2:252, 1988.

277. Bianco S, Pieroni MG, Refini RM, et al: Protective effect of inhaled furosemide on allergen-induced early and late asthmatic reactions. *N Engl J Med* 321:1069, 1989.

278. Karlsson J, Choudry NB, Zackrisson C, et al: A comparison of the effect of inhaled diuretics on airway reflexes in humans and guinea pigs. *J Appl Physiol* 72:434, 1992.

279. Robuschi M, Pieroni M, Refini M, et al: Prevention of antigen-induced early obstructive reaction by inhaled furosemide in (atopic) subjects with asthma and (actively sensitized) guinea pigs. *J Allergy Clin Immunol* 85:10, 1990.

280. Verdinai P, DiCarlo S, Baronti A, et al: Effects of inhaled furosemide on the early responses to antigen and subsequent change in airway reactivity of atopic patients. *Thorax* 45:377, 1990.

281. Broadstone RV, Robinson NE, Gray PR: Effects of furosemide on ponies with recurrent airway obstruction. *Pulm Pharmacol* 4:203, 1992.

282. Ali J, Wood JDH: Pulmonary vascular effects of furosemide on gas exchange in pulmonary edema. *J Appl Physiol* 57:169, 1984.

283. Baltopoulos G, Zakynthinos D, Dimopoulos A, et al: Effects of furosemide on pulmonary shunts. *Chest* 96:494, 1989.

284. Pascoe JR, McCabe AE, Franti CE, et al: Efficacy of furosemide in the treatment of exercise-induced pulmonary hemorrhage in Thoroughbred racehorses. *Am J Vet Res* 46:2000, 1985.

285. Sweeney CR, Soma LR, Maxson AD, et al: Effect of furosemide on the racing times of Thoroughbreds. *Am J Vet Res* 51:772, 1990.

286. Soma LR, Laster L, Oppenlander F, et al: Effects of furosemide on the racing times of horses with exercise-induced pulmonary hemorrhage. *Am J Vet Res* 46:763, 1985.

287. Breyer J, Jacobson RH: Molecular mechanisms of diuretic agents. *Annu Rev Med* 141:265, 1990.

288. Olsen SC, Coyne CP, Lowe BS, et al: Influence of cyclooxygenase inhibitors on furosemide-induced hemodynamic effects during exercise in horses. *Am J Vet Res* 53:1562, 1992.

289. Dikshit K, Vyden JK, Forrester JS, et al: Renal and extrarenal hemodynamic effects of furosemide in congestive heart fail-

ure after acute myocardial infarction. *N Engl J Med* 288:1087, 1973.

290. Bourland WA, Day DK, Williamson HE: The role of the kidney in the early nondiuretic action of furosemide to reduce left atrial pressure in the hypervolemic dog. *J Pharmacol Exp Ther* 202:221, 1977.

291. Manohar M: Flunixin meglumine does not negate the furosemide-induced reduction in pulmonary capillary blood pressure of maximally exercising Thoroughbreds. In Proceedings of the 40th Annual AAEP Convention, 1994, p 91.

4.2

Standing Chemical Restraint

John A. E. Hubbell, DVM, MS, ACVA
William W. Muir III, DVM, PhD, ACVA, ACVECC

The evolution of equine medicine has led to the incorporation of various diagnostic and therapeutic procedures into the daily routine of the equine practitioner. Many procedures are greatly facilitated if the horse remains motionless. Other procedures, especially those that involve invasive techniques, may require that analgesia be provided. On other occasions, it may be prudent to calm the horse before bringing it into close proximity of expensive equipment or simply to minimize the potential for someone getting hurt. There is no single drug that produces optimal conditions for all procedures. Often, combinations of drugs are employed when analgesia in addition to sedation is required. Some agents, because of their side effects, invalidate the results of diagnostic tests. Administration of xylazine, for example, causes increases in serum glucose levels and decreases in serum insulin levels. Acepromazine reduces the response to injected allergens when skin is tested for allergic reactions. The basis for safe and effective standing chemical restraint is an understanding of the basic and applied pharmacology of the agents employed. The pharmacology and clinical use of tranquilizers, sedatives, and analgesics are discussed in this chapter. The subjects of local, intravenous, and general anesthesia are covered in detail in other textbooks.

SEDATIVES AND TRANQUILIZERS

The goal of sedative and tranquilizer administration is to eliminate fear, produce a calming effect, reduce resistance to manipulation, and ideally eliminate pain. Classically, sedatives and tranquilizers are distinct groups of drugs based on their central nervous system (CNS) site of action. Sedatives are classically considered as agents that act at the cortical level; furthermore, sedatives, if given in sufficient quantity, produce CNS depression to the point at which hypnosis (artificial sleep) occurs. Tranquilizers act at subcortical levels, particularly at the reticular activating system, effectively filtering afferent and efferent nervous system activity. Increasing doses of tranquilizers produce greater degrees of calming but do not produce hypnosis. In practical use in animals, drugs acting at different levels of the CNS have been used to attain the same result. Thus, the distinction has become blurred, and the term "sedative-tranquilizer" has evolved.

Phenothiazine Tranquilizers

A large number of phenothiazine compounds have been formulated for a wide range of therapeutic uses, including tranquilization. Acepromazine, a potent phenothiazine derivative, is currently the most commonly used tranquilizer in veterinary medicine and the most commonly used phenothiazine tranquilizer in the horse.

Mode of Action. Phenothiazine tranquilizers act at the brain stem and other subcortical areas by inhibiting the action of CNS neurotransmitters, mainly dopamine.[1] Phenothiazine tranquilizers are excellent choices for preventing the excitatory and locomotor effects of opioids because of their ability to inhibit the CNS effects of dopamine. This inhibition of neurotransmitters causes calming, decreases in motor activity, and increases in the threshold to stimuli from the environment. Phenothiazine tranquilizers do not produce analgesia but may potentiate other drugs that are analgesic, such as butorphanol.

Pharmacology. Phenothiazines reduce sympathetic tone centrally and produce peripheral α_1-adrenoreceptor blockade. α_1-Adrenoreceptor blockade can produce hypotension and alters the vascular response to catecholamines. Most notably, prior administration of phenothiazines may block the usual vasoconstrictive response that follows administration of epinephrine. α_1-Adrenoreceptor blockade diminishes the effectiveness of epinephrine as a vasopressor and can potentiate hypotension because of epinephrine's β_2-adrenergic activity causing vasodilation of skeletal muscle blood vessels (epinephrine reversal). Phenothiazine-induced hypotension can be exacerbated in excited or stressed horses with high circulating concentrations of catecholamines. Hypotension-induced excitement may cause further release of epinephrine, compounding the problem. Phenothiazine-induced hypotension is best treated with intravenous fluids. Phenothiazine tranquilizers also have cardiac anti-arrhythmic and anti-fibrillatory activity.[2] Phenothiazine tranquilizers do not produce clinically significant respiratory depression. Respiratory rate is slowed, but tidal volume increases to compensate.[3] Although not significant when phenothiazine tranquilizers are administered alone, respiratory depression may become manifest when phenothiazines are used in combination with other drugs, particularly anesthetics.

Phenothiazine tranquilizers directly and indirectly produce a wide variety of effects on other organ systems. Packed cell volume and plasma proteins are reduced due to splenic sequestration.[4, 5] Serum glucose may increase, due to epinephrine release in response to induced hypotension. Platelet function has been shown to be inhibited in other species and thus is of potential concern. Phenothiazine tranquilizers reduce secretory and motor activity in the gastrointestinal tract. Phenothiazine tranquilizers have variable effects on the liver metabolism and renal excretion of other compounds, depending on the magnitude of their effect on blood flow. Phenothiazine tranquilizers alter reproductive function in other species, affecting ovulation, the synthesis and excretion of reproductive hormones, and the length of gestation. Phenothiazine tranquilizers produce paralysis of the retractor penis muscle and have produced priapism (persistent, abnormal erection of the penis). The incidence of priapism may be dose related. Treatment of priapism is essentially supportive and is not uniformly successful, although the administration of benztropine (0.01 to 0.02 mg/kg) has been occasionally therapeutic.[6] Benztropine is a synthetic compound that has anti-cholinergic and anti-histaminic effects. The effects of benztropine on priapism may be due to its acetylcholine antagonizing effects. It is recommended that phenothiazines be used with caution and at the minimal effective dose in stallions and geldings, particularly geldings receiving anabolic steroids.

Clinical Use. Phenothiazine tranquilizers produce calming in excitable horses that resist manipulation but in general do not profoundly affect behavior in aggressive or intractable horses. Phenothiazine tranquilizers rarely produce significant ataxia or muscle relaxation, thus horses remain stable for standing surgery and can be trailered. The onset of action following either intravenous or intramuscular administration is not immediate and is influenced by the environment in which the horse is held. The intensity of effect is enhanced by placing the horse in a quiet, familiar environment for 20 to 30 minutes following administration of therapy. The duration of action is dose dependent and often exceeds 6 hours. The degree and duration of flaccidity of the penis is an indication of the intensity of effect. Horses, even when calmed, are easily aroused, particularly if painful or if subjected to noisy or painful stimuli. Phenothiazine tranquilization is enhanced by a combination with sedatives and analgesics. Table 4–1 lists drugs and drug combinations that have been recommended for use in the horse.

Benzodiazepines

Benzodiazepines are anticonvulsants and produce muscle relaxation via CNS effects. Benzodiazepines have minor sedative properties in horses and are used occasionally as adjuncts to general anesthesia or as anticonvulsants. Benzodiazepines block chloride ion fluxes in the CNS thus hyperpolarizing membranes and inhibiting CNS function and enhancing the activity of gamma-aminobutyric acid and other inhibitory neurotransmitters.[7] Diazepam and midazolam are two benzodiazepines that have been used in the horse. The benzodiazepine, zolazepam, is only available as a component of the proprietary drug tiletamine zolazepam (Telazol), which has been used for short-term anesthesia and induction to inhalation anesthesia in horses.[8]

Pharmacology. Muscle relaxation and ataxia are the most prominent effects produced following the intravenous administration of diazepam to horses. Severe ataxia and recumbency are produced at higher doses (greater than 0.1 mg/kg, intravenously).[9] Diazepam appears to produce some calming at higher clinical doses in that the horses are less active and

Table 4–1. Recommended Intravenous Dosages of Drugs Used for Standing Chemical Restraint

Drug	Dose
Phenothiazine Tranquilizers	
Acepromazine	0.02–0.08 mg/kg
Promazine	0.5–1 mg/kg
Benzodiazepines	
Diazepam*	0.02–0.1 mg/kg
Midazolam*	0.01–0.05 mg/kg
α₂-Adrenoreceptor Agonists	
Xylazine	0.5–1 mg/kg
Detomidine	0.01–0.04 mg/kg
Chloral Derivatives	
Chloral hydrate	2–6 mg/kg
Opioids	
Butorphanol	0.01–0.05 mg/kg
Combinations	
Xylazine/acepromazine	0.6/0.02 mg/kg
Xylazine/butorphanol	0.6/0.01–0.02 mg/kg
Xylazine/morphine†	0.6/0.3–0.6 mg/kg

*Causes significant ataxia and muscle relaxation at these doses.
†Give xylazine 3 to 5 minutes prior to morphine.

may adopt a fixed gaze and stare. The cardiopulmonary effects of diazepam are negligible.

Clinical Use. Diazepam and midazolam are used primarily as anticonvulsants and as adjuncts to other drugs prior to general anesthesia. The degree of ataxia and muscle relaxation produced for a given level of sedation precludes their general use as sedatives. Horses given diazepam may demonstrate increased locomotor activity and become excited due to disorientation and their inability to maintain an upright posture. Ataxia following administration of diazepam may last for 2 hours or longer.

Butyrophenones

The use of butyrophenone tranquilizers has been reported in the horse.[10–12] Butyrophenones inhibit the excitatory effects of dopamine and norepinephrine centrally. Butyrophenone tranquilizers are potentially useful in a wide variety of species but can produce bizarre behavioral abnormalities, excitement, and extrapyramidal effects in horses that can be prolonged.[10] The use of butyrophenone tranquilizers is not recommended in the horse.

Pharmacology. Butyrophenones produce calming with minimal pulmonary and cardiovascular side effects. Hypotension, due to α₁-adrenergic blockade, can occur but is less pronounced than that which occurs following the administration

of phenothiazine tranquilizers. A wide variety of bizarre CNS side effects including apparent panic, vocalization, and profound stupor have been reported and are apparently dose independent.

Clinical Use. Although several butyrophenone tranquilizers (haloperidol, droperidol, lenperone, azaperone) have been investigated for use in horses, they cannot be recommended for use at this time based on their inconsistency of beneficial effects and their potential for untoward side effects.

α₂-Adrenoreceptor Agonists

α₂-Adrenoreceptor agonists produce sedation, muscle relaxation, and analgesia when administered intravenously or intramuscularly. The effects of α₂-adrenoreceptor agonists can be specifically antagonized by the administration of α₂-adrenoreceptor antagonists. Xylazine and detomidine are two α₂-adrenoreceptor agonists approved for use in the horse. Detomidine is approximately 100 times more potent than is xylazine and has a duration of action at least double that of xylazine.

Mode of Action. The effects of α₂-adrenoreceptor agonists are produced by stimulation of α₂-adrenoreceptors both centrally and peripherally. α₂-Adrenoreceptor stimulation reduces excitatory neurotransmitter concentrations by inhibiting the release of norepinephrine. The peripheral effects of α₂-adrenoreceptor agonists result from a combination of α₂- and weaker α₁-adrenoreceptor activity.

Pharmacology. α₂-Adrenoreceptor agonists produce decreases in heart rate and cardiac output and increases in arterial blood pressure, the magnitude and duration of which varies with dose, potency, and route of administration of the drug. Intravenous administration of xylazine causes transient increases in blood pressure followed by decreases.[13] Detomidine causes more pronounced increases in arterial blood pressure than does xylazine.[14] Decreases in heart rate are caused by increases in vagal tone and by decreases in central sympathetic output, which may produce sinus arrest or block and first- and second-degree heart block. Anticholinergics (atropine, glycopyrrolate) partially antagonize the bradycardic effects of α₂-adrenoreceptor agonists but do not restore cardiac output to pre-drug levels. Although xylazine increases the sensitivity of the myocardium to epinephrine-induced arrhythmias in other species, this does not occur in horses.[15] α₂-Adrenoreceptor agonists are respiratory depressants.[16, 17] Respiratory rate is most affected, but both the respiratory rate and tidal volume are decreased after the intravenous administration of larger doses. The arterial partial pressure of carbon dioxide may increase but usually remains within clinically acceptable values (less than 50 mm Hg). Oxygenation is impaired in part via decreases in respiratory rate and tidal volume but also because of decreases in respiratory compliance caused by relaxation of the muscles of the upper airway and by decreases in cardiac output leading to ventilation-perfusion abnormalities. The respiratory depressant activity of these drugs is seldom significant when the drugs are administered alone but may become significant when the drugs are used in combination with other drugs, particularly anesthetic drugs such as thio-barbiturates or ketamine that produce recumbency. α_2-Adrenoreceptor agonists cause decreases in gastrointestinal secretory and propulsive activity that can be profound and prolonged. Serum glucose is increased, and serum insulin levels are decreased in adults but not in foals.[18] α_2-Adrenoreceptor agonists induce a diuresis that is believed to be mediated by glucosuria and inhibition of renal tubular sodium resorption.[19] Increases in uterine tone occur, but there is no apparent effect on pregnancy.[20] Horses that are given α_2-adrenoreceptor agonists frequently sweat and may demonstrate patchy areas of piloerection.

Clinical Use. α_2-Adrenoreceptor agonists are used to provide standing chemical restraint for various procedures, to provide analgesia, and to act as sedatives prior to anesthesia. Horses typically assume a wide stance with the head extended and lowered. In male horses, some relaxation of the penis may occur and the lower lip becomes flaccid. Muscle relaxation and ataxia may be severe, particularly when large doses are given intravenously. If left unattended, horses tend to stagger forward and head press. α_2-Agonists can be used to calm excitable horses and in addition may blunt aggressive behavior. Despite their appearance, horses are arousable given a sufficient stimulus; therefore, care should be taken when handling or approaching these animals. The analgesia provided by α_2-agonists may be sufficient for minor surgery particularly on the head and neck, but a local anesthetic is often needed. Yohimbine and tolazoline are α_2-adrenoreceptor antagonists that can be given intravenously to reverse the effects of xylazine or detomidine. The dose of yohimbine in the horse is 0.04 to 0.08 mg/kg, intravenously. The dose range of tolazoline is 2.0 to 4.0 mg/kg, intravenously.

α_2-Adrenoreceptor agonists are widely used to treat abdominal pain (colic). These drugs have repeatedly been shown to be the most effective drugs for the relief of colic pain but are not without significant side effects.[21, 22] α_2-Adrenoreceptor agonists cause decreases in cardiac output, arterial partial pressure of oxygen (PaO_2), and intestinal motility in addition to relieving the pain.[23] The decreases in cardiac output, PaO_2, and motility have the potential to exacerbate the disease; thus, these agents should be used with discretion. The increased duration of action of detomidine is also of concern, because sustained analgesia may postpone surgery or re-evaluation of the patient. α_2-Adrenoreceptor agonists should be used in small incremental doses intravenously when evaluating and treating abdominal pain. This will minimize the duration of the decreases in motility and prompt frequent re-evaluation of the patient. Table 4–1 lists drug doses and drug combinations that have been recommended for use in the horse.

Chloral Hydrate

Chloral hydrate is a sedative hypnotic that can be used to produce useful sedation and general anesthesia in horses, but its use has been supplanted by the advent of newer intravenous and inhalation anesthetics. Chloral hydrate is not an analgesic at subanesthetic doses.

Pharmacology. Chloral hydrate produces dose-dependent cardiopulmonary depression. When used as a sedative, mini-

mal changes are produced. Respiratory depression, bradycardia, decreases in cardiac output, and first- and second-degree atrioventricular block can occur as doses are increased. Atrial flutter and fibrillation have been produced after the administration of anesthetic doses of chloral hydrate to adult horses.[24] The effect of sedative doses of chloral hydrate on pregnancy is unclear, but anesthetic doses have been associated with abortion probably due to hypoxia and hypotension. Chloral hydrate decreases gastrointestinal motility.

Clinical Use. Chloral hydrate is primarily used intravenously to produce sedation and mild hypnosis. This drug can be used orally but has a bitter taste and may irritate the gastrointestinal mucosa. Chloral hydrate, if inadvertently administered perivascularly, causes cellulitis that frequently results in sloughing of tissues. Chloral hydrate is seldom used alone but can be used to enhance the effects of other drugs. Chloral hydrate has been combined with pentobarbital and magnesium sulfate in proprietary combinations that are no longer available. The use of chloral hydrate has diminished greatly, because no proprietary solution is available. Chloral hydrate is a schedule IV controlled substance, thus accurate records must be kept regarding its use.

Opioid Analgesics

Opioids, generally referred to as narcotics, are used in the horse to produce analgesia and augment the sedation produced by other agents. A variety of schemes (agonist, partial agonist, agonist-antagonist, antagonist) have evolved in order to clarify the effects of opioid activity for clinical use. Currently, the drugs are best classified by identifying their activity at known clinically relevant opioid receptors. Opioids have the ability to induce excitement and increase locomotor activity in the horse.

Pharmacology. Opioid analgesics produce their effects by reversibly combining with opioid receptors both in the CNS and in other organs. While analgesia is the desired effect, opioids often produce side effects that are partly due to differences in potency at the various opioid receptor subtypes. These effects include sedation, respiratory depression, decreases in propulsive activity of the gastrointestinal tract, changes in cardiovascular function, and increases or decreases in locomotor activity. The clinical assessment of analgesic potency of opioids can be problematic, because some opioids produce analgesia without affecting mentation. Thus, although less painful, the horse may become more responsive to stimuli, such as touch and noise. Most opioids are combined with sedative-tranquilizers to reduce their response to environmental or physical stimuli when used to produce standing chemical restraint. The level of respiratory depression following the administration of opioids depends on the degree of CNS depression produced by the drug or drugs with which they are co-administered. Low doses of morphine, for example, cause transient hyperventilation even though morphine raises the respiratory center threshold to carbon dioxide (CO_2) and decreases the respiratory center sensitivity to CO_2. Transient hyperventilation is probably the result of morphine's differential effects on depressant and excitatory opioid receptors. The respiratory depressant effects of morphine can be produced if the horse is depressed or if drugs that cause depression are co-administered. Bradycardia, due to increases in vagal tone, can occur when morphine is given to depressed horses or is given in combination with agents that cause sedation. Increases in heart rate and blood pressure occur if horses become excited after administration of morphine. Opioid-induced CNS excitatory effects have been the basis for the illicit use of narcotics (particularly fentanyl and etorphine) in performance horses.

Clinical Use. The majority of opioids employed clinically in the horse are used in combination with sedative-tranquilizers. Some of these combinations are discussed in the next section. Butorphanol, a synthetic morphinan derivative, is marketed for use as an analgesic in horses. Butorphanol has an apparent lack of abuse potential and, therefore, does not require a narcotics license. It is a potent analgesic that produces ataxia after the intravenous administration of large doses but does not produce sedation.[25]

CLINICALLY USEFUL DRUG COMBINATIONS

Xylazine and Acepromazine

The intravenous use of a combination of xylazine and acepromazine is reported in the horse.[2] The combination of the two agents allows for a reduction of the dose of both agents. The advantages of the combination include a more rapid onset of effect than is seen with acepromazine and a longer duration of action than is seen with xylazine. For an apparently equal level of sedation, ataxia seems reduced. The cardiopulmonary effects of the intravenous administration of xylazine (0.55 mg/kg) and acepromazine (0.05 mg/kg) include decreases in heart rate, cardiac output, and respiratory rate. Central venous pressure and arterial blood pressure decrease. Respiratory variables do not change. These changes are similar to those seen after the administration of larger doses of xylazine.

Sedative-Tranquilizer and Butorphanol

Butorphanol is used in combination with xylazine to produce a short-duration (30 minutes) standing chemical restraint.[26] The cardiopulmonary changes are similar to those seen after administration of xylazine. The combination does not provide sufficient analgesia for a flank incision, thus a local block must be used if surgery is to be performed. Horses that are given xylazine and butorphanol may head press and occasionally make jerky movements of the head and neck. Butorphanol has been given in combination with detomidine but does not appear to enhance the restraint provided by detomidine alone. Butorphanol in combination with acepromazine in one study of preoperative sedation did not reduce the dose of guaiphenesin-thiamylal needed to produce recumbency.

Sedative-Tranquilizer Morphine

Morphine is used to produce analgesia and standing chemical restraint. Morphine is usually used in combination with xylazine but can be used in very small doses alone or in combination with acepromazine or detomidine.[27] When used in combination with the xylazine, it is advantageous to give xylazine first to ensure sedation prior to the administration of morphine. Following morphine administration, the horse assumes a "saw-horse" stance with the head down. Horses will head press or may stagger forward, thus a restraint is necessary. The placement of a nose twitch and elevation of the head will usually cause the horse to stand squarely on all four feet. Analgesia is produced, but the horses remain sensitive to touch; thus, administration of a local anesthetic should be incorporated if surgery is to be performed. The effects of morphine can be antagonized using naloxone. Naloxone is usually administered intravenously at a dose of 0.01 to 0.04 mg/kg. Because of the short duration of effect of naloxone, horses will occasionally, become hyperactive 2 to 6 hours following xylazine-morphine administration and naloxone reversal. This results because the sedative effects of the xylazine and the reversing effect of the naloxone have passed, allowing the excitatory effects of the morphine to appear. Administration of naloxone or a sedative-tranquilizer will quiet the horse until the effect of the morphine dissipates. Acepromazine is effective here because of its CNS anti-dopaminergic activity and its relatively long duration of action. Morphine is a schedule II narcotic; thus, it must be obtained by prescription and is subject to strict record-keeping requirements.

Other Combinations

The use of other opioids (e.g., etorphine, pentazocine, methadone, nalbuphine, meperidine, fentanyl, nalbuphine) in combination with sedative tranquilizers (acepromazine, promazine, xylazine, detomidine) has been reported in the horse.[28-33] The doses and combinations used are the result of a desire of practitioners to tailor the response to their individual needs. The pharmacologic effects produced by any combination are dependent on the drugs employed and also on the dose.

RECORD-KEEPING

The standards of modern veterinary practice dictate that the administration of any drug or treatment be recorded in a medical record. This is particularly true of sedative/tranquilizer, analgesic, and anesthetic drugs. The Drug Enforcement Agency has classified drugs according to their potential for abuse. Schedule II drugs include opioids, such as morphine, and must be ordered on special forms and stored in fixed, double-locked cabinets or safes. A log must be kept on each quantity of drug purchased, documenting the animal to which it was administered. Schedule III and IV drugs such as thiopental, tiletamine zolazepam, and diazepam do not have to be locked up, but their administration must be documented. Theft or loss of all scheduled drugs should be reported.

REFERENCES

1. Byck R: Drugs and the treatment of psychiatric disorders. In Goodman LS, Gilman A, eds: *Pharmacological Basis of Therapeutics.* New York, Macmillan, 1975, p 152.

2. Muir WW, Werner LL, Hamlin RL: Effects of xylazine and acetylpromazine upon induced ventricular fibrillation in dogs anesthetized with thiamylal and halothane. *Am J Vet Res* 36:1299, 1975.

3. Muir WW, Hamlin RL: Effects of acetylpromazine on ventilatory variables in the horse. *Am J Vet Res* 36:1439, 1975.

4. Demoor A, Desmet P, Van Den Hende C, et al: Influence of promazine on the venous hematocrit and plasma protein concentration in the horse. *Zentralbl Veterinarmed* 25:189, 1978.

5. Parry BW, Anderson GA: Influence of acepromazine on the equine haematocrit. *J Vet Pharmacol Ther* 6:121, 1983.

6. Wilson DV, Nickels FA, Williams MA: Pharmacologic treatment of priapism in two horses. *J Am Vet Med Assoc* 199:1183, 1991.

7. Harvey SC: Hypnotics and sedatives: Miscellaneous agents. In Goodman LS, Gilman A, eds.: *Pharmacological Basis of Therapeutics.* New York, Macmillan, 1975, p 124.

8. Hubbell JAE, Bednarski RM, Muir WW: Xylazine and tiletamine-zolazepam anesthesia in horses. *Am J Vet Res* 50:737, 1989.

9. Muir WW, Sams RA, Huffman RH, et al: Pharmacodynamic and pharmacokinetic properties of diazepam in horses. *Am J Vet Res* 43:1756, 1982.

10. Dodman NH, Waterman E: Paradoxical excitement following the intravenous administration of azaperone in the horse. *Equine Vet J* 11:33, 1979.

11. Lees P, Serrano L: Effects of azaperone on cardiovascular and respiratory functions in the horse. *Br J Pharmacol* 56:263, 1976.

12. Serrano L, Lees P: The applied pharmacology of azaperone in ponies. *Res Vet Sci* 20:316, 1976.

13. Muir WW, Skarda RT, Shehan WC: Hemodynamic and respiratory effects of a xylazine-acetylpromazine drug combination in horses. *Am J Vet Res* 40:1518, 1979.

14. Clarke KW, Taylor PM: Detomidine: A new sedative for horses. *Equine Vet J* 18:366, 1986.

15. Gaynor JS, Bednarski RM, Muir WW: The effect of xylazine on the arrhythmogenic dose of epinephrine in anesthetized horses. Proceedings of the 7th Veterinary Midwest Anesthesia Conference, Urbana, IL, June 8, 1991.

16. Garner HE, Amend JF, Rosborough JP: Effects of Bay Va 1470 on respiratory parameters in ponies. *VM/SAC* 66:921, 1971.

17. Short CE, Matthews N, Turner CL, et al: Cardiovascular and pulmonary function studies of a new sedative/analgesic (detomidine) for use in horses. *Proc Am Assoc Equine Pract* 30:243, 1986.

18. Thurmon JC, Neff-Davis C, Davis LE, et al: Xylazine hydrochloride-induced hyperglycemia and hypoinsulinemia in thoroughbred horses. *J Vet Pharmacol Ther* 5:241, 1988.

19. Trim CM, Hanson RR: Effects of xylazine on renal function and plasma glucose in ponies. *Vet Rec* 118:65, 1986.

20. Katila T, Oijala M: The effect of detomidine (Dormosedan) on the maintenance of equine pregnancy and foetal development: Ten cases. *Equine Vet J* 20:323, 1988.

21. Pippi NL, Lumb WV: Objective tests of analgesic drugs in ponies. *Am J Vet Res* 40:1082, 1979.

22. Muir WW, Robertson JT: Visceral analgesia: Effects of xylazine, butorphanol, meperidine, and pentazocine in horses. *Am J Vet Res* 46:2081, 1985.

23. Stick JA, Chou CC, Derksen FJ, et al: Effects of xylazine on equine intestinal vascular resistance, motility, compliance, and oxygen consumption. *Am J Vet Res* 48:198, 1987.

24. Detweiler DK: Experimental and clinical observations on auricular fibrillation in horses. In Proceedings of the annual meeting of the American Veterinary Medical Association, 1952, p 119.

25. Kalpravidh M, Lumb WV, Wright M, et al: Analgesic effects

26. Robertson JT, Muir WW: A new analgesic drug combination in the horse. *Am J Vet Res* 44:1667, 1983.

27. Muir WW, Skarda RT, Shehan WC: Hemodynamic and respiratory effects of xylazine-morphine sulfate in horses. *Am J Vet Res* 40:1417, 1979.

28. Schauffler AF: Acetylpromazine and methadone equal better equine restraint. *Mod Vet Pract* 50:46, 1969.

29. Davis LE, Sturm BL: Drug effects and plasma concentrations of pentazocine in domesticated animals. *Am J Vet Res* 31:1631, 1970.

30. Jenkins JT, Crooks JL, Charlesworth C: The use of etorphine-acepromazine (analgesic-tranquilizer) mixtures in horses. *Vet Rec* 90:207, 1972.

31. Alexander F, Collett RA: Pethidine in the horse. *Res Vet Sci* 17:136, 1974.

32. Nolan AM, Hall LW: Combined use of sedatives and opiates in horses. *Vet Rec* 114:63, 1984.

33. Taylor PM: Chemical restraint of the standing horse. *Equine Vet J* 17:269, 1985.

4.3

Considerations in Fluid and Electrolyte Therapy

Randolph H. Stewart, DVM, MS

The decision to include fluid and electrolytes in a therapeutic regimen should always involve the same basic intellectual process: (1) the recognition that a fluid or electrolyte derangement is present, (2) an estimate of the qualitative and quantitative aspects of the derangement, (3) the judgment that specific intervention is needed to correct the derangement, (4) the selection of the type and quantity of fluids and electrolytes to be administered as well as the route and rate of administration, and, finally, (5) an evaluation of the therapy and the decision to continue, discontinue, or alter therapy. This section seeks to discuss general principles of normal fluid and electrolyte physiology, the pathophysiologic consequences of disease states, and pertinent aspects of fluid selection and administration that provide the tools necessary to implement and evaluate a fluid therapy program. This discussion assumes that the reader is familiar with the general principles of behavior of physiologic solutions, including the concepts of osmotic pressure and the behavior of ions in solution. For a more thorough treatment of these principles, refer to other textbooks.[1-3]

Fluid Balance. All of the water contained within the body constitutes 60% to 70% of body weight and can be divided, for the purpose of discussion, into the intracellular and extracellular compartments.[4, 5] Intracellular fluid (ICF) is the fluid contained within cells and is composed of approximately 40% of body weight.[4] The extracellular fluid (ECF), which makes up approximately 20% to 30% of body weight,[6-8] can be further subdivided into plasma, interstitial fluid, lymph, and transcellular fluid. Plasma constitutes 4% to 6% of body weight[7, 8] and interstitial fluid, located in the tissues surrounding the cells, makes up approximately 15%. Transcellular fluids are epithelial secretions such as digestive secretions, sweat, and cerebrospinal, pleural, peritoneal, synovial, and intraocular fluids.[1]

It should be remembered that the content and properties of the fluids within any of these divisions are not uniform. Although the vascular compartment is a contiguous body of fluid, its content changes as it traverses the vascular circuit due to the addition or removal of oxygen, carbon dioxide, nitrogenous waste, and other substances. Interstitial fluid and intracellular fluid are contained within numerous small compartments and show even greater heterogeneity. However, for the sake of simplicity, we shall discuss each compartment as if it were a uniform body of fluid.

Since cell membranes are freely permeable to water, interstitial fluid and intracellular fluid share the same osmolarity. Plasma maintains a slightly higher osmolarity than does interstitial fluid, such that the osmotic pressure retaining fluid within the vascular space offsets the hydrostatic pressure moving fluid out.[1] For a substance to exert osmotic pressure between two adjacent fluid spaces it must be maintained at differing concentrations across a selectively permeable membrane. Sodium freely diffuses between plasma and the interstitial fluid; therefore, it is not effective for generating osmotic pressure between these fluid spaces. The substance responsible for the osmotic pressure between these spaces is protein, because it is fairly well contained within the vascular space.

The Na^+–K^+ pump located in the cell wall actively transports potassium into the cell and sodium out of the cell. These actions maintain high extracellular and low intracellular concentrations of sodium, as well as low extracellular and high intracellular concentrations of potassium. Sodium is, therefore, the main extracellular cation and potassium is the principal intracellular cation; additionally, sodium and potassium with their associated anions are the principal extracellular and intracellular osmolar agents, respectively. The relationship of extracellular and intracellular fluid volumes is thus dependent on the body's content of freely exchangeable sodium and potassium.

Consider the following scenarios and their basic effects on ICF and ECF. (Remember that the effects mentioned are those that occur prior to the moderating effects of fluid and electrolyte intake or excretion.)

Intake of Pure Water. The water would be distributed into both the ECF and ICF to maintain equivalent osmolarity between the fluid spaces; therefore, both compartments would increase in volume. Administration of pure water directly into the vascular space results in rapid movement of water into erythrocytes, causing them to rupture.

Intake of an Isotonic Sodium Chloride Solution. The sodium would be maintained in the ECF and, therefore, so would the water. Since the osmolarity of the ECF would be unchanged, there would be no reason for water to move into the cell. In fact, the equal osmolarities of the two fluid spaces would act to prevent such a movement. Only the ECF would increase in volume.

Intake of a Hypertonic Sodium Chloride Solution. Again

the sodium would be maintained within the ECF; however, the addition of this solution would increase the osmolarity of the ECF. The result would be a movement of water out of the cell into the ECF. Therefore, the ECF volume would increase, and the ICF volume would decrease.

Loss of an Isotonic Sodium Chloride Solution. Only the ECF would decrease in volume. Since the remaining ECF would have an osmolarity equivalent to the ICF, there would be no impetus for fluid movement out of the cell.

It is evident that the loss or gain of body fluid may affect the fluid compartments differently depending on the nature and concentration of particles within that fluid. Horses deprived of feed and water develop deficits of water, sodium, chloride, and potassium resulting in loss of both ECF and ICF volumes.[9] The loss of isotonic sodium-rich solutions, such as that seen with hemorrhage, results in a significant decrease in ECF volume without significant change in ICF volume.

Acid-Base Status. An electrolyte is a substance that dissociates into charged particles or ions in solution. For example, sodium chloride is an electrolyte that dissociates into sodium ions and chloride ions when placed in an aqueous solution. Ions that are totally dissociated under physiologic conditions are called fixed or "strong" ions.[10–12] Conversely, labile or "weak" ions remain in equilibrium between their associated and dissociated forms.[10–12] Sodium (Na^+), chloride (Cl^-), and potassium (K^+) are all strong ions.[10–12] Lactate also acts as a strong anion and plays an important role in the acid-base disturbances of pathologic conditions involving increased anaerobic glycolysis.[10, 11] Hydrogen ion (H^+), bicarbonate ion (HCO_3^-), proteins, and carbonate ion (CO_3^{2-}) are weak ions.[10, 11] For example, H^+ in physiologic solutions may combine with hydroxyl ion (OH^-) to form water, with HCO_3^- to form carbonic acid, or with weak acids such as protein or phosphates and is in equilibrium between its ionized state and these non-ionized states. The manner in which these ions interact and exert their influence on the acid-base status of physiologic solutions has been described by Stewart.[10, 11] A very brief synopsis of this approach to acid-base physiology follows.

Stewart states that there are three independent variables that determine the acid-base status of physiologic solutions. Independent variables are the components of a solution whose values can only be changed by adding them to or taking them from the solution. The dependent variables are the components of the solution whose values can change within the solution depending on the values of the independent variables.

The independent variables are: (1) the strong ion difference, (2) the total weak acid concentration, and (3) the PCO_2. The strong ion difference is the sum of the strong cation concentrations minus the sum of the strong anion concentrations. Upon review of the behavior of strong ion solutions, we find that the hydrogen ion concentration varies inversely with the strong ion difference (SID).

$$SID = [Na^+] - [Cl^-]$$

Using Na^+ and Cl^- (the primary strong cation and strong anion in extracellular fluid) we see that as sodium ion concentration [Na^+] increases or chloride ion concentration

[Cl⁻] decreases, the strong ion difference increases, the hydrogen ion concentration [H⁺] decreases, and the solution becomes more alkaline. The converse is also true. A decrease in the difference between the sodium and chloride concentrations results in an increase in the hydrogen ion concentration and the solution becomes more acidic.

Proteins, when considered as a whole, are weak acids and make up approximately 95% of the weak acids present in plasma. The other 5% consists primarily of phosphates. As we might expect, an increase in total proteins tends to make plasma more acidic and a decrease makes it more alkaline. The ionic charge due to plasma proteins appears to be entirely the result of charges on albumin.[13] The contribution of globulins to acid-base balance is negligible.[13]

The third independent variable that determines the acid-base status of physiologic solutions and the one with which we are most familiar is PCO_2. The effect of CO_2 is evident in the carbonic acid dissociation reaction:

$$CO_2 + H_2O \leftrightarrow H_2CO_3 \leftrightarrow H^+ + HCO_3^-$$

As the partial pressure of CO_2 increases, the equation shifts to the right, H^+ concentration increases, and the solution becomes more acidic. As PCO_2 decreases, the solution becomes more alkaline. Since CO_2 readily penetrates cell membranes, changes in PCO_2 affect all body fluids comparably. Following the onset of hypoventilation, the PCO_2 of ICF and ECF rapidly increases and results in an increased H^+ concentration and a decreased pH.

The dependent variables included in this concept of acid-base physiology are the concentrations of H^+, OH^-, HCO_3^-, CO_3^{2-}, weak acids in the dissociated state, and weak acids in the associated state. It is important to realize that these dependent variables are the result and not the cause of what is happening within the solution. H^+ and HCO_3^- in particular are often considered to be the substances that cause changes to take place in the acid-base status of a solution; however, Stewart's concept gives them more the appearance of indicators of that status.

In light of this evaluation of the behavior of physiologic solutions, we are led to consider how the body acts to regulate acid-base balance. Although protein concentration is an independent variable, it appears unlikely that control of acid-base balance by the body is maintained through manipulation of protein levels. This control is achieved through alterations in PCO_2 by the lungs (the respiratory component) and alterations in strong ion difference primarily by the kidney and to a lesser degree by the gastrointestinal tract (the non-respiratory component). Additionally, because most membranes are relatively impermeable to protein and highly permeable to CO_2, the mechanism for regulating acid-base across membranes must depend on the transport of strong ions. This includes interaction between ICF and ECF as well as between extracellular and transcellular fluids. An example would be the formation of gastric fluid containing a high Cl^- concentration and very low concentrations of strong cations, resulting in a very acidic solution with a negative strong ion difference.

Sodium. Sodium ion and its associated anions are the principal extracellular osmoles due to their relatively high concentration in the ECF.[2] ECF sodium *content* is the major determinant of ECF volume.[2] Sodium excess is usually associated with increased extracellular volume, resulting in ascites or edema. Conversely, sodium depletion is observed clinically as hypovolemia.[14] Plasma or ECF sodium *concentration,* however, is not a good indicator of sodium content or ECF volume; rather, it is an indicator of relative water balance.[15]

It has been determined that the sum of exchangeable sodium (Na_e^+) and exchangeable potassium ions (K_e^+) divided by the total body water is approximately equal to the plasma sodium concentration.[1, 2] This relationship can be illustrated as:

$$Plasma\ [Na^+] \approx (Na_e^+ + K_e^+)/TBW$$

From this relationship we can see that hyponatremia (low Na^+ concentration) may be related to Na_e^+ or K_e^+ loss alone or by water retention alone.[2] However, we find that as exchangeable sodium content increases or decreases, there is often a concomitant increase or decrease in the ECF component of total body water; therefore, the plasma sodium concentration is changed minimally if at all.

Potassium depletion may induce hyponatremia by any of three mechanisms. First, potassium loss from the cell results in the movement of sodium into the cell to maintain electroneutrality.[2] Second, potassium depletion results in a decrease in the intracellular osmolarity and, if there is not an equivalent decrease in the extracellular sodium, a movement of water out of the cell causing dilution of the plasma sodium. The third mechanism involves the possible hormonal response to potassium depletion. Antidiuretic hormone (ADH) secretion causes water retention in excess of sodium by increasing water reabsorption in the collecting tubules and collecting duct. The stimulus for ADH release by the posterior lobe of the pituitary is generated by the supraoptic nucleus as a response to a decrease in osmoreceptor cell size.[16] This size decrease may be caused by: (1) loss of free water from the body, (2) increased ECF osmolarity, or (3) loss of intracellular K^+ and decreased intracellular osmolarity—all of which result in a movement of free water out of the cell.[2] Therefore, potassium loss could trigger ADH release and a relative increase in water balance. Total body potassium depletion could, by these mechanisms, result in a hyponatremic condition that would not easily be corrected without supplementation of potassium.

Since plasma or serum sodium concentration is not a good indicator of total body sodium content or extracellular volume, it should be evaluated in light of physical examination findings that more directly reflect vascular and interstitial fluid volume, such as heart rate, pulse quality, capillary refill time, presence of edema, skin elasticity, and moistness of mucous membranes.

Potassium. The Na^+–K^+ pump located in the cell wall continuously moves potassium ions into the cell and sodium ions out of the cell; therefore, potassium is maintained at high intracellular levels and is primarily responsible for intracellular osmolarity. The plasma K^+ concentration is relatively low and is not a good indicator of intracellular or total body potassium content.[17–19] Hyperkalemia associated with acidosis may occur in the presence of normal or reduced total body potassium content.[12, 17] Hypokalemia occurs in association with alkalosis, elevated levels of plasma insulin, or total body potassium depletion.[12] The clinical signs associated with the deficit or excess of potassium ion reflect the very important role it plays in the excitability of nerve and muscle. The clinical effects of hypokalemia include cardiac arrhythmias, myocardial dysfunction, muscular weakness, and intestinal ileus.[12, 17, 20] A hyperkalemic syndrome in horses referred to as hyperkalemic periodic paralysis causes a myotonia characterized by muscle spasms and fasciculations followed by episodes of muscular weakness and recumbency as well as cardiac arrhythmias.[21, 22]

Measurement of intracellular potassium concentration in red blood cells as a means of evaluating total body potassium has been performed in horses.[18] This method appeared to offer an easy direct measurement of intracellular $[K^+]$ and its results appeared to correlate to disease states.[20, 23] However, a study on potassium depletion in horses caused by food deprivation showed erythrocyte potassium concentration to be a poor indicator of whole body potassium status.[19]

Estimation of total body K^+ may be made using plasma sodium concentration and volume estimates. The equation demonstrating the relationship of plasma sodium concentration, exchangeable sodium and potassium, and total body water (TBW) can be rearranged to provide a rough estimate of exchangeable potassium.[24]

$$K_e^+ \approx (\text{plasma } [Na^+] \times TBW) - Na_e^+$$

Exchangeable sodium may be estimated by multiplying plasma $[Na^+]$ by the extracellular volume. The exchangeable potassium for a 500-kg horse with a plasma $[Na^+]$ of 140 mEq/L, an estimated total body water of 300 L (60% of 500 kg) and an estimated ECF volume of 100 L (20% of 500 kg) can then be derived by:

$$K_e^+ \approx (\text{plasma } [Na^+] \times TBW) - (\text{plasma } [Na^+] \times ECF) \approx$$
$$\text{plasma } [Na^+] \times (TBW - ECF) \approx$$
$$140 \text{ mEq/L} \times (300 \text{ L} - 100 \text{ L}) \approx$$
$$28,000 \text{ mEq}$$

This turns out to be the same as multiplying the plasma sodium concentration by the estimated ICF volume. Remember to take possible fluid deficits into account when making an estimate.

The high roughage diet consumed by most horses provides a very high level of dietary potassium—a significant portion of which is excreted in its urine. This high urinary potassium excretion is only moderately reduced in horses that are deprived of food, and its continued loss results in depletion of total body potassium.[9] Healthy horses deprived of feed and water for 72 hours continued to excrete 350 to 750 mEq/day of potassium.[9] It is therefore important, when evaluating a fluid therapy plan for a horse with significantly reduced feed intake, to provide adequate potassium supplementation. Diarrhea and excessive salivary or sweat loss can also contribute to potassium depletion.[25, 26]

Chloride. Changes in chloride concentration with proportional changes in sodium are generally related to loss or gain of free water. These changes may also be associated with mild to moderate changes in acid-base status. For example, a proportional decrease in sodium and chloride concentra-

tions is associated with an increase in free water and dilution of the electrolyte content. If sodium concentration decreases from 144 mEq/L to 127 mEq/L and chloride concentration decreases from 102 mEq/L to 90 mEq/L, the strong ion difference decreases from 42 mEq/L to 35 mEq/L and a mild non-respiratory acidosis results. A similar effect is observed in the loss of free water with an increase in the strong ion difference and development of a non-respiratory alkalosis. This volume contraction alkalosis is observed occasionally in the very early stages of acute diarrhea.

Changes in plasma chloride concentration that are not accompanied by similar changes in sodium concentration cause more dramatic acid-base disturbances. Decreases in plasma chloride without proportional changes in sodium lead to non-respiratory alkalosis caused by an increase in the strong ion difference.[10, 11] This may be observed in conditions that result in the loss of a significant volume of chloride-rich fluid, such as gastric reflux, saliva, or sweat.[25-29] Similarly, acidosis associated with hyperchloremia results from a decrease in strong ion difference. Cases of renal tubular acidosis have been reported in horses associated with hyperchloremia and acidosis with or without hyponatremia.[30-32] In one report, the urinary fractional excretion of sodium in these horses was shown to be elevated.[31] When evaluated using the "strong ion difference" concept,[10, 11] renal tubular acidosis may be the result of an abnormality in the tubular reabsorption of sodium and chloride.

Effects of Volume Infusion. The desirable effects of intravenous fluid administration include an increase in circulating blood volume and pressure and enhanced tissue perfusion; however, the clinician should remain aware of the potential for less desirable consequences. The increase in venous pressure that results from rapid intravenous infusion has two important effects on fluid balance. The first of these effects is an increase in capillary hydrostatic pressure that induces an increased flow from the capillaries to the interstitium. The second effect is a decrease in interstitial fluid drainage resulting from decreased lymph flow.[33] This second effect is rarely considered, but the reason for its occurrence becomes obvious when you consider that the great lymphatic vessels empty into the venous circulation and, therefore, the systemic venous pressure is the lymphatic outflow pressure. The effect on lung water balance is particularly important in the critical care patient. Intravenous crystalloid infusion has been shown experimentally to promote pulmonary edema and pleural effusion via these mechanisms.[33-35] Neonates and patients with hypoproteinemia or left-sided heart dysfunction are at increased risk and should be monitored during volume infusion.

Clinical Indications for Therapy. The information necessary to determine the need for fluid therapy, the type of fluid used, and the route of administration can be acquired from a good history, a thorough physical examination, and a routine set of laboratory data. Discussion of the history should include the presence of diseases or activities associated with fluid and electrolyte disturbances such as colic, diarrhea, nasogastric reflux, hemorrhage, renal failure, and excessive sweating. Also included are the severity and duration of the condition as well as the appetite and water intake since the episode began. The history should not only assist in your estimation of past losses and current requirements of fluids and electrolytes but should also allow you to make reasonable estimates of ongoing losses and future requirements.

Depletion of the sodium-rich ECF is usually associated with clinical signs indicative of decreased plasma volume and decreased tissue perfusion, including increased heart rate, increased capillary refill time, decreased pulse pressure, and cold extremities. Conditions such as acute diarrhea, strangulating obstruction of the bowel, and hemorrhage usually entail loss of fluid primarily from the extracellular space. Severe ECF losses result in cardiovascular compromise and constitute a medical emergency; under these conditions, replacement of fluid volume with an isotonic sodium-containing solution is of prime importance and the evaluation of specific electrolyte imbalances becomes less important. Often, with the administration of an adequate volume of a physiologically balanced solution and in the presence of relatively normal kidney function, the body is able to correct even moderately severe electrolyte imbalances.

Decreased feed and water intake or chronic diarrhea may have associated depletion of total body potassium as well as sodium and loss of intracellular and extracellular water. Clinical signs include changes in skin turgor, dry tongue and mucous membranes, and sunken eyes.[14] These clinical signs begin to appear with fluid losses equalling 4% to 5% of body weight and become more severe as losses increase to 10% to 12% of body weight.

Packed cell volume (PCV) and total plasma or serum protein (TPP) and albumin concentrations are useful indicators of changes in plasma/ECF volume and are relatively easy to obtain. Since they tend to reflect the fluid volume within the vascular space, they are more closely correlated with changes in sodium content and ECF volume than TBW.[14] The problems associated with using these indices are that changes in the indices commonly occur independently of changes in vascular or extracellular volume and that erythrocytes or protein may be lost in conjunction with fluid loss. Horses are particularly susceptible to increases in PCV caused by splenic contraction due to excitement, pain, or stressful situations. Anemia may be present for a variety of reasons.

Increases in TPP may occur as a result of chronic antigenic stimulation and increased gamma globulin levels. Decreases in TPP or albumin are observed with protein loss externally or to enlarged transcellular fluid spaces or with decreased protein production. This occurs in protein-losing enteropathy, pleuritis, peritonitis, and end-stage hepatic failure. Hyperalbuminemia is a more reliable indicator of fluid deficit than are increases in TPP and PCV. PCV, TPP, and albumin determinations are all useful in evaluating fluid balance as long as one is cognizant of their limitations. Repeated measurements are even more useful as a determination of changes in fluid balance in response to therapy.

Therapeutic Plan. While formulating a fluid therapy plan one must keep in mind the daily maintenance requirements of the horse, the current deficits, and the pathologic processes that caused the deficits. The pathologic processes that might require fluid and electrolyte therapy for correction can, for the sake of this discussion, be considered in four general categories with considerable overlap between the groups: shock, decreased intake, increased loss, and conditions of maldistribution. More than one of these processes may be present in a single patient, and each one should be considered when developing a therapeutic plan.

Shock is the cascade of pathophysiologic events induced by tissue perfusion and oxygen delivery that are inadequate to meet the demands of tissue metabolism. Shock, in fact, may be considered to be the extreme example of the other three processes listed earlier; however, it remains a distinct entity conceptually. Shock may occur for several reasons, including loss of plasma volume due to hemorrhage or third space sequestration, decreased cardiac output caused by electrical or mechanical cardiac dysfunction, or maldistribution of blood flow as occurs in endotoxemia.[36] Regardless of the etiology, the shock state, if left untreated, usually progresses to multiple system failure and death.[36] Although several aspects of shock therapy are controversial, some form of fluid therapy is invariably required. Isotonic polyionic fluids have been the mainstay of shock treatment; however, studies have demonstrated the beneficial hemodynamic effects of hypertonic saline solutions (2,400 mOsm/L) in the treatment of experimentally induced shock and hypotensive states in horses.[37–39] The response to hypertonic saline is the result of several factors, including a fluid shift into the vascular space and a decrease in total peripheral vascular resistance.[37] One of the advantages of the use of hypertonic saline in horses is the relatively small volume (~ 2L for an adult horse) required for it to exert its effect. The beneficial effects of hypertonic saline last approximately 30 minutes and should be followed with conventional fluid therapy.

Decreased intake of food or water may occur because of management errors, anorexia, painful conditions such as laminitis, recumbency caused by neurologic or musculoskeletal diseases, or conditions in which the attending clinician limits intake. Regardless of the cause, there will be continuing urinary, fecal, and insensible losses of sodium, chloride, potassium, and water that are not being replaced. Patients in whom potassium depletion and intracellular volume contraction have occurred require potassium supplementation in order to ensure the effectiveness of fluid replacement; however, large potassium deficits are very difficult to correct using only intravenous fluids and may only be fully restored once the horse returns to eating substantial quantities of hay.[14] Oral administration of 40 g of potassium chloride up to three times per day in an adult horse should be considered.[14] Saline administration alone has been shown to be inadequate in correcting the water deficit created by food and water deprivation because it does not attend to the potassium depletion.[40] Also, the presence of hypoglycemia should be investigated and corrected in neonates that are unable or unwilling to nurse.

Diarrhea, reflux of gastric fluid, the sequestration of fluid in the gastrointestinal tract in colic, hemorrhage, polyuric renal failure, and excessive sweating all involve increased loss of fluid and electrolytes. The ECF space generally bears the brunt of rapid fluid loss and loses fluids containing primarily sodium and chloride. The goal of fluid replacement should, therefore, be restoration of extracellular volume with sodium-containing fluids. Horses suffering from exhaustion associated with profuse sweating are commonly chloride and potassium depleted as well as volume depleted.[28, 29] The volume depletion is evidence of sodium depletion regardless of the plasma sodium concentration. An effective solution to use in this case would be saline with the addition of potassium chloride (10 mEq/L), because it will provide chloride in greater amounts than a physiologically balanced solution as well as providing sodium and potassium.[28] These horses also benefit from oral potassium chloride administration. Exhausted horses with synchronous diaphragmatic flutter should have calcium solutions added to their fluid regimen, as needed.[28]

Fluid therapy may be required for conditions involving maldistribution of fluid or electrolytes. Several solutions have proved useful in treating hyperkalemic periodic paralysis, including 5% sodium bicarbonate (1 mEq/kg), 5% dextrose (4.4 to 6.6 mL/kg), and 23% calcium gluconate (0.2 to 0.4 mL/kg) diluted in 1 to 2 L of 5% dextrose.[21, 22] One aspect of the pathophysiology of exertional myopathy is believed to be maldistribution of blood flow and a local increase in lactate concentration.[41] A hypochloremic alkalosis has been associated with this disease; therefore, saline or a balanced electrolyte solution appear to be the best choices for therapy.[42] Sodium bicarbonate solution would be a poor choice in that the additional sodium load would tend to aggravate the alkalosis.

Early recognition of deficits and initiation of appropriate therapy are key determinants of the success of fluid and electrolyte therapy. The first concern is volume depletion. Patients showing signs of cardiovascular compromise should receive immediate attention with provisions made for volume replacement with a balanced solution. The same is true of horses that are persistently hyperthermic and have a recent history of intense exercise and profuse sweating. The ability of the horse's body to cool itself by removing heat from its core to its periphery is dependent on adequate circulating volume. Every effort should be made to cool the horse quickly, including volume replacement.

The next consideration is estimation of electrolyte imbalances and adjustment of the fluid formulation according to the specific needs of the patient. Estimation of sodium content is based on clinical signs of volume depletion or excess. The plasma sodium concentration is then used to determine the relative sodium:water balance. Hyponatremia indicates a relative water excess even in a horse that is volume depleted. The chloride is then evaluated according to the sodium concentration. An increase or decrease in plasma chloride concentration that is proportional to the increase or decrease in sodium concentration indicates only a free water abnormality. A chloride concentration that is not proportional to that of sodium is treated as a primary chloride abnormality.

Intravenous administration of sterile fluids provides the clinician with the greatest direct control over the rate and composition of fluid and electrolyte replacement, although there are some limitations as to content and volume. The potassium concentration of intravenous fluids is important because hyperkalemia should be avoided and there is some time lag for the administered potassium to be moved from the ECF to the ICF. Unless the horse is monitored closely during administration, the upper limit of potassium in intravenous fluids should be 15 to 20 mEq/L.[14] The administration of potassium in intravenous fluids should not exceed 0.5 mEq/kg of body weight/hr.

The volume and rate of administration of intravenous fluids are dependent mainly on the severity of the deficits. The maintenance fluid requirement for adult horses at rest is approximately 65 ml/kg/day or 26 to 30 L/day.[43] Calculations should include maintenance volume plus deficit replacement plus consideration of ongoing losses and oral intake, if any. It is not usually necessary that fluid and electrolyte replacement be immediate or total. Fluids may be formulated to replace mild to moderate deficits over a period of 2 to 3 days. Severe deficits, however, may be life-threatening and require more rapid replacement. Horses with severe volume depletion may receive 5 to 15 L/hr of sodium-containing fluids.[14]

The use of oral fluids administered via nasogastric tube or taken free choice should not be overlooked. They may be used alone or in conjunction with intravenous fluids. They are a great deal cheaper than sterile intravenous preparations, can be fairly easily administered in the field in relatively large volumes, and are particularly useful in less severe or chronic conditions. A horse with chronic diarrhea can often be adequately maintained by providing sodium bicarbonate and potassium chloride in its water.[44] When using oral electrolyte preparations, fresh water not containing supplemental electrolytes should always be available to the horse. Oral fluids should be isotonic or hypotonic and, when given via nasogastric tube, may be administered at the rate of 5 to 10 L every 30 to 60 minutes.[14] Hypertonic oral fluids draw ECF into the gastrointestinal tract and exacerbate the already existing volume depletion. Oral fluids should not be used in horses with gastrointestinal obstructions or gastric reflux.

Occasionally, one may consider administering fluids to horses via an enema. Little information is presently available concerning the effectiveness of enemas as a means of rehydrating horses. One study could not demonstrate rehydration in horses with furosemide-induced dehydration.[45] It is possible that the furosemide interfered with intestinal absorption of fluid and that other experimental models would give a more positive result.[45] Basic guidelines for use of enemas as a method of rehydration should include warm isotonic physiologically balanced solutions administered per rectum through soft flexible tubing. Care should be taken not to damage the rectum or small colon. The appropriate rate of fluid administration by this method is not well delineated; however, in the aforementioned study, horses weighing 298 to 323 kg were given 44 L of isotonic sodium chloride solution over 20 minutes with no reported adverse effects.[45]

REFERENCES

1. Rose BD: *Clinical Physiology of Acid/Base and Electrolyte Disorders,* ed 3. New York, McGraw-Hill, 1989.
2. Saxton DR, Seldin DW: In Kokko JP, Tannen RL, eds: *Fluids and Electrolytes.* Philadelphia, WB Saunders, 1986, p 3.
3. Guyton AC: *Textbook of Medical Physiology,* ed 7. Philadelphia, WB Saunders, 1986, p 348.
4. Gross DR: Drugs acting on fluid and electrolyte balance—physiologic basis. In Booth NH, McDonald LE, eds: *Veterinary Pharmacology and Therapeutics,* ed 6. Ames, IA, State University Press, 1988, p 537.
5. Judson GJ, Mooney GJ: Body water and water turnover rate in thoroughbred horses in training. In Snow DH, Persson SGB, Rose RJ, eds: *Equine Exercise Physiology.* Cambridge, Granta Editions, 1983, p 371.
6. Carlson GP, Harrold D, Rumbaugh GE: Volume dilution of

sodium thiocyanate as a measure of extracellular fluid volume in the horse. *Am J Vet Res* 40:587, 1979.

7. Kohn CW, Muir WW, Sams R: Plasma volume and extracellular fluid volume in horses at rest and following exercise. *Am J Vet Res* 39:871, 1978.

8. Carlson GP: Hematology and body fluids in the equine athlete: A review. In Gillespie JR, Robinson NE, eds: *Equine Exercise Physiology 2.* Davis, CA, ICEEP Publications, 1987, p 393.

9. Rumbaugh GE, Carlson GP, Harrold D: Urinary production in the healthy horse and in horses deprived of feed and water. *Am J Vet Res* 43:735, 1982.

10. Stewart PA: *How to Understand Acid-Base: A Quantitative Acid-Base Primer for Biology and Medicine.* New York, Elsevier, 1981.

11. Stewart PA: Modern quantitative acid-base chemistry. *Can J Physiol Pharmacol* 61:1444, 1983.

12. Mudge GH, Weiner IM: Agents affecting volume and composition of body fluids. In Gilman AG, Rall TW, Nies AS, et al, eds: *Goodman and Gilman's The Pharmacological Basis of Therapeutics,* ed 8. New York, Pergamon Press, 1990, p 682.

13. Figge J, Rossing TH, Fencl V: The role of serum proteins in acid-base equilibria. *J Lab Clin Med* 117:453, 1991.

14. Carlson GP: Fluid therapy. In Robinson NE, ed: *Current Therapy in Equine Medicine.* Philadelphia, WB Saunders, 1983, p 311.

15. Carlson GP: Fluid, electrolyte, and acid-base balance. In Kaneko JJ, ed: *Clinical Biochemistry of Domestic Animals.* New York, Academic Press, 1989, p 543.

16. Guyton AC: *Textbook of Medical Physiology,* ed 7. Philadelphia, WB Saunders, 1986, p 425.

17. Brobst D: Review of the pathophysiology of alterations in potassium homeostasis. *J Am Vet Med Assoc* 188:1019, 1986.

18. Muylle E, Van Den Hende C, Nuytten J, et al: Potassium concentration in equine red blood cells: Normal values and correlation with potassium levels in plasma. *Equine Vet J* 16:447, 1984.

19. Johnson PJ, Goetz TE, Foreman JH, et al: Effect of whole-body potassium depletion on plasma, erythrocyte, and middle gluteal muscle potassium concentration of healthy adult horses. *Am J Vet Res* 52(10):1676, 1991.

20. Muylle E, Nuytten J, Van Den Hende C, et al: Determination of red blood cell potassium content in horses with diarrhoea: A practical approach for therapy. *Equine Vet J* 16:450, 1984.

21. Cox JH, DeBowes RM: Episodic weakness caused by hyperkalemic periodic paralysis in horses. *Compend Contin Educ Pract Vet* 12:83, 1990.

22. Spier SJ, Carlson GP, Holliday TA, et al: Hyperkalemic periodic paralysis in horses. *J Am Vet Med Assoc* 197:1009, 1990.

23. Bain FT, Merritt AM: Decreased erythrocyte potassium concentration associated with exercise-related myopathy in horses. *J Am Vet Med Assoc* 196:1259, 1990.

24. Rose RJ: Electrolyte profiles in horses. *Vet Annual* 25:217, 1985.

25. Stick JA, Robinson NE, Krehbiel JD: Acid-base and electrolyte alterations associated with salivary loss in the pony. *Am J Vet Res* 42:733, 1981.

26. Eckersall PD, Aitchison T, Colquhoun KM: Equine whole saliva: Variability of some major constituents. *Equine Vet J* 17:391, 1985.

27. Rose RJ: Endurance exercise in the horse—A review. Part II. *Br Vet J* 142:542, 1986.

28. Carlson GP: Medical problems associated with protracted heat and work stress in horses. *Compend Contin Educ Pract Vet* 7:S542, 1985.

29. Carlson GP, Ocen PO: Composition of equine sweat following exercise in high environmental temperatures and in response to intravenous epinephrine administration. *J Equine Med Surg* 3:27, 1979.

30. Hansen TO: Renal tubular acidosis in a mare. *Compend Contin Educ Pract Vet* 8:864, 1986.

31. Ziemer EL, Parker HR, Carlson GP, et al: Renal tubular acidosis in two horses: Diagnostic studies. *J Am Vet Med Assoc* 190:289, 1987.

32. Ziemer EL, Parker HR, Carlson GP, et al: Clinical features and treatment of renal tubular acidosis in two horses. *J Am Vet Med Assoc* 190:294, 1987.

33. Gabel JC, Fallon KD, Laine GA, et al: Lung lymph flow during volume infusions. *J Appl Physiol* 60(2):623, 1986.

34. Allen SJ, Laine GA, Drake RE, et al: Superior vena caval pressure elevation causes pleural effusion formation in sheep. *Am J Physiol* 255 (Heart Circ Physiol 24):H492, 1988.

35. Laine GA, Allen SJ, Katz J, et al: Effect of systemic venous pressure elevation on lymph flow and lung edema formation. *J Appl Physiol* 61(5):1634, 1986.

36. Muir WW: Equine shock: The need for prospective clinical studies. *Equine Vet J* 19:1, 1987.

37. Schmall SM, Muir WW, Robertson JT: Haemodynamic effects of small volume hypertonic saline in experimentally induced haemorrhagic shock. *Equine Vet J* 22:273, 1990.

38. Bertone JJ, Gossett KA, Shoemaker KE: Effect of hypertonic vs isotonic saline solution on responses to sublethal *Escherichia coli* endotoxemia in horses. *Am J Vet Res* 51:999, 1990.

39. Dyson DH, Pascoe PJ: Influence of preinduction methoxamine, lactated Ringer solution, or hypertonic saline solution infusion or postinduction dobutamine infusion on anesthetic-induced hypotension in horses. *Am J Vet Res* 51:17, 1990.

40. Carlson GP, Rumbaugh GE: Response to saline solution of normally fed horses and horses dehydrated by fasting. *Am J Vet Res* 44:964, 1983.

41. Hodgson DR: Myopathies in athletic horses. *Compend Contin Educ Pract Vet* 7:S551, 1985.

42. Koterba A, Carlson GP: Acid-base and electrolyte alterations in horses with exertional rhabdomyolysis. *J Am Vet Med Assoc* 180:303, 1982.

43. Groenendyk S, English PB, Abetz I: External balance of water and electrolytes in the horse. *Equine Vet J* 20:189, 1988.

44. Rose RJ: A physiological approach to fluid and electrolyte therapy in the horse. *Equine Vet J* 13:7, 1981.

45. Hjortkjaer RK: Enema in the horse: Distribution and rehydrating effect. *Nord Vet Med* 31:508, 1979.

4.4

Hypertonic Saline in Management of Shock

Joseph J. Bertone, DVM, MS

Hypertonic (7.2%) sodium chloride solution (HSS) is effective in experimental hemorrhagic and endotoxic shock in horses and other species. HSS provides rapid restitution of vascular volume, cardiovascular performance, and metabolic function in several models of acute cardiovascular failure (shock).

INTRAVENOUS FLUID SUPPORT

The prognosis in shock is often directly related to the rapidity with which metabolic and cardiovascular homeostasis is re-established. Therefore, the goal of fluid support in acute circulatory failure is to rapidly increase or restore circulating vascular volume, cardiac output, and perfusion of vital organs and enhance the return of tissues to normalcy.

Resuscitation of horses in shock has relied on the intravenous administration of large volumes of isotonic fluids. Advantages of isotonic fluid support are the relative safety, vast quantity of clinical experience, and beneficial responses identified with its administration. The disadvantage of isotonic fluid support for adult, full-sized horses is associated with the large volume of fluids necessary to realize substantial benefits in acute circulatory failure. The volume of isotonic fluids required (50 to 100 mL/kg; 25 to 50 L) to achieve substantial responses, in the presence of shock, often exceeds that available to ambulatory clinicians. If the required volumes are available, safe administration under field conditions is often difficult to accomplish, and the associated benefits are relatively short lived. This is especially true when fluids cannot be continually administered. The short duration of responses to isotonic electrolyte solutions are a function of rapid dispersion of isotonic solutions into the extravascular space. Twenty to 60 minutes after receiving a bolus of isotonic electrolyte solution, vascular volume is increased by only 10% to 15% of the total volume of fluids administered. Beneficial responses are absent shortly after cessation of fluid administration. This is regardless of whether the patients are normal or in various stages of shock.[1] Substantial time is required to administer these large volumes, thus delaying rapid restoration of adequate circulatory volume and clinical improvement. This delay may also lengthen referral and preanesthetic periods. If rapid administration is achieved, complications (e.g., pulmonary edema, hypoproteinemia, anemia, edema) may occur. The expense of sterile isotonic fluids is also a consideration.

To alleviate the problems associated with large-volume isotonic fluid resuscitation, the ideal solution should: (1) have prolonged, beneficial responses, (2) be associated with rapidly achieved benefits, (3) be required in small volumes, (4) have no associated complications, and (5) be inexpensive. HSS appears to meet these criteria if used with care.

HYPERTONIC SALINE SOLUTION

Scientific literature indicates that HSS may offer a potential solution to the problems associated with isotonic fluid resuscitation under field or hospital circumstances.

The use of HSS was first identified in hemorrhagic shock models by Penfield in 1919.[2] He found that terminally shocked dogs had greater survival with HSS than with isotonic solution. A similar, but more detailed analysis was performed by Baue.[3] These data were for the most part ignored until the early 1970s. At this time the usefulness of these solutions was identified in clinical burn shock patients[4] and subsequently in experimental hemorrhagic shock in dogs when 2,400 mOsm/kg solutions were used at a rate of 4 mL/kg.[5] Other species in which HSS has been beneficial in the treatment of shock include pigs,[6] sheep,[7, 8] cats,[9, 10] calves,[11, 12] rabbits,[13] and humans.[14] It was identified in pigs that 7.5% NaCl was associated with greater responses and survival than other concentrations of saline.[6] The importance of NaCl versus other hypertonic solutions,[15] and subsequently the

greater durability of beneficial responses, was then elucidated.[6, 16, 17]

Beneficial Responses

HSS, when compared with isotonic solutions, in burned, hemorrhaged, and endotoxin-shocked animals, is associated with cardiovascular responses that include increased cardiac output, cardiac index,[9, 18–20] myocardial stroke work efficiency, and O_2 delivery.[21] Restoration of arterial pressure and decreased peripheral and pulmonary vascular resistance have been identified.[9, 18, 19, 21] There is some question with regard to effects of HSS on myocardial contractility. In vivo studies with HSS indicate that myocardial contractility is increased.[9, 12, 19] Intracranial pressure is protected in hemorrhaged subjects and in those with hemorrhage and cranial trauma.[22]

Some controversy exists over blood flow redistribution. HSS is associated with blood redistribution from peripheral tissues (skin and muscle) to the splanchnic vasculature,[20] but this may be species specific, because it does not occur in horses.

Pulmonary responses associated with HSS have been difficult to identify. There is no apparent effect of HSS on pulmonary mechanics and gas exchange indices.[11] HSS is associated with the return of mean pulmonary arterial pressure to baseline values in endotoxic shock.[18] Pulmonary lung water does not change with HSS resuscitation but increases when isotonic saline is administered in sufficient volumes to achieve similar increases in cardiac output.[8]

Administration of HSS is associated with greater increases in plasma volume than is explained by the volume of fluids administered. The increased plasma volume has been identified in normal[23] and shocked[24] horses. Increased plasma volume is reflected in the decreased packed cell volume and plasma total protein concentration evident with administration of HSS.[18, 23, 24]

Other responses associated with HSS include restoration of acid-base equilibrium[12, 20, 24] and increased plasma Na and Cl concentrations and osmolality.[18, 19] However, in normal horses, these responses seem to be attenuated or at least less predictable.[23] HSS is associated with increased urine output, decreased urine osmolality,[18, 19] and a substantial kaliuresis.[18] Intracellular water shifts and membrane potential aberrations, associated with hemorrhagic shock, are normalized with HSS.[7]

Mechanism of Action

HSS generates an osmotic extracellular plasma expansion and increased plasma volume. Other mechanisms that have been described include a pulmonary-mediated vascular response reflex. Data would indicate that intact pulmonary and vagal innervation and first passage of the HSS through the lung are required for the most beneficial response.[20] Some question as to the importance or the presence of this response have been raised.[9, 25]

HYPERTONIC SALINE SOLUTION IN EQUINE PRACTICE

Several studies have evaluated the effects of HSS in experimental shock; however, clinical application of HSS will require further evaluation. Until clinical evaluation is complete, clinicians should proceed cautiously. If HSS is used, isotonic fluids should follow within 1 to 2 hours.

Indications

HSS should be used in emergency situations in which rapid circulatory restoration may be necessary to sustain life and act as preanesthetic support for patients with cardiovascular compromise. Beneficial effects of HSS in horses in experimental hemorrhagic[19, 24] and endotoxic shock[18] have been identified. Acetylpromazine and halothane-induced hypotension are controlled with the administration of HSS.[26] The beneficial effects of HSS last for 90 to 180 minutes after administration in these models. These studies and studies in normal horses justify clinical trials in similar circumstances.[23] To date, clinical trials have not been completed but are underway. In the author's experience, and only measuring clinical parameters (i.e., pulse strength, mucous membrane color, mentation, stability at induction), the use of small-volume HSS has been associated with greater clinical improvement in patients than could be expected with similar volumes of isotonic solutions. For all clinical cases in which HSS has been used by the author and colleagues, administration has been followed by isotonic solutions.

HSS should be considered in severely burned patients. It has been proved to be efficacious for this purpose.[27]

Possible Indications

Other than the studies and conditions mentioned,[18, 19, 24, 26] HSS has not been critically evaluated under all circumstances that often require fluid therapy in equine medicine. Several situations and scenarios need to be addressed.

Neonatal Care. The ability of normal and septic foals to manage a sodium load is unclear. Preliminary studies indicate that the ability of normal and hemorrhaged foals to manage HSS may be similar to that of adults. Some clinical cases of foals in circulatory failure appear to respond well, and no adverse effects have been noted. However, volumes of isotonic fluids necessary to resuscitate foals should be readily available in most clinical situations. Therefore, the need of HSS in these situations is questionable. The author and colleagues have used HSS in the management of a ruptured bladder with desirable results.

Inflammatory Bowel Disease. Mechanisms for electrolyte abnormalities in enteritic conditions of horses remain unclear. In the case of salmonellosis, it appears that at least some component of the diarrhea is induced by hypersecretion of electrolytes. An initial bolus of HSS may be indicated not only to replace the loss of Na but also to achieve rapid restoration of cardiovascular function and perfusion to aid in lactic acid clearance. Clearly, this needs to be evaluated further.

Uncontrolled Hemorrhage. In an experimental model of uncontrolled hemorrhage, HSS was associated with more severe hemorrhage from the mesenteric vasculature than isotonic saline.[28] This may or may not be significant but should be considered in situations such as in uterine artery rupture, hepatic or renal hemorrhage secondary to a biopsy, meningeal or intracranial hemorrhage, or other forms of uncontrolled bleeding. Needless to say, in the case of uterine artery rupture, mares often need immediate support and the presence of continuing hemorrhage may be insignificant. Several mares that presented to the Ohio State University teaching hospital with uterine artery rupture have appeared to respond well to HSS when in apparently fatal volume depletion. Three mares were treated successfully with HSS at presentation. These mares suffered successive life-threatening bleeds days after presentation and were resuscitated successfully with HSS. In one mare, HSS administration was associated with increased arterial pressure and successful cesarean section.

Contraindications

There are several circumstances in which HSS should not be used. Further evaluation may prove otherwise, but for now the judicious approach will be to avoid the use of HSS in these conditions.

Exhaustion and Electrolyte Losses in Sweat. The use of HSS in conditions related to excessive prolonged exercise is not known. Equine sweat contains large quantities of K, Na, and Cl. The horses that become exhausted often display metabolic alkalosis in association with Cl losses. Intuitively, under these circumstances, electrolyte replacement may seem beneficial. However, HSS generates an extreme kaliuresis that may be deleterious in animals that are depleted of potassium by extreme sweat losses. These cases most often do not require aggressive resuscitation but do require persistent fluid replacement until the deficits are restored. The judicious approach is to use the experience of proven success with isotonic fluids and K and Ca supplementation.

Hyperosmotic States. HSS should not be used in any condition in which there is plasma hyperosmolality. Salt intoxication, water deprivation, heat prostration, and forms of renal disease may be associated with hyperosmolality. Infusion of hypertonic solutions under these circumstances may lead to neurologic deficits, arrhythmias, and other perturbations of hyperosmolality.

Renal Failure. Although a diuresis may be generated with HSS, if renal function is impaired, the ability to manage a salt load is also impaired. This may lead to worsening plasma hyperosmolality.

Adverse Reactions Associated with Hypertonic Saline Solution

With rapid infusion of HSS local hemolysis at the injection site and mild transient ataxia have been identified. Although, theoretically, arrhythmias may develop, none have been seen in experimental or clinical trials in any species.

Practical Application

HSS (7.2% to 7.5%) should be administered at 4 to 6 mL/kg. Commercial preparations of 7% NaCl are available.

Commercially prepared stock concentrates for the formulation of 0.9% NaCl may be formulated at eight times greater than the package instructions stipulate to achieve a final concentration of 7.2%. Care should be taken to identify the presence of preservatives and other electrolytes that may be present and may be toxic when concentrated. The entire volume should be administered in no less than 15 minutes. Always follow with isotonic solutions within 1 to 2 hours.

SUMMARY

Experimental data support the use of HSS as an effective, early, and aggressive form of support for circulatory failure in toxemia, hemorrhage, and burn and as a pre-inductant. HSS should be used in emergency situations in which rapid circulatory restoration may be necessary to sustain life. HSS may also be important in the maintenance of circulatory function during shipment to critical care facilities. Under any circumstances, if HSS is used, it should be followed within 2 hours with significant volumes of isotonic solutions (15 to 20 L). This is due to the substantial diuresis associated with HSS. Under certain circumstances, as described earlier, HSS may be contraindicated.

REFERENCES

1. Hauser CG, Shoemaker WC, Turpin I: Oxygen transport responses to colloids and crystalloids in critically ill surgical patients. *Surg Gynecol Obstet* 150:811, 1980.
2. Penfield WG: The treatment of severe and progressive hemorrhage by intravenous injection. *Am J Physiol* 48:121, 1919.
3. Baue AE, Tragus ET, Parkins WM: A comparison of isotonic and hypertonic solutions and blood on blood flow and oxygen consumption in the initial treatment of hemorrhagic shock. *J Trauma* 7:743, 1967.
4. Monafo WW, Chuntrasakul C, Ayvazian VH: Hypertonic sodium solutions in the treatment of burn shock. *Am J Surg* 126:778, 1973.
5. Velasco IT, Pontieri V, Rocha-E-Silva M, et al: Hyperosmotic NaCl and severe hemorrhagic shock. *Am J Physiol* 239:H664, 1980.
6. Traverso LW, Bellamy RF, Hollenbach SJ, et al: Hypertonic sodium chloride solutions: Effects on hemodynamics and survival after hemorrhage in swine. *J Trauma* 27:32, 1987.
7. Nakayama S, Kramer GC, Carlsen RC, et al: Infusion of very hypertonic saline in bled rats: Membrane potentials and fluid shifts. *J Surg Res* 38:180, 1985.
8. Nerlich M, Gunther R, Demling RH: Resuscitation from hemorrhagic shock with hypertonic saline or lactated Ringer's (effect on pulmonary and systemic microcirculation). *Circ Shock* 10:179, 1983.
9. Muir WW, Sally J: Small-volume resuscitation with hypertonic saline solution in hypovolemic cats. *Am J Vet Res* 50:1883, 1989.
10. Bitterman H, Triolo J, Lefer A: Use of hypertonic saline in the treatment of hemorrhagic shock. *Circ Shock* 21:271, 1987.
11. Constable PD, Schmall LM, Muir WW, et al: Respiratory, renal, hematologic and serum biochemical effects of hypertonic saline in endotoxic calves. *Am J Vet Res*. In press.
12. Constable PD, Schmall LM, Muir WW, et al: Small volume hypertonic saline (2400 mOsm/L) treatment of calves in endotoxic shock: Hemodynamic response. *Am J Vet Res* In press.
13. Mazzoni MC, Borgstrom P, Arfors KE, et al: Dynamic fluid redistribution in hyperosmotic resuscitation of hypovolemic hemorrhage. *Am J Physiol* 255:H629, 1988.
14. Shackford SR, Fortlage DA, Peters RM, et al: Serum osmolar and electrolyte changes associated with large infusions of hypertonic sodium lactate for intravascular volume expansion of patients undergoing aortic reconstruction. *Surg Gynecol Obstet* 164:127, 1987.
15. Rocha-E-Silva M, Velasco IT, Nogueira da Silva RI, et al: Hyperosmotic sodium salts reverse severe hemorrhagic shock: Other salts do not. *Am J Physiol* 253:H751, 1986.
16. Velasco IT, Rocha-E-Silva M, Oliveira MA, et al: Hypertonic and hyperoncotic resuscitation from severe hemorrhagic shock in dogs: A comparative study. *Crit Care Med* 17:261, 1989.
17. Kramer GC, Perron PR, Lindsey DC, et al: Small volume resuscitation with hypertonic saline dextran solution. *Surgery* 100:239, 1986.
18. Bertone JJ, Gossett KA, Shoemaker KE, et al: Effect of hypertonic vs isotonic saline solution on responses to sublethal *Escherichia coli* endotoxemia in horses. *Am J Vet Res* 51:999, 1990.
19. Schmall LM, Muir WW, Robertson JT: Haemodynamic effects of small volume hypertonic saline in experimentally induced haemorrhagic shock. *Equine Vet J* 22:273, 1990.
20. Rocha-E-Silva M, Negraes GA, Soares AM, et al: Hypertonic resuscitation from severe hemorrhagic shock: Patterns of regional circulation. *Circ Shock* 19:165, 1986.
21. Rowe GG, McKenna DH, Corliss RJ, et al: Hemodynamic effects of hypertonic sodium chloride. *J Appl Physiol* 32:182, 1972.
22. Prough DS, Johnson JC, Stump DA, et al: Effects of hypertonic saline versus lactated Ringer's solution on cerebral oxygen transport during resuscitation from hemorrhagic shock. *J Neurosurg* 64:627, 1986.
23. Bertone JJ, Shoemaker KE: Effect of hypertonic vs isotonic saline solution on plasma constituents of conscious horses. *Am J Vet Res.* In press.
24. Schmall LM, Muir WW, Robertson JT: Haematologic, serum electrolyte, and blood gas effects of small volume hypertonic saline in experimentally induced haemorrhagic shock. *Equine Vet J* 22:278, 1990.
25. Schertel ER, Valentine AK, Allen DA, et al: Isotonic saline and hemorrhagic shock: Role of the vagus. *FASEB J* 3:A713, 1989.
26. Dyson HH, Pascoe PJ: Influence of preinduction methoxamine, lactated Ringer solution infusion or postinduction dobutamine infusion on anesthetic-induced hypotension in horses. *Am J Vet Res* 51:17, 1990.
27. Caldwell FT, Bowser BH: Critical evaluation of hypertonic and hypotonic solutions to resuscitate severely burned children: A prospective study. *Ann Surg* 189:546, 1979.
28. Gross D, Landau EH, Assalia A, et al: Is hypertonic saline resuscitation safe in "uncontrolled" hemorrhagic shock? *J Trauma* 28:751, 1988.

4.5

Mode of Action of Equine Anthelmintics

Craig R. Reinemeyer, DVM, PhD

An anthelmintic is defined as a drug that causes the death or removal of helminth parasites (nematodes, cestodes, and trematodes). In horses, drugs with activity against bots are usually included in this classification, although *Gasterophi-*

lus is an arthropod, not a helminth. Anthelmintics (dewormers) are probably the most frequently administered of all equine drugs and are used therapeutically for specific syndromes or prophylactically for general parasite control and health maintenance.

Classification by Mode of Action. Numerous anthelmintics are currently approved for equine use, but closer examination reveals that these dewormers belong to only about a half-dozen distinct chemical families. Because drugs within a chemical family kill parasites by the same mode of action, the relationships among equine anthelmintics are most easily understood by studying their chemical families or modes of action.

Classification by Spectrum. A secondary system for classifying equine anthelmintics is based on the spectrum of target parasites removed by each drug. Dewormers for horses are commonly described as broad or narrow spectrum. An equine anthelmintic is termed "broad spectrum" if it is effective against large strongyles, cyathostomes (small strongyles), ascarids, and pinworms. Some authors use a more restrictive definition and require that an equine anthelmintic also kill bots to be considered broad spectrum.[1] A "narrow-spectrum" equine anthelmintic is essentially one that kills fewer types of nematodes than do broad-spectrum drugs.

The broad-spectrum anthelmintics currently marketed are usually more than 90% effective against the most prevalent and damaging equine parasites.[2, 3] Broad-spectrum compounds are therefore the most appropriate choices for routine, scheduled dewormings, which are often performed without the benefit of a specific diagnosis.

In the subsequent discussion, anthelmintics are classified both according to mode of action and to spectrum.

ANTHELMINTICS WITH NEUROMUSCULAR ACTIVITY

Internal parasites require neuromuscular coordination to feed and to maintain their position in an advantageous ecologic niche within the host.[4] Feeding activities are crucial, because even temporary interference with ingestion may lead to depletion of energy reserves, expulsion from the niche, and subsequent death.

Nematodes, which are the major internal parasites of horses, utilize acetylcholine and γ-aminobutyric acid (GABA) as excitatory and inhibitory neurotransmitters, respectively.[4] These two compounds also serve as neurotransmitters in arthropods and mammals. Because similar neurotransmitters are present in the host and target parasites, anthelmintics with neuromuscular activity should be administered carefully to prevent host toxicity.

Broad-Spectrum Neuromuscular Anthelmintics

Macrocyclic Lactones. This chemical family, also known as the avermectins, represents the newest group of compounds to exhibit anthelmintic activity in horses. The avermectins are fermentation products of the actinomycete *Streptomyces avermitilis*;[5] other macrocyclic lactones have been derived from various *Streptomyces* species and are currently in various stages of commercial research and development.[6] Ivermectin (Eqvalan, Zimecterin; Merck AgVet) is the only avermectin approved in the United States for use in horses (Table 4–2).

The avermectins exhibit a unique mode of action that has not been thoroughly characterized. At recommended dosages, the avermectins bind specifically and with high affinity to glutamate-gated chloride channels in the target invertebrates,[7] which increases neural membrane permeability to chloride ions.[8] At higher dosages, avermectins also enhance GABA-mediated neurotransmission.[5] In nematodes, the lethal effect of avermectins may be related to interference with crucial feeding mechanisms rather than to the classic concept of somatic paralysis and expulsion from the host.[9]

Ivermectin is extremely potent; the usual equine dosage is only 200 μg/kg. This level provides excellent activity against bots and most nematode parasites of horses,[10] including the larval stages of *Onchocerca*[11] and *Habronema*[12] that are associated with dermatologic lesions.

Ivermectin has a wide index of safety in horses, and 15 times the recommended dosage resulted in only mild signs of toxicity.[13] The specificity of ivermectin for invertebrate chloride channels may account for its mammalian safety. In addition, although mammals utilize GABA as a neurotransmitter, it is restricted to the central nervous system and ivermectin does not cross the blood-brain barrier.

Table 4–2. Equine Anthelmintics Affecting Neuromuscular Transmission

Chemical Family	Generic Name	Proprietary Name(s)	Sponsor
Broad Spectrum*, †			
Macrocyclic lactones	Ivermectin	Eqvalan; Zimecterin	Merck
Tetrahydropyrimidines	Pyrantel pamoate	Strongid-T, -P	Pfizer, Inc.
	Pyrantel tartrate	Strongid-C	Pfizer, Inc.
Narrow Spectrum†			
Piperazine	Piperazine		

*Ascarids, cyathostomes, large strongyles, and pinworms.
†Additional details about the spectrum of individual drugs are presented in the text.

Table 4–3. Equine Anthelmintic Formulations That Are Combinations of Drugs with Metabolic and Neuromuscular Modes of Action

Proprietary Name(s)	Activity		Sponsor
	Metabolic	Neuromuscular	
Benzelmin Plus	Oxfendazole	Trichlorfon*	Fort Dodge
Telmin-B	Mebendazole	Trichlorfon	Mallinckrodt

*Expands the spectrum to include bots.

Tetrahydropyrimidines. This chemical group exerts a cholinergic effect at the ganglionic level, resulting in muscular contraction and spastic paralysis of the nematode.[14] Pyrimidines are reportedly up to 100 times more potent than is acetylcholine in inducing muscular contraction.[15] Pyrimidines are relatively safe in mammals because they are not absorbed well from the gastrointestinal tract.

Pyrantel salts (see Table 4–2) are usually administered therapeutically, but pyrantel tartrate (Strongid C; Pfizer, Inc.) has a prophylactic regimen as well. The daily addition of 1.2 g/454 kg to the feed prevents strongyle and ascarid infections by killing newly ingested larvae in the lumen of the gut before they can enter host tissues.[16]

Narrow-Spectrum Neuromuscular Anthelmintics

Organophosphates. This chemical family phosphorylates the esterification site of the enzyme acetylcholinesterase, inhibiting its activity. Because acetylcholinesterase normally degrades the excitatory neurotransmitter acetylcholine, blocking its effect results in sustained muscular contraction and spastic paralysis.[17] Internal and external parasites utilize acetylcholine as a neurotransmitter, and both are similarly affected by organophosphates.

Organophosphates are volatile and are partially inactivated by the basic pH of the small intestine.[18] For this reason, most formulations are effective only against parasites of the anterior gut, namely bots and ascarids.[2] Pinworms are removed as well. A formulation of dichlorvos-impregnated resin pellets (Cutter Dichlorvos), however, releases dichlorvos slowly as it traverses the gut, providing additional efficacy against large and small strongyles in the large bowel.[2] At this writing, Cutter Dichlorvos is no longer marketed in the United States. The resin pellet formulation of dichlorvos arguably could be grouped with the broad-spectrum anthelmintics. Trichlorfon is an organophosphate used most commonly for bot control, either alone or in combination with broad-spectrum anthelmintics (Table 4–3).

Organophosphates have a narrower index of safety than do most other anthelmintics, because they also affect mammalian acetylcholinesterases.[18]

Piperazine. Piperazine exerts its effect by hyperpolarizing muscle membrane, thus blocking muscular contraction.[4] The net effect is flaccid paralysis of the nematode. Although relatively safe in horses, neurologic side effects have been reported after an accidental overdose (six times the normal dose) of piperazine.[19]

Piperazine is seldom used alone in horses because of its poor efficacy against large strongyles or migrating larvae.[2] It is usually added to other anthelmintics to enhance their activity against ascarids or cyathostomes.[3] Piperazine also provides a useful therapeutic option in herds with benzimidazole (BZD)-resistant cyathostomes.

ANTHELMINTICS WITH METABOLIC ACTIVITY

Numerous anthelmintics kill nematodes through disturbances of energy metabolism rather than by neuromuscular interference. All of the equine dewormers that affect energy metabolism are chemically related and apparently employ the same mode of anthelmintic activity.

Broad-Spectrum Metabolic Anthelmintics

Benzimidazoles. More equine anthelmintics belong to this chemical class than to any other. The various BZD drugs differ in solubility, absorption, and spectrum, but all apparently block the intracellular assembly of microtubules from tubulin subunits. To better understand the consequences of this mode of action, a brief discussion of the normal structure and function of tubulin and microtubules is warranted.

Tubulin is a soluble, intracellular protein that is synthesized in two forms known as α- and β-tubulin. Single molecules (monomers) of α- and β-tubulin combine to form dimers. Dimers are assembled into tubulin oligomers, which are the structural units of microtubules. Tubulin and microtubules exist in a state of equilibrium within the cell.[21] Microtubules are constantly remodeled, with tubulin molecules continually being added or removed.

Microtubules participate in many essential cellular functions, including motility, nutrient absorption, intracellular transport, and formation of the mitotic spindle during cell division. Microtubules also comprise essential structural components of organelles, including the cell membrane, nucleus, Golgi apparatus, ribosomes, and mitochondria.[21]

Disruption of the formation of microtubules affects many intracellular processes, potentially triggering a chain of biochemical and physiologic events that combine to destroy cellular homeostasis. These effects can be lethal to the organism.

BZDs exert their action by binding to tubulin and preventing its polymerization into microtubules. Because of the essential role of microtubules in mitosis and energy metabolism,

Table 4–4. Equine Anthelmintics Affecting Parasite Metabolism

Chemical Family	Generic Name	Proprietary Name(s)	Sponsor
Benzimidazoles			
	Fenbendazole	Panacur; Safeguard	Hoechst-Roussell
	Mebendazole	Telmin	Mallinckrodt
	Oxfendazole	Benzelmin	Fort Dodge
	Oxibendazole	Anthelcide E.Q.;	Pfizer, Inc.
	Thiabendazole	Equizole	Merck AgVet
Pro-benzimidazoles			
	Febantel	Rintal; Cutter	Bayer

BZDs are most effective in actively dividing cells, such as those found in developing nematode ova and larvae.[22]

BZDs do not consistently cause lethal changes in adult nematodes but nevertheless render target parasites susceptible to expulsion from their niche within the host.[21]

BZDs differ in their physical and pharmacologic properties. In general, the less soluble BZDs (e.g., fenbendazole, oxfendazole) persist longer in the host and are consequently more effective.[18] This is consistent with the observation that BZD efficacy is increased by extending the duration of exposure to the drug.[23] Expanded efficacy can be achieved by administering standard or elevated doses of BZDs over several consecutive days. This approach is the basis of several therapeutic regimens utilizing BZDs against migrating *Strongylus vulgaris* larvae in the horse.[24]

With few exceptions, the benzimidazoles currently approved for equine use in the United States (Table 4–4) have similar spectra of activity against target nematodes.[3] Most BZDs have a wide margin of safety up to 5 to 20 times the recommended dosage.[25]

Pro-Benzimidazoles. These compounds are pharmacologic precursors that are actively converted into BZDs within the host. Febantel (Rintal, Cutter; Bayer), for example, is metabolized by the horse into fenbendazole and then into oxfendazole.[26] Febantel is the only pro-BZD approved for horses in the United States, but the sponsor plans to withdraw it from the market in the near future. The practical utility of BZDs and pro-BZDs in many herds may be limited by anthelmintic resistance.

Equine Anthelmintics Not Currently Marketed

This discussion has omitted a few equine anthelmintics which, although approved, are not presently marketed in the United States. Interested readers are referred to an additional source for a current listing.[20]

RESISTANCE TO EQUINE ANTHELMINTICS

Clinicians and horse owners occasionally note the failure of an anthelmintic to perform as expected. Some of these failures can be attributed to suboptimal dosing, but an increasingly common cause is anthelmintic resistance. Anthelmintic resistance is defined as "a greater frequency of individuals within a population able to tolerate doses of a compound than in a normal population of the same species."[27]

Prevalence and Distribution of Resistance

Unequivocal cases of anthelmintic resistance in horses have all involved cyathostomes treated with BZDs, pro-BZDs, or phenothiazine.[3, 28, 29] Reports of cyathostomes resistant to piperazine or pyrantel are isolated, and a case of purported mebendazole resistance in large strongyles may have involved phenomena other than resistance.[30, 31]

Of the more than 40 species of cyathostomes infecting horses, BZD resistance has been observed in at least 12 species.[32, 33] This proportion includes the most prevalent and numerous species, however, which often comprise more than 95% of the total cyathostome population in a typical infection.[32]

BZD-resistant cyathostomes have been reported from multiple sites in Australia, North America, and Europe,[28] where surveys have demonstrated resistant worms on high proportions of farms.[34–36]

Nature of Benzimidazole Resistance

Resistant nematodes possess biochemical or physiologic adaptations that mitigate the effects of anthelmintics. Because resistance characteristics are hereditary, they are not present to the same extent in populations of susceptible parasites. Recent research comparing resistant and susceptible strains has identified a specific molecular mechanism that may determine BZD resistance in nematodes.[28]

Genetic heterogeneity enables nematodes to synthesize multiple isoforms of α- and β-tubulin (e.g., β_1, β_2), and the various tubulin isoforms have different physical and chemical properties.[21] The tubulin isoform patterns of BZD-susceptible and BZD-resistant *Haemonchus contortus* have been shown to be different, and the β-tubulins synthesized by resistant worms have fewer high-affinity BZD receptors.[28] In effect, the β-tubulins of resistant nematodes bind insufficient BZD to block microtubule polymerization, and normal cellular metabolism can be maintained in the face of anthelmintic treatment.

Side-Resistance. Nematodes develop resistance to chemical modes of action rather than to specific proprietary drugs. Accordingly, a population of worms resistant to one anthelmintic is likely to be resistant to other dewormers in the same chemical family. The phenomenon of resistance to a drug that is induced through selection by another drug with a similar mode of action is known as side-resistance.[27]

Cyathostomes exhibit side-resistance to the BZD and pro-BZD drugs.[28] Small strongyles that have developed BZD resistance subsequent to selection with thiabendazole or febantel will likely be resistant to most other BZDs, even those never previously used against that population. A notable exception seems to be oxibendazole, which remains effective against many BZD-resistant cyathostome populations.[3] Resistance to oxibendazole can develop, however, after frequent and exclusive use over a period of time.[37]

Selection for Resistance

Experimental evidence indicates that anthelmintic resistance is a polygenic trait.[38] The genes imparting resistance occur randomly within nematode populations but remain at low frequencies until the population encounters circumstances in which those genetic characteristics are advantageous. In the context of the present discussion, that circumstance (i.e., selection pressure) is anthelmintic treatment.

Selection Pressure. For an individual nematode, the benefit of resistance is survival of anthelmintic treatment. The advantage at the population level, however, is reproduction without competition from susceptible worms during the interval after treatment. This increases the ratio of resistant to susceptible progeny among the pre-parasitic stages in the environment, and reinfection from this pool increases the proportion of resistant adults within the host. Further selection repeats the cycle and amplifies the frequency of resistant genes in the general population.

The following factors modify the intensity of selection pressure from anthelmintic treatment:

Refugia. The portion of a population that is not exposed to a selection pressure is known as the *refugia*, which is essentially a reservoir of susceptible genes. The development of resistance is delayed by maintaining a large *refugia*.

Because all cyathostome stages within a horse are theoretically exposed to anthelmintic at the time of deworming, examples of *refugia* include pre-parasitic stages in the environment and parasitic stages in untreated horses. A large cyathostome refugia can be maintained by selective treatment of only certain horses in the herd and by treating only when the number of larvae in the environment (i.e., the risk of reinfection) is high. Adoption of these practices is unlikely, however, because both are contrary to usual equine parasite control recommendations.

Pharmacokinetics. Low anthelmintic concentrations, whether associated with the declining stages of a plasma concentration curve or from dosing at less than label recommendations, allow some nematodes to survive drug exposure.[38] Because the resistance status of individual nematodes differs quantitatively, sublethal dosing allows those with lower levels of resistance to survive, whereas the most resistant members of the population may be eliminated only by very high anthelmintic dosages. Accordingly, the use of suboptimal dosages and persistent anthelmintics with long half-lives theoretically increases the frequency of some resistance genes in the general population.

Frequency of Treatment. Frequent treatment minimizes the reproductive opportunities of susceptible worms, especially if treatments are administered at intervals less than the pre-patent period.[27] The latter statement has little application to horses, because the pre-patent periods for cyathostomes range from 6 weeks to more than 2 years.[32] Nevertheless, a survey in Australia[34] reported that BZD resistance was more common in herds treated at intervals of 16 weeks or less. A survey of parasite control practices in the United States found that more than 50% of owners dewormed their horses at least that often.[39] This suggests that resistance would be very common among cyathostome populations if horse owners used BZD anthelmintics exclusively.

Choice of Anthelmintic. To date, cyathostomes have developed widespread resistance only to BZD and pro-BZD drugs.[28] The use of non-BZD anthelmintics is less likely to select for resistance, but sustained susceptibility to alternate compounds is by no means guaranteed.

The frequency of rotation of anthelmintics presents a dilemma in that resistance can be selected both by exclusive use of a single anthelmintic class for more than one worm generation and by the use of multiple anthelmintics within a generation.[40] A cyathostome generation is approximately 1 year,[40] and a suitable compromise for equine parasite control seems to be rotation among drug classes at annual intervals.

Detection of Resistance

In experimental settings, anthelmintic resistance can be verified by controlled anthelmintic efficacy testing in which postmortem worm counts are compared between control animals and those treated with the anthelmintic in question.[41]

Less invasive in vitro techniques include the egg hatch assay (EHA), which exploits the ovicidal properties of BZDs.[42] In the EHA, nematode eggs are incubated in various concentrations of BZDs, and the concentration that blocks 50% of egg hatching (LC_{50}) is determined. Ova from resistant worms are able to hatch at higher BZD concentrations than are susceptible progeny, and this is reflected by higher LC_{50} values for resistant populations.[41]

A useful procedure for practitioners is the fecal egg count reduction (FECR) test.[41, 43] In this technique, baseline quantitative fecal egg counts are compared with counts performed 10 to 14 days after treatment with the anthelmintic in question. Calculations should be based on the mean egg counts (eggs per gram [EPG]) of several horses, and the same horses should be sampled on both dates. It is not necessary to test all horses in a group; a useful rule of thumb is to sample five horses, or 10% of the herd, whichever is greater. Percent efficacy is calculated by the following formula:

$$\text{Efficacy} = \frac{X_c - X_t}{X_c} \times 100$$

$$X_c = \text{mean EPG (pretreatment)}$$
$$X_t = \text{mean EPG (post-treatment)}$$

Currently marketed equine anthelmintics should decrease cyathostome egg counts by more than 90% to 95%.[2, 3] A mean egg count reduction of less than 90% for a group of horses is consistent with anthelmintic resistance.

Management of Resistance

Once resistance has been demonstrated in a population of cyathostomes, the use of anthelmintics with the same mode of action should be discontinued on the premises. In the absence of other selection pressures, anthelmintic resistance becomes a stable genetic characteristic of the worm population. In one study, avoiding BZD anthelmintics for 38 months did not result in reversion to BZD susceptibility.[44]

The selection of effective anthelmintics for BZD-resistant populations is limited to pyrantel, ivermectin, or oxibendazole.[45, 46] An alternative is piperazine, which requires administration by nasogastric intubation.[3]

Prevention of Resistance

All new horses should be treated and quarantined upon arrival at the farm to reduce the introduction of resistant strains of cyanthostomes.[40] Anthelmintics should be administered according to label directions, and doses should be based on recent, accurate body weights.

Annual rotation among anthelmintic classes is strongly recommended, but proper rotation requires thorough knowledge of the chemical classification of the various anthelmintics at hand.[40] Side-resistance dictates that rotation must be between drug classes and not merely among different drugs within the same class.

Decreasing the overall use of anthelmintics in horses would lessen selection for resistance but may have deleterious consequences for equine health. Nevertheless, alternative parasite control practices that reduce the dependency on anthelmintics should be encouraged. These practices include seasonal, strategic treatments,[45, 46] alternate species grazing,[47] and pasture hygiene.[48]

REFERENCES

1. Drudge JH, Lyons ET: *Internal Parasites of Horses with Emphasis on Treatment and Control.* Somerville, NJ, Hoechst-Roussel Agri-Vet Company, 1986, p 2.
2. Drudge JH, Lyons ET, Tolliver SC: Parasite control in horses: A summary of contemporary drugs. *Vet Med Small Anim Clin* 76:1479, 1981.
3. Wescott RB: Anthelmintics and drug resistance. *Vet Clin North Am*, 1986, p 367.
4. Rew RS: Mode of action of common anthelmintics. *J Vet Pharmacol Ther* 1:183, 1978.
5. Campbell WC: An introduction to the avermectins. *N Z Vet J* 29:174, 1981.
6. Takiguchi Y, Mishima H, Okuda M: Milbemycins, a new family of macrolide antibiotics: Fermentation, isolation and physicochemical properties. *J Antibiot* 33:1120, 1980.
7. Shoop WL, Mrozik H: Veterinary pharmacology in animal health discovery: Structure and activity of avermectins and milbemycins in animal health. *Proc Am Acad Vet Pharmacol Ther* 9:35, 1994.
8. Turner MJ, Schaeffer JM: Mode of action of ivermectin. In Campbell WC, ed. *Ivermectin and Abamectin.* New York, Springer-Verlag, 1989, p 73.
9. Geary TG, Sims SM, Thomas EM, et al: *Haemonchus contortus:* Ivermectin-induced paralysis of the pharynx. *Exp Parasitol* 77:88, 1993.
10. Campbell WC, Leaning WHD, Seward RL: Use of ivermectin in horses. In Campbell WC, ed. *Ivermectin and Abamectin.* New York, Springer-Verlag, 1989, p 234.
11. Herd RP, Donham JC: Efficacy of ivermectin against *Onchocerca cervicalis* microfilarial dermatitis in horses. *Am J Vet Res* 44:1102, 1983.
12. Herd RP, Donham JC: Efficacy of ivermectin against "summer sores" due to *Draschia* and *Habronema* infection in horses. *Proc Am Assoc Vet Parasitol* 26:8, 1981.
13. Pulliam JD, Preston JM: Safety of ivermectin in target animals. In Campbell WC, ed. *Ivermectin and Abamectin.* New York, Springer-Verlag, 1989, p 149.
14. Barragry T: Anthelmintics—a review. *N Z Vet J* 32:161, 1984.
15. Aubry ML, Cowell P, Davey MJ, et al: Aspects of the pharmacology of a new anthelmintic: Pyrantel. *Br J Pharmacol* 38:332, 1970.
16. DiPietro J: Daily anthelmintic therapy in horses. *Compend Contin Educ Pract Vet* 14:651, 1992.
17. Knowles CO, Casida JE: Mode of action of organophosphate anthelmintics: Cholinesterase inhibition in *Ascaris lumbricoides. J Agric Food Chem* 14:566, 1966.
18. Barragry T: Anthelmintics—review, Part II. *N Z Vet J* 32:191, 1984.
19. McNeil PH, Smyth GB: Piperazine toxicity in horses. *J Equine Med Surg* 2:321, 1978.
20. Courtney CH, Sundlof SF: *Veterinary Antiparasitic Drugs 1991: A Comprehensive Compendium of FDA-Approved Antiparasitic Drugs.* Gainesville, FL, Institute of Food and Agricultural Sciences, 1991, p 119.
21. Lacey E: The role of the cytoskeletal protein, tubulin, in the mode of action and mechanism of drug resistance to benzimidazoles. *Int J Parasitol* 18:885, 1988.
22. Kirsch R, Schleich H: Morphological changes in trichostrongylid eggs after treatment with fenbendazole. *Vet Parasitol* 11:375, 1982.
23. Hennessy DR: Manipulation of anthelmintic pharmacokinetics. In Anderson N, Waller PJ, eds. *Resistance in Nematodes to Anthelmintic Drugs.* Glebe, N.S.W., Australia, CSIRO Division of Animal Health, 1985, p 79.
24. Drudge JH, Lyons ET: Large strongyles—recent advances. *Vet Clin North Am*, 1986, p 263.
25. Seiler JP: Toxicology and genetic effects of benzimidazole compounds. *Mutation Res* 32:151, 1975.
26. Marriner SE, Bogan JA: Pharmacokinetics of fenbendazole in sheep. *Am J Vet Res* 42:1146, 1981.
27. Prichard RK, Hall CA, Kelly JD, et al: The problem of anthelmintic resistance in nematodes. *Austr Vet J* 56:239, 1980.
28. Prichard RK: Anthelmintic resistance in nematodes: Extent, recent understanding and future directions for control and research. *Int J Parasitol* 20:515, 1990.
29. Drudge JH, Elam G: Preliminary observations on the resistance of horse strongyles to phenothiazine. *J Parasitol* 47:38, 1961.
30. Lyons ET, Drudge JH, Tolliver SC, et al: Anthelmintic resistance in equids. In Boray JC, Martin PJ, Roush RT, eds. *Resistance of Parasites to Antiparasitic Drugs.* Rahway, NJ, Merck Agvet, 1990, p 67.
31. French DD, Klei TR: Benzimidazole-resistant strongyle infections: A review of significance, occurrence, diagnosis and control. *Proc Am Assoc Equine Pract* 19:313, 1983.
32. Reinemeyer CR: Small strongyles—recent advances. *Vet Clin North Am*, 1986, p 281.
33. Eysker M, Boersema JH, Kooyman FNJ, et al: Possible resis-

tance of small strongles from female ponies in The Netherlands against albendazole. *Am J Vet Res* 49:995, 1988.

34. Kelly JD, Webster JH, Griffin DL, et al: Resistance to benzimidazole anthelmintics in equine strongles. *Austr Vet J* 57:163, 1981.

35. Repeta DL, Birnbaum N, Courtney CH: Anthelmintic resistance on pleasure horse farms in Florida. *Proc Am Assoc Vet Parasitol* 36:39, 1991.

36. Bauer C, Merkt JC, Janke-Grimm G, et al: Prevalence and control of benzimidazole-resistant small strongles on German thoroughbred studs. *Vet Parasitol* 21:189, 1986.

37. Drudge JH, Lyons ET, Tolliver SC, et al: Use of oxibendazole for control of cambendazole-resistant small strongles in a band of ponies: A six-year study. *Am J Vet Res* 46:2507, 1985.

38. LeJambre LF: Genetic aspects of anthelmintic resistance in nematodes. In Anderson N, Waller PJ, eds. *Resistance in Nematodes to Anthelmintic Drugs.* Glebe, N.S.W., Australia, CSIRO Division of Animal Health, 1985, p 97.

39. Reinemeyer CR, Rohrbach BW: A survey of equine parasite control practices in Tennessee. *J Am Vet Med Assoc* 196:712, 1990.

40. Herd RP: Epidemiology and control of parasites in northern temperate regions. *Vet Clin North Am*, 1986, p 337.

41. Presidente PJA: Methods for detection of resistance to anthelmintics. In Anderson N, Waller PJ, eds. *Resistance in Nematodes to Anthelmintic Drugs.* Glebe, N.S.W., Australia, CSIRO Division of Animal Health, 1985, p 13.

42. LeJambre LF: Egg hatch as an in vitro assay of thiabendazole resistance in nematodes. *Vet Parasitol* 2:385, 1976.

43. Herd RP: Cattle practitioner: Vital role in worm control. *Compend Contin Educ Pract Vet* 13:879, 1991.

44. Uhlinger C, Johnstone C: Failure to reestablish benzimidazole susceptible populations of small strongles after prolonged treatment with non-benzimidazoles. *Equine Vet Sci* 4:7, 1984.

45. Herd RP, Willardson KL, Gabel AA: Epidemiologic approach to the control of horse strongles. *Equine Vet J* 17:202, 1985.

46. Herd RP: Parasite control in horses: Seasonal use of equine anthelmintics. *Mod Vet Pract* 67:895, 1986.

47. Eysker M, Jansen J, Kooyman FNJ, et al: Comparison of two control systems for cyathostome infections in the horse. *Vet Parasitol* 22:105, 1986.

48. Herd RP: Pasture hygiene: A nonchemical approach to equine endoparasite control. *Mod Vet Pract* 67:36, 1986.

4.6

Gastrointestinal Motility and Adynamic Ileus

Clara K. Fenger, DVM, PhD
Alicia L. Bertone, DVM, MS, PhD
Joseph J. Bertone, DVM, MS

Gastrointestinal motility is defined as any motor activity of the gastrointestinal tract. This activity may produce propulsion, retropulsion, mixing movement, or no movement of ingesta. Movement of ingesta correlates with coordinated progressive myoelectrical and motor events that extend over a length of the gastrointestinal tract. Transit time of ingesta varies with location within the tract and is partially controlled by intestinal motor events.[1-7] In the colon, patterns of electrical and motor activity vary among species more than do patterns in the small intestine. This variation is expected because of differences among species concerning diet and anatomy of the ascending colon. The adult horse is a non-coprophagic, monogastric herbivore that has a complex, voluminous, sacculated large colon. Therefore, longer retention time is needed in its large colon than is required for other monogastrics for microbial digestion and fermentation of fiber.[8]

PATTERNS OF INTESTINAL ACTIVITY

As with all muscles of the body, intestinal smooth muscle requires electrical stimulation to contract. If the sum of all the incoming impulses exceeds the threshold potential, a muscle action potential results. However, unlike much of the other muscles of the body, the smooth muscle of the intestinal tract has inherent rhythmicity. The membranes slowly depolarize, due to spontaneous, transient oscillations in the membrane potential that are mediated by fluctuations in sodium conductance. This rhythmic depolarization can occur at any given site in the tract and is referred to as electrical control activity or a slow wave. The slow wave begins at a pacemaker in the longitudinal layer, then radiates outward in the longitudinal layer and luminally to the circular layer, traveling from cell to cell along gap junctions.[9]

Slow waves bring the resting potential in these muscle layers closer to threshold potential. When incoming nervous activity is superimposed on slow waves, action potentials, or spike potentials (also known as electrical response activity), the result is muscle contraction synchronous with slow waves (Fig. 4–1). Electrical response activity occurs only during the depolarization of electrical control activity (slow waves), and therefore slow waves control the frequency of contractions and act as the small intestinal pacemaker.[10] Spike potentials do not occur during every slow wave. Extrinsic innervation does not change the basic rhythmicity of the slow wave but instead affects the number of spikes overlying the slow wave and therefore imparts on the force of contraction. Parasympathetic stimulation causes an increase in the force of contraction, whereas sympathetic stimulation decreases the force of contraction.

CONTROL OF MOTILITY

Several levels of neural control of the gastrointestinal tract exist. The enteric nervous system constitutes an intrinsic source of neural input and is made up of a complete network of neurons within the intestine that allow intrinsic control of motility (Fig. 4–2). This system includes the myenteric plexus, located between the longitudinal and circular muscles, and the submucosal plexus, located in the submucosa. Numerous receptors in the mucosa, submucosa, and muscular layers stimulate afferent fibers that may synapse in either plexus and amplify or modulate the response. These fibers may also synapse with efferent fibers that stimulate or inhibit tonic or propulsive contractions. This intrinsic nervous sys-

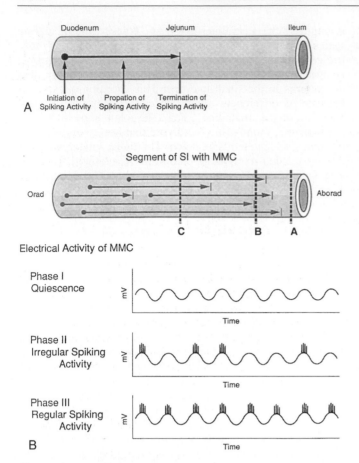

Figure 4–1. *A,* Schematic diagram of the propagation of an action potential in the small intestine. The *arrow* begins at the site of initiation and ends at the site of termination. *B,* Migrating myoelectric complex of the small intestine. Multiple action potentials will sweep aborally along a segment of bowel. The overall pattern will gradually progress toward the ileum. When measured at a fixed section of intestine, the electrical activity will show characteristic patterns. These patterns are described as quiescence, irregular spiking activity, and regular spiking activity and will correspond with the mechanical activity of quiescence, segmentation, and peristalsis, respectively.

tem is capable of integrating signals from the lumen and initiating action. Although the initiation of slow wave depolarization and even spiked potentials is of myogenic origin, the intramural plexuses are important for the coordination and duration of the spike potential. The intrinsic plexuses regulate the pattern of reciprocal excitation and inhibition necessary for migration of regular spiking activity.[10] The intrinsic nervous system therefore supports propulsive motility and local reflexes independent of extrinsic nerves.[11, 12] Continuity of structures in the small intestine, and therefore the intramural plexuses, is essential for the propagation of the myoelectric complex. In the large intestine, the role of continuity seems to be of less importance, and local factors such as the bulk of the contents may be more important in inciting motility.

The myenteric plexus consists of a repeating pattern of ganglia, which extends the length of the gastrointestinal tract. Originating from these ganglia are neurons that directly

stimulate the smooth muscle via acetylcholine release. The inherent rhythmicity of smooth muscle and superimposed cholinergic stimulation tend to produce a contractile state in the gastrointestinal tract. Modulatory neurons act to coordinate and limit muscular activity. The fundamental modulatory unit is a "driver" neuron, which fires in an oscillating pattern, activating "follower" neurons (see Fig. 4–2). Follower neurons are tonic inhibitors of smooth muscle function. The driver-follower mechanism, therefore, provides for smooth muscle relaxation and both prevents tonic contraction and limits propagation of intestinal contractions. Additional tonic inhibitory input is provided by the pre-synaptic α_2-adrenergic inhibition of cholinergic motor neurons. Removal of the sympathetic innervation, either by surgical or pharmacologic manipulation, results in an increase in smooth muscle activity. Therefore, the normal intestine relies on several mechanisms to provide tonic inhibition to the intestines. Both the intestinal smooth muscle and the inhibitory follower neurons have additional modulating neural inputs, including cholinergic motor neurons and peptidergic interneurons.[11, 12]

Many peptides are found in the plexuses and are likely to serve as neurotransmitters.[11] Vasoactive intestinal peptide (VIP) is inhibitory to intestinal smooth muscle, suggesting that it may be the neurotransmitter of follower neurons.[13] Acetylcholine,[14] somatostatin,[15, 16] and serotonin[17] all have some action that increases inhibitory follower neuron activity, thus suppressing motility. Opiates increase resting smooth muscle tone by inhibiting follower neuron activity,[18] but this effect is misleading. The overall smooth muscle tone is increased, increasing segmentation, but not peristalsis. The effect in horses, as in other species, is therefore constipative. Opiate antagonism stimulates propulsive motility, particularly in the hypomotile intestine.[19]

Autonomic extrinsic nerves modulate the intrinsic enteric nervous system. Pre-ganglionic parasympathetic nerves from the vagus synapse on ganglion cells of the myenteric plexus from the esophagus to the mid-colon and in the rectum, while those of the sacral nerves innervate the caudal half of the colon.[20] These fibers predominantly excite intestinal smooth muscle and inhibit sphincter tone.[11] Sympathetic input originates in the spinal cord between T_8 and L_3. The pre-ganglionic fibers synapse in the celiac and mesenteric ganglia. Post-ganglionic sympathetic fibers, primarily from the splanchnic nerve, synapse in the myenteric plexus and directly on smooth muscle cells of the blood vessels. Their primary effect is inhibition of smooth muscle activity and stimulation of sphincters, primarily via inhibition of the myenteric plexus. Sympathetic fibers also synapse on α_2-adrenergic receptors on the pre-synaptic axon terminals of parasympathetic fibers and inhibit acetylcholine release[11] (see Fig. 4–2). In addition, paracrine (local-acting) and endocrine (remote-acting) signals in the form of prostaglandins, motilin, and other peptides also modulate motility.

GASTRIC MOTILITY

Slow wave signals are generated by a pacemaker located on the greater curvature of the gastric antrum in the longitudinal muscle layer. The slow wave sweeps aborally over the fundus to the pylorus at a rate of two to five depolarizations

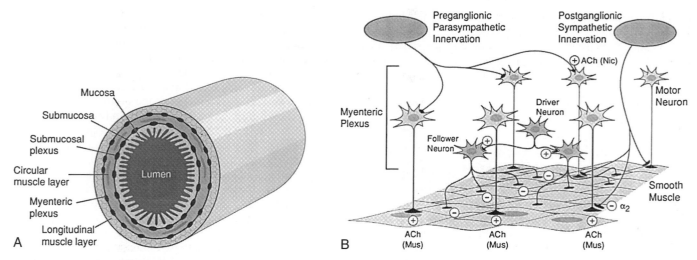

Figure 4–2. The enteric nervous system. *A*, General morphology of the intestinal tract. *B*, Myenteric plexus. Multiple inputs synapse on the enteric ganglia and the smooth muscle. Inhibition and stimulation of the intestinal smooth muscle is controlled by two systems. Stimulation is accomplished by intrinsic electrical properties of the muscle, creating the slow wave, and by intestinal motor neurons. The motor neurons act at muscarinic (Mus) receptors to stimulate smooth muscle. These neurons are stimulated by preganglionic parasympathetic innervation at nicotinic (Nic) receptors. Inhibition is provided by both extrinsic postganglionic sympathetic neurons and intrinsic "driver-follower" neurons. The driver neurons depolarize spontaneously, providing tonic inhibition to the smooth muscle via the inhibitory follower neurons. Extrinsic sympathetic innervation provides tonic inhibition at presynaptic α_2-adrenergic receptors on parasympathetic motor neurons.

per minute in the horse.[21, 22] The action potential or spiking activity accompanied by smooth muscle contraction is superimposed on the slow wave, with the frequency of spikes depending on the autonomic balance.[23] The sequence of gastric spiking activity begins with a quiescent stage, followed by variable intermittent spiking activity, and then becomes a prolonged regular spiking phase. Intermittent activity is associated with progressive motility, whereas prolonged spiking activity is associated with mixing.[24]

Gastric peristalsis occurs as a result of the biphasic gastric action potential, which follows the slow wave. Impulses begin at the pacemaker and travel aborally and luminally toward the circular muscle layer. The circular layer contracts, producing a constricted ring that travels distally along the path of the slow wave. The first phase of contraction of the gastric action potential pushes fluid contents through the relaxed pyloric sphincter, a phenomenon called "pyloric systole." Subsequently, the pyloric sphincter reflexly contracts, and the second phase of contraction proceeds against a closed pylorus resulting in retrograde flow, and mixing of stomach contents.[9] In this manner, the larger particles tend to remain in the cardia, while smaller particles and fluid empty rapidly.[23] Seventy-five percent of fluid should leave the stomach by 30 minutes after ingestion, while solid food takes considerably longer.[8]

SMALL INTESTINAL MOTILITY

Mechanical activity occurs at a slower rate in the caudal small intestine than cranially.[25] The slow wave frequency is initially about 15 depolarizations per minute and decreases aborally to 10 depolarizations per minute in the ileum.[22] This progressive decrease in slow wave frequency, in concert with

superimposed spiking activity, produces a gradient for the aboral movement of ingesta. Despite the fact that slow wave frequency is much lower for the stomach than the duodenum, there is seldom retrograde flow through the pylorus. Presumably, this is due to a significant pressure gradient of 3 to 4 cm H_2O from the stomach to the duodenum.

Electrical spiking activity of small intestine, which is superimposed on the slow wave during fasting, follows a coordinated pattern of impulses called the migrating myoelectric complex (MMC), which has migrating motor activity associated with it. The MMC begins at the duodenum, progresses aborally until termination at the ileum, and takes about 90 minutes (see Fig. 4–1). There are four phases of the MMC, which are associated with different types of motility. Phase 1 is a quiescent stage, characterized by slow wave activity without superimposed action potentials. Phase 2 consists of irregular spiking activity, which is associated with progressive motility, or peristalsis. This spiking activity increases in frequency to become phase 3, the phase of regular spiking activity; the accompanying motor activity being in the form of segmental contractions. This occupies 5% to 10% of the approximately 90-minute cycle.[26] The last phase, phase 4, is characterized by rapidly diminishing activity. Extrinsic innervation is important for the initiation of the MMC; however, once initiated, the MMC will continue despite denervation. The MMC of horses is similar to that seen in other species,[10, 24] except that it is not disrupted during feeding in horses, whereas it is in other species.[27]

Segmental contraction, seen with phase 3 of the MMC, is responsible for mixing of the ingesta and maximal exposure to the villous surfaces. However, segmental contraction does result in some net aboral transit due to the aboral gradient of the slow wave. Peristalsis (phase 2) causes circular muscle contractions to pass along the small intestine aborally. Stimulation of mechanoreceptors in the gut by intestinal distention enhances aboral peristalsis, which is mediated by the myenteric plexus. Because both segmentation and peristalsis are regulated by the enteric nervous system, they occur in extrinsically denervated gut. The extrinsic innervation, however, is important for initiation of electrical activity, modification of the frequency and strength of contraction, and coordination of movement of the different regions of the small intestine.[24]

LARGE INTESTINAL MOTILITY

The horse has a well-developed hindgut. A slow wave type of pacesetter has been demonstrated in the cecum, right ventral colon,[27, 28] and pelvic flexure[1] (Fig. 4–3). Four distinct types of electrical activity have been identified in the colon: (1) electrical control activity (slow waves), (2) discrete electrical response activity (short spike bursts; <5 sec), (3) continuous electrical response activity (long spike bursts; >5 sec), and (4) contractile electrical complex (oscillatory potential).[10, 26, 29–32] The electrical episodes that migrate orally or aborally over at least one half of the colon are defined as migrating colonic myoelectrical complexes.[29, 32] All other patterns of electrical activity are called colonic non-migrating myoelectrical complexes. In the horse, as in other species, colonic myoelectrical activity consists of similar patterns (long and short spike bursts).[33, 34] The slow wave frequency is more variable than in the small intestine. Long spike bursts migrate in both the oral and aboral directions and are the predominant myoelectrical activity in the pelvic flexure.[34] Myoelectrical events are correlated with motor events.[29, 32]

The cecum has frequent low-pressure contractions (2 to 3 mm Hg) that result in haustral changes or in the movement of feed material from one haustra to an adjacent haustra. Approximately once every 4 minutes, there are strong longitudinal muscle contractions that originate in the cecal apex and travel to the base, generating pressures of 20 to 50 mm Hg. These contractions move ingesta over longer distances and push it over the dorsal plica into the colon. Subsequently, the cecal base contracts and closes the cecocolic junction, which prevents reflux of ingesta from the colon into the cecum.[35] The cecal pacemaker at the cecal apex is responsible for aboral propulsion from the cecum to the right ventral colon.[27, 28] The total transit time for fluid in the cecum is approximately 5 hours,[35] and the retention time for particulate matter is approximately 20 hours.[36]

The pelvic flexure is regarded as having the ventral colon pacemaker and generates bidirectional depolarizations that initiate pressure waves. These pressure waves travel antegrade into the dorsal colon and retrograde into the ventral colon at the rate of 4 to 7 cm/sec.[1, 2] The right ventral colon has a similar motility pattern to that of the cecum, with frequent low-pressure haustral changes and a strong progressive contraction every 4 minutes. This progressive wave is coupled to the wave leaving the cecum.[35] There is also a low-pressure retrograde wave responsible for retaining ingesta in the ventral colon.[28] The coordination, or coupling of the different sections of large bowel, is under extrinsic control.[35] The cecum, ventral colon, dorsal colon, and small colon are all separate mixing pools. By the aforementioned mechanisms, retrograde flow is prevented between mixing pools, although it occurs within them. The resistance to flow through the large intestine increases through each functional barrier, so that the transverse colon provides the greatest impedance to flow. This mechanism appears to optimize the time that ingesta remains in the large bowel for fermentation. The disappearance times for fluid and particulate matter in the large colon are approximately 50 hours and 69 hours, respectively.[35]

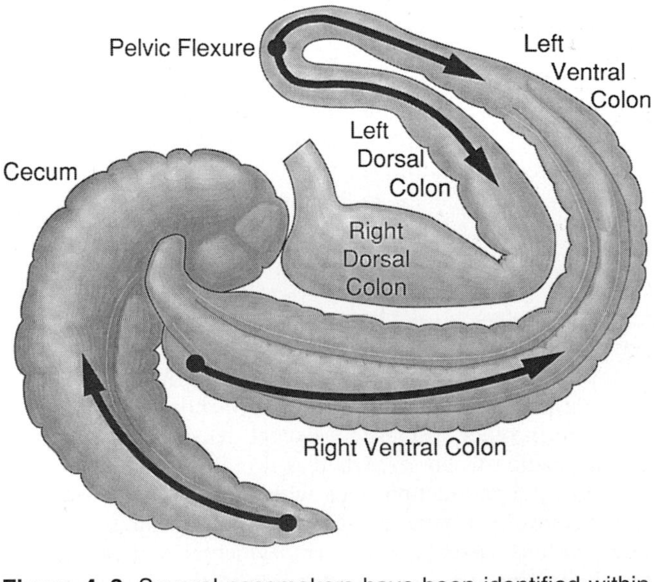

ENTERIC REFLEXES

Extrinsic innervation of the bowel is responsible for mediating protective enteric reflexes. The vagus-mediated gastrocolic and intestino-intestinal reflexes are comparable with those in other species.[10, 37] The gastrocolic reflex involves the stimulation of colonic motility in response to gastric distention. This reflex stimulates the emptying of the aboral tract in response to feed intake. The intestino-intestinal reflex is the reflex inhibition of the intestines in response to marked local distention. This prevents large increases in wall tension and potential rupture in response to intestinal obstruction.

The swallowing reflex, a vagus-mediated reflex causing receptive relaxation of the stomach during swallowing, is minimal in the horse. Therefore, horses must compensate for feed intake by a different and unique mechanism that allows immediate gastric emptying with stimulation of buccal receptors and is also a vagal reflex.[38] Retrograde power propulsion (vomiting) in response to local irritation is a protective reflex in many species that allows rapid removal of potential toxins by emesis. Horses are incapable of retrograde peristalsis of the stomach and esophagus and consequently cannot vomit. Regurgitation of gastric fluid occurs occasionally in conjunction with severe gastric dilatation in which it is presumed that intragastric pressure exceeds that created by

Figure 4–3. Several pacemakers have been identified within the musculature of the large colon. These pacemakers are responsible for both antegrade and retrograde flow.

the cardiac sphincter, resulting in the spontaneous reflux of gastric fluid.

In addition to the local motility patterns, the gastrointestinal tract exhibits coordination of individual segments. For example, when the stomach is in its quiescent phase, the orad jejunum is in phase 3 of the MMC (segmental contractions), and when the stomach is in its contractile state, the jejunum is in phase 2 of the MMC (peristalsis). Coordinated behavior of the gastrointestinal tract is essential for progressive motility.

EFFECTS OF FEEDING AND THE VOLUME OF INGESTA

After feeding, colonic motor activity increases in a bimodal pattern. The early response correlates to the gastrocecal reflex.[10] The later enterocolic reflex occurs when the ingesta is propelled through the ileocecal junction. A hormonal mediation of this reflex has been proposed. In the horse, a rise in colonic intraluminal pressure peaks occurs during the first hour of feeding.[2, 4] The degree of fullness of the cecum and large colon may be the main factor responsible for long spike burst activity in the equine colon and may function so locally as to only involve the intramural plexus in a specific segment. The general rise in pressure in the colon during feeding from distention of the viscus may stimulate motility.[10] This mechanism is complicated by the law of reflex relaxation[39] in which distention of a viscus and subsequent wall tension is abolished by relaxation of the smooth muscle. Therefore, changes in velocity of flow of ingesta are minimal until the distention capacity of the intestine is reached,[8] unless modulating input (neural) occurs.

ISCHEMIA

Ischemia and subsequent reperfusion are common injuries to segments of the equine intestinal tract because strangulation obstruction and thromboembolic infarction subsequent to *Strongylus vulgaris* larval migration are two major causes of equine colic.[40] Ischemia and hypoxia alter electrical and contractile activities of the intestine, depending on the duration, severity, and type (arterial or venous occlusion) of the insult. Partial ischemia induces a temporary increase in motility for less than 5 minutes, which is mediated by the intrinsic nerve supply.[41–43] This increase is followed by a progressive decrease in motor and electrical activity.[43] Ischemia may lower the intrinsic frequency or coupling of the slow waves, possibly as a result of hypoxic insult to the myenteric plexus.[43] Recovery of motility after recirculation depends on the duration and method of induction of ischemia.[41, 43] Venous occlusion creates a hemorrhagic obstruction to blood flow that produces severe edema and intestinal wall thickening. Loss of motility is more rapid in that model than in the arterial occlusion model in the horse.[41] Levels of circulating eicosanoids have been measured during strangulation obstruction in the horse in an attempt to isolate antagonists that could be used for treatment of the systemic effects of ischemia.[44] The role of increased eicosanoids in intestinal motility is not completely understood, but prostaglandins are an important local neuromodulator substance (see later).

In the horse, verminous arteritis in the cranial mesenteric artery with subsequent thrombosis and embolization have long been thought to lead to a reduction in the relative blood flow through the colic arteries. Experimental inoculation of ponies with infective *S. vulgaris* larvae did produce decreased fecal production, depression, and decreased small intestinal spiking activity during the migration phase.[1, 35, 45] In chronic infection, however, with marked reduction in blood flow through the colic arteries in these ponies, alteration in colonic intraluminal pressure peaks (motility indices) did not differ from that found in control ponies.[1, 35] The ability of the pony to accommodate to such massive arterial occlusion is related to the extensive collateral circulation (rete mirabile) that is peculiar to the equine species in this location (colic arteries).[1]

The significant increases in intestinal motility following partial ischemia and reperfusion may be detrimental. Motility (tonic contractions) can further decrease intestinal blood flow (particularly mucosal flow) by increasing intravascular/vascular resistance and at the same time increasing the muscle layer's oxygen consumption.[41]

DISTENTION AND OBSTRUCTION

The effects of luminal distention on local blood flow and motility depend on the degree and method of distention. The total blood flow and mucosal blood flow are reduced at 15 to 45 mm Hg intraluminal pressure, but flow to the muscle layer is increased.[41] Intraluminal pressures produced by obstruction do not usually exceed 20 mm Hg (because distention occurs slowly and "law of reflex relaxation" prevents increases in intraluminal pressure up to a point. Therefore, the effects of distention on blood flow to the gut and oxygen consumption are probably minimal in pathologic states.[41] In the horse, intraluminal pressures have been measured in clinical cases. Pressures higher than 15 mm Hg have a poor prognosis, and the horses did not survive resection and anastomosis.[46]

Experimental extraluminal obstruction of the equine jejunum induced continuous spiking activity as the predominant myoelectric pattern cranial to the obstruction in the distended segment of small intestine. Strain gauge deflection correlated with the height of myoelectric spike potentials. Average intraluminal pressures were in the range of 18 to 24 mm Hg; however, at the termination of regular spiking activity or during continuous spiking activity, pressure peaks increased to 30 to 60 mm Hg. Other studies have confirmed increased intestinal motility cranial to obstruction in horses.[44, 47] The increased motility cranial to the obstruction did not appear to be related to the distention because the increase in motility started immediately after the obstruction and may be caused by a direct irritant effect.[24] The increase in forceful contractions may impede blood flow while increasing the metabolic demands of the intestine.

In the pathologic state, ischemia and distention can lead to alteration in the ratio of mucosal to muscular blood flow and may alter total blood flow to the intestine, which stimulates tonic contraction of the intestinal tract. This can lead to a vicious cycle of further decreased blood flow owing to mechanical effects of contraction as well as increased cellular oxygen consumption and continued destruction of the intestinal tract.

DIARRHEA

Although intuitively it seems that hypermotility would be a factor in diarrhea, there is little evidence to suggest that hypermotility plays a major role in any disease associated with diarrhea.[48, 49] In most cases, there is decreased or incoordination of gastrointestinal motility.[48–50] The decreased motility promotes the overgrowth of bacteria and may play a role in bacteria-associated diarrheic syndromes. Some studies have implied that bacteria and enterotoxins can induce a hypermotility syndrome.[51, 52]

EXPERIMENTAL MODELS OF ILEUS

Adynamic ileus has been studied in horses using several different models. These models usually involve celiotomy and manipulation of the bowel. These techniques include rubbing the small intestine and exposing it to air and then drying the intestines to produce serosal desiccation.[24, 53] Ileus has also been produced in horses by surgical, pharmacologic, or nutritional manipulation to mimic intestinal distention. Lowe and associates inflated rubber balloons in ponies with surgically created colonic fistulas to simulate distention.[54] Alternatively, the colon of some ponies was obstructed by abruptly changing the feed from pelleted feed to coarser forage. Amitraz, an acaricide, has also been used to induce impactions in horses.[55]

ILEUS AND MECHANISMS OF MOTILITY DYSFUNCTION

Adynamic ileus is characterized by a lack of propulsive motility of the gastrointestinal tract[11] and can be associated with gastrointestinal diseases, such as obstruction,[56] duodenitis/proximal jejunitis,[57] and grass sickness.[58] Sepsis, peritonitis, pain, and intraperitoneal or extraperitoneal inflammation can also cause ileus,[12, 56] as can endotoxemia, which may accompany any of the aforementioned diseases.[59–61] This complication occurs commonly after abdominal surgery in horses and may be responsible for up to 44% of postoperative mortality.[62]

Clinical signs of ileus include colic, depressed appetite, and an absence of borborygmi due to persistently poor motility. Ileus may be accompanied by gastric reflux. When the small intestine is involved, a rectal examination may reveal distention of the small intestine, and nasogastric reflux is usually obtained. Large intestinal ileus will be characterized by distention of the large colon and cecum, which can be detected by a rectal examination and by percussion of a high-pitched ping over the cecum or colon in the right flank or the colon in the left flank. Secondary to intestinal distention, fluid accumulation, and appetite suppression is dehydration and electrolyte imbalance (particularly hypokalemia and hypocalcemia).[38] Therapy is directed primarily at supportive care and secondarily at pharmacologic manipulation of motility.

The lack of propulsive motility allows the accumulation of gas, chyme, and gut secretions within the lumen, causing distention[53] and high intraluminal pressure.[63] Depending on the site, this dilatation can involve the stomach, small intestine, colon, or the entire gastrointestinal tract and may result in colic or even gastric or colonic rupture. Local insults may lead to generalized inhibition of gastrointestinal motility owing to exaggerated inhibition via the intestino-intestinal reflex.[11] After abdominal surgery, gastrointestinal motility may be completely depressed for as long as 4 days.[64] In experimental models in both people and horses, the colon remains inactive longest, followed by the stomach.[24, 65] Clinical experience in horses suggests that the small intestine remains quiescent longest after small intestinal surgery.

Lack of propulsive motility could be the result of failure of intrinsic or extrinsic electrical activity, incoordination of regional contractile activity, or dissociation of electrical and mechanical events. In dogs with implanted electrodes, ileus created by celiotomy and rubbing of the bowel resulted in failure of propulsive motility with no change in the amplitude or frequency of the gastric, jejunal, and ileal slow waves.[53] In addition, the smooth muscle retains normal electrical properties in adynamic ileus.[56] Therefore, abnormal function during ileus is not caused by an abnormality in the smooth muscle itself; rather, there is a lack of action potentials and accompanying muscular contractions.

The MMC requires initiation by a command signal via extrinsic innervation but can progress normally without further extrinsic innervation.[11] After a celiotomy, the MMC pattern is disrupted, and electrical and sphere studies have indicated that the disturbance of the progressive motility after surgery appears to be due to failure of the MMC. In dogs, the MMC was completely inhibited for 24 hours after colon resection.[64] Disruption of the MMC is also observed during ileus in the horse subsequent to celiotomy and serosal desiccation.[24] These results suggest that ileus is accompanied by a decrease in the initiation and propagation of MMCs. Because signals normally can propagate independently of extrinsic innervation, there must be either active inhibition of the enteric nervous system by extrinsic innervation or an aberration in the enteric nervous system itself.

During ileus, electrical slow waves persist, but superimposed action potentials are diminished. The predominant type of neural activity that occurs during ileus is the continual firing of "follower" inhibitory neurons.[11] The follower neurons receive neural input from the "driver" neurons as well as from other sources, and the response is a summation of input from all these sources. This suggests that ileus is at least partly due to the active neural stimulation (or lack of inhibition) of these follower inhibitory neurons.[11]

One of the possible mechanisms for this persistent inhibition is high sympathetic tone[53, 66] via the suppression of neural networks that normally inhibit follower neurons.[11] The sympathetic nervous system is responsible for the normal intestino-intestinal inhibitory reflex.[66] Many studies have been performed to evaluate the role of the sympathetic nervous system in ileus. The administration of the β-antagonist propranolol and the α-antagonist phentolamine at the time of surgery significantly increased the percentage of time associated with phase 3 (segmentation) of the MMC, but the actual transit time of spheres was not changed.[53] In addition, disruption of sympathetic input in dogs and sheep by resection of the splanchnic nerve, and paravertebral anesthesia, respectively, prevented the postoperative inhibition of the MMC.[64] These findings suggest that although there is normally a balance between tonic inhibition and stimulation of the bowel, sympathetic activity predominates after surgery and has a role in the inhibition of the MMC. However, it is not completely responsible for the failure of propulsive motility.

Aberration of other gastrointestinal hormones and neurotransmitters may also contribute to reduce gastrointestinal motility. Gerring and Hunt studied the effect of adrenergic blockade on gastrointestinal coordination in ponies.[24] Their model of serosal desiccation produced a decrease in the percentage of coordinated migrating myoelectric complexes showing coordination from 100% before surgery to 22% postoperatively. With β-adrenergic blockade using propranolol, the degree of coordination did not change significantly. The addition of an α_2-antagonist, yohimbine, improved coordination to 53%. Because yohimbine competes with norepinephrine at α_2-receptors, these results suggest a role for α_2-receptors in gastrointestinal coordination. The results of other studies have shown that the norepinephrine inhibition of acetylcholine release within the enteric plexuses is mediated by *presynaptic* α_2-adrenergic receptors.[67] Although the adrenergic receptors in smooth muscle are both α and β_2, these receptors likely have no direct contribution to ileus, because smooth muscle properties are unaltered in ileus. Therefore, part of the normal inhibition of the follower neurons is likely via cholinergic neurons. The discharge of the parasympathetic neurons, which should suppress the inhibitory neurons in the normal state, is prevented by presynaptic inhibition at α_2-receptors. Because α_2-receptor blockade by yohimbine failed to restore all coordinated activity, additional factors must contribute to the development of adynamic ileus.

Epinephrine, which is often increased in the plasma of patients with ileus, has been investigated as a potential contributor to adynamic ileus. Circulating catecholamines have a direct inhibitory action on intestinal smooth muscle and are increased about five-fold during the first postoperative day.[56] However, the plasma concentration of epinephrine peaks a few hours after surgery and rapidly declines to presurgical values by 12 hours, thus declining well before any improvement in the ileus. Therefore, it is unlikely that circulating epinephrine is a primary contributor to ileus. Conversely, plasma concentrations of norephinephrine gradually increase and remain elevated for several days after surgery.[53] The plasma concentration of norepinephrine parallels overall sympathetic nervous activity.

Dopamine also contributes to postoperative ileus. Dopamine, which was added to strips of human colonic mucosa in vitro, directly inhibited longitudinal muscle activity and indirectly inhibited motility via the enteric nervous system in circular muscle.[65] The direct effect of dopamine on longitudinal muscle probably does not contribute to ileus, because the smooth muscle properties are unchanged during ileus. However, the effect of dopamine on the enteric nervous system and the presence of specific dopamine receptors throughout the gastrointestinal tract suggest a role for dopamine in ileus. Intravenous administration of dopamine in sheep causes an immediate inhibition of the MMC, followed by re-initiation of the MMC in the duodenum, which is an effect mediated by the vagus.[68] The inhibition of the MMC may be caused by a direct effect of dopamine on the enteric nervous system. The subsequent re-initiation of the MMC would then be caused by a vagus-mediated reflex. During adynamic ileus, the dopamine-related initial effect may predominate, whereas the vagal component is inhibited due to the presynaptic inhibition by the sympathetic effects at the α_2-receptors. The effect of dopamine is dependent on cholinergic neurotransmission,[69] which places the site of action at the presynaptic parasympathetics, such as for α_2-receptors.

Further evidence for the role of dopamine in the development of adynamic ileus is the response of the intestine to antidopaminergic drugs. In the serosal desiccation model of Gerring and Hunt,[24] the dopamine antagonist metoclopramide increased the percentage of coordinated migrating myoelectric complexes to 100%. Metoclopramide increased gastric emptying by enhancing the inherent antral contractions,[70] increasing local intestinal activity, and restoring aboral propulsion of ingesta in the orad intestine.[70] There is no specific stimulation of the cecum or colon by metoclopramide.[71, 72] This suggests that dopamine has a role in the pathophysiology of ileus, particularly in the stomach and small intestine. However, metoclopramide has other actions in addition to the anti-dopaminergic effect. It has some α_2-blocker activity and stimulates the release of acetylcholine. Therefore, the results of this study need to be interpreted carefully, because one of these other mechanisms may contribute to the action of this drug. In addition, the different studies use a wide range of dosages, which makes it difficult to draw comparisons.

Several researchers have evaluated the efficacy of cholinergic agents (muscarinic agonists and cholinesterase inhibitors) in postoperative ileus because of the role of parasympathethic innervation in the coordination of the gastrointestinal tract.[21, 24, 33, 73, 74] In the stomach, cholinergic agents such as neostigmine, bethanechol, and carbachol stimulate contraction and can cause violent contractile activity. However, they significantly delay gastric emptying of particulate matter.[74] These findings suggest that cholinergic agents have a direct effect on the motility but do not coordinate contraction with gastric emptying. Furthermore, neostigmine showed no effect on the MMC of the jejunum and actually decreased small intestinal propulsive motility.[33, 74] Despite this effect in the upper gastrointestinal tract, these agents exhibit a prokinetic, or progressive motility, effect on the cecum and large colon.[21, 33] These studies suggest that coordination is achieved by a finely controlled release of acetylcholine at parasympathetic terminals, rather than a global increase in parasympathetic tone. This fine control may be more important in the orad gastrointestinal tract than in the large colon.

In addition to these neural mechanisms, hormones may modulate ileus. Motilin is released at surgery with the manipulation of the large intestine. Motilin stimulates colonic activity, and its increase postoperatively is associated with the return of normal motility.[65] Prostaglandins also affect gastrointestinal motility. PGE_2 administered to normal horses mimics endotoxin-induced ileus.[61] PGE_1 and PGI_2 inhibit the motility of most of the gastrointestinal tract of the normal horse.[61, 75] $PGF_{2\alpha}$ stimulates gastric and colonic motility.[61] In a postoperative ileus model in rats, 16,16-dimethyl PGE_2 increased gastric emptying and small intestinal and colonic transit time.[76] Clearly, there are many contributing factors that balance and modulate ileus.

In summary, adynamic ileus in the horse is the lack of motility due to inhibition of the smooth muscle of the gastrointestinal tract. This inhibition is not caused by a loss of intrinsic ability of the smooth muscle to contract but rather is a result of the tonic discharge of inhibitory neurons, secondary to altered summation of pre-synaptic input.[11] Inhibition of the inhibitory neurons, which is normally provided by parasympathetic neurons, is suppressed by pre-synaptic inhibition at α_2-adrenergic receptors. The neurotransmitter, dopamine, also inhibits the parasympathetic nerves.[69] Therefore, drugs that act to block the α_2-adrenergic receptors, dopaminergic receptors, or enhance the release of acetylcholine at parasympathetic nerve terminals all improve gastrointestinal motility during ileus. In addition to these neural effects, other endogenous modulators such as motilin, serotonin, opiate peptides, and prostaglandins are likely to contribute to the clinical presentation of ileus.

REFERENCES

1. Sellers AF, Lowe JE, Drost CJ, et al: Retropulsion-propulsion in the equine large colon. *Am J Vet Res* 43:390, 1982.
2. Sellers AF, Lowe JE, Brondum J: Motor events in the equine large colon. *Am J Physiol* 237:E457, 1979.
3. Sellers AF, Lowe JE, Rendano VT: Equine colonic motility: Interactions among wall motion, propulsion and fluid flow. *Am J Vet Res* 45:357, 1984.
4. Ross MW, Donawick WJ, Sellers AF, et al: Normal and altered cecocolic motility patterns in ponies. *Vet Surg* 14:63, 1985.
5. Ross MW, Donawick WJ, Sellers AF, et al: Normal motility of the cecum and right ventral colon in ponies. *Am J Vet Res* 47:1756, 1986.
6. Bueno L, Fioramonti J, Ruckebusch Y: Rate of flow of digesta and electrical activity of the small intestine in dogs and sheep. *J Physiol* 249:69, 1975.
7. Sellers AF, Lowe JE: Review of large intestinal motility and mechanisms of impaction in the horse. *Equine Vet J* 18:261, 1986.
8. Argenzio RA: Functions of the equine large intestine and their interrelationship in disease. *Cornell Vet* 65:303, 1975.
9. Jensen D: Gastrointestinal motility and its regulation. In *The Principles of Physiology*, ed 2. New York, Appleton-Century-Crofts, 1980, p 774.
10. Ruckebusch Y: Motor functions of the intestines. *Adv Vet Sci Comp Med* 25:345, 1981.
11. Wood JD: Physiology of the enteric nervous system. In Johnson LR, ed. *Physiology of the Gastrointestinal Tract.* New York, Raven Press, 1987, p 67.
12. Livingston EH, Passaro EP: Postoperative ileus. *Dig Dis Sci* 35:121, 1990.
13. Angel F, Go VLW, Szurszewski JS: VIP is an inhibitory neurotransmitter in the muscularis mucosa of the canine gastric antrum. *Gastroenterology* 80:1101, 1981.
14. Hirst GD, McKirdy NC: A nervous mechanism for descending inhibition in guinea pig small intestine. *J Physiol (Lond)* 238:129, 1974.
15. Furness JB, Costa M: Actions of somatostatin on excitatory and inhibitory nerves in the intestine. *Eur J Pharmacol* 56:69, 1979.
16. Katayama Y, North RA: The action of somatostatin on neurones of the myenteric plexuses of the guinea-pig. *J Physiol (Lond)* 303:315, 1980.
17. Vermillion D, Gillespie J, Cooke AR, et al: Does 5-hydroxytryptamine influence purinergic inhibitory neurons in the intestine? *Am J Physiol* 237:E198, 1979.
18. Shimo Y, Ishii T: Effects of morphine on nonadrenergic inhibitory responses of the guinea-pig *Taenia coli. J Pharm Pharmacol* 30:496, 1978.
19. Roger T, Barden T, Ruckebusch Y: Colonic motor responses in the pony: Relevance of colonic stimulation by opiate antagonists. *Am J Vet Res* 46:31, 1985.
20. deGroat WC, Krier J: An electrophysiological study of the sacral parasympathetic pathway to the colon of the cat. *J Physiol (Lond)* 260:425, 1978.
21. King JN, Gerring EL: Actions of the novel gastrointestinal prokinetic agent cisapride on equine bowel motility. *J Vet Pharmacol Ther* 11:314, 1988.
22. Phaneuf LP, Ruckebusch Y: Physiological, pharmacological and therapeutic aspects of some gastrointestinal disorders in the horse. In Ruckebusch Y, ed. *Veterinary Pharmacology and Toxicology.* Boston, MTP Press, 1983, p 371.
23. Meyer JH, Thomson JB, Cohen MB, et al: Sieving of food by the canine stomach and sieving after gastric surgery. *Gastroenterology* 76:804, 1979.
24. Gerring EL, Hunt JM: Pathophysiology of equine postoperative ileus: Effect of adrenergic blockade, parasympathetic stimulation and metoclopramide in an experimental model. *Equine Vet J* 18:249, 1986.
25. MacHarg MA, Adams SB, Lamar CH, et al: Electromyographical, myomechanical and intraluminal obstruction of the jejunum in conscious ponies. *Am J Vet Res* 47:7, 1986.
26. Sarna SK: Cyclic motor activity; migrating motor complex. *Gastroenterology* 89:894, 1985.
27. Ross MW, Cullen KK, Rutkowski JA: Myoelectric activity of the ileum, cecum, and right ventral colon in ponies during interdigestive, nonfeeding, and digestive periods. *Am J Vet Res* 51:561, 1990.
28. Ross MW, Donawick WJ, Sellers AF, et al: Normal motility of the cecum and right ventral colon in ponies, Vol. 2. Proceedings of the 2nd Equine Colic Research Symposium, 1986, p 95.
29. Ruckebusch Y, Fioramonti J: Colonic myoelectrical spiking activity: Major patterns and significance in 6 different species. *Zentralbl Veterinarmed[A]* 27:1, 1980.
30. Fioramonti J, Bueno L: Electrical activity of the large intestine in normal and megacolon pigs. *Ann Rech Vet* 8:275, 1977.
31. Sarna SK: Myoelectric correlates of colonic motor complexes and contractile activity. *Am J Physiol* 250:G213, 1986.
32. Ferre JP, Ruckebusch Y: Myoelectrical activity and propulsion in the large intestine of fed and fasted rats. *J Physiol* 62:93, 1985.
33. Adams SB, Lamar CH, Masty J: Motility of the jejunum and pelvic flexure in ponies: Effects of six drugs. *Am J Vet Res* 45:795, 1984.
34. Lamar CH, Masty J, Adams SB, et al: Impedance monitoring of equine intestinal motility. *Am J Vet Res* 45:810, 1984.
35. Sellers AF, Lowe JE, Rendano VT, et al: The reservoir function of the equine cecum and ventral large colon—its relationship to chronic nonsurgical obstructive disease with colic. *Cornell Vet* 72:233, 1982.
36. Bertone AL, VanSoest PJ, Johnson DJ, et al: Large intestinal capacity, retention times and turnover rates of particulate ingesta associated with extensive large-colon resection in horses. *Am J Vet Res* 50:1621, 1989.
37. Ruckebush Y, Vigroux P: Étude électromyographique de la motricité du caecum chéz le cheval. *Cahiers Med Vet* 42:128, 1974.
38. Becht JL: Alterations in intestinal motility: Effects on therapeutics in the horse, Vol. 2. Proceedings of the 2nd Equine Colic Research Symposium, 1986, p 26.
39. Guyton AC: Movement of food through the alimentary tract.

In *Textbook of Medical Physiology,* ed 5. Philadelphia, WB Saunders, 1976, p 850.

40. Baker JR, Ellis CE: A survey of post mortem findings in 480 horses 1958–1980. 1: Causes of death. *Equine Vet J* 13:43, 1981.

41. Sullins KE, Stashak TS, Mero KN: Pathologic changes associated with induced small intestinal strangulation obstruction and nonstrangulating infarction in horses. *Am J Vet Res* 46:193, 1985.

42. Meissner A, Bowes KL, Sarna SK: Effects of ambient and stagnant hypoxia on the mechanical and electrical activity of the canine upper jejunum. *Can J Surg* 19:316, 1976.

43. Chou CC, Gallivan RH: Blood flow and intestinal motility. *Fed Proc* 41:2090, 1982.

44. Robertson-Smith RG, Adams SB, Bottoms GD: Intestinal motility and eicosanoid levels following jejunal strangulation/ obstruction and resection. *Vet Surg* 15:132, 1986.

45. Berry CR, Merritt AM, Burrows CF, et al: Evaluation of the myoelectrical activity of the equine ileum infected with *Strongylus vulgaris* larvae. *Am J Vet Res* 47:27, 1986.

46. Allen DA Jr, White NA, Tyler DE: Factors for prognostic use in equine obstructive small intestinal disease. *J Am Vet Med Assoc* 189:777, 1986.

47. Parks AH, Stick JA, Arden WA, et al: Effects of distension and neostigmine on intestinal vascular resistance, oxygen consumption and motility. *Am J Vet Res* 50:54, 1989.

48. Moon HW: Mechanisms in the pathogenesis of diarrhea: A review. *J Am Vet Med Assoc* 172:443, 1978.

49. Binder HJ, Donowitz M: A new look at laxative action. *Gastroenterology* 69:1001, 1975.

50. Ritchie JA: Colonic transport in the irritable colon syndrome. In Demling L, Ottenjann R, eds. *Gastrointestinal Motility.* New York, Academic Press, 1971, p 104.

51. Grady GF, Keusch GT: Pathogenesis of bacterial diarrheas. *N Engl J Med* 285:891, 1971.

52. Donaldson RM: The blind loop syndrome. In Sleisenger MH, Fordtran JS, eds. *Gastrointestinal Disease.* Philadelphia, WB Saunders, 1973, p 927.

53. Smith J, Keith KA, Weinshilboum RM: Pathophysiology of postoperative ileus. *Arch Surg* 112:203, 1977.

54. Lowe JE, Sellers AF, Brondum J: Equine pelvic flexure impaction: A model used to evaluate motor events and compare drug response. *Cornell Vet* 70:401, 1980.

55. Roberts MC: Development of a drug-induced impaction colic model in the horse, Vol. 2. Proceedings of the 2nd Equine Colic Research Symposium, 1986, p 88.

56. Nadrowski L: Paralytic ileus: Recent advances in pathophysiology and treatment. *Curr Surg* 40:260, 1983.

57. Johnston JK, Morris DD: Comparison of duodenitis/proximal jejunitis and small intestinal obstruction in horses: 68 cases (1977–1985). *J Am Vet Med Assoc* 191:849, 1987.

58. Bishop AE, Hodson NP, Major JH, et al: The regulatory peptide system of the large bowel in equine grass sickness. *Experientia* 40:801, 1984.

59. King JN, Gerring EL: Disruption of equine bowel motility by endotoxin—evidence of a role for prostaglandins and PAF (Abstract). *Br J Pharmacol* 97 (Proc Suppl):428P, 1989.

60. King JN, Gerring EL: Antagonism of endotoxin-induced disruption of equine gastrointestinal motility with the platelet-activating factor antagonist WEB 2086. *J Vet Pharmacol Ther* 13:333, 1990.

61. King JN, Gerring EL: The action of low dose endotoxin on equine bowel motility. *Equine Vet J* 23:11, 1991.

62. Edwards GB, Hunt JM: An analysis of the incidence of equine postoperative ileus and an assessment of the complications, Vol 2. Proceedings of the 2nd Equine Colic Research Symposium, 1986, p 307.

63. Allen D, White NA, Taylor DE: Factors for prognostic use in equine obstructive small intestinal disease. *J Am Vet Med Assoc* 189:177, 1986.

64. Bueno L, Fioramonti J, Ruckebusch Y: Postoperative intestinal motility in dogs and sheep. *Dig Dis* 23:682, 1978.

65. Rennie JA, Christofides ND, Mitchenere P, et al: Neural and humoral factors in postoperative ileus. *Br J Surg* 67:694, 1980.

66. Furness JB, Costa M: Adynamic ileus, its pathogenesis and treatment. *Med Biol* 52:82, 1974.

67. Suprenant A, North RA: μ-Opiod receptors and α_2- adrenoreceptors coexist on myenteric but not on submucous neurons. *Neuroscience* 16:425, 1985.

68. Bueno L, Fioramonti J: Dopaminergic control of gastrointestinal motility. In Ruckebusch Y, ed. *Veterinary Pharmacology and Toxicology.* Boston, MTP Press, 1983, p 283.

69. Thorner MO: Dopamine is an important neurotransmitter in the autonomic nervous system. *Lancet* 1:662, 1975.

70. Hunt JM, Edwards GB, Clarke KW: Incidence, diagnosis and treatment of postoperative complications in colic cases. *Equine Vet J* 18:264, 1986.

71. Ruckebusch Y, Roger T: Prokinetic effects of cisapride, naloxone and parasympathetic stimulation at the equine ileo-cecocolonic junction. *J Vet Pharmacol Ther* 11:322, 1988.

72. Sojka JE, Adams SB, Lamar CH, et al: Effect of butorphanol, pentazocine, meperidine, or metoclopramide on intestinal motility in female ponies. *Am J Vet Res* 49:527, 1988.

73. Kilbinger H, Weihrach TR: Drugs increasing gastrointestinal motility. *Pharmacology* 25:61, 1982.

74. Adams SB, MacHarg MA: Neostigmine methylsulfate delays gastric emptying of particulate markers in horses. *Am J Vet Res* 46:2498, 1985.

75. Hunt JM, Gerring EL: The effect of prostaglandin E_1 on motility of the equine gut. *J Vet Pharmacol Ther* 8:165, 1985.

76. Ruwart MJ, Klepper MS, Rush BD: Prostaglandin stimulation of gastrointestinal transit in post-operative ileus rats. *Prostaglandins* 19:415, 1980.

Chapter 5

Clinical Nutrition

Debra K. Rooney, PhD

Basic knowledge of the proper method for feeding horses is important to veterinarians in order that they may assist their clients with the determination of feed choices that are wholesome, economical, and tailored to the workload or intended use of the horses. In addition, many veterinarians operate a boarding or breeding facility and need to provide balanced rations to the horses in their care. In order to best help the client, the veterinarians should know the number, type, and use of the horses. Client preference regarding feeds is also important since the choice may be at least partially determined or governed by the amount of staff available and the ability of the staff to comply with detailed instructions.

The basic considerations for the amount and type of feed are determined by the age, size, and use or workload of the horses.[1, 2] Broodmares have different needs than growing horses, which are quite different from horses in heavy work. The nutritional management of orphaned foals and very sick neonates or adult horses with serious infectious diseases or neoplasia requires special dietary consideration.

FEEDS

Forages

The most common forms of forage fed to horses are pasture and hay. Silage, haylage, and "green chop" have also been used to a much lesser extent. The choice of forage type depends on several factors: land availability, fertility of the soil, storage capability, and climate. Regardless of the form, the quality of the forage fed will be dictated by the species, soil fertility, temperature, degree of rainfall, method of harvesting, and most important, the stage of maturity at harvest. The best-quality forages are cut before seed heads (boot stage in grasses) and blooms (bud stage for legumes) appear. This results in a higher proportion of leaves, a decrease in the poorly digestible cell wall content, and consequently a more nutritious product. Hay cubes are fed less often but can be useful when limited storage space is available.

Grasses

The grass species are generally divided into two groups: the cool-season and the warm-season grasses. The cool-season grasses include Kentucky bluegrass, smooth brome grass, orchardgrass, tall fescue, timothy, and oats. These grasses are grown predominantly in the northern half of the United States. These species are of greatest value in the spring and fall, providing a forage stand that is lush and high in nutritive value and palatability.

Kentucky Bluegrass. Long favored by horsepeople everywhere as the ideal pasture grass, bluegrass is highly palatable and winter-hardy, and is a ready volunteer, producing high yields in the cooler months. It seems to handle close grazing well. It does not, however, do well in the summer months or under heavy traffic. Kentucky bluegrass is used exclusively in pastures.

Smooth Brome Grass. Like bluegrass, brome grass forms a dense sod and is winter-hardy. Unlike bluegrass, it is heat- and drought-tolerant. Its good palatability, even when mature, makes it a good choice for pasture or hay when seeded with alfalfa. Brome grass does not tolerate overgrazing or frequent harvesting and is slow to regrow.

Orchardgrass. Another common grass species in the temperate zones, orchardgrass produces early growth, is more heat-, shade-, and drought-tolerant than most grasses, and recovers rapidly after harvest or grazing with good-quality growth. Its early maturity makes it very compatible in seedings with alfalfa. Orchardgrass is less winter-hardy than other species.

Tall Fescue. Of the grasses, this species is the most traffic- and drought-tolerant. It adapts to a wide range of soil and climate conditions and is persistent. Palatability is generally not high, but improves in the spring and following the first frost. The biggest drawbacks to using tall fescue in pastures are their high concentration of alkaloids and the more recent problems associated with endophyte infestations or fescue toxicosis that have serious consequences in broodmare bands.[3] The problem often affects broodmares in late pregnancy and young growing horses. The endophytic fungus *Acremonium coenophiolum* affects growing pasture and sometimes hay made from these pastures. (For additional information, see Chapter 19, Toxicological Problems.)

Timothy. The most well-known of the grasses and the most popular of the grass hays, timothy is winter-hardy, easy to establish, and widely adapted. It is generally a clean, dust-free hay, and readily consumed by horses. It is not a good pasture grass because of its low tolerance for heavy grazing or cutting and the production of an open, clumpy sod. Like most grasses, it is not as heat- or drought-tolerant as legumes.

Oat Hay. A popular forage in the western United States and Canada, oat hay is best if harvested when the grain is at the late milk or dough stage. When cut at the proper time, the protein content can be as high as 13%. A valid concern is the potential for nitrate poisoning if harvested at a very young stage[1] and testing for nitrate concentration is recommended if oat hay is going to be used as the predominant forage source. Concentrations of nitrate between 0.4% and 0.6% are considered safe for horses.[1] For further discussion, see Chapter 19.

The warm-season grasses, Bermudagrass, Bahiagrass, and pangola grass, do well in sandy soils, are more drought-tolerant, but are generally lower in digestibility than the cool-season grasses and often produce lower yields. These forages are found primarily in the southern coastal and southeastern regions of the United States. Most are used as pasture grasses. The exception is Bermudagrass, which can also serve as an easily harvested, high-yielding species for hay production.

Legumes

Alfalfa and clover are the predominant legume species. In some areas of the country, stands of birdsfoot trefoil and lespedeza (also called *Sericea*) are still grown. The deep-rooted characteristic of legumes is what contributes to their drought tolerance. Their high protein and calcium content is useful in improving the nutritional value of grass pastures. A disadvantage of legumes is their intolerance to heavy traffic, overgrazing, and poor drainage.

Alfalfa. Alfalfa has become the predominant legume grown in the United States. It is leafy and fine-stemmed, produces high yields, is resistant to many pests and diseases, and is high in digestibility and palatability. Despite these advantages, there are many wives' tales and myths that exist, making its use controversial. There are no data to support the long-held contention that the protein content makes it too "rich" for horses and, likewise, that it causes kidney damage. The high protein and mineral content of alfalfa will stimulate an increase in water intake and a concomitant increase in urine volume and nitrogen and calcium excretion. Alfalfa has also been called a "hot" feed, but research has shown that there is no difference in sweat production or body temperature in horses fed either alfalfa or timothy hay.[1]

The major concerns with alfalfa are the wide calcium-to-phosphorus ratios that can occur, the potential for overfeeding, and the problems with blister beetle infestation. Most alfalfa hays have calcium-to-phosphorus ratios between 3:1 and 5:1, but ratios as high as 15:1 have been observed.[1] Mature horses can tolerate ratios of the total diet as high as 6:1, but some mature horses have developed a propensity for dirt-eating or rock-chewing suggestive of pica at calcium-to-phosphorus ratios of 3:1. Ratios higher than 3:1 are not advised for young, growing horses.[2] When the use of alfalfa results in undesirable ratios, adding phosphorus to the diet

or reducing the amount of alfalfa by replacing it with a grass hay should narrow the ratio.

The digestible energy content of alfalfa is generally higher than other forages, making it much easier to overfeed. Fourteen pounds of alfalfa hay is equal in energy content to 18 lb of timothy hay. Horses fed high-quality alfalfa (>55% total digestible nutrients, TDN) at 2% of their body weight can become fat very quickly, consuming in some cases 50% more calories than required for maintenance. Less alfalfa can be fed and still meet the animal's needs. Supplying some grass hay should help to appease boredom if additional forage seems indicated.

Cantharidin toxicosis from the ingestion of blister beetles was first reported in horses in 1978.[4] (See Chapter 19 for a thorough discussion of cantharidin poisoning.)

Red and White Clover. Red clover is still preferred by some horsepeople, but has declined in popularity. When harvested properly, it can be as high in nutritive value as alfalfa. Because cutting clover at an earlier stage of maturity reduces yield, most is cut well beyond the bloom stage. This results in a coarse, thick-stemmed forage that becomes moldy, dark, and dusty when baled.

Red clover can also be infected by *Rhizoctonia legumini-cola*, a fungus that produces an alkaloid called slaframine, resulting in the condition known as "slobbers." Excessive salivation is the most consistent clinical sign, though abortion in a mare has also been reported.[5] Once the affected forage is removed, salivation ceases. White and ladino clovers, known for their high proportion of leaves, are used primarily as pasture forages. Neither is particularly winter-hardy or shade-tolerant.

Birdsfoot Trefoil. This legume is still grown in parts of the temperate zone, but has lost favor with many producers because it is difficult to establish, is weak-stemmed, and is slow to recover from grazing. The forage was named for the crow's foot-like seed pod that develops in the fall. Like the other legumes, it can be high in feeding value when harvested properly.

Alsike Clover and Sweet Clover. Alsike and sweet clover are not commonly fed to horses and for good reason. Mild to severe photosensitization reactions and hepatitis have been reported in horses consuming alsike clover.[6] The stemmy consistency of sweet clover makes it difficult to cure for hay, increasing its susceptibility to mold. Common molds such as *Penicillium* species can convert coumarin, a nontoxic substance in sweet clover, to dicumarol. Dicumarol interferes with the activation of vitamin K, making it a potent anticoagulant. These two forages should be avoided if at all possible.

Pasture

When well cared for, pasture is the most inexpensive and nutritious form of forage that can be fed. A combination of grasses and legumes are typically used, taking advantage of the drought-resistant, high-calcium content of the legumes and the traffic resistance and early growth characteristics of grasses. The "perfect" or "ideal" pasture is obtained by cultivating those species that have adapted to that area and are compatible with the soil and drainage conditions that are present. The best sources for this information are extension agencies or agronomy departments at universities.

Well-managed pastures can provide ample forage stocked at a rate of one horse per acre. Where space is limited or management is difficult, nearly 8 to 10 acres per horse may be needed. To maintain good, safe pastures, agronomists suggest (1) routine soil testing; (2) clipping to reduce weeds and stimulate new growth; (3) removal of toxic weeds; (4) rotation, if possible; (5) maintaining optimal stocking rates; (6) the proper mixture of grass and legume species; and (7) the spreading or removal of manure to prevent burning and increase the usable acreage.

Hay

Any hay can be the best hay for horses as long as it is cut at the proper stage of maturity. As forage matures, its nutrient content, especially the protein content and protein digestibility, decreases. The more youthful the plant, the higher the leaf content and the higher the nutritive value since 80% of the nutrients are found in the leaves. Quality hay will be free of mold, dust, and weeds, have few if any seed heads, be soft to the touch, and have a pleasant aroma. Probably the best determinant of quality is intake; horses will devour high-quality hays with relish.

Hay can be chopped, pelleted, cubed, or fed long-stem from the square or round bale. Alfalfa cubes are usually of very good quality due to the amount of leaf that is needed for cubing. There is generally less waste and storage space required. One disadvantage is the boredom that may occur since it takes less time to eat the cubes than the equivalent weight in long-stem hay. Choking is a frequently cited concern but would seem to be reserved for the greedy eater. Before purchasing cubes, ask for the name and address of the manufacturer, and inspect a sample for the presence of foreign materials such as twine, newspaper, or insects. Alfalfa pellets are also available but have their greatest use in mashes. The pellets tend to be more dusty and crumble more easily, increasing wastage. Because of their small size, they are consumed much more quickly. This may result in an increase in delinquent activities such as wood-chewing, cribbing, or consumption of bedding to appease the desire to chew if alfalfa pellets are the sole source of forage. Chopped hay has been shown to decrease the rate of consumption when mixed with grain[1] and has been used successfully in group-feeding situations to prevent overeating.

Grass Clippings

Fresh lawn or pasture trimmings can be fed to horses, but there are several provisos. Anyone who has prepared compost is familiar with the heat that is produced in the center of the pile as a result of the favorable microbial environment; that is, dark, moist, high in carbohydrate, and ultimately anaerobic.

Pockets of mold can develop within the mass that may have unfavorable consequences for the horse. This can be prevented by spreading out what the horse will consume in 30 to 60 minutes and discarding any remaining. Moreover, grass from well-tended yards may contain high concentra-

tions of nitrates from frequent fertilizer applications and should be fed judiciously.

Grains

Grains are fed to provide a more concentrated source of energy. Compared to some forages, such as grass hays, grains can provide 50% to 100% more digestible energy per pound and in a smaller volume. The feed grains vary in size, weight per unit volume, and nutrient content. For this reason, grains should be fed by weight and not volume (e.g., coffee can, scoop). Processes such as rolling, crimping, cracking, steam flaking, and popping can improve digestibility, particularly for foals and horses that have difficulty chewing or have poor teeth. The nutrient value of grains or grain mixtures can usually be obtained from the feed tag, or feed tables, or by requesting a nutrient analysis from the manufacturer or feed dealer. If a guaranteed analysis is not available, the veterinarian should encourage the client to have the feed analyzed.

Oats. Oats have long been the favorite and preferred grain of horsepeople. Oats contain approximately 10% fiber, the highest of the feed grains. Oats are therefore more "bulky" than the other grains, helping to reduce the risk of overconsumption. Protein content varies, from as low as 8% for "light" oats to as high as 12% for the heavy Swedish oats. When purchasing oats, they should be large, plump, and clean. The heavier the oat weight per bushel, the higher the energy content. Top-quality oats today can weigh as much as 42 lb/bushel, compared to the standard bushel weight of 32 lb. "Clipped" oats have had the ends of the hulls removed. Crimping or rolling is recommended only for foals and horses that cannot chew their food well.

The claim that oats make a horse "high" or excitable ("feeling their oats") is an old one and is unfounded. There are no known substances in oats to produce this effect other than extra calories making the horse feel more energetic.

Corn. The use of corn is increasing as the cost of oats becomes more prohibitive. Corn is energy-dense, containing approximately 1.5 Mcal/lb. Its reputation as a "hot" feed is unsubstantiated, other than through wives' tales, producing no more heat from digestion than any other grain and far less than hay. It is the heaviest grain per unit volume and therefore has the highest risk of being overfed if not managed properly. It is low in protein (8%–9%) and low in fiber (2%–3%) compared with the other feed grains, but is the only grain used commonly in horse feeds that contains vitamin A. Corn is also graded by weight, the top grade weighing a minimum of 56 lb/bushel. It is most often fed whole or cracked, but steam-rolled, steam-flaked, and steam-popped corns are gaining in popularity for use in textured ("sweet") feeds. Ground corn is not recommended because it is dusty. Corn may also be fed from the cob, but horses should be watched carefully as cobs have become lodged in the mouth and throat.

Of the grains, corn seems to have a greater potential for supporting mold growth. More recent concerns have involved outbreaks of aflatoxicosis and leukoencephalomalacia in horses, caused by toxins produced by *Aspergillus flavus* and *Fusarium moniliforme*, respectively.[7] In response, feed companies voluntarily began screening corn shipments for the presence of aflatoxins, reducing the threat of commercial feed contamination. It is not reasonable to stop the use of corn in feeds based on these isolated incidents. As with all grains, feed with an off odor or that is moldy in appearance should never be fed.

Barley. Barley is used more on the West Coast and in the far North. This grain is an excellent choice for horses. Its protein and digestible energy content falls between corn and oats. Because of the small size and tenacious seed coat, barley should be crimped or rolled to improve digestibility.

Sorghum or Milo. This southern-grown feed grain is not used widely as an energy source for horses. Like corn, it is high in energy, low in fiber and therefore the same cautions regarding overfeeding apply. It, too, should be rolled, crimped, or steam-flaked for improved digestibility.

Rye. Rye has been fed to horses, but is not commonly used today. It is similar in nutrient content to barley. The low palatability, concern of ergot poisoning, and the bounty of other more suitable grains have reduced its use in feeds.

Wheat. This grain is occasionally available for use as feed, though it is expensive. It is similar in nutrient content to barley. Because of its small size, processing by steam-crimping or rolling is highly recommended. Wheat has a reputation of forming doughy masses in the stomach and is generally limited to one third of the grain mix.

Protein Supplements

The level of protein required in the diet of horses is somewhat influenced by physiologic status (e.g., growth, maintenance, gestation), protein source, and feed intake. The plant protein sources are used most often in horse feeds. These include soybean, cottonseed, linseed, peanut, and sunflower meals. Soybean meal is by far the leading protein supplement in use. It contains 44% protein and is the highest in lysine (2.8%–3.0%), an essential amino acid. Soybeans must be toasted to inactivate trypsin inhibitors, but not overheated so as to reduce amino acid availability. Interestingly, soybean meal has been found to contain goitrogens, anticoagulant factors, and phytoestrogens. These do not appear to result in problems in horses.

Other seed meals are used to a much lesser degree and tend to be regional. Most of the cottonseed and peanut meal are used in the South. Though cottonseed can be a good protein source when supplemented with lysine,[8] the presence of gossypol, an antioxidant and cardiotoxin,[9] reduces its acceptability by horsepeople. Peanut meal is also limited in lysine, somewhat expensive, and risky to feed because it can be a source of aflatoxins.[10] Sunflower meal is low in lysine but higher in methionine.

Linseed meal is more commonly known for its ability to impart a sheen to the hair coat than as a protein supplement. Immature seed can contain the cyanogenic glycoside linamarin and its enzyme linase, both of which are destroyed by

heat-processing.[11] It is also low in lysine. Low production and expense have reduced its use in animal feeds.

Urea has also been used as a nonprotein nitrogen source for adult horses, but has no advantage over more common sources.[12, 13] Horses are not as efficient in the utilization of urea as are cattle and are much more tolerant to excessive levels.[14] Urea toxicity is less likely in horses because urea is absorbed by the gastrointestinal tract and excreted in the urine before reaching the hindgut, where the microbial population hydrolyzes urea to ammonia and carbon dioxide via urease. Urea toxicosis has been produced in ponies experimentally by oral dosing of 5 g urea per kilogram of body weight.[14] The clinical signs of urea toxicity are confined to the central nervous system, with muscle tremor, incoordination, and weakness. Death is the result of ammonia intoxication.

Byproduct Feeds

There are a variety of feedstuffs that are "waste" products of the feed and food industry. Some can add extra fiber and others can be used as energy sources. They include byproducts such as cottonseed hulls, peanut hulls, soybean hulls, wheat bran, wheat middlings, dried brewer's and distiller's grains, citrus pulp, and dried whey, to name but a few. Other byproducts may be available on a regional basis. One that is becoming increasingly popular is beet pulp. A byproduct of the sugar industry, beet pulp is added to textured feeds as a fiber source. The primary markets for these feeds have been racing horses and horses with hay allergies or respiratory diseases, most notably heaves. It is high in digestible energy and provides some dietary calcium. Though feeds containing

Table 5–1. Commonly Used Vitamin Sources in Horse Feeds

Vitamin	Source
Vitamin A	Vitamin A acetate
	Vitamin A palmitate
	Vitamin A propionate
	Beta carotene (precursor)
Vitamin D	Activated animal sterol (D_3)
	Cholecalciferol
	Ergocalciferol (D_2)
Vitamin E	α-Tocopherol acetate
	α-Tocopheryl acetate
Vitamin K	Menadione sodium bisulfite
Thiamine (B_1)	Thiamine hydrochloride
	Thiamine mononitrate
Riboflavin (B_2)	Riboflavin
Pyridoxine (B_6)	Pyridoxine hydrochloride
Niacin	Nicotinic acid
	Nicotinamide
Pantothenic acid	Calcium pantothenate
Biotin	*d*-Biotin
Folacin (folic acid)	Folacin
Cyanocobalamin (B_{12})	Cyanocobalamin
Choline	Choline chloride
Vitamin C	Ascorbic acid

beet pulp are bulky, horses do develop vices and bad habits from "grazing boredom" if some long-stem hay is also not made available.

Vitamin and Mineral Supplements

The National Research Council (NRC) recommendations for vitamins in horses are restricted to vitamins A, D, E, thiamine, and riboflavin. Table 5–1 lists the sources commonly used to supplement vitamins in most feeds. As ingredients, they vary in price, regional availability, solubility, potency, and stability.

For minerals, the sulfate forms are generally higher in availability than the carbonates or oxides. Newest additions to the trace mineral supplements are the chelated minerals. These are trace elements bound to amino acids, peptides, or polysaccharides, with the goal of decreasing the opportunity for mineral antagonisms and increasing absorption. Whether they are in fact superior to inorganic forms in either avail-

ability or efficacy remains to be determined in the horse. They are more expensive than the inorganic forms but may prove advantageous in improving the palatability of feeds containing high concentration of minerals. A list of mineral sources is provided in Table 5–2.

NUTRITION OF THE MATURE HORSE

The nutrient requirements of the mature horse can be met under most circumstances by feeding a good-quality hay, water, and a salt block supplemented with trace minerals. The rule of thumb of providing 2% of body weight per day in dry feed is still a good rule to follow. Contrary to the practices of most owners, grain is needed only when energy needs cannot be met by hay alone. This may be necessary when the exercise plane increases or there is a decrease in forage quality. Overnutrition from feeding excess grain and empirical supplementation of vitamins and minerals are of more concern today than are dietary deficiencies. A summary

Table 5–2. Commonly Used Mineral Sources in Horse Feeds

Mineral	Source	Mineral Content
Calcium, phosphorus	Limestone	38% Ca
	Dicalcium phosphate (dynafos)	20% Ca, 18% P
	Mono- and dicalcium phosphate (biofos)	18% Ca, 21% P
	Tricalcium phosphate	38% Ca, 18% P
	Monosodium phosphate (monofos)	22% P, 17% Na
	Sodium tripolyphosphate	25% P, 31% Na
Magnesium	Magnesium sulfate	20% Mg
	Magnesium oxide	28% Mg
Potassium	Potassium chloride	52% K
	Potassium sulfate	45% K
Sodium	Sodium chloride	39% Na, 61% Cl
Copper	Copper sulfate	25% Cu
	Copper oxide	80% Cu
	Copper carbonate	57% Cu
	Copper proteinate	10%–13% Cu
Manganese	Manganese sulfate	23% Mn
	Manganous oxide	77% Mn
	Manganous sulfate	32% Mn
	Manganese proteinate	15% Mn
Cobalt	Cobalt carbonate	49% Co
	Cobalt sulfate	38% Co
	Cobalt proteinate	9%–11% Co
Iron	Ferric carbonate	48% Fe
	Ferric chloride	21% Fe
	Ferric ammonium citrate	17% Fe
	Ferrous fumarate	33% Fe
	Ferric oxide	70% Fe
	Ferrous sulfate	20%–30% Fe
	Iron dextran	2%–5% Fe
Zinc	Zinc sulfate	22%–36% Zn
	Zinc oxide	80% Zn
	Zinc proteinate	15%–22% Zn
	Zinc methionine	Not available
Iodine	Ethylenediaminedihydroiodide	77% I
	Potassium iodide	76% I
	Calcium iodide	65% I
Selenium	Sodium selenite	45% Se

of the nutrient requirements for the mature horse is listed in Table 5–3.

Energy

The energy needs of the mature horse can vary. The digestible energy (DE) requirement for "field" maintenance allows for what is necessary to maintain body weight (BW) and daily, nonworking activity (searching for food, socialization). For horses under 600 kg, the DE can be calculated from the equation[15]:

$$0.03 \ (BW_{kg}) + 1.4 = \text{Mcal of DE per day}$$

For horses over 600 kg,

$$0.0383(BW_{kg}) - 0.000015(BW_{kg})^2 + 1.82 = \text{Mcal DE per day}$$

allows for the decrease in voluntary activity observed in the larger breeds.[2] Both of these estimates apply to horses maintained out-of-doors in pastures, paddocks, or dry lots. For stall-bound horses, the amount of energy expended for activity and thermoregulation has been reduced. The resting energy expenditure (REE) of horses in metabolism stalls calculated from

$$0.021 \ (BW_{kg}) + 0.975 = \text{Mcal DE per day}$$

is probably closer to the energy needs of most pleasure and halter horses.[15]

It is important for owners to periodically obtain the body weight and assess the condition of their horses to prevent undesirable weight gain. Cloth weight tapes provide a quick and reasonably accurate estimate. The body weight can also be calculated using the equations based on chest girth[16] (Table 5–4). For accuracy, this measurement should be taken at the base of the withers and pulled snugly without embedding the tape into the skin. Body condition scores should also be evaluated. Table 5–5 provides descriptions of body conditions rated on a scale of 1 to 9.[17] Horses, regardless of age, are best kept at a score of 4 to 5, where ribs can be barely seen but easily felt.

The requirements for work expenditure have been calculated using the weight of the horse, rider, and tack and the workload.[18, 19] For practical purposes, increases over

Table 5–3. Daily Nutrient Requirements of the Mature Horse*

Nutrient	Stall Rest	Maintenance	13 lb Alfalfa† 2 oz TM Salt‡	16 lb Grass† 1 lb PVM§
Digestible energy, Mcal	11	15	14	14
Crude protein, g	416	596	944	654
Calcium, g	18	18	65	30
Phosphorus, g	13	13	15	24
Potassium, g	23	23	145	121
Sodium, g	6	6	28	13
Magnesium, g	7	7	15	18
Copper, mg	60	60	65	126
Iron, mg	300	300	1,870	1,254
Manganese, mg	300	300	400	380
Zinc, mg	300	300	347	340
Cobalt, mg	1.5	1.5	5	3
Iodine, mg	1.5	1.5	2	2
Selenium, mg	1.5	1.5	7	2
Vitamin A, IU	20,500	20,500	130,000	137,070
Vitamin D, IU	1,770	1,700	10,620	12,706
Vitamin E, IU	295	295	60	210
Vitamin K, IU	NA	NA	NA	NA
Thiamine, mg	18	18	22	17
Riboflavin, mg	12	12	74	67
Niacin, mg	NA	NA	224	209
Folic acid, mg	NA	NA	22	15
Pyridoxine, mg	NA	NA	24	4
Pantothenic acid, mg	NA	NA	155	59
Biotin, mg	NA	NA	2	1
Cyanocobalamin, μg	NA	NA	NA	25

*Calculated for a 450-kg horse.
†Sun-cured in midbloom.
‡Trace mineral salt containing selenium 120 ppm.
§Average analysis for protein-vitamin mineral (PVM) pellet such as MannaPro Spur, Tizwhiz 30 Plus, Wayne Propel, Buckeye Gro'N Win.

Table 5–4. Equations for Calculating Body Weight From Chest Girth (CG) Measurements*†

Chest girth >66 in.:
Males	$0.14475\ (CG_{in.})$ = Body weight, lb
Females	$0.14341\ (CG_{in.})$ = Body weight, lb

Chest girth <66 in. (including foals):
Colts	$0.1387\ (CG_{in.})\ +\ 0.400$ = Body weight, lb
Fillies	$0.1382\ (CG_{in.})\ +\ 0.344$ = Body weight, lb

*Adapted from Willoughby DP: *Growth and Nutrition in the Horse.* Cranbury, NJ, AS Barnes, 1975.
†Use the adult formulas for mature ponies.

maintenance of 25% for pleasure and equitation; 50% for roping, cutting, and jumping; and 100% for distance training and polo should be a reasonable guide. Adjustments in feed intake should be based on body condition.

Protein

The protein requirement of the mature horse is roughly 1.3 g of crude protein per kilogram of body weight or 40 g/Mcal of DE.[2] However, because protein is not used as an important fuel source in horses, a level of 12% of dry matter is adequate for most horses. Quality of protein is less important for mature horses than it is for the growing horse, but it should not be overlooked. Despite a widespread belief, excess protein will not cause kidney damage in healthy horses. Feeding more protein than is necessary is expensive for the owner and only harmful to the pocketbook.

Minerals

For the mature horse, the major mineral needs are met with the consumption of good-quality feed to meet energy and protein needs. Trace mineral salt blocks are strongly recommended to provide the sodium, zinc, and iodine not found in most feeds. In areas where selenium is deficient, a salt block with added selenium is required. Unlike salt used for human consumption, most white salt blocks do not contain iodine and should be replaced with trace mineral blocks containing iodine. The label found on the block or brick will provide the mineral content.

Vitamins

A horse consuming good-quality hay or pasture receives all the necessary vitamins directly from the feed, body stores (fat-soluble vitamins), or by microbial synthesis in the hindgut. Naturally occurring B vitamin deficiencies have been reported only in cases where dietary or chemical antagonists were present.[20, 21] When poor-quality hay is fed, the addition of a commercial feed to supplement energy intake will provide the needed vitamins.

General Guidelines

Providing 1.5% to 2.0% of the body weight in feed per day will meet the needs of most horses. For grass hays, a 1,000-

Table 5–5. Body Condition Scores*

Score	Description
1 Poor	Animal extremely emaciated; spinous processes, ribs, tailhead, tuber coxae and ischii projecting prominently; bone structure of withers, shoulders, and neck easily noticeable; no fatty tissue can be felt
2 Very thin	Animal emaciated; slight fat covering over base of spinous processes; transverse processes of lumbar vertebrae feel rounded; spinous processes, ribs, tailhead, tuber coxae, and ischii prominent; withers, shoulders, and neck structure faintly discernible
3 Thin	Fat buildup about halfway on spinous processes; transverse processes cannot be felt; slight fat cover over ribs; spinous processes and ribs easily discernible; tailhead prominent, but individual vertebrae cannot be identified visually; tuber coxae appear rounded but easily discernible; tuber ischii not distinguishable; withers, shoulders, and neck accentuated
4 Moderately thin (ideal)	Slight ridge along back; faint outline of ribs discernible; tailhead prominence depends on conformation; fat can be felt around it; tuber coxae not discernible; withers, shoulders, and neck not obviously thin
5 Moderate	Back is flat (no crease or ridge); ribs not visually distinguishable but easily felt fat around tailhead beginning to feel spongy; withers appear rounded over spinous processes; shoulders and neck blend smoothly into body
6 Moderately fleshy	May have slight crease down back; fat over ribs spongy; fat around tailhead soft; fat beginning to be deposited along the side of withers, behind shoulders, and along the sides of neck
7 Fleshy	May have crease down back; individual ribs can be felt, but noticeable filling between ribs with fat; fat around tailhead soft; fat deposited along withers, behind shoulders, and along neck
8 Fat	Crease down back; difficult to feel ribs; fat around tailhead very soft; area along withers filled with fat; area behind shoulder filled with fat, noticeable thickening of neck fat deposited along inner thighs
9 Extremely fat	Obvious crease down back; patch fat appearing over ribs; bulging fat around tailhead, along withers, behind shoulders, and along neck; fat along inner thighs may rub together; flank filled with fat

*Data from National Research Council: *Nutrient Requirements of Horses.* Washington, DC, National Academy Press, 1989.

lb horse kept on dry lot or minimal pasture will need approximately 18 lb/day. If alfalfa hay is fed, only 14 lb is needed to provide the same amount of energy for "field" maintenance because of the higher energy content. If grain is fed, the ratio by weight of hay:grain should not exceed 50:50. Plenty of clean, fresh, cool water should be available at all times. Water intake appears to be directly related to dry matter intake.[22] Most horses consume a minimum of 1 L/Mcal of DE or 2 to 3 L/kg of dry feed.

NUTRITION OF THE STALLION AND BROODMARE

The Stallion

Nutritional management of the stallion differs little from that described for the mature horse. During breeding season, an increase in energy intake is generally needed to compensate for the increase in activity and stress. Adjustments in feed intake should be gradual. Feed should be increased to provide enough energy to maintain the stallion at the desired weight and condition. An average increase of 25% above maintenance may be needed. The usual energy requirement for stallions in the nonbreeding season is about 15 kcal/lb body weight and about 19 kcal/lb body weight during the breeding season.

Obesity is not an uncommon problem in stallions, particularly in the off season. This occurs when the quantity of feed fed is not reduced when activity level decreases, resulting in overfeeding. The consensus of stallion managers is that stallions kept in good body condition either through dietary control, exercise, or both are more sound, more responsive, and fertile, and remain healthier than stallions that are permitted to become obese. To help maintain optimal body weight during the breeding season, stallions should be turned out or exercised in hand for a few hours each day.

Contrary to popular belief, there is no evidence that extra minerals or vitamins are required for breeding stallions above those for maintenance. Stallions with access to well-managed pasture or that are receiving good-quality hay and trace mineral salt will derive little benefit from additional supplementation. The testicular degeneration reported in rats fed vitamin E–deficient diets has not been observed in horses and there is no evidence that vitamin E, A, or C supplementation will improve libido or prevent sterility in the stallion.[23, 24] However, there is no evidence that supplementation of these vitamins is harmful.

The Open Mare

Mares with a condition score of 5 or 6 should be fed according to the guidelines for the mature horse. Mares that have recently retired from athletic competition or may be in poor condition should be placed in a weight-gaining plane before breeding to increase the likelihood of conception and improve reproductive efficiency. Recent research indicated that "flushing," or increasing the energy intake approximately 10% to 15% above maintenance, increased the chance of conceiving and reduced the number of covers for mares with a body condition of 4 or lower.[17] There is no advantage to overfeeding the fat mare. Obesity has been cited as a contributing cause to angular limb deformities in

foals and reduced conception rates.[25, 26] As in stallions, there is no evidence to indicate that supplementation of other nutrients above requirements enhances reproductive performance.

The Pregnant Mare

The nonlactating mare in early and midgestation should be fed to meet maintenance requirements (Table 5–6). The early growth of the fetus is minimal and does little to increase nutrient demand. Often, mares are "fed for two" early in pregnancy, which can result in higher feed costs and, more commonly, undesirable weight gain. Recent research suggests that weight gain occurs during midgestation for use as a source of energy later in gestation,[26, 27] but there seems to be no advantage to gains greater than 12% to 15%. Additional calories and other nutrients to support lactation and athletic activity should be included in the dietary plan.

The greatest increase in fetal growth and nutrient demand occurs during the last 3 to 4 months of gestation[28–30] (Table 5–7), necessitating increases in most nutrients to support growth and development. Supplying the extra nutrients is confounded, however, by the reduction in digestive capacity as a result of the increasing size of the fetus. The solution is to increase the nutrient concentration and, in some cases, the quality of the feed.

The increases in energy intake for the last-trimester mare were based on the energy content of equine fetal growth in the last 3 months of gestation. Estimates of the DE requirements for broodmares are 1.11, 1.13, and 1.2 times the maintenance requirement for the 9th, 10th, and 11th month, respectively,[2] but may be higher for mares in poor condition.[31] For the 1,100-lb mare at field maintenance, this would be equal to an additional 1.64, 2.10, and 3.28 Mcal/day during months 9, 10, and 11, respectively. These increases can easily be met by an additional 11 lb of fresh pasture, 2 to 3 lb of hay per day, or 2 lb of grain, demonstrating that large quantities of feed are not required. In cases where grass hay is the primary forage, a proportional increase in concentrate to 20% to 30% and a decrease in roughage to 70% to 80% will usually provide the energy needed. Mares should be monitored as previously described to prevent undesired increases in condition score. Decreases in energy intake to encourage weight loss (>10%) in obese mares is not recommended owing to the potential risk of hyperlipemia.[32]

A 10% increase in protein intake has been recommended for protein accretion of the fetus.[2] In nearly all cases, the additional feed provided to meet energy needs will supply the extra protein. The effects of higher intakes of protein on fetal health have not been evaluated but the fact that many mares fed alfalfa consume nearly twice their requirement for protein and produce healthy, vigorous foals suggests that there should be little concern.

Recent studies of fetal growth, body composition, and postnatal development have provided some estimates of mineral needs during the last 3 to 4 months of pregnancy.[33] Data suggest that to provide for fetal mineral deposition, the calcium and phosphorus intake must increase by nearly 80% above maintenance; magnesium and potassium must increase by 25%.[2] Because most maintenance diets provide nearly

Table 5–6. Nutrient Requirements of the Gestating and Lactating Mare*

Nutrient	Early Gestation	Last Trimester	Lactation
Digestible energy, Mcal	15–19	17–22	26–32
Crude protein, g	600–760	750–1,000	1,300–1,700
Calcium, g	18–24	36–45	50–65
Phosphorus, g	13–18	27–35	32–45
Potassium, g	22–30	30–40	40–55
Magnesium, g	7–9	10–11	10–12
Sodium, g	6–15	7–16	8–18
Copper, mg	100–150	250–300	250–300
Iron, mg	400–500	400–500	400–500
Manganese, mg	400–500	600–700	600–700
Zinc, mg	400–500	700–800	700–800
Cobalt, mg	1–2	1–2	1–2
Iodine, mg	1–2	2–3	2–3
Selenium, mg	1–2	2–3	2–3
Thiamine, mg	27–30	30–35	35–40
Riboflavin, mg	18–20	20–22	22–24
Pyridoxine, mg†	—	—	—
Niacin, mg†	—	—	—
Pantothenic acid, mg†	—	—	—
Folic acid, mg†	—	—	—
Biotin, mg†	—	—	—
Cyanocobalamin, μg†	—	—	—

*Mares weighing 450 to 600 kg. Energy need may vary according to age, desired body condition, and milk production.
†No requirement established.

twice the NRC recommendation for calcium, phosphorus, and magnesium and nearly six times that for potassium, supplementation is rarely required. However, mares fed diets of grass hay and unfortified grain are likely to be deficient in both calcium and phosphorus. Current intake should be

Table 5–7. Length and Weight of Equine Fetuses for Gestational Age*

Age (days)	Crown-Rump Length (cm)†	Weight
60	6	17 g
90	16	160 g
120	25	700 g (1.5 lb)
150	35	1.6 kg (3.5 lb)
180	48	4.0 kg (9.0 lb)
210	60	10 kg (22 lb)
240	75	17 kg (37 lb)
270	85	20 kg (44 lb)
300	95	29 kg (64 lb)
330	100	42 kg (92 lb)
Average birth weight		42–55 kg (92–120 lb)

*Adapted from Bergin WC, Gier HT, Frey RA, et al: Developmental horizons and measurements useful for age determination of equine embryos and fetuses. In *Proceedings of the 13th Annual Meeting of the American Association of Equine Practitioners,* New Orleans, 1967, pp 179–196; and Platt H: Growth of the equine foetus. *Equine Vet J* 16:247–252, 1984.
†Straight line from tip of forehead to base of tail.

compared with the recommended levels in Table 5–6 to determine how much extra calcium or phosphorus is needed.

There has been a great deal of interest in work concerning trace mineral supplementation of the late-gestation broodmare and its role in the developmental orthopedic diseases (DODs) of foals.[34, 35] Though additional studies are needed, recent research has demonstrated that supplementation of copper to mares during the last 90 days of gestation and to their foals reduced the frequency of cartilage abnormalities in the foals when compared with mares and foals consuming NRC-recommended concentrations of copper.[35] It is also important to note that copper was not the only nutrient increased in this study. Manganese, zinc, and selenium concentrations were also increased between diets to prevent antagonisms, but nutrient ratios extrapolated from NRC recommendations were maintained. Therefore, adding copper or any mineral alone without evaluating the other minerals is not likely to be of benefit and is not recommended. Selenium and iodine are also of importance to the broodmare but caution should be exercised to avoid oversupplementation, particularly with iodine. Foals from mares fed from 35 to 48 mg of iodine per day were born with enlarged thyroid glands, characteristic of iodine toxicity.[36, 37] The levels of trace minerals listed in Table 5–6 are currently recommended by me for broodmare diets on farms where nutrition is believed to be a contributing factor to the occurrence of the DODs. In most situations, the recommendations given for early gestation may be sufficient.

Of the vitamins, A, E, and folate are of greatest concern. Studies have demonstrated that serum concentrations of these vitamins are higher in pastured horses and decrease when diets of hay and grain are fed,[38, 39] suggesting the potential for deficiencies. However, the decreases in serum concentrations were not associated with clinical evidence of vitamin deficiency, possibly owing to the mobilization of body stores. The total dietary vitamin intake should be evaluated before supplementation is recommended. The NRC recommendations should be followed.[2] Beta carotene (1 mg = 400 IU vitamin A) has been recommended as the vitamin A supplement of choice owing to its lower potential for toxicity when compared with vitamin A.[40] The authors also suggest that folate supplementation should not exceed 100 mg/day.[40]

The Lactating Mare

Energy requirements for the lactating mare depend largely on the volume of milk she is capable of producing. Production will also be influenced by the number of previous lactations, the stage of lactation, genetic potential, nutrient supply (most notably energy and water), and foal intake.

During the first 3 months of lactation, most mares can be expected to produce between 3.0% and 3.5% of body weight in fluid milk each day, pony mares slightly more at 4%.[41–43] Field experience suggests that maiden mares tend to have lower milk yields than multiparous mares. Peak lactation can be expected to occur between 6 and 10 weeks post partum[41, 44–46] but the peak of maximum production may vary and has occurred as early as 30 days.[41] As lactation continues, milk yields decline to approximately 2% of body weight.

Nutrient composition also changes during lactation (Table 5–8). Mare's milk becomes more nutrient-dilute as lactation progresses. Protein, fat, vitamin, and mineral content decreases and lactose increases.[41, 42, 47–50] The increase in lactose content is not high enough to offset the decreases in protein and energy-dense fat, resulting in a lower calorie content.

Recent analyses of mare's milk have further characterized its unique protein distribution and amino acid profile.[51, 52] Milk varies between species in its proportion of whey to casein.[53] The ratio in mare's milk is roughly 50:50 during lactation, though it is higher in whey content (85:15) during the early hours postpartum.[51] This is in contrast to bovine milk protein (whey:casein ratio of 16:82) which is primarily casein protein.[53, 54] Amino acid patterns are also quite different among species.[52] The amino acid patterns recently reported for cow, goat, sow, and mare's milk are summarized in Table 5–9. Unlike cow, goat, and sow milk, mare's milk protein is nearly two times higher in arginine, a finding suggested by a study that examined growth and plasma amino acid concentrations in foals receiving either mare's milk or a defined formula containing bovine protein.[55] The true importance of this high level of arginine remains to be determined. If the arginine is needed for optimal growth, the low level of arginine in bovine protein and, consequently, in most commercial milk replacers, may help to explain the less-than-optimal performance often observed in orphan foals compared with their nursing counterparts.[56, 57]

The nutrients in greatest demand are water and energy, followed by protein, calcium, and phosphorus. Water is the major constituent of mare's milk, being roughly 90%.[41, 42, 47] A 500-kg mare producing 15 kg of milk daily would have

Table 5–8. Nutritional Profile of Mare's Milk (Per Liter)*

Nutrient	Weeks		
	1–4	5–8	9–12
Gross energy, kcal	570	515	470
Protein, g	28.5	22	20.2
Fat, g	18.6	15.4	12.5
Lactose, g	65	67	66
Ash, g	5.3	4.8	3.0
Calcium, g	1.2	0.98	0.77
Phosphorus, g	0.6	0.5	0.4
Potassium, g	0.7	0.5	0.4
Sodium, g	0.2	0.2	0.15
Magnesium, g	0.09	0.07	0.05
Copper, mg	0.6	0.3	0.26
Iron, mg	0.9	0.7	0.5
Manganese, mg	1.1	1.2	1.1
Zinc, mg	2.6	2.5	2.2
Cobalt, mg	0.04	0.05	0.02
Iodine, mg	NA	NA	NA
Selenium, mg	0.008	0.005	NA
Vitamin A, IU†	40		
Vitamin D, IU†	<80		
Vitamin E, mg†	0.48		
Thiamine, mg†	0.32		
Riboflavin, mg†	0.61		
Pyridoxine, mg†	0.41		
Niacin, mg†	0.93		
Pantothenate, mg†	8.9		
Folic acid, μg†	82		
Biotin, μg†	8.8		
Choline, mg†	73		
Vitamin B_{12}, μg†	3.1		
Density, g/mL	1.03		

*Data from references 41, 42, 46–48.
†Data from Ross Products Division, Abbott Laboratories, Columbus, Ohio.

to increase her water intake nearly twofold to replenish this loss. Additional calories are also needed. Early in lactation, mare's milk contains approximately 560 kcal/kg of fluid milk.[41, 42, 47] Assuming that mares convert 60% of feed DE into milk gross energy,[2] an extra 792 kcal of DE must be consumed for every kilogram of milk produced, or an extra 11.9 Mcal in the case of the 500-kg mare, an increase of 72% above maintenance. Protein needs have been estimated to more than double from those of maintenance from 1.3 to 2.8 g of crude protein per kilogram of body weight.[2]

Calcium and phosphorus losses during lactation can be significant, making supplementation of these minerals essential. Mare's milk in early lactation contains 120 mg of calcium and 60 mg of phosphorus per kilogram of fluid milk, decreasing to 80 and 40 mg, respectively, in later weeks. Because only 40% to 50% of the calcium and phosphorus is available from dietary sources, supplementation of 240 mg of calcium and 150 mg of phosphorus per kilogram of milk seems likely. To date, there are no comprehensive studies on the effects of dietary calcium and phosphorus intake on milk mineral content or composition.

Table 5–9. Reported Amino Acid Composition of Selected Mammalian Milks*†

Amino Acid	Horse	Cow	Goat	Pig
Alanine	37 ± 2	32 ± 1	34 ± 5	36 ± 2
Arginine	60 ± 2	34 ± 1	29 ± 1	44 ± 1
Aspartic acid	95 ± 5	70 ± 5	75 ± 1	78 ± 5
Cystine	11 ± 2	9 ± 1	9 ± 1	16 ± 1
Glutamic acid	217 ± 8	208 ± 2	209 ± 15	208 ± 5
Glycine	16 ± 1	18 ± 1	18 ± 2	32 ± 1
Histidine	22 ± 2	24 ± 1	26 ± 1	24 ± 1
Isoleucine	39 ± 1	47 ± 1	48 ± 1	40 ± 2
Leucine	93 ± 3	99 ± 1	96 ± 3	89 ± 4
Lysine	73 ± 5	86 ± 2	80 ± 10	79 ± 3
Methionine	22 ± 1	26 ± 1	25 ± 2	22 ± 1
Phenylalanine	43 ± 2	50 ± 1	47 ± 1	43 ± 3
Proline	91 ± 8	100 ± 4	106 ± 8	117 ± 3
Serine	52 ± 8	56 ± 1	49 ± 5	51 ± 3
Threonine	39 ± 2	42 ± 1	49 ± 1	37 ± 1
Tyrosine	45 ± 4	47 ± 1	38 ± 1	39 ± 1
Valine	47 ± 2	52 ± 2	61 ± 1	46 ± 1

*Milligrams per gram of total amino acids.

†Adapted from Davis TA, Nguyen HV, Garcia-Bravo R, et al: Amino acid composition of human milk is not unique. *J Nutr* 124:1126–1132, 1994.

The trace mineral and vitamin content of mare's milk is available from a limited number of studies.[48–50, 58] Because no overt signs of vitamin deficiencies have been observed in nursing foals, it is assumed that sufficient quantities are available. All of the trace minerals are very low in milk (see Table 5–8). Increased efficiency of absorption and reliance on prenatal reserves are likely important in preventing the development of deficiencies until solid food intake begins.[48]

The point at which mare's milk and hepatic stores can no longer provide for the needs of the foal is not known. Growth rate of the foal and the pre- and postpartum nutrition of the mare are two likely determining factors. The fact that selenium-responsive, nutritional muscular dystrophy is most often seen in nursing foals[59] and the more recent evidence demonstrating a reduction in cartilage defects following trace element supplementation at 3 months of age[35] suggest that supplementation may be needed earlier for some minerals.

Generally, body condition score is the best gauge for determining the energy needs of the lactating mare. The habit of "feeding the stall" rather than the horse often results in underfeeding the good producers and overfeeding the poor producers. Mares that lose weight during lactation should be provided with either more energy, a higher quality of feed, or both, if clinical examination reveals no underlying cause. Mares that continue to gain weight during lactation are storing the energy as fat rather than channeling it toward milk production.

NUTRITION OF THE GROWING HORSE
Foals

The precocious nature of foals requires that they receive nutrients within hours of birth to survive. Body composition studies have shown that foals have little in energy reserves compared to the adult horse.[29, 33] A readily available food source is therefore needed to fuel organ systems, red blood cells, and to support thermoregulation and growth. These energy needs are met by frequent nursing,[60] an inherent ability for a high rate of water turnover,[42] and physiologic lengthening of the small intestine to increase available surface area for greater absorption.[61] This becomes of greater importance for the foals born of mares that are malnourished or that may have chronic placental insufficiency or uterine sepsis, all of which may result in small foals with low nutrient reserves.[62] Because of the increase in nutrient demand following injury or disease, supplying ample, balanced, and complete nutrition is critical for health, development, growth, and recovery.

Data collected from several studies have provided reasonable estimates for evaluating growth and growth rates of foals.[63–67] The greatest increase is in body weight. At birth, foals are approximately 11% of their adult body weight; normal birth weights for most light breeds are between 90 and 110 lbs. The period of most rapid growth is the first 30 days when birth weight generally doubles. Average daily gain for the first week is 1.6 kg/day, which decreases steadily with increasing age, to 1.2 kg/day by the fourth week. The reported body weights, rates of weight gain, and relationship to adult weight for growing foals are presented in Tables 5–10 and 5–11.

Foals are roughly 60% of their adult height at birth.[1] Accurate wither heights at birth are complicated by the tendon laxity frequently encountered in neonates, but most foals are between 38 and 42 in. in height. As with weight, growth rate in height is greatest the first week and then steadily declines. Wither heights, rates of height gain, and comparisons to adult measurements are shown in Tables 5–10 and 5–11.

Data collected from lactation and growth studies have provided some estimate of the energy, protein, calcium, and phosphorus needed to support early growth in healthy foals. Nursing foals consume approximately 150 kcal gross energy (GE)/kg of body weight during the first week.[42, 43, 46] This is equal to 13 to 14 qt of mare's milk per day for light horse foals or 15 to 17 qt/day for large warm blood or draft foals. Similarly, protein needs are high: 6 to 7 g/kg of body weight. As the foal ages, the growth rate slows and the energy and protein needed as a function of body weight decreases accordingly (Table 5–12). However, because the larger foal

Table 5–10. Reported Growth Rates for Healthy Foals*

Age	Weight (kg/day)	Height (cm/day)
First week	1.6	0.4
Second week	1.5	0.35
Birth–4 wk	1.4	0.32–0.33
4–8 wk	1.3	0.25–0.26
8–12 wk	1.1	0.20–0.25

*Data from references 63–65; D. A. Knight, Columbus, Ohio.

Table 5–11. Estimated Body Weight and Wither Height Ranges for Growing Horses of Light Breeds*

Age	Weight (kg)	Percent of Mature Weight†	Height (cm)	Percent of Mature Height†
Birth	50 ± 9	10	96 ± 5	60
14 days	73 ± 14	14	104 ± 5	65
1 mo	91 ± 14	18	109 ± 5	68
2 mo	136 ± 14	27	114 ± 5	71
3 mo	163 ± 14	33	119 ± 5	75
4 mo	191 ± 14	38	123 ± 5	76
5 mo	214 ± 14	43	127 ± 5	79
6 mo	240 ± 14	48	129 ± 5	81
9 mo	295 ± 23	59	142 ± 5	89
12 mo	340 ± 23	68	147 ± 5	92
18 mo	409 ± 23	82	152 ± 5	95

*Data from references 16, 56–60, 63–67; H. F. Hintz, Ithaca, NY; D. A. Knight, Columbus, Ohio.
†Age at maturity = 5 years (60 months).

has more total mass to support, the volume of milk needed to meet the requirements increases.

The calcium and phosphorus concentration of mare's milk appears to be adequate in meeting the early needs of the growing foal. Because foals gradually begin to consume hay and grain during the time they are nursing, it is not known at what point these mineral needs are no longer met by milk alone. It appears that trace element and fat-soluble vitamin stores are supplied for the short term by prenatal stores.[48–50] Trace element insufficiencies have been suggested to be responsible for some of the DODs present in growing foals and weanlings,[35, 68] requiring supplementation of these nutrients prior to weaning.[35]

From birth, the equine digestive tract undergoes anatomical and physiologic adaptions that favor the utilization of carbohydrate. Lactase, maltase, and sucrase activities have been measured in the small intestine of both fetuses and foals.[69] Fetal disaccharidase activity is low, but lactase begins to rise within a few hours of birth. Lactase continues to be the predominant disaccharidase in the equine small intestine until 3 to 4 months of age when the activity of maltase equals that of lactase. Maltase activity continues to rise, becoming the primary disaccharidase of the mature small intestine. As mentioned previously, the growth of various portions of the gastrointestinal tract seems to parallel these changes in enzyme activity.[61] Significant increases in the length and diameter of the small intestine occur within the first month, increasing the available villous surface area and making it possible for the foal to process increasing volumes of milk to meet its needs. During the next 5 months, there is continued growth of the small intestine but the greatest increases occur in the lengths of the cecum and large colon at a time when foals traditionally begin mimicking adult grazing behavior and increasing their intake of hay and grain.[70] From 6 months on, most of the growth occurs in the cecum and large intestine, allowing for the increased consumption and utilization of fibrous feeds.

The actual nutrient requirements of nursing foals have not been determined. From studies of foals 4 months and older, nutrient requirements have been estimated. The nutrient recommendations for foals from 4 to 6 months of age is shown in Table 5–13.

Feeding the Orphan Foal

Orphan foals can either be grafted onto a nurse mare or raised by hand. This decision is best made by evaluating several factors with the personnel who will share in the responsibility of caring for the foal.

Table 5–12. Estimated Calories and Volume of Mare's Milk Needed to 2 Months of Age by a Foal Weighing 55 kg at Birth

Age	Kilocalories	Volume		
		Qt	mL/hr	kcal/kg
Birth to 7 days	7,500	14	550	145–150
8–14 days	9,800	18	700	135–145
15–28 days	11,000	20	800	100–135
1–2 mo	12,500	23	900	80–100

Table 5–13. Nutrient Recommendations for the Foal, Weanling, and Yearling*

Nutrient	Foal†	Weanling	Yearling
Feed intake, % body weight	2.5–3.0	2.2–2.5	2.0–2.2
Digestible energy, Mcal	13–15	15–18	18–20
Crude protein, g	650–800	750–850	850–1,000
Calcium, g	35–45	40–50	40–50
Phosphorus, g	25–35	30–40	30–40
Potassium, g	10–15	15–20	20–25
Magnesium, g	4–5	5–6	6–7
Sodium, g	4–6	6–8	8–9
Copper, mg	100–150	150–180	175–200
Iron, mg	300–350	350–450	350–450
Manganese, mg	250–300	300–350	350–400
Zinc, mg	350–450	400–475	475–500
Cobalt, mg	0.5–1.0	0.5–1.0	0.5–1.0
Iodine, mg	0.5–1.0	0.5–1.0	1.0–2.0
Selenium, mg	1.0–1.5	1.0–2.0	1.0–2.0
Vitamin A, IU	15,000–20,000	20,000–25,000	25,000–30,000
Vitamin D‡	—	—	—
Vitamin E, mg	300–400	500–650	700–800
Vitamin K‡	—	—	—
Thiamine, mg	10–15	15–20	20–25
Riboflavin, mg	7–10	12–15	15–18
Pyridoxine, mg‡	—	—	—
Niacin, mg‡	—	—	—
Pantothenic acid, mg‡	—	—	—
Folic acid, mg‡	—	—	—
Biotin, μg‡	—	—	—
Cyanocobalamin, μg‡	—	—	—

*Horses with a mature weight of 400 to 500 kg.
†Foals from 4 to 6 months of age.
‡No requirement has been established.

The nurse mare has the advantage of being the most "natural" substitute. Nurse mares usually are purebred draft or draft crosses, mild in temperament, and provide the foal with an appropriate role model. Average cost at the time of this writing was between $10 and $15/day in the United States. It has been my experience that they are best recommended for farms where labor or technical expertise is limited and turn-out is a major portion of the management. However, there are some disadvantages. Nurse mares are not readily available in many parts of the country. Not all mares are immediately compatible with the orphan, especially if the mare has had sufficient time to bond to her own foal. In some cases, several mares may be needed before a successful graft takes place. The transient nature of nurse mares increases their exposure to infectious disease and the possibility of disease transmission to the privately owned broodstock. Moreover, most leasing agreements require that the nurse mare be returned in-foal, which may be difficult for farms without access to a stallion.

If a nurse mare is selected, ask for her foaling date and whether her foal is still at her side. A mare 4 to 6 weeks into lactation may not have the quality of milk to sustain a neonate and will have bonded to her own foal, making grafting difficult. It is also not uncommon for nurse mares to arrive at farms nearly devoid of milk because of stress or lack of mammary stimulation if her foal died or was prematurely removed. Reinduction of lactation is difficult and not always successful.

Hand-rearing is accomplished by teaching the foal to drink milk substitute from a bottle or, preferably, a bucket. Teaching a foal to drink from a bucket is preferable to bottle-feeding because it is less labor-intensive for the owner and allows the foal to drink milk on demand. Bucket-feeding may also help to prevent some of the behavioral problems frequently encountered with foals that have bonded to humans. While some of these behaviors are entertaining when the foal is small, a growing foal can cause serious injury to handlers if not reprimanded early. Foals older than 7 to 10 days of age are more difficult to train to bucket-feeding, possibly because the nursing reflex has been well established. It may be best to consider a nurse mare for these foals.

Several milk substitutes for foals are available (Table 5–14). Selection should be based on quality, performance, acceptability, and nutritional profile. Cow's milk, goat's milk and calf, lamb, and kid milk replacers also have been used. These substitutes are different from mare's milk in several respects and are not always nutritionally complete or balanced for foals (see earlier discussion on feeding the lactating mare). Though goat's milk has been advocated by subjective appraisal as a suitable replacer for foals, poor weight gains and metabolic acidosis were recently reported

Table 5–14. Comparison of Milk Substitutes and Formulas (per Liter)*

Nutrient	Mare	Goat	NutriFoal†	Foal-Lac‡	Kid Replacer§
Energy (kcal)	550	690	700	650	600
Protein, g	25	33	45	36	38
Carbohydrate, g	62	47	60	93	49
Fat, g	21	40	31	27	29
Calcium, g	1.4	1.4	2.0	1.7	0.9
Phosphorus, g	0.9	0.9	1.4	1.4	1.2
Ca/P ratio	1.5:1	1.5:1	1.4:1	1.2:1	0.75:1
Iron, mg	0.8	0.5	19	17	16
Copper, mg	0.5	0.2	7.0	5.0	2.0
Manganese, mg	1.3	0.1	10	13	5.0
Zinc, mg	3.0	4.0	18	15	12
Selenium, mg	0.007	0.01	0.05	Not known	Not known
Total solids, %	11	13	14	17	14
Osmolality (mOsm/kg water)	350	280	300	Not known	Not known
CHO source	Lactose	Lactose	Lactose	Lactose Maltodextrins, corn syrup	Lactose
Casein:whey ratio	50:50	86:14	50:50	Not known	Not known
Calories from:					
Protein (%)	20	18	26	19	25
Carbohydrate (%)	47	28	31	49	32
Fat (%)	33	53	43	32	43
NPCal/N ratio	105:1	107:1	75:1	107:1	75:1
Cal/N ratio	132:1	131:1	100:1	132:1	100:1

*Abbreviations: CHO, carbohydrate; NPCal/N ratio, nonprotein calories-to-nitrogen ratio.
†KenVet, Ashland, Ohio.
‡Pet-Ag, Inc, Elgin, Ill.
§As analyzed, Land O'Lakes, Inc., Fort Dodge, Iowa.

in neonatal foals fed goat's milk to provide 135 kcal/kg/day.[71] Products containing maltodextrins, corn syrups, oligosaccharides, and glucose polymers are not recommended for foals less than 3 weeks of age owing to the low level of maltase activity present in the foal's small intestine.[69] Carbohydrates that are not digested are fermented by the microbial population of the gut and may result in excessive gas production or an osmotic diarrhea.

Bucket-training begins by isolating the foal in a deeply bedded stall for approximately 2 to 4 hours after its last meal. This acts to stimulate appetite, making the foal more willing to accept the new diet. If the foal is dehydrated, an appropriate electrolyte solution should be offered first. The milk substitute should be prepared according to package directions. A wire kitchen whisk is recommended to aid in blending and speeding the mixing process. As with any change in diet, the foal should be offered roughly half of the recommended volume for the first day or two rather than alter the concentration. A standard 2-gal plastic or rubber bucket is ample for most foals. For the first attempt, a full bucket is recommended to make the milk more accessible to the foal. Encourage the foal to nurse from a finger or nipple and gently guide the foal to the bucket. Tipping the bucket slightly makes it easier for the foal's outstretched head to contact the milk surface. Several attempts separated by rest periods are usually required before the foal nurses from the bucket on its own. Most foals learn to drink within 12 hours but some take as long as 24 hours. Once the foal has consumed milk on its own, the bucket should be hung so that the rim is slightly higher than the point of the shoulder and the foal assisted when needed. If the foal fails to nurse within 4 hours, tube feeding may be necessary since the energy reserves are minimal.

Foals generally consume 20% to 30% of their body weight in milk each day or approximately 120 to 135 mL/lb of body weight for formulas with a caloric density of 500 to 650 kcal/L. As a general rule, most foals of light-horse breeding will need 4 or 5 gal of milk substitute each day; 6 to 8 gal for draft foals. Many foals can be fed two to four times a day. For foals requiring more observation, a more rigorous schedule of six to eight times a day with smaller volumes may be initiated, with the volume increased and number of feedings decreased as the foal's condition improves. Milk replacer should be mixed only as needed and not stored. Milk that has not been consumed after 12 hours should be discarded. All feeding equipment should be kept scrupulously clean to avoid bacterial growth and contamination.

Foals should be introduced to solid feeds as soon as possible. Once the foal has mastered drinking from a bucket, several handfuls of high-quality hay and 0.5 lb of milk-based pellets should be placed nearby. Few foals show any interest in these feeds, but their inherent curiosity allows them to become familiar with the aroma and texture. Increase the quantity of milk-based pellets as indicated by appetite, up to a maximum of 2 lb/day. Once this goal has been achieved, a balanced, high-quality 16% to 18% foal feed can be added. By 2 months of age, liquid milk feeding should be discontinued. Most foals are eating 2 to 2$\frac{1}{2}$ lb of concentrate and 2 to 3 lb of hay. By 4 to 5 months, milk-based pellets are no longer needed and can be replaced with the foal feed of choice. By 6 months, foals can consume 6 to 8 lb of foal feed and 4 to 5 lb of hay. Foals should be fed to the condition where ribs are palpable but not visible. Owners frequently confuse the presence of a "potbelly" with obesity. Potbellies in young horses can be the result of intestinal parasite burden, poor-quality feed, underfeeding, overconsumption of hay, or lack of exercise.

Ample exercise is necessary to encourage growth, proper musculoskeletal development, and ease boredom. Behaviors such as suckling the umbilical stump, prepuce, penis, stifle, or ears of other foals or animals are not uncommon and generally cease with time. Placing orphans with other weaned foals of similar age or with a placid, tolerant gelding or mare provides companionship and tutoring in equine "social skills."

Weanlings

For a young horse to grow and develop properly, the diet must be fed in sufficient quantity and contain the appropriate balance of nutrients (see Table 5–13). Weanlings will generally consume between 2.0% and 2.5% of their body weight in feed per day, depending on the quality and quantity of feed available and the desired growth rate. To meet their energy needs, younger weanlings should receive diets consisting of 30% to 40% grain and 60% to 70% hay. As weanlings increase in body size and digestive capacity, the proportion of grain to hay should shift in favor of more hay if the quality of the hay is high. By 12 months of age, a diet of 50% hay, 50% grain by weight is usually adequate. With the exception of exceptionally large, active individuals and the feeding of poor-quality hay, grain feeding in excess of 8 to 10 lb/day is not necessary or recommended.

Growth rates of weanlings from 6 to 12 months of age continue to decline. Weight gain decreases from 0.8 kg/day during the 6th month to 0.55 kg/day during the 12th month. Cumulative gain in wither height drops to 0.07 cm/day. The amount of digestible energy per kilogram of body weight needed to support growth decreases to 60 to 65 kcal.[2]

Daily exercise is important for skeletal growth, development, and appetite stimulation. Weanlings that are group-fed should have ample feed space provided to prevent dominance by any one youngster. Chopped hay can be mixed in with the grain to slow the feeding rate and increase the bulk, reducing the chance of grain engorgement and the risk of gastric dilatation and rupture.[2, 72] Individual feeding provides a greater opportunity for control of nutrient intake and supplementation when needed, but is more labor-intensive.

Overfeeding is a common problem in the management of growing horses. The reasons that young horses are overfed

are, presumably, to enhance growth rate and, in the case of show horses, to give them a "smoother" appearance. Several studies comparing the growth of weanlings fed energy and protein levels as high as 150% to 200% above the 1979 NRC recommendations have been conducted,[73–76] but differences in design make them difficult to compare. The most consistent effect of overfeeding is an increase in average daily weight of 12% to 36%. Average daily gains in wither height have been reported to not differ[73, 74] or to increase by 7% to 12%.[75, 76] In summary, there does not appear to be any advantage to feeding a weanling in excess of its needs.

The DODs physitis, osteochondrosis, and contracted tendons frequently occur and are diagnosed just prior to or after weaning,[77–79] though the initiation of the defect probably occurs much earlier.[35] Diet analysis and correction of any imbalances or inadequacies is recommended as a conservative treatment to prevent further lesion development.[79]

Yearlings

Diets for yearlings should contain the same balance and fortification established in the weanling program (see Table 5–13). Growth rate continues to slow; weight gain has decreased to 0.5 kg/day, wither height to 0.04 cm/day. Yearlings have attained nearly 90% of their adult height by 12 months, 95% by 18 months. Overfeeding in preparation for sale or show may aggravate existing disease or result in conditions that may not be manifested in the short term[76] and is therefore not recommended. The presence of physitis, osteochondrosis, or cervical vertebral stenotic myelopathy is not uncommon in this age group.[78, 80, 81] With the exception of physitis, changes in the diet at this stage are not likely to improve clinical outcome but may arrest further lesion development, and is recommended.[35]

PROBLEMS RELATED TO NUTRITION
Obesity

Obesity in horses is a condition that is currently not recognized as a medical problem, is rarely treated, but is likely to have as major an impact on the health and longevity of horses as it does in other species.[82–84] It would seem logical to expect that excess condition in horses is just as likely to aggravate bone and joint injuries, reduce exercise tolerance, decrease heat tolerance, increase susceptibility to disease, and adversely affect reproductive performance.

When is a horse considered to be obese? A person is considered to be obese if his or her body weight is 20% above the standard for height and frame; at 10% the person is simply overweight. There have been no criteria established for horses as there have been for dogs and cats.[84] Body condition scores of 6 to 9 describe horses with increasing degrees of fat deposition. In one study, an increase in body weight of 30 kg in a group of mares was associated with an elevation in condition score from moderately thin to fleshy.[17] This was only a 6% increase in body weight, indicating that different criteria may be needed for the horse. Subjective appraisal by body condition scores and breed standards should be used to provide a reasonable guide until more data are available.

The primary cause of obesity in horses is overfeeding or

supplying calories in excess of use. Ponies, pleasure horses, and broodstock seem to be affected most often. Horses on lush pasture and with little exercise (i.e., broodmares) can become quite heavy; this is understandably difficult to control. There may also be endocrine (i.e., hypothyroidism), metabolic, and genetic factors involved.

With the exception of halter horses or market yearlings, feeding horses to an overweight or obese state is not intended. The problem and its treatment is a matter of dietary management rather than the dietary constituents per se. Some factors involved in obesity may be the following:

1. *Lack of knowledge concerning energy content of feeds and feed-weight-per-unit volume.* Few, if any, owners know the energy content of feedstuffs. Most can tell you that corn is higher in energy than oats but not the actual difference. This lack of knowledge is further underscored by the habit of feeding grain and hay by the convenient unit rather than weight: the scoop, coffee can, quart, and cup for grain; flake, section, and bat for hay, regardless of quality or type.

2. *Overestimation of maintenance needs.* Few owners know or have ever measured the weight of their horse. If the horse is one of the light breeds, it is assumed to weigh "1,000 lb" and fed according to the recommendations for the 1,000-lb reference horse at maintenance. As discussed earlier, there are probably two levels of maintenance for most horses. The one referred to most often in feeding directions and textbooks has been discussed in the context of this chapter as "field" maintenance. For horses that spend a good deal of the time in stalls, feeding at this level may exceed their daily energy expenditure by as much as 30%.

3. *Inability to assess body condition.* Owners will rarely admit that their horses are carrying more weight than is ideal and most are probably not sure how to know. Little emphasis is placed on the value or the "how to" of evaluating body condition in horses. As an example, "hay bellies," more the result of poor-quality hay and little exercise, are often assumed to be a sign of obesity in horses, particularly young horses.

4. *Overestimation of exercise intensity.* An hour of leisurely trail riding at a walk and slow trot burns about 1 Mcal, resulting in minimal energy expenditure. Many owners feel this constitutes "work" and increase caloric intake. The presence of sweat is often viewed as evidence that the horse has "worked hard" and may be given extra feed to make up for this perceived increase in energy expenditure.

5. *Animal-human bond.* Like dogs and cats,[84] horses are frequently rewarded for compliance or their friendship by receiving feed: carrots, apples, horse treats, handfuls of grain, extra flakes of hay. Feeding establishes a direct relationship between owner and horse. The horse soon associates the presence of the owner with feed; the owner views the interest as affection and the relationship continues.

If no medical cause for excessive weight gain can be found, treatment by dietary means should be discussed with the owner. The current weight and condition score of the horse should be obtained. To encourage weight loss, a reduction in calories below expenditure is needed. A method that I have used with success begins with the formulation of a diet that will provide 70% of the horse's maintenance energy requirements *at its ideal weight*. Grass hay is suggested as the diet base because it is lower in digestible energy per kilogram than legume hay. It also weighs approximately half as much per unit of volume as alfalfa hay so more sections or flakes can be fed. This helps to reduce the concern of owners that they are "starving" their horse. Vitamins and minerals can be supplied by a supplement and trace mineral salt.

Exercise is an integral component of a weight loss program through stimulating the loss of fat rather than lean body mass. This may not be possible if the horse is lame or has respiratory compromise. Any increase in exercise, regardless of intensity, should be done slowly and monitored frequently.

It is also helpful to give the owner some idea of how long it will take for the horse's goal weight to be reached. In most cases, it will be a matter of 3 to 5 months. By giving the owner an honest appraisal, he or she will know what to expect and be more willing to comply. Periodic evaluations should be scheduled to monitor the horse's progress. Once the goal weight has been reached, the caloric intake should be adjusted for body maintenance and planned activity level.

Diarrhea

This discussion is limited to common "nutritional" diarrheas in the horse. They are usually more of a nuisance and unaesthetic than of clinical concern. There are no studies of their pathophysiology in the literature. Most likely, the diarrheas of dietary origin are osmotic and appear to result from an increase in carbohydrate fermentation and change in the microbial population. Osmotic diarrhea usually occurs when there is an excess of nonabsorbable, water-soluble, low-molecular-weight solutes present in the bowel, drawing water into the gut. This type of diarrhea is usually self-limiting if the horse is given time to adapt to the change.

Sudden and large increases in grain intake can result in diarrhea in some horses. An increase in rate of passage presents a large quantity of partially digested and undigested carbohydrate to the colon where it undergoes rapid fermentation by the hindgut microflora. The rise in lactate and volatile fatty acid (VFA) concentration results in an increase in osmolality of the colonic fluid, causing an influx of water into the colon. If lactate production exceeds the buffering capacity of the colon, mucosal damage may occur, increasing toxin absorption.[85]

Fresh pasture is high in water and soluble carbohydrate. The loose, watery feces seen after horses are turned out to pasture are likely caused by a combination of the fermentation of the available carbohydrate, a more rapid rate of passage reducing water absorption, the high water content of the ingesta overwhelming absorptive capability, and the lack of long fiber to produce formed feces.

The soft feces that develop when some horses are fed alfalfa hay happens most often when there has been an abrupt change from a grass hay to alfalfa hay or when there has been a dramatic improvement in the quality of the alfalfa hay. In this case, the diarrhea is probably due to the increased mineral content of alfalfa causing an osmotic diarrhea.[22] Fiber content has also decreased, reducing the dry matter content of the feces.

Show horses and racehorses frequently develop diarrhea during shipping or prior to performances. While it could be partly due to changes in feed and water, this diarrhea is more likely due to stress, resulting in excessive stimulation of the parasympathetic nervous system, increasing gut motility and mucous secretion. However, the most common stress-induced diarrhea in horses is associated with *Salmonella* species (see Chapter 2).

Colic

As with obesity, the nutritional causes and nutritional methods of prevention of colic are somewhat limited. In cases where poor-quality or tainted feed is accidentally fed, colic may result, and the owner should be cautioned more about dietary management than about the diet itself. The horse evolved as a continuous grazer, consuming small meals frequently.[70] Most horses today are raised in confinement, with little or no access to pasture, and are fed high-concentrate meals according to schedules devised by the owner.[70, 85] Hay is all too often underfed at stables and water is not always clean and readily available. Without hay to keep their grazing instinct satisfied, horses may begin to eat wood or bedding or develop other vices such as weaving or cribbing to assuage boredom.[70, 86] Only recently has evidence been provided to support the contention that current feeding practices alter physiologic responses and contribute to the occurrence of digestive upsets in the horse.[85]

There are several ways to reduce the risk of some colics by dietary means. A discussion of the current practices with the owner or manager will help to identify those of most importance and narrow the focus.

1. Provide sufficient quantities of free-choice, good-quality, long-stem hay. Horses fed hay ad lib. spend more time eating than horses fed pelleted feeds or all-grain diets.[86–88]
2. Increase the frequency of feeding and reduce the meal size.[85]
3. Avoid abrupt changes in hay or grain type or quantity.[1, 85]
4. Avoid abrupt changes in times of feeding or order of feeding.[85]
5. Reduce the grain meal by half when the feeding schedule has been interrupted.
6. To slow the feeding rate, offer hay first to reduce the initial hunger urge.[1]
7. Provide plenty of clean, fresh, cool water.

The Developmental Orthopedic Diseases

The DODs are conditions of the young, growing horse that occur when there has been a disturbance in the conversion of cartilage to weight-bearing bone. Included in this group are osteochondrosis, osteochondritis dissecans (OCD) of cartilaginous origin, acquired angular limb deformities, physitis, subchondral cystic lesions, some cervical vertebral stenotic myelopathies (CSMs), flexural deformities, and cuboidal bone malformations.[89]

Age at diagnosis is typically between birth and 2 years.[77, 79, 81] These diseases appear to occur predominantly in purebred horses, with Thoroughbreds, quarter horses, Standardbreds, and Arabians as the breeds most commonly affected.[89] Anecdotal and clinical data tend to support a higher inci-

dence of OCD and CSM in colts,[77, 89] but the gender distribution for the other conditions has not been reported.

The etiologic profile of the DODs is complex. The factors most frequently implicated are (1) genetic predisposition, (2) rapid growth rate, (3) nutrition, (4) biomechanics and conformation, (5) trauma, and (6) metabolic. It is probable that there is no one cause, but rather a combination of all or some of these factors.

Genetic Predisposition

There is a growing body of evidence to indicate that a heritable factor may be involved in some of these diseases.[90–93] A study of offspring produced by two wobbler stallions out of 12 wobbler mares did not result in neurologic lesions, but a high incidence of contracted tendons (30%), physitis (40%), and OCD (50%) was observed.[90] Radiographic screening of Standardbred trotting and Swedish Warmblood horses identified progeny from particular stallions that had a significantly ($P < .001$) higher frequency of OCD in the tibiotarsal joint than offspring of other stallions.[92] These observations have been confirmed by a more recent study where the incidence of tibiotarsal osteochondrosis was as high as 30% for the progeny of two stallions.[93] The authors point out that neither of these stallions had radiographic evidence of the disease, suggesting that progeny testing may be the best method of identifying genetically unsuitable broodstock.

Growth Rate

Energy, protein, and the effects of overfeeding these nutrients on accelerating growth rate have long been implicated as the most likely cause of cartilage and bone disease in young horses,[77, 94] but only anecdotal data exist.

Increases in energy and protein intake have resulted in greater weight gains compared with controls[75, 76] but not when compared with gains inferred from available growth data for young horses.[63, 65–67, 95] Acceleration of vertical growth (wither height) by overfeeding has been less consistent.[73–76] Increased weight gains have been associated with a higher occurrence of conformational defects in yearlings fed ad lib.[76] and radiographic evidence suggestive of physitis in weanlings,[95] but do not appear to be related to contracted tendons[75] or be necessary for the development of osteochondrosis.[35, 91]

Nutrition

There are several nutrients or dietary factors that may be directly or indirectly involved. It is likely that the balance and quantity of all dietary elements are critical for nutritional intervention.

Energy and Protein

Endocrine aberrations in response to the overfeeding of energy were implicated in studies where starch intakes of 4.5 g/kg of body weight were shown to result in a transient (60 minute) increase in postprandial circulating levels of triiodothyronine (T_3) and consequent decreases in thyroxine (T_4) concentration compared with starch intakes of 2.5 to 3.5 g/kg of body weight.[96, 97] Biochemical changes in normal-appearing cartilage from foals with dexamethasone-induced bone lesions[98] were presumed to be characteristic of OCD and some similarities were found in cartilage from weanlings consuming high starch diets.[73] Because T_4 is required for cartilage maturation, this led to the hypothesis that lesions of osteochondrosis may result from a high carbohydrate–induced, hypothyroid state.[97] T_3 and T_4 have similar biological effects.[99] T_3 has been shown to stimulate chondrocyte maturation and hypertrophy and increase alkaline phosphatase activity in porcine physeal cartilage.[100] Alkaline phosphatase secretion by matrix vesicles in the hypertrophic zone is considered a preparatory step in cartilage mineralization though its precise role is unclear.[101, 102] Therefore, it would seem that increases in T_3 would accelerate cartilage maturation and endochondral ossification rather than retard it. Moreover, the concentrations of circulating T_3 and T_4 and insulin reported for the high carbohydrate group were well within the normal range for horses between the ages of 4 months and 5 years.[103] It also should be noted that the weanlings in these studies received their entire caloric intake in two meals. The endocrine response would seemingly be different with the more standard management practice of continuous access to hay or pasture interspersed with two or three grain meals.

High dietary protein has been linked with high energy in increasing growth rate,[77] and has been reported to increase renal calcium excretion, resulting in negative calcium balance.[104] Increase in dietary protein above the requirement in a later study did not increase gains in height or weight, nor were any detrimental effects on calcium absorption observed.[105]

Calcium and Phosphorus

The importance of calcium and phosphorus in proper bone formation is well known. Low dietary calcium or phosphorus can result in an excess of uncalcified bone and widening of the metaphyseal cartilage.[2] Nutritional secondary hyperparathyroidism, or "big head," and other skeletal abnormalities occur in the presence of low dietary calcium and adequate to high phosphorus.[106, 107] Because calcium is absorbed primarily in the small intestine and phosphorus in both the small and large intestine,[108] excess dietary phosphorus will interfere with calcium by competing for the absorptive site. Physitis, once referred to as rickets, has also been linked to improper calcium and phosphorus balance,[78] though there are no scientific data to prove the relationship.

Conversely, excess dietary calcium and hypercalcitonemia have recently been proposed to cause osteochondrosis in horses[109] based on data from an earlier overnutrition study in Great Dane puppies in which many nutrients (especially vitamin D) were excessive.[110] Studies have demonstrated that young ponies[108] and horses[111] respond to high calcium intake by decreasing intestinal absorption and increasing calcium excretion in the urine and feces and uptake by bone. No deleterious effects attributed to calcium have been noted at two[35, 75] to five[112] times the requirement when adequate phosphorus (ratio of at least 2:1) was present.

It is unlikely that high calcium per se is responsible for DOD, but its effect on other nutrients should be considered. Alfalfa is becoming the predominant forage fed to horses.[1] The calcium content of alfalfa can be between 2 and 10 times higher than that of grass or mixed hay.[2] If alfalfa hay is fed with commercial feeds designed for grass hay, a higher-than-desirable intake of calcium could result[113] and be of concern in the presence of high dietary vitamin D. Excess dietary calcium can interfere with the absorption of zinc[114–116] and manganese,[117] two trace elements that are cofactors in cartilage metabolism.

Trace Minerals

Low dietary concentrations of copper, manganese, or zinc have been shown to result in cartilage and bone abnormalities in several species,[118–123] including the horse.[35, 68, 124] Their primary roles are as constituents of metalloenzymes involved in cartilage synthesis or calcification.[119, 121, 125]

As early as 1946, copper supplementation was shown to prevent the development of angular limb deformities and articular surface erosions in young show calves.[126] In 1949, articular cartilage defects were observed in normally growing foals fed diets containing 8 ppm copper, but not when 18 ppm was provided.[127] The relationship between copper and cartilage abnormalities in foals was further supported by reports of a copper-responsive osteodysgenesis[128, 129] and the presence of severe cartilage ulcerations in hypocupremic foals.[124] Subsequently, copper supplementation to mares in late gestation and to their foals was found to significantly reduce the number and type of cartilage lesions in the foals when compared with the number of lesions in foals that, with their dams, had been fed diets containing copper concentrations in accordance with the NRC recommendation.[35] Though it is well known that copper is a component of lysyl oxidase, the enzyme responsible for the cross-linking of hydroxylysyl residues in collagen synthesis,[130] the mechanism of copper's apparent effect is not known. It is possible that other biochemical roles for copper in cartilage synthesis and calcification remain to be identified. A 1993 study[68] that should prompt further investigation described biochemical changes in the cartilage of foals fed low copper diets.

Manganese deficiency causes enlarged joints and perosis in growing chicks.[121, 131] The primary cartilage defect in chicks appears to result from a decrease in proteoglycan synthesis due to a lack of glycosyltransferases, manganese-containing metalloenzymes.[121] Angular limb deformities, congenital fractures, and tendon contractures in foals have been associated with low manganese concentrations in pastures, but the precise biochemical or structural cause was not identified.[132, 133]

A decrease in osteoblastic activity with an increase in cartilage matrix was observed in chicks on zinc-deficient diets.[119] Consequently, the activity of alkaline phosphatase, a zinc metalloenzyme, was shown to be reduced in zinc deficiencies.[134] Alkaline phosphatase concentration and activity are high in the resting zone and in matrix vesicles of the zone of hypertrophy.[101, 135] Though initially its primary role was thought to be via the hydrolysis of pyrophosphate, an inhibitor of cartilage calcification,[136] it now appears alkaline phosphatase activity is quite diverse in cartilage matrix, cleaving a variety of phosphate-containing substances crucial to the initiation of calcification.[101, 102]

Zinc is inherently low in most feedstuffs, with an average concentration of 20 to 25 ppm.[2] This is below the NRC dietary recommendation of 40 ppm. Moreover, the presence of dietary antagonists may further inhibit absorption. Soybean meal is frequently used as the protein source in diets for young horses.[1, 2] Bean and seed meals are known to contain high levels of phytate which has been shown to interfere with zinc availability, particularly in the presence of high calcium.[114, 116] This could be of concern when a forage high in calcium, such as legumes, are fed.

Biomechanics and Conformation

Excessive compression of growth plates has been shown to result in focal areas of cartilage thickening and, when severe and prolonged, eventual thinning, premature vascular invasion, and closure of the plate.[137, 138] When the compression was removed, mineralization and calcification were restored. It is believed that the primary lesions resulted from a cessation of blood flow to the cartilage, reducing nutrient delivery. The focal, cone-shaped thickenings observed in rabbit cartilage undergoing compression have been reported in metaphyseal cartilage of foals and weanlings,[35, 139] but their pathologic significance in young horses is not known.

Young horses that are heavily muscled, carrying excess condition, and that have some degree of limb malalignment seem to be more prone to the development of the firm, metaphyseal enlargement of the distal radius, metacarpus, or metatarsus referred to as physitis.[78, 95, 140, 141] Foals that are toed-in with offset knees also seem more vulnerable.[140] Thinning of physeal cartilage with columnar disorganization and the formation of bone bridges has been associated with epiphyseal compression and the formation of exostoses in young horses with clinical evidence of physitis.[141]

Trauma

Any damage that compromises vascular penetration and nutrient delivery will affect cartilage growth and maturation. Trauma is likely to be responsible for the separation of defective tissue, as in osteochondritis dissecans, but is not believed to be the primary cause.[142] It seems unlikely that trauma accounts for a majority of the cases of DOD seen, but its presence cannot be overlooked.

Metabolic

Cartilage growth and endochondral ossification are orchestrated by the initial or subsequent release of several hormones. Growth hormone, somatomedin C, insulin, T_4, parathyroid hormone, calcitonin, vitamin D, estrogen, and testosterone can either stimulate or suppress chondrocyte proliferation, sulfate incorporation, proteoglycan synthesis, or calcification.[135, 143] In hypothyroid foals, evidence of faulty endochondral ossification, such as osteochondrosis, delayed physeal closure, and ossification of the carpal and tarsal bones, has been described.[144, 145]

NUTRITIONAL SUPPORT OF THE SICK HORSE

There continues to be growing interest in the development of nutritional support protocols for the hospitalized veterinary patient. The adverse effects of inadequate nutritional support are well documented and may be a contributing factor to poor response of traditional therapies. Early, aggressive nutritional intervention of critically ill or injured patients will help to prevent unnecessary depletion of nutrient stores, promote repair, reduce the number and severity of secondary complications, improve the response to antibiotic treatment, and increase the chances of a favorable outcome.

Metabolic Consequences of Starvation vs. Disease

Recognizing the differences in the metabolic response of the body to starvation and to disease is critical for understanding the importance of nutritional intervention. In starvation, the goal of the body is to economize, to do what is necessary to lengthen life in the face of low or no food supplies. The decrease in circulating insulin following food deprivation results in a reduction of the conversion of T_4 to T_3, lowering the metabolic rate and reducing energy expenditure. Glucagon is released in response to the hypoglycemia, triggering hepatic glycogenolysis to supply the needed glucose. This source is quickly depleted, making amino acids from body protein the predominant sources of glucose in the early phase of starvation. Fats are also mobilized as energy sources, producing fatty acids and glycerol. In the starving horse, most of the fatty acids and glycerol are reesterified to triglycerides and transported out as very-low-density lipoprotein (VLDL).[146] Analysis of the composition of VLDL produced in the fasted state show that it is higher in cholesterol and lower in protein than the VLDL in fed ponies[147] and may explain the hypercholesterolemia observed during fasting. VLDL is transported to the peripheral tissues where it is cleaved by membrane-bound lipoprotein lipase, providing free fatty acids as energy substrates. Some of the glycerol is used for glucose production, and fatty acids channeled for ketone production can be used by brain and heart as an alternative energy source, sparing glucose and, ultimately, body protein. When this occurs, stored body fat becomes the main source of fuel, though protein losses still continue at a slower rate. Other effects of starvation include (1) decreased synthesis of albumin, transferrin, and fibrinogen; (2) shrinking of the intestinal villi and decreased digestive enzyme synthesis and activity; (3) depression of immune response mechanisms, including antibody synthesis, phagocytosis, and neutrophil activation, and (4) muscle atrophy and weakness from continued degradation of muscle protein. Once fat stores have been depleted, protein becomes the primary fuel source. Continued protein degradation results in multiple organ failure, and, ultimately, death.

The body's response to stress is much different than is its response to starvation. The attempt to conserve is reversed in the presence of trauma and disease. D. P. Cuthbertson[148] has described the response to stress in two phases: the "ebb" phase and the "flow" phase. The ebb phase is characterized as the period immediately following injury when there is a

Table 5–15. Features of the Physical Examination Suggesting Poor Nutritional Status*

1. Cutaneous
   a. Thin, shiny skin
   b. Drying and scaling of skin
   c. Easily pluckable hair
   d. Decubitus ulcers
   e. Follicular hyperkeratosis
   f. Nonhealing surgical wounds
2. Mucous membranes
   a. Pallor or redness of buccal mucosa, gums
   b. Atrophy of lingual papillae
3. Musculoskeletal and neurologic
   a. Joint laxity
   b. Physitis
   c. Growth retardation
   d. Flexural deformities (<1 yr old)
   e. Weakness and atrophy
   f. Ataxia
4. Abdominal and other organs
   a. Hepatomegaly
   b. Ascites
   c. Small bowel distention, gas or fluid
   d. Lymphadenopathy, tumors
5. General appearance
   a. Edema
   b. Obesity
   c. Cachectic appearance

*Adapted from Butterworth CE Jr: Some clinical manifestations of nutritional deficiency in hospitalized patients. In *Proceedings of the Second Ross Conference on Medical Research: Nutritional Assessment—Present Status, Future Directions and Prospects.* Columbus, Ohio, Ross Laboratories, 1981, p 2.

loss, functions such as wound healing and host defense may be sacrificed to support tissues of highest priority for sustaining life.

Enteral Feeding

Candidates for Nutritional Support

Not all patients require enteral nutritional support. Most horses that were well nourished prior to the onset of acute, short-term disease will resume eating within a short period (3–4 days). It is not uncommon, however, for the disease process of some horses to worsen, prolonging the inappetence and initiating the catabolic state described earlier. The criteria of Butterworth,[150] modified for horses and listed in Tables 5–15 and 5–16, are suggested to help identify likely candidates for nutritional support.

Horses that have been anorectic for more than 3 days will generally be normo- or hypoglycemic, hypertriglyceridemic, hypercholesterolemic, and hyperbilirubinemic (Table 5–17). Though hypertriglyceridemic horses are usually hypophagic, the converse is not always true.[151] The appearance of opaque sera is suggestive of hyperlipemia, a serious condition requiring immediate medical and nutritional intervention. Azotemia may or may not be present, but may exacerbate the development of hyperlipemia.[151] Horses that have been ill for some time often have low packed cell volumes but normal mean corpuscular hemoglobin concentrations and mean corpuscular volumes, indicative of the anemia of inflammatory disease.[152]

If there is no reason to suspect that the absorptive capacity of the digestive tract has been reduced, enteral feeding should be chosen. This route is the most physiologic as well

decrease in peripheral vascular perfusion, cardiac instability, and hypometabolism. Once resuscitation has been successful and perfusion has been restored, the hypermetabolism, amino acid mobilization from skeletal muscle, and marked increases in gluconeogenesis associated with the flow phase of the stress response begin. There are several hormones that act as key effectors in the flow phase. Catecholamines are released in response to stress, causing an increase in the metabolic rate and the β-adrenergic-stimulated release of glucagon to elevate glucose production. A rise in adrenocorticotropic hormone (ACTH) also occurs, promoting a subsequent increase in glucocorticoid secretion and providing an additional stimulus for glucagon, continuing to drive amino acid mobilization from skeletal muscle and lipolysis. Tumor necrosis factor and interleukin-1, two of several cytokines produced by T cells and macrophages during the acute phase response, initiate the induction of fever by a direct effect on the hypothalamus, thereby increasing energy expenditure approximately 7% for every degree Fahrenheit rise in body temperature.[149] Hyperglycemia is frequently observed in septic patients in the face of normal or increased insulin secretion, possibly due to a combination of cortisol-driven gluconeogenesis and an increased peripheral insulin resistance.[149] Additional demands for glucose and amino acids are also incurred for tissue repair and acute phase protein synthesis. Without protein and energy intake to ameliorate some of the

Table 5–16. Features of the Clinical History Suggesting Nutritional Risk*

1. Recent weight loss of 10% or more of usual body weight
2. Restricted oral intake of nutrients or IV infusions of simple solutions only for the preceding 10 days or more
3. Protracted nutrient losses as a result of:
   a. Diarrhea, malabsorption syndromes
   b. Surgical absence of portions of the GI tract
   c. Draining fistulas, abscesses, wounds, burns
4. Increased metabolic needs due to:
   a. Extensive burns, infection, trauma
   b. Fever
   c. Lactation, recent pregnancy, recent surgery or trauma
5. Use of drugs with antinutrient or catabolic properties, such as:
   a. Corticosteroids
   b. Immunosuppressants
   c. Antitumor agents
   d. Miscellaneous (e.g., antibiotics, antacids, anticonvulsants)
6. Chronic disease or impaired function of any major organ system

*Adapted from Butterworth CE Jr: Some clinical manifestations of nutritional deficiency in hospitalized patients. In *Proceedings of the Second Ross Conference on Medical Research: Nutritional Assessment—Present Status, Future Directions and Prospects.* Columbus, Ohio, Ross Laboratories, 1981, p 2.

Table 5–17. Some Reported Serum Chemistry Changes in Fed, Fasted, and Sick Horses*

Measurement	Fed	Fasted (88 hr)	Sick	
			Anorectic	Hyperlipemic
Triglycerides, mg/dL	23 ±7	160 ±50	158 ±66	1,567 ±972
Free fatty acids, mg/dL	0.5 ±0.5	23 ±10	—	23 ±8
Total lipids, mg/dL	330 ±10	510 ±125	730 ±860	1,773 ±769
Cholesterol, mg/dL	99 ±9	84 ±10	172 ±134	242 ±114
Blood urea nitrogen, mg/dL	26	18	23 ±11	177 ±179
Creatinine, mg/dL	1.6	No change	No change	10 ±7
Total bilirubin, mg/dL	0.5	3.5–3.7	4.1 ±2.7	1.8 ±1.4

*Data from Naylor JM, Kronfield DS, Acland H: Hyperlipemia in horses: Effects of undernutrition and disease. *Am J Vet Res* 41:899, 1980.

as the simplest, easiest, safest, and least expensive method of providing nutritional support.

Nutritional Formulas

The first "blenderized" enteral diet for hospitalized horses, pioneered by Naylor et al.[153] (Table 5–18), provided clinicians with a means by which to meet the energy and protein needs of their equine patients. Unfortunately, this diet and other "home-brews" are not only difficult to procure, mix, deliver, and store but can often be energy-dilute because of the large volume of water needed to deliver them and they may lack nutritional balance and adequacy. Since then, other diets for enteral feeding have been tested or developed. Pelleted horse feeds designed to supply both the grain and forage components of the diet are generally used as the base for slurries.[154] They have the advantage of being nutritionally balanced, less expensive, and widely available when compared to the alfalfa-casein-dextrose mixture. The pelleted feed chosen should be age- and nutrient-appropriate for the horse that is being fed. These diets can also be tailored to

meet specific needs. To increase energy density, vegetable oil may be added. Increases in protein may be accomplished by adding alfalfa meal, finely ground soybean meal, or a modular component used for human liquid diets. Adding raw eggs to increase protein is not advised because of the risk of salmonella contamination. As with the Naylor diet, large volumes of water are needed to reduce viscosity for hand-pumping or funneling via tube.

Commercially available liquid diets fed to hospitalized human patients have also been used successfully as the sole source of nutritional support in a variety of clinical cases.[155, 156] Proteins of high quality such as casein, whey, or soy protein isolate are most frequently used as the protein source. The fat sources are all vegetable in origin. Many formulas contain a combination of one or more of the vegetable oils with medium-chain triglycerides (MCTs). MCTs are prepared from the fractionation of coconut oil and are 6 to 10 carbons in length.[157] MCTs are more water-soluble, requiring little lipase activity or conjugation to bile salts for absorption to occur. They are hydrolyzed more rapidly than long-chain triglycerides and are transported directly into the

Table 5–18. Composition of and Feeding Schedule for the "Naylor Diet"*

Constituents†	Day						
	1	2	3	4	5	6	7
Electrolyte mixture, g†‡	230	230	230	230	230	230	230
Water, L	21	21	21	21	21	21	21
Dextrose, g	300	400	500	600	800	800	900
Dehydrated cottage cheese, g§	300	450	600	750	900	900	900
Dehydrated alfalfa meal, g	2,000	2,000	2,000	2,000	2,000	2,000	2,000
Energy, Mcal‖	7.4	8.4	9.4	10.4	11.8	11.8	12.2

*From Naylor JM, Freeman DE, Kronfield DS: Alimentation of hypophagic horses. *Compendium Continuing Educ Pract Vet* 6:S93, 1984.
†These allowances should be divided and administered in three feedings daily. Maintenance requirements for a 450-kg horse are 13 Mcal of digestible energy and 580 mg of crude protein.
‡Ten g NaCl, 15 g NaHCO₃, 75 g KCl, 60 g K₂HPO₄, 45 g CaCl₂ + 2H₂O, 25 g MgO.
§Dehydrated cottage cheese—82% crude protein with less than 2% lactose (American Nutritional Laboratory, St Louis, MO) or casein (Sigma Chemical, St Louis, MO).
‖Megacalories of digestible energy.

Table 5–19. Total Feed Required per Day to Meet a 500 kg Adult Horse's Maintenance Requirements*

Ingredient	Amount/Recipe	×	No. Recipes Needed/Day	=	Total Ingredients Needed/Day
Alfalfa/casein/dextrose slurry					
Alfalfa meal	454 g	×	5.9	=	2679 g alfalfa meal
Casein	204 g	×	5.9	=	1204 g casein
Dextrose	204 g	×	5.9	=	1204 g dextrose
Electrolyte mixture	52 g	×	5.9	=	307 g electrolyte mixture
Water	5 L	×	5.9	=	30 L water
Pellet–vegetable oil slurry					
Complete pelleted horse feed	454 g	×	10.7	=	4860 g complete pellet
Corn oil	46 g	×	10.7	=	492 g (535 ml) corn oil
Water	3 L	×	10.7	=	32 L water

*Total ingredients needed for 1 day are determined by multiplying the amount per recipe by the total recipes per day.

blood via the portal system, making them a readily available energy source.[155] The carbohydrate sources are primarily starch hydrolysates (e.g., maltodextrins, oligosaccharides), which are absorbed rapidly, and by being more complex help to reduce osmotic load. Because these formulas were designed to meet the nutrient needs of humans, they do not meet all of the horse's vitamin and mineral requirements and should not be used in long-term feeding situations. As a direct result of these efforts, an enteral formula designed exclusively for use in horses has recently become available (NutriPrime, KenVet, Ashland, Ohio). Though the cost per day for these liquid diets is somewhat higher than conventional slurries, the complete nutrient profile, consistent nutrient composition, ease of administration, and sterile packaging are noteworthy advantages. The ingredients and nutritional composition of some of the prepared formulas, including the equine diet, are given in Tables 5–19, 5–20, and 5–21.

Nutrient Requirements

The purpose of enteral support is to provide the necessary nutrients for maintenance and healing until sufficient quantities can be obtained by voluntary oral intake. Though the specific nutrient needs of the sick horse are not known, data pooled from human and animal studies have provided reasonable estimates for use in equine cases. The basal energy requirement rather than that for resting maintenance is the foundation for calculating the energy expenditure in sick humans and animals. Horses requiring medical attention are generally at "stall rest" in a controlled environment, reducing the energy need for physical activity and thermoregulation. The resting energy requirement of horses in metabolism stalls can be calculated from the formula 21 kcal (BW_{kg}) + 975 kcal.[15] This is roughly 70% of that needed for field maintenance, equal to 11 Mcal/day for a 500-kg horse. The basal energy requirement is but one part of the resting energy value. Another significant component is the heat of fermentation produced by microbial action in the hindgut. When feed intake decreases, there will be less fresh substrate available for the microbes, reducing substrate turnover. Microbial fermentation will gradually decrease and less heat will be produced. The energy for digestion, absorption, and product formation will also have decreased, lowering energy losses even further. Therefore, the horse's actual energy requirement at rest may be closer to 55% to 60% of field maintenance. Until more data are available, the increases in energy expenditure resulting from illness or injury are applied to the resting energy estimate through the use of "injury factors" (Table 5–22). If more than one factor is involved, the highest multiplier is used.

Nitrogen balance studies have been used to determine the protein needs of hospitalized human patients.[158, 159] Protein catabolism increases dramatically, with nitrogen losses in burned and septic patients increasing by nearly 250%. Without sufficient protein or caloric intake, protein is metabolized

Table 5–20. Quantity of Diets Required per Day to Meet Daily Energy Requirement*

Diet	Energy Required	Energy per Recipe or Liter of Diet	Recipes or Liters Needed per Day
Alfalfa/casein/dextrose slurry	16.4 Mcal	2.77 Mcal/recipe	16.4/2.77 = 5.9 recipes
Pellet–vegetable oil slurry	16.4 Mcal	1.53 Mcal/recipe	16.4/1.53 = 10.7 recipes
Osmolite HN	16.4 Mcal	1.06 Mcal/L	16.4/1.06 = 15.5 L
EquiCal	16.4 Mcal	1.00 Mcal/L	16.4/1.00 = 16.4 L

*Daily energy requirement for a 500-kg adult horse = 16.4 Mcal of digestible energy.

Table 5–21. Nutrient Profile of Enteral Diets Supplying Daily Maintenance Energy Requirements for a 500-kg Adult Horse

Nutrient	Requirements*	Alfalfa-Casein-Dextrose Slurry	Pellet–Vegetable Oil Slurry	Osmolite HN†	Equical‡
Energy (DE), Mcal	16.4	16.4	16.4	16.4	16.4
Protein, g	656	1,710	682	688	742
Calcium, g	20	81	32	11.7	32.8
Phosphorus, g	14	41	20	11.7	22.4
Sodium, g	8.2	16.2	10	14.4	25.9
Potassium, g	25	159	—	24.2	29.3
Magnesium, g	7.5	97	10	4.7	10.4
Copper, mg	82	35	122	23.6	120.8
Zinc, mg	328	100	438	264	414
Iron, mg	328	984	389	211	414
Selenium, mg	0.82	0.9	1.5	—	1.2

*From National Academy of Sciences: *Nutrient Requirements of Horses,* ed 5. Washington, DC, National Academy of Sciences, National Research Council, 1989.
†Ross Products Division, Abbott Laboratories, Columbus, Ohio.
‡Marketed as NutriPrime, KenVet, Ashland, Ohio.

for energy instead of being used for protein synthesis and repletion. The calories-to-nitrogen (Cal/N) or nonprotein calories-to-nitrogen (NPCal/N) ratio is therefore used to estimate the protein requirement. A Cal/N ratio between 130:1 and 180:1 or an NPCal/N ratio between 100:1 and 150:1 is considered optimal for most stressed human patients.[159] The lower ratios are recommended for septic or severely traumatized patients. Until more data are available, these ratios seem reasonable for sick horses as well. For practical purposes, there should be 5 g of protein for every 100 kcal.

Increases in vitamin and mineral needs above those needed for maintenance do not appear to be necessary unless drug-nutrient interactions affect micronutrient status.

Method of Delivery

Feeding solutions are generally delivered by gravity flow or by hand pump. Nasogastric intubation or cervical esophagostomy are the preferred routes.[160] As with liquid diets, the soft pouches and gravity feeding sets developed for human hospitals have been relatively easy to adapt for veterinary use.[156]

Feeding Tubes

Nasogastric tubes for enteral support of mature horses are generally 200 to 250 cm (80–100 in.) in length. The internal diameter (ID) should not be less than 14F to obtain a reasonable flow rate. Tubes should be placed either in the stomach or in the distal esophagus. Gastric reflux is more likely to occur when large-bore tubes are passed into the stomach.[158] The tube should be secured to the halter or, in the case of esophagostomy, taped to the neck. A muzzle may be necessary to prevent the horse from dislodging the tube. The tube should be removed prior to the reintroduction of solid food as it may double back into the oral cavity where it can be chewed in half.

Large-bore, thick-walled rubber and polyvinylchloride (Tygon) stomach tubes used for drenching and gastric decompression are commonly used. One drawback, however, is that they become stiff and brittle when exposed to digestive fluids. Local irritation and ulceration of the nasal septum, larynx, and pharynx are also a major concern if these tubes must be left in place. The smaller bore (6–8 mm ID) versions of these tubes have been used for short-term support but suffer from excess pliability, making them difficult to place and subject to kinking.

Table 5–22. Activity and Injury Formulas Suggested for Use in Horses*†

Activity		Injury	
Stall rest	1.2 × REE	Minor trauma or surgery	1.3 × REE
Walking, grazing	1.7 × REE	Skeletal trauma	1.3–1.4 × REE
		Sepsis, cancer	1.5–1.7 × REE
		Major burn	1.7–2.0 × REE

*Adapted from Long CL, Schaffel N, Geiger JW, et al: Metabolic response to injury and illness: Estimation of energy and protein needs from indirect calorimetry and nitrogen balance. *JPEN J Parenter Enteral Nutr* 3:452, 1979.
†REE (resting energy expenditure) = 21 kcal (BW$_{kg}$) + 975 kcal.

Polyurethane and silicone tubes dominate the human enteral tube market. These materials offer several advantages in that they are softer, less irritating, and do not harden. Most are also radiopaque. Silicone stomach tubes designed for horses are available (BIVONA, Inc., Gary, Ind.) but are rather large and thick-walled, making flow rate difficult to control. A polyurethane, 18F, 98-in. enteral feeding tube for adult horses is currently available (KenVet).

Rate of Delivery

Bolus delivery, or the rapid administration of formula by hand pump or syringe, is used most often. While this method certainly saves time, it can result in diarrhea, abdominal pain, and distention, especially during the period of diet introduction.

Continuous and intermittent feeding will become more popular as the use of enteral support increases. In intermittent feeding, a prescribed volume is infused by gravity drip over a longer period of time (60–120 minutes) at set intervals (every 2 or 3 hours) rather than continuously. Many of the complications that occur with bolus feeding in humans have been reduced by slower and more controlled rates of delivery.

Guidelines for Feeding the Sick Horse

1. The horse should be adequately hydrated and any electrolyte or acid-base abnormalities should be corrected before initiating enteral feeding.

2. Estimate the horse's energy needs using the *current* body weight rather than the ideal body weight. The *initial* goal is to prevent further weight loss. Estimate protein needs.

3. Select the formula or slurry to be used and calculate the volume needed to meet the energy needs. Extra protein, if needed, can be added with protein modules (i.e., ProMod, Ross Laboratories, Columbus, Ohio; Casec, Mead Johnson Nutritionals, Evansville, Ind.).

4. Design the feeding schedule such that the maximum volume per feeding when the full-volume goal is reached is 3 to 4 qt. A minimum of four to six feedings is usually required. Tolerance is best when small feedings are delivered frequently.

5. The stomach tube or indwelling nasogastric tube should be placed. The proper position of the tube should be verified before each feeding. Horses must remain standing or in sternal recumbency during feeding to prevent reflux and aspiration.

6. Some horses may need to be brought up to full-volume feeding slowly. For young horses, postsurgical cases, or horses that have been anorectic for 5 days or more, feed 25% of the full-feeding volume on the first day. Increase to 50% on the second or third day and then to 75% if tolerance has been acceptable. Though energy needs have been estimated, the actual calories needed to maintain body weight will vary from horse to horse. Some may maintain their weight when fed at 75% of the calculated full-feeding volume. If this occurs, no further increases in formula volume may be needed. Otherwise, increase to 100% as dictated by body weight and tolerance.

7. The tube should be flushed with warm water *before* feeding to verify placement and patency and *after feeding* to rinse out formula and prevent clogging. If the tube cannot be flushed, formula exits from the nostril, or the horse is in distress, do not feed!

8. Feeding volumes of 3 to 4 qt have been delivered by bolus safely over a 10- to 15-minute period. Slower rates (feeding over a 30–60-minute period) are recommended during the adaptation period to reduce the risk of intolerance.

9. Between feedings, horses should be muzzled to prevent removal of the tube but allow for free-choice water consumption.

10. Feces production and volume will vary depending on the diet that is used. Loose feces are not uncommon and are of little concern if not accompanied by other signs of organic disease. The liquid enteral preparations are low residue diets, resulting in small, soft fecal balls with mucus of low frequency and volume. If the horse becomes depressed, febrile, colicky, or dehydrated, feeding should be stopped.

11. Continuous or intermittent gravity drip of liquid enteral formula is strongly recommended for horses that may have reduced absorptive capability (i.e., prolonged inappetence, humane rescues). In some of these horses, a combination of enteral and parenteral support may be most effective until gastrointestinal function is restored.

Clinical Monitoring

Laboratory work should be reviewed as needed to monitor clinical status. There are no definitive indices to assess the quality of nutritional intervention in horses. Serum triglycerides, cholesterol, and bilirubin generally respond quickly to refeeding, falling back to within normal ranges in 24 to 48 hours. Because of the peripheral insulin resistance that occurs in hypermetabolic states, blood glucose concentrations should be monitored closely in the early stages for the development of hyperglycemia. In this instance, formula volume should be decreased to reduce glucose intake.

Reintroducing Solid Feed

Once the disease process has been brought under control, most horses begin to show interest in hay and grain. Energy formerly used for battling disease is rechanneled to support increased voluntary activity, resulting in little, if any, change in estimates for energy need. The initial goal, however, is to merely substitute the enteral formula for solid feeds before any increases in energy intake are implemented. As recommended for any feeding program, the addition of these proprietary feeds should be done gradually to allow the digestive tract time to adjust to the "new" substrates. Using feeds that the horse is familiar with will further encourage eating. Select hay that is leafy and has a fresh aroma to encourage consumption. The type of hay is not critical, though alfalfa tends to be higher in leaf content and therefore higher in energy and protein than most grass hays or clover hay. Begin by offering 3 to 5 lb/day for the first 3 to 4 days, reducing the amount of enteral formula by roughly 1 qt for every pound of hay consumed. Grain should be added only when energy needs cannot be met with hay alone. If there has been a decrease in lean body mass, repletion by increasing energy intake above the requirement with no increase in muscular activity will result in the deposition of fat instead of muscle. Repletion of all nutrients is best accomplished gradually.

Drug-Nutrient Interactions

Drugs that are commonly used in veterinary medicine can have a profound effect on the nutritional status of the animal, either through suppression of appetite or by a direct pharmacologic effect. This is not to suggest that the use of drugs should be questioned if nutritional status will be affected, but a more thorough understanding of their interactions will assist the clinician in addressing the nutritional needs of the patient more accurately.

Several drugs have been shown to affect the senses of taste and smell in humans. If this also occurs in horses, many horses may refuse to consume feeds that are normal constituents of their diet. Table 5–23 lists the drugs commonly used in equine medicine and the effects that these drugs have been reported to have in human patients.

When should medications be administered to horses that are tube-fed? Since most pharmacologic data suggest that absorption occurs most rapidly in the fasted state, the recommendation that drugs be given either 2 hours before or 2 hours after a feeding seems appropriate. Using liquid preparations of certain drugs when available rather than grinding or crushing tablets for administration prevents clogging of the tube, necessitating tube removal and replacement.

Complications of Enteral Feeding

Aspiration of formula into the lungs can be one of the most serious complications of enteral feeding. It is advisable to verify tube placement before and after each feeding, check for gastric residuals prior to feeding, and be certain that the head and neck are raised during administration of the diet. If a gastric residual volume equal to or greater than 50% of the normal feeding volume is obtained, the feeding should be withheld and the cause of the decrease in gastric emptying should be evaluated. Gastric emptying rates are reduced in sepsis, peritonitis, or following abdominal surgery.[161] Certain drugs also may reduce the gastric emptying rate.

Because the composition of most enteral formulas makes them ideal growth media for bacteria, care in preparation and handling is essential. Though not a major cause of clinical problems in the human hospital setting, secondary infections attributable to bacterial contamination of formula have been reported.[162, 163] Many bacteria have been isolated, including *Escherichia coli, Enterobacter, Klebsiella*, and *Salmonella*, to name but a few. Sterile commercial preparations

---

Table 5–23. Drug-Nutrient Interactions Reported in Humans

Drug	Gastrointestinal	Metabolic	Laboratory Values*
Amikacin sulfate		Anorexia, polydipsia, salivation	↑ BUN, creatinine
Amoxicillin	Diarrhea	Anemia, affects taste	↑ AST
Ampicillin			↑ AST, ALT
Cimetidine (Tagamet)	Diarrhea, gastric secretion		↑ Creatinine, AST, ALT, ALP
Erythromycin	Diarrhea, cramps	Jaundice	↑ ALP, bilirubin, AST, ALT
Betamethasone valareate–gentamicin sulfate (Gentocin)		Anorexia, polydipsia	↑ BUN, AST, ALT, LDH, bilirubin, creatinine; ↓ Mg, Na, K, Ca
Metoclopramide (Reglan)	Diarrhea		
Metronidazole (Flagyl)	Diarrhea, epigastric distress	Anorexia, alters taste	
Moxalactam		Decreases bacterial synthesis of vitamin K	↑ AST, ALT, BUN, creatinine, ALP
Penicillin G, procaine, penicillin G benzathine	Diarrhea, gastritis	Alters taste, anorexia	
Pyrimethamine (Daraprim)		Interferes with folate metabolism; anorexia	
Ranitidine (Zantac)	Constipation, abdominal pain		
Rifampin	Epigastric distress, cramps, diarrhea	Anorexia, alters taste	↑ AST, ALT, GGT, creatinine
Sucralfate (Carafate)	↓ Absorption of vitamins A, D, E, and K; constipation		↑ AST, ALP, BUN, bilirubin, uric acid
Sulfamethoxazole-trimethoprim (Bactrim)	Diarrhea, ↓ absorption of folate and vitamin K	Anorexia	↑ Creatinine, BUN, AST, ALT, bilirubin
Tetracycline	↓ Absorption of Ca, Fe, Mg, Zn, and amino acids; diarrhea	Anorexia, ↓ vitamin K synthesis by bacteria	↑ ALP, BUN, bilirubin, AST, ALT

*Abbreviations: AST, aspartate aminotransferase; ALT, alanine aminotransferase; ALP, alkaline phosphatase; BUN, blood urea nitrogen; LDH, lactic dehydrogenase; GGT, γ-glutamyltransferase.

can be contaminated at mixing or from the hospital environment and many home-brews may be inherently contaminated. To reduce this risk, the formula should be prepared in a reasonably clean environment and administered as soon as possible after preparation. Prepare only enough formula for one feeding if bolus-fed; do not mix a 12- to 24-hour quantity, even if it is to be stored under refrigeration. All utensils should be thoroughly washed and rinsed. Enteral feeding bags and administration sets should be rinsed until the wash solution is clear and disposed of after 24 to 48 hours.

Gastrointestinal complications such as bloating, colic, and diarrhea can occur during the first few days of enteral feeding and can have a variety of causes: an adaptation period that is too short, bolus feeding, rapid administration, large infrequent feedings, carbohydrate intolerance, or the cause may be nondietary, such as antibiotic therapy. These complications can generally be avoided by taking a conservative approach to enteral feeding, developing a reasonable adaptation schedule to guarantee compliance, feeding small volumes slowly and frequently, and returning to a previously tolerated rate and volume until tolerance is reestablished. The commonly encountered, antibiotic-induced diarrhea usually resolves quickly once the drugs are discontinued. However, if the microfloral population has been significantly reduced, additional time may be needed for these microbes to become reestablished.

Parenteral Support

Parenteral nutrition is the administration of nutrients by intravenous infusion. If desired, all of the horse's nutritional needs can be supplied by the intravenous route. The goals of parenteral support are the same as those for enteral: providing energy and protein to prevent catabolism of body protein and promote repair. This method of nutritional support is of value when use of the gastrointestinal tract is contraindicated for more than 5 to 7 days. Lack of access to the gastrointestinal tract (e.g., pharyngeal obstruction), severe diarrhea, malnutrition, massive small bowel resection, intestinal obstruction or prolonged ileus, continual gastric reflux, and a high risk of aspiration are situations when parenteral support is appropriate.[164] As with human patients, the decision to use parenteral nutrition must be made carefully on a case-by-case basis owing to the expense, time, and expertise required for mixing, administering, and monitoring, as well as the potential risks involved.[165] However, knowledge of the potential complications and their causes, careful monitoring, and prompt treatment by attentive, dedicated staff have made parenteral nutrition a successful adjunct to veterinary care.

Admixtures

Admixtures used in parenteral nutrition are generally composed of sterile solutions of dextrose, amino acids, and electrolytes. Fat can also be added in the form of a lipid emulsion if greater caloric density is needed. Like enteral solutions, these mixtures are ideal growth media for bacteria and must be used within 12 hours or less after mixing. To prevent contamination, solutions should be mixed using aseptic techniques in a designated area, preferably with a laminar flow hood. If solutions must be stored after final mixing, they should be refrigerated immediately and used within 12 to 24 hours.

Dextrose (glucose) is the carbohydrate used in most, if not all, parenteral mixtures. To increase the caloric density, several concentrations of dextrose are available, but care must be taken because of the hypertonicity of such solutions. Fifty percent dextrose solutions are used most often in equine parenteral support, with an osmolarity of 2,525 mOsm/L. For most standard formulas, the dextrose concentration should not exceed 30% of the final mixture or 60% of the total volume infused.

Crystalline amino acid solutions are the main source of nitrogen in parenteral mixtures. They contain both essential and nonessential amino acids at various concentrations, with solutions containing 8.5% amino acids used most commonly. Again, as with concentrated dextrose solutions, these products are high in osmolarity, approximately 800 mOsm/L. Because of the lability of the essential amino acid tryptophan, these solutions should be stored at room temperature and protected from light. Amino acid solutions are available with added electrolytes in the free-base rather than chloride form, reducing the risk of hyperchloremia. Final amino acid concentrations of most standard admixtures should not exceed 4.5%. Amino acid solutions must be mixed first with the dextrose solution before being added to lipid. The high pH of these solutions will break the emulsion if added directly to it.

Lipid emulsions are often used to increase the energy density and nonprotein nitrogen calories of a solution and supply the essential fatty acids linoleate and linolenate. Though high in caloric density at 9 kcal/g, these solutions have the added advantage of being isotonic. All are composed of soybean oil or a combination of soybean and safflower oil, with egg yolk phospholipids and glycerin acting as the emulsifying agents. Lipid emulsions can be "piggybacked" into the main line below the filter or added into premixed dextrose–amino acid solutions to provide an "all-in-one" mixture. They are the most expensive component of the admixture. Lipid emulsions should not constitute more than 50% of the total calories to prevent the suppression of the immune response reported both in vitro and in vivo.[166-168] Products available for parenteral admixtures are listed in Table 5–24.

Guidelines for Delivery

As with enteral feeding, all fluid, electrolyte, and acid-base abnormalities must be corrected before initiating any feeding. Energy goals for parenteral support are similar as for enteral. Some admixtures that have been used in both partial and total parenteral support are listed in Table 5–25.

A central venous line (i.e., jugular) is preferred to using a peripheral vein because of the large volume of fluid required and the risk of thrombogenesis when hypertonic solutions are infused into small vessels. For mature horses, 16-gauge Silastic or polyurethane catheters, 5 to 7 in. in length, have been recommended.[164, 169] Catheters should be placed according to the manufacturer's guidelines using strict aseptic techniques.[169] Once a line is established, it is best to dedicate

Table 5–24. Products for Parenteral Alimentation

A. Dextrose Solution

Concentrate (g/dL)	Osmolarity (mOsm/L)	Calories (kcal/L)	Maintenance Requirement (L)[a]
2.5	126	85	71
5.0	253	170	35
10.0	505	340	18
20.0	1,010	680	9
50.0	2,520	1,700	4

B. Lipid Emulsions

Product	Concentration (g/dL)	Osmolarity (mOsm/L)	Calories (kcal/L)
Intralipid[b]	10 (20)	280 (330)	1,100 (2,000)
Liposyn[c]	10 (20)	276 (340)	1,100 (2,000)

C. Crystalline Amino Acids

Product (Without Electrolytes)	Concentration (g/dL)	Total Nitrogen (g/L)	Osmolarity (mOsm/L)
Aminosyn[d]	8.5 (10.0)	13.4 (15.7)	850 (1,000)
Travasol[e]	8.5 (10.0)	14.3 (16.8)	860 (1,060)

D. Supplements

Multivitamin Concentrate (M.V.C. 9 + 3)[f]				Trace Elements (M.T.E. 5 [1-mL vial])[g]	
Ascorbic acid	100 mg	Niacin	40 mg	Zinc	5 mg
Vitamin A	3,300 IU	Pantothenic acid	15 mg	Copper	1 mg
Vitamin D	200 IU	Vitamin E	101 IU	Manganese	0.5 mg
Thiamine (B₁)	3.0 mg	Biotin	60 μg	Chromium	10 μg
Riboflavin (B₂)	3.6 mg	Folic acid	400 μg	Selenium	20 μg
Pyridoxine (B₆)	4.0 mg	Vitamin B₁₂	5 μg		

[a]Maintenance for 50-kg foal = 120 kcal/kg/day = 6,000 kcal.
[b]Intralipid, KabiVitrum Inc., Alameda, Calif.
[c]Liposyn, Abbott Laboratories, North Chicago, Ill.
[d]Aminosyn, Abbott Laboratories, North Chicago, Ill.
[e]Travasol, Baxter Healthcare Corp., Deerfield, Ill.
[f]M.V.C. 9 + 3. Multivitamin concentrate, Lypho Med Inc., Melrose Park, Ill.
[g]M.T.E. 5. Trace element additive, Lypho Med Inc., Melrose Park, Ill.

this line for parenteral feeding only to reduce the risk of contamination. This may not always be possible or practical. If a single line is necessary, aseptic technique is essential.[170] Stopcocks should not be used so that a closed system is maintained. At no time should blood be drawn through this line.

Gradual introduction of parenteral feeding solutions reduces the risk of complications. For adult horses, compute the desired goal, including injury factors, and prepare a mixture to infuse over the first 24 hours that will provide roughly half of the patient's caloric needs. Most starter solutions can be formulated using dextrose and amino acids. Lipids can be added as an energy source when hyperglycemia cannot be resolved by decreases in rate alone. The composition and rate of flow are adjusted according to metabolic tolerance and nutrient need.

Complications of Parenteral Feeding

Monitoring procedures for the adult equine may be patterned after those suggested for foals (Table 5–26). When lipid emulsions are included in the parenteral solution, blood samples should be checked for evidence of lipemia. Serum triglycerides should be less than 150 mg/dL. If this occurs, decreasing the rate of administration or administering heparin or insulin should improve clearance.

Hyperglycemia, glucosuria, and rebound hypoglycemia are conditions that can occur. The insulin resistance and reduced glucose utilization seen in sepsis, shock, and major trauma lead to the hyperglycemic state. Careful monitoring of blood and urinary glucose concentrations and gradual weaning onto solutions over 24 to 36 hours can reduce the likelihood of occurrence. Serum and urine glucose should

Table 5–25. Suggested Admixtures for Parenteral Nutrition of Horses*

| | MLS | | | | | | Grams/kg BW | | | | |
	Dextrose (50%)	Amino Acids (8.5%)	Amino Acids (10%)	Lipid (10%)	Lipid (20%)	Kilocalories (per kg BW)	CHO	Protein	Lipid	NPNCal/ N Ratio	% Calories	
Partial Support/ Starter Regimen												
Foals (45–50 kg)												
Protocol A												
Step 1	1000	—	1000	500	—	53	10	2	1	140:1	68	18
Step 2	1200	—	1500	1000	—	75	12	3	2	130:1	59	26
Protocol B	1500	1000	—	—	—	58	17	2	—	178:1	78	—
Horses (450 kg)	4500	3500	—	—	—	20	5	0.7	—	153:1	86	—
Total Parenteral Support												
Foals (45–50 kg)												
Protocol A	1500	—	1500	1500	—	94	15	3	3	175:1	53	13
Protocol B	1000	1500	—	—	1000	90	11	3	4	172:1	42	45
Horses (450 kg)												
Protocol A	5000	4000	—	6000	—	34	5	0.75	1.3	255:1	35	56
Protocol B	4500	7000	—	—	3500	36	5	1.3	1.5	146:1	46	38

1 g dextrose = 3.4 kcal; 1000 mL dextrose = 1700 kcal (500 g)
1 g amino acids = 4 kcal; 1000 mL 8.5% solution = 340 kcal (85 g)
1 g lipid emulsion = 11 kcal; 1000 mL 10% solution = 1100 kcal (100 g)
*Data from Hansen TO: Nutritional support—Parenteral feeding. In Koterba AM, Drummond WH, Kosch PC, eds: *Equine Clinical Neonatology.* Philadelphia, Lea & Febiger, 1990, p 747; Spurlock SL: *A Practical Approach to Parenteral Nutrition in the Equine Patient.* Deerfield, Ill, Baxter Healthcare; and Hansen TO, White NA, Kemp DT: Total parenteral nutrition in four healthy adult horses. *Am J Vet Res* 49:122, 1988.

be monitored at least two to three times per day, more often during introduction. When glucose concentrations greater than 200 mg/dL are present, the flow rate should be decreased until tolerance is achieved. Substituting some of the carbohydrate calories for fat calories also reduces the glucose load.

Rebound hypoglycemia occurs when there is a sudden cessation of glucose delivery without providing an alternative source of enteral carbohydrate calories. This can be prevented by slowly decreasing the rate of infusion by half for 12 hours while gradually increasing enteral support. Further decreases should be taken in accordance with patient response.

Azotemia and hyperammonemia are complications of pro-

Table 5–26. Monitoring Procedures for Parenteral Alimentation*

Observation†	Initial Monitoring Frequency	Monitoring After Stabilization
Vital signs	q.4h.	q.8h.
Catheter, vein inspection	q.8h.	q.8h.
Intake-output	q.8h.	q.8h.
Weight	Daily	Daily
Urine glucose	q.6–8h.	q.8–12h.
Serum glucose	q.6–12h.	q.24h.
Serum electrolytes	q.24h.	1–2/wk
Creatinine/BUN	q.24h.	2/wk
Triglycerides, cholesterol	Baseline	Weekly
Liver enzymes (GGT, LDH, SAP)	Baseline	Weekly
Liver function tests (bilirubin)	Baseline	Weekly
Packed cell volume, total protein	q.12–24h.	q.2–3d.
White blood cell differential	Baseline	Weekly
Fibrinogen	Baseline	Weekly

*From Vaala WE: Nutritional management of the critically ill neonate. In Robinson NE, ed: *Current Therapy in Equine Medicine,* vol 3. Philadelphia, WB Saunders, 1992, p 748.
†Abbreviations: BUN, blood urea nitrogen; GGT, γ-glutamyltransferase; LDH, lactic dehydrogenase; SAP, serum alkaline phosphatase.

tein metabolism that have been reported. Providing insufficient calories from nonprotein sources results in the amino acids being used for energy instead of protein synthesis. Assessing serum ammonia and blood urea nitrogen (BUN) concentrations during total parenteral nutrition (TPN) administration is recommended. The most common electrolyte abnormalities are hypokalemia and hypomagnesemia.[164, 171] Increased tissue synthesis increases the requirement for both minerals. Moreover, potassium may also be lost during glucose-induced osmotic diuresis.[172] Supplementation should be followed by laboratory assessment to monitor status.

One of the common and serious mechanical complications that can develop in parenteral delivery is the development of venous thrombosis.[169, 173] The risk can be reduced by selecting catheters made of Silastic elastomers or the newer polyurethanes. Studies in both human and veterinary medicine have documented the low thrombogenicity of these materials compared with polyethylene, polyvinylchloride, or Teflon.[164, 169, 174]

Transition to Enteral Feeding

The transition to liquid or solid diets from parenteral delivery should be accomplished gradually over a period of 3 to 5 days to allow for the stimulation of gut activity and digestive enzyme synthesis. Maintaining both systems of feeding for a short period also guards against short-term nutrient deprivation should inappetence return. A survey of transitional feeding practices in the human hospital setting indicated that parenteral nutrition was most often terminated when 50% to 75% of the calories are met orally.[175] This would appear reasonable for horses. The speed of progress will be based largely on gastrointestinal tolerance. There are no established transition protocols for horses. A conservative approach may be taken by feeding 25% of caloric needs by the oral route in small, frequent meals and reducing the volume infused isocalorically at the expense of lipid. Advance daily in 25% increments as tolerance permits. It is probably reasonable to discontinue parenteral feeding when the horse has received 75% of its caloric needs enterally for at least 36 to 48 hours with no complications.

NUTRITIONAL MANAGEMENT OF THE PREMATURE OR COMPROMISED FOAL

Approximately half of the length and two thirds of fetal weight gain occur during the last 3 to 4 months of gestation.[28] The high metabolic rate and nutrient needs of the foal present many nutritional challenges. A premature or dysmature foal has been denied the benefit of intrauterine growth and nutrient transfer and therefore may not have the nutrient reserves of a full-term foal. In many cases, providing nutritional support can mean the difference between a positive and negative outcome.

Nutrient Requirements

The nutritional requirements of the sick foal have not been defined and lack of relevant data in the human pediatric literature provides little guidance. The issue of whether sick foals should or can be fed to support growth has not been resolved, though most would agree obtaining growth is a preferred goal. For healthy, preterm infants, growth rates similar to those of full-term infants during the last 30 days in utero are desired. In foals, growth rates comparable to those of equine fetuses during the last 30 days of gestation (0.5–0.7 kg/day) occur at 90 to 100 kcal DE/kg in healthy foals[28, 176] and may be a reasonable starting point for premature and sick foals. Additional increases may be needed for metabolic alterations induced by disease or trauma, but whether they are analogous to the injury factors applied to adults is not known. Caloric intakes between 120 and 160 kcal DE/kg have been reported to provide acceptable responses with minimal complications.[177]

Though only limited data were available, weight gains of foals receiving parenteral nutrition were found to be negatively correlated with the NPCal/N ratio, reemphasizing the need for a balance between protein and energy in order to achieve proper utilization.[175] Nursing foals consume 6 to 7 g of protein per kilogram of body weight during the first 2 weeks of life.[42] The NPCal/N ratio in mare's milk is approximately 105:1, slightly below that of several milk substitutes and much lower than that of most parenteral admixtures suggested for foals.[164, 171] The current recommendations for the foal are higher than those for the human infant, especially considering their preciosity and rapid growth. Ratios less than 176:1,[164, 176] and perhaps closer to the ratio of mare's milk, may be of greater benefit, but more studies are needed.

Between birth and 4 months of age, estimates of calcium and phosphorus accretion in foals appear to be 10 g/kg and 5 g/kg of gain, respectively.[2, 50] If these values are taken as minimal and allowing for lower dietary availabilities from inorganic sources and reported endogenous losses, calcium and phosphorus requirements for neonates are at least 20 to 25 g/day and 10 to 16 g/day, respectively.[2] For foals gaining as little as 0.8 kg/day, extrapolation of these data suggests at least 18 g of calcium and 9 g of phosphorus would be needed for neonates.

Vitamin and trace mineral needs must, again, be estimated from the paucity of data in healthy foals and the nutrient content of mare's milk. Assuming that the foal would consume approximately 14 qt of milk per day during the first week, the vitamin and trace mineral intake in Table 5–27, seems to be a reasonable starting place.

Enteral Support

It is generally accepted that enteral nutrition should be attempted whenever possible. Lactase activity is present in the fetal small intestine during the last trimester, reaching its peak at 2 days post partum,[69] suggesting that a premature foal may have digestive capability. Intermittent enteral feeding most closely mimics the "natural" state, stimulating gastrointestinal enzyme and hormone activity and increasing small intestinal villous growth. There are fewer complications associated with enteral feeding (though some do exist), less monitoring is required, and it is less expensive than providing nutrients parenterally.

Table 5–27. Estimated Daily Trace Mineral and Vitamin Intake from Mare's Milk During First Week of Life

Trace minerals	Iron	10 mg
	Copper	7.0 mg
	Manganese	17 mg
	Zinc	40 mg
	Selenium	0.09 mg
Vitamins	Thiamine	4.2 mg
	Riboflavin	4.9 mg
	Pyridoxine	5.4 mg
	Niacin	12.3 mg
	Pantothenate	117.5 mg
	Folic acid	1,082 μg
	Biotin	116 μg
	Choline	964 mg
	B_{12}	40.9 μg
	Myo-inositol	984 mg

Formulas

Mare's milk should be used whenever possible. Because the goal is ultimately to return the foal to the mare, hand-milking the mare provides food for the foal and will help to maintain lactation. Mare's milk has no discernible odor and has the appearance of 2% low fat cow's milk. Any milk that appears abnormal should not be fed. The milk should be strained through a gauze sponge to remove hair, dirt, and other debris before storing, and be kept under refrigeration.

Unfortunately, not all mares will tolerate hand-milking and some will stop lactating despite continual and frequent evacuation of the udder. Supplementation with other substitutes is usually necessary. Because of increased endogenous losses, incomplete absorption, and the lower digestibility of nutrient sources compared to what nature provides, pediatric researchers have found that the concentration of most nutrients in infant formulas must be higher, especially those for the preterm infant.[178] This may very well be applicable to compromised foals. The milk substitutes designed for the healthy orphan have traditionally been used for sick foals, but their efficacy has been highly variable and many are too nutrient-dilute for sick foals when smaller feeding volumes are indicated.[179] A new nutrient-dense, equine neonatal formula is now available for such foals (NutriFoal, KenVet). This formula is similar in caloric distribution to goat's milk but has added protein to meet the needs of the young foal. (For the nutrient content, see Table 5–14). The casein-to-whey ratio and addition of the amino acid arginine results in an amino acid pattern similar to that of mare's milk protein. Minerals, vitamins, carnitine, and taurine have been added at levels to maintain nutrient balance.

Method of Delivery

For bottle-feeding, most foals prefer the soft lamb nipples over the large, wide-bore calf nipples. When nasogastric delivery is needed, polypropylene enteral nutrition bags or flexible 1-L containers are ideal for the smaller volumes needed for foals. An attached in-line drip chamber and clamp permits control of the formula flow.

Stallion catheters (¼ in. outer diameter, OD) and foal stomach tubes (⅜ in. OD) of polyvinylchloride or silicone have traditionally been used. Small-diameter (12F), polyurethane enteral feeding tubes adapt well for use in foals (Flexiflo Nasoenteric Feeding Tube # 475, Ross Products Division, Abbott Laboratories, Columbus, Ohio). A stylet provides enough rigidity to prevent kinking during placement. A U tube placed at the nares helps to keep the tube in place. Foals have been fed for as long as 14 days with no signs of discomfort, irritation, or ulceration.[180] The Y-connector with side port should be capped when not in use. The tube is secured by tape or by butterfly suture to the foal's muzzle.

Rate of Delivery

For most foals in intensive care, intermittent or continuous drip will result in the fewest complications. Foals that become colicky or bloated following even the smallest bolus feedings can usually tolerate slower, continuous infusions quite well. As the foal's physical condition and gastrointestinal tolerance improve, larger bolus feedings may be attempted. Advancement to bolus feedings should be done gradually by keeping the same per-feeding volume and slowly decreasing the time over which it is given. For example, if a foal is fed intermittently by infusing 1,350 mL over a 3-hour period every 4 hours, advance the feeding to 1,350 mL over a 2-hour period every 4 hours. If tolerance is maintained for 24 to 48 hours, advance until the desired bolus schedule is attained.

Guidelines for Enteral Feeding of the Compromised Foal

1. The hydration, electrolyte, and acid-base status of the foal should be corrected before initiating feeding.

2. Obtain the foal's weight and estimate its energy needs. Start at 100 kcal/kg, with a goal of 120 to 150 kcal/kg.

3. Estimate the protein needs. Maintain an appropriate NPCal/N or Cal/N ratio.

4. Select the formula to be used and calculate the volume needed.

5. The indwelling nasogastric tube should be placed using the approved clinic procedure and the manufacturer's guidelines. If the tube becomes dislodged, it is best not to attempt to reinsert the stylet into the dwelling tube. Remove the tube, reinsert the stylet, and replace the tube. As with adults, the proper placement of the tube must be verified, preferably by radiography or endoscopy.

6. Foals should be standing (if able) or in sternal recumbency during feeding. This will help to prevent gastric reflux, reducing the risk of aspiration pneumonia, a common and frequently fatal complication of sick foals.

7. The sicker the foal, the more intolerant it will generally be to feedings. In some cases, intolerance caused by early aggressive feeding is difficult to reverse. The conservative approach is best. Begin with half the desired volume and increase gradually after at least 24 hours, using tolerance as a guide. Intermittent or continuous feeding is recommended over bolus delivery. Start at 100 mL/hr and increase to 300 mL/hr as quickly as tolerance allows.

8. Check for gastric residuals before feeding. Gastric emptying is reduced in sepsis. If a volume greater than or equal to the designated feeding volume is present, do not feed and investigate possible causes.

9. The tube should be flushed before feeding to verify patency and placement. If there is resistance to flushing, formula exits from the foal's nostril(s), or the foal is in distress, do not feed. Flush the tube after feeding to rinse out formula and prevent clogging.

10. After rinsing the tube, cap the feeding port to prevent air from entering the tube and formula from siphoning out.

11. Colic, constipation, and diarrhea are common problems that are not always diet-related. Though feeding should be discontinued until the cause has been identified, prolonged gut rest (greater than 24–36 hours) may further compromise the foal. Parenteral support should be reserved for those foals for which all attempts to feed enterally have been unsuccessful.

12. If the goal is to put the foal back on the mare, encourage suckling from the mare or a bottle to develop the suckle reflex as soon as the foal is able. If the foal is to be hand-reared, teach the foal to drink from a shallow container and raise as suggested for an orphan.

13. Owners should be cautioned not to overfeed the foal in an effort to "catch up" with others of similar age. Premature and sick foals need time to continue recovery, even after release. Overfeeding will not be rewarding! Foals should be fed according to their current age and weight rather than to the weight of age-matched "normal" foals.

Parenteral Support

Suggested parenteral solutions for use in foals are summarized in Table 5–25.[171, 181] Initial caloric goals vary from 55 to 100 kcal/kg and are dictated primarily by the clinical status of the foal, for example, the sicker the foal, the lower the initial goal should probably be to minimize complications. Protein goals in current protocols range from 2 to 3 g/kg of body weight. Fat intake from mare's milk early in lactation ranges from 5 to 6 g/kg of body weight, slightly higher than the 2 to 4 mg/kg of most parenteral solutions. Other supplements added to the solution include vitamins, trace minerals, and potassium chloride for foals not receiving enteral feedings. In humans, potassium and protein coexist in body tissues in a relatively constant ratio. Catabolic patients can lose as much as 3 mEq of potassium in the urine for each gram of protein that is lost. Without adequate potassium, protein synthesis will be depressed.[182] Osmotic diuresis that occurs during hyperglycemia and diuretic-induced diuresis can also increase potassium lost through urine.[162, 183] To counter these losses, 40 to 60 mEq of potassium has been added per liter of parenteral solution for foals.[183] Calcium and phosphorus concentrations of admixtures fed to foals will not be adequate to meet the needs of growing foals. Calcium gluconate (25–50 mEq/L) and potassium phosphate (5–15 mEq/L) can safely be added to provide part of the needs until enteral feeding is possible.[183] Additional calcium supplementation to the admixture runs the risk of mineral precipitation.

Care should be taken to begin infusions slowly and increase gradually. The goal infusion rate may not be achieved for 12 to 24 hours, depending on the foal. Patient tolerance to the parenteral mixture can be monitored by using the schedule in Table 5–26.[184] Weaning foals from parenteral support should be done in conjunction with the introduction of enteral feeding. Rebound hypoglycemia should not be a problem as long as sufficient enteral calories are provided. Parenteral support is best withdrawn over a 2- to 3-day period and followed with 1 to 2 L of 5% dextrose to aid in reestablishing glucose control mechanisms.[183]

Advances in volume or the inclusion of lipid emulsions should be based on metabolic tolerance. As in human infants, lipid emulsions are not recommended for foals with hyperbilirubinemia, as this may further compromise bilirubin transport.

REFERENCES

1. Hintz HF: *Horse Nutrition—A Practical Guide.* New York, Arco, 1983.
2. National Research Council: *Nutrient Requirements of Horses.* Washington, DC, National Academy Press, 1989.
3. Putnam MR, Bransby DI, Schumacher J, et al: Effects of fungal endophyte *Acremonium coenephialum* in fescue pasture on pregnant mares and foal viability. *Am J Vet Res* 52:2071–2074, 1991.
4. Schoeb TR, Panceria RJ: Blister beetle poisoning in horses. *J Am Vet Med Assoc* 173:75, 1978.
5. Sockett DC, Baker JC, Stowe CM: Slaframine (*Rhizoctonia leguminicola*) intoxication in horses. *J Am Vet Med Assoc* 181:606, 1982.
6. Traub JL, Potter KA, Bayly WM, et al: Alsike clover poisoning. *Modern Vet Pract*, April:307, 1982.
7. Masri MD, Olcott BM, Nicholson SS, et al: Clinical, epidemiologic and pathologic evaluation of an outbreak of mycotoxic encephalomalacia in south Louisiana horses. *Proc Am Assoc Equine Pract* 33:367, 1987.
8. Moise L, Wysocki A: The effect of cottonseed meal on growth of young horses. *J Anim Sci* 53:409, 1981.
9. Morgan SE: Gossypol as a toxicant in livestock. *Vet Clin North Am Food Anim Pract* 5:251, 1989.
10. Hintz HF: Molds, mycotoxins and mycotoxicosis. *Vet Clin North Am Equine Pract* 6:421, 1990.
11. McDonald P, Edwards RA, Greenhalgh JFD: *Animal Nutrition.* New York, Wiley, 1988, p 16.
12. Nelson DD, Tyznik WJ: Protein and nonprotein nitrogen utilization in the horse. *J Anim Sci* 32:68, 1971.
13. Hintz HF, Schryver HF: Nitrogen utilization in ponies. *J Anim Sci* 34:592, 1972.
14. Hintz HF, Lowe JE, Clifford AJ, et al: Ammonia intoxication resulting from urea ingestion by ponies. *J Am Vet Med Assoc* 157:963, 1970.
15. Pagan JD, Hintz HF: Equine energetics I. Relationship between body weight and energy requirements in horses. *J Anim Sci* 63:815, 1986.
16. Willoughby DP: *Growth and Nutrition in the Horse.* Cranbury, NJ: AS Barnes, 1975.
17. Henneke DR, Potter GD, Kreider JL, et al: Relationship between condition score, physical measurement, and body fat percentage in mares. *Equine Vet J* 15:371, 1983.
18. Anderson CE, Potter GD, Kreider JL, et al: Digestible energy requirements for exercising horses. *J Anim Sci* 56:91, 1983.
19. Pagan JD, Hintz HF: Equine energetics. II. Energy expenditure in horses during submaximal exercise. *J Anim Sci* 63:822, 1986.

20. Cymbaluk NF, Fretz PB, Loew FM: Amprolium-induced thiamine deficiency in horses. *Am J Vet Res* 39:255, 1978.
21. Bertone JJ, Hintz HF, Schryver HF: Effect of caffeic acid on thiamin status in ponies. *Nutr Rep Int* 30:281, 1984.
22. Fonnesbeck PV: Consumption and excretion of water by horses receiving all hay and hay-grain diets. *J Anim Sci* 27:1350, 1968.
23. Ralston SL, Rich GA, Squires EL, et al: Effect of vitamin A supplementation on seminal characteristics and vitamin A absorption in stallions. *Equine Vet Sci* 6:203, 1986.
24. Rich GA, McGlothlin ED, Lewis LD, et al: Effect of vitamin E supplementation on stallion seminal characteristics and sexual behavior. *Proc Equine Nutr Physiol Soc* 10:545, 1987.
25. Mason TA: A high incidence of angular limb deformities in a group of foals. *Vet Rec* 109:93, 1981.
26. Powell DM, Lawrence LM, Parett DF, et al: Body composition changes in broodmares. In *Proceedings of the 11th Equine Nutrition Physiology Society Symposium*, Stillwater, Okla, May 18–20, 1989, p 91.
27. Lawrence LM, DiPetro J, Ewert K, et al: Changes in body weight and condition of gestating mares. *J Equine Vet Sci* 12:355, 1992.
28. Bergin WC, Gier HT, Frey RA, et al: Developmental horizons and measurements useful for age determination of equine embryos and fetuses. *Am Assoc Equine Pract* 23:179, 1967.
29. Meyer H, Ahlswede L: The interuterine growth and body composition of foals and the nutrient requirements of pregnant mares. *Anim Res Dev* 8:86, 1976.
30. Platt H: Growth of the equine foetus. *Equine Vet J* 16:247, 1984.
31. Kronfeld DS: Feeding on horse breeding farms. *Proc Am Assoc Equine Pract* 24:461, 1978.
32. Jeffcott LB, Field JR: Current concepts of hyperlipaemia in horses. *Vet Rec* 116:461, 1985.
33. Meyer H, Ahlswede L: Über das uterine Wachstum und die Korpuszusammensetzung von Fohlen sowie den Nährstoffbedarf tragender Stuten. *Über Tierernährung* 4:263, 1976.
34. Knight DA, Gabel AA, Reed SM, et al: Correlation of dietary mineral to incidence and severity of metabolic bone disease in Ohio and Kentucky. In *Proceedings of the 31st Annual Meeting of the American Association of Equine Practitioners*, 1985, p 445.
35. Knight DA, Weisbrode SE, Schmall LM, et al: The effects of copper supplementation on the prevalence of cartilage lesions in foals. *Equine Vet J* 22:426, 1990.
36. Baker HJ, Lindsey JR: Equine goiter due to excess dietary iodine. *J Am Vet Med Assoc* 153:1618, 1968.
37. Driscoll J, Hintz HF, Schryver HF: Goiter in foals caused by excessive iodine. *J Am Vet Med Assoc* 173:858, 1975.
38. Roberts MC: Serum and red cell folate and serum vitamin B$_{12}$ levels in horses. *Aust Vet J* 60:106, 1983.
39. Maenpää PH, Koskinen T, Koskinen E: Serum profiles of vitamins A, E and D in mares and foals during different seasons. *J Anim Sci* 66:1418, 1988.
40. Donoghue S, Meacham TN, Kronfeld DS: A conceptual approach to optimal nutrition of brood mares. *Vet Clin North Am Equine Pract* 6:383, 1990.
41. Gibbs PG, Potter GD, Blake RW, et al: Milk production of quarter horse mares during 150 days of lactation. *J Anim Sci* 54:496, 1982.
42. Oftedal OT, Hintz HF, Schryver HF: Lactation in the horse: Milk composition and intake by foals. *J Nutr* 113:2169, 1983.
43. Doreau M, Boulot S, Martin-Rosset W, Robelin: Relationship between nutrient intake, growth and body composition of the nursing foal. *Reprod Nutr Dev* 26:683, 1986.
44. Flade E: Milchleistung und Milchqualität bei Stuten. *Arch Tierzucht* 9:381, 1955.
45. Neseni R, Flade E, Heidler G, et al: Milchleistung und Milch-

46. Bouwman H, van der Schee W: Composition and production of milk from Dutch warmblooded saddle horse mares. *Z Tierphysiol Tierernahrung Futtermittelkd* 40:39, 1978.
47. Ullrey DE, Struthers RD, Hendricks DG, et al: Composition of mare's milk. *J Anim Sci* 25:217, 1966.
48. Ullrey DE, Ely ET, Covert RL: Iron, zinc and copper in mare's milk. *J Anim Sci* 38:1276, 1974.
49. Stowe HD: Vitamin A profiles of equine serum and milk. *J Anim Sci* 54:76, 1982.
50. Schryver HF, Oftedal OT, Williams J, et al: Lactation in the horse: The mineral composition of mare milk. *J Nutr* 116:2142, 1986.
51. Zicker SC, Lonnerdal B: Protein and nitrogen composition of equine (*Equus caballus*) milk during early lactation. *Comp Biochem Physiol* 108A:411–421, 1994.
52. Davis TA, Nguyen HV, Garcia-Bravo R, et al: Amino acid composition of human milk is not unique. *J Nutr* 124:1126–1132, 1994.
53. Jenness, R: The composition of milk. In Larson BL, Smith UR, eds: *Lactation: A Comprehensive Treatise*, vol 3. New York, Academic Press, pp 3–107.
54. Jenness R: Composition and characteristics of goat milk: Review 1968–1979. *J Dairy Sci* 63:1605–1630, 1980.
55. Buffington CA, Knight DA, Kohn CW, et al: Effect of protein source in liquid formula diets on food intake, physiologic values, and growth of equine neonates. *Am J Vet Res* 53:1941–1946, 1992.
56. Wilson JH: Feeding considerations for neonatal foals. In *Proceedings of the 33rd Annual Meeting of the American Association of Equine Practitioners*, New Orleans, Nov 29–Dec 2, 1987, pp 823–829.
57. Naylor JM, Bell R: Raising the orphan foal. *Vet Clin North Am Equine Pract* 1:169–178, 1985.
58. Breedveld L, Jackson SG, Baker JP: The determination of a relationship between copper, zinc and selenium levels in mares and those of their foals. In *Proceedings of the 10th Equine Nutrition Physiology Society Symposium*, Fort Collins, Colo, June 11–13, 1987, p 159.
59. Moore RM, Kohn CW: Nutritional muscular dystrophy in foals. *Compendium Continuing Educ Pract Vet* 13:476, 1991.
60. Carson K, Wood-Gush D: Behaviour of Thoroughbred foals during nursing. *Equine Vet J* 15:257, 1983.
61. Smyth GB: Effects of age, sex, and post mortem interval on intestinal lengths of horses during development. *Equine Vet J* 20:104, 1988.
62. Koterba AM: Prematurity. Section one: Identification, assessment and treatment. In Koterba AM, Drummond WH, Kosch PC, eds: *Equine Clinical Neonatology*, Philadelphia, Lea & Febiger, 1990, p 55.
63. Green DA: A study of the growth rate in thoroughbred foals. *Br Vet J* 125:539, 1969.
64. Reed KR, Dunn NK: Growth and development of the Arabian horse. In *Proceedings of the Fifth Equine Nutrition Physiology Society Symposium*, 1977, p 76.
65. Hintz HF, Hintz RL, Van Vleck LD: Growth rate of thoroughbreds. Effect of age of dam, year and month of birth, and sex of foal. *J Anim Sci* 48:480, 1979.
66. Green DA: A review of studies on the growth rate of the horse. *Br Vet J* 117:181, 1961.
67. Knight DA, Tyznik WJ: The effect of artificial rearing on the growth of foals. *J Anim Sci* 60:1, 1985.
68. Hurtig M, Green SL, Dobson H, et al: Correlative study of defective cartilage and bone growth in foals fed a low copper diet. *Equine Vet J* (suppl 16):66–73, 1993.
69. Roberts MC: The development and distribution of mucosal

enzymes in the small intestine of the fetus and young foal. *J Reprod Fertil* 23:717, 1975.

70. Houpt KA: Ingestive behavior. *Vet Clin North Am Equine Pract* 6:332, 1990.

71. Wilson JH, Schneider CJ, Drummond WH, et al: Metabolic acidosis in neonatal foals fed goat's milk. In *Proceedings of the Second International Conference on Veterinary Perinatology*, Cambridge, England, 1990, p 62.

72. Carter GK: Gastric diseases. In Robinson NE, ed: *Current Therapy in Equine Medicine*, vol 2. Philadelphia, WB Saunders, 1987, p 41.

73. Glade MJ, Belling TH Jr: Growth plate cartilage metabolism, morphology and biochemical composition in over- and underfed horses. *Growth* 48:473, 1984.

74. Glade MJ, Belling TH Jr: A dietary etiology for osteochondrotic cartilage. *J Equine Vet Sci* 6:151, 1986.

75. Szczurek EM, Jackson SG, Rooney JR, Baker JP: Influence of confinement, plane of nutrition and low heel on the occurrence of acquired forelimb contracture. In *Proceedings of the 10th Equine Nutrition Physiology Society Symposium*, Fort Collins, Colo, June 11–13, 1987, p 19.

76. Cymbaluk NF, Christianson GI, Leach DH: Longitudinal growth analysis of horses following limited and ad libitum feeding. *Equine Vet J* 22:198, 1990.

77. Stromberg B: A review of the salient features of osteochondrosis in the horse. *Equine Vet J* 11:211, 1978.

78. Turner AS: Diseases of bones and related structures. In Stashak TS, ed: *Adams' Lameness in Horses*. Philadelphia, Lea & Febiger, 1987, p 317.

79. Beard W, Knight D: Developmental Orthopedic Disease. In Robinson NE, ed: *Current Therapy in Equine Medicine*, vol 3. Philadelphia, WB Saunders, 1992, p 105.

80. Papageorges M, Gavin PR, Sande RD, et al: Radiographic and myelographic examination of the cervical vertebral column in 306 ataxic horses. *Vet Radiol* 28:53, 1987.

81. Stewart RH, Reed SM, Weisbrode SE: The frequency and severity of osteochondrosis in cervical stenotic myelopathy in horses. *Am J Vet Res* 52:873–879, 1991.

82. Strauss RJ, Wise L: Operative risks of obesity. *Surg Gynecol Obstet* 146:286, 1978.

83. Bray GA: Complications of obesity. *Ann Intern Med* 103:1052, 1985.

84. Lewis LD, Morris ML Jr, Hand MS: *Small Animal Clinical Nutrition*, vol 3. Topeka, Kan, Mark Morris, 1987, p 6-1.

85. Clarke LL, Roberts MC, Argenzio RA: Feeding and digestive problems in horses. *Vet Clin North Am Equine Pract* 6:433, 1990.

86. Willard JG, Willard JC, Wolfram SA, et al: Effect of diet on cecal pH and feeding behavior of horses. *J Anim Sci* 45:87, 1977.

87. Sweeting MP, Houpt CE, Houpt KA: Social facilitation of feeding and time budgets in stabled ponies. *J Anim Sci* 160:369, 1985.

88. Sweeting MP, Houpt KA: Water consumption and time budgets of stabled ponies (*Equus caballus*) geldings. *Appl Anim Behav Sci* 17:1, 1987.

89. McIlwraith CW, ed: *Proceedings from Panel on Developmental Orthopedic Diseases*. Amarillo, Tex, American Quarter Horse Association, 1986.

90. Wagner PC, Grant BD, Watrous BJ, et al: A study of the heritability of cervical vertebral malformation in horses. *Proc Am Assoc Equine Pract* 31:43, 1985.

91. Wagner PC: Genetic factors in pathogenesis. In McIlwraith, ed: *Proceedings from Panel on Developmental Orthopedic Diseases*. Amarillo, Tex, American Quarter Horse Association, 1986, pp 34–37.

92. Hoppe F, Philipsson J: A genetic study of osteochondritis dissecans in Swedish horses. *Equine Pract* 7:7, 1985.

93. Schougaard H, Falk Ronne J, Philipsson J: A radiographic survey of tibiotarsal osteochondrosis in a selected population of trotting horses in Denmark and its possible genetic significance. *Equine Vet J* 22:288, 1990.

94. Stromberg B, Rejno S: Osteochondrosis in the horse. I. A clinical and radiologic investigation of osteochondritis dissecans of the knee and hock joint. *Acta Radiol Suppl* 358:139, 1978.

95. Thompson KN, Jackson SG, Rooney JR: The effect of above average weight gains on the incidence of radiographic bone aberrations and epiphysitis in growing horses. In *Proceedings of the 10th Equine Nutrition Physiology Society Symposium*, Fort Collins, Colo, June 11–13, 1987, p 5.

96. Glade MJ, Reimers TJ: Effects of dietary energy supply on serum thyroxine, triiodothyronine and insulin concentrations in young horses. *J Endocrinol* 104:93, 1985.

97. Biesik LM, Glade MJ: Changes in serum hormone concentrations in weanling horses following gastric infusion of sucrose or casein. *Nutr Rep Int* 33:651, 1986.

98. Glade MJ, Krook L, Schryver HF, et al: Morphologic and biochemical changes in cartilage of foals treated with dexamethasone. *Cornell Vet* 73:170, 1983.

99. Guyton AC: The thyroid metabolic hormones. In Guyton AC, ed: *Textbook of Medical Physiology*, ed 7. Philadelphia, WB Saunders 1986, p 900.

100. Burch WM, Lebovitz HE: Triiodothyronine stimulates maturation of porcine growth-plate cartilage in vitro. *J Clin Invest* 70:496, 1982.

101. Lewinson D, Toister Z, Silbermann M: Quantitative and distributional changes in the activity of alkaline phosphatase during the maturation of cartilage. *J Histochem Cytochem* 30:261, 1982.

102. Ali SY: Calcification of cartilage. In Hall BK, ed: *Cartilage, vol 1. Structure, Function and Biochemistry*. New York, Academic Press, 1983, p 343.

103. Chen CL, Riley AM: Serum thyroxine and triiodothyronine concentrations in neonatal foals and mature horses. *Am J Vet Res* 42:1415, 1981.

104. Glade MJ, Beller D, Bergen J, et al: Dietary protein in excess of requirements inhibits renal calcium and phosphorus reabsorption in young horses. *Nutr Rep Int* 31:649, 1985.

105. Schryver HF, Meakim DW, Lowe JE et al: Growth and calcium metabolism in horses fed varying levels of protein. *Equine Vet J* 19:280, 1987.

106. Schryver HF, Hintz HF, Craig PH: Calcium metabolism in ponies fed a high phosphorus diet. *J Nutr* 101:1257, 1971.

107. Krook L, Lowe JE: Nutritional secondary hyperparathyroidism in the horse. *Pathol Vet* 1 (suppl 1):1, 1964.

108. Schryver HF, Hintz HF, Lowe JE: Calcium and phosphorus in the nutrition of the horse. *Cornell Vet* 64:493, 1974.

109. Krook L, Maylin GA: Fractures in Thoroughbred race horses. *Cornell Vet* 78 (suppl 11):1, 1988.

110. Hedhammar A, Wu FM, Krook L, et al: Overnutrition and skeletal disease. An experimental study in Great Dane dogs. *Cornell Vet* 64 (suppl 5):1, 1974.

111. Whitlock RH, Schryver HF, Krook L, et al: The effects of high dietary calcium for horses. *Proc Am Assoc Equine Pract* 16:127, 1970.

112. Jordan RM, Myers VS, Yoho B, et al: Effect of calcium and phosphorus levels on growth, reproduction, and bone development in ponies. *J Anim Sci* 40:78, 1975.

113. Kronfeld DS, Meacham TN, Donoghue S: Dietary aspects of developmental orthopedic disease in young horses. *Vet Clin North Am* 6:451, 1990.

114. O'Dell BL, Yohe JM, Savage JE: Zinc availability in the chick as affected by phytate, calcium and ethylenediaminetetraacetate. *Poultry Sci* 43:415, 1964.

115. Likuski HJA, Forbes RM: Mineral utilization in the rat. IV.

Effects of calcium and phytic acid on the utilization of dietary zinc. *J Nutr* 85:230, 1965.

116. Norrdin RW, Krook L, Bond WG, et al: Experimental zinc deficiency in weanling pigs on high and low calcium diets. *Cornell Vet* 63:264, 1973.

117. Davis GK: Effects of high calcium intakes on the absorption of other nutrients. *Fed Proc* 18:1119, 1959.

118. Baxter JH, Van Wyk JJ, Follis RH: A bone disorder associated with copper deficiency. II. Histological and chemical studies on the bones. *Bull Johns Hopkins Hosp* 93:25, 1953.

119. Westmoreland N, Hoekstra WG: Pathological defects in epiphyseal cartilage of zinc-deficient chicks. *J Nutr* 98:76, 1969.

120. Lema O, Sandstead HH: Zinc deficiency, effect on collagen and glycoprotein synthesis and bone mineralization. *Fed Proc* 29:297, 1970.

121. Leach RM: Role of manganeses in mucopolysaccharide metabolism. *Fed Proc* 30:991, 1971.

122. Smith BP, Fisher GL, Poulos PW, et al: Abnormal bone development and lameness associated with copper deficiency in young cattle. *J Am Vet Med Assoc* 166:682, 1975.

123. Strause L, Saltman P, Glowacki J: The effect of deficiencies of manganese and copper on osteoinduction and/or resorption of bone particles in rats. *Calcif Tissue Int* 41:145, 1987.

124. Bridges CH, Womack JE, Harris ED, et al: Considerations of copper metabolism in osteochondrosis of suckling foals. *J Am Vet Med Assoc* 185:173, 1984.

125. Rucker RB, Parker HE, Rogler JC: Effect of copper deficiency on chick bone collagen and selected bone enzymes. *J Nutr* 98:57, 1969.

126. Washburn LE: Skeletal abnormality of probable nutritional-endocrine origin observed in cattle receiving antirachitogenic rations. *J Anim Sci* 5:395, 1946.

127. Cupps PT, Howell CE: The effects of feeding supplemental copper to growing foals. *J Anim Sci* 8:286, 1949.

128. Egan DA, Murrin MP: Copper-responsive osteodysgenesis in a thoroughbred foal. *Irish Vet J* 27:61, 1973.

129. Carbery JT: Osteodysgenesis in a foal associated with copper deficiency. *N Z Vet J* 26:280, 1984.

130. Chou WS, Savage JE, O'Dell BL: Relation of monoamine oxidase activity and collagen cross-linking in copper-deficient and control tissues. *Proc Soc Exp Biol Med* 128:948, 1968.

131. Bolze MS, Reeves RD, Lindbeck FE, et al: Influence of manganese on growth, somatomedin and glycosaminoglycan metabolism. *J Nutr* 115:352, 1985.

132. Cowgill UM, States SJ, Marburger JE: Smelter smoke syndrome in farm animals and manganese deficiency in northern Oklahoma. *USA Environ Pollut (Series A)* 22:259, 1980.

133. Donoghue S: Nutritionally-related bone diseases. *Proc Am Assoc Equine Pract* 26:65, 1980.

134. Westmoreland N, Hoekstra WG: Histochemical studies of alkaline phosphatase in epiphyseal cartilage of normal and zinc-deficient chicks. *J Nutr* 98:83, 1969.

135. Iannotti JP: Growth plate physiology and pathology. Pathologic fractures in metabolic bone disease. *Orthop Clin North Am* 21:1–17, 1990.

136. Fleisch H, Neuman WF: Mechanism of calcification: Role of collagen polyphosphates and phosphatase. *Am J Physiol* 20:671, 1962.

137. Trueta J, Trias A: The vascular contribution to osteogenesis. IV. The effect of pressure upon the epiphyseal cartilage of the rabbit. *J Bone Joint Surg [Br]* 43:800–813, 1961.

138. Frost HM: A chondral modeling theory. *Calcif Tissue Int* 28:181, 1979.

139. Firth EC, Poulos PW: Blood vessels in the developing growth plate of the equine distal radius and metacarpus. *Res Vet Sci* 33:159, 1982.

140. Bramlage LR: Clinical manifestations of disturbed bone formation in the horse. In *Proceedings of the 33rd Annual Meeting at the American Association of Equine Practitioners*, New Orleans, 1985, p 135.

141. Rooney JR: Epiphyseal compression in young horses. *Cornell Vet* 53:567–574, 1963.

142. McIlwraith CW: Diseases of joints, tendons and related structures. In Stashak TS, ed: *Adams' Lameness in Horses*. Philadelphia, Lea & Febiger, 1987, p 396.

143. Pool RR: Developmental orthopedic diseases in the horse: Normal and abnormal bone formation. *Proc Am Assoc Equine Pract* 33:143, 1987.

144. McLaughlin BG, Doige CE: A study of ossification of carpal and tarsal bones in normal and hypothyroid foals. *Can Vet J* 23:164, 1982.

145. Vivrette SL, Reimers TJ, Krook L: Skeletal disease in a hypothyroid foal. *Cornell Vet* 74:373, 1984.

146. Morris MD, Zilmersmit DB, Hintz HF: Hyperlipoproteinemia in fasting ponies. *J Lipid Res* 13:383, 1972.

147. Bauer JE: Plasma lipids and lipoproteins of fasted ponies. *Am J Vet Res* 44:379, 1983.

148. Cuthbertson DP: The metabolic response to injury and its nutritional implications: Retrospect and prospect. *JPEN J Parenter Enteral Nutr* 3:108, 1979.

149. Jacobs DO, Black PR, Wilmore DW: Hormone-substrate interactions. In Rombeau JL, Caldwell MD, eds, *Clinical Nutrition, Enteral and Tube Feeding*, ed 2. Philadelphia, WB Saunders, 1990, p 43.

150. Butterworth CE Jr.: Some clinical manifestations of nutritional deficiency in hospitalized patients. In *Proceedings of the Second Ross Conference on Medical Research: Nutritional Assessment—Present Status, Future Directions and Prospects*. Columbus, Ohio, Ross Laboratories, 1981, p 2.

151. Naylor JM, Kronfeld DS, Acland H: Hyperlipemia in horses: Effects of undernutrition and disease. *Am J Vet Res* 41:899, 1980.

152. Stone MS, Freden GO: Differentiation of anemia of inflammatory disease from anemia of iron deficiency. *Comp Contin Educ* 12:963, 1990.

153. Naylor JM, Freeman DE, Kronfeld DS: Alimentation of hypophagic horses. *Compendium Continuing Educ Pract Vet* 6:S93–S99, 1984.

154. Burkholder WJ, Thatcher CD: Enteral nutrition support of sick horses. In Robinson NE, ed: *Clinical Therapy in Equine Medicine*, vol 3. Philadelphia, WB Saunders, 1992, p 724.

155. Sweeney RW, Hansen TO: Use of a liquid diet as the sole source of nutrition in six dysphagic horses and as a dietary supplement in seven hypophagic horses. *J Am Vet Med Assoc* 197:1030, 1990.

156. Golenz MR, Knight DA, Yvorchuk-St Jean KE: Use of a human enteral feeding solution for supportive therapy of an esophageal laceration and hyperlipemia in a miniature horse. *J Am Vet Med Assoc* 200:951, 1992.

156a. Moore BR, Abood SK, Hinchcliff KW: Hyperlipemia in 9 miniature horses and miniature donkeys. *J Vet Intern Med* 8:376, 1994.

156b. Rivas LS, Reed SM, Kohn CA: Use of an enteral feeding tube in the management of long-term hypophagia in horses. *American Association of Equine Practitioners, Proceedings*, 41:47–48, 1995.

157. Bach AC, Babayan VK: Medium-chain triglycerides: An update. *Am J Clin Nutr* 36:950, 1982.

158. Long CL, Crosby F, Geiger JW: Parenteral nutrition in the septic patient: Nitrogen balance, limiting plasma amino acids and calorie to nitrogen ratio. *Am J Clin Nutr* 29:380, 1976.

159. Long CL, Schaffel N, Geiger JW, et al: Metabolic response to injury and illness: Estimation of energy and protein needs from indirect calorimetry and nitrogen balance. *JPEN J Parenter Enteral Nutr* 3:452, 1979.

160. Stick JA, Derksen FJ, Scott EA: Equine cervical esophagos-

tomy: Complications associated with duration and location of feeding tubes. *Am J Vet Res* 42:727, 1981.

161. Nimmo WS: Drugs, diseases and altered gastric emptying. *Clin Pharmacokinet* 1:189, 1974.

162. DeLeeuw IH, Vandewoude MF: Bacterial contamination of enteral diets. *Gut* 27(suppl 1):56, 1986.

163. Allwood MC: Microbial contamination of parenteral and enteral nutrition. *Acta Chir Scand* 507:383, 1981.

164. Spurlock SL, Ward MV: Parenteral nutrition in equine patients: principles and theory. *Compendium Continuing Educ Pract Vet* 13:461, 1991.

165. Ang SD, Daly JM: Potential complications and monitoring of patients receiving total parenteral nutrition. In Rombeau JL, Caldwell MD, eds: *Parenteral Nutrition*, ed 2. Philadelphia, WB Saunders, 1990, p 331.

166. Nugent KM: Intralipid effects on reticuloendothelial function. *J Leukoc Biol* 36:123, 1984.

167. Skeie B, Askanazi J, Rothkopf MM, et al: Intravenous fat emulsions and lung function: A review. *Crit Care Med* 16:183, 1988.

168. Salo M: Inhibition of immunoglobulin synthesis *in vitro* by intravenous lipid emulsion (Intralipid). *JPEN J Parenter Enteral Nutr* 14:459, 1990.

169. Spurlock SL, Spurlock GH: Risk factors of catheter-related complications. *Compendium Continuing Educ Pract Vet* 12:241, 1990.

170. Forlaw L, Torosian MH: Central venous catheter care. In Rombeau JL, Caldwell MD, eds: *Parenteral Nutrition*, ed 2. Philadelphia, WB Saunders, 1990, p 316.

171. Hansen TO: Nutritional support: Parenteral feeding. In Koterba AM, Drummond WH, Kosch PC eds: *Equine Clinical Neonatology*. Philadelphia, Lea & Febiger, 1990, p 747.

172. Walker WA, Hendricks KM: Nutritional support in patients with altered intestinal function. In *Manual of Pediatric Nutrition*. Philadelphia, WB Saunders, 1985, p 121.

173. Deem DA: Complications associated with the use of intravenous catheters in large animals. *Calif Vet* 6:19, 1981.

174. Welch GW, McKell DW, Silverstein P, et al: The role of catheter composition in the development of thrombophlebitis. *Surg Gynecol Obstet* 138:426, 1974.

175. Krey SH, Murray RL: Modular and transitional feedings. In Rombeau JL, Caldwell MD, eds: *Parenteral Nutrition*, ed 2. Philadelphia, WB Saunders, 1990, p 141.

176. Spurlock SL, Donoghue S: Weight change in foals supported with parenteral nutrition. In *Proceedings of the Second International Conference on Veterinary Perinatology*, Cambridge, England, 1990, p 61.

177. Koterba AM, Drummond WH: Nutritional support of the foal during intensive care. *Vet Clin North Am Equine Pract* 1:35, 1985.

178. Ziegler EE, Biga RL, Fomon SJ: Nutritional requirements of the premature infant. In Suskind RM, ed: *Textbook of Pediatric Nutrition*. New York, Raven Press, 1981, p 29.

179. Vaala WE: Diagnosis and treatment of prematurity and neonatal maladjustment syndrome in newborn foals. *Compendium Continuing Educ Pract Vet* 8:S211, 1986.

180. Kohn CW, Knight DA, Yvorchuk-St Jean KE: A preliminary study of tolerance of healthy foals to a low residue enteral feeding solution. *Equine Vet J* 23:374, 1991.

181. Spurlock SL: *A Practical Approach to Parenteral Nutrition in the Equine Patient*. Deerfield, Ill, Baxter Healthcare, 1995.

182. Cannon PR, Grazier LE, Hughes RH: Influence of potassium on tissue protein synthesis. *Metabolism* 1:49–57, 1952.

183. Vaala WE: Nutritional management of the critically ill neonate. In Robinson NE, ed: *Current Therapy in Equine Medicine*, vol 3. Philadelphia, WB Saunders, 1992, p 741.

184. Spurlock SL, Ward MV: Parenteral nutrition. In Robinson NE, ed: *Current Therapy in Equine Medicine*, vol 3. Philadelphia, WB Saunders, 1992, p 737.

Chapter 6

Respiratory System

Dorothy M. Ainsworth, DVM, PhD, **|** David S. Biller, DVM, MS

Disorders of the respiratory system may be second to those of the musculoskeletal system in limiting the athletic performance of the horse. Major economic losses are sustained when the training programs of horses are interrupted because of respiratory diseases. Thus, early detection of respiratory problems is essential for the rapid return of performance animals to training protocols, but it is even more important in the prevention of secondary complications which may ultimately terminate the horse's career prematurely.

DIAGNOSTIC APPROACH TO RESPIRATORY DISORDERS
History

Questions should be directed to the person most familiar with the horse's performance and medical history. Accurately defining the problem, devoid of subjective impressions, can be the most difficult part of the history taking!

Age and Breed. The age and breed of the animal exhibiting respiratory-related signs may provide clues to the nature of the problem. Congenital defects (nasal septal deviations, choanae atresia, subepiglottic cysts, and hypoplastic lungs) are typically evident at birth, while other conditions, such as chronic bacterial pneumonia (*Rhodococcus equi*), may not be evident until the foal is older (1 to 3 months of age). Viral and bacterial upper respiratory tract infections tend to occur in the weanling and yearling, whereas conditions such as pleuropneumonia or exercise-induced epistaxis are more commonly found in the performance horse older than 2 years of age. In contrast, heaves, or recurrent airway disease, is primarily diagnosed in the more mature horse. Considering the breed of the horse is also important in the investigation of respiratory disorders. For example, Arabian foals with chronic infections should be evaluated for combined immunodeficiency syndrome, a heritable condition in which both cell-mediated and humoral limbs of the immune system are deficient. In addition, solitary defects in the humoral immune

system also predispose to the development of chronic respiratory and enteric infections. Selective IgM deficiency tends to occur more frequently in Arabians and quarter horses,[1] whereas agammaglobulinemia has been documented in Thoroughbreds and standardbreds.[2, 3]

Environment. The type of environment that the horse was or is presently exposed to should be ascertained. For example, is the horse stabled at a racetrack where population turnover is high and the potential for viral respiratory outbreaks is increased, or is the horse a sole inhabitant of a small pasture, seldom exposed to other horses? Is there a history of endemic infections on the farm, as often occurs with *Streptococcus equi* outbreaks? Can the environment in which the horse is maintained be responsible for the development of the respiratory disease? The type of diet (hay, pelleted rations, pasture), the nature of the bedding materials (straw, peat, shavings), and the amount of time the horse spends stabled are important considerations in establishing the allergic nature of some respiratory disorders such as heaves. Respiratory conditions that appear to be correlated with seasonal or environmental changes may have allergic components. The deworming and vaccination schedules should also be ascertained. Young horses are at risk for developing verminous pneumonia secondary to *Parascaris equorum* migration. Nematode eggs are able to survive for prolonged periods of time once established on a pasture. If the horse is a performance animal and at high risk for the development of upper respiratory tract infections, one should determine how frequently equine influenza and equine herpesvirus type 1 (EHV-1) and type 4 (EHV-4) vaccinations are administered.

Prior Medical Problems. Has the horse had a previous history of illness or trauma that might be related to the present complaint? Viral respiratory conditions often precede the development of bacterial pneumonia. Sequelae to *S. equi* infections include internal abscessation, guttural pouch empyema, and retropharyngeal abscesses, which may ultimately affect the respiratory system in various ways. Trauma may be implicated in the development of diaphragmatic hernias, pneumothorax, or tracheal injury and subsequent stricture formation.

Present Problem. Questions are directed at defining the exact problem, at establishing the chronicity of the disorder and the rapidity of its development. Was the problem insidious in onset or is it an acute disorder of less than 2 weeks' duration? Was the onset associated with a "stressful" event such as a race or a prolonged van ride? Were there any major alterations in husbandry practices? For example, is the horse now pastured with donkeys or mules (lungworms)? Were there new arrivals on the farm that were not adequately quarantined? The effect of the respiratory complaint on the expected athletic performance is also determined. Are clinical signs evident during eupneic (resting) breathing or do they only become noticeable during the hyperpnea of exercise? Has the horse received any medication and was there any improvement in the clinical condition? Amelioration of signs during therapy suggests that the previous treatment protocols were not of sufficient duration or that an underlying immunodeficiency exists.

Thus, the history remains an important initial step in determining the nature and cause of the respiratory problem and should be thorough.

The Physical Examination

Prior to examination of the horse, it is helpful to simply step back and evaluate the horse's demeanor and mental status (alert or depressed), posture, and manner of movement. Has it adopted a particular stance (extended head and neck) or is it reluctant to move because of pain (pleurodynia)? Are there obvious changes in the pattern of breathing from the normal eupneic state (Table 6–1)? Is the breathing pattern rapid and shallow? Is there a pronounced expiratory effort accompanied by nostril flaring? The normal respiratory rate of the adult horse varies from 8 to 15 breaths per minute, with a slightly noticeable abdominal component during expiration (an active process in the horse).

Abnormalities of the respiratory system are further evidenced by the production of unusual sounds associated with respiration; the presence of a cough; a nasal or ocular discharge; the existence of lymphadenopathy; epistaxis; facial, pharyngeal, or cervical swellings; and cyanotic mucous membranes. Ataxia or reluctance to move, the presence of ventral thoracic or limb edema, foul odors associated with breathing, and a history of weight loss may all occur with respiratory disorders.

The air flow from both nostrils is assessed to rule out potential obstructions or masses within the nasal cavity. Atheromas, which may restrict air flow, especially during exercise, can be detected with palpation of the false nostrils. Any peculiar breath odors can be detected at this time. Percussion of the frontal and maxillary sinuses, performed by gently tapping over the sinuses while the horse's mouth is held slightly open, may reveal dullness due to accumulations of fluid or inflammatory products, but the absence of a percussable change does not eliminate sinus disorders. Evidence of swelling in the intermandibular space (lymphadenopathy) or in the pharyngeal (guttural pouch or retropharyngeal disorders) and cervical areas (accessory lungs[4]) is determined. Palpation of the larynx and trachea is routinely performed and should not elicit paroxysmal coughing episodes in the normal horse. Evidence of muscle atrophy or prior surgeries (laryngoplasty, laryngotomy, myotomy) are also detected during the physical examination of the upper respiratory tract. Check for patency of the jugular veins (thrombophlebitis and secondary pulmonary abscessation) or for evidence of perivascular injections which may contribute to upper respiratory tract obstructions by their involvement of the recurrent laryngeal nerve or vagosympathetic trunks.

A complete physical examination should then be conducted with attention paid to all organ systems (and not simply focused on the respiratory system). In respiratory emergencies, an abbreviated initial examination is conducted and efforts are directed at patient stabilization until that time when a more thorough physical can be conducted.

Auscultation of the Lung Fields

Evaluation of the thoracic cavity should be performed in a quiet area, free of distractions and conversation! Examine the horse both during quiet breathing and while it is hyperpneic (by use of a rebreathing bag). The examination should be conducted in a systematic fashion. Standardization of lung sound terminology has been advocated to obtain a better appreciation of the pathophysiology of the disorder as well as to improve communication among colleagues.

Normal breath sounds are the sounds produced by turbulent air movement through the tracheobronchial tree and will vary in intensity and quality depending upon the portion of the lung field auscultated. They are quietest over the middle and diaphragmatic lung lobes, where the term *vesicular sounds* has been used, but are loudest over the trachea and the base of the lung, where they are referred to as *bronchial*

Table 6–1. Breathing Patterns

Eupnea   The normal quiet and seemingly effortless breathing pattern adopted by the healthy horse at rest. Both inspiration and expiration in the horse are active processes.

Tachypnea   A breathing pattern characterized by rapid frequency and shallow depth or small tidal volume.

Hyperpnea   A breathing pattern characterized by an increase in the depth and rate of breathing, as might be found during exercise.

Apnea   A period of time in which there is no discernible respiratory effort and air flow has ceased. May accompany sleep-related disorders or excessive ventilation (hypocapnia-induced apnea).

Hypoventilation   A pattern of breathing that alters gas exchange sufficiently to cause hypercapnia or elevations of arterial carbon dioxide tension.

Hyperventilation   A pattern of breathing that increases alveolar ventilation and results in arterial hypocapnia.

Dyspnea   A breathing pattern that appears to reflect difficulty in breathing. The animal appears to be distressed and an increased work of breathing is obvious.

sounds.[5–7] In the normal horse, breath sounds may be more easily heard on the right side than the left. There may be considerable variation between normal patients in the intensity of the breath sounds. For example, vesicular sounds are often barely audible during eupneic (normal) breathing in the obese patient and are perceived as soft rustling sounds. However, breath sounds may be easily heard in the thin or young animal because its chest wall attenuates sounds less effectively than that of the obese horse. The intensity of breath sounds also increases with increases in air flow velocity. Thus, breath sounds are accentuated in febrile or excited animals or in animals hyperpneic from a variety of causes (exercise, hypoxia, acidemia). However, auscultatory findings do not always correlate well with the degree of alveolar ventilation.[6] This is especially evident in cases of lung consolidation where transmission of breath sounds from adjacent areas gives the false impression that that region is well ventilated.[6] Breath sounds may also become more difficult to hear in cases of (1) alveolar overinflation in which the aerated tissue of the lung is a poor conduction medium of sound or (2) pneumothorax and pleural effusions in which the sound is reflected at the pleural surface (acoustic impedance).[6]

Adventitious lung sounds are abnormal sounds superimposed upon the normal breath sounds and have been described as crackles or wheezes. Crackles are short, explosive, discontinuous sounds that have been likened to the sound of salt thrown in a hot frying pan or the sound of cellophane being crumpled. They are usually of low intensity and heard during the inspiratory phase of respiration. Their production has been attributed to the sudden equalization of pressure in two compartments after airways have reopened. Crackles are heard in cases of interstitial pneumonia and pulmonary edema (restrictive pulmonary diseases), as well as in cases of bronchopneumonia or airway diseases (obstructive disorders). Crackles may also be produced by breathing 100% oxygen as the nitrogen stent maintaining alveolar distention is eliminated.[8] Crackles are also heard in cases of subcutaneous emphysema. Wheezes are musical sounds thought to arise from the vibration of airway walls or tissue masses in close contact with the airway walls and may be heard during either inspiration or expiration. Wheezes may be monophonic or polyphonic, the latter indicative of multiple sites of airway obstruction. Pleuritic friction rubs have been described as "sandpaper-like sounds" generated by the movement of the visceral and parietal pleurae across each other. They may (infrequently) be detected in the early stages of "dry" pleuritis, prior to the effusive stage.

Percussion of the Thorax

Percussion is achieved by methodically tapping over the intercostal spaces of the thoracic cavity using a plexor and pleximeter (foals) or a large spoon and neurologic hammer (adults) and evaluating the nature of the sound produced. Aerated tissues produce a sound described as resonant compared to fluid-filled structures (bowel, heart) which produce a dull sound. As the sound quality changes during percussion from dorsoventrad or craniocaudad, a small mark or piece of tape is placed at the transitional site. The limits of the percussed field are compared with those of the normal horse.

The cranial limit is the shoulder musculature, the dorsal limit is the back musculature, and the caudoventral limits are the 17th intercostal space at the level of the tuber coxae, the 16th intercostal space at the level of the tuber ischii, the 13th intercostal space at the midthorax, the 11th intercostal space at the level of the scapulohumeral articulation, and the 6th intercostal space at the olecranon.[9] The technique of percussion is not painful and resentment by the horse may be indicative of a thoracic disorder (pleurodynia). The most common finding in equine respiratory cases is ventral dullness suggestive of pleural effusion, pleural thickening, lung consolidation, or pericardial effusion. Occasionally, expanded borders may be percussed suggestive of alveolar overinflation, which may accompany recurrent airway disease.

Endoscopy

Fiberoptic endoscopy provides an invaluable means of assessing the upper respiratory and proximal lower respiratory tract of the horse. It is helpful in (1) establishing the origin of respiratory noises that accompany laryngeal hemiplegia, dorsal displacement of the soft palate, aryepiglottic fold entrapment, rostral displacement of the palatopharyngeal arches, tracheal collapse or stenosis, and pharyngeal narrowing; (2) establishing the existence of congenital defects such as subepiglottic cysts, cleft palate, or choanae atresia; (3) localizing the site of exudate or hemorrhage formation as might occur with guttural pouch mycosis or empyema, ethmoidal hematoma, pulmonary epistaxis, retropharyngeal abscessation, and chronic pulmonary disease; and (4) extracting foreign bodies from the tracheobronchial tree. With the development of equine performance centers, videoendoscopic examination of the upper respiratory tract during maximal exercise (12–14 m/sec) is now becoming routine and is well tolerated by most performance horses. Dynamic collapse of the upper airway structures may be visualized while the horse performs at maximal exercise intensities. Accumulations of mucopurulent exudate within the pharynx or the trachea during exercise are suggestive of chronic pulmonary disease. Endoscopy is also a useful means of obtaining tracheobronchial aspirates (guarded swabs or catheters), thus eliminating the potential complications that may accompany percutaneous aspirations.[10] A number of different fiberoptic endoscope models are available but an 11-mm (outer diameter, OD) endoscope is usually used in adult horses and a smaller, 7.8-mm (OD) pediatric scope is recommended for foals. The reader is referred to an excellent source on equine endoscopy for further details.[11]

Sampling of Respiratory Tract Secretions

Centesis of the Paranasal Sinuses. This should be performed when radiographic examination reveals fluid lines or soft tissue densities. The contents of the sinuses may be aspirated by using aseptic technique and local anesthesia. Sedation of the horse may be indicated. A Steinmann pin is useful for the initial puncture of the sinus. The rostral maxillary sinus is entered at a site 2.5 cm dorsal to the facial crest and 2.5 cm caudal to the infraorbital foramen. The caudal maxillary sinus (which communicates with the frontal sinus) is entered at a site 2.5 cm dorsal to the facial crest and 2.5 cm rostral to the medial canthus. Aspirates should be submitted for cytologic examination and bacterial culture.

Guttural Pouch Catheterization and Culture of the Exudate. Catheterization is useful in cases of empyema or distention of the pouches by accumulations of exudate. While the horse is sedated, a fiberoptic endoscope is passed into the guttural pouch using either the biopsy instrument or a Chambers catheter as a guidewire for the endoscope. A culture of the exudate may be obtained with a triple-guarded catheter or protected swab. Caution must be exercised in the selection of patients. Horses suspected of having guttural pouch epistaxis should be catheterized very carefully as the blood clot may become dislodged, predisposing them to a fatal hemorrhagic episode. In some cases it may be best to not catheterize the pouch.

Sampling of Tracheobronchial Secretions. Several techniques have been advocated for obtaining tracheobronchial samples. The site of the collection sample (tracheal vs. bronchoalveolar) will depend upon the nature of the respiratory disorder being investigated. For example, the appropriateness of using tracheal samples to evaluate chronic pulmonary disorders has recently been challenged since little correlation between tracheal and bronchoalveolar lavage cytology or between tracheal and pulmonary histopathologic findings was found to exist.[12, 13] In contrast, a good correlation between bronchoalveolar lavage cytology and pulmonary histopathologic findings has been determined by Fogarty.[14] Bronchoalveolar lavage is indicated in the investigation of chronic pulmonary disorders, but may be performed in conjunction with transtracheal aspirates if an infectious process cannot be dismissed. Representative cytologies from bronchoalveolar lavage studies of normal horses are shown in Table 6–2. Sedation of horses prior to bronchoalveolar lavage is recommended. Using either a fiberoptic endoscope (permitting direct visualization of the lung segment to be lavaged) or using a thick-walled flexible tube with a cuffed end (which is passed blindly into the distal airways), 100 to 300 mL of physiologic saline solution is instilled within the pulmonary segment. Approximately 50% to 75% of the fluid can be retrieved and examined cytologically.

In the absence of a suitable method for collecting bronchoalveolar lavage fluid aseptically, tracheobronchial aspirates remain the method of choice for investigation of infectious lower respiratory tract disorders. Collection of culture samples by fiberoptic endoscopy simplifies the procedure and eliminates some of the complications formerly associated with the transtracheal technique, such as cellulitis and pneumomediastinum. Both guarded tracheal swabs[17] and the protected aspiration catheter of Darien[10] are convenient and reliable techniques for obtaining representative samples.

Characterization of the normal bacterial isolates from tracheobronchial aspirates in healthy horses has been well documented.[18] When examining a horse with suspected respiratory disease, one must evaluate culture results in the light of the cytologic findings and clinical examination. For example, the tracheobronchial aspirates of approximately 8% of normal horses (either pastured or stabled) were found to be culture-positive for *Klebsiella*, β-hemolytic streptococci, *Pasteurella* species, and *Pseudomonas aeruginosa*. However, for a microorganism to be implicated in a lower airway disorder, one would expect (1) to obtain a moderate to heavy growth of the organism on culture, (2) to identify organisms within phagocytic cells, and (3) to have evidence of degenerative neutrophils. In contrast, anaerobes, which are a normal component of the flora of the upper respiratory tract (cranial to the larynx), are not normally grown from aspirates of healthy horses, which emphasizes their importance when recovered from respiratory cases. Based upon their studies, Sweeney and colleagues[18] have also described a group of transient bacterial flora of questionable pathogenicity such as *Enterobacter, Bacillus, Acinetobacter,* α-hemolytic streptococci (except for *Streptococcus pneumoniae* type 3), and *Staphylococcus epidermidis,* which may be isolated from tracheobronchial aspirates. In contrast, *S. pneumoniae* is gaining recognition as a potential pathogen of the respiratory tract in horses.[19–21] Fungal hyphae may be found either free or engulfed within mononuclear cells.

Radiography

Radiographs remain a useful diagnostic aid in the investigation of upper respiratory tract disorders, permitting (1) the detection of soft tissue masses (abscesses, granulomas, neoplasia, hematomas, polyps) or fluid accumulations within the paranasal sinuses, the nasal cavity proper, the guttural pouches, and the retropharyngeal areas; and (2) the evaluation of orofacial deformations secondary to congenital nasal septal or premaxillary deviations or fractures secondary to trauma. Assessment of the anatomical dimensions of the pharyngeal and laryngeal structures (thickened soft palate, hypoplastic epiglottis, hyoid bone fractures) can also be done radiographically. When nasal or sinus disorders are suspected, both lateral and dorsoventral views should be taken. Oblique views may also be helpful in accentuating

---

Table 6–2. Differential Counts in Bronchoalveolar Lavage Fluid (% of Total WBC Count ± SE or SD)

Neutrophils	Macrophages	Lymphocytes	Eosinophils	Mast Cells	Epithelial	Reference
8.9 ± 1.2	45.0 ± 2.8	43.0 ± 2.7	<1.0	1.2 ± 0.3	3.5 ± 0.7	12
5.0 ± 4.0	72 ± 10	18 ± 3.0	2.0 ± 4.0	1.0 ± 1.4	—	14
6.2 ± 5.0	70.3 ± 15.2	7.6 ± 3.9	1.0 ± 1.4	0.6 ± 1.4	14.3 ± 13.4	15
6.2 ± 2.4	48.5 ± 2.5	35.3 ± 2.5	2.5 ± 0.9	5.2 ± 0.8	2.3 ± 1.4	16

the area of interest. Proper restraint and positioning of the cassette can usually be achieved with xylazine, detomidine, or butorphanol sedation.

Radiographic evaluation of the equine thorax remains preferable to ultrasonography for the detection of diffuse parenchymal disease such as interstitial pneumonia, pulmonary edema, and chronic airway disorders, or for the detection of mediastinal or deep parenchymal abscesses.[22] Three to four overlapping lateral radiographs are needed to image the thorax of the standing horse. However, compared with human or small animal medicine, where there are well-established correlations between the pulmonary disorder and the radiographic findings, the radiographic changes in equine respiratory disorders tend to be rather nonspecific. In addition, many pulmonary diseases, such as bronchitis, exercise-induced pulmonary hemorrhage, and chronic recurrent airway disease, are often associated with normal radiographs.[23]

Four types of patterns have been described radiographically and include alveolar (airspace), interstitial, bronchial, and vascular patterns. It is important for the reader to gain some appreciation for the type of radiographic lung patterns in order to more fully understand the disease mechanisms. Alveolar patterns are represented by opaque areas that coalesce and completely obliterate the vessels and bronchi. This type of pattern occurs with pulmonary edema, hemorrhage, lung consolidation, or neoplastic infiltration. Air bronchograms are rarely seen in the adult horse with respiratory disease. Interstitial patterns are the most commonly found patterns associated with a variety of conditions. This pattern causes a blurring of the edges of the pulmonary vessels, a diffuse increase in lung opacity, and variable reticular, linear, or nodular opacities.[23, 24] A reticular pattern is found with viral, bacterial, or parasitic pneumonia; pulmonary edema; or fibrosis. An irregular linear pattern is seen with resolving bronchopneumonia and a nodular pattern occurs with abscesses, granulomas, or metastasis. Bronchial patterns alone are not commonly found but usually occur in association with interstitial patterns. Paired linear opacities or numerous small circular opacities represent thickening of the large and medium-sized airways or of the septa around the lobules. This pattern is found in cases of equine bronchitis and bronchiolitis. A vascular pattern is due to variations in the size, shape, and number of the pulmonary vessels and may be seen in horses following exercise or in horses with left-to-right cardiac shunts.

Extraparenchymal disorders evident radiographically include the presence of free pleural fluid or the presence of free gas (pneumothorax) represented by the separation of the right or left or both caudal lung lobes from the dorsal and dorsolateral body wall by a free-air density.

Ultrasonography

Diagnostic, therapeutic, and prognostic evaluation of peripheral parenchymal lung or pleural disorders may be assisted by thoracic ultrasonography. Unlike thoracic radiography, which requires technology limited to specialty practices or veterinary medical teaching hospitals, ultrasonography is a method readily available to the practicing veterinarian. It is considered to be superior to thoracic radiography in the detection of pleural effusion, pulmonary consolidation, or

abscess formation[22] and should be performed when clinical examination or thoracic percussion reveals pain and areas of dullness within the thorax. In ultrasonography, piezoelectric crystals housed within a transducer transmit sound waves at high frequencies through soft tissues. When a change in the tissue density occurs, the sound waves are reflected, detected by the piezoelectric crystals, and an image is produced.[25] The depth of penetration and the degree of image resolution is a function of the frequency of sound generation (e.g., 3-MHz vs. 7.5-MHz transducer) as well as of the relationship of the beam direction to the structures to be imaged.

Normal lung tissue reflects the ultrasound beam, producing an echogenic pulmonary periphery (thin white line) and reverberation artifacts or concentric equidistant echoes. Normal pleural fluid appears as an anechoic (black) area separating the parietal pleura from the lung tissue and a small amount of pleural fluid is commonly detected in the ventral thorax of racehorses.[26] In respiratory disorders, accentuated amounts of anechoic or hypoechoic (gray) pleural fluid may be detected. The character of the pleural fluid, the presence of fibrin or gas, the degree of loculation, and the existence of pleural adhesions can be determined during the examination.[27] Pulmonary abscesses appear ultrasonographically as encapsulated cavitated areas filled with fluid or echogenic (white) material, while areas of pulmonary consolidation appear as dense patterns of homogeneous internal echoes with a gray-tone quality.[27] Depending upon the degree of consolidation, bronchial and vascular structures may become more easily visualized on the sonogram.[25] Mediastinal masses may also be visualized using ultrasonography. Detection of caudal mediastinal masses is improved when there is concurrent pleural effusion, as the aerated caudal lungs impair examination. Masses located in the cranial mediastinum can often be visualized at the third right intercostal space in the absence of pleural effusions.[25] Thus, ultrasonography is useful for (1) the localization of fluid lines or areas of pulmonary consolidation, abscessation, and thoracic neoplasia; (2) the proper selection of thoracocentesis or biopsy sites; and (3) the placement of indwelling catheters in fluid pockets with loculation.

Diagnostically, there are certain limitations inherent in the technique of ultrasonography. A deep parenchymal lesion may not be detected if the overlying aerated lung reflects the ultrasound beam. In addition, cases of pneumothorax may be difficult to identify because the free air in the dorsal thorax and the aerated ventral lung appear ultrasonographically similar.[22] Ultrasonography is also used prognostically. The detection of free gas echoes (associated with anaerobic bacterial infections), extensive fibrinous tags, or areas of loculations within the pleural fluid are associated with a poorer prognosis requiring a more extensive therapeutic regimen.[28] For further information, the reader is referred to several reviews describing the technique of ultrasonography and the normal findings.[22, 26, 27, 29]

Thoracocentesis

Sampling of the pleural fluid by means of thoracocentesis is utilized for diagnostic, prognostic, and therapeutic benefits. Abnormal pleural fluid accompanies numerous respiratory disorders, including pulmonary abscessation (pleuropneumonia), chronic pneumonia, systemic mycoses, neoplasia (lymphosarcoma, gastric squamous cell carcinoma), pulmonary granulomas, and equine infectious anemia.[30] The technique is easily performed at the sixth or seventh intercostal space approximately 10 cm dorsal to the olecranon by aseptically inserting a teat cannula through an anesthetized site in the intercostal space, just cranial to the border of the rib. To reduce the amount of air aspirated into the pleural cavity, a three-way stopcock is attached to the cannula. Both sides of the thorax should be sampled and the aspirate submitted for cytologic and microbiological examination. Up to 100 mL of pleural fluid may be obtained, although smaller amounts (10–30 mL) are more routine.[30] Normal pleural aspirates contain less than 10,000 nucleated cells per microliter, 60% of which are neutrophils, and up to 3 g/dL of protein. Samples should be cultured both aerobically and anaerobically. Fluid with a putrid odor is associated with anaerobic bacteria and carries a less favorable prognosis for the horse.[31] The type of fluid, for example, an exudate vs. a transudate, is helpful in the diagnosis. Transudates contain less than 3.0 mg/dL of protein with a pleural fluid:serum protein ratio of less than 0.5, and have a specific gravity of less than 1.016. Exudates contain greater than 3.0 mg/dL of protein, have pleural fluid:serum protein ratios greater than 0.5, and specific gravity greater than 1.016.

Nuclear Medicine Imaging

Scintigraphy, or nuclear medicine imaging, is a specialized technique available at some university and practice facilities. Using gamma-emitting radioisotopes such as krypton 81m or technetium 99m, pulmonary ventilation and perfusion can be assessed in the horse.[32, 33] Aerosolized technetium particles generated by a nebulizer are inhaled by the horse breathing through a closed circuit. Aerosolized particles are of sufficiently small diameter to be deposited in the alveoli and small airways. Thus, their distribution mirrors ventilation. The sites of deposition within the lung fields are recorded by a gamma camera. For the perfusion scan, technetium-labeled macroaggregated albumin is injected intravenously. The large protein particles lodge in the blood capillaries of the lung enabling imaging of the pulmonary perfusion by the gamma camera. Hence, lung scintigraphy permits evaluation of regional ventilation:perfusion ($\dot{V}/\dot{Q}$) relationships not possible radiographically or ultrasonographically. Scintigraphic images may provide additional insights into the diagnosis and pathogenesis of such disorders as chronic obstructive pulmonary disease or exercise-induced pulmonary hemorrhage (EIPH) or in the evaluation of the horse with poor performance.[34, 35] For example, in horses with EIPH, there appears to be a perfusion deficit in the caudodorsal lung lobe which results in a high ventilation:perfusion area.[34] Horses with chronic obstructive pulmonary disease may produce several patterns, including ventilation:perfusion deficits in the costophrenic angle (caudoventral diaphragmatic margin), ventilation deficits in the mid-dorsal lung area, or patterns similar to those seen in EIPH.[36] In addition to the assessment of pulmonary ventilation and perfusion, tracheal mucus transport can be evaluated scintigraphically by intratracheal injection of technetium. This is performed by timed assessment of the movement of the radioactive

bolus over a given tracheal distance.[37, 38] Normal values for the unsedated horse range from 16.6 to 20.7 mm/min. Further studies are needed to examine alterations in tracheal mucus transport during disease. For further information, the reader is referred to additional reviews.[36]

Pulmonary Function Testing

The idea of pulmonary function testing in the resting horse is not new, having been well described in a review by Willoughby and McDonell.[39] Measurements of lung volumes, pleural (esophageal) pressure changes, and air flow rates, coupled with nitrogen washout studies and arterial blood gas determinations, have been utilized in the assessment of horses with chronic pulmonary disease (small airway disease). Pulmonary function tests require that a cooperative subject wear a tightly fitting breathing apparatus to which an air flow meter has been attached. Pleural pressure changes occurring during each breath are estimated by catheters placed in the midesophagus, exteriorized through the nares, and attached to pressure transducers. By integrating the air flow rates, the inspiratory and expiratory volumes are obtained. Additional parameters obtained from measurements of air flow include inspiratory and expiratory times, breathing frequency, and peak air flow rates. In general, the simple measurement of tidal volume, breathing frequency, or minute volume (the product of tidal volume and breathing frequency) provide limited information regarding the functionality of the lung, as these values tend to be maintained near normal limits until the respiratory disease is quite advanced.[40]

Measures of lung distensibility (dynamic compliance) and airway obstruction (pulmonary resistance) provide more meaningful information regarding pulmonary health. Dynamic compliance (C_{dyn}) is measured by dividing the tidal volume by the change in pleural pressure occurring between the start and end of inhalation. Pulmonary resistance (R_L) is measured by several different techniques depending upon whether the resistance is measured at peak air flow or at specific ventilatory volumes (e.g., 50% tidal volume). Generally, it is obtained by dividing the air flow by the change in pleural (esophageal) pressure. Alterations in these two values can provide information on the nature of the lung disorder. For example, in obstructive disorders of the tracheobronchial tree, usually dynamic compliance decreases and pulmonary resistance increases. A decrease in dynamic compliance in the absence of a change in pulmonary resistance suggests that the lung parenchyma has been stiffened by alveolar disease or by obstruction of the peripheral bronchioles. (Recall that peripheral bronchioles, owing to their immense cross-sectional area, contribute little to the resistance of breathing until the disorder is well advanced.) Conversely, an increase in pulmonary resistance in the absence of a change in dynamic compliance suggests that the obstruction exists in the upper airway, trachea, or bronchus.[41]

Pulmonary function testing of *exercising* horses and its use in the assessment of the "poor performer" is a relatively new approach in equine respiratory physiology. With the availability of high-speed treadmills and the ability to measure high flow rates during exercise,[42] analysis of tidal volume, breathing frequency, dynamic compliance, lung resistance, end-expiratory lung volume, and flow-volume and pressure-volume loops may provide additional insights into the cause of the poor performance. However, these measurements require the use of catheters that have adequate frequency response times and that are exactly in phase with ventilatory measuring devices. In addition, breathing masks must be constructed in such a way to prevent resistance to air flow or rebreathing of expired carbon dioxide. Lastly, measurements of inertance, previously ignored in respiratory mechanics measurements at rest, may become an important consideration in the calculation of respiratory mechanics during high-intensity exercise. Yet once these difficulties are overcome, the measurements will undoubtedly improve our diagnostic capabilities in the assessment of respiratory tract disorders in the performance horse. We may address such important questions as whether the horse with subclinical bronchitis or bronchiolitis experiences mechanical limitation of expiratory flow rates at exercise intensities much less than the normal or whether hyperinflation of the lung due to small airway disease predisposes to the development of diaphragmatic fatigue.

Lung Biopsy

A histopathologic diagnosis of certain lower respiratory tracts may prove useful in the therapeutic management of certain lung disorders. The methodology and application of this technique in equine medicine was described by Raphel and Gunson[43] and is usually without major complications. A biopsy instrument is inserted aseptically through the seventh or eighth intercostal space, approximately 8 cm above a horizontal line through the scapulohumeral articulation. The technique is not recommended in patients that are tachypneic, dyspneic, or exhibiting uncontrollable coughing or in horses suffering from bleeding disorders or compromised cardiopulmonary function. Hemoptysis occurred in 10% of the cases but was self-limiting.

DISORDERS OF THE UPPER RESPIRATORY TRACT

Sinus Disorders

Sinusitis

Anatomical Considerations. There are six pairs of sinuses that communicate with the nasal cavity in the horse: the dorsal, middle, and ventral conchal and the maxillary, frontal, and sphenopalatine.[44] The conchal sinuses, extensions of the turbinates, communicate with either the frontal (dorsal conchal) or maxillary sinuses (middle and ventral conchal). However, most clinically important conditions involve the maxillary and frontal sinuses.[45] The sinuses are lined by a respiratory epithelium—pseudostratified ciliated columnar—interspersed with goblet cells and underlying serous glands.[46]

The maxillary sinus is divided into a rostral and caudal compartment by a bony oblique septum. In most horses, the division is complete so that there is no communication between the two compartments. Each compartment communicates with the middle nasal meatus by the nasomaxillary opening, a narrow slit that is easily occluded during in-

flammation of the mucosa. This process leads to retention of exudate within the sinuses. In horses less than 5 years of age, the last three cheek teeth—the first, second, and third molars—occupy most of the maxillary sinus. As the horse ages and the residual root decreases, the sinus cavity enlarges. The larger frontal sinus communicates with the caudal compartment of the maxillary sinus via the frontomaxillary opening, thus establishing a natural drainage route of the frontal sinus with the nasal cavity.[47]

Etiology. Primary sinusitis or empyema reflects accumulation of exudate within the sinus cavities and is a sequela of viral or bacterial upper respiratory tract infections. Streptococcal (and rarely staphylococcal) organisms are the usual bacterial isolates.[48–50] Secondary sinusitis (empyema) of the maxillary sinus is usually associated with dental disorders such as fractured teeth, patent infundibula, and alveolar periostitis. The first molar is the most commonly involved tooth. However, secondary sinusitis may follow traumatic head injuries or the development of congenital paranasal cysts. The latter are usually found in the maxillary sinus but have also been identified in the frontal sinus.[50, 51] Neoplasms associated with secondary sinusitis include squamous cell carcinoma (most common), osteogenic sarcoma, lymphosarcoma, myxoma, osteoma, sarcoids, neurofibroma, and mast cell tumor.[49, 52, 53] Although relatively rare, fungal granulomas induced by *Cryptococcus neoformans* and *Coccidioides immitis* may cause secondary sinusitis.[54, 55] Progressive hematomas may also occur in the maxillary sinus.[52]

Clinical Signs. Clinical signs depend upon the inciting agent, its location, and the chronicity of the disorder. A unilateral nasal discharge suggests unilateral sinus involvement; a bilateral nasal exudate suggests that both the right and left sinuses are involved. Sinusitis secondary to dental disease or invasive neoplastic masses is characterized by a purulent foul-smelling and persistent nasal discharge, while a serosanguineous exudate is more typical of sinus cysts, slowly growing neoplasms, and certain stages of mycotic granulomas and hematomas. Inflammatory reactions of the skin, subcutaneous tissues, teeth, and bones may produce facial asymmetry. When sinus inflammation extends into the periorbital region, exophthalmos may ensue. Other clinical signs associated with sinusitis include difficult breathing, epistaxis, headshaking, weight loss, and neurologic signs if the sinusitis extends through the cribriform plate and causes meningoencephalitis.[45, 49]

Diagnosis. Diagnosis is based upon the history of the disorder, the age of the animal, and the nature of the clinical signs. Percussion of the sinuses may reveal dullness. Endoscopic examination helps to eliminate other potential sources of nasal discharge and demonstrates the presence of an exudate from the turbinate area proximal to the ethmoids. This strongly suggests that the exudate originates from the sinus compartment. Confirmation of the sinus disorder may be achieved by sinuscopy. A thorough oral examination of the upper dental arcade should always be conducted even if it requires short-acting anesthesia. The presence of fractured or displaced teeth, receding gum lines, exudate around a specific tooth, or patent infundibula are indications that den-

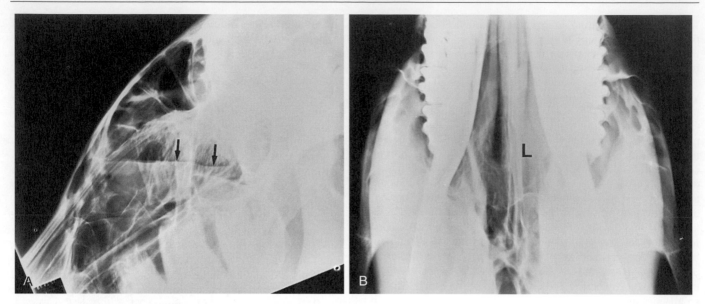

Figure 6–1. Five-year-old Thoroughbred with a 7-month history of left-sided nasal discharge. **A,** Air-fluid interface *(arrows)* in the caudal maxillary sinus on the lateral radiograph secondary to dental disease and consistent with maxillary sinusitis. **B,** Note increased soft tissue opacity in the left (L) maxillary sinus on the dorsoventral radiograph.

tal disease is the cause of the disorder.[45] Both lateral and dorsoventral radiographs are helpful in the diagnosis of sinusitis and may demonstrate single or multiple horizontal fluid-air interfaces, abnormalities of the teeth, lytic changes within the sinuses, or a combination of these[56] (Figs. 6–1 and 6–2). Neoplastic lesions may present radiographically as either loculated or diffuse soft tissue densities.[57] Culture and cytology of the sinus fluid or biopsy of the tissue mass is helpful in the diagnosis, although differentiating between a

neoplastic or dysplastic process or inflammatory reaction may be difficult.[57] Tumors may vary in consistency but usually have gelatinous areas mixed with combinations of cysts and solid tissue (fibrous tissue).[57]

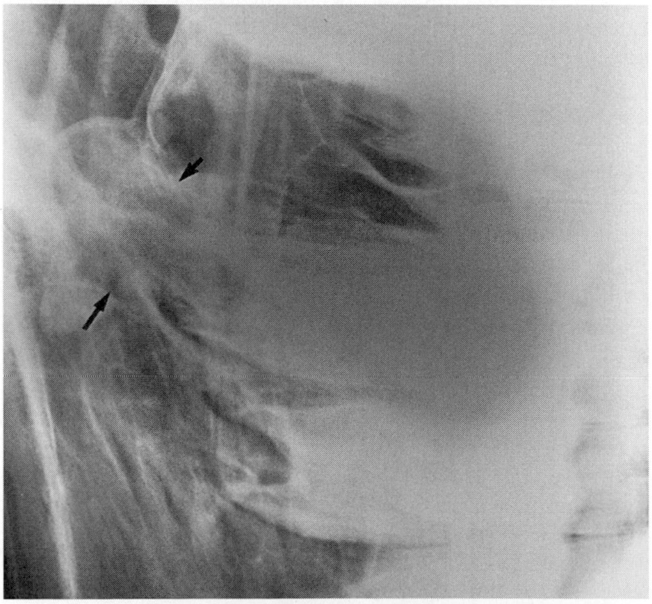

Treatment. Treatment requires surgical removal of the affected teeth, tumorous or granulomatous tissue, and establishment of adequate drainage. Extensive flushing of the sinuses has been recommended until the trephine sites have healed.[45] Surgical removal of paranasal cysts has been associated with a favorable prognosis,[51] whereas fungal granulomas warrant a poorer prognosis. Because of the potential public health danger, it has been recommended that horses with fungal granulomas be euthanized. Neoplastic lesions have a poor prognosis and a low rate of success is apparently achieved with either surgical resection or ablation owing to extensive infiltration of the neoplasm or recurrence of the tumor.[53, 57]

Ethmoid Hematomas

Definition. Ethmoid hematomas are encapsulated expansive angiomatous masses which appear to develop from the mucosal lining of the ethmoid conchae[58] but may also originate from the walls of the maxillary and frontal sinus. The inciting factor in their development is not known. Some have speculated that they develop secondary to chronic infection, repeated episodes of hemorrhage, or congenital or neoplastic conditions.[59] They appear bilaterally in 50% of the cases and are more prevalent in older horses.[58–60]

Clinical Signs. Clinical signs include intermittent unilateral discharge consisting of either frank blood, or serous or mucopurulent exudates. Stertorous breathing due to obstruction of nasal air flow may also occur.[58, 59] Other clinical signs

Figure 6–2. Lateral oblique radiograph of midmaxillary cheek teeth. The fourth cheek tooth had been previously removed. Sclerotic bony reaction *(arrows)* is noted surrounding the root of the third cheek tooth.

include facial swelling, exophthalmos, malodorous breath, headshaking, and coughing.[61]

Diagnosis. Diagnosis is based upon the clinical signs, endoscopic examination, and radiographic evaluation. A diagnosis is confirmed by histopathologic study of the removed tissue. On endoscopy, a yellow, yellow-green, yellow-gray, red to red-purple smooth glistening mass originating from the ethmoid region is observed.[58, 59] Petechial hemorrhages or surface erosions may also be noted. The mass may protrude beyond the nasal septum (and in those cases may cause a bilateral nasal discharge). Radiographs reveal a space-occupying soft tissue density with smooth margins. Single or multilobular rounded opacities may be observed radiographically in the ventral aspect of the caudal maxillary sinus superimposed upon the ethmoid turbinates. The ethmoid hematoma may in some cases extend dorsally into the frontal sinus[56] (Fig. 6–3).

Treatment. Treatment is surgical ablation by curettage, cryosurgery, or photoablation. The removal is associated with extensive hemorrhage and blood transfusions may be required during surgery; a preoperative crossmatch is warranted. A tracheotomy may be required postoperatively if extensive packing of the nasal cavity with rolled gauze is performed. Antimicrobials and anti-inflammatory agents are indicated. Following removal, approximately 30% to 50% of the hematomas recur,[58, 59] although in a recent retrospective study by Greet,[60] recurrence of the ethmoidal hematomas was noted only in 22% of the cases. Postoperative complications have been reported and include facial wound dehiscence, suture periostitis, facial bone sequestration, persistent nasal discharges, fungal sinus plaque formation, and encephalitis.[62]

Guttural Pouch Disorders

Anatomical Considerations. The guttural pouches are caudoventral diverticula of the auditory tube whose functions remain undefined! Each pouch, the capacity of which approximates 300 mL, is divided into a medial and lateral compartment by the invagination of the stylohyoid bone. The mucosal lining of each pouch is secretory, being covered by ciliated pseudostratified epithelium with goblet cells and glands.[63] The mucosal lining is generally thinner than that found in the nasopharynx. It also contains small aggregates of subepithelial lymphocytic tissue.[46] Thus, disorders of the guttural pouch may be manifested by catarrh. However, more important, disorders often induce dysfunctions of the surrounding neural structures, cranial nerves VII, IX, X, XI, and XII and the sympathetic trunk, or manifest as involvement of vascular structures, the internal carotid artery, the external carotid artery, and the maxillary artery.

Guttural Pouch Tympany

Definition. This is a nonpainful distention of the guttural pouch with air, visualized as an external swelling in the parotid region. It is primarily seen in young foals, although horses up to 20 months of age may be evaluated for this disorder.[64] It appears to be more prevalent in fillies than in colts.

Pathogenesis. The cause of the air accumulation within the pouch is not known. It has been proposed that an abnormal mucosal flap at the pharyngeal orifice functions as a unidirectional valve, trapping air or fluid within the pouch. However, it would appear to be more of a functional defect than an anatomical defect as no abnormality is visualized endoscopically or during surgical exploration.[65]

Clinical Signs. Clinical signs depend upon the degree of distention. If marked, the foal may exhibit stertorous breathing, nasal discharge, dysphagia, respiratory distress, or evidence of pneumonia secondary to aspiration. Regurgitation of milk from the nostrils may also be evident.[66] Endoscopic examination may reveal collapse of the nasopharyngeal area secondary to distention of the pouches.

Diagnosis. Diagnosis is confirmed by radiographic examination of the skull and pharynx. A large air-filled guttural pouch with or without fluid accumulation is noted (Fig. 6–4). The distinction as to whether the problem is unilateral or bilateral can be difficult. Aspiration of air from one guttural pouch should nearly correct the problem if a unilateral tympany exists. Dorsoventral radiographic views may also be helpful in detecting bilateral involvement.

Treatment. Guttural pouch tympany requires surgical correction. For unilateral tympany, surgical ablation of the median septum separating the two guttural pouches is performed. Bilateral involvement may necessitate resection of the excessive plica salpingopharyngeal flap.[67] As many cultures of the pouches yield β-hemolytic streptococci and the potential for the development of aspiration pneumonia exists, administration of antimicrobials is justified.[64] The prognosis for uncomplicated cases of guttural pouch tympany is favorable.

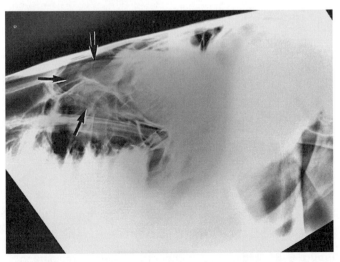

Figure 6–3. Ethmoidal hematoma. Note focal increased soft tissue opacity *(arrows)* adjacent to the ethmoids.

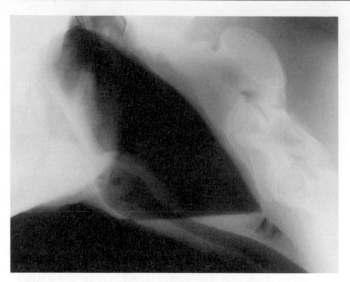

Figure 6–4. Guttural pouch tympany. Lateral radiograph of a 5-month-old Arabian colt demonstrating a markedly distended gas-filled guttural pouch.

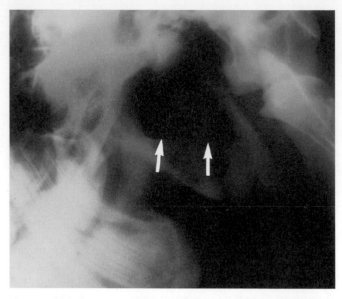

Figure 6–5. Guttural pouch empyema. Lateral radiograph showing a fluid line *(arrows)* or air-fluid interface within the guttural pouch.

Guttural Pouch Empyema

Definition. Empyema is an accumulation of exudate within the guttural pouches and it is usually a sequela of upper respiratory tract infections (streptococcal species). It may also result from the rupture of abscessed retropharyngeal lymph nodes into the pouches[66] or may accompany cases of guttural pouch tympany. The condition may be unilateral or bilateral.

Clinical Signs. Clinical signs include a white nonodorous nasal discharge (either unilateral or bilateral), lymphadenopathy, painful distention in the parotid region, stertorous breathing, dysphagia, and occasionally epistaxis.[66] Inspissation of the material may occur with chronic infections, forming masses called chondroids.

Diagnosis. Diagnosis is confirmed by radiographic examination. Radiographs demonstrate a fluid line or an opacity in the pouch (Fig. 6–5). Inspissated material may also be evident radiographically (Fig. 6–6). On endoscopic examination, a purulent material may be seen at the pharyngeal orifice of the eustachian tubes and within the medial or lateral compartments of the guttural pouches. Distortion of the pharynx may occur if distention is significant.

Treatment. Treatment may entail both medical and surgical modalities. Lavage of the guttural pouch with saline solutions and administration of systemic antimicrobials is an initial first step in therapeutic management. Surgery may be elected if medical therapy is unsuccessful or if the material within the guttural pouches is inspissated.[66]

Guttural Pouch Mycosis

Definition. This condition is manifest by the development of fungal plaques on the mucosal walls of the guttural pouches. The plaques are usually found at two sites, with the majority of them on the roof of the medial compartment and less frequently on the lateral wall of the lateral compartment of the pouch. The plaques are closely associated with the underlying vascular structures, the internal and external carotid arteries.[68]

Pathogenesis. The events leading to the formation of fungal plaques are not known. Some workers have suggested that aneurysmal dilatations of the vasculature, visualized radiographically,[69] may provide a suitable environment for fungal organisms to proliferate. Fungal colonization leads to erosion

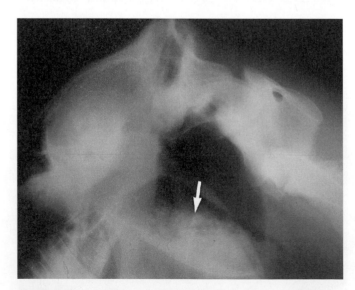

Figure 6–6. Guttural pouch chondroids. Lateral radiograph demonstrating irregular soft tissue opacities in the ventral guttural pouch outlined by gas *(arrow).*

of the underlying mucosa and vascular structures or inflammatory reactions of the surrounding nerves.

Clinical Signs. Clinical signs depend upon the integrity of the neural and vascular structures surrounding the guttural pouch. Horses may exhibit episodes of spontaneous epistaxis, dysphagia, nasal catarrh, laryngeal hemiplegia, Horner's syndrome, abnormal head extension, swelling in the parotid region, facial paralysis, mycotic encephalitis, and atlanto-occipital joint infections.[70]

Diagnosis. Diagnosis may be more difficult than has previously been advocated. The stress of handling the horse may precipitate fatal epistaxis. Attempts to visualize the interior of the pouch may be unsuccessful if blood obscures the visual field of the endoscope. There is the additional risk of dislodging a blood clot which had effected hemostasis.[68] Radiographs of the guttural pouch show evidence of fluid accumulation, of osteolytic changes in the stylohyoid bone, or suggestions of mycotic plaque formation. Angiographic demonstration of aneurysms of the internal or external carotid artery and endoscopic confirmation of secondary neuropathies support the diagnosis of guttural pouch mycoses.

Treatment. Treatment is dependent upon surgical occlusion of the affected vessels. Several different techniques have been advocated[68, 71–73] although complications, including ischemic optic neuropathy, have been reported.[74] Lane[68] has recommended that surgical treatment be combined with topical therapy (natamycin irrigation of the guttural pouch) and supportive care. Horses that have secondary neuropathies may need to be enterally supported via nasogastric intubation or esophagostomy. Medical treatment alone, with topical or parenteral antimycotic drugs, is not efficacious in eliminating the mycotic plaques.

Pharyngeal and Laryngeal Disorders
Lymphoid Hyperplasia

Definition. Acute inflammation of the pharynx accompanies upper respiratory tract infections from equine influenza, equine herpesvirus type 1, equine herpesvirus type 4, and *Streptococcus equi*.[75] Acute pharyngitis may also occur with prolonged placement of a nasogastric tube. Chronic inflammation of the pharynx, also termed *pharyngeal lymphoid hyperplasia, lymphoid follicular hyperplasia,* and *pharyngeal folliculitis,* is a condition frequently observed in young performance horses 2 to 3 years of age.[76]

Etiology. The cause of chronic pharyngitis is not known but probably is multifactorial. Many horses have a history of upper respiratory tract infections causing some clinicians to speculate that lymphoid hyperplasia is a sequela of chronic antigenic stimulation. The condition has been experimentally reproduced with inoculation of EHV-1 and EHV-2.[75, 77] However, the severity of the pharyngeal lymphoid hyperplasia is not correlated with the level of EHV-1 titers or with the isolation of EHV-2.[78] *Streptococcus zooepidemicus, Bordetella bronchiseptica,* and *Moraxella* species have been isolated from nasopharyngeal swabs of affected horses, but

their role in the development of the lymphoid hyperplasia is also unknown.[79, 80] In one study, the pharyngeal flora were similar in normal control horses and in those exhibiting grade I lymphoid hyperplasia. As the severity of the pharyngitis increased, the number of bacterial organisms that were isolated (colony-forming units per gram of swab material) also increased.[80]

Epidemiology. There appears to be an inverse relationship between the age of the horse and the prevalence of pharyngeal lymphoid hyperplasia. Approximately 60% to 90% of 2-year-olds exhibit a grade II or more (Table 6–3). Between 35% and 65% of 3- and 4-year-olds and 10% to 20% of 5-year-olds still show grade II or greater lymphoid hyperplasia. With aging, lymphoid follicles regress and tend to disappear.

Clinical Signs. Some horses may show a nasal discharge and mild submandibular lymphadenopathy. A cough may be induced with manipulation of the larynx. Unless severe, it has not been associated with poor performance or alterations in arterial blood gases.[81, 82]

Diagnosis. Endoscopically, one observes raised hyperemic and edematous follicles distributed throughout the nasopharyngeal walls. Some follicles may have an ulcerated edge to them; others may appear thickened and fibrotic. A gradation scheme based upon the severity of the nodule formation was proposed by Raker[83] and is outlined in Table 6–3. On histopathologic examination, there is a lymphocytic proliferation and necrosis,[81] the degree of which does not readily distinguish the grades observed endoscopically.[79]

Treatment. In the absence of a clear understanding of the pathogenesis of this disorder, numerous therapeutic modalities have been tried, including rest and topical administration of antimicrobial and anti-inflammatory solutions (nitrofurazone, dimethyl sulfoxide (DMSO) solution, and prednisolone acetate) or topical application of caustic agents

---

Table 6–3. Grading Scheme for Lymphoid Hyperplasia*

Grade I: A small number of inactive, white follicles scattered over the dorsal pharyngeal wall. The follicles are small and inactive, a normal finding in horses of all ages.

Grade II: Many small white and inactive follicles over the dorsal and lateral walls of the pharynx to the level of the guttural pouch. Numerous follicles that are larger, pink, and edematous are interspersed throughout.

Grade III: Many large pink follicles and some shrunken white follicles are distributed over the dorsal and lateral walls of the pharynx, in some cases extending onto the dorsal surface of the soft palate and into the pharyngeal diverticula.

Grade IV: More numerous pink and edematous follicles packed close together covering the entire pharynx, the dorsal surface of the soft palate and epiglottis, and the lining of the guttural pouches. Large accumulations appear as polyps.

*From Raker CW: The nasopharynx. In Mansmann RA, McAllister ES, eds: *Equine Medicine and Surgery.* Santa Barbara, Calif, Veterinary Publications, 1982, p 747.

to cauterize the follicles (50% trichloroacetic acid).[79] Other treatments include electrocautery and cryosurgery to induce the formation of a diphtheritic membrane which eventually sloughs within 2 weeks. Horses may be returned to training approximately 6 weeks later.[84]

Dorsal Displacement of the Soft Palate

Definition. During breathing, the soft palate normally occupies a position ventral to the epiglottis. This position is abruptly reversed during swallowing as the palate moves dorsally and the epiglottis covers the adducted arytenoid cartilages and vocal folds. These muscle activities insure that food or saliva is directed dorsally into the esophagus and not into the trachea.[85] The positioning of the palate is complex, controlled in part by the palatine, the tensor, and the levator muscles, which are innervated by the trigeminal, vagus, and glossopharyngeal nerves, respectively.[81] Intermittent or persistent malpositioning of the soft palate dorsal to the epiglottis is termed *dorsal displacement of the soft palate, soft palate paresis, soft palate elongation, soft palate hypertrophy,* and *dissociation.*[84, 86]

Etiology. Several mechanisms have been proposed to account for the displacement of the soft palate and include the untoward effects of inflammatory lesions of the pharynx (lymphoid hyperplasia, pharyngeal cysts), larynx (epiglottic hypoplasia, chondritis), and palate (ulcers, cysts) on the correct anatomical positioning of the soft palate.[79] Inflammatory lesions may predispose to the generation of excessive negative intrapharyngeal pressures causing dynamic collapse of the pharynx with subsequent laryngopalatal dissociation,[84] although recent data suggest that peak pharyngeal or tracheal pressures during maximal exercise are not different from normal horses which do not displace their soft palate.[87] Swallowing or opening of the mouth during exercise may also promote elevation of the soft palate above the epiglottis, allowing displacement to occur.[81] Another hypothesis suggests that excessive flexion of the head with narrowing of the nasopharyngeal opening predisposes to displacement by creating excessive negative pressure within the pharynx.[88] Others propose that epiglottic shortening and caudal retraction of the larynx by the sternothyrohyoideus muscle allows malpositioning of the soft palate.[85] Prior to the actual displacement, there appears to be a lowering of the pharyngeal roof, an elevation of the rostral portion of the soft palate, and a caudal retraction of the larynx.[79] Recent data suggest that many of these hypotheses are unfounded.

Pathogenesis. With dorsal displacement of the soft palate, there is a reduction in the cross-sectional area of the nasopharynx. This increases the resistance to air flow and may completely occlude the passageway, temporarily inducing asphyxia. This displacement creates an abnormal noise during both inspiration and expiration as the soft tissues vibrate.[81, 86] Because of the obstruction, air flow may be diverted through the mouth during expiration. A recent study of 10 horses exercising on a high-speed treadmill found that the time of displacement relative to exercise intensity was variable, occurring in two horses at peak speed, in two horses prior to obtaining peak speed, and in six horses as they started to slow down during the exercise protocol.[87] The time of displacement relative to the breathing-swallowing cycle was also variable, with displacement occurring during inspiration in three horses, during expiration in three horses, and was associated with a swallow in four horses.[87]

Clinical Signs. The production of sounds is loudest during expiration, resembling a gurgling noise. Exercise intolerance is a common complaint in the performance horse.

Diagnosis. Diagnosis is based upon a history of exercise intolerance, a description of respiratory stridor, and endoscopic evidence that the soft palate is displaced immediately after exercise. It is important to note that many horses examined at rest will appear normal. During endoscopic examination of the horse, sedation should be avoided. Endoscopy while the horse is exercised on a treadmill provides definitive evidence of the displacement. The serrated edges of the epiglottis and the vascular pattern are no longer visualized during the displacement. Some horses may also exhibit ulcerative lesions on the soft palate. Radiographs of the larynx may demonstrate a hypoplastic epiglottis, that is, one less than 7 cm in length. A thorough examination of the lower respiratory tract (e.g., auscultation, endoscopy) should be performed on these horses to rule out concomitant pulmonary disease.

Treatment. Treatment is variable and includes both medical and surgical approaches. One or two tongue ties may be used in an attempt to prevent caudal retraction of the larynx and subsequent displacement of the soft palate. A short course of nebulization therapy using a solution of 350 mL of liquid nitrofurazone (Furacin), 125 mL of DMSO, and 500 mg of prednisolone acetate (30 min/day for 7–10 days) may be helpful in cases of pharyngeal inflammation.[81] Other modalities include partial sternothyrohyoideus myectomy to prevent caudal retraction of the larynx, and staphylectomy; resection of the caudal margin of the soft palate, to increase the size of the ostium intrapharyngeum[86]; and epiglottic augmentation by injection of Teflon into the epiglottal submucosa.[89] The last procedure is performed through a ventral laryngotomy and may be combined with staphylectomy or sternothyrohyoideus myectomy.[84] Dorsal displacement of the soft palate is a difficult condition to treat: the success rate for the myectomy and staphylectomy approaches 50% to 60%.[90]

Rostral Displacement of the Palatopharyngeal Arches

Definition. In the horse, the soft palate terminates caudally at the confluence of the palatopharyngeal arches which cover the esophageal orifice.[86] In rostral displacement, the caudal pillars of the soft palate appear to be displaced forward, overlying the apices of the arytenoid cartilages. The condition was first described by Cook[91] in 1974, and has been subsequently diagnosed by others.

Etiology. The displacement of the palatopharyngeal arches is associated with malformation of the thyroid cartilage, and the cricopharyngeal and cricothyroid muscles. Goulden and colleagues[92] have speculated that the anomaly results from developmental defects of the fourth branchial arch, which normally forms the thyroid cartilage.

Pathogenesis. Both cartilaginous and muscular defects have been found in this condition. There is a deformation of the thyroid cartilage, a lack of the cricothyroid articulation, and often an absence or agenesis of the cricothyroid and cricopharyngeal muscles.[92, 93] Abnormal pharyngeal configurations prevent normal deglutition, predisposing to the development of aspiration pneumonia.

Clinical Signs. The condition may be present from birth. In severe cases, horses exhibit dysphagia, nasal discharge of food material, persistent coughing, belching, and abnormal inspiratory noise during exercise.[91, 92]

Diagnosis. The diagnosis is based upon the clinical signs and history but is confirmed with endoscopic examination. The rostrally displaced palatopharyngeal arches obscure the normal view of the arytenoid cartilages. Postmortem examination or surgical exploration of the larynx confirms the presence of developmental defects.

Treatment. There is no treatment since this represents a major deformation of the laryngeal structures. Most horses are euthanized.

Aryepiglottic Fold Entrapment

Definition. The aryepiglottic fold is the mucous membrane that extends from the lateral aspect of the arytenoid cartilages to the ventrolateral aspect of the epiglottis. Here it blends with the subepiglottic mucosa and the glossoepiglottic fold. In aryepiglottic fold entrapment, this membrane is either elevated over the margin of the epiglottis or it envelops the entire rostral aspect of the epiglottis.[86, 94]

Etiology. The cause is not completely understood. It may result from congenital epiglottic hypoplasia or it may be secondary to inflammation of the upper respiratory tract structures, including the palatopharyngeal arch and epiglottis.

Epidemiology. Aryepiglottic entrapment is predominantly seen in standardbred and Thoroughbred racehorses, with males and females equally affected.[95]

Pathogenesis. Ballooning of the entrapping membranes during respiration decreases the cross-sectional area of the pharynx and effectively obstructs the air flow.

Clinical Signs. Most horses will present with a complaint of exercise intolerance and make abnormal respiratory sounds such as choking or coughing during exercise. Since entrapment may be an intermittent finding, the persistence of the entrapment during exercise should be confirmed by endoscopic examination during exercise or immediately following completion of exercise.

Diagnosis. Diagnosis is based upon endoscopic examination.

The normal serrated margin of the epiglottis and the dorsal vascular pattern are obscured. The shape of the epiglottis can still be appreciated. Ulceration of the free margin of the fold and erosion of the entrapped epiglottis may be apparent.[79, 86] Hypoplasia of the epiglottis may be diagnosed both endoscopically and radiographically. The entrapment may also be visualized on lateral radiographs (Fig. 6–7).

Treatment. Surgical correction of the entrapment is required. A number of different approaches have been advocated. Resection or division of the tissue may be accomplished (1) under general anesthesia via pharyngotomy, laryngotomy, or by an oral approach; (2) transendoscopically, using a contact neodymium:yttrium-aluminum-garnet (Nd:YAG) laser; or (3) transnasally, using a hooked bistoury.[95, 96] Augmentation of the hypoplastic epiglottis by Teflon submucosal injections has been advocated to increase the bulk of the epiglottis and thus offset some of the structural defects which may predispose to entrapment.[89] This procedure is performed through a ventral laryngotomy.

Pharyngeal Cysts

Definition. Cysts are fluid-filled structures that have been found in the subepiglottic tissues and the dorsal nasopharynx, and within the soft palate.[97, 98] Depending upon their location, they may represent embryonic remnants of the thyroglossal and craniopharyngeal ducts. They are usually considered congenital in origin. Acquired cysts are associated with secretory cells and may occur secondary to obstruction or inflammation of the mucous glands.[85, 98] The cysts are usually lined by pseudostratified cuboidal or columnar epithelium or by squamous epithelium, and often contain mucoprotein.[98]

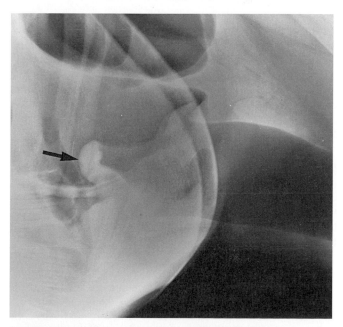

Figure 6–7. Seven-year-old male standardbred with an entrapped epiglottis. Lateral radiograph of the larynx demonstrates a rounded distal end to the epiglottis (arrow). The epiglottis also appears shortened.

Clinical Signs. Horses may exhibit exercise intolerance, abnormal respiratory noises, coughing, nasal discharge, dysphagia, and lower respiratory tract signs consistent with aspiration pneumonia. Dorsal displacement of the soft palate may coexist.

Diagnosis. Diagnosis is confirmed by visualization of smooth-walled structures 1 to 5 cm in diameter. Subepiglottic cysts may distort the appearance of the epiglottis, causing it to assume a more upright position in the pharynx.[81] Endoscopic differentiation between subepiglottic and soft palatal cysts may be difficult. Lateral radiographs of the pharynx and larynx may be useful in distinguishing cysts from conformational defects of the epiglottis.

Treatment. Treatment is surgical resection of the cyst via a ventral midline laryngotomy. Some cysts may be accessible via Nd:YAG laser techniques, eliminating the need for general anesthesia. Broad-spectrum antimicrobials are indicated because of the potential for development of aspiration pneumonia and should be initiated immediately. A course of 7 to 10 days may be indicated postoperatively, depending upon the involvement of the lower respiratory tract structures.

Arytenoid Chondritis

Definition. *Arytenoid chondritis* is an abnormal enlargement of the arytenoid cartilages, the cause of which has not been determined. Trauma and infection or inflammation have been cited as potential causes.[81]

Epidemiology. This is primarily a disease of horses performing at high speeds. While the racing Thoroughbred or standardbred is primarily affected, it has been found in a Hackney pony, Clydesdale, and Dutch Warmblood.[99]

Pathogenesis. The inflammatory lesions obstruct air flow through the larynx by physical enlargement of the arytenoids and subsequent narrowing of the rima glottis, by inflammation of the surrounding muscles of the larynx and pharynx which physically prevents arytenoid movement, or by impairment of the cricoarytenoid articulation. In most cases the condition is progressive and debilitating and thus a guarded to poor prognosis should be given.[98]

Clinical Signs. Clinical signs include exercise intolerance and inspiratory noises produced during exercise. A cough can be easily elicited with tracheal compression, and palpation of the larynx suggests that the cartilages are less resilient than normal.[100] If the chondritis is severe, dyspnea at rest may be evident.

Diagnosis. Diagnosis is based upon endoscopic examination. Ulcerations in the mucous membranes over the medial aspect of the corniculate processes, granulomas that project into the laryngeal lumen and induce defects on the medial aspect of the contralateral cartilage, and distortions of the corniculate processes may be found.[81, 99] With the progression of signs, the arytenoids may become more vertical. Other abnormalities, such as aryepiglottic entrapment or dorsal displacement

of the soft palate, may be seen. Radiographs may reveal excessive mineralization of laryngeal cartilages.

Treatment. Treatment includes both medical and surgical approaches. Rest, nonsteroidal anti-inflammatory therapy, antimicrobials, and throat sprays or nebulization may be utilized in some cases.[99] In more advanced cases, surgical resection of the affected cartilage is performed. Several techniques have been advocated. Arytenoidectomy involves removal of the corniculate and arytenoid cartilages, including the muscular processes. Partial arytenoidectomy (with ventriculectomy and cordectomy) involves resection of the laryngeal saccule, vocal fold, and arytenoid cartilage, excluding the muscular process and the rostral strip of the corniculate.[101] This is usually performed on horses with advanced uni- or bilateral disease in which the cartilage is thick and dense.[99] Subtotal arytenoidectomy involves removal of the arytenoid cartilage except for the muscular process.[102]

Laryngeal Hemiplegia

Definition. Laryngeal hemiplegia is a disorder in which there is paresis or paralysis of the laryngeal musculature preventing efficient abduction and adduction of the arytenoid cartilages. The recurrent laryngeal nerve innervates all of the intrinsic muscles of the larynx with the exception of the cricothyroideus. Paralysis of the cricoarytenoideus dorsalis prevents phasic abduction of the arytenoid cartilages during inspiration or maintained abduction of the cartilages during exercise. Denervation of the arytenoideus transversus, cricoarytenoideus lateralis, ventricularis, and vocalis prevents adduction of the arytenoids and slackening of the vocal folds.[85]

Etiology. In the majority of cases there is no known cause for the laryngeal paralysis; thus it has been termed idiopathic laryngeal hemiplegia (ILH). Most of the clinically detectable cases of ILH involve the left recurrent laryngeal nerve. Several theories have been advanced to explain the recurrent laryngeal neuropathy and include (1) mechanical compression or stretch of the left recurrent laryngeal nerve as it courses over the aortic arch, (2) bacterial- or viral-induced neuropathies, and (3) vitamin deficiencies.[103] In some cases, laryngeal hemiplegia has been known to occur secondary to perivascular or perineural injections, organophosphate intoxication,[103, 104] lead poisoning, plant poisoning, guttural pouch mycosis, neoplasia, traumatic accidents to the neck, and paralaryngeal abscessation.[103, 105]

Epidemiology. ILH is generally considered to be a disorder of larger-breed horses, rarely reported in Arabians and ponies. Clinical signs usually occur after 3 years of age at a time when work is initiated. However, left laryngeal asymmetry has been observed endoscopically in foals.[106] Males are reported to be more commonly affected than females, although the physical size difference may be an important consideration in this regard as ILH is more frequently seen in larger horses (>160 cm in height) with long necks and narrow chests.[103] ILH has been reported more frequently in certain family lines of horses, thus causing some to propose it to be a heritable disorder.[107, 108] However, the exact mode of transmission remains uncertain.

Pathogenesis. In ILH there is distal degeneration of the nerve fibers in the left recurrent laryngeal nerve and subsequent atrophy of the intrinsic laryngeal musculature.[109, 110] There are also similar, although less severe changes in the right recurrent laryngeal nerve of hemiplegic horses. Mild involvement of other peripheral long nerve fibers, for example, of the distal hindlimb, have also been seen.[111] The finding of bilateral recurrent neuropathy, along with changes in other peripheral nerves, is inconsistent with the hypothesis that neuropathy is a sequela of compression or stretching of the nerve as it courses along the aortic arch. The findings, however, are not inconsistent with the development of a distal axonopathy secondary to an energy-dependent disorder, an antioxidant disorder, or a filamentous neuropathy.[111]

Pathophysiology. Inadequate abduction of the arytenoids provides an inspiratory resistance to air flow. In experimentally induced hemiplegia, a significant increase in inspiratory or expiratory resistance at rest is not evident. However, during moderate exercise intensities, a significant increase in inspiratory resistance and a subsequent inspiratory air flow limitation develops.[112] The effect of this limitation on gas exchange has been evaluated. During eupneic breathing, there are no detectable alterations in gas exchange. However, during exercise, there is a worsening of the physiologic hypercapnia and hypoxemia normally found.[113, 114] The ensuing hypoxemia may contribute to the exercise intolerance. The inspiratory resistance increases the work of breathing and *may* predispose to the development of respiratory muscle fatigue.

Clinical Signs. Most horses with unilateral laryngeal hemiplegia present with a history of exercise intolerance and the production of an inspiratory noise described as either a whistle or a roar. In contrast, horses with bilateral laryngeal paralysis may present in respiratory distress and require emergency tracheostomies. In cases of bilateral paralysis secondary to toxins (e.g., organophosphate overdose), clinical signs may not be apparent for several weeks following the toxic insult.[115]

Diagnosis. Physical examination and palpation of the larynx may detect atrophy of the cricoarytenoideus dorsalis muscle. The slap test has been used to evaluate the adductor function of the intrinsic laryngeal muscles. In normal horses, when the saddle area of the horse is slapped, contralateral arytenoid cartilage adduction occurs. This adduction is detected either endoscopically or by palpation of the larynx during the procedure. This reflex is absent in horses with idiopathic recurrent laryngeal neuropathy.[116] However, the demonstration of a normal laryngeal reflex when the horse is at rest does not indicate that the horse is completely free of laryngeal hemiplegia.[107] Ultimately, the diagnosis is usually made by an endoscopic examination wherein one observes asymmetric positioning or range of motion of the arytenoid cartilages and relaxation of the vocal folds on the affected side. A proposed grading scheme is provided in Table 6–4 and may aid in the decision for surgical intervention. For example, horses with grade IV can be expected to benefit from surgery, whereas horses with grades I and II are usually not compromised during exercise and thus are not good surgical

---

Table 6–4. Grading Scheme for Laryngeal Anatomy*

Grade I: Synchronous full abduction and adduction of left and right arytenoid cartilages

Grade II: Asynchronous movement such as hesitation, flutters, adductor weakness of the left arytenoid during inspiration or expiration, or both, but full abduction induced by swallowing or nasal occlusion

Grade III: Asynchronous movement of the left arytenoid during inspiration or expiration, or both, but full abduction not induced and maintained by swallowing or nasal occlusion

Grade IV: Marked asymmetry of the larynx at rest and lack of substantial movement of the left arytenoid

*From Ducharme NG, Hackett RP: The value of surgical treatment of laryngeal hemiplegia in horses. *Compendium Contin Educ Pract Vet* 13:472, 1991.

---

candidates. Horses with grade III are considered suspect, some of these horses demonstrating dynamic collapse of the airway and thus requiring surgical intervention. Ideally, endoscopic examination of the horse during treadmill exercise should be performed to ascertain the importance of slight asymmetry at rest in the production of exercise intolerance.

Treatment. Surgical correction of the flow obstruction is necessary. Laryngoplasty, use of a prosthesis to maintain the affected arytenoid in abduction, is most commonly used. Complications associated with the surgery include chronic infection of the prosthesis, formation of a suture sinus, ossification of cartilage, dysphagia, esophageal obstruction, pneumonia, intralaryngeal granulomatous polyps, right-sided laryngospasm during exercise, laryngeal edema, chondritis, and coughing.[117] Ventriculectomy, surgical ablation of the lateral ventricles in an effort to induce adhesions between the vocal cords and laryngeal walls, has also been performed, either singly or in conjunction with the laryngoplasty. Prosthetic laryngoplasty prevents the increase in inspiratory resistance and flow limitation during moderate exercise.[113] However, ventriculectomy alone fails to alleviate the increased inspiratory impedance during exercise.[115] Attempts to restore laryngeal abduction in experimentally induced laryngeal hemiplegia by transplantation of nerve-muscle pedicle (cervical nerve 2, the omohyoid) transplants were recently evaluated.[117] However, endoscopic evaluation revealed only a 30% restoration of normal arytenoid abduction at rest in 25% of the ponies. Similarly, either implantation of the cut end of the second cervical nerve into the left cricoarytenoideus muscle or anastomosis of the first cervical nerve to the abductor branch of the left recurrent laryngeal nerve in ponies with left laryngeal hemiplegia resulted in minimal restoration of abduction.[118, 119]

In horses with bilateral laryngeal paralysis, tracheostomy may be required until resolution or lessening of paralysis occurs. Affected horses should not be stressed or subjected to undue movements. Broad-spectrum antimicrobial and anti-inflammatory therapy should be instituted.

Streptococcus equi *Infections* (Strangles)

Etiology. *Streptococcus equi,* a gram-positive bacterium of the Lancefield Group C, is the causative agent of strangles. It is not a normal inhabitant of the equine upper respiratory tract and does not require prior viral infections for successful colonization and infection.[120] Based upon morphologic features of the bacterial colony, there are two strains of the organism which differ in virulence. The typical and highly virulent encapsulated *S. equi* have golden honey-colored mucoid colonies on blood agar, whereas the atypical *S. equi* exhibit a matt appearance of their colony within 24 hours of incubation.[121]

Epidemiology. The infection occurs primarily in horses 1 to 5 years old, but is not restricted to this age group.[122] Morbidity is nearly 100% in susceptible populations while mortality is typically quite low if appropriate therapy is instituted.[122, 123] Horses with strangles may shed the organism for several weeks following clinical recovery, with one survey detecting organisms for up to 10 months after exposure.[124] A 6-week course of shedding may be more typical. The organism survives only for short periods in the environment unless protected in moist discharges.[125]

Pathogenesis. The organism is inhaled or ingested after direct contact with the mucopurulent discharges from infected horses or contaminated equipment. *S. equi* adheres to the epithelial cells of the buccal and nasal mucosa of horses. Adherence is neutralized by antibodies to the organism; thus protection may be afforded by preventing the adhesion.[126] There are two features of the organism that are important in its pathogenicity: (1) the hyaluronic acid capsule possesses a strongly negative charge and apparently repels phagocytic cells, and (2) M protein, a cell wall antigen, protects the cell from ingestion by polymorphonuclear leukocytes. The M antigen is also important for adherence of the organism to the epithelium.[127] Thus the organism is able to replicate relatively unchecked.

Clinical Signs. The incubation period is between 2 and 6 days. Horses are febrile, have a serous and then mucopurulent nasal discharge, and evidence of intermandibular or retropharyngeal lymphadenopathy. Lymph nodes are initially firm but become fluctuant before rupturing 7 to 10 days after the onset of signs. Lymphadenopathy may become so severe that dysphagia and dyspnea develop, requiring supportive care, including tracheostomy. The average duration for the course of the syndrome is 23 days.[120]

Clinical Pathology. A neutrophilic leukocytosis, hyperfibrinogenemia, and an anemia of chronic infection are seen in cases of strangles.

Diagnosis. Diagnosis is usually based upon the typical clinical signs, upon culture of the draining lymph nodes or nasal and pharyngeal swabs. Lymph node cultures yield higher isolation rates.[120]

Treatment. Treatment is a function of the stage of the disease. Sweeney et al.[120] outlined a treatment protocol which is described below:

1. If horses exhibit signs of *S. equi* infection without abscessation of the lymph nodes, then the progression of the disease can be arrested by the use of penicillin G therapy. Horses should be isolated during their treatment protocol.

2. If horses exhibit evidence of lymph node abscessation, then administration of penicillin will slow the progression of lymph node abscessation and is generally contraindicated. Hence, unless the horse is febrile, anorectic, depressed, or dyspneic, then hot packing the area(s) is done to promote abscess formation. Once achieved, the abscess should be lanced and flushed with a 2% tamed iodine solution. Horses are treated in isolation.

3. If horses are exposed to the organism, then penicillin therapy is indicated to prevent seeding of the pharyngeal lymph nodes. Antimicrobial therapy should be continued for as long as the horse remains exposed to the organism.

4. If the horse develops any complications, then supportive care, in addition to high levels of intravenous penicillin, should be provided. This may include intravenous fluid therapy, a tracheostomy, nonsteroidal anti-inflammatory drugs, and feeding via the nasogastric tube.

Sequelae. The reader is referred to excellent reviews of the potential complications of *S. equi* infections.[120, 128] Complications include:

1. Internal abscessation of the mesentery or of parenchymatous organs. The causes of internal abscessation are not known, although inadequate antimicrobial therapy during respiratory catarrh and lymphoid abscessation may be contributory.[129] The horse may present with a history of intermittent colic, periodic pyrexia, anorexia, depression, and weight loss. Diagnostic techniques, including rectal palpation, thoracic radiography, thoracocentesis, abdominocentesis, and ultrasonography, should be directed at determining the location of the abscess. However, cases of internal abscessation can be difficult to differentiate from other causes of weight loss and colic, including neoplasia. Both processes (internal abscessation and neoplasia) may induce similar abnormalities in the peritoneal fluid (leukocytosis and hyperproteinemia) and differentiation between the two processes may not be possible unless exfoliated neoplastic cells are identified.[130] Hematologic and serum biochemical abnormalities in cases of internal abscessation include (a) leukocytosis due to neutrophilia and monocytosis, (b) hyperfibrinogenemia, (c) hyperproteinemia due to hyperglobulinemia (despite the presence of hypoalbuminemia),[129] and (d) hypocalcemia.[130] However, these changes are not unique to abscesses and may not be found in horses with intra-abdominal abscesses.[130] Thus, the diagnosis of internal abscessation represents a medical challenge. Once confirmed, long-term penicillin therapy is indicated and may be required for several months. Clinical signs, rectal palpation, repeated abdominocentesis, and multiple complete blood counts (CBCs) can be used to monitor the progress of therapy.

2. The development of purpura hemorrhagica. This is an aseptic vasculitis that is usually seen in the mature horse following a second natural exposure to *S. equi* infection or following vaccination after having been previously exposed

to a natural in[____] [____]rpura are variable and ra[____] [____] a severe and fatal form. Horses with purpura have pitting edema of the limbs, head, and trunk and petechiation and ecchymoses of the mucous membranes.[128] Horses may also have colic secondary to edema and hemorrhage of the bowel. The vasculitis may progress to the point of skin sloughing and death may ensue secondarily from pneumonia, renal failure, or gastrointestinal disorders.[128]

3. Guttural pouch empyema (see earlier discussion).

4. Septicemia and the development of infectious arthritis, pneumonia, and encephalitis. This warrants a poor prognosis.[131]

5. Retropharyngeal abscessation. Horses may present with acute upper respiratory tract obstruction, dyspnea, or dysphagia. Endoscopy of the nasopharynx demonstrates collapse of the nasopharynx, deviation of the larynx, or drainage of purulent material into the nasopharynx when external pressure is applied to the parotid region.[132] Radiographs demonstrate a distortion or compression of the guttural pouches, pharynx, and trachea. The retropharyngeal abscess may rupture into the pharynx and cause a secondary pneumonia or it may rupture dorsally into the guttural pouches.[128, 132]

6. Laryngeal hemiplegia occurs when abscessed lymph nodes encroach upon the recurrent laryngeal nerve.[133]

7. Tracheal compression secondary to abscessation of the cranial mediastinal lymph nodes has also been reported. The horse may present in respiratory distress or exhibit stertorous breathing. Laryngeal hemiplegia may be an additional complication if the abscess compressing the trachea involves the recurrent laryngeal nerves.[133]

8. Endocarditis or myocarditis secondary to abscess formation.

9. Agalactia in periparturient mares.

10. Suppurative necrotic bronchopneumonia, which may result in death.

Prevention. Several vaccines are available but do not guarantee the prevention of strangles in vaccinated horses.[123] Failure to prevent the disease is not due to absence of antibody formation. Indeed, vaccinated ponies exhibit strong serum bactericidal activity, but these antibodies are not necessarily protective. It appears that nasopharyngeal immunity plays a significant role in the resistance to infection and that protection may follow intranasal vaccination.[126] Vaccines currently available include Equibac II (killed suspension of *S. equi* in aluminum hydroxide gel), Strepvax (concentrated M protein extract of *S. equi*), and Strepguard (purified enzyme extract of *S. equi*).

Viral Infections of the Upper Respiratory Tract

Many different viral agents have been isolated from the upper respiratory tract of both clinically normal and ill horses. The exact role of many of these viruses in the production of rhinitis, pharyngitis, tracheitis, or pneumonitis is uncertain. Viruses of known pathogenicity to the horse that produce upper respiratory tract disease include equine influenza virus, EHV-1 and EHV-4, and equine arteritis virus.

Equine Influenza

Etiology. The influenza viruses are enveloped myxoviruses containing single-stranded RNA. Based upon the internal nucleoproteins and matrix antigens, influenza viruses have been classified as three types—A, B, and C. Types B and C infect only humans, but type A infects many different species, including humans, horses, swine, and avian species.[134] Natural cross-species infections have occurred between humans and swine and experimental infection of humans with equine influenza virus (subtype 2) is possible, although natural infections do not occur.[135] Type A is further classified into subtypes based upon the surface antigens, the hemagglutinin (H) and neuraminidase (N), with two subtypes being recognized as infectious for the horse: subtypes H7N7 and H3N8. Subtype H7N7 was first isolated in Prague in 1956 and has been called equine-1 influenza (A/equine/Prague/56), while subtype H3N8 was first isolated in Miami in 1963 and was designated as equine-2 influenza (A/equine/Miami/63). Several variants of subtype 2 (antigenic drift) have been identified and include A/equine/Fontainebleau/79 and A/equine/Kentucky/81.[134] Compared to the human influenza virus, the equine influenza virus is relatively stable antigenically, not experiencing major "antigenic shifts." This has been postulated to be the result of the shorter life span of horses relative to humans and the lower mutation pressure placed upon the equine influenza viruses because of low specific antibody titers.[135]

Epidemiology. Influenza most commonly affects 2- and 3-year-old horses. It may be the most common cause of respiratory illness in racehorses, with some tracks experiencing influenza outbreaks two to three times within a racing season.[136] This may reflect poor ventilation systems and lack of adequate immunization protocols. The reservoir of equine influenza virus between epizootics remains unknown. Some speculate that the virus is maintained in the horse population itself and that asymptomatic carriers shed virus when stressed. Alternatively, the virus may be harbored in other species such as birds, which are asymptomatic but shed the virus in their feces.[135]

Pathogenesis. The incubation period is 1 to 3 days with the virus infecting the upper respiratory tract and the lungs to a lesser extent. Healthy respiratory tract epithelium is ciliated and contains mucus that forms a protective layer over the cell surface. This normally acts as a mechanical barrier between air and tissue and contains antibody and protein substances that deter the attachment of viral particles to the epithelium.[137] Neuraminidase activity of the viral particles alters the efficiency of the mucociliary apparatus, allowing the virions to attach via hemagglutinin antigens to epithelial cells. Replication within the respiratory tract epithelium is followed by cell necrosis and desquamation. Since complete epithelial cell regeneration takes 3 weeks, impairment of the mucociliary elevator predisposes to the development of secondary bacterial infections. Both humoral and cellular immunity are important in providing protection against viral disease: IgA blocks viral penetration but is not bactericidal; IgM and IgG, found predominantly in the lower respiratory tract, opsonize the virus particles and enhance phagocytosis.[138]

Clinical Signs. Signs of influenza appear 3 to 5 days following exposure to the virus. Horses exhibit a sudden onset of fever (103°–105°F), which may be biphasic; a serous nasal discharge; anorexia; depression; and a dry deep cough. Some horses exhibit myalgia, myositis, and limb edema, and are thus reluctant to move.[135, 138] A mild form of azoturia (myoglobinuria) has been seen in some cases. Intermandibular lymphadenopathy, as well as endoscopic evidence of pharyngitis and tracheitis, may be found. A mild bronchitis with minimal changes in lung sounds may occur. From experimental studies, inoculation with A/equine-1 produces a milder (subclinical) syndrome unless the animal is stressed prior to infection, whereas A/equine-2 usually generates the typical clinical signs. The course of the infection usually lasts 2 to 10 days in uncomplicated cases. In young foals, influenza is quite severe, producing signs of viral pneumonia, which may lead to death within 48 hours. Secondary bacterial infections are common. Horses remain infectious for 3 to 6 days after the last signs of illness.

Clinical Pathology. Horses may initially exhibit a lymphopenia followed by a monocytosis.

Diagnosis

Viral Isolation. The chances of viral isolation are greater when samples are collected early in the course of the outbreak, within the first 24 hours.[136] Pharyngeal swabs or samples of nasal mucus should be submitted along with serum to improve the chances of accurate diagnosis.

Serology. Several diagnostic methods for detecting influenza virus antibodies in the horse are utilized and include complement fixation, hemagglutination inhibition, single radial hemolysis, viral neutralization, and enzyme immunoassay.[139] Both acute and convalescent serum samples are needed to establish a definitive diagnosis, and although viral neutralizing antibodies may be detected within a week of infection, it may take up to 28 days to exhibit a rise in hemagglutination titers.[135]

Treatment. Treatment is primarily symptomatic, insuring that the horse continues to maintain adequate hydration and is not subjected to undue stresses. Nonsteroidal anti-inflammatory drugs may be indicated to reduce the fever, eliminate the myalgia, and improve the appetite. The risk is that the horse will be returned to strenuous exercise before the horse has been rested a sufficient length of time. Horses that suffer severe infections may be unfit for competition for 50 to 100 days after infection. During the infection, frequent examinations of the respiratory tract are indicated to detect the development of secondary complications such as pneumonia, pleuropneumonia, and myocarditis.

Prevention. Regular vaccination significantly reduces the population at risk. In fact, it has been suggested that at least 70% of the equine population (horses, ponies, donkeys) should be vaccinated to prevent epidemics of influenza.[140] Currently available adjuvant vaccines maintain protective levels of antibody for 12 weeks. Vaccines contain both subtypes of influenza virus and some of their variants (e.g., A/equine-2/KY 81). It is recommended that young horses that are early in their athletic career be vaccinated more frequently (at 4–6-month intervals) than horses who have received regular boosters for years. Older, regularly vaccinated animals are given booster vaccinations at 9- to 12-month intervals, especially if they seldom attend shows or competitions.[140] Inactivated vaccines are effective in eliminating virus shedding upon reexposure to the virus.[141] Future efforts to produce a more efficacious vaccine may be directed at (1) producing temperature-sensitive viruses which, when inoculated intranasally, are unable to replicate but still induce local immune reactions, or (2) synthesizing recombinant vaccines (e.g., equine-avian recombinant). There are some undesirable side effects of vaccination, including fever, depression, pain, swelling at the vaccine site, and muscular stiffness, but these usually resolve within 1 or 2 days.[136]

Sequelae. Secondary bacterial pneumonia and pleuropneumonia are potential complications that may follow viral respiratory diseases in horses that have not been adequately rested before being returned to training or that have undergone other potentially stressful events such as long trailer rides. Myocarditis, pericarditis, and cardiac arrhythmias are other possible sequelae to influenza infections.

Equine Herpesvirus Types 1 and 4

Etiology. There are two strains of this DNA herpesvirus, type 1 and type 2, associated with respiratory disease in the horse. Type 1 has also been associated with several other clinical syndromes in the horse, including abortions, myeloencephalitis, and neonatal deaths. Type 2 has recently been referred to as EHV-4.[142]

Epidemiology. Respiratory disease occurs mainly in foals, weanlings, and yearlings. Since immunity to reinfection is short, most horses are reinfected during their breeding or racing careers. Reexposure usually results in mild or inapparent infections, except in the case of broodmares in which reinfection may lead to abortion in the last trimester. Perinatal disease (respiratory distress) is usually evident within 18 to 24 hours, with foals dying within 24 to 72 hours.[143] It has been assumed that EHV-1 may persist within a herd because of latent infections and recrudescence occurring during periods of stress or immunosuppression. However, the exact site of viral or proviral persistence is not known.[78]

Pathogenesis. Infection occurs via inhalation of the virus or contact with infected tissues. The virus is relatively delicate and does not survive in the environment; thus close contact appears to be important for transmission.[143] Virions invade and replicate within the nasal, pharyngeal, and tonsillar epithelium. Mononuclear cells phagocytose viral particles and carry them to other tissue sites where replication of virions continues (viremic phase). Infection is not confined to the upper respiratory tract. Burrell[78] has shown that two thirds of EHV-1 infections produce lower respiratory tract inflammation, as evidenced by mucopus 2 to 12 weeks after the initial infection, and experimental inoculation produces herpetic lesions in all parts of the respiratory tract.[143]

Clinical Signs. Clinical signs of rhinopneumonitis appear 1 to 3 days following infection and are indistinguishable from influenza. Horses are febrile and exhibit a dry cough and a serous nasal discharge, which may become mucopurulent with secondary bacterial infections. Horses develop rhinitis, pharyngitis, and tracheitis detectable endoscopically.

Clinical Pathology. An epidemiologic survey by Mason and colleagues[144] during an outbreak of EHV-1 infection on a racetrack in Hong Kong revealed an increase in the monocyte counts (>500 cells/µL) during the first 5 days of clinically apparent infections.[144]

Diagnosis. Viral isolation may be attempted from citrated blood samples. Virus has been recovered from mononuclear cells for up to 2 weeks post infection or from nasopharyngeal swabs. Serology is useful in the diagnosis by demonstration of a fourfold increase in titers. Antibodies against EHV-1 can be detected by virus neutralization, immunoassay, complement fixation, and a radial immunodiffusion enzyme assay.[145] Postmortem examination of foals who died from EHV-1 infection reveals interstitial pneumonia, pleural and peritoneal effusions, hypoplasia of the thymus and spleen, focal necrosis of the liver, and viral inclusion bodies within the hepatic parenchyma. Similar pathologic findings are observed in aborted fetuses.

Treatment. Treatment is supportive, minimizing stresses and insuring adequate rest. Return to training sessions before complete healing may predispose to the development of pleuropneumonia.

Prevention. Currently available vaccines are produced from both EHV-1 and EHV-4 and although the vaccine does not prevent infection, the severity of clinical signs is reduced.

Other Herpesviruses. EHV-2 is a slowly replicating virus recovered from clinically normal horses as well as from those exhibiting respiratory tract disease.[146] Many adult horses are seropositive for EHV-2. Foals that are infected experimentally with EHV-2 develop pharyngitis and lymphoid hyperplasia; thus EHV-2 has been implicated as an etiologic agent of chronic lymphoid hyperplasia in young horses.[146] EHV-2 has also been isolated from 2- to 3-month-old foals exhibiting respiratory distress. In some of these outbreaks, EHV-2 was the only agent isolated from the respiratory tract,[147, 148] although a mixed culture of *Streptococcus zooepidemicus* and *Rhodococcus equi* was also isolated from the transtracheal aspirates.[149] Some authors have speculated that if the foals are under stress or infected with a large dose of virus during a period in which maternal antibodies are waning, then the virus may invade the cells of the immune system and cause further immunosuppression. This would increase the susceptibility of the foal to secondary infections by other viral and bacterial agents.[148]

EHV-3 is the cause of equine coital exanthema, producing vesicular lesions on the vulva of mares. It has been isolated from the upper respiratory tract of a foal exhibiting herpetic lesions in the nostril, but no other signs of respiratory disease.[150]

Equine Viral Arteritis

Etiology. Equine arteritis virus is an enveloped single-stranded RNA virus. It is also a nonarthropod-borne togavirus, with apparently only one serotype recognized at this time.[151]

Epidemiology. Prior to the 1984 epizootic of equine viral arteritis (EVA) in Kentucky, little attention was paid to this virus.[152] Most infections were assumed to be transmitted by inhalation until the important role of venereal transmission was demonstrated in those outbreaks. The virus is maintained within the equine population by both long-term and short-term stallion carriers, the duration of the carrier status ranging from several weeks to years. A carrier state has not been identified in mares.[152] It is presumed that primary exposure to the virus is via the venereal route. Viral shedding into the respiratory tract allows secondary horizontal transmission of the virus to occur.

Pathogenesis. With intranasal challenge (aerosolization of virions), replication occurs within the macrophages of the lung and the bronchial lymph nodes. From there, the virus is disseminated throughout the horse by hematogenous routes, infecting mesenteric lymph nodes; spleen; liver; kidneys; nasopharyngeal, pleural, and peritoneal fluid; and urine.[152] The virus induces a necrotizing arteritis, a panvasculitis. Abortions occur from the 10th to the 34th day following exposure, but the mechanism is not known. Unlike other togaviruses, EVA has not been associated with teratologic abnormalities in fetuses or foals. The virus is also transmitted venereally and can be isolated from swabs of the rectal and vaginal mucosa during the febrile periods.

Clinical Signs. Clinical signs are variable, ranging from severe disease to subclinical infections. The variation may be a function of both host factors, such as age and immune status, and virus factors, including the virulence, the amount of infective virus, and the route of infection.[153] The incubation period ranges from 3 to 14 days (6–8 days if venereally transmitted). Horses are febrile (105 °F) for 1 to 5 days, anorectic, depressed, and may cough. In addition to a serous nasal discharge, congestion of the nasal mucosa, and intermandibular lymphadenopathy, there is conjunctivitis, lacrimation, and, less frequently, corneal opacification. Edema of the sheath, scrotum, ventral midline, limbs, and eyelids occurs secondary to the vasculitis. Other signs may include respiratory distress, stiffness, soreness, diarrhea, icterus, skin rash on the neck, and papular eruptions on the inside of the upper lip. Most horses recover uneventfully with the exception of a sporadic death in a young foal.[152]

Clinical Pathology. Pathologic study reveals leukopenia and profound lymphopenia.

Diagnosis. EVA is a reportable disease. Although virus may persist in the buffy coat for up to 36 days post infection, viral isolation can be difficult.[153] Citrated blood samples should be submitted. Viral particles may be isolated from nasopharyngeal and conjunctival swabs as well as from semen from an infected stallion. Serologic diagnosis should also be attempted. Virus neutralization, complement fixation, immunodiffusion, and immunofluorescence are techniques used to demonstrate increase in antibody titers. A fourfold or greater rise in titer or a change in status from seronegative to seropositive can be used to indicate a recent infection. Postmortem examinations of aborted fetuses do not show signs of arteritis, as seen in adults. There is evidence of edema, excessive pleural fluid, and petechiation on the mucosal surfaces of the respiratory and gastrointestinal tracts. But focal necrosis of the liver or intranuclear inclusions are not features of the disease.[151]

Treatment. Treatment is primarily symptomatic, maintaining the horse's hydration status and providing analgesics (nonsteroidal anti-inflammatories) as needed. Horses should be isolated for 3 to 4 weeks to minimize the chances of transmission.

Prevention. Vaccination of seronegative stallions with a commercially available modified live vaccine is credited with preventing the establishment of carrier states in the stallion or with further increases in the carrier state during the 1984 epizootic in Kentucky. Stallions were bred only to mares that were vaccinated or seropositive from previous natural exposure to EVA. Following vaccination, clinical immunity was found to develop rapidly and to last for 1 to 3 years.[152] Primary vaccination does not prevent reinfection and limited shedding of virus. Vaccination is not recommended for use in pregnant mares or in foals less than 6 weeks of age.

Equine Rhinovirus

Equine rhinovirus types 1 and 2 are RNA viruses that have been reported to cause mild respiratory disease in young horses, although the role of these viruses in the production of respiratory disorders is controversial. Most horses exhibit antibodies to the rhinoviruses and they can be isolated from normal horses as well as from those showing signs of respiratory disease.[154] The viruses have been implicated as a cause of pharyngitis. No vaccine is currently available.

Tracheal Disorders

Definition. Inflammations, obstructions, compressions, lacerations, and containment of foreign bodies are the predominant disorders of the trachea in the horse.[136, 155–158] Tracheitis often accompanies viral upper respiratory tract diseases (see earlier discussion) and is manifested as areas of hyperemia and epithelial desquamation. Lacerations are usually secondary to trauma, while compressions may be the result of extraluminal masses such as streptococcal abscesses or neoplasms like lymphosarcoma or lipomas. Intraluminal obstructions may follow fibrotic stricture formation secondary to trauma, tracheostomy, or pressure necrosis from inflated cuffs of endotracheal tubes, or may be due to granulomatous reactions within the trachea.[136, 155] Foreign bodies, such as twigs, are probably inhaled during deglutition. Tracheal collapse may represent a congenital defect in miniature horses and ponies.[159, 160]

Clinical Signs. Clinical signs are variable and range from stertorous breathing and dyspnea to chronic and persistent coughing and bilateral nasal discharge with a foul odor. Paroxysmal bouts of coughing may also be induced with mild manipulation of the trachea.

Diagnosis. The diagnosis is made on physical examination or endoscopic evaluation of the trachea. A history of a previous tracheal surgery or traumatic episode will alert the diagnostician to the possibility of an intraluminal obstruction or stricture. Foreign bodies may be visualized on examination but may require radiographs to delineate the extent of their involvement. Radiographic examination of the thorax should also be performed to determine if a concomitant pneumonia, pneumomediastinum, or pneumothorax exists.

Treatment. Treatment is directed at the primary cause. Primary inflammations secondary to viral infections are not treated unless a persistent fever and a secondary bacterial tracheitis and pneumonia develop. Foreign bodies are extracted but may require tracheotomy to retrieve them if the endoscope is not long enough. In the adult horse, a 2-m endoscope is necessary to reach the level of the carina located at the fifth to sixth intercostal space. Extraluminal masses require careful drainage or excision, with the potential for spread of infection into the mediastinum to develop. Horses with *Streptococcus equi* infections should be isolated from other Equidae. Rupture of the trachea may require temporary tracheotomy distal to the rupture to insure patency of air flow. A 2-week course of broad-spectrum antimicrobial therapy may be indicated, especially if the mucociliary clearance mechanism is compromised. Complications such as subcutaneous emphysema, cellulitis, and pneumomediastinum usually resolve over a 2-week period.[161] Horses with tracheal defects have a poor to guarded prognosis for return to athletic potential.

THE NORMAL LUNG
Anatomy

The lungs of the horse differ from those of other domestic species in that they lack deep interlobar fissures and distinct lung lobes. Superficially, however, the left lung consists of a cranial and caudal lobe while the right lung contains a cranial, intermediate, and caudal lobe.[162] The intrathoracic trachea bifurcates into the right and left mainstem bronchi at the level of the fifth or sixth intercostal space and enters the hilum of each lung. At its division from the trachea, the right bronchus assumes a straighter, more horizontal position relative to the left bronchus, a configuration which may predispose to the development of right-sided pulmonary disorders. Each bronchus divides into lobar, segmental, and subsegmental bronchi with the eventual formation of bronchioles. In the distal part of the bronchial tree, the terminal bronchioles lead into poorly developed respiratory bronchioles or open directly into alveolar ducts.[162, 163] The tracheobronchial lining consists of tall columnar, pseudostratified epithelium interspersed with serous and goblet cells. The goblet cells and the underlying submucosal mucous glands function to produce mucus consisting of an outer gel and an inner sol layer.[164] Mucus serves to prevent epithelial dehydration, contains protective factors that guard against infectious agents, and is an integral part of the mucociliary apparatus. The rapid beating of the cilia move mucus and any particulate matter to the pharynx to be swallowed. Approximately 90% of material deposited on the mucinous layer is cleared within 1 hour.

Ciliated cells decrease in frequency with successive divisions of the airways so that at the level of the bronchioles the epithelium is composed predominantly of low ciliated and taller nonciliated Clara cells.[165] Glands are also absent at this level.[164] The bronchiolar epithelium becomes contiguous with that of the alveoli, which are characterized by two distinct cell types. Type I pneumocytes cover the majority of the alveolar surface with thin cytoplasmic extensions 0.2 to 0.5 μm thick.[164] Type II cells are cuboidal and contain the characteristic lamellar cytoplasmic inclusions thought to constitute surfactant components. Type II cells are also considered to be "stem cells," replacing the type I cells when damaged.

Lymphocytes are scattered throughout the pulmonary epithelium. They are also associated with the bronchioles and bronchi and occur in discrete nodules or patches.[166] These cells, along with alveolar macrophages, provide an integral component of the pulmonary immune surveillance system. Macrophages are derived from blood monocytes via the interstitium and are continuously cleared from the alveoli. They are the predominant cell type recovered from the bronchoalveolar lavage in normal horses (see Table 6–2). Pulmonary interstitial macrophages have recently been shown to rapidly ingest particles introduced within the pulmonary circulation.[167] The ability of these macrophages to localize antigenic particles within the pulmonary vasculature may predispose the equine lung to the development of acute pulmonary inflammation (e.g., during endotoxemia).

Additional cells within the lung parenchyma include the subepithelial and free mast cell. These cells bear IgE on their cell surface and release biogenic amines in response to specific antigen stimulation. They appear to be important in the pathogenesis of several equine pulmonary disorders, including heaves and lungworm infections.

Tracheobronchial secretions consist of substances secreted from mucous and serous glands as well as serum transudates. The principal component of the secretions is water, with approximately equal amounts of protein, carbohydrate, lipid, and inorganic material.[164] Contained within the protein fraction of the tracheobronchial secretions are albumin, IgA, IgG (the predominant immunoglobulin in the lower lung), lysozyme, lactoferrin, haptoglobulin, transferrin, and complement components.[164]

Vascular Supply

There are two sources of blood flow to the lung. The major source of blood is via the pulmonary circulation, a low-pressure, low-resistance system. Its serves primarily to deliver blood to the alveoli for participation in gas exchange but also provides nutrients to the alveolar constituents. The distribution of the pulmonary arterial flow to the various lung regions is largely dependent upon mechanical forces—gravity and pulmonary arterial, pulmonary venous, and alveolar pressures.[168] In the standing horse, a vertical perfusion gradient of the lung has been demonstrated,[169] the most dorsal part of the equine lung being less well perfused than the ventral dependent regions. The distribution of pulmonary blood flow is also influenced by vasoactive compounds such as catecholamines, histamine, and eicosanoids, as well as by changes in alveolar oxygen and carbon dioxide. Alterations in pulmonary vascular resistance may help to match ventilation with perfusion, and optimize gas exchange.

The bronchial circulation, the second source of blood flow to the lungs, provides nutrient support to the lymphatics and vascular and airway components.[163] It provides arterial blood to the pleural surface and anastomotic connections with the alveolar capillary bed derived from the pulmonary circulation.[163] The magnitude of the anastomotic flow will depend upon the relative pressure in the bronchial and pulmonary microvasculature, as well as upon the alveolar pressure. Thus in the dorsal part of the lung, where pulmonary arterial flow is relatively poor, blood flow from the bronchial circulation may be favored.[170] The degree of anastomotic bronchial blood flow through the alveolar capillaries will also increase with systemic arterial hypoxemia and alveolar hypoxia.[168] The bronchial circulation undergoes hypertrophy (angiogenesis) in response to such inflammatory pulmonary diseases as chronic bronchitis, bronchiolitis, and bronchiectasis.

Innervation

Innervation to the pulmonary structures is supplied by the autonomic nervous system. This nervous system influences (1) airway smooth muscle tone, (2) secretion of mucus from the submucosal glands, (3) transport of fluid across airway epithelium, (4) permeability and blood flow in the bronchial circulation, and (5) release of mediators from mast cells and other inflammatory cells.[171] In the horse, the autonomic nervous system can be functionally classified into three categories: (1) the parasympathetic, (2) sympathetic, and (3) nonadrenergic noncholinergic (NANC) pathways.[172] The vagus nerve is an integral component of both the parasympathetic and NANC systems. It not only contains the efferent fibers of these pathways, which help to alter airway resistance, lung volume, and compliance, but also contains the afferent fibers whose central input regulates the pattern of breathing. When parasympathetic fibers within the vagus nerve are stimulated (i.e., the efferent limb), acetylcholine is released from the postganglionic fibers and combines with the muscarinic receptors of the airway smooth muscle to cause bronchoconstriction. Yet because atropinization (antagonism of muscarinic receptors) does not normally change airway resistance, the parasympathetic system appears to exert little influence on resting airway tone in the *healthy* horse.[173] However, vagal efferents are important in reflex bronchoconstriction during pulmonary disease.

As described earlier, the vagus nerve also contains afferent nerve fibers which transmit information detected by three types of pulmonary mechanoreceptors: (1) the slowly adapting receptors, (2) the rapidly adapting receptors, and (3) the nonmyelinated C fibers. This information is relayed to the central respiratory neurons located within the ventral medulla and pons. Changes in breathing depth and frequency occur in response to mechanical deformations or chemical stimulation of these receptors. Thus, the tachypneic breathing pattern that occurs in response to inhalation of irritant substances is mediated by these receptors. Stimulation of these receptors also influences airway smooth muscle tone,[174] inducing reflex bronchoconstriction in response to inhaled irritants.

In the lung, sympathomimetic effects are mediated through α- and β-adrenergic receptors. Postsynaptic fibers course from the sympathetic ganglion to airway smooth muscle where released norepinephrine interacts with both α- and β-receptors. Postganglionic sympathetic fibers also innervate parasympathetic ganglia. The released norepinephrine inhibits cholinergic neurotransmission.[172] There are, however, numerous β$_2$-adrenergic receptors distributed throughout the pulmonary parenchyma that lack innervation by the sympathetic fibers.[171] Circulating catecholamines are probably important in activating these receptors and in causing subsequent bronchodilation. It is of interest that β$_2$-adrenergic stimulation does not alter airway diameter in the healthy horse,[175] but does increase airway caliber in horses with recurrent airway disease. β-Agonists also promote ion transport and water secretion across human airway epithelium (in vitro) and may cause similar effects in vivo in the horse. This would benefit mucociliary clearance by increasing the sol component of the mucus. In addition, β-agonists stimulate surfactant secretion by type II pneumocytes, inhibit antigen-induced mast cell degranulation, and modulate cholinergic neural transmission.[171] Such effects remain to be demonstrated in the horse, however.

α-Adrenergic receptors also exist in the equine lung, but their stimulation induces bronchoconstriction only in heavey and not in normal ponies.[176] This finding suggests that, in health, these receptors are probably relatively unimportant in the regulation of bronchomotor tone.

An additional autonomic pathway, the nonadrenergic noncholinergic inhibitory system, has also been demonstrated in the equine lung and its fibers course within the vagus nerve.[172] Although the mediators involved in neural transmission have not been definitively identified, there is some speculation that vasoactive intestinal peptide (VIP) or peptide histidine isoleucine (PHI), or both, may be the neurotransmitters.[177] Stimulation of this pathway causes a 50% reduction in smooth muscle tone and thus exerts a vasodilating effect.[178] Interestingly, horses with recurrent airway disease appear to lack NANC innervation in the bronchioles and this dysfunction may contribute to the airway hyperactivity observed.[172]

Lymph Drainage

Lymph drainage from the lung is accomplished by (1) the deep lymphatics, which begin at the level of the alveolar ducts and run with the conducting airway and arteries toward the hilar lymph nodes, and (2) the superficial lymphatics, which drain the visceral pleura through a plexus converging on the hilum.[164]

Pulmonary Physiology
Gas Exchange

The major function of the lung is gas exchange—diffusion of oxygen and elimination of carbon dioxide. During eupnea,

an adult horse breathes at a frequency of about 12 breaths per minute and a tidal volume near 6.5 L.[179] This represents a total minute ventilation of 77 L/min, or over 100,000 L/day! During this same period, the resting horse consumes approximately 2.1 L/min of oxygen (3,000 L/day) and produces approximately 1.7 L/min of carbon dioxide (2,400 L/day).[180] Thus the lung provides an important means by which normal arterial oxygen and carbon dioxide tensions and arterial pH are maintained. In the absence of lung disease, pulmonary arterial oxygenation (PaO_2) is dependent upon the inspired fraction of oxygen (normally 0.21) and the effective level of alveolar ventilation. This is approximated by a version of the alveolar gas equation:

$$PAO_2 = PIO_2 - (PACO_2)/R$$

where PaO_2 is the alveolar oxygen tension, PiO_2 is the inspired oxygen tension, PaCO_2 is the alveolar carbon dioxide tension, and R is the respiratory exchange quotient (the ratio of CO_2 production to O_2 consumption). Because there is admixture of venous blood with the pulmonary arterial circulation, alveolar oxygen tension exceeds arterial oxygen tension by approximately 10 mm Hg.

In the absence of alterations in inspired oxygen tensions, arterial hypoxemia (PaO_2 <85 mm Hg) may result from basically four processes, including (1) hypoventilation, (2) diffusion impairment, (3) ventilation:perfusion ($\dot{V}/\dot{Q}$) inequality, and (4) shunts.[181]

Alveolar and thus arterial CO_2 levels are dependent upon the rate of CO_2 elimination relative to its production, given by the following equation:

$$PACO_2 \approx \dot{V}CO_2/\dot{V}A$$

where $\dot{V}CO_2$ is the rate of CO_2 production and $\dot{V}A$ is alveolar ventilation. *Hypoventilation* is defined as inadequate CO_2 elimination relative to production, resulting in an elevated PaCO_2 (hypercapnia, hypercarbia). Hypoventilation can result from a variety of abnormalities. A convenient diagnostic approach follows the control of breathing from (1) the respiratory center in the medulla, (2) the efferent nerves (phrenic), (3) the "bellows" (diaphragm and chest wall muscles), (4) the pleural space, and (5) the airways. Some examples include (1) drug administration (barbiturates, diazepam, xylazine); (2) diseases of the brainstem secondary to infection (encephalitis), trauma, hemorrhage, or neoplasia; (3) diseases of the respiratory muscles, including botulism, trauma, or fatigue; (4) pleuritis and space-occupying lesions; and (5) choke and upper airway obstruction.

In patients suffering from hypoventilation, arterial oxygenation will improve with oxygen administration (by increasing PiO_2), but the most efficacious mode of correcting the hypercapnia and consequent hypoxemia is by mechanical ventilation. Diffusion impairment occurs when there is inadequate time for equilibration of alveolar oxygen tensions with pulmonary capillary oxygen tensions. Under normal resting conditions, equilibration of oxygen tensions occurs within 0.25 second, approximately one third of the contact time of the blood in the pulmonary circulation.[181] There is some evidence suggesting that in the exercising horse, the arterial hypoxemia that normally develops at high exercise intensities is in part due to the decrease in time available for oxygen diffusion.[182, 183] During rest, diffusion impairment is unlikely to occur. Arterial hypoxemia due to diffusion impairment can be corrected by administration of supplemental oxygen.

$\dot{V}/\dot{Q}$ inequalities are the primary cause of arterial hypoxemia and occur when alveolar ventilation and pulmonary blood flow are mismatched despite the existence of several reflexes which normally tend to prevent this problem. For example, a fall in the $\dot{V}/\dot{Q}$ ratio causes alveolar hypoxia, which induces pulmonary vasoconstriction and decreases perfusion to that lung region. (But this reflex also increases pulmonary vascular resistance and thus the work of the right side of the heart.) A second reflex is hypocapnic bronchoconstriction. When the $\dot{V}/\dot{Q}$ ratio increases, regional ventilation of those lung units is reduced by smooth muscle constriction.[184] $\dot{V}/\dot{Q}$ inequalities interfere with both oxygen and carbon dioxide transfer so that both hypoxemia and hypercapnia may ensue. Usually the consequent hypercapnia increases chemoreceptor drive and thus increases alveolar ventilation, which restores normocapnia. However, because of the shape of the oxyhemoglobin dissociation curve, the increase in oxygen tension in the normal alveoli due to the hyperventilation does not significantly increase the oxygen content of the blood coming from these units.[184] Several factors can exacerbate the hypoxemia of $\dot{V}/\dot{Q}$ inequalities, including hypoventilation (sedation) and decrements in cardiac output (mechanical ventilation with positive end-expiratory pressure, PEEP).[181] $\dot{V}/\dot{Q}$ inequalities will respond to oxygen therapy, although this may lead to increases in arterial carbon dioxide tension by (1) a reduction of the chemoreceptor (hypoxic) drive, (2) an increase in $\dot{V}/\dot{Q}$ inequalities, and (3) a shift in the carboxyhemoglobin dissociation curve to the right, decreasing its affinity for carbon dioxide.[184] Mechanical ventilation may be indicated in severe $\dot{V}/\dot{Q}$ inequalities if hypercapnia is progressive.

Passage of blood through abnormal cardiovascular communications (atrial septal defects, ventricular septal defects, patent ductus arteriosus) or through pulmonary capillaries within the walls of atelectatic or fluid-filled alveoli is the cause of shunts and consequent hypoxemia. It may be considered as one extreme of $\dot{V}/\dot{Q}$ inequality ($\dot{V}/\dot{Q}=0$) and is resistant to correction by oxygen therapy.[184] In shunts due to pulmonary disease, mechanical ventilation and PEEP are used to increase end-expiratory lung volume and thus the alveolar surface area available for gas exchange. The incremental increase in end-expiratory lung volume may also help to redistribute the excessive extravascular lung water from the alveoli to the interstitium.

Metabolic Functions

The entire cardiac output passes through the pulmonary circulation, thus providing an ideal means by which hormones and drugs may be metabolized to inactive compounds. Indeed, relative to the hepatic blood flow (approximately 25% of the cardiac output), the lung's contribution to the total body clearance of drugs or xenobiotics may be significant.[185] The lung contains hydrolytic enzymes that cleave peptides such as bradykinin and angiotensin I, thus serving to either inactivate (bradykinin) or to bioactivate (angiotensin) compounds. The enzymatic activity responsi-

ble is concentrated within the caveolae of the pulmonary capillary endothelium or in pouchings in the plasma membranes of these cells.[185] Other pulmonary enzymes exist which are capable of cleaving phosphate groups from nucleotides (adenosine triphosphate [ATP], diphosphate [ADP], and monophosphate [AMP]), of oxidizing steroid hormones (testosterone), of inactivating prostaglandins E and F, and of metabolizing biogenic amines such as 5-hydroxytryptamine, norepinephrine, and tyramine.[168, 185, 186]

Defense Against Infection

The "sterile" environment of the lung is the result of several mechanisms, including the mucociliary apparatus, which clears particulate debris from the lung at a rate of approximately 17 mm/min,[187] and vagally mediated reflexes, which serve to initiate coughing and concomitant bronchoconstriction. However, the predominant line of defense against noxious agents and bacteria is provided by the alveolar macrophages of the distal airways and alveoli. Recent investigations have shown depression in alveolar macrophage function following exercise or long van rides.[188–190] Macrophage function is also depressed during viral infections. (See Disorders of the Lower Respiratory Tract, which follows.) Helping to maintain immunosurveillance and the sterile pulmonary environment are polymorphonuclear cells, responding to chemotactic stimuli, and lymphocytes.

DISORDERS OF THE LOWER RESPIRATORY TRACT

Bacterial Pneumonia

Etiology. Pneumonia caused by gram-positive organisms in the equine adult is usually due to β-hemolytic *Streptococcus zooepidemicus,* an opportunist and a normal inhabitant of the equine upper respiratory tract. Rarely, *Streptococcus equi, Staphylococcus aureus,* and perhaps *Streptococcus pneumoniae* (α-hemolytic) are associated with pneumonia.[191–194] *Nocardia* organisms have also been isolated from horses with pulmonary infections, but these are relatively rare and appear to require derangements of the defense mechanisms.[195] Mixed bacterial infections are not uncommon in equine pneumonia. The gram-negative organisms that have been isolated from pneumonic horses include *Escherichia coli* and *Pasteurella, Klebsiella,* and *Bordetella* species. (*Pseudomonas* species do not appear to be a significant pathogen in equine pneumonia. Isolation of this organism from tracheobronchial aspirates suggests contamination of the aspirate by equipment.) The necrotizing effects of the gram-negative organisms are enhanced by anaerobes such as *Bacteroides fragilis* and *Bacteroides melaninogenicus.*

Pathogenesis. Bacterial pneumonia often follows viral infections or other stressful events such as general anesthesia, athletic events (races), transportation, overcrowding, poor nutrition, or following exposure to inclement weather. In addition, pneumonia may follow aspiration of bacteria due to dysfunction of the larynx and pharynx occurring (1) with primary neuropathies of the 9th and 10th cranial nerves, (2) with primary myopathies of the pharyngeal, laryngeal, or esophageal musculature (vitamin E and selenium deficiency, botulism, megaesophagus), or (3) as a consequence of laryngeal surgery or esophageal obstruction. An excellent review of pulmonary viral-bacterial interactions is available,[196] but basically viral-induced modifications of respiratory tract defenses include (1) enhanced susceptibility to bacterial attachment and colonization following damage to the epithelial cells, (2) diminished mucociliary clearance and thus reduced physical translocation of bacterial particles deposited on the bronchial ciliated epithelium, and (3) decreased surfactant levels due to viral destruction of alveolar type II cells with collapse of airways. This creates an anaerobic environment that impairs macrophage function. Lack of an aerobic environment may predispose to macrophage dysfunction. In addition, the alveolar exudate that accompanies viral pneumonitis may provide a nutrient medium for bacterial multiplication. The stress of exercise or transportation has been shown to have a depressant effect on alveolar macrophage function.[188–190] In addition, by physically restraining the horse's head (as might occur during transportation) and preventing postural drainage, bacterial colonization of the lower respiratory tract is enhanced.[197] Thus, impaired pulmonary defense mechanisms promote bacterial colonization and the development of pneumonia.

Clinical Signs. Clinical signs associated with pneumonia include intermittent fever, tachypnea or respiratory distress, nasal discharge, coughing, and inappetence. Submandibular lymphadenopathy may be apparent in streptococcal pneumonia (*Streptococcus equi*) as bronchopneumonia is often a sequela of this upper respiratory tract infection. A foul-smelling nasal discharge is suggestive of an anaerobic component. Clinical signs exhibited in individual cases may be variable. In addition, exercise intolerance and weight loss may also be apparent.

Diagnosis. The diagnosis is based upon the clinical signs and history. Auscultation of the thorax reveals increased harsh expiratory sounds, crackles, and wheezes. Fluid may be auscultated within the trachea and manipulation of the trachea or larynx may induce a cough. Clinical pathologic data supportive of a bacterial pneumonia includes a leukocytosis with an absolute neutrophilia, with or without the appearance of immature neutrophils. Neutropenia may also be evident if gram-negative organisms are involved. A hyperfibrinogenemia (>500 mg/dL), hyperglobulinemia, and anemia of chronic inflammation are compatible with the diagnosis of bacterial pneumonia. Thoracic radiographs demonstrate radiopacity in the anteroventral thorax and a loss of clarity in the lung fields caudal to the heart. Air bronchograms are usually not found in the adult horse with bacterial pneumonia (Fig. 6–8). Tracheobronchial aspirates yield degenerative neutrophils, damaged epithelial cells, and microorganisms. The presence of squamous epithelial cells would support a diagnosis of aspiration pneumonia, provided that the tracheal catheter was not misplaced in the pharynx during sampling. Both aerobic and anaerobic cultures should be performed on the sample.

Treatment. Treatment should be directed at the causative organism, but in the absence of microbiology results broad-spectrum antimicrobials should be administered. Appropriate

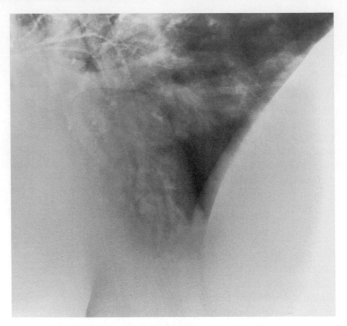

Figure 6–8. Two-year-old Thoroughbred with pneumonia. A, patchy area of pulmonary consolidation is noted in the ventral dependent portion of the lung silhouetting the heart and diaphragm.

therapy might include intravenous aqueous sodium or potassium penicillin and an aminoglycoside or third-generation cephalosporin (Table 6–5). The aminoglycosides are efficacious against most gram-negative aerobes, but lack efficacy against anaerobes. However, metronidazole is effective against most anaerobes, including the penicillin-resistant *Bacteroides fragilis*. Metronidazole should be included in the treatment protocol when a foul odor or nasal discharge is noted on physical examination of the horse. Aminoglycosides should be used judiciously in animals that have renal

Table 6–5. Antimicrobials Commonly Used in the Treatment of Respiratory Conditions

Antimicrobial	Dosage		
Ampicillin sodium	11–22 mg/kg	IV, IM	t.i.d., q.i.d.
Amikacin	7 mg/kg	IV, IM	t.i.d.
Ceftiofur	4.4 mg/kg	IV, IM	q.i.d.
Chloramphenicol	50 mg/kg	PO	q.i.d.
Erythromycin estolate	10–25 mg/kg	PO	t.i.d., q.i.d.
Gentamicin	2.2 mg/kg	IV, IM	t.i.d.
Kanamycin	5.0 mg/kg	IM	t.i.d.
Metronidazole	15–25 mg/kg	PO	q.i.d.
Oxytetracycline	5.0 mg/kg	IV	b.i.d.
Penicillin G			
Sodium	22,000 IU/kg	IV	q.i.d.
Potassium	22,000 IU/kg	IV	q.i.d.
Procaine	22,000 IU/kg	IM	b.i.d.
Rifampin	5–10 mg/kg	PO	b.i.d.
Trimethoprim-sulfadiazine	15–20 mg/kg	PO, IV	b.i.d.

compromise or are dehydrated. Depending upon the culture sensitivity results, potentiated sulfonamides may also be administered. With gram-negative infections and the potential for endotoxemia, small doses of flunixin meglumine 0.25 mg/kg t.i.d. may be given to inhibit arachidonic acid metabolism.

Other treatment modalities that have been advocated include nebulization, the use of bronchodilators, and expectorants, although the efficacy of these pharmacologic agents has not been thoroughly examined. Supportive care should be provided with the goal of minimizing stress and insuring adequate ventilation and hydration status. Ideally, horses should be bedded on paper or on other materials relatively free of dusts or molds and fed forages of excellent quality and free of molds. Attention should also be directed at correcting the primary cause of the pneumonia. Depending upon the chronicity of the pneumonia, clinical improvement should be noted in 48 to 72 hours. The prognosis can be excellent if the pneumonia is treated aggressively, but the owner should be forewarned of potential complications, including pulmonary abscessation and septic pleuropneumonia. These conditions carry a less favorable prognosis.

Preventive measures which help deter the development of pneumonia include (1) adequate immunization protocols with vaccination against equine influenza virus, EHV-1 and EHV-2, every 2 to 3 months (in the performance horse); (2) the minimization of stresses such as long van rides in which the head is constantly restrained; and (3) the use of excellent management or husbandry methods which minimize dust or noxious gas accumulations within the stall, prevent exposure to inclement weather, and provide adequate nutritional planes for the horse.

Pleuropneumonia

Etiology. This condition most often occurs in conjunction with pneumonia and pulmonary abscessation, but it may also occur secondary to thoracic trauma, neoplasia, and esophageal rupture. Pleuritis may also occur as a primary disease, as discussed later.[198]

Epidemiology. Several different studies have examined the occurrence of pleuropneumonia. Schott and Mansmann,[199] in a review of 46 cases of pleural effusion, found that approximately two thirds of the cases had effusion associated with pleuropneumonia or lung abscessation.[199] In their survey, survival rates were higher in acute cases. Raphel and Beech[200] found that approximately 74% of the horses with pleural effusion had pleuritis secondary to pneumonia or lung abscessation.

Pathogenesis. The factors causative of equine pleuropneumonia are not known but are undoubtedly the same factors that suppress the pulmonary defense mechanisms and predispose to the development of bacterial pneumonia, as discussed earlier. These include such conditions as surgery or anesthesia, transportation over long distances, laryngeal or pharyngeal dysfunction, pulmonary epistaxis, and strenuous exercise.[200] The indiscriminate use of corticosteroids with direct suppression of the pulmonary defense mechanisms or the administration of nonsteroidal anti-inflammatory agents

masking early viral respiratory infections may promote the development of pleuropneumonia. The distribution of the pulmonary lesions is usually cranioventral with the right cranial and middle lung lobes more severely afflicted. These findings are consistent with a bronchopneumonia secondary to inhalation or aspiration rather than from hematogenous routes.[201] In addition, bacterial isolates from clinical cases are typically organisms constituting the normal bacterial flora of the pharynx—*Streptococcus zooepidemicus; E. coli; Klebsiella, Pasteurella,* and *Bordetella* species; and anaerobic *Bacteroides* species.

Clinical Signs. Pleuropneumonia has been classified into four stages based upon the length of time that the disease has been present[202]:

Stage I (preacute): Horses are febrile and depressed, have a slight nasal discharge, and may exhibit pleurodynia, pleural friction rubs, and ventral dullness of the thorax on auscultation and percussion.

Stage II (acute): Horses exhibit inappetence, recurrent fever, pleural friction rubs, and ventral thoracic dullness. The clinical course ranges from 2 days to 2 weeks.

Stage III (chronic): Horses are sick for at least 2 weeks, often have positive fluid cultures, and require indwelling chest tubes or repeated thoracic drainage.

Stage IV (endstage): Horses are ill for periods greater than 4 weeks and exhibit chronic weight loss, depression, and anemia with hyperfibrinogenemia. There is a severe bacterial pneumonia with bronchopleural fistulas or large abscesses full of debris and a scarred pleura. Horses may also exhibit substernal or limb edema, intermittent colic, tachypnea, and dyspnea.

Diagnosis. Diagnosis is based, individually or severally, upon (1) auscultation, in which there is a decrease or absence of air movement in the ventral thorax, (2) percussion of a possible fluid line in the ventral thorax, (3) presentation of fluid during thoracocentesis, (4) radiographic evidence of a fluid line, or (5) ultrasonographic confirmation of a fluid line, lung consolidation, pulmonary abscessation, or fibrinoid tags.[203]

On auscultation of the thorax, vesicular sounds may only be heard dorsally, with an absence of sounds ventrally. Bronchial or tracheal sounds may be heard if lung consolidation exists. Cardiac sounds radiate over a wider area of the lung field than normal, a finding distinct from clinical cases of pericarditis. Upon percussion of the chest, a painful response may be elicited (pleurodynia) and an area of dullness or decreased resonance is detected.

Ultrasound is the diagnostic technique of choice in cases of pleuropneumonia or pleural effusion. The reader is referred to the discussion on ultrasonography under Diagnostic Approach to Respiratory Disorders. Briefly, using ultrasonography, free or loculated fluid, pleural thickening, pulmonary abscessation, and concurrent pericarditis can be accurately detected. In a study by Reimer and colleagues,[28] free gas echoes within pleural or abscess fluid correlated with the presence of anaerobic infections. Thus, ultrasonography may provide an etiologic diagnosis in cases of pleuropneumonia. In addition, ultrasonography enables accurate placement of the catheter during thoracocentesis and insures pro-

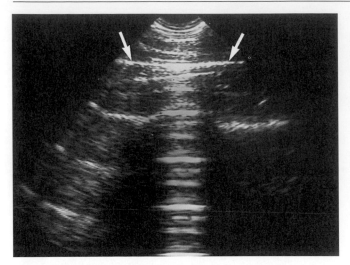

Figure 6–9. Normal thoracic ultrasound. Ultrasound demonstrates a highly echogenic interface *(arrows)* between the chest wall and normal lung. A reverberation artifact is noted deep to the chest wall–lung interface.

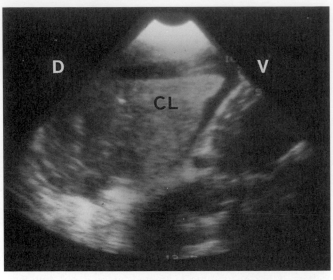

Figure 6–11. Ultrasound of ventrally consolidated lung (CL) surrounded by a small amount of pleural effusion. V, ventral; D, dorsal.

ductive yields (Figs. 6–9 to 6–13). However, radiography remains a useful technique in the evaluation of pleuropneumonia, permitting detection of a concomitant pneumothorax or assessment of abscesses located deep to aerated lung tissue.

Thoracocentesis of both sides of the chest is indicated unless concurrent coagulopathies exist. Fluid should be submitted for cytologic examination and for aerobic and anaerobic culture. Pleural fluid in healthy horses contains less than 10,000 cells per microliter, approximately 60% of which are neutrophils, and a total protein of less than 3 g/dL. In cases of pleuropneumonia, pleural fluid white blood cell (WBC) counts and protein are elevated and glucose levels may be

low (<40 mg/dL). The fluid may exhibit a foul odor if anaerobes are contributing to the infection, but the absence of an odor should not dismiss the possibility of an anaerobic component. Isolation of an anaerobe is associated with a poor prognosis (33% survival rate).[204] A tracheobronchial aspirate should always be performed to improve recovery of the bacterial organisms involved in the lung disease.

Treatment. Treatment is directed at (1) removing excessive pleural fluid, (2) administering systemic antimicrobial and

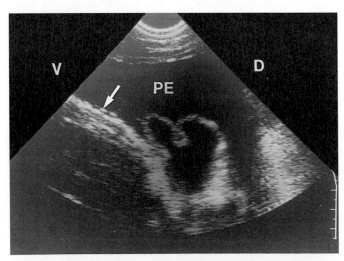

Figure 6–10. Ultrasound of pleural effusion. Anechoic *(black)* area represents pleural effusion (PE). The echogenic *(white)* tortuous fibrin strand is attached to the parietal pleura of the diaphragm. V, ventral; D, dorsal; *arrow,* diaphragm.

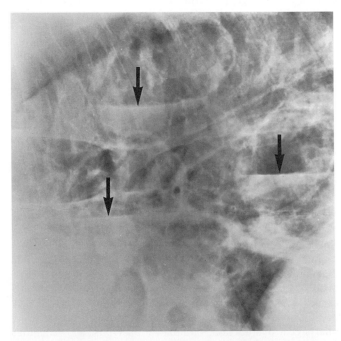

Figure 6–12. Nine-year-old saddle horse. Multiple cavitating pulmonary abscesses are present within the lungs. *Arrows,* air-fluid interfaces within the abscesses.

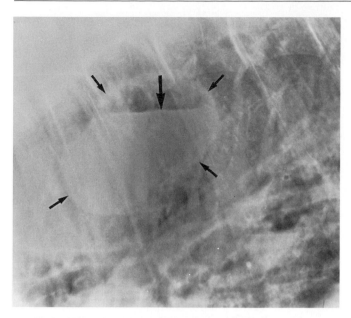

Figure 6–13. A large air-capped pulmonary abscess. *Small arrows,* abscess; *large arrow,* air-fluid interface.

analgesic therapy, and (3) providing supportive care. Oxygen therapy may be indicated if the horse remains dyspneic after thoracic drainage or is hypoxemic. Aminophylline 5 mg/kg PO t.i.d. and furosemide 1 mg/kg IV may also be indicated for bronchodilation and mobilization of fluid.

Indwelling chest tubes should be considered if large volumes of foul-smelling fluid with microorganisms are obtained or if a poor response to intermittent drainage occurs.[199] Rapid removal of large volumes of fluid from the chest should be avoided to guard against the development of hypovolemia.

Appropriate antimicrobial therapy is based upon the results of the culture and sensitivity, but pending results, broad-spectrum intravenous antibiotics should be administered. Penicillin is the drug of choice if anaerobes other than *Bacteroides fragilis* are encountered. Potentiated sulfonamides and aminoglycosides are not efficacious against anaerobic bacteria but can be used in combination with penicillin in mixed bacterial infections. Metronidazole is routinely used against anaerobes, especially *B. fragilis.*[202] Erythromycin and rifampin both attain good concentrations in the lung and pleural fluid as well as within phagocytic cells, but expense may preclude their use in adult animals. Antimicrobial therapy should be continued until the horse is gaining weight, the foul odor is gone, and hematologic values return to normal. This may entail a course of therapy of 2 to 6 months with limited exercise (hand walking) and avoidance of stress. Refractory cases should be reevaluated using the techniques of ultrasonography, thoracocentesis, or transtracheal aspiration to determine if drug resistance has developed, if additional pathogens are involved, or if untoward sequelae have occurred (see below). In refractory cases, unilateral rib resection with mechanical debridement of large abscesses may become necessary. Initial attempts at drainage using a large-bore chest tube (24F) directed through the capsular wall of the abscess followed by suction of the

abscess contents should be considered prior to rib resection. Lavage of the contents of the abscess may improve removal of the purulent material. Care should be taken to prevent spillage of the contents into the pleural cavity. Additional therapeutic modalities that have been recommended include the use of antithrombotic agents such as subcutaneous heparin 40 IU/kg b.i.d,[205] although these are not routinely used by us.

Long-term medical treatment of pleuropneumonia may induce such complications as venous phlebitis or thrombosis, or both, secondary to intravenous catheter placement; cellulitis or pneumothorax following thoracocentesis; and diarrhea due to antimicrobial and anti-inflammatory therapy or endotoxemia. With minor changes in the therapeutic approaches, most of these complications will resolve and not impede the eventual return to health of the horse. However, more serious sequelae of infectious pleuropneumonia have been described in detail by Byars and colleagues.[206, 207] In a survey of 153 horses presenting to their veterinary hospital over a 4-year period with pleuropneumonia, they detailed the development of cranial thoracic masses (7.2%), bronchopleural fistulas (6.5%), pericarditis (2.6%), and laminitis (1.3%).

Cranial thoracic masses should be suspected when horses exhibit tachycardia, jugular distention, forelimb extension (pointing), and caudal displacement of the heart. The presence of empyema, loculations, or encapsulated abscesses cranial to the heart can be confirmed by ultrasonography. In the majority of cases, medical therapy is effective at reducing the abscess, and thus this conservative approach should initially be elected. Additional therapeutic modalities include the administration of a diuretic (furosemide) and a chronotropic agent (digitalis) to improve cardiac performance. However, refractory cases may require ultrasound-guided drainage of the abscess performed under short-term anesthesia (xylazine-ketamine combination).

Bronchopleural fistulas develop when necrotic pulmonary tissue sloughs, providing a direct communication of the airways with the pleural cavity. Diagnosis is confirmed by visualization of the airways following pleuroscopy or by the intratracheal appearance of contrast media injected into the pleural cavity. Bronchopleural fistulas may eventually close as the pulmonary tissue adheres to the chest wall or as the airways close.

Pleural Effusion

Etiology. Accumulation of fluid within the pleural space may also be the result of neoplastic infiltrates such as lymphosarcoma, gastric squamous cell carcinoma, myxoma, adenocarcinoma, and myeloma.[199, 208, 209] Pleural effusion accompanies a number of other conditions, including thoracic trauma, pericarditis, peritonitis, viral respiratory diseases, mycoplasmal infections, congestive heart failure, liver disease, diaphragmatic herniation, hypoproteinemia, equine infectious anemia, pulmonary granulomas, chylothorax, and fungal pneumonia.[199, 205, 210–212]

Diagnosis. Thoracocentesis is helpful. Neoplastic cells or fungal elements may be detected on cytology. Transudates are usually associated with congestive heart failure, liver fibrosis, hypoalbuminemia, or early neoplastic processes. Exudates occur with infections and intra-abdominal diseases, while modified transudates are often found in neoplastic conditions.[205] A Coggins test and titers against *Coccidioides immitis, Cryptococcus neoformans,* and *Mycoplasma felis* should also be performed.

Treatment. Treatment is directed at the primary cause, but neoplastic conditions and pleural effusions associated with an endstage organ failure carry a poor prognosis.

Fungal Pneumonia

Epidemiology. Fungal pneumonia in the horse as a primary entity is relatively uncommon.

Etiology. Organisms involved include *Coccidioides immitis, Cryptococcus neoformans,* and *Histoplasma capsulatum.*[213, 214] Opportunistic organisms such as *Aspergillus, Mucor, Rhizopus,* and *Candida* may also cause fungal pneumonia and are likely to exist in the compromised host.[215] Thus, factors that contribute to the development of pulmonary mycotic infections include suppression of the host immune system, immunodeficiency, overzealous administration of antibiotics, and exposure to large numbers of mycotic organisms.[216]

Clinical Signs. In primary fungal pneumonia, horses may present with a chronic cough, anorexia and weight loss, and nasal discharge.[213, 214] Many horses with fungal pneumonia will have more serious primary problems such as colitis, peritonitis, septicemia, or endotoxemia.[215, 216] In such cases it has been hypothesized that pulmonary lesions are a sequela of mycotic invasion of the intestinal tract or immunocompromise and tissue devitalization secondary to severe acute enterocolitis.[217]

Diagnosis. Tracheobronchial aspirates may reveal degenerated neutrophils, yeast cells, and often bacteria. Diagnosis should not be based on the results of tracheal aspirates alone, as fungal elements may be recovered from the tracheal washings of normal horses.[18] Radiographs may reveal circular masses with or without fluid lines. The demonstration of high titers against *Coccidioides immitis* or *Cryptococcus neoformans* provides further support of the diagnosis. However, high titers against *Aspergillus* are not diagnostic, as many normal horses maintain high immunoglobulin levels to this organism.[215] The diagnosis may be confirmed with lung biopsy and by the presence of other systemic alterations. Cases of immunosuppression or immunocompromise should be investigated by quantitation of immunoglobulin levels and by mitogen stimulation tests.

Treatment. Treatment against the primary fungal pathogens is not recommended because of the potential public health hazards. With secondary fungal pneumonia, treatment should be directed to the primary cause.

Mycoplasmal Pneumonia

Mycoplasma organisms have been isolated from the upper respiratory tract and the lower airway of clinically normal horses as well as of horses with respiratory disease, but the role of these organisms in inflammatory conditions of the respiratory tract is not known.[210, 218] Experimental induction of pleuritis has been demonstrated following intrapleural inoculation with *M. felis* and its isolation from horses with pleuritis has also been documented.[219]

Pulmonary Edema

Etiology. Increases in lung water are associated with a number of conditions, including anaphylaxis, aspiration pneumonia, near-drowning, congestive heart failure, rupture of the mitral valve chordae tendineae, monensin toxicity, septicemia, endotoxemia, and intravenous fluid volume overload.[220–224]

Pathogenesis. Accumulation of fluid within the lung interstitium and alveoli is a function of capillary and interstitial oncotic pressures, capillary and interstitial hydrostatic pressures, and the integrity of the capillary endothelium. Permeability changes in the alveolar epithelium and capillary endothelium may occur following aspiration of water, feed, or medications. Permeability changes in the capillary endothelium accompany septicemia and endotoxemia. Alterations in hydrostatic pressure occur with congestive heart failure or with left heart dysfunction.

Clinical Signs. Horses are dyspneic and tachypneic, and may exhibit coughing. A red-tinged or yellow frothy material may be evident at the nares. Fever may be a component of the syndrome depending upon the primary cause of the pulmonary edema.

Diagnosis. Diagnosis depends upon the physical findings and history. Crackles may be detected on auscultation and fluid may be auscultated within the trachea. Loud murmurs or cardiac arrhythmias may be auscultated in cases of pulmonary edema secondary to cardiac dysfunction (left heart failure, mitral valve insufficiency). Radiographs reveal an interstitial pattern, although an alveolar pattern due to ventral consolidation of the lung fields may follow aspiration pneumonia.

Treatment. Treatment should be directed at the primary cause. The rate of delivery of intravenous fluids should be slowed. Plasma may be administered if hypoproteinemia exists. Furosemide at 1 mg/kg IV helps to mobilize lung extravascular water. Oxygen therapy may be beneficial, although mechanical ventilation may be difficult in adult horses. Depending upon the extent of the hypoxemia and the severity of ventilation:perfusion inequalities, nasal insufflation of oxygen may be beneficial. Broad-spectrum antimicrobials and nonsteroidal anti-inflammatory drugs are indicated in aspiration pneumonia and septicemia. Digoxin is used in cases of congestive heart failure, although mitral valve insufficiency secondary to chordae tendineae rupture carries a poor prognosis.

Heaves

Definition. This is a naturally occurring respiratory disease typified by periods of acute airway obstruction followed by periods of remission. It has been termed *chronic obstructive* *pulmonary disease, chronic pulmonary disease, chronic airway reactivity, hyperactive airway disease, broken wind,* and *hay sickness.* Pulmonary function testing demonstrates a decrease in lung compliance, an increase in lung resistance, an increase in the work of breathing, and the development of arterial hypoxemia, usually in the absence of hypercapnia.[39, 225, 226] During airway obstruction, affected horses are hyperresponsive to nonspecific stimuli such as histamine, methacholine, and water.[227]

Epidemiology. The condition is seen worldwide, with affected horses tending to be older, with a mean age of 8 years.[228, 229]

Etiology. There is still much debate concerning the cause of heaves. Many consider it to be a hypersensitivity reaction to dusts or molds commonly found in poorly cured hay or straw. The condition is relatively rare in horses kept outdoors on pasture. The two most frequently implicated molds are *Aspergillus fumigatus* (fungus) and *Micropolyspora faeni* (a thermophilic actinomycete).[230] A similar condition has also been described in the southeastern United States. However, these horses appear to react to pasture-associated allergens or dusts and improve only when stabled.[231] Other factors implicated in the development of heaves include viral infections, hypersensitivity to chickens,[232] possibly lungworm infections, and a genetic predisposition.[228]

Pathogenesis. The condition is characterized by periods of airway obstruction (primarily of the bronchioles) due to smooth muscle contraction and accumulations of mucous plugs, cellular debris, and exudate. The inhalation of the allergen may induce a type I or type III immune reaction with release of mediators from inflammatory cells and activation of the parasympathetic system. A type I reaction involves antibody-induced degranulation of mast cells. This mechanism is supported by bronchoalveolar lavage cytology: when heavy ponies are challenged with aerosolized *M. faeni,* fewer mast cells are recovered in the bronchoalveolar lavage fluid compared with normal non-heavy ponies.[233] A type III reaction has been implicated in the pathogenesis of heaves because circulating IgG concentrations increase approximately 7 days following challenge with molds. A type III allergic reaction with influx of neutrophils and release of cytokines which induce airway inflammation has also been proposed.[232] However, when clinically normal ponies are challenged with aerosolized *M. faeni,* neutrophil counts increase in their bronchoalveolar lavage, without altering airway reactivity.[233] Perhaps the difference between healthy and heavy ponies is in the state of neutrophil activation and subsequent mediator release.[234]

Because atropine administration to heavy horses provides some clinical improvement, an important role of the parasympathetic system in mediating airway reactivity has been implicated. It would appear that the airway smooth muscle of heavy ponies is hyperresponsive to normal amounts of acetylcholine. However increased vagal reflex activity or an augmented release of acetylcholine as a result of inflammatory mediators cannot be dismissed and requires further investigation.[234]

Clinical Signs. Horses present with a chronic cough, a mucopurulent nasal discharge, and an accentuated expiratory effort. Hypertrophy of the external oblique muscle due to continued recruitment is evident (heave line). The respiratory rate may be normal or increased (tachypnea). Exercise intolerance, weight loss, and cachexia may also be evident in severe cases. Horses are usually afebrile.

Diagnosis. Diagnosis is based upon the clinical signs and history of a seasonal disorder associated with husbandry alterations such as new hay or bedding or having recently been stabled. Auscultation reveals inspiratory or expiratory wheezes, crackles, or "tracheal rattles." Percussion may be normal or an expanded lung field may be detected. Endoscopic examination reveals excessive mucopurulent exudate within the trachea. A bronchoalveolar lavage supports a *nonseptic* inflammatory reaction with increases in mucus and the percentage of intact neutrophils. Albumin and immunoglobulin levels within the bronchoalveolar lavage may not increase.[233] Gram-positive organisms may be retrieved by tracheobronchial aspirates if a concurrent septic inflammation exists. Pollen, fungal hyphae, and Curshmann's spirals (inspissated mucus plugs) may also be seen. Thoracic radiography may demonstrate an increase in the interstitial and bronchial pattern throughout the lung fields. However, these changes may be difficult to interpret relative to the normal aging changes that occur. Exudate within the trachea may also be detected on thoracic radiograph (Fig. 6–14). Intradermal skin testing has been advocated by some, but its usefulness is questionable. Theoretically, heavy horses should react if sensitized to a given allergen, but some clinically normal horses react to the allergens and some heavy horses do not.[228, 230] Usually, there are no abnormalities detected in the leukogram or clinical chemistries.

Pathology. Postmortem examination reveals a diffuse bronchiolitis with goblet cell metaplasia, airway smooth muscle hypertrophy, excess mucus, and inflammatory cells in the small airways. Eosinophilic infiltration around the bronchi-

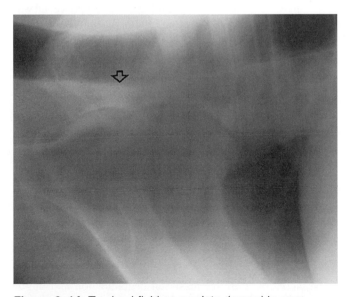

Figure 6–14. Tracheal fluid or exudate *(arrow)* is seen ventrally in the trachea at the level of the thoracic inlet.

oles is a variable finding, present in approximately one third of the horses examined by Gerber.[229] Varying degrees of alveolar emphysema and atelectases can also be found, as well as evidence of fibrosis of the alveolar septa.[235] The larger airways—the bronchi and trachea—may also show variable changes, including epithelial hyperplasia with loss of ciliated cells, goblet cell hyperplasia, and inflammatory cell infiltration.[236]

Treatment. Elimination of the source of the mold or dust can be the most beneficial step in the treatment regimen, but also the most difficult management change to effect. Horses may be fed pelleted alfalfa or a complete pelleted feed. This may be the most important recommendation.[237] The transition from hay to complete feed is made gradually over a 3- to 4-week period. Unless the condition is exacerbated by pasture, horses should be kept outside, blanketed in the winter, and allowed access to a three-walled shelter affording protection from the wind and rain. If the horse is stabled, the stall should be bedded in shredded paper, shaving, peat moss, or clay to eliminate dusts and molds. The surrounding stalls should be bedded similarly.

Medical management has also been indicated in these cases. Corticosteroids are efficacious in reducing the inflammatory reaction in the lungs, whereas nonsteroidal antiinflammatory drugs provide no benefit. Prednisone may be given initially at 1.0 mg/lb orally once daily in the morning for 1 week, 0.5 mg/lb once daily for 1 week, 0.25 mg/lb once daily for 1 week, and then 0.25 mg/lb one time every other day for a week with the objective of weaning the horse off the glucocorticoid.

Bronchodilators have also been recommended. There are three types of compounds used to relax airway smooth muscle: the β-adrenergics, the methylxanthines, and the anticholinergics. The $β_2$-adrenergic compounds include clenbuterol, terbutaline, and albuterol. Experimental investigations with clenbuterol suggest that when given at a dose of 0.8 μg/kg once daily by mouth, it may be efficacious in alleviating some of the signs of heaves.[238] In addition to a direct smooth muscle effect, clenbuterol may also stabilize mast cells, increase mucociliary clearance, and improve airway secretions.[238] An oral dose of terbutaline has not been established and potential side effects include sweating, tremors, and excitement.[237] The methylxanthines include aminophylline (theophylline), which dilates smooth muscle by increasing cyclic AMP (cAMP) levels intracellularly. cAMP also inhibits degranulation of mast cells and subsequent mediator release. Aminophylline may be given at 2 to 3 mg/lb PO t.i.d. However, in a recent study, aminophylline 12 mg/lb IV provided clinical improvement in only 50% of the cases.[239] The third class of compound used to effect smooth muscle dilatation includes the anticholinergics, of which atropine and glycopyrrolate are representatives. Atropine provides clinical improvement when administered IV at 0.02 mg/kg, but the duration of effect is short-lived (2 hours) and it may be associated with ileus and abdominal pain as well as a thickening of airway secretions.[239] Glycopyrrolate has been reported to be efficacious at a dose of 0.007 mg/kg.[240]

Disodium cromoglycate, is considered efficacious by some, acting to stabilize mast cell degranulation and inhibit the vagal efferent component of histamine response. A suggested dose from the study of McPherson and Thomson was 80 mg once daily for 4 days by nebulization.[230] Mucolytics (acetylcysteine, dembrexine) and mucokinetics (iodides, bromhexine) may provide some relief.[241] Antimicrobials are indicated if microorganisms are isolated on the tracheobronchial aspirate.

Prevention. Recommendations are difficult to make considering that much remains unknown about the pathogenesis of the disorder. Routine immunizations against the viral respiratory pathogens and good management practices are logical suggestions.

Lungworms

Etiology. Lungworm infections in the equine species are caused by *Dictyocaulus arnfieldi*. Infections in the donkey and mule are asymptomatic, but provide a source of viable eggs for clinically apparent infections in the horse and pony.

Epidemiology. Lungworm infections have been diagnosed by recovery of larvae in live animals or by recovery of the worms in the lungs of dead animals. Using this approach, one study reported that approximately 68% to 80% of the donkeys, 29% of the mules, and 2% to 11% of the horses were infected with *D. arnfieldi*.[242, 243]

Pathogenesis. Donkeys are considered as possible reservoirs for the parasite in horses, but there are instances of lungworm infections in horses in which no contact with donkeys could be established, suggesting horse-to-horse transmission.[243] Infective larvae are ingested, migrate through the gut wall, and are carried to the lungs via the lymphatics where, in hosts in which infections are patent, the larvae mature to egg-laying adults in the bronchi toward the periphery of the lobes. The prepatent period is approximately 2 to 3 months. Eggs are transported out of the lungs by the mucociliary apparatus, swallowed, and excreted in the feces where they become infective by 4 days.[244] First-stage larvae have survived for at least 49 days but do not survive over the winter.[245] In horses and ponies, larval development in the lungs is retarded (fifth stage), but airway inflammation and exudate accumulation still occur.

Clinical Signs. Horses exhibit chronic coughing and an increased expiratory effort. Auscultation reveals crackles and wheezes, especially over the dorsal and caudal parts of the lung fields.[246] Signs are often indistinguishable from those associated with heaves.

Diagnosis. Endoscopic examination may reveal a mild lymphoid follicular hyperplasia and copious amounts of exudate in the trachea and bronchioles. Tracheobronchial aspirates or bronchoalveolar lavage may contain a predominance of eosinophils and is suggestive of a lungworm infection, although other conditions may also be accompanied by increased eosinophil counts. A peripheral eosinophilia is a variable finding in these horses.[247] Definitive diagnosis is by identification of *D. arnfieldi* in the sediment of centrifuged mucus, although this may be difficult.[245] The Baermann technique should be performed, although patent infections in the horse are rare (2%).[248] Donkeys to which the horse has been exposed should also be tested. Diagnosis most often depends upon the clinical signs, the history of exposure to donkeys, and the response to anthelmintic therapy.

Treatment. Ivermectin 200 μg/kg is effective against *D. arnfieldi* in both controlled studies and field evaluations and did not cause any detrimental side effects.[248]

Prevention. Horses should not be pastured with donkeys or mules unless they are confirmed to be free of lungworms.

Exercise-Induced Pulmonary Hemorrhage

Etiology. The cause is not known. Several theories have been advanced concerning its development and are discussed under the Pathogenesis.

Epidemiology. EIPH has been detected in most breeds of horses undergoing strenuous athletic events. Its prevalence is estimated to be between 44% and 75% in the Thoroughbred, 26% in the standardbred, 62% in the racing quarter horse, 50% in racing Appaloosas, 68% in steeplechasers, 67% in timber racing horses, 40% in 3-day eventers, 10% in pony club event horses, and 11% in polo ponies.[249–253] The prevalence of EIPH increases with the age of the horse. There is no clear correlation between EIPH and the location of stables, the condition of the track, or the track type.[254] There does not appear to be a geographical variation in the prevalence of EIPH.

Pathogenesis. The mechanisms responsible for the development of EIPH have not been determined. Several theories have been advanced. Robinson and Derksen[255] have proposed that poor collateral ventilation in the horse coupled with small airway disease (and thus altered time constants for alveolar filling) predisposes to the development of underventilated lung regions. Extreme fluctuations in the alveolar pressure of these underventilated regions may produce parenchymal tearing or alveolar capillary rupture. Small airway disease has been detected in a large percentage of horses with EIPH[256] but its prevalence in racehorses not demonstrating EIPH has yet to be determined. Clarke[257] has speculated that visceral constraint of the diaphragm may predispose to the development of greater mechanical forces or stresses in the dorsal thorax. Thus, in the caudodorsal lung, these mechanical forces are borne over a relatively narrow area and may allow parenchymal tearing or rupture to occur. Another theory of the pathogenesis of EIPH has recently been proposed by O'Callaghan and colleagues[256]: small airway disease, possibly of viral origin, coupled with maximal exercise, induces a localized hypoxia, which initiates bronchial angiogenesis. The local hypoxia also initiates pulmonary vasoconstriction with a greater proportion of bronchial blood flow now being directed to the alveolar capillary bed through bronchial anastomotic connections. The exact site of hemorrhage is not certain but may occur at the advancing margin of the new vascular growth of the bronchial vessels. The accumulation of blood and cellular infiltrates may alter lung compliance and resistance further, exacerbating hypoxia and maintaining the cycle of events.[256]

Clinical Signs. Evidence of frank blood occurs in less than 10% of the horses with EIPH. The effect of EIPH on racing performance is variable. A clear association between finishing position in a race and the prevalence of EIPH in Thoroughbreds or standardbreds has not been demonstrated.[258] Often horses will continue to perform at levels judged to be adequate. In other cases, horses may slow or stop and some may exhibit difficult or labored breathing, coughing, or excessive swallowing.[259]

Diagnosis. Endoscopic examination of the upper respiratory tract and detection of frank blood within the trachea is the usual method of diagnosis. Optimal time for endoscopic examination is within 90 minutes of a race or workout. However, EIPH is not a consistent finding; it may not be apparent in a given horse examined on different occasions after the same level of exercise.[78] Transtracheal aspirates or bronchoalveolar lavage reveals hemosiderophages, intact and degenerating neutrophils, some with intracellular bacteria, and erythrocytes.[260] Radiographs may demonstrate increases in interstitial patterns, a radiopaque region in the caudal lung lobe, and possible dorsal displacement of the major pulmonary vessels[260] (Fig. 6–15).

Treatment. Rest has been recommended, but it is likely that pulmonary hemorrhage will recur once the horse resumes training.[259] The finding of concomitant small airway disease in several studies suggests that minimization of allergens should be attempted. However, the practicality of this approach on a racetrack is questionable. Antimicrobials may be indicated as the hemorrhage provides an excellent medium for bacterial growth to occur. Furosemide 250 to 300 mg, given 4 hours prior to the race, has also failed to prevent the development of EIPH in horses that were previously EIPH-negative.[261, 262] Other compounds, such as bioflavonoids, advocated for their purported enhancement of capillary integrity, have not been efficacious in the prevention of EIPH.[261] Cromoglycate, which is believed to stabilize mast cell membranes, also is not efficacious in the prevention of EIPH.[263]

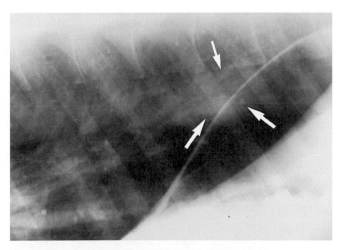

Figure 6–15. Focal area of increased interstitial pulmonary opacity *(arrows)* in the dorsal caudal lung field representing exercise-induced pulmonary hemorrhage.

Prevention. The efficacy of treatment regimens in the prevention of EIPH under race conditions has been difficult to determine even when speed handicapping methods are employed. Variables such as the administration of drugs unknown to the investigators, or the inability to diagnose or reproduce EIPH within a given horse on consecutive days, makes interpretation of these studies difficult. And yet controlled studies conducted on a treadmill probably do not accurately simulate race conditions, so that false conclusions may also be drawn.

Interstitial and Bronchointerstitial Lung Diseases

Definition. Although traditionally considered to be a chronic disorder, interstitial pneumonia encompasses both acute and chronic inflammatory responses occurring predominantly within the alveolar walls and the interstitial tissues of the lung.[264] Interstitial lung disease includes, then, a heterogeneous group of disorders characterized by damage to the alveolar walls and loss of functional alveolar capillary units. When this disorder also involves the conducting airways, the term *bronchointerstitial pneumonia* is used.

Etiology. Most of the recognized spontaneously occurring interstitial pneumonias in animals are caused either by toxins or infectious or parasitic agents. Toxic lung injury in the horse has been documented following consumption of crofton weed, pyrrolizidine alkaloids, and *Perilla* ketones.[264–266] Interstitial pneumonia is also a feature of viral infections, silicosis, and possibly oxygen therapy.[267, 268] Other cases of interstitial pneumonia may not have a well-defined cause.[269–271] Rarely, granulomatous interstitial pneumonia may also occur in tuberculosis.[272] Involvement of the airways, as well as the interstitium (bronchointerstitial pneumonia), has also been described in both adult horses and in foals 1 to 2½ months of age.[272–274] The cause of this disorder has not been determined, although several different agents, including toxins, viruses (EHV-2), and *Pneumocystis carinii* infections, have been proposed.

Pathophysiology. In interstitial pneumonia, the inciting agent initiates damage to pulmonary epithelial or endothelial cells with coagulative necrosis of the alveoli occurring. The acute or exudative phase is characterized by pulmonary congestion, interstitial edema, and alveolar flooding. The fibrin, protein-rich fluid, cellular debris, and inflammatory cells (neutrophils and macrophages) form characteristic hyaline membranes. During this acute phase (day 1–5), horses exhibit respiratory distress. The exudative phase is followed by a proliferative stage in which the type II cells, the pulmonary stem cells, replace damaged type I pneumocytes. Interlobar septa widen due to the proliferation of fibroblasts and inflammatory cell infiltration by neutrophils and macrophages.[264] The changes described by Prescott[273] and Ainsworth[274] and their colleagues in foals with bronchointerstitial pneumonia were similar to those described above with the exception that terminal bronchioles were also affected. This was evidenced by epithelial necrosis and the appearance of multinucleated syncytial cells within both the alveoli and bronchioles. Primary bronchioles or bronchi were not af-

fected. Because the pulmonary lesions closely resembled those found in respiratory syncytial or parainfluenza 3 virus infections in cattle, Prescott and associates suggested that bronchointerstitial pneumonia in the foal may be secondary to EHV-2 infection contracted during a time of declining maternal antibody levels.[273] However, virus isolation procedures on the foals examined did not support this hypothesis.

Based upon the detection of *P. carinii* organisms on histopathologic examination, Ainsworth and co-workers proposed that bronchointerstitial pneumonia (and the consequent respiratory distress in foals) may be secondary to this protozoal (fungal) organism complicating *Rhodococcus equi* infections.[274] The question of whether (1) the bacterial organism produces an immunosuppressive state allowing the pneumocystosis to then occur or whether (2) a primary immunosuppressive state occurs initially, permitting both the bacterial and protozoal pneumonia to develop simultaneously, could not be determined in their study. Buergelt and colleagues[270] described lesions affecting both the alveoli and terminal airways in both adult horses and in foals with clinical presentations of respiratory distress. Although *P. carinii* was noted in a single foal, they concluded that the pulmonary histopathologic findings were more compatible with toxin-induced injury, although the historical data were not able to support their hypothesis.

Clinical Signs. Clinical signs are variable depending upon the stage of the pneumonia and the causative agent. In the acute phase, horses may present in respiratory distress: they are tachypneic, may be hypoxemic, and may or may not be febrile.[266, 267] They may have underlying bacterial infections as evidenced by nasal discharge and cough.[274] Horses may also present with signs similar to those exhibited by heavey horses with an increased respiratory rate and a marked expiratory effort. They are afebrile and exhibit a cough and nasal discharge.[269–271] In chronic disorders, horses may exhibit exercise intolerance[268] or simply have a history of weight loss and anorexia.[272]

Diagnosis. The diagnosis is based upon clinical signs, history, and radiographic examination and in some cases isolation of an infectious agent. Radiographs demonstrate pulmonary infiltrate with discrete and diffuse nodules, suggestive of chronic granulomatous interstitial pneumonia or an increase in the interstitial pattern of the lung (Fig. 6–16). Serum titer levels may indicate a high titer to equine influenza virus.[267] The diagnosis of interstitial pneumonia secondary to *Mycobacterium tuberculosis* is confirmed by isolation of the acid-fast organisms at postmortem examination or from lung biopsy. Bronchoalveolar lavage may be necessary to isolate *P. carinii*. Intradermal skin testing is not a reliable diagnostic test in the horse.[272] Silicosis, also a rare finding in the horse, is diagnosed by using x-ray diffraction techniques on lung tissue specimens.[268]

Pathology. The lung changes will be a function of the stage and the causative agent. Postmortem examination may reveal diffuse pulmonary fibrosis and hypercellularity of alveolar septa and scarring of the interlobular septa and parts of the pleura. Severe chronic bronchitis and bronchiolitis may also be evident if concurrent airway disease exists, but this is

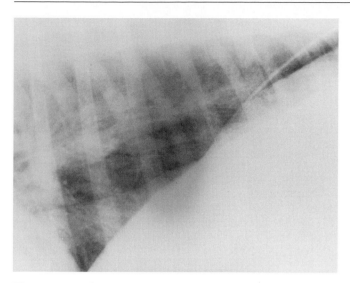

Figure 6–16. Overall increase in interstitial pulmonary opacity representing pneumonia.

typically not a feature of interstitial pneumonia.[270] Multifocal granulomas may be detected.[268, 271, 272]

Treatment. The prognosis is poor for the majority of these horses presenting with respiratory distress and interstitial pneumonia. Of six adult horses presenting to a veterinary clinic for chronic respiratory disease, only one horse improved.[270]

Tumors of the Respiratory System

Etiology. The most frequently encountered tumors in equine postmortem surveys include sarcoids, squamous cell carcinomas, fibromas, melanomas, papillomas, fibrosarcomas, and lymphosarcomas.[275, 276] Yet neoplastic involvement of the respiratory system, either the pulmonary parenchyma or thoracic structures per se, remains relatively rare in horses, occurring at a prevalence rate of 0.15 to 0.62.[277, 278] Primary lung tumors that have been reported include granular cell tumor (myoblastoma),[279, 280] bronchial myxoma, and pulmonary carcinoma.[275, 281] The incidence of granular cell tumor ranges from 3 in 2,000 to 3 in 40,000 cases, with most tumors involving the right lung.[282, 283] Metastatic tumors include (1) adenocarcinoma, with primary sites of origin in the kidney, uterus, thyroid, and ovary[278] and (2) hemangiosarcoma,[284] with the primary tumor originating in the hindlimb musculature. Although hemangiosarcomas are reported to be most common in older horses, leading to rapid clinical deterioration,[285, 286] three cases of hemangiosarcoma have occurred in relatively young horses (ages 3, 3, and 6½ years). Yet hemangiosarcoma remains relatively rare, occurring in 2 in 1,322 horses in a study by Sundbery and associates[276] and in 1 in 4,739 cases in a survey reported by Hargis and McElwain.[287] Neoplasms of the thoracic cavity include lymphosarcoma, pleural mesothelioma, thymoma, pulmonary chondrosarcoma, gastric squamous cell carcinoma, and hemangiosarcoma.[288, 289] With the exception of lymphosarcoma, most thoracic neoplasms reflect metastatic processes.[278]

Diagnosis. Most tumors are diagnosed at postmortem examination unless signs referable to the respiratory system become obvious. In some reports horses exhibited signs that were initially compatible with allergic airway disease, pleuropneumonia, and pulmonary epistaxis.[279, 289, 290] Endoscopic examination may reveal the presence of masses occluding the bronchi, as in the case of primary granular cell tumors and bronchogenic carcinomas.[279–281] Transtracheal aspirates, thoracic radiography, and thoracocentesis may be helpful in the diagnosis.[278] Radiographic or ultrasonographic evidence of multifocal interstitial densities (2–3 cm in diameter), tracheal elevation, or mediastinal densities are suggestive of neoplasia.[281] Pleural effusions with elevated erythrocyte counts, total protein concentrations, and reactive mesothelial cells have been found in cases of hemangiosarcoma.[289]

Treatment. The prognosis is poor for neoplastic conditions and most patients are euthanized.

REFERENCES

Diagnostic Approach

1. Rumbaugh GE, Ardans AA: Immunologic diseases. In Robinson NE, ed.: *Current Therapy in Equine Medicine.* Philadelphia, WB Saunders, 1983, p 321.
2. Banks KL, McGuire TC, Jerrells TR: Absence of B lymphocytes in a horse with primary agammaglobulinemia. *Clin Immunol Immunopathol* 5:282, 1976.
3. Deem DA, Traver DS, Thacker HL, et al: Agammaglobulinemia in a horse. *J Am Vet Med Assoc* 175:469, 1979.
4. Davis DM, Honnas CM, Hedlund CS, et al: Resection of a cervical tracheal bronchus in a foal. *J Am Vet Med Assoc* 198:2097, 1991.
5. Kotlikoff MI, Gillespie JR: Lung sounds in veterinary medicine part I. Terminology and mechanisms of sound production. *Compendium Continuing Educ Pract Vet* 5:634, 1983.
6. Kotlikoff MI, Gillespie JR: Lung sounds in veterinary medicine part II. Deriving clinical information from lung sounds. *Compendium Continuing Educ Pract Vet* 6:462, 1984.
7. Viel L, Harris FW, Curtis RA: Terminology of lung sounds in large animal veterinary medicine. In Deegen E, Beadle RE, eds: *Lung Function and Respiratory Diseases.* Stuttgart, Hippiatrika, 1986, p 87.
8. Forgacs P: *Lung Sounds.* London, Bailliere Tindall, 1978, p 7.
9. Roudebush P, Sweeney CR: Thoracic percussion. *J Am Vet Med Assoc* 197:714, 1990.
10. Darien BJ, Brown CM, Walker RD, et al: A tracheoscopic technique for obtaining uncontaminated lower airway secretions for bacterial culture in the horse. *Equine Vet J* 22:170, 1990.
11. Traub-Dargatz JL, Brown CM: *Equine Endoscopy.* St. Louis, Mosby–Year Book, 1990.
12. Derksen FJ, Brown CM, Sonea I, et al: Comparison of transtracheal aspirate and bronchoalveolar lavage cytology in 50 horses with chronic lung disease. *Equine Vet J* 21:23, 1989.
13. Larson VL, Busch RH: Equine tracheobronchial lavage: Comparison of lavage cytologic and pulmonary histopathologic findings. *Am J Vet Res* 46:144, 1985.
14. Fogarty U: Evaluation of a bronchoalveolar lavage technique. *Equine Vet J* 22:174, 1990.
15. Mair TS, Stokes CR, Bourne FJ: Cellular content of secretions obtained by lavage from different levels of the equine respiratory tract. *Equine Vet J* 19:458, 1987.

16. Viel L: Structural-functional correlations of the lung in horses with small airway disease. In Deegen E, Beadle RE, eds: *Lung Function and Respiratory Diseases in the Horse.* Stuttgart, Hippiatrika, 1986, p 41.
17. Sweeney CR, Sweeney RW, Benson CE: Comparison of bacteria isolated from specimens obtained by use of endoscopic guarded tracheal swabbing and percutaneous tracheal aspiration in horses. *J Am Vet Med Assoc* 195:1225, 1989.
18. Sweeney CR, Beech J, Roby KAW: Bacteria isolated from tracheobronchial aspirates of healthy horses. *Am J Vet Res* 46:2562, 1985.
19. Burrell MH, Mackintosh ME: Isolation of *Streptococcus pneumonia* from the respiratory tract of horses. *Equine Vet J* 18:183, 1986.
20. Mackintosh ME, Grant ST, Burrell MH: Evidence for *Streptococcus pneumonia* as a cause of respiratory disease in young Thoroughbred horses in training. In Powell DG, ed: *Equine Infectious Diseases V: Proceedings of the Fifth International Conference,* Lexington, University of Kentucky Press, 1988, p 41.
21. Benson CE, Sweeney CR: Isolation of *Streptococcus pneumonia* Type 3 from equine species. *J Clin Microbiol* 20:1028, 1984.
22. Reimer JM: Diagnostic ultrasonography of the equine thorax. *Compendium Continuing Educ Pract Vet* 12:1321, 1990.
23. Lamb CR, O'Callaghan MW: Diagnostic imaging of equine pulmonary disease. *Compendium Continuing Educ Pract Vet* 11:1110, 1989.
24. King GK: Equine thoracic radiography part II. Radiographic patterns of equine pulmonary and pleural diseases using air-gap rare-earth radiography. *Compendium Continuing Educ Pract Vet* 3:S283, 1981.
25. Reef VB: Ultrasonographic evaluation. In Beech J, ed: *Equine Respiratory Disorders.* Philadelphia, Lea & Febiger, 1991, p 69.
26. Rantanen NW: Diseases of the thorax. *Vet Clin North Am Equine Pract* 2:49, 1986.
27. Reef VB, Boy MG, Reid CF, et al: Comparison between diagnostic ultrasonography and radiography in the evaluation of horses and cattle with thoracic disease: 56 cases (1984–1985). *J Am Vet Med Assoc* 198:2112, 1991.
28. Reimer J, Reef VB, Spencer PA: Ultrasonography as a diagnostic aid in horses with anaerobic bacterial pleuropneumonia and/or pulmonary abscessations: 27 cases (1984–1986). *J Am Vet Med Assoc* 194:278, 1989.
29. Allen AK, Stone LR: Equine diagnostic ultrasonography: Equipment selection and use. *Compendium Continuing Educ Pract Vet* 12:1307, 1990.
30. Bennett DG: Evaluation of pleural fluid in the diagnosis of thoracic disease in the horse. *J Am Vet Med Assoc* 188:814, 1986.
31. Sweeney CR, Divers TJ, Benson CE: Anaerobic bacteria in 21 horses with pleuropneumonia. *J Am Vet Med Assoc* 187:721, 1985.
32. O'Callaghan MW, Hornof WJ, Fisher PE, et al: Ventilation imaging in the horse with 99mtechnetium-DPTA radioaerosol. *Equine Vet J* 19:19, 1987.
33. Attenburrow DP, Portergill MJ, Vennart W: Development of an equine nuclear medicine facility for gamma camera imaging. *Equine Vet J* 21:86, 1989.
34. O'Callaghan MW, Hornof WJ, Fisher PE, et al: Exercise-induced pulmonary haemorrhage in horses: Results of a detailed clinical post-mortem and imaging study. VII. Ventilation/perfusion scintigraphy in horses with EIPH. *Equine Vet J* 19:423, 1987.
35. O'Callaghan MW, Kinney LM: Pulmonary scintigraphy in horses with chronic obstructive pulmonary disease. *Comp Resp Soc* 8:78, 1989.
36. O'Callaghan MW: Scintigraphic imaging of lung disease. In Beech J, ed: *Equine Respiratory Disorders.* Philadelphia, Lea & Febiger, 1991, p 129.
37. Nelson R, Hampe DW: Measurement of tracheal mucous transport rate in the horse. *Am J Vet Res* 44:1165, 1983.
38. Willoughby RA, Ecker G, Riddolls L, et al: Mucociliary clearance in the nose and trachea of horses. *Comp Resp Soc* 8:36, 1989.
39. Willoughby RA, McDonell WN: Pulmonary function testing in horses. *Vet Clin North Am* 1:171, 1979.
40. Robinson NE: The physiologic basis of pulmonary function tests. *Proc ACVIM* 10:403, 1992.
41. Robinson NE: Tests of equine airway function. *Proc ACVIM* 10:284, 1992.
42. Art T, Anderson L, Woakes AJ, et al: Mechanics of breathing during strenuous exercise in thoroughbred horses. *Respir Physiol* 82:279, 1990.
43. Raphel CF, Gunson DE: Percutaneous lung biopsy in the horse. *Cornell Vet* 71:439, 1981.

Upper Respiratory Tract Disorders

44. Hillman DJ: The Skull. In Getty R, ed: *Sisson and Grossman's the Anatomy of the Domestic Animals.* Philadelphia, WB Saunders, 1975, p 318.
45. Scott EA: Sinusitis. In Robinson NE, ed: *Current Therapy in Equine Medicine.* Philadelphia, WB Saunders, 1987, p 605.
46. Pirie M, Pirie HM, Wright NG: A scanning electron microscopic study of the equine upper respiratory tract. *Equine Vet J* 22:333, 1990.
47. King AS, Riley VA: *A Guide to the Physiological and Clinical Anatomy of the Head.* Liverpool, University of Liverpool, 1980.
48. Honnas CM, Pascoe JR: Paranasal sinuses. In Smith BP, ed: *Large Animal Internal Medicine.* St. Louis, Mosby–Year Book, 1990, p 555.
49. Freeman DE: In Beech J, ed: *Equine Respiratory Disorders.* Philadelphia, Lea & Febiger, 1991, p 275.
50. Beard WL, Robertson JT, Leeth B: Bilateral congenital cysts in the frontal sinuses of a horse. *J Am Vet Med Assoc* 196:453, 1990.
51. Lane JG, Longstaffe JA, Gibbs C: Equine paranasal sinus cysts: A report of 15 cases. *Equine Vet J* 19:537, 1987.
52. Leyland A, Baker JR: Lesions of the nasal and paranasal sinuses of the horse causing dyspnoea. *Br Vet J* 131:339, 1975.
53. Boulton CH: Equine nasal cavity and paranasal sinus disease: a review of 85 cases. *J Equine Vet Sci* 5:268, 1985.
54. Roberts MC, Sutton RH, Lovell DK: A protracted case of cryptococcal nasal granuloma in a stallion. *Aust Vet J* 57:287, 1981.
55. Reed SM, Boles C, Dade AW, et al: Localized equine nasal coccidioidomycosis granuloma. *J Equine Med Surg* 3:119, 1979.
56. O'Callaghan MW: Bleeding from the nose. In Brown CM, ed: *Problems in Equine Medicine.* Philadelphia, Lea & Febiger, 1989, p 107.
57. Hilbert BJ, Little CB, Klein K, et al: Tumours of the paranasal sinuses in 16 horses. *Aust Vet J* 65:86, 1988.
58. Pascoe J: Ethmoid hematoma (progressive ethmoidal hematoma, hemorrhagic nasal polyps). In Smith BP, ed: *Large Animal Internal Medicine.* St. Louis, Mosby–Year Book, 1990, p 557.
59. Specht TE, Colahan PT, Nixon AJ, et al: Ethmoidal hematoma in nine horses. *J Am Vet Med Assoc* 197:613, 1990.
60. Greet TRC: Outcome of treatment in 23 horses with progressive ethmoidal haematoma. *Equine Vet J* 24:468, 1992.
61. Freeman DE: Paranasal sinuses. In Beech J, ed: *Equine Respiratory Disorders.* Philadelphia, Lea & Febiger, 1991, p 275.

62. Cook WR, Littlewort MCG: Progressive haematoma of the ethmoid region in the horse. *Equine Vet J* 6:101, 1974.

63. Habel RE: *Applied Veterinary Anatomy*. Ithaca, NY, RE Habel, 1975, p 57.

64. McCue PM, Freeman DE, Donawick WJ: Guttural pouch tympany: 15 cases (1977–1986). *J Am Vet Med Assoc* 194:1761, 1989.

65. Freeman DE: Guttural pouches. In Beech J, ed: *Equine Respiratory Disorders*. Philadelphia, Lea & Febiger, 1991, p 305.

66. Freeman DE: Diagnosis and treatment of diseases of the guttural pouch (part 1). *Compendium Continuing Educ Pract Vet* 2:S3, 1980.

67. Mason TA: Tympany of the eustachian tube diverticulum (guttural pouch) in a foal. *Equine Vet J* 4:153, 1972.

68. Lane JG: The management of guttural pouch mycosis. *Equine Vet J* 21:321, 1989.

69. Colles CM, Cook WR: Carotid angiography in the horse. *Vet Rec* 113:483, 1983.

70. Church S, Wyn-Jones G, Parks AH, et al: Treatment of guttural pouch mycosis. *Equine Vet J* 18:362, 1986.

71. Freeman DE, Donawick WJ: Occlusion of the internal carotid artery in the horse by means of a balloon-tipped catheter: Evaluation of a method designed to prevent epistaxis caused by guttural pouch mycosis. *J Am Vet Med Assoc* 176:232, 1980.

72. Freeman DE, Donawick WJ: Occlusion of the internal carotid artery in the horse by means of a balloon-tipped catheter: Clinical use of a method to prevent epistaxis caused by guttural pouch mycosis. *J Am Vet Med Assoc* 176:236, 1980.

73. Greet TRC: Outcome of treatment of 35 cases of guttural pouch mycosis. *Equine Vet J* 19:483, 1987.

74. Hardy J, Robertson JT, Wilkie DA: Ischemic optic neuropathy and blindness after arterial occlusion for treatment of guttural pouch mycosis in two horses. *J Am Vet Med Assoc* 196:1631, 1990.

75. Blakeslee JR, Olsen RG, McAllister ES, et al: Evidence of respiratory tract infection induced by equine herpesvirus type 2 in the horse. *Can J Microbiol* 21:1940, 1975.

76. McAllister ES, Blakeslee JR: Clinical observations of pharyngitis in the horse. *J Am Vet Med Assoc* 170:739, 1977.

77. Prickett ME: The pathology of disease caused by equine herpesvirus-1. In *Proceedings of the Second International Conference on Equine Infectious Diseases*. Princeton, NJ, Veterinary Publications, 1969, p 24.

78. Burrell MH: Endoscopic and virological observations on respiratory disease in a group of young Thoroughbred horses in training. *Equine Vet J* 17:99, 1985.

79. Baker GJ: Diseases of the pharynx and the larynx. In Robinson NE, ed: *Current Therapy in Equine Medicine*. Philadelphia, WB Saunders, 1987, p 607.

80. Hoquet H, Higgins R, Lessard P, et al: Comparison of the bacterial and fungal flora in the pharynx of normal horses and horses affected with pharyngitis. *Can Vet J* 26:342, 1985.

81. Robertson JT: Pharynx and larynx. In Beech J, ed: *Equine Respiratory Disorders*. Philadelphia, Lea & Febiger, 1991, p 331.

82. Bayly WM, Grant BD, Breeze RG: Arterial blood gas tension and acid base balance during exercise in horses with pharyngeal lymphoid hyperplasia. *Equine Vet J* 16:435, 1984.

83. Raker CW: The Nasopharynx. In Mansmann RA, McAllister ES, eds: *Equine Medicine and Surgery*. Santa Barbara, Calif, Veterinary Publications, 1982, p 747.

84. Dean PW: Upper airway obstruction in performance horses. *Vet Clin North Am* 7:125, 1991.

85. Koch C: Diseases of the larynx and pharynx of the horse. *Compendium Continuing Educ Pract Vet* 11:S73, 1980.

86. Haynes PF: Dorsal displacement of the soft palate and epi-

87. Hackett RP, Ducharme NG, Rehder RS: Use of the highspeed treadmill in management of horses with dorsal displacement of the soft palate (abstract). *Proc AAEP* 38, 1993.

88. Heffron CJ, Baker GJ: Observations on the mechanism of functional obstruction of the nasopharyngeal airway in the horse. *Equine Vet J* 11:142, 1979.

89. Tulleners EP, Hamir A: Epiglottic augmentation in the horse: A pilot study (abstract). *Vet Surg* 19:79, 1990.

90. Harrison IW, Raker CW: Sternothyrohyoideus myectomy in horses: 17 cases (1984–1985). *J Am Vet Med Assoc* 193:1299, 1988.

91. Cook WR: Some observations on diseases of the ear, nose and throat in the horse, and endoscopy using a flexible fibreoptic endoscope. *Vet Rec* 94:533, 1974.

92. Goulden BE, Anderson LJ, Davies AS, et al: Rostral displacement of the palatopharyngeal arch: A case report. *Equine Vet J* 8:95, 1976.

93. Kleig HF, Deegen E, Stockhofe N, et al: Rostral displacement of the palatopharyngeal arch in a seven-month-old Hanoverian colt. *Equine Vet J* 21:382, 1989.

94. Boles C, Raker CW, Wheat JD: Epiglottic entrapment of arytenoepiglottic folds in the horse. *J Am Vet Med Assoc* 172:883, 1978.

95. Tulleners EP: Transendoscopic contact neodymium:yttrium aluminum garnet laser correction of epiglottic entrapment in standing horses. *J Am Vet Med Assoc* 196:1971, 1990.

96. Honnas CM, Wheat JD: Epiglottic entrapment: A transnasal surgical approach to divide the aryepiglottic fold axially in the standing horse. *Vet Surg* 17:246, 1988.

97. Stick JA, Boles C: Subepiglottic cyst in three foals. *J Am Vet Med Assoc* 77:62, 1980.

98. Haynes PF, Beadle RE, McClure JR, et al: Soft palate cysts as a cause of pharyngeal dysfunction in two horses. *Equine Vet J* 22:369, 1990.

99. Tulleners EP, Harrison IW, Raker CW: Management of arytenoid chondropathy and failed laryngoplasty in horses: 75 cases (1979–1985). *J Am Vet Med Assoc* 192:670, 1988.

100. Haynes PF, Snider TG, McClure JR, et al: Chronic chondritis of the equine arytenoid cartilage. *J Am Vet Med Assoc* 177:1135, 1980.

101. Ducharme NG, Hackett RP: The value of surgical treatment of laryngeal hemiplegia in horses. *Compendium Continuing Educ Pract Vet* 13:472, 1991.

102. Speirs VC: Laryngeal surgery—150 years on. *Equine Vet J* 19:377, 1987.

103. Cahill JI, Goulden BE: The pathogenesis of equine laryngeal hemiplegia—a review. *N Z Vet J* 35:82, 1987.

104. Rose RJ, Hartley WJ, Baker W: Laryngeal paralysis in Arabian foals associated with oral haloxon administration. *Equine Vet J* 13:171, 1981.

105. Barber SM: Paralaryngeal abscess with laryngeal hemiplegia and fistulation in a horse. *Can Vet J* 22:389, 1981.

106. Hillidge CJ: Interpretation of laryngeal function tests in the horse. *Vet Rec* 118:535, 1986.

107. Cook WR: Diagnosis and grading of hereditary recurrent laryngeal neuropathy in the horse. *J Equine Vet Sci* 8:432, 1988.

108. Gerber H: The genetic basis of some equine diseases. *Equine Vet J* 21:244, 1989.

109. Cole CR: Changes in the equine larynx associated with laryngeal hemiplegia. *Am J Vet Res* 7:69, 1946.

110. Duncan ID, Griffiths IR, McQueen A, et al: The pathology of equine laryngeal hemiplegia. *Acta Neuropathol* 27:337, 1974.

111. Cahill JI, Goulden BE: Equine laryngeal hemiplegia. Part I. A light microscopic study of peripheral nerves. *N Z Vet J* 34:161, 1986.

112. Derksen FJ, Stick JA, Scott EA, et al: Effect of laryngeal hemiplegia and laryngoplasty on airway flow mechanics in exercising horses. *Am J Vet Res* 47:16, 1986.

113. Bayly WM, Grant BD, Modransky PD: Arterial blood gas tensions during exercise in a horse with laryngeal hemiplegia, before and after corrective surgery. *Res Vet Sci* 36:256, 1984.

114. Shappell KK, Derksen FJ, Stick JA, et al: Effects of ventriculectomy, prosthetic laryngoplasty, and exercise on upper airway function in horses with induced left laryngeal hemiplegia. *Am J Vet Res* 49:1760, 1988.

115. Duncan ID, Brook D: Bilateral laryngeal paralysis in the horse. *Equine Vet J* 17:228, 1985.

116. Greet TRC, Jeffcott LB, Whitwell KE, et al: The slap test for laryngeal adductory function in horses with suspected cervical spinal cord damage. *Equine Vet J* 12:127, 1980.

117. Ducharme NG, Horney FD, Partlow GD, et al: Attempts to restore abduction of the paralyzed equine arytenoid cartilage I. Nerve-muscle pedicle transplants. *Can J Vet Res* 53:202, 1989.

118. Ducharme NG, Horney FD, Hulland TJ, et al: Attempts to restore abduction of the paralyzed equine arytenoid cartilage II. Nerve implantation (pilot study). *Can J Vet Res* 53:210, 1989.

119. Ducharme NG, Viel L, Partlow GD, et al: Attempts to restore abduction of the paralyzed equine arytenoid cartilage III. Nerve anastomosis. *Can J Vet Res* 53:216, 1989.

120. Sweeney CR, Benson CE, Whitlock RH, et al: *Streptococcus equi* infection in horses—part I. *Compendium Continuing Educ Pract Vet* 9:689, 1987.

121. Prescott JF, Srivastava SK, deGannes R, et al: A mild form of strangles caused by an atypical *Streptococcus equi*. *J Am Vet Med Assoc* 180:293, 1982.

122. Sweeney CR: *Streptococcus equi*. In Smith B, ed: *Large Animal Internal Medicine*. St. Louis, Mosby–Year Book, 1990, p 519.

123. Sweeney CR, Benson CE, Whitlock RH, et al: Description of an epizootic and persistence of *Streptococcus equi* infections in horses. *J Am Vet Med Assoc* 194:1281, 1989.

124. George JL, Reif JS, Shideler RK, et al: Identification of carriers of *Streptococcus equi* in a naturally infected herd. *J Am Vet Med Assoc* 183:80, 1983.

125. Timoney JF: Protecting against "strangles": A contemporary view. *Equine Vet J* 20:392, 1988.

126. Galan JE, Timoney JF: Mucosal nasopharyngeal immune responses of horses to protein antigens of *Streptococcus equi*. *Infect Immun* 47:623, 1985.

127. Barnum DA: Streptococcus. In Gyles C, Thoen CO, eds: *Pathogenesis of Bacterial Infections in Animals*. Ames, Iowa State University Press, 1986, p 3.

128. Sweeney CR, Benson CE, Whitlock RH, et al: *Streptococcus equi* infection in horses—part 2. *Compendium Continuing Educ Pract Vet* 9:845, 1987.

129. Rumbaugh GE, Smith BF, Carlson GP: Internal abdominal abscesses in the horse: A study of 25 cases. *J Am Vet Med Assoc* 172:304, 1978.

130. Zicker SC, Wilson WD, Medearis I: Differentiation between intra-abdominal neoplasms and abscesses in horses, using clinical and laboratory data: 40 cases (1973–1988). *J Am Vet Med Assoc* 196:1130, 1990.

131. Yelle MT: Clinical aspects of *Streptococcus equi* infection. *Equine Vet J* 19:158, 1987.

132. Todhunter RJ, Brown CM, Stickle R: Retropharyngeal infections in five horses. *J Am Vet Med Assoc* 187:600, 1985.

133. Rigg DL, Ramey DW, Reinertson EL: Tracheal compression secondary to abscessation of cranial mediastinal lymph nodes in a horse. *J Am Vet Med Assoc* 186:283, 1985.

134. Wood JM: Antigenic variation of equine influenza: a stable virus. *Equine Vet J* 20:316, 1988.

135. Higgins WP, Gillespie JH, Holmes DR, et al: Surveys of equine influenza outbreaks during 1983 and 1984. *J Equine Vet Sci* 6:15, 1986.

136. Kemen MJ, Frank RA, Babish JB: An outbreak of equine influenza at a harness horse racetrack. *Cornell Vet* 75:225, 1985.

137. McChesney AE: Viral respiratory infections of horses: Structure and function of lungs in relation to viral infection. *J Am Vet Med Assoc* 166:76, 1975.

138. Paradis MR: Equine viral infections (respiratory). In Smith B, ed: *Large Animal Internal Medicine*. St. Louis, Mosby–Year Book, 1990, p 524.

139. Garine B, Plateau E, Gillet-Forin S: Serological diagnosis of influenza A infections in the horse by enzyme immunoassay. Comparison with the complement fixation test. *Vet Immunol Immunopathol* 13:357, 1986.

140. Baker DJ: Rationale for the use of influenza vaccines in horses and the importance of antigenic drift. *Equine Vet J* 19:93, 1986.

141. Mumford JA, Hannant D, Jessett DM: Experimental infection of ponies with equine influenza (H3N8) viruses by intranasal inoculation or exposure to aerosols. *Equine Vet J* 22:93, 1990.

142. Bryans JT, Allen GP: Herpesviral disease of the horse. In Wittman G, ed: *Herpes virus disease of cattle, horses and pigs*. Boston, Kluvar, 1989, p 176.

143. Campbell TM, Studdert MJ: Equine herpesvirus type 1 (EHV1). *Vet Bull* 53:135, 1983.

144. Mason DK, Watkins KL, McNie JT, et al: Haematological measurements as an aid to early diagnosis and prognosis of respiratory viral infections in thoroughbred horses. *Vet Rec* 126:359, 1990.

145. Gradil C, Joo HS: A radial immunodiffusion enzyme assay for detection of antibody to equine rhinopneumonitis virus (EHV-1) in horse serum. *Vet Microbiol* 17:315, 1988.

146. Blakeslee JR, Olsen RG, McAllister ES, et al: Evidence of respiratory tract infection induced by equine herpes virus type 2 in the horse. *Can J Microbiol* 21:1940, 1977.

147. Palfi V, Belak S, Molnar T: Isolation of equine herpesvirus type 2 from foals showing respiratory symptoms. Brief report. *Zentralbl Veterinarmed* [B] 25:165, 1978.

148. Fu ZF, Johnson AJ, Horner GW, et al: Respiratory disease in foals and the epizootiology of equine herpesvirus type 2 infections. *N Z Vet J* 34:152, 1986.

149. Ames TR, O'Leary TP, Johnston GR: Isolation of equine herpesvirus type 2 from foals with respiratory disease. *Compendium Continuing Educ Pract Vet* 8:664, 1986.

150. Crandell RA, Davis ER: Isolation of equine coital exanthema virus (equine herpes virus 3) from the nostril of a foal. *J Am Vet Med Assoc* 187:503, 1985.

151. Mumford JA: Preparing for equine arteritis. *Equine Vet J* 17:6, 1985.

152. Timoney PJ, McCollum WH: Equine viral arteritis. *Can Vet J* 28:693, 1987.

153. Traub-Dargatz JL, Ralston SL, Collins JK, et al: Equine viral arteritis. *Compendium Continuing Educ Pract Vet* 7:S490, 1985.

154. Hofer B, Steck F, Gerber H: Virological investigations in a horse clinic. In Bryans JT, Gerber H, eds: *Proceedings of Fourth International Conference on Equine Infectious Disease*. Princeton, NJ, Veterinary Publications, 1978, p 475.

155. Mair TS, Lane JG: Tracheal obstructions in two horses and a donkey. *Vet Rec* 126:303, 1990.

156. Kirker-Head CA, Jakob TP: Surgical repair of ruptured trachea in a horse. *J Am Vet Med Assoc* 196:1635, 1990.

157. Urquhart KA, Gerring EL, Shepherd MP: Tracheobronchial foreign body in a pony. *Equine Vet J* 13:262, 1981.

158. Brown CM, Collier MA: Tracheobronchial foreign body in a horse. *J Am Vet Med Assoc* 182:280, 1983.

159. Simmons TR, Petersen M, Parker J, et al: Tracheal collapse due to chondrodysplasia in a miniature horse foal. *Equine Pract* 10:39, 1988.

160. Martin JE: Dorsoventral flattening of the trachea in a pony. *Equine Pract* 3:17, 1981.

161. Freeman D: Trachea. In Beech J, ed: *Equine Respiratory Disorders*. Philadelphia, Lea & Febiger, 1991, p 392.

The Normal Lung

162. Hare WCD: Equine respiratory system. In Getty R, ed: *Sisson and Grossman's the Anatomy of the Domestic Animals*. Philadelphia, WB Saunders, 1975, p 498.

163. McLaughlin RF, Tyler WS, Canada RO: A study of the subgross pulmonary anatomy in various mammals. *Am J Anat* 108:149, 1961.

164. Breeze R, Turk M: Cellular structure, function and organization in the lower respiratory tract. *Environ Health Perspect* 55:3, 1984.

165. Pirie M, Pirie HM, Cranston S, Wright NG: An ultrastructural study of the equine lower respiratory tract. *Equine Vet J* 22:338, 1990.

166. Mair TS, Batten EH, Stokes CR, et al: The histological features of the immune system of the equine respiratory tract. *J Comp Pathol* 97:575, 1987.

167. Frevert CW, Warner AE, Adams ET, et al: Pulmonary intravascular macrophages are an important part of the mononuclear phagocyte system in the horse (abstract). *J Vet Intern Med* 5:145, 1991.

168. Taylor AE, Rehder K, Hyatt RE, et al: *Clinical Respiratory Physiology*. Philadelphia, WB Saunders, 1989, p 65.

169. Amis TC, Pascoe JR, Hornof W: Topographic distribution of pulmonary ventilation and perfusion in the horse. *Am J Vet Res* 45:1597, 1984.

170. Robinson NE: Exercise induced pulmonary haemorrhage (EIPH): Could Leonardo have got it right? (editorial). *Equine Vet J* 19:370, 1987.

171. Barnes PJ: Neural control of human airways in health and disease. *Am Rev Respir Dis* 134:1289, 1986.

172. Derksen FJ, Broadstone RV: Bronchodilation therapy and the autonomic nervous system in horses with airway obstruction. *Proc ACVIM* 9:47, 1991.

173. Derksen FJ, Robinson NE, Slocombe RF: Ovalbumin induced allergic lung disease in the pony: Role of vagal mechanisms. *J Appl Physiol* 53:719, 1982.

174. Sant'Ambrogio G: Nervous receptors of the tracheobronchial tree. *Annu Rev Physiol* 49:611, 1987.

175. Derksen FJ, Scott JS, Slocombe RF, et al: Effect of clenbuterol on histamine-induced airway obstruction in ponies. *Am J Vet Res* 48:423, 1987.

176. Scott JS, Garon HI, Broadstone RV, et al: Alpha-1 adrenergic induced airway obstruction in ponies with recurrent pulmonary disease. *J Appl Physiol* 52:562, 1982.

177. Sonea I, Bowker RM, Broadstone R, et al: Presence and distribution of vasoactive intestinal peptide-like and peptide histidine isoleucine-like immunoreactivity in the equine lung (abstract). *Am Rev Respir Dis* 143:A355, 1991.

178. Robinson NE, Wilson R: Airway obstruction in the horse. *J Equine Vet Sci* 9:155, 1989.

179. Koterba AM, Kosch PC, Beech J, et al: Breathing strategy of the adult horse (*Equus caballus*) at rest. *J Appl Physiol* 64:337, 1988.

180. Art T, Anderson L, Woakes AJ, et al: Mechanics of breathing during strenuous exercise in thoroughbred horses. *Respir Physiol* 82:279, 1990.

181. West JB: *Pulmonary Pathophysiology*. Baltimore, Williams & Wilkins, 1982, p 19.

182. Bayly W, Grant BD, Breeze RG, et al: The effects of maximal exercise on acid-base balance and arterial blood gas tension in thoroughbred horses. In Snow DH, Persson SGB, Rose RJ, eds: *Equine Exercise Physiology*. Cambridge, England, Granta, 1983, p 400.

183. Wagner PD, Gillespie JR, Landgren GL, et al: Mechanism of exercise-induced hypoxemia in horses. *J Appl Physiol* 66:1227, 1989.

184. Dantzker DR: Physiology and pathophysiology of pulmonary gas exchange. *Hosp Pract* 21:135, 1986.

185. Roth RA: Biochemistry, physiology and drug metabolism—implications regarding the role of the lungs in drug disposition. *Clin Physiol Biochem* 3:66, 1985.

186. Gillis CN, Pitt BR: The fate of circulating amines within the pulmonary circulation. *Am Rev Physiol* 44:269, 1982.

187. Nelson R, Hampe DW: Measurement of tracheal mucous transport rate in the horse. *Am J Vet Res* 44:1165, 1983.

188. Wong CW, Thompson HL, Thong YH, et al: Effect of strenuous exercise on chemiluminescence response of equine alveolar macrophages. *Equine Vet J* 22:33, 1990.

189. Huston LH, Bayly WM, Liggitt HD, et al: Alveolar macrophage function in Thoroughbreds after strenuous exercise. In Gillespie JR, Robinson NE, eds: *Equine Exercise Physiology*, vol 2. Davis, Calif, ICEEP Publications, 1987, p 243.

190. Bayly WM: Stress and equine respiratory immunity. *Proc ACVIM* 8:505, 1990.

Lower Respiratory Tract Disorders

191. Warner A: Bacterial pneumonia in adults. In Smith BP, ed.: *Large Animal Internal Medicine*. St. Louis, Mosby–Year Book, 1990, p 489.

192. Spurlock SL, Spurlock GH, Donaldson LL: Consolidating pneumonia and pneumothorax in a horse. *J Am Vet Med Assoc* 192:1081, 1988.

193. Mackintosh ME, Grant ST, Burrell MH: Evidence for *Streptococcus pneumoniae* as a cause of respiratory disease in young Thoroughbred horses in training. In Powell DG, ed: *Equine Infectious Diseases V: Proceedings of the Fifth International Conference*. Lexington, University of Kentucky Press, 1988, p 41.

194. Benson CE, Sweeney CR: Isolation of *Streptococcus pneumoniae* Type 3 from equine species. *J Clin Microbiol* 20:1028, 1984.

195. Biberstein EL, Jang SS, Hirsh DC: *Nocardia asteroides* infection in horses: A review. *J Am Vet Med Assoc* 186:273, 1985.

196. Jakab GJ: Viral-bacterial interactions in pulmonary infection. *Adv Vet Sci Comp Med* 155, 1982.

197. Racklyeft DJ, Love DN: Influence of head posture on the respiratory tract of healthy horses. *Aust Vet J* 67:402, 1990.

198. Arthur RM: Lower respiratory disease in thoroughbred racehorses. *J Equine Vet Sci* 9:253, 1989.

199. Schott HC, Mansmann RA: Thoracic drainage in horses. *Compendium Continuing Educ Pract Vet* 12:251, 1990.

200. Raphel CF, Beech J: Pleuritis secondary to pneumonia or lung abscessation in 90 horses. *J Am Vet Med Assoc* 181:808, 1982.

201. Pipers FS: Pathophysiology of pleuropneumonia in the equine. *Proc ACVIM* 7:573, 1989.

202. Bernard-Strother S, Mansmann RA: Diagnosis and treatment of anaerobic bacterial pleuropneumonia in six horses. *Compendium Continuing Educ Pract Vet* 7:S341, 1985.

203. Purdy CM: Septic pleuritis in a horse. *Compendium Continuing Educ Pract Vet* 7:S361, 1985.

204. Sweeney CR, Divers TJ, Benson CE: Anaerobic bacteria in 21 horses with pleuropneumonia. *J Am Vet Med Assoc* 187:721, 1985.

205. Semrad SD, Byars TD: Pleuropneumonia and pleural effusion: diagnosis and treatment. *Vet Med* 84:627, 1989.

206. Byars TD, Dainis CM, Seltzer KL, et al: Cranial thoracic

masses in the horse: A sequel to pleuropneumonia. *Equine Vet J* 23:22–24, 1991.

207. Byars TD, Becht JL: Pleuropneumonia. *Vet Clin North Am* 7:63, 1991.

208. Wrigley RH, Gay CC, Lording P, et al: Pleural effusion associated with squamous cell carcinoma of the stomach of a horse. *Equine Vet J* 13:99, 1981.

209. Foreman JH, Weidner JP, Parry BW, et al: Pleural effusion secondary to thoracic metastatic mammary adenocarcinoma in a mare. *J Am Vet Med Assoc* 197:1193, 1990.

210. Ogilvie TH, Rosendal S, Blackwell TE, et al: *Mycoplasma felis* as a cause of pleuritis in horses. *J Am Vet Med Assoc* 182:1374, 1983.

211. Burbidge HM: Penetrating thoracic wound in a Hackney mare. *Equine Vet J* 14:94, 1982.

212. Mair TS, Pearson H, Waterman AE, et al: Chylothorax associated with a congenital diaphragmatic defect in a foal. *Equine Vet J* 20:304, 1988.

213. Pearson EG, Watrous BJ, Schmitz JA, et al: Cryptococcal pneumonia in a horse. *J Am Vet Med Assoc* 183:577, 1983.

214. Kramme PM, Ziemer EL: Disseminated coccidioidomycosis in a horse with osteomyelitis. *J Am Vet Med Assoc* 196:106, 1990.

215. Sweeney CR: Fungal pneumoniae. In Smith BP, ed: *Large Animal Internal Medicine*. St. Louis, Mosby–Year Book, 1990, p 516.

216. Hattel AL, Drake TR, Anderholm BJ, et al: Pulmonary aspergillosis associated with acute enteritis in a horse. *J Am Vet Med Assoc* 199:589, 1991.

217. Slocombe RF, Slauson DO: Invasive pulmonary aspergillosis of horses: An association with acute enteritis. *Vet Pathol* 25:277, 1988.

218. Antal T, Szabo I, Antal V, et al: Respiratory disease of horses associated with mycoplasma infection. *J Vet Med B* 35:264, 1988.

219. Rosendal S, Blackwell TE, Lumsden JH, et al: Detection of antibodies to *Mycoplasma felis* in horses. *J Am Vet Med Assoc* 188:292, 1986.

220. Mansmann RA: Lower respiratory tract infections. In Mansmann RA, McAllister ES, eds: *Equine Medicine and Surgery*. Santa Barbara, Calif, Veterinary Publications, 1982, p 776.

221. Humber KA: Near drowning of a gelding. *J Am Vet Med Assoc* 192:377, 1988.

222. Austin SM, Foreman JH, Goetz TE: Aspiration pneumonia following near-drowning in a mare: A case report. *J Equine Vet Sci* 8:313, 1988.

223. Sembrat R, DiStazio J, Reese J, et al: Acute pulmonary failure in the conscious pony with *Escherichia coli* septicemia. *Am J Vet Res* 39:1147, 1978.

224. Brown CM, Bell TG, Paradis MR, et al: Rupture of the mitral chordae tendineae in two horses. *J Am Vet Med Assoc* 182:281, 1983.

225. Muylle E, Oyaert W: Lung function tests in obstructive pulmonary disease in horses. *Equine Vet J* 5:37, 1973.

226. Derksen FJ, Scott J, Robinson NE, et al: Intravenous histamine administration in ponies with recurrent airway obstruction (heaves). *Am J Vet Res* 46:774, 1985.

227. Derksen FJ, Robinson NE, Scott JS, et al: Aerosolized *Micropolyspora faeni* antigen as a cause of pulmonary dysfunction in ponies with recurrent airway obstruction (heaves). *Am J Vet Res* 49:933, 1988.

228. Genetzky RM, Loparco FV: Chronic obstructive pulmonary disease in horses—pt 1. *Compendium Continuing Educ Pract Vet* 7:S407, 1985.

229. Gerber H: Chronic pulmonary disease in the horse. *Equine Vet J* 5:26, 1973.

230. McPherson EA, Thomson JR: Chronic obstructive pulmonary disease in the horse. 1. Nature of the disease. *Equine Vet J* 15:203, 1983.

231. Beadle RE: Summer pasture–associated obstructive pulmonary disease. In Robinson NE, ed: *Current Therapy in Equine Medicine*. Philadelphia, WB Saunders, 1983, p 512.

232. Beech J: Diagnosing chronic obstructive pulmonary disease. *Vet Med* 84:614, 1989.

233. Derksen FJ, Scott JS, Miller DC, et al: Bronchoalveolar lavage in ponies with recurrent airway obstruction (heaves). *Am Rev Respir Dis* 132:1066, 1985.

234. Robinson NE, Wilson R: Airway obstruction in the horse. *J Equine Vet Sci* 9:155, 1989.

235. Kaup FJ, Drommer W, Damsch S, et al: Ultrastructural findings in horses with chronic obstructive pulmonary disease (COPD) II: Pathomorphological changes of the terminal airways and the alveolar region. *Equine Vet J* 22:349, 1990.

236. Kaup FJ, Drommer W, Deegen E: Ultrastructural findings in horses with chronic obstructive pulmonary disease (COPD) I: Alterations of the larger conducting airways. *Equine Vet J* 22:343, 1990.

237. Beech J: Managing horses with chronic obstructive pulmonary disease. *Vet Med* 84:620, 1989.

238. Genetzky RM, Loparco FV: Clinical efficacy of clenbuterol with COPD in horses. *J Equine Vet Sci* 5:320, 1985.

239. Pearson EG, Riebold TW: Comparison of bronchodilators in alleviating clinical signs in a horse with chronic obstructive pulmonary disease. *J Am Vet Med Assoc* 194:1287, 1989.

240. Goetz TE: Successful management of equine chronic obstructive pulmonary disease. *Vet Med* 79:1073, 1984.

241. Matthews AG, Hackett IJ, Lawton WA: The mucolytic effect of Sputolosin in horses with respiratory disease. *Vet Rec* 122:106, 1988.

242. Lyons ET, Tolliver SC, Drudge JH, et al: Parasites in lungs of dead equids in Kentucky: Emphasis on *Dictyocaulus arnfieldi*. *Am J Vet Res* 46:924, 1985.

243. Lyons ET, Tolliver SC, Drudge JH, et al: Lungworms (*Dictyocaulus arnfieldi*): Prevalence in live equids in Kentucky. *Am J Vet Res* 46:921, 1985.

244. Clayton HM: Lung parasites. In Robinson NE, ed: *Current Therapy in Equine Medicine*. Philadelphia, WB Saunders, 1983, p 520.

245. George LW, Tanner ML, Roberson EL, et al: Chronic respiratory disease in a horse infected with *Dictyocaulus arnfieldi*. *J Am Vet Med Assoc* 179:820, 1981.

246. Clayton HM, Duncan JL: Natural infection with *Dictyocaulus arnfieldi* in pony and donkey foals. *Res Vet Sci* 31:278, 1981.

247. Beech J: Equine lungworms. In Smith BP, ed: *Large Animal Internal Medicine*. St. Louis, Mosby–Year Book, 1990, p 529.

248. Lyons ET, Drudge JH, Tolliver SC: Ivermectin: Treating for naturally occurring infections of lungworms and stomach worms in equids. *Vet Med* 80:58, 1985.

249. Pascoe JR, Ferraro GL, Cannon JH, et al: Exercise-induced pulmonary hemorrhage in racing thoroughbreds: A preliminary study. *Am J Vet Res* 42:701, 1981.

250. Raphel CF, Soma L: Exercise-induced pulmonary hemorrhage in Thoroughbreds after racing and breezing. *Am J Vet Res* 46:1123, 1982.

251. Hillidge CJ, Lane TJ, Whitlock TW: Exercise-induced pulmonary hemorrhage in the racing appaloosa horse. *J Equine Vet Sci* 5:351, 1985.

252. Hillidge CJ, Lane TJ, Johnson EL, et al: Preliminary investigations of exercise-induced pulmonary hemorrhage in racing quarter horses. *Equine Vet Sci* 4:21, 1984.

253. Voynick BR, Sweeney CR: Exercise-induced pulmonary hemorrhage in polo and racing horses. *J Am Vet Med Assoc* 188:301, 1986.

254. Mason DK, Collins EA, Watkins KL: Exercise-induced pulmonary hemorrhage in horses. In Snow DH, Persson SGB,

Rose RJ, eds: *Equine Exercise Physiology.* Granta Editions, Cambridge, Burlington Press, 1983, p 57.

255. Robinson NE, Derksen FJ: Small airway obstruction as a cause of exercise-associated pulmonary hemorrhage: An hypothesis. *Am Assoc Equine Pract* 26:421, 1980.

256. O'Callaghan MW, Pascoe JR, Tyler WS: Exercise-induced pulmonary haemorrhage in the horse: Results of a detailed clinical, post mortem and imaging study. VIII. Conclusions and implications. *Equine Vet J* 19:428, 1987.

257. Clarke AF: Review of exercise induced pulmonary haemorrhage and its possible relationship with mechanical stress. *Equine Vet J* 17:166, 1985.

258. Sweeney CR: Exercise-induced pulmonary hemorrhage. In Robinson NE, ed: *Current Therapy in Equine Medicine,* vol 2. Philadelphia, WB Saunders, 1987, p 603.

259. Pascoe J: EIPH. In Smith BP, ed.: *Large Animal Internal Medicine.* St. Louis, Mosby–Year Book, 1990, p 542.

260. Pascoe JR, O'Brien TR, Wheat JD, et al: Radiographic aspects of exercise-induced pulmonary hemorrhage in racing horses. *Vet Radiol* 24:85, 1983.

261. Sweeney CR, Soma LR: Exercise-induced pulmonary hemorrhage in Thoroughbred horses: Response to furosemide or hesperidin-citrus bioflavinoids. *J Am Vet Med Assoc* 185:195, 1984.

262. Sweeney CR, Soma LR, Maxson AD, et al: Effects of furosemide on the racing times of thoroughbreds. *Am J Vet Res* 51:772, 1990.

263. Hillidge CJ, Whitlock TW, Lane TJ: Failure of inhaled disodium cromoglycate aerosol to prevent exercise-induced pulmonary hemorrhage in racing Quarter Horses. *J Vet Pharmacol Ther* 10:257, 1987.

264. Dungworth DL: Interstitial pulmonary disease. *Adv Vet Sci Comp Med* 26:173, 1982.

265. O'Sullivan BM: Crofton weed (*Eupatorium adenophorum*) toxicity in horses. *Aust Vet J* 55:19, 1979.

266. Breeze RG, Laegreid WW, Bayly WM, et al: *Perilla* ketone toxicity: A chemical model for the study of equine restrictive lung disease. *Equine Vet J* 16:180, 1984.

267. Turk JR, Brown CM, Johnson GC: Diffuse alveolar damage with fibrosing alveolitis in a horse. *Vet Pathol* 18:560, 1981.

268. Schwartz LW, Knight HD, Malloy RL, et al: Silicate pneumoconiosis and pulmonary fibrosis in horses from the Monterey-Carmel peninsula. *Chest* 80:82s, 1981.

269. Winder C, Ehrensperger R, Hermann M, et al: Interstitial pneumonia in the horse: Two unusual cases. *Equine Vet J* 20:298, 1988.

270. Buergelt CD, Hines SA, Cantor G, et al: A retrospective study of proliferative interstitial lung disease of horses in Florida. *Vet Pathol* 23:750, 1986.

271. Derksen FJ, Slocombe RF, Brown CM, et al: Chronic restrictive pulmonary disease in a horse. *J Am Vet Med Assoc* 180:887, 1982.

272. Peel JE: Tuberculosis. In Robinson NE, ed: *Current Therapy in Equine Medicine.* Philadelphia, WB Saunders, 1983, p 29.

273. Prescott JF, Wilcock BP, Carman PS, et al: Sporadic, severe bronchointerstitial pneumonia of foals. *Can Vet J* 32:421, 1991.

274. Ainsworth DM, Weldon AD, Beck KA, et al: The recognition of *Pneumocystis carinii* in foals with respiratory distress. *Equine Vet J* 25:103, 1993.

275. Bastianello SS: A survey on neoplasia in domestic species over a 40-year period from 1935 to 1974 in the Republic of South Africa IV. Tumours occurring in Equidae. *Onderstepoort J Vet Res* 50:91, 1983.

276. Sundbery JP, Burnstein T, Page EH, et al: Neoplasms of Equidae. *J Am Vet Med Assoc* 170:150, 1977.

277. Cotchin E, Baker-Smith J: Tumours in horses encountered in an abattoir survey. *Vet Rec* 97:339, 1975.

278. Sweeney CR, Gillette DM: Equine thoracic neoplasia. In Smith BP ed: *Large Animal Internal Medicine.* St. Louis, Mosby–Year Book, 1990, p 522.

279. Nickels FA, Brown CM, Breeze RG: Myoblastoma equine granular cell tumor. *Mod Vet Pract* 61:593, 1980.

280. Turk MAM, Breeze RG: Histochemical and ultrastructural features of an equine pulmonary granular cell tumour (myoblastoma). *J Comp Pathol* 91:471, 1981.

281. Schultze AE, Sonea I, Bell TG: Primary malignant pulmonary neoplasia in two horses. *J Am Vet Med Assoc* 193:477, 1988.

282. Misdorp W, Nauta-van Gelder HL: Granular-cell myoblastoma in the horse. A report of 4 cases. *Pathol Vet* 4:384, 1968.

283. Parodi AL, Tassin P, Rigoulet J: Myoblastome à cellules granuleuses. Trois nouvelles observations à localisation pulmonair chez le cheval. *Rec Med Vet* 150:489, 1974.

284. Valentine BA, Ross CE, Bump JL, et al: Intramuscular hemangiosarcoma with pulmonary metastasis in a horse. *J Am Vet Med Assoc* 188:628, 1986.

285. Waugh SL, Long GG, Uriah L, et al: Metastatic hemangiosarcoma in the equine: report of two cases. *J Equine Med Surg* 1:311, 1977.

286. Frye FL, Humphrey DK, Brown SI: Hemangiosarcoma in a horse. *J Am Vet Med Assoc* 182:287, 1983.

287. Hargis AM, McElwain TF: Vascular neoplasia in the skin of horses. *J Am Vet Med Assoc* 184:1121, 1984.

288. Rebhun WC, Bertone A: Equine lymphosarcoma. *J Am Vet Med Assoc* 184:720, 1984.

289. Freestone JF, Williams MM, Norwood G: Thoracic haemangiosarcoma in a 3-year-old horse. *Aust Vet J* 67:269, 1990.

290. Johnson JE, Beech J, Saik JE: Disseminated hemangiosarcoma in a horse. *J Am Vet Med Assoc* 193:1429, 1988.

Chapter 7

Cardiovascular Diseases

John D. Bonagura, DVM I Virginia B. Reef, DVM

Identification, evaluation, and treatment of the horse with cardiovascular (CV) disease presents a significant challenge to the veterinarian. CV lesions are quite common in horses. Often these lesions are minor and well tolerated; however, CV disease can be clinically significant, manifested as exercise intolerance, arrhythmia, weakness, systemic infection, congestive heart failure (CHF), or sudden death. Since the horse is a species renowned for its physiologic murmurs and arrhythmias,[1-3] the findings of a CV examination may be confusing. Moreover, the impact of a cardiac lesion on a performance animal that is so dependent on circulatory function can be difficult to quantify.

Equine cardiology has advanced significantly over the past three decades. Much of the important groundwork in clinical equine cardiology can be attributed to the studies of Detweiler and colleagues,[1, 4-6] Hamlin, Smith, and Smetzer,[7-15] and Holmes and his graduate students.[2, 16-39] The initial information that these cardiologists provided about normal function, auscultation, and electrocardiography of the equine heart was very accurate, and it is still common to make clinical decisions based on the data that they provided. Due to the great size of the mature horse, traditional diagnostic studies such as radiography have played a smaller role in the assessment of heart diseases. Recent laboratory developments, including Holter electrocardiography, Doppler echocardiography, and functional exercise testing, are becoming increasingly important in the assessment of CV disease. These diagnostic studies allow both the detection and quantitation of a variety of anatomical and physiologic disturbances of the heart and circulation.

There are no comprehensive studies of CV *disease prevalence*. Holmes observed that 2.5% of hospitalized horses were in atrial fibrillation.[16] Else and Holmes noted myocardial fibrosis in 14.3% of horses examined at necropsy and evidence of chronic valvular disease in approximately 25% of the hearts examined.[17-19] Various CV lesions were considered to be important in 8.5% of 480 consecutive losses in a necropsy study conducted by Baker and Ellis.[40] CV diseases have been suggested to be the third most common cause of poor performance following musculoskeletal and respiratory diseases.[41, 42] Occult cardiac disease or cardiac arrhythmias may be an important reason for unexplained sudden death.[43-51] Certainly, most clinicians encounter manifestations of CV disease or dysfunction on a regular basis.

The assessment of CV disease in a horse is predicated on a competent clinical examination and on the clinician's knowledge and ability to evaluate data from various diagnostic studies. Incomplete information may impede an accurate communication of risks to the client and delay a proper course of management. A review of the currently available information regarding the diagnosis and therapy of CV diseases is the focus of this chapter. The authors assume that the reader is familiar with basic CV anatomy, physiology, and electrophysiology, and these topics have been reviewed elsewhere.[7, 14, 52-58] Pertinent aspects of clinical cardiac anatomy and physiology relevant to causes of equine heart diseases are described. Important studies essential in the diagnosis of CV disease are reviewed. Subsequent sections are designed to provide the student and practicing veterinarian with a framework for understanding the pathophysiology, clinical identification, and management of important congenital and acquired conditions of the heart and major vessels. Instrumental to each discussion are clinically relevant aspects of diagnosis and therapy. Clinical aspects of circulatory shock are described in this text. The reader is referred elsewhere for the management of cardiopulmonary arrest.[59, 60]

ANATOMICAL CORRELATES OF CARDIOVASCULAR DISEASES

Many diagnostic techniques, including cardiac auscultation, cardiac catheterization, and echocardiography, are predicated on an understanding of cardiac anatomy and physiology. Furthermore, the causes of CV disease can be subdivided into anatomical and physiologic (functional) diagnoses as well as etiologic considerations (Tables 7–1 and 7–2).

The CV system is divided into two separate circulations—systemic and pulmonary. The systemic circulation has a greater venous capacitance, ventricular pumping pressure, arterial pressure, and vascular resistance.[54, 57] Despite these differences, the functions of these two circulations are intertwined. Systemic and pulmonary circulations are arranged in series; therefore, disordered function of either side can affect the contralateral circulation. Cardiac output (CO) from the left ventricle must be equal to that of the right ventricle, because ventricular filling depends on venous return from the contralateral circulation. Isolated left ventricular (LV) failure increases pulmonary venous pressure. The resultant pulmonary hypertension imparts a pressure load on the right ventricle and is a common cause of right ventricular (RV)

Table 7–1. Cardiac Diagnoses

Anatomic Diagnosis

Cardiac malformation
Valvular (endocardial) disease
Myocardial disease
Pericardial disease
Cor pulmonale (pulmonary disease leading to secondary heart
 disease)
Disorder of the impulse forming or conduction system
Vascular disease

Physiologic Diagnosis

Systemic—pulmonary shunting
 Left to right
 Right to left
Valvular stenosis or insufficiency
Myocardial failure
Diastolic dysfunction
Cardiac rhythm disturbance
Cardiac syncope
Heart insufficiency or failure (limited cardiac output)
Congestive heart failure
Shock
Sudden cardiac death
Cardiopulmonary arrest

Etiologic Diagnosis

Malformation (genetic)
Degenerative disease
Metabolic or endocrine disease
Neoplasia
Nutritional disorder
Inflammatory disease
 Infective or parasitic
 Noninfective
  Immune mediated
  Idiopathic
Ischemic injury
Idiopathic disorder
Iatrogenic disease
Toxic injury
Traumatic injury

failure. Leftward bulging of the ventricular septum, secondary to RV dilatation, can impair filling of the left ventricle.

The heart consists of various active and passive components[57]; therefore, different methods and techniques are needed to evaluate these structures and their associated functions. For normal heart action to proceed, there must be coordination of electrical activity, muscular contraction and relaxation, and valve motion. When reviewing heart anatomy, and subsequently cardiac pathology, it is useful to consider the normal development of the heart and the anatomical integrity of the pericardium, myocardium, endocardium and valves, specialized impulse-forming and conduction systems, and blood vessels.[58]

Pericardial Disease

The pericardium limits cardiac dilatation, acts as a barrier against contiguous infection, and contributes to the diastolic properties of the heart. The pericardial space is formed by the reflection of the two pericardial membranes, the parietal pericardium and the visceral pericardium (the epicardium), and normally contains such a small amount of serous fluid that it cannot be seen by echocardiography. Pericardial effusion, tamponade, and constriction can greatly decrease ventricular filling and diastolic function. Pericardial diseases, as well as mass lesions impinging on the systemic veins or the heart, can lead to right-sided CHF.

Pericardial effusion can develop as a primary disorder or secondary to pleuropneumonia. Infective pericarditis can produce an effusion that is sufficient to cause cardiac tamponade or eventual constriction of the heart.[61–68] Sterile, idiopathic pericardial effusion has also been reported in horses. The volume of effusion can be substantial and can lead to cardiac decompensation.[69] Cardiac mass lesions and intrapericardial tumors have been reported sporadically.[70–73] Cranial mediastinal tumors (lymphosarcoma) or abscesses secondary to pleuropneumonia can also compress the heart and mimic pericardial disease.[74] Clinical aspects of pericardial disease are discussed later in this chapter.

Myocardial Disease

The myocardium forms the bulk of the atrial and ventricular muscular walls. The right atrium, which is larger than the left atrium, communicates with the RV inlet through the right atrioventricular (AV) or tricuspid valve. The right ventricle, appearing crescent-shaped on cross-sectional echocardiographic studies, is functionally U-shaped with the inlet at the right hemithorax and the outlet, pulmonary valve, and main pulmonary artery located on the left side of the chest. The thicker (by approximately 2.5 to 3 times) ventricular septum and attached LV wall is circular in cross-section when viewed by echocardiography and is functionally V-shaped with an inlet and outlet separated by the cranioventral (septal or "anterior") leaflet of the left AV, or mitral, valve (Fig. 7–1). The aorta originates in the LV outlet, continuous with the ventricular septum cranially and the septal mitral leaflet caudally, and exits from the center of the heart and to the right of the main pulmonary artery. Ventricular or atrial dilatation are recognized echocardiographically or at necropsy by distention and rounding of the affected chambers. Persistent embryologic openings in the cardiac septa are known as septal defects, with the ventricular septal defect (VSD) representing the most common cardiac anomaly in most practices (see Table 7–2).

The myocardium may dilate or hypertrophy in response to increased work due to another structural cardiac lesion or as a consequence of a noncardiac disorder. Lesions causing systolic pressure overload lead to concentric hypertrophy.[75] More common are lesions such as incompetent valves that cause ventricular volume overload with dilatation and eccentric ventricular hypertrophy. Increased cardiac work also occurs in response to exercise, severe anemia, and infections. In these situations, compensatory increases in CO, sympathetic activation, and peripheral vasodilation occur in order to maintain oxygen delivery to the tissues.[76, 77]

The overall prevalence of myocardial disease is unknown; however, multifocal areas of fibrosis are commonly found at necropsy.[17, 18, 78–80] Whether these areas indicate prior inflammation or ischemic necrosis caused by intramural coronary disease is uncertain. Cases of multifocal or diffuse

Table 7–2. Causes of Cardiovascular Disease

Congenital Cardiac Malformation

Simple systemic to pulmonary shunts (left to right)
  Atrial septal defect
  Ventricular septal defect
    Right ventricular inlet (subcristal) VSD
    Right ventricular outlet (supracristal) VSD
    Defects of the muscular ventricular septum
  Patent ductus arteriosus
Patent foramen ovale (permitting right to left shunting)
Valvular dysplasia
  Pulmonic stenosis (bicuspid pulmonary valve)
  Pulmonary atresia (leading to a right to left shunt)
  Tricuspid stenosis/atresia (leading to a right to left shunt)
  Aortic stenosis/insufficiency (bicuspid or quadricuspid valve)
Subaortic rings with stenosis
Tetralogy of Fallot
  Pulmonary atresia with VSD (pseudotruncus arteriosus)
Double-outlet right ventricle
Subaortic stenosis
Hypoplastic left heart
Other complex malformations

Valvular Heart Disease Causing Valve Insufficiency or Stenosis

Congenital valve malformation
Semilunar valve fenestrations causing valve insufficiency
Degenerative (fibrosis) or myxomatous disease causing valve
  insufficiency
Bacterial endocarditis causing valve insufficiency ± stenosis
Rupture of a chorda tendinea causing mitral or tricuspid valve
  insufficiency
Rupture of a valve leaflet causing flail leaflet and valve
  insufficiency
Noninfective valvulitis
Valvular regurgitation secondary to dilatation of the heart or a great
  vessel
Valve prolapse

Myocardial Disease

Idiopathic dilated cardiomyopathy—ventricular dilatation and
  myocardial contractility failure
Myocarditis
Myocardial fibrosis
  Ischemic (?embolic) myocardial fibrosis
  Parasitic (Strongylus) embolization

Myocardial Disease (Continued)

Myocardial degeneration/necrosis
  Toxic injury (e.g., monensin)
  Nutritional deficiencies (e.g., selenium deficiency)
Myocardial neoplasia
  Lymphosarcoma
  Melanoma
  Hemangioma/hemangiosarcoma
  Pulmonary carcinoma

Pericardial Disease

Pericardial effusion ± cardiac tamponade
  Infective—bacterial or viral
  Idiopathic pericardial effusion
  Constrictive pericardial disease
  Mass lesion (intrapericardial or extrapericardial) compressing the
    heart

Pulmonary Hypertension and Cor Pulmonale

Pulmonary hypertension secondary to left-sided heart disease
Pulmonary vascular disease secondary to left to right shunt
Immature pulmonary circulation
Primary bronchopulmonary disease
Alveolar hypoxia with reactive pulmonary arterial vasoconstriction
Severe acidosis
Pulmonary thromboembolism

Cardiac Arrhythmias (see Table 7–15)

Atrial arrhythmias
Junctional (nodal) arrhythmias
Ventricular arrhythmias
Conduction disturbances

Vascular Diseases

Congenital vascular lesions
Rupture of the aorta, pulmonary artery, or systemic artery
Aneurysm of the aortic sinus of Valsalva
Aortic or aortoiliac degenerative disease
Arteritis
  Infective
  Immune mediated
Thrombophlebitis
Pulmonary embolism
Mass lession or tumor obstructing blood flow

VSD, ventricular septal defect.

---

myocarditis have been observed. Myocardial inflammation and myocardial failure can lead to cardiac arrhythmias and heart failure.[1, 3, 81] Idiopathic dilated cardiomyopathy develops sporadically and is recognized echocardiographically or by nuclear studies as a dilated, hypokinetic left or right ventricle.[82, 83] Ingestion of monensin can cause mild to severe myocardial injury.[84–86] Neoplastic infiltration is considered rare.[45, 71, 72, 87] Myocardial contraction is dictated by electrical activity of the myocardium; accordingly, cardiac arrhythmias—especially atrial fibrillation—can limit CO and cause exercise intolerance in performance animals (see later). Clin-

ical aspects of myocardial disease are discussed later in this chapter.

Valvular and Endocardial Diseases

The cardiac chambers are lined by the endocardium, which also covers the four cardiac valves and is continuous with the endothelium of the great vessels. Normal valves govern the one-way flow of blood in the heart by preventing regurgitation of blood from higher to lower pressure zones. The AV inlet valves—the tricuspid and the mitral—are anchored by

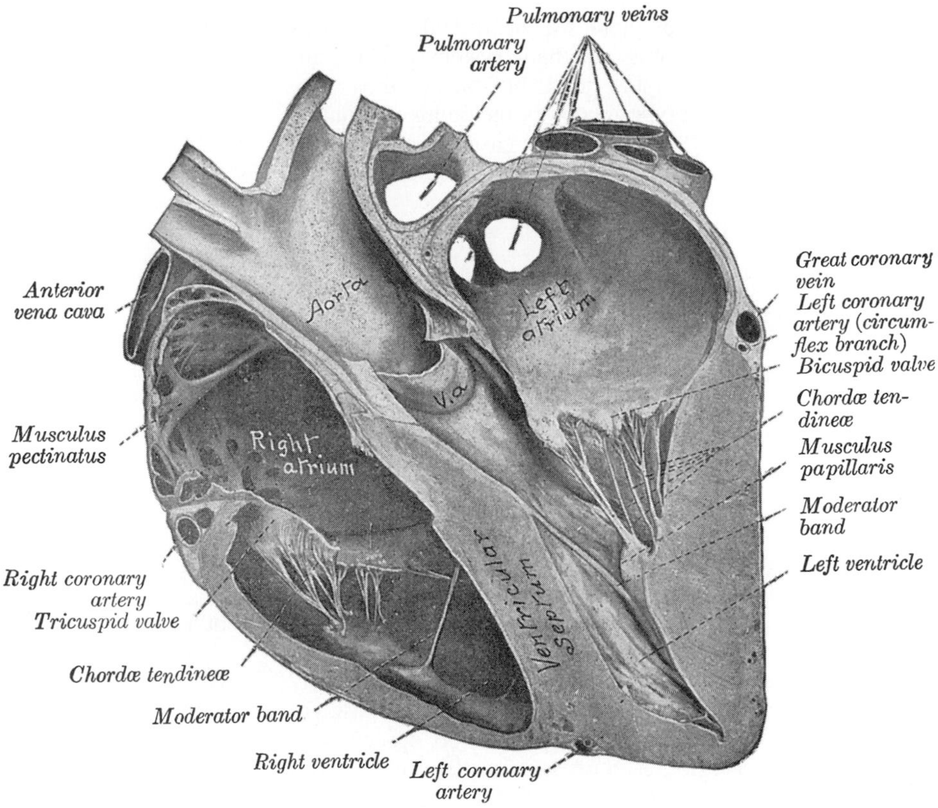

Figure 7–1. Sagittal view of the equine heart. The relative thicknesses of the ventricles, the position of the atria relative to the ventricles, and the relationship of the left ventricular inlet and outlet are evident. The bicuspid valve referred to in this figure is the mitral valve. Note the relatively circular appearance of the left atrium and the relationship of the septal cusp of the mitral valve to the left ventricular inlets and outlets. These aspects are important when examining the heart by echocardiography. (v.a., segment of aortic valve.) (From Sisson S, Grossman JD: *Anatomy of the Domestic Animals,* ed 4. Philadelphia, WB Saunders, 1953.)

the collagenous chordae tendineae and papillary muscles and are supported by a valve "annulus" and the caudal atrial walls (Fig. 7–2; see also Fig. 7–1).[58] The mitral valve consists of two major cusps and several accessory cusps.[34] The tricuspid valve is the largest valve and consists of three well-defined leaflets. Lesions of any portion of the AV valve apparatus or dilatation of the ventricle can lead to valvular insufficiency (see Table 7–2). The aortic and pulmonary valves each consist of three leaflets that close during diastole to protect the ventricles from the higher arterial blood pressures. The left and right main coronary arteries originate within the aortic valve sinuses (of Valsalva).

Valvular disorders are common. Congenital valve stenosis, dysplasia, or atresia are recognized sporadically in foals.[1, 3, 88–102] Degenerative diseases of the aortic, mitral, and tricuspid valves are quite common in mature horses,[11, 12, 17–19, 38, 103] and endocarditis can develop on any cardiac valve[1, 3, 104–112] (see Table 7–2). Valvular lesions of obscure etiology, including nonseptic valvulitis, have been recognized in a few cases. Tricuspid regurgitation, of unknown etiology, is often detected in performance animals, particularly Standardbred and National Hunt horses.[113, 113a] Mitral regurgitation (MR) due to rupture of a chorda tendinea is not uncommon and has been observed in both foals and mature animals.[32, 114–116] Clinical aspects of valvular heart disease are discussed later in this chapter.

Disease of the Impulse-Forming and Conduction Systems

The specialized cardiac tissues consist of the sinoatrial (SA) node, internodal pathways, AV node, bundle of His, bundle branches, fascicles, and Purkinje system (Fig. 7–3). The SA node, a relatively large, crescent-shaped structure, is located subepicardially at the junction of the right auricle and cranial vena cava. Well-documented sinus node disease, while suggested,[117] is rare; in contrast, vagal-induced sinus arrhythmias are common.[14, 117–119] The equine atrial muscle mass is large and predisposes the horse to development of re-entrant rhythms and atrial fibrillation.[120] The AV node, situated in the ventral atrial septum, and the bundle of His, which continues on into the bundle branches, are sites for AV block, both physiologic (vagal), and infrequently, pathologic in nature. Conduction is slow across the AV node.[121–123] The His-Purkinje system in the ventricular septum and ventricular myocardium can act as substrates for junctional and ventricular ectopic impulses and tachycardias. Because the horse has relatively complete penetration of Purkinje fibers to the ventricular free walls—except for a small portion of the LV free wall—the substantial equine ventricles are electrically activated in a relatively short time (~110 msec).[9]

The autonomic nervous system extensively innervates the heart and influences cardiac rhythms.[1, 3, 124–130] Interplay between the sympathetic and parasympathetic branches normally controls heart rate and rhythm in response to changes in arterial blood pressure.[14, 131] The vagus innervates supraventricular tissues extensively and probably affects proximal ventricular tissues to a minor extent. Vagal influence is generally depressive to heart rate, AV conduction, excitability, and myocardial inotropic (contractile) state. However, because vagotonia shortens the action potential and refractory period of atrial myocytes, high vagal activity may be a predisposing factor in the development of atrial fibrillation.[132] Innervation of the stimulatory sympathetic nervous system is extensive throughout the heart and has effects opposite to those of the parasympathetic system. β_1-Adrenergic receptors dominate in the heart, but presumably, there are other autonomic subtype receptors including β_2- and α-adrenergic receptors.[133] The notable increase in heart rate that attends exercise is related to increased sympathetic efferent activity and withdrawal of parasympathetic tone.[14] Increases in heart rate to 220 to 240 beats/min are not uncommon with maximal exercise.[134–138] The exact role of dysautonomia in the genesis of cardiac arrhythmias has not been determined; however, infusion of autonomic receptor agonists and antagonists can be associated with direct or baroreceptor-induced changes in heart rate and rhythm.[139–142] Cardiac arrhythmias are discussed later in this chapter.

Vascular Diseases

The arteries and veins consist of three layers: adventitia, media, and intima. The overall structure and function of each layer varies with the vessel and location. Vascular receptors[7, 54, 57, 133] and anatomical lesions influence vascular resistance and blood flow. α-Adrenoreceptors dominate in the systemic vasculature, and blood pressure is generally raised by vasoconstriction following stimulation of postsynaptic α-adrenergic receptors by norepinephrine, epinephrine, or infused α-adrenergic receptor agonists like phenylephrine.[143, 144] The presence of vasodilator β_2-adrenergic receptors is clinically relevant, insofar as infused β_2-agonists

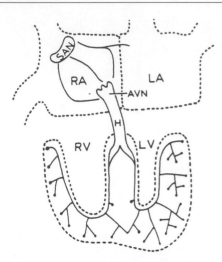

Figure 7–3. Schematic demonstrating the anatomy of the impulse forming and the conduction system. The sinoatrial node (SAN), right atrium (RA), left atrium (LA), atrioventricular node (AVN), bundle of His (H), and the bundle branches continuing into the Purkinje system in the right ventricle (RV) and the left ventricle (LV) are shown. (Courtesy of Dr. Robert L. Hamlin.)

cause vasodilation in circulatory beds that contain high β-agonist adrenergic receptor density. Many vascular beds also dilate following the production of local vasodilator substances released during exercise, stress, or metabolic activity.[54, 57] Dopaminergic receptors, when present in vascular walls, may be stimulated to cause vasodilation provided vasoconstricting α-adrenergic activity does not dominate. Stimulation of histamine (H_1) receptors or serotonin (5-HT) receptors causes arteriolar dilatation, venular constriction, and increased capillary permeability.[57] Infusion of calcium salts causes arterial vasoconstriction,[145] whereas administration of calcium channel antagonists (e.g., verapamil) causes vasodilation of vascular smooth muscle.

Various vascular lesions have been reported (see Table 7–2). Rupture of the aorta, pulmonary artery, or middle uterine artery is devastating and typically lethal.[1, 3, 20, 44, 146–148] Although parasitic arteritis may predispose to vascular injury, the cause of most vascular lesions, including aortic-iliac thrombosis, is unknown.[149–154] Causes of vasculitis include *Strongylus vulgaris* infestation of the cranial mesenteric artery, infective thrombophlebitis of the jugular veins, equine viral arteritis, and suspected immune-mediated disease.[78, 80, 155] Clinical features of vascular disease are discussed later in this chapter.

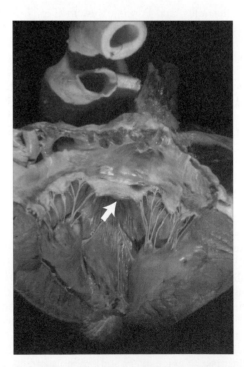

Figure 7–2. Anatomy of the left atrioventricular (mitral) valve. Opened left atrium and left ventricle viewed from the caudal perspective. Note the large anterior (cranioventral or septal) leaflet in the center of the figure. Chordae tendineae attach the valve to the papillary muscles. The ventricle has been cut so that the multiple cusps of the posterior (caudodorsal or mural) leaflet are observed to the left and the right of the anterior leaflet.

CLINICAL CARDIOVASCULAR PHYSIOLOGY

The clinician must appreciate elementary aspects of normal heart function in order to understand changes in the pulses and auscultation and hemodynamic alterations that develop in heart disease and CHF. Central to this are the electrical-mechanical correlates of Wiggers' cardiac cycle.[133]

Cardiac Cycle

The association between electrical and mechanical events of the heart first described by Wiggers has been reviewed in standard physiology textbooks (Fig. 7–4).[54, 57, 133] From a study of this cycle, it is evident that cardiac electrical activity precedes pressure and volume changes; therefore, arrhythmias can have deleterious hemodynamic effects, especially during exercise, illness, or anesthesia. Understanding the cardiac cycle and considering the interrelated events during the course of an examination provides the clinician with critical information regarding cardiac rhythm and the health of the heart. Relevant aspects of this cycle are now considered.

The P wave of the electrocardiogram (ECG) occurs as a result of electrical activation of the atria, late in ventricular diastole, and after the ventricles have been passively filled. During the ensuing atrial contraction the *atrial sound* (S_4) is generated and the ventricle is filled to a slightly greater extent (termed the end-diastolic volume). The increase in atrial pressure, the atrial "a" wave, is reflected up the systemic venous system causing a normal *jugular pulse* in the ventral cervical region. The magnitude of the atrial contribution to ventricular filling is greatest at high heart rates; therefore, atrial tachyarrhythmias such as atrial fibrillation have a most serious impact during exercise.

The QRS complex heralds ventricular systole. After depolarization of the ventricular myocytes, calcium enters the cell to trigger shortening of the myofilaments and develop tension, an event that can be enhanced by digitalis glycosides or with catecholamines such as dobutamine. These changes lead to an abrupt increase in ventricular wall tension and intraventricular pressure. The AV valves close once atrial pressure is exceeded (generating the high-frequency *first heart sound*; S_1), the intraventricular pressure increases (*isovolumetric period*) and subsequently the semilunar valves

open.[25, 27] The contracting heart twists slightly during systole, and the left ventricle strikes the chest wall caudal to the left olecranon causing the *cardiac impulse* or "apex beat." This early systolic movement, coincident with opening of the aortic valve, is a useful timing clue for cardiac auscultation. The delay between the onset of the QRS and the opening of the semilunar valves, termed the *pre-ejection period,* can be measured by echocardiography and is an index of ventricular myocardial contractility such that positive inotropic drugs shorten the pre-ejection period. Blood is ejected into the pulmonary and systemic arteries with an initial velocity that generally peaks at 1 m/sec and can be measured by Doppler echocardiography.[156, 156a] The aortic ejection time usually exceeds 400 msec in a horse at rest, and reductions of either ejection velocity or ejection time are suggestive of reduced LV function. A *functional systolic ejection murmur* is often heard during ejection. Such murmurs, by definition, must begin after the first sound and end before the second sound. The *arterial pulse* can be palpated during systole, but the actual timing of the pulse depends on the proximity of the palpation site relative to the heart. At the end of the *ejection period,* as ventricular pressures fall below those of the corresponding arteries, the semilunar valves close producing the high-frequency *second heart sound*(s) (S_2) and the incisura of the arterial pressure curves.[15, 25, 27] The pulmonary valve may close either after or before the aortic valve.[1, 4, 157] Asynchronous valve closure may lead to audible splitting of S_2, which is normal but can be extreme in some horses with lung disease. During the ejection period the ventricular volume curve graphs a marked reduction from the end-diastolic volume: this volume ejected is defined as the *stroke volume*. The ratio of the stroke volume to the end-diastolic volume is the *ejection fraction,* a commonly used index of systolic heart function. Contraction of the ventricles causes the atrial pressures to decline leading to the x-descent of the

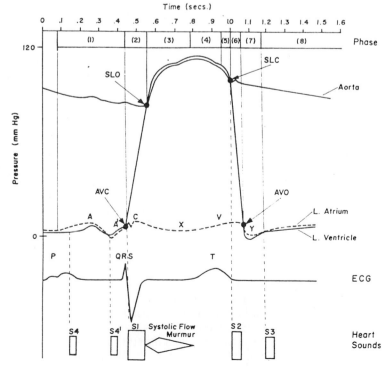

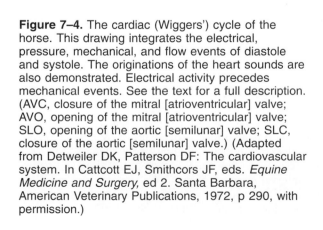

Figure 7–4. The cardiac (Wiggers') cycle of the horse. This drawing integrates the electrical, pressure, mechanical, and flow events of diastole and systole. The originations of the heart sounds are also demonstrated. Electrical activity precedes mechanical events. See the text for a full description. (AVC, closure of the mitral [atrioventricular] valve; AVO, opening of the mitral [atrioventricular] valve; SLO, opening of the aortic [semilunar] valve; SLC, closure of the aortic [semilunar] valve.) (Adapted from Detweiler DK, Patterson DF: The cardiovascular system. In Cattcott EJ, Smithcors JF, eds. *Equine Medicine and Surgery,* ed 2. Santa Barbara, American Veterinary Publications, 1972, p 290, with permission.)

atrial pressure curve and a brief systolic collapse of the jugular vein. Subsequent to atrial filling during ventricular systole, a positive pressure wave, the v wave, occurs in the atrial pressure curves. Severe tricuspid regurgitation accentuates this wave and may lead to pathologic systolic pulsations in the jugular furrow. The last event in true ventricular systole is the decline in ventricular pressure (isovolumetric relaxation) that occurs at the initiation of ventricular relaxation and just before the AV valves open.

Ventricular diastole can be subdivided into three phases: rapid ventricular filling, diastasis, and atrial contraction.[54, 57, 133] The ventricles have relaxed so that atrial pressure exceeds the corresponding ventricular pressure; the AV valves open; and rapid, passive filling ensues with a peak velocity of about 0.5 to 1 m/sec but varies directly with the heart rate.[156] The ventricular pressures increase only slightly during this phase, whereas the ventricular volume curves change dramatically from the venous return. Rapid filling may be associated with a *functional protodiastolic murmur*, which is concluded by the *third heart sound* (S_3), the low-frequency vibrations caused by termination of rapid ventricular filling. The loss of atrial volume and corresponding decline in the atrial pressure (the "y" descent) is reflected in the jugular furrow as the vein collapses. Following rapid filling, a period of greatly reduced low-velocity filling, diastasis, ensues. This period may last for seconds during sinus bradycardia or pronounced sinus arrhythmia, and with markedly exaggerated pauses, the jugular vein may begin to fill prominently. The last phase of diastole is the contribution to ventricular filling caused by the atrial contraction. A functional *presystolic murmur* has been associated with this period between the fourth and first heart sounds.

Assessment of Ventricular Function

The ability of the ventricles to eject blood depends on both systolic and diastolic ventricular function as well as heart rate and rhythm (Table 7–3). The most commonly used measurements of overall ventricular performance and circulatory function are invasively or noninvasively determined arterial blood pressure, rate of ventricular pressure change, CO, stroke volume, ejection fraction, LV shortening fraction, central venous pressure, pulmonary artery or wedge pressures, and arteriovenous oxygen difference (A-V DO$_2$).[26, 28, 33, 82, 158–171] CO, the amount of blood pumped by the left (or right) ventricle in 1 minute (L/min), is the product of ventricular stroke volume (mL/beat) multiplied by the heart rate (beats/min). Cardiac index refers to the CO divided by (indexed to) the body surface area. CO coupled to systemic vascular resistance determines the mean arterial blood pressure: an increase in either variable raises mean arterial pressure. Values for CO vary widely with the size and activity of the horse and are often influenced by drug therapy or anesthesia.[140, 172–183] A noninvasive estimate of CO can also be obtained using Doppler techniques.[170, 170a, 170b]

Ventricular stroke volume depends on myocardial contractility and loading conditions (preload and afterload).[26, 28] While traditionally considered to be independent determinants of myocardial function, these variables are all interconnected and influence force, velocity, and duration of ventricular contraction.[133] Ultimately, the availability of calcium to

---

Table 7–3. Determinants of Cardiac Function

Systolic Function—Determinants of Ventricular Stroke Volume

Preload [+]—ventricular end-diastolic volume
    Determinants of diastolic function (see below)
    Plasma volume
    Venous pressure/venous return
Myocardial inotropism [+]—"contractility" of the myocardium
    Sympathetic activity
    Myocardial disease
    Drugs (positive or negative inotropic agents)
    Myocardial perfusion
Ventricular afterload [−]—wall tension required to eject blood
    Aortic impedance
    Vascular resistance
    Ventricular volume (tension increases with dilatation)
    Ventricular wall thickness (thin walls have higher tension)
Cardiac lesions increasing workload or affecting stroke volume [−]
    Valvular regurgitation (common)
    Valvular stenosis (rare)
    Septal defects and shunts

Diastolic Function—Determinants of Ventricular Filling

Pleural/mediastinal factors (pressure, mass lesions)
Pericardial function (intrapericardial pressure, constriction)
Ventricular wall distensibility (chamber and myocyte compliance)
Venous pressure and venous return (must be matched with compliance)
Heart rate and ventricular filling time (shortened by tachycardia)
Myocardial perfusion (ischemia impairs relaxation)
Atrial contribution to filling (lost in atrial fibrillation)
Cardiac rhythm (arrhythmias can alter atrioventricular contraction sequencing)
Atrioventricular valve function

Cardiac Output

Cardiac output = Stroke volume [+] × heart rate [+]

Arterial Blood Pressure

Arterial blood pressure = Cardiac output [+] × vascular resistance [+]

[+], increases physiologic variable; [−], decreases or reduces physiologic variable.

---

the sarcomere is modulated by the inotropic state, the initial myocardial stretch (preload), and the tension that must be generated in order to eject blood into the vascular system (afterload).

Myocardial contractility is increased by catecholamines, calcium, and digitalis glycosides.[139, 145, 176, 184–186] Contractility is difficult to measure in the clinical setting but can be estimated by observing directional changes in ejection fraction (which is also load-dependent) or by Doppler echocardiographic techniques including shortening fraction, pre-ejection period, ejection time, aortic acceleration, and velocity time integral (Figs. 7–5 and 7–6).

Ventricular fiber length or preload is a positive determinant of ventricular systolic function that depends on venous

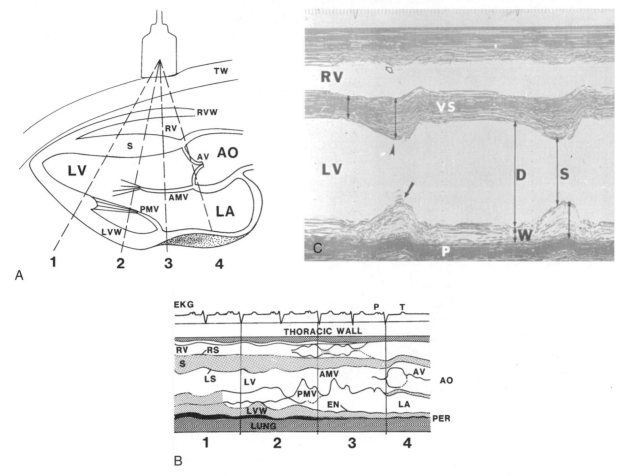

Figure 7–5. Ventricular function and echocardiography. *A,* Derivation of the M-mode echocardiogram. The lines demonstrate typical paths of M-mode recording planes (1 = ventricular/papillary muscle; 2 = chordae tendineae; 3 = anterior mitral valve (AMV); 4 = aortic root and left atrium/auricle). The drawing at the bottom of the figure *(B)* demonstrates the appearance of the M-mode echocardiogram at each level. (PER, pericardium; RS/LS, right and left sides of the ventricular septum; PMV = posterior mitral valve; EN = endocardium; LVW = left ventricular wall.) *C,* M-mode echocardiogram demonstrating the method of measuring left ventricular shortening fraction (LVSF) = D − S/D in which: D, diastolic dimension; S, systolic dimension. Note the prominent thickening of the walls during systole. The end-systolic excursion of the left ventricular wall is shown *(arrow).* (W, left ventricular wall; VS, ventricular septum.)

return and ventricular size and distensibility. The normal ventricle depends greatly on preload so that an increase in preload increases stroke volume. Dehydration, venous pooling, loss of atrial contribution to filling (atrial fibrillation), and recumbency all reduce ventricular filling and decrease stroke volume. When hypotension develops consequent to decreased ventricular filling, intravenous crystalloid is usually administered to increase venous pressure and preload. Increased ventricular preload can be observed in horses with heart disease. Moderate to severe valvular insufficiency and CHF increase ventricular filling pressure and preload.[32, 38, 77, 114, 187, 187a] The increased ventricular diastolic dimension serves as a compensatory mechanism that maintains forward stroke volume in the setting of a failing ventricle or regurgitant heart valve.

Ventricular preload can be estimated by determining ventricular end-diastolic volume or size, as measured by echocardiography, or by measuring venous filling pressures.[187a] The measurement of venous filling pressures (central venous pressure, pulmonary diastolic or wedge pressure) provides

an accurate gauge of preload provided that ventricular compliance (distensibility) is normal and ventilation is relatively stable. Myocardial ischemia, which stiffens the ventricle, and pericardial diseases, which restrict the ventricle, both reduce ventricular compliance; in such cases, the venous filling pressures may not accurately reflect changes in ventricular preload.

Ventricular *afterload* is represented by the tension that must be developed in the ventricular walls prior to ejection of blood into the arteries. Increases in systemic arterial resistance, aortic blood pressure, and aortic impedance usually increase afterload and resist ventricular shortening. This decreases stroke volume, unless ventricular force of contraction is increased to compensate for the load. Afterload is difficult to measure clinically, and while systemic arterial blood pressure is not identical to afterload, it is often used to estimate directional changes in afterload. LV failure, alveolar hypoxia-induced pulmonary vasoconstriction, and atelectasis are important clinical causes of increased RV afterload. Arterial vasodilators such as hydralazine decrease LV afterload.[180]

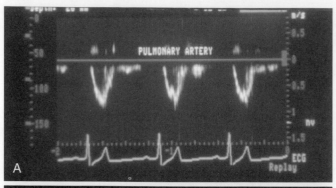

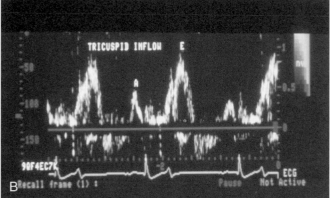

Figure 7–6. Pulsed wave Doppler recording. *A,* Flow velocity profile in the proximal pulmonary artery. Velocity (m/sec) is shown along the Y axis (right side) and the time along the X axis. Flow patterns can be timed relative to the electrocardiogram. The area under the triangular systolic curve (the velocity time integral) and the rate of development of maximal velocity (acceleration) can be measured as indices of systolic function. In addition, the pre-ejection period (the delay between the initial activity of the QRS complex and the onset of ejection) and the ejection time can be determined from the velocity spectrum and accompanying electrocardiogram. *B,* Velocity profile across the tricuspid valve demonstrating two peaks of diastolic filling—early rapid filling (E) and late filling from atrial contraction (A). (*B,* Courtesy of Dr. Karen Long Blissitt.)

Ventricular *synergy* refers to the normal method of ventricular activation and contraction. Normal electrical activation causes a burst of activation of great mechanical advantage.[7] Cardiac arrhythmias, especially ventricular rhythm disturbances, can cause dyssynergy with a resultant decrease in stroke volume. Coronary occlusions leading to ischemic myocardial necrosis also cause dyssynergy but are quite rare.[43, 80, 188]

Structural and functional competency of the cardiac valves and ventricular septa influence ventricular systolic function. Valve insufficiency or obstruction may seriously reduce ventricular stroke volume unless there is adequate compensation from ventricular dilatation and hypertrophy or heart rate reserve. Many septal defects are well tolerated at rest and during moderate exercise; however, large defects can lead to substantial shunting and volume overload with limited LV stroke volume. Cardiomegaly, arrhythmias, or CHF may ensue.

Ventricular *diastolic function* determines ventricular filling and preload.[54, 57, 133] Factors that affect diastolic function are indicated in Table 7–3. When diastolic function is abnormal, there is often greater heart rate dependency for maintenance of CO. A common cause of diastolic dysfunction is restriction or compression of the heart due to pericardial disease. Ventricular diastolic function is affected by arrhythmias. Persistent tachycardia impairs diastolic function by shortening the time allowed for ventricular filling and coronary perfusion. With atrial fibrillation, the atrial contribution is lost. Junctional and ventricular arrhythmias prevent normal AV sequencing. Ventricular chamber dilatation or hypertrophy decrease ventricular compliance and require higher ventricular distending pressures for filling. LV diastolic dysfunction as a consequence of severe RV dilatation or hypertrophy can be explained by bulging of the ventricular septum into the left ventricle, which impedes left-sided filling. This is observed clinically with constrictive pericardial disease and pulmonary hypertension.

Objective measures of diastolic function are very complicated, and no good clinical indicators of diastolic function are currently available. However, diastolic dysfunction may be assumed when one of the aforementioned conditions is recognized.

Imbalance between *myocardial oxygen demand* and delivery can reduce ventricular systolic and diastolic function and may affect cardiac rhythm. Myocardial oxygen demand is augmented by increasing myocardial inotropic state, heart rate, and ventricular wall tension (related to preload and afterload).[133] Oxygen delivery depends on coronary anatomy and vasomotion (degree of vessel constriction), diastolic arterial blood pressure, diastolic (coronary perfusion) time, and metabolic activity of the myocardium.[57, 189–197] Normal coronary flow is highest to the LV myocardium in the ventricular septum and LV wall.[197] The immediate subendocardial layer of myocardium is probably most vulnerable to ischemic injury,[14] and altered ventricular depolarization may develop secondary to an imbalance in myocardial oxygen delivery. This may account in part for the ST-T depression and changes in the T waves observed in hypotensive animals and in normal horses during sinus tachycardia. Coronary vasomotion is effective in augmenting coronary perfusion even at high heart rates (up to 200/min in ponies); however, coronary autoregulation is not as effective if diastolic perfusing pressure decreases in the aorta.[190, 191, 194]

The clinician may use the [arterial blood pressure] × [heart rate] "double product" as an estimate of myocardial oxygen demand.[133] Persistent ST-segment depression or elevation, especially at normal heart rates, suggests deficient myocardial perfusion.

CARDIOVASCULAR EXAMINATION OF THE HORSE

General Approach

A general approach to the recognition and diagnosis of heart disease and an assessment of its severity is summarized in Table 7–4. Undoubtedly, history and auscultation are the most important initial evaluation procedures in the CV examination of the horse. With the exception of subtle abnormalities in ventricular function, normal cardiac auscultation in a horse with good exercise tolerance practically precludes significant heart disease. The initial CV physical examina-

Table 7-4. Clinical Examination of the Equine Cardiovascular System

History and Physical Examination*

Work history and identification of possible hemodynamic dysfunction
Heart rate and rhythm
Examination of the arterial and venous pulses, refill, and pressure
Inspection of the mucous membranes
Evaluation for abnormal fluid accumulation: pulmonary, pleural, peritoneal, and subcutaneous
Auscultation of the heart and lungs
Measurement of arterial blood pressure (indirect method)

Electrocardiography

Heart rate, rhythm, and conduction sequence
P-QRS-T complexes: configuration, amplitude, duration, and axis
Post-exercise and exercise electrocardiography†
Holter (tape-recorded) electrocardiogram†‡

Echocardiography

M-mode echocardiography—cardiac dimensions and systolic ventricular function; cardiac anatomy and valve motion; estimation of cardiac output
Two-dimensional echocardiography—cardiac anatomy and systolic ventricular function; identification of lesions; estimation of cardiac output
Doppler echocardiography‡—identification of normal and abnormal flow; estimation of intracardiac pressures; estimation of cardiac output
Post-exercise echocardiography—identification of regional or global wall dysfunction or valve dysfunction exacerbated by exercise

Thoracic Radiography

Evaluation of pleural space, pulmonary parenchyma, and lung vascularity
Estimation of heart size (more beneficial in foals)

Clinical Laboratory Tests

Complete blood count and fibrinogen to identify anemia or inflammation
Serum biochemical tests including electrolytes, renal function tests, and muscle enzymes—these studies may be useful for assessment of arrhythmias, identification of low cardiac output (azotemia), and recognition of myocardial cell injury (cardiac isoenzymes of creatine kinase or lactic dehydrogenase)
Serum protein to identify hypoalbuminemia and hyperglobulinemia
Arterial pH and blood gas analysis to evaluate pulmonary and renal function and to assess acid-base status
Urinalysis to identify renal injury from heart failure or endocarditis
Blood cultures for bacteremia and diagnosis of endocarditis
Serum/plasma assays for digoxin, quinidine, and other drugs

Radionuclide Studies§

Detection of abnormal blood flow or lung perfusion; assessment of ventricular function

Cardiac Catheterization and Angiocardiography§

Diagnosis of abnormal blood flow and identification of abnormal intracardiac and intravascular pressures

Adapted from Bonagura JD: Clinical evaluation and management of heart disease. *Equine Vet Educ* 2:31–37, 1990.
*Most important part of the cardiac evaluation.
†May be needed to identify paroxysmal atrial fibrillation.
‡Generally done after referral.
§Uncommonly performed.

tion should include a thorough auscultation of the heart at all valve areas, auscultation of both lung fields, palpation of the precordium, evaluation of the arterial pulses (head and limbs), inspection of the veins, and evaluation of the mucous membranes for pallor, refill time, and cyanosis, which may develop in foals secondary to a right to left cardiac shunt (see Table 7–4). An accurate resting heart rate and respiratory rate should also be recorded.

It is worth emphasizing that most *serious* cardiac disorders can be detected initially by physical examination and a stethoscope. Sustained or recurrent cardiac arrhythmias are easily discovered through cardiac auscultation and palpation of the arterial pulse, and diagnosis of the rhythm can be verified through electrocardiography. Pericarditis and cardiac tamponade are usually characterized by muffled heart sounds, pericardial friction rubs, and RV failure. Significant myocardial disease is usually associated with heart failure, arrhythmias, or a cardiac murmur, especially in advanced cases wherein ventricular dilatation causes secondary insufficiency of the mitral or tricuspid valves. The presence of a cardiac murmur is the essential finding that leads one to suspect degenerative or infective valvular disease or a congenital heart malformation.[3, 89]

Laboratory studies and echocardiography are additional tests that are particularly useful in recognizing the underlying basis and severity of CV disease. Mild or subtle CV disease may require a detailed examination, including exercise testing,[198–202] before abnormalities can be objectively detected.

History

CV disease may be suspected from the history or may be an unexpected finding during the course of a routine examination.[2, 3, 81, 127, 169, 203–206] The horse with CHF may be examined for generalized venous distention, jugular pulsations, or edema whereas other problems such as an arrhythmia or murmur can be incidental findings, which are detected during a routine physical, pre-purchase, or insurance examination. Once an abnormality has been detected, a complete CV examination is aimed at determining the significance of the CV lesion in terms of safety, performance capabilities, and expected longevity.

The horse with clinically apparent CV disease may have subtle performance problems that are only apparent at peak performance levels. Slowing in the last quarter to three

---

Table 7–5. Cardiovascular Associations of Poor Performance

Arrhythmias

Atrial premature complexes
Ventricular premature complexes
Atrial fibrillation
Supraventricular tachycardia
Ventricular tachycardia
Advanced second-degree atrioventricular block
Complete third-degree atrioventricular block

Congenital, Valvular, or Myocardial Heart Diseases Associated with Murmurs

Ventricular septal defect
Mitral regurgitation
Tricuspid regurgitation
Aortic regurgitation
Cardiomyopathy with secondary atrioventricular valvular regurgitation

Occult Heart Disease

Pericardial disease
Cardiomyopathy or myocarditis

Vascular Disorders

Aortoiliac thrombosis
Jugular vein thrombophlebitis
Aortic root rupture
Pulmonary artery rupture

---

eighths of a race is a common historical complaint. In many cases, performance may deteriorate by only 2 to 3 seconds. In other horses, particularly in cases of atrial fibrillation, racing performance may decline greatly by 20 to 30 seconds or more. Horses with CV disease may have excessively high heart and respiratory rates during and after exercise and may take a longer than normal time to return to a resting rate. Such horses take longer to "cool out." Coughing, either at rest or during exercise, and exercise-induced pulmonary hemorrhage are reported in some horses with heart disease. CV disease must always be considered along with musculoskeletal, respiratory, metabolic, and neurologic problems in the differential diagnosis of poor performance (Table 7–5).[41, 42, 204–204b] Other performance-related problems with CV disease can include weakness, ataxia, collapse, and sudden death[40, 43–51, 147] (Table 7–6).

Auscultation

Clinical Method. Auscultation is a very accurate method for cardiac diagnosis, but effective auscultation requires an understanding of anatomy, physiology, pathophysiology, and sound. There is extensive clinical experience regarding cardiac auscultation in the horse,[1–4, 10, 11, 15, 22, 25, 27, 32, 38, 113, 113a, 125, 127, 169, 203–216c] and recent experience with Doppler echocardiography has refined the clinician's understanding of heart sounds and murmurs.[216b, c] A prerequisite for auscultation is an appreciation of the normal heart sounds, the genesis of

which has already been described (see Clinical Cardiovascular Physiology). The examiner must be familiar with the causes and clinical features of murmurs and arrhythmias (Tables 7–7 to 7–9) and the areas for auscultation (Figs. 7–7 and 7–8).[2–4, 10, 11, 15, 25, 27, 157, 207, 209, 211, 216] Auscultation is best carried out in a very quiet area because extraneous noise makes detection of soft to moderate murmurs quite difficult. The arterial pulse and the precordium should be palpated before commencing auscultation. Both stethoscope chest pieces—the diaphragm (applied tightly) and the bell (applied lightly)—should be used.

All auscultatory areas should be examined. The locations of the cardiac valve areas can be identified using the following method:

- The left thoracic wall cardiac impulse (left apical beat),

Table 7–6. Causes of Sudden Cardiovascular Death

Electrical Disorders of the Heart (Arrhythmias)

Ventricular tachycardia/flutter/fibrillation
Complete atrioventricular block
Asystole

Toxic Injury to the Heart

Acute myocardial failure
Anesthetics
Drug- or toxin-induced arrhythmia
Toxic plants
Myocardial toxins
Systemic toxin secondarily affecting the heart

Cardiac Tamponade

Bacterial pericarditis
Idiopathic pericarditis
Viral pericarditis
Trauma

Hemorrhage

Rupture of the heart (with cardiac tamponade)
Rupture of the aorta or pulmonary artery ($\pm$ cardiac tamponade)
Arterial rupture
   Middle uterine artery
   Mesenteric, omental, or other large arteries
Severe pulmonary hemorrhage
Rupture of the spleen or liver
Brain hemorrhage

Embolism

Carotid air embolism
Coronary embolism or thrombosis

Electrocution

Lightning
Alternating current electrocution

Cardiac Trauma

Cardiac catheterization or needle puncture of a ventricle leading to ventricular fibrillation
Penetrating thoracic wound

Table 7–7. Auscultation of Cardiac Arrhythmias

Rhythm	Heart Rate/min	Heart Sounds	Auscultation
Sinus Mechanisms			
Sinus rhythm	Variable	S4-1-2 (3)*	Rate and rhythm depend on autonomic tone
Sinus arrest/block	<26/min	S4-1-2 (3)	Irregular, long pauses
Sinus bradycardia	<26/min	S4-1-2 (3)	Generally regular unless escape rhythm develops
Sinus arrhythmia	25–50/min	S4-1-2 (3)	Irregular, cyclical change in heart rate; often variable interval between S4–S1; often associated with second-degree atrioventricular block or sinus bradycardia
Sinus tachycardia	>50/min	S4-1-2-3	Typically regular, but second-degree atrioventricular block may develop if sympathetic tone decreases
Sustained Atrial Tachyarrhythmias			
Atrial tachycardia and atrial flutter	>30/min	S1-2 (3)	Ventricular regularity and rate depend on atrioventricular conduction sequence sympathetic tone; consistent S4 absent; variable-intensity S1
Atrial fibrillation	>30/min	S1-2 (3)	Ventricular response irregular; rate related to sympathetic tone; heart rates consistently above 60/min suggest significant underlying heart disease or heart failure; consistent S4 is absent
Ectopic Rhythms			
Junctional rhythm	26–200	S1-2 (3)	Heart rate usually regular idionodal rhythms or junctional tachycardia; heart rate depends on the mechanism and sympathetic tone; inconsistent S4; variable intensity sounds
Ventricular rhythm	26–200	S1-2 (3)	Heart rate may be regular during monomorphic, unifocal ectopic rhythm or irregular during polymorphic or multifocal ectopic activity; the heart rate depends on the mechanism (e.g., escape rhythm versus ventricular tachycardia); variable intensity and split heart sounds may be heard
Premature atrial and junctional beats	Varies	Early S1–S2	Intensity of S1 may be louder or softer than normal; the sounds are not usually split; less than compensatory pause following the premature beat
Premature ventricular beats	Varies	Early S1–S2	Intensity of S1 often variable and ventricular beats may be softer than normal; heart sounds may be split from asynchronous ventricular activation heart sounds; compensatory pause typical following a premature beat
Atrioventricular Blocks			
Incomplete (first- and second-degree)	<50	S4-1-2 (3)	Heart rate variable; cyclical arrhythmia, variable S4–S1 interval; some variation in heart sounds
Complete (third-degree)	<26	S4/S1-2 (3)	Ventricular escape rhythm, usually regular; independent atrial (S4) sounds; variable-intensity heart sounds

*( ) = may be heard.

located under the left elbow, identifies the ventral region of the LV inlet; mitral sounds and murmurs usually project to this location as well as radiating dorsally into the left atrium; S_1 is best heard at this location.

- The aortic valve area is located dorsally and one or two intercostal spaces cranial to the left apical impulse; S_2 is loudest at this point, and aortic murmurs are heard well over this valve; the murmur of mitral regurgitation may also radiate dorsally and cranially to this area.
- Because of the central location of the aortic valve and the dextrad orientation of the ascending aorta, aortic flow murmurs and the murmur of aortic regurgitation can be heard bilaterally, just medial to the triceps muscles.

- The pulmonic valve is located slightly cranioventral (generally one intercostal space) to the aortic valve; the pulmonary component of S_2 is loudest at this point.
- The main pulmonary artery is dorsal to the pulmonic valve, very high on the left base; murmurs that radiate into the pulmonary artery are heard best at this location.
- The tricuspid valve area is located over a wide area on the right hemithorax, dorsal to the sternum and just cranial to the mitral valve; sounds and murmurs associated with tricuspid disease are usually heard best over the right hemithorax and typically radiate dorsocraniad into the right atrium and sometimes to the extreme left cranial hemithorax.

Table 7–8. Auscultation of Heart Sounds and Common Cardiac Murmurs

Auscultatory Finding	Timing	Point of Maximal Intensity (Valve Area)
Normal Heart Sounds		
First heart sound	Onset systole	Left apex (mitral valve)
Second heart sound	End systole	Left base (aortic valve)
Pulmonic component	End systole	Left base (pulmonic valve)
Third heart sound	Early dystole	Left apex (mitral valve)
Fourth (atrial) sound	Late dystole	Ventricular inlet (left)
Functional Murmurs*		
Systolic ejection murmur	Systole	Left base (aortic/pulmonary valves)
Early (proto-)diastolic	Dystole	Ventricular inlets (left/right)†
Late diastolic (presystolic)		Ventricular inlets (left/right)†
Valvular Regurgitation‡		
Mitral regurgitation	Systole	Left apex (mitral valve)§
Tricuspid regurgitation	Systole	Right hemithorax (tricuspid valve)
Aortic regurgitation	Dystole	Left base (aortic valve)
Pulmonary insufficiency	Dystole	Left base (pulmonic valve)
Ventricular septal defect‖	Systole	Right sternal border/left cardiac base (pulmonic valve)
Patent Ductus Arteriosus	Continuous	Dorsal left base over the pulmonary artery

Modified from Bonagura JD: Clinical evaluation and management of heart disease. *Equine Vet Educ* 2:31–37, 1990.

Only typical features are considered: "apex" refers to the ventral part of the heart, at the point of the palpable cardiac impulse (apex beat); "base" refers to the craniodorsal part of the heart over the outlet valves (aortic, pulmonic) where the second heart sound is most intense.

*The exact causes of functional (flow) murmurs have not been proved; however, systolic murmurs have been recorded within the aorta and pulmonary artery using intravascular phonocardiography. The systolic ejection murmur, which begins after the first heart sound and ends before the second heart sound, is the most commonly identified murmur; the protodiastolic murmur extends from the second to the third heart sound; the presystolic murmur is quite short and spans the fourth and first heart sounds. Functional murmurs may be musical.

†Ventricular inlets refer to the parts of the thorax overlying the ventricular inflow tracts and include the areas just dorsal to the mitral and tricuspid valve areas and extend ventrally to the apical regions of the ventricles.

‡Most cases of valvular regurgitation are evident throughout systole or diastole and extend into the second heart sound (holosystolic or pansystolic) or first heart sound (holodiastolic or pandiastolic); however, late systolic murmurs, which may be related to valve prolapse and minor chordal ruptures, have been identified with mitral or tricuspid valve insufficiency, and the murmur of aortic insufficiency may not always be holodiastolic. Documented reports of valve stenosis are quite rare. Murmurs of atrioventricular valve insufficiency are generally heard over the affected valve, project prominently towards the respective ventricular apex, and also radiate dorsally, following the regurgitant jet into the atrium. Occasionally, murmurs of tricuspid valve disease are prominent at the extreme left cranial heart border.

§The murmur of mitral regurgitation often radiates well into the aortic valve area and dorsally into the left atrium.

‖Murmurs caused by defects in the right ventricular inlet septum are heard best below the tricuspid valve and above the right sternal border and generate a softer systolic ejection murmur of relative pulmonic stenosis over the left cardiac base; murmurs from defects in the right ventricular outlet septum may be loudest over the pulmonary valve; flow across very large nonrestrictive defects can be relatively soft.

It is worthwhile to concentrate first on the individual heart sounds when assessing the heart rhythm, because the generation of cardiac sounds depends on the underlying electrical rhythm and heart murmurs are timed relative to the heart sounds. The atrial sound (S_4) is heard after the P wave. The first and second heart sounds (S_1 and S_2) encompass systole, indicating the presence of a QRS complex. A murmur detected between the first and second sounds is termed *systolic*. In contrast, a murmur heard after S_2 is designated as *diastolic*. The distinctive atrial sound (S_4) is absent in arrhythmias like atrial fibrillation. Normal variation in the PR interval causes gradual changes in the S_4–S_1 interval. Absence of a QRS complex, which occurs with second-degree AV block, causes a pause in which the first and second heart sounds are absent. The heart sounds and precordial movements can also be palpated, especially over the left thoracic wall. Frequently the cardiac movements and low-frequency vibrations corresponding to the atrial contraction (S_4), onset of ventricular contraction (S_1), and closure of the semilunar valves (S_2) can be detected. With ventricular volume overloading, an accentuated apex beat and third sound (S_3) will be palpated especially after a prolonged diastole. Cardiac enlargement or displacement of the heart by an intrathoracic mass may lead to an abnormal location of the cardiac impulse. A loud cardiac murmur is often associated with a palpable high frequency vibration or *thrill*.

Heart Sounds. Heart sounds should be easy to auscultate on both sides of the thorax, although there is some variability based on body type. Heart sounds are louder over the left hemithorax than over the right thoracic wall. All four heart sounds are generally detected in the standing horse, but all may not be heard at the same location (Fig. 7–9).[4, 25, 27] The ventricular filling sound (S_3) is most localized and variable and may be difficult to detect unless the bell is placed lightly

Table 7–9. Causes of Cardiac Murmurs

Cardiac Murmur	Lesion Identified by Echocardiography, Cardiac Catheterization, or Necropsy
Functional murmurs*	No identifiable lesions
Congenital heart disease murmurs	Defect(s) in the atrial or ventricular septa; patent ductus arteriosus; atresia/stenosis of the tricuspid or pulmonic valve; valve stenosis; other malformations of the heart
Mitral regurgitation	Degenerative thickening of the valve; bacterial endocarditis; mitral valve prolapse into left atrium; rupture of a chorda tendinea; dilated-hypokinetic ventricle (dilated cardiomyopathy); valvulitis; malformation
Tricuspid regurgitation	Same as mitral regurgitation; also pulmonary hypertension from severe left heart failure, chronic respiratory disease, or (?) chronic training†; malformation
Aortic regurgitation	Degenerative thickening of the valve; congenital fenestration of the valve; bacterial endocarditis‡; aortic prolapse into a ventricular septal defect or the left ventricle; flail aortic valve leaflet; valvulitis; malformation; ruptured aorta or aortic sinus of Valsalva
Pulmonary insufficiency	Bacterial endocarditis‡; pulmonary hypertension; flail pulmonic valve leaflet; valvulitis; malformation; rupture of the pulmonary artery
Murmur associated with vegetative endocarditis	Insufficiency of the affected valve‡

Modified from Bonagura JD: Clinical evaluation and management of heart disease. *Equine Vet Educ* 2:31–37, 1990.

*Functional murmur may be innocent (unknown cause) or physiologic (suspected physiologic cause). Functional murmurs are very common in foals and trained athletes (athletic murmur); associated with fever and high sympathetic nervous system activity (pain, stress, sepsis); and are often heard in anemic horses. Functional murmurs are very dependent on the physiologic state and can be altered by changing the heart rate. Such dynamic auscultation is very useful in detecting functional murmurs.

†"Silent" regurgitation across a right-sided cardiac valve can be identified in some horses by Doppler echocardiography; this is probably a normal finding of no clinical significance.

‡Anatomical stenosis is generally caused by a large vegetation and should also be associated with a diastolic murmur of valvular insufficiency; increased flow across the valve, even in the absence of a true stenosis, may generate a murmur of "relative" valvular stenosis (e.g., with aortic regurgitation there may be a systolic ejection murmur due to an increased stroke volume).

over the left apex. The intensity of the heart sounds should be consistent when the rhythm is regular; variation of heart sound intensity occurs with arrhythmias (irregular cardiac filling) and with volume-overloaded ventricles. Muffled heart sounds are heard with pericardial effusions or pericardial abscesses (in affected horses, the muffling may only be on one side of the thorax) but also occur in some horses with large pleural effusions and cranial mediastinal masses. Accentuation of all heart sounds, especially the third sound, may be detected with volume-loaded ventricles or with marked sympathetic activity.

The first heart sound varies after prolonged diastolic periods and often becomes louder (and sometimes softer). The intensity of the first heart sound varies whenever the rhythm is irregular, but this in itself is not diagnostic of an abnormality. Splitting of the first heart sound, if pronounced, may indicate abnormal ventricular electrical activation or ventricular premature complexes. Close splitting of the first sound may be more obvious when there is atrial fibrillation, and in the absence of an atrial sound, the split S_1 may be misinterpreted as a closely timed S_4–S_1 complex.

The second sound is loudest normally over the aortic valve area and may be audibly split over the pulmonic valve area.[1, 4, 157] This sound can be very soft or absent following a premature beat, and it may be obscured by a holosystolic murmur. Audible splitting of S_2 occurs commonly in normal horses, varies with heart rate or respiration, and only infrequently is associated with pulmonary hypertension. The relative closure of the semilunar valves probably varies with the heart rate and pulmonary artery pressure,[4, 157] although the pulmonic component is most often detected after the aortic component in the healthy, resting horse. If the pulmonary component of the second sound develops a tympanic quality, becoming equal to or louder than the aortic component of S_2, the clinician should suspect pulmonary hypertension. Identification of a loud pulmonic S_2 is a useful clinical finding in cases of right-sided heart failure because it often

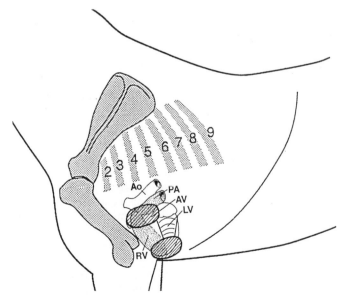

Figure 7–7. General areas for cardiac auscultation—left side. The typical flow murmur is loudest over the craniodorsal base (upper oval). Murmurs of mitral regurgitation often project loudly to the left apex (lower oval), although dorsal radiation is also common. (From Bonagura JD, Muir WW: The cardiovascular system. In Muir WW, Hubbell JAE, eds. *Equine Anesthesia*. St Louis, Mosby-Year Book, 1991, with permission.)

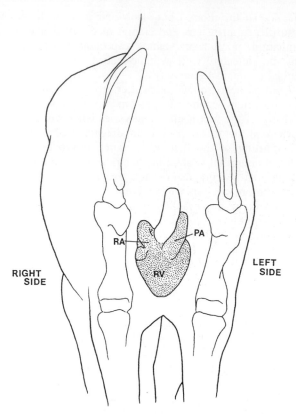

Figure 7–8. Cranial view of the heart demonstrating the U shape of the right ventricle. The tricuspid valve and the right ventricular inlet are located on the right side, whereas the outlet and pulmonary artery are on the left side. Murmurs of tricuspid regurgitation and perimembranous ventricular septal defects are typically loudest over the right hemithorax, whereas flow murmurs and those due to subaortic or subpulmonic septal defects are loudest over the left cardiac base. (From Bonagura JD, Muir WW: The cardiovascular system. In Muir WW, Hubbell JAE, eds. *Equine Anesthesia.* St Louis, Mosby-Year Book, 1991, with permission.)

indicates that a lesion on the *left* side of the heart has led to pulmonary hypertension and right-sided CHF.

Diastolic sounds are normal.[4, 10, 11, 15, 209] The atrial sound (S_4) should be detected in virtually all horses, and this sound may be quite loud in some cases. Isolated atrial sounds are normally auscultated at slow resting heart rates; however, multiple isolated S_4 sounds indicate high-grade AV block. The ventricular sound (S_3) is normal but may become very loud in ventricular failure or subsequent to ventricular dilatation.

Other sounds may be detected with heart disease. Systolic clicks may be detected uncommonly over the great vessels where they are thought to be benign. A systolic click that is heard best over the left apex may be a marker for mitral valve disease or prolapse of the valve into the left atrium. Constrictive pericardial disease may lead to a loud ventricular filling sound, a ventricular "knock." In addition to muffling of sounds, pericarditis is often associated with a pericardial friction rub. These rubs are classically triphasic and are detected during three portions of the cardiac cycle (systole, early diastole, late diastole). These portions must be distin-

guished from pleural friction rubs, which are occasionally associated with the cardiac cycle. In these horses, the pleural rub tends to be heard only during one or two phases of the cardiac cycle.

Heart Rate and Rhythm. Heart rate can change rapidly and dramatically, varying with autonomic efferent traffic and level of physical activity. Changes in the rate and rhythm are reflected in cardiac auscultation and palpation of the pulse (see Table 7–7).[212] The normal arterial pulse and cardiac rhythm is regular or cyclically irregular. Heart rate varies between 28 and 44 beats/min, although slightly slower heart rates can be detected in some very fit racehorses and higher heart rates may be present in foals, yearlings, draft horses,[217] and healthy but nervous horses. An elevated resting heart rate is commonly detected with fever, pain, hypovolemia, severe anemia, infection, or shock. Persistent, otherwise unexplained tachycardia is also present in heart failure wherein the resting heart rate usually exceeds 60 beats/min.

Physiologic arrhythmias associated with high resting vagal tone must be differentiated from pathologic arrhythmias, because relaxed and fit horses have many bradyarrhythmias that are normal. The most common of these is second-degree AV block, which is reported in 15% to 18% of normal horses at rest and has been detected in up to 44% of normal horses with 24-hour continuous electrocardiographic monitoring.[124, 128, 130, 218, 218a, 219] This arrhythmia is most common in fit racehorses or in other high-performance animals and disappears with exercise or excitement or after administration of atropine. Sinus arrhythmia also occurs in fit high-performance horses and is usually associated with sinus bradycardia and resting heart rates of 24 to 28 beats/min. Sinus arrhythmia may wax and wane with respiration; however, synchronization with ventilation is not a consistent finding in the horse. SA block and SA arrest occur sporadically in fit horses. Because these physiologic arrhythmias are associated with high vagal tone, it is typical for the heart rate to range from a low-normal value to bradycardia. Maneuvers that reduce vagal activity and increase sympathetic tone can be undertaken to ensure that the rhythm becomes normal. Successful methods include leading the horse through three or four tight circles, jogging, or lunging. It should be recognized, however, that some horses redevelop physiologic AV block within 15 to 60 seconds following completion of such maneuvers. If the arrhythmia persists after exercise, or if the auscultatory findings suggest another arrhythmia (see Table 7–7), an ECG should be obtained.

The arrhythmias associated with heart disease occur most often with normal to increased heart rates, with the exception of advanced second-degree and complete (third-degree) AV block (Table 7–7).[1, 3, 5, 16, 212, 220–222] Atrial premature beats are characterized by a regular cardiac rhythm, which is suddenly interrupted by an earlier than normal beat(s). Since the sinus node is reset during an atrial premature beat, the following pause is usually incomplete or less than compensatory. Premature atrial beats can also be blocked in the AV node, leading to a sudden pause in the rhythm. A ventricular premature beat is followed by a fully compensatory pause unless the extrasystole is interpolated between two normal sinus beats. Pulse deficits (more first sounds than arterial pulses) are expected with premature beats.

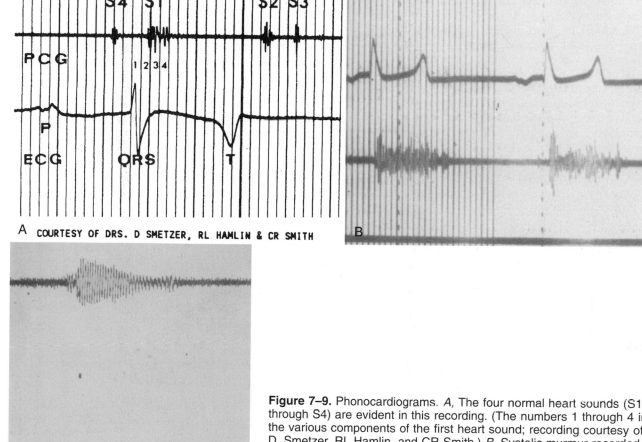

Figure 7–9. Phonocardiograms. *A,* The four normal heart sounds (S1 through S4) are evident in this recording. (The numbers 1 through 4 indicate the various components of the first heart sound; recording courtesy of Drs. D. Smetzer, RL Hamlin, and CR Smith.) *B,* Systolic murmur recorded from a yearling with a ventricular septal defect. (P waves on the electrocardiogram are negative in this tracing.) *C,* Decrescendo, musical, holodiastolic murmur recorded from a horse with aortic regurgitation. The murmur begins in early diastole (after the T wave) and ends at the QRS complex.

Atrial fibrillation is characterized by an irregularly irregular rhythm, with beats occurring sooner than expected, and pauses in the rhythm with no consistent underlying diastolic interval. The atrial contraction and hence the fourth sound are absent in atrial fibrillation. Infrequently, atrial fibrillation develops with recurring periodicity of cycle lengths that can cause difficulty in distinguishing this abnormal rhythm from second-degree AV block.[121, 123, 132] Another diagnostic pitfall can be the presence of a split first sound, because the clinician may mistake this for a closely timed S_4–S_1 complex.

Atrial tachycardia, on the other hand, may develop regular AV conduction and rapid regular rhythm. Junctional and ventricular tachycardias are usually manifested by a rapid regular rhythm, unless the arrhythmia is multiform, in which case the heart may sound irregular, such as in atrial fibrillation. Owing to associated AV dissociation or abnormal ventricular activation, the heart sounds may be split or variable in intensity.

Cardiac Murmurs. Cardiac murmurs are audible manifestations of blood flow in the heart and blood vessels. Although most heart murmurs are physiologic, other murmurs provide evidence of heart disease and may require further investigation. Most innocent or *functional* cardiac murmurs are caused by vibrations that attend the *ejection* of blood from the heart during systole or the *rapid filling* of the ventricles during diastole.[2, 12, 15, 22, 125, 169, 203, 210, 216, 223] Causes of abnormal murmurs include incompetent cardiac valves, septal defects, vascular lesions, and (rarely) valve stenosis (see Tables 7–8 and 7–9). The continuous murmur of patent ductus arteriosus is considered to be a normal finding in full-term foals for up to 3 days after parturition.[177, 208, 216, 224] It is almost always possible to distinguish the physiologic from the pathologic murmur provided that careful auscultation is undertaken. To be successful and to efficiently select animals requiring additional studies, the clinician must describe timing, quality, grade, point of maximal murmur intensity, and radiation of a murmur (see Table 7–8), as well as the effect of changing heart rate on the sounds. When a murmur does represent underlying cardiac pathology, the overall significance of the hemodynamic abnormality should include consideration of the work history, general physical examination, presence or absence of heart enlargement or cardiac failure, and results of ancillary tests such as echocardiography, electrocardiography, and exercise performance (or testing).

Functional or *physiologic heart murmurs* are very common and are not attributed to cardiac pathology. Such murmurs may be related to the large size and tremendous inflow and outflow volumes of the equine heart.[223] Physiologic causes of functional murmurs include fever, high sympathetic activity (e.g., colic, exercise), moderate to severe anemia, and peripheral vasodilation. These murmurs are typically soft (grades 1 to 3/6), localized, short, and labile. Increasing heart rate usually increases the intensity and duration of a functional murmur, although in some horses the murmur becomes less intense. Functional murmurs are neither holosystolic nor holodiastolic. Murmurs associated with organic heart disease, in contrast, are often quite long and change minimally, if at all, with increases in heart rate.

The most common functional murmur is the systolic ejection murmur heard over the aortic and pulmonic valves and their respective arteries at the left cardiac base (see Figs. 7–7 and 7–8).[4] As the functional ejection murmur is generated by flow into the great vessels, its duration cannot be truly holosystolic inasmuch as the murmur begins after S_1 and must end before S_2. Nonetheless, in some horses, the functional ejection murmur can be quite loud (grades 4 of 6) and may seem to be holosystolic (especially at higher heart rates). Remarkable changes in functional murmur intensity may be detected from one day to another. A loud functional murmur can radiate caudally and may be confused with mitral regurgitation. The clinician should not mistake a functional aortic ejection murmur for the murmur of aortic stenosis, which is an exceedingly rare defect in the horse.

Functional diastolic murmurs are also common, especially in the Thoroughbred breed. These murmurs are generally soft and are detected over the LV or RV inlets—from the dorsal atrium to the ventricular apex. The functional protodiastolic murmur is an early diastolic murmur detected between S_2 and S_3. The murmur may be musical or even "squeaky" and typically accentuates with increased heart rate.[4] The presystolic functional murmur is heard between S_4 and S_1 and may sound like a "rub" or long heart sound following the atrial contraction.

The most commonly detected murmurs associated with structural heart disease are those generated by tricuspid regurgitation, mitral regurgitation, ventricular septal defect, and aortic regurgitation. Typical causes and auscultatory features of these murmurs are indicated in Tables 7–8 and 7–9 and also later in this chapter. When a cardiac murmur indicative of valvular disease or a congenital cardiac defect is detected, additional studies are required. Certainly, the history should be reassessed, because the horse with excellent performance and good exercise tolerance is unlikely to have severe heart disease. Auscultation, however, is insufficient to distinguish trivial from significant heart disease in the poorly performing horse or in a horse with a cardiac arrhythmia. Echocardiography is helpful in these cases to quantify heart size and objectively assess ventricular function. Underlying lesions such as a valve vegetation, ruptured valve chorda tendinea, or dilated cardiomyopathy can be identified or discounted. Doppler echocardiography can document abnormal blood flow and can pinpoint the cause of a murmur. This type of objective information cannot be obtained as easily or effectively by other noninvasive methods. Other methods of assessing the significance of heart murmurs are thoracic radiography, exercise testing, radionuclide angiography, and cardiac catheterization. Cardiac catheter-

ization has been largely replaced by Doppler echocardiography.

Pulmonary Auscultation. Auscultation of the lungs should reveal normal breath sounds with the horse at rest, while ventilating into a rebreathing bag, and after exercise. Decreased or absent airway sounds or large airway sounds in the ventral portions of the thorax indicate a pleural effusion, a common finding in biventricular or right-sided heart failure. Moist or bubbling (fluid) sounds or crackles (i.e., rales) are uncommonly auscultated in the lungs of horses with pulmonary edema and left-sided heart failure. Instead, tachypnea associated with harsh bronchovesicular breath sounds is usually heard, since horses with chronic left-sided CHF seem to develop more interstitial than alveolar pulmonary edema. When alveolar edema does develop, respiratory distress may be severe, and free fluid may be auscultated in the trachea. On rare occasion, primarily with peracute left-sided heart failure, froth will be visible at the nares and the horse will cough and expel large quantities of pulmonary edema (Fig. 7–10). Such horses demonstrate severe respiratory distress (marked tachypnea and dyspnea), anxiety, and agitation.

Examination of the Peripheral Vasculature

An evaluation of the peripheral vasculature is part of a cardiovascular work-up and should include examination of the arteries and veins in the head, forelimbs, and hindlimbs. When possible, arterial blood pressure should also be measured. The genesis of the arterial and venous pulse has been previously described. The heart sounds should be correlated with both the jugular and arterial pulses. Heart rate and rhythm, as well as altered hemodynamic states, can be identified by palpating the facial artery pulse. The arterial pulse can be described as normal,

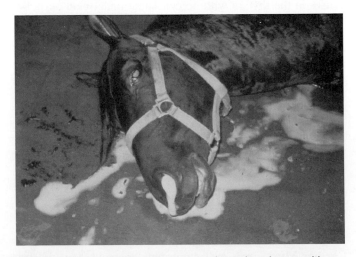

Figure 7–10. Peracute pulmonary edema in a horse with a ruptured chorda tendinea. The photo was obtained immediately after euthanasia. It is important to note that tracheal froth is often a postmortem artifact, particularly when observed hours after death.

hypokinetic (weak), hyperkinetic, or variable. Irregularity often indicates a cardiac arrhythmia. Abnormalities of arterial pressure and perfusion may cause changes in mucous membrane color and capillary refill time. Refill time is prolonged during hypotension or peripheral vasoconstriction; conversely, it may be shortened when there is vasodilation.

Normal quality *arterial pulses* should be palpable in the facial, median, carotid, great metatarsal, coccygeal, and digital arteries. Thready or hypokinetic arterial pulses are detected in CHF and in diseases associated with cardiovascular collapse, such as endotoxemia, or after profuse hemorrhage. Thready arterial pulses may also be detected only in the hindlimbs with aortoiliac thrombosis. Bounding, hyperkinetic arterial pulses are palpable with aortic regurgitation, patent ductus arteriosus, and aortic to pulmonary or aortic to right-sided heart fistulas. Marked variation in the intensity of the pulse usually occurs with arrhythmias, particularly atrial fibrillation and multiform ventricular tachycardia. A pulse deficit occurs when developed LV pressure does not exceed aortic pressure. Deficits are likely to be palpated in association with arrhythmias, particularly premature beats or following very short diastolic periods.

Palpation of the arterial pulse is a crude indication of the *arterial blood pressure,* representing the difference between peak systolic and diastolic pressures, the rate of rise of arterial pressure, and the physical characteristics of the artery and surrounding tissues. Arterial blood pressure can be measured directly by arterial puncture or cannulation or indirectly using various auscultatory, Doppler, or oscillometric techniques.[37, 52, 139, 166, 181, 225–244] Percutaneous placement of an arterial catheter in the facial or transverse tibial artery is frequently used to monitor pressure invasively in critically ill or anesthetized horses. Indirect methods have been used successfully to monitor pressure in the coccygeal artery; however, these methods are less sensitive in hypotensive animals and may lag in response during rapid changes in blood pressure.[227, 239, 240] Attention must be directed to placement and diameter of the occluding cuff when indirect methods are used,[234] and the optimal width of the cuff (bladder) is between approximately one quarter to one fifth of the circumference of the tail when measuring pressure in the middle coccygeal artery.[229, 231] The arterial pulse wave itself varies, depending on the site of measurement, and the distal arterial systolic pressure may be higher, and the diastolic pressure lower, than the corresponding aortic pressures.

Arterial blood pressure monitoring includes determination of systolic, diastolic, and mean pressures. Arterial pressure is determined by the interplay between CO and vascular resistance (see Table 7–3). Marked increases in CO, during exercise for example, lead to significant increases in arterial blood pressure with systolic pressures exceeding 200 mm Hg.[158, 245, 246]

Normal reported values for indirect arterial pressure are 111.8 mm Hg systolic (ranging from 79 to 145 mm Hg) and 67.7 diastolic (ranging from 49 to 106 mm Hg).[225, 227–238, 240] The values obtained at the coccygeal artery are slightly lower than central arterial pressures, but this is not a problem when monitoring an individual horse. Blood pressure is lowest in neonates and rises during the first month of life to the normal adult range.[166, 239] There is some variation among breeds. Draft breeds tend to have lower pressures than do racehorses, and Standardbreds have lower pressures than do Thoroughbreds.[237] Arterial pressures fluctuate slightly with ventilation and significantly if there are positive pressure ventilation or cyclic changes in heart rate. Posture imposes a significant influence on arterial pressure, since raising the head from the feeding position necessitates a higher aortic pressure in order to maintain cerebral perfusion pressure. Obviously, when the head is lowered, the hydrostatic pressure imposed during raising of the head is minimized. Mean arterial pressure measured in the middle coccygeal artery can vary approximately 20 mm Hg with the changing head position.[232]

The systolic arterial pressure is generated by the left ventricle and is consequently affected by the interplay between the stroke volume, aortic compliance, and previous diastolic blood pressure. Arterial *pulse pressure,* the difference between systolic and diastolic values, is greatly dependent on stroke volume and the peripheral arteriolar resistance that determines the run-off of diastolic pressure. Pulse pressure determines the intensity of the palpable peripheral arterial pulse. Ventricular failure reduces pulse pressure, whereas abnormal diastolic run-off (aortic insufficiency, generalized vasodilation) widens the pulse pressure. Diastolic and mean pressures are better estimates of perfusion pressure; these variables are increased by arteriolar vasoconstriction or by higher CO.

The cutaneous veins should be examined for distensibility, refill, thrombosis, and estimated venous pressure. *Jugular pulsations* are normally observed in the thoracic inlet and up to the ventral one third (10 cm) of the neck. These pulsations are reflections of right atrial pressure changes (discussed previously) and are visible along the entire length of the jugular vein when the head is lowered below the level of the heart. The carotid arterial pulse may be transmitted through the jugular furrow and mimic an abnormal systolic pulse wave in the jugular vein if the vein is distended. Occluding the jugular vein ventrally can demonstrate if the pulses are actually originating in the right atrium, since venous pulse transmission, or prominent collapse, will be prevented by light digital pressure over the vein. Pronounced jugular pulsations may be observed occasionally in excited but otherwise normal horses with high sympathetic tone. In some of these cases, the venous collapse is the prominent movement and the "pulse" is simply normal venous filling. The jugular vein in normal horses is collapsed, but the veins in the limbs and on the torso are visible and somewhat filled. Venous pressure in the jugular vein is normally less than 10 cm of water.

Abnormal jugular pulses are observed with arrhythmias causing AV dissociation, with diseases of the tricuspid valve, and with RV failure. An abnormal jugular pulse is one that extends proximally up the jugular vein for more than 10 cm in systole (with the horse's head held in a normal position) or that demonstrates retrograde filling from the heart when the vein is occluded dorsally. Doppler studies of the jugular vein can distinguish a prominent pulse caused by retrograde flow from an apparent pulse caused by prominent collapse and normal filling. Generalized venous distention, often accompanied by subcutaneous edema, is characteristic of heart failure (Fig. 7–11). Distention of only the veins cranial to the thoracic inlet should indicate a cranial mediastinal mass or abscess with obstruction of the cranial vena cava and not CHF.[74] Prolonged refill of the saphenous vein indicates the

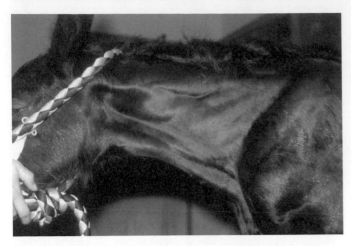

Figure 7–11. Jugular venous distention in a Shire foal with biventricular congestive heart failure caused by congenital heart disease.

possibility of aortoiliac thrombosis and decreased arterial supply to the affected limb.[149–154, 247, 248] Distended veins that are very firm on palpation, with marked distention of the more proximal veins, indicate probable venous thrombus.[249]

Congestive Heart Failure

CHF is relatively uncommon; however, the diagnosis of this pathophysiologic state can generally be made during a complete physical examination. Important clinical findings include persistent tachycardia (typically heart rate higher than 60/min), jugular distention and pulsation, abnormal arterial pulses, fluid retention (ventral subcutaneous edema, pleural effusion, or pulmonary edema), and loss of body condition (Fig. 7–12). LV failure secondary to valvular or myocardial heart disease causes pulmonary venous congestion with pulmonary interstitial, or, uncommonly, alveolar

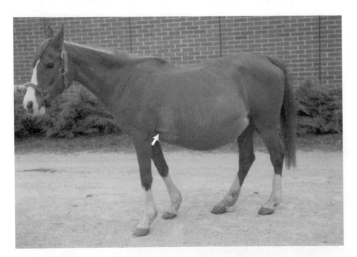

Figure 7–12. Ascites, ventral edema, and weight loss are evident in this mare with right-sided congestive heart failure. The distended lateral thoracic vein *(arrow)* is evident caudal to the triceps.

edema. Tachypnea associated with lung edema of left-sided CHF is frequently misdiagnosed as pneumonia. Lethargy, exercise intolerance, collapse (or syncope), anorexia, depression, and weight loss may also be detected with CHF or cardiac insufficiency. Heart failure is discussed more fully later in this chapter.

DIAGNOSTIC AND LABORATORY STUDIES

Exercise Testing

Exercise testing is an increasingly important part of the complete CV evaluation. While the sensitivity, specificity, and specific endpoints of the exercise test (as it pertains to detection of organic heart disease) are as yet undefined, exercise studies will likely become an important method for detecting subtle CV disease. As most horses have to function as athletes, some form of exercise testing should be included in the pre-purchase CV examination, unless the animal is too young to perform or is to be used solely for breeding. Even in these situations, evaluation of a foal, weanling, or yearling after a period of free exercise is optimal; furthermore, it should be determined that a stallion has sufficient stamina to perform in the breeding shed. Thus, the CV system should be evaluated at rest and immediately after exercise, and under the anticipated form of exercise required by the prospective owner. Increasingly, standardized treadmill testing is used to detect subtle clinical abnormalities that limit peak performance.[135, 198–202, 250, 251] Treadmill exercise is also important when evaluating the horse with a history of collapse or syncope, because the cardiac response to exercise should be evaluated without risk to a rider.

Changes in heart rate with exercise have been well studied.[135, 198–202, 250, 251] The normal horse develops sinus tachycardia associated with exercise, with the maximal heart rate depending on the level of exercise performed. At heart rates of less than 100 to 120 beats/min, SA node discharge is very labile and subject to psychologic influences. Once exercise has commenced, the heart rate should accelerate and then stabilize at a level appropriate for the work being performed. As a general guideline: heart rates of 70 to 120 beats/min are normal at the trot, 120 to 150 beats/min at the canter, 150 to 180 beats/min at a hand gallop, and more than 180 beats/min when galloping. The maximal heart rate for most horses is between 210 and 240 beats/min, although some animals develop higher rates. There is a linear relationship between heart rate and the velocity or work effort of exercise when the heart rate is between 120 and 210 beats/min. Heart rate usually recovers rapidly and falls to less than 100 beats/min upon the cessation of exercise. The recovery of heart rate to the resting level is influenced by many factors, including the humidity, ambient temperature, training fitness, work performed, psychologic factors, and state of cardiovascular health. After maximal work, such as a race, an hour may pass before the heart rate completely recovers to the resting rate. An inappropriately high heart rate for a given level of exercise may simply denote a healthy, but unfit, horse; however, this finding can also indicate the presence of CV, pulmonary, or musculoskeletal disease. Information about the heart rate is particularly useful when a horse has the heart rate monitored routinely during exercise.

Exercise-induced arrhythmias are a concern because disturbances in rhythm have been suspected to be a cause of sudden death.[46, 48–51] During the recovery period following exercise, horses have large fluctuations in sympathetic and parasympathetic tone. Arrhythmias are quite common during this time, even if the heart rhythm was normal at rest and during exercise. Marked sinus arrhythmias, supraventricular ectopia, and ventricular premature beats are most frequently detected in the immediate post-exercise period. When arrhythmias are detected during a routine post-exercise examination, an exercising ECG obtained by radiotelemetry is necessary to determine if the arrhythmia is present during exercise. A heart rate monitor may be used to provide an indication of arrhythmias during exercise; however, the detection of erratic heart "blips" or "beeps" does not adequately characterize the arrhythmia. With the exception of vagally mediated arrhythmias, resting or post-exercise arrhythmias are considered abnormal, although they are not always clinically significant. In some horses, a maximal performance is required to elicit abnormal cardiac rhythms. When performance problems are detected only at the peak of exercise, a treadmill exercise test to exhaustion should be performed in an attempt to investigate if cardiac arrhythmias are a cause of the poor performance. This is particularly important if CV disease is suspected from the history or clinical examination.

Electrocardiography

Normal Cardiac Cell Electrical Activity. Myocytes in the atria and ventricles are excitable, and some of the specialized cardiac tissues are capable of spontaneous depolarization independent of extrinsic innervation. The processes responsible for generation of electrical activity in the heart are due to ion fluxes across the cell membrane.[54, 133] This electrical activity is represented by the ECG. A general understanding of cellular activity, generation, and spread of the cardiac electrical impulse; effects of autonomic innervation; and electrocardiographic lead systems is required to interpret the equine ECG.

The partially selective nature of the cardiac cell membrane and the presence of various cell membrane pumps lead to a situation in which ions are partitioned unequally across the cell membrane.[54] This results in very high potassium and relatively low sodium concentrations intracellularly when compared with the extracellular fluid. Other ions including chloride and magnesium, but most notably calcium, are important to cellular electrical activity. Calcium is essential for cardiac contraction. Sudden changes in cardiac cell membrane permeability or conductance to sodium, calcium, and potassium are responsible for the processes of depolarization, muscular contraction, and repolarization. These processes, in turn, are affected by serum electrolyte concentration, acid-base status, autonomic traffic, myocardial perfusion and oxygenation, heart disease, and drugs. The basic cellular processes of depolarization, calcium influx, and repolarization form the basis for, respectively, the P and QRS complexes of the ECG, myocardial contraction, and the ST-T wave of the ECG.

The resting membrane potential is determined primarily by the partitioning of potassium ions and proteins across the cell membrane and the relative impermeability of the membrane to sodium. *Depolarization* of atrial and ventricular myocytes and Purkinje fibers is caused by a fast current related to a rapid influx of extracellular sodium into the cell.[56, 133, 219] This process is represented by phase 0 of the cardiac cell action potential recording (Fig. 7–13). Cardiac tissues depolarized in this manner normally conduct electrical impulses at high velocity. In contrast, the cells of the SA and AV nodes, as well as ischemic cells, demonstrate less negative diastolic membrane potentials. These cells depend on a slow inward current that is carried mostly by calcium ions for activation to occur. Because of this property, cells in the SA node, AV node, and ischemic tissue conduct electrical impulses very slowly and can be involved in abnormal automatic mechanisms or re-entrant pathways that promote cardiac arrhythmias. Anti-arrhythmic drugs act differently on tissues that are "fast" versus "slow" current dependent (see Cardiac Arrhythmias later in this chapter).

The influx of extracellular calcium into the cell during phase 2 of the action potential triggers the release of intracellular calcium from the sarcoplasmic reticulum. Increases in cytosolic calcium cause myocardial contraction. Hypoxia, acidosis, and many drugs can affect myocardial contractility by interfering with calcium entry into cells, with the release of calcium from the sarcoplasmic reticulum, or with the binding of calcium to contractile filaments.[54, 76, 133] Conversely, digitalis glycosides, dobutamine, and dopamine increase calcium influx and myocardial contractility.

Cellular *repolarization* is initiated by a decrease in the cell membrane conductance to sodium and calcium coincident with increased conductance to potassium. As intracellular potassium moves out of the cell, along its concentration gradient, phase 3 of the cardiac action potential occurs. Hypoxia and abnormalities in serum potassium or calcium alter this process, especially hyperkalemia, which actually accelerates repolarization and shortens the ST-T wave of the ECG. This occurs because hyperkalemia *increases* membrane permeability to potassium and the high intracellular

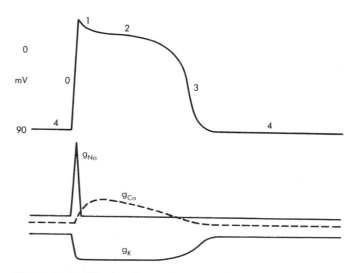

Figure 7–13. The cardiac action potential. The phases of depolarization and repolarization as well as membrane conductance (g) to important ions are demonstrated (see the text for details). (From Berne RM, Levy MN: *Cardiovascular Physiology.* St. Louis, CV Mosby, 1986, with permission.)

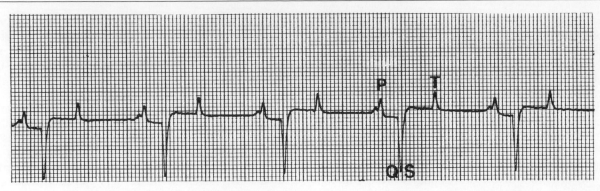

Figure 7–14. A normal equine base-apex lead electrocardiogram (25 mm/sec; 1 cm = 1 mV). The waveforms are indicated. The QRS complex often lacks an R-wave in this lead (QS complex). The T wave is very labile and may be negative, biphasic, or positive. Increases in heart rate or sympathetic tone usually lead to positive T waves in this lead.

potassium (exceeding 100 mmol/L) is more than adequate to drive potassium out of the cell (because extracellular potassium rarely exceeds 10 mmol/L).

Spontaneous depolarization or automaticity is a property of select cardiac tissues. Such activity is most prominent in the SA node but may also be encountered in cells around the AV node and in cells within the Purkinje network. Normal automaticity is observed during phase 4 of the cardiac action potential. Spontaneous *pacemaker activity* is generated in normal pacemaker tissues by the background inward sodium current and a time-related decrease in membrane permeability to potassium ion efflux.[133] A gradual depolarization process, modified markedly by vagal and sympathetic traffic, allows the cell to attain threshold, initiating phase 0 and depolarization. Depression of normal SA automaticity or increased activity in other tissues in the atria, Purkinje system, or in cells around the AV node may lead to an abnormal or "ectopic" cardiac rhythm. When the principal abnormality resides in depression of SA node function or blockage of the impulse in the AV node, the slow discharge of a subsidiary pacemaker is termed an escape mechanism. The normal purpose of these latent cardiac pacemakers is to rescue the heart from extreme bradycardia or asystole. However, ectopic pacemakers are often enhanced by drugs, inflammation, sympathetic activity, electrolyte disturbances, or ischemia, leading to *ectopic* rhythms that manifest as premature complexes or tachycardias. Other electrophysiologic mechanisms, including re-entry and myocardial fibrillation, account for the development of other arrhythmias.

Genesis of the Electrocardiogram. The SA node is located near the right auricle; therefore, initial cardiac muscle depolarization develops across the right atrium (see Fig. 7–3). Activation waves spread through the atrial myocardial cells to the left atrium and also in the direction of the AV node. Specialized atrial muscle cells composed of internodal pathways and Bachman's bundle facilitate transmission of current across the atria.[13, 252] These specialized pathways—as well as the SA node—differ from normal atrial muscle, are relatively resistant to high serum potassium concentrations, and are still functional during hyperkalemia.

Conduction continues across the AV tissues by first entering the AV node. The conduction across the AV nodal cells,

between the low right atrium and the bundle of His, is very slow and subject to physiologic blockade owing to vagal efferent activity.[122] Conduction proceeds at a greater velocity through the bundle of His and bundle branches. Propagation of the impulse through the ventricles is enhanced by the rapidly conducting Purkinje system that penetrates relatively completely through the ventricular myocardium.[8, 9]

Autonomic traffic affects these processes. Parasympathetic activity depresses SA nodal activity, enhances intra-atrial

---

Table 7–10. Electrocardiographic Leads

Frontal Plane Leads

Bipolar leads
    Lead I   = Left foreleg [+] − right foreleg [−]
    Lead II = Left rear leg [+] − right foreleg [−]
    Lead III = Left rear leg [+] − left foreleg [−]
Unipolar augmented limb leads
    Lead aVR = Right foreleg [+] − left foreleg and left rear leg [−]
    Lead aVL = Left foreleg [+] − right foreleg and left rear leg [−]
    Lead aVF = Left rear leg [+] − right foreleg and left foreleg [−]

Precordial Leads

Base-apex monitor lead
    [+] electrode over the left apex compared with the [−] electrode over the right jugular furrow*
Precordial V leads†
    [+] electrode over the selected precordial site; the lead is named based on the location of the exploring (V or C) electrode
    Lead V3—near the left apex
    Lead V10—over the dorsal spinous processes (interscapular)

---

*The most common method of obtaining the base-apex lead is to place the left foreleg electrode over the left apex, the right foreleg electrode over the jugular furrow (or at the top of the right scapular spine), and the select lead I on the electrocardiograph. This lead is an excellent choice to monitor the cardiac rhythm.

†Precordial leads other than V10 (over the dorsal spine) are not commonly used.

conduction by shortening atrial action potential duration, and slows AV nodal conduction. Conversely, sympathetic efferent traffic increases heart rate and shortens AV conduction time.[133] Sympathetic activity also increases cellular excitability, predisposes to some cardiac arrhythmias, and increases myocardial oxygen consumption by augmenting the heart rate, force of myocardial contraction, and myocardial wall tension. Parasympathetic efferent traffic dominates in the resting, standing horse and frequently fluctuates with changes in blood pressure. The pronounced sinus arrhythmia and second-degree AV block so often encountered in normal horses is caused by changing vagal tone and serves to regulate arterial blood pressure at rest.[52]

The ECG graphs the time-voltage activity of the heart. The average electrical potential generated by the heart muscle is recorded throughout the different phases of the cardiac cycle with time displayed along the X axis and electrical potential inscribed vertically (Fig. 7–14). The normal waveforms are the P wave (atrial depolarization), PR interval (mainly due to AV nodal conduction), QRS complex (ventricular depolarization), and ST-T wave (ventricular repolarization). A prominent atrial repolarization wave (Ta wave) is often noted in the PR segment of the equine ECG, particularly at faster heart rates. The QT interval represents total electrical activation-repolarization time.

Clinical Electrocardiography. The clinical application of electrocardiography to the horse has been studied extensively.[6, 8, 9, 13, 21, 31, 35, 36, 53, 126, 166, 219, 253–265] The principles of recording and interpreting the equine ECG are similar to those used for humans, dogs, and other species.[3, 266] The lead systems employed are identical, although some modified leads, such as the base apex lead, have been found to be useful in monitoring the cardiac rhythm of the horse and a number of semi-orthogonal lead systems have been evaluated experimentally. The modified Einthoven's lead system consisting of leads frontal planes I, II, III, $_a$VR, $_a$VL, and $_a$VF and lead V_{10} is commonly used (Table 7–10).

The value of continuous 24-hour (Holter) ECG monitoring is being realized (Fig. 7–15). In one study it was observed that many horses that were historically and clinically without evidence of cardiac disease had supraventricular or (less often) ventricular arrhythmias.[218] Holter monitoring can be performed with contact electrodes using a bipolar lead system similar to that used for the equine heart rate monitors. Electrodes are usually placed over the left saddle area and sternum and are kept moist and in contact with the horse using a surcingle and padding material. This type of continuous 24-hour rhythm monitor can be quite useful to evaluate the horse with a history of syncope or an arrhythmia, but in which an arrhythmia cannot be induced during resting, exercise, and post-exercise ECG examinations. Holter recordings also assist the clinician to characterize the frequency of arrhythmias during a 24-hour period as well as response to therapy.

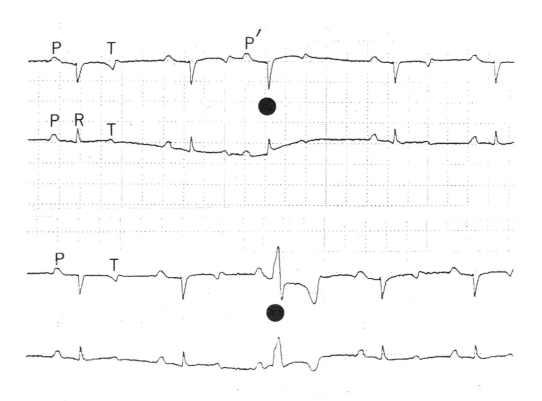

Figure 7–15. Examples of extrasystoles. Atrial (P'-top) and ventricular (bottom) extrasystoles in a mare with heart failure, sinus tachycardia, and premature beats. The recordings are from a 24-hour tape recorded (Holter) electrocardiogram. Two transthoracic leads are recorded simultaneously. The waveforms are indicated. The dark circles indicate the premature complexes. The PR interval of the atrial premature complex is longer owing to physiologic refractoriness in the atrioventricular node. The ventricular ectopic follows the sinus P wave (late diastolic) but discharges the ventricle before the sinus impulse can cause a normal QRS complex. The T wave of the ventricular extrasystole is abnormal (secondary T wave change); 25 mm/sec paper speed.

The orientation, amplitude, and duration of the ECG waveforms depend on many factors, including the age of the horse,[208, 267] the lead examined, the size of the cardiac chambers, the degree of training, and even the phase of ventilation.[268, 269] The principal use of the ECG is to diagnose the rhythm, because the ECG is less sensitive for detecting cardiomegaly, especially mild to moderate heart enlargement. A normal ECG does not exclude heart disease; moreover, the ECG is not a test of myocardial function. A systematic approach to ECG analysis should be undertaken and compared with reference values (Table 7–11).

Atrial depolarization generates the P wave. Normal activation proceeds from right to left and craniad to caudad, leading to positive P waves in left-right lead I and also in craniocaudal leads II and aVF.[13, 270] The normal P wave is notched or bifid; however, single peaked, diphasic, and polyphasic P waves may be encountered in normal horses. A negative/positive P wave is often recorded if the focus of pacemaker activity shifts to the caudal right atrium near the coronary sinus (Fig. 7–16). The initial peak of the common bifid P wave is reportedly caused by depolarization of the middle and caudal one third of the right atrium.[8] The second peak represents activation of the atrial septum and the medial surface of the left atrium. The P wave peaks can be subdivided with P_1 reported to be as high as 0.25 mV (mean of 0.14) and the second peak, P_2 reported to be as high as 0.5 mV (mean of 0.28).[266] There are differences among breeds of horses. The P wave morphology can change cyclically with waxing and waning of vagal tone during sinus arrhythmia. During tachycardia, the P wave shortens, becomes more peaked, and is followed by a prominent atrial repolarization (T_a) wave. Such features make the diagnosis of atrial enlargement by electrocardiography very difficult.

The time required for conduction across the AV node and His-Purkinje system is determined by measuring the PR interval. Because physiologic AV block is so common, there is significant variation in the PR interval even within the same horse; thus, normal maximal values for the PR interval are difficult to state. Values that persistently exceed 0.5 second are probably abnormal. Variation in the PR interval is not usually related to changes in ventilation[30] but is often correlated with changes in blood pressure.[52]

The morphology of the QRS complex is variable. The relatively complete penetration of the conduction system into the free walls of the ventricle causes these chambers to be activated simultaneously with a burst of depolarization, which cancels much of the divergent electromotive forces.[8, 9] Consequently, the normal electrical axis may vary and the amplitude of the QRS complex can be quite small in the frontal plane leads. A prominent dorsally oriented vector causes a prominent positive terminal deflection in lead V_{10}, while the [−]right base to [+]left apex lead exhibits a prominent S wave (Fig. 7–17). The normal slur in the ST segment makes determination of QRS duration difficult in many horses. The mean amplitude for the R wave in lead II for normal racehorses is about 0.8 to 1.1 mV.[1, 3, 6, 219, 255, 266, 271] Clinical experience suggests that R wave amplitudes exceeding 2.2 mV in lead II or 1.7 mV in lead I are abnormal. Occasionally, the R wave amplitude in a normal horse exceeds even these limits.

Table 7–11. Electrocardiography: Approximate Limits for Normal Frontal Plane Leads

Variable	Maximal Value	Comments
Heart rate	40/min	Resting mature horses; higher in foals, colts, and ponies
Cardiac rhythm	—	Sinus mechanisms, sinus arrhythmia, vagal-induced first- and second-degree AV block*
P wave	0.16 sec	Atrial repolarization (Ta wave) may make measurement difficult
PR interval	0.48 sec	Varies; longer when there is high vagal tone
QRS complex	0.14 sec	May vary with the size of the heart (often longer in the base-apex lead)
QT interval	0.575 sec	Inversely related to the heart rate
R wave lead I	0.85 mV	
R wave leads 2, aVF	2.3 mV	
Frontal axis	0–100 degrees	Axis is variable in foals and yearlings

*When evaluating the electrocardiographic rhythm, consider the following points:
  Technical aspects—paper speed, calibration, and lead(s)
  Artifacts—electrical, motion, twitching, and muscle tremor
  Heart rate/minute—atrial and ventricular
  Cardiac rhythm—atrial, atrioventricular conduction sequence, and ventricular conduction
  Arrhythmias
  Site or chamber of abnormal impulse formation, myocardial fibrillation, or conduction disturbance
  Rate of abnormal impulse formation
  Conduction of abnormal impulses
  Patterns or repeating cycles
  P wave—morphology, duration, amplitude, and variation
  PR interval—duration, variation, and conduction block (of P wave)
  QRS—morphology, duration, and amplitude
  Frontal plane mean electrical axis
  ST segment—depression or elevation
  T wave—changes in morphology or size; QT interval
  Miscellaneous—electrical alternans, synchronous diaphragmatic contraction

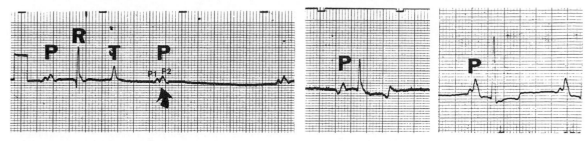

Figure 7–16. P waves of the horse are demonstrated. On the left is a normal, bifid P-wave morphology with two distinct peaks (designated as P1 and P2). There is also a physiologic second-degree atrioventricular block *(arrow)*. The center panel demonstrates a negative/positive P wave of "coronary sinus" origin. This is a normal variation. The right panel shows increased amplitude P waves recorded in a horse after conversion from atrial fibrillation. The second peak is particularly large. This may indicate atrial enlargement; however, such voltage criteria correlate poorly with cardiomegaly in horses. Echocardiography is a more accurate method for evaluating atrial size. Lead 2 recordings at 25 mm/sec paper speed.

The frontal plane leads can be inspected to estimate the mean electrical axis of depolarization, the "average" wave of depolarization (Fig. 7–18). This determination is usually reported by direction using a quadrant orientation (right or left; craniad or caudad) or is stated in degrees (lead I is 0 degrees; lead II is 60 degrees; lead aVF is 90 degrees; lead III is 120 degrees; lead aVR is [−]150 degrees; and lead aVL is [−]30 degrees). The general direction of the QRS axis can be quickly estimated by surveying the height of the R waves in the frontal leads and selecting the lead with the greatest net-positive QRS complex. The axis in foals and yearlings is variable and frequently oriented craniad while the frontal axis in most mature horses is directed left-caudad. Abnormal axis deviations have been observed with cardiomegaly, cor pulmonale, conduction disturbances, and electrolyte imbalance.[255]

Following the ventricular activation, repolarization of the ventricles is recorded. This period is measured from the end of the QRS complex (the "J point") and extends to the end of the T wave.[21, 261, 272] The T wave vector is most often directed toward lead III, resulting in a positive T wave in lead III and a negative or isoelectric T wave in most resting horses.[266] Although some clinical surveys have suggested that abnormalities of the ST-T indicate cardiac dysfunction in performance animals, marked deviation of the ST segment and increased amplitude of the T wave are anticipated even in normal horses following exercise or excitement-induced tachycardia. There is simply no unanimity of opinion regarding T waves in horses. Progressive J point or ST segment deviation in the horse with hypovolemia or shock may indicate myocardial ischemia, whereas enlargement of the T wave may develop with myocardial hypoxia or hyperkalemia.

Diagnosis and management of cardiac arrhythmias are discussed later in this chapter.

Thoracic Radiography

There are severe limitations to the use of thoracic radiography in the evaluation of the equine heart due to the large size of the mature horse and the ability to obtain only a standing lateral thoracic radiograph in all except the smallest neonatal foals.[83] While recumbent lateral, and on occasion, ventrodorsal or dorsoventral projections can be obtained on small neonatal foals, the stress of restraint or requirement for heavy sedation often makes such positioning contraindicated. Thoracic radiographs may be useful to identify areas of pulmonary or pleural disease and assist in the differential diagnosis of respiratory problems.

Gross changes in cardiac size and shape may be detected in a lateral thoracic radiograph of a foal or horse with significant cardiomegaly.[83, 137] A normal thoracic radiograph does not necessarily indicate that the heart is normal in size. Mild to moderate increases in the size of the cardiac chamber may go undetected, particularly in adult horses. Generalized enlargement of the cardiac silhouette is seen in cases of pericardial effusion or CHF (Fig. 7–19). Dorsal displacement of the trachea may be detected in some horses with left atrial (LA) and LV enlargement. In some horses with LA enlargement, the caudodorsal border of the cardiac silhouette bulges caudally. Increased contact between the ventral border of the heart and the sternum may be detected with RV enlargement but is usually difficult to appreciate. A 50% decrease in the spinotracheal angle (the angle between the

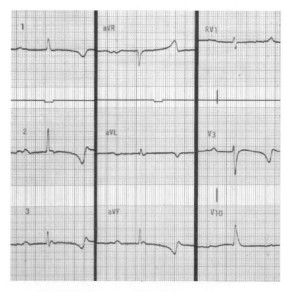

Figure 7–17. Multiple lead recordings in a normal horse. Note the varying configuration of the P-QRS-T complexes across the leads.

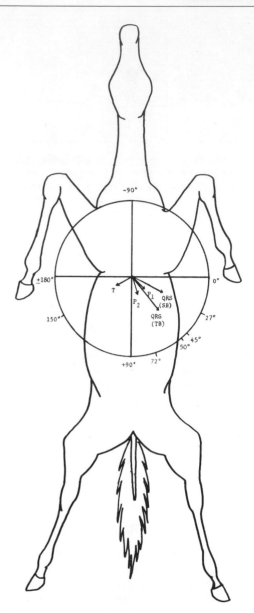

Figure 7–18. Diagram of the normal frontal plane lead axis. The predominant vectors for the QRS complex in Standardbred (SB) and Thoroughbred (TB) horses are indicated. The orientation of the two components of the normal P wave (P1 and P2, see Fig. 7–16) differ slightly. (From Fregin GF: The cardiovascular system. In Mansmann RA, McAllister ES, Pratt PW, eds. *Equine Medicine and Surgery.* Santa Barbara, American Veterinary Publications Inc., 1982, with permission.)

particularly in the hilar regions; the characteristic air bronchograms are more readily identified there when alveolar edema is present.

Angiocardiography is only practical in foals less than 250 lb and usually requires general anesthesia, which may be contraindicated in the foal with a severely compromised cardiovascular system. Both selective and nonselective positive contrast angiocardiograms have been performed in foals and adult horses (see Fig. 7–19),[89, 274, 275] but these techniques have been replaced by echocardiography at most institutions.

Nuclear medicine imaging has been developed in equine referral institutions and is likely to become more widespread in the future as it provides another method of assessing cardiac function. First-pass nuclear angiocardiography is most widely used and permits the visualization of the cardiac chambers during sequential phases of the cardiac cycle.[83]

Echocardiography

Ultrasound is the mechanical vibration of sound waves within a medium at frequencies greater than 20,000 cycles/sec (hertz = Hz). These inaudible sound waves follow the laws of optics, can be transmitted through tissue, and can also be refracted and reflected. This last property permits the clinician to image the heart and other organs. Examination of the equine heart requires the use of crystals that vibrate at a frequency of 2 to 5 megahertz (MHz). Echocardiography is the application of ultrasound diagnostics to the heart.[276–278] The technique is important in the evaluation of cardiac pathology[82, 103, 104, 107, 156, 157, 163–167, 170, 248, 276–299] and can be used in the assessment of the fetal heart.[300] The essential principle of echocardiography is straightforward: When ultrasound is directed into the chest and toward the heart, some of the sound energy reflects back to the transducer. This occurs because tissue interfaces with different acoustic impedance, such as collagen and blood, are encountered by the echobeam and ultrasound is reflected from these tissue interfaces. A hand-held transducer acts to both send and receive ultrasound.[301, 302] The echocardiograph computer is capable of determining the spatial orientation and distance of the returning echoes, processing the signals, and displaying an image of the heart. The image is usually displayed, by convention, with that part of the heart closest to the transducer at the top of the display and adjacent to the transducer artifact. Two imaging modalities, the M (motion)-mode and two-dimensional (B-mode or cross-sectional) formats are in general use. If Doppler studies are included, blood flow can be detected relative to the two-dimensional and M-mode images (Table 7–12, Fig. 7–20; see also Fig. 7–6).[156, 297] M-mode, two-dimensional, contrast echo, and Doppler studies can also be used to estimate ventricular function, CO, drug therapy, and cardiac mass.[292, 293, 303]

The M-mode echocardiogram is a single-crystal icepick image of the heart (see Fig. 7–6).[304] The movement of the cardiac structures (vertical axis) is displayed over time along the horizontal axis. The ECG waveforms provide a timing reference, and the depth of the cardiac structures from the transducer (Y axis) is displayed in centimeters. Visualization of the characteristic movements of cardiac structures permits the experienced viewer to evaluate and quantify cardiac anatomy and function (see Fig. 7–20). The high sampling

dorsal border of the trachea and the ventral border of the adjacent thoracic vertebrae) was demonstrated in young horses with cardiomegaly due to congenital cardiac disease.[83] Evaluation of the pulmonary vasculature and pulmonary parenchyma is also difficult and very dependent upon radiographic technique. Enlarged pulmonary vessels and increased radiolucency of the pulmonary parenchyma associated with pulmonary overcirculation (as with septal defects) can occasionally be observed; the opposite is also true. Pulmonary edema causes generalized increased radiopacity,

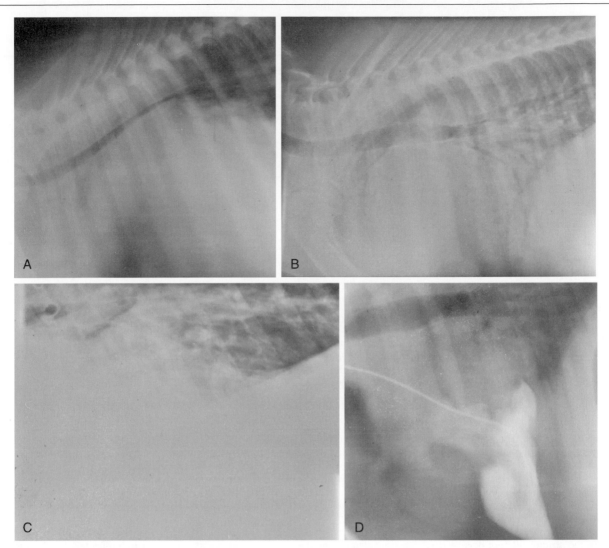

Figure 7–19. Thoracic radiography. *A,* Marked cardiomegaly in a quarter horse foal with complex congenital heart disease, including multiple ventricular septal defects. *B,* Cardiomegaly and alveolar pulmonary edema in a filly with mitral regurgitation and left-sided congestive heart failure. *C,* Increased pulmonary density and pleural effusion in a Standardbred gelding with atrial fibrillation, atrioventricular valvular regurgitation, myocardial failure, and biventricular congestive heart failure. *D,* Angiocardiogram obtained from an Arabian foal with pulmonary atresia and a large ventricular septal defect (pseudotruncus arteriosus). Contrast medium was injected in the left ventricle, and this medium opacifies a dilated, overriding aorta. Right to left shunting across the ventricular septal defect results in dilution of contrast medium.

rate of the M-mode study makes it excellent for visualizing rapidly vibrating structures, such as the oscillating septal (anterior) mitral leaflet in aortic regurgitation.[103]

The two-dimensional echocardiogram generates a cardiac field by mechanically or electrically sweeping one or more piezoelectric crystals across the heart (Fig. 7–21).[82, 287, 289, 291, 293, 296, 297] The operator must hand-direct the imaging probe to achieve a suitable image plane. The pie-shaped image obtained has both depth and breadth but has no significant thickness. Accordingly, different image planes must be used to interrogate the three-dimensional heart. These imaging planes are designated long-axis (sagittal), short axis (coronal), apical (when the transducer is near the left apex), and angled (hybrid) views. The two-dimensional field is constantly updated to visualize cardiac motion in real time, and this is done at sampling rates of 20 to 60 frames/

sec. Thus, the study is typically recorded on videotape for subsequent playback and analysis.

Doppler echocardiography relies on the Doppler principle to measure the direction and velocity of red blood cells (RBCs) in the heart (Fig. 7–22; see also Fig. 7–6).[156, 170, 276, 305–308b] In Doppler echocardiography, a portion of the ultrasound emitted by the transducer strikes moving RBCs. These targets cause ultrasound to be reflected back to the transducer. Since the RBCs constitute a moving "source" of (reflected) ultrasound, the returning sound waves attain a frequency that is slightly different from that originally transmitted (the "carrier frequency"). When the echocardiograph unit records the Doppler frequency shift, calculation of RBC velocity and direction relative to the transducer is possible. The information is displayed as a Doppler spectrum showing time along the horizontal axis, direction relative to a zero

Table 7–12. Interpretation of Doppler and Echocardiographic Studies

Cardiac Rhythm

Arrhythmias will alter cardiac motion and velocity signals

Identification of Atria, Cardiac Septa, Ventricles, Inlet and Outlet Valves, Great Vessels, Veins

Presence, absence, hypoplasia, or atresia of anticipated structures
Identification of cardiac mass lesions and thrombi
Identification of obvious lesions (e.g., septal defect, thick valve)

Cardiac Mensuration

Ventricular dilatation or hypertrophy
Atrial enlargement
Aortic/pulmonary artery dilatation or attenuation
Abnormally small chamber or great vessel

Global Left Ventricular Systolic Function

Subjective analysis of radial shortening (short-axis view)
M-mode fractional shortening (normal usually between 32% and 55%)
Reduced fractional shortening: rule out dilated cardiomyopathy, myocarditis, myocardial necrosis (e.g., monensin); atrial fibrillation (mild
    depression); prolonged ventricular tachycardia; general anesthesia and sedative drugs can decrease fractional shortening
Increased fractional shortening: rule out volume overload (especially mitral regurgitation or aortic regurgitation), sympathetic activity,
    recent exercise

Mitral/Tricuspid Valves

Identification of valve cusps, support apparatus, motion during cardiac cycle
Reduced opening or leaflet separation (M-mode E-F slope): rule out stenosis, vegetation, decreased AV flow, aortic regurgitant jet-striking
    septal mitral leaflet
Increased echogenicity: rule out vegetation, degenerative thickening, dysplasia
Diastolic mitral fluttering: rule out aortic insufficiency
Diastolic tricuspid valve fluttering: rule out ventricular septal defect, ruptured aortic sinus aneurysm
Systolic mitral fluttering: rule out AV insufficiency
Chaotic motion: rule out arrhythmias, ruptured chordae tendineae
Prolapse into the atrium: rule out degenerative disease, ruptured chordae tendineae, connective tissue disorder, bacterial endocarditis,
    malformation
Premature (diastolic) closure: rule out severe semilunar valve insufficiency or long PR interval
Delayed (systolic) closure: rule out LV failure (high end-diastolic pressure)
Increased mitral E point to septal distance: rule out LV dilatation, cardiac failure, aortic regurgitant jet-striking valve
Cleft: rule out endocardial cushion defect

Aortic/Pulmonic Valves

Identification of valve leaflets, motion during cardiac cycle
Narrowing of the LV or RV outflow tracts: rule out stenosis, hypertrophy
Diastolic fluttering: rule out semilunar valve insufficiency
Systolic fluttering: normal or high-flow state
Increased echogenicity (focal or diffuse): rule out bacterial vegetation, degeneration, congenital lesion
Prolapse into ventricle: rule out endocarditis, subaortic septal defect
Lack of systolic separation: rule out low cardiac output, arrhythmia, stenosis, endocarditis
Premature (midsystolic) closure: rule out outflow tract obstruction, ventricular septal defect
Systolic doming: rule out congenital valve fusion/stenosis, endocarditis

Left Ventricular Wall and Chamber

Hypertrophy: rule out hypertension, laminitis, aortic or subaortic stenosis, hypertrophic cardiomyopathy
Dilatation: rule out causes of volume overload, cardiomyopathy, valvular disease, left to right shunts, AV fistula
Hypokinesis: rule out myocardial failure, anesthesia, myocarditis, myocardial necrosis
Hyperkinesis: rule out mitral or aortic insufficiency, volume overload (e.g., left to right shunts), sympathetic stimulation, hypertrophic
    cardiomyopathy, ± stenosis
Dyskinesis: rule out cardiomyopathy, ischemia, infarct, thrombotic disease, toxic insult (e.g., ionophore)
Giant papillary muscle: rule out hypertrophy, AV valve dysplasia
Hypo/hyper-echogenicity: normal (variation), infarct, fibrosis, dissection, septal defect

Table 7–12. Interpretation of Doppler and Echocardiographic Studies (Continued)

Ventricular Septal Wall

Hypertrophy: rule out aortic or pulmonic stenosis, pulmonary/systemic hypertension, tetralogy of Fallot, truncus arteriosus
Hyperkinesis: as per LV chamber
Hypokinesis: as per LV chamber, rule out RV pressure or volume overload
Paradoxic or flattened motion: rule out moderate to severe RV volume or pressure overload, such as atrioseptal defect, tricuspid regurgitation, pulmonary hypertension
Echo "dropout": rule out septal defect, aneurysm
Discontinuity of septum and aortic root: rule out septal defect, tetralogy of Fallot, pulmonary artery atresia, truncus arteriosus

Right Ventricular Wall and Chamber

Hypertrophy: rule out pulmonary hypertension, pulmonic stenosis, tetralogy of Fallot
Dilatation: rule out tricuspid insufficiency, chronic RV pressure overload, atrial septal defect

Left Atrium

Decreased size: rule out right-to-left shunting, hypovolemia
Dilatation: rule out mitral regurgitation or stenosis, cardiomyopathy, left heart failure, left to right shunts
Increased density: rule out thrombus or tumor

Right Atrium

Dilatation: rule out tricuspid regurgitation or stenosis, cardiomyopathy, right heart failure, atrial septal defect
Increased density: rule out tumor, thrombus

Atrial Septal Wall

Marked "bowing": rule out volume overload of one atrium
Echo "dropout": rule out septal defect

Pulmonary Artery

Absence: rule out atresia
Dilatation: rule out pulmonic stenosis, intracardiac left to right shunt, patent ductus arteriosus, pulmonary hypertension from any causes including left-sided congestive heart failure

Aorta

Decreased diameter: rule out low cardiac output
Dilatation: rule out subaortic or aortic stenosis, tetralogy of Fallot, pulmonary artery atresia, patent ductus arteriosus, systemic hypertension, truncus arteriosus, aortic insufficiency
Aneurysm: rule out congenital lesion or secondary to endocarditis or vascular disease

Pericardium

Rule out pericardial effusion, constriction, or mass lesion
Rule out pulmonary/mediastinal abscess

Doppler Flow Studies (Color Coded, Pulsed Wave, Doppler, Continuous Wave Doppler)

Estimation of cardiac output (flow-velocity integral × vessel cross-sectional area × heart rate)
Estimation of ventricular function (from aortic and pulmonary artery peak velocity and acceleration time)
Estimation of intracardiac pressures (from continuous wave velocity measurements across incompetent, stenotic valves or septal defects)
Detection of valvular regurgitation (abnormal direction, turbulent flow signals)
Detection of valvular stenosis (abnormal high-velocity, turbulent flow signals)
Detection of intracardiac shunting (abnormal turbulent flow signals)

Modified from Bonagura JD, Herring DS, Welker F: Echocardiography. *Vet Clin North Am Equine Pract* 1:311, 1985.
AV, atrioventricular; LV, left ventricle; RV, right ventricle.

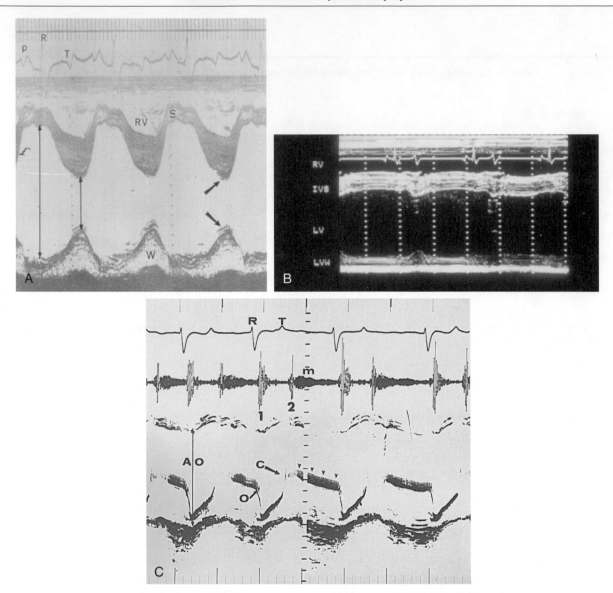

Figure 7–20. M-mode echocardiograms with simultaneous electrocardiograms. *A,* M-mode tracing demonstrating a hyperdynamic left ventricle in a horse with acute mitral regurgitation. This is typical of volume overloading with preserved ventricular function; furthermore, the reduced resistance to ejection of blood into the left atrium enhances ventricular shortening. The maximal systolic excursions of the septum and left ventricular wall (W) are indicated by *arrows.* Diastolic and systolic internal dimensions are indicated at the left. *B,* Recording through the ventricles demonstrating decreased contractility with a reduced left ventricular shortening fraction. This pattern of contraction can be caused by myocarditis, myocardial injury (e.g., monensin), idiopathic dilated cardiomyopathy, chronic volume overload, or administration of negative inotropic drugs. Calibrations are 1 cm every 1 sec. *C,* Recording from a horse with aortic regurgitation and atrial fibrillation, demonstrating fine diastolic fluttering of an aortic valve leaflet *(small arrows).* The aortic root (AO), valve opening (O), and valve closing (C) are indicated. The murmur (m) of aortic regurgitation is evident in the phonocardiogram above. First (1) and second (2) heart sounds are labeled. Diastolic fluttering of the mitral valve (most common), aortic valve, ventricular septum, or walls of the aortic root may be observed in horses with this hemodynamic abnormality. The M-mode sampling rate (approximately 1,000 pulses/sec) is ideal for detecting these high-frequency events.

baseline, and RBC velocity along the Y axis. Measurement of direction and velocity in a discrete area of the heart or circulation is obtained by the pulsed Doppler mode, of which color-coded Doppler is a more refined example. Color coding permits superimposition of the pulsed-wave Doppler flow information onto the two-dimensional image (Fig. 7–23). Color-coded Doppler is particularly useful in horses, because a large area of the heart can be readily screened

for flow disturbances. Pulsed Doppler techniques provide accurate information about the exact location of RBC velocity but are limited in ability to measure high velocity before the signal begins to be displayed in the incorrect direction, a problem called signal "aliasing."[170] For quantifying abnormal high-velocity flow, a continuous wave Doppler system is used. Continuous wave Doppler has virtually unlimited ability to record very high velocity but

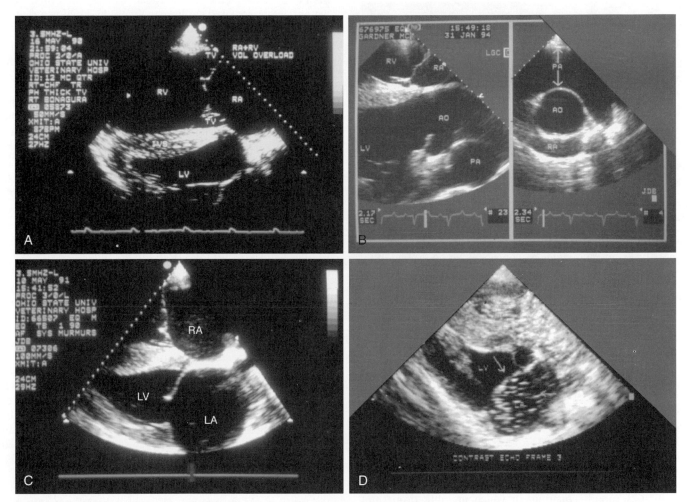

Figure 7–21. Two-dimensional echocardiograms. *A,* Long-axis image from the right thorax in a 12-year-old quarter horse gelding demonstrating marked right ventricular and right atrial dilatation secondary to tricuspid regurgitation and elevated pulmonary artery pressure. The pulmonary hypertension in this case was caused by a tumor that obstructed flow in the main pulmonary artery. The ventricular septum is flat and bulges slightly into the left ventricle. *B,* Images of the ascending aorta and pulmonary artery obtained from the right hemithorax *(left panel)* and left cranial hemithorax. An evaluation of the pulmonary artery diameter, relative to the aorta, is useful when identifying pulmonary hypertension. *C,* Bi-atrial dilatation in a Thoroughbred colt with mitral regurgitation, pulmonary hypertension, atrial fibrillation, and congestive heart failure. Both atria are rounded and appear "turgid." The cause of mitral disease in this case was idiopathic lymphocytic-plasmacytic mitral valvulitis. *D,* Contrast echocardiogram demonstrating right to left shunting at the level of the foramen ovale in a foal with severe respiratory disease. The saline generates echocontrast, opacifies the right atrium and right ventricle, and is observed to fill the left atrium *(arrows)* although the left ventricle has not yet been opacified. This technique is easy and practical for demonstrating right to left shunts across the cardiac septa.

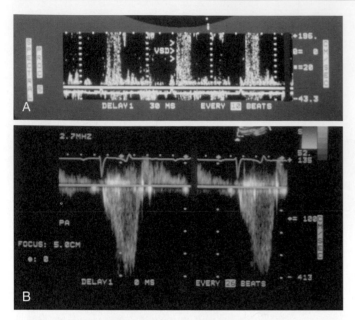

Figure 7–22. Spectral Doppler echocardiograms. *A,* Pulsed wave Doppler study from a horse with a ventricular septal defect. The baseline of zero flow has been shifted to the bottom. A high-velocity, turbulent systolic jet is recorded but cannot be faithfully quantified. The signal wraps around the baseline (signal alias). Calibration dots are 20 cm/sec. *B,* A continuous wave Doppler study from a filly with tetralogy of Fallot. The high-velocity flow pattern across the stenotic pulmonary artery is recorded as a negative signal below the zero baseline. Calibration dots are 1 m/sec. The jet velocity exceeds 4 m/sec.

with less accurate spatial discrimination than pulsed wave Doppler. High-velocity flow is encountered as RBCs are ejected from high to lower pressure zones across incompetent valves, stenotic valves, and intra- and extracardiac shunts (provided that there is a pressure difference across the defect). The pressure difference between the source and the sink of a high-velocity jet can be estimated by the modified Bernoulli equation, in which pressure drop (mm Hg) $= 4V^2$, and the maximal velocity, V (in m/sec), are recorded by continuous wave Doppler. If, for example, a peak velocity of 4.8 m/sec is recorded across a ventricular septal defect in a yearling, and if the systolic systemic arterial blood pressure is determined noninvasively to be 125 mm Hg, the estimated RV systolic pressure would be calculated as follows:

Pressure drop $= [4 \times 4.8^2] = 92$ mm Hg
Estimated LV systolic pressure $= 125$ mm Hg
Estimated RV systolic pressure $= 125 - 92 = 33$ mm Hg

This would indicate a very restrictive septal defect that would allow minimal left to right shunting and would be unlikely to cause difficulties for the horse except at high workloads.

Echocardiography is most useful in the evaluation of heart murmurs, pericardial diseases, heart failure, and cardiac arrhythmias; moreover, these studies have the potential to identify other lesions of the thorax that may masquerade as

heart disease.[74, 309] The source of a pathologic cardiac murmur and the impact of a cardiac lesion on the size and function of the heart can be accurately determined by combining the imaging of M-mode and two-dimensional echocardiography with Doppler studies. A normal echocardiogram and Doppler study in a horse with a cardiac murmur is a favorable finding, suggesting a functional basis for the murmur. Conversely, identification of an abnormal flow pattern with associated cardiomegaly or abnormal ventricular function may indicate a high risk or limitation for work. As with all diagnostic studies, there can be ambiguous results, particularly regarding the tricuspid valve, because physiologic tricuspid regurgitation, silent to auscultation, is detectable by Doppler studies in many clinically normal horses. Contrast echocardiography,[281] whereby saline is used to delineate the path of blood flow, is especially useful for the detection of right to left shunts in foals (see Fig. 7–21). Reference values for ventricular chamber size, wall thickness, and LV shortening fraction have been published,[165–165d, 296, 297] and representative data[165, 297] are given in Table 7–13. Clinical applications of echocardiography are illustrated later in this chapter.

Cardiac Catheterization

Cardiac catheterization has been largely replaced by Doppler echocardiography, inasmuch as anatomical, flow, and pressure estimates can be obtained noninvasively and more readily by ultrasound studies. There are some indications for cardiac catheterization, particularly for accurate measurement of pulmonary artery pressure and cardiac output. Hemodynamic variables that can be measured or calculated by catheterization include arterial blood pressure, pulmonary arterial and pulmonary artery occlusion (capillary wedge) pressure, intracardiac pressures, central venous pressure, CO, systemic and pulmonary vascular resistances, and arteriovenous oxygen difference. Normal values for these variables depend on the methods used for measurement, the head and body position of the horse, and the effects of administered tranquilizers, sedatives, or anesthetic agents.[23, 24, 158, 225, 227–229, 231, 232, 310–321]

Systemic arterial pressure is closely linked to left ventricular function. Measurement of arterial blood pressure has been described previously (see earlier in this chapter). Peak systolic pressures in the aorta and left ventricle should be essentially equal, and a substantial difference between these values would indicate an obstruction to outflow. LV diastolic pressure reflects diastolic function and the ability of the ventricle to empty its stroke volume. The reported diastolic pressure is usually the end-diastolic pressure (typically 12 to 24 mm Hg in standing animals), which is higher than the early (often subatmospheric) minimal diastolic LV pressure. Horses and ponies have higher ventricular end-diastolic pressures than do either humans or dogs.[23, 26, 158, 322] Exercise is a physiologic cause of increased left atrial and ventricular end-diastolic pressures.[193, 314, 315, 323] Elevation of resting LV end-diastolic pressure generally indicates either reduced myocardial contractility, ventricular failure, LV volume overload, myocardial restriction, or increasing ventricular wall stiffness.

The pulmonary arterial pressures can be obtained by percutaneous placement of a flow-directed catheter from the jugular vein to the pulmonary artery. It may be possible to inflate the balloon tip to transiently occlude the pulmonary

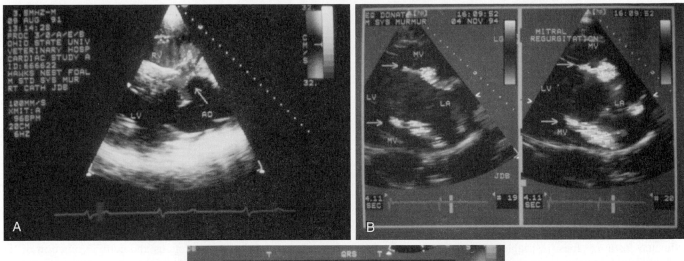

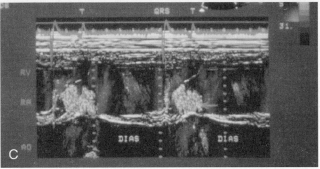

Figure 7–23. Color-coded Doppler echocardiograms. These black and white reproductions of color Doppler echocardiograms demonstrate the mapping of blood flow through the heart. *A,* Perimembranous ventricular septal defect in a foal *(arrow).* The flow pattern was coded red and aliased as the velocity increased across the defect. *B,* Two mitral regurgitation jets *(arrows)* in an aged horse with degenerative mitral valve disease. Early *(left)* and late *(right)* systole are shown. *C,* Color M-mode study from a horse with tricuspid regurgitation. The bright systolic flow pattern, following the QRS of the electrocardiogram, was mapped as turbulence in the color study.

Table 7–13. Reference Values for Equine Echocardiography

Measurement	Mean* (cm)	SD*	Mean† (cm)	SD†
Left ventricle (diastole) R/L	11.90/12.25	0.71/0.72	11.06	1.34
Left ventricle (systole)	7.35	0.72	6.11	0.91
	7.71	0.52		
Left ventricular wall (diastole)	2.39	0.26		
Left ventricular wall (systole)	3.96	0.93		
Ventricular septum (diastole)	3.02	0.39	3.06	0.6
Ventricular septum (systole)	4.55	0.55	4.81	0.71
Right ventricle (diastole)	3.83	0.91		
Right ventricle (systole)	2.71	1.00		
Right ventricular wall (diastole) from the left side	1.44	0.24		
Aorta (diastole)	8.50	0.51	7.31	
Left ventricular shortening fraction R/L	38.76	4.59	44.1	6.4
	37.01	3.91		
Body weight (kg)	517		445	

*Data from Long KJ, Bonagura JD, Darke PG: Standardised imaging technique for guided M-mode and Doppler echocardiography in the horse. *Equine Vet J* 24:226, 1992. (26 Thoroughbred horses).

†Data from Lescure F, Tamzali Y: Reference values for echocardiography applied to sport horses (English Thoroughbreds and French riding horses). *Rev Med Vet* 135:405, 1984. R/L, from right/left side.

artery and "wedge" the distal catheter tip. Such pulmonary capillary "wedge" pressures can be used to estimate pulmonary capillary and venous pressures.[177, 310, 311, 315, 317] The pulmonary artery pressures in standing mature horses are considerably lower than are those of the aorta because of the lower resistance encountered in the pulmonary vascular tree. Mean pulmonary artery pressure is higher in the newborn foal and decreases significantly during the first 2 weeks of life owing to decreased pulmonary arteriolar resistance.[177] Normal pulmonary arterial pressures are approximately 35 to 38 systolic/14 to 22 diastolic. Pulmonary pressures increase dramatically with increased CO as encountered during exercise.[246, 311, 315, 324] The pressure that must be developed in the pulmonary artery depends not only on pulmonary arteriolar resistance but (unlike the systemic circulation) also on the pulmonary capillary resistance. Pulmonary function can influence both of these variables. Alveolar hypoxia and acidosis cause reactive pulmonary arterial vasoconstriction, raising pulmonary pressures.[325] This reaction may be particularly important in newborn foals.[326] LV function directly influences pulmonary artery pressure since elevation of LA and pulmonary venous pressure places a direct burden on the pulmonary artery and right ventricle.[158] LV failure leads invariably to secondary pulmonary hypertension that can be very severe, often with pulmonary pressures exceeding 100 mm Hg. Presumably, other factors such as reactive vasoconstriction (from lung edema) or anatomical changes in the pulmonary vascular tree must develop to sustain such high resistances. In other cases, the cause of pulmonary hypertension may not be evident.[327] Accordingly, elevated pulmonary artery pressures must be assessed in light of pulmonary wedge (or LV end-diastolic) pressure,[187, 187a] as well as of CO. When pulmonary artery pressure is increased, RV and RA pressures must be high to overcome this pressure load, and if pulmonary hypertension is chronic, right-sided heart failure can ensue.

The pulmonary occlusion or wedge pressure is an estimate of LV filling pressure and should approximate LV end-diastolic pressure, provided that there are no obstructions in the pulmonary veins or at the mitral valve. Pulmonary artery wedge pressure can be estimated by the pulmonary artery diastolic pressure provided that the heart rate is normal and pulmonary arterial vasoconstriction (as might occur with hypoxia) is minimal. The pulmonary artery diastolic pressure does not fully equilibrate with the wedge pressure during tachycardia or if there is pulmonary vasoconstriction and a significant pressure gradient between the pulmonary artery diastolic and wedge pressures.[315, 317] The wedge pressure is reduced in hypovolemia and is increased during exercise,[315, 321] left-sided heart failure,[187a] severe MR, or after overinfusion of crystalloid or depression of LV function.

The RV systolic pressure is lower than that of the left ventricle and usually varies from 40 mm Hg up to 60 mm Hg in standing horses. A small gradient (usually 10 to 15 mm Hg) may be measured between the ventricle and pulmonary artery during systole in normal animals. RV end-diastolic pressure is usually between 10 and 14 mm Hg. The RA and central venous pressures influence RV end-diastolic pressure and preload. Hydrostatic venous blood pressure will become higher or lower causing corresponding changes in the RV end-diastolic pressure if the horse's head is raised or lowered.[234] Pathologic elevations in RV diastolic pressure

are encountered with pericardial disease, pulmonary hypertension, right-sided valvular disease, and RV failure (Fig. 7–24). Elevated RV systolic pressure is recorded in pulmonary hypertension from any cause, with large VSDs, and with RV outflow obstruction such as that caused by pulmonary valve vegetative endocarditis.[112]

Mean RA and central venous (vena caval) pressures estimate RV filling pressure and represent a balance between blood volume, venomotor tone, body position, and heart function.[328] Central venous pressure increases significantly in recumbent horses, especially during general anesthesia. Values frequently double from the standing pre-anesthetic measurement and central venous pressure determinations of 20 to 30 cm of water are not uncommon.[313, 328] A single measurement of central venous pressure or of the RA pressure profile is of little value. Trends are most important in assessment of the volume status and cardiac function of the animal. The "x" descent of the RA pressure waveform may be replaced by a positive "c-v" wave in the setting of significant tricuspid regurgitation; this pressure wave corresponds to a prominent jugular pulsation observed by inspection of the neck.

CO can be measured by thermodilution techniques, arteriovenous oxygen difference, Doppler studies, or other methods.[171–173, 179, 329–333] Determination of CO is most often done when monitoring the effects of fluid and drug therapy on the circulation in critical care situations, and it represents a key variable in the evaluation of oxygen delivery to tissues. Reported values range from approximately 72 to 88 mL/min/kg in standing horses or ponies. Noninvasive estimation of CO can be achieved using Doppler echocardiography.[170a, 170b, 305] The mixed venous (pulmonary artery) oxygen content (units = mL oxygen/dL blood) can be used as an indirect estimate of CO. Mixed venous samples obtained from pulmonary arterial catheters are superior to venous samples obtained from either the jugular or peripheral veins.[260] As CO increases, the tissues extract less oxygen from each aliquot of blood; consequently, the venous oxygen content increases.[179] The tissue extraction of oxygen increases and

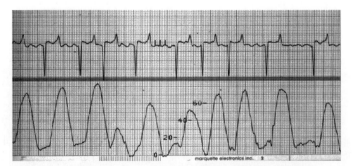

Figure 7–24. Recording of intravascular pressure during cardiac catheterization. Right ventricular pressure recordings from a Thoroughbred yearling with atrial fibrillation, pulmonary hypertension, and biventricular congestive heart failure. The pressure waveforms vary owing to ventilation and the arrhythmia. Peak pressures exceed 70 mm Hg. In the absence of pulmonic stenosis or a large ventricular septal defect, this indicates pulmonary hypertension. The ventricular end-diastolic pressure is also elevated and is compatible with heart failure.

the oxygen content decreases, thus widening the systemic-venous O_2 difference, when CO decreases. Oximetry determinations can also be used to detect intracardiac or extracardiac shunting, for example, to identify a left to right shunting VSD.

Systemic and pulmonary vascular resistances cannot be measured in the intact animal but are calculated using a variation of Poiseuille's law. The general formula for calculation of resistance is:

Systemic vascular resistance =
$$\frac{\text{Mean arterial pressure} - \text{mean atrial pressure}}{\text{cardiac output}}$$

The CO is usually measured in liters per minute by thermodilution. The pressures used are [mean aortic − mean right atria] for the systemic vascular resistance and [mean pulmonary artery − mean pulmonary wedge] for the pulmonary vascular resistance. Correction values may be added to convert resistance to c-g-s units.[318] Since mean arterial pressure is similar between horses of different size, vascular resistance will normally be higher in smaller horses and ponies. Mechanisms that increase systemic vascular resistance include sympathetic activation, activation of the renin-angiotensin system, and the release of other vasoactive hormones into the blood including arginine vasopressin (antidiuretic hormone) and epinephrine.[54]

Laboratory Studies

CV disorders may develop as a consequence of systemic or metabolic diseases such as electrolyte disturbances or septicemia. Conversely, circulatory failure or CV infections may alter routine laboratory tests. Prerenal azotemia and hyponatremia, for example, may be detected in the horse with CHF, especially after diuretic therapy. A routine complete blood count and fibrinogen, biochemical profile, and urinalysis are indicated in horses with arrhythmias, heart failure, or when there is clinical evidence of endocarditis, pericarditis, or vasculitis or pleuropneumonia (pleural effusion). Additional studies including blood cultures, blood gas tensions, other electrolytes (e.g., magnesium), oxygen saturation, cytology and culture of pericardial effusates, and myocardial isoenzymes of creatine kinase or lactate dehydrogenase may be useful in selected cases.

An overview of the studies useful in assessment and management of CV diseases is found in Table 7–4. Monitoring of serum or plasma drug concentrations, especially quinidine and digoxin, are also helpful when monitoring treatment in a cardiac patient.

CONGESTIVE HEART FAILURE
Causes of Heart Failure

CHF is a clinical syndrome characterized by limited CO, increased neurohumoral activity, sodium retention, accumulation of edema in tissues, and transudation of fluid into serous body cavities. Most cardiac lesions in horses are not severe enough to lead to CHF, and this syndrome is not common in equine practice. Nevertheless, CHF can develop

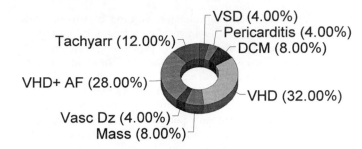

Figure 7–25. A graph demonstrating the overall causes of congestive heart failure (CHF) in 25 horses at a referral teaching hospital as a percentage of the total number of cases of equine CHF. (Tachyarr = tachyarrhythmia; DCM = dilated cardiomyopathy; VHD = valvular heart disease; VHD+AF = valvular heart disease and atrial fibrillation; Vasc Dz = vascular disease; VSD = ventricular septal defect; Mass = mass lesion.) (Data from Ohio State University Veterinary Hospital.)

in foals and mature horses as a consequence of severe degenerative valvular disease, valvulitis, dilated cardiomyopathy, myocarditis or myocardial necrosis (e.g., monensin toxicosis), bacterial endocarditis, pericardial effusion or constriction, congenital malformation, vascular rupture, or pulmonary artery obstruction. The most common cause of CHF in horses is valvular heart disease—often complicated by atrial fibrillation (Fig. 7–25). In addition to structural lesions of the heart and blood vessels, primary electrical disturbances, particularly sustained AV dissociation caused by junctional or ventricular tachycardia, can reduce myocardial function, decrease CO, and lead to CHF.[273] This is especially likely when the heart rate exceeds 100/min for many days. Resolution of CHF in such cases may be possible if antiarrhythmic therapy is successful.

The neurohumoral and renal abnormalities that characterize CHF have not been extensively studied in horses but are probably similar to those reported in other species.[77] These should include increased sympathetic activity, renal retention of sodium and water, and predominance of vasoconstricting hormones such as angiotensin and vasopressin over vasodilating prostaglandins and atrial natriuretic peptide. Probably the most characteristic hemodynamic feature of CHF is the increase in venous pressures that can be identified by physical examination or by cardiac catheterization.

Clinical Recognition of Heart Failure

CHF may develop suddenly or gradually. Peracute LV failure can occur following rupture of mitral valve chordae tendineae or consequent to acute bacterial endocarditis of the mitral or aortic valve. Heart failure may progress rapidly in a foal with a large ventricular septal defect as the pulmonary vascular resistance falls in the weeks following birth. Chronic valvular regurgitation may after many years lead to CHF, although most horses with degenerative valvular disease do not develop CHF. Some lesions, which might otherwise be well tolerated, can cause heart failure if there are increased demands for CO. Examples of such demands include strenuous work, severe anemia, or persistent fever.

Pregnancy is another example: the volume expansion and increased demands for CO in the latter stages of gestation may precipitate CHF in a mare with previously compensated heart disease. Development of atrial fibrillation in a horse with underlying structural disease, such as dilated cardiomyopathy or mitral regurgitation, can precipitate CHF. Such cases are distinguished from the more typical case of atrial fibrillation by the presence of persistent, resting tachycardia and identification by echocardiography of structural lesions and cardiomegaly.

The clinical features of CHF are easily recognized, and determination of the underlying cause of heart disease is not difficult if careful auscultation is combined with available diagnostic methods, particularly echocardiography and ultrasound examination of body cavities.[77, 334–337] Isolated right-sided CHF occurs infrequently—failure due to tricuspid valve endocarditis is an example. Generalized venous distention is a sign of right-sided CHF, as is the finding of generalized ventral, preputial, pectoral, and limb edema. Isolated limb edema, which is so common in hospitalized horses, is not a sign of CHF. Nor is ventral edema in the absence of generalized venous distention indicative of CHF—this finding should prompt consideration of other disorders such as vasculitis. Scrutiny of the jugular veins makes recognition of right-sided CHF straightforward, because these horses demonstrate elevated jugular venous pressure and often pathologic jugular pulses and filling. Pericardial effusion, cranial mediastinal lymphosarcoma,[338] and cranial thoracic masses must be distinguished from RV failure caused by pulmonary hypertension, tricuspid or pulmonic valve disease, cardiomyopathy, or MR or AR. These conditions can generally be identified by two-dimensional echocardiography. The diagnosis of isolated left-sided heart failure, which causes pulmonary venous congestion and pulmonary edema, can be more difficult. In these cases, heart sounds may be somewhat difficult to evaluate owing to loud airway sounds or crackles; accordingly, an erroneous diagnosis of pneumonia may be entertained. Echocardiographic examination of the horse in left-sided CHF will identify dilatation and rounding of the left atrium and dilatation of the pulmonary artery caused by pulmonary hypertension and may demonstrate anatomical lesions of the aortic root, ventricular septum, left heart valves, or chordae tendineae. Fulminant left-sided CHF can lead to coughing and expectoration of edema—a grave sign in most horses. Biventricular CHF is most commonly observed in horses. The clinical signs of advanced biventricular heart failure include persistent resting tachycardia (usually > 60 beats/min), subcutaneous edema, tachypnea (perhaps from interstitial lung edema), pleural effusion, pericardial effusion, ascites, jugular distention, and abnormal jugular pulsations. Chronic CHF is frequently characterized by lethargy and also by loss of body condition.

It is important to understand that *chronic* left-sided CHF in the horse is likely to cause interstitial lung edema and pulmonary hypertension. The magnitude of pulmonary hypertension is often impressive, with systolic pulmonary artery pressures exceeding 100 mm Hg in many cases. The mechanisms by which the lung accommodates such severe and chronic elevations in pulmonary venous pressures without development of alveolar edema are only speculative to date, but the possibility that pulmonary vascular resistance

may increase out of proportion to the increased wedge pressure should be investigated (this occurs in some human patients with chronic left-sided heart failure caused by mitral stenosis). Thus, the clinician should anticipate signs of right-sided CHF even when the primary lesion can be identified on the left side of the heart. This finding can be attributed to RV dilatation and tricuspid regurgitation, which are caused by increased pulmonary vascular resistance. Clinical findings of severe pulmonary hypertension caused by left-sided CHF include a loud, tympanic, pulmonary component of the second heart sound (heard cranioventral to the aortic valve area), a systolic murmur and jugular pulse of tricuspid insufficiency, and dilatation of the pulmonary artery, which can be identified by two-dimensional echocardiography. Further scrutiny will identify LA dilatation and a lesion of the left heart valves or the left ventricle. Investigation of the exact cause of CHF involves integration of physical examination findings with routine diagnostic studies, such as electrocardiography and echocardiography. Thoracic radiographs may be helpful and can demonstrate increased pulmonary vascularity, pulmonary infiltration near the hilus, pleural effusion, and rounding or enlargement of the cardiac silhouette. Echocardiography is essential to identify structural lesions of the pericardium, valves, and blood vessels and to quantify cardiomegaly and ventricular function. Doppler echocardiography can document abnormal flow patterns and predict pulmonary artery pressures (using the Bernouilli relationship) provided that the velocity of any tricuspid regurgitation or pulmonary insufficiency jets can be faithfully recorded. The ECG is needed to evaluate cardiac arrhythmias.

Therapy for Congestive Heart Failure

Therapy for CHF may be feasible for valuable breeding stallions and mares, mares that develop CHF during gestation, or horses and ponies kept as pets.[334] Before therapy can commence, an accurate diagnosis is needed. For example, pericardiocentesis (not cardiac drugs) would be appropriate initial management of cardiac tamponade; thereafter, surgical drainage of the effusion (using drainage tubes) or a pericardiectomy could be considered.[65, 67–69] Antibiotics would be essential in the treatment of bacterial endocarditis or infective pericarditis. Sustained junctional and ventricular tachyarrhythmias may lead to low CO and a potentially reversible cardiomyopathy. Anti-arrhythmic therapy with quinidine, magnesium sulfate solution, lidocaine, propafenone, or procainamide may be effective for treatment of some of these arrhythmias, and with resumption of normal rhythm, CHF may be reversed.

Furosemide[184, 339, 339a, 339b] and digoxin[184, 186, 334, 340–348] are the mainstays for both short- and long-term management of CHF (Table 7–14). Hydralazine therapy[180] might be considered in the initial management of severe MR caused by ruptured chordae tendineae or endocarditis, because systemic arterial dilatation can greatly reduce the mitral regurgitant fraction. There is no published information about the use of angiotensin-converting enzyme inhibitors for treatment of CHF in horses, and the cost would probably be prohibitive. Diuretic dosage must be titrated to mobilize edema and prevent its recurrence and improve respiratory effort when pulmonary edema is evident. The dosage should be con-

Table 7–14. Drug Therapy of Heart Disease

Drug	Formulation	Dosage Forms	Indications	Usual Dose
Digoxin	Lanoxin	Lanoxin 0.25 mg/mL, 2-mL vials; Lanoxin tablets 0.5 mg	CHF, atrial tachyarrhythmias, control of rapid ventricular response in atrial fibrillation/flutter	IV maintenance dose for treatment of CHF: 0.22 mg/100 kg body weight, q12hr Oral maintenance dose for chronic therapy of CHF or for control of ventricular rate response in atrial fibrillation: 1.1–1.75 mg/100 kg body weight, q12hr IV maintenance dose for control of ventricular rate response in atrial fibrillation (neither CHF nor renal failure are present)—0.22–0.375 mg/100 kg body weight, q12hr IV loading dose: 0.44 to 0.75 mg/100 kg body weight, q12hr × 2 doses (uncommonly used)
Procainamide	USP Pronestyl	100 or 500 mg/mL for injection; 500-mg capsules	Ventricular arrhythmias, atrial arrhythmias	25–35 mg/kg q8hr per os 1 mg/kg/min IV to a maximum of 20 mg/kg
Lidocaine	Xylocaine without epinephrine	2% solution, 20 mg/mL concentration	Ventricular tachycardia	0.5 mg/kg very slowly IV; can repeat in 15 minutes
Verapamil	USP, Calan, Isoptin	2-mg vials	Supraventricular tachycardia	0.025 to 0.05 mg/kg IV q 30 minutes; can repeat to 0.2 mg/kg total dose
Propranolol	USP Inderal	1-mg vials	Unresponsive tachyarrhythmias	0.03 mg/kg IV
Propafenone	Rhythmol	150- and 300-mg tablets	Sustained ventricular tachycardia; atrial fibrillation	2 mg/kg per os q8hr
Bretylium tosylate	Bretylium	500 mg/10 mL vials	Life-threatening or refractory ventricular arrhythmias	3–5 mg/kg IV
Furosemide	Lasix Furosemide USP	5% solution, 50 mg/mL	Edema	1–2 mg/kg as needed
Dobutamine	Dobutrex	200-mg vials for infusion	Cardiogenic shock, hypotension, complete AV block (emergency therapy)	1–5 μg/kg/min
Hydralazine	Apresoline Hydralazine USP	50-mg tablets	Mitral regurgitation	0.5–1.5 mg/kg q12hr
Quinidine sulfate (oral); gluconate (IV)	USP Cardioquin Quinaglute	50-g jars of quinidine sulfate powder, USP; tablets; quinidine gluconate for injection, 80 mg/mL for injection	Atrial arrhythmias, ventricular arrhythmias	22 mg/kg per os 1–10 mg/kg IV, total dose (see Table 7–17 for details)
Magnesium SO$_4$	USP (filter)	Dissolve 20–25 g in sterile water; filter	Ventricular tachycardia	IV infusion at 1 g/min to effect, up to a maximum of 25 g
Dexamethasone	Azium Azium SP	Injection, 4 mg/mL	Ventricular tachycardia, complete AV block	0.1 mg/kg to 0.22 mg/kg IV or IM
Glycopyrrolate or atropine	Robinol Atropine USP	0.2 mg/L 0.4 mg/L	Sinus bradycardia, vagal-induced arrhythmias	0.005 to 0.01 mg/kg IV
Sodium bicarbonate	Bicarbonate sodium, USP	Approximately 1 mEq/mL, available in ampules or bottles	Hyperkalemia, atrial standstill; quinidine toxicosis	1 mEq/kg IV; can be repeated
Phenylephrine HCl	Neo-Synephrine	10 mg/mL	Arterial hypotension, excessive vasodilation, quinidine toxicosis	0.01 mg/kg to effect

CHF, congestive heart failure; IM, intramuscular; IV, intravenous.

trolled to prevent pre-renal azotemia or electrolyte disturbances. Diuretic therapy may eventually be discontinued in some horses. Depending on urgency and ability to monitor ECG rhythm, digoxin can be administered initially as a loading dose or by using either an intravenous or oral maintenance regimen. The reported elimination half-life of digoxin has not been consistent (7.2 to 28 hours) and probably relates to the clinical state of the animals studied. As expected, oral doses of digoxin are relatively higher because of lower bioavailability (20%).[349] Long-term digoxin therapy involves once or twice daily oral administration, usually mixed with molasses and some grain (see Table 7–14). Chronic digitalization should be monitored by measuring serum digoxin concentration and evaluating a blood sample drawn 8 to 12 hours after the previous dose. Therapeutic values for the trough plasma level are generally considered to be between 1 and 2 ng/mL. Periodic cardiac examinations, measurements of serum biochemistries (creatinine, electrolytes), and recordings of ECG rhythm strips will be warranted during any long-term course of therapy.

For horses with cardiomyopathy or valvular disease, or in pregnant mares with CHF, the development of atrial fibrillation may precipitate CHF. Furosemide and digoxin can effectively control CHF in these animals as well. Quinidine is generally contraindicated in such animals, although horses may sometimes convert after the resolution of CHF by medical therapy. Reasonable long-term control of CHF may be achieved, thus permitting a comfortable existence for the horse and—in the case of breeding animals—continued reproductive service.

Prognosis in CHF is always guarded when irreversible structural heart disease is the cause of failure; thus, the long-term outcome for these animals is poor. Of course, the horse with CHF requires rest to reduce demands on the heart and should never be worked or ridden owing to the risk of pulmonary artery rupture or syncope. Valuable horses may be used for breeding; however, pregnant mares are likely to be difficult to control in the later stages of gestation.

CONGENITAL HEART DISEASE

The prevalence of congenital heart disease in the overall equine population is unknown. In one survey of causes for neonatal death or euthanasia in 608 cases, the prevalence of congenital heart disease was 3.5%.[93] A number of cardiac malformations have been identified.[1, 3, 47, 88–102, 108, 204, 279, 281, 286, 335, 350–362] While some defects are lethal to the neonate, others are compatible with life but limit peak performance or reproductive value. Most cardiac malformations involve shunting of blood, and isolated malformations leading to valvular stenosis or incompetency are relatively uncommon. Rare lesions such as subaortic stenosis,[360] double-outlet right ventricle,[363] transposition of the great vessels,[90, 99] bicuspid pulmonary valve, pulmonary stenosis,[102] persistent fetal circulation,[364] hypoplastic left heart syndrome,[91, 92] endocardial fibroelastosis,[47] and aortic origin of the pulmonary artery will not be discussed. Some of the more frequently recognized defects[365] are described later.

The clinician should be familiar with the development of the heart in order to understand the clinical findings of congenital heart malformations. During cardiac development, the atria and ventricles begin as a common chamber. The fetal common AV canal is partitioned by growth of cardiac septa that lead eventually to a four-chambered heart. The atria are partitioned by two septa: septum I (primum), which forms the first septum, and septum II (secundum), which later develops to the right of septum I. The foramen ovale, a slit-like passageway for blood between these septa, permits right to left atrial shunting in the fetus but closes functionally and subsequently anatomically in the neonate provided that the LA pressures exceed those of the right atrium. Echocontrast studies have indicated that, in the full-term foal with normal lungs, the foramen ovale is functionally closed within the first 24 to 48 hours of life. However, this passage can remain open if right-sided pressures remain high, as with neonatal respiratory distress syndrome. The ventricular septum is formed by a variety of cardiac primordia. Eventually, the ventral portion of the atrial septum connects to the upper ventricular septum by growth and differentiation of the endocardial cushions. The ventricular outlets are initially a single vessel—the truncus arteriosus—but this vessel is later partitioned and aligned to outflow from the respective ventricles. Because pulmonary circulation to the collapsed lung is minimal in the fetus, most of the pulmonary flow is diverted across the ductus arteriosus. Within the first few days of life, the lungs must expand; pulmonary resistance and pressures must fall; pulmonary blood flow must increase to equal systemic flow; and the ductus arteriosus and foramen ovale must functionally close.

Lesions Causing Systemic to Pulmonary Shunting

A defect in closure or partitioning of the ductus arteriosus, truncus arteriosus, ventricular septum, atrial septa, or endocardial cushions produces a patency or shunt between the systemic and pulmonary circulations. These forms of congenital heart disease are encountered either as an isolated lesion or as a component of more complex disorders like the tetralogy of Fallot. The pathophysiology of a simple systemic to pulmonary shunt is straightforward, and these principles are applicable to any communication, namely, the direction and volume of shunting depends on the caliber (or "restrictiveness") of the orifice and the relative resistances between the systemic and pulmonary circulations. Typically, blood shunts from left to right, but any condition that increases right-sided pressures will hinder this flow and may cause the shunt to reverse. Thus, if an atrial septal defect (ASD) or VSD is complicated by an obstruction at or distal to the level of the shunt, right to left shunting may develop. Causes of higher right-sided resistance include tricuspid atresia or stenosis, pulmonic stenosis, hypoplasia or atresia, and pulmonary hypertension.

Uncommonly, a horse with a large left to right shunt develops pulmonary vascular injury and high pulmonary vascular resistance: This can lead to severe pulmonary hypertension. Irreversible anatomical changes may develop in the pulmonary arteries, producing a fixed, high-resistance system. Consequently, resistance to RV outflow increases and RV systolic and diastolic pressures can increase to systemic levels. Reversed shunting—right to left—can thus develop and lead to a situation known as "Eisenmenger's physiology." The result is persistent arterial hypoxemia, cyanosis, polycythemia, poor growth, and exercise intolerance.

Ventricular Septal Defect

The cause of a VSD in most cases is unknown; although, a genetic basis is very likely in the Arabian breed.[89, 359] Uncomplicated VSD is also quite common in Standardbred horses. No other data delineate the etiopathogenesis of spontaneous septal defects in equidae. Most VSDs are located dorsally on the ventricular septum, below the aortic valve and communicate just ventral to the septal tricuspid leaflet. Such defects are called "inlet," "perimembranous," or "subcristal" defects (Figs. 7–26 and 7–27). Subaortic defects that communicate with the outlet portion of the RV septum are called "outlet," "subpulmonic," or "supracristal" defects. Muscular or multiple ("swiss cheese") defects are uncommon but have been observed. A VSD may be partially occluded by the septal leaflet of the tricuspid valve or from prolapse of an aortic valve leaflet into the defect. Aortic prolapse is more commonly observed in malalignment defects wherein the aortic root overrides the ventricular septum. Such prolapsing also causes aortic valve incompetency. Large defects that obliterate the supraventricular crest (crista supraventricularis) are not uncommon, particularly with tetralogy of Fallot or pulmonary atresia.

The pathophysiology of the isolated VSD is influenced by many factors (Fig. 7–28). Owing to the higher LV than RV pressures, left to right shunting develops and oxygen saturation in the RV outflow tract and the pulmonary artery demonstrates a "step-up" when compared with that in the right atrium.[355] Because much of the shunt volume pumped by the left ventricle is ejected immediately into the pulmonary artery, the left (not the right) ventricle does most of the extra volume of work. Additionally, as pulmonary flow increases, there is increased venous return to the left atrium and left ventricle such that LV diastolic pressure may increase. LV failure can develop in situations of marked left

to right shunting, although this is most likely to occur early in life, as pulmonary vascular resistance declines. The degree of RV hypertrophy and enlargement varies, depending on the size of the septal defect, pulmonary vascular resistance, and pulmonic valve function. Very large, nonrestrictive defects cause the two ventricles to behave as a common chamber, allowing ventricular pressures to equilibrate, and lead to severe RV hypertrophy. Blood then follows the path of least resistance. If the pulmonary valve and the vascular resistance are normal, tremendous left to right shunting is likely to occur leading to left or biventricular heart failure. If pulmonary vascular resistance increases, then left to right shunting will be diminished and bidirectional shunting may be observed. In the horse with tetralogy of Fallot, pulmonary atresia, or pulmonary vascular disease, the high right-sided resistance allows a net right to left cardiac shunt.[89, 352, 354]

The clinical features of VSD are variable. A mature horse may be presented for poor performance or with atrial fibrillation. More commonly, a murmur is detected incidentally during the physical examination for another problem or during a pre-purchase examination. Foals may be symptomatic for pulmonary edema or arterial hypoxemia. Because most defects communicate with the RV inlet septum, the most consistent physical examination finding is a harsh, holosystolic murmur that is loudest just below the tricuspid valve and above the right sternal border. An ejection murmur (one to two grades softer) of relative pulmonic stenosis is usually evident over the left base. The second heart sound may be split. The severity of the defect cannot be judged based on murmur intensity. In some cases, a small defect may be quite loud; whereas, a large, less restrictive defect may be loud or associated with only a soft flow murmur of relative pulmonic stenosis. When a diastolic murmur of aortic regurgitation is present, prolapse of an aortic cusp should be suspected and the lesion is likely to be relatively large.

Diagnostic studies confirm the lesion and help to assess the hemodynamic burden.[286, 352a, 355] Thoracic radiography demonstrates pulmonary overcirculation, LA and ventricular

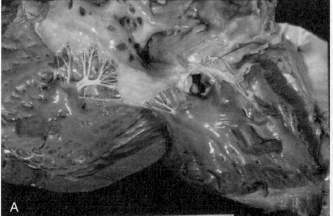
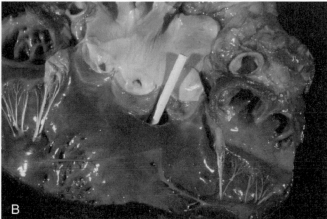

Figure 7–26. Pathology of ventricular septal defects. *A,* Opened right ventricle from a mare demonstrating a perimembranous septal defect opening just beneath the septal leaflet of the tricuspid valve. Aortic valve cusps can be observed through the defect. Congestive heart failure occurred late in life, after the development of atrial fibrillation. *B,* A large ventricular septal defect in a horse. A probe is placed through the defect. Note the dorsal location immediately beneath the right and the non-coronary cusps of the aortic valve. Ostia of both coronary arteries are also evident.

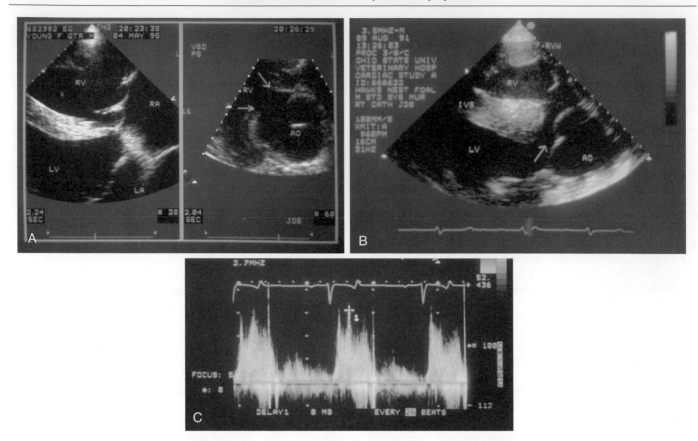

Figure 7–27. Echocardiograms demonstrating ventricular septal defects (see also Figs. 7–22*A*, 7–23*A*, and 7–31). *A,* This subaortic ventricular septal defect is not evident from the long axis image *(left panel)* but is seen in the short axis tomogram *(arrows).* This quarter horse gelding also had pulmonic stenosis. The elevated right ventricular pressures have led to marked right ventricular enlargement with bulging of the septum toward the left ventricle. *B,* Malalignment and a perimembranous septal defect associated with prolapse of an aortic valve leaflet across the defect *(arrow).* (RVW, right ventricular wall.) *C,* A continuous wave Doppler study recorded from a filly with a large, relatively unrestrictive ventricular septal defect. The maximal velocity of 3.1 m/sec predicts a pressure difference of less than 40 mm Hg.

dilatation, and cardiomegaly. Echocardiography successfully delineates the VSD in virtually all cases (see Fig. 7–27).[355a, 362] Doppler studies can be used to identify the high-velocity jet crossing the defect. If the VSD is an isolated defect, the velocity will be directly proportional to the pressure difference, and a high velocity, exceeding 4.5 m/sec, suggests a restrictive defect (see Doppler echocardiography, earlier). Color-coded Doppler or contrast echocardiography can be utilized to demonstrate shunting. Cardiac catheterization and angiocardiography can document the anatomical

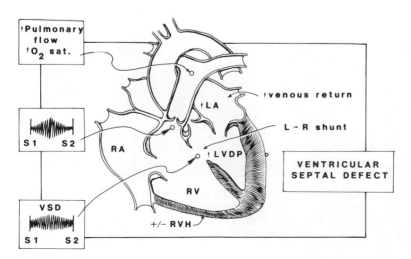

Figure 7–28. Pathophysiology of ventricular septal defects. See text for details. (RVH = right ventricular hypertrophy; LVDP = left ventricular diastolic pressure.) (From Bonagura JD: Congenital heart disease. *In* Bonagura JD [ed]: *Cardiology.* New York, Churchill Livingstone, 1987.)

lesions and estimate the degree of shunting but are rarely used today. An oxygen saturation "step-up" is recorded in the right ventricle at the level of the defect. Ventricular diastolic pressures are elevated with ventricular failure or severe diastolic overload. Pulmonary hypertension and elevated RV systolic pressure are evident in some cases related to left heart failure, excessive pulmonary flow, pulmonary vascular injury, or a combination of factors. Aortic regurgitation may be observed by Doppler studies.

Potential outcomes of VSDs include: (1) tolerance of the lesion; (2) partial or complete closure of a VSD by adherence of the septal tricuspid leaflet, RV hypertrophy, or aortic valve prolapse; (3) progressive aortic regurgitation due to valve prolapse or acute aortic regurgitation due to valve rupture; (4) development of CHF; (5) development of atrial fibrillation; (6) development of pulmonary hypertension; or (7) reversal of the shunt with development of arterial hypoxemia and cyanosis. It is difficult to predict the survival or work potential without detailed Doppler studies; however, defects estimated as less than 2.5 cm in diameter by two-dimensional echocardiography and shunts of greater than 4.5 m/sec velocity uncommonly lead to complications early in life other than limiting athletic ability. The horse with a small, highly restrictive defect may perform at a reasonable standard in the show ring, as a hunter-jumper, or even as a racehorse.

Therapy for VSD is rarely considered. In the authors' opinion, breeding of affected animals should be discouraged, especially in Arabian horses. Medical therapy for CHF or atrial fibrillation can be considered in selected cases.

Atrial Septal Defect and Endocardial Cushion Defect

ASDs and endocardial cushion defects are uncommon in foals. As indicated earlier, ASDs may involve the primum or secundum portion of the atrial septum or consist of a patent foramen ovale. Abnormal atrial septal patency is more likely to be observed with complex congenital cardiac defects, particularly when there is tricuspid or pulmonary atresia.[88, 89, 94, 366, 367] An ASD may be clinically insignificant, with no auscultatable murmur, unless associated with more complex congenital cardiac defects. In the case of a large ASD, flow is from left to right through the defect, resulting in a RA and RV volume overload and pulmonary overcirculation. Such defects are visible echocardiographically, and Doppler echocardiography can confirm the direction of the shunt and estimate its severity. Persistent atrial fibrillation has been observed in conjunction with ASD. Isolated defects, if not too large, are compatible with a moderate to good exercise capacity, since left to right shunting probably decreases as the systemic to pulmonary vascular resistance ratio declines.

Endocardial cushion defects are rarely seen and usually lead to CHF or atrial fibrillation at an early age. This developmental defect typically consists of a large ASD of the primum septum, located ventral to the fossa ovalis, a common and often incompetent AV valve leaflet, and a smaller defect in the basilar portion of the interventricular septum. The ventricles may be partitioned normally, unequally with one rudimentary ventricular chamber, or not at all, main-

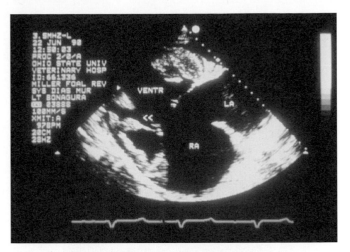

Figure 7–29. Echocardiogram demonstrating a primum atrial septal defect in a foal with complex congenital heart disease that included a common (left) ventricle, rudimentary (right) ventricle, and double-outlet ventricle. The septal defect is evident between the four cardiac chambers. The dorsal secundum septum *(right)* is present as well as the apical ventricular septum *(left)*.

taining a common ventricle. In such cases, a "double inlet–double outlet" ventricle may be present characterized by a common AV canal and single large AV valve. The clinical signs of the affected foal are variable. The foal with an unobstructed outlet to the pulmonary arteries will be hemodynamically similar to one with a large VSD. When a common ventricle is present, cyanosis may be observed. An echocardiographic evaluation of affected foals reveals an ASD involving the primum portion of the atrial septum, possibly a VSD involving the membranous and basilar portion of the interventricular septum, and malformed AV valves (Fig. 7–29). Doppler echocardiography reveals the AV valvular regurgitation and the intracardiac shunts. CHF may supervene; regardless, the prognosis for affected foals is grave.

Patent Ductus Arteriosus

Patent ductus arteriosus (PDA) is a rare isolated congenital cardiac defect in foals and is detected most frequently in combination with other, more complex congenital cardiac defects.[177, 224, 368, 369] The ductus arteriosus is a fetal vessel, derived from the left sixth aortic arch, which permits shunting from the pulmonary artery to the descending aorta in the fetus. At birth the ductus arteriosus normally constricts, in response to increased local oxygen tension and inhibition of prostaglandins. It is functionally closed 72 hours after birth in the vast majority of foals. If the ductus arteriosus does not close, a left to right shunt from the aorta to pulmonary artery occurs. Although there may be some hereditary predisposition to the development of this congenital lesion in other species, this lesion is so rare as an isolated congenital defect that this is not a significant concern. Premature foals, foals with persistent pulmonary hypertension, and foals whose dams have been given prostaglandin inhibitors may be more susceptible to the development of a PDA.

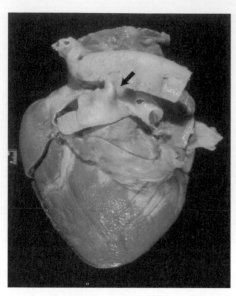

Figure 7–30. A postmortem demonstration of the ductus arteriosus *(arrow)*, between the descending aorta and the pulmonary artery, in a foal with complex congenital heart disease.

The clinical signs depend on the magnitude of the shunting through the PDA, which is determined by its resistance and that of the pulmonary circulation. Physical examination findings (with a left to right PDA) include a continuous machinery murmur and thrill, usually loudest over the main pulmonary artery (craniodorsal to the aortic valve area), and bounding arterial pulses.

Echocardiography will reveal pulmonary artery, LA, and LV volume overload. The severity of these findings depends on the magnitude of the shunt. Direct visualization of the PDA is not always possible by two-dimensional echocardiography, because the ductus arteriosus may be hidden from view by the overlying lung. Ductal flow is best identified from the left hemithorax by Doppler echocardiographic examination of the main pulmonary artery. Doppler studies demonstrate continuous high-velocity, turbulent flow, toward the main pulmonary artery (Fig. 7–30). Cardiac enlargement and increased pulmonary vascularity may be detected in neonatal foals with a PDA as well as radiographic evidence of pulmonary edema if the foal has developed CHF. Cardiac catheterization reveals elevated pulmonary artery and capillary wedge pressures and increased pulmonary arterial oxygen saturation. When PDA is diagnosed, the heart should be evaluated carefully for other congenital cardiac disease before surgical correction is attempted, because complex congenital malformations are the rule in foals with a PDA, and not the exception. Late complications of this lesion include rupture of the pulmonary artery.[369]

Lesions Causing Pulmonary to Systemic Shunting

Congenital cardiac anomalies associated with pulmonary to systemic shunting are invariably complex congenital cardiac diseases and are associated with a grave prognosis. The major factors determining the magnitude and direction of such shunts are the size of the communications between the chambers or vessels, the relative resistances and pressure differences between the chambers and vessels, ventricular outflow resistance, the diastolic compliance of the chambers and vessels, and the systolic function of the respective ventricles. For pulmonary to systemic shunting to occur, systemic pressures must develop in the right-sided cardiac chambers or vessels. Complex cyanotic congenital cardiac anomalies occur infrequently in foals, but most commonly in the Arabian breed.[3, 88–90, 94, 98, 99, 101, 354, 359, 363, 370]

Tetralogy of Fallot

The tetralogy of Fallot is one of the more common complex congenital cardiac anomalies in foals (Fig. 7–31).[89, 101] Tetralogy of Fallot is characterized by a VSD, RV outflow tract obstruction, cranial and rightward positioning (overriding) of the aorta, and RV hypertrophy. The severity of clinical signs in affected foals has to do with the size of the VSD and the degree of RV outflow tract obstruction, which is often due to a hypoplastic pulmonary artery, rather than a valvular pulmonic stenosis. Although it is possible for horses to live for a number of years with this lesion, most affected animals are humanely destroyed due to the poor prognosis for life. In some horses, a PDA is also present (pentalogy of Fallot) and serves to reduce symptoms by increasing pulmonary flow and LV filling. The condition must be distinguished from other cyanotic heart conditions, such as double-outlet right ventricle.[371]

Affected foals are usually smaller than normal, lethargic, and intolerant of exercise. Auscultation usually reveals a loud systolic murmur over the pulmonic valve area and a slightly softer systolic murmur over the right hemithorax. Cyanosis is most evident after exercise and may not be evident at rest. Polycythemia is usually mild, even when arterial oxygen tensions fall to 50 to 70 mm Hg. Echocardio-

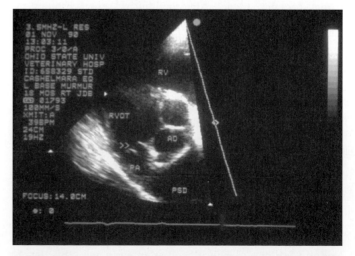

Figure 7–31. A two-dimensional echocardiogram from a filly with tetralogy of Fallot. A large ventricular septal defect is present between the right ventricular outflow tract (RVOT) and the subaortic region (Ao, aortic valve cusp observed in the oblique plane). The pulmonary artery eventually widens into a poststenotic dilatation (PSD). Shunting is bidirectional in this case.

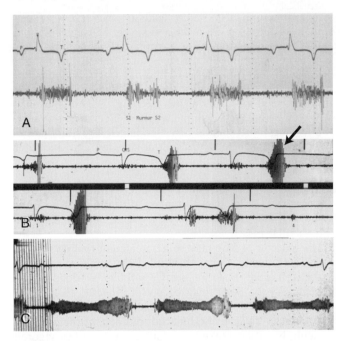

Figure 7-32. Phonocardiograms of cardiac murmurs due to valvular heart disease. *A,* A holosystolic murmur of mitral regurgitation in a horse with chronic valvular degeneration. *B,* A variable, late systolic murmur of mitral regurgitation related to mitral valve prolapse. The murmur has a crescendo and peaks at end-systole *(arrow).* Heart sounds are indicated. The murmur obscures the second sound. *C,* A holodiastolic, vibratory murmur of aortic regurgitation with presystolic accentuation is recorded. The accentuation is probably related to atrial contraction, altered ventricular volume and pressure, and an incremental increase in regurgitant volume.

graphic evaluation is diagnostic and reveals a large, unrestrictive VSD, RV outflow tract obstruction, malalignment and overriding of the aortic root, and RV hypertrophy. An injection of saline or other intravenous agent into the jugular vein results in a positive contrast echocardiogram, and the path of blood through the heart can be traced. Color flow and pulsed wave Doppler echocardiography can also be used to delineate the shunt and ventricular outflow obstruction. Affected foals have a poor to grave prognosis for life and should not be used or bred if they survive to adulthood.

Pulmonary Atresia and Persistent Truncus Arteriosus

These conditions may be virtually indistinguishable clinically and lead to similar clinical signs and outcome.[88, 89, 354, 372] Pulmonary hypoplasia and atresia are rare but have been observed most often in Arabian foals (see Fig. 7-31). This malformation represents the exaggerated form of tetralogy of Fallot. The RV outlet is atretic, the right ventricle hypertrophied, a large VSD is present in most cases, and the fetal truncus arteriosus has been partitioned unequally so that the aorta is markedly dilated and the pulmonary trunk is either atretic or severely hypoplastic (see Fig. 7-31). Without careful ultrasound studies or necropsy dissection,

the dilated aorta can be mistaken for a true persistent truncus arteriosus, hence the moniker "pseudotruncus arteriosus." Pulmonary blood flow must be derived from a PDA or from systemic collaterals via the bronchial arteries. This is in contrast to persistent truncus arteriosus, wherein the fetal truncus arteriosus never partitions and both ventricles continue to develop, communicating with the truncus arteriosus via a large VSD. Pulmonary blood flow in persistent truncus arteriosus arises from one or more pulmonary arteries, which arise from the truncus arteriosus. Foals with these conditions are often severely affected by hypoxia caused by a large right to left shunt. The magnitude of pulmonary blood flow is inversely related to the severity of systemic arterial hypoxemia, and if pulmonary flow is high, development to maturity is possible.

One important differential diagnosis for cyanotic heart conditions is tricuspid atresia,[97, 99, 359, 373] a malformation that dictates right to left shunting at the atrial level and leads to severe cyanosis. Affected foals rarely survive to weanling age owing to the severity of the right to left shunt. Foals are stunted and exhibit severe exercise intolerance and sinus tachycardia (> 100 beats/min). Arterial oxygen tension is often very low (40 to 60 mm Hg).

An ultrasound examination is the diagnostic method of choice in cyanotic heart disease. Each of these conditions, as well as many other complex malformations, may be recognized by echocardiography. Although the antemortem differentiation of pulmonary atresia and persistent truncus arteriosus may be difficult, the distinction is mainly academic. Contrast or Doppler echocardiography can characterize the abnormal blood flow patterns encountered in each of these conditions. The prognosis for life is grave.

ACQUIRED VALVULAR HEART DISEASE

Healthy cardiac valves maintain normal antegrade flow in the heart and prevent regurgitation of blood from high-pressure into low-pressure chambers. Diseased cardiac valves, which can be stenotic or incompetent, impair normal blood flow and place an increased workload on the heart. Although most stenotic lesions are congenital and quite rare, acquired valvular incompetency is commonly detected in horses.[12, 32, 38, 96, 97, 99, 103–107, 109, 112, 114–116, 285, 359, 373–386] Some lesions, notably bacterial endocarditis, cause valve incompetency but may also induce an acquired valvular stenosis. Important causes of valvular dysfunction are summarized in Table 7-2. Valvular incompetency and bacterial endocarditis are the valvular problems that are most often encountered by the equine practitioner and will be the focus of this section.

The severity of valvular regurgitation is highly dependent on the cross-section of the patent valve area, the pressure gradient across the valve, and the time allowed for regurgitation to occur. The movement of blood from a high to low pressure is associated with a high-velocity jet that is proportional to the pressure drop measured from source to sink. The production of these high-velocity jets leads to disturbed flow (including turbulence) and cardiac murmurs, the hallmark clinical feature of valvular heart disease (see Fig. 7-32). Doppler echocardiography is well suited for identification of these flow disturbances and is the clinical gold standard for verification of abnormal valvular function. The intensity of an insufficiency murmur is related not only to disturbed flow and physical characteristics of the thorax but also to the regurgitant volume. This is readily demonstrable in cases of "silent" tricuspid regurgitation wherein Doppler studies demonstrate a small regurgitant jet but auscultation is normal. Such valvular leaks—especially on the right side of the heart—are at this time considered within limits of normal, because they are commonly observed in healthy, high-performance horses as well as in normal individuals of other species. This is one reason why Doppler studies should not be performed outside of the context of a clinical examination. While the intensity of a heart murmur can be graded by the examiner (see earlier in this chapter), it is not possible to grade the severity of regurgitation by auscultation alone. Relatively loud murmurs may be associated with regurgitant volumes that are inconsequential to an individual horse. Thus, while valvular heart disease is best identified by auscultation (see Table 7–8), the clinical relevance of a valvular incompetency must be assessed by considering the animal's age, history, exercise capacity, and use and results of echocardiography.[216a–c, 308a, b] Commonly detected acquired valvular conditions are considered in this section.

Mitral Regurgitation

MR is one of the more common pathologic murmurs detected in horses.[3, 32, 34, 38, 56, 82, 114–116, 285, 377] The anatomical basis of mitral valve incompetency can be any of the following lesions: degenerative thickening, bacterial endocarditis, ruptured chordae tendineae, prolapse, myocardial disease with secondary cardiomegaly, noninfective mitral valvulitis, and congenital malformation of the valve (Figs. 7–33 and 7–34; see also Tables 7–8 and 7–9). Degenerative, fibrotic thickening of the mitral valve has been observed at necropsy in mature horses and is probably the basis of the mild to moderate MR observed in most horses.[17, 19] Ruptured mitral valve chordae tendineae can develop in animals of any age, including foals.[32, 114–116] Chordal ruptures (often involving the

accessory mitral cusps) may lead to severe loss of cusp support, resulting in pre-acute and severe MR and fulminant CHF. Conversely, small chordal ruptures, which may require diligent echocardiographic studies to visualize, can be associated with mitral prolapse or chronic MR without failure, including the musical, late-systolic crescendo murmur sometimes detected with this lesion (see Fig. 7–32). The mitral valve can be infected with the resultant ulceration or vegetation leading to substantial MR (see later). The authors have observed MR due to severe mitral scarring and thickening in weanlings and young horses. The cause of this is unknown but is thought to be nonsuppurative valvulitis, perhaps related to an immune-mediated process. Cardiomyopathy and myocarditis can lead to secondary dilatation of the mitral annulus or alteration of the papillary muscle support, permitting valvular insufficiency.

The murmur of MR may be an incidental finding detected during a routine examination. When MR is mild to moderate, neither left atrial dilatation nor LV volume overload may be present, and the horse may be performing satisfactorily. In other cases, however, MR is definitely associated with poor performance or exercise-induced pulmonary hemorrhage, particularly in the horse used for racing or other vigorous work. Some horses with MR develop atrial fibrillation. As with aortic regurgitation, if fever, weight loss, and lameness have occurred, the possibility of bacterial endocarditis should be entertained. Chordal rupture may cause severe left-sided CHF with pulmonary edema. This may progress to biventricular failure, or the horse may become severely limited by pulmonary dysfunction, even to the point of expectoration of edema (see Fig. 7–10). Chronic, hemodynamically significant MR from any cause can lead to pulmonary hypertension and secondary biventricular CHF, with clinical signs of right-sided CHF dominating the clinical presentation (see earlier in this chapter).[38, 114]

MR is identified by auscultation, which typically reveals a grade 2 to 5/6 holosystolic murmur. The murmur is detected most intensely over the left apex and mitral valve area (see Figs. 7–7 and 7–32). Often the murmur is loud

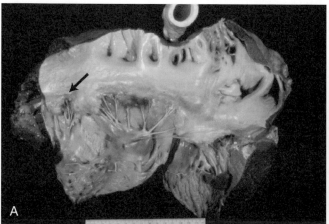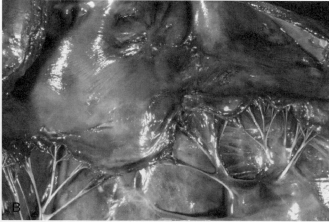

Figure 7–33. Postmortem lesions of mitral regurgitation (see also Fig. 7–40A). *A,* The opened left ventricle and left atrium are viewed from the caudal perspective. There is mild mitral valve fibrosis leading to thickening and incompetency. A jet lesion is evident *(arrow)* as well as modest left-sided heart enlargement. *B,* Chronic suppurative valvulitis due to chronic endocarditis has led to scarring, thickening, and distortion of the mitral valve. This horse developed severe left-sided congestive heart failure. Noninfective valvulitis is also recognized sporadically in horses, particularly in younger animals.

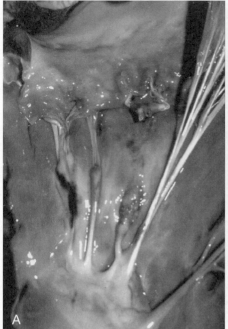
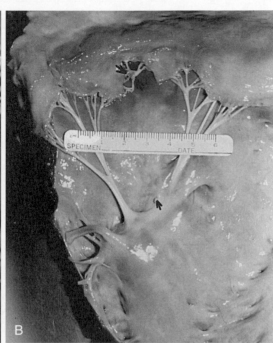

Figure 7–34. Rupture of the mitral valve chordae tendineae. *A,* Acute rupture of a chorda tendinea in a horse with lymphocytic plasmacytic valvulitis. The flail mitral cusp has actually twisted owing to loss of support. The ventral portion of the tear is obvious adjacent to intact chords. *B,* Chronic rupture of a chorda tendinea in a horse. Note the contraction of the scarred segments *(arrow).*

over or dorsal to the aortic valve, probably owing to the proximity of the septal mitral leaflet to the aortic valve or cranial projection of the regurgitant jet. The typical murmur is quite long (holosystolic or pansystolic), extending into the second sound.[38] This may cause the listener to misinterpret the third sound as the second, thus preventing a full appreciation of the significance of the murmur. Often the third sound is very loud, indicating volume overload or increased LV diastolic pressure. The murmur virtually always radiates dorsally, and often quite diffusely, but can also be projected caudally or cranially to the aortic valve area. Most moderate to loud murmurs of MR can also be heard well over the right chest, although the intensity is less. Since many horses with MR also have concomitant tricuspid regurgitation, echocardiographic examination and Doppler studies may be needed to differentiate bilateral AV valve insufficiency from isolated MR with radiation to the right. Variants of the MR murmur include the mid-to-late systolic crescendo murmur (see Fig. 7–32), which may be caused by minor chordal rupture or some other reason for mitral valve prolapse. In contrast with the typical situation of MR, wherein the regurgitation is worsened by LV dilatation, the murmur of mitral valve prolapse occurs after the left ventricle has begun ejection and decreased its volume, and valve support has become inadequate. This allows a mitral cusp to prolapse and regurgitation to begin in mid-systole. This type of murmur may be quite musical. Atrial fibrillation or premature beats may be detected, particularly in advanced cases.

Echocardiography and Doppler studies play a pivotal role in the assessment of the horse with MR (Fig. 7–35) and are indicated to examine the valve anatomy, the severity of MR, and the size and function of the atria and ventricles.[216a–c,] [378, 380] Severe MR causes LV volume overload with rounding of the LV apex and eventually increased end-diastolic dimension (see Table 7–13); however, in primary valvular disease, the myocardial function is normal to exuberant because

ventricular afterload is decreased by the incompetent valve (see Fig. 7–5B). The left atrium may take on a more circular, almost turgid, appearance when MR is hemodynamically significant, and the internal atrial dimension usually exceeds 13.5 cm by two-dimensional echocardiography. With acute or chronic MR, the lobar and main pulmonary artery may be dilated as a consequence of pulmonary hypertension, presumably related to increased LA pressure, interstitial lung edema, or both. The underlying cause of MR may be obvious from the echocardiography examination. Dilated cardiomyopathy is characterized by reduced LV shortening fraction. Mild to moderate thickening of the mitral valve leaflets is suggestive of degeneration or nonbacterial valvulitis. Prolapse of the mitral valve cusps has been observed in horses with MR, but the true limits of "normal" prolapse require further study. Lesions due to vegetative endocarditis cause the valves to appear irregularly thickened or shortened. Chordal rupture is recognized by observing chaotic flutter of a mitral structure (a flail leaflet), prolapse of a portion of the valve into the atrium, or the chordal remnant (it is usually contracted) flipping into the atrium during systole (see Fig. 7–35).[115, 116] High-frequency systolic vibrations of the mitral valve may be seen on the M-mode study in horses with a musical murmur of MR. Pulsed or continuous wave or color-flow Doppler studies can identify the mitral regurgitant jet (see Fig. 7–35). In most horses, this examination must be performed from the left cardiac window. High-velocity or turbulent jets may be difficult to find without a complete and thorough examination of the mitral valve. When color-flow Doppler demonstrates both a wide origin of the regurgitant jet and a pattern of diffuse distribution of turbulence deep into the left atrium, the likelihood of hemodynamically significant MR is greater.

The prognosis for horses with MR is variable and, as discussed earlier, is related to clinical findings, work history, and results of echocardiographic studies. Abnormalities ob-

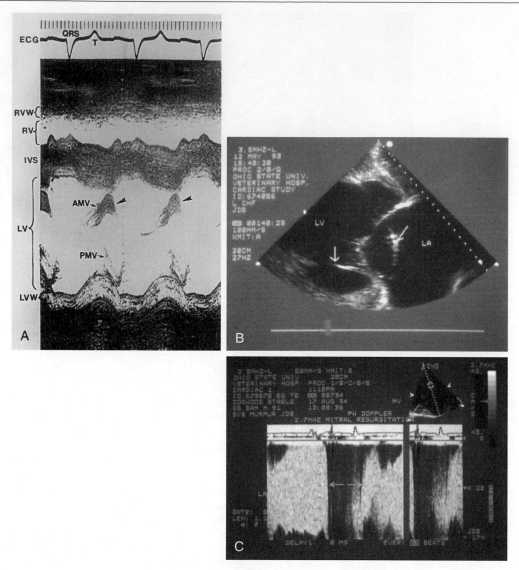

Figure 7–35. Echocardiograms recorded from horses with mitral regurgitation. *A,* M-mode study demonstrating marked thickening of the anterior mitral valve (AMV) leaflet *(arrows).* This would be compatible with endocarditis or severe valvulitis. (RVW, right ventricular wall; LVW, left ventricular wall.) *B,* Flail mitral leaflet *(right arrow)* in a horse with multiple chordae ruptures. The prolapsed portion of the mitral valve forms a curved echodense line in the dilated left atrium, whereas the other valve portions are to the left of this echocardiogram. A normal chord is evident *(left arrow). C,* Pulsed wave Doppler study recorded from the left atrium demonstrating a turbulent, high-velocity, aliased systolic jet of mitral regurgitation in a Thoroughbred horse. The duration of the event is shown *(arrows).*

served during echocardiography, including lesions of the mitral valve leaflets, the degree of LA and LV volume overloading, global LV function, and Doppler findings, should be considered when formulating the prognosis. Certainly, when MR is associated with CHF, atrial fibrillation, endocarditis, chordal rupture, marked cardiomegaly, severe valvular thickening, dilated cardiomyopathy, or pulmonary hypertension, the prognosis for life or performance is poor. The detection of pulmonary artery dilatation indicates significant pulmonary hypertension and the possibility of pulmonary artery rupture; therefore, such a horse should not be ridden or driven due to the low, but concrete risk of sudden death. Fortunately, many mature horses with MR appear to perform very well, suggesting that the incompetency is not always clinically important. Whether progressive exercise intolerance will develop in the future depends on the horse's

use and on the progression of the underlying mitral lesion. In most cases of MR caused by valve degeneration, the progression appears to be slow and gradual. Thus, MR associated with degenerative changes of the mitral valve leaflets in mature or older horses without clinical signs of heart disease carries a favorable prognosis for life, and performance may be well maintained. The analogous situation in a colt or filly should be less encouraging, and the presence of even mild to moderate LA dilatation implies a poor overall prognosis. The significance of apparently mild MR in the high performance horse or racehorse may be difficult to discern. Treadmill exercise may demonstrate a higher heart rate for a given level of work than might otherwise be expected, and this finding may be suggestive of a cardiac limitation to performance. Regardless of cause or severity of the condition, the horse diagnosed with MR merits follow-up examinations to evaluate progression of this hemodynamic burden and to detect the development of CHF, pulmonary hypertension, or cardiac arrhythmias. Treatment of MR involves management of complications such as heart failure, endocarditis, or arrhythmias. These topics are covered elsewhere in this chapter.

Aortic Regurgitation

Aortic regurgitation is a common valvular insufficiency.[1, 3, 12, 17, 18, 96, 103, 148, 375, 378a, 379, 380] Degeneration of the aortic valve is by far the most common reason for aortic regurgitation, although other potential causes are bacterial endocarditis, congenital valvular disease, VSD (see earlier in this chapter), noninfective valvulitis, idiopathic prolapse, and ruptured aortic sinus aneurysm (see Tables 7–8 and 7–9). The idiopathic degenerative nodular lesions and fibrous bands responsible for aortic regurgitation in older horses have been well described by Bishop and associates[375] (Fig. 7–36). Small fenestrations of the valve are often identified at necropsy but have uncertain clinical significance.

In most horses, aortic regurgitation is an incidental finding detected during a routine physical, pre-purchase, or insurance examination. Most horses with this murmur are older than 10 years of age, and the murmur is very common in aged horses, a testament to the degenerative nature of the lesion. Careful auscultation in a quiet area may identify a very soft diastolic murmur in a younger horse, and it is not uncommon to identify a small jet of aortic regurgitation by Doppler studies in mature horses with no identifiable murmur. When a prominent murmur of aortic regurgitation is identified in a younger animal, other causes should be considered. Poor performance is an infrequent presenting complaint in horses with aortic regurgitation, because most will continue at their prior performance level, provided that no other clinical or cardiac abnormalities are present. Intermittent fevers, weight loss, or lameness should prompt consideration of endocarditis. CHF is infrequently observed in conjunction with severe aortic regurgitation or the combination of aortic regurgitation with mitral disease or atrial fibrillation.

Aortic regurgitation is identified by cardiac auscultation, which reveals a holodiastolic murmur, with the point of maximal intensity over the aortic valve area, and radiation to the right and toward the left cardiac apex. The murmur may vary greatly in intensity. The quality is typically harsh and decrescendo ("blowing"), but there may be presystolic accentuation (see Fig. 7–32C) or the quality may be musical, "cooing," or buzzing. A precordial thrill is palpated over the aortic valve area when the murmur is loud. Atrial fibrillation, atrial premature depolarizations, and ventricular extrasystoles have infrequently been associated with aortic regurgitation. The quality of the arterial pulses is a good indicator of the severity of the isolated aortic regurgitation.[103] Bounding arterial pulses indicate a significant LV volume overload and moderate to severe aortic regurgitation. A systolic ejection murmur is often present, particularly when the regurgitant volume is large. This can be explained by ejection of a greater-than-normal stroke volume across the aortic valve. There is no compelling evidence that the degenerative aortic valve is anatomically stenotic. A complete echocardiographic examination including Doppler echocardiography is useful for further evaluation of horses with aortic regurgitation, particularly when the pulse is abnormal or cardiac-related clinical signs are suspected.

A number of echocardiographic abnormalities may be identified in horses with aortic regurgitation (Fig. 7–37).[82, 96, 103, 104, 148, 216a–c, 378a] Thickening of the aortic valve leaflets is common. Prolapse of one of the aortic valve cusps may be observed. Fenestrations of the aortic valve leaflets, flail aortic leaflet, aortic sinus aneurysm, or the thick, irregular, echogenic lesions of bacterial endocarditis are rarely detected. High-frequency diastolic vibrations of the septal leaflet of the mitral valve are commonly observed on M-mode recordings, related to the high-velocity regurgitant jet entering the LV outflow tract. Similar vibrations may also be detected on the intraventricular septum when the regurgitant jet is directed toward this structure. High-frequency fluttering of the aortic valve leaflets or aortic walls may be detected with

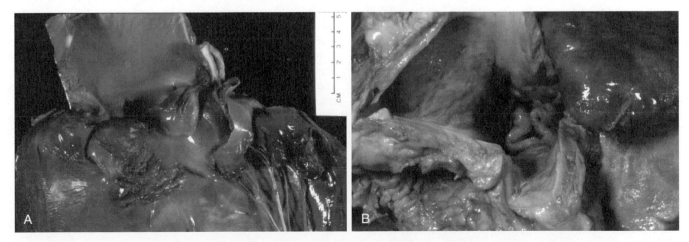

Figure 7–36. Postmortem lesions of aortic regurgitation (see also Fig. 7–40B). *A,* A segment of the left ventricular outflow tract and the ascending aorta. Linear bands are evident on the two valves shown, and a large jet lesion is also observed below the valves. This is a typical lesion in aged horses. *B,* The aortic valve viewed from the ascending aorta. There is severe thickening caused by noninfective valvulitis and scarring.

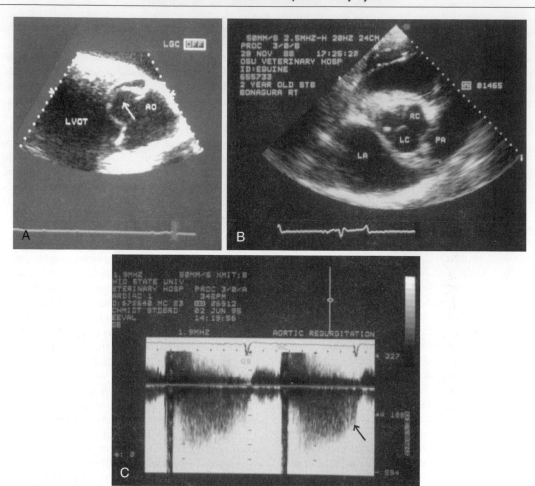

Figure 7–37. Echocardiograms recorded from horses with aortic regurgitation (see also Fig. 7–20C). *A,* Aortic valve prolapse *(arrow)* in a 12-year-old Standardbred gelding. *B,* A well-circumscribed, echodense "bead" on the noncoronary cusp of the aortic valve in a 2-year-old Standardbred colt. This short-axis image plane is recorded across the base of the heart. This may represent a congenital or acquired lesion. *C,* Continuous wave Doppler recording from the same horse as seen in Figure 7–37*A,* demonstrating a turbulent diastolic signal that ends at the QRS complex *(arrow).*

fenestrations, flail leaflet, or musical murmurs. Dilatation of the aortic root (even exceeding 10 cm) may be observed in horses with aortic regurgitation. Premature mitral closure and increased mitral valve E-point to septal separation may be consequences of mild aortic regurgitation with a suitably oriented jet that impinges on the valve or develop when severe aortic regurgitation causes ventricular dilatation and elevated ventricular end-diastolic pressure. In the latter case, other markers of severe insufficiency will be evident including ventricular dilatation; rounding of the LV apex; a strong, long, and wide-origin Doppler signal of aortic regurgitation; and a short pressure half-time. The LV volume overload that develops with aortic regurgitation leads to increased ventricular internal diameter at end-diastole, increased shortening fraction, and decreased free-wall thickness.[103] If myocardial failure develops, the end-systolic dimension may be increased, despite normal shortening fraction. Rounding of the LV apex and an exaggerated or swinging septal motion represent subjective observations of volume overloading on real-time two-dimensional echocardiographic examination.

The clinical significance and prognosis of aortic regurgita-tion is most accurately based on the history, physical examination, and echocardiogram. As most cases of aortic regurgitation are associated with a slow degeneration of the aortic valve leaflets, and this occurs in older horses without other cardiac problems, the prognosis for life and performance is usually good. Such animals typically have minimal echocardiographic abnormalities or only mild echocardiographic signs of volume overload. The findings of flail aortic valve leaflet, endocarditis, or echo markers of moderate to severe volume overload or myocardial failure indicate a poor prognosis for life and performance. Periodic re-examinations are indicated for horses with moderate to severe aortic regurgitation. The development of secondary MR, atrial fibrillation, or CHF should be anticipated in horses with severe volume overload.

Tricuspid Regurgitation

Tricuspid regurgitation may be the most frequently detected pathologic murmur in the horse, although there is virtually nothing written about this common disorder. The anatomical basis of tricuspid valve incompetency can be any of the following lesions: idiopathic, degenerative thickening, non-infective tricuspid valvulitis, bacterial endocarditis, pulmonary hypertension (including left-sided failure), ruptured chordae tendineae, myocardial disease with secondary cardiomegaly, and congenital malformation of the valve. Tricuspid regurgitation is relatively common in horses of racing age;[113a, 380] however, the anatomical correlate to this incompetency is uncertain. Degenerative, fibrotic thickening of the tricuspid valve in mature horses may lead to mild to moderate tricuspid regurgitation. When compared with the mitral condition, ruptured tricuspid valve chordae tendineae are uncommon[380] and better tolerated. The tricuspid valve can be infected by bacteria, and in some cases this is likely to be secondary to an injudicious or septic jugular venipuncture or catheterization. Pulmonary hypertension, cardiomyopathy, and myocarditis can lead to secondary dilatation of the tricuspid annulus or alteration of the papillary muscle support permitting valvular insufficiency. Tricuspid malformation does occur but seems more commonly associated with stenosis or atresia of the valve (see earlier in this chapter).[94, 99, 359]

The systolic murmur of tricuspid regurgitation may be an incidental finding detected during a routine examination. The murmur becomes more problematic when identified in a horse that is performing poorly. Many horses with tricuspid regurgitation race very well; therefore, the clinician should first exclude other likely reasons for poor performance before incriminating the tricuspid valve. Of course, if chronic hemodynamically significant tricuspid regurgitation has developed, then peak work effort will suffer and even right-sided CHF may develop. The latter situation is not common unless the tricuspid regurgitation is secondary to pulmonary hypertension or bacterial endocarditis.

Auscultation of the horse with tricuspid regurgitation typically reveals a grade 2 to 5/6 holosystolic murmur with the point of maximal intensity over the right hemithorax at the tricuspid valve area (see Fig. 7–8, Tables 7–8 and 7–9). The murmur can be holosystolic, decrescendo, or telesystolic. While the timing and intensity may at times remind the examiner of a functional murmur, the location of greatest murmur intensity argues against that possibility. The murmur usually radiates dorsally and at times to the extreme left cranial thorax. Atrial fibrillation or atrial premature beats are present in some horses with tricuspid regurgitation, particularly when the right atrium is dilated or the regurgitant jet is large.

Echocardiography including Doppler studies is useful in the assessment of tricuspid regurgitation (Fig. 7–38). Examinations of the tricuspid valve are typically performed from the right hemithorax, because the tricuspid valve and RV inlet are closer to the right thoracic wall; however, an extreme left cranial transducer location can also be successful for examining tricuspid flow. Since there are a number of potential reasons for tricuspid incompetency, careful attention must be directed to the valve and its support apparatus, the size of the pulmonary artery, and the left side of the heart. Doppler echocardiographic estimates of tricuspid regurgitant volume should be done if available. As with mitral regurgitation previously described, moderate to severe tricuspid regurgitation leads to RA and RV volume overload; however, it is more difficult to quantify these chamber volumes owing to their complex geometry. The underlying cause of tricuspid regurgitation may be obvious from the examination, although it is emphasized that a clear-cut lesion of the tricuspid valve leaflet is often not be detected. The two-dimensional echocardiography study is valuable, however, because valve thickening, prolapse, vegetations, chordal rupture, regurgitation secondary to RV dilatation, and pulmonary hypertension can usually be diagnosed or excluded. Doppler studies can identify the tricuspid regurgitant jet.[216a–c] In trivial or "silent"

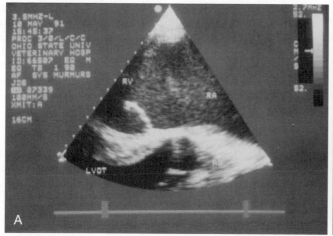
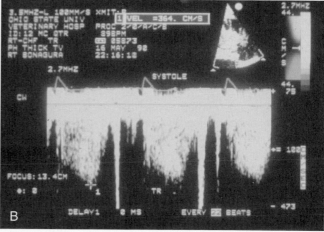

Figure 7–38. Echocardiograms from horses with tricuspid regurgitation (see also Fig. 7–23*C*). *A,* Two-dimensional echocardiogram demonstrating probable valve thickening, marked right atrial distention, and spontaneous right atrial contrast in a horse with severe tricuspid regurgitation, atrial fibrillation, and congestive heart failure (1-cm calibrations at the left of the sector; LVOT = left ventricular outflow tract). *B,* Continuous wave Doppler recording of a high-velocity tricuspid regurgitation jet from a horse with tricuspid regurgitation caused by pulmonary artery obstruction, secondary to a mass lesion. The high velocity of regurgitation, over 3.6 m/sec, indicates that elevated right ventricular pressure is driving the regurgitant jet. In this case, the high pressure is caused by supravalvular pulmonary stenosis due to the tumor. Tricuspid regurgitation jets associated with normal right ventricular pressures are typically less than 2.6 m/sec.

tricuspid regurgitation, this jet is typically oriented toward the aorta when evaluating the valve from the right hemithorax. When the jet is very wide at its origin, or projects more centrally into the right atrium, cardiomegaly seems more common. The RV systolic pressure can be estimated by faithfully recording the peak jet velocity. When the jet velocity is less than 2.5 m/sec, pulmonary hypertension is not present. Jets exceeding 3.2 to 3.4 m/sec are generally indicative of pulmonary hypertension (provided that there is no outflow obstruction or VSD [see Fig. 7–38]). The presence of pulmonary hypertension should also prompt careful examination of the left heart, because the main cardiac lesion may be centered over the mitral valve, aortic valve, or LV muscle.

The prognosis for horses with tricuspid regurgitation is generally quite favorable.[380] As with MR, the presence of tricuspid regurgitation is more likely to cause concern if there is right-sided cardiomegaly, pulmonary hypertension, or atrial fibrillation. Abnormalities detected during echocardiography of the tricuspid valve leaflets may be instructive because the visualization of a vegetation would indicate a poor prognosis for performance and a guarded prognosis for life. The width of the regurgitant jet at its origin and recent performance history are useful in developing a prognosis for life and future work, because tricuspid regurgitation may not be a limiting factor in many performance animals. It would be interesting to determine if exercise and the associated pulmonary hypertension worsen the degree of tricuspid regurgitation. Perhaps increased use of exercise testing and post-exercise echocardiography will provide answers to this question. Periodic re-examinations are indicated with tricuspid regurgitation to follow the progression of the lesion and to detect cardiomegaly or cardiac arrhythmias if they develop.

Pulmonary Insufficiency

Clinically significant pulmonic insufficiency is uncommon and occurs most frequently with pulmonary hypertension associated with primary MR or other causes of left-sided heart failure. A rare cause of this is rupture of the pulmonary valve.[381] Murmurs of pulmonic regurgitation are usually undetectable unless the regurgitant volume is large or is driven by pulmonary hypertension; however, it can be identified using pulsed-wave and color-flow Doppler echocardiography. Dilatation of the pulmonary artery may be detected echocardiographically when pulmonic insufficiency is caused by pulmonary hypertension (Fig. 7–39). Bacterial endocarditis and congenital abnormalities of the valve leaflets (bicuspid or quadricuspid) have been observed, but these are rare causes of pulmonary insufficiency.[112, 352] Trivial and clinically silent, physiologic pulmonic insufficiency can often be detected by Doppler studies; however, this is a normal finding.

When severe pulmonic regurgitation does develop, it is generally a consequence of left-sided heart failure and is accompanied by clinical signs of biventricular failure, including increased respiratory rate and effort. Signs of right-sided CHF occur as a consequence of pulmonary hypertension, pulmonic regurgitation, RV volume overload, and tricuspid regurgitation. If a murmur of pulmonic regurgitation is detected, it is usually holodiastolic and a decrescendo murmur, with the point of maximal intensity at the pulmonic valve area, radiating toward the right cardiac apex. The

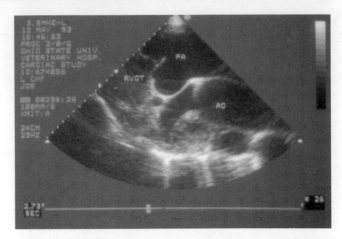

Figure 7–39. Left cranial, oblique image plane echocardiogram demonstrating a dilated pulmonary artery (PA). The cause was pulmonary hypertension secondary to left-sided congestive heart failure. The ascending aorta (Ao) and right ventricular outflow tract (RVOT) are indicated; however, this plane is not suitable for evaluating other structures.

prognosis for life and performance is usually poor in these cases.

Bacterial Endocarditis

Bacterial endocarditis is caused by invasion of the heart valves or endocardium by bacteria. Endocarditis is not common in horses but occurs sporadically in most populations.[82, 103–112, 115, 294, 309, 374, 376, 382–386] Horses of any age may be affected, although the pathogenesis may differ in younger animals or in those that are immunosuppressed. Numerous bacteria have been associated with bacterial endocarditis. The offending microorganism likely depends on the environment, portal of entry (e.g., gastrointestinal tract, skin, lung, oral cavity, or surgical wound), and the effects of prior antibiotic therapy that may select for resistant strains. *Streptococcus* sp. and *Actinobacillus equuli* have been isolated most frequently, whereas *Rhodococcus equi*, *Pasteurella* sp., *Candida parapsilosis*, *Erysipelothrix rhusiopathiae*, meningococci, *Staphylococcus aureus,* and other organisms have also been isolated.[108, 109, 111, 376, 385, 386]

The pathogenesis involves bacterial invasion from the bloodstream and colonization of the heart valve or endocardial surfaces. Bacteremia is a prerequisite for development of this condition. Direct invasion of a previously normal valve by virulent bacteria, or in the context of overwhelming sepsis, represents the most likely pathogenic mechanism involved in foals with bacterial endocarditis. Disruption of the endocardial surface by jet lesions associated with congenital intracardiac shunts may also predispose to endocarditis, although this mechanism is not well established in horses. Pre-existing valvular heart disease with endocardial changes or high-velocity jets may represent risk factors for bacterial colonization in older horses. The most common sites of bacterial endocarditis are the aortic and mitral valves, although endocarditis lesions have been reported on all cardiac valves. Mural endocarditis lesions have also been reported but occur much less frequently.[69, 227, 239, 300] The combination of bacterial injury, exposure of valve collagen, thrombosis, and host leukocyte response contributes to the development of a vegetation (Fig. 7–40), which consists microscopically of bacteria, platelets, fibrin, leukocytes, and varying degrees of granulation or fibrosis. Bacteria may not be evident at necropsy, especially if antimicrobial therapy has sterilized the vegetation.

The pathophysiology of endocarditis in horses is probably similar to that in other species. A host response, as well as the primary cardiac lesions, contributes to the morbidity of this disease. Cardiac manifestations include valvular injury leading to regurgitation and less often to stenosis; secondary cardiomegaly; myocarditis from extension of the infection or through coronary embolization; myocardial infarction if emboli are shed to the coronary arteries; arrhythmias from cardiomegaly or myocarditis; and myocardial depression from bacteremia. Recurrent or chronic bacteremia, and hence fever, is characteristic of endocarditis. Metastatic infection, distant thrombosis and infarction, and immune-mediated host responses can occur. Distant infection or immune complex disease can lead to multisystemic clinical signs, including arthritis, osteomyelitis, vasculitis, or nephritis. Right-sided

thrombi can lead to pulmonary thrombi, infarction, or lung abscess (see Fig. 7–40).[112, 374]

Clinical features of endocarditis are variable. Affected horses usually have a history of intermittent fever, weight loss, depression, anorexia, lethargy, and often intermittent lameness (Fig. 7–41). A predisposing condition or a concurrent infection may be evident, including jugular vein thrombophlebitis, strangles, or an abscess. In most horses there is no history of previous illness and no evidence of concurrent infection. The physical examination often reveals fever, and some horses may be tachypneic. The fever is often intermittent. Murmurs of mitral or aortic valvular insufficiency are most commonly detected; those of tricuspid regurgitation are less common. Systolic murmurs caused by valve destruction must be differentiated from the physiologic flow murmurs that are heard so often in febrile horses (see Table 7–8). Murmurs of valvular stenosis may also be detected with bacterial endocarditis but occur infrequently.[112] Some horses with bacterial endocarditis have no auscultatable murmurs or the quality or intensity of the murmur changes over a number of days. Atrial fibrillation, atrial or ventricular premature depolarizations, and ventricular tachycardia have been

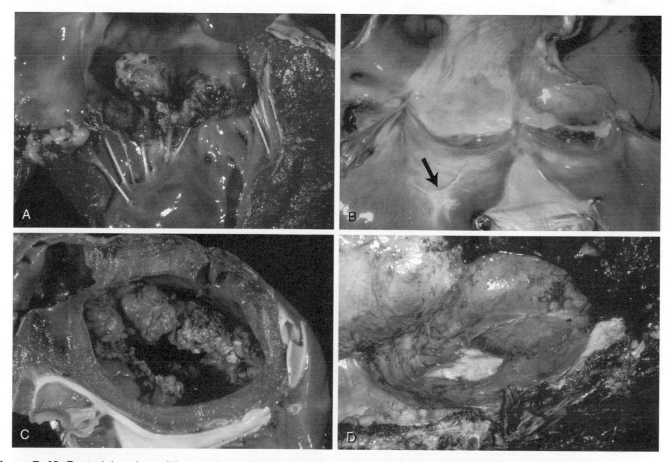

Figure 7–40. Bacterial endocarditis—postmortem lesions. *A,* Severe mitral valve endocarditis in a yearling. *B,* Focal aortic valve endocarditis is evident in this view of the left ventricular outlet and the ascending aorta. The septal mitral leaflet is at the lower right, and a jet lesion *(arrow)* can be observed in the left ventricular outflow tract. Above the mitral leaflet, in the center of the left coronary cusp, is a raised, irregular vegetation that caused aortic regurgitation. *C,* Tricuspid valve vegetation in a weanling. Although less common than mitral or aortic vegetations, right-sided endocarditis is a definite risk in horses, particularly in animals subjected to repeated jugular venous catheterization. *D,* A lung abscess in a horse following pulmonary valve endocarditis. The center of the abscess is incised and reveals caseous exudate. Systemic embolization and metastatic infection are recognized complications of valvular infections.

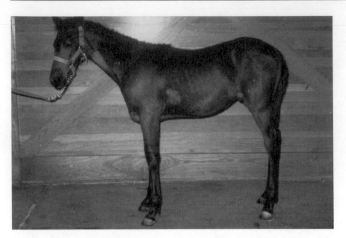

Figure 7–41. Weight loss, loss of condition, and ventral edema in this weanling with endocarditis and right-sided congestive heart failure (see also Fig. 7–40C).

observed with bacterial endocarditis.[106, 111] Swelling of the joints or tendon sheaths may be noted.

Laboratory studies obtained from horses with bacterial endocarditis may reveal anemia, hyperproteinemia, elevated fibrinogen, and leukocytosis with a mature neutrophilia. Multiple blood cultures should be performed when bacterial endocarditis is suspected. The result of blood cultures may be negative, however, particularly after antimicrobial therapy. A positive blood culture is more likely to be obtained if multiple samples are drawn at different times of the day during or after febrile episodes.

Diagnosis of bacterial endocarditis should be considered in any horse that presents with a fever of unknown origin and the aforementioned clinical signs. Endocarditis is most likely when the cause of fever cannot be isolated to another body system and concurrent cardiac disease is suspected. The diagnosis is confirmed with positive blood cultures in the setting of compatible clinical findings or by echocardiographic detection of vegetative lesions on the valve leaflets or endocardial surface (Fig. 7–42). Vegetative lesions usually

appear echocardiographically as thickened, echogenic to hyperechoic masses with irregular or "shaggy" edges. The lesion adheres to the endocardium (and therefore more with the valve), and the valve leaflet usually demonstrates diffuse thickening as well. With time, the lesion may contract or develop a smoother contour. Rupture of the chordae tendineae or avulsion of a valve leaflet may also be detected echocardiographically, and this complication is not uncommon in mitral or tricuspid valve endocarditis. Pulsed-wave and color-flow Doppler echocardiography can be used to confirm that the valve is incompetent or (rarely) stenotic. Valvular regurgitation often progresses because of continued damage to the valve leaflets associated with ongoing bacterial infection or subsequent to fibrosis associated with a bacteriologic cure.

Treatment of bacterial endocarditis should consist of high levels of bactericidal antibiotics, administered parenterally, and ideally based on culture and sensitivity patterns of blood culture isolates. Drugs that penetrate fibrin well, particularly potassium penicillin (22,000 to 44,000 IU/kg every 6 hours), are reasonable initial choices because bacteria may be sequestered in fibrin and may be unavailable to leukocytes. Intravenous therapy is preferred in the initial stages of treatment. To extend the antimicrobial spectrum, gentamicin sulfate (3.3 mg/kg, intravenously every 8 hours) may be administered. Erythromycin (20 mg/kg every 6 hours intravenously or orally) or rifampin (5 to 10 mg/kg every 12 hours orally) may be useful in some cases. Initial therapy should be broad spectrum, until the results of the blood culture are known, or when a positive blood culture cannot be obtained. Therapy should extend to at least 4 weeks and as long as 8 weeks. The duration and type of long-term therapy depend on numerous factors, and the bacterial isolate, clinical response, cost, and potential toxicosis of the antimicrobials must all be weighed in these decisions.

A poor expectation for survival is appropriate as the initial prognosis in any case of established bacterial endocarditis. Even in the absence of significant valvular regurgitation, there may be difficulty in achieving a bacteriologic cure, or progressive valvular damage may occur as the vegetation heals and scars the valve. Although some horses have been

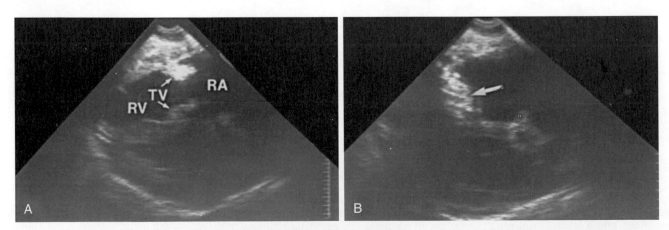

Figure 7–42. Two-dimensional echocardiogram of tricuspid valve endocarditis *(arrows)*, acquired rupture of the chordae tendineae, and flail tricuspid valve. The movement of the valve from diastole *(A)* to systole *(B)* is evident and is typical of a valvular involvement. The valve is highly echogenic and very thick, which is typical of chronic infection. (RA, right atrium; RV, right ventricle; TV, tricuspid valve.)

treated successfully for bacterial endocarditis,[382] overall, there is a low likelihood of long-term survival with continued use of the horse as a performance animal or in breeding. The absence of an obvious echocardiographic lesion is a favorable prognostic sign provided that a bacteriologic cure can be obtained. Progressive cardiomegaly, CHF, rupture of the pulmonary artery, atrial fibrillation, or sudden death have been reported in horses affected with endocarditis. Accordingly, periodic follow-up examination, including echocardiograms, should be performed in successfully treated cases.

PERICARDIAL DISEASE

Pericardial diseases occur uncommonly and are usually associated with pericardial effusion and fibrinous pericarditis.[61–70, 73, 74, 105, 107, 277, 294, 387–391] Pericarditis and pericardial effusion may be idiopathic, bacterial, viral, or traumatic in origin or associated with cardiac or pericardial neoplasia. Pericardial hernias have also been seen but are rare. Not all cases of pericarditis are septic; sterile suppurative, mixed, and eosinophilic effusates have been recognized,[67, 69, 391, 391a] although the possibility of an infectious etiology should be considered until proven otherwise. The pathogenesis of non-infective pericarditis is unknown. The pathophysiology of pericardial disease in the horse can be ascribed to cardiac compression (tamponade), constriction with impairment of filling, or the presence of a mass lesion having an impact on the heart. Other clinical signs may be referable to the underlying cause, including infection or neoplasia. The clinical syndrome of pericardial effusion with tamponade is characterized by impairment of RV filling, increases in ventricular filling pressures (Fig. 7–43), reduced systemic arterial blood pressure, and signs of right-sided CHF.

The history usually includes systemic signs of illness, such as fever, colic, lethargy, depression, anorexia, tachypnea, ventral edema, and weight loss. External thoracic trauma or penetration by a gastric foreign body may lead to

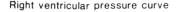

Right ventricular pressure curve

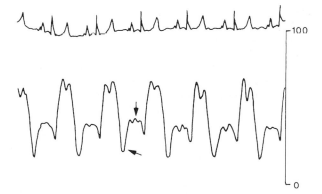

Figure 7–43. Pressure tracing demonstrating elevated right ventricular end-diastolic pressure in a horse with constrictive pericarditis and heart failure. There is a quick rise from the nadir of pressure *(lower arrow)* to a plateau *(upper arrow)*, which is typical of constrictive disease and ventricular filling that is limited to early diastole.

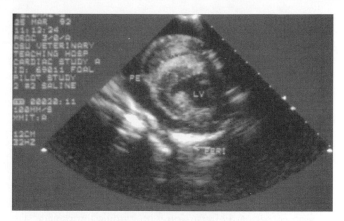

Figure 7–44. Two-dimensional echocardiogram demonstrating a small to moderate pericardial effusion (PE) in a foal. The echo-free space surrounds both ventricles in this short-axis tomogram. The brightly echodense parietal pericardium is readily observed (PERI).

bacterial inoculation of the pericardial space.[62, 66, 388] A recent history of an upper or lower respiratory tract infection is not uncommon. Physical examination abnormalities include tachycardia, muffled heart sounds, tachypnea, jugular and generalized venous distention, fever, pericardial friction rub, ventral edema, pleural effusion, thready pulses, and ascites. Arterial blood pressure may be decreased in cardiac tamponade.

Laboratory studies are contributory to the diagnosis. Clinical laboratory abnormalities are not specific, but the most frequently detected abnormalities include anemia, hyperproteinemia, hyperfibrinogenemia, and a neutrophilic leukocytosis. Other hematologic abnormalities may be observed related to inflammation, CHF, or organ hypoperfusion. Thoracic radiographs usually reveal a globoid cardiac silhouette or pleural effusion and may reveal interstitial pulmonary infiltrates and enlarged pulmonary vessels. The ECG usually demonstrates decreased amplitude of the QRS complexes. If the effusion is large and the heart is swinging, electrical alternans may be observed. Pericarditis may elevate the ST segment, but this change may occur simply as a result of tachycardia. Sinus tachycardia is typical, although ventricular or atrial premature complexes may be detected. The echocardiographic examination is diagnostic, because an anechoic or hypoechoic fluid space is detected between the pericardium and epicardial surface of the heart (Fig. 7–44). Fibrin tags are frequently seen on the parietal and visceral pericardial surfaces and on the epicardial surfaces of the heart. Diastolic collapse of the right ventricle or systolic collapse of the right atrium are diagnostic of cardiac tamponade. Associated pleural effusion is easily detected by ultrasound and is an expected finding. Extracardiac mass lesions, which can mimic pericardial disease, can also be excluded by echocardiography.[74] Right-sided heart catheterization is rarely needed to establish the diagnosis of tamponade or constriction; however, when done, this procedure is characterized by increased central venous pressure, elevated RV diastolic pressure, and possibly by a diastolic dip and plateau appearance to the RV waveform (see Fig. 7–43).[68]

Cytologic evaluation of the pericardial effusion is essential to distinguish septic, aseptic, or neoplastic pericardial effusion. Fluid can be obtained in the course of needle pericardiocentesis or during the placement of an indwelling catheter for pericardial lavage and drainage. Bacterial culture and sensitivity of the aspirated fluid should be performed so that antimicrobial therapy can be guided in cases of septic pericarditis. *Streptococcus* sp. have most frequently been reported with pericarditis, but *Actinobacillus equii, Pseudomonas aeruginosa, Pasteurella* sp., and mycoplasma have been isolated, and equine influenza and viral arteritis have been associated with fibrinous pericarditis.

The treatment of pericardial diseases varies, depending on the cause and clinical situation. Pericardiocentesis or catheter drainage is appropriate in all cases of infective pericardial effusion or pericardial effusion with cardiac tamponade. Because the development of cardiac tamponade depends not only on the volume of pericardial fluid but also on the rate at which it accumulates, the clinician's urgency should be guided by echocardiographic or clinical signs of cardiac tamponade. Tamponade is an indication for aggressive drainage of the pericardial sac. Echocardiography can be used to safely localize a site for pericardiocentesis and choose an appropriate length of needle, catheter, or drainage tube. Pericardiocentesis should be performed after locally anesthetizing the intercostal muscles and pleura. Electrocardiographic monitoring should be performed continuously during the procedure to monitor for cardiac puncture or in case ventricular arrhythmias develop. Pericardiocentesis is usually performed within the left fifth intercostal space, above the level of the lateral thoracic vein, although it can also be performed at the right hemithorax. Drainage is achieved using a large-bore catheter, teat cannula, or chest tube; the latter is recommended for repeated drainage and lavage of the pericardial sac and is most successful for aggressive management of septic or idiopathic fibrinous pericarditis. After insertion of an indwelling catheter, pericardial lavage and direct instillation of antimicrobials, combined with systemic antimicrobials, have been shown to be effective in the treatment of septic pericarditis.[67] Pericardial lavage should be continued for several days, until there is little accumulation of pericardial fluid (< 1 liter) over 12 hours, clinical signs have improved and the cytologic character of the fluid becomes less inflammatory. If the cytologic analysis and culture are negative for bacteria, anti-inflammatory doses of dexamethasone may be used for treatment of idiopathic, nonseptic, effusive pericarditis.[69, 391] Surgery is a rarely used option for treatment of pericardial disease but would be most appropriate for constrictive or constrictive-effusive pericarditis.[68]

The prognosis for survival and maintenance of performance in horses affected by pericardial disease is guarded, because the condition may become chronic. The potential of eventual constrictive or fibrotic pericardial disease is greatest with infective or inflammatory pericardial conditions so that early success may be tempered by later complications of the disease.[69] The best prognosis of horses with fibrinous pericarditis is when treatment includes repeated drainage and lavage. Horses treated by catheter drainage should be carefully followed and re-evaluated by echocardiography. The prognosis for cardiac or pericardial neoplasia is quite poor.

MYOCARDIAL DISEASE

Myocardial disease probably occurs more frequently than has been previously recognized, although there are few published reports regarding these disorders.[71, 75, 78, 80, 85, 87, 379, 392–395] Myocardial injury potentially can be induced by drugs, myocardial toxins (e.g., ionophore antibiotics), ischemia, hypoxia, infective agents, parasite migration, heavy metals, trauma, metabolic or nutritional imbalance or can occur by extension from a pre-existing infection (pericarditis, pericardial abscess, or endocarditis) or tumor (melanoma, lipoma, lymphosarcoma, hemangiosarcoma, mesothelioma) (Fig. 7–45; see also Table 7–2).[396] Idiopathic, dilated cardiomyopathy has also been recognized in the horse. In horses that have sustained many days of ventricular or supraventricular tachycardia, reversible myocardial failure can occur. Myocardial function in such cases can only be assessed a number of days following conversion to sinus rhythm.

Clinical Features of Myocardial Diseases

The general manifestations of myocardial disease, regardless of the underlying injury, can be attributed to the following *pathophysiologic disorders*: (1) reduced LV or RV ejection fraction, (2) decreased ventricular compliance, (3) ventricular dilatation with secondary mitral or tricuspid valve incompetency, or (4) the development of electrical disturbances. The overall cardiac disability varies greatly among affected horses. Some horses have no detectable clinical signs, whereas other horses demonstrate exercise intolerance, life-threatening arrhythmias, low-output CHF, or sudden death. While it is tempting to diagnose myocardial disease in the setting of any cardiac rhythm disturbance, many cardiac rhythm abnormalities appear to be more "functional" disturbances, without an obvious anatomical substrate. As such, arrhythmias are often observed in the setting of electrolyte, autonomic, or metabolic imbalance; sepsis; toxemia; hypoxia; ischemia; or iatrogenesis. Persistent ventricular premature depolarizations or ventricular tachycardia seem to be more commonly associated with primary myocardial disease than are atrial premature depolarizations, atrial tachycardia, or atrial fibrillation; nevertheless, atrial rhythm disturbances can also indicate structural myocardial disease.

The onset of signs may lag behind the initial myocardial insult, especially in cases of chronic injury or myocarditis. A typical scenario is that of a horse previously treated for an illness that now appears to have resolved. Problems become evident once the horse begins rigorous training. The trainer may complain that the horse is unable to achieve faster speeds or may stop or suddenly slow during hard training. The affected horse may take a long time to "cool out" after a workout. In more severe cases, marked exercise intolerance, weakness, ataxia, or collapse may occur. Respiratory distress, pulmonary edema, cyanotic mucous membranes, prolonged capillary refill time, and a rapid thready pulse may be detected after exercise. In fulminant cases, fever, tachycardia, arrhythmias, murmurs, pulmonary or ventral edema, and respiratory distress are reported. Sudden death may occur without premonitory signs.

Results of the *clinical examination* in horses with myocardial disease are inconsistent. Resting physical examination findings can range from no abnormalities to tachycardia, tachypnea, frequent premature beats, an irregular rhythm, systolic murmurs of AV valvular insufficiency, or CHF (see

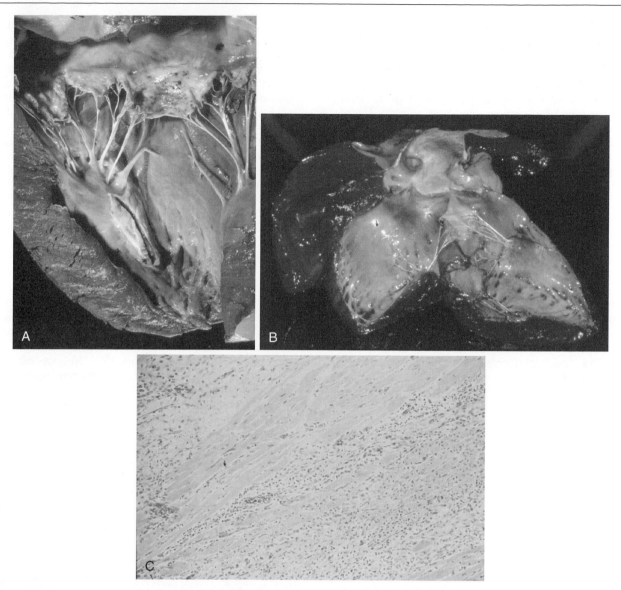

Figure 7–45. Myocardial diseases. *A,* An opened left ventricle revealing an (incised) large, oval area of subendocardial and myocardial fibrosis in a mare. No etiologic agent was found. *B,* Marked left ventricular dilatation and subendocardial fibrosis in a horse with idiopathic dilated cardiomyopathy. The white discoloration of the left ventricle and left atrium may be a consequence of chronic distention or represent fibrosis secondary to another injury. The opened right ventricle (to the left) is dilated but is not discolored. *C,* Myocardial lymphosarcoma. A substantial myocardial infiltration is evident in this photomicrograph.

earlier in this chapter). A post-exercise examination often detects an abnormally rapid heart rate, which remains persistently high after exercise is discontinued. An exercise ECG typically records an inappropriately high heart rate for the level of work being performed. Atrial or ventricular arrhythmias may be observed. Resting echocardiography usually reveals a low normal or low shortening fraction or LV segmental wall abnormalities. Marked increases in left ventricular or left atrial spontaneous contrast may be observed with very poor myocardial function, although this is not a specific finding. Abnormal areas of myocardial echogenicity have been observed, but myocardial tissue characterization by echocardiography has not been well established in horses. Post-exercise echocardiography demonstrates an unexpected reduction of the LV shortening fraction in some affected horses. If myocardial muscle enzymes are measured, ele-

vated myocardial fractions of creatine phosphokinase (CPK [CK-MB]) or lactate dehydrogenase (LDH) may be identified. While further studies are needed regarding these isoenzymes in horses, such elevations could indicate active myocardial cell injury or recent myocardial necrosis (normal values do not rule out the presence of significant myocardial injury). Atrial and ventricular premature depolarizations or atrial fibrillation may be detected. Due to the extreme variability of clinical and laboratory findings, the presumptive diagnosis of myocardial disease must be made after considering all findings, including the history, physical examination, echocardiogram, ECG, and laboratory tests.

Treatment of horses affected by myocardial disease is primarily supportive and depends on the myocardial insult and the consequences of the myocardial disease. All horses should be rested, preferably in a stall, until their myocardial function, ECG, and cardiac isoenzymes return to normal or stabilize and remain stable for several weeks. A minimum of 4 weeks' rest (and usually more) is needed before the horse is returned to work. Antiarrhythmic therapy should be administered if indicated for potentially life-threatening arrhythmias (see later in this chapter). When CHF has developed, digoxin and furosemide should be prescribed as described in the section on CHF (earlier in this chapter). Digitalization should be done cautiously in horses with ventricular extrasystoles, because the arrhythmia may be aggravated and is not indicated in monensin toxicosis (see later). Treatment of frequent premature supraventricular or ventricular depolarizations with an antiarrhythmic agent can be effective; however, the arrhythmia may return as soon as the drug is discontinued. If noninfective myocarditis is believed to be the cause of the arrhythmia or clinical signs, corticosteroid therapy may be indicated, although its use is controversial. When the principal manifestation of myocardial disease is electrical (i.e., frequent premature depolarizations with otherwise normal myocardial function), the prognosis is fair to good for resolution of the arrhythmias. Horses with decreased myocardial function by echocardiography or with CHF must be given a guarded prognosis for life and a poor prognosis for future performance. It is notable, however, that some horses with acute onset of CHF associated with myocardial dysfunction have recovered completely and returned to their prior performance level or have been able to serve successfully as breeding animals. Such horses most likely suffered from acute myocarditis that resolved spontaneously or following anti-inflammatory therapy.

Myocarditis

Myocardial inflammation, or myocarditis, is difficult to diagnose, although the diagnosis is often entertained in horses with cardiac arrhythmias or abnormal myocardial function, particularly when cardiac signs occur after another illness. Often the prior disorder is a viral (influenza) respiratory infection or an infection caused by *Streptococcus* sp. Immune-mediated myocarditis may be the cause of such inflammations. Whereas the clinical association between these problems seems well founded, definitive cause-and-effect proof is still lacking owing to the difficulty of obtaining myocardial biopsies. Myocarditis may also follow parasitic migration or extension from an inflamed pericardium or heart valve. Hematogenous spread to the heart may be another mechanism for myocarditis. Severe necrotizing myocarditis can lead to signs of myocardial dysfunction indicated earlier. The signs, treatment, and prognosis for myocardial dysfunction caused by myocarditis have been previously described.

Toxic Injury of the Myocardium

A number of toxins are potentially injurious to the myocardium. Ionophore antibiotics are the most notorious of these causes of myocardial necrosis.[84-86] Horses are uniquely sensitive to this class of drugs, which is used as a coccidiostat in poultry production and as a growth promoter in steers. Monensin toxicosis has occurred most frequently, but salinomycin and lasalocid have also resulted in myocardial injury

and death in horses.[397] The myocardial injury results from the ability of these compounds to transport cations across cell membranes, with each of the ionophores having a particular affinity for a different cation. Exposure of horses to the ionophore antibiotics has usually occurred through accidental contamination of equine feedstuffs at the mill or through accidental giving of poultry or cattle feeds to horses. In most outbreaks, a batch of feed of recent acquisition was fed to the animals. Otherwise, myocardial injury from feeding can occur with ingestion of blister beetles (cantharidin)[393, 394] or Japanese yew. Myocardial necrosis has also been observed following endotoxemia, particularly with clostridial infection, salmonellosis, and torsion of the large colon.

Clinical signs of horses with ionophore toxicity vary with the specific type, quantity, and concentration of ionophore ingested and the pre-existing health and body condition of the exposed horses. A wide range of clinical signs has been observed by one of the authors (VBR) in exposed horses ranging from none to clinical signs involving almost all body systems. Weakness, lethargy, depression, anorexia, ataxia, colic, diarrhea, profuse sweating, and recumbency have been seen. The cardiac findings are similar to those previously described for myocardial diseases. If sudden death occurs, it is usually within 12 to 36 hours of ingestion of the contaminated feed. Polyuria and hematuria have also been reported in ponies. A diagnosis of ionophore toxicity is based on the detection of the ionophore in the feed or stomach contents of exposed horses. Various clinicopathologic abnormalities are observed with monensin toxicity, including decreased serum calcium, potassium, magnesium, and phosphorus; increases in serum urea, creatinine, unconjugated bilirubin, aspartate aminotransferase, CPK, and LDH. Isoenzyme patterns of CPK and LDH have indicated cardiac, skeletal, and RBC damage.[84, 86] Elevated packed cell volume and total solids have been associated with dehydration. Echocardiographic evaluation of affected horses has revealed marked decreases in shortening fraction with segmental wall motion abnormalities that range from mild to severe. Horses that exhibit decreased shortening fraction and dyskinesis shortly after exposure to monensin do not survive. Horses with mild decreases in shortening fraction survive and may be useful breeding animals, but most do not return to previous performance levels. Horses with normal echocardiograms not only survive but typically return to work at their previous level. Postmortem findings range from no visible lesions in horses with normal echocardiograms to severe myocardial necrosis and fibrosis in those with decreased shortening fraction or ventricular dyskinesis. A single dose may lead to death from cardiac arrhythmias prior to the development of myocardial necrosis. Postmortem lesions have been described elsewhere but include myocardial pallor and signs of CHF.[84, 86]

Treatment for affected horses is largely symptomatic (see earlier), unless very recent exposure is known. Vitamin E has been suggested to have a protective effect in other species and may be beneficial in affected horses. Digoxin and probably calcium channel blockers are contraindicated in acutely affected horses. If ingestion of the contaminated feedstuff is recent, treatment with activated charcoal or mineral oil is indicated to reduce absorption of the ionophore. Intravenous fluid and electrolyte replacement therapy may be indicated, as well as antiarrhythmic, for any life-threatening arrhythmias. Stall rest in a quiet environment for up to 8 weeks after exposure is most important, because echocardiograms recorded after trivial exercise or excitement can result in marked decreases in fractional shortening and increased myocardial dyskinesis.

Dilated Cardiomyopathy

Dilated cardiomyopathy is a disorder of the myocardium characterized by global reduction of LV systolic function that cannot be explained by valvular, vascular, or congenital heart disease. The inciting cause of dilated cardiomyopathy is generally undetermined, although myocarditis or prior toxic injury is often suspected. The clinical signs are similar to those described earlier for myocardial diseases. Symptomatic therapy with digoxin and diuretics may temporarily stabilize CHF and lead to transient improvement, but most horses deteriorate in the 3 to 12 months after the diagnosis and subsequently are humanely destroyed. Echocardiography is diagnostic, revealing cardiomegaly with biatrial and biventricular dilatation and depressed shortening fraction (see Fig. 7–20A). Neither the history nor postmortem examination reveals the cause, and generally only diffuse or multifocal myocardial degeneration, necrosis, and fibrosis are observed.

Dilated cardiomyopathy can also be caused by vitamin E and selenium deficiency and is observed primarily in fast-growing foals from mares with a marginal or deficient selenium status raised in selenium-deficient areas. Affected foals are usually younger than 6 months of age and present with an acute onset of weakness, recumbency, respiratory distress, pulmonary edema, tachycardia, murmurs, and arrhythmias. The prognosis for foals affected with the myocardial manifestations of white muscle disease are poor, and most die within 24 to 48 hours after the onset of clinical signs. Laboratory abnormalities in affected foals include marked elevations of CK (including the MB fraction in foals with myocardial involvement), AST, and LDH as well as hyperkalemia, hyponatremia, and hypochloremia. Myoglobinuria may occur. Echocardiography demonstrates the severity of myocardial involvement. Whole blood selenium, RBC glutathione peroxidase, and vitamin E levels may be helpful in the diagnosis; however, tissue samples provide a more accurate indication of selenium stores. Treatment with vitamin E and selenium may be successful in some foals, but typically the myocardial necrosis is extensive and incompatible with life. Postmortem findings reveal pale streaking of the myocardium with intramuscular edema, myodegeneration, myocardial necrosis, and fibrosis or calcification. Prevention of white muscle disease is important in selenium-deficient areas. Supplementation of pregnant mares should occur during gestation based on individual blood and tissue selenium levels and should be continued during lactation, because more selenium is passed to the foal through the milk than across the placenta.

VASCULAR DISEASES

Diseases of the arteries and veins can be congenital or acquired. Acquired disorders include a variety of conditions ranging from subclinical to devastating.[20, 44, 147–155, 247, 248, 398, 399] Thrombophlebitis is probably the most common vascu-

lar problem encountered. Arteriosclerosis and thrombosis also occur in the arterial system and are often associated with parasite migration in the gastrointestinal arteries (particularly the cranial mesenteric artery) and at the aortic quadrifurcation. Rupture of the great vessels has been reported. Aortic rupture occurs most commonly in older breeding stallions, and pulmonary artery rupture is a consequence of longstanding pulmonary hypertension and left heart failure. AV communications occur uncommonly and may develop after vascular rupture or subsequent to growth of vascular tumors. Pulmonary vascular disease and associated hypertension may place a load on the right ventricle, a condition called "corpulmonale." However, there is no compelling evidence at this time to incriminate corpulmonale as an important common cause of heart disease. Idiopathic pulmonary hypertension has been reported as a cause of atrial fibrillation in horses; however, the left heart dysfunction was not completely excluded in the reported cases.[327] Tumors of the great arteries and veins are rare.[400] Catheter embolization is reported periodically and has been amenable to surgical and percutaneous catheter retrieval.[401] Venous aneurysms,[402] vascular and lymphatic malformations,[403] and angiomatous lesions are rare.[403a]

An echocardiographic observation that has been suggested to be abnormal in some horses is the development of intravascular, spontaneous contrast within the blood vessels and cardiac chambers.[283, 298] This observation is common during ultrasound examinations and is also dependent on the operator with respect to gain and contrast settings (Fig. 7–46). Intracardiac, intraluminal echo contrast is especially likely when there are low flow rates in the heart due to bradycardia, arrhythmia, or myocardial failure. It is also prominent when endocarditis is present. Lesions, partial thrombosis, or even venipuncture of the jugular vein can lead to generation of spontaneous echo contrast in systemic veins and the right side of the heart. These echogenic particles become more

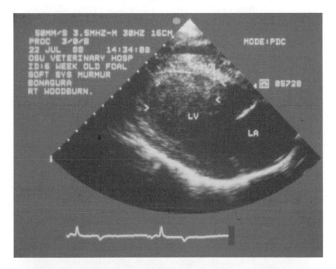

Figure 7–46. Spontaneous contrast in the apex of the left ventricle of a foal. The echodensities were noted to swirl in real time. Compare this with the density within the left atrium. Bradycardia, low cardiac output, and rouleaux formation are thought to be contributory to this finding (see also Fig. 7–38A).

obvious if CO suddenly increases. The overall significance (if any) of isolated intravascular contrast cannot be stated with certainty, and although it has been suggested to indicate abnormal platelet function in some cases,[283, 298] it probably represents a normal phenomenon in many horses.

Thrombophlebitis

Thrombophlebitis, inflammation, and thrombosis of a vein, are most commonly caused by intravenous catheterization or intravenous injection (Fig. 7–47).[249, 249a] The jugular veins are most often affected. Thrombophlebitis can develop in the absence of pre-existing vessel trauma subsequent to coagulation disorders. Clinical signs of phlebitis are straightforward, including swelling over the affected vein, heat, and pain on palpation of the involved tissues. Thrombotic occlusion of the affected vein results in distention of the veins and possibly subcutaneous edema, proximal or cephalad to the affected area. Marked swelling, heat, and pain on palpation, combined with fever, hyperfibrinogenemia, or a neutrophilic leukocytosis, indicates infection of the thrombus.[273]

The diagnosis of thrombophlebitis is based on the detection of the previously described clinical signs and can be confirmed with two-dimensional and duplex Doppler ultrasonography.[249a] Ultrasonographic examination of the affected vein reveals filling of the vein lumen with an anechoic, hypoechoic, hyperechoic (gas), or echogenic homogeneous material that partially or completely occludes the vessel (Fig. 7–48). Flow may be evaluated by pulsed-wave or color-coded Doppler studies or by contrast venography, using saline as an echogenic contrast agent. Flow across the thrombus, or drainage proximal and distal to the area of thrombosis, can be assessed (distal areas of collateral circulation may still enter the vein). Ultrasonographic evaluation of the affected vein may also reveal thickening of the vessel wall, perivascular swelling, tracts extending from the vein to the subcutaneous tissues or skin, or subcutaneous abscesses. Cavitation in the center of a thrombus is suggestive of infection, and an aspirate should be obtained from this cavitated region and cultured.

Infections with multiple organisms should be anticipated

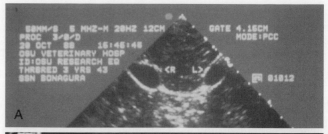
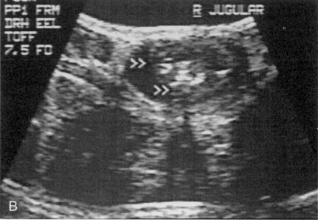

Figure 7–48. Vascular imaging—jugular veins. *A*, Ultrasound image of normal jugular veins. The echolucent lumina of the right and left veins are indicated. The image is just off transverse. *B*, Image of a mixed, echogenic thrombus *(arrows)* in the right jugular vein. Doppler studies could be used to evaluate the flow across this area.

in cases of infective thrombophlebitis, and high doses of broad-spectrum antimicrobials should be administered until culture and sensitivity results of the aspirate are obtained. Metronidazole (15 mg/kg every 6 hours) should be considered if anaerobic infection is suspected. Flunixin (1 mg/kg every 12 hours) may be added to reduce inflammation. Local therapy including hot compresses, topical ichthammol, or dimethyl sulfoxide may be helpful in the treatment of thrombophlebitis. If antimicrobial therapy is unsuccessful, surgical resection of the affected vein may be indicated. A careful evaluation of the communicating large veins and the heart should be performed on horses with suspected septic jugular vein thrombophlebitis. Bacterial endocarditis may develop secondary to embolization of infective thrombus or bacteremia.

Recanalization of an affected vein often occurs and is detected by ultrasound as blood dissecting between the vessel wall and the thrombus. Occasionally, loculation may be detected within the ends of the thrombus. Such loculation may result in persistent fibrous webs within the vein that restrict venous return. Venous stricture may also occur secondary to longstanding thrombophlebitis. Complete fibrous occlusion of the jugular vein (see Fig. 7–47) may impede venous return from the head such that if adequate collateral circulation does not develop, impaired venous drainage of the upper airways may limit performance.

Aortoiliac Thrombosis

Aortoiliac thrombosis is an uncommon, but potentially serious, disorder. The gross appearance, histologic features, and

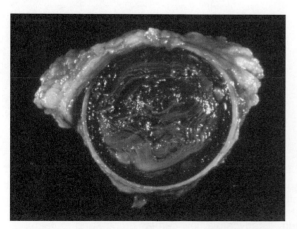

Figure 7–47. Thrombosis of a jugular vein secondary to iatrogenic thrombophlebitis.

clinical findings of this vaso-occlusive disorder have been reviewed extensively by Azzie, Maxie, and Physick-Sheard[149, 151, 153, 154, 247] and the interested reader is directed to these reports. Arteriosclerotic and atherosclerotic aortic lesions have also been observed at other sites (Fig. 7–49). Suggested etiologies of arterial disorders such as these include *Strongylus vulgaris* infection, systemic infections, embolization, and vasculitis. There is no convincing evidence that aortoiliac thrombosis is consistently caused by strongylus infection, and Azzie[151, 153] has presented substantial data to refute this contention. The quadrifurcation of the terminal aorta and the iliac arteries is involved, including their proximal branches. The vessels are occluded partially to completely by multifocal fibrous tissue, laminated thrombi, or fibrous plaques.[149] Histologic lesions include organized, fibrous connective tissue, hemosiderin-laden macrophages, irregular vascular channels, and disruption of the intimal and internal elastic lamina. The lesions are generally devoid of fat.[149]

This problem occurs infrequently, but clinically it can be associated with severe performance problems, including reproductive failure.[404] The typical features, which are well described by Azzie, include exercise-associated unilateral hindlimb lameness, ataxia, or collapse.[151, 153, 154] Aortoiliac thrombosis has also been diagnosed as a cause of breeding failure in stallions. Physical examination of an affected horse at rest may reveal weak metatarsal arterial pulses or delayed saphenous refill in the affected limb. The temperature of the limb in the resting animal is usually normal, unless complete arterial occlusion has occurred, in which case the limb is

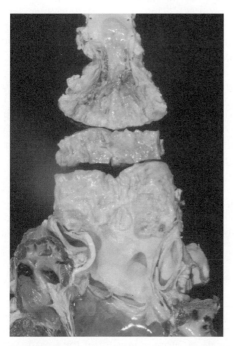

Figure 7–49. Severe atheromatous change with secondary *Streptococcus* infection of the proximal aorta. The intimal and subintimal change begins just distal to the coronary ostia. Representative sections of the ascending aorta are shown. *Strongylus vulgaris* was not found. The most distal segment was necrotic and severely narrowed flow across the region.

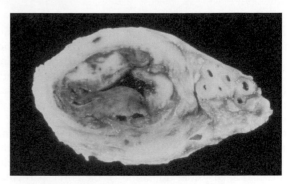

Figure 7–50. Verminous arteritis and thrombosis in the cranial mesenteric artery caused by *Strongylus vulgaris.*

cold and painful and may become edematous. Exercise in affected animals results in an exercise-associated gait abnormality (lameness, ataxia, or weakness) with a decreased or absent metatarsal and digital pulse and delayed or absent saphenous refill. The horse may be quite uncomfortable and reluctant to bear weight on the affected limb. Marked hyperpnea, other signs of distress, and profuse, generalized sweating are often present with trembling of the affected limb. A rectal examination may reveal fremitus, a weak or absent pulse, or aneurysmal dilatation of the affected artery or arteries. These abnormalities may be more evident after exercise and may help to confirm the diagnosis.

The diagnosis can be confirmed by ultrasonographic evaluation of the terminal aorta and iliac arteries with a high-frequency (5 or 7.5 MHz) rectal transducer.[150, 152, 248] Essential abnormalities include a hypoechoic to echogenic mass protruding into the arterial lumen. An estimation of the degree of obstruction can be made based on the percentage of the artery occluded. Many cases are longstanding, and hyperechoic areas, even tissues sufficiently echo-dense to cast acoustic shadows, may be imaged within the aortic or iliac thrombus: These findings suggest mature scar tissue and calcification.

The prognosis for this disorder is guarded. No controlled studies have evaluated therapy for this condition, though prior experience, including a recent case survey,[405a] suggests no treatment consistently improves outcome. Various treatments have been reported including intravenous sodium gluconate, larvicidal dewormings, phenylbutazone, low molecular weight dextran, and a controlled exercise program. Early diagnosis is essential if therapy is to be beneficial. Treatment is aimed at improving collateral circulation and preventing additional thrombus formation.

Parasitic Infection

The migrating larval forms, particularly L4, of *S. vulgaris,* are known causes of arterial disease, particularly involving the aorta and the cranial mesenteric artery and its branches (Fig. 7–50). Lesions have been described as far forward as the bulbous aorta and the aortic sinuses in infected horses. Rounded fibrous plaques and mural thrombi have been reported in the thoracic and cranial abdominal aorta in 9.4% of horses examined immediately after slaughter by Cranley and McCullagh.[78] These investigators reported a statistical association between the occurrence of proximal aortic *S. vulgaris* lesions and the presence of focal ischemic lesions in the myocardium. They hypothesized that these lesions were consequent to microembolism from parasitic lesions. With the advent of ivermectin and other new anthelmintics, and aggressive deworming programs currently recommended by practicing veterinarians, heavy *S. vulgaris* larval migration damage occurs less frequently. Migration of *S. vulgaris* L4 larvae must be considered in horses with poor deworming histories, high potential of exposure, high fecal egg counts, and palpable abnormalities on rectal examination, as well as fremitus and aneurysmal dilatation of the aorta, particularly in the region of the cranial mesenteric artery or iliac system. An ultrasonographic evaluation of the cranial mesenteric artery is possible and can be used to confirm the diagnosis of thrombosis in these vessels (Fig. 7–51).[405, 405a] Treatment should consist of larvicidal deworming, combined with a rigorous individual and environmental parasite control program.

Arteriovenous Fistulas

Arteriovenous fistulas occur uncommonly and are most often detected with large vascular tumors (hemangiomas, hemangiosarcomas) or as a rare congenital defect or post-traumatic sequela.[406] Classic features include a continuous thrill and murmur over the affected area, localized edema, slowing of the heart rate after occlusion of the shunt, and signs of increased CO if the shunt flow is great. A diagnosis can be made with Doppler ultrasound, including pulsed-wave and color-flow Doppler to demonstrate continuous and pulsatile flow from the artery, through the associated communication, into the distended veins. A complete cardiovascular examination should be performed because a large arteriovenous communication could lead to cardiac failure. Treatment depends on the underlying cause. No treatment may be indicated with small, uncomplicated arteriovenous communications. Large vascular neoplasms are usually inoperable at the time when they are diagnosed or complicated by the possibility of metastasis.

Arterial Rupture

Rupture of the aorta or its branches or of the pulmonary artery are reported sporadically.[20, 44, 105, 108, 146–148, 398] Rupture of the aortic root has been commonly reported in older horses, usually older breeding stallions but may also occur in older mares. Rupture typically involves the right aortic sinus (of Valsalva). The aortic root can rupture into the right atrium, right ventricle, or intraventricular septum.[44] Dystrophic changes in the media of the aorta have been reported, and the hypertension associated with breeding has been implicated as a cause of aortic root rupture. Aneurysms of the right sinus of Valsalva have also been reported and are related to congenital defects in the media of the aorta near the right coronary sinus.[148] Rupture of the middle uterine artery can lead to fatal peripartum hemorrhage.[146] Ruptures of the extrapericardial aorta or other blood vessels leading to fatal hemorrhage or a systemic to pulmonary shunt have been reported.[20, 40, 46, 48, 51, 147]

Rupture of an artery is often a catastrophic event, and most diagnoses are made at the necropsy floor. Antemortem diagnosis of an aortic sinus of Valsalva aneurysm is possible

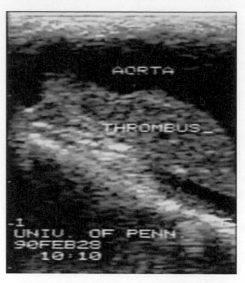

Figure 7–51. An ultrasound image of a distal aortic thrombosis obtained by transrectal probe. The thrombus and patent portion of the aorta are indicated.

by echocardiography. Once diagnosed, these animals should not be used for any athletic endeavor other than breeding, because rupture of the aneurysm could occur at any time. When aortic root rupture or rupture of a sinus of Valsalva aneurysm communicates with the right atrium or right ventricle, right-sided heart failure can occur. The aortic-cardiac fistula causes a continuous heart murmur. Cardiac arrhythmias (usually ventricular tachycardia) may also develop if dissection progresses into the intraventricular septum. The prognosis for life in these horses is generally grave, depending on the site and size of the communication. Some horses survive with supportive treatment for CHF.

Pulmonary artery rupture is most often caused by chronic pulmonary hypertension and pulmonary artery dilatation. This is most commonly detected in conjunction with severe chronic MR but may be seen in any horse with severe pulmonary hypertension, regardless of the cause. The potential for pulmonary artery rupture should be considered whenever a large dilated main pulmonary artery or left and right pulmonary artery is detected echocardiographically. Affected horses should be considered unsafe for riding or driving and should not be used, except for breeding, due to the possibility of sudden death (Fig. 7–51; see also Fig. 7–39). Focal medial calcification of the pulmonary artery is not uncommon at necropsy.[407]

CARDIAC ARRHYTHMIAS

Cardiac arrhythmias are disturbances in heart rate, rhythm, or conduction and can be classified based on atrial and ventricular rate, anatomical origin of the impulse, method of impulse formation, and conduction sequence. A wide variety of cardiac arrhythmias have been recognized. Of principal concern to the clinician are the hemodynamic consequences of arrhythmias (reduced pressure, flow, perfusion) and the potential for further electrical instability (myocardial fibrillation, sudden death).

The electrophysiologic basis of cardiac arrhythmias will not be discussed here, and the interested reader is referred elsewhere for descriptions of abnormal automaticity, re-entry, reflection, entrainment, and other cellular mechanisms of arrhythmogenesis.[408] Cardiac arrhythmias will be classified based on the anatomical origin of the manifest ECG mechanism (Table 7–15). The reader should be aware that some arrhythmias, especially those originating in the AV junction, may mimic either atrial rhythm disturbances or "high" ventricular rhythms. For purpose of discussion we have elected to distinguish "atrial" from "junctional"; however, the term "supraventricular" may also be applied to these rhythm disturbances. The clinical evaluation of the horse with an arrhythmia is reviewed in Table 7–16.

Sinus Rhythms

A number of physiologic sinus rhythms are recognized.[1, 3, 212, 256, 409, 410] These can be explained by the impact of autonomic

---

Table 7–15. Cardiac Rhythms of the Horse

Sinus Mechanisms*

Normal sinus rhythm
Sinus arrhythmia
Sinoatrial block/arrest
Sinus bradycardia
Sinus tachycardia

Atrial Rhythm Disturbances

Atrial escape complexes†
Atrial premature complexes
Atrial tachycardia—nonsustained and sustained
Atrial flutter
Atrial fibrillation
Re-entrant supraventricular tachycardia

Junctional Rhythm Disturbances

Junctional escape complexes†
Junctional escape rhythm† (idionodal rhythm)
Junctional premature complexes
Junctional ("nodal") tachycardia
Re-entrant supraventricular tachycardia

Ventricular Rhythm Disturbances

Ventricular escape complexes†
Ventricular escape rhythm† (idioventricular rhythm)
Ventricular premature complexes
Accelerated ventricular rhythm (idioventricular tachycardia)
Ventricular tachycardia
Ventricular flutter
Ventricular fibrillation

Conduction Disturbances

Sinoatrial block*
Atrial standstill (hyperkalemia)
Atrioventricular blocks: first-degree*; second-degree*; third-degree (complete)
Ventricular pre-excitation

*Generally physiologic.
†Escape complexes develop secondary to another rhythm disturbance.

Table 7–16. Evaluation of the Horse with a Cardiac Arrhythmia

General medical history, past illnesses, past and current medications

Work history and exercise tolerance

General physical examination

Physical examination—evidence of congestive heart failure
  Subcutaneous edema
  Jugular venous distention/pulsations
  Pulmonary edema
  Pleural/peritoneal effusion
  Weight loss, poor condition

Auscultation of the heart
  Assessment of heart sounds (rhythm, third heart sound)
  Assessment of heart murmurs

Resting electrocardiogram
  Heart rate and cardiac rhythm
  Analysis of P-QRS-T waveforms

Post-exercise electrocardiogram
Exercise (or treadmill) electrocardiogram

Clinical laboratory studies
  Complete blood count (rule out anemia, infection)
  Blood culture (in cases of suspected endocarditis)
  Serum electrolytes (particularly potassium and possibly magnesium)
  Serum biochemical tests (especially renal function)
  Skeletal muscle enzymes (cardiac isoenzymes)
  Red blood cell potassium
  Fractional excretion of potassium

Echocardiogram/Doppler echocardiogram
  Examine for cardiomegaly or reduced myocardial function
  Identify predisposing cardiac lesions and abnormal flow

Serum/plasma concentrations of cardioactive drugs
  Serum digoxin concentration
  Plasma quinidine concentration

Response to medications

Adapted from Bonagura JD: Clinical evaluation and management of heart disease. *Equine Vet Educ* 2:31–37, 1990.

---

nervous system traffic on the SA node (Fig. 7–52). Normal horses at rest demonstrate vagal-mediated sinus bradycardia, sinus arrhythmia, or sinus block or arrest; yet, fear or a sudden stimulus may provoke sympathetically driven sinus tachycardia. Exercise leads to pronounced sinus tachycardia with heart rates often exceeding 200/min. AV conduction, as a general rule, tends to follow sinus activity. During sinus tachycardia, the PR interval shortens, while during periods of progressive SA slowing the PR interval prolongs. Usually, second-degree AV block, type I (Wenckebach), follows a progressive prolongation of the PR interval. Sinus rate and AV conduction usually change in parallel[6]; however, some horses appear to control blood pressure during high sinus tachycardia by blocking impulses in the AV node.[1] Second-degree AV block is more likely in a standing horse, in a horse that has suddenly stopped submaximal exercise, or after a brief surge of sinus tachycardia in an anxious animal.

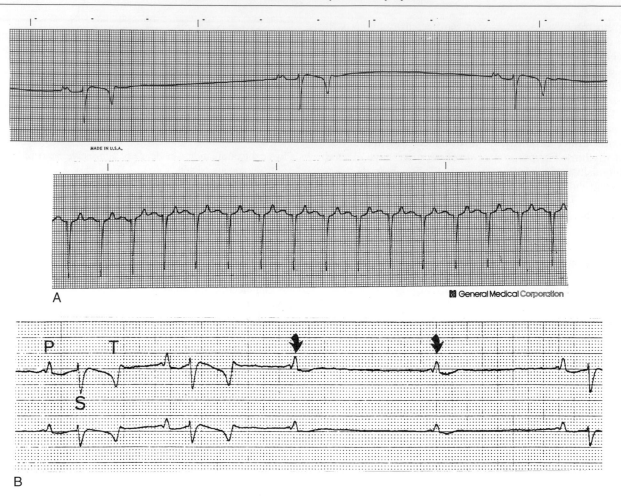

Figure 7–52. Sinus rhythms. *A,* Sinus bradycardia *(top)* and tachycardia *(bottom).* Base-apex lead, 25 mm/sec. *B,* Sinus arrhythmia with second-degree atrioventricular block *(arrows).* An ambulatory electrocardiogram is shown; transthoracic leads recorded at 25 mm/sec.

Sinus rate and rhythm must be carefully monitored in the critically ill or anesthetized horse since heart rate is a major determinant of CO and arterial blood pressure. Sedative drugs and anesthetics can cause sinus bradycardia. Anesthetic drugs or hypoxia can depress sinus node function as can traction on an abdominal viscus. Concurrent depression of the sinus node with stimulation of latent pacemakers in the coronary sinus or AV junction can lead to ectopic rhythms in the anesthetized horse. Conversely, an increasing sinus rate may indicate inadequate depth of anesthesia, pain, or hypotension. When sinus tachycardia is identified, the cause must be sought and treated. The possibilities of pain, hypotension, and sepsis should be considered and managed when appropriate.

Sinus bradycardia is generally a benign rhythm in standing horses; however, when encountered during sedation or anesthesia sinus bradycardia or arrest may cause CO to decrease and result in significant hypotension. Treatment of symptomatic sinus bradycardia can include the infusion of catecholamines (dobutamine, dopamine, epinephrine) or the administration of anticholinergic drugs (atropine, glycopyrrolate; see Table 7–14). Dopamine or dobutamine can be infused to increase heart rate and arterial blood pressure; however, reflex AV block may develop in some horses.[139, 143, 184] Exces-

sive administration of catecholamines causes sinus tachycardia and ectopic beats. Anticholinergic drugs may not be effective in the setting of anesthetic-induced depression of SA function, particularly if vagal efferent traffic is low. Gastrointestinal complications including ileus and colic may develop after anticholinergic drug therapy; thus, it should not be chosen for trivial rate problems.

Atrial Arrhythmias

Rhythms originating in the atria are common. These disturbances often develop as "functional" disorders with no overt structural cardiac lesion. Autonomic imbalance (including high sympathetic activity), hypokalemia, beta-agonists, infections, anemia, and colic can cause atrial premature complexes. Of course, atrial rhythm disturbances are quite common when there are structural lesions of the valves, myocardium, or pericardium. Myocarditis after viral or bacterial infection may precipitate atrial arrhythmias in some horses. Atrial premature complexes can precipitate sustained atrial arrhythmias, such as atrial tachycardia, atrial flutter, and atrial fibrillation. The large size of the equine atria and the frequent presence of microscopic atrial fibrotic lesions predispose the horse to these sustained arrhythmias. The high resting vagal tone present in most horses serves to shorten the duration of the action potential of atrial myocytes and also facilitates development of sustained atrial tachyarrhythmias, which probably depend on re-entry.

Atrial arrhythmias are the most common abnormal rhythms detected (Figs. 7–53 and 7–54).[5, 16, 30, 37, 39, 111, 120, 121, 123, 125, 126, 132, 220–222, 273, 280, 327, 377, 411–421] Atrial premature complexes are the least complex of these rhythm disturbances and may be clinically insignificant or associated with exercise intolerance or other signs of cardiac disease. In contrast, atrial tachycardia, atrial flutter, and atrial fibrillation are likely to be clinically significant. The overall importance of atrial premature complexes is often difficult to ascertain. Routine ECG rhythm strips recorded from over 950 horses and interpreted by one of the authors (JDB) in conjunction with Dr. Michael S. Miller, indicated that atrial arrhythmias, overall, were present in less than 3% of the horses studied. However, when clinically normal horses were examined by Holter monitor by one of us (VBR), atrial premature complexes were recorded in 28% of the horses. Thus, it appears that the incidence of atrial arrhythmias depends not only on the population examined but also on the methods used. It is also clear that these rhythm disturbances should be assessed in light of other clinical findings.

Atrial Premature Complexes

Atrial premature complexes are detected by auscultation and are documented by an ECG. Auscultation usually reveals a regular sinus rhythm that is interrupted by an obviously premature beat (see Table 7–7). Premature atrial contractions may be fully interpolated (there is continuation of the regular sinus rhythm after the premature atrial contraction) or there may be a pause, if the sinus node is reset. The ECG is characterized by a premature (usually narrow) QRS complex, which is preceded by an abnormal, premature P′ wave that is often buried within the preceding T wave. Often the P′R interval is longer than normal (physiologic first-degree AV block), and in other cases the P′ wave is nonconducted (physiologic second-degree AV block; see Fig. 7–53). Care must be taken not to overdiagnose atrial premature complexes. Sinus arrhythmia and sinus bradycardia often lead to variations in the P-P intervals, and there is often a "wandering atrial pacemaker" that gradually alters the P wave morphology. Exercise or excitement will abolish such physiologic rhythms.

Atrial premature complexes, as a general rule, are more likely to be clinically significant in the following circumstances: if they (1) are frequent at rest, (2) are associated with nonsustained or sustained runs of atrial tachycardia, (3)

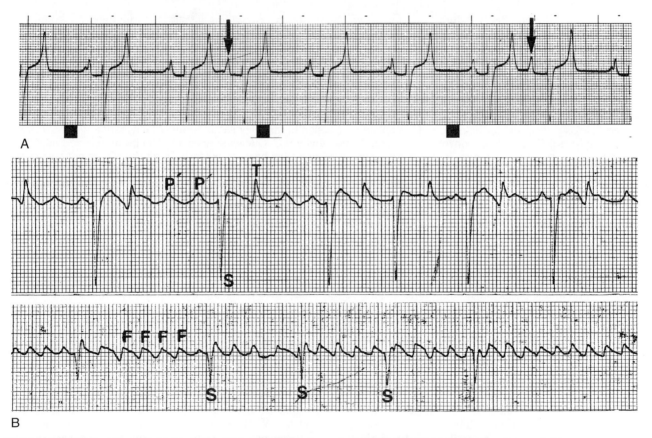

Figure 7–53. Electrocardiograms with atrial rhythm disturbances. *A,* Premature atrial complexes *(arrows).* Note the premature P waves of different morphology, the slightly prolonged PR interval indicating atrioventricular nodal refractoriness, and the normal-appearing QRS complex indicating a supraventricular origin. There is a slight conduction aberrancy in the second premature QRS complex (see also Fig. 7–15). *B,* Sustained atrial tachyarrhythmias. The top picture shows atrial tachycardia with rapid, regular P waves (P′) and a variable ventricular rate response to conducted P waves. The base-apex lead is 25 mm/sec. The lower trace shows atrial flutter (F) with variable ventricular response (S). Lead 3 recorded at 25 mm/sec.

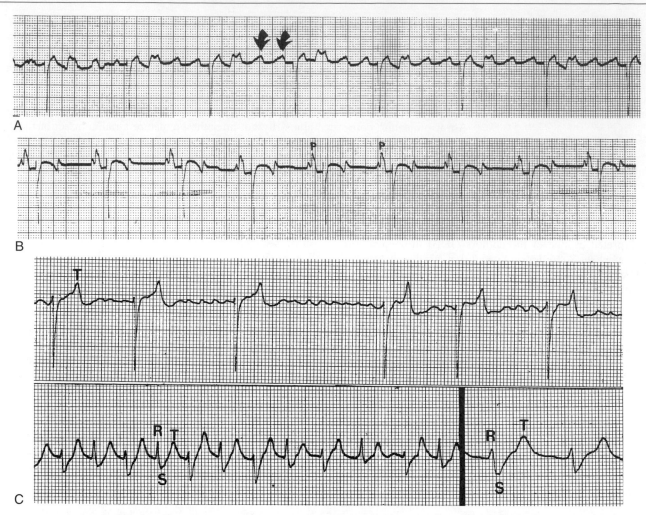

Figure 7–54. Quinidine therapy of atrial arrhythmias. *A* and *B,* Successful conversion of atrial fibrillation using a combination of digoxin and quinidine (see text for details). *A,* Incomplete conversion of atrial fibrillation to atrial tachycardia with rapid, regular atrial activity *(arrows)*. *B,* Results of conversion to normal sinus rhythm. *C,* Quinidine toxicosis can be manifested as abnormalities on the electrocardiogram. In this horse, atrial fibrillation *(top;* base-apex lead, 25 mm/sec) was not converted. The lower recording shows persistent atrial fibrillation with a rapid atrioventricular conduction response, electrical alternans, and widening of the QRS complex (lead 2 at 25 mm/sec; right panel at 50 mm/sec). The rapid rate response is related to the vagolytic effect of quinidine. The electrical alternans is not uncommon with supraventricular tachycardias with rapid ventricular responses and indicates varying conduction into the ventricle. The widened QRS is a sign of quinidine toxicosis. An idiosyncratic reaction leading to polymorphous ventricular tachycardia has also been recognized (see Fig. 7–56).

are related to poor performance (while other causes are excluded), (4) precipitate paroxysmal atrial flutter or fibrillation, or (5) develop in conjunction with other signs of cardiac disease. Documentation of atrial arrhythmias *during* exercise may be critical for determining if paroxysmal atrial tachycardia or fibrillation is likely to be the cause of poor performance. Clinical judgment must be used; however, because supraventricular premature complexes are most likely to occur in the immediate post-exercise period, probably associated with autonomic imbalance. If these post-exercise arrhythmias are not associated with clinical signs and are not detected during exercise, they are unlikely to be clinically significant. Cardiac rhythm monitoring during exercise may be necessary to be certain. In summary, routine electrocardiography, clinical chemistry, hematology, echocardiography, exercising electrocardiography, post-exercise electrocardiography, and continuous 24-hour electrocardiographic monitoring may all play a role in the complete evaluation of a horse suspected of having intermittent cardiac arrhythmias.

Isolated atrial premature complexes generally are not treated. The hemodynamic consequences of these rhythm disturbances is minor, unless sustained abnormal activity develops. Consideration of antiarrhythmic therapy might be appropriate if frequent atrial extrasystoles are documented to precipitate atrial fibrillation. In such cases, either quinidine or procainamide (though both therapies are somewhat impractical for chronic use) or digoxin could be contemplated. While digoxin is easiest to administer long term, the effectiveness of such treatment has not been established except in the setting of CHF. Maintenance of normal serum potassium may be important in suppressing atrial ectopic activity. In cases of suspected immune-mediated myocarditis, anti-inflammatory doses of dexamethasone might be considered as empirical therapy.

Atrial Tachycardia

Atrial tachycardia, a sustained, ectopic, abnormal atrial tachyarrhythmia, occurs infrequently. Atrial tachycardia may be sustained or nonsustained (paroxysmal) and is precipitated by an atrial premature complex. The atrial rate is rapid and regular; however, since many of the ectopic P′ waves are blocked physiologically in the AV node, an irregular ventricular rate response often results. Atrial rates of 120 to 300 beats/min are typical in horses with sustained atrial tachycardia. At lower atrial rates, 2:1 AV conduction may yield a regular, relentless heart rate. At the higher atrial rates, the rhythm may be indistinguishable from atrial flutter. Differentiation of atrial tachycardia from flutter is not critical because both arrhythmias carry the same clinical significance and are treated identically. Sustained atrial tachycardia is most often recognized during treatment of horses with quinidine sulfate. Prior to conversion of atrial fibrillation to sinus rhythm, atrial tachycardia may be observed; thus, this rhythm indicates a partial therapeutic effect of quinidine on the atrial myocardium. When this atrial tachycardia occurs as an isolated finding, structural or underlying myocardial disease should be suspected and the horse should be considered predisposed to the development or recurrence of atrial fibrillation. Treatment is the same as that described for atrial fibrillation.

Atrial Flutter

Atrial flutter is even less common than atrial tachycardia and represents a form of atrial circuit movement or macro-reentry. The clinical circumstances and assessment of this rhythm disturbance are identical to those of atrial tachycardia. The ECG in atrial flutter is characterized by a very rapid, abnormal, but regular atrial activity that is usually manifested as a "saw-toothed" ECG baseline. The atrial frequency often exceeds 300/min. The RR intervals are usually irregular due to variable AV conduction, and there are fewer QRS and T complexes than flutter waves (see Fig. 7–53). The ventricular rate depends on the refractory period of the AV node and on the strength of the atrial stimulus. Treatment of atrial flutter is similar to that for horses with atrial fibrillation.

Atrial Fibrillation

Atrial fibrillation is the most common atrial arrhythmia associated with poor performance and exercise intolerance.[5, 16, 39, 121, 123, 220–222, 377, 411, 412, 415, 421] CO at rest is normal in most horses with atrial fibrillation[418]; yet, maximal CO during exercise is limited because the atrial contribution to filling is most important at higher heart rates. Undoubtedly, the already high LA pressure present in heavily exercising horses[314, 315] is further increased by the loss of active atrial transport function. As expected, exercise intolerance is most common in high-performance horses (racehorses, advanced combined training horses, polo ponies, and some Grand Prix jumpers) and less common in show hunters and in pleasure, dressage, and endurance horses. Exercise-induced pulmonary hemorrhage, respiratory distress, CHF, ataxia or collapse, and myopathy have all been reported with atrial fibrillation; conversely, the arrhythmia is often detected as an incidental finding.[222, 377]

Atrial fibrillation may be paroxysmal or sustained. Paroxysmal atrial fibrillation is often associated with a single episode of poor performance, with the horse often decelerating suddenly during a race.[39, 412] The arrhythmia usually disappears spontaneously within 24 to 48 hours. Paroxysmal atrial fibrillation may be associated with transient potassium depletion, particularly in horses treated with furosemide or bicarbonate solutions, and is most often unrelated to other clinical or echocardiographic abnormalities of cardiac disease. Sustained atrial fibrillation may be less common than paroxysmal atrial fibrillation but is easier to diagnose as the arrhythmia is sustained. It is also emphasized that many horses with sustained atrial fibrillation have no other evidence of significant underlying cardiac disease. Table 7–17 summarizes those factors that interact in the prognosis of a horse with atrial fibrillation. Of these, CHF represents the overall worst prognostic indicator. Atrial fibrillation is most common in adult horses and has been reported infrequently in foals, weanlings, yearlings, or ponies.[111, 417, 422] Several studies indicate a higher incidence in Standardbreds, draft horses, and Warmblood horses compared with the general hospital population. Atrial fibrillation also occurs commonly in horses with advanced mitral or tricuspid insufficiency or CHF. In these horses, treatment should be aimed at controlling CHF.

Atrial fibrillation is characterized on auscultation by an irregularly irregular heart rhythm, variable intensity heart sounds, and an absent fourth heart sound (see Table 7–7). Arterial pulses vary in intensity, and pulse deficits may be present. The ECG is characterized by an absence of P waves; instead, fibrillation or "f" waves are seen in the baseline. These "f" waves may be coarse (large) or fine (small), and the number of atrial impulses/minute cannot be counted but usually exceeds 500. The QRS-T complexes are normal in morphology and duration, but ventricular rate response is quite irregular, although periodicity may be observed infrequently.[121] As for all atrial tachyarrhythmias, the ultimate ventricular rate response depends on the refractory period of the AV node and the strength of the atrial stimuli. In the otherwise healthy horse in atrial fibrillation, vagal tone will be high and sympathetic tone low when standing; consequently, the ventricular rate will be close to normal or slightly increased (30 to 40 beats/min). If sympathetic activity is increased for any reason, or if vagal activity is blocked (as occurs with quinidine sulfate therapy), the ventricular rate response will increase as the AV nodal refractory period shortens. This explains the clinician's simple, but very useful, dependence on measuring pretreatment, resting heart rate in horses with atrial fibrillation.[222, 377] Since the horse with structural heart disease will be more likely to require sympathetic support to maintain CO and arterial blood pressure, persistent resting tachycardia, higher than 60 beats/min, is associated with a poorer prognosis.

Laboratory studies in horses with atrial fibrillation are usually normal. Infrequently, a horse is found to have low serum potassium, fractional excretion of potassium, or RBC potassium. Chest x-rays are usually normal unless there is concurrent pulmonary disease, and this study is not a high-yield procedure in horses without compatible signs of lung disease or structural heart disease. The echocardiogram is usually normal, unless there is concurrent valvular or ventricular myocardial disease. It is not uncommon for an otherwise normal horse to demonstrate a slightly reduced LV

Table 7–17. Management of Atrial Fibrillation

General Examination of the Horse (see Table 7–4)

Identification of Negative Prognostic Factors

Congestive heart failure
Consistently elevated resting heart rate
Dilated cardiomyopathy
Mitral, tricuspid, or aortic valve regurgitation with cardiomegaly
Long history of atrial fibrillation
Prior bouts of atrial fibrillation
Unresponsive to therapeutic doses of quinidine

Horse Without Heart Failure

Recommended Method: Initial Oral Dosing at 2-Hour Intervals

- Initiate therapy with quinidine sulfate via nasogastric tube, 22 mg/kg body weight, q2hr, to a total cumulative dose of 88 to 132 mg/kg, or until conversion or toxicosis occurs
- When the aforementioned treatment fails to achieve conversion to normal sinus rhythm, continue quinidine therapy at a dose of 22 mg/kg q6hr for an additional 2 to 4 days, monitoring plasma quinidine concentration
- Digoxin should be administered concurrently during quinidine therapy in the following situations: (1) if the vagolytic effect of the drug causes significant acceleration in ventricular rate response, (2) if resting heart rate exceeds 90 to 100/min, (3) if the horse exhibits low "resting" vagal tone (e.g., a nervous animal), or (4) beginning on the second day of quinidine therapy if conversion has not yet occurred
- An oral maintenance dose range of digoxin for control of ventricular rate response in atrial fibrillation is 1.1 to 1.5 mg/100 kg body weight, q12hr*; alternatively, an IV maintenance dose of digoxin can be administered at 0.22 to 0.375 mg/100 kg body weight, q12hr*
- Monitor plasma levels of quinidine if possible; therapeutic levels associated with conversion to normal/sinus rhythm are 2 to 5 μg/mL†
- Monitor plasma levels of digoxin to avoid digoxin toxicity.

Alternative Therapy: IV Dosing

- IV quinidine gluconate 1 mg/kg IV, every 5 to 10 minutes, to a maximum of 10 mg/kg cumulative dose
- This treatment is most frequently used for conversion of atrial fibrillation of recent onset (<7 days), during anesthesia, or when nasogastric delivery is difficult or impossible

Toxicosis

- Monitor the electrocardiogram for response and toxicosis (increasing ventricular rate response, increasing QRS duration, or pro-arrhythmic effect causing ventricular tachycardia)
- If toxicosis develops (see text), discontinue therapy until all signs resolve, and initiate oral therapy using the q6hr method as described earlier
- Consider a 24-hour Holter electrocardiogram on the day after conversion to evaluate for recurrent atrial arrhythmias

Rest the Horse

For 1 to 2 weeks if possible (in racing horses, training can begin 48 hours after conversion)

Re-evaluate the Horse

For atrial arrhythmias both prior to starting training and during training

Horse with Heart Failure

- Very low probability for return to serious work; however, successful therapy may permit breeding or keeping the animal as a pet
- Establish diuresis with furosemide (1 mg/kg, IV or IM, q12hr) as needed to control edema. Maintenance furosemide therapy is continued at 0.5 to 1 mg/kg, per os, q12 to 24 hr; titrate the daily dose to effect
- Digitalize the horse to control heart rate and treat heart failure
    An IV maintenance dose for treatment of CHF, 0.22 mg/100 kg body weight, q12hr,* can be used to initiate therapy until clinical signs of CHF have been controlled (alternative: begin therapy using the oral maintenance dose below)
    An oral maintenance dose of 1.1 to 1.75 mg/100 kg body weight, q12hr,* is administered chronically
- Monitor the serum digoxin concentration (therapeutic trough levels = 1 to 2 ng/mL)
- Monitor serum electrolytes, blood urea nitrogen, and serum creatinine
- Monitor the resting heart rate, clinical signs, and electrocardiogram

---

*When a dosage range is given, generally begin at the lower end of the dose.
†The potential for quinidine-digoxin drug interaction elevating the serum digoxin should be considered (see text).
CHF, congestive heart failure; IM, intramuscular; IV, intravenous.

---

shortening fraction (usually 24% to 32%), which returns to normal once the horse has been converted to sinus rhythm.[423, 424] This decrease in fractional shortening is probably multifactorial in origin but is related in part to decreased preload from loss of the atrial contribution to ventricular filling. Doppler studies are useful in evaluating horses with concurrent valvular disease.

An excellent prognosis for conversion (>95% conversion rate) may be given for horses with a heart rate of less than or equal to 60 beats/min, murmurs less than or equal to grade 3/6, and atrial fibrillation of less than 4 months' duration.[377] Recurrences affect approximately 25% of these horses. Horses with longer duration of atrial fibrillation or significant other cardiac disease may be more difficult to convert to sinus rhythm (80% conversion) and have a higher recurrence rate (60% recurrence). Horses can usually be returned to training within 24 to 48 hours after conversion, once plasma quinidine concentrations are undetectable. Horses with heart rates in excess of 60 beats/min should be carefully evaluated for heart failure or structural disease and should probably not be treated with quinidine prior to a complete evaluation.

Conversion of atrial fibrillation to sinus rhythm using quinidine sulfate has been successful in many horses and using a variety of treatment plans (see Fig. 7–54).[220, 222, 413, 414, 416, 418, 419, 421] General recommendations for therapy, including alternative treatments, are summarized in Table 7–17. Intravenous quinidine gluconate can be successful in conversion of horses with no other significant cardiac disease and atrial fibrillation of recent onset.[425] If this treatment is not successful or the suspected duration is longer than 1 month, conversion with quinidine sulfate, administered via nasogastric intubation, should be attempted. Quinidine sulfate should be administered via nasogastric tube at a dosage of 22 mg/kg every 2 hours until the horse converts or develops initial signs of toxicosis. Toxicosis or a cumulative dose of 88 to 132 mg/kg should be considered endpoints for therapy and if conversion has not occurred, a plasma sample should be obtained for determination of quinidine plasma concentration and therapy temporarily discontinued for at least 6 hours. Therapeutic plasma quinidine concentrations for conversion from atrial fibrillation to sinus rhythm are 2 to 5 μg/mL. Subsequent quinidine sulfate administration should be based on the most recent plasma concentration. The mean quinidine elimination half-life after an oral 10-g dose is 6.65 hours. Thus, after the loading regimen every 2 hours, treatment intervals can be prolonged to every 6 hours (approximately every half-life). These treatment intervals can be continued until the horse shows toxic signs or converts to sinus rhythm, or the owner elects to discontinue treatment. If conversion to sinus rhythm has not occurred after 24 hours of therapy, digoxin at 0.011 mg/kg orally twice a day may be added to the treatment regimen for 24 to 48 hours. Combination therapy beyond 48 hours may be associated with elevated digoxin concentrations and should be continued only while monitoring serum digoxin concentrations.[425a] Even horses that do not convert on the "standard" administration regimen every 2 hours may convert after the initiation of an every 6-hour interval or the combined use of quinidine with digoxin.[423] The value of using such a treatment plan every 6 hours is that steady-state levels are reached, there is sufficient time to attain myocardial concentrations, and quinidine toxicity is less frequent when compared with the every 2-hour regimen.

Conversion of horses with atrial fibrillation generally results in a return to their previous performance level.[222, 377] Horses with repeated episodes of atrial fibrillation are often converted numerous times with quinidine sulfate treatment. Most horses that experience a recurrence of atrial fibrillation do so within 1 year of initial conversion, but periods as long as 6 years have occurred between episodes of atrial fibrillation in some horses. If the duration of sinus rhythm becomes shorter, repeated treatments may no longer be practical and a career change may be indicated. Some horses eventually become refractory to quinidine sulfate, probably due to progressive atrial fibrosis or underlying myocardial disease.

Careful clinical and continuous electrocardiographic mon-

itoring should be performed on horses with atrial fibrillation during conversion to sinus rhythm. The QRS duration should be monitored and compared with the pretreatment QRS duration before each additional treatment is administered. Prolongation of the QRS duration to greater than 25% of the pretreatment value is an indication of quinidine toxicity and should prompt discontinuation of therapy. The simplest ECG change is an acceleration of AV nodal conduction related to the vagolytic effect of quinidine. Rapid supraventricular tachycardias with ventricular rate responses of 300 beats/min have been seen in several horses receiving quinidine sulfate. These horses have been treated with intravenous digoxin at 0.002 mg/kg to slow the ventricular response rate, intravenous replacement fluids to improve perfusion, intravenous sodium bicarbonate at 1 mEq/kg to bind any free plasma quinidine, and if needed, a phenylephrine drip to restore blood pressure if there is critical hypotension. Ventricular arrhythmias (torsades de pointes, multiform ventricular tachycardia, and ventricular complexes) have also been detected with quinidine toxicosis (see Fig. 7–54). Intravenous sodium bicarbonate is also indicated in these horses to bind free circulating quinidine, while intravenous magnesium sulfate (up to 25 g in a 450- to 500-kg horse) is the treatment of choice for quinidine-induced ventricular arrhythmias. Lidocaine HCl may also be used if needed.

Clinical markers of quinidine toxicosis include ataxia, diarrhea, colic, hypotension due to vasodilation, and edema. Upper respiratory tract stridor, probably an idiosyncratic reaction, is infrequently observed. These adverse effects may prompt discontinuation of therapy or altering treatment intervals. Depression, tachycardia, paraphimosis, convulsions, CHF, laminitis, urticaria, and sudden death have also been reported associated with quinidine sulfate administration, although these are fortunately quite rare. Most adverse reactions to quinidine sulfate are associated with higher plasma concentrations of the drug (>5 μg/mL) and can be avoided with careful clinical and electrocardiographic monitoring. Particularly nervous horses, or those prone to the vagolytic effects of quinidine, may benefit from pre-treatment with digoxin at 0.011 mg/kg orally b.i.d. to blunt the ventricular rate response. When the ventricular rate response exceeds 100 beats/min in any horse undergoing quinidine sulfate conversion, digitalization should be considered, particularly if there are no other signs of quinidine toxicosis (that would indicate an excessive plasma concentration).

Junctional Arrhythmias

Cardiac arrhythmias that originate within the AV conducting tissues, the ventricular specialized conducting tissues, or myocardium are classified as "junctional" (AV nodal or bundle of His) or ventricular in origin. Unlike sinus or atrial arrhythmias, these arrhythmias are not preceded by a conducted P wave. Junctional and ventricular rhythms often lead to dissociation between the SA (P wave) activity and that of the ventricle (QRS-T), resulting in AV dissociation. AV dissociation in these cases develops because the premature AV junctional or ventricular depolarization causes interference to the conduction of normal SA impulses.

It may be difficult to distinguish between junctional and ventricular arrhythmias and to determine the exact location of the abnormal impulse formation. The differentiation of junctional and ventricular rhythms can sometimes be made by inspection of the QRS complex. Junctional impulses are more likely to result in a narrow, relatively normal-appearing QRS complex with normal initial activation and electrical axis, because they originate above the ventricular myocardium. Complexes of ventricular origin, by contrast, are conducted abnormally and more slowly, resulting in a widened QRS, an abnormal QRS orientation, and abnormal T waves. However, junctional tachycardias may be conducted aberrantly, resulting in a bizarre and wide QRS complex. When sustained, both types of rhythms cause AV dissociation with an independent atrial rhythm superimposed on the ectopic ventricular rhythm. The normal heart contains potential cardiac pacemakers within the AV and ventricular specialized tissues. These potential pacemakers may become manifest during periods of sinus bradycardia or AV block. Such complexes are termed escape complexes or, if the junctional or ventricular complexes are linked together, *escape rhythms.* Escape rhythms are characterized by slow ventricular rates, often in the realm of 15 to 25 beats/min. These normal pacemakers may be enhanced under certain conditions, including the administration of anesthesia or catecholamines.

Preanesthetic drugs like xylazine and detomidine and anesthetic drugs (halothane) suppress SA function, resulting in sinus bradycardia or periods of sinus arrest while enhancing the effects of catecholamines on latent junctional and ventricular pacemakers (Fig. 7–55). Such accelerated idioventricular (or idionodal) rhythms generally have little clinical significance other than to prompt the reduction of anesthetic dosages or promote administration of vagolytic drugs to increase the SA rate. Specific antiarrhythmic drug suppression of escape rhythms is generally not necessary and is contraindicated since these rhythms serve as rescue mechanisms for the heart.

Junctional complexes that arise early relative to the normal cardiac cycle are designated as *premature* junctional complexes. These complexes may occur as single or repetitive events and can resemble ectopic rhythms that might originate in the atria. Repetitive ectopic complexes that occur in short bursts or runs are termed nonsustained or paroxysmal tachycardias. Sustained junctional tachycardias may also occur and can lead to CHF.

The clinical significance of an occasional junctional pre-

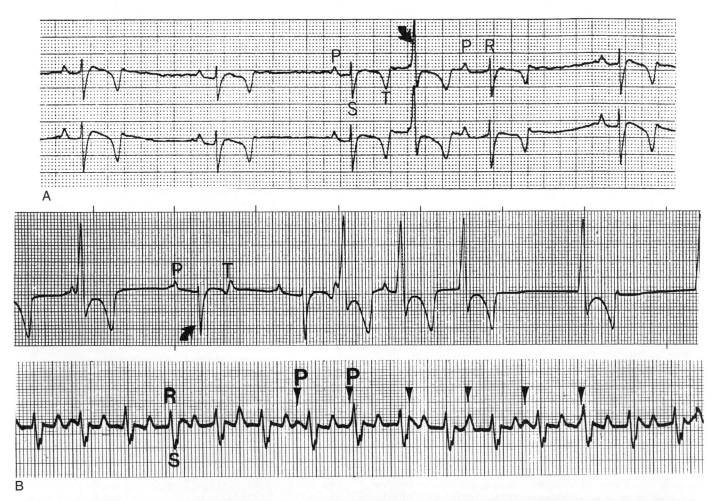

Figure 7–55. Ventricular extrasystoles (see also Fig. 7–15). *A,* The ectopic complex *(arrow)* is interpolated between two sinus beats. The prolonged PR interval following the premature complex is due to partial penetration of the atrioventricular node (concealed conduction) and physiologic refractoriness to the next impulse (ambulatory electrocardiogram recorded at 25 mm/ sec). *B,* Ventricular rhythms. The top tracing demonstrates an idioventricular tachycardia in a postoperative gastrointestinal surgery case. Sinus complexes *(arrow)* are followed by ventricular ectopic beats at varying rates (base-apex lead at 25 mm/ sec). The lower tracing demonstrates atrioventricular dissociation caused by a sustained high ventricular (or junctional) ectopic rhythm. The atria are discharged independently by the sinus node *(arrowheads*; lead 2 at 25 mm/sec).

mature complex is difficult to ascertain. Persistent or repetitive junctional or ventricular rhythms are indicative of heart disease, systemic disease, or a drug-induced abnormality of cardiac rhythm. The best management choice is uncertain inasmuch as some junctional rhythms behave more like atrial tachyarrhythmias, whereas others cause AV dissociation and appear to act like ventricular ectopic impulses. Because the mechanism responsible for junctional tachycardias can be either abnormal automaticity or re-entry (circuit) movement using the AV node, empirical therapy is usually required to control sustained arrhythmias. If there is obvious AV dissociation, then quinidine would seem a reasonable first choice. If the mechanism is uncertain but is clearly supraventricular, then intravenous digoxin, intravenous verapamil, or propranolol may either silence the rhythm or slow the rate.

Ventricular Arrhythmias

Ventricular arrhythmias are less common than atrial arrhythmias but are more likely to be associated with underlying cardiac disease or a multisystemic disorder.[130, 218, 264, 426–432] Ventricular arrhythmias may be observed with severe toxemia or sepsis or primary gastrointestinal disorders including proximal enteritis and large bowel disorders; with electrolyte (potassium, magnesium) or metabolic disorders, hypoxia, or ischemia; or associated with halothane anesthesia. Drugs, myocardial toxins such as the ionophores, viral or bacterial myocarditis, endocarditis, or pericarditis may all lead to significant ventricular arrhythmias. The approach to the horse with ventricular arrhythmias should emphasize ruling out the noncardiac causes, correcting them (if possible), and then following if necessary with a complete CV examination, including electrocardiography and echocardiography. Cardiac isoenzymes should be considered to identify cardiac injury, although it may be problematic to separate primary from secondary causes of cardiac isoenzyme elevation (see Table 7–16). Ventricular ectopic rhythms are classified as indicated in Table 7–15.

Ventricular Premature Complexes

Ventricular premature complexes are characterized by an ectopic, premature complex usually followed by a compensatory pause, because the next sinus impulse is blocked by the refractory AV conduction system. If the sinus rate is slow or the ventricular premature depolarization is closely coupled to the preceding normal sinus beat, it may be interpolated between two normal beats. Ventricular ectopic impulses are characterized by QRS and T waves that are wide and often bizarre in appearance (Fig. 7–56). Of course, the premature QRS bears no relationship to any preceding P waves, though genesis of ventricular ectopics may be dependent on underlying cardiac cycle length. The morphology of the ventricular premature complex may be uniform or multiform. The relationship of a ventricular extrasystole to the preceding sinus QRS-T is expressed by the "coupling interval" between them. Often the coupling interval is fixed, although it may vary minimally[432] or markedly in cases of ventricular parasystole. A very short coupling interval may place the ectopic QRS on the preceding T wave, a phenomenon called "R on T" and related to increased ventricular vulnerability for fibrillation. Ventricular premature complexes occurred in

14% of clinically normal horses during routine 24-hour continuous electrocardiographic monitoring.[218] The distribution pattern of ventricular ectopics may include haphazard distribution, bigeminy, couplets (pairs of ventricular premature complexes), or runs of ventricular ectopics. Runs of accelerated ventricular rhythm, usually developing at relatively slow heart rates, are not uncommon in horses with ventricular ectopic activity. Infrequently, protected, totally independent ventricular rhythms typical of parasystole are recorded by Holter ECG. Runs of ventricular ectopics at a rapid rate—ventricular tachycardia—are more likely to be hemodynamically and electrically unstable, particularly when they develop at rates higher than 100/min (see later).

When premature ventricular beats are identified by auscultation, an ECG should be obtained, and a workup similar to that outlined in Table 7–15 should be undertaken. Occasional premature ventricular complexes, as with occasional supraventricular premature complexes, may be clinically insignificant and not require treatment. Rest is highly recommended for horses with frequent ventricular premature complexes. In the majority of horses with premature ventricular complexes, the arrhythmia seems to resolve spontaneously after 4 to 8 weeks of rest. The horse may then be able to return successfully to its prior performance level. Antiarrhythmic therapy is usually successful in abolishing ventricular premature complexes, but most return when the antiarrhythmic agent is discontinued, unless the underlying problem has been resolved. Dexamethasone and other anti-inflammatory drugs may also be helpful in abolishing ventricular premature complexes, but their use is controversial and they should certainly not be administered to horses with a recent or current infection.

Ventricular Tachycardia

Ventricular tachycardia is an ectopic ventricular rhythm characterized by either a regular or irregular ventricular rate (Fig. 7–57; see also Fig. 7–56). Ventricular tachycardia is recognized clinically by the increased heart rate, often exceeding 100 beats/min, and the loud, sometimes booming heart sounds that may be detected. Arterial pulses are typically weak or variable in intensity. Multiform ventricular tachycardia is characterized by an irregular rhythm and is usually associated with more clinical signs of CV disease than uniform (unifocal) ventricular tachycardia. With multiform ventricular tachycardia, heart sounds are more likely to vary in intensity and arterial pulses are likely to be abnormal. Jugular pulsations may be detected due to AV dissociation. Syncope is associated with higher rates of ventricular tachycardia (180 beats/min or higher). Respiratory distress and pulmonary edema may develop from systolic and diastolic dysfunction. Sustained junctional or ventricular tachycardias (>120 beats/min) may lead to CHF.[273, 428a]

Ventricular tachycardia may be life threatening if R on T complexes are detected; the arrhythmia is rapid (>180 to 200 beats/min); multiform ventricular tachycardia is detected; or polymorphic tachycardia with torsades de pointes is present.[432] Immediate treatment of CV collapse may be required.[348] Intravenous lidocaine or quinidine is usually chosen for emergencies, although both drugs have been associated with sudden death. Quinidine is a myocardial depressant, and lidocaine causes central nervous system excitation in horses; thus, the risks:benefits of treatment should

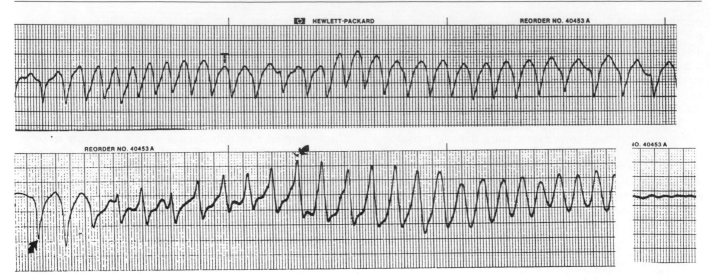

Figure 7–56. Sustained, very rapid ventricular tachycardia *(top)* of varying rate that develops into a polymorphic ventricular rhythm with varying morphology complexes (torsades de pointes). The horse died of cardiac arrest *(lower right panel)*. The *arrows* indicate QRS complexes of varying polarity (25 mm/sec).

be carefully weighed. Emergency treatment includes lidocaine at 0.25 to 0.5 mg/kg as a bolus or quinidine gluconate at 1.1 to 2.2 mg/kg intravenously as a bolus. Magnesium sulfate is an alternative antiarrhythmic that can be effective in both normomagnesemic and hypomagnesemic horses. Intravenous magnesium sulfate may be administered in 2 g or larger boluses or as a rapid drip, up to a total dosage of 25 g/450 to 500 kg. Other antiarrhythmics, including IV or oral procainamide[433] or propafenone,[434] may be tried in refractory ventricular arrhythmias (Table 7–14). A period of rest (4 to 8 weeks) followed by electrocardiographic and echocardiographic re-evaluation (including an exercising ECG) is indicated for follow-up of horses that have developed sustained ventricular tachycardia. A substantial number of these horses can be successfully returned to performance after treatment with antiarrhythmics or anti-inflammatory drugs and rest.

Conduction Disturbances

Once a cardiac electrical impulse is formed, it is conducted rapidly throughout the heart. The sequence of cardiac electric activation is usually dictated by the specialized conducting tissues in the atria, the AV node, the bundle of His, the bundle branches, and the Purkinje fiber system. This conduction system permits orderly activation of atrial and ventricular muscle and facilitates effective mechanical activity of the heart. A variety of conduction disorders are recognized, including SA nodal exit block, atrial standstill (usually due to hyperkalemia), AV block, bundle branch block, and ill-defined ventricular conduction disturbances (Figs. 7–58 and 7–59).[36, 129, 409, 435–439]

Rarely, accelerated conduction occurs in the heart, which involves a pathway around the normally slow-conducting AV node and results in early excitation of the ventricles.[440] These syndromes are termed pre-excitation and have various associated labels related to similar human disorders (e.g., Wolff-Parkinson-White). The pre-excitation syndromes are usually characterized by short PR intervals and widened QRS complexes. Some examples of these conduction disorders will be illustrated.

Atrioventricular Conduction Block

Delays in AV conduction are the most common conduction disorders. These delays are classified as first-, second-, and third-degree (or complete). *First-degree AV block* occurs when the PR (or PQ) interval exceeds a certain value (while the atrial impulse still transmits through the AV conduction system and activates the ventricle, causing a QRS). Some P waves are not conducted to the ventricles during *second-degree AV block,* which results in occasional P waves not followed by a QRS-T complex. *Third-degree* or *complete AV*

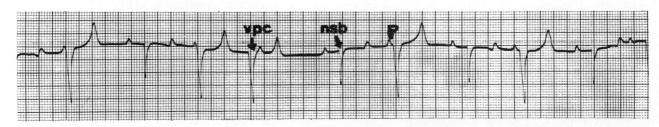

Figure 7–57. Frequent ventricular ectopic contractions (vpc) are noted in a horse previously treated for ventricular tachycardia. There are normal sinus beats (nsb) and widened ventricular ectopic complexes evident.

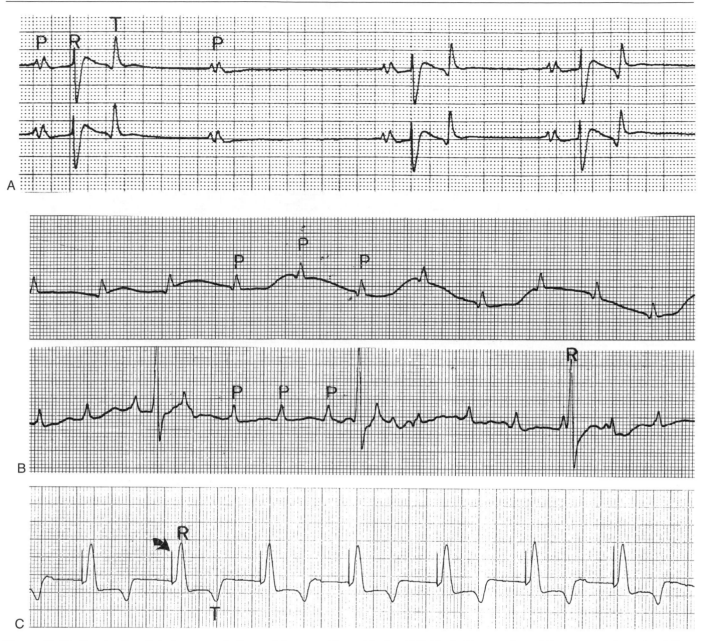

Figure 7–58. Conduction disturbances. *A,* Second-degree atrioventricular (AV) block. Nonconducted P waves and varying PR intervals are evident (base-apex lead at 25 mm/sec). *B,* The tracings are from a horse with third-degree AV block. The upper strip demonstrates multiple blocked P waves. The lower tracing shows nonconducted P waves and ventricular escape complexes (base-apex lead at 25 mm/sec). *C,* Permanent transvenous ventricular pacing in a miniature donkey with a complete AV block. A pacemaker spike *(arrow)* precedes each paced ventricular complex.

block is characterized by an absence of atrial to ventricular conduction. P waves are never followed by or related to QRS complexes, and to prevent ventricular asystole, a junctional or ventricular escape rhythm must develop below the level of the AV block.

First- and second-degree AV block are considered normal variations. These rhythms are most often associated with high vagal tone and may be seen with sinus bradycardia or sinus arrhythmia. Second-degree AV block can usually be abolished with exercise, stress, or vagolytic drugs such as atropine or glycopyrrolate. Complete AV block is indicative of organic heart disease, severe drug toxicity, or rarely very high vagal activity. Generally speaking, third-degree AV

block caused by vagal-efferent traffic is short-lived. Intraventricular conduction blocks, such as bundle branch block, are less common and more difficult to diagnose. Widening of the QRS complex and axis deviation are typical features. These abnormalities may also be found after atrial premature complexes, from overdosage with quinidine sulfate, or secondary to supraventricular tachycardias with rapid ventricular response.

Sudden development of high-grade or complete AV block may require the administration of atropine or a catecholamine, or rapid transvenous insertion of a pacing wire into the right ventricle. Chronic third-degree AV block requires treatment with a pacemaker; such a pacemaker has been successfully placed

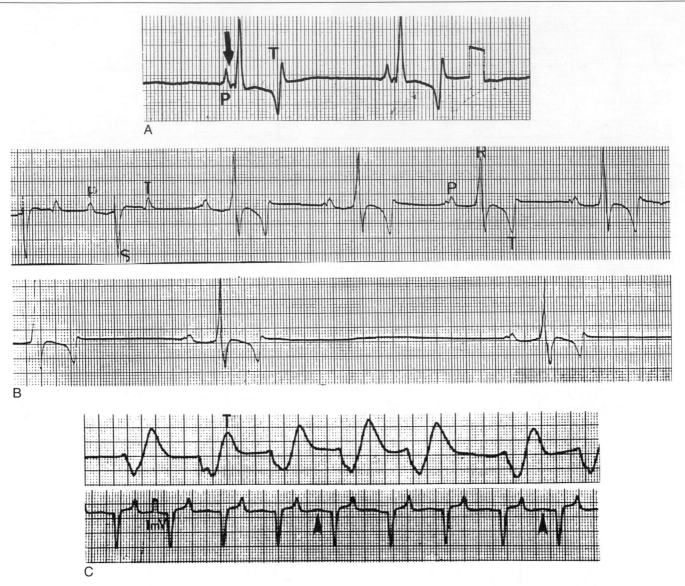

Figure 7–59. Conduction disturbances. *A,* Ventricular pre-excitation. The short PR interval *(arrow)* and small deflection in the PR segment (delta wave) are indicative of an accessory pathway around the atrioventricular node with premature activation of a portion of the ventricle (delta wave and initial portion of the QRS). The large QRS and secondary T-wave changes can be explained by the loss of normal cancellation of ventricular electrical forces. *B,* A sinus arrhythmia and intraventricular conduction disturbance. Note the sudden change and widening of the ventricular conduction pattern, despite the relatively consistent PR interval. This probably represents a bundle branch block, although this diagnosis is difficult to make in horses (base-apex lead at 25 mm/sec). *C,* Hyperkalemia in a foal with a ruptured bladder. The top strip demonstrates atrial standstill (no P waves), marked widening of the QRS complexes, and large T waves with a relatively shortened ST segment. The lower tracing shows the effects after initial medical therapy for hyperkalemia, which included treatment with saline and sodium bicarbonate. Note the normalization of the QRS complexes and the appearance of low-amplitude P waves *(arrows).* (Tracing courtesy of Dr. Ron Hilwig.)

epicardially and transvenously in several horses and miniature (Jerusalem) donkeys (Figs. 7–58 and 7–60).

Pre-excitation

Pre-excitation, or accelerated AV conduction, has been reported sporadically,[440] but the clinical significance of this electrocardiographic abnormality has yet to be determined in this species. Ventricular pre-excitation in humans and in dogs is often due to an anomalous conducting pathway around the AV node, which serves as a path for re-entrant supraventricular tachycardias. These rhythm disturbances may cause hypotension and syncope. Whether pre-excitation syndromes are important has yet to be determined. Nevertheless, ECG traces occasionally show evidence of ventricular pre-excitation and are characterized by a P-QRS-T relationship but with an extremely short PR interval, early excitation of the ventricle characterized by a slurring of the initial QRS complex (a delta wave), and an overall widening of the QRS complex.

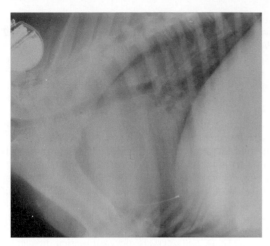

Figure 7–60. A lateral radiograph of a permanent transvenous pacing system in a miniature donkey. The pacemaker is evident at the upper left of the radiograph. The thin transvenous pacing wire extends from the device through the jugular vein and vena cava and into the right ventricular apex.

Hyperkalemia

Hyperkalemia can cause significant depression of atrial, AV, and ventricular conduction and can shorten ventricular repolarization. Serum potassium is most likely to be markedly elevated following oliguria, rupture of the ureter during shock, in foals with ruptured bladder and uroperitoneum, or after excessive intravenous potassium replacement. Experimentally, changes in the ECG are usually evident at potassium serum concentrations greater than 6 mEq/L with severe changes evident when serum concentrations are between 8 and 10 mEq/L.[129, 441–444] Broadening and flattening of the P wave are the most consistently observed change. Either inversion or enlargement (tenting) of the T waves is also likely.[70] Marked widening of the QRS complex may be noted as near-lethal concentrations of potassium are approached. Ventricular asystole or fibrillation can develop. The QT interval is not a reliable indicator of induced hyperkalemia, and other electrolyte/acid-base alterations, including serum calcium and sodium, influence the effect of hyperkalemia on the heart.

Therapy for hyperkalemia includes correction of the underlying problem; infusion of saline; and administration of sodium bicarbonate (initial dose 0.25 to 0.5 mEq/kg) and possibly calcium chloride. While controversial, the administration of regular insulin in conjunction with dextrose infusion may be considered in cases of life-threatening hyperkalemia. Potassium follows glucose intracellularly and lowers the extracellular potassium concentration.

REFERENCES

1. Detweiler DK, Patterson DF: The cardiovascular system. In Catcott EJ, Smithcors JF, eds. *Equine Medicine and Surgery,* ed. 2. Santa Barbara, American Veterinary Publications, 1972, p 277.
2. Holmes JR: The equine heart: Problems and difficulties in assessing cardiac function on clinical examination. *Equine Vet J* 1:10, 1968.
3. Fregin GF: The cardiovascular system. In Mansmann RA, McAllister ES, Pratt PW, eds. *Equine Medicine and Surgery.* Santa Barbara, American Veterinary Publications, 1982.
4. Patterson DF, Detweiler DK, Glendinning SA: Heart sounds and murmurs of the normal horse. *Ann N Y Acad Sci* 127:242, 1965.
5. Detweiler DK: Auricular fibrillation in horses. *J Am Vet Med Assoc* 126:47, 1955.
6. Detweiler DK: Electrocardiogram of the horse. *Fed Proc* 11:34, 1952.
7. Smith CR, Hamlin RL: Regulation of the heart and blood vessels. In Swenson MJ, ed. *Dukes' Physiology of Domestic Animals.* Ithaca, NY, Comstock Publishers, 1970, p 169.
8. Hamlin RL, Smetzer DL, Smith CR: Analysis of QRS complex recorded through a semiorthogonal lead system in the horse. *Am J Physiol* 207:325, 1964.
9. Hamlin RL, Smith CR: Categorization of common domestic mammals based on their ventricular activation process. *Ann N Y Acad Sci* 127:195, 1965.
10. Smetzer DL, Smith CR, Hamlin RL: The fourth heart sound in the equine. *Ann N Y Acad Sci* 127:306, 1965.
11. Smetzer DL, Smith CR: Diastolic heart sounds of horses. *J Am Vet Med Assoc* 146:937, 1965.
12. Smetzer DL, Bishop S, Smith CR: Diastolic murmur of equine aortic insufficiency. *Am Heart J* 72:489, 1966.
13. Hamlin RL, Smetzer DL, Senta T, et al: Atrial activation paths and P waves in horses. *Am J Physiol* 219:306, 1970.
14. Hamlin RL, Klepinger WL, Gilpin KW, et al: Autonomic control of heart rate in the horse. *Am J Physiol* 222:976, 1972.
15. Smetzer DL, Hamlin RL, Smith CR: Cardiovascular sounds. In Swenson MJ, ed. *Dukes' Physiology of Domestic Animals.* Ithaca, NY, Comstock Publishers, 1970, p 159.
16. Holmes JR, Darke PGG, Else RW: Atrial fibrillation in the horse. *Equine Vet J* 1:212, 1969.
17. Else RW, Holmes JR: Cardiac pathology in the horse. I: Gross pathology. *Equine Vet J* 4:1, 1972.
18. Else RW, Holmes JR: Cardiac pathology in the horse. II: Microscopic pathology. *Equine Vet J* 4:57, 1972.
19. Else RW, Holmes JR: Cardiac pathology in the horse. III: Clinical correlations. *Equine Vet J* 4:195, 1972.
20. Holmes JR, Rezakhani A, Else RW: Rupture of a dissecting aortic aneurysm into the left pulmonary artery in a horse. *Equine Vet J* 5:65, 1973.
21. Holmes JR, Rezakhani A: Observations on the T wave of the equine electrocardiogram. *Equine Vet J* 7:55, 1975.
22. Holmes JR: Prognosis of equine cardiac conditions. *Equine Vet J* 9:181, 1977.
23. Brown CM, Holmes JR: Haemodynamics in the horse. 2: Intracardiac, pulmonary arterial, and aortic pressures. *Equine Vet J* 10:207, 1978.
24. Brown CM, Holmes JR: Haemodynamics in the horse. I: Pressure pulse contours. *Equine Vet J* 10:188, 1978.
25. Brown CM, Holmes JR: Phonocardiography in the horse. 2: The relationship between the external phonocardiogram and internal pressure and sound. *Equine Vet J* 11:183, 1979.
26. Brown CM, Holmes JR: Assessment of myocardial function in the horse. 2: Experimental findings in resting horses. *Equine Vet J* 11:248, 1979.
27. Brown CM, Holmes JR: Phonocardiography in the horse. 1: The intracardiac phonocardiogram. *Equine Vet J* 11:11, 1979.
28. Brown CM, Holmes JR: Assessment of myocardial function in the horse. 1: Theoretical and technical considerations. *Equine Vet J* 11:244, 1979.
29. Holmes JR: Sir Frederick Smith Memorial Lecture. A superb transport system—the circulation. *Equine Vet J* 14:267, 1982.
30. Miller PJ, Holmes JR: Effect of cardiac arrhythmia on left ventricular and aortic blood pressure parameters in the horse. *Res Vet Sci* 35:190, 1983.

31. Holmes JR: Equine electrocardiography: Some practical hints on technique. *Equine Vet J* 16:477, 1984.

32. Holmes JR, Miller PJ: Three cases of ruptured mitral valve chordae in the horse. *Equine Vet J* 16:125, 1984.

33. Miller PJ, Holmes JR: Computer processing of transaortic valve blood pressures in the horse using the first derivative of the left ventricular pressure trace. *Equine Vet J* 16:210, 1984.

34. Miller PJ, Holmes JR: Observations on structure and function of the equine mitral valve. *Equine Vet J* 16:457, 1984.

35. Miller PJ, Holmes JR: Interrelationship of some electrocardiogram amplitudes, time intervals and respiration in the horse. *Res Vet Sci* 36:370, 1984.

36. Miller PJ, Holmes JR: Beat-to-beat variability in QRS potentials recorded with an orthogonal lead system in horses with second degree partial A-V block. *Res Vet Sci* 37:334, 1984.

37. Miller PJ, Holmes JR: Relationships of left side systolic time intervals to beat-by-beat heart rate and blood pressure variables in some cardiac arrhythmias of the horse. *Res Vet Sci* 37:18, 1984.

38. Miller PJ, Holmes JR: Observations on seven cases of mitral insufficiency in the horse. *Equine Vet J* 17:181, 1985.

39. Holmes JR, Henigan M, Williams RB, et al: Paroxysmal atrial fibrillation in racehorses. *Equine Vet J* 18:37, 1986.

40. Baker JR, Ellis CE: A survey of post mortem findings in 480 horses 1958 to 1980. 1: Causes of death. *Equine Vet J* 13:43, 1981.

41. Reef VB: Clinical approach to poor performance in horses. *Proc Am Coll Vet Intern Med* 566, 1989.

42. Morris EA, Seeherman HJ: Clinical evaluation of poor performance in the racehorse: The results of 275 evaluations. *Equine Vet J* 23:169, 1991.

43. Cronin MTL, Leader GH: Coronary occlusion in a thoroughbred colt. *Vet Record* 64:8, 1952.

44. Rooney JR, Prickett ME, Crowe MW: Aortic ring rupture in stallions. *Vet Pathol* 4:268, 1967.

45. Pascoe RR, O'Sullivan BM: Sudden death in a Thoroughbred stallion. *Equine Vet J* 12:211, 1980.

46. Platt H: Sudden and unexpected deaths in horses: A review of 69 cases. *Br Vet J* 138:417, 1982.

47. Hughes PE, Howard EB: Endocardial fibroelastosis as a cause of sudden death in the horse. *Equine Practice* 6:23, 1984.

48. Gelberg HB, Zachary JF, Everitt JI, et al: Sudden death in training and racing Thoroughbred horses. *J Am Vet Med Assoc* 187:1354, 1985.

49. Kiryu I, Nakamura T, Kaneko M, et al: Cardiopathology of sudden death in the race horse. *Heart Vessels Suppl* 2:40, 1987.

50. Lucke VM: Sudden death (Editorial). *Equine Vet J* 19:85, 1987.

51. Brown CM, Kaneene JB, Taylor RF: Sudden and unexpected death in horses and ponies: An analysis of 200 cases. *Equine Vet J* 20:99, 1988.

52. Geddes LA, Hoff HE, McCrady JD: Some aspects of the cardiovascular physiology of the horse. (Baylor University College of Medicine) *Cardiovasc Res Center Bull* 3:80, 1965.

53. Miller MS, Bonagura JD: Genesis of the equine electrocardiogram and indications for electrocardiography in clinical practice. *J Equine Vet Sci* 5:23, 1985.

54. Guyton AC: The circulation. In Guyton AC, ed. *Textbook of Medical Physiology.* Philadelphia, WB Saunders, 1986, p 205.

55. Jones WE: *Equine Sports Medicine.* Philadelphia, Lea & Febiger, 1988.

56. Bonagura JD, Muir WW: The cardiovascular system. In Muir WW, Hubbell JAE, eds. *Equine Anesthesia.* St Louis, Mosby–Year Book, 1991, p 39.

57. Shepherd JT, Vanhoutte PM: *The Human Cardiovascular System.* New York, Raven Press, 1992.

58. Sisson S, Grossman JD: *Anatomy of the Domestic Animals,* ed 4. Philadelphia, WB Saunders, 1953.

59. Muir WW: Cardiopulmonary resuscitation and the prevention of hypotensive emergencies in horses. *Proc Am Assoc Equine Pract* 30:117, 1984.

60. Muir WW: Anesthetic complications and cardiopulmonary resuscitation in the horse. In Muir WW, Hubbell JAE (eds). *Equine Anesthesia.* St Louis, Mosby–Year Book, 1992, p 461.

61. Rainey JW: A specific arthritis with pericarditis affecting young horses in Tasmania. *Aust Vet J* 20:204, 1944.

62. Wagner P, Miller R, Merritt F, et al: Constrictive pericarditis in the horse. *J Equine Med Surg* 1:242, 1977.

63. Dill SG, Simoncini DC, Bolton GR, et al: Fibrinous pericarditis in the horse. *J Am Vet Med Assoc* 180:266, 1982.

64. Wagner PC: Pericarditis. In Robinson NE, ed. *Current Therapy in Equine Medicine.* Philadelphia, WB Saunders, 1983, p 149.

65. Reef VB, Freeman D, Gentile D: Successful treatment of pericarditis in a horse. *J Am Vet Med Assoc* 185:94, 1984.

66. Bertone JJ, Dill SG: Traumatic gastropericarditis in a horse. *J Am Vet Med Assoc* 187:742, 1985.

67. Bernard W, Reef V, Clark ES, et al: Pericarditis in horses: Six cases (1982–1986). *J Am Vet Med Assoc* 196:468, 1990.

68. Hardy J, Robertson JT, Reed SM: Constrictive pericarditis in a mare: Attempted treatment by partial pericardiectomy. *Equine Vet J* 24:151, 1992.

69. Freestone JF, Thomas WP, Carlson GP, et al: Idiopathic effusive pericarditis with tamponade in the horse. *Equine Vet J* 19:38, 1987.

70. Carnine BL, Schneider G, Cook JE, et al: Pericardial mesothelioma in a horse. *Vet Pathol* 14:513, 1977.

71. Baker D, Kreeger J: Infiltrative lipoma in the heart of a horse. *Cornell Vet* 77:258, 1987.

72. Dill SG, Moise NS, Meschter CL: Cardiac failure in a stallion secondary to metastasis of an anaplastic pulmonary carcinoma. *Equine Vet J* 18:414, 1986.

73. Birks EK, Hultgren BD: Pericardial haemangiosarcoma in a horse. *J Comp Pathol* 99:105, 1988.

74. Byars TD, Dainis CM, Seltzer KL, et al: Cranial thoracic masses in the horse: A sequel to pleuropneumonia. *Equine Vet J* 23:22, 1991.

75. Rugh KS, Garner HE, Sprouse RF, et al: Left ventricular hypertrophy in chronically hypertensive ponies. *Lab Anim Sci* 37:335, 1987.

76. Braunwald E, Sonnenblick EH, Ross J Jr: Mechanisms of cardiac contraction and relaxation. In Braunwald E, ed. *Heart Disease: A Textbook of Cardiovascular Medicine.* Philadelphia, WB Saunders, 1992, p 351.

77. Braunwald E: Pathophysiology of heart failure. In Braunwald E, ed. *Heart Disease: A Textbook of Cardiovascular Medicine.* Philadelphia, WB Saunders, 1992, p 393.

78. Cranley JJ, McCullagh KG: Ischaemic myocardial fibrosis and aortic strongylosis in the horse. *Equine Vet J* 13:35, 1981.

79. Dudan F, Rossi GL, Luginbuhl H: Cardiovascular study of the horse: Relationships between vascular and tissue lesions in the myocardium, vol. 2. *Schweiz Arch Tierheilkd* 126:527, 1984.

80. Dudan F, Rossi GL, Luginbuhl H: Cardiovascular study in the horse: Relationship between vascular and myocardial lesions, vol. 3. *Schweiz Arch Tierheilkd* 127:319, 1985.

81. Bonagura JD: Equine heart disease: An overview. *Vet Clin North Am Equine Pract* 1:267, 1985.

82. Bonagura JD, Herring DS, Welker F: Echocardiography. *Vet Clin North Am Equine Pract* 1:311, 1985.

83. Koblik PD, Hornof WJ: Diagnostic radiology and nuclear cardiology: Their use in assessment of equine cardiovascular disease. *Vet Clin North Am Equine Pract* 1:289, 1985.

84. Amend JF, Nicholson RL, Freeland LR, et al: Clinical toxicology of an antibiotic ionophore (monensin) in ponies and horses; diagnostic markers and therapeutic considerations. In *Comparative Veterinary Pharmacology, Toxicology and Therapy.* Lancaster, UK, 1986, pp 381–389.

85. Mollenhauer HH, Rowe LD, Witzel DA: Effect of monensin on the morphology of mitochondria in rodent and equine striated muscle. *Vet Hum Toxicol* 26:15, 1984.

86. Amend JF, Mallon FM, Wren WB, et al: Equine monensin toxicosis: Some experimental clinicopathologic observations. *Compend Contin Educ Pract Vet* 2:S172, 1980.

87. Sweeney RW, Hamir AN, Fisher RR: Lymphosarcoma with urinary bladder infiltration in a horse. *J Am Vet Med Assoc* 199:1177, 1991.

88. Rooney JR, Franks WC: Congenital cardiac anomalies in horses. *Vet Pathol* 1:454, 1964.

89. Bayly WM, Reed SM, Leathers CW, et al: Multiple congenital heart anomalies in five Arabian foals. *J Am Vet Med Assoc* 181:684, 1982.

90. McClure JJ, Gaber CE, Watters JW, et al: Complete transposition of the great arteries with ventricular septal defect and pulmonary stenosis in a Thoroughbred foal. *Equine Vet J* 15:377, 1983.

91. Tadmor A, Fischel R, Tov AS: A condition resembling hypoplastic left heart syndrome in a foal. *Equine Vet J* 15:175, 1983.

92. Musselman EE, LoGuidice RJ: Hypoplastic left ventricular syndrome in a foal. *J Am Vet Med Assoc* 185:542, 1984.

93. Crowe MW, Swerczek TW: Equine congenital defects. *Am J Vet Res* 46:353, 1985.

94. Physick Sheard PW, Maxie MG, Palmer NC, et al: Atrial septal defect of the persistent ostium primum type with hypoplastic right ventricle in a Welsh pony foal. *Can J Comp Med* 49:429, 1985.

95. Reef VB: Cardiovascular disease in the equine neonate. *Vet Clin North Am Equine Pract* 1:117, 1985.

96. Clark ES, Reef VB, Sweeney C, et al: Aortic valve insufficiency in a one-year-old colt. *J Am Vet Med Assoc* 191:841, 1987.

97. Reef VB, Mann P: Echocardiographic diagnosis of tricuspid atresia in 2 foals. *J Am Vet Med Assoc* 191:225, 1987.

98. Sojka JE: Persistent truncus arteriosus in a foal. *Equine Pract* 9:19, 1987.

99. Zamora CS, Vitums A, Nyrop KA, et al: Atresia of the right atrioventricular orifice with complete transposition of the great arteries in a horse. *Anat Histol Embryol* 18:177, 1989.

100. Leipold HW, Saperstein G, Woollen NE: Congenital defects in foals. In Smith BP, ed. *Large Animal Internal Medicine*. St. Louis, CV Mosby, 1990, p 137.

101. Cargile J, Lombard C, Wilson JH, et al: Tetralogy of Fallot and segmental uterine aplasia in a three-year-old Morgan filly. *Cornell Vet* 81:411, 1991.

102. Hinchcliff KW, Adams WM: Critical pulmonary stenosis in a newborn foal. *Equine Vet J* 23:318, 1991.

103. Reef VB, Spencer P: Echocardiographic evaluation of equine aortic insufficiency. *Am J Vet Res* 48:904, 1987.

104. Bonagura JD, Pipers FS: Echocardiographic features of aortic valve endocarditis in a dog, a cow, and a horse. *J Am Vet Med Assoc* 182:595, 1983.

105. Brown CM: Acquired cardiovascular disease. *Vet Clin North Am Equine Pract* 1:371, 1985.

106. Buergelt CD, Cooley AJ, Hines SA, et al: Endocarditis in six horses. *Vet Pathol* 22:333, 1985.

107. Rantanen NW: Diseases of the heart. *Vet Clin North Am Equine Pract* 2:33, 1986.

108. Travers CW, van den Berg JS: Pseudomonas spp. associated vegetative endocarditis in two horses. *J S Afr Vet Assoc* 66:172–176, 1995.

109. Dedrick P, Reef VB, Sweeney RW, et al: Treatment of bacterial endocarditis in a horse. *J Am Vet Med Assoc* 193:339, 1988.

110. Hamir AN, Reef VB: Complications of a permanent transvenous pacing catheter in a horse. *J Comp Pathol* 101:317, 1989.

111. Collatos C, Clark ES, Reef VB, et al: Septicemia, atrial fibrillation, cardiomegaly, left atrial mass, and *Rhodococcus equi* septic osteoarthritis in a foal. *J Am Vet Med Assoc* 197:1039, 1990.

112. Nilfors L, Lombard CW, Weckner D, et al: Diagnosis of pulmonary valve endocarditis in a horse. *Equine Vet J* 23:479, 1991.

113. Patteson MW, Cripps PJ: A survey of cardiac auscultatory findings in horses. *Equine Vet J* 25:409, 1993.

113a. Patteson M, Blissitt K: Evaluation of cardiac murmurs in horses 1. Clinical examination. *In Practice* 18:367–373, 1996.

114. Brown CM, Bell TG, Paradis MR, et al: Rupture of mitral chordae tendineae in two horses. *J Am Vet Med Assoc* 182:281, 1983.

115. Reef VB: Mitral valvular insufficiency associated with ruptured chordae tendineae in three foals. *J Am Vet Med Assoc* 191:329, 1987.

116. Marr CM, Love S, Pirie HM, et al: Confirmation by Doppler echocardiography of valvular regurgitation in a horse with a ruptured chorda tendinea of the mitral valve. *Vet Rec* 127:376, 1990.

117. Kiryu K, Kaneko M, Kanemaru T, et al: Cardiopathology of sinoatrial block in horses. *Jpn J Vet Sci* 47:45, 1985.

118. Matsui K, Sugano S, Amada A: Heart rate and ECG response to twitching in Thoroughbred foals and mares. *Nippon Juigaku Zasshi* 48:305, 1986.

119. Matsui K, Sugano S: Relation of intrinsic heart rate and autonomic nervous tone to resting heart rate in the young and the adult of various domestic animals. *Jpn J Vet Sci* 51:29, 1989.

120. Moore EN, Spear JF: Electrophysiological studies on atrial fibrillation. *Heart Vessels Suppl* 2:32, 1987.

121. Meijler FL, Kroneman J, van der Tweel I, et al: Nonrandom ventricular rhythm in horses with atrial fibrillation and its significance for patients. *J Am Coll Cardiol* 4:316, 1984.

122. Meijler FL: Atrioventricular conduction versus heart size from mouse to whale. *J Am Coll Cardiol* 5:363, 1985.

123. Meijler FL, van der Tweel I: Comparative study of atrial fibrillation and AV conduction in mammals. *Heart Vessels Suppl* 2:24, 1987.

124. Raekallio M: Long term ECG recording with Holter monitoring in clinically healthy horses. *Acta Vet Scand* 33:71, 1992.

125. Mill J, Hanak J: Diagnosis of heart valve defects, arrhythmia and functional disorders of cardiac conduction in competition horses and racehorses. *Arch Exp Veterinarmed* 39:319, 1985.

126. Tschudi P: Electrocardiography in the horse. 2: Disorders of impulse formation and impulse conduction. *Tierarztl Prax* 13:529, 1985.

127. Littlewort MCG: The equine heart in health and disease. In Mansmann RA, McCallister ES, Pratt PW, eds. *Equine Medicine and Surgery*. Santa Barbara, American Veterinary Publications, 1982.

128. Reef VB: Heart murmurs, irregularities and other cardiac abnormalities. In Brown C, ed. *Problems in Equine Medicine*. Philadelphia, Lea & Febiger, 1992.

129. Bonagura JD, Miller MS: Common conduction disturbances (ECG in the horse). *J Equine Vet Sci* 6:23, 1986.

130. Reef VB: Twenty-four hour rhythm monitoring. In Mayhew I, ed. *Equine Medicine and Surgery IV*. Santa Barbara, American Veterinary Publications, 1991, p 213.

131. Slinker BK, Campbell KB, Alexander JE, et al: Arterial baroreflex control of heart rate in the horse, pig, and calf. *Am J Vet Res* 43:1926, 1982.

132. Meijler FL: Atrial fibrillation: A new look at an old arrhythmia. *J Am Coll Cardiol* 2:391, 1983.

133. Opie LH: *The Heart: Physiology and Metabolism*. New York, Raven Press, 1991.

134. Evans DL, Rose RJ: Determination and repeatability of maximum oxygen uptake and other cardiorespiratory measurements in the exercising horse. *Equine Vet J* 20:94, 1988.

135. Evans DL, Rose RJ: Cardiovascular and respiratory responses in Thoroughbred horses during treadmill exercise. *J Exp Biol* 134:397, 1988.

136. Landgren GL, Gillespie JR, Fedde MR, et al: O$_2$ transport in the horse during rest and exercise. *Adv Exp Med Biol* 227:333, 1988.

137. Littlejohn A, Snow DH: Circulatory, respiratory and metabolic responses in Thoroughbred horses during the first 400 meters of exercise. *Eur J Appl Physiol* 58:307, 1988.

138. Marsland WP: Heart rate response to submaximal exercise in the Standardbred horse. *J Appl Physiol* 24:98, 1968.

139. Donaldson LL: Retrospective assessment of dobutamine therapy for hypotension in anesthetized horses. *Vet Surg* 17:53, 1988.

140. Swanson CR, Muir WW, Bednarski RM, et al: Hemodynamic responses in halothane-anesthetized horses given infusions of dopamine or dobutamine. *Am J Vet Res* 46:365, 1985.

141. Trim CM, Moore JN, White NA: Cardiopulmonary effects of dopamine hydrochloride in anaesthetized horses. *Equine Vet J* 17:41, 1985.

142. Whitton DL, Trim CM: Use of dopamine hydrochloride during general anesthesia in the treatment of advanced atrioventricular heart block in four foals. *J Am Vet Med Assoc* 187:1357, 1985.

143. Hinchcliff KW, McKeever KH, Muir WW: Hemodynamic effects of atropine, dobutamine, nitroprusside, phenylephrine, and propranolol in conscious horses. *J Vet Intern Med* 5:80, 1991.

144. Hardy J, Bednarski RM, Biller DS: Effect of phenylephrine on hemodynamics and splenic dimensions in horses. *Am J Vet Res* 55:1570, 1994.

145. Gasthuys F, De Moor A, Parmentier D: Cardiovascular effects of low dose calcium chloride infusions during halothane anaesthesia in dorsally recumbent ventilated ponies. *Zentralbl Veterinarmed* 38:728, 1991.

146. Rooney JR: Internal hemorrhage related to gestation in the mare. *Cornell Vet* 54:11, 1964.

147. van der Linde Sipman JS, Kroneman J, et al: Necrosis and rupture of the aorta and pulmonary trunk in four horses. *Vet Pathol* 22:51, 1985.

148. Roby KA, Reef VB, Shaw DP, et al: Rupture of an aortic sinus aneurysm in a 15-year-old broodmare. *J Am Vet Med Assoc* 189:305, 1986.

149. Maxie MG, Physick-Sheard PW: Aortic-iliac thrombosis in horses. *Vet Pathol* 22:238, 1985.

150. Reef VB, Roby KAW, Richardson DWE: Use of ultrasonography for the detection of aortic-iliac thrombosis in horses. *J Am Vet Med Assoc* 190:286, 1987.

151. Azzie MAJ: Clinical diagnosis of equine aortic iliac thrombosis and its histopathology as compared with that of the strongyle aneurysm. *Proc Am Assoc Equine Pract* 18:43, 1972.

152. Edwards GB, Allen WE: Aorto-iliac thrombosis in two horses: Clinical course of the disease and use of real-time ultrasonography to confirm diagnosis. *Equine Vet J* 20:384, 1988.

153. Azzie MAJ: Aortic/iliac thrombosis of Thoroughbred horses. *Equine Vet J* 1:113, 1969.

154. Physick-Sheard PW, Maxie MG: Aortoiliofemoral arteriosclerosis. In Robinson NE, ed. *Current Therapy in Equine Medicine.* Philadelphia, WB Saunders, 1983, p 153.

155. Reef VB: Vasculitis. In Robinson NE, ed. *Current Therapy in Equine Medicine II.* Philadelphia, WB Saunders, 1992, p 312.

156. Reef VB, Lalezari K, Boo J, et al: Pulsed-wave Doppler evaluation of intracardiac blood flow in 30 clinically normal Standardbred horses. *Am J Vet Res* 50:75, 1989.

156a. Blissitt KJ, Bonagura JD: Pulsed wave Doppler echocardiography in normal horses. *Equine Vet J* 19(Suppl):38–46, 1995.

157. Welker FH, Muir WW: An investigation of the second heart sound in the normal horse. *Equine Vet J* 22:403, 1990.

158. Rugh KS, Garner HE, Miramonti JR, et al: Left ventricular function and haemodynamics in ponies during exercise and recovery. *Equine Vet J* 21:39, 1989.

159. Beglinger R, Becker M: Comparative study of the contractility measurement max. dp/dt in the horse, cow, swine, dog, cat and man. *Schweiz Arch Tierheilkd* 126:265, 1984.

160. Hillidge CJ, Lees P: Left ventricular systole in conscious and anesthetized horses. *Am J Vet Res* 38:675, 1977.

161. Koblik PD, Hornof WJ, Rhode EA, et al: Left ventricular ejection fraction in the normal horse determined by first-pass nuclear angiocardiography. *Vet Radiol* 26:53, 1985.

162. Hillidge CJ, Lees P: Studies of left ventricular isotonic function in the conscious and anaesthetised horse. *Br Vet J* 133:446, 1977.

163. Robine FJ: Morphological and functional measurements on the equine heart by means of two-dimensional echocardiography. *Tierarztl Hochsc* 143, 1990.

164. Pipers FS, Hamlin RL: Echocardiography in the horse. *J Am Vet Med Assoc* 170:815, 1977.

165. Lescure F, Tamzali Y: Reference values for echocardiography applied to sport horses (English Thoroughbreds and French riding horses). *Rev Med Vet* 135:405, 1984.

165a. Patteson MW, Gibbs C, Wotton PR, et al: Echocardiographic measurements of cardiac dimensions and indices of cardiac function in normal adult thoroughbred horses. *Equine Vet J* 19(Suppl):18–27, 1995.

165b. Patteson MW, Gibbs C, Wotton PR, et al: Effects of sedation with detomidine hydrochloride on echocardiographic measurements of cardiac dimensions and indices of cardiac function in horses. *Equine Vet J* 19(Suppl):33–37, 1995.

165c. Slater JD, Herrtage ME: Echocardiographic measurements of cardiac dimensions in normal ponies and horses. *Equine Vet J* 19(Suppl):28–32, 1995.

165d. Stadler P, Robine F: B-Mode echocardiographic measurement of heart dimensions in warm-blooded horses without heart disease. *Pferdeheilkunde* 12:35–43, 1996.

166. Lombard CW, Evans M, Martin L, et al: Blood pressure, electrocardiogram and echocardiogram measurements in the growing pony foal. *Equine Vet J* 16:342, 1984.

167. Stewart JH, Rose RJ, Barko AM: Echocardiography in foals from birth to three months old. *Equine Vet J* 16:332, 1984.

168. van Aarde MN, Littlejohn A, Van der Walt JJ: The ratio of cardiopulmonary blood volume to stroke volume as an index of cardiac function in horses. *Vet Res Commun* 8:293, 1984.

169. Reef VB: Evaluation of the equine cardiovascular system. *Vet Clin North Am Equine Pract* 1:275, 1985.

170. Goldberg SJ, Allen HD, Marx GR, et al: *Doppler Echocardiography.* Philadelphia, Lea & Febiger, 1988.

170a. Young LE, Blissitt KJ, Clutton RE, et al: Feasibility of transesophageal echocardiography for evaluation of left ventricular performance in anaesthetised horses. *Equine Vet J* 19(Suppl):63–70, 1995.

170b. Young LE, Blissitt KJ, Clutton RE, et al: Temporal effects of an infusion of dopexamine hydrochloride in horses anesthetized with halothane. *Am J Vet Res* 58:516–523, 1997.

171. Wetmore LA, Derksen FJ, Blaze CA, et al: Mixed venous oxygen tension as an estimate of cardiac output in anesthetized horses. *Am J Vet Res* 48:971, 1987.

172. Hillidge CJ, Lees P: Cardiac output in the conscious and anaesthetised horse. *Equine Vet J* 7:16, 1975.

173. Muir WW, Skarda R, Milne D: Estimation of cardiac output in the horse by thermodilution techniques. *Am J Vet Res* 37:697, 1976.

174. Thomas DP, Fregin GF, Gerber NH, et al: Effects of training on cardiorespiratory function in the horse. *Am J Physiol* 245:R160, 1983.

175. Evans DL: Cardiovascular adaptations to exercise and training. *Vet Clin North Am Equine Pract* 1:513, 1985.

176. Swanson CR, Muir WW: Dobutamine-induced augmentation of cardiac output does not enhance respiratory gas exchange in anesthetized recumbent healthy horses. *Am J Vet Res* 47:1573, 1986.

177. Thomas WP, Madigan JE, Backus KQ, et al: Systemic and pulmonary haemodynamics in normal neonatal foals. *J Reprod Fertil Suppl* 35:623, 1987.

178. Ward DS, Fessler JF, Bottoms GD: In vitro calibration and surgical implantation of electromagnetic blood flow transducers for measurement of left coronary blood flow and cardiac output in the pony. *Am J Vet Res* 48:1120, 1987.

179. Weber JM, Dobson GP, Parkhouse WS, et al: Cardiac output and oxygen consumption in exercising Thoroughbred horses. *Am J Physiol* 253:R890, 1987.

180. Bertone JJ: Cardiovascular effects of hydralazine HCl administration in horses. *Am J Vet Res* 49:618, 1988.

181. Gasthuys F, De Moor A, Parmentier D: Haemodynamic changes during sedation in ponies. *Vet Res Commun* 14:309, 1990.

182. Hinchcliff KW, McKeever KH, Schmall LM, et al: Renal and systemic hemodynamic responses to sustained submaximal exertion in horses. *Am J Physiol* 258:R1177, 1990.

183. Schmall LM, Muir WW, Robertson JT: Haemodynamic effects of small volume hypertonic saline in experimentally induced haemorrhagic shock. *Equine Vet J* 22:273, 1990.

184. Muir WW, McGuirk SM: Pharmacology and pharmacokinetics of drugs used to treat cardiac disease in horses. *Vet Clin North Am Equine Pract* 1:335, 1985.

185. Gasthuys F, De Moor A, Parmentier D: Influence of dopamine and dobutamine on the cardiovascular depression during a standard halothane anaesthesia in dorsally recumbent, ventilated ponies. *Zentralbl Veterinarmed* 38:494, 1991.

186. Brumbaugh GW, Thomas WP, Enos LR, et al: A pharmacokinetic study of digoxin in the horse. *J Vet Pharmacol Ther* 6:163, 1983.

187. Nuytten J, Deprez P, Picavet T, et al: Heart failure in horses: Hemodynamic monitoring and determination of LDH1 concentration. *J Equine Vet Sci* 8:214, 1988.

187a. Fruhauf B, Stadler P, Deegen E: Evaluation of pulmonary wedge pressure in horses with and without left-heart abnormalities detected by echocardiography. *Pferdeheilkunde* 12:544–550, 1996.

188. Rugh KS, Garner HE, Hatfield DG, et al: Ischaemia induced development of functional coronary collateral circulation in ponies. *Cardiovasc Res* 21:730, 1987.

189. Parks CM, Manohar M: Distribution of blood flow during moderate and strenuous exercise in ponies *(Equus caballus)*. *Am J Vet Res* 44:1861, 1983.

190. Parks C, Manohar M, Lundeen G: Regional myocardial blood flow and coronary vascular reserve in unanesthetized ponies during pacing-induced ventricular tachycardia. *J Surg Res* 35:119, 1983.

191. Parks CM, Manohar M: Transmural coronary vasodilator reserve and flow distribution during severe exercise in ponies. *J Appl Physiol* 54:1641, 1983.

192. Hamlin RL, Levesque MJ, Kittleson MD: Intramyocardial pressure and distribution of coronary blood flow during systole and diastole in the horse. *Cardiovasc Res* 16:256, 1982.

193. Manohar M: Transmural coronary vasodilator reserve and flow distribution during maximal exercise in normal and splenectomized ponies. *J Physiol Lond* 387:425, 1987.

194. Manohar M, Parks C: Transmural coronary vasodilator reserve in ponies at rest and during maximal exercise. In Persson SGB, Rose RJ, eds. *Equine Exercise Physiology.* Cambridge, England, Granta, 1983, p 91.

195. Parks CM, Manohar M: Transmural distribution of myocardial blood flow during graded treadmill exercise in ponies. In Persson SGB, Rose RJ, eds. *Equine Exercise Physiology.* Cambridge, England, Granta, 1983, p 105.

196. Parks CM, Manohar M: Regional blood flow changes in response to near maximal exercise in ponies: A review. *Equine Vet J* 17:311, 1985.

197. Reddy VK, Kammula RG, Graham TC, et al: Regional coronary blood flow in ponies. *Am J Vet Res* 37:1261, 1976.

198. Thornton JR: Exercise testing. *Vet Clin North Am Equine Pract* 1:573, 1985.

199. Evans DL, Rose RJ: Dynamics of cardiorespiratory function in standardbred horses during different intensities of constant-load exercise. *J Comp Physiol* 157:791, 1988.

200. Foreman JH, Bayly WM, Grant BD, et al: Standardized exercise test and daily heart rate responses of thoroughbreds undergoing conventional race training and detraining. *Am J Vet Res* 51:914, 1990.

201. Rose RJ, Hendrickson DK, Knight PK: Clinical exercise testing in the normal thoroughbred racehorse. *Aust Vet J* 67:345, 1990.

202. Seeherman HJ, Morris EA: Comparison of yearling, two-year-old and adult thoroughbreds using a standardised exercise test. *Equine Vet J* 23:175, 1991.

203. Glendinning SA: The clinician's approach to equine cardiology. *Equine Vet J* 9:176, 1977.

204. Mitten LA: Cardiovascular causes of exercise intolerance. *Vet Clin North Am Equine Pract* 12:473, 1996

204a. Lillich JD, Gaughan EM: Diagnostic approach to exercise intolerance in racehorses. *Vet Clin North Am Equine Pract* 12:555, 1996.

204b. Fregin GF: Medical evaluation of the cardiovascular system. *Vet Clin North Am Equine Pract* 8:329–346, 1992.

205. Littlewort MCG: Cardiological problems in equine medicine. *Equine Vet J* 9:173, 1977.

206. Glazier B: Clinical aspects of equine cardiology. *Practice* 9:98, 1987.

207. Littlewort MCG: The clinical auscultation of the equine heart. *Vet Rec* 74:1247, 1962.

208. Rossdale PD: Clinical studies on the newborn thoroughbred foal. II: Heart rate. *Br Vet J* 123:521, 1967.

209. Vanselow B, McCarthy M, Gay CC: A phonocardiographic study of equine heart sounds. *Aust Vet J* 54:161, 1978.

210. Littlejohn A, Button C: When is a murmur not a murmur? *J S Afr Vet Assoc* 53:130, 1982.

211. Kammerer H: Auscultation of the horse's heart, using a new stethoscope. *DTW Dtsch Tierarztl Wochenschr* 90:521, 1983.

212. McGuirk SM, Muir WW: Diagnosis and treatment of cardiac arrhythmias. *Vet Clin North Am Equine Pract* 1:353, 1985.

213. Reef VB: The significance of cardiac auscultatory findings in horses—insight into the age-old dilemma. *Equine Vet J* 25:393, 1993.

214. Reimer J: Performing cardiac auscultation on horses. *Vet Med* 88:660, 1993.

215. Gerring EL: Auscultation of the equine heart. *Equine Vet Educ* 2:22, 1990.

216. Machida N, Yasuda J, Too K: Auscultatory and phonocardiographic studies on the cardiovascular system of the newborn thoroughbred foal. *Jpn J Vet Res* 35:235, 1987.

216a. Reef VB: The significance of cardiac auscultatory findings in horses: Insight into the age-old problem. *Equine Vet J* 25:393–394, 1993.

216b. Reef VB: Heart murmurs in horses: Determining their significance with echocardiography. *Equine Vet J* 19(Suppl):71–80, 1995.

216c. Blissitt KJ, Bonagura JD: Colour flow Doppler echocardiography in horses with cardiac murmurs. *Equine Vet J* 19(Suppl):82–85, 1995.

217. Hintz HF, Collyer C, Brant T: Resting heart rates in draft horses. *Equine Pract* 11:7, 1989.

218. Reef VB: Frequency of cardiac arrhythmias and their significance in normal horses. *Proc Am Coll Vet Intern Med* 506, 1989.

218a. Raekallio M: Long term ECG recording with Holter monitoring in clinically healthy horses. *Acta Vet Scand* 33:71–75, 1992.

219. Bonagura JD, Miller MS: Electrocardiography. In Jones WE, ed. *Equine Sports Medicine*. Philadelphia, Lea & Febiger, 1985, p 89.

220. Bertone JJ: Atrial fibrillation in the horse: Diagnosis, prognosis, treatment. *Equine Pract* 6:6, 1984.

221. Bertone JJ, Wingfield WE: Atrial fibrillation in horses. *Compend Contin Educ Pract Vet* 9:763, 1987.

222. Deem DA, Fregin GF: Atrial fibrillation in horses. *J Am Vet Med Assoc* 180:261, 1982.

223. Li JK: Laminar and turbulent flow in the mammalian aorta: Reynolds number. *J Theor Biol* 135:409, 1988.

224. Machida N, Yasuda J, Too K, et al: A morphological study on the obliteration processes of the ductus arteriosus in the horse. *Equine Vet J* 20:249, 1988.

225. Glen JB: Indirect blood pressure measurement in anesthetised animals. *Vet Rec* 87:349, 1970.

226. Amend JF, Garner H, Rosborough JP, et al: Hemodynamic studies in conscious domestic ponies. *J Surg Res* 19:107, 1975.

227. Ellis PM: The indirect measurement of arterial blood pressure in the horse. *Equine Vet J* 7:22, 1975.

228. Johnson JH, Garner HE, Hutcheson DP: Ultrasonic measurement of arterial blood pressure in conditioned thoroughbreds. *Equine Vet J* 8:55, 1976.

229. Geddes LA, Chaffee V, Whistler SJ, et al: Indirect mean blood pressure in the anesthetized pony. *Am J Vet Res* 38:2055, 1977.

230. Kvart C: An ultrasonic method for indirect blood pressure measurement in the horse. *J Equine Med Surg* 3:16, 1979.

231. Latshaw H, Fessler JF, Whistler SJ, et al: Indirect measurement of mean blood pressure in the normotensive and hypotensive horses. *Equine Vet J* 11:191, 1979.

232. Parry BW, Gay CC, McCarthy MA: Influence of head height on arterial blood pressure in standing horses. *Am J Vet Res* 41:1626, 1980.

233. Taylor PM: Techniques and clinical application of arterial blood pressure. *Equine Vet J* 13:271, 1981.

234. Parry BW, McCarthy MA, Anderson GA, et al: Correct occlusive bladder width for indirect blood pressure measurement in horses. *Am J Vet Res* 43:50, 1982.

235. Muir WW, Wade A, Grospitch B: Automatic noninvasive sphygmomanometry in horses. *J Am Vet Med Assoc* 182:1230, 1983.

236. Parry BW, Anderson GA: Importance of uniform cuff application for equine blood pressure measurement. *Equine Vet J* 16:529, 1984.

237. Parry BW, McCarthy MA, Anderson GA: Survey of resting blood pressure values in clinically normal horses. *Equine Vet J* 16:53, 1984.

238. Fritsch R, Bosler K: Monitoring circulation in the horse during sedation and anesthesia by indirect blood pressure measurement. *Berl Munch Tierarztl Wochenschr* 98:166, 1985.

239. Franco RM, Ousey JC, Cash RS, et al: Study of arterial blood pressure in newborn foals using an electronic sphygmomanometer. *Equine Vet J* 18:475, 1986.

240. Fritsch R, Hausmann R: Indirect blood pressure determination in the horse with the Dinamap 1255 research monitor. *Tierarztl Prax* 16:373, 1988.

241. Gasthuys F, Muylle E, De Moor A, et al: Influence of pre-medication and body position during halothane anaesthesia on intracardial pressures in the horse. *Zentralbl Veterinarmed* 35:729, 1988.

242. Abrahamsen E, Hellyer PW, Bednarski RM, et al: Tourniquet-induced hypertension in a horse. *J Am Vet Med Assoc* 194:386, 1989.

243. Wens HM: Catheterization of the heart by J.B.A. Chauveau in 1861. *Tierarztl Umschau* 44:90, 1989.

244. Hellyer PW, Dodam JR, Light GS: Dynamic baroreflex sensitivity in anesthetized horses, maintained at 1.25 to 1.3 minimal alveolar concentration of halothane. *Am J Vet Res* 52:1672, 1991.

245. Bayly WM, Gabel AA, Barr SA: Cardiovascular effects of submaximal aerobic training on a treadmill in standardbred horses, using a standardized exercise test. *Am J Vet Res* 44:544, 1983.

246. Physick-Sheard PW: Cardiovascular response to exercise and training in the horse. *Vet Clin North Am Equine Pract* 1:383, 1985.

247. Tillotson PJ, Kooper PH: Treatment of aortic thrombus in a horse. *J Am Vet Med Assoc* 149:766, 1966.

248. Tithof PK, Rebhun WC, Dietze AE: Ultrasonographic diagnosis of aorto-iliac thrombosis. *Cornell Vet* 75:540, 1985.

249. Dickson LR, Badcoe LM, Burbidge H, et al: Jugular thrombophlebitis resulting from an anesthetic induction technique in the horse. *Equine Vet J* 22:177, 1990.

249a. Gardner S, Reef VB: Ultrasonographic evaluation of 46 horses with jugular vein thrombophlebitis (1985–1988). A retrospective study. *J Am Vet Med Assoc* 199:370, 1991.

250. Rose RJGE, Lovell DK: Symposium on exercise physiology. *Vet Clin North Am Equine Pract* 1:437, 1985.

251. Poggenpoel DG: Measurements of heart rate and riding speed on a horse during a training programme for endurance rides. *Equine Vet J* 20:224, 1988.

252. Glomset DJ, Glomset ATA: A morphologic study of the cardiac conduction system in ungulates, dog, and man. Part I: The sinoatrial node. *Am Heart J* 20:389, 1940.

253. Lannek N, Rutqvist L: Normal area of variation for the electrocardiogram of horses. *Nord Vet Med* 3:1094, 1951.

254. Landgren S, Rutqvist L: Electrocardiogram of normal cold blooded horses after work. *Nord Vet Med* 5:905, 1953.

255. White NA, Rhode EA: Correlation of electrocardiographic findings to clinical disease in the horse. *J Am Vet Med Assoc* 164:46, 1974.

256. Hilwig RW: Cardiac arrhythmias in the horse. *J Am Vet Med Assoc* 170:153, 1977.

257. Hanak J, Zert Z: Some ECG characters in thoroughbred horses, common to parents and their offspring. *Vet Med (Praha)* 27:87, 1982.

258. Hanak J, Jagos P: Electrocardiographic lead system and its vector verification. *Acta Vet Brno* 52:67, 1983.

259. Littlejohn A, Button C, Bowles F: Studies on the physiopathology of chronic obstructive pulmonary disease in the horse. VIII: Mean modal vectors of the P wave and the QRS complex. *Onderstepoort J Vet Res* 50:119, 1983.

260. Stewart JH, Rose RJ, Davis PE, et al: A comparison of electrocardiographic findings in racehorses presented either for routine examination or poor racing performance. In Persson SGB, Rose RJ, eds. *Equine Exercise Physiology*. Cambridge, England, Granta, 1983, p 135.

261. Costa G, Illera M, Garcia-Sacristan A: Electrocardiographical values in non-trained horses. *Zentralbl Veterinarmed* 32:196, 1985.

262. Matsui K: Fetal and maternal heart rates in a case of twin pregnancy of the thoroughbred horse. *Nippon Juigaku Zasshi* 47:817, 1985.

263. Miller MS, Bonagura JD: Atrial arrhythmias. *J Equine Vet Sci* 5:300, 1985.

264. Bonagura JD, Miller MS: Electrocardiography. What is your diagnosis? Junctional and ventricular arrhythmias. *J Equine Vet Sci* 5:347, 1985.

265. Tschudi P: Electrocardiography in the horse. 1: Principles and normal picture. *Tierarztl Prax* 13:181, 1985.

266. Fregin GF: The equine electrocardiogram with standardized body and limb positions. *Cornell Vet* 72:304, 1982.

267. Tovar P, Escabias MI, Santisteban R: Evolution of the ECG from Spanish bred foals during the post natal stage. *Res Vet Sci* 46:358, 1989.

268. Grauerholz H: Influence of respiration on the QRS complex of the ECG in clinically healthy horses and in horses with respiratory problems. *Berl Munch Tierarztl Wochenschr* 103:293, 1990.

269. Grauerholz H, Jaeschke G: Alterations induced by training in reference vectors of the electrocardiographic QRS complex of young trotting horses. *Berl Munch Tierarztl Wochenschr* 103:329, 1990.

270. Illera JC, Hamlin RL, Illera M: Unipolar thoracic electrocardiograms in which P waves of relative uniformity occur in male horses. *Am J Vet Res* 48:1697, 1987.

271. Fregin GF: Electrocardiography. *Vet Clin North Am Equine Pract* 1:419, 1985.

272. Matsui K, Sugano S: Species differences in the changes in heart rate and T-wave amplitude after autonomic blockade in thoroughbred horses, ponies, cows, pigs, goats and chickens. *Jpn J Vet Sci* 49:637, 1987.

273. Bonagura JD: Diagnosis of cardiac arrhythmias. In Robinson NE (ed): *Current Therapy in Equine Medicine,* 4th ed. Philadelphia, WB Saunders, pp. 240–250.

274. Carlsten J, Kvart C, Jeffcott LB: Method of selective and non-selective angiocardiography for the horse. *Equine Vet J* 16:47, 1984.

275. Scott EA, Chaffee A, Eyster GE, et al: Interruption of aortic arch in two foals. *J Am Vet Med Assoc* 172:347, 1978.

276. Bonagura JD: Equine echocardiography. *Br Vet J* 150:503, 1994.

276a. Bonagura JD, Blissitt KJ: Echocardiography. *Equine Vet J* 19(Suppl):5–17, 1995.

277. Marr CM: Equine echocardiography—sound advice at the heart of the matter (Review). *Br Vet J* 150:527, 1994.

278. Reef VB: Advances in echocardiography. *Vet Clin North Am Equine Pract* 7:435, 1991.

279. Pipers FS, Hamlin RL, Reef VB: Echocardiographic detection of cardiovascular lesions in the horse. *J Equine Med Surg* 3:68, 1979.

280. Wingfield WE, Miller CW, Voss JL, et al: Echocardiography in assessing mitral valve motion in 3 horses with atrial fibrillation. *Equine Vet J* 12:181, 1980.

281. Bonagura JD, Pipers FS: Diagnosis of cardiac lesions by contrast echocardiography. *J Am Vet Med Assoc* 182:396, 1983.

282. Gerlis LM, Wright HM, Wilson N, et al: Left ventricular bands: A normal anatomical feature. *Br Heart J* 52:641, 1984.

283. Rantanen NW, Byars TD, Hauser ML, et al: Spontaneous contrast and mass lesions in the hearts of race horses: Ultrasound diagnosis—preliminary data. *J Equine Vet Sci* 4:220, 1984.

284. Yamaga Y, Too K: Diagnostic ultrasound imaging in domestic animals: Two-dimensional and M-mode echocardiography. *Jpn J Vet Sci* 46:493, 1984.

285. Kvart C, Carlsten J, Jeffcott LB, et al: Diagnostic value of contrast echocardiography in the horse. *Equine Vet J* 17:357, 1985.

286. Pipers FS, Reef VB, Wilson J: Echocardiographic detection of ventricular septal defects in large animals. *J Am Vet Med Assoc* 187:810, 1985.

287. Reef VB: Electrocardiography and echocardiography in the exercising horse. In Robinson NE (ed): *Current Therapy in Equine Medicine,* 4th ed. Philadelphia, WB Saunders, 1997, pp 234–239.

288. Bertone JJ, Paull KS, Wingfield WE, et al: M-mode echocardiographs of endurance horses in the recovery phase of long-distance competition. *Am J Vet Res* 48:1708, 1987.

289. Carlsten JC: Two-dimensional, real-time echocardiography in the horse. *Vet Radiol* 28:76, 1987.

290. O'Callaghan MW: Echocardiography. In Robinson E, ed. *Current Therapy in Equine Medicine.* Philadelphia, WB Saunders, 1987, p 139.

291. Stadler P, D'Agostino U, Deegen E: Real-time, two-dimensional echocardiography in horses. *Pferdeheilkunde* 4:161, 1988.

292. Voros K, Holmes JR, Gibbs C: Left ventricular volume determination in the horse by two-dimensional echocardiography: An in vitro study (Comments). *Equine Vet J* 22:398, 1990.

293. Voros K, Holmes JR, Gibbs C: Anatomical validation of two-dimensional echocardiography in the horse. *Equine Vet J* 22:392, 1990.

294. Reef VB: Advances in echocardiography. *Vet Clin North Am Equine Pract* 7:435, 1991.

295. Reef VB: Equine pediatric ultrasonography. *Compend Contin Educ Pract Vet* 13:1277, 1991.

296. Voros K, Holmes JR, Gibbs C: Measurement of cardiac dimensions with two-dimensional echocardiography in the living horse. *Equine Vet J* 23:461, 1991.

297. Long KJ, Bonagura JD, Darke PG: Standardised imaging technique for guided M-mode and Doppler echocardiography in the horse. *Equine Vet J* 24:226, 1992.

298. Mahony C, Rantanen NW, DeMichael JA, et al: Spontaneous echocardiographic contrast in the thoroughbred: High prevalence in racehorses and a characteristic abnormality in bleeders. *Equine Vet J* 24:129, 1992.

299. Reef VB: Echocardiography. In Mayhew I, ed. *Equine Medicine and Surgery IV.* Santa Barbara, American Veterinary Publications, 1991.

300. Adams Brendemuehl C, Pipers FS: Antepartum evaluations of the equine fetus. *J Reprod Fertil Suppl* 35:565, 1987.

301. Reimer J: Cardiac evaluation of the horse—using ultrasonography. *Vet Med* 88:748, 1993.

302. Reef VB: Echocardiographic examination in the horse: The basics. *Compend Contin Educ Pract Vet* 12:1312, 1990.

303. O'Callaghan MW: Comparison of echocardiographic and autopsy measurements of cardiac dimensions in the horse. *Equine Vet J* 17:361, 1985.

304. Stadler P, Rewel A, Deegen E: M-mode echocardiography in dressage horses, class S jumping horses and untrained horses [German]. *Zentralbl Veterinarmed [A]* 40:292, 1993.

305. Stadler P, Weinberger T, Deegen E: Pulsed Doppler-echocardiography in healthy warm-blooded horses. *Zentralbl Veterinarmed [A]* 40:757, 1993.

306. Stadler P, Kinkel N, Deegen E: Evaluation of systolic heart function in the horse with pw-doppler echocardiography compared with thermodilution. *Dtsch Tierarztl Wochenschr* 101:312, 1994.

307. Long KJ: Doppler echocardiography—clinical applications. *Equine Vet Educ* 5:161, 1993.

308. Long KJ: Doppler echocardiography in the horse. *Equine Vet Educ* 2:15, 1990.

308a. Blissitt KJ, Bonagura JD: Colour flow Doppler echocardiography in normal horses. *Equine Vet J* 19(Suppl):47–55, 1995.

308b. Marr CM, Reef VB: Physiologic valvular regurgitation in clinically normal young racehorses: Prevalence and two-dimensional colour flow Doppler echocardiographic characteristics. *Equine Vet J* 19(Suppl):56–62, 1995.

309. Rantanen NW: Diseases of the thorax. *Vet Clin North Am Equine Pract* 2:49, 1986.

310. Erickson BK, Erickson HH, Coffman JR: Pulmonary artery and aortic pressure changes during high intensity treadmill exercise in the horse: Effect of furosemide and phentolamine. *Equine Vet J* 24:215, 1992.

311. Goetz TE, Manohar M: Pressures in the right side of the heart and esophagus (pleura) in ponies during exercise before and after furosemide administration. *Am J Vet Res* 47:270, 1986.

312. Hall LW: Cardiovascular and pulmonary effects of recumbency in two conscious ponies. *Equine Vet J* 16:89, 1984.

313. Hall LW, Nigam JM: Measurement of central venous pressure in horses. *Vet Rec* 97:66, 1975.

314. Jones JH, Smith BL, Birks EK, et al: Left atrial and pulmonary arterial pressures in exercising horses (Abstract). *Physiologist* 35:A2020, 1992.

315. Manohar M: Pulmonary artery wedge pressure increases with high-intensity exercise in horses. *Am J Vet Res* 54:142, 1993.

316. Manohar M: Right heart pressures and blood-gas tensions in ponies during exercise and laryngeal hemiplegia. *Am J Physiol* 251:H121, 1986.

317. Milne DW, Muir WW, Skarda RT: Pulmonary artery wedge pressure blood gas tensions and pH in the resting horse. *Am J Vet Res* 36:1431, 1975.

318. Orr JA, Bisgard GE, Forster HV, et al: Cardiopulmonary measurements in nonanesthetized resting normal ponies. *Am J Vet Res* 36:1667, 1975.

319. Schatzmann U, Battier B: Factors influencing central venous pressure in horses. *Dtsch Tierarztl Wochenschr* 94:147, 1987.

320. Sheridan V, Deegen E, Zeller R: Central venous pressure (CVP) measurements during halothane anaesthesia. *Vet Rec* 90:149, 1972.

321. Smith BL, Jones JH, Pascoe JR, et al: Why are left atrial pressures high in exercising horses (Abstract)? *Physiologist* 35:225, 1992.

322. Hillidge CJ, Lees P: Influence of general anaesthesia on peripheral resistance in the horse. *Br Vet J* 133:225, 1977.

323. Manohar M: Furosemide attenuates the exercise-induced increase in pulmonary artery wedge pressure in horses. *Am J Vet Res* 54:952, 1993.

324. Davis JL, Manohar M: Effect of splenectomy on exercise-induced pulmonary and systemic hypertension in ponies. *Am J Vet Res* 49:1169, 1988.

325. Bisgard GE, Orr JA, Will JA: Hypoxic pulmonary hypertension in the pony. *Am J Vet Res* 36:49, 1975.

326. Drummond WH, Sanchez IR, Kosch PC, et al: Pulmonary vascular reactivity of the newborn pony foal. *Equine Vet J* 21:181, 1989.

327. Gelberg HB, Smetzer DL, Foreman JH: Pulmonary hypertension as a cause of atrial fibrillation in young horses: Four cases (1980–1989). *J Am Vet Med Assoc* 198:679, 1991.

328. Klein L, Sherman J: Effects of preanesthetic medication, anesthesia, and position of recumbency on central venous pressure in horses. *J Am Vet Med Assoc* 170:216, 1977.

329. Fisher EW, Dalton RG: Determination of cardiac output of cattle and horses by the injection. *Br Vet J* 117:141, 1961.

330. Staddon GE, Weaver BMG, Webb AI: Distribution of cardiac output in anaesthetised horses. *Res Vet Sci* 27:38, 1979.

331. Steffey EP, Dunlop CI, Farver TB, et al: Cardiovascular and respiratory measurements in awake and isoflurane-anesthetized horses. *Am J Vet Res* 48:7, 1987.

332. Dunlop CI, Hodgson DS, Chapman PL, et al: Thermodilution estimation of cardiac output at high flows in anesthetized horses. *Am J Vet Res* 52:1893, 1991.

333. Mizuno Y, Aida H, Hara H, et al: Comparison of methods of cardiac output measurements determined by dye dilution, pulsed Doppler echocardiography and thermodilution in horses. *J Vet Med Sci* 56:1, 1994.

334. Brumbaugh GW, Thomas WP, Hodge TG: Medical management of congestive heart failure in a horse. *J Am Vet Med Assoc* 180:878, 1982.

335. Glazier DB: Congestive heart failure and congenital cardiac defects in horses. *Equine Pract* 8:20, 1986.

336. Bonagura JD: Clinical evaluation and management of heart disease. *Equine Vet Educ* 2:31, 1990.

337. Bonagura JD: Congestive heart failure in the horse: Proceedings of the Eleventh Annual Veterinary Medical Forum. *Am Coll Vet Intern Med* 614, 1993.

338. Garber JL, Reef VB, Reimer JM: Sonographic findings in horses with mediastinal lymphosarcoma—13 cases (1985–1992). *J Am Vet Med Assoc* 205:1432, 1994.

339. Hinchcliff KW, Muir WW: Pharmacology of furosemide in the horse: A review. *J Vet Intern Med* 5:211, 1991.

339a. Harkins JD, Hackett RP, Ducharme NG: Effect of furosemide on physiological variables in exercising horses. *Am J Vet Res* 54:2104–2109, 1993.

339b. Manohar M, Hutchens E, Coney E: Furosemide attenuates the exercise-induced rise in pulmonary capillary blood-pressure in horses. *Equine Vet J* 26:51–54, 1994.

340. Francfort P, Schatzmann HJ: Pharmacological experiments as a basis for the administration of digoxin in the horse. *Res Vet Sci* 20:84, 1976.

341. Pedersoli WM, Belmonte AA, Purohit RC, et al: Pharmacokinetics of digoxin in the horse. *J Equine Med Surg* 2:384, 1978.

342. Button C, Gross DR, Johnston JT, et al: Digoxin pharmacokinetics, bioavailability, efficacy, and dosage regimens in the horse. *Am J Vet Res* 41:1388, 1980.

343. Pedersoli WM, Ravis WR, Belmonte AA, et al: Pharmacokinetics of a single, orally administered dose of digoxin in horses. *Am J Vet Res* 42:1412, 1981.

344. Muir WW, McGuirk S: Cardiovascular drugs: Their pharmacology and use in horses. *Vet Clin North Am Equine Pract* 3:37, 1987.

345. Pearson EG, Ayers JW, Wood GL, et al: Digoxin toxicity in a horse. *Compend Contin Educ Pract Vet* 9:958, 1987.

346. Staudacher G: Individual glycoside therapy using serum concentration determination in heart insufficiency of horses. *Berl Munch Tierarztl Wochenschr* 102:1, 1989.

347. Gasthuys F, De Moor A, Parmentier D: Influence of digoxin followed by dopamine on the cardiovascular depression during a standard halothane anaesthesia in dorsally recumbent, ventilated ponies. *Zentralbl Veterinarmed* 38:585, 1991.

348. Marr CM: Treatment of cardiac arrhythmias and cardiac failure. In Robinson NE (ed): *Current Therapy in Equine Medicine,* 4th ed. Philadelphia, WB Saunders, pp 250–255.

349. Sweeney RW, Reef VB, Reimer JM: Pharmacokinetics of digoxin administered to horses with congestive heart failure. *Am J Vet Res* 54:1108, 1993.

350. Glazier DB, Farrelly BT, O'Connor J: Ventricular septal defect in a 7-year-old gelding. *J Am Vet Med Assoc* 167:49, 1975.

351. Greene HJ, Wray DD, Greenway GA: Two equine congenital cardiac anomalies. *Irish Vet J* 29:115, 1975.

352. Critchley KL: An interventricular septal defect, pulmonary stenosis and bicuspid pulmonary valve in a Welsh pony foal. *Equine Vet J* 8:176, 1976.

352a. Seahorn TL, Hormanski CE: Ventricular septal defect and atrial fibrillation in an adult horse—a case-report. *J Equine Vet Sci* 13:36–38, 1993.

353. Huston R, Saperstein G, Leipold HW: Congenital defects in foals. *J Equine Med Surg* 1:146, 1977.

354. Vitums A, Bayly WM: Pulmonary atresia with dextroposition of the aorta and ventricular septal defect in three Arabian foals. *Vet Pathol* 19:160, 1982.

355. Lombard CW, Scarratt WK, Buergelt CD: Ventricular septal defects in the horse. *J Am Vet Med Assoc* 183:562, 1983.

355a. Reef VB: Evaluation of ventricular septal defects in horses using two-dimensional and Doppler echocardiography. *Equine Vet J* 19(Suppl):86–95, 1995.

356. Johnson JW, DeBowes RM, Cox JH, et al: Diaphragmatic hernia with a concurrent cardiac defect in an Arabian foal. *J Equine Vet Sci* 4:225, 1984.

357. Zamora CS, Vitums A, Foreman JH, et al: Common ventricle with separate pulmonary outflow chamber in a horse. *J Am Vet Med Assoc* 186:1210, 1985.

358. Koblik PD, Hornof WJ: Use of first-pass nuclear angiocardiography to detect left-to-right cardiac shunts in the horse. *Vet Radiol* 28:177, 1987.

359. Wilson RB, Haffner JC: Right atrioventricular atresia and ventricular septal defect in a foal. *Cornell Vet* 77:187, 1987.

360. King JM, Flint TJ, Anderson WI: Incomplete subaortic stenotic rings in domestic animals—a newly described congenital anomaly. *Cornell Vet* 78:263, 1988.

361. Cox VS, Weber AF, Lima A, et al: Left cranial vena cava in a horse. *Anat Histol Embryol* 20:37, 1991.

362. Reef VB: Echocardiographic findings in horses with congenital cardiac disease. *Compend Contin Educ Pract Vet* 1:109, 1991.

363. Vitums A: Origin of the aorta and pulmonary trunk from the right ventricle in a horse. *Vet Pathol* 7:482, 1970.

363a. Reimer JM, Marr CM, Reef VB, et al: Aortic origin of the right pulmonary artery and patent ductus arteriosus in a pony foal with pulmonary hypertension and right-sided heart failure. *Equine Vet J* 25:466–468, 1993.

364. Cottrill CM, O'Connor WN, Cudd T, et al: Persistence of foetal circulatory pathways in a newborn foal. *Equine Vet J* 19:252, 1987.

365. Lombard CW: Cardiovascular diseases. In Koterba A, ed. *Equine Clinical Neonatology.* Philadelphia, Lea & Febiger, 1990, pp 240–261.

366. Ecke P, Malik R, Kannegieter NJ: Common atrioventricular canal in a foal. *N Z Vet J* 39:97, 1991.

367. Taylor FGR, Wotton PR, Hillyer MH, et al: Atrial septal defect and atrial fibrillation in a foal. *Vet Rec* 128:80, 1991.

368. Glazier DB, Farrelly BT, Neylon JF: Patent ductus arteriosus in an eight-month-old foal. *Irish Vet J* 28:12, 1974.

369. Buergelt CD, Carmichael JA, Tashjian RJ, et al: Spontaneous rupture of the left pulmonary artery in a horse with patent ductus arteriosus. *J Am Vet Med Assoc* 157:313, 1970.

370. Vitums A, Grant BD, Stone EC, et al: Transposition of the aorta and atresia of the pulmonary trunk in a horse. *Cornell Vet* 63:41, 1973.

371. Chaffin MK, Miller MW, Morris EL: Double outlet right ventricle and other associated congenital cardiac anomalies in an American miniature horse foal. *Equine Vet J* 24:402, 1992.

372. Steyn PF, Holland P, Hoffman J: The angiocardiographic diagnosis of a persistent truncus arteriosus in a foal. *J S Afr Vet Assoc* 60:106, 1989.

373. Button C, Gross DR, Allert JA, et al: Tricuspid atresia in a foal. *J Am Vet Med Assoc* 172:825, 1978.

373a. Reppas GP, Canfield PJ, Hartley WJ, et al: Multiple congenital cardiac anomalies and idiopathic thoracic aortitis in a horse. *Vet Record* 138:14–16, 1996.

374. Innes JM, Berger J, Francis J: Subacute bacterial endocarditis with pulmonary embolism in a horse. *Br Vet J* 106:245, 1950.

375. Bishop SP, Cole CR, Smetzer DL: Functional and morphologic pathology of equine aortic insufficiency. *Vet Pathol* 3:137, 1966.

376. McCormick BS, Peet RL, Downes K: *Erysipelothrix rhusiopathiae* vegetative endocarditis in a horse. *Aust Vet J* 62:392, 1985.

377. Reef VB, Levitan CW, Spencer PA: Factors affecting prognosis and conversion in equine atrial fibrillation. *J Vet Intern Med* 2:1, 1988.

378. Stadler P, Weinberger T, Kinkel N, et al: B-mode-, M-mode- and Dopplersonographic findings in mitral valve insufficiency (MVI) in horses. *J Vet Med* 39:704, 1992.

378a. Stadler P, Hoch M, Fruhauf B, et al: Echocardiography in horses with and without heart murmurs in aortic regurgitation. *Pferdeheilkunde* 11:373–383, 1995.

379. Marcus LC, Ross JN: Microscopic lesions in the hearts of aged horses and mules. *Vet Pathol* 4:162, 1967.

380. Johnson JE, Reef VB: Tricuspid valvular insufficiency associated with a ruptured chorda. *J Am Vet Med Assoc* In Press.

381. Reimer JM, Reef VB, Sommer M: Echocardiographic detection of pulmonic valve rupture in a horse with right-sided heart failure. *J Am Vet Med Assoc* 198:880, 1991.

382. Hillyer MH, Mair TS, Holmes JR: Treatment of bacterial endocarditis in a Shire mare. *Equine Vet Educ* 2:5, 1990.

383. Keen P: The use of drugs in the treatment of cardiac disease in the horse. *Equine Vet Educ* 2:81, 1990.

384. Ball MA, Weldon AD: Vegetative endocarditis in an Appaloosa gelding. *Cornell Vet* 82:301, 1992.

385. Ewart S, Brown C, Derksen F, et al: *Serratia marcescens* endocarditis in a horse. *J Am Vet Med Assoc* 200:961, 1992.

386. Pace LW, Wirth NR, Foss RR, et al: Endocarditis and pulmonary aspergillosis in a horse. *J Vet Diagn Invest* 6:504, 1994.

387. Ryan AF, Rainey JW: A specific arthritis with pericarditis affecting horses in Tasmania. *Aust Vet J* 21:146, 1945.

388. Bradfield T: Traumatic pericarditis in a horse. *Southwestern Vet* 23:145, 1970.

389. Buergelt CD, Wilson JH, Lombard CW: Pericarditis in horses. *Compend Contin Educ Pract Vet* 12:872, 1990.

390. Voros K, Felkai C, Szilagyi Z, et al: Two-dimensional echocardiographically guided pericardiocentesis in a horse with traumatic pericarditis. *J Am Vet Med Assoc* 198:1953, 1991.

391. Robinson JA, Marr CM, Reef VB, et al: Idiopathic, aseptic, effusive, fibrinous, nonconstrictive pericarditis with tamponade in a standardbred filly. *J Am Vet Med Assoc* 201:1593, 1992.

391a. Morley PS, Chirinotrejo M, Petrie L, et al: Pericarditis and pleuritis caused by *Mycoplasma felis* in a horse. *Equine Vet J* 28:237–240, 1996.

392. Reef VB: Myocardial disease. In Robinson NE, ed. *Current Therapy in Equine Medicine.* Philadelphia, WB Saunders, 1992, p 393.

393. Shawley RV, Rolf LLJ: Experimental cantharidiasis in the horse. *Am J Vet Res* 45:2261, 1984.

394. Schmitz DG: Cantharidin toxicosis in horses. *J Vet Intern Med* 3:208, 1989.

395. Guarda F, Rattazzi C: Pathology of cardiac ventricular aneurysms in the horse. *Schweiz Arch Tierheilkd* 136:76, 1994.

396. Weldon AD, Step DL, Moise NS: Lymphosarcoma with myocardial infiltration in a mare. *Vet Med* 87:595, 1992.

397. Doonan GR, Brown CM, Mullaney TP, et al: Monensin poisoning in horses—an international incident. *Can Vet J* 30:165, 1989.

398. Lester GD, Lombard CW, Ackerman N: Echocardiographic detection of a dissecting aortic root aneurysm in a thoroughbred stallion. *Vet Radiol Ultrasound* 33:202, 1992.

399. Spier S: Arterial thrombosis as the cause of lameness in a foal. *J Am Vet Med Assoc* 187:164, 1985.

400. Lombardo de Barros CS: Aortic body adenoma in a horse. *Aust Vet J* 60:61, 1983.

401. Hoskinson JJ, Wooten P, Evans R: Nonsurgical removal of a catheter embolus from the heart of a foal. *J Am Vet Med Assoc* 199:233, 1991.

402. Hilbert BJ, Rendano VT: Venous aneurysm in a horse. *J Am Vet Med Assoc* 167:394, 1975.

403. King JM: Anomalous epicardial lymphatics. *Vet Med* 88:512, 1993.

403a. Platt H: Vascular malformations and angiomatous lesions in horses: A review of 10 cases. *Equine Vet J* 19:500, 1987.

404. McDonnell SM, Love CC, Martin BB, et al: Ejaculatory failure associated with aortic-iliac thrombosis in two stallions. *J Am Vet Med Assoc* 200:954, 1992.

405. Wallace KD, Selcer BA, Tyler DE, et al: In vitro ultrasonographic appearance of the normal and verminous equine aorta, cranial mesenteric artery, and its branches. *Am J Vet Res* 50:1774, 1989.

405a. Dyson SJ, Worth L: Aortoiliacofemoral thrombosis. In Robinson NE (ed): *Current Therapy in Equine Medicine* (4th ed). Philadelphia, WB Saunders, pp 267–268.

406. Parks AH, Guy BL, Rawlings CA, et al: Lameness in a mare with signs of arteriovenous fistula. *J Am Vet Med Assoc* 194:379, 1989.

407. Cranley JJ: Focal medial calcification of the pulmonary artery: A survey of 1066 horses. *Equine Vet J* 15:278, 1983.

408. Zipes DP: Genesis of cardiac arrhythmias: Electrophysiological consideration. In Braunwald E, ed. *Heart Disease: A Textbook of Cardiovascular Medicine.* Philadelphia, WB Saunders, 1992, p 588.

409. Gabriel F, Lekeux P: Cardiac arrhythmias encountered in 159 Belgian riding horses. *Ann Med Vet* 130:205, 1986.

410. Hilwig RW: ECG of the month: Sinus tachycardia in a gelding. *J Am Vet Med Assoc* 182:1074, 1983.

411. Amada A, Kiryu K: Atrial fibrillation in the race horse. *Heart Vessels Suppl* 2:2, 1987.

412. Amada A, Kurita H: Five cases of paroxysmal atrial fibrillation in the racehorse. *Exp Rep Equine Hlth Lab* 12:89, 1975.

413. Bertone JJ, Traub Dargatz JL, Wingfield WE: Atrial fibrillation in a pregnant mare: Treatment with quinidine sulfate. *J Am Vet Med Assoc* 190:1565, 1987.

414. Cipone M, Venturoli M: Atrial fibrillation in five horses: Changes in the ECG during quinidine therapy. *Summa* 3:53, 1986.

415. Glazier DB, Nicholson JA, Kelly WR: Atrial fibrillation in the horse. *Irish Vet J* 13:47, 1959.

416. Glendinning SA: The use of quinidine sulfate for the treatment of atrial fibrillation in horses. *Vet Rec* 77:951, 1965.

417. Machida N, Yasuda J, Too K: Three cases of paroxysmal atrial fibrillation in the thoroughbred newborn foal. *Equine Vet J* 21:66, 1989.

418. Muir WW, McGuirk SM: Hemodynamics before and after conversion of atrial fibrillation to normal sinus rhythm in horses. *J Am Vet Med Assoc* 184:965, 1984.

419. Oka Y: Studies on uses of quinidine sulfate for treatment of atrial fibrillation in heavy horses (Abstract of Thesis). *Jpn J Vet Res* 33:89, 1985.

420. Petch MC: Atrial fibrillation: Bad news for man and horse? *Equine Vet J* 18:3, 1986.

421. Rose RJ, Davis PE: Treatment of atrial fibrillation in three racehorses. *Equine Vet J* 9:68, 1977.

422. Irie T: A study of arrhythmias in thoroughbred newborn foals immediately after birth. *Jpn J Vet Res* 38:57, 1990.

423. Reef VB, Reimer JM, Spencer PA: Treatment of atrial fibrillation in horses—new perspectives. *J Vet Intern Med* 9:57, 1995.

424. Stadler P, Deegen E, Kroker K: Echocardiography and therapy of atrial fibrillation in horses. *DTW Dtsch Tierarztl Wochenschr* 101:190, 1994.

424a. Marr CM, Reef VB, Reimer JM, et al: An echocardiographic study of atrial fibrillation in horses: Before and after conversion to sinus rhythm. *J Vet Intern Med* 9:336–340, 1995.

425. Muir WW, Reed SM, McGuirk SM: Treatment of atrial fibril-

lation in horses by intravenous administration of quinidine. *J Am Vet Med Assoc* 197:1607, 1990.

425a. Parraga MA, Kittleson MD, Drake CM: Quinidine administration increases steady state serum digoxin concentration in horses. *Equine Vet J* 19(Suppl):114–119, 1995.

426. Miller PJ, Rose RJ, Hoffman K, et al: Idioventricular tachycardia in a horse. *Aust Vet J* 64:55, 1987.

427. Cornick JL, Seahorn TL: Cardiac arrhythmias identified in horses with duodenitis/proximal jejunitis: Six cases (1985–1988). *J Am Vet Med Assoc* 197:1054, 1990.

428. Nielsen IL: Ventricular tachycardia in a thoroughbred racehorse. *Aust Vet J* 67:140, 1990.

428a. Traub-Dargatz JL, Schlipf JW Jr, Boon J, et al: Ventricular tachycardia and myocardial dysfunction in a horse. *J Am Vet Med Assoc* 205:1569–1573, 1994.

429. Cornick JL, Hartsfield SM, Miller M: ECG of the month: Premature ventricular complexes in an anesthetized colt. *J Am Vet Med Assoc* 196:420, 1990.

430. Pfister R, Seifert-Alioth C, Beglinger R: Location of the ectopic focus of the ventricular extrasystoles in the horse. *Schweiz Arch Tierheilkd* 126:165, 1984.

431. Vrins A, Doucet M, DeRoth L: Paroxysmal ventricular tachycardia in a horse. *Med Vet Quebec* 19:79, 1989.

432. Reimer JM, Reef VB, Sweeney RW: Ventricular arrhythmias in horses: 21 cases (1984–1989). *J Am Vet Med Assoc* 201:1237, 1992.

433. Ellis EJ, Ravis WR, Malloy M, et al: The pharmacokinetics and pharmacodynamics of procainamide in horses after intravenous administration. *J Vet Pharmacol Ther* 17:265, 1994.

434. Puigdemont A, Riu JL, Guitart R, et al: Propafenone kinetics in the horse: Comparative analysis of compartmental and noncompartmental models. *J Pharmacol Methods* 23:79, 1990.

435. Gasthuys F, Parmentier D, Goossens L, et al: A preliminary study on the effects of atropine sulphate on bradycardia and heart blocks during romifidine sedation in the horse. *Vet Res Commun* 14:489, 1990.

436. Reef VB, Clark ES, Oliver JA, et al: Implantation of a permanent transvenous pacing catheter in a horse with complete heart block and syncope. *J Am Vet Med Assoc* 189:449, 1986.

437. Nihouannen JC, Sevestre J, Dorso Y, et al: Implantation of a cardiac pacemaker into horses. I: Equipment and techniques. *Rev Med Vet* 135:91, 1984.

438. Yamamoto K, Yasuda J, Too K: Arrhythmias in newborn thoroughbred foals. *Equine Vet J* 24:169, 1992.

438a. Yamaya Y, Kubo K, Amada A, et al: Intrinsic atrioventricular conductive function in horses with a 2nd-degree atrioventricular block. *J Vet Med Sci* 59:151, 1997.

439. Nihouannen JC, Sevestre J, Dorso Y, et al: Implantation of a cardiac pacemaker into horses. II: Postoperative monitoring of a pacemaker with epicardial and myocardial electrodes in a pony. *Rev Med Vet* 135:165, 1984.

440. Muir WW, McGuirk SM: Ventricular preexcitation in two horses. *J Am Vet Med Assoc* 183:573, 1983.

441. Glazier DB, Littledike ET, Evans RD: Electrocardiographic changes in induced hyperkalemia in ponies. *Am J Vet Res* 43:1934, 1982.

442. Castex AM, Bertone JJ: ECG of the month: Sinus tachycardia and hyperkalemia in a horse. *J Am Vet Med Assoc* 194:654, 1989.

443. Hardy J: ECG of the month: Hyperkalemia in a mare. *J Am Vet Med Assoc* 194:356, 1989.

444. Epstein V: Relationship between potassium administration, hyperkalaemia and the electrocardiogram: An experimental study. *Equine Vet J* 16:453, 1984.

Chapter 8

Musculoskeletal Disease

Patricia A. Harris, MRCVS, PhD,
with contributions by Ian G. Mayhew, BVSc, PhD

One of the reasons that the horse has been so successful in its partnership with humans is its ability to run and jump. Effective locomotion depends on the coordination of various body systems. Ultimately, however, movement depends on the skeletal muscles.

STRUCTURE

Mammalian skeletal muscle consists of approximately 75% water, 18% to 22% protein, 1% carbohydrate, and 1% mineral, with a variable lipid content. Depending on the breed and type, between 44% and 53% of the live weight of a mature 500-kg horse has been estimated to be muscle.[1] Fusiform, multinucleated cells called myofibers constitute 75% to 90% of the volume of muscle. In addition, fibroblasts, capillaries, adipose cells, nerves, and connective tissue fibers are present to a varied extent depending on the muscle. Golgi tendon organs are found in the major tendinous origins and insertions. The nerve that supplies a muscle usually enters it, accompanied by blood vessels, close to the midpoint, at the neurovascular hilum.

Each myofiber is bounded by a complex membrane called the sarcolemma or, more correctly, the plasmalemma, which invaginates into the muscle fiber at numerous points to form the T, or transverse, tubules. These T tubules terminate within the muscle cell in close proximity to sacs of the cell's sarcoplasmic reticulum, forming a structure known as the triad. The plasmalemma is surrounded by a basement membrane, which in turn is closely attached to a layer of connective tissue called the endomysium. This is continuous with the perimysium, which surrounds groups or bundles of muscle fibers. This in turn is continuous with the epimysium, which surrounds the whole muscle. Satellite cells, which consist of a simple cell membrane around a nucleus with a minimum of cytoplasm and mitochondria, lie in shallow indentations on the myofiber surface between the plasmalemma and the basement membrane. The nuclei of the satellite cells and the myofiber are oriented to the long axis of the muscle fiber. The muscle fiber nuclei lie at the periphery just below the plasmalemma.

Each myofiber contains many myofibrils, the basic contractile units of the muscle. These are rodlike structures composed of a series of contractile units called sarcomeres. Sarcomeres are made up of the myofilaments, actin and myosin, together with rods of tropomyosin, complexes of troponin T (binds tropomyosin), troponin I (inhibits actomyosin adenosinetriphosphatase, ATPase) and troponin C (binds calcium). An electron micrograph of several myofibrils is shown in Figure 8–1. The thicker myosin filaments (forming the so-called A band, which is the broadest band—in Fig. 8–1 it has a narrow, darker gray strip running down its middle) interdigitate with the thin actin filaments. Transverse links of alpha actin form the very dark (almost black) Z lines. Because of the differing way these structures absorb light under the microscope, the regular alternation of A bands and Z lines in adjacent myofibrils produces the microscopic striated appearance characteristic of skeletal muscle fibers.

Within a myofiber, the number, size, and shape of the mitochondria vary with the muscle, site of sampling, and to a certain extent the fiber type.[2-4]

MUSCLE CONTRACTION

In order to understand the pathophysiology of muscle disorders it is of value first to define the sequential steps that lead to contraction.

Excitation

This involves the conduction of a nerve impulse to the motor end plate located in a deep primary cleft or fold of the plasmalemma. Acetylcholine is released, which transmits the impulse across the myoneural or neuromuscular junction to the end-plate region of the plasmalemma. The binding of acetylcholine molecules to specific receptor proteins produces a conformational change in these receptors, which, in turn, results in the opening of ion channels. The resultant ionic fluxes lead to a slight local depolarization: the miniature end-plate potential. Sufficient release of acetylcholine will result in full depolarization. Depolarization ceases with the diffusion of acetylcholine from the receptors and hydrolysis by acetylcholine esterase. The action potential generated is propagated across the plasmalemma in all directions and is carried deep into the muscle fiber by the T tubule system.

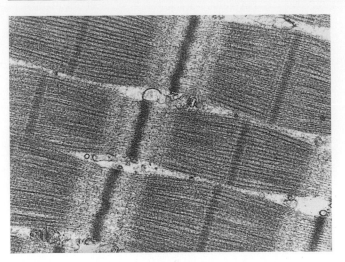

Figure 8–1. Electron micrograph of several muscle myofibrils (×45,000).

Excitation-Contraction Coupling

This starts with the arrival of the action potential at the triad region. The release of calcium from the neighboring cisterns or sacs of the intracellular sarcoplasmic reticulum is triggered by the rapid transmembrane sodium flux. Calcium interaction with troponin C results in the tropomyosin molecules being able to move and unmask part of the actin filament: the G-actin monomers.

Contraction

In this energy-dependent step there is a conformational change in the myosin filament so that the myosin globular heads move to a new position and combine with the newly unmasked G-actin monomers at a 90-degree angle. The force for contraction is then believed to be generated by the movement of this cross-bridge head to a 45-degree angle. This results in a sliding of the myofilaments relative to one another and a shortening of the sarcomere. The hydrolytic products of adenosine triphosphate (ATP) then detach from the myosin head. This enables the cycle to recommence, as the addition of new ATP to the myosin molecule results in the rapid dissociation of the actin and myosin filaments.[5, 6] Sustained contraction occurs with the rapid repetition of this mechanicochemical cycle.[6] All the myofibrils within a fiber contract simultaneously, resulting in contraction of that fiber. In type I fibers (see Fiber Type) calcium released from the mitochondria may also play a part in excitation-contraction coupling.

Relaxation

Energy-dependent resorption of calcium by the sarcoplasmic reticulum results in the release of calcium from troponin C, restoration of the resting configuration of the troponin-tropomyosin complexes, and disruption of the linkage between the myosin and actin filaments. Further details on muscle structure and contraction are available.[5–8]

Source of Energy for Contraction

The energy for contraction is provided by hydrolysis of ATP to adenosine diphosphate (ADP) and inorganic phosphate. This is catalyzed by ATPase, which is associated with the myosin molecule.

ATP is not stored in large amounts in the muscle fiber and has to be derived from the metabolism of fats, carbohydrates, and creatine phosphate stores, either aerobically or anaerobically. Aerobic production occurs in the muscle mitochondria by the oxidation of either fatty acids mobilized from the triglyceride fat stores in muscle and fat depots, or glucose from liver and muscle glycogen stores. In the sarcoplasm the oxidation of glucose through acetyl coenzyme A (acetyl-CoA) also produces ATP through substrate phosphorylation of ADP.

Anaerobic production occurs in the aqueous sarcoplasm through substrate phosphorylation of ADP by either creatine kinase, using the creatine phosphate stores, or glycolysis, utilizing glucose derived from liver and muscle glycogen stores producing lactic acid.

The rate-limiting factor in the extramuscular supply of glucose to working muscles under normal circumstances appears to be glucose uptake by the myofiber. However, with prolonged exercise the supply of glucose from the stores within the liver may become limited and the rate of glycogenesis within the liver may become an important factor. At very high intensity exercise it is possible that there may be inhibition of glucose phosphorylation within the muscle, due to inhibition of hexokinase by glucose-6-phosphate, which will affect the rate of glucose utilization. The rate-limiting factor in the supply of free fatty acids (FFA) to the muscle appears, at least initially, to be the rate of FFA release from adipose tissue. Once the necessary enzymes have been activated and so on, so that there is adequate mobilization and supply, the rate-limiting factors seem to be the mechanisms for transport and uptake of FFA into the muscle and the mitochondria. It is possible that, especially with high-intensity exercise, the rate of beta-oxidation within the mitochondria may become a limiting factor.

FIBER TYPE

Differentiation

Myofibers differ according to their metabolic and functional characteristics and have therefore been classified in several different ways according to the specific properties examined. The most common method of differentiation relies on the different contractile properties and involves the measurement of myofibrillar ATPase activity (the enzyme responsible for the breakdown of ATP at the actin-myosin cross-bridges). Staining for this enzyme distinguishes, at pH 9.4, two distinct fiber types. The slow-twitch type I fibers have a low activity at this pH and so appear lighter in color than the fast-twitch type II fibers (Fig. 8–2). The type II fibers can be further divided by preincubation at a more acidic pH into types IIA, IIB, and IIC (the pH values required for this differentiation vary with the laboratory but are around 4.5 and 4.3). Work is currently in progress at various centers to develop and refine antibody techniques for the identification of fiber types. These techniques may clarify some of the issues concerning fiber types in the horse, may overcome many of the practical difficulties of myosin ATPase staining, and may be adaptable to automatic tissue analysis systems.

The metabolic properties of the myofibers can also be used to differentiate the fiber types. Most commonly they are divided into those with a low oxidative ability (with, e.g., a high concentration of the sarcoplasmic enzyme glycogen phosphorylase) or a high oxidative ability (with high concentrations of the mitochondrial enzymes such as succinic dehydrogenase. The type I fibers are highly oxidative. The type IIA fibers are also highly oxidative, but the type IIB fibers have low oxidative properties.[9–11]

It should, however, be appreciated that, although there are fundamental contractile and metabolic differences between the type I and type II fibers, within the type II fiber group itself there is most probably a gradation of types. This is why, even within a single muscle biopsy, using different staining methods, different percentages of the type IIA, B, and C fibers can be reported, and explains why details of staining procedures used for differentiation need to be given in any study.

Innervation

Two types of motor nerve fiber are found (Table 8–1). Each motor neuron may innervate a few or several hundred myofibers. Each myofiber, however, is only innervated by a branch of one motor neuron. The type of motor neuron determines the physiologic and biochemical nature and thus the type of myofiber. The large phasic motor nerve fibers innervate the type II myofibers, whereas the small tonic fibers innervate the type I fibers.

Sensory axon endings contact the muscle spindles, which are a bundle of specialized intrafusal muscle fibers, and generate nerve impulses in response to the absolute length of the muscle or to changes in that length. Discharges are relayed directly to the ipsilateral spinal motor neurons that innervate the muscle in which the spindle is located, re-

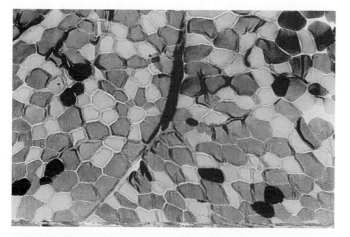

Figure 8–2. Preincubation at a pH of 4.5 of a needle muscle biopsy sample taken at a depth of 4 cm from the middle gluteal muscle of a 2-year-old racehorse. Type I fibers are darkly stained, type IIA are lightly stained, and type IIB are intermediate in staining intensity. In the area shown about 5% are type I fibers. (Courtesy of D. Sewell).

Table 8–1. Fiber Type Innervation

	Fiber Type Characteristics	
	I	II
Cell bodies	Small	Large
Conduction velocities	Slow	Fast
Discharge	Tonic	Phasic/fast
Action potential frequency	Low	High

sulting in a "reflex arc." Two types of sensory neurons innervate each spindle: the primary endings are from the large-diameter group IA afferents while the less elaborate secondary endings are from the smaller group II afferent axons. The intrafusal fibers also receive motor neuron innervation from small gamma motor neurons. This helps to keep the spindle taut when the muscle contracts, which in turn enables the sensory endings to respond to a wide range of muscle lengths.

A sensory nerve ending wraps around each Golgi tendon organ. These are found at the ends of the muscle fibers and are formed from a common tendon to which a number of muscle fibers are attached. The sensory nerve responds to tension generated by the contraction of any of these muscle fibers and the discharge is relayed to the ipsilateral alpha motor neurons where it is inhibitory. This forms another reflex arc responding to muscle tension.

Characteristics

Type I fibers tend to depend largely on aerobic metabolism of glucose and fatty acids for their energy. They are capable of prolonged activity but slower contraction responses. The type II fibers derive energy mainly from anaerobic glycolysis with glycogen as the main substrate. These fibers become more rapidly fatigued but are capable of rapid contraction and therefore are found in the highest proportions in muscle groups that move limbs rapidly. A summary of the characteristics of the different fiber types is given in Table 8–2.

Fiber Recruitment

Under neural control an orderly selection of fibers occurs with increasing demands. When just maintaining posture or walking, only the nerves supplying the slow-twitch type I, and possibly a few of the fast-twitch high-oxidative type IIA fibers, will be used. As the speed or intensity of work increases, more and more fibers will be recruited. Thus, at a medium trot, approximately 50% will be contracting, while at the gallop, most or all fibers will be involved. The fibers are recruited in a set order: type I, type IIA, and then type IIB.

Table 8–2. Fiber Type Characteristics

		Type II*	
	Type I	A	B
Physiologic Characteristics			
Speed of contraction/twitch	Slow	Fast	Fast
Fatigability	Low	Intermediate	Rapid
Maximum tension developed	Low	High	High
Histochemical Properties			
Myofibrillar ATPase stain pH 9.4	Light	Dark	Dark
Preincubation at a pH of			
≈ 4.5	Dark	Light	Medium
≈ 4.3	Dark	Light	Light
Oxidative capacity	High	Intermediate-high	Low
Enzymes for glucose breakdown	Intermediate	High	High
Enzymes for free fatty acid breakdown	High	Intermediate	Low
No. of capillaries	High	Intermediate	Low
Glycogen content	Low	High	High

*Type IIC fibers have been described following acid preincubation with staining intensities between the light type IIA and medium type IIB fibers.

Distribution

The proportions of fiber types present within a muscle vary according to the muscle, the breed, and the age, as well as the individual.[7, 9–17] In some muscles (in particular, the middle gluteal muscle, which is most commonly sampled) the distribution also depends on the sampling site, as there is a nonhomogeneous distribution of fiber types.[9, 10, 16, 18] It has, however, been suggested that within a specific muscle of an individual, the variation in fiber types is small if samples are taken from the same site or an identical contralateral site under controlled conditions.[16, 19]

The type IIC fibers are found in relatively large numbers in very young animals, but are rare in the mature horse, in which they are usually referred to as transitional fibers. These fibers have been suggested to be either a stage in the development of new fibers from satellite cells or fibers in direct transition from one fiber type to another.[9, 20]

Effect of Training

It has been suggested that the relative proportions of type I and type II fibers are under genetic control and that under normal training conditions cannot significantly be altered.[20, 21] Changes in the relative proportions of type IIA and IIB fibers have, however, been reported, although there has been some controversy regarding this interconversion.[7, 22–24] In general, it has been suggested that training results in an increase in the ability of a fiber to utilize oxygen, that is, more mitochondria with a decrease in the utilization of muscle glycogen and blood glucose plus a greater reliance on fat oxidation, as well as a decrease in the amount of lactate produced per given intensity of exercise.

Variable results have been reported on the effects of exercise on fiber size and capillarization. The extent and nature of the changes appear to depend on the duration, intensity, and type of exercise involved, as well as the age of the animal. Further information on the effect of training on muscle is available.[7, 9, 21–28]

Relationship to Performance

It has been suggested that a relationship exists between performance and the proportion of type I and type II fibers and their subtypes.[20, 22, 29, 30] Performance, however, depends on many factors, just one of which may be the genetic endowment of fiber type distribution, coupled with the beneficial effects of appropriate training. Given the heterogeneity of muscle, basing any performance characterization solely on the relative proportions of the fibers is therefore likely to be misleading.[20, 22]

MUSCLE DEVELOPMENT AND GROWTH

Mammalian skeletal muscle develops from the embryonic myotomes. Some myoblasts remain as single cells but retain their mitotic ability and form the satellite cells. Fusion of the remaining mononuclear myoblasts to form multinucleated myotubules is believed to be the way that muscle fibers develop in the fetus. Smaller secondary myotubules then form on the surface of these large primary myotubules. Initially, these share a common basement membrane but soon become separate. It has been suggested that the primary myotubules develop slow-twitch (type I) fiber characteristics while the secondaries develop fast-twitch (type II) characteristics. Genetic, hormonal, and nutritional factors may influence the number of these primary and secondary myotubules.[31-34] Near to the time of birth and for a period afterward, a proportion of the secondary fibers that lie closest to the primary fiber may become modified to form type I fibers,[35] although by this stage innervation of the fibers with their specific nerve types should already have occurred. It has, therefore, been suggested that there can be an "unplugging" from one neural type to another during development in response to motor stimulation. However, there is still much confusion regarding fiber differentiation.[31, 36]

Tertiary and later generations of myotubules form between the first- and second-degree myotubules. This is accompanied by the concurrent maturation of the established myotubules to myofibers, including migration of the nuclei to a peripheral position and synthesis of contractile proteins. Established fibers then increase in both diameter and length. This process is associated with the fusion of mononuclear satellite cells with the fibers. Postnatal increases in fiber diameter are associated with the addition of myofilaments and an increase in the number of myofibrils (perhaps derived from the satellite cells). Increases in length occur by the formation of extra sarcomeres together with a slight increase in mean sarcomere length. In the horse it has been suggested that training may cause an increase in the absolute number of fibers,[24, 27] but this is disputed as it is believed that the number of cells in most muscles is established very early on in life.[7, 22] Other work has supported the idea that the increase in muscle volume, associated with growth and training, does not depend on an increase in the number of fibers but on the hypertrophy of each muscle fiber.[37]

PATHOLOGIC CHANGES

General Response of Muscle to Injury

Muscle responds to injury or damage in a limited number of ways. There is growing evidence that all myopathic conditions share a common final pathway of muscle fiber degeneration,[38] although the number and type of fibers affected and the degree of damage may vary. A failure to prevent or control the influx of calcium ions or inadequate removal of calcium ions may initiate muscle damage, as the increase in intracellular calcium concentration may induce hypercontraction of myofibers and myofibrillar lysis.[38, 39] In addition, calcium sequestration into the mitochondria could result in metabolic disturbances.[38, 39]

The exact nature of these calcium-activated degenerative pathways is still unknown. It has recently been suggested that a key step may be calcium-induced membrane phospholipid hydrolysis via the activation of phospholipase enzymes, resulting in the production of tissue-damaging metabolites. Other processes, however, involving nonenzymatic lipid peroxidation may also be activated. During exercise there is an increased flow of oxygen. At the same time there is an overall depletion of ATP sources. The resultant metabolic stress to the cells leads in turn to a markedly increased rate of oxygen free radical production. This may exceed the cells' scavenger and antioxidant defense systems, leading to a loss of cell viability and damage. This could initiate skeletal muscle damage caused especially by exhaustive exercise. It is possible that either the increase in free radical activity

can lead to a failure of calcium homeostasis and consequent muscular damage or, alternatively, calcium overloading may lead to an activation of free radical–mediated processes. Little evidence has been produced to support the latter idea,[40] although it is still possible that activation of free radical–mediated processes occurs independently in skeletal muscle following excessive contractile activity, and so on. Free radical–induced skeletal muscle damage may also be especially important when there has been a period of ischemia followed by reperfusion.[41]

Often, therefore, the pathologic feature that enables one muscle disorder to be distinguished from another is not the presence or absence of specific lesions but a combination of the distribution, character, and age of the lesions; the presence or absence of certain cell types and parasites; as well as lesions in other organs. Segmental necrosis of muscle fibers, for example, can be seen in a variety of muscle disorders, in particular those associated with myoglobinuria. Determining the cause of this type of necrosis can be very difficult, especially in the horse. In man, using specific staining procedures for enzymes may be beneficial in determining whether an enzyme deficiency is involved, for example, phosphorylase deficiency in McArdle's disease. The presence of lesions in other organs can also be of value, for example, with chronic alcoholism marked changes in the liver will also be present. The nature of any cellular infiltrate may also be of interest, for example, in trichinosis an eosinophilic and neutrophilic infiltration of any necrotic sarcoplasm may be present. In most cases of segmental necrosis there is only a limited secondary involvement of the interstitial tissues or blood vessels. With vascular injury and regional necrosis (following arterial or venous occlusion, hemorrhage, or trauma), the necrosis of the muscle fibers is only part of a more extensive lesion involving the interstitial tissue and blood vessels.

Other, more general, pathologic changes that can be found in muscle include changes in fiber volume, number and shape, malformation, degeneration or proliferation of organelles, and disruption of the basic architecture of the fiber. Aggregates of inflammatory cells, reactive changes in vessel walls, occlusion of blood vessels, and increased amounts of fibrous tissue are other possible pathologic findings. In some conditions, such as tetanus, however, no marked changes have been identified. Further information on the types of changes that occur is available.[35, 42, 43]

Various histologic stains have been developed that can be used to highlight the different morphologic changes and inclusions that occur.[11, 43-45] Thus, periodic acid–Schiff (PAS), for example, will highlight glycogen stores within a cell as well as membrane structures containing mucopolysaccharide, glycoproteins, mucoproteins, glycolipids, or phospholipids. Histochemical staining for fiber type enables the pathologic changes to be recognized as affecting all fibers or those of one type only. This can be extremely important, for example, when looking for evidence of reinnervation when fiber type grouping occurs.

Histochemical staining can also aid in the detection of enzyme deficiencies and indicate the storage of various atypical metabolic compounds.[43, 46, 47, 47a] These procedures can be combined with a morphometric examination of the muscle[2] to provide further information. Immunocytochemical studies have been used, especially in man, in the investigation of neuromuscular disorders.[43] These help to localize specific enzymes and certain intracellular and extracellular muscle components such as the various collagen and myosin types, complement, and fibronectin. These techniques have not been used extensively in the horse. Electron microscopic studies enable the ultrastructural reactions of muscle fibers to be investigated. Little work has been carried out in the horse, but this is a developing field in human medicine.[48]

Atrophy and Hypertrophy

Atrophy may be defined as a decrease in muscle fiber diameter or cross-sectional area. It can occur in a variety of circumstances, including denervation, disuse, and cachexia, as well as in many muscle diseases, secondary to circulatory disturbances, and extensive myolysis. Within 2 or 3 weeks, following peripheral denervation, up to two thirds of the originally supplied muscle mass may be lost, although this may not always be obvious clinically owing to the continued presence of superficial and intramuscular fat deposits. The changes that can be seen histologically in the denervated muscle[35] will affect the muscle fiber type supplied by the affected nerve. In disuse atrophy due to tenotomy, for example, there appears to be a preferential atrophy of type I fibers, often with hypertrophy of type II fibers. In contrast, with cachexia and malnutrition, generally it is the type II fibers that are affected, especially in the essentially postural muscles.[35]

Not all muscles will show the same degree of atrophy, even within one disease process. In cachexia, the back and thigh muscles tend to be the first to be affected, and the loss of muscle is usually symmetric, with a concurrent loss of fat deposits. A localized asymmetric atrophy tends to be seen with paralysis, immobilization, and denervation.[35]

As indicated above, hypertrophy may occur through training. A compensatory hypertrophy also may occur in the fibers surrounding an area where fibers have been lost or have markedly decreased in size, for example, with chronic denervation atrophies and in advanced cachectic atrophy. Often, very large fibers are seen histologically in such conditions, with evidence of incomplete longitudinal division.[35]

Repair After Denervation and Injury

Following Denervation

Reinnervation can occur in two ways. Firstly, with axonotmesis, where the axons are damaged but the Schwann cell and endoneural fibrous sheaths remain, axons from the proximal part of the damaged nerve may reestablish connections with empty residual Schwann cell sheaths in the distal portion of the original nerve. Initially, atrophy of scattered muscle fibers can be seen, but after reinnervation, if this occurs within a certain time period, a proportion of the muscle fibers will be restored to their normal size and functional capability. Even if the affected muscle is not fully restored, other surrounding unaffected muscles may be able to compensate so that overall function is maintained. A slight gait abnormality may, however, remain. The second type of reinnervation tends to occur when some nerve fascicles are completely severed or when the lesion is located a great distance away from the muscle. This occurs, for example, when lesions have involved the motor neuron cell bodies and nerve roots. In these circumstances, collateral reinnervation from adjacent unaffected axons can occur. As the nerve type characterizes the muscle type, this will result in regrouping of muscle fibers so that with successive episodes of denervation and reinnervation clusters of fibers of the same histochemical type will be found rather than the normal checkerboard pattern. This is referred to as fiber type grouping.

Following Injury to the Muscle

Regeneration, where there has been a break in the continuity of the muscle fiber, differs considerably from that described above. In such cases repair involves multiplication of nuclei, formation of new internal structures and organelles followed by fusion and alignment into an integrated unit. It seems that regeneration can only take place if parts of the affected fiber remain intact. If this is so, recovery can be very quick. Regeneration can occur either at the healthy end of the severed fiber (continuous or budding regeneration) or by fusion of the mononuclear myoblasts lying free in the tissue to form a myotube, which develops in a similar way to fetal fibers (discontinuous or embryonic regeneration). The origin of these myoblasts is disputed. Some workers believe they are derived from undamaged sarcoplasmic nuclei, others that they come from satellite cells.[44] If the scaffolding, basement membrane, and supporting tissues remain intact, and the initiating disease process subsides, these new fibers will tend to orient in a similar way to the original fibers. This type of regeneration is usually seen with segmental necrosis, where there has been necrosis of the whole diameter of the fiber, often involving several sarcomeres, but there is preservation of the basement membrane. Fibroblastic and vascular reactions are minimal in this type of regeneration.

Trauma, hemorrhage, infection, and infarction can result in complete disorientation of the regenerating fibers with marked proliferation of fibroblasts and vessels, as this type of damage tends to result in destruction of the muscle fibers as well as the interstitial tissue.

AIDS TO THE DIAGNOSIS OF SKELETAL MUSCLE DISORDERS

The clinical signs seen with muscle disorders are relatively few and rather nonspecific, but include pain on deep palpation, fatigue with light exercise, tenderness to touch, atrophy, hypertrophy, contracture of joints, degrees of weakness, and the presence of discolored urine. In the majority of instances, clinical signs alone are of limited diagnostic value and the use of other techniques is required. These can include muscle histology, muscle histochemistry, thermography, electromyography (EMG), and, most commonly in equine medicine, plasma-serum biochemical investigations.

Muscle Biopsy

Muscle biopsy samples can be obtained by surgical excision under general or local anesthesia[49] or, more commonly, by percutaneous needle biopsy.[9, 12, 50] Obviously, owing to the variation in fiber composition with sample site in certain muscles, the position and depth of sampling are important. Good specimen preparation is also vital to prevent artifacts such as ice crystals, sarcomere shortening, and fiber kinking.[9, 43, 51]

Muscle biopsy allows the morphologic, biochemical, and physiologic properties of the myofibers, as discussed above, to be examined with the animal still alive and with minimal fuss, especially if obtained by percutaneous needle biopsy, for which chemical sedation is rarely required. Typical sites used for percutaneous biopsy include the semimembranosus, the biceps femoris, and, most commonly, the gluteal muscles. A small area of skin over the gluteal muscle is closely shaven, washed, and cleaned. Local anesthetic is injected subcutaneously along the proposed line of incision and into the connective tissue or fascia overlying the muscle. Anesthetic is not injected into the muscle itself. An incision is then made through the skin and fascia and the biopsy needle is inserted to a predetermined depth (Fig. 8–3). Using the "Tru-Cut" principle, a small piece of muscle can be caught and removed with the needle. The incision is left unsutured.

The exact site used for the biopsy tends to vary slightly with the investigator. We, for example, routinely sample approximately 15 cm from the tuber coxae on a line drawn from the proximal aspect of the tuber coxae to approximately the fourth caudal vertebra.

Thermography

An infrared thermographic scanner converts the skin's radiated thermal energy to electrical signals that can be amplified and displayed on a video screen. By using isotherm colors of known temperature, it is therefore possible to obtain two-

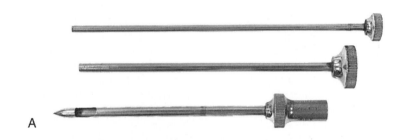

A

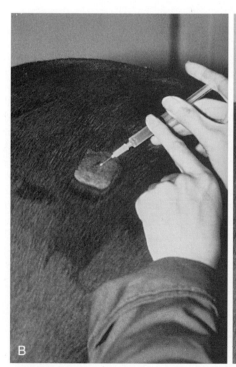

B

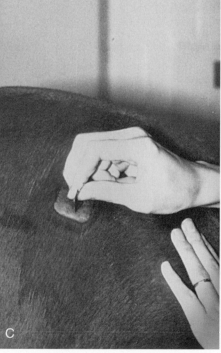

C

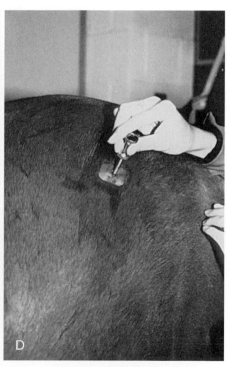

D

Figure 8–3. A, Percutaneous muscle biopsy needle, often referred to as a Bergstrom biopsy or Stille-Eschmann cannula, available with 4-mm, 5-mm, and 6-mm internal diameters. **B,** A small area (approximately 2.5 cm) of skin over the gluteal muscle (two thirds of the distance on a line from the tail head to the tuber coxae) is closely shaven, cleaned, and prepared in a sterile manner, and 1.5 mL of local anesthetic (lidocaine 2% with epinephrine) is injected subcutaneously along the proposed line of incision and into the connective tissue or fascia overlying the muscle. No anesthetic is injected into the muscle tissue itself. **C,** An incision is made through the skin and fascia using a no. 23 scalpel blade. **D,** The biopsy needle is inserted into the muscle to a predetermined depth (indicated by an indelible mark on the shaft of the biopsy needle). Using the Tru-Cut principle, a small piece of muscle (up to 100 mg) can be caught and removed with the needle. The incision is left unsutured.

dimensional, graphical, and quantitative information regarding the precise temperature of the skin surface. This technique can be used noninvasively as a means of detecting changes in skin temperature resulting primarily from changes in peripheral blood flow. The latter can be affected by local alterations of blood flow due to inflammation, atrophy, and neoplasia and also by neurologic lesions, particularly of the autonomic supply to the skin.

Abnormalities have been found in exercise-exacerbated focal thoracolumbar gait abnormalities, as well as disuse atrophy.[52] The technique has been particularly useful in documenting hindlimb muscle strain as a cause of lameness in horses. However, this technique is not in widespread use.

Electromyography

Needle electromyography is the study of the electrical activity of muscles. A recording needle electrode is placed into the muscle and the electrical activity is amplified, recorded on an oscilloscope, and projected audibly into a loudspeaker. The electrical status of muscle membranes depends on the integrity of the whole motor unit. Thus, an EMG evaluates the function of the ventral motor horn cell, its axon, axon terminals, and neuromuscular junctions, as well as the muscle fibers it innervates.

Investigations are usually carried out in two phases. Firstly, an assessment of the electrical potentials associated with physical disruption of muscle membranes resulting from insertion of the needle in the muscle is made. These insertional potentials, if relayed through a loudspeaker, tend to sound like short bursts of loud static. They vary among muscles, probably due to differences in the size and number of motor units present.

The second phase involves the assessment of electrical potentials when the needle electrode is at rest in the muscle. Normally, electrical silence occurs with cessation of needle movement, unless the needle is located near to a nerve branch or the end-plate zone when miniature end-plate potentials are recorded continuously; these sound like a low intensity "shhhh. . . ." Insertional activity may persist after needle movement has stopped. This is commonly seen with denervation and is due to increased excitability of the muscle fiber membranes. In relaxed, diseased muscles, different types of abnormal electrical activity have been recognized. *Positive sharp waves* are slow monophasic waves, rapid in onset, often with a slow decay to the baseline, which occur repeatedly with a variable amplitude (100 μV–20 mV). Their cause is uncertain, although they are often seen with denervation and may represent a nonpropagated depolarization region in the muscle fibers near to the tip of the electrode. When occurring in trains, these positive sharp waves sound like a waning "brrrr. . . ."

Fibrillation potentials are electrical signals generated by a single muscle fiber. Long random volleys of mono- or bi- (occasionally tri-) phasic potentials of short duration (0.5–5.0 ms), with an amplitude of usually less than 200 μV, are commonly seen in denervation (depending on the stage). Constant and repetitive fibrillation potentials, which sound like rain on a tin roof or the sizzling of frying eggs, can be found especially in the early stages of denervation. Fibrillation potentials can also be seen in myopathic disorders where

segmental muscle necrosis may have caused, for example, the separation of a muscle fiber and its nerve supply.

Myotonic discharges, which are high-frequency (up to 1,000 Hz) repetitive discharges with a waxing and waning of the potentials seen and heard with a characteristic, musical, dive-bomber, or more precisely, revving motorcycle-like sound, can be found in myotonia if the exploring EMG electrode is moved or the muscle is externally percussed. *Bizarre high-frequency discharges* (often referred to as pseudomyotonia) may produce a dive-bomber-like sound. There is no true waxing and waning, although the amplitude and frequency of the potentials may change abruptly to mimic a revving motorcycle-like sound. The discharges are often in couplets or triplets and are likely to terminate abruptly. These, or similar discharges, can be seen in longstanding denervations, ventral horn cell disease, polymyositis, and certain myopathies. Unlike the myotonic discharges, pseudomyotonic discharges may be abolished by curare and therefore are believed to originate presynaptically.

Fasciculations, often seen in association with visible muscle twitching, are due to the spontaneous contraction of some or all of the constituent fibers of a motor unit. They are seen primarily with any cause of weakness (myasthenia), either local or generalized, and especially in neurogenic disorders, as well as in tetanus and certain debilitating and metabolic disorders. In addition, the electrical activity induced by electric stimulation of nerves or associated with voluntary or induced muscle contraction can be assessed.

Further information on EMG is available in the literature[53–56] and in Chapter 9.

Scintigraphy

Bone-seeking radiopharmaceuticals have been used to detect and localize skeletal muscle involvement, especially in "poor performance" cases, but are likely to be of limited routine value in the field.[56a] The accumulation in damaged muscle may be related to the deposition of calcium in the damaged fibers, binding by tissue hormones or enzyme receptors, tagging to denatured proteins, and/or altered capillary permeability. Uptake of labeled phosphates appears to occur only when muscle damage is ongoing and not in areas of repair. Three main types of muscle uptake were identified in one study of horses with skeletal muscle damage: a diffuse, severe, and generalized uptake; bilateral symmetrical uptake involving muscle groups that perform synergistic functions; and asymmetrical radioisotope uptake in one or more muscle groups on one side of the animal.[56a] The reasons for the various patterns have not been fully elucidated.

Urinalysis: Myoglobinuria

Myoglobin (molecular weight, 16,500) is essential for the transport of oxygen into and within muscle cells. Most mammalian muscles contain about 1 mg myoglobin per gram of fresh tissue, and it has been suggested that acute destruction of at least 200 g of muscle must occur before serum myoglobin levels are raised sufficiently for it to be found in the urine.[57] In humans, myoglobinuria occurs in a wide variety of conditions, including myocardial infarction, crush and burn injuries, malignant hyperthermia, idiopathic and exertional rhabdomyolysis, and certain genetic metabolic abnormalities.[42, 45, 57–59] In the horse, myoglobinuria has been seen, for example, in equine rhabdomyolysis,[60, 61] white muscle disease in foals,[62] and postanesthetic myositis.[63]

Any cause of hemolysis in the horse can result in hemoglobinuria. In addition, hemoglobinuria has been reported in horses with acorn poisoning,[64] hepatic and renal disease,[65] and equine rhabdomyolysis.[66, 67] The presence of both hemoglobin and myoglobin in the urine from animals suffering from equine rhabdomyolysis is very rare in our experience. It may occur in animals suffering from a concurrent disease or condition that causes hemolysis. Alternatively, it may be caused by a variant of the equine rhabdomyolysis syndrome (ERS) with a different pathophysiology. It has also been suggested that hemoglobin may be present after exhaustive exercise.[67]

Unfortunately, stored urine, concentrated urine, and urine containing myoglobin, hemoglobin, or other porphyrins can all appear similar in color[57, 69, 70] (Fig. 8–4). Therefore, myoglobinuria cannot be distinguished by color alone and other methods are required. The orthotoluidine-impregnated strips commonly used by veterinary surgeons (e.g., BM-Test-8 (Boehringer Ingelheim Pharmaceuticals, Ridgefield, Conn.) are very sensitive to the presence of both myoglobin and hemoglobin.[60, 71] The differential salting out of hemoglobin with ammonium sulfate has been shown to give false results in man[69, 57, 58, 72] and the horse.[71] Visual inspection of the serum or plasma may indicate the cause of the pigmenturia. The low affinity of myoglobin for haptoglobin means that myoglobin is excreted at plasma concentrations around 0.2 g/L, whereas hemoglobin will only appear in the urine at plasma concentrations greater than 1.0 g/L. At this concentration a pink discoloration of the plasma occurs indicating that hemoglobin is present.[49, 57, 58]

Spectroscopy has been used to differentiate between the oxyforms of myoglobin and hemoglobin but it will not identify oxymyoglobin when oxyhemoglobin is also present.[72] In fresh urine oxymyoglobin is rapidly converted to its met form and in older urine samples both oxyforms will

have been spontaneously converted to their met-forms. These can be reduced chemically, but this can result in a denaturation of the proteins. In humans, because methemoglobin and metmyoglobin have almost identical absorption spectra, spectrophotometry has been stated not to be able to distinguish one from the other if both are present in the same sample.[72] The same has been shown for the horse.[71] Ultrafiltration has also been shown to be unreliable in the horse, perhaps due to the higher viscosity of equine urine compared to human.[71]

On electrophoretic separation on cellulose acetate, myoglobin migrates as a β_2-globulin and hemoglobin as an α_2-globulin. This method can distinguish the two proteins in urine containing high concentrations (>125 μg/mL) of either protein, provided no other proteins, apart from albumin, are present. Immunoassays are the most sensitive and specific tests, and can be used for the detection of small amounts of myoglobin in blood and urine.[71, 73, 74]

Sequelae of acute tubular necrosis and acute renal failure have been associated with myoglobinuria in man[68] and the horse[49, 66] (see Chapter 16).

Plasma and Serum Enzyme Activities

A change in the plasma activity of any enzyme can occur for a variety of reasons, including alteration in the permeability of the enclosing cell membrane, cell necrosis, impaired removal or clearance of the enzyme, and increased synthesis, as well as impaired synthesis. Decreases in plasma enzyme activities are not usually a consequence of a loss of activity due, for example, to aging, and there is often no one specific organ of elimination, although most occur via the liver, kidneys, and lungs. Therefore, under most circumstances, the elimination rate of an enzyme from the plasma remains fairly constant and it is the rate of influx to the plasma that is the crucial factor.

Increases most commonly occur owing to a defect in the integrity of the membrane containing the enzyme.[75, 76] This defect may be due to partial or complete disruption of the cell or a change in the membrane resulting in a transient increase in permeability. A complete explanation for the pattern of release of intracellular constituents from diseased muscles cannot be given here. Most of the enzymes that can be detected in increased concentrations in the blood with the various muscle disorders are the major "soluble" (sarcoplasmic) enzymes, although the mitochondrial form of aspartate aminotransferase (AST) can also be found with severe injury. Intensification of cell function, as would occur during exercise or as a reaction to cell damage, results in increased substrate utilization, which in turn may result in a greater membrane permeability. It is not, however, clear whether the increase in substrate permeation of the boundary surfaces themselves is sufficient to allow incidental escape of cell enzymes or whether a reduction in the energy potential is needed before cells "leak." It is, therefore, often very difficult to distinguish between borderline physiologic and borderline pathologic changes in enzyme plasma activities.

It has been suggested that considerable enzyme efflux can occur even when the light and electron microscope cannot detect with any certainty changes in cell structure. In Duchenne's muscular dystrophy, for example, it has been

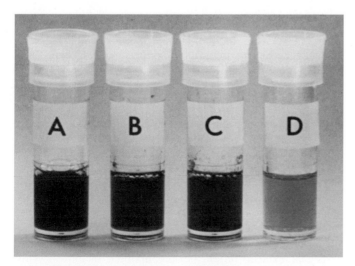

Figure 8–4. Four urine samples: (A) with 3 mg/mL hemoglobin; (B) with 3 mg/mL myoglobin; (C) stored for 1 month at 18°C; (D) Control: fresh urine.

suggested that there is a change in the structure of the plasmalemma at the molecular level, which leads to a selective passage of cellular constituents based partly on molecular weight.[76] Under general circumstances the rate of efflux of an enzyme most likely depends not only on molecular weight and intracellular localization but also on its binding to various intracellular structures, as well as its relative concentration intracellularly and extracellularly. No explanation for the marked differences in half-lives of the various plasma muscle enzymes reported for man and the horse has been given.

The enzymes found to be of most use in evaluating the muscular system are, in the horse, creatine kinase (CK, EC 2.7.3.2), AST (EC 2.6.1.1), and lactate dehydrogenase (LDH, EC 1.1.1.27).

Creatine Kinase

In the horse, CK is found mainly in skeletal muscle, the myocardium, and the brain.[77] There appears to be little or no exchange of CK between the cerebrospinal fluid and plasma. A significant increase in total plasma CK activity is, therefore, due to cardiac or skeletal muscle damage. Creatine kinase (80,000 Da) does not enter the blood stream directly after its release from the muscle cells but transits through the lymph via the interstitial fluid. The total circulating CK quantity in the horse has been estimated to correspond to the CK quantity found in approximately 1 g of muscle and a three- to fivefold increase in plasma CK activity corresponds to the apparent myolysis of around 20 g of muscle.[77a]

In humans there appear to be two monomers of CK, designated M and B. The enzyme is dimeric and three possible primary forms exist: MM, MB, and BB. In simplified terms, MM is found mainly in skeletal muscle, BB in the brain and epithelial tissues, and MB in the myocardium. In humans the measurement of MB activities has been used as a sensitive test for the diagnosis of myocardial infarction.[78] It has, however, been suggested that chronic skeletal muscle damage can also result in the characteristic "myocardial infarction" pattern.[79]

In the horse there has been some confusion over CK isoenzymes with workers reporting different electrophoretic bands and tissue activities, perhaps because of the different techniques used.[80–83] In one study it was found that the heart and skeletal muscle both contained predominantly the MM dimer; the brain (and pancreas and kidney), mainly the BB dimer; and the intestine, both the MB and BB dimers.[82] This work suggested, therefore, that in the horse, CK isoenzymes on their own could not be used to differentiate between skeletal and cardiac muscle damage. The plasma half-life of CK in the horse is very short (108 minutes,[84] 123 ± 28 min with a plasma clearance of 0.36 ± 0.1 mL/kg per min)[77a] in contrast to reports of 12 hours in humans.[85]

Aspartate Aminotransferase

AST is found mainly in skeletal muscle, liver, and heart, although lower activities are present in several other tissues. It is, therefore, not tissue-specific.[75, 77, 86] Two isoenzymes have been identified by electrophoresis: MAST (found exclusively in the mitochondria) and CAST (originating from the cytoplasm or sarcoplasm). The ratio of cytosolic to mitochondrial enzyme in horse serum is significantly greater than that found in man and many other mammals.[87] In the horse, although the ratio of these two forms varies between tissues, there appears to be no tissue-specificity for either isoenzyme. Therefore, it has been concluded that the examination of sera for AST isoenzyme activities cannot indicate the tissue source,[88] although large increases in MAST are unlikely to be found in the serum unless severe muscular injury has occurred.[88] Some workers have reported an apparently unique form of the enzyme in the sera from "azoturia" cases.[88] The plasma half-life of AST in the horse is 7 to 10 days,[84] far longer than the 11.8 hours in man.[85]

Lactate Dehydrogenase

LDH is a tetrapeptide made up of combinations of two different peptides, H (heart) and M (muscle), which form the five isoenzymes referred to as LDH_1 to LDH_5, that is, H_4, MH_3, M_2H_2 M_3H, and M_4, respectively.

Like AST, LDH is found in most tissues and is therefore not organ-specific. However, tissues contain various amounts of the LDH isoenzymes and the isoenzyme profile, obtained by electrophoretic separation, has been used to identify specific tissue damage.[89] For the most part, LDH_5 (plus some LDH_4) is found in the locomotor muscles, the liver contains mainly LDH_3 (with some LDH_4 and LDH_5), the heart contains mainly LDH_1 (with LDH_2 and LDH_3), and all types have been found in certain nonlocomotor muscles.[80, 83] Training has been shown to increase the percentage of LDH_1 to LDH_4 and decrease that of LDH_5 in skeletal muscle.[90] Nonhemolyzed samples should be used for LDH determinations, as red blood cells (RBCs) contain relatively large amounts of LDH.

Use of Exercise Tests

Certain physiologic changes can result in a transient alteration in cell membrane permeability. Hypoxia, catecholamines, hypoglycemia, changes in pH, and altered ionic concentrations have been reported as causing such a change in membrane permeability.[86, 91, 92] Many of these are believed to act by decreasing the amount of ATP available for the maintenance of cell integrity. This becomes especially important during exercise.[92]

Measuring the CK and AST activities before and after a controlled period of exercise has been suggested as an aid to the diagnosis of certain muscle disorders. A major difficulty has been to establish exactly the "normal" enzyme response to exercise. There has been much confusion in the literature regarding this, partly caused by the differences in the intensity and duration of the exercise undertaken, the varying sampling intervals used in the reports, and the inclusion of individuals with possible muscular problems. The majority of workers have suggested that an increase in CK activities occurs with hard exercise,[93–95] whereas with slower work, others have shown no significant increase. This suggests that intensity could be an important factor.[96, 97] This was supported by work in dogs, which showed that CK activities correlated with the intensity of muscular activity.[98] Another study in the horse,[99] however, suggested that CK elevations did not vary according to the intensity of the work, and it was proposed[100] that the duration of exercise was a more important factor. A recent study suggested that when the duration of exercise was kept constant, the intensity of the exercise did, in fact, have an effect on the extent of CK activity increase.[101] However, this investigation did not look at the effects of exercise duration on the CK response.

Although no significant increase in CK activity was found following trotting exercise in conditioned animals by one worker, significant increases were recorded when the same exercise was performed after one or more days' rest.[96, 96a] Increases in AST activities of 35% have been reported following a 1,500-m canter,[102] and 50% following strenuous exercise in previously rested animals.[93] Most other workers have found little increase in AST following different types of exercise.[84, 87, 100, 103]

Therefore, the effects of exercise on plasma muscle enzyme activities may depend on the fitness of the animal and the intensity and duration of the exercise, as well as the environment.[67, 80, 100] In horses, as in humans, there may be large intersubject variability in the postexercise rise in CK activities to be taken into account.[77a] Plasma volume changes may affect the activities recorded, especially if measured immediately after exercise. A test that would enable fit and unfit horses to be tested equally has been proposed, which involves riding the horse over a given distance at a speed that produces a steady heart rate of 200 beats per minute.[104] However, it is very difficult to exercise at an exact heart rate, and many veterinary surgeons do not have access to heart rate monitors. This has meant that veterinary surgeons tend to use the same "exercise test" in all animals regardless of their fitness.

As discussed above, the physiologic increase in CK activity following exercise is believed to be due to a change in cell membrane permeability, possibly caused by hypoxia, although other factors are likely to be involved. Hypoxia may occur at lower workloads in unconditioned horses and these may be expected to show higher postexercise activities than a fit horse given the same work. It has been suggested that the magnitude of the exercise-induced rise decreases with training.[84, 99, 100] Some workers have found no significant changes in the AST and CK responses to exercise during a training program,[97] whereas others have found that following an endurance ride the fittest animals (indicated by speed of the heart rate recovery following an endurance ride) had lower increases in CK activities.[103] The magnitude of exercise-induced changes in CK activities has been shown to increase with detraining.[101] It was concluded from this study that increases of more than 100% in AST activity following exercise are likely to be abnormal regardless of the intensity of the exercise or the fitness of the animal.[101] Also, if a short submaximal exercise test is carried out, the serum CK and AST activities at 2 hours post exercise should not rise to more than 250% and 50% of the preexercise values, respectively, regardless of fitness.[101]

It has been stressed that, although exercise might result in statistically significant changes in CK and AST activity, these may not always be of biological or clinical significance.[105, 105a] The clinical history and clinical presentation must always, for example, be taken into consideration when interpreting enzyme values. For example, a young racehorse given its first gallop will often have activity changes greater

than those described above (e.g., from a preexercise level of 40 IU/L to a 2-hour postexercise level of 350 IU/L), although this is unlikely to be of clinical significance. However, in cases of recurrent equine rhabdomyolysis, similar changes may indicate ongoing subclinical muscular damage. In humans it has been suggested that there is no relationship between CK activity and the amount of muscle damage after an eccentric exercise bout, reflecting that CK activity is a manifestation of muscle damage rather than a direct indicator of its severity.[77a]

Currently, we recommend a submaximal exercise test, which is varied for each horse. The intensity and duration of this test should be chosen according to the fitness of the horse and the exercise program it is undertaking, with the aim of giving the horse strenuous exercise without overexerting it. A normal response to such a test is illustrated in Table 8–3.

Other Factors Affecting AST and CK Activities

Gender and Age

A group of Thoroughbreds were sampled over a 9-month period and it was found that the 2-year-old fillies showed more marked fluctuations in AST and CK activities than the 3-year-old fillies and colts. Unfortunately, no 2-year-old colts were studied.[106] In a later study of sixty-six 2- and 3-year-old Thoroughbred racehorses in training, it was found that fillies were more likely to have high CK and AST activities than colts, and 2-year-olds were more likely to have raised ASTs than the 3-year-olds.[107] The effect of age on the incidence of raised muscle enzyme activities was thought not to have been caused by the natural loss of 2-year-olds from training with high enzyme activities, especially as several of these raced and won.[107] It may be that certain animals have physiologically higher plasma activities, or their muscle enzymes are more slowly removed from the circulation. Alternatively, they may be more sensitive to the various insults that cause permeability changes in muscle fiber membranes. Age or training, or a combination of both, could have a dampening effect on muscle membrane changes. In dogs

---

Table 8–3. Criteria for a Normal Response to a Submaximal Exercise Test Designed for a Given Individual Horse*

1. Pre-exercise:
   CK activity <100 IU/L (laboratory resting reference range, 0–49 IU/L)
   AST activity <300 IU/L (laboratory resting reference range, 150–230 IU/L)
2. Not more than a doubling of the resting CK activity at 2–4 hr post exercise
3. Return to baseline CK activities at 24 hr post exercise
4. Not more than a 50% increase in AST activity
5. No clinical signs of stiffness

*Abbreviations: CK, creatine kinase; AST, aspartate aminotransferase.

a significant decrease in CK activities has been reported with age, but there was no difference between males and females.[107a] In one study no correlation was found between plasma progesterone concentrations and the fluctuations in CK/AST activities.[106] However, a later study showed that when fillies with high median AST activities were removed from the study group a highly significant relationship was found between progesterone and AST, but not CK activities, and estradiol showed a significant effect on CK but not on AST activities.[96a] In rats CK release after exercise or in vitro electrical stimulation has been shown to be greater in males than in females.[107b] Estradiol has been suggested to have a protective effect and to attenuate CK influx.[96a, 107b] However, further work on the role of such hormones in CK and AST activities in the horse is needed before conclusions can be drawn.

Time of Year and Training

Several workers have suggested that AST plasma activities increase in the early stages of training and then decrease as training progresses.[108, 109] Time of year has been shown not to have a significant effect on the number of animals with normal or with high AST and CK activities.[107] However, an increase in mean activities to a peak in April and May followed by a decrease to a low in September was shown in a group of Thoroughbred racehorses in the Northern Hemisphere.[107] The very high mean activities found in April, May, and June were accompanied by very high standard deviations, which made definitive conclusions difficult. Such large standard deviations were also found in another study on Thoroughbreds in training.[110] On an individual basis, a change in AST activities does not always seem to occur with training.[111] Changes in the serum levels of AST isoenzyme concentrations have not been thought to be good indicators of peak fitness or slight overtraining.[87]

In a recent study of AST activities in a small number of barren and pregnant standardbred mares, evidence for a diurnal rhythm was apparently found, with the lowest activities occurring in the early hours (4–6 AM) and the maximal ones at night (10–12 PM). The mean levels increased from September-November until March. A circannual cyclicity was found, but the pattern differed between the two groups. In the barren animals the arcophase appeared to occur in the second half of January, whereas for the pregnant animals it occurred in September (approximately month 5 of pregnancy). The error fields were, however, quite broad.[112]

Relationship to Performance

It has been stated that elevated CK and AST activities decrease a horse's chance of winning.[113] However, a group of 500 standardbred trotters with a recent history of equine rhabdomyolysis and raised plasma muscle enzyme activities had a significantly better racing record compared with a large group of apparently unaffected horses.[114] Fifty percent of the horses with high median AST activities raced and won at least once in another study.[107] It is, however, obviously not possible to determine if they would have given better performances or won in better classes if they had not had such raised activities.

Sampling Technique

It has been shown that incorrect venipuncture techniques can have an effect on plasma CK activities.[105a]

CLASSIFICATION OF MYOPATHIES

Coordinated movement as well as resting muscle tone relies on the interaction between the central nervous system (CNS) and the motor units with input from the Golgi tendon organs (responding to muscle tension) and the muscle spindle apparatus (monitoring muscle length). Pathologic alterations in skeletal musculature can be induced by lesions in the neurons and their end plates (neurogenic myopathies) or in the muscle fibers themselves (myogenic myopathies). The term *primary myopathy* has been given to "any disorder which can be attributed to primary morphological, biochemical or electrical changes occurring in the muscle fibers or in the interstitial tissues of voluntary musculature and in which there is no evidence that such changes are in any way secondary to changed function in the central or peripheral nervous system."[115] Differences in the histologic appearance of neurogenic and myopathic myopathies have been reported in man[44, 47] and the horse.[116] However, longstanding neurogenic disorders may show features typical of a myopathy.

Classification of primary myopathies with regard to pathologic changes only is difficult, if not impossible, because skeletal muscle has limited ways to respond to a variety of insults. The most useful basis for classification may, therefore, be etiology. Various systems have been suggested for the horse[67, 117] in which disorders have been divided into congenital, exertional, neurologic, and endocrinologic categories. An alternative way is to classify according to the underlying pathophysiology, that is, disorders of excitation, action potential propagation, etc. Owing to our limited knowledge of the pathophysiology of the various equine skeletal muscle disorders, this system is of limited use. Tables 8–4 and 8–5 show how the various equine skeletal disorders might be classified under these two systems, using current information.

This chapter concentrates on the myopathic myopathies and follows the etiologic classification system shown in Table 8–4.

TRAUMA

Physical injuries to muscle can occur following external trauma that results, for example, in lacerations to the skin and underlying muscle. Alternatively, violent contraction or overexertion, with or without external trauma, may result in muscle rupture or tearing. The changes seen within the muscle depend on the extent of the damage to the muscle and surrounding tissue.[35]

Fibrotic Myopathy
Pathophysiology

This tends to be a chronic progressive disorder. It may occur following excessive exercise, over a long period that has resulted in the tearing and stretching of muscle fibers.[56] It has also been seen in quarter horses and stock horses following maneuvers such as sliding stops, in which the large thigh muscles are contracting while the stifle and hock are

---

Table 8–4. Classification According to Etiology

Neurogenic—may be hereditary or environmental in origin, acquired or congenital

A. Disorders of anterior horn cells
B. Disorders of motor nerve roots
C. Peripheral neuropathies
D. Disorders of neuromuscular transmission
    1. Botulism
    2. Tetanus

Myopathic

A. Traumatic, e.g., fibrotic myopathy
B. Inflammatory
    1. Idiopathic
    2. Intramuscular injection of irritant drugs
        a. Oxytetracycline
        b. Phenylbutazone
        c. Iron, etc.
C. Infectious
    1. Bacterial, e.g., clostridial infection
    2. Viral, e.g., influenza; possibly part of the equine rhabdomyolysis syndrome
    3. Parasitic, e.g., sarcocysts
D. Toxic
    1. Plants, e.g., *Cassia occidentalis*
    2. Drugs, e.g., monensin
E. Hormonal
    Myopathy associated with:
    1. Hyperadrenocorticalism
    2. Hypothyroidism; possibly part of the equine rhabdomyolysis syndrome
F. Autoimmune
    ?Purpura hemorrhagica
G. Circulatory
    1. Localized postanesthetic myositis
    2. ?Generalized postanesthetic myositis
    3. Aortic-iliac thrombosis
H. Genetic
    1. Hyperkalemic periodic paralysis
    2. ?Myotonia
    3. Metabolic myopathies, e.g.
        a. ?Equine rhabdomyolysis syndrome
        b. ?Glycogen storage disease
        c. ?Malignant hyperthermia
I. Nutritional
    1. Vitamin E/selenium-responsive
    2. Malnutrition
J. Exercise-related
    Postexhaustion syndrome
K. Cachectic atrophy
L. Disuse atrophy
M. Malignancy
N. Multifactorial
    1. Equine rhabdomyolysis syndrome
    2. Congenital developmental defects
O. Miscellaneous/idiopathic
    1. Atypical myoglobinuria
    2. Postanaesthetic myasthenia

Table 8–5. Classification According to Pathophysiology

A. Disorders of excitation
    1. Disorders affecting nerve cells, axons, and terminals
    2. Functional disorders of the neuromuscular junction, e.g., botulism, certain drug-induced disorders
B. Disorders of action potential propagation
    1. Periodic paralysis
    2. Myotonic disorders
C. Disorders of excitation contraction coupling
    1. Abnormalities of calcium, parathyroid hormone
    2. ?Malignant hyperthermia
    3. Corticosteroid myopathy
D. Disorders of contraction: not recognized in the horse
E. Disorders of energy supply: suspected but not proved in the horse
    1. Glycogen storage disease
    2. Lipid storage disorders
    3. Hypothyroidism
    4. Mitochondrial disorders
F. Direct action on muscle fibers/structures
    1. Hypothyroidism
    2. Certain drug-related myopathies
    3. Certain nutritionally related disorders, e.g., vitamin E/selenium deficiency
    4. Trauma
    5. Disuse atrophy
G. Miscellaneous/multifactorial
    Equine rhabdomyolysis syndrome

---

extending,[117, 118] and in horses tied by a halter and shank, which pull back suddenly.[119] Congenital cases have also been described, perhaps due to periparturient trauma,[119] as well as cases secondary to intramuscular injection.[120] The semitendinosus muscle is the most frequently affected but adhesions to the semimembranosus and biceps femoris are common. The gracilis muscle may also be involved. The biceps brachii muscle can be affected.

The pathophysiologic process appears to involve trauma (external or work-related) followed by inflammation, muscle fiber atrophy, and replacement by fibrous tissue. Occasionally, mineral deposits form in the affected tissues, in which case the condition has been referred to as an ossifying myopathy.[120]

The clinical signs have been suggested to occur due to a mechanical disturbance, by the scar tissue, of the normal pattern of muscular contraction. Alternatively, an altered gamma efferent loop with an abnormal setting of the muscle spindle trigger may allow the early unchecked contraction of caudal thigh muscles during the late swing phase of the stride.[52]

Clinical Signs

Fibrotic myopathy has been described as a nonpainful mechanical lameness associated with a distinct gait abnormality.[119] The condition can be unilateral or bilateral and the affected limb(s) is pulled back and down before the end of the protraction phase so that the foot is slammed down, resulting in a louder sound on impact than that of an unaffected limb. This results in a shortened cranial or swing phase and a lengthened weight-bearing phase,[119] which has been referred to as a "goose-stepping" gait. The condition tends to be most obvious at the walk. If the biceps brachii muscle is involved, the horse shows a shortened cranial phase of the thoracic limb with a tendency for the foot to land at the toe in a similar way to those animals affected by the navicular syndrome. Occasionally the area of muscle damage can be identified due to a dimpling or depression in the skin overlying the muscle. The lameness tends to be unresponsive to routine anti-inflammatory therapy.

Diagnosis

The diagnosis is based on the clinical signs and history, although the muscles may appear abnormally firm on palpation. In one report two congenital cases did not have palpable thickening of the muscle or tendon and there was no evidence of scar formation.[121] Histologically, a band of dense collagenous connective tissue may be found or irregular, jagged pieces of mineral. Diagnostic ultrasound has been useful in some cases to confirm the diagnosis and to determine whether mineralization is present in addition to the fibrosis.

One of the main differentials is stringhalt, although in this condition the leg is hyperflexed during the cranial or swing phase and the stepwise caudal jerking movement does not occur just before the foot hits the ground.[118]

Treatment and Prognosis

Resection of the fibrotic band or a semitendinosus myotenectomy has been tried as well as a simplified semitendinosus tenotomy.[67, 120, 121] Some improvement in gait may occur in some cases, although it is unlikely that complete absence of lameness will result. The long-term prognosis is poor as the condition tends to recur following surgery, which may not be surprising as muscle repair following resection tends to be by fibrosis. Postoperative problems with wound healing also appear to be common.[120] Transection of the semitendinosus tendon insertion on the tibia distal to the myotendonosus junction has been said to result in much less postoperative trauma, which may help to decrease the potential for recurrence[121] and full recovery has been anecdotally reported in a few cases. It may, therefore, be preferable to perform a less radical excision and combine this with passive postoperative flexion-and-extension physiotherapy. Surgery is unlikely to be of value if the biceps brachii is involved.[117]

Gastrocnemius Muscle Rupture
Pathophysiology

Rupture of the gastrocnemius muscle has been found in animals attempting to get up following a long period of recumbency (e.g., post anesthesia, postpartum paralysis). It has also been seen in animals that rear and fall over backward, and very occasionally following overextension. In foals, cases have been reported following the foal's first attempt to rise, especially if there is poor muscle tone or poor coordination. The condition has been seen in dystocia and in foals where there have been manual attempts to straighten a fixed tibiotarsal joint.[122, 123] If the rupture occurs in the tendon of insertion it may result in avulsion of a portion of the tuber calcanei. If it occurs in the muscle a hematoma may form, which may calcify.

Clinical Signs and Laboratory Findings

The condition can occur unilaterally or bilaterally; the animal will be unable to stand if it is bilateral. The affected hock(s) is excessively flexed due to the loss of the extensor influence of the gastrocnemius. Heat, swelling, and pain are normally evident in the initial stages. The plasma muscle enzyme activities also tend to be elevated, at least initially.[122, 123]

Treatment

Support in a sling with the affected limb immobilized in an extended position has been recommended,[122] but the prognosis is guarded.

Serratus Ventralis Rupture

This is only rarely seen either secondary to dorsal impact trauma over the withers and neck region or possibly after jumping a high fence or jumping off a raised platform. Animals are usually bilaterally affected. The thorax drops between the paired scapulae so that the dorsal borders are above the thoracic spinous processes. The croup is often higher than the withers. This is a very painful condition and radiographs are needed to eliminate the possibility of dorsal spinous process fracture.

The prognosis is poor. Recommended treatment is a prolonged period in a sling if the horse is temperamentally suited to such a restriction.[124]

"Sore" and "Pulled" Muscles

"Pulled" muscles (i.e., muscle tears or strains resulting in some disruption of muscle architecture and occasionally the formation of a hematoma) often present clinically during or immediately following exercise. Depending on the extent of the trauma and the muscle groups involved, obvious swelling and apparent pain on palpation may or may not be present. Plasma CK and AST activities may or may not be significantly elevated. Definitive diagnosis may be difficult especially in chronic cases. Faradic stimulation, scintigraphy, thermography, and diagnostic ultrasound are some of the more common techniques used to diagnose a "pulled" muscle. Treatment tends to be a combination of rest and physiotherapy (e.g., manipulation, faradism, ultrasound). "Pulled" muscles should perhaps be differentiated from the "overexerted" or "sore muscle" in which the associated damage tends to be at the cellular level involving structural damage of the contractile elements. Delayed onset muscular soreness (DOMS) is a commonly recognized condition in humans. The soreness tends to increase in intensity over the initial 24 hours and peaks around 24 to 72 hours, and hence its name. It is not certin that DOMS occurs in the horse, although it has been suggested when a stiff gait, palpable soreness, and a reluctance to move, as well as raised hydroxyproline concentrations, are observed 24 hours after exercise. Free radicals may be involved in the pathophysiology of both acute and delayed onset postexercise muscular soreness. Treatment of DOMS in humans varies from rest to light exercise with or without analgesia and the external application of heat. In the horse continued exercise may be contraindicated in two of the main differentials for muscle soreness: muscle strains and the equine rhabdomyolysis syndrome (see below). In humans the best prevention for DOMS is previous appropriate training.

INFECTIOUS AGENTS

Infectious agents (bacteria, viruses, and parasites) can affect skeletal muscles. Some produce essentially inflammatory reactions (myositis), whereas others give rise to, often mild, degenerative changes (i.e., myopathy). The differentiation can be difficult, especially in subacute and chronic cases, as an inflammatory reaction often induces secondary degenerative changes and vice versa.

Bacterial
Gas Gangrene and Malignant Edema

These occur with wound infections where strains of clostridia, C. septicum, C. perfringens, C. novyi, C. sordelli, and C. chauvoei, are the principal pathogens. Germination of spores and vegetative growth occur when suitable local anaerobic conditions (alkaline pH, low oxidative reduction potential, etc.) exist following castration, parturition injuries, stake wounds, and in particular, intramuscular injections.[125] Toxin production results in the destruction of the cellular defense mechanisms and marked tissue necrosis.

Affected animals may be found recumbent or dead. In less acute cases, lameness often occurs, which can be very severe. Painful muscular swellings may be present and crepitation may be felt. The overlying skin may initially appear hot and be discolored but may progress to become cool to the touch and insensitive. Affected animals are usually extremely depressed with systemic signs of a profound toxemia. The prognosis is poor as the condition often progresses rapidly with ataxia, recumbency, coma, and death.

Diagnosis is usually made from the clinical signs and history. The finding of a nonclotting, malodorous fluid on needle aspiration (with or without gas) can be indicative of clostridial infection. Anaerobic culture and fluorescent antibody identification of the organism in tissue specimens have been recommended for a definitive diagnosis.[126]

Clinicopathologic changes tend to be nonspecific and similar to those seen in other septic-toxic conditions. Although raised plasma muscle enzyme activities may be found, they often do not appear to be in proportion to the degree of muscle damage.[126] In gas gangrene there tends to be extensive disintegration of muscle tissue, with serosanguineous exudate and bubbles of gas present. Malignant edema is more typically a cellulitis with sparing of the muscle fibers, although this may sometimes progress to gangrene.[35, 126]

Antibiotics, in particular penicillin (20,000–40,000 IU/kg

IV t.i.d. or q.i.d.—some clinicians have recommended these to be initially given intravenously at high doses around 44,000 IU/kg every 2–4 hours), either on its own or in combination with metronidazole (20–25 mg/kg PO t.i.d. or 20 mg/kg IV b.i.d. or t.i.d.), in addition to surgical debridement or fenestration, or both, to remove necrotic tissue and disrupt the anaerobic environment, have been used to treat such conditions.[126] Long-term antibiotic therapy is usually required. Antibiotic therapy should be continued until infection has resolved and for a minimum of 7 days. In many instances, for example diffuse cellulitis extending down fascial planes, therapy may be required for several weeks. Supportive fluid therapy and analgesics are often necessary. Corticosteroids should be used with caution, although initial short-term therapy may be beneficial. The prognosis in most cases is poor.[125] Survival appears to be most frequent with C. perfringens infections, although extensive skin sloughing may occur, which, in its turn, may necessitate euthanasia. Chronic cases of bacterial myositis may result in muscle wasting.

Suppurative Myositis: Abscessation

This may be hematogenous in origin or result from penetrating wounds, intramuscular injections, or from an extension of an infective focus in an adjacent or distant structure. Streptococcus equi is a frequent cause. Early on there is an ill-defined cellulitis, which may either heal or progress to the classic organized abscess or, in the case of certain staphylococci, may extend, resulting in extensive muscle damage. Abscesses may slowly heal, expand, or fistulate to the surface. Once fistulated they may collapse and heal, usually with scar tissue, or persist as chronic granulomas (especially Staphylococcus aureus in the neck and pectoral region).[35] Corynebacterium pseudotuberculosis may also be isolated from large abscesses in various muscles, in particular, the pectorals.

There appears to be a marked geographical variation in the clinical signs seen with C. pseudotuberculosis infection. On a worldwide basis, ulcerative lymphangitis, usually with sores, abscesses, fever, lameness, anorexia, and lethargy, which may progress to chronic lameness and weight loss, is the most common condition. In the western United States, especially in the more arid parts, the organism tends to be associated with ventral midline, inguinal, and pectoral abscesses. The condition has been referred to as "pigeon fever" (after the swollen pectorals giving the appearance of a pigeon's breast), or alternatively as "dryland distemper" or "Colorado strangles" (after its geographical distribution).

Cases can occur at any time of the year, although they are more common toward the end of summer and in the fall and early winter. One or a number of animals within a group may be affected. Outbreaks in a number of animals at one establishment have been reported. The organism can survive in the soil and enters the body via lesions in the skin or mucous membranes and spreads via the lymphatics. It has been suggested that insect vectors may be involved. Clinical signs vary with the stage of the condition and the site of the abscess(es).[26a] The affected animal can be pyrexic and anorectic during the maturation phase of the abscess. Ventral pitting edema, lameness, and depression may also be seen.

Weight loss may occur. If the abscesses are located in the axillary or inguinal regions the affected animal can be very lame and is more likely to be intermittently febrile. Such cases can be difficult to diagnose as it may take weeks or even months for the abscesses to develop fully. Raised white blood cell counts and fibrinogen levels may be found, although in the more chronic stages little clinicopathologic changes tend to be seen. *C. pseudotuberculosis* infections seem to be less likely than staphylococcal or streptococcal abscesses to result in raised white blood cell counts or fibrinogen levels. The abscesses typically form deep in the muscle beds and can be very large with thick capsular walls filled with a nonodorous light tan pus. The differential diagnosis includes seromas, tumors, and other bacterial abscesses. The diagnosis can be confirmed by ultrasound or culture of any aspirated fluid. Abscesses in the axillary region, in particular, can be difficult to locate, even with ultrasound. A synergistic hemolysis inhibition test is available, which can detect antibodies to the organism, but the intensity of the antibody response depends on a number of factors, including the thickness of the capsule surrounding the abscess and the chronicity of the infection. For example, animals with chronic thick-walled abscesses that have been recently lanced can have low or zero detectable circulating antibody levels, perhaps because these have been utilized in combating the massive toxin release. The test can, however, for example, be very helpful in determining whether internal *C. pseudotuberculosis* abscessation should be included in the differential diagnosis of certain cases.

The treatments recommended include encouraging the maturation process via hot poultices, lancing, flushing, and draining. In some cases surgical intervention may be required to adequately expose the abscess. There is some controversy over the use of antibiotics, especially with respect to the timing of administration. It may depend on the stage of abscessation. The antibiotics commonly recommended, however, include procaine penicillin 20,000 IU/kg IM b.i.d. or potassium penicillin 40,000 IU/kg IV q.i.d., sulfadiazine-trimethoprim, and erythromycin. Rifampicin is often recommended to be used in combination with penicillin (to avoid resistance developing) at 2.5 to 5.0 mg/kg PO b.i.d. Antibiotic therapy once initiated should ideally be maintained for several weeks.

Prognosis is guarded; a certain number of cases do not completely resolve following treatment. Some may recur once antibiotic therapy is stopped; others may recur months later. In a few cases internal abscessation may occur, often resulting in chronic weight loss and sometimes ventral edema, ascites, dyspnea, recurrent colic, exercise intolerance, recurrent pyrexia, etc. Abortion also can be a sequela.[127]

It has been recommended that contamination of paddocks, via a draining lesion, be avoided and that contaminated bedding be dealt with appropriately. Good fly control can also be beneficial.

Systemic Infections

Degenerative lesions may occur in muscle with acute systemic infections. The widespread lesions tend not to be visible grossly and consist of a variable degree of segmental degeneration.[35]

Parasitic Diseases

Sarcocystis

This protozoal parasite has a two-host obligatory development. It is found in horse muscle as part of the intermediate host infection. Sporocysts are eaten with herbage contaminated by carnivore feces. Sporozoites are released and migrate to various sites. The second or third generation of schizonts develops within the muscle fibers as thin-walled cysts. Entry into muscle fibers can result in extensive fiber degeneration and marked enzyme release if there is a heavy infestation. Enlargement of the cysts over the next 100 days or so can result in further muscular damage and lameness. Although three *Sarcocystis* species (*S. bertrami, S. equicanis,* and *S. feyeri*) have been recognized, there is some controversy as to whether the three are distinct species.[35] A high postmortem prevalence of sarcocysts and evidence of transplacental infection have been reported,[128] suggesting that inapparent infection is probably quite common. A light and electron microscope study of sarcocysts in the horse has been undertaken.[129]

There is some dispute as to whether sarcocysts cause clinical muscle disease in the horse.[35] Twelve out of 91 horses presenting with a history of chronic muscle problems were found to be positive for sarcocysts on muscle biopsy in one study.[130] It was not found possible to separate the group of animals with sarcocysts from the others on the basis of laboratory findings, history, or clinical signs. Weight loss, lethargy, difficulty in chewing and swallowing, generalized muscle weakness, and fasciculations have been reported in one case with widely distributed sarcocysts, and the clinical signs were attributed to the sarcocyst infestation.[131]

Chronic illness in an experimentally infected pony has also been reported[132] and a sarcocystis species appears to be involved in equine protozoal myeloencephalitis.[133]

Trichinella spiralis

This nematode can be found as an encysted larva in a bulging glassy segment of a muscle fiber in animals whose feed has contained porcine muscle tissue. It is, therefore, rare. There is usually one per fiber and the larva can be up to 100 μm long. Degeneration (plus regeneration) may occur in neighboring muscle fibers. The larva can live for many years, but if the parasitized segment degenerates, the larva is exposed and soon dies. This in turn results in an acute inflammation, predominantly eosinophilic.[35, 115] The parasitic infection appears to be asymptomatic.

TOXICOSES

There are only a few available and palatable toxic compounds that cause muscle fiber degeneration in the horse. (For additional information, see Chapter 19.)

Plants (e.g., *Cassia*)

Cassia occidentalis (coffeeweed, senna) is toxic to the horse and can cause ataxia, incoordination, recumbency, and death with liver and muscle damage. However, natural ingestion of this plant seems to be rare.[134]

Ionophores (e.g., Monensin)

Pathophysiology

Monensin is a carboxylic ionophorous antibiotic fermentation product derived from *Streptomyces cinnamonensis*. It is used as a coccidiostat for poultry and as a feed additive for cattle in which it increases feed utilization by altering rumen fermentation. Access to ruminant feed or accidental contamination of horse feed in a mill producing both cattle and horse feed are the most common reasons for intoxication.

A possible explanation for the pathophysiology of monensin is that the lipid-soluble monensin sodium complex releases sodium once across the cell membrane in exchange for a proton. The protonated monensin then leaves the cell to pick up more sodium and the cycle repeats. Small concentrations of monensin may also result in an increase in intracellular potassium, whereas large concentrations tend to decrease the level. The increase in intracellular sodium stimulates the Na^+, K^+-ATPase pump, and indirectly results in an increase in calcium. This increase in intracellular calcium may then result in the release of certain factors such as catecholamines which, in turn, may be responsible for some of the clinical signs seen, especially in relation to the heart. When the mitochondria become saturated with the calcium they have taken up, the process of oxidative phosphorylation will be disturbed and the supplies of ATP will decrease. Swelling and disruption of the mitochondria will then follow, resulting in release of the stored calcium. This may potentiate or precipitate catecholamine-induced cardiac arrhythmias. The calcium may also result in a brief period of extreme contraction of the muscle (due to effects on actin-myosin binding) as well as by release of various cellular lytic enzymes. The rapid onset of cardiac or skeletal muscle necrosis may result from the energy deficiency resulting from these lytic processes. Other tissues, less dependent on ATP, may not show such severe signs.[135, 115, 136] In the muscle, swelling and disintegration of mitochondria are the first visible lesions, although it has been reported that monensin does not cause mitochondrial structural defects in cultured muscle cells.[137] Further work is therefore needed to determine if other substances or metabolites of monensin are involved in the pathophysiology in vivo.[135]

Clinical Signs

The horse is very sensitive to monensin, being susceptible to 2 to 3 mg/kg body weight (cf. cattle, 20–34 mg/kg) for crystalline monensin. (The LD_{50} for mycelial monensin has been estimated to be 1.38 ± 0.19 mg/kg body weight.) This may be because horses do not clear monensin from the bloodstream as rapidly as cattle, and in addition equine heart muscle is known to be very sensitive to the effects of catecholamines.[135] Following ingestion of a single toxic dose, signs of lethargy, muscular weakness, and stiffness, often with recumbency, occur within 24 hours. In the early stages a progressive hypokalemia resulting in cardiac conduction disturbances has been reported.[136] The cardiovascular signs that may be present include tachycardia with possible arrhythmias, prominent jugular pulse, congested or pale mucous membranes, cold extremities, weak pulse, and profuse sweating. Tachypnea, hyperpnea, or dyspnea may be seen.

Early on, affected animals may show signs of colic, including sweating, increased pulse, and increased or absent borborygmus. Reduced amounts of feces or no feces may be passed. Animals may be anorectic. Myoglobinuria and muscle tremor may also be seen, together with progressive ataxia and signs of CNS malfunction. Depending on the dose ingested (and the individual), death may occur within 24 hours. Hindlimb muscles tend to be involved most severely.[35, 115, 135] Progressive cardiac insufficiency plus weight loss and sometimes renal failure are more common with chronic toxicity. In such cases the symptoms related to skeletal muscle involvement may disappear, although poor performance and muscular weakness may be apparent if asked to perform. Signs of chronic toxicity may not be noticed for weeks after ingestion of the compound has stopped.[138] The amounts of monensin to be ingested and the time course in which it causes signs of chronic monensin toxicity are controversial.

Laboratory Findings

In the peracute cases, which die within 24 hours, a progressive hemoconcentration associated with an increased urine output and a decreased urine specific gravity has been reported, together with elevated urea and creatinine concentrations.[136]

CK and AST activities may be moderately to markedly elevated, primarily due to skeletal muscle damage. Interestingly, the increase in total LDH activities noted appears (at least initially) to be due to the LDH_1 and LDH_2 isoenzymes. It has been suggested that this may be related to increased erythrocyte fragility and hemolysis. Elevations in alkaline phosphatase activities have also been found, apparently due to an increase in the bone isoenzyme.[136] Hemoglobinuria or myoglobinuria or both may occur.

Sodium concentrations do not appear to change markedly, whereas calcium tends to decrease initially, within the first 12 to 24 hours by about 10% to 15%, and then recovers. Hypokalemia tends to occur in the first 24 hours with a decrease of 1 to 2 mmol/L followed by a return to normal by 36 hours. In chronic toxicity the findings are often non-specific and tend to reflect the various organ involvement. In one study of 32 horses presenting with a history of unthriftiness and poor performance following prior ingestion of monensin-contaminated feed, low bilirubin values were found with increased alkaline phosphatase activities. In four cases elevated LDH_5 activities were also found.[138]

Histology

In animals that die peracutely, gross lesions may not be found. In less acute cases the gross changes are not pathognomonic for monensin toxicosis and can include edema, hydropericardium, hydrothorax, ascites, hemorrhages, and pale areas in the heart or diaphragm[135, 137, 138]. It can be difficult to differentiate this condition histologically from vitamin E/selenium deficiency or the equine rhabdomyolysis syndrome.[35]

Diagnosis

The clinical signs and history of access to monensin are important in the diagnosis. The finding of high monensin concentrations in feed and stomach contents may confirm the diagnosis. The ingestion of blister beetles (*Epicauta* species) can cause cardiomyopathy and needs to be excluded from the differential diagnosis, as does ERS.

Treatment and Prognosis

Intensive isotonic polyionic fluid therapy with additional potassium has been recommended for the treatment of the hypovolemic peracute case. Although this may support the animal during the initial crisis, the prognosis is guarded because the longer-term actions of monensin, particularly on the heart, may still cause death.[136, 138]

Activated charcoal or mineral oil administered orally may help to decrease further monensin resorption. Purgatives that act by stimulating the vagal system should be avoided because of the risk of causing arrhythmias in an already damaged heart. Similarly, intravenous calcium may not be advisable and the cardiac glycosides should be avoided as they may work synergistically with monensin, resulting in extensive cardiac muscle damage.

Miscellaneous Toxicoses

Selenium, iron, thallium, and perhaps sulfur and cobalt may cause muscle disease when fed above certain levels. Metals such as iron may act by affecting vitamin E/selenium status or lipid peroxidation.[35] Bracken (*Pteridium aquilinum*), horsetail (*Equisetum arvense*), and rock fern (*Cheilanthes sieberi*), if ingested, may induce a thiamine deficiency with signs of anorexia, gait disturbances, staggering, lack of coordination, lethargy, a weak, irregular pulse, and muscular tremors.[139]

AUTOIMMUNE DISEASE
Purpura Hemorrhagica

This condition has been described in greater detail in Chapter 11. Purpura hemorrhagica may cause muscular lesions secondary to intramuscular bleeding.[140] Skeletal muscle necrosis with fragmentation and swelling of the muscle fibers and a cellular infiltration may be seen histologically. Classically, the lesions are believed to be caused by a type III hypersensitivity vasculitis. In humans there is, however, a suggestion that certain bacteria share similar immunodeterminants with muscle so that antibodies produced against the bacteria may also affect the muscle directly, causing necrosis.[141]

CIRCULATORY DISORDERS
Postanesthetic Myositis

It has been reported that postanesthetic muscle damage may occur in around 6% of anesthetized horses[141a]; postanesthetic myopathy may be divided into two forms: localized (the more common form) and generalized.

Localized
Pathophysiology

The localized form has been suggested to occur as a consequence of undergoing anesthesia combined with the position-

ing of the horse during the anesthesia, which results in direct pressure to the muscle or perfusion disturbances. Damage may occur due to increases in pressure within the osteofascial compartments, resulting in a local relative ischemia. In this context compartment is defined as a muscle or group of muscles enclosed within a low-compliance envelope of fascia and sometimes periosteum.[142] This is comparable to the compartmental syndrome described in humans. Venous occlusion tends to result in a greater inflammatory response and more extensive fibrous tissue repair than arterial occlusion. Support for this theory comes from several workers[142–145] as sufficiently high intramuscular pressures have been reported during anesthesia to compromise capillary blood flow and possibly affect neural transmission. Postanesthetic compartmental syndrome per se has only rarely been reported in the horse, perhaps because the compartmental pressures decrease rapidly when a horse stands.[145a]

Various other findings, such as an increase in the lactate concentration of blood draining from the dependent muscle, a significant postischemic hyperemia in the dependent muscles, and an increase in the plasma levels of thromboxane and prostaglandin E_2 have been reported.[146] The damage may in fact be a result of the reperfusion of the ischemic muscles rather than the ischemia per se, as it has been proposed that strong oxidants are generated during reperfusion, which may initiate membrane lipid peroxidation and muscle damage.[146]

The suggested risk factors associated with the development of this condition have included the weight and fitness of the animal (it is reported to occur more commonly in large, fit horses); the positioning; the nature of the supporting surfaces' padding; the duration of the operation (the longer it proceeds, the greater the risk); and the type of drugs or anesthetic used.

In one study the intramuscular pressure was measured with a catheter in the lowermost limb of 11 laterally recumbent horses, and the effect of position and padding was noted. The highest pressure readings (up to 92 mm Hg) were found with no padding when the limb in contact with the table was kept perpendicular to the body and the free limb was unsupported. The lowest pressure (11 mm Hg) was measured with padding when the limb in contact with the table had been pulled forward and the free limb was supported.[144] Muscle pressures were not correlated with weight in this study, but animals with greater muscle mass appeared to have higher muscle pressures.

Halothane anesthesia has been shown to result in a decreased blood flow to muscle (0.40 mL/min/100 g muscle) compared with that seen in unanesthetized muscle (1.20 mL/min/100 g muscle).[147] A predisposition to ischemia has also been suggested to occur with certain disease states that may cause an underlying hypotension, as this will also result in a decrease in muscle perfusion. However, in one study no correlation between body weight, halothane vaporizer concentration, intracompartmental muscle pressures, cardiac output, blood pressure, and the development of postanesthetic forelimb lameness was found, although prolonging the anesthetic time appeared to increase the degree or severity of lameness.[142] Since then, two studies have looked at the effect of maintaining horses for a relatively long period of time (3½–4 hours) under normotensive anesthesia (with a mean arterial blood pressure around 80–95 mm Hg) or hypotensive anesthesia, as a result of increasing the inspired halothane concentration (with a mean arterial blood pressure around 50–65 mm Hg). This work suggested that hypotension, as a result of a high concentration of halothane, may predispose to postanesthetic myositis even when protective padding is used.[148, 149] There appears to be no increase in the incidence of problems when repeated episodes of normotensive anesthesia are undertaken, even when halothane is used.[148]

The intracompartmental pressures of the upper (or noncompressed) extensor carpi radialis and the long head of the triceps muscle bellies were found to be much lower than the lower (or compressed) muscle values in one of the studies.[149] There were, however, no significant differences between the intracompartmental pressures recorded under normotensive or hypotensive anesthesia for the noncompressed muscles.[149] This suggested that reduced delivery of blood during hypotensive anesthesia to noncompressed muscles does not alter intracompartmental muscle pressures. A statistically significant decrease in the intracompartmental pressure of the downside extensor carpi radialis, but not in the long head of the triceps, was seen under hypotensive anesthesia. The critical closing pressure has been quoted as being 25 to 30 mm Hg[149, 150] for capillary blood flow and the downside intracompartmental pressures were higher than this level under both normotensive and hypotensive anesthesia.[149] Marked postanesthetic myositis, however, was not seen following normotensive anesthesia. This suggests that downside intracompartmental pressures alone are not useful indicators of the likely development of postanesthetic myositis.[151]

Usually the signs are seen in the limb that is down (compressed) when in lateral recumbency. In the forelimbs the triceps, deltoids, and occasionally the brachiocephalic and cranial pectoral muscles tend to be affected. In the hindlimbs, usually the biceps and vastus lateralis are affected. The flank muscles and masseter muscles may also be involved. Occasionally, however, the upper limb may be affected if its circulation is compromised.[151] One study investigated the effect of limb position on the cephalic venous pressure and the triceps compartmental pressure in the upper limb of anesthetized normotensive ponies.[151] It was found that when the upper limb was in the position often used to allow surgical access to the lower limb (i.e., leg parallel to the floor and pulled back with reasonable force), considerably higher venous pressures were recorded compared with the limb in the neutral position (i.e., leg raised so that it was parallel to the floor and at right angles to the spine). The intracompartmental pressures were only found to be significantly increased when the upper limb was flexed horizontally, hard forward (i.e., with the leg parallel to the floor, fully flexed at the carpus, and pushed forward with reasonable force), which is a potential alternative leg position allowing surgical access to the lower limb. This position also resulted in significantly higher venous pressures than the neutral limb position, which suggests that it would not be advisable for clinical use. This work suggested that impaired venous drainage may be a contributory factor in the development of postanesthetic myositis, at least with respect to the upper limb.[153] The position that appeared to provide adequate surgical access to the lower limb and yet had low compartmental and venous pressures was the flexed horizontal forward position (i.e., leg parallel to the floor, fully flexed at the carpus, and pushed gently forward).

When in dorsal recumbency it is the gluteal and occasionally the longissimus dorsi muscles that tend to be affected. Although in one study it was the adductor, pectineus, and gracilis muscles that were involved, this was attributed to arterial hypotension coupled with partial occlusion of the artery primarily supplying these muscles (the medial circumflex femoral artery) perhaps due to the hindlimbs being passively flexed.[152]

Clinical Signs

Clinical signs are normally seen during the initial recovery period but may occasionally be delayed for 1 hour or more. The condition may be first suspected if the recovery is prolonged or there are repeated unsuccessful attempts to stand. Signs attributable to damage to one muscle group, one peripheral nerve, or mixtures of muscle groups and peripheral nerve(s), may be seen. Affected muscle groups tend to be hot and may be swollen. Palpation is often resented and the animal is usually reluctant to bear weight on the affected limb. Signs of severe pain with sweating may be observed. Classically, with forelimb muscle involvement, the affected animal stands as if the radial nerve has been paralyzed, but it can use the extensor muscles. If the hindlimbs are involved, there may just be knuckling of the fetlock; if the quadriceps femoris is involved, the stifle and hock may buckle and the animal may not be able to rise, especially if both hindlimbs are involved. Signs may persist for several days, even in uncomplicated cases.

In some cases, isolated raised painful plaques may be the only abnormality seen or these may be found in combination with forelimb or hindlimb dysfunction. These swellings are usually found over the table contact hip, rib, or facial area and may be due to inadequate padding, trauma due to the positioning devices, or the weight of the patient.[149]

On occasion, after recovery from general anesthesia, a horse will demonstrate considerable discomfort with continued treading of the feet by sweating, holding its limbs (usually the hindlimbs) in abnormal positions, and kicking out. The syndromes appear nonresponsive to even large doses of opioid and other analgesics, and serum CK activities are not raised within the subsequent 48 to 96 hours and no myoglobinuria results. It is assumed that these syndromes are a form of paresthesia ("pins and needles") due to sensory neuropraxis, but there is a strong clinical similarity to the condition of postanesthetic neuromyopathy.

Generalized

Pathophysiology

The generalized form of postanesthetic myositis may occur during an operation when it may, at least in some instances, be caused by a condition similar to malignant hyperthermia in humans. Alternatively, signs may be seen during recovery, with many of the muscle groups affected being independent of positioning.

The cause is again uncertain, but it has also been suggested to be a result of local ischemia that becomes more generalized owing to hypotension, sensitivity of the muscle cells to anesthetic drugs, or depolarizing muscle relaxants (suxamethonium), or a combination of these. In the two studies that looked at the effect of hypotensive anesthesia, cases of generalized myositis occurred during recovery.[148, 149] In vitro examination of muscle using an adapted human contracture test (used for the identification of malignant hyperthermia susceptibility) has shown increased sensitivity to caffeine and halothane in samples taken from certain susceptible Equidae.[153]

Clinical Signs

The condition may occur at any time during anesthesia. The temperature, pulse, and respiratory rates increase and the muscles may fasciculate and contract. The horse may resist assisted ventilation and appear rigid. Death can occur.

Postoperative cases also tend to occur regardless of the length of the anesthesia and the positioning. Signs of extreme pain are seen and often the affected animal is unable to rise. The muscles may be rigid and excessive sweating usually occurs. Signs of colic with myoglobinuria may be present, as well as fluid disturbances.

Differentiation from postanesthetic myelopathy may need to be made. In this condition signs can range from difficulty in standing to paraplegia with flaccid paralysis and analgesia involving the pelvic limbs. In addition, loss of sensation and spinal reflexes over several contiguous segments may be found (see Chapter 9).

Both Forms

Laboratory Findings

Plasma and serum CK, AST, and LDH activities are usually raised in both forms. Raised plasma muscle enzyme activities may help differentiate those animals with overt muscular damage from those with conditions similar to paresthesia (possibly caused by a reduced blood supply to sensory nerve endings). Fluid and electrolyte disturbances may also be present. Hypocalcemia, hypomagnesemia, hyperphosphatemia, metabolic acidosis, hyperkalemia, and hyperglycemia have been reported. Myoglobinuria may occur, and renal function may be compromised.

Histology

Histologically, severely affected muscle shows loss of striation, swollen fibers, and a variation in fiber diameter. Fragmentation, target fibers, and signs of supercontracture may also be found.

Treatment

The aim of any treatment regimen is to relieve pain, prevent further damage, correct fluid and electrolyte disturbances, and maintain renal function. The treatment usually given is similar to that given for ERS (discussed later), although if a metabolic acidosis is present, intravenous sodium bicarbonate administration may be required. If the condition occurs during an operation, the anesthetic should, whenever possible, be stopped or alternative intravenous agents used. The horse should be rapidly cooled and intravenous fluids plus analgesics should be given as required. Initial fluid infusion

rates of up to 10 to 20 ml/kg/hour have been recommended, slowing to 4 to 5 ml/kg/hour. Analgesics that have been used include the NSAIDs and the opioids. Diazepam and glyceryl guaiacolate to help reduce muscle spasm may be of value but should be used with caution due to possible induced ataxia, and therefore increased problems with standing. Sedation may also be required in certain cases. The alpha-2 agonists (xylazine/detomidine/romifidine) may help provide good sedation and muscle relaxation but may exacerbate any ataxia, and by promoting sweating, hypoinsulinemia, and hyperglycemia, together with an increased urine output, may further exacerbate fluid loss. These agents' vasoconstrictive effect together with their effect on cardiac output may further compromise tissue blood flow. Their use in the more violent cases may be necessary although they should still be used with caution and, if appropriate, with concurrent opioids. Acetylpromazine in combination with opioids may provide good sedation with minimal ataxia, and the vasodilatory effect may help improve tissue flow (providing circulatory volume is maintained and hypovolemia does not occur).

Intravenous and then oral dantrolene sodium has been suggested to be of benefit.[154] Dantrolene of 1 mg/kg body weight PO has been reported to successfully treat postoperative cases. Recent work on the pharmacokinetics of dantrolene[153] has, however, suggested that higher doses are likely to be needed to establish and maintain effective blood levels (based on human efficacy studies), that is, an intragastric dose of 2.5 mg/kg every hour after a loading dose of 10 mg/kg.[154] Alternatively, an intravenous loading dose of 1.9 mg/kg has been suggested to achieve a more immediate therapeutic effect.[153] Dantrolene is not licensed for use in horses, is expensive, and is potentially hepatotoxic. Transient weakness and ataxia have been associated with intravenous administration. Care should therefore be taken with its use until more information is available on its efficacy, the actual blood levels required in the horse, the dose required to reach such levels, and the possible side effects of such doses.

Prevention

Correct positioning to prevent restriction of venous drainage or arterial input and the use of appropriate padding are recommended. Foam padding, for example, has been reported to be inferior to air mattresses or waterbeds.[150] Positioning is very important and various recommendations have been made: for example, the upper limb should be elevated and pressure on the lower triceps reduced by pulling the leg forward.[144] In lateral recumbency the hind legs should be kept parallel or above parallel to the table and sufficiently separated to promote venous drainage. In dorsally recumbent horses, rather than letting the hindlimbs position themselves passively, they should be supported in slight extension by a hoist. Problems with hindlimb adductor myopathies do not always develop with passive positioning. Pulling back of the hind limbs should be avoided. If the hind limbs are required to be drawn back in full extension, for example for certain arthroscopic examinations, the surgical time should be kept to a minimum to reduce the risk of quadriceps myopathy. The flexed horizontal forward position, that is, with the uppermost (noncompressed forelimb) parallel to the floor, fully flexed at the carpus, and pushed gently forward, would appear to be preferable when carrying out surgery that needs access to the medial aspect of the lower carpus and distal radius.[151]

Some suggest withholding grain feed for 48 to 72 hours prior to the anesthetic. It has been the clinical impression of a number of people that heavily muscled and fitter horses are at an increased risk, in particular those presenting with athletic-induced sports injuries. These impressions have not been supported by the clinical studies to date.

Blood pressure should be maintained at more than 80 mm Hg (mean arterial blood pressure) to maintain muscle perfusion. The amount of halothane used should be kept to a minimum. Intraoperative fluids and inotropes may be valuable.

Prophylactic dantrolene has been recommended, especially if there is a history of similar problems. Various doses have been used. For example, in the United Kingdom intragastric administration at 2 to 4 mg/kg has been recommended, whereas higher doses (10 mg/kg) have been used in the United States.[154] Little work, however, has been carried out on the efficacy of such measures, partly because it is difficult to predict which animals will be affected by this condition.

Prognosis

The prognosis will depend partially on the extent of the muscle damage and the treatment instituted as well as the temperament of the individual in certain cases. Affected animals often recover completely, especially if the condition is localized to one muscle group. Occasionally, the animal may be left with residual muscle atrophy, fibrosis, and scarring. Death can occur with massive areas of ischemic myonecrosis and intrafascicular nerve fiber degeneration post mortem. Euthanasia may be required on humane grounds. Further discussion of the pathophysiology, treatment, and prevention of anesthetic myoneuropathy is available in the literature.[63, 67, 117, 118, 152–154]

Aortic-Iliac Thrombosis
Pathophysiology

The cause of this syndrome is still disputed.[155, 156] The theory commonly given is that the thrombi result from damage to the intima by migrating *Strongylus vulgaris* larvae. Signs of verminous arteritis in the affected vessels (such as larvae, eosinophils, other inflammatory cells) have not, however, been reported,[156] and the larvae do not tend to migrate as far caudally as the thrombi are found. Also, the condition is apparently more common in racehorses, which tend to be kept under a high standard of management, including a regular worming regimen. However, in horses not asked to perform maximally, the condition may not be clinically apparent and, therefore, underdiagnosed. An alternative suggestion is that *S. vulgaris* larvae could be an indirect cause of the condition via the formation of thromboemboli, which become organized and result in arterial occlusion and further thrombosis.[155, 156] Hormonal, nutritional, and mechanical factors, as well as prior infections with strangles or influenza,

have been proposed as predisposing factors to thrombus formation.[156–158]

The internal iliac arteries are more closely bound to fascia than many other arteries. This, coupled with the large forces generated during movement that act on this region, could increase the risk of injury to these vessels. In affected animals intimal plaques ascribed to intimal *S. vulgaris* migrations have been reported in various branches of the abdominal aorta. However, similar thickenings in brachial, carotid, and cerebral arteries (sites in which strongylus migrations are unlikely) have been reported in both control and affected horses.[156] Repair of spontaneous damage occurring to the arterial endothelium at areas of turbulence or arterial branching may, for example, result in plaque formation and eventually a thrombus. It has been postulated, therefore, that aortic-iliac thrombosis is similar to the human condition arteriosclerosis obliterans, a form of arteriosclerosis causing intermittent claudication.[156] Individual variation in the aortic quadrification or vascular repair mechanisms could explain why certain animals are predisposed to the development of this condition.

Clinical Signs

In affected animals, following exercise, ischemia of the muscle usually occurs due to circulatory interference. This is usually reversible, as the blood flow may be adequate when at rest or at light work. The clinical signs vary in severity according to the degree of vascular occlusion, the vessels affected, and the extent of collateral circulation. The lameness tends to become more severe as exercise continues. Very mild cases may, however, be missed as they appear normal when the horse is pulled up after a disappointing performance. Poor performance, intermittent hindlimb lameness, transient lameness or weakness with exercise, a tendency to drag the toe and occasionally to knuckle over, gradual shortening of the stride leading to a transient inability to move, have all been reported in clinical histories of affected animals. A peracute condition with paraplegia, shock, and death has also been recognized.

Both hindlimbs may be affected, although usually one more than the other. Post exercise, the superficial veins on the more affected limb may appear relatively collapsed (due to delayed filling) compared with the distended vessels on the more "normal" limb. It may take up to 90 seconds for the superficial veins of the affected limb(s) to fill after intense exercise compared with about 10 seconds in normal horses. The affected limb often feels cooler than expected, especially around the gaskin, and may not sweat. A reduced digital pulse may be felt. The animal may sweat profusely on the body, head, and neck and sometimes will cow-kick or shake the affected limb (perhaps because of paraesthesias following reduced blood supply to sensory nerve endings). Within 20 to 30 minutes full recovery tends to have occurred.

On palpation of the peripheral pulses *at rest,* abnormalities may be detected, including a flattened, weak, and prolonged contour to the pulse distal to the site of obstruction, while proximally the pulse may be normal or increased in strength. Alternatively, certain pulses may be absent.

The condition has been reported in both males and females, although a greater incidence of clinical problems has been reported in the male. One of the reasons for this difference in incidence may be a more efficient collateral circulation in females.[156] The mean age of affected animals was 5.2 years in one study.[156]

Laboratory Findings

Plasma and serum muscle enzyme activities are usually within normal range both before and after exercise. In severe cases with marked muscle damage, however, increases in CK have been reported.[156]

Postmortem and Histologic Findings

On postmortem examination the affected vessels tend to be enlarged and a large thrombotic mass is usually present at the aortic quadrification (Fig. 8–5). This may be attached to, and therefore possibly originate from, organized masses in the internal and external iliac arteries. These may extend to the popliteal artery's bifurcation, but rarely do they extend far into the tibial arteries or the muscular branches of the femoral artery.

Histologically, the affected muscles show signs of ischemia. Damaged fibers and supporting structures tend to be removed with little sign of inflammation or fibrosis.[155]

Diagnosis

Diagnosis is established from the clinical signs and either palpation of the thrombus per rectum or ultrasonic demonstration of the thrombus. In affected animals rectal examination often reveals no abnormality, with signs such as a decreased arterial pulse or an unusual firmness of a vessel being easily missed. It is also possible for the obstruction to be fairly peripheral, which may in fact result in an increase in the pulse proximally. Ultrasonography is therefore the definitive method for diagnosis. A linear array ultrasound probe with a frequency of 5.0 or 7.5 MHz has been recommended.[159, 160]

The differential diagnosis includes ERS, cervical vertebral

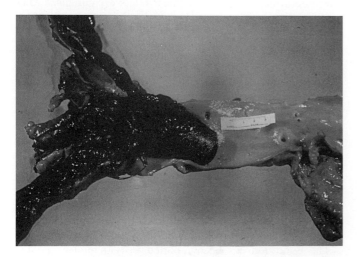

Figure 8–5. Aortic-iliac thrombosis.

malformation, and degenerative joint disease of the tarso-metatarsal joints. Perineural and intra-articular anesthesia will help to eliminate lameness originating from the distal limb.

Treatment

Treatment for aortic-iliac thrombosis is directed toward either elimination of the thrombus or development of collateral circulation. At present, an effective drug, selectively able to break down mature thrombi, is not available, and surgical intervention in the horse is precluded.

Sodium gluconate 450 mg/kg body weight by slow IV infusion has been recommended,[161] but there has been no evidence to show that sodium gluconate has any effect on a mature thrombus.[156] Giving prednisolone sodium succinate 100 mg 30 minutes prior to the sodium gluconate may help to eliminate the systemic reactions frequently associated with this drug.[155, 156] Other suggested protocols include monthly administration of ivermectin (Eqvalan MSD-AGVET) and twice-daily doses of oral phenylbutazone at 2.2 mg/kg body weight for 3 months.[159] Any improvement in such cases may in fact be due to the development of an effective collateral circulation.

Prognosis

The prognosis for horses severely affected with this condition is poor and a hereditary predisposition has been suggested,[155] although there is little supporting evidence.

GENETIC DISORDERS
Myotonia
Pathophysiology

In humans, several myotonic myopathies are recognized.[162, 163] Myotonia is seen clinically as the "delayed relaxation of skeletal muscle after a voluntary contraction or a contraction induced by an electrical or mechanical stimulus."[164] The defect is thought to be at the level of the sarcolemma or transverse tubular system because neuromuscular blockade does not eliminate myotonic contractions. However, this does not rule out the possibility of involvement of neural elements of the motor unit in certain forms of the clinical condition.[165]

During repetitive muscle stimulation there is a tendency for a decrease in the resting potential to occur, due to a buildup of potassium ions in the T tubules. The persistent afterdepolarization so produced could be adequate to open the surface sodium conductance channels and initiate a new action potential. If the sarcolemma generates multiple uncontrolled action potentials in response to a normal stimulus at the neuromuscular junction, a substantial contraction will result. Normally this does not occur because of the high permeability of the T-tubule membrane to chloride; as the membrane becomes positive the Cl^- ions move out, speeding up repolarization. In humans and the goat some forms of myotonia (myotonia congenita) are associated with a reduced transmembrane chloride conductance.[163, 164]

In the horse no membrane chloride defect has been found

in those animals tested, but at least one form of the condition, like that in humans, persists in the face of neuromuscular blockade.[166, 167] Prolonged in vitro muscle relaxation times have been found by one group of workers in affected horses.[168] These in vitro findings were apparently normalized by the administration of phenytoin. The authors suggested that this action may be related to phenytoin's sodium channel blocking effect and possibly a calcium channel blocking action.

It is probably advisable, at the present time, not to try and classify the equine myotonic conditions according to human definitions. Most of those cases examined to date appear to have some of the features of more than one human type, rather than fitting neatly into any one human category. However, three cases have recently been reported of a severe, progressive neuromuscular disorder that more closely resembles myotonic dystrophy in humans.[168a]

Clinical Signs

Stiffness of gait with prolonged contraction of the affected muscle seen following local mechanical (finger flick) stimulation are the hallmarks of clinical myotonia (Fig. 8–6). There may be at least three forms of myotonia found in the horse.[118, 165, 168] The first is characterized by the presence of myotonic discharges on EMG but no overt primary muscular problems. This has been seen in quarter horses used for general purposes and does not appear to be progressive.

The second form is characterized by the early onset of a progressive deterioration in muscle function. Signs are usually seen in the first 6 months of life. Initially, lameness associated with stiffness and hypertrophy of the affected muscles may be seen. The lack of fluid, smooth movement is most pronounced after rest and diminishes with exercise. In the majority of cases the abnormality is confined to the hindquarters, and the head, neck, and forelimbs may appear unaffected, although all four limbs may be involved.[169] No other body systems seem to be involved. In many cases the animals progressively become weaker and may have difficulty getting up in the later stages, although the clinical course may vary. It has been suggested, based on the clinical, electrophysiologic, and pathologic findings,[165] that animals suffering from this form most resemble the human myotonia congenita or undefined myotonia.[168a]

A third, severe, and progressive form has recently been reported in young horses in which signs may be apparent as early as 1 month of age. This form appears to be characterized initially by generalized myotonia with hypertonicity of the larger proximal limb muscles, which progresses fairly rapidly to muscle stiffness, atrophy, and weakness.[168a] In one of the cases, testicular hypoplasia, early cataract formation, and mild glucose intolerance were also found, suggesting multisystemic involvement. This myotonic dystrophy-like form appears to be associated with specific histologic changes.[168a]

Laboratory Findings

CK and AST activities may be elevated, but these increases are often not sustained throughout the course of the disease and tend to be unpredictable.

Histology

Not all muscles that exhibit the classic myotonic discharges (see Diagnosis) show histologic changes. Fiber size variation, changes in number and size of the individual fiber types, increased numbers of central nuclei, and clustering together of fiber types with signs of necrosis and degeneration have been reported.[5, 165, 165, 170] Differences in the histologic findings may reflect different forms of the condition.[165]

Diagnosis

The diagnosis is based on the clinical signs and the classic waning ("dive-bomber") or waxing and waning ("revving motorcycle") sounds of the EMG trains of high-frequency discharges (Fig. 8–7). These are seen on insertion of the electrode and on voluntary, mechanical, or chemical stimulation of the affected muscle. Following percussion or stimulation, positive sharp waves and fibrillation potentials may be seen. These abnormal discharges ultimately subside when the muscle has been at *complete* rest for some time, although they can be initiated readily after the patient is given neuromuscular blockade (e.g., curarization).

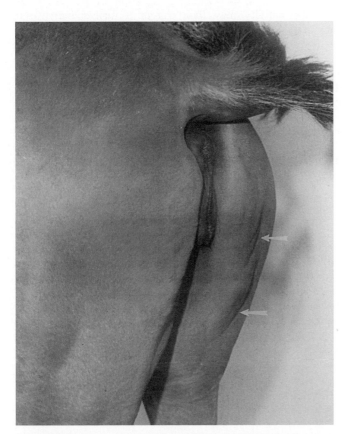

Figure 8–6. Prominent muscle groups of the hindquarters and a knot of sustained muscular contraction following mechanical stimulation in a foal suffering from clinical myotonia.

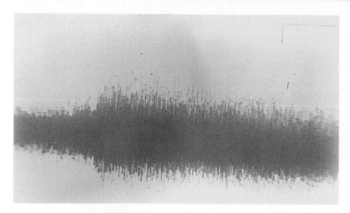

Figure 8–7. Prolonged myotonic discharges present on needle electromyographic examination. These high-frequency discharges sound very much like a revving motorcycle but there was no true waxing and waning. Instead, the amplitude and frequency of the discharges change suddenly (as shown), altering the tone heard. These discharges are not abolished with either suxamethonium or tubocurarine under general anesthesia.

Treatment

In humans, many drugs have been used, in particular quinine, procainamide, taurine, and phenytoin (diphenylhydantoin). Most of these decrease muscle excitability by blocking sodium movement, although they do not increase the chloride fluxes.[171] In humans the duration of the EMG relaxation time after maximum voluntary effort has been shown to be the only reliable indicator of muscle excitation and response to therapy.[163] This is impractical in the horse.

Various drugs have been used in the horse, including acepromazine, xylazine, thiopentone, pancuronium bromide, quinidine, and phenytoin, but no significant improvement has been reported.[172, 173] Prolonged in vitro times to 90% muscle relaxation were found in two cases of myotonia[168]; these were apparently normalized by the administration of phenytoin to the affected animals. However, no obvious clinical improvement or significant effect on EMG was noted with the relatively short duration of therapy.[168] The long-term effects of phenytoin on the clinical signs or progressive nature of the condition is not yet known.

Prognosis

The prognosis is poor for those suffering from the progressive type of myotonia, although mildly affected animals may improve as they get older.

Inheritance

In humans, apart from chondrodystrophic myotonia, the conditions are primarily autosomal dominant. This is also true in the goat. A familial tendency has been reported in dogs, but in horses too few animals have been investigated to arrive at any conclusion.

Hyperkalemic Periodic Paralysis

Pathophysiology

In humans three types of periodic paralysis are recognized—hypokalemic, hyperkalemic, and normokalemic. These are believed to be caused by an abnormality in membrane permeability or a defective cation pump, which results in an altered electrochemical gradient across the sarcolemma. This in turn results in a change in the resting membrane potential and the threshold potential, which means that the muscle fiber will be more, or less, excitable.[5]

Hyperkalemic periodic paralysis (HYPP) in humans has been extensively studied and shown to be inherited as an autosomal dominant trait, as has paramyotonia congenita. HYPP is characterized by intermittent attacks of weakness or paralysis, which can be variably precipitated by a number of factors including potassium intake, fasting, cold, and rest after exercise. Paramyotonia congenita typically presents as a cold-induced myotonia. Both conditions have been linked to the human adult skeletal muscle sodium gene on chromosome 17q. The genetic mutation responsible for HYPP in humans affects a gene at the SCN4A locus that encodes the alpha subunit of the adult human skeletal muscle voltage-dependent sodium channel.[173a] In sufferers there is believed to be an increase in membrane sodium conductance due to a defective subpopulation of the voltage-dependent sodium channels failing to inactivate and remaining open or repeatedly opening. A small rise in the serum potassium concentration due to clinical variation, ingestion of potassium, or muscular activity may then trigger a further increase in membrane sodium conductance, depolarization of the muscle membrane, and movement of potassium out of the muscle. As the membrane depolarization develops the membrane may become hyperexcitable and show myotonic behavior. Then, with further depolarization of the muscle, it may become unexcitable and paralysis may occur.[171, 173a]

The plasma potassium concentrations of normal horses undergoing intensive exercise can reach the levels recorded during an episode of this condition without any of the associated clinical signs.[101] This suggests that the elevated potassium alone is not responsible for the clinical signs.

Clinical Signs

In the horse the condition is currently believed to be present only in pure or part-bred quarter horses, paints, Appaloosas, and other horses carrying bloodlines that trace back to the sire Impressive. The animals tend to be very well muscled. Between episodes, the majority (see below) appear to be clinically normal and can be highly successful show horses, although one affected stallion seemed to show pelvic limb weakness.[174] Prolapse of the membrana nictitans may be the initial sign with or without facial muscle spasm and generalized muscle tension. Sustained contraction of the muscles of the muzzle and drooling may be seen. Heart rate and respiratory rate are often normal or only slightly elevated. Whole body sweating has often been reported. Muscle fasciculations tend to be a common sign and are usually prominent in the shoulders, flanks, and neck area. Myotonia may be clinically apparent.[114, 174, 175] Although the horse may remain standing, it may not be able to lift its head and may show intermittent buckling at the knees and hocks. In mild cases, however, the only signs observed may be mild muscle fasciculations or twitching similar to signs seen with shivering. Recumbency may occur in some cases with diminished tendon reflexes, although the animals tend to remain conscious and alert. The duration of episodes is usually short (20 minutes to 4 hours, typically 30 minutes to 1 hour). Death can occur during an episode, usually from cardiac arrest and/or respiratory failure.

Some horses have been reported to have altered vocalization and audible respiratory stridor, which may indicate laryngeal spasm or paralysis. In a survey of 69 homozygous horses over 90% were reported to suffer some degree of abnormal airway noise, often between episodes.[175a] This tended to be an inspiratory stridor and was continuous in 21% of those evaluated. Exercise, excitement, and stress were possible triggering factors. Twenty-four animals had been scoped and 9 had pharyngeal collapse, 10 had laryngeal spasm, 9 had pharyngeal edema, and 6 manifested a displaced soft palate. Clinically, homozygously affected animals tend to show exercise intolerance, whereas heterozygous animals may tolerate exercise well.[175a]

In affected animals, clinical episodes have usually been seen before they reach 3 years of age.[175b] However, there appears to be a wide variation in the clinical expression of the condition, with some affected animals showing either very mild or apparently no clinical signs. It has been suggested that the variability in clinical signs may occur due to a higher expression of mutant channels in the muscle of horses with symptoms than those that are asymptomatic. The homozygous animals tend to have the most severe clinical signs. Muscle fiber diameter or fiber type is not believed to be related to clinical expression, and overall it has been suggested that management factors may have the major influence.[175a]

Laboratory Findings

Between episodes serum potassium is normally within acceptable limits, but can be elevated. During an attack serum potassium is raised (5.0–11.7 mmol/L),[176] although episodes in affected animals without associated hyperkalemia have been reported both with "natural" as well as KCl-induced episodes.[176a, 176b] Therefore, the absence of hyperkalemia does not necessarily preclude a diagnosis of HYPP. Sodium and calcium concentrations may be decreased. Hemoconcentration may be seen. Serum CK and AST activities may be normal or mildly increased.[118, 174, 175] Recovery from an episode is associated with a decrease in serum potassium.

Histology

In humans periodic paralysis conditions are sometimes referred to as vacuolar myopathies. The vacuoles, visible on light microscopy, have been suggested to arise from the coalescence of dilated components of sarcoplasmic reticulum or from fusion of T-system networks or focal fiber destruction.[177]

In the horse no abnormalities were found on light microscopy in one case.[175] In another study of eight horses, either no abnormalities were seen or mild intracellular vacuolation

of the type IIB fibers with occasional degenerative changes were found.[176]

Electromyography

An EMG should be carried out to determine if there is concurrent myotonia. Numerous abnormalities, even between episodes, have been reported,[176, 176a, 176b] including increased insertional activity and spontaneous activity. Complex repetitive discharges have been reported to be the most consistent finding, although myotonic potentials, fibrillation potentials, and positive sharp waves can occur. Interestingly, the amount of abnormal spontaneous EMG activity can fluctuate substantially on repeated examinations.

EMG findings of spontaneous activity and high-frequency myotonic or pseudomyotonic discharges were found to be as reliable as KCl challenge testing in detecting HYPP-positive horses in one study and could be carried out more quickly and safely. The sensitivity and specificity of EMG findings were suggested to be around 90% in this study, although it was suggested that a combination of the KCl challenge and EMG testing might be advantageous.[175b]

Muscle Characteristics

Affected animals have been said to have a lower intracellular potassium concentration and a higher intracellular water volume than normal horses, although few details are available.[176] Using whole-fiber intercostal muscle biopsies, the mean resting membrane potentials of five affected horses were found to be significantly closer to the threshold potential when compared with unaffected animals.[176] It was concluded that this may indicate a defect in membrane transport.

Diagnosis

In affected humans 2 to 10 g of potassium chloride given just after exercise when in the fasted state will provoke episodes. In the horse a test dose of 88 to 160 mg/kg potassium chloride can be given as an isotonic solution in water, via a stomach tube, after a 12-hour fast to induce an attack and determine serum potassium concentrations. Much larger doses given to normal animals have no clinical effects and there is less increase in serum potassium (mean peak concentration of 5.97 mmol/L).[174] Such a test should not be carried out without a thorough physical examination and laboratory testing to rule out conditions such as cardiac disease, renal disease, and impaired adrenocortical function. It is advisable when undertaking this test to have the drugs at hand that may help abort an attack (see Treatment). However, it has been reported that KCl challenge testing using doses up to 0.16 g/kg body weight can give false negative results and up to 0.2 g/kg may be needed, especially in the older horse,[175b] but the risk of potential problems increases with the higher doses.

The differential diagnosis includes other causes of collapse, including syncope, narcolepsy or cataplexy, and seizures, as well as other electrolyte disorders, neurologic dysfunction, and vitamin E/selenium–responsive myopathy.[118]

A DNA blood test has been developed and is currently available to identify horses that are heterozygous or homozygous for HYPP. Approximately 29,000 horses had been tested by the end of 1995. Of these, 64% were found to be normal, 35% heterozygous, 1% homozygous (S. Spier, personal communication, 1995). False positives apparently have not yet been identified, although some positive animals, as discussed earlier, have not shown clinical signs although they have responded positively to KCl challenge or show typical changes on electromyography. A test that would predict at an early age which animals are prone to suffer significant clinical episodes would obviously be of value.

Treatment

For mild cases (i.e., nonrecumbent but with muscle fasciculations) it has been suggested that the horse be lightly exercised, although caution is advised, since falling over is a potential risk. Feeding a readily absorbable source of carbohydrate (oats are commonly recommended or light Karo syrup for glucose supplement) to promote insulin-induced reuptake of potassium has also been suggested in addition to giving acetazolamide by mouth (3 mg/kg). Such procedures are often "routinely" undertaken by responsible and experienced owners of affected animals.

During more severe or induced episodes, especially when recumbency occurs, 5% dextrose with sodium bicarbonate (with or without insulin) has been used to try to decrease serum potassium. Intravenous calcium has also been reported to be of benefit, both in humans and horses.[174, 175, 177] Treatment with slow IV administration of 23% calcium gluconate 0.2 to 0.4 mL/kg diluted in 1 to 2 L of 5% dextrose; 5% dextrose 4.4 to 6.6 mL/kg; or bicarbonate 1 to 2 mEq/kg have been recommended.[176] If required, potassium-free isotonic fluids are used.

Glucocorticoids may be contraindicated in susceptible horses because they have been shown to induce episodes in humans.[174] The inhalation of β-adrenergic agents has aborted acute attacks in humans, but the use of such drugs has not been reported in the horse.[177, 178]

Prognosis

In humans the prognosis is fairly good, although a permanent myopathy and weakness may occur. This also seems to be the case in the horse, although in at least one case the condition progressed, necessitating euthanasia.[174] In a recent report it was suggested that "the chances of a paralytic episode occurring while the horse is being ridden appear unlikely. However, because episodes of paralysis are unpredictable, we recommend that only persons experienced with the symptomatology handle and ride affected horses and to use caution if any abnormal clinical signs are observed."[175a]

Inheritance

Initial studies with an affected stallion and mare produced three offspring by embryo transfer. All three had suffered at least one episode associated with hyperkalemia by 2 months of age. Further studies by these investigators confirmed that the mode of inheritance was the same in horses as in humans.[176] It has since been confirmed that the condition is inherited as an autosomal dominant trait.[178a] Linkage analysis

shows complete segregation. Gene frequency has been reported in one study to be 0.02.[175a] Recently it has been shown that a single amino acid substitution (Phe to Leu) in the gene controlling the equine sodium channel was responsible for the condition.[178a, 178b]

Prevention

In man, preventive therapy consists of frequent meals with a high carbohydrate content, avoidance of fasting or of exposure to cold or overexertion, and the use of diuretics such as acetazolamide or chlorthiazide, which promote kaliuresis.

Small doses of albuterol, a β-adrenergic agent, have also been recommended in humans.[178] This compound is believed to work by stimulating the Na^+, K^+-pumps, thus enhancing potassium transport across the muscle cell membrane. Tocainide, a frequency-dependent antiarrhythmic drug, may prevent the weakness caused by the myotonia.[177]

In the horse, acetazolamide has been used with apparent success, 3.85 mg/kg given PO q.i.d. for 3 days, then 2.2 mg/kg PO b.i.d. for maintenance.[174, 176] Hydrochlorothiazide 250 mg b.i.d. was used in another case, again with apparent success, although in addition no alfalfa hay was fed.[175] Other recommendations include feeding oat or timothy hay rather than alfalfa, which helps to decrease total potassium intake. Feeding grain twice a day, providing access to salt, and regular mild exercise may also be beneficial. A regular feeding and exercise schedule should be established. Rapid changes in diet, fasting, or water deprivation should be avoided. Turnout to pasture or into a paddock can be beneficial.

NUTRITIONAL DISORDERS

Nutritionally Associated Myodegeneration: Vitamin E and Selenium

Pathophysiology

The selenium-containing enzyme glutathione peroxidase (GSHPx), together with vitamin E, helps to protect cells against free radicals,[179] which are formed by the reduction of molecular oxygen and during normal oxidative processes, for example,

$$O_2 \xrightarrow{\text{enzyme}} O_2^- \text{ (superoxide)}$$

A free radical (or reactive oxygen species [ROS]) is any chemical substance that has an unpaired electron in its outer orbital. The presence of this electron makes the free radical inherently unstable. Superoxide radicals, for example, in solution form hydrogen peroxide by dismutation:

$$2O_2^- + 2H^+ \xrightarrow{\text{(superoxide dismutase)}} H_2O_2 + O_2$$

The superoxide radical can also react with hydrogen peroxide and hydrogen ions to produce the very potent hydroxyl radical (HO·).

$$H^+ + O_2^- + H_2O_2 \longrightarrow O_2 + H_2O + HO·$$

The hydroxyl radicals in turn can react with almost any organic molecule to produce other organic radicals via chain reactions.

Free radical reactions are responsible for a number of key biochemical events, including mitochondrial electron transport, prostaglandin synthesis, phagocytosis, degradation of catecholamines, etc. Under controlled circumstances they are therefore necessary for life, but when uncontrolled they may result in a number of degenerative disease processes because they can cause the irreversible denaturation of essential cellular proteins. The exposed polyunsaturated fatty acids, for example, within the phospholipid structure of the membrane can be attacked (lipid peroxidation), resulting in structural damage and the formation of further hydroperoxides. The cellular membrane damage in turn may result in the release of liposomal enzymes and further damage. The free radicals can also cause damage to hyaluronic acid and collagen and result in enhanced prostaglandin production. They can also uncouple oxidative phosphorylation and inactivate certain enzymes. A system of natural antioxidant defenses is present within the body to counteract such free radical–induced damage, including glutathione peroxidase and vitamin E. GSHPx acts to reduce the production of hydroxyl radicals by reducing hydroperoxides to alcohols as part of a cyclic system re-forming glutathione. Within the RBCs the enzyme acts as an integral part of the system protecting against the conversion of hemoglobin to methemoglobin by hydroperoxides. Vitamin E acts as a scavenger of free radicals. Vitamin C may assist by reducing the tocopheroxyl radicals formed by this scavenging. In addition, vitamin E helps to block lipid peroxidation and may also form an important part of the membrane structure due to its interaction with membrane phospholipids. Other naturally occurring antioxidant defenses include chelators that bind to and decrease the concentrations of transition metals (e.g., iron).

Vitamin E and selenium deficiencies have been implicated in muscular problems in several species, especially sheep and pigs.[115, 180] In the horse, a myopathy attributed to vitamin E and selenium deficiency has been reported in foals from birth to 9 months of age.[181] This is often referred to as white muscle disease. In older animals, maxillary myositis, polymyositis, and dystrophic myodegeneration have also been attributed to such a deficiency.[182] However, there is some controversy over the role of vitamin E and selenium in such conditions. In foals, the syndrome has apparently been well documented in geographic areas of known selenium deficiency and inadequate vitamin E intake,[173]although it has been noted that many foals raised in such areas may have decreased GSHPx activities and low blood selenium concentrations without being affected.[183]

Free Radicals, Vitamin E, and Muscle Damage

Two common sources of free radicals during exercise are increased activity of xanthine oxidase during anaerobic degradation of purine nucleotides and the partial reduction of oxygen during oxidative phosphorylation within the mitochondria. The precise mechanisms leading to muscle damage and fatigue during exercise are uncertain although it is possible that free radicals or ROS may play an important role. Following strenuous exercise, free radical production may exceed the capacity of the cell's natural defense mechanisms, leading to muscular damage.

For many years it has been appreciated that the human genetic muscular dystrophies share many characteristics with the vitamin E and selenium deficiency myopathies in animals, although treatment of patients with vitamin E has not so far been shown to be of benefit. However, with increased speculation that free radical–mediated damage may be a factor in the etiology of the processes involved, a wide range of techniques has been developed to evaluate them, but to date no single method has been developed as the optimal way to study free radical processes. Perhaps because of the various techniques used and differing criteria used for the choice of patients, few consistent abnormalities have been reported, especially with respect to the measurement of antioxidant levels in blood or tissue.[184] The glutathione redox ratio has been suggested to be one of the most sensitive indices of oxidative stress, although inconsistent reports of the effects of exercise on the glutathione system in humans have been reported, perhaps due to the varying fitness of the subjects and differences in the exercise intensity used.[184a] A recent study in the horse has suggested that exercise can induce changes in biochemical parameters (including the glutathione redox ratio) that are indicative of oxidative stress in the fit horse and this is exacerbated during exercise at high temperatures and humidity.[184a]

Vitamin E has, however, been shown to have an apparent protective effect on experimental damage to rat skeletal muscle. Recent work has suggested that it may be acting via a non-antioxidant mechanism with the hydrocarbon chain being the important mediator of the effects seen.[185] There has been shown to be an apparent protective effect of supranormal extracellular vitamin E concentrations on normal rat muscle, and exacerbation of exercise-induced damage to skeletal muscle by vitamin E deficiency has been reported. It has therefore been suggested that nutritional modification of skeletal muscle, perhaps by reduction of the unsaturation of skeletal muscle membranes or enhancement of the antioxidant status of muscles, or a combination of both, may help to prevent or reduce calcium-induced skeletal muscle damage.[40] Artificial methods to reduce oxidant damage during exercise include the administration of exogenous sources of naturally occurring antioxidant defenses (e.g., vitamin E) and limiting the formation of free radicals by minimizing the formation of inosine monophosphate (IMP) from purine degradation during exercises. (See also Pathological Changes. General Response of Muscle to Injury.)

Type I and type IIA fibers are the fibers most likely to result in excess free radical formation, since they are the most oxidative fibers as well as the ones that contain the most intracellular lipid stores. Selective type I fiber degeneration is found in vitamin E/selenium–responsive nutritional myopathies of sheep and pigs.[38]

Foals affected by this condition have been shown to have a significantly higher proportion of type IIC fibers and lower proportions of type I and type IIA fibers than healthy foals of comparable age.[186] It was suggested that these type IIC fibers include both the undifferentiated fibers normally seen in foals and a proportion of previous type I and type IIA fibers, which appear as type IIC owing to degenerative or regenerative processes. Some differences in the pathologic processes do, however, appear to exist between the equine vitamin E/selenium deficiency–associated conditions and those in other species. Vitamin E deficiencies in calves and chicks show mitochondrial alterations very early on in the condition. In vitamin E/selenium–deficient lambs and chickens, the earliest changes are seen in small vessels, connective tissue, and neuromuscular elements. In the horse the changes appear to affect the myofibrils first. Morphologic changes in mitochondria and the sarcoplasmic reticulum seem only to be seen in fibers with advanced lesions.[186, 187]

Factors that may predispose to a vitamin E and selenium deficiency have been suggested to include rancid feed, the addition of fish or plant oil to the feed, prolonged storage of grain (e.g., dry grain loses tocopherol activities far more slowly than moist grain), poor-quality hay, and lush pastures.[117] Pastures associated with acid, poorly aerated soils, soils with a high sulfur content, or volcanic rock are more likely to be selenium-deficient. Cases are more likely to be seen in areas with low (<0.05 ppm) plant selenium content. Dietary levels of selenium may, however, be misleading, not only because other factors are likely to be involved in the pathogenesis of the condition but also because the biological availability of the various "types" of selenium have not been determined. In addition, high, but nontoxic, levels of copper, silver, tellurium, and zinc could possibly interfere with selenium availability and therefore induce typical lesions in animals on diets containing amounts of selenium usually considered to be adequate.

It is probable that other factors such as "stress" (including managemental regimens and environment), as well as increased physical activity, may be important for clinical signs to become apparent in the face of a deficiency. This may explain why two similar groups of animals receiving the same dietary intake can show different clinical responses to the amounts of vitamin E and selenium present. Acute selenium toxicity in the adult horse may also be associated with myodegeneration plus pulmonary edema, gastroenteritis, hepatic degeneration, and necrosis.[187, 188]

Name

This nutritionally associated condition is often described in the literature as a muscular dystrophy. *Muscular dystrophy* is defined in human medicine as a group of progressive genetically determined primary myopathies. They are usually not present at birth and the neural and vascular components are not initially involved. Regeneration of muscle cells is absent or inadequate and there is replacement of muscle cells with fat and fibrous tissue. This differs from the nutritionally associated disease in horses, which should not, therefore, be called a muscular dystrophy.

Clinical Signs

These vary, depending on the distribution of the muscular lesions and the extent of the damage. Signs are most commonly seen in animals under 2 months of age and can occur peracutely and progress rapidly. Death may occur immediately, possibly from a fatal arrhythmia, or after a few hours from exhaustion and circulatory collapse. The

myocardium, diaphragm, and respiratory muscles are usually involved, leading to heart failure, dyspnea, and pulmonary edema. Occasionally, painful subcutaneous swellings may be found, in particular over the rump, ventral abdominal wall, and nuchal crest. These are more common in older foals. In older animals sudden postexercise recumbency may occur with death within a few hours caused by pulmonary edema and myocardial failure.[118]

In less acute cases, weakness is a common finding, as well as stiffness and lethargy. The body temperature can vary from subnormal to increased. The affected animal may become recumbent and unable to rise. Hindlimb muscles often appear to be sore on palpation. Dysphagia is often the first sign noted due to involvement of the tongue plus the pharyngeal and sometimes the masticatory muscles, and in some cases probably contributes to the development of pneumonia. Regurgitation, starvation, and ptyalism are other possible complications. If the heart is involved, tachycardia, arrhythmias, systolic murmurs, and respiratory distress may also be found. Myoglobinuria has been reported in a number of cases. A swollen tongue or tachypnea alone is an unusual presenting sign. A 10-month-old aborted fetus with histologic lesions typical of this condition has been reported.[183]

The condition appears to occur in any breed and does not appear to have a sex predilection. Recovery can occur often within days or weeks of the presenting signs.[183] Signs may be seen in an individual animal or several animals within a group.

Laboratory Findings

In the acute form, AST and CK activities are markedly elevated. In the recovery stages the values may be only slightly elevated or within the normal range. Increased CK and AST activities have also been found in about 25% of the mares of affected foals and in 20% of clinically normal foals in the same stables.[189] This was suggested to reflect the existence of subclinical lesions in these animals.

It has been suggested that because selenium is only incorporated into erythrocytes during erythropoiesis, the GSHPx activity of RBCs is a better indicator of long-term selenium status than serum selenium values (although plateauing of GSHPx values is found above a certain selenium intake, i.e., when blood selenium levels of around 0.12 μg/mL serum or 0.16 μg/mL whole blood are reached). Low GSHPx, selenium, and vitamin E values have been reported in affected animals. In our laboratory, for example, GSHPx values of more than 30 IU/mL of RBCs would be expected in stabled animals fed a balanced diet. Values above 25 IU/mL may be expected in grazing animals on an adequate intake; values below 20 IU/mL tend to be associated with animals on a deficient intake. Values above 1.5 μg/mL for vitamin E have been reported as being normal,[127] although far lower values have been reported in clinically normal animals.[190] Reference values vary according to the laboratory and care has to be taken with the collection of samples, especially for vitamin E determination, as contact with rubber, for example, may interfere with analysis. It has even been suggested that single serum sample assays cannot be used as an indicator of vitamin E status in the individual horse because of the high variability in values between animals and within the same animal.[190] Decreased GSHPx, selenium, or vitamin E levels cannot be used to confirm the condition because, as stated earlier, supposedly low values have been found in apparently normal animals. Normal vitamin E levels have been reported in some affected foals[189]; this may, however, reflect the recent ingestion of colostrum, which would tend to elevate the concentration. Many of these foals' dams had low serum vitamin E concentrations (<200 µg/dL), and it is possible that the affected foals' levels were low prior to suckling.

The liver plays a role in selenium storage, and liver selenium concentrations of three foals (119 ± 5 µg/kg ppm) were found to be statistically lower than those of foals with other diseases (162 ± 20 µg/kg) in one report.[189] The skeletal muscle selenium concentrations of affected animals seemed to be higher compared with the other foals in this study. Liver selenium concentrations on a wet weight basis have been reported to be adequate at 0.300 to 1.000 ppm, marginal at 0.161 to 0.299 ppm, and deficient at 0.160 ppm or less.[127]

Myoglobinuria was confirmed by acetate electrophoresis in one case.[183] In other cases, the diagnosis of myoglobinuria appears to have been made either visually or via a positive reaction to orthotoluidine agent in a test strip. Hyperlipemia has been reported in some cases with and without signs of steatitis post mortem.[35, 182]

Electrolyte disturbances include hyperkalemia, hyponatremia, and hypochloremia. Such findings seem to be associated with a poorer prognosis. Metabolic acidosis may be present and the blood urea nitrogen is often elevated; this may, at least in part, be due to prerenal factors. Alterations in the hemogram may be seen depending on the presence or absence of complications such as aspiration pneumonia.

In foals suspected of suffering from this condition a full hematologic and clinical chemistry profile with a urinalysis is advisable. In very young foals, especially those with dysphagia or poor sucking reflex, it is also advisable to check IgG levels.

Postmortem Findings

Macroscopically, in peracute neonatal cases, often very little is seen. In acute cases the muscle may appear pale and streaks may be present representing areas of coagulative necrosis next to less affected tissue. Generally, all muscle groups of the pelvic and thoracic limbs are affected. The muscles of mastication, the diaphragm, tongue, pharynx, and as cervical musculature are commonly involved. The distribution is usually bilateral and symmetric. In subacute cases yellow-white streaks may be found in the heart and muscle, representing calcification.[187] Steatitis, yellow fat deposits, and fat necrosis have also been described in some but not all cases.[183]

Histology

The typical signs at various stages of the condition have been described.[187] During the first few days, extensive floccular, granular, and severe hyaline degeneration of myofibers may be seen. After about a week, phagocytosis of necrotic tissue is seen with endomysial thickening due to edema, mononuclear infiltration, and proliferation of fibroblasts. By 2 weeks, epimyseal connective tissue has proliferated. Early regenerating fibers can be seen coexisting with signs of myodegeneration.

Diagnosis

At present diagnosis is based on the following:

1. Appropriate clinical signs, for example, weakness, stiffness (but patients can still be bright and alert, at least in the early stages)
2. Elevated AST and CK activities, especially in the acute stages
3. Lowered blood selenium and GSHPx values
4. Response to vitamin E and selenium administration

The differential diagnosis (Table 8–6) can be quite extensive depending on the signs shown by the affected animal. However, few of the conditions listed in Table 8–6 result in marked elevations of muscle enzyme activities or myoglobinuria. It is very important to differentiate this condition from colic, for which it may initially be mistaken because the animal cannot get up and tends to fall around, thrashing its limbs.[182] Foals with botulism usually have decreased muscle tone.

Treatment

Reduction of physical activity and prompt administration of vitamin E and selenium are usually recommended. Injections of vitamin E and selenium are usually required but because of the potential for anaphylactoid reactions, the intravenous route should be avoided. Deep intramuscular injections should be given, although it should be noted that intramuscular injections may give rise to muscle soreness and have been

---

Table 8–6. Differential Diagnosis of Nutritionally Related Myodegeneration

1. Botulism
2. Medullary diseases, e.g., herpesvirus type 1, myelitis
3. Spinal cord diseases
4. Cerebellar diseases
5. Tetanus
6. Suppurative meningitis
7. Rabies
8. Trauma
9. Septic polyarthritis
10. Various causes of dysphagia (e.g., cleft palate, ulcers, peripheral damage to certain cranial nerves)
11. Various causes of dyspnea (e.g., pneumonia, cardiac disease, etc.)
12. Colic
13. Polymyositis
14. Equine rhabdomyolysis syndrome
15. Atypical myoglobinuria
16. Purpura hemorrhagica
17. Tick paralysis
18. Muscular dystrophy
19. Equine motor neuron disease

associated with abscess formation. Care regarding possible toxicity should therefore be taken. The level of 200 μg/kg has been cited as a toxic dose for foals.[138] Nasogastric feeding may be preferable in the dysphagic, anorectic, or recumbent foal.[127] Fluid therapy is often needed to combat dehydration and electrolyte disturbances, as well as to maintain urine output and prevent myoglobin-associated renal damage. Fluids with high potassium content should not be used when hyperkalemia is present, although care should be taken that once the animal has been rehydrated and its acid-base status restored, hypokalemia does not occur, especially if the animal is dysphagic.

Anti-inflammatory agents may be helpful to reduce the pain and swelling but need to be used with caution in foals because of their ulcerogenic properties. Antibiotic therapy may be advisable if the animal is dysphagic or shows signs of respiratory distress, pneumonia, and so forth. Selenium deficiency by itself may result in immunosuppression,[127] which may be compounded by the complete or partial failure of passive transfer.

Prevention

Vitamin E and selenium supplementation is suggested, either orally or by injection. It is, however, probably preferable to feed a constant daily level, especially as injectable preparations have been associated with fatalities.

Various amounts are recommended in the literature, such as 1.5 to 4.4 mg/kg α-tocopherol acetate daily for adult standardbred horses on a low vitamin E diet.[191] There are at least eight different tocopherols with vitamin E activity. α-Tocopherol has the greatest activity and accounts for 70% to 90% of total biological activity. The supplementary form of vitamin E is usually α-tocopherol acetate, which is not an antioxidant and is therefore much more stable to moisture, heat, and oxygen. It is converted to active tocopherol during digestion and absorption from the gut. It has been recommended that 5 mg of additional vitamin E be added for every 1% of blended fat. This may be very important with respect to endurance horses. The value of vitamin E injections has been questioned, especially as the amounts within the injectable preparations are low.[183] Feeding good-quality, properly stored hay and grain, and allowing access to good-quality green forage may help to maintain vitamin E intake.

Feeding 1 mg/day of oral selenium has been said to maintain blood selenium values above the level associated with myodegeneration in horses and foals.[192] Only limited amounts of selenium cross the placenta, which may explain why clinical cases may be seen in offspring of supplemented mares.[193] The milk from mares that have been supplemented appears to contain more selenium than milk from unsupplemented animals, but the amount present is small, as selenium is not concentrated in milk. Organic selenium supplementation appears to be more beneficial than inorganic. Therefore, while many recommend, especially in deficient areas, that mares be supplemented from late gestation through lactation, others prefer to supplement the foals at birth[192] and 2 and 6 weeks later,[183, 192] although this may not prevent the cases seen at birth or in the first few days of life. Others recommend that, in problem areas, a selenium injection should be given at birth and then every 2 to 3 months during the first 6 months of life.[188] Still others recommend injecting every 5 to 10 days.[127]

In pigs, it has been suggested that selenium may be teratogenic. This has not been observed in mares but it has been recommended that selenium injections not be given in an early pregnancy. The levels recommended for oral supplementation of mares during pregnancy have varied from allowing free access to a trace mineralized salt containing 15 to 30 ppm selenium or feeding a ration containing 0.5 ppm selenium (on a dry matter basis). Alternatively feeding at a higher level (0.1–0.2 ppm), equivalent to the 1 mg/day mentioned earlier, has been recommended.[127] Special care has to be taken with selenium administration as toxicity can occur. The single minimum lethal dose of oral sodium selenite (Na_2SeO_3) has been given as 3.3 mg/kg in the adult and results in a variety of clinical signs including severe dyspnea, incoordination, diarrhea, recumbency, and death within a few hours. There is evidence to suggest that whereas a gradually reduced selenium uptake occurs with increased oral supplementation, giving large single oral doses of selenium does not seem to be advantageous and daily administration seems preferable. Increases in GSHPx activity in the blood should not be expected for 2 to 3 weeks after selenium supplementation. It should be noted again that GSHPx values tend to plateau before toxic levels of selenium are reached and it may take several months for levels to decrease following cessation of supplementation.

Prognosis

The prognosis is guarded, especially if the animal is recumbent or if treatment has been delayed. Prognosis also seems to be less favorable in animals with acid-base and electrolyte disturbances.

EXERCISE-RELATED DISORDERS
Exhausted Horse Syndrome
Pathophysiology

The exhausted horse syndrome tends to occur when horses have been pushed past their performance limits. It is believed to have a complex etiology involving a combination of fluid and electrolyte losses, depletion of energy stores, and extremes of environmental conditions. The syndrome, therefore, is usually seen in association with 3-day events and long-distance rides.[118, 194] A brief summary of some of the possible contributing factors is given here. More detailed information is available.[195–198]

The amount of sweat produced by an exercising horse depends on the environmental conditions, nature of the work, and the animal's fitness. Under favorable climatic conditions, sweat loss can be on the order of 5 to 8 L/hr on long-distance rides. In hot, humid conditions, where sweating is partially ineffective, sweat production can be as high as 10 to 15 L/hr. This means that an endurance horse can lose 25 to 30 L or more if conditions are unfavorable. A racehorse performing at top speed, under average conditions, for a sprint may lose between 1 and 5 L. Sweat production seems to only decrease after extreme water loss. When the sweat loss is low, much of the loss can be made up by absorption of water from the large intestine. However, if water losses are between 5% and 10% of body weight, a decrease in circulatory volume occurs. This tends to occur after about 3 hours of exercise with moderate sweating, but much sooner at rates of 10 to 15 L/hr.

Sweat has been shown to contain low concentrations of calcium and phosphate, but is hypertonic to plasma with respect to sodium, potassium, and chloride. During exercise the horse appears to be able to maintain, initially at least, its plasma electrolyte concentrations at the expense of other body compartments. This is especially true for sodium where it is believed that the contents of the gastrointestinal tract may provide an important reservoir. Decreases of up to 6 mmol/L of sodium have been reported during endurance rides in hot weather. These are likely to be the result of marked sodium and water losses followed by partial replacement of the water deficit by drinking. Sodium concentrations may, in fact, increase in those animals that are not allowed to drink or that refuse to drink. During severe sweating muscle tissue may be the source of potassium replacement. Apart from the high losses of potassium in sweat, potassium status is further compromised by the concomitant sodium deficiency, as potassium absorption from the gastrointestinal tract is decreased as potassium replaces sodium in the digestive secretions.

Hypochloremia is commonly found following endurance rides, which reflects the fact that chloride losses in sweat represent a much greater proportion of the body's chloride stores. Chloride is the major anion absorbed in the kidney, and in its absence bicarbonate is resorbed.

The most consistent acid-base alteration associated with endurance in hot environments is metabolic alkalosis, which appears to be associated with the hypochloremia and hypokalemia caused by the heavy sweating and may not, therefore, be seen in cooler conditions. Hypocalcemia has sometimes been observed in endurance horses. This might result from calcium losses in sweat or from disturbances of calcium homeostasis. These have been suggested to include energy deficiency, alkalosis, or competition with sodium and potassium exchange in the skeleton.

Many endurance horses may, even with frequent access to water, develop clinical signs of slight to moderate dehydration during the course of a ride, as well as signs due to some disturbance in electrolyte status. The combination of dehydration and sodium depletion results in a decreased plasma volume shown by raised packed-cell volume (PCV), total protein, blood viscosity, etc. This, in turn, may result in inadequate tissue perfusion and inefficient oxygen and substrate transport. These in their turn may result in impaired renal function. Alterations in acid-base balance plus calcium, magnesium, and potassium depletion may contribute to the development of gastrointestinal tract stasis or ileus, as well as muscle cramps, synchronous diaphragmatic flutter, etc. If very severe losses of water and electrolytes occur, then sweat production may decrease, resulting in even less effective thermoregulation.

Clinical Signs and Laboratory Findings

Some of the signs seen with this condition and the associated laboratory findings are shown in Table 8–7. Signs may last for several days.

Table 8–7. Clinical Signs and Laboratory Findings in the Exhausted Horse*

Clinical Signs†	Laboratory Findings
Depression	Metabolic alkalosis
Dehydration, anorexia, decreased thirst	Paradoxical aciduria
Elevated respiratory and heart rates	Hypokalemia, hyponatremia, hypochloremia
Raised temperature	Increase in CK, AST, LDH activities
Poor sweating response	Proteinuria
Poor jugular distention, increased CRT, decreased pulse pressure	Azotemia
Decreased intestinal sounds, laminitis	Lipidosis
Muscle cramps	Signs of hepatic failure
Synchronous diaphragmatic flutter	

*Abbreviations: CK, creatine kinase; AST, aspartate aminotransferase; LDH, lactic dehydrogenase.
†Not all signs are present in all cases.

Various guidelines have been given in the literature to help distinguish the "exhausted" horse from the nonexhausted but often tired horse. The pulse and respiratory rates may be similar in both cases at the end of the ride but in the nonexhausted horse the rates will tend to return toward normal far quicker, for example, to a heart rate of less than 60 to 70 beats per minute (bpm) with a respiratory rate of less than 40 per minute within 25 to 30 minutes, unless the ambient temperature is high. In the exhausted horse the pulse rate tends to remain high, for example, greater than 70 bpm at 30 minutes' post exercise, with a respiratory rate more than half the pulse rate and a persistently elevated rectal temperature.[118, 188, 198]

Treatment

Horses that appear depressed with persistently elevated pulse and respiratory rates may respond to rest, cooling out, and access to salt, feed, and water. If no improvement is seen within 30 minutes, fluid therapy is often needed. In the more severe case of a horse that refuses to eat or drink, prompt and vigorous fluid therapy is needed. Fluids are required primarily to restore circulating blood volume as well as to correct electrolyte deficits and provide a source of readily metabolizable energy. Five to 8 L can be given orally every 30 minutes to 1 hour, if required, but should be stopped if any discomfort or gastric reflux becomes apparent. Hypertonic solutions should not be given. In severely affected animals, up to 10 to 20 L/hr of IV fluids plus stomach tubing may be needed. Saline, Ringer's solution, etc. can be used, although potassium chloride should be added to provide around 10 mmol/L. Once the horse starts eating hay, the potassium supplementation can stop. Glucose can be given either as 5% dextrose saline, or 50% dextrose can be added to Ringer's solution to deliver between 50 and 100 g/hr (concurrent insulin administration has been recommended).

Slow administration of calcium may also be of value. Sodium bicarbonate administration is not, however, indicated. Other therapeutic agents to control pain and anxiety may be required although the nonsteroidal anti-inflammatory agents (NSAIDs) and phenothiazine derivatives should be used with extreme caution in the face of dehydration. It has also been recommended that corticosteroid administration be avoided unless absolutely necessary.

Cold-water body sprays and alcohol baths, particularly over the head and neck region, should be used to cool the patient, without chilling. Care has to be taken not to induce muscle spasms by pouring very cold water over large muscle masses. In recumbent, hyperthermic patients, cold-water enemas, delivered via a handheld rectal tube and gravity-fed, should be given. Further information is available.[194–198]

Prevention

It can be of value to train an endurance horse to drink electrolyte-rich water. This may help to partially restore electrolyte concentrations during a race. However, plain water should always be available as an alternative. It is not possible to restore all losses at once, and caution should be taken, as during exercise the circulation is drawn away from the gut to the muscles and there is probably a reduced rate of absorption. It is possibly best to feed a suitable diet before exercise and then give small amounts of electrolytes plus water during the ride.

Various suggestions have been made as to the optimal nature of any electrolyte supplement. From one to four times more sodium than potassium has been recommended, for example. Sodium bicarbonate has often been suggested as part of an electrolyte mix, but as most endurance horses tend to become alkalotic, this may, in fact, be counterproductive and is not recommended. Additional sodium and potassium chloride over a few days after competition may be helpful but often is unnecessary if the basic diet is acceptable.[197–199]

MALIGNANCY
Muscle Tumors

Primary tumors of skeletal muscle are rare, malignant tumors being twice as frequent as benign ones. Rhabdomyosarcomas of the limbs, head, or neck appear as hard, spherical masses deep in the muscle. A significant proportion appears to occur in sites of earlier muscle fiber destruction and repair.[35] Frequently, young animals less than 2 years old are affected. Other primary tumors, benign and malignant, including lipomas, liposarcomas, fibromas, fibrosarcomas, myxomas, and hemangiosarcomas can occur in muscles. Metastatic spread to the muscles, especially of malignant melanomas, angiosarcomas, and tumors of the lymphoreticular system, also may occur.[35]

Muscle Wasting with Malignant Disease

Owing to a combination of cachexia, malnutrition, disuse, infection, and old age, muscle weakness and occasionally muscle necrosis may develop with malignancies involving other body systems.

MULTIFACTORIAL DISORDERS
Equine Rhabdomyolysis Syndrome
Name

There is much confusion regarding the naming of this condition. Some have referred to it as azoturia or Monday morning disease, others as tying-up, myositis, set-fast, or chronic intermittent rhabdomyolysis.[200] Others have suggested that the tying-up syndrome and equine rhabdomyolysis syndrome are distinct but similar conditions.[87, 201] Today, the majority of workers accept that they are probably different clinical manifestations of the same syndrome referred to as equine rhabdomyolysis or equine exertional rhabdomyolysis.[61, 202] The term *equine rhabdomyolysis syndrome* is preferred because the clinical signs, presentation, and so forth vary considerably, even within an individual; it is unlikely that a single pathophysiologic process can explain all manifestations, and not all cases are associated with *exertion.*

Pathophysiology

In the past ERS was described in the literature under diseases of the liver, kidney, blood, or muscle.[203] It has also been attributed to infection, cold weather, intoxication, nervous irritation, calcium deficiency, excess of glycogen, lactic acid poisoning, an increase in RBCs, and an unbalanced alkali reserve.[203] A good description of some of these older theories has been given.[204] Some are still popular, but others—as the infectious agent,[205] faulty fat metabolism,[206] and viscosity theories[207]—have few supporters today.

Any theory as to the pathophysiology of this syndrome needs to take into account that the condition can be of variable clinical severity (even within an individual sufferer); is often recurrent with a variable interval between episodes; and can affect one individual within a group all on the same management feeding and exercise regimen. Between episodes many sufferers are able to perform as required. Exercise is a very common triggering factor, although the nature and type of any preceding exercise varies between and often within individual sufferers.

It is likely that there is an underlying abnormality that predisposes to the syndrome. A triggering factor, most commonly exercise, may then be necessary to initiate the clinical signs. The pathophysiology of this condition is not clear and it is likely that the predisposing factor(s) and triggering factor(s) are not identical for each animal affected. Possible predisposing factors include the following.

Carbohydrate Overloading

In 1914–1915 it was recorded that when oats were scarce and raw sugar was fed as a substitute, there was an increase in the incidence of metabolic diseases, especially "azoturia."[208] It was postulated that excessive glycogen buildup resulted in an overproduction of lactic acid on exercise. Injecting lactic acid or potassium lactate into the hindlimbs of mice was found to produce a cramplike condition with muscle degeneration.[208] Many years later clinical stiffness was produced by multiple small injections of concentrated lactic acid into the backs of horses.[209] Myositis was evident histologically. However, it is likely that these effects would result from the injection of any highly irritant substance.

Support for the carbohydrate overloading theory mainly arose from two studies,[210, 211] in which the condition was reproduced by feeding horses 3 kg of molasses daily and then exercising them after a rest period. In 1974[202] it was reported that 4 of 12 animals studied had raised muscle lactate levels 15 minutes to 1 hour after an attack of equine rhabdomyolysis. However, the levels found in this study were low compared to those seen in muscle of normal unaffected animals after racing.[212] It has also been pointed out that if lactic acid accumulation were responsible for the muscle degeneration, a state of lactic acidosis would be expected and yet this is often not seen.[38, 213] As most histologic studies have shown the involvement of only a small proportion of muscle fibers, it is possible that high lactate accumulation in these fibers could be missed[214] and such a limited involvement of fibers might not cause an appreciable rise in blood lactate.

The theory of glycogen overloading has been modified over the years. It has been proposed that any factor that increases the rate of glycogen utilization or muscle glycogen deposition would predispose to equine rhabdomyolysis, as would decreased circulation to the muscle, because during exercise glycogen would be broken down more rapidly than it could be completely oxidized,[188] resulting in the rapid production of excessive lactic acid. This, in turn, would cause local tissue damage and vasospasm resulting in a decreased circulation and a further reduction in lactic acid removal. Some workers have stated that increased muscle glycogen stores have not been detected histochemically,[67] although others have reported that subsarcolemmal glycogen deposits can be found in biopsies from some equine rhabdomyolysis sufferers.[215] It has been shown that after a day of racelike work it takes several days to restore the muscle glycogen content.[216] Therefore, it is difficult to understand how glycogen overloading could occur in racing animals given a single day of rest. However, very high resting glycogen concentrations have been found in the muscles of some affected horses.[101, 217] In one of these studies, near maximal exercise resulted in depletion of the muscle glycogen levels in affected animals to concentrations similar to those found in the control animals. Resynthesis, however, occurred quickly so that within 24 hours the initial high resting values were reestablished. It was concluded, however, that neither intramuscular glycogen accumulation per se nor a rapid rate of anaerobic glycolysis with excessive lactate accumulation was the cause of the muscle damage.[217] (See also under Metabolic Pathway Abnormalities.)

Anecdotally in the United Kingdom, decreasing the energy and, in particular, the soluble carbohydrate intake seems to reduce the incidence of ERS in some but not all cases. More work is needed on the role of diet in this condition.

Local Hypoxia

Histologically, the type II muscle fibers appear to be predominantly affected.[38, 202, 217a] These fibers are larger and have greater glycogen stores and fewer capillaries surrounding them than the slow-twitch fibers.[20, 22] Local hypoxia during exercise could provide the stimulus for increased lactate production in these highly glycolytic fibers.[202] However, equine rhabdomyolysis often occurs at the start of light exercise when the fast-twitch fibers are unlikely to have been recruited. In addition, the condition is not usually seen in horses with impaired circulation caused by a subacute to chronic aortic-iliac thrombosis.

Postexercise muscle biopsies from three recurrent sufferers with raised CK, AST, and myoglobin concentrations following being exercised submaximally on the treadmill showed randomly scattered swollen vacuolated type IIA and IIB fibers on light microscopy. Approximately 6% were affected. On electron microscopy myofibrillar disruption, irregular sarcomeres, and enlarged rounded mitochondria with degenerate cristae together with dilated sarcoplasmic reticulum were found. The researchers suggested that the scattered pattern of fibronecrosis meant that the rhabdomyolysis was likely to have been specifically induced within particular motor units, implying a more specific etiology than general hypoxia or general lactic acidosis.[217a] Interestingly, glycogen overloading in humans is associated with an increased uptake of intracellular water. The consequent increase in fiber size has been suggested to result in reduced capillary perfusion and thereby a local hypoxia due to increased intramuscular pressure.

Thiamine Deficiency

Thiamine acts as a coenzyme in the oxidative decarboxylation of pyruvate. A deficiency of thiamine could result in the accumulation of pyruvic and lactic acid in tissues. Thiamine deficiency has been induced in the horse and resulted in a mixture of clinical signs including loss of appetite, weight loss, bradycardia, peripheral and central nervous system disturbances, and muscular weakness together with elevated serum sorbitol dehydrogenase (SDH) and CK activities.[218] "Azoturia" has been suggested to be the result of a disturbance in carbohydrate metabolism, which could be overcome by the feeding of thiamine.[219] A nutritional myopathy with clinical signs similar to equine rhabdomyolysis has been said to have been produced by feeding horses a diet of polished rice, casein, and fish oils.[60] This was attributed to thiamine deficiency. More probably, the cause was the myopathic effects of the high content of unsaturated fatty acids in the oils and low vitamin E/selenium status.[60]

Vitamin E and Selenium Deficiency

A relationship between equine rhabdomyolysis and vitamin E/selenium deficiency has been claimed as a result of the reported success of supplementation in preventing further attacks.[220] Most workers, however, have failed to produce any scientific evidence to support these findings. Muscle biopsy samples from equine rhabdomyolysis cases, for example, have shown no deficiency in vitamin E or selenium levels.[221] No relationship between low blood GSHPx activity and high AST levels has been found[222] and the feeding of additional vitamin E has been shown not to decrease the frequency of high AST activities.[223] The claim that vitamin E and selenium prevent or cure equine rhabdomyolysis has been refuted.[224] A group of horses fed apparently low dietary levels of vitamin E for 4 months demonstrated no apparent clinical signs, nor were clinically abnormal levels of CK or AST recorded, and the animals' performance in standardized exercise tests were not compromised.[225]

In a survey of 144 animals believed to suffer from the rhabdomyolysis syndrome, five had lowered GSHPx activities.[101, 224] In addition, these five animals also had abnormal urinary fractional electrolyte excretion values (see Electrolyte Imbalances). Appropriate oral electrolyte and selenium supplementation resulted in no further clinical episodes. However, it is not possible to determine if this recovery would have occurred if either of the measures had been undertaken alone.

Metabolic Pathway Abnormalities

In humans there are several genetically determined conditions that produce signs similar to equine rhabdomyolysis. At least six different enzymatic defects affecting the ability to metabolize glycogen to pyruvate and lactate have been characterized.[225a] McArdle's disease (lack of muscle phosphorylase) and Tarui's disease (lack of phosphofructokinase) result in cramps on exercise and myoglobinuria after strenuous activity. In these conditions the muscle glycogen is not available for anaerobic metabolism during periods of decreased oxygen supply. The diagnosis is therefore based on the absence of a rise in blood lactate concentration following ischemic forearm exercise.[57, 226] A major deficiency in the carbohydrate glycolytic pathway, as is found in McArdle's disease, can be discounted in most cases of equine rhabdomyolysis, as the clinical signs would tend to be present whenever the animal was exercised. This is in contrast to the more usual intermittent nature of equine rhabdomyolysis, although it is possible that a few isolated cases may occur that are due to such a defect. A predisposition to equine rhabdomyolysis based on an abnormal activity level of 20 intracellular enzymes, including phosphorylase, was not found in one study of 22 affected animals.[227] Workers in Davis, California, however, have identified a metabolic defect in muscle energy production in a group of Arabian horses that became very tired after exercise with signs of stiffness, although no actual muscle damage could be found. Abnormally high plasma concentrations of lactic acid were found following exercise.[217] A glycogen storage disorder characterized by an abnormal accumulation of an intensely PAS-positive material has been identified in muscle biopsies from 28 horses with exercise-induced rhabdomyolysis in the United States.[47a] The number of affected fibers varied from 1 per sample to 40% of all fibers, and on electron microscopy the acid mycopolysaccharide inclusions were found to consist of beta glycogen particles and filamentous material. The biopsies also showed numerous subsarcolemmal vacuoles, especially in the type II fibers. Six of the 14 horses tested had a phosphofructokinase activity of less than 50% that of the controls. Two of the affected horses undertook a number of standardized treadmill exercise tests. The maximum speed attainable by those with this polysaccharide storage myopathy was 9 or 10.5 m/sec versus 12 m/sec in the controls. The oxygen consumption at maximum speed was approximately 50% that of healthy horses at their maximal speed and the rate of lactate accumulation was far lower in the affected animals. This suggested abnormal glycolytic metabolism consistent with an impaired activity of the Embden-Meyerhof pathway (glucose 1-phosphate to pyruvate), resulting in an insufficient amount of pyruvate for oxidation or anaerobic conversion to lactate. In humans, an inherited deficiency in the M subunit of the phosphofructokinase enzyme is responsible for the polysaccharide storage myopathy associated with exercise-induced rhabdomyolysis. The horse appears to have histologic and electron microscopic findings in common with this condition in humans, although the biochemical abnormality may differ, as the glycolytic activity appears to be only partially impaired in the horse. Further work is needed to clarify this condition. Another metabolic defect in carbohydrate metabolism resulting in rhabdomyolysis, poor performance, and abnormal hind limb movement in Percheron and Belgian draft horses has been reported but few details are available at present.

Loosely coupled oxidative phosphorylation has been reported in certain skeletal muscle mitochondria in some muscle samples from affected animals.[228] It was suggested that this may have been caused by a mitochondrial energy crisis. However, such uncoupling can also be seen in samples from normal athletes post exercise[214] and may not be related to a pathologic condition.

A clinical condition almost identical to equine rhabdomyolysis is found in carnitine palmitoyltransferase deficiency. This enzyme is involved in mitochondrial oxidation of long-chain fatty acids.[171, 229] However, in humans this deficiency most commonly occurs in males and tends to be precipitated by fasting prior to exercise. The respiratory muscles are often involved and signs are not usually seen with short bursts of intense activity.[45] An apparent carnitine palmitoyltranferase I and II deficiency (relative to humans) appears to be present in all horses, not just horses that suffer from this syndrome.[230] It is also thought unlikely that a systemic or a myopathic carnitine deficiency is the cause of equine rhabdomyolysis.[230]

Other, less severe enzyme abnormalities could occur in equine rhabdomyolysis. Several new conditions have been recognized in humans that can result in exercise intolerance and recurrent discolored urine post exercise.[45] It has, in fact, been suggested that most forms of myoglobinuria in humans occur as a result of a metabolic defect, when not caused by crush injuries or alcoholism.[45, 225a] Whether any similar deficient states occur in horses with equine rhabdomyolysis is not yet known.[227]

Hormonal Disturbances

Reproductive Hormones. It has been suggested that young fillies are more likely to have high plasma muscle enzyme activities and are more prone to attacks of equine rhabdomyolysis than colts or geldings.[60] As early as the 1870s it was claimed that equine rhabdomyolysis tended to affect mares, especially during estrus.[231] This suggested that reproductive hormones may be important as triggering factors for the condition, although no correlation between the stage of estrus cycle and the occurrence of raised muscle enzyme activities was found in one study.[106] A preliminary study showed that the extent of any hormonal influence on urinary electrolyte excretion appeared to vary considerably among individuals, and suggested that there could be marked changes in an individual's electrolyte urinary excretion during the estrous cycle despite a constant dietary intake.[231a] Particularly it fed an electrolyte-deficient or imbalanced diet, such changes could have a significant effect on that individual's electrolyte status, and this could be a contributory factor to the occurrence of ERS in certain individuals (see below). Further work is needed, however, to substantiate this work.

Hypothyroidism. It is well recognized that muscular problems are a common symptom of hypothyroidism in humans.[232, 233] In mild cases, fatigue may be the only presenting symptom, although the more severe cases can be accompanied by overt muscle cell damage, elevated resting plasma CK activities and sometimes raised myoglobin levels.[234] Poor racing performances and certain myopathies have been related to mild secondary hypothyroidism,[235] although this conclusion has been challenged.[236] Oral thyroxine (T_4) supplementation has been suggested to improve performance or decrease the incidence of myopathies in these hypothyroid cases.[67, 235] However, there is still considerable debate as to whether hypothyroidism is involved in the pathogenesis of exertional myopathies in the horse.[61]

Resting T_4 concentrations were found not to differ significantly between animals believed to be suffering from the rhabdomyolysis syndrome and those suffering from a variety of other conditions. However, some rhabdomyolysis sufferers may have a lowered response to thyrotropin-releasing hormone (TRH).[101] This may reflect a decreased thyroid reserve, but too few cases have been investigated to date.

Cortisol. Low blood cortisol levels have been implicated in the pathophysiology of this condition.[114] Horses with acute signs of equine rhabdomyolysis have been reported to have a reduced serum cortisol response to adrenocorticotropin (ACTH).[114]

Malignant Hyperthermia

A similarity between equine rhabdomyolysis and the genetically influenced condition of malignant hyperthermia in humans and the porcine stress syndrome has been suggested.[154, 237–239] Malignant hyperthermia occurs on exposure to a triggering factor such as stress, excitement, anxiety, exercise, volatile anesthetic agents, and depolarizing muscle relaxants. In response to these factors there is an abnormal release of calcium from the sarcoplasmic reticulum. This results in hyperthermia, metabolic and respiratory acidosis, and muscle damage.[239, 240] The clinical signs vary from slight muscle cramping to a fulminant, fatal form. Even in susceptible individuals the reaction may not always occur immediately or on first exposure to an anesthetic. An adaptation of the human diagnostic halothane-caffeine contracture test has been described for use in the horse.[153, 239] In a preliminary study it was found that two of the five horses that had suffered repeated bouts of rhabdomyolysis that were tested had contractures similar to those expected from persons susceptible to malignant hyperthermia.[239] There is little evidence, however, to indicate that the majority of cases of rhabdomyolysis suffer from malignant hyperthermia. Malignant hyperthermia may, however, play a role in equine anes-

thetic-induced hyperthermia and myopathy, as discussed earlier.[153, 239]

Viral Etiology

Muscle pain or myalgia has been accepted as a common symptom in the acute phase of influenza and other viral illnesses in man, although there are only a few reports of severe muscular involvement.[45, 241, 242] Myalgia, together with myoglobinuria, has been found with herpesvirus infections.[45] In the horse it has often been claimed that certain animals are stiff and unwilling to work during or after an attack of the "virus."[243] Also, viral infection has been reported as being one of the predisposing factors to equine rhabdomyolysis.[194]

A clinical investigation was carried out into an outbreak of muscle stiffness and poor performance in a flat-racing stable of Thoroughbreds.[244] Over a third of the horses showed signs of muscular stiffness over a 2-month period and 64% at one or more of the sampling times had obviously elevated CK and AST activities. Serology was highly suggestive of an equine herpesvirus type 1 (EHV-1) infection. The possibility of a viral etiology, at least in outbreaks of stiffness in racing yards, should be evaluated in more depth. However, the muscular involvement associated with viral disease may be a separate condition rather than a variation of ERS. Muscle could be directly affected by the virus, resulting in an increased susceptibility to exercise-induced damage. Alternatively, the increase in blood viscosity that is found post infection could result in an impaired blood flow and decreased oxygen delivery to the peripheral tissues.[245]

In humans it has been suggested that there may be a metabolic effect on mitochondria, perhaps involving fatty acid oxidation.[246] There is, however, uncertainty regarding the causes of the postviral fatigue syndrome in humans and its effects on the muscular system.[247]

Electrolyte Imbalances

Several workers have implicated electrolyte disturbances as a predisposing cause of this syndrome[66, 248, 249] and sodium, potassium, or calcium supplementation, individually or combined, has been recommended for prevention.[22]

Electrolyte imbalances are difficult to detect simply and routinely.[101] An alternative is to use the urinary fractional electrolyte (FE) excretion test, which has been shown to be a practical means of assessing certain alterations in electrolyte status,[101, 249, 250] although there are limitations to its use.[101] The FE test was carried out in 144 horses believed to have suffered repeated attacks of this syndrome.[101, 251] One hundred horses had FE results outside the established reference range for the diet they were being fed. Of these 100 horses, 72 suffered no further attacks of the condition after being fed either the appropriate electrolyte supplementation (Table 8–8) based on the FE results or a diet believed to provide an adequate and balanced electrolyte intake. These results suggest that for *some* horses an electrolyte abnormality may be involved in the pathophysiology of the condition, although the exact nature of this involvement is not known. The FE test, however, must be applied and interpreted with care,[251a] and the different feeding practices among countries

Table 8–8. Examples of Supplementation Given to 400- to 500-kg Horses Based on Fractional Electrolyte (FE) Excretion Test Results*

FE Values	Supplementation
Low Na$^+$	2 oz (56 g)/day NaCl
Low Na$^+$ and K$^+$	2 oz (56 g) NaCl + 10 oz (28 g) KCl/day for 2 wk, then 2 oz (56 g) NaCl/day
High	Decrease bran intake if it is fed, + 2 oz (56 g) CaCO$_3$/day, or an alternative source(s) of calcium
High Na$^+$	Lower Na$^+$ intake (e.g., change source of hay if grown near the coast)

Normal values: FE$_{Na^+}$ = 0.04–0.8; FE$_{K^+}$ = 35–80; FE$_{PO_4}$ = 0–0.2

*Data from Harris P, Colles C: The use of creatine clearance ratios in the prevention of equine rhabdomyolysis: A report of four cases. *Equine Vet J* 20:459, 1988.

may mean that electrolyte supplementation based on the FE test may have more or less relevance.

A group of recurrent ERS sufferers in one study were shown to have lower muscle potassium concentrations on a dry weight basis than the control group. The ERS sufferers also tended to have lower %K FE values, although the differences were not significant.[168a] In vitro twitch characteristics of muscle samples from recurrent sufferers differed from a control group in one study having particularly prolonged relaxation times, which could be a result of abnormal calcium fluxes.[168]

In the horse most reports on the clinical effects of calcium and phosphorus imbalances have concentrated on the resultant skeletal abnormalities[252–256] and only the effects of severe potassium and sodium depletion have been described.[257, 258] In all of these conditions the signs were either permanently present or could consistently be induced by a triggering factor, such as exercise. The same cannot always be said for equine rhabdomyolysis and the most likely explanation of the role of electrolytes in equine rhabdomyolysis may involve transient alterations in ionic concentrations or fluxes across the muscle cell membrane. The intracellular concentrations of sodium and potassium are predominantly maintained by the Na$^+$,K$^+$-pump. Changes in the number or efficiency of these pumps would result in an alteration in the maximum capacity of the cell to perform active Na$^+$, K$^+$ transport.[259] The potassium, calcium, magnesium, thyroid, energy status, and training stage may all affect the concentration and efficiency of these pumps.[68, 259–262] In addition, suppression of the pumps could result in a severe impairment in the capacity to clear potassium from plasma, which is of special importance during exercise and following potassium absorption from the gastrointestinal tract.[262, 263] Altered potassium distribution has been suggested to affect functional properties such as membrane potential, action potential, and excitation-contraction coupling in muscle fibers.[264]

Possible Triggering Factors

Possible contributory triggering factors may include temperament, management, nutrition, concurrent disease, weather, time of year, hormonal imbalances, and so on. The final triggering factor is usually movement. Cases following transportation have been reported.

Epidemiology

Unfortunately, few extensive surveys into the epidemiology of this syndrome have been undertaken, although some underlying factors have been implicated. These are now discussed.

Environmental Conditions

Inclement weather has often been cited as causing an increase in incidence, as has the time of year.[200, 203] Compared to the submission of samples from non-equine rhabdomyolysis sufferers in a recent survey over a 2-year period in the United Kingdom, significantly more samples were submitted from equine rhabdomyolysis sufferers in the period November to February than during other times of the year.[101, 265]

Sex

It has been suggested that fillies and mares, especially those with a history of nymphomania or granulosa cell tumors, are more commonly affected than colts.[61] Young fillies in training in particular appear to be more susceptible.[60] A recent epidemiological survey carried out in the United Kingdom confirmed that females are more likely than males to suffer from this condition, particularly in the 0- to 2-year-old and 5- to 6-year-old age groups.[101, 265] However, an equal sex ratio was reported in another study.[118]

Genetic Factors

A familial predisposition has been postulated.[60] When the homogeneity of 15 blood group systems was compared, sufferers of equine rhabdomyolysis were shown to differ significantly from a control population of standardbreds.[114] Of the 29 reported cases of polysaccharide storage myopathy (PSM) recently reported, 24 had available pedigrees. Of these animals, 20 were found to be related to one stallion and 13 were related to a second stallion. The two stallions had a linked common blood line. It therefore has been suggested that there may be a familial basis for this condition and although heritability has not been proven, it is a possibility.

No breed incidence has been reported in the literature, although it has been suggested that heavily built horses have a higher incidence of muscle-related problems.[238] In a recent survey in the United Kingdom[265] it was shown that the syndrome can occur in many breeds and types. There was an apparent bias to the Thoroughbred, perhaps reflecting the location and clientele of the referral center and the popularity of this breed for competitive riding in the United Kingdom.[101, 265] Four percent of owners in this survey knew of a sufferer related to their own animal.

Exogenous or Endogenous Cortisol

In 37% of cases in one study the clinical signs developed 3 to 5 days after treatment with corticosteroids and it was suggested that most horses were subjected to a stress condition prior to development of the myopathy.[202] Prior treatment with steroids was not a recognized factor in a recent survey in the United Kingdom.[101, 265]

Sufferers of Polysaccharide Storage Myopathy

The animals that have been demonstrated to have polysaccharide storage myopathy tend to have a calm and sedate manner. Most of those investigated to date have suffered numerous episodes, typically commencing at the start of training, but a few have suffered only one or two episodes a year. The clinical signs tend to vary in severity from mild to severe, and fatalities have been reported. To date more mares than geldings have been diagnosed as suffering from this condition.

Miscellaneous Factors

Fat, poorly conditioned animals of any age have been suggested to be more susceptible to the condition[266] although this has not been our finding. Foaling and release to pasture in the spring have been anecdotally noted to be associated with the condition. Traditionally, equine rhabdomyolysis was seen in susceptible animals that had been rested without a reduction in feed intake. This type of case now appears to be less commonly reported.

Clinical Signs

The clinical signs of equine rhabdomyolosis tend to occur intermittently during or after exercise but they have been reported in nonexercising animals.[101, 203] Clinical signs vary from a slight stiffness or shortening of the stride to a total inability to move, and sometimes recumbency. Death can occur. Usually the croup, loin, and thigh muscle groups are involved bilaterally, although proximal muscles of the forelimb(s) and other muscle groups may be clinically affected on their own or in combination. The affected muscles may become swollen and appear firm on palpation, which may be resented. Discolored urine is not usually present in mildly affected animals.

The syndrome has been divided by one worker into three forms[230]: (1) a mild acute form, which occurs after exercise once the animal has returned to its stall or box; (2) an intermediate form, which occurs after 20 to 30 minutes of exercise, when the animal may become recumbent and demonstrate myoglobinuria on return to its box; and (3) a severe form, which occurs after 10 to 20 minutes of exercise when the affected animal is often unable to move and usually becomes recumbent. The last has a poor prognosis. The severity of the condition cannot always, however, be related to the intensity or duration of the triggering exercise. Therefore, it may be preferable to divide the condition according to the severity of the stiffness and the auxiliary signs (Table 8–9). This is the grading currently used by us.

Little information is available on the prevalence of cardiac muscle involvement in this condition. In one study functional disturbances of the heart were found clinically and confirmed by histopathologic lesions in 85% of the cases.[267]

Polysaccharide Storage Myopathy

These animals tend to show limited exercise tolerance, which becomes especially marked at higher speeds. The animals commonly are reported to stretch out after exercise, and dimpling of the flank and muscle fasciculations may be seen. They tend to have persistently elevated CK activities following 15 minutes lunging even if only very mild clinical signs are observed. The CK activities can be higher the following day and in some may be persistently elevated even between episodes.[47a]

Diagnosis

Many conditions have been included in the differential diagnosis of equine rhabdomyolysis (Table 8–10). Originally the diagnosis was thought to be simple[268] but recently even the so-called pathognomonic sign of discolored urine[77] has been recognized in other conditions, such as acorn poisoning.[64] The diagnosis is further complicated because gastrointestinal disturbances (colic) and other conditions may occur before, during, or after an attack of equine rhabdomyolysis.[61, 269, 270]

Laboratory Findings

The clinical diagnosis relies on an accurate clinical history followed by a thorough physical examination. Laboratory investigations often are required to confirm the provisional diagnosis and to monitor recovery. Various aids have been used in the diagnosis, the most important of which are the serum and plasma muscle enzyme activities. In addition, analysis of muscle biopsy tissue, EMG, and urinalysis may be of value. In fatal cases a postmortem examination should confirm the diagnosis.

Plasma and Serum Muscle Enzyme Activities

Increases in total plasma and serum CK and AST activities in equine rhabdomyolysis were first reported in the

Table 8–9. Equine Rhabdomyolysis Syndrome Graded According to Clinical Severity*†

Clinical Signs	Grade				
	1	2	3	4	5
Mobility	Slight stiffness, shortened stride	Reluctant to move	Unable to move	Unable to move, may become transiently recumbent	Rapidly becomes recumbent
Muscle	NAD NAD	Often	± Firm and swollen, resents palpation	Firm and swollen, may not resent palpation	Firm ± wasting
Exessive sweating	−	±	+	+ +	+ +
Pulse and respiratory rates elevated above expected levels	−	±	+	+ +	+ + +
Signs normally attributed to GI tract disturbances	−	±	+	+ +	+ + +
Discolored urine	−	±	+	+ +	+ + +
Comments	Easily confused with other conditions			Pain in response to palpation	GI tract stasis can occur; shock may develop; death may occur

*Data from Harris PA: Equine rhabdomyolysis syndrome. *Equine Pract* 11:3, 1989.
†Key: NAD, no abnormality detected; GI, gastrointestinal; −, absent; ±, sometimes present; +, usually present; + +, prominent; + + +, severe.

1960s.[87, 271] It has been suggested that although AST activities would increase slightly with mild muscle inflammation and liver disease, much higher values were likely to be found in acute equine rhabdomyolysis.[272] Significant increases in plasma LDH have also been reported in equine rhabdomyolysis.[77, 272] A selective elevation of LDH_4 and LDH_5 was reported by one group,[273] but there was also some elevation of LDH_3, LDH_2, and LDH_1.

The time at which peak circulating activities of these enzymes may be found following an attack of equine rhabdomyolysis has been reported as 3 to 15 hours for CK and 24 hours for LDH and AST. The time to return to the preattack activities has been given as 1 to 7 days for CK, 5 to 10 days for LDH, and 2 to 4 weeks for AST, depending on the extent of the initial increase[49, 77, 87, 101, 273] (Fig. 8–8). These differences allow the simultaneously measured AST and CK activities to be used to indicate whether the muscular damage is active or resolving. A combination of total and isoenzyme activities may also be useful. An increase in the CK MM and LDH_5 isoenzymes appears more likely to occur in equine rhabdomyolysis cases with a quick recovery time, whereas those with an increase in CK MM plus CK MB with LDH_1 and LDH_5 have a poor prognosis according to one report.[274]

The rise in enzyme activities may be proportional to the degree of muscle fiber damage[114] as well as the clinical severity.[49] However, some cases of grade 2 clinical severity (see Fig. 8–8) have been found to have markedly higher CK and AST activities than cases showing signs typical of a higher grade of clinical severity[101] (Fig. 8–9). A partial explanation may be that animals have different pain thresholds and the nature or temperament of the horse may be important.[67] Also, damage to certain muscle groups may be more painful than damage to others. Some affected horses

Taber 8–10. Differential Diagnosis of Equine Rhabdomyolysis*

Anthrax
Castration sequelae
Colic
Cystitis
Spinal cord disease ("wobbles")
Hernia
Iliac thrombosis
Inguinal/popliteal lymphadenitis
Laminitis
Nephritis
White muscle disease
Pleuritis
Acorn poisoning
Postexhaustion syndrome
Tetanus
"Back" problems
Proximal limb lamenesses
Monensin poisoning

*Data from references 66, 67, 194, 206, 283, 300.

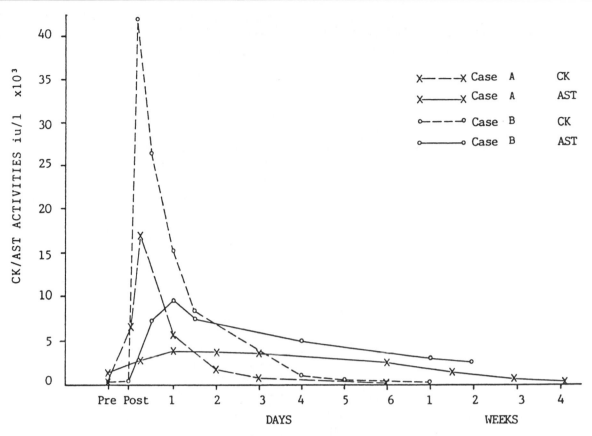

Figure 8–8. Plasma aspartate aminotransferase (*AST*) and creatine kinase (*CK*) activity changes following two cases of the equine rhabdomyolysis syndrome. Both cases suffered an episode of grade 2 clinical severity.

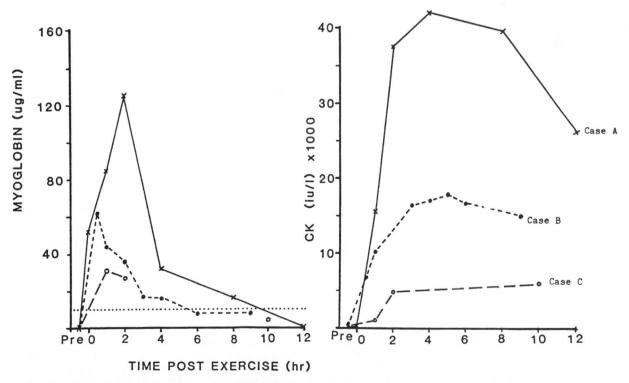

Figure 8–9. Changes in serum myoglobin and creatine kinase values in three cases of equine rhabdomyolysis. Cases *A* and *B* are the same as depicted in Figure 8–8 and had suffered grade 2 clinical severity episodes. Case *C* had suffered a grade 3 clinical severity episode.

may suffer localized, limited but severe in nature, muscular involvement, resulting in a high clinical grade episode without markedly elevated activities. Another possibility is that some animals suffer a mild but generalized pathologic increase in cell permeability, which results in a marked increase in plasma muscle enzyme activities but little overt muscular damage and pain.

Using muscle enzyme activities alone to make a diagnosis of equine rhabdomyolysis has been questioned. Problems with diagnosis can arise when either elevated plasma enzyme activities without clinical signs, or clinical signs without increased activities, are found. Mild clinical signs can be missed[84, 87] and it is possible that a more detailed examination of the stride length and limb positioning of those animals with high activities and no clinical signs may reveal abnormalities not obviously apparent. Several apparently healthy endurance animals have been reported to have elevated resting plasma enzyme activities.[275] Following endurance rides, high CK activities were found in some animals that returned toward baseline values within 24 hours without clinical signs of muscular damage.[275] The increase in CK in these cases could not be correlated with poor performance or postexercise signs of fatigue. These elevated levels possibly reflect an altered state of muscle metabolism caused by the endurance exercise. Such changes appear to be confined to individuals and do not appear to be a general finding. This suggests that the physiologic or pathologic processes involved are unique to the individual(s) rather than being linked to endurance riding alone. Certainly high plasma CK and AST activities have been recorded in endurance horses suffering from equine rhabdomyolysis, and other workers have shown that those horses with an optimal rate of heart rate recovery have lower increases in plasma CK.[103] It may be that animals with raised activities that return toward baseline values 24 hours post exercise may just be showing a normal variation in the physiologic response to exercise. Alternatively, this may reflect an increased sensitivity of the cell membrane to those processes that cause an alteration in its permeability. If the latter be the case, such a response may be abnormal and could indicate a predisposition to muscular damage or equine rhabdomyolysis. There may be physiologic variations among individuals in the way CK is cleared, for example.

Clinical signs without raised enzyme activities may represent a misdiagnosis (see Table 8–11). Another possibility is that in some cases there is insufficient muscle mass damage to cause a significant rise in plasma enzyme activities, even though the damage is sufficient to cause overt signs of myopathy and pain. There may also be a condition, akin to severe muscle cramps in humans, with a completely different pathophysiology that results in spasm of muscles without the cellular damage associated with equine rhabdomyolysis.

Measuring plasma CK and AST activities before and after a controlled period of exercise has been suggested as an aid to diagnosis.[67] A prolonged submaximal exercise test may be of more value in precipitating marked changes in CK activities and overt attacks of rhabdomyolysis.[217] Changes in activities need to be compared with those of normal horses exercised and sampled in the same manner, because of the physiologic exercise-induced rise in CK activities.

The results of any exercise test have also to be interpreted along with the clinical history and the type of exercise undertaken. Often between clinical attacks, a sufferer of this syndrome will have a normal response to an exercise test.[101] Therefore, a normal exercise test does not eliminate the condition from the differential diagnosis.

Other Enzyme Changes

Changes in other serum enzyme activities during and after an attack of equine rhabdomyolysis have been examined by several workers. In a group of relatively mild cases, the levels of SDH and γ-glutamyltransferase (GGT) remained within their normal ranges.[273] However, fairly marked increases in SDH have been reported in more severe cases,[77] although this was partially attributed to concurrent kidney damage. Aldolase has been found to be a sensitive indicator of muscle damage but less specific than CK, as it can be influenced by liver damage.[77]

Blood Acid-Base and Electrolyte Balance

The acid-base status and electrolyte balance appear to be similar in animals that are affected by this condition and apparently also in normal animals that have undergone the same intensity and duration of exercise.[230] A metabolic alkalosis has, therefore, been found in animals that suffer attacks after submaximal exercise.[213] Significantly lower RBC potassium concentrations have been reported in horses that have had signs of a myopathy (stiffness plus raised CK activities) within 48 hours of the blood sample being collected.[276] It was suggested that either an alteration in potassium balance was related to the pathogenesis of the myopathies or this occurred secondary to the process that caused the myopathies. Decreases in RBC potassium values have, however, been found following intensive exercise in several healthy animals. There is also considerable dispute over whether these anuclear RBCs are representative of the whole-body status. Further work is needed to investigate this area in more detail.

Plasma Urea and Glucose

Plasma urea concentrations are elevated when renal compromise occurs secondary to an episode of equine rhabdomyolysis. It should be noted, however, that plasma urea levels can be significantly elevated following exercise, especially long-distance rides, in horses unaffected by this condition. Significantly higher preexercise and 1-hour postexercise blood glucose concentrations were found in a group of affected animals compared with a control group.[230]

Plasma Myoglobin

Myoglobin was found to peak earlier than CK in the plasma of clinical rhabdomyolysis sufferers[101, 202a] (see Fig. 8–9). The levels of plasma myoglobin recorded were similar to those found by other workers[73, 74] and it has been suggested that myoglobin is a good indicator of muscle necrosis.[74, 202a] The rapid disappearance of myoglobin from the plasma soon after an attack of rhabdomyolysis may be explained by its rapid elimination by the kidney.[277]

Table 8–11. Therapeutic Agents Likely to Be of Benefit in the Equine Rhabdomyolysis Syndrome

Analgesics

Care must be taken if condition complicated by other disease processes

1. Phenylbutazone   ⎫ Most commonly used, but care needed if renal compromise has occurred because of potential
2. Flunixin meglumine ⎬ nephrotoxicity
3. Meclofenamic acid ⎭
4. Butorphanol

Sedatives, Tranquilizers

1. Phenothiazine derivatives (*Note:* α-blockade could lead to hypovolemia and shock)
2. Xylazine
3. Detomidine
4. Diazepam

Corticosteroids

May be of use during initial acute stages to (a) perhaps stabilize cellular membranes; (b) relax capillary sphincters, which
  may help improve tissue perfusion; but possibly only indicated in more severe cases

Fluids

Very important, especially in grades 3, 4, and 5

1. Oral fluids: probably adequate only for grade 3
2. Oral and IV fluids may be needed for grades 4 ad 5
3. Type depends on exercise given prior to the episode: usually balanced electrolyte solutions IV plus half-strength oral
   supplement PO.
4. In severe cases (grades 4 and 5); advisable to regularly check electrolyte and acid-basc status
5. Probably maintain fluid therapy until urine is free of pigmentation
6. Diuretics should be avoided (may potentiate alkalosis and exacerbate electrolyte abnormalities)

Histology

A focal distribution of hyaline degeneration (mainly in the fast-twitch type II fibers) with an insignificant inflammatory reaction and slight calcification was shown in one of the most extensive studies.[202] In another investigation, evidence of segmental muscle fiber degeneration was found in biopsies taken 24 hours after clinical signs of soreness and raised enzyme activities had been seen.[38] Additionally, in this study the gluteus medius muscle fibers in affected animals were found to be larger in cross-sectional area than those of control horses and there was a preferential degeneration of type II fibers.[38] Other histologic findings include increased perimysial and endomysial connective tissue, ring fibers, and subsarcoplasmic masses.[66, 202a, 215] Not all workers have found such diagnostic histologic lesions, even in chronic cases.[278] Also, certain lesions found in equine rhabdomyolysis can be seen in other conditions.[215]

The various morphologic and enzymatic changes that occur following an attack have been reported in depth.[227, 230] Such techniques are, however, unlikely to be used by veterinary practitioners in their diagnosis. In addition, there are several problems inherent in relying on muscle biopsy samples for a definitive diagnosis. Firstly, the relatively small sample size, the nonhomogeneous distribution of lesions, and the differences in the extent and location of the damage to the biopsied muscle mean that pathologic lesions may not always be seen in such biopsies. This has been found by workers using biopsies taken from the middle gluteal,[227] semimembranosus,[235] and omobrachialis[239] muscles. Secondly, between attacks it is unlikely that any diagnostic abnormality would be seen on a routine light microscopic study of the muscles. Even during an episode the type of pathologic lesion found may not be diagnostic of the underlying condition. These problems have also been reported in humans when specific and more complicated histochemical stains are not used or electron microscopy is not carried out.[44, 45]

Polysaccharide Storage Myopathy

Confirmation of the presence of the recently identified polysaccharide storage myopathy is via examination of biopsy material from the gluteal, semimembranosus, or biceps femoris muscle.[47a]

Postmortem Findings

The gross postmortem changes tend to be extensive, and are most likely to be found in the dorsal and central lumbar masses, the gluteals, and the quadriceps. Sometimes the affected muscles show little obvious abnormalities "other than moderate swelling and distinct pallor with an increased amount of interstitial fluid."[35] Other muscles may have patchy areas of grayish-yellow friable tissue, often with small hemorrhagic spots.[35] Hyaline myocardial degeneration may be found in some case.[35, 38] Renal changes with pigmented, tubular casts are frequently found.

Urinalysis

The presence of dark or coffee-colored urine was described in the earliest reports of this condition and there were many theories as to its cause. By the end of the nineteenth century it was suggested that the dark color was caused by the products of muscle degeneration[279] and this was later confirmed.[210] Visible darkening of the urine was suggested to occur if the concentration of myoglobin exceeded about 40 mg/100 mL.[60] However, a similar discoloration can occur with hemoglobin (see Fig. 8–4) and it has been suggested that some patients with equine rhabdomyolysis void hemoglobin in addition to myoglobin,[66, 67] although this is very rare in our experience.

Renal damage may occur due to circulatory disturbances and the precipitation of myoglobin in the renal tubules. Urinary FE excretion values, together with other urinary indices such as osmolarity, may help to detect early renal damage.[67, 272, 280]

Miscellaneous Findings

An altered phospholipid distribution in the semimembranosus muscle of horses with rhabdomyolysis has been found.[281] The authors could not determine if this was a cause or a consequence of the condition.

Electromyography

The EMG abnormalities seen in chronic myositis and equine rhabdomyolysis include fibrillation potentials and abnormal sharp waves.[67, 215] At present this technique is rarely used for the diagnosis of equine rhabdomyolysis.

Outcome and Prognosis

Initial Prognosis

The prognosis has been stated to vary from excellent for mild cases to grave for horses that become recumbent or develop renal complications.[49] Apparent transient femoral and peroneal paralysis has been reported a few days after attacks of equine rhabdomyolysis.[282]

Long-term Prognosis

Certain isoenzyme combinations have been suggested to reflect a poorer prognosis with the development of chronic complications, while other combinations carry a better prognosis.[273, 274] It has been reported that loss of muscular power can remain for a long time[283] and in some cases fibrosis may occur leading to gait abnormalities and disfigurement,[284] although persistent muscle dysfunction is unlikely if the attacks are mild, even if they are repeated.[67] The repair of damaged muscle fibers tends to be by myoblastic regeneration and hypertrophy.[38]

Young horses may be more likely to suffer recurrent attacks, but the frequency usually decreases with age.[284] However, a less optimistic outlook has been expressed[200] to the extent that it has been recommended that if there are multiple cases within a family, the animals should not be used for breeding.[67]

Overall, in cases where the potential contributory triggering factors can be identified and where appropriate management and nutritional safeguards can be instituted, further episodes may not occur. The risk of recurrence may be decreased further if the horse returns to work without a second episode. However, especially when there appears to be no common set of triggering factors, appropriate changes in diet and management have been undertaken, and the episodes occur once back in full work. An animal that suffers repeated episodes is more likely to suffer another episode at some indeterminable point in the future. The return to work after an episode appears to be a "high risk" time for a repeat episode.

Treatment

It can be very difficult to differentiate between rhabdomyolysis and other nontraumatic, postexertional conditions, especially overexertion and pulled muscles and tendons. Mild cases of all these conditions may respond favorably to walking. However, forced walking can increase the severity of rhabdomyolysis by exacerbating the muscle damage. Complete rest is therefore advisable unless it is certain that mild overexertion, for example, is the cause. Transporting affected animals in trailers may also precipitate a more severe episode because of the muscular effort required to maintain position.

The feed intake should be reduced, in severe cases to just grass, hay, and water. If necessary, low-energy, low-protein compounded cubes can be fed. The animals should be kept warm and dry. If they become recumbent, it is advisable to allow them to lie quietly in a well-padded stall with access to water, feed, etc. Animals should not be forced to rise, but assisted to do so as soon as possible. In all instances it is of particular importance to check the hydration status to see that water intake is adequate and that urination is normal. In some cases urinary catheterization may be required (see Chapter 16).

Initial Therapy

Treatment is undertaken to limit further muscular damage and to reduce pain and anxiety. If necessary, fluids and electrolytes should be given to maintain adequate hydration and kidney function. The treatment required will vary with the individual and the clinical severity, for example, in mild cases (i.e., clinical severity grade 1 and sometimes grade 2), analgesics are not always needed, nor is fluid therapy.

The commonly recommended therapeutic agents are shown in Table 8–11. As each theory on the possible pathogenesis of ERS is introduced, new treatments have evolved to correct the supposed abnormality.

Sodium Bicarbonate. There is a great deal of controversy regarding the role of lactic acid in this syndrome. In fact, many patients have been shown to have a metabolic alkalosis. Therefore, it is not advisable to administer sodium bicarbonate unless the acid-base status is known. It is suggested that bicarbonate should not be given unless the plasma bicarbonate concentration is less than 15 mEq/L.[188]

Vitamin E and Selenium. Most workers have found no correlation between vitamin E and selenium status and ERS. However, it has been suggested that these two substances may have some value in treatment in view of their action against tissue-damaging free radicals.[101] Vitamin E–selenium combinations should not be injected intravenously.

Methocarbamol. This is a muscle relaxant that supposedly acts to decrease pain by reducing muscle spasms. However, animals can become ataxic and depressed and workers have found it of little value.[61, 284, 285]

Thiamine. A dose of 500 mg has been recommended.[188] Brewer's yeast 28 g/day has also been suggested as an alternative source of B vitamins. There is, however, no evidence for the validity of using thiamine or of its efficacy.

Dantrolene. See Prevention.

Miscellaneous Therapy. ACTH, other B vitamins, dimethyl sulfoxide (DMSO), and sodium salicylate have also been suggested.[61, 187, 272] A serotonin S$_2$ antagonist (R 50 970, metrenperone), has been reported to be of value both clinically and histologically in a group of horses with chronic myopathies[286] and it was suggested that serotonin is involved in the pathologic changes and the poor performance observed in such cases. The cause of the chronic myopathies in this report was not, however, ascertained.

Further Therapy

The nature of the treatment needed after the initial stages and the speed at which the animal can return to work depend on the severity of the episode and the clinical history. Often no treatment is needed in the convalescent period, although in more severely affected cases oral NSAIDs may be of value.

After a period of stall rest (the length of which depends on the severity of the attack), the animal, whenever possible, should be turned out into a small paddock (lush pastures with high soluble carbohydrate content should be avoided) before any riding or walking exercise is given. The animal should be moving freely in the stable, with no signs of pain or discolored urine and no resentment of muscle palpation before turn out. Very occasionally sedation may be required when initially turning out. The animal should not be allowed to become chilled. The length of time between turn out and the start of ridden exercise will vary from days to weeks according to the individual circumstances. In recurrent sufferers it may be advisable to rest the horse until AST and CK levels have returned to within the normal resting range, or at least until the CK activities are less than half the peak recorded. Longeing is not advisable in the early stages of return to work. Exercise should be increased gradually and the feed adjusted accordingly.

As balanced a diet as possible should be fed, which should

have limited energy provided from soluble carbohydrate sources. The use of cereal grains, especially oats, at least in large amounts, should be avoided as far as possible. Intake levels should be low initially, and the diet should deliver initially a lower energy intake than theoretically required by the animal and the energy intake in general should be kept behind the anticipated workload. Therefore, recommended diets tend to be more fiber than cereal based. The use of fat/oil as an additional energy source has been of anecdotal success in a number of cases, in combination with other appropriate management changes. Care should be taken that the intake of minerals (especially sodium in heavily sweating animals), trace elements, and vitamins is sufficient for the long term if feeding less than manufacturer's recommended intakes. In recurrent sufferers it may be of benefit to carry out an "exercise test" after a week and again after 4 weeks. At each stage samples should be collected before and 2 to 6 hours post exercise. The exercise undertaken should be considered as a hard workout, but should not be overstrenuous, and the horse must have worked at a similar intensity and for a similar duration in the recent past. No significant increase in AST or CK activities (see above) following such an "exercise test" would suggest that detectable muscular damage was not occurring with each exercise bout. It does not, however, mean that the animal will not suffer an episode of rhabdomyolysis in the near future. Checking Fe values after being on a balanced diet for a minimum of 2 weeks may be of value.

Prevention

Management

The history of the first reported cases[231] typically stated that the clinical signs occurred after the animal had been exercised following a period of rest, that is, classic Monday morning disease in heavy draught horses. With the decline of the heavy horse and an increasing awareness of good horse management, fewer such cases are seen. However, cases are occasionally reported in saddle horses and racehorses if they are rested without any decrease in feed intake. Therefore, the first stage of any preventive regimen is to ensure a well-balanced and controlled exercise and feeding regimen. A balanced diet should be fed according to the workload, and periods of inactivity should be accompanied by decreased feed intake.

Subjectively, regular exercise often appears to be of benefit, prolonged periods out on grass can also be of value, and some animals may benefit from being ridden while turned out on grass. Sometimes a change in the exercise pattern seems to be of value. Anecdotally, keeping a blanket over the lumbar area in cold weather has been recommended.

Prophylactic Agents

Thyroxine has been recommended when hypothyroidism has been detected,[235] although the optimal way to determine equine thyroid status is at present unclear. It has, however, been suggested that continuous monitoring should be carried out as the "hypothyroid" condition could spontaneously resolve.[67] It has also been stated that even if the thyroid status is not known it could be beneficial to administer levothyroxine at 0.01 mg/kg or iodinated casein 6 to 14 mg/kg.[61, 285] However, at least 10 mg of levothyroxine appears to be needed to increase the circulating T_4 and triiodothyronine (T_3) levels of resting horses (approximately 500 kg in weight).[287] Five to 10 mg/day given orally to sufferers with a reduced response to TRH has subjectively appeared to be beneficial in some cases (Harris, unpublished data). However, further evaluation is required, and efficacy remains unproven. The potential negative effects of suddenly ceasing high level thyroxine supplementation in the horse have not been fully evaluated.

Dantrolene. Dantrolene has been used in human medicine to treat and help prevent malignant hyperthermia. In this condition there appears to be an abnormal release of calcium from the sarcoplasmic reticulum resulting in prolonged contracture, hyperthermia, metabolic and respiratory acidosis, and muscle damage. Dantrolene is believed to decrease the rate of calcium release from the sarcoplasmic reticulum and to affect charge movement in the T-tubule system. It has been used in humans to treat recurrent exertional rhabdomyolysis.[288]

Although dantrolene sodium has been suggested for the treatment of equine rhabdomyolysis, it is more commonly used in prevention. Giving 2 mg/kg/day diluted in normal saline by a stomach tube for 3 to 5 days and then every third day for a month has been recommended.[61, 289] A lower daily dose (300 mg) may be equally beneficial[289] and perhaps preferable because the drug is hepatotoxic.[61] One regimen of 500 mg per os for 3 to 5 days, then 300 mg every third day for a period of time, has been used by the authors. The time period will depend on the circumstances and the individual effect on the liver, but prolonged treatment is not recommended. Monitoring of hepatic status and function is recommended because the effects on the liver seem to be individually variable. Up to 1 g of dantrolene, given with a small feed 1½ to 2 hours prior to exercise for 3 to 5 days has been used with apparent success in racehorses in the United Kingdom, but in some cases the horses may have been suffering from overexertion, for example, rather than the rhabdomyolysis syndrome. No controlled studies have been undertaken. In addition, it has been suggested that such doses are unlikely to reach therapeutic levels.[154] The drug appears not to be as bioavailable in the horse as in humans and is cleared more quickly.[154] It is unlikely to be of such use in these animals that suffer episodes infrequently. Care must be taken with its use, and efficacy remains uncertain.

Sodium Bicarbonate. The addition of alkali syrup or sodium bicarbonate to the feed of horses prone to equine rhabdomyolysis has often been carried out by owners, trainers, and veterinary surgeons. Thus, 2 to 4 oz, for example, has been recommended to be fed daily to help prevent "azoturia."[290] One patient, which had suffered repeated attacks despite vitamin E, selenium, dantrolene, corticosteroids, ACTH, promazine, and flunixin administration, apparently improved clinically with the feeding of sodium bicarbonate, although marked increases in CK activities still occurred with exercise.[278] It has been suggested that the sodium bicarbonate acts to facilitate the removal of hydrogen ions from the cell, to increase the buffering protection on both sides of the muscle cell membrane, and to increase the efflux of lactate from muscle into the blood.[278, 291] However, work in humans has shown that bicarbonate has little effect on intramuscular buffering as the sarcolemma is impermeable to bicarbonate ions.[292] The efficacy of sodium bicarbonate in the prevention of equine rhabdomyolysis has not been proved. It is a possibility that any beneficial effect is due to the sodium content, and care may be needed if sufficient sodium bicarbonate is added to affect the cation–anion balance of the diet especially if the animal is likely to suffer periods of dehydration.

Vitamin E and Selenium. Many workers have reported beneficial effects, especially in problem cases, from the administration, either orally or parenterally, of vitamin E and selenium.[220, 293] It has been noted that the beneficial effects of these compounds are often difficult to assess as they are often given in addition to changes in diet and exercise.[270] It is possible that any effect is due to limitation/prevention of free radical induced muscle damage. Oral administration is preferable to intermittent injection.

Electrolytes. Recent work has suggested that for some animals the feeding of an appropriate electrolyte supplement based on the results of an FE test may be of value in preventing episodes.[251, 251a] Because many horse diets are imbalanced with respect to their electrolyte intake, it is likely that many apparently normal animals may have abnormal FE values. It is possible that some animals are better able to adjust to such diets than others, or that they present with different clinical problems. Ideally, affected horses· should be fed a balanced and adequate diet and investigative steps taken, as illustrated in Figure 8–10.

It is very difficult to prove the efficacy of any preventive measure recommended for this condition. First, the intermittent nature of the syndrome means that it is difficult to determine if the animal would have suffered further episodes if the electrolyte supplementation or other preventive agent had not been given. Second, there is no test or indicator that can, without controversy, confirm that an animal is, has, or will suffer from this condition. Third, there are ethical problems in reproducing the condition, especially in referred clinical cases, by asking the owners to stop feeding an apparently beneficial supplement. In one study[251] eight of the 72 cases that were apparently helped by supplementation had their supplementation stopped. In all cases this resulted in the recurrence of the syndrome. Restoration of the advised supplementation resulted in no further attacks. This work does *not,* however, confirm the role of electrolyte imbalances in the syndrome, but it does suggest that the correction of any imbalance may be of value in prevention.

Phenytoin. This has been used with some success.[168] Differences in the in vitro muscle twitch parameters of surgically removed muscle tissue have been demonstrated in animals suffering from the rhabdomyolysis syndrome and in control animals. Administration of phenytoin resulted, in some cases, in a clinical improvement as well as normalization of the in vitro twitch characteristics. This may be related to the possible effects of phenytoin on neurotransmitters at the neuromuscular junction, on the release of calcium from

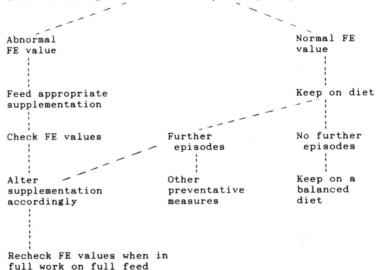

```
                    FEED   ADEQUATE  AND  BALANCED  DIET
                (for  at  least  2  weeks   prior   to  sampling)



          Collect paired urine and heparinized blood samples

          1    Urine  should  be  a  freely  voided  sample.  In
               mares/fillies  only,  catheterisation  is  acceptable  if  a
               brief  trot  is  given  first.

          2    Samples  should  be  collected  at  least  5  days  after  a
               rhabdomyolysis  episode.

          3    Plasma  should  be  separated  as  soon  as  possible  after
               collection.



          Determine  fractional  electrolyte  excretion  (FE)  values  for
                        Na,  K,  Cl,  Ca,  Mg,  PO4
          (N.B.  Ca  and  Mg  via  Atomic  absorption  spectophotometry)


          Abnormal                                    Normal FE
          FE value                                    value


          Feed appropriate                            Keep on diet
          supplementation


          Check FE values          Further            No further
                                   episodes           episodes


          Alter                    Other              Keep on a
          supplementation          preventative       balanced
          accordingly              measures           diet


          Recheck FE values when in
          full work on full feed
```

Figure 8–10. Protocol for the use of the fractional electrolyte excretion test in clinical cases of the equine rhabdomyolysis syndrome.

the sarcoplasmic reticulum, or on sodium fluxes across the plasmalemma. The following preventive protocol has been recommended.[118] Initial oral dosing should start at 10 to 12 mg/kg b.i.d. for several days unless side effects are seen (such as tranquilization or seizures). Blood concentrations of phenytoin should then be checked and the dose adjusted to maintain blood levels at 5 to 10 μg/mL 4 to 6 hours post administration. In some cases a larger dose in the morning should be given with a smaller dose at night. Occasionally, administration is needed only once a day. Other suggested regimens include 8 to 12 mg/kg b.i.d. for 3 days, then 10 mg/kg t.i.d. for a week. Then start training, with or without continued treatment (5 to 6 mg/kg t.i.d.). The clearance of the drug varies among individuals, although 3 to 5 days has been reported as the time usually needed for the drug to become undetectable by existing laboratory methodology.[118] This should not, however, be taken as the definitive withdrawal period for all animals. It is advisable that other medications not be given concurrently as there is a risk of drug interaction and the potentiation of toxicity.[118] The investigative techniques used[118] are, however, highly inva-

sive and owing to the possible side effects of phenytoin this is often not practical as a routine measure. Further work in more cases followed over a longer period of time is needed before a true indication of the efficacy of this drug can be given.

Dimethylglycine (DMG). Dimethylglycine has been used as a nutritional supplement for horses with the aim of delaying fatigue by decreasing lactate production. It has also been reported to decrease the incidence of the rhabdomyolysis syndrome given at doses of around 1 mg/kg. However, recent studies have shown no beneficial cardiorespiratory or metabolic effects in the horse.[294] It is possible that the drug acts via a different mechanism to assist affected horses. However, again there have not been any scientifically documented reports as to its efficacy in this condition.

Methylsulfonylmethane (MSM). This drug is an oral additive that has been suggested to be a natural alternative to the steroidal and nonsteroidal anti-inflammatory agents. The exact mechanism of its action has not been elucidated and its use in this syndrome has yet to be shown clinically or scientifically. It is possible that it may be of more benefit therapeutically (instead of NSAIDs) than preventively. Its efficacy is unproven. The most common dosage is 5 to 15 g by mouth.

Miscellaneous Drugs. Small doses of phenothiazine tranquilizers, e.g., acepromazine (ACP) 0.01 to 0.02 mg/kg given about 30 minutes before exercise have been suggested to decrease the incidence of equine rhabdomyolysis, especially in anxious horses.[61] It has been suggested that ACP acts either as a vasodilator, resulting in increased blood flow, or as a tranquilizer, perhaps modifying the release of catecholamines. However, recent work showed that ACP did not alter circulating catecholamine levels measured either in anticipation of exercise or in the immediate postexercise period.[295] However, the study reported lower lactate concentrations at 2 and 30 minutes post exercise in the ACP-treated animals compared to the control group. In addition, there was a delayed return of RBC-potassium levels to normal concentrations after exercise. The authors suggested that ACP could act by either decreasing the production or increasing the clearance lactate. Alternatively, by influencing electrolyte movements ACP may alter neuromuscular activity.[295] Further work in this area is required. Diazepam 0.25 mg/kg IV has also been beneficial, primarily in horses that appear particularly anxious.

Other. Certain herbal preparations have anecdotally appeared to be of benefit in a number of cases. A wide variety of other preventive agents has been suggested over the years, including B vitamins and sodium salicylate.

Polysaccharide Storage Myopathy

Suggested preventive regimens for this condition are based on increasing the oxidative capacity of the skeletal muscle through gradual training and the provision of a high-fat diet. It has been recommended that the diet should be changed to one with a good quality grass hay, no grain or sweet feed, and the addition of a fat source if required, plus a balanced vitamin and mineral mix and additional selenium and vitamin E supplementation. Daily lunging or riding is recommended as is daily turn out.[47a]

Conclusion

Except for those individuals suffering from polysaccharide storage myopathy, to date, no single theory can explain why ERS occurs in one particular animal rather than others kept under identical management. Predisposing factor(s) and triggering factor(s) are unlikely to be identical in each case. Therefore, it is likely that affected animals may require different treatment and preventive measures and the methods that work for one may be of no value in others.

Examining the theory of electrolyte imbalances, for example, a variety of predisposing factors could result in a disturbance in the ionic balance of the cell, which could then result in cellular damage. Hypothyroidism, sodium depletion, potassium and calcium disturbances, or muscle ischemia

could each be important in different animals, but they could all result in the common endstage of rhabdomyolysis. An individual variation in electrolyte absorption or utilization, resulting in an individual animal having an inadequate electrolyte balance despite an apparently adequate diet, could be a partial explanation of why one animal out of a group (all kept under the same management regimen) is affected by this condition.

Research has been hampered by the lack of a diagnostic marker, the condition's intermittent nature and clinical variability, and inability to reproduce and reliably initiate the condition in large numbers of animals. Conclusions have often been based on only one or two cases. Finally, the relatively low incidence, low mortality, and intermittent nature of the syndrome means that the owner or trainer is often reluctant to pay for intensive investigations.

It may be beneficial if future work concentrates on ionic fluxes within muscle cells. Methods of quantifying abnormalities in ionic transport mechanisms could be of value. For example, rapid methods of determining the number of Na^+,K^+-pumps in muscle biopsy tissue have been developed and could be applied to muscle from clinical cases.[296]

A means of determining whether raised CK or AST activities post exercise, without clinical signs, is indicative or not of muscle damage or a predisposition to equine rhabdomyolysis is required. One possible method could involve the measurement of plasma and serum myoglobin. At present, myoglobin determinations are not available routinely and no work has been undertaken to look at the changes that may be seen with overexertion and pulled muscles, and so forth. In humans, carbonic anhydrase III (CA-III) has been suggested to be a more specific marker of skeletal muscle damage than myoglobin or CK and has been used to indicate skeletal muscle damage in rhabdomyolysis.[297] In the future the simultaneous measurement of myoglobin (released by all fiber types) as well as CA-III (released predominantly by type I fibers, at least in humans) may enable those animals with damage to the type II fibers (predominantly affected in equine rhabdomyolysis) to be detected. CA-III is present in high concentrations in the liver and thymus, and in humans the concentration has been seen to increase in the serum after long-distance running or intensive exercise.[298] This may preclude its use in the horse. Serum from clinically normal horses has been shown to have a very variable concentration of CA-III, which may also preclude the use of this test in the horse,[298] but further work is needed.

A specific diagnostic indicator or marker or a group of diagnostic criteria is needed to be able to state with confidence that animals showing such a factor or factors are suffering from this condition. It appears that the syndrome may differ between the young horse in training and the mature animal. In addition, the pathophysiology of episodes that occur consistently after hard exercise may be quite different from those that occur at rest or after light exercise. Thus it may be useful in the future to divide cases of equine rhabdomyolysis into subtypes depending on certain clinical criteria. The recent finding of a subgroup of sufferers with a specific pathophysiologic process gives support to the possibility that in the future cases of equine rhabdomyolysis may be divided into subtypes depending on certain clinical criteria or pathophysiologic process.

In summary, much more work is needed so that this

quotation from 1917 by Steffin, which applies today, is not still relevant in another 80 years. "No one disease of horses has been the subject of so many theories, theoretical treatments and hypothetical suggestions as this one."

Arthrogryposis

Arthrogryposis is a congenital developmental defect characterized by muscle contracture and fixation of various joints in extension and flexion. The primary defect in the majority of cases is believed to be in the skeletal or nervous system. Occasionally, it may be in the muscles. In such cases the muscles may show degenerative changes or atrophy and an increase in adipose and fibrous tissue. These changes may also be seen secondary to neurogenic defects and there is difficulty in distinguishing primary neuropathic from primary myopathic forms of the disease. This has resulted in patients being referred to as suffering from neuromuscular arthrogryposis[299] (Fig. 8–11). In one case, for example, a foal was born following an uncomplicated delivery with a single hindlimb fixed in a flexed position. This animal showed loss of the lower motor neuron cell bodies in the ventral horn of the spinal cord in segments L3–S4, as well as lesions in the peripheral nerves and muscles of the affected limb.[299] In humans the majority of cases are thought to be neurogenic with the majority arising from undefined

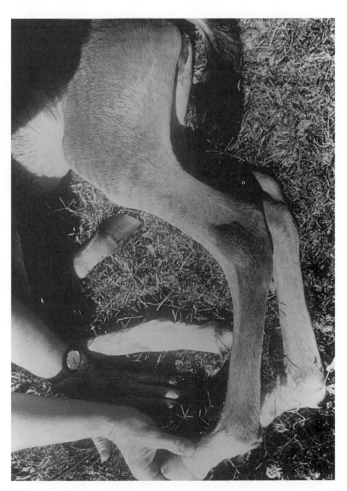

Figure 8–11. Arthrogryposis in a foal.

disturbances of the anterior horn cells. Skeletal malformations and connective tissue disorders are rare causes. The infrequent primary myopathic forms have been associated with various muscular dystrophies or myotonia, and strong hereditary factors.[299]

The cause of the primary abnormality in the horse is unknown, although genetic and environmental factors, such as unfavorable intrauterine conditions, uterine malpositioning, and maternal ingestion of locoweed or hybrid Sudan pasture, have been suggested.[35, 115, 299–302] In the horse, detailed examination of neuromuscular tissues has rarely been carried out and the majority of cases have simply been suggested to be skeletal in origin. Therefore, the relative importance of the primary neuropathic or myopathic condition is unknown.

The extent of the condition varies with involvement of one to four limbs and may include the axial skeleton. Often the more severely affected animals are born dead. Dystocia often occurs. Milder cases can occur. For example, foals may be born with an apparent inability to straighten one fetlock. Muscle loss tends not to be apparent in such cases, but affected muscles appear to have lost sarcomeres from the end of the myofibers (possibly due to prolonged flexion of the joint(s) in late gestation). Constant tension seems to result in the restoration of these sarcomeres.[35]

The recommended symptomatic treatment of arthrogryposis of any cause has included the use of splints, casts, and physiotherapy, as well as surgery,[303] the last having been very successful in human infants and calves.

MISCELLANEOUS IDIOPATHIC DISORDERS
Atypical Myoglobinuria

Sudden death from ERS is comparatively rare and usually occurs in an animal that has undergone some degree of exertion prior to the attack. Severe and often fatal attacks of a condition with similarities to ERS have been reported in the United Kingdom in groups of animals out at pasture with no history of sudden exertion.[304] The condition has been referred to as "atypical myoglobinuria."

Pathophysiology

Factors common to many of the atypical myoglobinuria cases include adverse climatic conditions prior to the outbreak and the availability of tree bark, often on dead wood. This atypical syndrome characteristically affects a group of horses over a short period of time, and therefore the possible predisposing trigger or etiologic factor(s) has been thought to be of an environmental or toxic nature. No consistent abnormality in selenium or GSHPx values has been seen. One case appeared to have a low liver vitamin E concentration, although another animal affected in the same outbreak had an apparently normal value.[304] In some, but not all cases, *Trichoderma* fungi were isolated from grass and wood taken from the fields grazed by the affected horses. Mycotoxins have therefore been suggested as being of possible significance.

No known access to toxins such as monensin or salinomycin was shown in any case. Oak trees with acorns were not always present and the gastrointestinal signs associated with acorn poisoning were not seen.[65] Spraying with an atrazine herbicide had occurred prior to one outbreak.[305] The simazine residues found were not thought to be at toxic levels and the clinical signs reported were not those seen with triazene herbicide toxicity, that is, severe colic, cessation of eating and drinking, and a dog-sitting posture.[304]

The cause of these atypical myoglobinuria cases has, therefore, not been identified. In patients that died, the precise cause of death was uncertain, but damage to the heart and diaphragm in association with biochemical alterations, such as hypocalcemia, may have been important. Renal failure may be a contributory cause, but is unlikely to be the primary cause of death. Further work needs to be undertaken to provide a better understanding of the pathogenesis.

More detailed investigation may reveal that a toxic factor is involved or, alternatively, may lead to the conclusion that this is just another variant of ERS.

Clinical Signs

The condition is most frequently found in horses and ponies at pasture that is often of low quality. One or more animals in a group may be affected. There is usually a sudden onset of stiffness that is unrelated to exertion, and this is soon followed by severe myoglobinuria. Temperature, pulse, and respiration rates are generally within the normal range. No age, sex, or breed predilection has been found, but too few cases have been investigated. Of cases that have been well documented, the rate of progression is rapid and mortality is high. Despite profound weakness and recumbency, many of the affected animals do not appear to be in any distress or pain, and they eat and drink well, even when recumbent. CK activities are markedly elevated and advanced myodegeneration of all muscles, including the heart, may be present.[304]

Histology

Myodegeneration indistinguishable from that seen in ERS at the light microscope level has been found (although fiber preference was not determined) together with myocardial lesions in some cases.[299] Large hyperchromatic hepatocyte nuclei were found in some liver sections together with patchy vacuolation and infiltration of neutrophils into the portal areas. Pink proteinaceous granular material tended to be present in the kidney tubules and within Bowman's capsule.[304] Skeletal abnormalities may not be obvious on gross postmortem examination.

Laboratory Findings

High CK activities (often > 50,000 IU/L) due to myodegeneration are found. AST levels also tend to be markedly elevated. Very high SDH values (up to 288 IU/L; laboratory reference range, 0.4–1.5 IU/L) were found in several cases in one investigation.[299] Hypocalcemia may occur, especially in the terminal stages. Myoglobin is usually present in a sufficiently high concentration in the urine to be detectable by electrophoresis on cellulose acetate.

Treatment

As the cause of the condition is unknown, symptomatic treatment is recommended, including intensive fluid therapy. This should be based on biochemical monitoring. The calcium status should be monitored, in particular, as horses may become hypocalcemic. Feeding a readily available source of calcium may be of benefit in some cases.

Postanesthetic Myasthenia

This has been reported in three horses.[306] The condition could be a form of botulism or a drug-induced myasthenia. The characteristic signs were a difficult recovery from anesthesia, lack of any facial expression, flaccid tongue, mydriasis, an inability to raise the head, and dysphagia. All three patients recovered totally with supportive care.

Polymyopathy

An aged pony mare developed a slowly progressive stiffness of gait that varied in severity. She was reluctant to move or eat and there was general loss of muscle bulk. The condition responded temporarily to NSAIDs. Needle EMG revealed a diffuse polymyopathy. Muscle histopathologic study revealed shrinkage, fragmentation, loss of muscle fibers, replacement of muscle bundles with adipose tissue, and some evidence of myofiber regeneration. The cause of the condition was unknown. Other cases of polymyopathy of unknown cause have been suspected in horses and await documentation and further categorization.

REFERENCES

1. Gunn HM: Muscle, bone and fat proportions and muscle distribution of thoroughbreds and other horses. In Gillespie JR, Robinson NE, eds: *Equine Exercise Physiology,* vol 2. Davis, Calif, ICEEP, 1987, p 253.
2. Hoppeler H, Jones JH, Linstedt SL, et al.: Relating maximal oxygen consumption to skeletal muscle mitochondria in horses. In Gillespie JR, Robinson NE, eds: *Equine Exercise Physiology,* vol 2. Davis, Calif, ICEEP, 1987, p 278.
3. Kayar SR, Hoppeler H, Essen-Gustavsson B, et al.: The similarity of mitochondrial distribution in equine skeletal muscles of differing oxidative capacity. *J Exp Biol* 137:253, 1988.
4. Kayar SR, Hoppeler H, Mermod L, et al.: Mitochondrial size and shape in equine skeletal muscle: A three dimensional reconstruction study. *Anat Rec* 222:233, 1988.
5. Andrews TM: Metabolic disorders of muscle. In Elkeles RS, Tavill AS, eds: *Biochemical Aspects of Human Diseases,* Oxford: Blackwell, 1983, p 157.
6. Cardinet GH: Skeletal muscle function. In Kaneko JJ, ed: *Clinical Biochemistry of Domestic Animals,* ed 4., San Diego, Academic Press, 1989, p 462.
7. Bechtel PJ, Lawrence LM: The muscles and athletic training. In Jones WE, ed: *Equine Sports Medicine,* Philadelphia, Lea & Febiger, 1989, p 121.
8. Barchi RL: The pathophysiology of excitation in skeletal muscle. In Walter J, ed: *Disorders of Voluntary Muscle,* Edinburgh, Churchill Livingstone, 1988, p 372.
9. Snow DH: Skeletal muscle adaptations: A review. In Snow

DH, Persson SGB, Rose RJ, eds: *Equine Exercise Physiology,* Cambridge, England, Granta Es, 1983, p 160.

10. Van den Hoven R, Wensing TL, Breukink HJ, et al.: Variation of fiber types in the triceps brachii, longissimus dorsi, gluteus medius and biceps femoris of horses. *Am J Vet Res* 46:939, 1985.

11. Andrews FM, Spurgeon TL: Histochemical staining characteristics of normal horse skeletal muscle. *Am J Vet Res* 47:1843, 1986.

12. Snow DH, Guy PS: Percutaneous needle biopsy in the horse. *Equine Vet J* 8:150, 1976.

13. Raub RR, Bechtel PJ, Lawrence LM: Variation in the distribution of muscle fiber types in equine skeletal muscles. *J Equine Vet Sci* 5:34, 1985.

14. Raub RH, Kline KK, Lawrence LM, et al.: Distribution of muscle fiber type in fetal equine gluteus medius muscle. *J Equine Vet Sci* 6:148, 1986.

15. Lopez-Rivero J, Aguera E, Vivo J, et al.: Histochemical and morphological study of the middle gluteal muscle in Arabian horses. *J Equine Vet Sci* 10:144, 1990.

16. Snow DH, Guy PS: Muscle fiber type composition of a number of limb muscles in different types of horse. *Res Vet Sci* 28:137, 1980.

17. Kline KH, Bechtel PJ: Changes in the metabolic profile of equine muscle from birth through one year of age. *J Appl Physiol* 68: 1399, 1990.

18. Kline KH, Bechtel PJ: Changes in the metabolic profile of the equine gluteus medius as a function of sampling depth (abstract). *Comp Biochem Physiol* 91A:815, 1988.

19. Hodgson DR, Rose RJ: Effects of a nine month endurance training programme on muscle composition in the horse. *Vet Rec* 121:271, 1987.

20. McMiken D: Muscle fiber types and horse performance. *Equine Prac* 8:6, 1986.

21. Hodgson DR, Rose RJ, DiMauro J, et al.: Effects of training on muscle composition in horses. *Am J Vet Res* 47:12, 1986.

22. Hodgson DR: Muscular adaptations to exercise and training. *Vet Clin North Am Equine Pract* 1:533, 1985.

23. Lindholm A, Essen-Gustavsson B, McMiken D, et al.: Muscle histochemistry and biochemistry of thoroughbred horses during growth and training. In Snow DH, Persson SGB, Rose RJ, eds: *Equine Exercise Physiology,* Cambridge, England, Granta, 1983, p 211.

24. Henkel P: Training and growth induced changes in the middle gluteal muscle of young standardbred trotters. *Equine Vet J* 15:134, 1983.

25. Essen-Gustavsson B, Lindholm A, McMiken D, et al.: Skeletal muscle characteristics of young standardbreds in relation to growth and early training. In Snow DH, Persson SGB, Rose RJ, eds: *Equine Exercise Physiology,* Cambridge, England, Granta, 1983, p 200.

26. Gottlieb-vedi M: *Circulating and Muscle Metabolic Responses to Draught Work of Varying Intensity and Duration in Standardbred Horses,* thesis, Uppsala, Sweden, 1988.

27. Essen-Gustavsson B, McMiken D, Karlstrom K, et al.: Muscular adaptation of horses during intensive training and detraining. *Equine Vet J* 21:27, 1989.

28. Foreman JH, Bayly WM, Allen JR, et al.: Muscle responses of thoroughbreds to conventional race training and detraining. *Am J Vet Res* 51:909, 1990.

29. Snow DH, Guy PS: Fiber type and enzyme activities of the m. gluteus medius in different breeds of horse. In Poortmans J, Niset G, eds: *Biochemistry of Exercise IVB.* Baltimore, University Park Press, 1981, p 275.

30. Wood CH, Ross TT, Armstrong JB, et al.: Variations in muscle fiber composition between successfully and unsuccessfully raced quarter horses. *J Equine Vet Sci* 8:217, 1988.

31. Davies AS: Muscle growth and innervation. In Alley MR, ed: *Diseases of Muscle and Peripheral Nerve. Proceedings of the 13th Annual Meeting of the New Zealand Society of Veterinary and Comparative Pathology,* 1983, p 10.

32. Cullen MJ, Landon PN: The ultrastructure of the motor unit. In Walton J, ed: *Disorders of Voluntary Muscle.* Edinburgh, Churchill Livingstone, 1988, p 27.

33. Hooper ACB: Quantitative aspects of postnatal changes in muscle mass (abstract). *J Anat* 161:223, 1988.

34. Stickland NC: Prenatal muscle development and its effect on postnatal growth. *J Anat* 161:223, 1988.

35. Hulland TJ: Muscles and tendons. In Jubb KVF, Kennedy PC, Palmer N, eds: *Pathology of Domestic Animals,* ed 3., Orlando, Fla, Academic Press, 1985, p 139.

36. Draeger A, Weeds AG, Fitzsimons RB: Primary, secondary and tertiary myotubes in developing skeletal muscle: A new approach to the analysis of human myogenesis. *J Neurol Sci* 81:19, 1987.

37. Uehara N, Sawazaki H, Mochizuki K: Changes in the skeletal muscles volume in horses with growth. *Jpn J Vet Sci* 47:161, 1985.

38. McEwen SA, Hulland TJ: Histochemical and morphometric evaluation of skeletal muscle from horses with exertional rhabdomyolysis (tying-up). *Vet Pathol* 23:400, 1986.

39. Wrongemann K, Pena SDJ: Mitochondrial calcium overload: A general mechanism for cell necrosis in muscle disease. *Lancet* 1:672, 1976.

40. Jackson MJ: Intracellular calcium, cell injury and relationships to free radicals and fatty acid metabolism. *Proc Nutr Soc* 49:77, 1990.

41. Oredsson S, Plate G, Qwvarfordt P: Allopurinol—a free radical scavenger reduces reperfusion injury in skeletal muscle. *Eur J Vasc Surg* 5:47, 1991.

42. Astrom KE, Adams RD: Pathological changes in disorders of skeletal muscle. In Walton J, ed: *Disorders of Voluntary Muscle.* Edinburgh, Churchill Livingstone, 1988, p 153.

43. Sewry CA, Dubowitz V: Histochemical and immunocytochemical studies in neuromuscular diseases. In Walton J, ed: *Disorders of Voluntary Muscle.* Edinburgh, Churchill Livingstone, 1988, p 241.

44. Swash M, Schwartz MS: *Biopsy Pathology of Muscle.* London, Chapman & Hall, 1984.

45. Dubowitz V: *Muscle Biopsy: A Practical Approach,* ed 2. London, Bailliere Tindall, 1985.

46. Van den Hoven R, Meyer AEFH, Wensing TL, et al.: Enzyme histochemical features of equine gluteus muscle fibers. *Am J Vet Res* 46:1755, 1985.

47. Van den Hoven R, Meyer AEFH, Breukink HJ, et al.: Enzyme histochemistry on muscle biopsies as an aid in the diagnosis of diseases of the equine neuromuscular system: A study of six cases. *Equine Vet J* 20:46, 1988.

47a. Valberg SJ: Exertional rhabdomyolysis and polysaccharide storage myopathy in Quarter horses. *Proceedings of the Forty-First Annual Convention of the American Association of Equine Practitioners,* pp 228–230, 1995.

48. Cullen MJ, Hudgson P, Mastaglia FL: Ultrastructural studies of diseased muscle. In Walton J, ed: *Disorders of Voluntary Muscle.* Edinburgh, Churchill Livingstone, 1988, p 284.

49. Hammel EP, Raker CW: Myopathies. In Catcott EJ, Smithcoors JF, eds: *Equine Medicine and Surgery,* ed 2. Wheaton, Ill, American Veterinary, 1972 p 575.

50. Lindholm A, Piehl K: Fibre composition enzyme activity and concentrations of metabolites and electrolytes in muscles of standardbred horses. *Acta Vet Scand* 15:287, 1974.

51. Mermod L, Hoppeler H, Rayer SR, et al.: Variability of fiber size, capillary density and capillary length related to horse muscle fixation procedures. *Acta Anat* 133:89, 1988.

52. Mayhew IG: *Large Animal Neurology: A Handbook for Veterinary Clinicians.* Philadelphia, Lea & Febiger, 1989.

53. Steinberg HS: A review of electromyographic and motor nerve conduction velocity techniques. *J Am Anim Hosp Assoc* 15:613, 1979.

54. Sims MH: Electrodiagnostic techniques in the evaluation of diseases affecting skeletal muscle. *Vet Clin North Am Small Anim Pract* 13:145, 1983.

55. Barwick PD, Fawcett PRW: The clinical physiology of neuromuscular disease. In Walton J, ed: *Disorders of Voluntary Muscle.* Edinburgh, Churchill Livingstone, 1988, p 1015.

56. Oliver JE, Hoerlein BF, Mayhew IG: *Veterinary Neurology.* Philadelphia, WB Saunders, 1987.

56a. Morris E, Seeherman HJ, O'Callaghan MW: Scintigraphic identification of rhabdomyolysis in horses. *Proceedings of the Thirty-Seventh Annual Convention of the American Association of Equine Practitioners,* pp 315–324, 1991.

57. Rowland LP, Penn AS: Myoglobinuria. *Med Clin North Am* 56:1233, 1972.

58. Boulton FE, Huntsman RG: The detection of myoglobin in urine and its distinction from normal and variant hemoglobins. *J Clin Pathol* 24:816, 1971.

59. Schiff HB, MacSearraigh ETM, Kallmeyer JC: Myoglobinuria, rhabdomyolysis and marathon running. *Q J Med* 47:463, 1978.

60. McLean JG: Equine paralytic myoglobinuria ("azoturia"): A review. *Aust Vet J* 49:41, 1973.

61. Hodgson DR: Myopathies in the athletic horse. *Compendium Continuing Educ Pract Vet* 7:551, 1985.

62. Wilson TM, Morrison HA, Palmer NC, et al.: Myodegeneration and suspected selenium/vitamin E deficiency in horses. *J Am Vet Med Assoc* 169:213, 1976.

63. Klein L: A review of 50 cases of post operative myopathy in the horse—Intrinsic and management factors affecting risk. *Proc Am Assoc Equine Pract* 24:89, 1978.

64. Anderson GA, Mount ME, Vrins AA, et al.: Fatal acorn poisoning in a horse. Pathologic findings and diagnostic considerations. *J Am Vet Med Assoc* 24:1105, 1983.

65. Coffman J: Testing for renal disease. *Vet Med Small Anim Clin* 75:1039, 1980.

66. Arighi M, Baird JD, Hulland TJ: Equine exertional rhabdomyolysis. *Compendium Continuing Educ Pract Vet* 6:5726, 1984.

67. Waldron-Mease E, Raker CW, Hammel EP: The muscular system. In Mansmann RA, McAllister ES, Pratt PW, eds: *Equine Medicine and Surgery,* ed 3. Santa Barbara, Calif, American Veterinary, 1982, p 923.

68. Knochel JP: Rhabdomyolysis and myoglobinuria. *Annu Rev Med* 33:435, 1982.

69. Carlson GP, Harrold DR, Ocen PO: Field laboratory evaluation of the effects of heat and work stress in horses. *Proc Am Assoc Equine Pract* 21:314, 1975.

70. Coffman J: *Equine Clinical Chemistry and Pathophysiology.* Kansas City, Kansas, Veterinary Medicine, 1981, p 181.

71. Kent JE, Harris PA: Myoglobinuria: Methods for diagnosis. In Blackmore DJ, ed: *Animal Clinical Biochemistry,* Cambridge, England, Cambridge University Press, 1988, p 191.

72. Kelner MJ, Alexander NM: Rapid separation and identification of myoglobin and hemoglobin in urine by centrifugation through a microconcentrator membrane. *Clin Chem* 31:112, 1985.

73. Watanabe M, Ireda S, Kameya T, et al.: Evaluation of myoglobin determination for the diagnosis of tying-up syndrome in racehorses in Japan. *Exp Rep Equine Health Lab* 15:79, 1978.

74. Valberg S, Holmgren N, Jonsson L, et al.: Plasma AST, CK and myoglobin responses to exercise in rhabdomyolysis susceptible horses (abstract). *Can J Sport Sci* 13:34, 1988.

75. Boyd JW: The mechanisms relating to increases in plasma enzymes and isoenzymes in diseases of animals. *Vet Clin Pathol* 12:9, 1985.

76. Pennington RJT: Biochemical aspects of muscle disease. In Walton J, ed: *Disorders of Voluntary Muscle.* Edinburgh, Churchill Livingstone, 1988, p 455.

77. Gerber H: The clinical significance of serum enzyme activities with particular reference to myoglobinuria. *Proc Am Assoc Equine Pract* 14:81, 1968.

77a. Volfinger L, Lassourd V, Michaux JM, et al: Kinetic evaluation of muscle damage during exercise by calculation of amount of creatine kinase released. *Am J Physiol* 266:R434–R441, 1994.

78. Lang H, Wurzburg V: Creatine kinase, an enzyme of many forms. *Clin Chem* 28:1439, 1982.

79. Keshgegian AA: Serum creatine kinase MB isoenzyme in chronic muscle disease. *Clin Chem* 30:575, 1984.

80. Anderson MG: The effect of exercise on the lactic dehydrogenase and creatine kinase isoenzyme composition of horse serum. *Res Vet Sci* 20:191, 1976.

81. Fujii Y, Ikeda S, Watanabe H: Analysis of creatine kinase isoenzyme in racehorse serum and tissues. *Bull Equine Res Inst* 17:21, 1980.

82. Argiroudis SA, Kent JE, Blackmore DJ: Observations on the isoenzymes of creatine kinase in equine serum and tissues. *Equine Vet J* 14:317, 1982.

83. Sighieri C, Longa A, Mariani AP, et al.: Preliminary observations on the creatine kinase isoenzymes in equine blood serum by polyacrylamide-gel isoelectrofocusing. Influence of physical exercise. *Arch Vet Ital* 36:45, 1985.

84. Cardinet GH, Littrell JF, Freedland RA: Comparative investigations of serum creatine phosphokinase and glutamic-oxaloacetic transaminase activities in equine paralytic myoglobinuria. *Res Vet Sci* 8:219, 1967.

85. Posen S: Turnover of circulating enzymes. *Clin Chem* 16:71, 1970.

86. Cornelius CE, Burnham LG, Hill HE: Serum transaminase activities of equine thoroughbred horses in training. *J Am Vet Med Assoc* 142:639, 1963.

87. Rudofsky R, Rej U, Magro A, et al.: Effects of exercise on serum aminotransferase activity and pyridoxal phosphate saturation in thoroughbred racehorses. *Equine Vet J* 22:205, 1990.

88. Jones S, Blackmore DJ: Observations on the isoenzyme of aspartate aminotransferase in equine tissues and serum. *Equine Vet J* 14:311, 1982.

89. Littlejohn A, Blackmore DJ: Blood and tissue content of the iso-enzymes of lactate dehydrogenase in the thoroughbred. *Res Vet Sci* 25:118, 1987.

90. Guy PS, Snow DH: The effect of training and detraining on lactate dehydrogenase isoenzymes in the horse. *Biochem Biophys Res Commun* 75:863, 1977.

91. Raven PB, Conners TJ, Evonuk E: Effects of exercise on plasma lactate dehydrogenase isoenzymes and catecholamines. *J Appl Physiol* 29:374, 1970.

92. Cerny FJ, Haralambie G: Exercise-induced loss of muscle enzymes. In Knuttgen HG, Vogel JA, Poortmans J, eds: *Biochemistry of exercise,* vol 13. Champaign, Ill, Human Kinetics, 1983, p 441.

93. Milne DW: Blood gases, acid-base balance and electrolyte enzyme changes in exercising horses. *J S Afr Vet Assoc* 45:345, 1974.

94. Hambleton PL, Slade LM, Hamar DW, et al.: Dietary fat and exercise conditioning effect on metabolic conditioning reduced exercise-induced increases in parameters in the horse. *J Anim Sci* 51:1330, 1980.

95. Poso AR, Soveri T, Oksanen HE: The effect of exercise on blood parameters in standardbred and Finnish bred horses. *Acta Vet scand* 24:170, 1983.

96. Shelle JE, Van Huss WD, Rook JS, et al.: Blood parameters as a result of conditioning horses through short strenuous exercise bouts. In *Proceedings of the Ninth Equine Nutritional Physiology Symposium,* Mich, 1985, p 206.

96a. Serrantoni M, Harris PA, Allen WR: Muscle enzyme activities in the plasma of Thoroughbred fillies in relation to exercise and stage of oestrous cycle. *Submitted for publication,* 1996.

97. Milne DW, Skarda RJ, Gabel AA, et al.: Effects of training on biochemical values in standardbred horses *Am J Vet Res* 37:285, 1976.

98. Heffron JJA, Bomzon L, Pattinson RA: Observations on plasma creatine phosphokinase activity in dogs. *Vet Rec* 98:338, 1970.

99. Aitken MM, Anderson MG, Mackenzie G, et al.: Correlations between physiological and biochemical parameters used to assess fitness in the horse. *J S Afr Vet Assoc* 45:361, 1975.

100. Anderson MG: The influence of exercise on serum enzyme levels in the horse. *Equine Vet J* 7:160, 1975.

101. Harris PA: *Aspects of the Equine Rhabdomyolysis Syndrome,* thesis, Cambridge University, 1988.

102. Codazza D, Maffeo G, Redaelli G: Serum enzyme changes and haemato-chemical levels in thoroughbreds after transport and exercise. *J S Afr Vet Assoc* 45:331, 1974.

103. Rose RJ, Purdue RA, Hensley W: Plasma biochemistry alterations in horses during an endurance ride. *Equine Vet J* 9:122, 1977.

104. Bayly WM: Exercise testing at the race track. *Int Conf Equine Sports Med* 102:123, 1986.

105. Freestone JF, Kamerling SG, Church G, et al.: Exercise induced changes in creatine kinase and aspartate aminotransferase activities in the horse: Effects of conditioning, exercise tests and acepromazine. *J Equine Vet Sci* 9:275, 1989.

105a. Fayolle P, Lefebre H, Braun JP: Effects of incorrect venepuncture on plasma creatine kinase activity in dogs and horses. *Br Vet J* 148:161–162, 1992.

106. Frauenfelder HC, Rossdale PD, Ricketts SW: Changes in serum muscle enzyme levels associated with training schedules and stage of the oestrous cycle in thoroughbred racehorses. *Equine Vet J* 18:371, 1986.

107. Harris PA, Greet TRC, Snow DH, et al.: Some factors influencing plasma AST/CK activities in thoroughbred racehorses. *Equine Vet J* 9(suppl):66, 1990.

107a. Aktas M, Auguste D, Concorddet D, et al.: Creatine kinase in dog plasma: Preanalytical factors of variation, reference values and diagnostic significance. *Research in Veterinary Science* 56:30–36, 1994.

107b. Amelink GL, Koot RW, Erich WBM, et al.: Sex linked variation in creatine kinase release and its dependence on oestradiol can be demonstrated in an *in-vitro* rat skeletal muscle preparation. *Acta Physiol Scand* 138:115–124, 1990.

108. Cardinet GH, Fowler ME, Tyler WS: The effects of training, exercise and tying-up on serum transaminase activities in the horse. *Am J Vet Res* 24:980, 1963.

109. Mullen PA, Hopes R, Sewell J: The biochemistry, haematology, nutrition and racing performance of two year old thoroughbreds throughout their training and racing season. *Vet Rec* 104:90, 1979.

110. Judson GJ, Mooney GJ, Thornbury RS: Plasma biochemical values in thoroughbreds in training. In Snow DH, Persson SGB, Rose RJ, eds: *Equine Exercise Physiology.* Cambridge, England, Granta, 1983, p 354.

111. Snow DH, Harris PA: Enzymes as markers for the evaluation of physical fitness and training of racing horses. *Adv Clin Enzymol* 6:257, 1988.

112. Flisinka-Bojanowska A, Komosa M, Gill J: Influence of pregnancy on diurnal and seasonal changes in glucose level and

113. Sommer H: Blood profile testing in racehorses. *Equine Pract* 5:21, 1983.

114. Lindholm A: Pathophysiology of exercise induced diseases of the musculoskeletal system of the equine athlete. In Gillespie JR, Robinson NE, eds: *Equine Exercise Physiology,* vol 2. Davis, Calif, ICEEP, 1987, p 711.

115. Goedegebuure SA: Spontaneous primary myopathies in domestic mammals: A review. *Vet Q* 9:155, 1987.

116. Cardinet GH, Holliday TA: Neuromuscular diseases of domestic animals: A summary of muscle biopsies from 159 cases. *Ann N Y Acad Sci* 317:290, 1979.

117. Turner S: Diseases of bones and related structures. In Stashak TS, ed: *Adams' Lameness in Horses,* ed 4. Philadelphia, Lea & Febiger, 1987, p 293.

118. Beech J: Myopathies in horses. In *Proceedings from Equine Seminar 1988.* Foundation for Continuing Education of the New Zealand Veterinary Association, publication no. 117, 1988, p 101.

119. Clayton HM: Cinematographic analysis of the gait of lame horses V: Fibrotic myopathy. *Equine Vet Sci* 8:297, 1988.

120. Turner AS, Trotter GW: Fibrotic myopathy in the horse. *J Am Vet Med Assoc* 184:335, 1984.

121. Bramlage LR, Reed SM, Embertson RM: Semitendinosus tenotomy for treatment of fibrotic myopathy in the horse. *J Am Vet Med Assoc* 186:565, 1985.

122. Sprinkle FP, Swerczek TW, Ward Crowe M: Gastrocnemius muscle rupture and hemorrhage in foals. *Equine Pract* 7:10, 1985.

123. Schneider JE, Guffy MM, Leipold HW: Ruptured flexor muscles in a neonatal foal. *Equine Pract* 8:11, 1986.

124. Stashak TS: Lameness. In Stashak TS, ed: *Adams' Lameness in Horses,* ed 4. Philadelphia, Lea & Febiger, 1987, p 486.

125. Valberg SJ, McKinnon AO: Clostridial cellulitis in the horse: A report of five cases. *Can Vet J* 25:67, 1984.

126. Rebhun WC, Shin SJ, King JM, et al.: Malignant edema in horses. *J Am Vet Med Assoc* 187:732, 1988.

126a. Aleman M, Spier S, Wilson WD: Retrospective study of *Corynebacterium pseudotuberculosis* infection in horses: 538 cases (1982–1993). *Proceedings of the Fortieth Annual Convention of the American Association of Equine Practitioners,* p 117, 1994.

127. Miers KC and Ley WB: *Corynebacterium pseudotuberculosis* infection in the horse: Study of 117 clinical cases and consideration of etiopathogenesis. *J Am Vet Med Assoc* 177:250, 1980.

128. Edwards GT: Prevalence of equine sarcocysts in British horses and a comparison of two detection methods. *Vet Rec* 115:265, 1984.

129. Tinling SP, Cardinet GH, Blythe LL, et al.: A light and electron microscopic study of sarcocysts in a horse. *J Parasitol* 66:458, 1980.

130. Fransen JLA von, Degryse ADAY, Van Mol KAC, et al.: Sarcocysts und chronische Myopathien bei Pferden. *Berl Munch Tierarztliche Wochenschr,* 100:229, 1987.

131. Freestone JF, Carlson GP: Muscle disorders in the horse: A retrospective study. *Equine Vet J* 1991, in press.

132. Fayer R, Hounsel C, Giles RC: Chronic illness in a sarcocystis infected pony. *Vet Rec* 113:216, 1983.

133. Dubey JP, Davis SW, Speer CA, et al.: *Sarcocystis neurona* n.sp *(Protozoa: apicomplexa):* The etiologic agent of equine protozoal myeloencephalitis. *J Parasitol* 1991, in press.

134. Martin BW, Terry MK, Bridges CH, et al.: Toxicity of *Cassia occidentalis* in the horse. *Vet Hum Toxicol* 23:416, 1981.

135. Hatch RC: Poisons having unique effects. In Booth NH, McDonald LE, eds: *Veterinary Pharmacology and Therapeutics.* Ames, Iowa State University Press, 1988, p 1132

136. Amend JF, Mallon FM, Wren WB, et al.: Equine monensin toxicosis. Some experimental clinicopathologic observations. *Compendium Continuing Educ Pract Vet* 2:S173, 1980.

137. Mollenhauer HH, Rowe LD, Witzel DA: Effect of monensin on the morphology of mitochondria in rodent and equine striated muscle. *Vet Hum Toxicol* 26:15, 1984.

138. Muylle E, Vandenhende C, Oyaert W, et al.: Delayed monensin sodium toxicity in horses. *Equine Vet J* 13:107, 1981.

139. Hintz HF: Bracken fern. *Equine Pract* 12:6, 1990.

140. King AS: Studies on equine purpura hemorrhagica. Article no. 3—morbid anatomy and histology. *Br Vet J* 105:35, 1949.

141. Krisher K, Cunningham MW: Myosin: A link between streptococci and heart. *Science* 227:413, 1985.

141a. Richey MT, Holland MS, McGrath CJ, et al.: Equine postanesthetic lameness: A retrospective study. *Veterinary Surgery* 19:392, 1990.

142. Lindsay WA, McDonell W, Bignell W: Equine post-anesthetic forelimb lameness: Intracompartmental muscle pressure changes and biochemical patterns. *Am J Vet Res* 41:1919, 1980.

143. White N: Post anesthetic recumbency myopathy in horses. *Compendium Continuing Educ Pract Vet* 4:S44, 1982.

144. White NA, Suarez M: Changes in triceps muscle intracompartmental pressure with repositioning and padding of the lowermost thoracic limb of the horse. *Am J Vet Res* 47:2257, 1986.

145. Serteyn D, Coppers P, Mottart E, et al.: Myopathie postanesthésique équine: Mesure de paramètres respiratoires et hémodynamiques. *Ann Med Vet* 131:123, 1987.

145a. Norman WM, Williams R, Dodman NH, Kraus AE: Postanesthetic compartmental syndrome in a horse. *J Am Vet Med Assoc* 195:502, 1989.

146. Serteyn D, Mothart E, Deby C, et al.: Equine postanesthetic myositis: A possible role for free radical generation and membrane lipoperoxidation. *Res Vet Sci* 48:42, 1990.

147. Weaver BMQ, Lunn CEM: Muscle perfusion in the horse. *Equine Vet J* 16:66, 1984.

148. Grandy JL, Steffey EP, Hodgson DS, et al.: Arterial hypotension and the development of post anesthetic myopathy in halothane-anesthetized horses. *Am J Vet Res* 48:192, 1987.

149. Lindsay WA, Robinson GM, Brunson PB, et al.: Induction of equine postanesthetic myositis after halothane-induced hypotension. *Am J Vet Res* 50:404, 1989.

150. Lindsay WA, Pascoe PJ, McDonnell WN, et al.: Effect of protective padding on forelimb intracompartmental muscle pressures in anesthetized horses. *Am J Vet Res* 46:688, 1985.

151. Taylor PM, Young SS: The effect of limb position on venous and compartmental pressure in the forelimb of ponies. *J Assoc Vet Anesthesiology* 17:35, 1990.

152. Dodman NH, Williams R, Court MH, et al.: Postanesthetic hind limb adductor myopathy in five horses. *J Am Vet Med Assoc* 193:83, 1988.

153. Hildebrand SV, Arpin D, Howitt GA, et al.: Muscle biopsy to differentiate normal from malignant hyperthermia suspect horses and ponies. *Vet Surg* 17:172, 1988.

154. Court MH, Engelking LR, Dodman NH, et al.: Pharmacokinetics of dantrolene sodium in horses *J Vet Pharmacol Ther* 10:218, 1985.

155. Azzie MAJ: Aortic iliac thrombosis of thoroughbred horses. *Equine Vet J* 1:113, 1969.

156. Maxie MG, Physick-Sheard PW: Aortic-iliac thrombosis in horses. *Vet Pathol* 22:238, 1985.

157. Merillat LA: Thrombosis of the iliac arteries in horses. *J Am Vet Med Assoc* 104:218, 1944.

158. Mayhew IG, Kryger MD: Aortic-iliac-femoral thrombosis in a horse, *Vet Med Small Anim Clin* 70:1281, 1975.

159. Tithof PK, Rebhun WC, Dietze AE: Ultrasonographic diagnosis of aorto-iliac thrombosis. *Cornell Vet* 75:540, 1985.

160. Reef VB, Roby KAW, Richardson DW, et al.: Use of ultrasonography for the detection of aortic-iliac thrombosis in horses. *J Am Vet Med Assoc* 190:286, 1987.

161. Branscomb BL: Treatment of arterial thrombosis in a horse with sodium gluconate. *J Am Vet Med Assoc* 152:1643, 1968.

162. Griggs RC: The myotonic disorders and the periodic paralyses. In Griggs RC, Moxley RT, eds: *Advances in Neurology,* vol 17. New York, Raven Press, 1977, p 143.

163. Harper PS: The myotonic disorders. In Walton J, ed: *Disorders of Voluntary Muscle.* Edinburgh, Churchill Livingstone, 1988, p 569.

164. Barchi RL: The pathophysiology of excitation in skeletal muscle. In Walton J, ed: *Disorders of Voluntary Muscle.* Edinburgh, Churchill Livingstone, 1988, p 372.

165. Hegreberg GA, Reed SM: Skeletal muscle changes associated with equine myotonic dystrophy. *Acta Neuropathol* 80:426, 1990.

166. Farnbeck GC: Myotonia. In Mansmann RA, McAllister ES, Pratt PW, eds: *Equine Medicine and Surgery,* ed 3. Santa Barbara, Calif, American Veterinary, 1982, p 935.

167. Bradley R, McKerrell RE, Barnard EA: Neuromuscular disease in animals. In Walton J, ed: *Disorders of Voluntary Muscle.* Edinburgh, Churchill Livingstone, 1988, p 910.

168. Beech J, Fletcher JE, Lizzo F, et al.: Effect of phenytoin on the clinical signs and *in vitro* muscle twitch characteristics in horses with chronic intermittent rhabdomyolysis and myotonia. *Am J Vet Res* 49:2130, 1988.

168a. Beech J, Lindborg S: Potassium concentrations in muscle, plasma and erythrocytes and urinary fractional excretion in normal horses and those with chronic intermittent exercise-associated rhabdomyolysis. *Res Vet Sci* 55:43–51, 1993.

169. Jamison JM, Baird JD, Smith Maxie LL, et al.: A congenital form of myotonia with dystrophic changes in a Quarterhorse. *Equine Vet J* 191:353, 1987.

170. Hammel EP, Marks H: Presented at Fifth International Congress on Neuromuscular Disease, Marseilles, 1982.

171. Edwards RHT, Jones DA: Diseases of skeletal muscle. In Peachey CD, ed: *Handbook of Physiology,* sect 10. Md, American Physiological Society, 1983, p 633.

172. Roneus B, Lindholm A, Jonsson L: Myotoni hos hast. *Svensk Vet Tidn* 35:217, 1983.

173. Hegreberg GA, Reed SM: Muscle changes in a progressive equine myotonic dystrophy. *Fed Proc* 46:728, 1987.

173a. McClatchey AI, Trofatter J, McKenna-Yasek D, et al.: Dinucleotide repeat polymorphisms at the SCN4A locus suggest allelic heterogeneity of hyperkalemic periodic paralysis and paramyotonia congenita. *Am J Hum Genet* 10:896–901, 1992.

174. Cox JH: An episodic weakness in four horses associated with intermittent serum hyperkalemia and the similarity of the disease to hyperkalemic periodic paralysis in man. *Proc Am Assoc Equine Pract* 31:383, 1985.

175. Steiss JE, Naylor JM: Episodic muscle tremors in a quarter horse—Resemblance to hyperkalemic periodic paralysis. *Can Vet J* 27:332, 1986.

175a. Spier S, Valberg V, Carr EA, et al.: Update on hyperkalaemic periodic paralysis. *Proceedings of the Forty-First Annual Convention of the American Association of Equine Practitioners,* pp 231–233, 1995.

175b. Naylor JM, Jones V, Berry SL: Clinical syndrome and diagnosis of hyperkalaemic paralysis in Quarter horses. *Equine Vet J* 25:227–232, 1993.

176. Spier SJ, Carlson GP, Pickar J, et al.: Hyperkalemic periodic paralysis in horses: Genetic and electrophysiologic studies. *Proc Am Assoc Equine Pract* 35:399, 1989.

176a. Stewart R, Bertone JJ, Yvorchuk-St Jean K, et al.: Possible normokalaemic variant of hyperkalemic periodic paralysis in two horses. *J Am Vet Med Assoc* 203:421–424, 1993.

176b. Robinson JA, Naylor JM, Crichlow EC: Use of electromyography for the diagnosis of equine hyperkalaemic periodic paresis. *Canad J Vet Res* 54:495–500, 1990.

177. Engel AG: Metabolic and endocrine myopathies. In Walton J, ed: *Disorders of Voluntary Muscle.* Edinburgh, Churchill Livingstone, 1988, p 811.

178. Bendheim PE, Reale EO, Berg BO: β-Adrenergic treatment of hyperkalemic periodic paralysis. *Neurology* 35:746, 1985.

178a. Rudolph JA, Spier SJ, Bryns G, Hoffman EP: Linkage of hyperkalaemic periodic paralysis in Quarter horses to the horse adult skeletal muscle sodium channel gene. *Animal Genetics* 23:241–250, 1992.

178b. Rudolph JA, Spier SJ, Bryns G, et al.: Periodic paralysis in Quarter horses: A sodium channel mutation disseminated by selective breeding. *Nature Genetics* 2:144–147, 1992.

179. Hitt ME: Oxygen-derived free radicals: Pathophysiology and implications. *Compendium Continuing Educ Pract Vet* 10:939, 1988.

180. Blood DC, Henderson JA, Radostits OM: Metabolic diseases. In Blood DC, Henderson JA, eds: *Veterinary Medicine. A Textbook of the Diseases of Cattle, Sheep, Pigs and Horses.* Philadelphia, Lea & Febiger, 1979, p 846.

181. Hamir AN: White muscle disease in a foal. *Aust Vet J* 59:57, 1982.

182. Owen LR, Moore JN, Hopkins JB, et al.: Dystrophic myodegeneration in adult horses. *J Am Vet Med Assoc* 17:343, 1977.

183. Dill SG, Rebhun WC: White muscle disease in foals. *Compendium Continuing Educ Pract Vet* 7:S627, 1985.

184. Jackson MJ, Jones DA, Edwards RHT: Techniques for studying free radical damage in muscular dystrophy. *Med Biol* 62:135, 1984.

184a. Mills PC, Smith NC, Casas I, et al.: Effects of exercise intensity and environmental stress on indices of oxidative stress and iron homeostasis during exercise in the horse. *In press,* 1996.

185. Phoenix J, Edwards RHT, Jackson MJ: The effect of vitamin E analogues and long carbon chain compounds on calcium-induced muscle damage. A novel role for alpha-tocopherol. *Biochem Biophys Acta* 1097:212, 1991.

186. Roneus B, Essen-Gustavsson B: Muscle fiber types and enzyme activities in healthy foals and foals affected by muscular dystrophy. *J Am Vet Med Assoc* 33:1, 1986.

187. Roneus B, Jonsson L: Muscular dystrophy in foals. *Zentralbl Veterinarmed [A]* 31:441, 1984.

188. Lewis LD: The role of nutrition in musculoskeletal development and disease. In Stashak TS, ed: *Adams' Lameness in Horses,* ed 4. Philadelphia, Lea & Febiger, 1987, p 282.

189. Higuchi T, Ichijo S, Osame S, et al.: Studies on serum selenium and tocopherol in white muscle disease of foals. *Jpn J Vet Sci* 51:52, 1989.

190. Craig AM, Blythe LL, Lassen ED, et al.: Variations of serum vitamin E, cholesterol, and total serum lipid concentrations in horses during a 72 hr period. *Am J Vet Res* 50:1527, 1989.

191. Roneus BO, Hakkarainen RVJ, Lindholm CA, et al.: Vitamin E requirements of adult standardbred horses evaluated by tissue depletion and repletion. *Equine Vet J* 18:50, 1986.

192. Maylin GA, Rubin DS, Lein DH: Selenium and vitamin E in horses. *Cornell Vet* 70:272, 1980.

193. Roneus B: Glutathione peroxidase and selenium in the blood of healthy horses and foals affected by muscular dystrophy. *Nord Vet Med* 31:350, 1982.

194. Carlson GP: Medical problems associated with protracted heat and work stress in horses. *Compendium Continuing Educ Pract Vet* 5:542, 1985.

195. Fowler ME: Veterinary problems during endurance trail rides. *Proc Am Assoc Equine Pract* 25:460, 1979.

196. Carlson GP: Thermoregulation fluid and electrolyte balance. In Snow DH, Persson SGB, Rose RJ, eds: *Equine Exercise Physiology.* Cambridge, England, Granta, 1983, p 291.

197. Smith CA, Wagner PC: Electrolyte imbalances and metabolic disturbances in endurance horses. *Compendium Continuing Educ Pract Vet* 7:S575, 1985.

198. Carlson GP: The exhausted horse syndrome. In Robinson NE, ed: *Current Therapy in Equine Medicine,* vol 2. Philadelphia, WB Saunders, 1987, p 482.

199. Meyer H: Nutrition of the equine athlete. In Gillespie JR, Robinson NE, eds: *Equine Exercise Physiology,* vol 2. Davis, Calif, ICEEP, 1987, p 644.

200. Meginnis P: Myositis (tying-up) in race horses. *J Am Vet Med Assoc* 130:237, 1957.

201. Brennan BF, Marshak RR, Keown GH, et al.: The tying up syndrome—a panel discussion. *Proc Am Assoc Equine Pract* 5:157, 1959.

202. Lindholm A, Johannson HE, Kjaersgaard P: Acute rhabdomyolysis ("tying-up") in standardbred horses. A morphological and biochemical study. *Acta Vet scand* 15:325, 1974.

203. Udall DH: Azoturia. In Udall DH, ed: *The Practice of Veterinary Medicine,* ed 3. Ithaca, NY: Udall, 1939, p 296.

204. Duccilot J, ed.: *Traité pathologie médicale des animaux domestique,* ed 4. Belgium, Gembloux, 1995, p 835.

205. Roman B, Martin H: The muscular changes in azoturia. *Cornell Vet* 16:286, 1926.

206. Badame GF: The "tying-up" syndrome. *Proc Am Assoc Equine Pract* 19:353, 1973.

207. McCracken RW, Steffen MR: New and successful treatment for azoturia. *Am J Vet Med* 7:429, 1912.

208. Hertha K: Ursachen, Verhütung und Behandlung der Hämoglobinämie des Pferdes. *Manatsschn Tierheilkd* 32:165, 1921; *Cornell Vet* 14:165, 1924.

209. Jeffcott LB, Dalin G, Drevemo S, et al.: Effect of induced back pain on gait and performance of trotting horses. *Equine Vet J* 14:129, 1982.

210. Carlstrom B: Über die Atiologie und Pathogenese der Kreuzlahmuns des Pferdes (Hämglobinämia paralytica). *Skand Arch Physiol* 61:161, 1931.

211. Carlstrom B: Über die Atiologie und Pathogenese der Kreuzlahmung des Pferdes (Hämoglobinämia paralytica). *Skand Arch Physiol* 63:164, 1932.

212. Snow DH, Harris RC, Gash SP: Metabolic response of equine muscle to intermittent maximal exercise. *J Appl Physiol* 58:1689, 1985.

213. Koterba A, Carlson GP: Acid base and electrolyte alterations in horses with exertional rhabdomyolysis. *J Am Vet Med Assoc* 180:303, 1982.

214. Harris PA, Snow DH: Tying up the loose ends of equine rhabdomyolysis (editorial). *Equine Vet J* 18:346, 1986.

215. Andrews FM, Spurgeon TL, Reed SM: Histochemical changes in skeletal muscles of four male horses with neuromuscular disease. *Am J Vet Res* 47:2078, 1986.

216. Snow DH, Harris RC, Marlin DJ, et al.: Glycogen repletion following different diets. In Gillespie JR, Robinson NE, eds: *Equine Exercise Physiology,* vol 2. Davis, Calif, ICEEP, 1987, p 701.

217. Valberg S: Personal communication,

217a. Valberg S, Jonsson L, Lindholm A, Holmgren N: Muscle histopathology and plasma aspartate aminotransferase, creatine kinase and myoglobin changes with exercise in horses with recurrent exertional rhabdomyolysis. *Equine Vet J* 25(1):11–16, 1993.

218. Schryver HF, Hintz HF: Vitamins. In Robinson NE, ed: *Current Therapy in Equine Medicine,* ed 1. London, WB Saunders, 1983, p 84.

219. Patton JW: A new conception of azoturia. *Vet Med* 39:10, 1944.

220. Hill HE: Selenium–vitamin E treatment of tying up in horses. *Mod Vet Pract* 43:66, 1962.

221. Roneus BO, Hakkarainen RVJ: Vitamin E in serum and skele-

tal muscle tissue and blood glutathione peroxidase activity from horses with azoturia–tying up syndrome. *Acta Vet Scand* 26:425, 1985.

222. Lindholm A: Glutathione peroxidase, selenium and vitamin E in blood and in relation to muscle dystrophy and tying-up in the horse. Presented at 12th Linderstrom-Lang Conference, Langarvatri, Iceland, IVB Symposium no. 110, 1982, p 62.

223. Lindholm A, Asheim A: Vitamin E and certain muscular enzymes in the blood serum of horses. *Acta Agric Scand suppl* 19:40, 1973.

224. Snow DH, Gash SP, Rice D: Field observations on selenium status, whole blood glutathione peroxidase and plasma gamma-glutamyl transferase activities in thoroughbred race horses. In Gillespie JR, Robinson NE, eds: *Equine Exercise Physiology,* vol 2. Davis, Calif, ICEEP, 1987, p 494.

225. Petersson KH, Hintz HF, Schryver HF, et al.: The effect of vitamin E on membrane integrity during submaximal exercise. In Sune GB, Person SGB, Lindholm A, et al, eds: *Equine Exercise Physiology,* vol 3. Davis, Calif, ICEEP, 1991, p 315

225a. DiMauro S, Tsujino S: Glycogenoses. *In.* Engel AG, Banker BQ (eds). *Myology.* New York: McGraw-Hill, pp 1554–1576, 1994.

226. Rennie MJ, Edwards RHT: Carbohydrate metabolism of skeletal muscle and its disorders. In Randle PJ, Skeiner DF, Whelan WJ, eds: *Carbohydrate Metabolism and Its Disorders,* vol 3. London, Academic Press, 1981, p 75.

227. Van den Hoven R, Wensing T, Breukink HJ, et al.: Enzyme histochemistry in exertional myopathy. In Gillespie JR, Robinson NE, eds: *Equine Exercise Physiology* vol 2. Davis, Calif, ICEEP, 1987, p 796.

228. Van den Hoven R, Breukink HJ, Wensing T, et al.: Loosely coupled skeletal muscle mitochondria in exertional rhabdomyolysis. *Equine Vet J* 18:418, 1986.

229. Layzer RB, Havel RJ, McUroy MB: Partial deficiency of carnitine palmityltransferase. Physiologic and biochemical consequences. *Neurology* 30:627, 1980.

230. Van de Hoven R: *Some Histochemical and Biochemical Aspects of Equine Muscles with Special Respect to Equine Exertional Myopathy,* thesis, University of Utrecht, Netherlands, 1987.

231. Williams W: Azoturia. In Williams W, ed: *The Principles and Practice of Veterinary Medicine,* ed 2. Edinburgh, Maclachlan & Sherwood; New York, William Wood, 1879, p 413.

231a. Kinslow P, Harris P, Gray, Allen WR: Influence of the oestrous cycle on electrolyte excretion in the mare. *Equine Vet J Suppl* 18:388–391, 1995.

232. Evered DC, Ormston BJ, Smith PA, et al.: Grades of hypothyroidism. *Br Med J* 1:657, 1973.

233. DeGroot LJ, Larsen PR, Refetoff S, et al.: *The Thyroid and Its Diseases.* ed 5. Chichester, England, Wiley, 1984, p 571.

234. Docherty I, Harrop JS, Hine KR, et al.: Myoglobin concentration, creatine kinase activity and creatine kinase B subunit concentrations in serum during thyroid disease. *Clin Chem* 30:42, 1984.

235. Waldron-Mease E: Hypothyroidism and myopathy in racing thoroughbreds and standardbreds. *J Equine Med Surg* 3:124, 1979.

236. Morris DD, Garcia M: Thyroid-stimulating hormone response test in healthy horses and effect of phenylbutazone on equine thyroid hormones. *Am J Vet Res* 44:503, 1983.

237. Waldron-Mease E: Correlation of post-operative and exercise-induced equine myopathy with the defect malignant hyperthermia. *Proc Am Assoc Equine Pract* 24:95, 1978.

238. Manley SV, Kelly AB, Hodgson D: Malignant hyperthermia-like reactions in three anesthetized horses. *J Am Vet Med Assoc* 183:85, 1983.

239. Hildebrand SV, Arpin D, Cardinet GH: Exertional rhabdomy-

olysis related to malignant hyperthermia using the halothane-caffeine contracture test. In Gillespie JR, Robinson NE, eds: *Equine Exercise Physiology,* vol. 2. Davis, Calif, ICEEP, 1987, p 786.

240. Gronert GA: Malignant hyperthermia. *Anesthesiology* 53:395, 1980.

241. Savage DCL, Forbes M, Pearce GW: Idiopathic rhabdomyolysis. *Arch Dis Child* 46:594, 1971.

242. Dietzman DE, Shaller JG, Ray CG, et al.: Acute myositis associated with influenza B infection. *Pediatrics* 57:255, 1976.

243. McQueen JL, Davenport FM, Keeran RJ, et al.: Studies of equine influenza in Michigan 1963. *Am J Epidemiol* 83:280, 1966.

244. Harris PA: Outbreak of the equine rhabdomyolysis syndrome in a racing yard. *Vet Rec* 127:468, 1990.

245. Carlson GP: Blood chemistry body fluids and hematology. In Gillespie JR, Robinson NE, eds: *Equine Exercise Physiology,* vol 2. Davis, Calif, ICEEP, 1987, p 393.

246. Currie S: The inflammatory myopathies. In Walton J, ed: *Disorders of Voluntary Muscle.* Edinburgh, Churchill Livingstone, 1988, p 588.

247. David AS, Wessely S, Pelosi AJ: Post viral fatigue syndrome: Time for a new approach. *Br Med J* 296:696, 1988.

248. Carlson GP, Nelson T: Exercise related muscle problems in endurance horses. *Proc Am Assoc Equine Pract* 22:223, 1976.

249. Coffman JR, Amend JF, Garner HE, et al.: A conceptual approach to pathophysiologic evaluation of neuromuscular disorders in the horse. *J Equine Med Surg* 2:85, 1978.

250. Genetzky RM, Loparco FV, Ledet AE: Clinical pathologic alterations in horses during water deprivation test. *Am J Vet Res* 48:1007, 1987.

251. Harris PA, Snow DH: Role of electrolyte imbalances in the pathophysiology of the equine rhabdomyolysis syndrome. Third ICEEP Conference, Sweden, 1991, in press.

251a. Harris PA, Gray J: The use of the urinary fractional electrolyte excretion test to assess electrolyte status in the horse. *Equine Vet Educ* 4(4):162–166, 1992.

252. Krook L: Dietary calcium-phosphorus and lameness in the horse. *Cornell Vet* 58(suppl):59, 1968.

253. Jordan RM, Myers VS, Yoho B, et al.: Effect of calcium and phosphorus levels on growth, reproduction and bone development of ponies. *J Anim Sci* 40:78, 1975.

254. Knight DA, Gabel AA, Reed SM, et al.: Correlation of dietary mineral to incidence and severity of metabolic bone disease in Ohio and Kentucky. *Proc Am Assoc Equine Pract* 31:445, 1985.

255. Krook L, Maylin GA: Fractures in thoroughbred race horses. *Cornell Vet* 78(suppl 11):7, 1988.

256. Mason DK, Watkins KL, McNie JT: Diagnosis, treatment and prevention of nutritional secondary hyperparathyroidism in thoroughbred racehorses in Hong Kong. *Equine Pract* 10:10, 1988.

257. Lindner A, Schmidt M, Meyer H: Investigations on sodium metabolism in exercised Shetland ponies fed a diet marginal in sodium. In Snow DH, Persson SGB, Rose RJ, eds: *Equine Exercise Physiology.* Cambridge, England, Granta, 1983, p 311.

258. Meyer H, Gurer C, Lindner A: Effects of a low K^+ diet on K^+ metabolism, sweat production and sweat composition in horses. In *Proceedings of the Ninth Equine Nutrition Physiology Symposium,* Mich 1985, p 130.

259. Dorup I, Skajaa K, Clausen T, et al.: Reduced concentrations of potassium, magnesium and sodium-potassium pumps in human skeletal muscle during treatment with diuretics. *Br Med J* 296:455, 1988.

260. Akaike N: Sodium pump in skeletal muscle central nervous

system induced by α-adrenoreceptors. *Science* 213:1252, 1981.

261. Hardveld C van, Clausen T: Effect of thyroid status on K⁺ stimulated metabolism and Ca exchange in rat skeletal muscle. *Am J Physiol Endocrology Metab* 247:E421, 1984.

262. Kjeldsen K: Determination of muscle tissue, Na, K-pump concentration, its regulation and relation to muscle function and potassium homeostasis (abstract). *Can J Sport Sci* 13:21P, 1988.

263. Kjeldsen K, Everts ME, Clausen T: Effects of semistarvation and potassium deficiency on the concentration of (³H) ouabain-binding sites and sodium and potassium contents in rat skeletal muscle. *Br J Nutr* 56:519, 1986.

264. Fong CN, Atwood HL, Jeejeebhoy KN, et al.: Nutrition and muscle potassium: Differential effect in rat slow and fast muscles. *Can J Physiol Pharmacol* 65:2188, 1987.

265. Harris PA: The equine rhabdomyolysis syndrome in the United Kingdom. Epidemiological and clinical descriptive information. *Br Vet J* 1991, in press.

266. Stuck EK, Reinertson EL: Equine exertional myopathy. *Iowa State Univ Vet* 49:56, 1987.

267. Grodski K: Elektrokardiogram w miesniochwacie pora zennym koni. *Pol Arch Wet* 8:505, 1984; *Vet Bull* 35:8379, 1965.

268. Steffen MR: Azoturia. In Campbell DM, ed: *Special Equine Therapy. Veterinary Medicine Series no. 14,* Chicago, American Veterinary, 1917, p 101.

269. Shideler RK: Post-colic azoturia (a case report). *Vet Med Small Anim Clin* 64:431, 1969.

270. White KK: Exertional myopathy. In Robinson NE, ed: *Current Veterinary Therapy in Equine Medicine.* Toronto, WB Saunders, 1983, p 101.

271. Gerber H: Aktivität Bestimmungen von Serumenzymen in der Veterinärmedizin. III C. Bestimmungen der SGOT-, SGPT-, und SCPK Aktivität bei Myopathien and Cardiopathien des Pferdes. *Schweiz Arch Tierheilkd* 106:478, 1964.

272. Andrews FM, Reed SM: Diagnosis of muscle disease in the horse. *Proc Am Assoc Equine Pract* 32:95, 1986.

273. Yamaoka S, Ikeda S, Watanabe H, et al.: Clinical and enzymological findings of tying-up syndrome in thoroughbred racehorses in Japan. *Exp Rep Equine Health Lab* 15:62, 1978.

274. Fujii Y, Watanabe H, Yamamoto T, et al.: Serum creatine kinase and lactate dehydrogenase isoenzymes in skeletal and cardiac muscle damage in the horse. *Bull Equine Res Inst* no. 20:87, 1983.

275. Kerr MG, Snow DH: Plasma enzyme activities in endurance horses. In Snow DH, Persson SGB, Rose RJ, eds: *Equine Exercise Physiology.* Cambridge, England, Granta, 1983, p 432.

276. Bain FT, Merritt AM: Decreased erythrocyte potassium concentration associated with exercise-related myopathy in horses. *J Am Vet Med Assoc* 196:1259, 1990.

277. Rozman MJ, Peterson JA, Adams EC: Differentiation of haemoglobin and myoglobin by immunochemical methods. *Invest Urol* 1:518, 1964.

278. Robb EJ, Kronfeld DS: Dietary sodium bicarbonate as a treatment for exertional rhabdomyolysis in a horse. *J Am Vet Med Assoc* 188:602, 1986.

279. Fronher: Über rheumatische Hämoglobinamie beim Pferde und ihr Verhältnis zur paroxysmalen Hämoglobinurie des Menschen. *Arch Tierheilkd* 10:296, 1884.

280. Grossman BS, Brobst DF, Kramer JW, et al.: Urinary indices for differentiation of prerenal azotemia and renal azotemia in horses. *J Am Vet Med Assoc* 180:284, 1982.

281. Fletcher JE, Beech J, Rosenberg H, et al.: Altered phospholipid distribution in skeletal muscle of horses with chronic intermittent rhabdomyolysis ("tying-up"). *Fed Proc* 46:810, 1987.

282. Wegmann E: Peroneal paralysis associated with myopathy in a horse. *Mod Vet Pract* 66:1007, 1985.

283. Gresswell JB, Gresswell AG: Azoturia. In Gresswell JB, Gresswell AG, eds: *A Manual of the Theory and Practice of Equine Medicine,* ed 2., London, Bailliere Tindall; New York, Williams Jenkins, 1890, p 189.

284. Dwyer RM: The practical diagnosis and treatment of metabolic conditions in endurance horses. *Equine Pract* 8:21, 1986.

285. Hodgson DR: Exertional rhabdomyolysis. In Robinson NE, ed: *Current Veterinary Therapy in Equine Medicine,* London, WB Saunders, 1987, p 487.

286. Ooms LAA, Degryse AAY, Fransen JLA, et al.: Treatment of chronic myopathies in horses with the serotonin S₂-antagonist R 50 970: A preclinical study. *Drug Dev Res* 8:219, 1986.

287. Chen CL, McNulty ME, McNulty PK, et al.: Serum levels of thyroxine and triiodothyronine in mature horses following oral administration of synthetic thyroxine (synthyroid). *J Equine Vet Sci* 4:5, 1984.

288. Haverkort-Poels PJE, Joosten EMG, Ruitenbeek W: Prevention of recurrent external rhabdomyolysis by dantrolene sodium. *Muscle Nerve* 10:45, 1987.

289. Waldron-Mease E: Update on prophylaxis of tying-up using dantrolene. *Proc Am Assoc Equine Pract* 25:379, 1979.

290. Adams OR: Azoturia. In Adams OR, ed: *Lameness in Horses,* ed 3. Philadelphia, Lea & Febiger, 1974, p 285.

291. Lawrence LM, Muler PA, Bechtel PJ, et al.: The effect of sodium bicarbonate ingestion on blood parameters in exercising horses. In Gillespie JR, Robinson NE, eds: *Equine Exercise Physiology,* vol 2. Davis, Calif, ICEEP, 1987, p 448.

292. Parry-Billings M, Maclaren DPM: The effect of sodium bicarbonate and sodium citrate ingestion on anaerobic power during intermittent exercise. *Eur J Appl Physiol* 55:524, 1986.

293. Mansmann RA, Podkonjak KR, Jackson PD, et al.: Panel report: Tying-up in horses. *Mod Vet Pract* 63:919, 1982.

294. Rose RJ, Schlierf HA, Knight PK, et al.: Effects of N,N-dimethylglycine on cardiorespiratory function and lactate production in thoroughbred horses performing incremental treadmill exercise. *Vet Rec* 125:268, 1989.

295. Freestone JF, Wolfsheimer KJ, Kamerling SG, et al.: Exercise-induced hormonal and metabolic changes in thoroughbred horses: Effects of conditioning and acepromazine. *Equine Vet J* 23:219, 1991.

296. Dorup I, Skajaa K, Clausen T: A simple and rapid method for the determination of the concentrations of magnesium sodium, potassium and sodium, potassium pumps in human skeletal muscle. *Clin Sci* 74:241, 1988.

297. Syrjala H, Vuori J, Huttunen K, et al.: Carbonic anhydrase III as a serum marker for diagnosis of rhabdomyolysis. *Clin Chem* 36:696, 1990.

298. Nishita T, Matsushita H: Carbonic anhydrase III in equine tissues and sera determined by a highly sensitive enzyme-immunoassay. *Equine Vet J* 22:247, 1990.

299. Mayhew IG: Neuromuscular arthrogryposis multiplex congenita in a thoroughbred foal. *Vet Pathol* 21:187, 1984.

300. Pritchard JT, Voss JL: Fetal ankylosis in horses associated with hybrid Sudan pasture. *J Am Vet Med Assoc* 150:871, 1967.

301. McIlwraith CW, James LF: Limb deformities in foals associated with ingestion of locoweed by mares. *J Am Vet Med Assoc* 181:255, 1982.

302. Vandeplassche M, Simoens P, Bouters RN de vos, et al.: Aetiology and pathogenesis of congenital torticollis and head scolioses in the equine foetus. *Equine Vet J* 16:419, 1984.

303. Leitch M: Musculoskeletal disorders in neonatal foals. *Vet Clin North Am* 1:189, 1985.

304. Whitwell KE, Harris PA, Farrington PG: An outbreak of atypical myoglobinuria. *Equine Vet J* 20:357, 1988.

305. Egyed MN, Nathan A, Eilat A, et al.: Poisoning in sheep and horses caused by the ingestion of weeds sprayed with simazine and aminotriazole. *Refuah Vet* 32:59, 1975.

306. Mayhew IG, McKay RJ: Nervous system. In Mansmann RA, McAllister ES, Pratt PW, eds: *Equine Medicine and Surgery,*

ed 3. Santa Barbara, Calif, American Veterinary, 1982, p 1245.

307. Harris P, Colles C: The use of creatinine clearance ratios in the prevention of equine rhabdomyolysis: A report of four cases. *Equine Vet J* 20:459, 1988.

308. Harris PA: Equine rhabdomyolysis syndrome. *Equine Pract* 11:3, 1989.

Chapter 9

Neurologic Disease

9.1

Neurologic Examination

Stephen M. Reed, DVM, Dip ACVM

The assessment of the central nervous system in horses may seem a difficult task; however, with careful examination and by following a craniocaudal approach, it is not difficult. In my opinion a craniocaudal approach is the most logical and efficient. The examination focuses on the neuroanatomical localization of the lesion or lesions and should be completed as part of the physical examination. Subtle neurologic deficits may be hidden by musculoskeletal disease or missed because of lack of knowledge or understanding of these disorders. To accomplish a complete and accurate neurologic examination the veterinarian must feel comfortable with the format he or she has chosen to evaluate the nervous system as well as have knowledge of which musculoskeletal disorders are commonly associated with neurologic disease. Problems such as osteochondrosis of the stifle, hock, and shoulder joints often occur concurrently in horses with cervical vertebral stenotic myelopathy (CVM). Examples of typical histories in horses presented for neurologic examination are previous medial patellar desmotomy or bilateral bog spavin in early life. Osteochondrosis of the distal tibia or femur and contracted tendons are examples of conditions that may occur simultaneously. Bilateral bog spavin is often associated with osteochondrosis of the distal tibia or other sites in the tibiotarsal joint. Patellar desmotomy to correct upward fixation of the patella may be necessary because of either a conformational problem of the stifle joint or as a result of abnormal joint proprioception or quadriceps weakness secondary to neurologic disease. This problem is more commonly associated with neurologic disease than many veterinarians realize, and the gait deficits caused by these lamenesses often mimic neurologic disease.

The goals of a neurologic examination are to establish whether or not a neurologic problem is present and to determine the anatomical localization of the problem. It is ideal to be able to account for all clinical signs with a single lesion; however, if this is not possible, the presence of multifocal disease or multiple diseases should be considered. Following anatomical localization, a decision is made about what additional testing is necessary to determine the underlying cause of the clinical signs. Cervical radiography, cerebro-spinal fluid (CSF) analysis, and electrodiagnostic testing may be useful in locating and determining the cause of the lesions.

My examination always begins at the head and proceeds to the tail, although some segments of the neurologic examination are performed as part of the physical examination. The examiner should proceed in a consistent fashion, and should record his or her findings in an orderly manner so as to avoid any part of the examination being omitted. A sample format is shown in Figure 9–1. The craniocaudal approach may be used for all animals, whether ambulatory or recumbent.

The examination procedure has been described.[1–10] I follow the format developed by Mayhew,[1] which divides the examination into five categories. These are the head and mental status, gait and posture, neck and forelimbs, trunk and hindlimbs, and tail and anus. The functional divisions of the nervous system include the sensory, integration, and motor systems.

At the start of the examination it can be helpful for the veterinarian to know the age, sex, breed, and use of the horse, although these are not essential. This information is useful because horses of various breeds behave differently. It is important to ask the owner about any unusual behavior the horse has exhibited, as well as the date of onset of the behavior. Age is helpful because problems such as CVM and cerebellar abiotrophy begin at a young age, usually less than 1 year. These problems occur more often in certain breeds. For example, CVM is most common in Thoroughbreds and cerebellar abiotrophy is most often observed in Arabians.

EXAMINATION

The evaluation of the head should include observation of the horse at rest and during motion, along with palpation, postural reactions, cranial nerve function, cervicofacial reflexes, and evaluation of sensation. Evaluation of the head includes observation of the horse's behavior and mental status. This portion of the examination can be partially completed prior to handling the horse. A close and careful examination is necessary to evaluate the head and neck posture and its coordination, and identify abnormalities of the cranial nerves. Initial consideration includes the horse's environmental awareness. A normal horse appears bright and alert, and responds appropriately to external stimuli. While the horse is being caught, the examiner can look for unusual behaviors such as yawning, abnormal or aimless wandering, seizures or circling or head tilt, as well as begin to assess

NEUROLOGIC EXAMINATION

Date: _____
Sire _____
Dam _____
Dam's sire _____

History _____
_____
_____
_____

General observations _____
_____
_____
_____

CRANIAL NERVE EXAM:

Menace (2, 7)	_____	_____	Facial symmetry:	
Pupil size (2,3, sym.)	_____	_____	Temporal/masseter (5)	_____
Pupil symmetry (3, sym.)	_____	_____	Expressive muscles (7)	_____
PLR (2, 3)	_____	_____	Palpebral reflex (5, 7)	_____
Doll's eye (8, 3, 4, 6)	_____	_____	Retractor oculi (5, 6)	_____
Ocular position (8, 3, 4, 6)	_____	_____	Gag reflex (9, 10)	_____
Pathologic nystagmus	_____	_____	Tongue (12)	_____

Symmetry of neck/body (muscle mass, scoliosis, etc.) _____
_____

Manipulation of the neck   L/R _____
                            up/down _____
Spontaneous involuntary movements (tremor, myoclonus, myotonia, etc.) _____

Description of gait (at walk and trot) _____
_____
_____

Circling	large L	_____	
	R	_____	
	small L	_____	
	R	_____	
Backing		_____	
Up/down an incline		_____	
Elevation of head		_____	
Proprioception	LF	_____	RF _____
	LR	_____	RR _____
Sway reaction	fore	_____	
	rear	_____	
	tail pull	_____	

Grading System—write in grading according to deLahunta
   0 = No gait deficits
   1 = Deficits barely perceptible—worsened with head elevation
   2 = Deficits noted at a walk
   3 = Deficits noted at rest, walking; nearly falls with head elevation
   4 = Falls or nearly falls at normal gaits
   5 = Recumbent patient

Figure 9–1. Example of a neurologic examination form. *PLR,* pupillary light response.

the vision and hearing of the horse. If the horse shows behavior abnormalities, such as head-pressing or aggressiveness, these should be noted. If the examiner suspects rabies, then precautions should be taken to avoid unnecessary and potentially dangerous exposure.

Lesions of the reticular activating system or the cerebral hemispheres could result in severe signs such as coma or obtundation of consciousness. Horses that have a serious systemic illness may also appear very depressed or stuporous. The level of consciousness is recorded as alert,

Gait and posture (graded 0 to +4)

		Motor		Sensory
	Weakness	Spasticity		Ataxia
LF	_____	_____		_____
RF	_____	_____		_____
LR	_____	_____		_____
RR	_____	_____		_____

Reflexes   Anal   _____

              Patellar   _____

              Triceps   _____

              Other   _____

Nociceptive (withdrawal) _____

Tail tone _____

Autonomic   Urinary   _____

               Rectal   _____

               Sweating   _____

Cutaneous sensation _____

Assessment/comments _____

Lesion localization _____

Tentative DX _____

CSF		Cells	Protein	Culture	Cytology
	L/S	_____	_____	_____	_____
	A/O	_____	_____	_____	_____

Radiographs _____

Myelogram _____

Comments _____

Figure 9–1 *Continued*

depressed, stuporous, comatose, or semicomatose. An animal that is depressed may react to its environment in an inappropriate or unresponsive fashion. Stuporous horses may appear to be asleep unless stimulated with pain, light, or noise.

Head posture and coordination are controlled by the cerebellar and vestibular regions of the brain and brainstem in response to sensory input from receptors in the head, limbs, and body. It is helpful to examine head and neck posture with the horse at rest, while eating, and while moving. Careful examination of the vestibular region is important because many horses develop a head tilt as a result of head trauma, an inner ear infection, or a guttural pouch infection. A head tilt is characterized by the poll deviated about the muzzle and needs to be distinguished from abnormal or unusual turning of the head, as may occur with damage to the region of the forebrain or injury to the cervical vertebrae. Additional signs that may accompany vestibular disease or injury include nystagmus, ipsilateral weakness, and facial nerve paralysis.

Postural abnormalities of the head and neck can sometimes be difficult to distinguish from head tilt. Horses with torticollis of the head and neck may have a congenital abnormality of the vertebrae or may have injured the muscles of the neck region. Careful examination, including palpation, should help identify fractures of the cervical vertebrae or painful muscles caused by trauma or an injection reaction. In some horses radiographs of the cervical vertebrae may be useful to confirm a fracture or osteomyelitis. Blindness can sometimes lead to an abnormal head or neck posture.

The cerebellum helps regulate rate and range of motion.

With damage to this area a horse will often show fine resting tremors of the head which worsen with intentional movements.[3] This tremorous movement of the head and neck may be observed in the newborn or very young foal, but is not normal in older foals and adult horses. In young Arabians and a few other breeds, a condition of cerebellar abiotrophy has been reported.[1, 3] Horses with this condition show a hypermetric gait, failure to blink when exposed to bright light, and absence of a menace response.

After the horse's alertness, mental attitude, head and neck posture, and coordination have been evaluated, the examiner should closely examine the cranial nerves. In the past I have recommended that the examiner follow the cranial nerve examination in a road map form. This is necessary to ensure that a subtle lesion along the brainstem is less likely to be missed. The examination is accomplished by evaluating facial symmetry, facial sensation (including sensation inside the nares), head posture, eyes, nose, mouth, jaw tone, pharynx, and larynx. To determine if an animal can smell is usually not important, but determining if it can see, hear, breathe, and swallow is critical.

The examination of the eyes should include evaluation of the animal's blink or menace response, its ability to negotiate in a strange environment, pupillary light response, and in some cases a funduscopic examination. If a horse has a lesion of the eye or optic nerve, it will result in complete or partial ipsilateral blindness. To develop contralateral blindness the horse would have to have a lesion in the optic tract or the lateral geniculate nucleus.[1]

The examination of the face should include evaluation of pupil size and symmetry. These are under control of the autonomic nervous system and will be affected by environmental light and level of fear or excitement. To test the pupillary response a light should be directed in each eye and the constriction of the pupil noted. It is often difficult to identify a consensual response in the horse when working alone. A swinging light test has been described.[1] Moving the light from side to side takes advantage of the ipsilateral light response being stronger than the consensual response. This procedure can be performed by a single examiner.

One possible cause of asymmetric pupils in a horse is Horner's syndrome. This syndrome includes ptosis of the upper eyelid, miosis of the pupil, and protrusion of the third eyelid (nictitating membrane). In addition, the horse will have unilateral facial sweating, increased facial temperature, and hyperemia of the nasal and conjunctival membranes. The presence of these signs should alert the examiner to the possibility of a previous perivascular injection, or a guttural pouch infection, or damage to the sympathetic nerves in the vagosympathetic trunk, which courses from the cranial thoracic spinal cord through the thoracic inlet and upward to the orbit.[5]

Loss of symmetric positioning of the eyes or the presence of abnormal deviation (i.e., strabismus) occurs when a horse has injured either the third (oculomotor), fourth (trochlear), or sixth (abducens) cranial nerve or the connections between the eighth (vestibulocochlear) cranial nerve and these nuclei in the brainstem along the medial longitudinal fasciculus. Deviations of the eyes may be seen with head trauma or midbrain lesions or can be a variation of normal in newborn foals.

The nuclei along the fifth (trigeminal) cranial nerve are among the largest nuclei along the brainstem of the horse. This nerve contains both motor and sensory branches which supply innervation to the muscles of mastication and sensation to the skin and mucous membranes of the head. Injury to this nerve leads to dropped jaw and ipsilateral loss of, or decreased sensation to, the side of the face and the inside of the nares.

Damage to the seventh (facial) and eighth cranial nerves is common in horses. Injury to the seventh cranial nerve results in unilateral facial paralysis. This nerve contains branches which supply the ears, eyelids, and nares. Thus injury to this nerve may affect all or only part of these structures. The most easily recognized sign is deviation of the nares toward the unaffected side coupled with drooping of the eyelid and ear on the affected side. Because this nerve also innervates the salivary and lacrimal glands, loss of or damage to this nerve may cause dry eye and decreased salivation.

Eighth cranial nerve deficits are easy to recognize, since unilateral injury to this nerve results in a head tilt toward the affected side. The eighth cranial nerve is important to hearing as well as to control of balance. Projections from this nerve pass to the medulla and cerebellum. A horse that has damage to this nerve will often appear disoriented and have a head tilt toward the side of the lesion along with abnormal position of the limbs and body and horizontal nystagmus. If the lesion involves the peripheral portion of the vestibular system, then the fast phase of the nystagmus will be directed away from the side of the lesion. If the lesion involves the central portion of the vestibular system, the nystagmus may appear vertical, rotary, or horizontal and may not always appear the same, depending on head position.

Horses that have peripheral damage to the vestibular system will usually compensate for the deficits in a short time by use of visual and proprioceptive input. Therefore, it is judicious to avoid the use of a blindfold in cases of suspected vestibular disease. This will hamper the horse's ability to compensate and it may become dangerous. However, blindfolding a horse with a suspected vestibular disease, but no longer showing an obvious head tilt, may sometimes be helpful in localizing the lesion.

Within the medial compartment of the guttural pouch along the caudodorsal and lateral walls are the ninth (glossopharyngeal) cranial nerve and a branch of the vagus nerve. When a horse develops a guttural pouch infection these nerves may be damaged, resulting in loss of innervation to the pharyngeal muscles. The clinical signs include dysphagia on the same side as the damaged nerve. If the infection is severe enough to involve the internal carotid nerve, which contains postganglionic sympathetic fibers to the structures of the head and eye, Horner's syndrome results. As mentioned earlier, the signs include ptosis of the upper eyelid, enophthalmus resulting in prolapse of the third eyelid, miosis of the pupil, and sweating along the side of the face.

Other diseases which should be considered when evidence of Horner's syndrome is noted during a neurologic examination include injury or infarction to the cranial thoracic spinal cord, avulsion of the brachial plexus, a hematoma, or tumor invading the sympathetic trunk in the region of the caudal, cervical, or cranial thoracic sympathetic trunk. Mycosis of the guttural pouch can cause damage to the internal carotid nerve or the cranial cervical ganglion along the caudodorsal wall of the guttural pouch. Finally, an injury to, or neoplasia of, the structures within or just behind the orbit may also cause Horner's syndrome.

The presence of focal sweating in a horse indicates involvement of the peripheral pre- or postganglionic sympathetic neurons. Identification of this problem can also aid in the anatomical localization of a neurologic lesion.[1]

Intact innervation to the larynx and pharynx is important, especially if the horse is to be used as an athlete. The easiest means to evaluate this region is by endoscopic examination of the pharyngeal and laryngeal regions. Throat latch palpation and a laryngeal adductory slap test can be performed. Endoscopic examination is helpful and important to a complete evaluation. The innervation of the pharynx and larynx is via the ninth, tenth (vagus), and eleventh (accessory) cranial nerves and the connections of these nerves in the caudal medulla oblongata.

Following careful examination of the mental status and behavior of the horse, as well as of the head, neck, and cranial nerves, the examiner should look for asymmetry of the muscles of the trunk, pelvic region, tail, and anus. Identification of focal sweating, focal muscle atrophy, or increased or decreased pain responses is helpful in localizing signs. In addition, the horse has two cervical reflexes. The cervicofacial reflexes result in a local twitch and drawing back of the lips ("smile" reflex) when the skin along the side of the neck down to the region of the second cervical vertebra is pricked. Below the region of the second cervical vertebra a local response should be observed.[11]

To evaluate the tail and anus one should begin by observing the tail carriage at rest and with the horse in motion. The normal tail carriage is straight down but with free movement in all directions. Some normal horses will allow the tail to be lifted with very little resistance, whereas other horses will strongly resist and clamp the tail. The usual response to anal stimulation is to clamp the tail and squat down, although with prolonged stimulation the horse may relax and eventually raise its tail.

Evaluation of Gait

The evaluation of a horse's gait should include examination of postural reactions in all horses and may include evaluation of spinal reflexes in young or very small horses. Although they may appear very weak and ataxic, foals are ambulatory within hours after birth, making it possible to evaluate gait. Because postural reactions are sometimes difficult to interpret in horses, it is essential to use gait abnormalities to help localize a lesion. I nearly always place the feet and limbs in an unusual position and observe the response of the horse. Gait abnormalities that are commonly observed in horses with neurologic disease include ataxia, spasticity, and weakness or paresis.

The evaluation of gait is critical because subtle neurologic gait deficits often go unrecognized or may sometimes be incorrectly considered insignificant. The examination should be conducted with the horse observed at a walk and trot both in a straight line and while turning. In some horses it is helpful to observe the horse negotiate over small obstacles such as a curb. When possible the examiner should observe the horse turned free and walking up and down an incline. Elevation of the head and walking on a slope may exaggerate a subtle deficit and make it more noticeable.

This portion of the examination should be conducted with the animal at rest to observe its posture, while walking, while trotting, and sometimes while the horse is being ridden. The examiner should pay attention to which limbs show abnormal posture or abnormal movements and must be able to determine whether the horse has a painful, mechanical musculoskeletal problem rather than a neurologic gait deficit. The examiner must identify the presence of weakness, ataxia, and spasticity in each limb.

The important centers for posture and coordination in the brainstem and spinal cord have been briefly described. These centers are located in the regions of C6–T2 and L4–S2 in the spinal cord, along with coordination centers in the brainstem. Horses that demonstrate a very wide base stance at rest often have a lesion of the cerebellum or vestibular system, or may have conscious proprioceptive abnormalities.

To evaluate an animal's gait, begin by observing the horse at a walk and trot. At a walk the examiner can walk alongside, in step with first the rear- and then the forelimbs. This allows the examiner to more easily determine the stride length and foot placement. A weak limb will often have a low arc and longer stride length.

The horse should also be observed walking in a circle, on a slope, and with its head elevated. These procedures help to demonstrate if the horse is showing persistent irregular movements with its limbs. Horses with a musculoskeletal problem have been described as being regularly irregular, whereas a horse with neurologic gait deficits shows fewer consistent mistakes when positioning its limbs. Although it is helpful to have a chance to observe the horse running free in a paddock or round pen and while being ridden, this is not always possible. There are certain legal ramifications a veterinarian must consider before asking a person to ride a horse during the examination.

Additional tests which may be helpful during a neurologic examination include blindfolding the horse, walking it over a curb or other obstacle, and walking it with its head and neck extended. The strength and ability of the horse to correct body positions can be evaluated by performing a sway test. This test is accomplished by application of lateral pressure at the shoulder, hip, and tail while the horse is standing and walking. Pressure should be applied several times while the horse is walking to catch the limb in various stages of weight-bearing. Observing a horse while it is backing is important. When a normal horse is backing it should lift each leg and place it in a coordinated and appropriate location. Horses with neurologic abnormalities often place the limbs in very wide-based positions or will lean back and be reluctant or refuse to move. It may also step on the rear feet with the front feet.

The horse should be observed closely while being turned in a tight circle. Abnormal wide outward excursions of the rearlimb (circumduction) may be identified during this procedure. Additional tests to assess proprioceptive function include a standing sway test where pressure is applied to the side of the shoulder. The horse should initially press into the examiner, then lean away, and finally it should step away with the offside limb. I also cross the limbs over the opposite fore- or rearlimb to determine if the horse recognizes and tolerates these unusual limb positions. Following this I lift one front limb and force the horse to hop on the opposite front limb in a modified postural reaction.

The examiner should carefully observe the movements of each limb to determine if a deficit is present and assign a grade to the deficit. The system I use is a modification of the grades described by deLahunta[3] and Mayhew.[1] The severity is graded between 0 and 5. Grade 0 is assigned when there are no gait deficits. A grade 1 deficit requires careful observation to be certain the gait abnormality is caused by a neurologic dysfunction. Grade 2 deficits are moderate but obvious to most observers as soon as the horse begins to move, but are still mild to moderate in severity. Grade 3 deficits are very obvious and are exaggerated during the negotiation of a slope or with head elevation. Grade 4 gait deficits may cause a horse to fall or nearly fall. When attempting to walk, an animal with these severe deficits often displays abnormal positioning while standing in its stall. Grade 5 horses are recumbent.

Weakness is used to describe knuckling, stumbling, or buckling and can sometimes be characterized by toe-dragging while walking. Weakness may be associated with either an upper motor neuron or lower motor neuron lesion. In the case of a lower motor neuron or peripheral nerve injury or illness, the horse will show muscle atrophy and sensory loss. Ataxia is typified by abnormal foot placement and wide swaying of the foot and limb, especially while turning.

The gait abnormalities along with the findings from other parts of the neurologic examination allow the examiner to determine the neuroanatomical site of the problem. The severity of the clinical signs also helps to evaluate the extent or severity of the problem.

Horses with an obscure or unusual gait which might be lameness should be reexamined after use of local anesthetics to block selected peripheral nerves or following treatment with intra-articular medications. The use of nonsteroidal anti-inflammatory drugs for a period of 1 to 2 days may also alleviate pain and help to distinguish between a lameness and a neurologic gait deficit.

It is important to realize that many horses that have minimal (grade 1 or mild grade 2) deficits can often race or perform other athletic activities.[12] The examining veterinarian has the responsibility of separating a neurologic from a musculoskeletal gait deficit and helping the owner determine the usefulness of the horse. For example, a horse with gait deficits up to grade 3 may be useful as a broodmare or breeding stallion if the horse is handled by careful, knowledgeable horsepersons who understand the risks and have a facility that can accommodate a horse in need of special management. Stallions with this degree of impairment may require assistance when mounting and dismounting mares. If the breed association allows artificial insemination, the stallion may be easier to manage.

Localizing the Lesion

At the conclusion of the examination the veterinarian needs to determine if a neurologic abnormality exists and where it is located. If the horse showed no evidence of abnormal behavior, seizures, or abnormal mental status, and showed no cranial nerve deficits, the lesion is most likely caudal to the foramen magnum.

The most difficult lesions to localize are in the brainstem unless the signs include cranial nerve deficits or depression. Horses with brainstem lesions often show signs of weakness and ataxia similar to horses with a lesion in the cervical spinal cord. Two of the most common brainstem lesions in horses involve the seventh and eighth cranial nerves. Vestibular disease or injury may be a sequela of head trauma or an inner ear infection. Facial nerve paralysis may result from trauma to the nerve root origin in the brainstem or where the nerves course along the neck and face to the ears, eyelids, and nares. These problems may occur in horses infected with *Sarcocystis* parasites.

Specific cranial nerve involvement such as head tilt, facial nerve paralysis, or loss of facial sensation can result from trauma, guttural pouch infection, osteomyelitis of the stylohyoid bone, or equine protozoal encephalomyelitis. In addition, cranial nerve deficits may occur with polyneuritis equi and equine motor neuron disease.

Cerebellar lesions are characterized by a failure to blink to bright light, lack of a menace response, and a head tremor that worsens with intentional movements. This disease is an abiotrophy and is seen most frequently in Arabian horses.

Cervical spinal cord disease includes gait and proprioceptive deficits in all four limbs with no signs of brain, brainstem, or cranial nerve deficits. It should be noted that horses with cervical vertebral stenotic myelopathy may have mild pelvic limb deficits with minimal or barely detectable signs in the thoracic limbs.[13]

Horses with signs of neurologic gait deficits confined to the pelvic limbs have a neuroanatomical localization caudal to T2. When examining a horse with a lesion caudal to T2 it is important to carefully check the tail and anus for involvement of the peripheral nerves or spinal cord segments in this region.

Horses that have peripheral nerve injury, equine motor neuron disease, or polyneuritis equi will show evidence of weakness, muscle atrophy, and in some cases selected areas of sensory loss. Primary muscle diseases such as exertional rhabdomyolysis, myotonia (either congenita or dystrophica), and hyperkalemic periodic paralysis are covered elsewhere in this book. These conditions can sometimes mimic a neurologic problem.

Description of Normal Gaits

The reader is reminded that a walk is a natural four-beat gait in the horse. At this gait the normal horse has three feet on the ground at all times. Therefore, the walk is a very stable gait. Overtracking and interference may occur if the conformation of the horse is abnormal (e.g., with long limbs and a short body) and not as a result of neurologic disease.[8] The trot is also a useful gait to observe when performing a neurologic examination in the face of subtle gait deficits. In this two-beat symmetric movement the diagonal limbs are in contact with the ground at the same time. If the horse is examined while on hard pavement the trot is the most helpful gait to distinguish a lameness from a neurologic gait deficit. Normally the pace is a gait that results in significant truncal sway as the legs on the same side of the body strike the ground simultaneously. In horses that have neurologic disease it is common to identify ataxia with truncal sway, which is often accompanied by pacing. In horses with subtle ataxia, pacing is observed when horses are walked with the head held in an extended position. Whenever a horse is observed to pace it bears close observation, as this may be an indication of an underlying neurologic disorder.

The gallop is a high-speed four-beat gait which often seems to be easier to perform than walking in a tight circle or moving at a slow trot. Therefore, some horses with a neurologic gait deficit may perform better at high speed. When accelerating or slowing down, abnormalities may be detected and it is important to observe the horse carefully for this is the time when an ataxic horse is most unsafe.

Abnormal gaits associated with stringhalt, upward fixation of the patella, and fibrotic myopathy deserve careful attention. Horses that show these gait abnormalities have a mechanical lameness, although the exact cause is unknown and may sometimes be associated with underlying neurologic disease.

Stringhalt often begins as an abrupt onset of excessive flexion of one or both rearlimbs. In some horses the condition may worsen and result in frequent episodes of the foot hitting the abdomen. The condition has been reported for a long time and in some areas of the world may occur as an outbreak.[14] The clinical syndrome is similar to the movement of a horse with a tibial neurectomy with unopposed flexion of the hock and extension of the digit. In the case of Australian stringhalt there may be involvement of the forelimbs and neck muscles. It is mentioned in this chapter only because it is my opinion that when this gait is observed the examiner should be certain no other signs of neurologic gait deficits exist. As most readers know, the primary condition can usually be corrected by performance of a tenectomy of the lateral digital extensor tendon, including a portion of the muscle belly. The underlying cause of the disease may be a sensory neuropathy, a myopathy, or primary spinal cord disease. As has been described, the defect likely affects the neuromuscular spindle as well as the efferent and afferent pathways controlling muscle tone.[7]

Fibrotic myopathy is a result of scar tissue formation following injury to the semitendinosus and semimembranosus muscles. The characteristic foot placement coupled with the abrupt rearward movement of the affected limb may be confused with a spastic gait caused by spinal cord injury or disease. With careful examination it is not likely that a horse suffering from fibrotic myelopathy will go undiagnosed.

Upward fixation of the patella in horses with neurologic disease may be a result of weakness in the quadriceps muscle group. This weakness is thought to occur because of a lack of use of these muscles or may be due to abnormal transmission of proprioceptive information to and from the muscles and joint capsule as a result of damage to the spinal cord.

Horses with profound ataxia often pace when they walk. This is often accompanied by circumduction of the outside rearlimb while turning. These signs are suggestive of general proprioceptive deficits. If the horse has these deficits while walking it is a good idea to observe the horse walking with its head elevated as well as on a slope. These maneuvers often exaggerate a subtle problem.

If the horse shows signs only in the trunk and pelvic limbs, the neuroanatomical localization of the lesion is between T2 and S2 or involves the nerves and muscles of the pelvic limbs. However, the examiner needs to realize that horses with cervical spinal cord lesions often demonstrate signs in the pelvic limbs that are one grade worse than over the thoracic limbs. Therefore, a very mild cervical spinal cord or brainstem lesion could show minimal or no thoracic limb signs with grade 1 or very subtle signs in the pelvic limbs.

It is helpful to palpate the horse over its back, rump, and muscles of the rearlimbs, being careful to detect any muscle atrophy. I routinely stimulate the horse over the side of its body and observe for any twitching of the cutaneous trunci muscles. It is usually accompanied by a cerebral response and requires a fairly severe lesion to detect areas of analgesia.

A sway reaction performed while the horse is both standing and walking is also necessary to assess the pelvic limb strength and proprioceptive functions. In addition, strength may be evaluated by slow but deliberate and forceful pressure along the back and sacral muscles. A normal horse should reflexly arch its back upward, whereas a horse with rearlimb weakness may be unable to withstand this pressure and its rearlimbs may even buckle.

Examination of the tail and anus must be completed as part of the neurologic examination to determine whether damage has occurred to the sacrococcygeal nerve and muscle segments. A normal perineal reflex results in contraction of the anus and clamping of the tail in response to light stimulation of the skin in this region. Cauda equina neuritis or polyneuritis equi, trauma, and iatrogenic injury resulting from an alcohol tail block are some disorders that may affect this area.

The evaluation of the major peripheral nerves in the horse is also an important part of the neurologic examination. The important points to remember are that damage to a peripheral nerve can result in both sensory and motor deficits in the area supplied by the nerve and that focal muscle atrophy will follow within a short time after damage to one of these nerves. The examiner is referred to other portions of this book for a more detailed anatomical description of these nerves in the horse; however, a dropped elbow joint with radial nerve paralysis, inability to fix the stifle with femoral nerve paralysis, and atrophy of the supraspinatus and infraspinatus muscles (sweeney) with damage to the suprascapular nerve are classic examples of what to expect with peripheral nerve injuries.[1–3]

CONCLUSION

To conclude the description of the neurologic examination, the reader is reminded that for a horse to be a good athlete it must gather information from muscles, tendons, and nerves; process this information in the brain, brainstem, and spinal cord; and relay this information to the musculoskeletal system. All of this must be accomplished in a very short time to perform very complex maneuvers at a high rate of speed. When this is to be performed in a setting involving many other horses or when a rider or driver is involved, the horse needs to be able to control these movements in a coordinated fashion to protect itself, other horses, and especially people. While it is not necessary to have every neuron, spinal tract, and glial cell working to be athletic, it is very important that the veterinarian be able to distinguish between a musculoskeletal lameness and a neurologic condition that may make the horse unsafe for use and dangerous to itself or the rider.

Beyond this, it is important for veterinarians to recognize which musculoskeletal and neurological conditions occur together in order to better assist the prospective buyer with the decision about whether or not to purchase the horse. When these things are recognized and understood, the horse with subtle neurologic gait deficits caused by trauma, infection, or compression may yet be a safe and useful athlete.

REFERENCES

1. Mayhew IG: *Large Animal Neurology. A Handbook for Veterinary Clinicians.* Philadelphia, Lea & Febiger, 1989, pp 15–49.
2. Blythe LL: Neurologic examination of the horse. *Vet Clin North Am Equine Pract* 3:255–281, 1987.
3. deLahunta A: *Veterinary Neuroanatomy and Clinical Neurology,* ed 2. Philadelphia, WB Saunders, 1983, pp 389–401.
4. Mayhew IG: *Large Animal Neurology. A Handbook for Veterinary Clinicians.* Philadelphia, Lea & Febiger, 1989, p 221.
5. Matthews HK, Andrews F: Performing a neurologic examination in a standing or recumbent horse. *Vet Med Equine Pract* 1229–1240, 1990.
6. Andrews FM, Matthews HK: Localizing the source of neurologic problems in horses. *Vet Med Equine Pract* 1107–1120, 1990.
7. Mayhew IG: Equine neurologic examination. *Prog Vet Neurol* 1:40–47.
8. Mayhew IG: Neurological and neuropathological observations on the equine neonate. *Equine Vet J Suppl* 28–33.
9. Woods JR: Neurological examination of the horse. *OVMA* 24:13–18, 1972.
10. Mayhew IG: Neurologic examination of the horse with a discussion of common diseases and syndromes. Presented at the 24th Annual Convention of the Association of Equine Practitioners, Dec 1978.
11. Rooney JR: Two cervical reflexes in the horse. *J Am Vet Med Assoc* 162, 1973.
12. Clayton H: Locomotion. In Jones WE, ed: *Equine Sports Medicine.* Philadelphia, Lea & Febiger, 1989, pp 149–189.
13. Yeager MJ, Middleton DL, Render JA: Identification of spinal cord lesions through the use of Zenker's fixation and radiography. *J Vet Diagn Invest* 1:264–266, 1989.
14. Robertson-Smith RG, Jeffcott LB, Friend SCE, et al: An unusual incidence of neurological disease affecting horses during a drought. *Aust Vet J* 62, 1985.

9.2

Cerebrospinal Fluid Evaluation

Frank M. Andrews, DVM, MS

Cerebrospinal fluid (CSF) evaluation has diagnostic importance in evaluating neurologic disease in horses. Collection and analysis of CSF is indicated when making or confirming a diagnosis of neurologic disease, but this is not without limitations. CSF values may be normal in an animal with severe neurologic deficits because the lesion is extradural, it is early or late in the course of disease, the CSF is collected too far away from the lesion, or with diseases involving the ventral roots and peripheral nerve. Even with its limitations it provides valuable information about the central nervous system (CNS). However, it must be emphasized that CSF evaluation is another piece of the diagnostic puzzle and together with the history, physical examination, neurologic examination, and other ancillary procedures may help in the diagnosis and prognosis of neurologic disease in horses.

FORMATION, FLOW, AND FUNCTION OF CEREBROSPINAL FLUID

Cerebrospinal fluid is an actively transported ultrafiltrate of plasma that bathes the CNS.[1] The CSF is located in the ventricles of the brain and subarachnoid space of the spinal canal (Fig. 9–2) and originates from the choroid plexus and ependymal lining of the ventricles.[2] CSF flows from the ventricular system up over the cerebral hemispheres and through the subarachnoid space surrounding the spinal cord.[1] Pulsation of blood in the choroid plexuses forces the CSF in a caudad direction. The rate of CSF production varies from 0.017 mL/min in cats to 0.5 mL/min in humans,[3] and is independent of the blood hydrostatic pressure. The rate of CSF production has not been determined for horses. Osmotic and hypertonic solutions such as mannitol and dimethyl sulfoxide, when added to blood, decrease CSF production and decrease CSF pressure and edema.[1]

Collections of arachnoid villi (arachnoid granulations) are located in the venous sinus or the cerebral vein and absorb CSF. CSF absorption is directly related to the pressure gradient between the CSF and venous sinus. When CSF pressure exceeds venous pressure, these villi act as one-way ball valves forcing CSF flow to the venous sinus.[4]

CSF functions to suspend the brain and spinal cord for protection, regulate intracranial pressure, and maintain the proper ionic and acid-base balance.[1]

CEREBROSPINAL FLUID COLLECTION

Techniques for collection of CSF in horses have been described in detail elsewhere.[1, 5] CSF may be collected from the lumbosacral site in a standing horse sedated with an intravenous injection of xylazine 0.2 to 0.5 mg/kg or butorphanol 0.01 to 0.02 mg/kg, or a combination of both drugs. Alternatively, CSF can be collected from the atlanto-occipital site of an anesthetized horse. In foals and recumbent adult horses, CSF can be collected while the animal is restrained and heavily sedated with xylazine 1.0 mg/kg IV and butorphanol 0.2 mg/kg IV. If the lesion is localized to an area above the foramen magnum (at least cranial to C2), CSF collected from the atlanto-occipital site will be more diagnostic. If the lesion is localized to an area below the foramen magnum (caudal to C2), CSF collected from the lumbosacral site will be more diagnostic. This is because of the craniocaudal circulation of CSF. Collecting CSF from both sites at the same time and comparing the findings may be helpful in cases in which neuroanatomical localization of the lesion is difficult.[5]

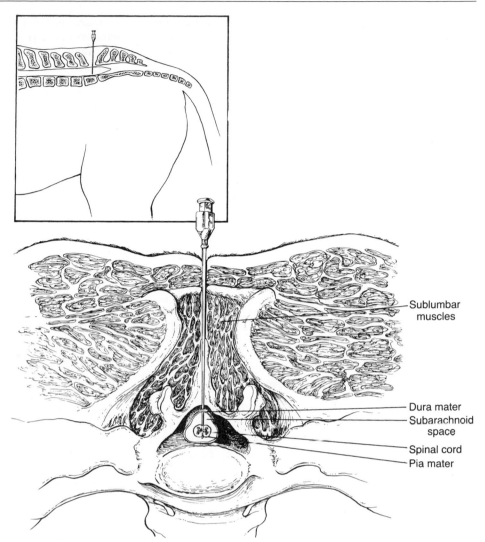

Figure 9–2. Lumbosacral spinal fluid collection from a horse showing the various tissue layers that the spinal needle must pass through in order to obtain a sample. Note that the spinal fluid is being collected ventral to the spinal cord in the subarachnoid space. *Inset,* Lateral view of spinal needle placement in the lumbosacral space for collection of cerebrospinal fluid. (From Andrews FM, Adair HS III: Anatomy and physiology of the nervous system. In Auer JA: *Equine Surgery.* Philadelphia, WB Saunders, 1992, p 536; modified from deLahunta A: *Veterinary Neuroanatomy and Clinical Neurology,* ed 2. Philadelphia, WB Saunders, 1983, p 43.)

CEREBROSPINAL FLUID EXAMINATION

Reference values for CSF in horses have been reported,[6–11] but each laboratory should determine its own reference ranges. CSF determinations that are helpful in evaluating horses with neurologic diseases include pressure, appearance, cellular content, protein concentration (total protein, albumin, IgG), enzyme activity (creatinine kinase, CK; aspartate aminotransferase, AST; lactate dehydrogenase, LDH), and lactic acid concentration.

Pressure

Opening CSF pressure can be measured prior to withdrawing CSF by attaching a manometer tube with a three-way stopcock to a properly placed spinal needle, allowing the CSF to rise within.[12] Since the cranial and vertebral cavities are enclosed in a rigid bony compartment, changes in blood pressure or volume can cause a concomitant increase in CSF pressure. Thus, increased CSF pressure may occur from venous compression or jugular occlusion. Venous compression causes increased blood volume in the cranial cavity and compression of the CSF space, leading to increased CSF pressure. Jugular occlusion can be used clinically to increase CSF pressure and facilitate collection of CSF fluid.[13] The jugular compression maneuver, or Queckenstedt's phenomenon, can be used to help diagnose compressive lesions, neoplastic lesions, or an abscess along the spinal cord.[1] With compression and obliteration of the subarachnoid space by a compressive lesion in the cervical or thoracic spinal cord, jugular vein compression will not cause a CSF pressure increase in the lumbosacral site.[1]

Increased CSF pressure may occur following injury; systemic changes in blood pressure; and in the presence of an intracranial space-occupying mass, such as a tumor, abscess, hemorrhage, or edema. An adequate airway after injury and during surgery must be provided to prevent hypoxia-mediated cytotoxic cerebral edema and vasogenic cerebral edema.[14] Cytotoxic edema is caused by inadequate cerebral oxygenation and leads to neuronal, glial, and endothelial cell swelling. This is especially important during long surgical procedures or recumbency in which there may be respiratory hypoxia and poor alveolar ventilation (hypercapnia). Hypercapnia increases cerebral blood flow in the cranial cavity and CSF pressure and may worsen existing cerebral edema.[1]

Increased CSF volume may occur in hydrocephalus. *Hy-*

drocephalus is defined as an increased volume of CSF and can be classified as compensatory or obstructive.[15] Compensatory hydrocephalus is an accumulation of CSF in areas where brain tissue has been destroyed and may occur from brain injury or inflammation. *Hydranencephaly* is destruction of brain tissue from a viral or other infectious agent and results in severe accumulation of CSF.[15] CSF pressure in compensatory hydrocephalus is usually not increased.[1]

Obstructive hydrocephalus is an accumulation of CSF in the ventricles from an obstruction to CSF outflow or absorption. Cerebral aqueduct malformation may lead to obstruction of ventricular CSF outflow.[1] Inflammatory lesions, especially of the arachnoid villi, result in decreased absorption of CSF and increased CSF pressure.[1] The white matter is more severely affected than the gray matter in obstructive hydrocephalus, but the cerebral cortex is usually spared.[1] CSF pressure in obstructive hydrocephalus is usually increased. The presence of an abnormally high opening pressure that drops by 25% to 50% after removing 1 to 2 mL of fluid suggests a space-occupying intracranial mass or spinal cord compression cranial to the site of collection.[12] The removal of more fluid would risk causing tentorial herniation.[12]

Appearance

The appearance of CSF can be evaluated immediately after collection. Normal CSF is clear, colorless, and does not clot, and newsprint is visible through it.[16] CSF may be red-tinged from blood contamination after a traumatic tap or from preexisting trauma to the CNS. In the case of a traumatic tap, the CSF will usually clear if allowed to flow for several seconds (about 0.5–1.0 mL). With preexisting trauma and secondary hemorrhage, the supernatant of CSF after centrifugation will be xanthochromic.

Other causes of CSF xanthochromia include increased protein concentration (150 mg/dL)[16] and direct bilirubin leakage from serum in horses with high serum bilirubin concentration.[1] Also, indirect bilirubin may leak across a damaged blood-brain barrier (BBB). Clots in the CSF are abnormal and may be caused by increased amounts of fibrinogen due to inflammation.[1]

Turbid CSF may indicate an increased number of white blood cells (WBCs >200/μL), an increased number of red blood cells (RBCs >400/μL), epidural fat, bacteria, fungal elements, or amebic organisms.[1] Cytologic evaluation and cultures can help differentiate causes of turbidity.

Cytology

A standard hemocytometer can be used to obtain a complete blood count. Also, the use of a sedimentation chamber requiring 0.5 to 1.0 mL of CSF is a rapid method for cytologic evaluation.[17] Cell counts and cytologic evaluation must be done within 30 minutes to avoid degeneration. If cell counts or cytologic evaluation cannot be done immediately, then a portion of the sample can be mixed with equal volumes of 50% ethanol to preserve cellular characteristics.[12] CSF from normal horses and foals usually contains fewer than 10 WBCs per microliter. However, much variation can be seen in CSF WBC counts in horses.[9, 10]

There appears to be no difference in CSF WBC counts in samples taken from the atlanto-occipital space.[10] However, one study did show a slightly higher total WBC count in CSF taken from the lumbosacral site, but WBC counts in all of those horses were less than 10/μL.[6]

Small mononuclear cells (70%–90%) and large mononuclear cells (10%–30%) predominate in horse CSF.[9] Rarely, neutrophils may be seen in horse CSF.[9] Increased CSF large mononuclear phagocytes are seen in horse CSF in diseases of axonal degeneration.[9] Increased CSF neutrophils can be seen in encephalomyelitis, bacterial meningitis, parasitism, and diseases with extensive inflammation.[9, 17, 18] Occasionally, in severe inflammatory diseases of the neurologic system or parasitism, eosinophils may be seen.[9, 17, 18] In some cases cytologic evaluation of CSF may reveal specific etiologic agents causing neurologic disease such as fungal organisms,[16] bacteria, or tumor cells. While CSF cytology may support a diagnosis of neurologic disease, it may not yield a specific etiologic diagnosis.

Protein Concentration and Composition

Normal total protein values range from 20 to 124 mg/dL, depending on the measuring method used[1, 6, 10] (Table 9–1). Total protein concentration is higher in lumbosacral (LS) CSF when compared with atlanto-occipital (AO) CSF[6] (see Table 9–1). A difference of 25 mg/dL of protein between the AO and LS spaces may suggest a lesion closer to the space with greater spinal fluid protein.[10] Proteins in the CSF are derived from the peripheral blood and include albumin, IgG, and possibly other globulins. Increased CSF albumin and IgG concentrations may occur with damage to the BBB or increased intrathecal production of IgG. CSF albumin and IgG concentrations can be determined by electrophoresis and radial immunodiffusion (RID), respectively, and compared with serum concentrations.[6] Special low-level RID plates (VMRD, Inc., Pullman, Wash.) are available to quantify CSF IgG concentration. The albumin quotient ([Albc]/[Albs] × 100) and IgG index ([IgGc]/[IgGs] × [Albs]/[Albc]) can be calculated to determine BBB permeability and intrathecal IgG production[6] (see Table 9–1). Increased intrathecal IgG production (increased IgG index) may occur in inflammatory spinal cord disease such as equine protozoal myeloencephalitis (EPM), bacterial meningitis, some tumors, and equine motor neuron disease. Increased BBB permeability (increased albumin quotient) may occur in equine herpesvirus type 1 (EHV-1), secondary to a necrotizing vasculitis.[7] Determining BBB integrity is also important in planning therapy. If the BBB is damaged, pharmacologic agents, such as penicillin, that do not normally penetrate the BBB will penetrate a disrupted BBB and attain bactericidal CSF concentration.

CSF Enzyme Determination

CSF enzyme activity may be increased in neurologic disease. CK and AST activity may be increased in diseases with myelin degeneration and neuronal cell damage such as EPM, polyneuritis equi, equine degenerative myelopathy, and equine motor neuron disease. Increased CK activity may also occur in conditions that alter BBB permeability, such

Table 9–1. CSF Values [Mean ± SD (Range)] from Atlanto-Occipital (AO) and Lumbosacral (LS) Spaces of Normal Healthy Adult Horses*

	AO Space	LS Space
RBC (per μL)	51.0 ± 160 (0–558)	36.8 ± 59.7 (0–167)
WBC (per μL)	0.33 ± 0.49 (0–1)	0.83 ± 1.11 (0–3)
Total protein (mg/dL)†	87.0 ± 17.0 (53 ± 11.6) (59–118) (35–74)	93.0 ± 16.0 (58.0 ± 11.0) (65–124) (39–78)
CSF albumin (mg/dL)	35.8 ± 9.7 (24–51)	37.8 ± 11.2 (24–56)
Albumin quotient	1.4 ± 0.4 (1.0–2.0)	1.5 ± 0.4 (1.0–2.0)
CSF IgG (mg/dL)	5.6 ± 1.4 (3–8)	6.0 ± 2.1 (3–10)
IgG index	0.19 ± 0.046 (0.12–0.27)	0.19 ± 0.5 (0.12–0.26)
CK (IU/L)	0–8	0–8
LDH (IU/L)	0–8	0–8
AST (IU/L)	4–16	0–16
Glucose (mg/dL)	35%–70% of blood glucose	
Lactate (mg/dL)	1.92 ± 0.12	2.30 ± 0.21
Sodium (mEq/L)	140–150	140–150
Potassium (mEq/L)	2.5–3.5	2.5–3.5

*RBC, red blood cell count; WBC, white blood cell count; CK, creatine kinase; LDH, lactic dehydrogenase; AST, aspartate aminotransferase.
†Total protein concentration next to the mean ± SD in parentheses is the value expected using a total protein standard.

as EHV-1. In diseases in which the BBB is damaged, serum CK can leak into the CSF and increase CSF CK activity. This increased CK activity is not associated with damaged myelin.

Increased CK activity may also suggest other diseases of the CNS. In one study, CK activity (>1 IU/L) was most often associated with EPM in horses, and it may be helpful in differentiating compressive spinal cord disease from EPM.[19] Furthermore, persistently increased CSF CK activity may be associated with a poor prognosis in horses with EPM.[19] LDH activity may be increased in spinal lymphosarcoma.

Lactic Acid Concentration

CSF lactic acid concentration may be an indicator of neurologic disease (see Table 9–1). CSF lactic acid concentration increases in eastern equine encephalomyelitis (4.10 ± 0.6 mg/dL), head trauma (5.40 ± 0.9 mg/dL), and brain abscess (4.53 mg/dL).[20] Lactic acid concentration may be the only CSF parameter increased in horses with brain abscess.[20]

SUMMARY

Normal CSF findings do not always rule out the presence of neurologic disease. Normal CSF values can be seen with lesions outside the CNS not bathed in the CSF, such as extradural, ventral root, and peripheral nerve lesions. Normal

CSF values may also occur early or late in the disease process and in CSF samples taken away from the site of the lesion. Acute neurologic disease, especially if multifocal, may not have sufficient time to cause significant damage to the BBB and alter CSF constituents, whereas in chronic CNS disease the BBB may be repaired and functional, but with nervous tissue replaced by fibrous tissue. Fibrosis of nervous tissue may result in significant neurologic gait deficits and normal CSF constituents. CSF taken away from the site of the lesion will show normal findings despite significant neurologic gait deficits. For example, CSF in a horse with a cervical spinal cord abscess may show a suppurative inflammation in the LS CSF and a normal AO CSF. This discrepancy is due to the caudad flow of CSF.

CSF may be helpful in supporting the diagnosis of neurologic disease in horses and is part of the diagnostic workup. As an ancillary diagnostic test, it should be used in conjunction with, and not as a substitute for, a thorough history, physical examination, neurologic examination, and other diagnostic tests.

REFERENCES

1. deLahunta A: *Veterinary Neuroanatomy and Clinical Neurology.* Philadelphia, WB Saunders, 1983.
2. Milhort TH: The choroid plexus and cerebrospinal fluid production. *Science* 166:1514, 1969.
3. Blood DC, Henderson JA, Radostits O: *Veterinary Medicine,* ed 5. Philadelphia, Lea & Febiger, 1979.

4. Tripathi R: Tracing the bulk outflow of cerebrospinal fluid by transmission and scanning electron microscopy. *Brain Res* 80:503, 1974.

5. Mayhew IG: *Large Animal Neurology.* Philadelphia, Lea & Febiger, 1989.

6. Andrews FM, Maddux JM, Faulk DS: Total protein, albumin quotient, IgG, and IgG index determinations in horse cerebrospinal fluid. *Prog Vet Neurol* 1:197–204, 1990.

7. Blythe LL, Mattson DE, Lassen ED, et al: Antibodies against equine herpesvirus 1 in the cerebrospinal fluid of horses. *Can Vet J* 26:218, 1985.

8. Wilson JW: Clinical application of cerebrospinal fluid creatine phosphokinase determination. *J Am Vet Med Assoc* 171:2000, 1977.

9. Beech J: Cytology of equine cerebrospinal fluid. *Vet Pathol* 20:553–562, 1983.

10. Mayhew IG, Whitlock RH, Tasker JB: Equine cerebrospinal fluid: Reference values of normal horses. *Am J Vet Res* 38:1271, 1977.

11. Rossdale PD, Falk M, Jeffcott LB, et al: A preliminary investigation of cerebrospinal fluid in the newborn foal as an aid to the study of cerebral damage. *J Reprod Fertil Suppl* 27:593, 1979.

12. Hayes TE: Examination of cerebrospinal fluid in the horse. *Vet Clin North Am Equine Pract* 3:283–291, 1987.

13. George LW: Cerebrospinal fluid examination. In Smith BP, ed: *Large Animal Internal Medicine.* St Louis, Mosby–Year Book, 1990, pp 901–904.

14. Fishman RA: Brain edema. *N Engl J Med* 293:706, 1975.

15. Greene HJ, Leipold HW, Vestwebor J: Bovine congenital defects: Variations of internal hydrocephalus. *Cornell Vet* 64:596, 1974.

16. Andrews FM, Matthews HK, Reed SM: The ancillary techniques and tests for diagnosing equine neurologic disease. *Vet Med* 85:1325–1330, 1990.

17. Jamison JM, Prescott JF: Bacterial meningitis in large animals—part I. *Compend Contin Educ Pract Vet* 9:399–406, 1987.

18. Darian BJ, Belknap J, Niefield J: Cerebrospinal fluid changes in two horses with central nervous system nematodiasis (*Micronema deletrix*). *J Vet Intern Med* 2:201–205, 1988.

19. Furr MO, Tyler RA: Cerebrospinal fluid creatine kinase activity in horses with central nervous system disease: 69 cases (1984–1989). *J Am Vet Med Assoc* 197:245–248, 1990.

20. Green EM, Green S: Cerebrospinal fluid lactic acid concentration: Reference values and diagnostic implications of abnormal concentrations in adult horses. In McGuirk SM, ed: *Proceedings of the American College of Veterinary Internal Medicine,* Blacksburg, Va, ACVIM, 1990, pp 495–499.

9.3

Electrodiagnostic Aids and Selected Neurologic Diseases

Frank M. Andrews, DVM, MS

Localizing lesions to and within the nervous system can, in some cases, be difficult utilizing only clinical and neurologic examinations. Generally, neurologic disease is characterized by changes in cell electrical activity; since electrical activity has both amplitude and frequency, it can be measured by electronic equipment. The observed electrical activity may be helpful in defining and localizing lesions of the nervous system.

Electromyography (EMG), auditory brainstem response (ABR) testing, and electroencephalography (EEG) are electrodiagnostic aids that may be helpful in the localization, diagnosis, and prognosis of neurologic disease in horses. Needle EMG and nerve conduction studies are helpful in localizing and defining diseases of the lower motor neuron or motor unit. ABR testing is helpful in localizing lesions to cranial nerve VIII and auditory pathways along the brainstem. EEG is helpful in diagnosing focal and diffuse intracranial lesions. The use of these diagnostic aids as an extension of the neurologic examination, separately or collectively, can provide valuable information about nervous system function and help in the diagnosis of neurologic disease. These techniques are relatively noninvasive and in many cases can be done on the awake horse, with mild sedation. Even when these techniques do not provide the information necessary to arrive at a diagnosis, they may provide a more complete understanding of the disease process.

ELECTROMYOGRAPHY

Needle EMG is the graphic recording of muscle cell electrical activity during contraction or at rest from a recording electrode placed in the muscle. Electrical activity is recorded by means of an amplifier on an oscilloscope.[1–3] Nerve conduction studies consist of stimulating a peripheral nerve with electrical current and recording the resultant physiologic electrical activity from other segments of the nerve or from the muscles innervated by those nerves.[4] Together, EMG and nerve conduction studies may help in the localization, diagnosis, and prognosis of diseases of the lower motor unit. The motor unit consists of the ventral horn cell bodies (located in the ventral horn of the spinal cord), its axon, the peripheral nerve, the myoneural junction, and the muscle fibers it innervates (Fig. 9–3).

Electromyographic Examination

A history and physical and neurologic examination should always precede the EMG examination. These aid in localizing the lesion, shorten the examination time, and minimize trauma to the horse. Initially, horses are examined standing, under mild sedation. Tranquilization with xylazine 0.2 to 0.5 mg/kg IV or xylazine and butorphanol 0.2 to 0.5 mg/lb and 2 to 10 mg IV, respectively, can be used. Examination of the awake horse aids in evaluating individual motor unit action potentials (MUAPs), summated MUAPs, and interference pattern. Normal and abnormal MUAPs can be evaluated and their amplitude measured. Unfortunately, in the awake horse an interference pattern (many MUAPs) can sometimes obscure abnormal low-amplitude EMG potentials. In this case, further examination may require general anesthesia.

In the needle EMG examination, the exploring electrode should be thrust briskly into the muscle and held until the

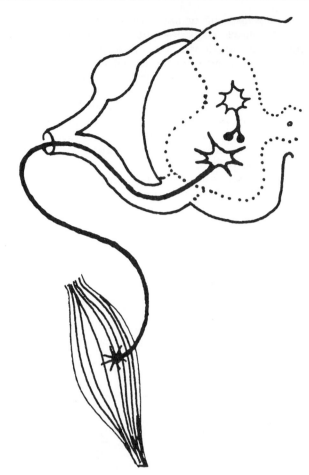

Figure 9–3. Illustration of the motor unit, including the ventral horn cell in the spinal cord, ventral root, peripheral nerve, neuromuscular junction, and muscle.

animal completely relaxes. To enable relaxation, the animal can be forced to bear weight on the opposite limb. Once relaxation has occurred, the resting activity or any postinsertional activity of the muscle can be evaluated. At least four areas and depths of smaller skeletal muscles and six to eight areas and depths of larger skeletal muscles should be evaluated when possible. A systematic examination should be done in order not to miss a lesion. Needle EMGs can be done in many of the major extrinsic muscles of the horse (Table 9–2). Also, needle EMGs can be done on facial, laryngeal, esophageal, pectoral, and external anal sphincter muscles when indicated by neurologic examination. Nerve conduction studies and muscle biopsy specimens may be collected to further define suspected lesions or confirm a diagnosis.

Nerve Conduction Studies

The evaluation of nerve conduction velocities requires knowledge of the topographic anatomy of nerves and muscles, plus a stimulator capable of delivering up to 150 V at durations of 0.1 to 3 ms at variable frequencies, up to 100 Hz. Most standard EMGs have built-in stimulators with adequate parameters to do nerve conduction studies. The peripheral nerve to be assessed can be located either by

palpation or by anatomical landmarks and then stimulated. The resultant muscle contraction can be palpated or observed, and the evoked muscle action potential, which has a thumping sound, can be viewed on the oscilloscope.

Nerve conduction studies are difficult to do in horses and therefore are not routinely done. However, the technique for radial and median nerve conduction studies in the horse has been reported.[5, 6] Nerve conduction studies must be done under general anesthesia and may be used to evaluate the speed of conduction of large myelinated motor nerves. The horse should be placed in lateral recumbency with the affected side up. The appropriate motor nerve is stimulated by monopolar needle electrodes inserted at or near the nerve and an evoked motor unit action potential (MUAP) from an innervated muscle is recorded (Figs. 9–4 and 9–5). Contraction of appropriate muscles may be visualized or palpated and needle electrodes inserted until a repeatable response is obtained. The unaffected limb may be used as a control.

In horses, radial nerve recordings can be obtained from the extensor carpi radialis and abductor digiti longus (extensor carpi obliquus) muscles[5, 6] (Fig. 9–4). Median nerve recordings can be obtained from the humeral and radial heads of the deep digital flexor tendon[5, 6] (Fig. 9–5). Facial nerve recording can be obtained from the levator nasolabialis

Table 9–2. Muscles, Nerves, and Nerve Roots Evaluated During Routine Electromyographic Examination of Horses

Muscles	Peripheral Nerve	Spinal Nerve Root
Rear Limb		
Long digital extensor	Peroneal nerve	L6–S1
	Tibial nerve	S1–2
Gastrocnemius	Tibial nerve	S1–2
Deep digital flexor	Ischiatic nerve	L5–S2
Semimembranosus	Femoral nerve	L3–L5
Vastus lateralis	Caudal gluteal, ischiatic, and peroneal nerves	L6–S2
Biceps femoris		
Middle gluteal	Cranial and caudal gluteal nerves	L5–S2
Paravertebral		
Paravertebral muscles (segmentally)	Dorsal branches of ventral spinal nerves (L6–C1)	L6–C1
Thoracic Limb		
Subclavius	Pectoral nerve	C6–C7, T1
Supraspinatus	Suprascapular nerve	C6–8
Infraspinatus		
Deltoideus	Axillary nerve	C6–8
Biceps brachii	Musculocutaneous nerve	C6–8
Triceps	Radial nerve	C7–T1
Extensor carpi radialis	Radial nerve	C7–T1
Superficial digital flexor	Ulnar nerve	C8–T2
Deep digital flexor	Ulnar and median nerve	C7–T1, T2

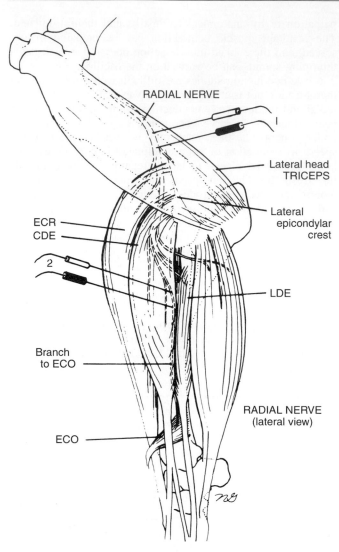

Figure 9–4. Illustration of anatomy and electrode placement used in radial nerve conduction velocities. *ECR,* extensor carpi radialis; *ECO,* extensor carpi obliquus. (From Henry RW, Diesem CD, Wiechers MD: Evaluation of equine radial and median nerve conduction velocities. *Am J Vet Res* 40:1406–1410, 1979.)

muscle by stimulating the buccal branch of the facial nerve just ventral to the facial crest.[7] Usually, a supramaximal stimulus can be obtained at 70 to 90 V for 0.1-ms duration. Nerve conduction studies can be helpful in diagnosing radial nerve, median nerve, and possibly facial nerve injury.

NORMAL ELECTROMYOGRAPHIC POTENTIALS

Normally occurring EMG potentials and nerve stimulation studies are described next. The muscle can be examined at rest, under submaximal contraction, maximal contraction, and secondary to direct nerve stimulation.

Insertional Activity

Insertional activity consists of short bursts of high-amplitude, moderate-to-high frequency (<200 Hz) electrical activ-

ity following insertion or movement of the exploring electrode in the muscle (Figs. 9–6 and 9–7). In normal skeletal muscle this activity stops a few milliseconds following cessation of needle movement. Insertional activity may be due to mechanical stimulation, muscle fiber injury,[3, 8, 9] or depolarization of muscle fibers directly adjacent to the EMG needle.[1] Positive sharp waves and fibrillation potentials observed during, or associated with, needle insertion that stop after cessation of needle movement are considered normal. Damage to muscle fibers by needle insertion is probably the source of these potentials. However, positive sharp waves and fibrillation potentials persisting after needle insertion are considered abnormal and may suggest early muscle denervation.[3]

Resting Activity (Postinsertional Baseline)

Resting activity is observed in relaxed muscle and is characterized by electrical silence. A flat line is observed on the oscilloscope. When the needle comes to rest near a nerve

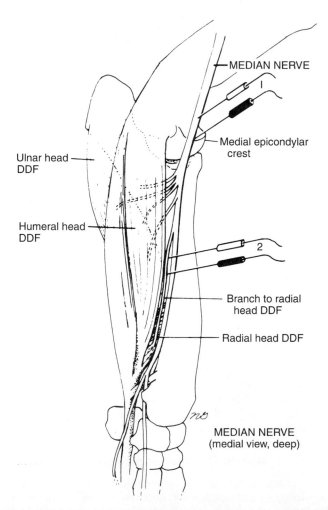

Figure 9–5. Illustration of anatomy and electrode placement used in median nerve conduction velocities. (From Henry RW, Diesem CD, Wiechers MD: Evaluation of equine radial and median nerve conduction velocities. *Am J Vet Res* 40:1406–1410, 1979.)

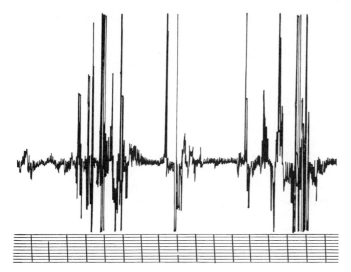

Figure 9–6. Normal insertional activity in the infraspinatus muscle. Gain = 0.500 mV/division; time = 10 ms/division.

twig or end plate, the needle may irritate small intramuscular nerve terminals which results in the production of two characteristic potentials, end-plate noise and end-plate spikes. End-plate noise produces a rippling of the baseline and a low-pitched continuous noise (Fig. 9–8). End-plate spikes, on the other hand, are high-amplitude intermittent spikes and make a popping sound (Fig. 9–8). End-plate noise and

spikes can occur alone or together. The origin of end-plate noise is thought to be extracellularly recorded miniature end-plate potentials (MEPPs),[10, 11] whereas end-plate spikes are thought to be single muscle fiber contractions secondary to needle electrode irritation of the nerve terminals.[11] In humans these potentials are associated with dull pain,[3] and repositioning the needle often eliminates their activity.

Motor Unit Action Potentials

MUAPs are voluntary or reflex muscle contractions observed after insertion of the needle electrode. They represent the sum of a number of single muscle fiber potentials belonging to the same motor unit. MUAPs are usually mono-, bi-, and triphasic. Since individual muscle fibers fire nearly synchronously the prefixes refer to the number of phases above and below the baseline (Fig. 9–7). A few polyphasic potentials (greater than four phases) may be seen in normal muscle, but usually do not exceed 5% to 15% of the population of MUAPs observed.[3] MUAPs have an amplitude ranging from 500 to 3000 μV, and a duration ranging from 1 to 15 ms. Examination of the awake horse enhances the evaluation of the amplitude and number of phases of MUAPs in the muscle.

These MUAPs may be seen when the animal is forced to bear weight on or retract a limb, resulting in contraction of that explored muscle. In lightly stimulated muscle, single MUAPs may be seen, as single motor units are recruited (see Fig. 9–7). As muscle contraction becomes more intense, more motor units are recruited, and the greater frequency of MUAPs appears on the oscilloscope. Once the screen is filled with MUAPs, an interference pattern is observed. Clinically, the number of phases and the duration of MUAPs are of greater importance than amplitude, since amplitude may be influenced by species, the muscle explored, the horse's age, and electrode position.[9] Furthermore, MUAP duration has been shown to increase with age in humans.[12]

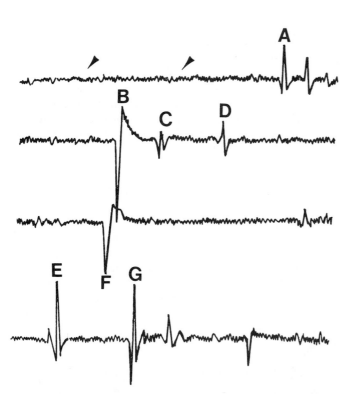

Figure 9–7. Electromyograph of the middle gluteal muscle showing normal resting activity *(arrowheads)*, fasciculation potentials *(A, E, G)*, fibrillation potentials *(C)*, positive sharp waves *(B, F)*, and a small motor and action potential *(D)*.

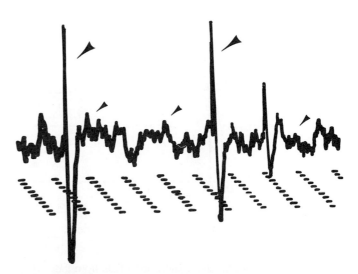

Figure 9–8. Electromyograph from triceps brachii muscle showing end-plate spikes *(large arrowheads)* and end-plate noise *(small arrowheads)*. Gain: 0.500 mV/stairstep; time: 10 ms/division.

EVOKED MUSCLE POTENTIALS

Stimulation of a mixed motor and sensory nerve results in two observed potentials: the direct evoked muscle action potential (M wave) and the reflex evoked muscle action potential (H wave). The M wave is the direct muscle action potential resulting from orthodromic conduction of direct nerve stimulation (Fig. 9–9). The M wave is the most commonly used potential in veterinary medicine. This wave is usually biphasic or triphasic and is larger than the H wave. The amplitude of these evoked potentials is dependent upon the number of motor units activated, as well as upon the size of the muscle, predominant fiber type, and type of recording electrode used.[4] With monopolar electrodes, amplitudes observed in the horse range from 5 to 60 mV for a 2- to 10-ms duration. Normal amplitudes and durations have been reported for several muscles in the horse.[5, 6] The time required for the potential to travel down the motor nerve, cross the neuromuscular junction, travel down the muscle membrane, and stimulate a response in the muscle is called the latency. When two points along the motor nerve are stimulated, the distance between the stimulating electrodes can be measured (in millimeters) and divided by the difference in latencies (in milliseconds). Normal median and radial nerve conduction velocities are 60 to 80 m/sec.[5, 6] Normal facial nerve conduction velocities are 55 to 70 m/sec.[7]

ABNORMAL ELECTROMYOGRAPHIC POTENTIALS

Spontaneous activity in a relaxed muscle after cessation of needle movement may be clinically significant. Diseases affecting the motor unit can lead to altered muscle electrical activity, such as prolonged or decreased insertional activity, postinsertional activity, altered waveforms, and complex repetitive discharges. Some abnormal EMG potentials are described next.

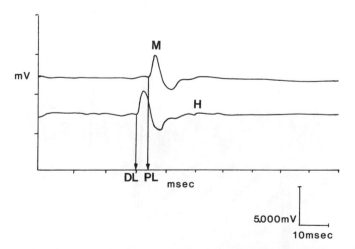

Figure 9–9. Evoked muscle action potentials from the levator nasolabialis muscle after direct stimulation of the buccal branch of the facial nerve illustrating the M wave and H wave. Nerve conduction velocity = 66.0 m/sec. *DL*, distal latency; *PL*, proximal latency.

Prolonged or Decreased Insertional Activity

Prolonged electrical activity continuing 1 to 10 ms after needle insertion and placement in the muscle is considered abnormal and is probably due to hyperirritability and instability of the muscle fiber membrane.[9] This activity is most prominent 4 to 5 days after denervation in dogs.[13] Increased or prolonged insertional activity usually precedes the onset of other denervation potentials (fibrillation potentials and positive sharp waves) and may suggest early denervation atrophy.[9] However, prolonged insertional activity may also be seen in myotonic disorders and myositis.[13]

Decreased insertional activity (decreased amplitude, duration, or both) may be associated with a decreased number of functioning muscle fibers and may suggest a longstanding neuropathy or myopathy. Infiltration of connective tissue and fat in the muscle can lead to a decreased number of muscle fibers, which can decrease insertional activity. Complete fibrosis of the muscle may result in loss of insertional activity. Insertional activity may also be absent when muscle fibers are functionally inexcitable, as occurs during attacks of familial periodic paralysis[3, 14] or if a faulty needle electrode is used, or if the EMG needle comes to rest in a normal muscle.[3]

Polyphasic Motor Unit Action Potentials

Polyphasic MUAPs (myopathic potentials) are MUAPs of increased frequency (greater than four phases) and decreased amplitude and duration (Fig. 9–10). These are observed during submaximal muscle contraction, and result from an increased number of action potentials for a given strength of contraction. Myopathic potentials result from a diffuse loss of muscle fibers,[15] and indicate the need for extra motor units to perform the work normally done by fewer motor units.[16] Myopathic potentials are polyphasic and most often seen in primary myopathies such as myotonia-like syndromes, periodic paralysis, myositis, botulism, and myasthenia gravis-like syndromes.[9] They have also been reported in steroid-induced myopathies, Cushing's syndrome, and membrane defect myopathies.[9]

Neuropathic Motor Unit Action Potentials

Neuropathic potentials are MUAPs of decreased frequency and longer duration than myopathic potentials and may be seen during minimal and maximal muscle contraction (see Fig. 9–10). Thus fewer MUAPs of increased amplitude are observed than expected for the strength of contraction. This is more noticeable during maximal contraction and produces a "sputtering" or "motorboat" sound. Neuropathic potentials are probably due to a decreased number of functioning axons firing during maximal muscle contraction. These potentials are most often present in primary neuropathies in which collateral reinnervation has occurred.[16]

Fibrillation Potentials

Fibrillation potentials are the most commonly observed abnormal spontaneous electropotential in EMG (see Fig. 9–7).

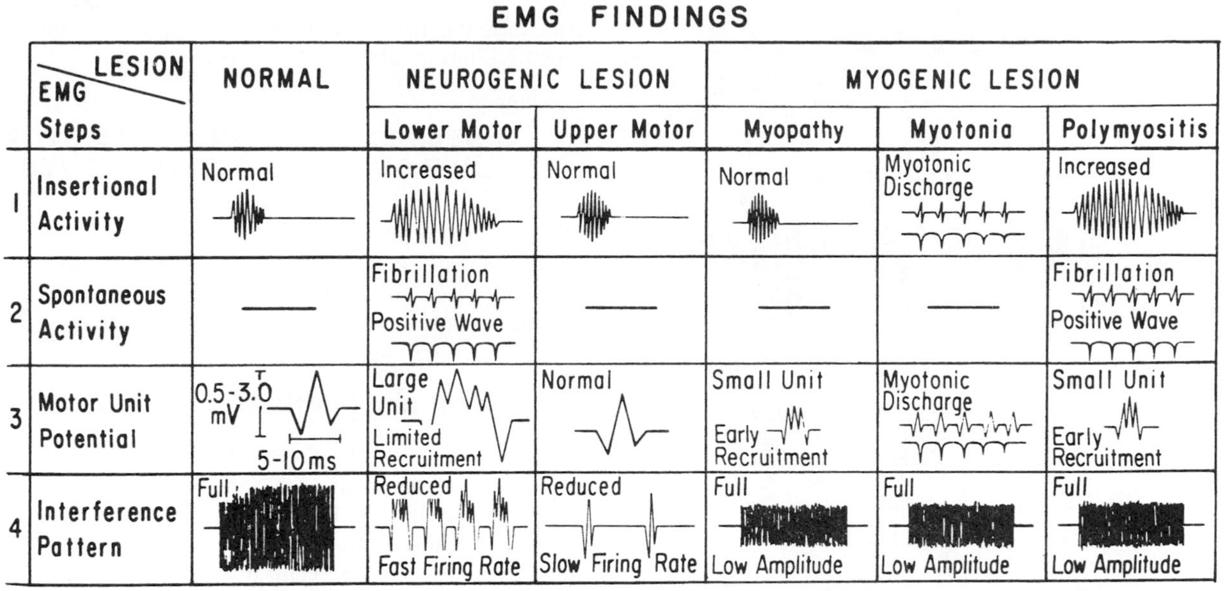

EMG FINDINGS

LESION EMG Steps	NORMAL	NEUROGENIC LESION		MYOGENIC LESION		
		Lower Motor	Upper Motor	Myopathy	Myotonia	Polymyositis
1 Insertional Activity	Normal	Increased	Normal	Normal	Myotonic Discharge	Increased
2 Spontaneous Activity	—	Fibrillation Positive Wave	—	—	—	Fibrillation Positive Wave
3 Motor Unit Potential	0.5-3.0 mV 5-10ms	Large Unit Limited Recruitment	Normal	Small Unit Early Recruitment	Myotonic Discharge	Small Unit Early Recruitment
4 Interference Pattern	Full	Reduced Fast Firing Rate	Reduced Slow Firing Rate	Full Low Amplitude	Full Low Amplitude	Full Low Amplitude

Figure 9–10. Differential EMG findings in neurogenic and myogenic conditions. (Modified from Kimura J: *Electrodiagnosis in Diseases of Nerve and Muscle: Principles and Practice.* Philadelphia, FA Davis, 1984, p 263.)

These spontaneous discharges sound like "frying eggs," "crinkling cellophane," or "frying bacon" and have an initial positive deflection of 100 to 300 μV in amplitude and 2 to 4 ms in duration. They are diphasic or triphasic in waveform. Fibrillation potentials strongly suggest denervation, but have been observed in polymyositis, muscular dystrophy, and botulism.[1, 17] Their origin is uncertain, but fibrillation potentials are thought to be spontaneous discharges from acetylcholine-hypersensitive denervated muscle fibers,[1, 17] or may be secondary to muscle necrosis,[18] muscle inflammation, and focal muscle degeneration. A few fibrillation potentials have been observed in normal healthy muscle, but they are usually not reproducible in other areas of the muscle.

The onset of fibrillation potentials following denervation depends upon the size of the animal. The larger the animal the later the onset of fibrillation potentials[19]; they have been reported between days 5 and 16 postdenervation in dogs[20] and humans.[18] We have observed fibrillation potentials 4 to 10 days after nerve injury in horses. Fibrillation potentials were often seen in conjunction with positive sharp waves. They increase, then decrease in amplitude as the muscle atrophies, with activity ceasing upon complete muscle atrophy. Fibrillation potentials occurring alone denote a more severe disease process than the presence of positive sharp wave potentials alone.[17] Fibrillation potentials are helpful in evaluating the length of time muscle denervation has been present and are important in diagnosing denervation prior to clinical muscle atrophy. They can also be used as a prognostic indicator: by monitoring fibrillation frequency and amplitude changes with serial examinations, the extent and progress of denervation can be assessed. Also, a decrease in fibrillation potentials followed by the recording of MUAPs may indicate reinnervation and may suggest a favorable prognosis.[18]

Positive Sharp Waves

Positive sharp waves are potentials in which the primary deflection is in the downward direction, followed by a lower-amplitude longer-duration negative deflection (see Fig. 9–7). This waveform has been described as resembling a saw tooth.[3] Positive sharp waves occur with muscle denervation and muscular diseases such as myositis, exertional rhabdomyolysis (tying-up syndrome),[21] and spinal shock.[16] Sometimes positive sharp waves are observed in association with or shortly after insertional activity and persist after electrode placement. If more than two positive sharp waves occur after insertional activity, it may indicate early denervation. Positive sharp waves may occur in denervated muscle secondary to chronic exertional rhabdomyolysis,[21] myotonia,[21] equine protozoal myeloencephalitis (EPM), laryngeal hemiplegia,[22] suprascapular nerve injury (sweeney),[23] and compressive myelopathies. Positive sharp waves often precede or appear along with fibrillation potentials in denervated muscle. These potentials can be observed singly or in trains (Fig. 9–11) and may sound like a "machine gun." Their origin is uncertain but may be associated with hyperexcitable muscle cell membranes.[17]

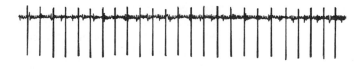

Figure 9–11. Electromyograph showing trains of positive sharp waves. Gain: 500 V/stairstep.

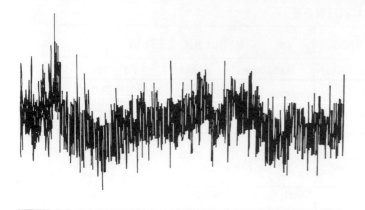

Figure 9–12. Electromyograph showing waxing and waning myotonic potentials. Gain: 500 V/stairstep.

Fasciculation Potentials

Fasciculation potentials are spontaneous discharges from a group of muscle fibers representing either the whole or part of a motor unit[3, 17] (see Fig. 9–7). Their source has not been determined yet, but evidence suggests they originate from neural discharges in the spinal cord or along the peripheral nerve.[24, 25] They can be seen in diseases of anterior horn cells and irritative-type lesions of root or peripheral nerve, such as radiculopathies and nerve entrapments in humans.[13] Little significance is placed on isolated fasciculation potentials in horses. However, fasciculation potentials in the presence of fibrillation potentials or positive sharp waves may indicate lower motor neuron disease and may be seen in suprascapular nerve entrapment (sweeney) in horses.

Complex Repetitive Discharges vs. Myotonic Potentials

Complex repetitive discharges (bizarre high-frequency potentials) and myotonic potentials are less frequently observed in horses. Both of these potentials are repetitive MUAPs induced by insertion of the needle electrode or percussion of muscle. Bizarre high-frequency potentials tend to be shorter in duration and end abruptly when compared with myotonic discharges. Bizarre high-frequency potentials sound like a machine gun. On the other hand, myotonic potentials often wax and wane in amplitude, last 4 to 5 seconds,[2, 3, 9] and sound like a "dive-bomber," hence the nickname "dive-bomber potential"[1, 9] (Fig. 9–12). Both myotonic and bizarre high-frequency potentials are thought to be associated with hyperexcitability of the muscle cell membrane.[1] Bizarre high-frequency potentials may be seen in diseases of the lower motor unit such as muscular dystrophy,[1, 9, 21] steroid-induced myopathy,[9] polymyositis,[26] chronic denervation,[26] and hyperkalemic periodic paralysis.[14] Myotonic potentials may be seen in myotonia congenita,[21] myotonia dystrophica,[21] and may be seen in hyperkalemic periodic paralysis in humans, which may reflect abnormal muscle chloride or potassium conductance.[3] Myotonic potentials have also been seen in horses with hyperkalemic periodic

paralysis, but some were obscured by concurrent complex repetitive discharges.[14]

DISEASES AFFECTING THE MOTOR UNIT AND PERIPHERAL NERVES

Diseases of the motor unit and peripheral nerves can lead to changes in skeletal muscle electrical activity or nerve conduction velocity, or both. In these diseases EMG may be a useful diagnostic aid in localizing the lesion.

Focal and Multifocal Myelopathies

Compressive cervical myelopathies, cervical stenotic myelopathy (wobbler syndrome), and EPM are common causes of neurologic signs in the horse. These conditions are characterized by damage to the sensory pathways and in some instances damage to the ventral horn cells of the spinal cord, a component of the motor unit. Physical examination may reveal muscle atrophy and sweating over affected muscles. Needle EMG of the cervical axial musculature in horses presented with truncal, forelimb, and hindlimb ataxia, with-

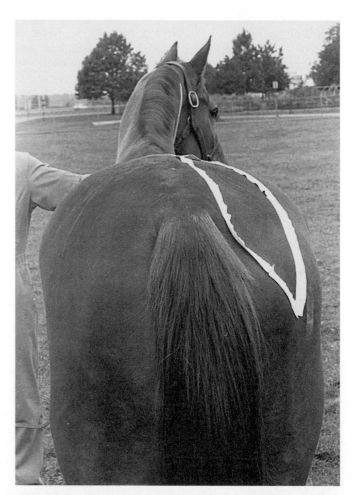

Figure 9–13. Horse with gluteal muscle atrophy secondary to protozoan myelitis showing distribution of abnormal EMG potentials.

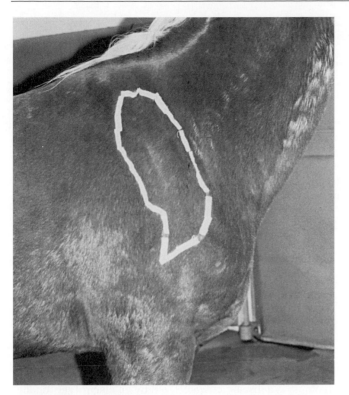

Figure 9–14. Horse with suprascapular nerve injury with characteristic EMG distribution of fibrillation potentials and positive sharp waves in supraspinatus and infraspinatus muscles.

out cranial nerve deficits, may reveal increased insertional activity, fibrillation potentials, and positive sharp waves indicating compression of the ventral horn cells or ventral roots.[27] Abnormal postinsertional activity at the level of the spinal cord compression may allow the clinician to focus the radiographic examination.

In cases of EPM, needle EMG may reveal fibrillation potentials, positive sharp waves, and abnormal insertional activity in affected limb muscles in horses presented for obscure lameness. Also, horses presented with muscle asymmetry (Fig. 9–13) can be examined via needle EMG to determine the extent of muscle involvement. This may lead to early diagnosis of EPM, so that treatment can be prescribed. Also, serial needle EMG examination may be helpful in monitoring the response to treatment and prognosis.

Radial and Suprascapular Nerve Injury

Damage to the peripheral nerves leads to muscle atrophy of the innervated muscle. Damage to the radial and suprascapular nerves can occur with trauma to the cranial aspect of the shoulder. Needle EMG and nerve conduction studies are helpful in evaluating the extent of damage to these and other peripheral nerves. Also, needle EMG and nerve conduction studies may be able to differentiate lost or reduced limb function due to nerve damage from painful conditions. Muscle groups that have atrophied owing to disuse (disuse atrophy) caused by a painful condition will show no postinsertional activity on needle EMG examination.

Positive sharp waves and fibrillation potentials in the triceps brachii and extensor carpi radialis muscles may suggest radial nerve injury. Positive sharp waves and fibrillation potentials in the supraspinatus and infraspinatus muscles may suggest suprascapular nerve injury (Fig. 9–14). Postinsertional activity in these muscle groups and the lateral head of the triceps suggests damage to the brachial plexus (Fig. 9–15). Thus, needle EMG may be helpful in differentiating suprascapular nerve injury (see Fig. 9–14) from brachial plexus injury (see Fig. 9–15). Visible evidence of muscle atrophy may not be present until several weeks after injury. To confirm a radial nerve injury, the radial nerve conduction velocity (NCV) can be calculated (Fig. 9–16). If the NCV is less than 60 m/sec or markedly less than the opposite limb, radial nerve injury may be suspected. Also, radial nerve

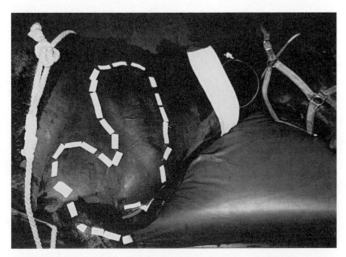

Figure 9–15. Horse with brachial plexus injury showing characteristic distribution of EMG charges, including fibrillations and positive sharp waves. Note the involvement of the supraspinatus, infraspinatus, triceps brachii, extensor carpi radialis, and pectoral muscles.

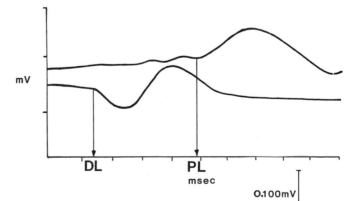

Radial Nerve Conduction Velocities

mV

DL   PL

msec

0.100mV

10msec

Figure 9–16. Evoked muscle action potential from the extensor carpi radialis muscle showing decreased amplitude and decreased nerve conduction velocity, suggestive of radial nerve injury. *DL,* distal latency; *PL,* proximal latency.

injury may lead to a decreased amplitude and duration of the evoked muscle action potential (see Fig. 9–16).

Needle EMG and nerve conduction studies may also be helpful in determining success of nerve decompression surgery. Once the nerve is surgically decompressed, serial needle EMG examinations may be helpful in determining if permanent nerve damage has occurred and the extent of return of nerve function.

Laryngeal Hemiplegia

Laryngeal hemiplegia (LH) has been described extensively in the literature as denervation of the intrinsic laryngeal musculature, specifically the recurrent laryngeal nerve.[5] One difficulty with this condition is that current diagnostic techniques (endoscopy, inspiratory stridor with exercise) are limited to recognizing LH after onset of clinical signs.[28] However, fibrillation potentials and positive sharp waves in the dorsal cricoarytenoid muscle on needle EMG examination may appear prior to clinical signs. Thus, needle EMG may be useful in the early detection of LH in horses.[22] Spontaneous EMG activity, including fibrillation potentials, positive sharp waves, or bizarre high-frequency discharges, have been reported in the dorsal cricoarytenoid muscle of horses affected with laryngeal hemiplegia.[22] Fibrillation potentials and positive sharp waves are the most common abnormal electrical potential observed in horses with LH.[22] Decreased insertional activity and bizarre high-frequency discharges were reported at a lesser frequency.[22]

Myopathies, Myositis, and Myotonia

Needle EMG may be helpful in evaluating horses presented for signs of primary muscle disease, such as muscle tremors, muscle fasciculations, muscle stiffness, weakness, and percussion dimpling. Myopathies are generally classified into inflammatory or degenerative types.[29] Degenerative myopathies are characterized by an intact motor unit, but a loss of viable muscle fibers. This results in an increased number of polyphasic MUAPs with decreased duration (see Fig. 9–10). Inflammatory myopathies (myositis) are characterized by a subacute or acute degeneration of muscle fibers with active infiltrates of inflammatory cells. The characteristic potentials are increased insertional activity, low-voltage brief MUAPs, fibrillation potentials, and positive sharp waves (see Fig. 9–10). Needle EMG is a valuable aid in the diagnosis and localization of both focal and diffuse myopathies. Primary myopathies such as exertional rhabdomyolysis and myositis can be differentiated from myotonia and myotonia-like syndromes by needle EMG examination[21] (see Fig. 9–10). Furthermore, fibrillation potentials and positive sharp waves have been observed on EMG examination in horses with chronic myositis, exertional rhabdomyolysis, shivers, and hyperkalemic periodic paralysis.[14, 21] After the needle EMG examination is finished, muscles with postinsertional activity may be further evaluated by muscle biopsy and evaluated microscopically.[21, 30]

Myotonia

Myotonia is a disease characterized by an electrolyte conductance deficit in the skeletal muscle membrane.[3] Fibrillation potentials, positive sharp waves, a train of positive sharp waves, and myotonic potentials may be observed on EMG examination in horses with myotonia congenita[21] and myotonia dystrophica.[31] Characteristic electrophysiologic findings include waxing-and-waning, high-frequency spontaneous and induced myotonic discharges (dive-bomber potentials) in many muscle groups, including the middle gluteal and semitendinosus muscles[21, 31] (see Fig. 9–12). Needle EMG may be used to confirm the diagnosis of myotonia, to distin-

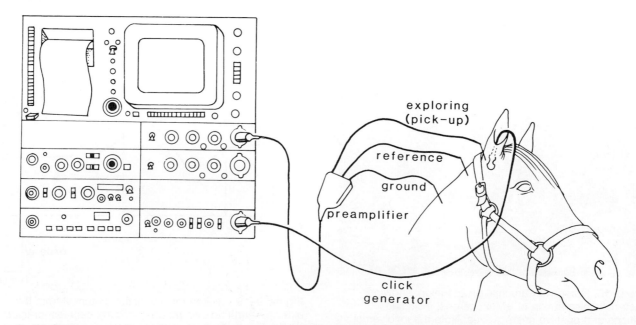

Figure 9–17. System used for auditory brainstem response testing in the horse. (From Rolf SL, Reed SM, Melnick W, et al: Auditory brainstem response testing in anesthetized horses. *Am J Vet Res* 48:910–914, 1987.)

guish this condition from pseudomyotonia, and to localize areas for muscle biopsy (see Fig. 9–10). Myotonia and myotonia-like syndromes may also present as tremors or even seizure activity. EMG along with a thorough physical and neurologic examination can help differentiate seizures from primary myopathy.

AUDITORY BRAINSTEM RESPONSE TESTING

Auditory brainstem response testing is a method of recording potentials arising from the eighth cranial nerve and its projections in response to acoustic stimulation via surface or subcutaneously placed electrodes. The ABR is those evoked potentials, or waves, arising within the first 10 ms after delivery of an acoustic stimulus (clicks) (Fig. 9–17). In humans, ABR is recognized as consisting of from five to seven waves, generally designated I through VII. Of these, waves I through V are the most common. In dogs and cats fewer waves are observed.[32, 33] In people and animals, there is correspondence between these waves and certain anatomical generator sites[33–39]: (1) wave I is generated by bipolar neurons of the eighth cranial nerve, (2) wave II may also be generated partly by the eighth cranial nerve, (3) waves II through V probably reflect more generalized activity in the auditory system in the medulla and pons and may represent neural activity ipsilateral and contralateral to the stimulated ear. A wide range of clinical applications of ABR in humans have been well described.[19, 34, 37, 39–46] However, its use in the horse has been limited.[47, 48] ABR testing is a method of assessing not only auditory function but a variety of neurologic disorders involving the brainstem. It is unaffected by the state of arousal of the test subject and responses are not degraded by sedation or general anesthesia.[37, 45]

Horses can be examined either awake, with or without mild sedation, or anesthetized (see Electromyography). If the horse is tested awake, each ear is stimulated and the resultant waveforms are recorded independently. If the patient is anesthetized, the uppermost ear is examined first, then the horse is turned, and the lower ear is done.

Interpretation of Auditory Brainstem Response Testing

Five peaks are commonly observed and are considered analogous to waves I through V seen in humans[4, 35, 37, 39–44, 49, 50] (Fig. 9–18). Mean latencies have been reported previously in horses under general anesthesia.[51] As has been observed in dogs and cats,[32, 33] latencies of the waves decrease as stimulus intensity increases. The ABR can be used clinically in horses with head tilts (Fig. 9–19) to verify the presence of hearing loss (Fig. 9–20), middle or inner ear infections, and stylohyoid osteomyelitis. It may also be helpful in the diagnosis and prognosis of traumatic, infectious, or inflammatory brainstem lesions such as vascular infarcts or anomalies, ischemic fibrocartilaginous emboli, basisphenoid bone fracture, and protozoal encephalomyelitis. Quantitative and qualitative characteristics of the ABR-generated waveforms can be assessed. Persistent prolonged latencies suggest retrocochlear or conductive abnormalities.[37] Interaural latency differences of wave V may suggest unilateral brainstem

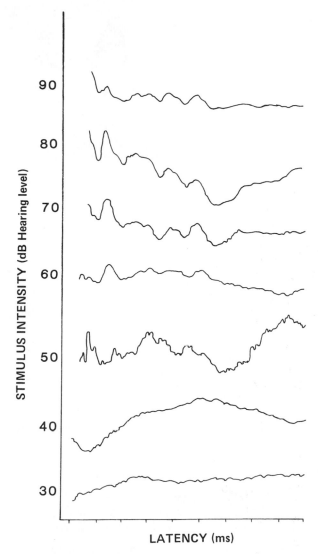

Figure 9–18. Mean latency waves at 136 −dB, sound pressure level (SPL) through 87 dB SPL. Five waves are present except at 40 of 80 dB SPL. (From Rolf SL, Reed SM, Melnick W, et al: Auditory brainstem response testing in anesthetized horses. *Am J Vet Res* 48:910–914, 1987.)

disease, except when cochlear disease is present. Qualitative ABR changes are of greater use in equine medicine, as quantitative measures of normal and abnormal horses are limited. In human beings qualitative changes such as peak presence, waveform morphologic characteristics, and response stability are of greater use in the diagnosis of central disorders, particularly acoustic neuromas and demyelinating diseases.[37]

The limitations of ABR include a dependence on cochlear function; susceptibility to extraneous noise, which may affect waveform morphology; and the limits of the machinery in excluding 60-cycle interference.

ELECTROENCEPHALOGRAPHY

Electroencephalography is the graphic recording of electrical activity arising from the cerebral cortex. The origin of this electrical activity is not known, but it is thought to arise

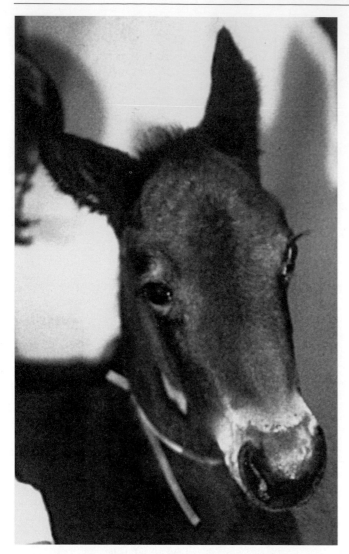

Figure 9–19. Photograph of foal with a right head tilt and dropping of the right ear. Auditory brainstem response (see Fig. 9–20) shows a hearing loss in the left ear, the presumed cause of his head tilt. The right ear was normal.

from pyramidal cell dendrites located within a 2-mm depth of the cerebral cortex. This electrical activity may be modified by deeper structures such as the brainstem, reticular activating system, and thalamus. EEG is an extension of the neurologic examination and is a valuable tool for determining the presence of a cerebral disease, localizing it, determining its extent (focal or diffuse), differentiating between inflammatory and degenerative changes, and establishing a prognosis.

EEG has been used and reviewed extensively in humans[52, 53] and small animals,[8, 49] but little work has been done in the horse.[54] In this discussion a brief description of the use, interpretation, and limitations of EEG is presented so that a better understanding regarding its use may be gained.

Normal EEG Patterns

The EEG should be evaluated for symmetry, waveform, morphology, frequency, and amplitude. The bipolar montage,

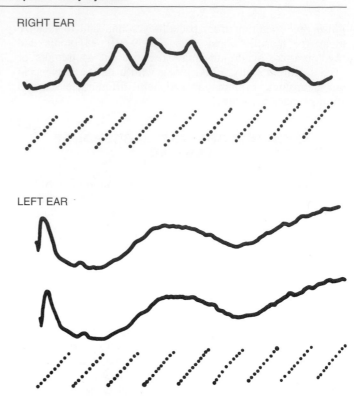

RIGHT EAR

LEFT EAR

Figure 9–20. Auditory brainstem response of the foal in Figure 9–19 showing normal right ear and abnormal left ear.

as discussed earlier, allows comparison of cortex to cortex. The potentials generated by the left occipital (LO) region can be compared with those of the right occipital (RO) cortex; the potentials generated by the left frontal (LF) cortex region can be compared with those of the right frontal (RF) area; and the potentials generated by the left side (LF-LO)

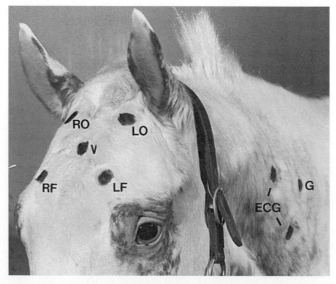

Figure 9–21. Photograph of horse illustrating bipolar montage for electroencephalography. *RO,* right occipital; *LO,* left occipital; *RF,* right frontal; *LF,* left frontal; *V,* vertex; *G,* ground; *ECG,* electrocardiogram position.

Table 9–3. Amplitudes and Frequencies Observed in Electroencephalographic (EEG) Patterns in Normal Horses and Horses with Tranquilization

	EEG Patterns	
	Voltage (μV)	Frequency (Hz)
Normal (awake)	8–15	18–30
	10–40	5–10
Xylazine HCl	10–80	10–15
(Rompun)	5–30	25–405
	10–90	0.5–4.05
Acetylpromazine	5–40	25–405
	5–10	1–4

can be compared with those of the right side (RF-RO) (Fig. 9–21). Normal EEG potentials in the horse consist of a dominant waveform in the awake alert horse of low voltage (8–15 μV) and fast activity (18–30 Hz) (Table 9–3). Usually this activity is superimposed over a low-to-medium voltage (10–40 μV) and slow activity (5–10 Hz) (see Table 9–3). Muscle artifact occasionally interrupts the baseline, when the animal shakes its head, moves its eyes, or twitches the facial muscles.

Abnormal EEG Patterns

Diseases of the cerebral cortex can alter frequency, amplitude, and symmetry of EEG patterns. Low voltage–fast activity and spikes may be seen with ongoing irritative processes such as seizures or inflammation (Fig. 9–22). High voltage–slow activity indicates death of neurons in such diseases as brain abscess (Fig. 9–23) and neoplasia. However, low voltage–fast activity and high voltage–slow activity are not pathognomonic for any disease process, but suggest the various disease states discussed above. Localized EEG changes indicate focal cortical disease such as infarcts, hemorrhage, early tumor, or abscessation (see Fig. 9–23), whereas generalized EEG changes may indicate a diffuse cortical or subcortical disease such as infection (see Fig. 9–22), trauma, space-occupying lesions (hydrocephalus, tumor), idiopathic epilepsy, or a systemic metabolic illness (hepatic encephalopathy). Serial recordings may be helpful in following therapy and the progress of disease. Generally,

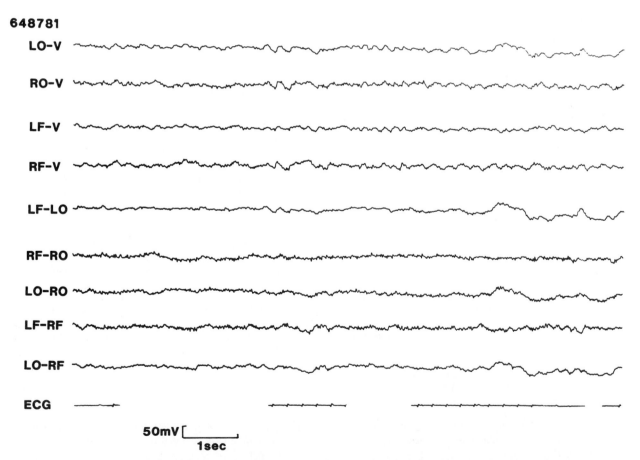

Figure 9–22. Electroencephalograph from a horse with cryptococcal meningitis showing generalized low-voltage high-frequency activity and frequent spikes. For abbreviations, see Figure 9–21.

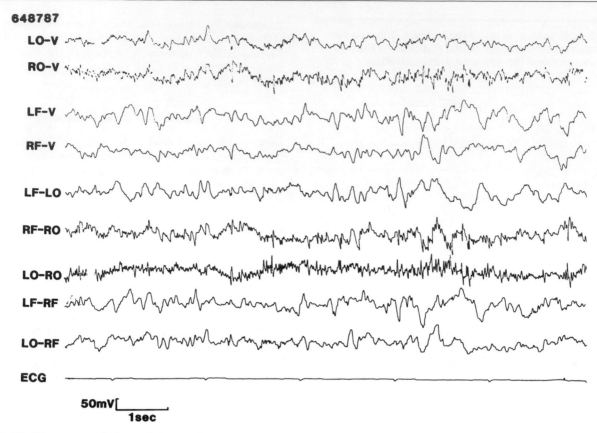

648787

LO–V

RO–V

LF–V

RF–V

LF–LO

RF–RO

LO–RO

LF–RF

LO–RF

ECG

50mV[
1sec

Figure 9–23. Electroencephalograph from a horse with a space-occupying mass in the left frontal area of the brain. Note generalized high-voltage low-frequency wave and asymmetry of left cortex.

artifacts such as ocular movement and facial muscle twitches produce asymmetric and symmetric low voltage–slow activity, whereas hypothyroidism may produce symmetric low voltage–medium-to-slow activity.[49] The difficulty in EEG in the horse is differentiating artifact (muscle movement, eye movement, headshaking, EEG artifact) from true EEG changes. It must be reemphasized that the EEG alone is only one part of the diagnostic workup. The EEG examination should always be interpreted in conjunction with the history, clinical signs, and neurologic examination.

REFERENCES

1. Chrisman DC, Burt JK, Wood PK, et al: Electromyography in small animal neurology. *J Am Vet Med Assoc* 160:311–318, 1972.
2. deLahunta A: *Veterinary Neuroanatomy and Clinical Neurology,* ed 2. Philadelphia, WB Saunders, 1983, pp 65–66.
3. Kimura J: *Electrodiagnosis in Diseases of Nerve and Muscle: Principles and Practice.* Philadelphia, FA Davis, 1984.
4. Sims MH: Electrodiagnostic techniques in the evaluation of diseases affecting skeletal muscle. *Vet Clin North Am Small Anim Pract* 13:145–162, 1983.
5. Henry RW, Diesem CD, Wiechers MD: Evaluation of equine radial and median nerve conduction velocities. *Am J Vet Res* 40:1406–1410, 1979.
6. Henry RW, Diesem CD: Proximal equine radial and median motor nerve conduction velocity. *Am J Vet Res* 42:1819–1822, 1981.
7. Andrews FM: Facial nerve conduction velocities in the horse (unpublished data).
8. Klemm WR: *Animal Electroencephalography.* New York, Academic Press, 1969.
9. Klemm WR: *Applied Electronics for Veterinary Medicine and Small Animal Physiology.* Springfield, Ill, Charles C Thomas, 1976.
10. Buchthal F, Rosenfalck P: Spontaneous electrical activity of human muscle. *Electroencephalogr Clin Neurophysiol* 20:321, 1966.
11. Weiderholt WC: End plate noise in electromyography. *Neurology* 20:214, 1970.
12. Buchthal F: *An Introduction to Electromyography.* Copenhagen, Scandinavia University Books, 1957.
13. Kugelberg E, Petersen I: Insertion activity in electromyography with notes on denervated muscle response to constant current. *J Neurol Neurosurg Psychiatry* 12:268–273, 1949.
14. Spier SJ, Carlson GP, Holiday TA, et al: Hyperkalemic periodic paralysis in horses. *J Am Vet Med Assoc* 197:1009–1017, 1990.
15. Warmolts JR, Engel WK: A critique of the "myopathic" electromyogram. *Trans Am Neurol Assoc* 95:173–177, 1970.
16. Buchthal F, Guild C, Rosenfalck D: Multielectrode study of the territory of a motor unit. *Acta Physiol Scand* 39:83–104, 1957.
17. Chrisman CL: Electromyography in small animals. In Ettinger S, ed: *Textbook of Veterinary Internal Medicine.* Philadelphia, WB Saunders, 1975.
18. Feinstein B, Pattle RE, Weddell G: Metabolic factors affecting fibrillation in denervated muscle. *J Neurol Neurosurg Psychiatry* 8:1–11, 1945.
19. Thompson DS, Woodward JB, Ringel SP, et al: Evoked potential abnormalities in myasthenic dystrophy. *Electroencephalogr Clin Neurophysiol* 56:453–456, 1983.

20. Inada S, Sugaro S, Ibaraki T: Electromyographic study on denervated muscles in the dog. *Jpn J Vet Sci* 25:327–336, 1963.

21. Andrews FM, Spurgeon TL, Reed SM: Histochemical changes in skeletal muscles of four male horses with neuromuscular disease. *Am J Vet Res* 47:2078–2083, 1986.

22. Moore MP, Andrews FM, Reed SM, et al: Electromyographic evaluation of horses with laryngeal hemiplegia. *J Equine Vet Sci* 8:424–427, 1988.

23. Andrews FM: Indication and use of electrodiagnostic aids in neurologic disease. *Vet Clin North Am Equine Pract* 3:293–322.

24. Denny-Brown D, Pennybacker JB: Fibrillation and fasciculation in voluntary muscle. *Brain* 61:311, 1938.

25. Wettstein A: The origin of fasciculations in motor neuron disease. *Ann Neurol* 5:295, 1979.

26. Farnbach GC: Clinical electrophysiology in veterinary neurology, Part 1: Electromyography. *Compend Contin Educ Pract Vet* 11:791–797, 1980.

27. Mayhew IG, deLahunta A, Whitlock RH: Spinal cord disease in the horse. *Cornell Vet* 68(suppl):44–70, 1978.

28. Cook WR: The diagnosis of respiratory unsoundness in the horse. *Vet Rec* 77:516, 1965.

29. Kornegay JN, Gorageaz EJ, Dawe DL, et al: Polymyositis in dogs. *J Am Vet Med Assoc* 176:431, 1980.

30. Andrews FM, Reed SM, Johnson G: Indications and techniques for muscle biopsy in the horse. *Proc Am Assoc Equine Pract* 35:357–366, 1989.

31. Reed SM, Hegreberg GA, Bayly WM, et al: Progressive myotonia in foals resembling human dystrophia myotonia. *Muscle Nerve* 2:291–296, 1988.

32. Achor LJ, Starr A: Auditory brainstem response in the cat. I. Intracranial and extracranial responses. *Electroencephalogr Clin Neurophysiol* 48:155–173, 1980.

33. Marshall AE: Brainstem auditory-evoked response of the non-anesthetized dog. *Am J Vet Res* 46:966–973, 1985.

34. Fria TJ: The auditory brainstem response: Background and clinical applications. *Monogr Contemp Audiol* 2:1–5, 1980.

35. Glattke TJ, Runge CA: Comments on the origin of short latency auditory potentials. In Beasley DS, ed: *Audition in Childhood: Method of Study.* San Diego, College Hill Press, 1984.

36. Hashimoto I, Ishiyama Y, Yoshimoto T, et al: Brainstem auditory evoked potentials recorded directly from human brainstem and thalamus. *Brain* 103:841–859, 1981.

37. Hosford-Dunn H: Auditory brainstem response audiometry: Applications in central disorders. *Otol Clin North Am* 18:257–284, 1985.

38. Jewett DL, Williston JS: Auditory evoked potential for far fields averaged from the scalp of human beings. *Brain* 94:681–696, 1971.

39. Keranishvili ZS: Sources of the human brainstem auditory evoked potential. *Scand Audiol* 9:75–82, 1980.

40. Anziska BJ, Cracco RQ: Short latency somatosensory evoked potentials in brain-dead patients. *Arch Neurol* 37:222–225, 1980.

41. Cushman MZ, Rossman RN: Diagnostic features of the auditory brainstem response in identifying cerebellopontine angle tumors. *Scand Audiol* 12:35–41, 1983.

42. Greenberg RP, Becker DP, Miller JD, et al: Evaluation of brain function in severe human head trauma with multimodality evoked potentials. Part 2: Localization of brain dysfunction and correlation with post-traumatic neurological conditions. *J Neurosurg* 47:761–768, 1975.

43. Jabbari B, Schwartz DM, MacNeil B, et al: Early abnormalities of brainstem auditory evoked potentials in Friedreich's ataxia: Evidence of primary brainstem dysfunction. *Neurology* 33:1071–1074, 1983.

44. Jay WM, Hoyd CS: Abnormal brainstem auditory-evoked po-

tentials in Stelling-Turk-Duane retraction syndrome. *Am J Ophthalmol* 89:814–818, 1980.

45. Robinson D, Rudge P: The use of the auditory evoked potential in the diagnosis of multiple sclerosis. *J Neurol Sci* 45:235–244, 1980.

46. Starr A, Achor J: Auditory brainstem response in neurological disease. *Arch Neurol* 32:761–768, 1975.

47. Marshall AE, Byars TD, Whitlock RH, et al: Brainstem auditory evoked response in the diagnosis of inner ear injury in the horse. *J Am Vet Med Assoc* 178:282–286, 1978.

48. Marshall AE: Brainstem auditory-evoked response in the non-anesthetized horse and pony. *Am J Vet Res* 46:1445–1450, 1985.

49. Redding RW, Knecht CD: Neurologic examination. In Ettinger S, ed: *Textbook of Veterinary Internal Medicine,* vol 1. Philadelphia, WB Saunders, 1975, pp 303–332.

50. Stockard JE, Stockard JJ, Westmoreland BF, et al: Brainstem auditory-evoked responses: Normal variation as a function of stimulus and subject characteristics. *Arch Neurol* 36:823–831, 1979.

51. Rolf SL, Reed SM, Melnick W, et al: Auditory brainstem response testing in anesthetized horses. *Am J Vet Res* 48:910–914, 1987.

52. Elul R: Specific site of generation of brain waves. *Physiologist* 7:125, 1964.

53. Gibbs FA, Gibe EL: *Atlas of Electroencephalography,* 3 vols. Reading, Mass, Addison Wesley, 1958, 1959, 1964.

54. Mysinger PW, Redding RW, Vaughan JT, et al: Electroencephalographic patterns of clinically normal sedated, and tranquilized newborn foals and adult horses. *Am J Vet Res* 46:3641, 1985.

9.4

Seizures, Narcolepsy, and Cataplexy

Frank M. Andrews, DVM, MS
Hilary K. Matthews, DVM

SEIZURES

Seizures are clinical manifestations of rapid excessive electrical discharges from the cerebral cortex that result in involuntary alterations of motor activity, consciousness, autonomic functions, or sensation.[1–5] Seizures may be referred to as "fits," "attacks," "strokes," "convulsions," or "epilepsy."[2] A true seizure, however, refers to a specific clinical event regardless of cause or morphology. Epilepsy refers to reoccurring seizures with nonprogressive intracranial alterations, which may be genetic or acquired.[2] True inherited epilepsy probably does not occur in horses.[2] Convulsions, on the other hand, refer to seizures accompanied by tonic-clonic muscle activity and loss of consciousness. Convulsions may include a generalized seizure.

Seizures in horses can be classified into three broad forms based on clinical signs: partial seizure, generalized seizure, and status epilepticus. A partial seizure involves a discrete area of the cerebral cortex and results in localized clinical signs, such as facial or limb twitching, compulsive running in a circle, or self-mutilation.[2, 3] A partial seizure may be observed after cervical myelography, anesthesia, and cranial trauma, and may spread throughout the cerebral cortex and produce a secondary generalized seizure.[2, 3] A generalized seizure involves the entire cerebral cortex, and results in generalized tonic-clonic muscle activity over the whole body, with loss of consciousness. Generalized seizures are the most common form of seizures observed in adult horses and foals.[2, 3] Status epilepticus is characterized by generalized seizures occurring in rapid succession and is uncommon in horses.[2]

Pathogenesis

Adult horses have a high seizure threshold. Severe damage must occur to the brain before adult horses have seizures. Foals, on the other hand, have a lower seizure threshold and are more susceptible to conditions causing seizures.[6] Seizures may be caused by either intracranial or extracranial factors[2] (Tables 9–4 and 9–5). The most common causes of seizures in foals under 2 weeks of age are neonatal maladjustment syndrome, trauma, and bacterial meningitis[6] (see Table 9–4). The most common causes of seizures in foals less than 1 year of age are trauma and idiopathic epilepsy in Arabian foals[2, 3] (see Table 9–4). The most common causes of seizures in adult horses older than 1 year of age are brain trauma, hepatoencephalopathy, and toxicity[2] (see Table 9–5). Tumors, especially pituitary adenoma, may cause seizures and blindness in horses older than 7 years[2] (see Table 9–5).

The pathophysiologic mechanisms of seizures are not thoroughly known. Current research has focused on intracellular neuronal and synaptic events that initiate excessive and prolonged neuronal depolarization, known as "paroxysmal depolarization shift."[7, 8] Several mechanisms are thought to cause paroxysmal depolarization shifts and seizures. These include increased excitatory neural transmitters, decreased inhibitory neural transmitters (γ-aminobutyric acid, GABA), alteration in neural transmitter receptor sites, or a derangement in the neuron's internal cellular metabolism.[7, 8] The most widely held hypothesis for seizure initiation is development of excitatory postsynaptic potentials (EPSPs).[7, 9] Seizures may develop because there is a summation of synchronous EPSPs in large groups of neurons which may be precipitated by an increase in excitatory neurons, a decrease in inhibitory neurons, or a decrease in inhibitory neurotransmitters, or any combination of these.[7, 9] Once a "critical mass" of neurons has fired, an uncontrolled spread of electrical activity may occur over the cerebral cortex and precipitate a generalized seizure. Head trauma and decreased cerebral blood supply have been implicated in creating seizure foci. Head trauma may result in cerebral cortical hypoxia, which in turn may lead to necrosis of inhibitory neurons. Since cerebral inhibitory neurons are more sensitive to hypoxia than excitatory neurons, a loss of inhibitory neurons allows the spread of these EPSPs and seizure development.[10]

Inhibitory neurons surround excitatory neuron groups and check areas of intense stimulation. Decreased inhibitory neurotransmitters in these areas, such as GABA, have been implicated in seizure formation in animals. Application of penicillin directly to the brain of laboratory animals sup-

Table 9–4. Known and Suspected Causes of Seizures in Horses Less Than 1 Year of Age

	Differential Diagnosis		
Classification	Extracranial	Intracranial	Diagnostic Aids*
Anomalies (congenital)		Hydrocephalus	
		Hydranencephaly	1–6, 8
		Benign epilepsy	11
Metabolic	Hypoxia, hyponatremia, hypoglycemia, hyperkalemia		2, 3, 4, 8, 11
Toxic	Organophosphates	Moldy corn	2–6
	Strychnine	Locoweed	9–11
	Metaldehyde		
Traumatic		Brain trauma	2–4
		Lightning	5, 6, 8, 10, 11
Vascular		Neonatal maladjustment syndrome (vascular accidents)	2–6
Infectious	Septicemia	Bacterial meningitis	2–4
	Endotoxemia	Cerebral abscesses	5–9
	Fever	Rabies	11
	Tetanus	Viral encephalitis	
	Botulism		

*Key: *1*, breed; *2*, onset; *3*, clinical course; *4*, physical examination; *5*, neurologic examination; *6*, clinical pathology–CSF analysis; *7*, serology; *8*, radiology (CT scan, ultrasound, radiographs); *9*, toxicology; *10*, electrodiagnostics (EEG, EMG); *11*, pathology.

Table 9–5. Known and Suspected Causes of Seizures in Horses Greater Than 1 Year of Age

| | Differential Diagnosis | | |
Classification	Extracranial	Intracranial	Diagnostic Aids*
Metabolic	Hepatoencephalopathy, hypomagnesemia, hypocalcemia, uremia, hyperlipidemia		2–6, 11
Toxic	Organophosphates		2–6
	Strychnine	Moldy corn	9, 11
	Metaldehyde	Locoweed	
		Bracken fern	
		Lead, arsenic, mercury	
		Rye grass	2–6
Traumatic		Brain trauma	8, 10, 11
Vascular		*Strongylus vulgaris*	2–4
		Cerebral thromboembolism	5, 6, 11
		Intracarotid injection	
Tumor		Neoplasia	2–5
		Hemarthroma	6, 8, 10, 11
		Cholesterol granuloma	
Infectious		Cerebral abscess	
		Rabies	1, 3–6
		Tetanus	7, 8, 12, 13
		Arbovirus encephalitides	
		Mycotic cryptococcosis	
		Protozoal myelitis	

*Key: *1*, breed; *2*, onset; *3*, clinical course; *4*, physical examination; *5*, neurologic examination; *6*, clinical pathology–CSF analysis; *7*, serology; *8*, radiology (CT scan, ultrasound, radiographs); *9*, toxicology; *10*, electrodiagnostics (EEG, EMG); *11*, pathology.

presses GABA and induces seizures.[11] These seizures can be blocked by use of other agents that potentiate inhibitory neurotransmitters. Phenobarbital and pentobarbital potentiate inhibitory neural transmitters, such as GABA, and block seizure foci caused by penicillin and hypoxia.

Alterations in the neuronal cell microenvironment may lead to seizure generation. Systemic and local neuronal electrolyte abnormalities may disturb excitatory neuron homeostasis and lead to spontaneous and excessive action potentials.[7] Intracellular potassium released during neuronal activity may reach sufficient concentration to move the resting membrane potential toward the threshold and generate a seizure focus.[12] Spontaneous action potentials generated by alteration in intracellular potassium concentration may spread to other parts of the cerebral cortex causing a generalized seizure.

Furthermore, alterations in one intracellular neuronal electrolyte may alter the homeostasis of other intracellular electrolytes. This is supported by the observation of increased intracellular potassium concentration, together with decreased intracellular calcium and chloride concentrations, in the long-duration changes in excitability known to occur during interictal epileptogenesis and the transition from interictal to ictal activities.[13, 14]

Also, alterations in sodium conductance have been implicated in causing seizures.[15] Rapid influxes of sodium into

the neuron may lead to hyperexcitability of the neuron and rapid firing. Phenytoin, a hydantoin derivative, blocks these rapid influxes of sodium into neurons and suppresses repetitive firing by hyperexcitable neurons.[15] Thus, there may be a complex interaction between these electrolytes and the internal cell homeostasis that precipitates seizure formation.

Clinical Signs and Diagnosis

Seizure activity is manifested clinically in a variety of ways depending on the area and the extent of the cerebral cortex involved. In partial seizures, asymmetric twitching of a limb, facial twitching, excessive chewing, compulsive running, or self-mutilation may occur.[2] A localized seizure may develop into a generalized seizure.

In a generalized seizure, three distinct clinical periods may be observed. Just prior to the seizure (aura), horses may exhibit signs of anxiety and uneasiness. During the seizure (ictus), horses may become recumbent, unconscious, and have symmetric clonic muscle contractions (contractions and relaxations of muscles occurring in rapid succession), followed by symmetric tonic muscle contractions (continuous unremitting muscle contractions).[2, 3] Horses may also show deviation of eyeballs, dilated pupils, ptyalism, trismus or jaw clamping, opisthotonos, lordosis or kyphosis, violent paddling movements of the limbs, uncontrolled urination and defecation, and excessive sweating.[2] A generalized seizure may last from 5 to 60 seconds.[2] After the seizure (postictus), horses may show depression and blindness from hours to days.[2, 3]

Diagnosis of seizure is based on history, clinical signs, and ancillary diagnostic tests to determine an underlying cause, whenever possible (see Tables 9–4 and 9–5). In all paroxysmal, involuntary neurologic events, seizures should be considered first unless the cause is proved otherwise. Careful questioning of the owner can reveal information about the event, the time of day, relationship to feeding, date, unusual environmental circumstances (stimuli such as thunderstorms, fireworks, changes in housing), recent trauma, febrile episodes, exposure to drugs or toxins, recent behavioral changes, and the seizure history of the dam, sire, and other siblings. It is important to rule out other conditions that mimic seizures, including painful conditions (colic, limb fractures, exertional myopathy), hyperkalemic periodic paralysis, and syncope. In these conditions horses do not lose consciousness but remain bright and alert. Horses with hyperkalemic periodic paralysis may show prolapse of the nictitating membranes of the eye, and muscle fasciculations, but remain anxious, alert, and have normal pain perception.[16, 17] This condition occurs in quarter horse and quarter horse crosses, 2 to 3 years of age.[16, 17] Serum potassium concentration in these horses ranges from 5.5 to 9.0 mEq/L during or shortly before collapse.[16, 17]

Narcolepsy and cataplexy can be confused with seizures. Most narcoleptic horses (except for some ponies) remain standing with the head hanging close to the ground.[18] If recumbency occurs, loss of muscle tone and rapid eye movement (REM) sleep may follow.[18] Cardiac arrhythmias or severe murmurs may precipitate syncopal episodes. Auscultation of the heart may help determine the presence of severe murmurs, and electrocardiography (ECG) may help determine the presence of arrhythmias. Icteric mucous membranes may be seen in horses with hepatoencephalopathy and diarrhea may be seen in horses after toxin ingestion.

A complete neurologic examination should be done to determine the presence of other neurologic signs. The neurologic examination should be done during the interictal period, as an immediate postictal examination may reveal depression, weakness, blindness, crossed extensor reflex, and may lead to false anatomical localization of lesions.[1–3]

Cerebrospinal fluid (CSF) from the cisterna magna may be helpful in determining the cause of seizures. Increased CSF protein, red blood cell count, white blood cell count, and abnormal differential white blood cell count may be helpful in determining the cause of the seizure.[1–3] Also, increased CSF lactic acid concentration may be seen in horses with cerebral abscess.[19]

Skull radiographs may help determine the presence of traumatic skull fractures. Bone scan may reveal nondisplaced skull fractures. A fundic examination may reveal papillary edema, detached retina, or active inflammation that may suggest trauma or an infectious cause. Electroencephalography (EEG) and a computed tomography (CT) scan may be helpful in localizing and determining the cause of a seizure.[20–22] If an underlying cause cannot be found, then a diagnosis of idiopathic epilepsy may be made.[2, 3]

Treatment

Treatment of horses having seizures must be based on medical considerations, client considerations, owner preference and compliance, and the long-term expense of medication. Starting anticonvulsant therapy should be based on the frequency and severity of the horse's seizures. Guidelines for anticonvulsant therapy may be extrapolated from treatment guidelines used in humans and small animals.[23] Generally, anticonvulsant therapy is indicated in status epilepticus (which occurs rarely in adult horses, and uncommonly in foals): one seizure occurring every 2 months; clusters of seizures more than three to four times per year; or several multiple seizures occurring over 1 to 3 days.[23] Also, foals with idiopathic epilepsy that have several seizures over 1 to 3 days may require short-term (1–3 months) anticonvulsant therapy.[2, 3] The chronic use of anticonvulsants in horses is rare. Therapy guidelines are listed in Table 9–6.[2–4] Maintenance therapy should be decreased slowly to determine if continued therapy is needed. The goals of anticonvulsant therapy are to reduce the frequency, duration, and severity of seizures without intolerable side effects. The complete elimination of a seizure may not be possible. The best initial treatment for seizures in horses is diazepam and phenobarbital sodium. Each horse must be treated as an individual and the treatment dosages tailored to fit the individual.

Adult horses and foals in seizure may also benefit from dimethyl sulfoxide (DMSO) 1 g/kg given IV as a 10% solution, with lactated Ringer's solution or 5% dextrose. DMSO scavenges free oxygen radicals released in damaged tissue and helps maintain cerebral blood flow by reducing thromboxane production, which may result in vasoconstriction and platelet aggregation.[24]

Corticosteroids may be effective initially as an anticonvulsant therapy. A single dose of dexamethasone 0.1 to 0.2 mg/kg IV should be given initially and the horse should be reevaluated the next day.[25] Corticosteroids may stabilize neuronal membranes and decrease seizure foci. Corticosteroids and DMSO may be synergistic.

Several drugs are contraindicated in seizures and they include acetylpromazine, xylazine, and ketamine. Although acetylpromazine has been used to control seizures in foals, it is risky because of its ability to lower the seizure threshold.[2, 3] Xylazine decreases cerebral blood flow and increases intracranial pressure, which may exacerbate cerebral hypoxia and worsen seizures. However, it may be necessary to give xylazine in an emergency situation until a more appropriate drug becomes available. Ketamine increases cerebral blood flow, oxygen consumption, and intracranial pressure, and may exacerbate seizures.

NARCOLEPSY

Narcolepsy is a rare incurable sleep disorder of the central nervous system characterized by uncontrolled episodes of loss of muscle tone (cataplexy) and sleep.[1, 3, 4] The disease has been reported in Suffolk and Shetland foals (the fainting disease),[26] Welsh ponies, a miniature horse, and in the Thoroughbred, quarter horse, Morgan, appaloosa, and standardbred.[1, 3, 4, 27] A familial occurrence is thought to exist in affected Suffolk and Shetland pony foals.[3]

Table 9–6. Anticonvulsant Drugs Used to Treat Seizure Disorders in Horses

Regimen	Drug	50-kg Foal	450-kg Horse
Initial therapy (including status epilepticus)	Diazepam	5–20 mg IV	25–100 mg IV
	Pentobarbital	150–1,000 mg IV	To effect
	Phenobarbital	250–1,000 mg IV	2–5 g IV
	Phenytoin	50–250 mg IV or PO q4h	—
	Primidone	1–2 g PO	—
	Chloral hydrate ($\pm$ MgSO$_4$, barbiturate)	3–10 g IV	15–60 g IV
	Xylazine*	25–100 mg IV or IM	300–1,000 mg IV or IM
	Guaifenesin ($\pm$ barbiturate)	To effect	40–60 g
	Carbamazine	250–500 mg	
	Triazolam	1 g	
Maintenance therapy	Phenobarbital	100–500 mg PO b.i.d.	1–5 g PO b.i.d.
	Phenytoin	50–250 mg PO b.i.d.	500–1,000 mg PO t.i.d. (low therapeutic index)
	Primidone	1 g PO, s.i.d., or b.i.d.	

*Should be used only in an emergency situation until an appropriate anticonvulsant agent can be started.

Pathophysiology

Four components of narcolepsy are seen in man and include excessive daytime sleepiness associated with short periods of REM sleep; cataplexy; hypnagogic hallucinations; and sleep paralysis.[4, 28] Cataplexy or sudden collapse with complete inhibition of skeletal muscle tone is seen in horses with narcolepsy.[1, 3, 4] Respiratory and cardiac muscles are spared.[1]

The normal sleep cycle consists of two stages. Slow wave sleep (non-REM, or NREM sleep), mediated by serotonin, occurs first and originates from the midline raphe of the pons.[1, 29] Slow wave sleep is followed by fast wave (REM) sleep, which is mediated by norepinephrine. These centers are located in the locus ceruleus of the pons.[1, 29] Both slow and fast wave sleep act through the ascending and descending activation system of the reticular formation.[1] In fast wave sleep, when REM occurs, the locus ceruleus activates the medial reticular formation nucleus, whose axons descend the spinal cord to inhibit the lower motor neurons of the somatic efferent system. This inhibition produces atonia.[1, 30, 31] EEG recordings during fast wave sleep are characterized by low-amplitude, fast activity.[1] Electromyographic (EMG) recordings during fast wave sleep show no recordable muscle tone.[1]

With narcolepsy and cataplexy, there may be a biochemical abnormality of the brainstem or sleep-wake center responsible for the disease. A recent study showed that decreased concentrations or turnover of serotonin, dopamine, or norepinephrine may play a role in narcolepsy and cataplexy.[1, 32] Also, a cholinergic mechanism, mediated by acetylcholine, may play a role.[33] No morphologic lesion has been found to cause sleep dysrhythmia.[3]

Cataplectic episodes are not usually associated with exercise. Petting or stroking of the head and neck, hosing with cold water after exercise, leading out of a stall, the initiation of eating or drinking, and stall rest may precipitate a cataplectic episode.[4]

The onset of narcolepsy or cataplexy occurs at approximately 6 months of age.[1] However, adult onset has been described.[4] A predictable pattern of duration and frequency of attacks is set within the first 1 to 2 weeks following the onset of disease.[1]

Clinical Signs

Clinical signs of narcolepsy vary from mild muscle weakness to complete collapse.[1, 3, 4] Adult horses may drop their heads, buckle at the knees, and stumble.[1, 3, 4] If forced to walk, the horse may be ataxic. Pony breeds are more likely to become recumbent.[4] Horses and ponies that collapse may show absent spinal reflexes and REM sleep.[1, 3, 4] Occasional sudden contraction of a limb or trunk muscle can occur resulting in a spasmodic motion. Episodes may last from a few seconds to 10 minutes.[1, 3, 4] Eye and facial responses, normal cardiovascular function, and normal respiratory function are maintained during the attack.[3] Horses can be aroused from the attack with varying degrees of difficulty and most recover and rise quietly without incident.[3] Affected horses are neurologically normal between attacks.[1, 4]

Diagnosis

Diagnosis of narcolepsy is based on history, clinical signs, pharmacologic testing, and the absence of other diseases. A complete blood count and serum biochemical profile may help determine underlying systemic and metabolic abnormalities. Cerebrospinal fluid is normal in affected horses.[4] EEG and needle EMG during an attack may reveal fast waves of REM sleep and the absence of postinsertional activity of resting muscle.[1]

A provocative test is useful in diagnosing narcolepsy or cataplexy in horses. Physostigmine salicylate, an anticholinesterase drug, 0.06 to 0.08 mg/kg slow IV and 0.05 to 0.1 mg/kg slow IV will precipitate a cataplectic attack within 3 to 10 minutes after administration in affected horses.[3, 4, 27]

This compound crosses the blood-brain barrier.[4] Careful monitoring of the horse after physostigmine administration is necessary because of untoward effects such as colic and cholinergic stimulation.

Atropine sulfate, a muscarinic blocker, 0.04 to 0.08 mg/kg IV or 20 to 60 mg IV reduces the severity of cataplectic attacks minutes after administration, and can prevent their reoccurrence for 3½ to 30 hours following administration.[3, 4] Response to atropine sulfate supports a possible cholinergic mechanism for causing cataplexy. Horses given atropine sulfate must be monitored for ileus and colic.

Neostigmine, a cholinesterase inhibitor, 0.005 mg/kg IV, does not cross the blood-brain barrier and therefore has no effect on cataplectic attacks. However, neostigmine may help rule out conditions causing muscle weakness such as myasthenia-like syndromes and botulism. Horses with muscle weakness will show increased muscle tone and a favorable response to neostigmine.

Differential Diagnosis

Other causes of acute collapse in the horse should be considered. Acute collapse without warning is characteristic of cardiovascular collapse or syncope. Atrial fibrillation, ruptured chordae tendineae, myocardial infarction, myocardial fibrosis, aortic endocarditis, and pericarditis have been associated with syncope in horses. Cerebral hypoxia may occur in these conditions which may lead to coma, with or without signs of cardiac failure. Seizures should be considered in ruling out acute collapse. Botulism (shaker foal syndrome, forage poisoning), myasthenia-like syndrome, postanesthetic neuromyopathy, exertional rhabdomyolysis, and metabolic causes such as hyperthermia, shock, hypoglycemia, hypocalcemia, hypo- or hyperkalemia, endotoxemia, anaphylaxis, and snakebite should also be considered. Also, horses with hyperkalemic periodic paralysis may have attacks similar to those seen in horses with narcolepsy. These horses typically have muscle tremors and may become recumbent with hyporeflexia, but are alert and anxious. Attacks in horses with hyperkalemic periodic paralysis may last up to 15 minutes and the horse will usually stand without incident. Diagnosis of this condition is based on clinical signs, serum potassium concentration, potassium chloride provocation, and EMG findings.[16, 17]

A cataplectic state may be induced in neonatal foals by tight whole-body restraint. This response is thought to be an inherent in utero mechanism that prevents violent movements, especially during parturition.

Treatment and Prognosis

Imipramine, a tricyclic, antidepressant drug, is used to control narcolepsy and cataplexy.[1, 3, 4] The drug blocks the uptake of serotonin and norepinephrine, and decreases REM sleep.[4] Imipramine can be used at a dose of 0.55 mg/kg IV or 250 to 750 mg PO.[3, 4] Oral administration produces inconsistent results.[4] As mentioned previously, atropine sulfate can provide relief from acute attacks for up to 30 hours, but its use must be weighed against the adverse gastrointestinal side effects it causes.

The prognosis for narcolepsy or cataplexy is variable.

Some newborn Thoroughbreds and miniature horses may have severe attacks, but recover fully.[3] In Shetland and Suffolk ponies, the disease may persist throughout life, as is true with the adult-onset form.[1, 3, 4] In horses 1 to 3 years of age, several episodes may occur, but are without permanent consequence.[3]

REFERENCES

1. deLuhunta A: *Veterinary Neuroanatomy and Clinical Neurology,* ed 2. Philadelphia, WB Saunders, 1983, pp 88–89, 326–343.
2. Mayhew IG: Seizure disorders. In Robinson NE, ed: *Current Therapy in Equine Medicine.* 1983, pp 344–349.
3. Mayhew IG: *Large Animal Neurology: A Handbook for Veterinary Clinicians.* Philadelphia, Lea & Febiger, 1989, pp 113–125, 133–139.
4. Sweeny CR, Hansen TO: Narcolepsy and epilepsy. In Robinson NE, ed: *Current Therapy in Equine Medicine,* ed 2. Philadelphia, WB Saunders, 1987, pp 349–353.
5. Lane SB, Bunch SE: Medical management of recurrent seizures in dogs and cats. *J Vet Intern Med* 4:26–39, 1990.
6. Collatos C: Seizures in foals: Pathophysiology, evaluation, and treatment. *Compend Contin Educ Pract Vet* 12:393–400, 1990.
7. Prince D: Neurophysiology of epilepsy. *Annu Rev Neurosci* 1:395–415, 1978.
8. Delgado-Escueta AV, Ward AA, Woodbury DM, et al: New wave of research in the epilepsies. *Adv Neurol* 44:3–55, 1986.
9. Ayala GF, Dichter M, Gumnit RJ, et al: Genesis of epileptic interictal spikes: New knowledge of cortical feedback systems suggests neurophysiological explanation of brief paroxysms. *Brain Res* 52:1–17, 1973.
10. Russo ME: The pathophysiology of epilepsy. *Cornell Vet* 71:221–247, 1981.
11. Ajmone-Marsan C: Acute effects of topical epileptogenic agents. In Jasper HH, Ward AA Jr, Pope A, eds: *Basic Mechanisms of the Epilepsies.* Boston, Little, Brown, 1969, pp 299–328.
12. Fertiziger AP, Ranck JB: Potassium accumulation in interstitial space during epileptiform seizures. *Exp Neurol* 26:571–585, 1970.
13. Prince DA: Cortical cellular activities during cyclically occurring inter-ictal epileptiform discharges. *Electroencephalogr Clin Neurophysiol* 31:469–484, 1971.
14. Heinemann U, Lux HD, Gutnick MJ: Extracellular free calcium and potassium during paroxysmal activity in the cerebral cortex of the cat. *Exp Brain Res* 27:237–243, 1977.
15. Adler EM, Selzer ME: Cellular pathophysiology and pharmacology of epilepsy. In Asbury AK, McKhann GM, McDonald WI, eds: *Diseases of the Nervous System.* Philadelphia, WB Saunders, 1986, pp 982–999.
16. Cox JH: An episodic weakness in four horses associated with intermittent serum hyperkalemia and the similarity of the disease to hyperkalemic periodic paralysis in man. *31st Proc Am Assoc Equine Pract* 383–391, 1985.
17. Spier S, Carlson GP, Pikar J, et al: Hyperkalemic periodic paralysis in horses: Genetic and electrophysiologic studies. *35th Proc Am Assoc Equine Pract* 399–402, 1989.
18. Sweeney CR, Hansen TO: Narcolepsy and epilepsy. In Robinson NE, ed: *Current Therapy in Equine Medicine,* ed 2. Philadelphia, WB Saunders, 1987, pp 349–353.
19. Green EM, Green S: Cerebrospinal fluid lactic acid concentration: Reference values and diagnostic implications of abnormal concentrations in adult horses. In McGuirk SM, ed: *Proceedings of American College of Veterinary Internal Medicine,* Blacksburg, Va, ACVIM, 1990, pp 495–499.

20. Andrews FM: Indications and use of electrodiagnostic aids in neurologic disease. *Vet Clin North Am* 3:293–322, 1987.
21. Allen JR, Barhee DD, Crisman MV, et al: Diagnosis of equine pituitary tumors by computed tomography. Part 1. *Compend Contin Educ Pract Vet* 10:1103–1107, 1988.
22. Allen JR, Crisman MV, Barhee DD, et al: Diagnosis of equine pituitary tumors by computed tomography. Part II. *Compend Contin Educ Pract Vet* 10:1196–1201, 1988.
23. Selcer RR, Selcer ES: A practical approach to seizure management in dogs and cats. *Prog Vet Neurol* 1:147–156, 1990.
24. Blythe LL, Craig AM, Christensen JM, et al: Pharmacokinetic disposition of dimethyl sulfoxide administered intravenously to horses. *Am J Vet Res* 47:1739–1743, 1986.
25. Andrews FM, Matthews HK, Reed SM: Medical, surgical, and physical therapy for horses with neurologic disease. *Vet Med* 85:1331–1333, 1990.
26. Sheather AL: Fainting in foals. *J Comp Pathol Ther* 37:106–113, 1924.
27. Sweeney CR, Hendricks JC, Beech J, et al: Narcolepsy in a horse. *J Am Vet Med Assoc* 183:126–128, 1983.
28. Katherman AE: A comparative review of canine and human narcolepsy. *Compend Contin Educ Pract Vet* 11:818, 1980.
29. Henley K, Morrison AR: A reevaluation of the effects of lesions of the pontine tegmentum and locus coeruleus on phenomena of paradoxical sleep in the cat. *Acta Neurobiol Exp* 34:215, 1974.
30. Sakai K, Sastre JP, Salvert D, et al: Tegmentoreticular projections with special reference to the muscular atonia during paradoxical sleep in the cat: An HRP study. *Brain Res* 176:233, 1979.
31. Jones BF: Elimination of paradoxical sleep by lesions of the pontine gigantocellular tegmental field in the cat. *Neurosci Lett* 13:385, 1979.
32. Faull K, Foutz AS, Holman RB, et al: Assays of monoamine metabolites in CSF samples from control and narcoleptic canines. In *Proceedings of the Fourth International Catecholamine Symposium,* 1978.
33. Delashaw JB, Foutz AS, Guillemineult C, et al: Cholinergic mechanisms and cataplexy in dogs. *Exp Neurol* 66:745, 1979.

9.5

Spinal Cord, Vertebral, and Intracranial Trauma

Hilary K. Matthews, DVM

SPINAL CORD AND VERTEBRAL TRAUMA

Spinal cord and vertebral trauma are not uncommon findings in equine practice and should be considered in any acute case of neurologic disease. Clinical signs in traumatic injuries reflect the neuroanatomic location and range from inapparent to severe incapacitating tetraparesis or tetraplegia. Commonly, trauma occurs because of falling or colliding with a large stationary object such as a jump, fence, or another horse, and may be caused by a penetrating injury.

Neurologic signs are usually observed immediately after the accident, but may occur weeks to months after the initial insult because of delayed damage to the spinal cord caused by instability, arthritis, or bony callus formation.

An age-related distribution in the location of trauma has been noted.[1] Foals and young horses are more susceptible to vertebral trauma than adult horses, especially in the cranial cervical and caudal thoracic areas.[1] There is an increased incidence of luxations, subluxations, and epiphyseal separations in young horses.[1] This may be because cervical vertebral growth plate closure does not occur until 4 to 5 years of age.[1,2] Adult horses are more prone to caudal cervical (C5–7) and caudal thoracic injuries and considerable force is required for injury.[1] Table 9–7 lists the location, type of trauma, inciting incident, and clinical signs associated with the common types of vertebral trauma.

Pathophysiology

Spinal cord damage secondary to trauma is a dynamic process. The development of spinal cord damage does not coincide with the clinical picture, as pathologic changes may progress in severity for approximately 1 week, even in the face of clinical improvement.[3] Classically, initial spinal cord trauma results in changes in the center, or gray matter, of the cord.[3] The reason for this is not entirely clear, but is most likely related to the rich blood supply and increased metabolic requirements for oxygen and glucose of the nerve cell bodies in the gray matter.[3] The increased vascular and cell content of the gray matter may make it more susceptible to traumatic insult. Initial edema and gray matter hemorrhage in the central cord will progress outward to include central necrosis, white matter edema, and demyelination of the entire spinal cord.[3] The degree of progression is directly related to the initial amount of trauma sustained.[3,4]

Following spinal cord trauma, there is a reduction in blood flow to the cord.[3,4] Initial hemorrhage is followed by an inflammatory reaction and an increased circulation time.[3] Impairment to the spinal cord arterial blood supply causes ischemia and necrotic changes in the cord.[3] Venous outflow obstruction in the spinal cord also occurs, leading to cavitation in the central gray matter.[3] Reduction in blood flow to the spinal cord decreases the rate of aerobic metabolism owing to development of a hypoxic state.[4] Also, injury produces vasospasm, which is responsible for the release of vasoactive monoamines such as norepinephrine.[5] Norepinephrine is thought to be responsible for the early hemorrhage and necrosis.[5] However some investigators dispute the role of norepinephrine in the pathogenesis of spinal cord damage, as increased concentrations of norepinephrine have not been found in experimental models of spinal cord trauma.[6] Calcium, iron, and copper released as a result of trauma may be associated with free radical peroxidation of the myelinated neuronal membranes.[7]

Release of prostaglandins E_2 (PGE_2) and F_2 (PGF_2) following trauma may be associated with vasospasm and a decrease of oxidative phosphorylation, furthering local spinal cord ischemia.[1,4] Direct endothelial damage from trauma decreases prostacyclin production and release.[4] Prostacyclin (PGI_2) is responsible for vasodilation and platelet disaggregation.[4] Without prostacyclin, vessel constriction and platelet

Table 9–7. Common Types of Vertebral Trauma*

Level of Injury	Age	Type of Vertebral Trauma	Common Traumatic Incident	Syndrome
Cervical	Foal to yearling	Fracture of dens, luxation C1–2	Hyperflexion (e.g., somersault)	Tetraparesis, respiratory depression, death
Cervical	Young adult	Epiphyseal fracture	Hyperextension	Tetraparesis to tetraplegia
Cervical	Adult	Compression fracture	Head-on collision	Tetraparesis to tetraplegia
Cranial thoracic	Usually young	Fracture of dorsal spinous process	Flipping over backward	Often none
T2–S1	Any	Transverse fracture of vertebral arch, with dislocation	Somersaulting or falls	Paraparesis
Sacroiliac subluxation	Adult	Subluxation	Falls or slipping on ice	None
Sacral fracture	Any	Compression	Fall over backward or dog-sitting when backed	Urinary and fecal incontinence with or without posterior paresis; paralysis of the tail and anus

*From Reed SM: Spinal cord trauma. In Robinson NE, ed: *Current Therapy in Equine Medicine,* ed 2. Philadelphia, WB Saunders, 1987, p 375.

aggregation ensue, further decreasing blood flow.[4] Additionally, the release of endogenous opioids as a result of trauma, especially dynorphin and other k-receptor opioids, contributes to secondary injury by decreasing blood flow in the microcirculation.[8]

Initial spinal cord hemorrhage results in ischemic hypoxia.[4] This state is responsible for altered cell metabolism resulting in decreased aerobic metabolism and a shift to anaerobic metabolism, which is a less efficient method of energy production.[4, 7] Anaerobic metabolism results in lactic acid accumulation, causing acidosis in nervous tissue, thus decreasing glucose and oxygen consumption.[4, 7] Lactic acid stimulates prostaglandin production, adenosine diphosphate release, platelet aggregation, thromboxane A_2 release, vasospasm, vasoconstriction, and the inhibition of neurotransmitter release.[4]

In hypoxic states, the Na^+–K^+-ATPase (adenosine triphosphatase)–dependent cell pump is inhibited or damaged, resulting in the cell's inability to maintain its electrical polarity.[4, 7] Damage to the Na^+–K^+-ATPase pump allows for accumulation of potassium extracellularly and sodium intracellularly. This mechanism is important in the development of edema.[4]

Neurologic Evaluation

Clinical signs observed can be neuroanatomically localized to the affected area. Damage is worse in the large myelinated motor and proprioceptive fibers compared to the smaller or nonmyelinated nociceptive fibers.[1] Therefore, ataxia and loss of proprioception and motor function will occur prior to the loss of deep pain.[1]

Initial evaluation of the patient should be directed toward stabilization and correction of any life-threatening problems such as airway obstruction, hemorrhage, cardiovascular collapse, pneumothorax, and open head injury. In addition,

major long-bone fractures must be identified, as these may be the limiting factor for survival of the horse. A systematic neurologic evaluation, as described in Chapter 9.1, should then be performed in order to localize the site of injury.[9, 10] Figure 9–24 shows the steps in evaluating and neuroanatomically localizing the lesion in the nervous system in a recumbent horse.[9]

Spinal shock (areflexia caudal to the lesion) and Schiff-Sherrington syndrome (extensor hypertonus in otherwise normal thoracic limbs with a cranial thoracic lesion) are infrequent and short-lived findings in the horse.[11, 12] Both carry a grave prognosis.

Ancillary diagnostic aids that may be beneficial include radiography, scintigraphy, cerebrospinal fluid (CSF) analysis, nerve conduction velocities (NCVs), electromyography (EMG), and computed tomography (CT).[13, 14] Radiography may demonstrate fractures, luxations, subluxations, and vertebral compression. Scintigraphy is helpful in diagnosing nondisplaced or occult fractures and soft tissue lesions.[15] Common CSF findings following spinal cord trauma include xanthochromia and mild-to-moderate increased total protein concentrations.[1, 12] CSF analysis may be normal, especially in very acute or chronic cases.[12] The use of NCV and EMG testing thoroughly evaluates the lower motor neuron and aids in lesion localization. However, changes in the EMG may not develop until 4 to 5 days following nerve damage.[16] Currently, CT is the diagnostic aid of choice in humans to evaluate acute spinal cord trauma.[14] The use of CT in equine practice is currently limited to a few referral clinics, but if available, it is very helpful in identifying the nature and extent of spinal cord lesions.

Treatment and Prognosis

The goals of treatment are to stop the cascade of cellular events initiated by the traumatic insult. Specifically, im-

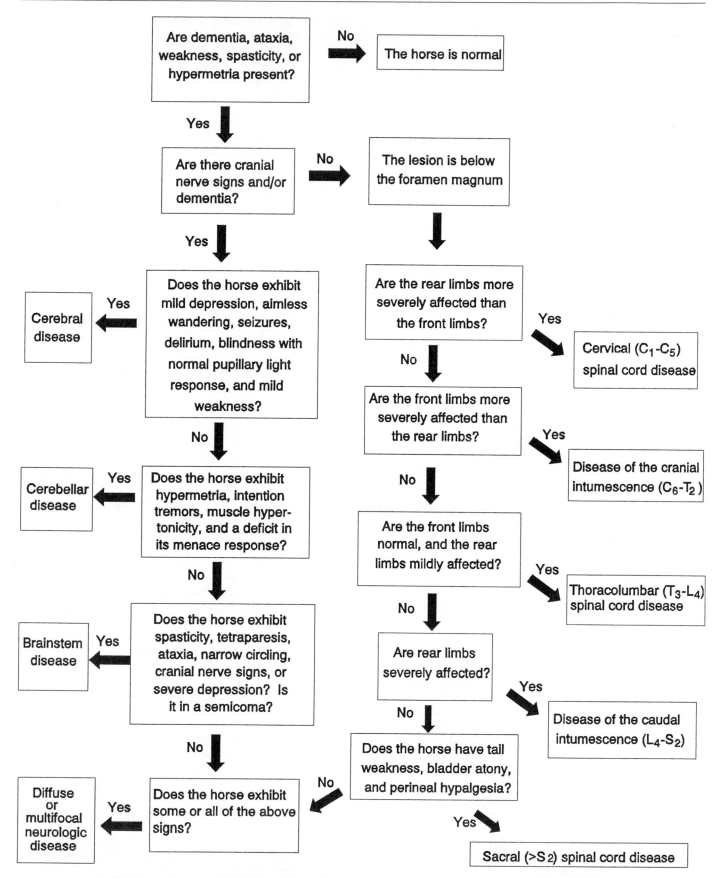

Figure 9–24. Flow chart for localizing a lesion in the nervous system in a recumbent horse.

provement in spinal cord blood flow; reduction in hemorrhage, edema, and membrane lipid peroxidation; and neural tissue preservation are the goals of treatment.

Corticosteroids (CS), alone or in combination with other drugs, are the classic drugs of choice for acute spinal cord trauma. Reported dosages of dexamethasone for horses range from 0.1 to 0.25 mg/kg IV q.6–24h. for 24 to 48 hours.[1, 12] A favorable response is expected within 4 to 8 hours after CS administration.[1] Horses on CS therapy should be monitored closely for the development of laminitis. If improvement in clinical signs is observed, the horse may be placed on oral prednisone therapy (0.5–1.0 mg/kg tapered over 3–5 days) to decrease the chance of laminitis. Potential beneficial effects of CS include maintenance of normal blood glucose concentrations while maintaining electrolyte balance, reduction in the spread of morphologic damage, and the prevention of the loss of axonal conduction and reflex activity.[4] They also preserve vascular membrane integrity and stabilize white matter neuronal cell membranes in the presence of central hemorrhagic lesions.[4] Their anti-inflammatory properties are useful in reducing edema and fibrin deposition, and their ability to reverse sodium and potassium imbalance due to edema and necrosis is beneficial.[4] However, some reports dispute the usefulness of CS in the treatment of acute spinal cord trauma.[17, 18]

Recently, new work with the use of high-dose methylprednisolone sodium succinate (MP) following spinal cord trauma has produced encouraging results.[19, 20] MP is a synthetic glucocorticoid with 4 times more anti-inflammatory activity and 0.8 times less mineralocorticoid action compared with cortisol.[21] It is 40% to 60% bound to plasma proteins and has 2.4-hour and 12- to 36-hour plasma and biological half-lives, respectively.[21]

Beneficial effects of MP on neural tissue include inhibition of lipid peroxidation, eicosanoid formation, and lipid hydrolysis, including arachidonic acid release, maintenance of tissue blood flow and aerobic energy metabolism, improved elimination of intracellular calcium accumulation, reduced neurofilament degradation, and improved neuronal excitability and synaptic transmission.[19, 21]

The results of the recent multicenter randomized, double-blind, placebo-controlled study in humans compared the effects of MP, naloxone, and a placebo on the neurologic outcome of acute spinal cord injury patients.[19, 20] MP was administered as a 30-mg/kg bolus followed by infusion at 5.4 mg/kg/hr for 23 hours. Naloxone was administered as a 5.4-mg/kg bolus followed by infusion at 4 mg/kg/hr for 23 hours.[19] This study, known as the Second National Acute Spinal Cord Injury Study (NASCIS II), then followed the patients' recovery for 1 year. At 6 months, patients receiving MP within 8 hours of injury had significant improvement in motor function, sensation, and touch compared with the other groups.[19] This finding was true for patients with complete and incomplete lesions. At 1 year, the MP group had significant improvement in motor function compared with the other groups.[20] Complications, such as wound infection and gastrointestinal bleeding, were not statistically different among the treatment groups.[19, 20] Mortality was approximately 6% among all groups.[19, 20]

The beneficial effects of MP were only seen in patients treated within 8 hours of injury. This is probably because lipid peroxidation and hydrolysis and release of vasoactive products of arachidonic acid breakdown begin and peak within 8 hours of injury.[22] Apparently, it is the cell membrane anti-lipid peroxidation effect of MP that is most beneficial.[19, 21] The dose of MP used exceeds that necessary for activation of steroid receptors, suggesting that MP acts through mechanisms that are unrelated to steroid receptors.[19, 21]

On the basis of this study, the investigators concluded that high-dose MP treatment within 8 hours of spinal cord injury improved neurologic recovery.[19, 20] The use of naloxone in spinal cord injury was not recommended.[19, 20] The usefulness of high-dose MP treatment for spinal cord trauma in the horse remains to be investigated. Based on the results of this human trial and other animal trials, MP seems to be a promising drug for treatment of spinal cord injury.

Dimethyl sulfoxide (DMSO) 1 g/kg IV as a 10% to 20% solution for 3 consecutive days followed by three treatments every other day has been found to be of benefit in acute spinal cord trauma.[1, 12] The pharmacokinetics of DMSO in horses indicates that twice-daily dosing is necessary to maintain adequate blood levels.[23] Reported benefits of DMSO include increased brain and spinal cord blood flow, decreased brain and spinal cord edema, increased vasodilating PGE_1, decreased platelet aggregation, decreased PGE_2 and PGF_2, protection of cell membranes, and trapping of hydroxyl radicals.[4, 24] The exact mechanism of DMSO remains unknown. This treatment remains controversial as some researchers have found no positive effects on neurologic outcome from the use of DMSO.[14, 25]

Osmotic diuretics such as 20% mannitol administered at 2 g/kg IV may be helpful in decreasing spinal cord edema.[1] This drug should not be used continuously as its hypertonic nature may create dehydration, urine retention, and hypotension. Adequate patient hydration must be maintained when osmotic agents are used. Some investigators and clinicians have found these agents to be of little benefit in spinal cord trauma.[4, 12]

The use of more experimental compounds such as naloxone,[4] a narcotic receptor antagonist, and thyrotropin-releasing hormone (TRH),[26] a functional narcotic antagonist, has been effective in improving neurologic signs following experimental spinal cord trauma. These compounds may block or antagonize endogenous opioids released as a result of trauma. Reported experimental dosages for naloxone are in the range of 1.5 mg/kg. However, in light of the NASCIS II study, the use of naloxone is no longer advocated.[19, 20]

In one study, TRH at 2 mg/kg followed by 2 mg/kg/hr for 4 hours significantly improved the neurologic outcome in experimental spinal cord trauma in cats.[26] The effects of TRH have reportedly been better than those of naloxone or CS.[27] More work is needed to define the role of these compounds in the treatment of spinal cord trauma.

The use of nonsteroidal anti-inflammatory drugs (NSAIDs) such as flunixin meglumine and phenylbutazone may decrease the inflammation associated with a traumatic episode. These compounds work by inhibiting cyclooxygenase, which converts arachidonic acid to inflammatory mediators (endoperoxides). They probably do not alter the course of the neurologic disease.

Antibiotics are not always necessary in the treatment of vertebral or spinal cord trauma.[1, 12] However, they are indicated in treating open fractures and secondary complications associated with a recumbent horse, such as pneumonia and decubital sores. Antibiotic choice should be based on culture and sensitivity testing. Good empirical choices for broad-spectrum coverage include trimethoprim-sulfamethoxazole at 30 mg/kg PO or IV q.12h. or penicillin at 22,000 IU/kg IM q.12h. or IV q.6h. in combination with gentamicin at 2.2 mg/kg IM or IV q.8h. Appropriate monitoring for aminoglycoside toxicity should be undertaken with their use.

Nutritional support also plays a role in the outcome following neurologic injury. In humans, it has been found that neurologic recovery from head injury occurs faster in patients receiving early adequate nutritional support.[28] If the horse is able to eat, and the gastrointestinal tract is functioning normally, water and good-quality hay should be available at all times. Small amounts of grain should be fed three to four times a day to boost caloric intake. The amount of grain fed should be based on the horse's condition and ability to tolerate grain feeding. Horses with a poor appetite or those unable to swallow may have to be tube-fed using a gruel of alfalfa and complete feed pellets. The pellets are soaked in water, usually for 8 to 12 hours, until they have a soupy consistency. They can then be pumped into the horse's stomach via a nasogastric tube. Approximately 1 gal of gruel fed three to four times per day is necessary. Horses that cannot tolerate this procedure, severely depressed or comatose horses, and horses not maintainable with other feeding methods are candidates for total parenteral nutrition (TPN). The procedure for performing TPN in horses has been described elsewhere.[29]

Physical therapy is important in the rehabilitative process in spine-injured horses. Controlled exercise allows the unaffected parts of the nervous system to compensate for the affected parts by increasing strength and conscious proprioception. Exercise is especially helpful in improving weakness, ataxia, spasticity, and hypermetria. In recumbent horses, massage, therapeutic ultrasound, and hydrotherapy of affected muscle groups for 10 to 15 minutes at least twice a day is important. These measures help combat necrosis and muscle atrophy of the horse's dependent muscle groups. Passive flexion and extension of all limbs is helpful in maintaining full range of motion in recumbent horses.[30]

Surgical intervention is warranted when there is need for stabilization, fracture repair, or evidence of a compressive lesion, and has been described elsewhere.[31–33] Surgery should also be considered when there is lack of response to medical treatment. The use of medical treatment to stabilize the patient should always be instituted before surgery is performed.

Prognosis is based on response to therapy and is directly related to the time from injury to the institution of treatment. Horses that show rapid neurologic improvement have a fair-to-good prognosis. Recumbent horses or horses suffering from fractures or luxations have a guarded-to-poor prognosis.[12] Horses that have lost deep pain sensation have a functional or anatomical spinal cord transection and have a grave prognosis.[12] The longer the time from loss of deep pain to treatment, the poorer the prognosis. Partial or complete recovery of horses with spinal cord trauma may take weeks to months, so time and nursing care are required.

INTRACRANIAL TRAUMA

Head trauma in horses, which may or may not be associated with a fracture, is due to many of the same incidents that cause spinal cord trauma. In addition, penetrating wounds, kicks to the head, and rearing up and falling over backward, often resulting in fractures of the basisphenoid and basioccipital bones,[34] may result in intracranial trauma. Other common fractures seen in association with head injuries include mandibular, maxillary, orbital, periorbital rim, and incisive bone fractures.[35, 36] Clinical signs seen as a result of trauma reflect the extent and location of the injury.

Pathophysiology

Following a traumatic insult to the brain, a cycle of events occurs, including membrane disruption, ischemia, hypoxia, edema, and hemorrhage. The degree of these is dependent on the type and extent of the initial injury. Microvascular collapse often ensues as a result of swelling, petechial hemorrhage, and extraluminal blood clots.[37] Hemorrhage, neural changes, and microvascular changes commonly extend beyond the site of injury.[37]

The traumatic insult is also responsible for an increased permeability of brain capillary endothelial cells resulting in vasogenic edema.[38] This is the most common type of edema found following head trauma.[35] Cerebral white matter is especially vulnerable to vasogenic edema, possibly owing to its low capillary density and blood flow.[38] This type of edema results in increased extracellular fluid accumulation.[38] The edema fluid is a plasma filtrate high in plasma proteins.[37] Vasogenic edema displaces cerebral tissue and increases intracranial pressure.[38] This process may result in brain herniation. The elevated intracranial pressure will further decrease cerebral perfusion pressure.[38]

Cytotoxic edema will develop as a result of swelling of the cellular elements of the brain (neurons, glia, and endothelial cells).[38] The cells swell because of failure of the Na^+–K^+-ATPase pump in the presence of hypoxia.[38] Sodium and thus water accumulate in cells.[38] This type of edema occurs in gray and white matter and will decrease the extracellular fluid volume.[38] If capillary endothelial cells are edematous, the capillary lumen size will diminish, creating an increased resistance to arterial flow.[38] Capillary permeability is usually not affected in cytotoxic edema.[38] Major decreases in cerebral function occur with cytotoxic edema, with stupor and coma being common signs.[38]

Many of the mechanisms decreasing blood flow in spinal cord trauma also apply to cerebral trauma. Blood flow interruption is responsible for disruption in ion homeostasis (especially calcium, sodium, and potassium), and a switch to anaerobic glycolysis resulting in lactic acid production and acidosis.[36, 39] Cell membrane lipid peroxidation with subsequent prostaglandin and thromboxane synthesis, formation of oxygen radicals, and energy failure also ensue.[36, 39] Because of the high metabolic rate and oxygen demand of the brain, disruption of blood flow and normal energy-supplying processes leads to impaired nerve cell function and even cell death.[36]

The types of cranial trauma from least to most severe are concussion, contusion, laceration, and hemorrhage.[35, 36] Concussion is a short-term loss of consciousness and is primarily due to a direct blow to the head. It is often reversible and occurs without an anatomical lesion.[35, 36] Contusion is associated with vascular and nervous tissue damage without major structural disruption.[35, 36] Contusions may be on the same or opposite side of the injury and result from blows or sudden accelerations or decelerations of the head.[35] Contusion may result in intraparenchymal hemorrhage with later cavitation.[35] Cerebral hemorrhage and laceration result from penetrating wounds (gunshots) and fractures in addition to the above-mentioned injuries. Cerebral hemorrhage in horses may be epidural, subdural (rare), intracerebral, or subarachnoid (common).[35, 40] Hematoma formation is of special concern because of the potential for devastating expansion within the rigid calvarium, as can occur with edema.[35, 40] These processes displace brain tissue, with herniation, pressure necrosis, and brainstem compression possible sequelae.[35, 36, 40]

Neurologic Evaluation

Clinical signs associated with head trauma range from inapparent to recumbency with profound depression, dementia, and tetraparesis. As with spinal cord trauma, life-threatening injuries should be attended to first, and then a complete neurologic examination performed. Serial neurologic examinations are vital to ensure proper treatment and to predict prognosis. Reflex and nociceptive testing should be performed to rule in or out a concurrent spinal cord injury. As with spinal cord trauma, concurrent long-bone fractures, which may limit the outcome, must be identified. Table 9–8 provides an outline for localizing the level of brain injury based on the neurologic findings.[35]

Some horses may be intractable following a traumatic incident and sedation may be necessary for examination. It should be remembered that xylazine and detomidine transiently cause hypertension, which may potentiate intracranial

hemorrhage.[35, 40] However, a recent study found xylazine to cause a minor decrease in cerebrospinal pressure in normal, conscious horses.[41] Although no studies were performed on horses with cerebral trauma, it is believed that xylazine is a safe sedative to use in head trauma.

Severe brainstem injuries can be associated with apneustic or erratic breathing and reflect a poor prognosis.[35, 36] Bilaterally dilated and unresponsive pupils indicate an irreversible brainstem lesion. Horses with bilaterally miotic pupil size should be routinely monitored, as a change to dilated and unresponsive indicates a progression of the lesion and the need for immediate medical treatment.[35] This carries a grave prognosis.

General physical examination is important in cranial trauma as fractures and other concurrent injuries are not uncommon and require identification and treatment. Physical findings as a result of cranial trauma include blood coming from the nostrils, mouth, and ears, or CSF draining from the ear (basilar fractures).[34, 35] With severe head trauma, a brain-heart syndrome can develop consisting of cardiac arrhythmias, increased serum levels of heart-specific enzymes (the BB isoenzyme of creatine kinase and hydroxybutyrate dehydrogenase), myocardial necrosis, and sudden death due to heart failure.[40]

Ancillary diagnostic aids helpful in further defining cranial trauma include radiography to identify fractures, and CSF analysis.[13] Cisternal CSF collection is contraindicated if increased intracranial pressure is suspected because of the possibility of brain herniation through the foramen magnum. Lumbosacral collection may be a safer alternative but can be normal despite a traumatic episode, especially in the acute phase, and because the sample is not obtained closest to the lesion, it may not reflect the changes that have occurred.[40] As with spinal cord trauma in humans, CT is also the

Table 9–8. Signs Characteristic of Focal Brain Injury*

Levels	Consciousness	Motor Function	Pupils	Other Signs
Cerebrum	Behavior change, depression, coma	Circling	Normal	Blindness
Cerebellum		Ataxia and hypermetria, intention tremor		Menace response deficit without blindness
Diencephalon (thalamus)	Depression to stupor	Normal to mild tetraparesis, "aversive syndrome"†	Bilateral, nonreactive pupils with visual deficit	None
Midbrain	Stupor to coma	Hemiparesis, tetraparesis or tetraplegia	Nonreactive pupils, mydriasis, anisocoria	Ventrolateral strabismus
Pons	Depression	Ataxia and tetraparesis, tetraplegia	Normal	Head tilt, abnormal nystagmus, facial paralysis, medial strabismus
Rostral medulla oblongata (including inner ear)	Depression	Ataxia or hemiparesis to tetraplegia	Normal	Same
Caudal medulla oblongata	Depression	Ataxia, hemiparesis to tetraparesis, abnormal respiratory patterns	Normal	Dysphagia, flaccid tongue

*From Reed SM: Cranial trauma. In Robinson NE, ed: *Current Therapy in Equine Medicine,* ed 2. Philadelphia, WB Saunders, 1987, p 379.
†Deviation of the head and eyes with circling toward the side of a unilateral lesion.

diagnostic aid of choice in cases of head trauma.[14, 42] If available, CT is an invaluable diagnostic aid.

Treatment and Prognosis

The use of CS and DMSO for the reasons discussed under Spinal Cord and Vertebral Trauma are beneficial in the treatment of cranial trauma. The dosages used in horses with intracranial trauma are the same as in spinal cord trauma. The neuroprotective effects of high-dose MP treatment may also be applicable to head injury.[21] Further research on the use of MP treatment in head trauma patients is needed to verify its usefulness.

Osmotic diuretics such as 20% mannitol 0.25 to 2.0 mg/kg IV over 20 minutes and glycerol 0.5 to 2.0 mg/kg IV q.6–12h. for 24 hours are effective in combating cerebral edema and increased intracranial pressure.[35, 40] These have a rapid onset of action (10–20 minutes) and work because of their hyperosmolar nature.[43] Caution should be exercised in the use of these compounds as they can cause further hemorrhage by decreasing edema and allowing space for more bleeding.[38] Also, leakage of these hypertonic solutions into the tissue may increase cerebral edema.[38] Horses receiving osmotic diuretics should be adequately hydrated. The use of osmotic substances is warranted in any horse with worsening mental status, abnormal pupillary size or inequality indicating transtentorial herniation, or development of paresis.[42, 43]

Experimentally, furosemide has reportedly been found effective in decreasing intracranial pressure.[44] A 1-mg/kg bolus IV dose was given at 5-hour intervals and a 0.5-mg/kg/hr dose was given IV for 4 hours, 1 hour after the initial bolus.[44] Normal hydration status is required before furosemide is administered. Furosemide may also be used concurrently with mannitol to increase the duration of intracranial pressure reduction provided by mannitol, and to diminish the potential for rebound intracranial pressure elevation.[45]

Other methods to lower intracranial pressure include elevation of the head by 30 degrees if no cervical fractures are present.[46] Hyperventilation to lower the partial pressure of carbon dioxide to 26 to 28 mm Hg in humans decreases cerebral blood flow, thus lowering intracranial pressure.[42] Hyperventilation may be considered in cases of increased intracranial pressure in horses. Proper hyperventilation requires monitoring of arterial blood gases, and may require use of neuromuscular blockers if the horse is not comatose and is resisting the ventilator.

Barbiturate treatment or coma may decrease cerebral metabolism, thereby providing a protective effect against cerebral ischemia.[7, 35, 42] Barbiturates may also limit lipid peroxidation.[7, 35] However, the actual benefits of barbiturate use on the neurologic outcome remain controversial. The effects of barbiturates on lowering intracranial pressure are enhanced by concurrent hyperventilation.[36] An exact dosage regimen for barbiturate treatment in horses has not been investigated, but 5 to 10 mg/kg IV to effect is reported to be useful.[36] The major side effect of barbiturates is hypotension, especially if mannitol and furosemide have been administered, so they must be used with caution and adequate blood pressure monitoring. In my opinion, the use of barbiturates should be reserved for those cases where elevated intracranial pressure is refractory to other treatments.

Fluid therapy in cases of intracranial trauma is often needed to maintain hydration and blood pressure. Isotonic crystalloid fluids administered in typical shock doses of 40 to 90 mL/kg/hr may produce worsening of cerebral edema and increased intracranial pressure.[47, 48] Comparison of isotonic crystalloid fluids with hypertonic saline solutions for fluid support of head trauma patients in shock has shown hypertonic saline to be the fluid of choice.[47] Hypertonic saline is associated with significant decreases in intracranial pressure and cerebral water content compared with isotonic fluid treatment.[48] Hypertonic saline administered early in the treatment of shock associated with head trauma may enhance return of cerebral blood flow and cell membrane function.[48] Effects of hypertonic saline are due to its ability to move water out of cells, and to decrease tissue pressure and cell size by osmotic plasma expansion.[48, 49] These effects result in a lowering of intracranial pressure and cerebral water content. The beneficial effects of hypertonic saline prevail even with subsequent administration of isotonic fluids.[48, 50] A recent study compared 1.8% sodium chloride with hypotonic Ringer's lactate as 24-hour maintenance fluids following experimental cerebral injury.[51] The 1.8% saline provided the above beneficial effects as well as adequate cardiovascular support, suggesting hypertonic saline may be the maintenance fluid of choice in head injury.[51]

Hypertonic saline may be given to head trauma horses in shock as a 5% or 7% sodium chloride solution in a 4- to 6-mL/kg bolus IV dose over 15 minutes.[49] Isotonic fluids may then be used for maintenance if needed. Monitoring central venous pressure to keep it in the normal range of −5 to −7 cm H_2O is important in comatose horses to avoid overhydration. Contraindications to the use of hypertonic saline include dehydration, ongoing hemorrhage, hypernatremia, renal failure, hyperkalemic periodic paralysis, and hypothermia.[49]

The use of carbohydrate-containing intravenous solutions should be avoided early in the treatment of head trauma patients.[35, 52, 53] Glucose suppresses ketogenesis, and may increase lactic acid production by the traumatized brain, limiting the availability of nonglycolytic energy substrates.[52] Carbon dioxide liberated from glucose metabolism causes vasodilation and worsening of cerebral edema.[35, 53]

Antibiotic treatment is usually warranted in cases of head trauma, especially when fractures are involved.[35, 40] The presence of hemorrhage increases the possibility of septic meningitis. Broad-spectrum antimicrobials, such as those listed for spinal cord trauma, are effective. Owing to disruption of the blood-brain barrier, other antimicrobials probably penetrate into the central nervous system, and therefore their use may also be efficacious.

It is not unusual for horses sustaining cranial trauma to develop seizures. The drug of choice in controlling seizures is diazepam. Doses range from 5 mg (foals) to 25 to 100 mg (horses) IV, repeated as necessary to control seizure activity.[35, 40] Intractable seizures may necessitate general anesthesia. Agents useful for general anesthesia include guaifenesin, chloral hydrate, barbiturates, and gas anesthesia. Ketamine should not be used as part of a balanced anesthesia regimen as it increases cerebral blood flow and intracranial pressure.[54]

Adequate nutritional support as discussed for spinal cord trauma also applies to head-injured horses. Additionally, the

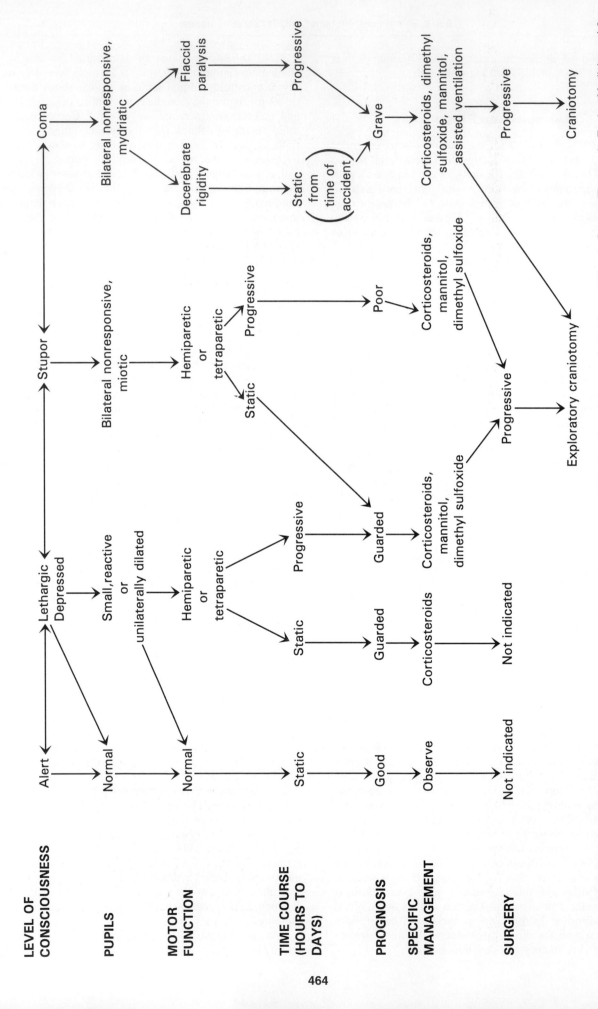

LEVEL OF CONSCIOUSNESS

PUPILS

MOTOR FUNCTION

TIME COURSE (HOURS TO DAYS)

PROGNOSIS

SPECIFIC MANAGEMENT

SURGERY

Figure 9–25. Flow chart for management of cranial trauma. (From Reed SM: Spinal cord trauma. In Robinson NE, ed: *Current Therapy in Equine Medicine*, ed 2. Philadelphia, WB Saunders, 1987, p 379; modified from Kirk KW, ed: *Current Veterinary Therapy VII*, WB Saunders, 1980, p 819.)

use of thiamine 1 g IM for 5 days may be of benefit in treating head injuries. Thiamine aids breakdown of lactic acid and is a necessary coenzyme in brain energy pathways.[30]

Emergency surgical treatment (although not commonly performed) is warranted in open cranial fractures and in the face of deterioration despite medical therapy. The surgical techniques for these procedures have been described elsewhere.[33, 55] Once the patient is stabilized, repair of less life-threatening fractures can be considered. Figure 9–25 summarizes medical and surgical therapies for cranial trauma.[35]

As with spinal cord trauma, the prognosis for cranial trauma is dependent on early treatment and is gauged by response to treatment. Basilar fractures and severe brainstem injuries carry a grave prognosis.[34] Recumbency, tetraparesis, and severe dementia carry a poor-to-grave prognosis.[35] Time, good nursing care, and adequate nutritional support, especially in the recumbent horse, are vital for a positive outcome.

REFERENCES

1. Reed SM: Spinal cord trauma. In Robinson NE, ed: *Current Therapy in Equine Medicine,* ed 2. Philadelphia, WB Saunders, 1987, p 374.
2. Wagner PC: Diseases of the spine. In Mansmann RA, McAllister ES, eds: *Equine Medicine and Surgery.* Santa Barbara, Calif, American Veterinary Publications, 1982, p 1148.
3. Ducker TB, Kindt GW, Kempe LG: Pathological findings in acute experimental spinal cord trauma. *J Neurosurg* 35:700, 1971.
4. de la Torre JC: Spinal cord injury. Review of basic and applied research. *Spine* 6:315, 1981.
5. Osterholm JL, Matthews GJ: Altered norepinephrine metabolism following experimental spinal cord injury. *J Neurosurg* 36:336, 1972.
6. de la Torre JC, Johnson CM, Harris LH, et al: Monoamine changes in experimental head and spinal cord trauma: Failure to confirm previous observations. *Surg Neurol* 2:5, 1974.
7. Rucker NC: Management of spinal cord trauma. *Prog Vet Neurol* 1:397, 1990.
8. Faden AI: Neuropeptides and central nervous system injury. *Arch Neurol* 43:501, 1986.
9. Matthews HK, Andrews F: Performing a neurologic examination in a standing or recumbent horse. *Vet Med* 85:1229, 1990.
10. Mayhew IG: *Large Animal Neurology. A Handbook for Veterinary Clinicians.* Philadelphia, Lea & Febiger, 1989, p 15.
11. deLahunta A: *Veterinary Neuroanatomy and Clinical Neurology,* ed 2. Philadelphia, WB Saunders, 1983, p 185.
12. Mayhew IG: *Large Animal Neurology. A Handbook for Veterinary Clinicians.* Philadelphia, Lea & Febiger, 1989, p 266.
13. Andrews F, Matthews HK, Reed SM: The ancillary techniques and tests for diagnosing equine neurologic disease. *Vet Med* 85:1325, 1990.
14. Gilman S: Advances in neurology. *N Engl J Med* 326:1608, 1992.
15. Twardock AR, Baker GJ, Chambers MD: The impact of nuclear medicine as a diagnostic procedure in equine practice. *Compend Contin Educ Pract Vet* 13:1717, 1991.
16. Griffith IR, Duncan ID: The use of electromyography and nerve conduction studies in the evaluation of lower motor neuron disease or injury. *J Small Anim Pract* 19:329, 1978.
17. Eidelberg E, Stulen E, Watkins CJ, et al: Treatment of experimental spinal cord injury in ferrets. *Surg Neurol* 6:243, 1976.
18. Hedeman LS, Shellenberger MK, Gordon JH: Studies in experimental spinal cord trauma. *J Neurosurg* 40:44, 1974.
19. Bracken MB, Shepard MJ, Collins WF, et al: A randomized, controlled trial of methylprednisolone or naloxone in the treatment of acute spinal-cord injury, *N Engl J Med* 322:1404, 1990.
20. Bracken MB, Shepard MJ, Collins WF, et al: Methylprednisolone or naloxone treatment after acute spinal cord injury: 1-year follow-up data. *J Neurosurg* 76:23, 1992.
21. Hall ED: The neuroprotective pharmacology of methylprednisolone. *J Neurosurg* 76:13, 1992.
22. Braughler JM, Hall ED: Correlation of methylprednisolone levels in cat spinal cord with its effects on $(NA^+ + K^+)$-ATPase, lipid peroxidation, and alpha motor neuron function. *J Neurosurg* 61:290, 1984.
23. Blythe LL, Craig AM, Christensen JM, et al: Pharmacokinetic disposition of dimethyl sulfoxide administered intravenously to horses. *Am J Vet Res* 47:1739, 1986.
24. Brayton CF: Dimethyl sulfoxide (DMSO): A review. *Cornell Vet* 76:61, 1986.
25. Hoerlein BF, Redding RW, Hoff EJ, et al: Evaluation of dexamethasone, DMSO, mannitol and solcoseryl in acute spinal cord trauma. *J Am Anim Hosp Assoc* 19:216, 1983.
26. Faden AI, Jacobs TP, Smith MT: Thyrotropin-releasing hormone in experimental spinal injury: Dose response and late treatment. *Neurology* 34:1280, 1984.
27. Faden AI, Jacobs TP, Smith MT, et al: Comparison of thyrotropin-releasing hormone, naloxone and dexamethasone treatments in experimental spinal injury. *Neurology* 33:673, 1983.
28. Young B, Ott L, Twyman D, et al: The effect of nutritional support on the outcome from severe head injury. *J Neurosurg* 67:668, 1987.
29. Spurlock SL, Ward MV: Parenteral nutrition in equine patients: Principles and theory. *Compend Contin Educ Pract Vet* 13:461, 1991.
30. Andrews FA, Matthews HK, Reed SM: Medical, surgical, and physical therapy for horses with neurological disease. *Vet Med* 85:1331, 1990.
31. Nixon AJ: Surgical management of equine cervical vertebral malformation. *Prog Vet Neurol* 2:183, 1991.
32. Wagner PC, Bagby GW, Grant BD, et al: Surgical stabilization of the equine cervical spine. *Vet Surg* 8:7, 1979.
33. Stashak TS, Mayhew IG: The nervous system. In Jennings PB, ed: *The Practice of Large Animal Surgery.* Philadelphia, WB Saunders, 1984, p 983.
34. Stick JA, Wilson T, Kunac D: Basilar skull fractures in three horses. *J Am Vet Med Assoc* 176:338, 1980.
35. Reed SM: Intracranial Trauma. In Robinson NE, ed: *Current Therapy in Equine Medicine,* ed 2. Philadelphia, WB Saunders, 1987, p 377.
36. Reed SM: Management of head trauma in horses. *Compend Contin Educ Pract Vet* 15:270, 1993.
37. Hekmatpanah J, Hekmatpanah CR: Microvascular alterations following cerebral contusion in rats: Light, scanning, and electron microscope study. *J Neurosurg* 62:888, 1985.
38. Fishman RA: Brain edema. *N Engl J Med* 293:706, 1975.
39. Raichle ME: The pathophysiology of brain ischemia. *Ann Neurol* 13:2, 1983.
40. Mayhew IG: *Large Animal Neurology. A Handbook for Veterinary Clinicians.* Philadelphia, Lea & Febiger, 1989, p 139.
41. Moore RM, Trim C: Effect of xylazine on cerebrospinal fluid pressure in conscious horses. *Am J Vet Res* 53:1558, 1992.
42. White RJ, Likavec MJ: The diagnosis and initial management of head injury. *N Engl J Med* 327:1507, 1992.
43. Sternback GI: Evaluation and initial management of blunt head injury. *Hosp Physician* 28:16, 1992.
44. Albright LA, Latchaw RE, Robinson AG: Intracranial and

systemic effects of osmotic and oncotic therapy in experimental cerebral edema. *J Neurosurg* 60:481, 1984.

45. Feldman Z, Kanter MJ, Robertson CS, et al: Effect of head elevation on intracranial pressure, cerebral perfusion pressure, and cerebral blood flow in head-injured patients. *J Neurosurg* 76:207, 1992.

46. Borel C, Hanley D, Diringer MN, et al: Intensive management of severe head injury. *Chest* 98:180, 1990.

47. Crowe DT: Triage and trauma management. In Murtaugh RJ, Kaplan PM, eds: *Veterinary Emergency and Critical Care Medicine.* St Louis, Mosby–Year Book, 1992, p 77.

48. Gunnar W, Jonasson O, Merlotti G, et al: Head injury and hemorrhagic shock: Studies of the blood brain barrier and intracranial pressure after resuscitation with normal saline solution, 3% saline solution, and dextran-40. *Surgery* 103:398, 1988.

49. Bertone JJ: Hypertonic saline in the management of shock in horses. *Compend Contin Educ Pract Vet* 13:665, 1991.

50. Prough DS, Johnson JC, Poole GV, et al: Effects on intracranial pressure of resuscitation from hemorrhagic shock with hypertonic saline versus lactated Ringer's solution. *Crit Care Med* 13:407, 1985.

51. Shackford SR, Zhuang J, Schmoker J: Intravenous fluid tonicity: Effect on intracranial pressure, cerebral blood flow, and cerebral oxygen delivery in focal brain injury. *J Neurosurg* 76:91, 1992.

52. Robertson CS, Goodman JC, Narayan RK, et al: The effect of glucose administration on carbohydrate metabolism after head injury. *J Neurosurg* 74:43, 1991.

53. Feldman NJA, Fish S: Resuscitation fluid for a patient with head injury and hypovolemic shock. *J Emerg Med* 19:465, 1991.

54. Lassen NA, Christensen MS: Physiology of cerebral blood flow. *Br J Anaesth* 48:719, 1976.

55. Blackford JT, Blackford LA: Surgical treatment of selected musculoskeletal disorders of the head. In Auer J, ed: *Equine Surgery.* Philadelphia, WB Saunders, 1992, p 1075.

9.6

Vestibular Disease

Bonnie Rush Moore, DVM, MS

The vestibular system is a special proprioceptive system responsible for maintenance of balance and reflex orientation to gravitational forces. This system functions to maintain appropriate eye, trunk, and limb position in reference to movements and positioning of the head.[1, 2]

THE VESTIBULAR APPARATUS

The afferent unit of the vestibular system is composed of the receptor organ within the inner ear and the vestibulocochlear nerve (the eighth cranial nerve). The vestibulocochlear nerve processes both auditory and vestibular input through a common physiologic mechanism. Acoustic stimuli and acceleration forces result in mechanical deformation of hair cells in both the cochlea and vestibular receptor organs which transform physical forces into electrical impulses.[3] The inner ear is located in the petrous temporal bone and consists of the bony and membranous labyrinth. The membranous labyrinth is suspended within the bony labyrinth by perilymph, fluid similar to and likely derived from cerebrospinal fluid.[2] The membranous labyrinth is made up of the cochlea, the saccule, the utricle, and the three semicircular canals.[4] The cochlea is responsible for auditory functions and has no input to the vestibular system.[5] Endolymph fills the membranous labyrinth and is derived from blood vessels along one side of the cochlea.[2]

The three semicircular canals are oriented at right angles to one another, which allows for detection of rotation in any plane at any angle. At one end of each semicircular canal is a dilatation of the canal called the ampulla. A ridge of connective tissue called the crista is located on one side of the ampulla. The internal surface of the crista is lined with hair cells (neuroreceptor cells) and sustentacular cells (support cells) which are oriented perpendicular to the flow of endolymph.[2, 6] These cells are covered with a gelatinous protein-polysaccharide material called the cupula, which extends across the lumen of the ampulla.[5] Rotation of the head in any plane causes endolymph to flow in one or more of the semicircular ducts. Each hair cell has 40 to 80 stereocilia and a single modified kinocilium. Movement of endolymph causes the cupula to move across the stereocilia. Deformation of the stereocilia by the flow of endolymph toward the kinocilia results in increased neuronal activity of the vestibular nerve. Inhibition of vestibular neurons occurs with deviation of stereocilia away from kinocilia.[5] The semicircular canals are responsible for dynamic equilibrium and respond only to changing forces such as acceleration and deceleration, but not to constant velocity or stationary positioning.[2] Changing forces at a rate of 1 degree/sec^2 can be detected by the semicircular canals.[5]

A similar receptor organ called the macula is located in the wall of both the saccule and the utricle. The organ consists of a 2-mm oval plaque of dense connective tissue, lined by neuroepithelial cells and covered with a gelatinous substance, termed the *otolithic membrane.* Calcium carbonate crystals called statoconia (otoliths) lie on the otolithic membrane and their movement initiates stimulation of the vestibular neurons.[7] The macula sacculi is vertically oriented and the macula utriculi is horizontally oriented. Gravitational forces continuously affect the position of otoliths in at least one of the maculae, supplying constant information regarding the static position of the head.[8] These receptor organs can detect changes in head position of one-half degree from the stationary plane.[5] The maculae of the saccule and utricle also detect linear acceleration and deceleration and are responsible for maintenance of static equilibrium.[8]

The hair cells of the crista ampullaris and maculae synapse with sensory neurons of the vestibular nerve. The cell bodies of these bipolar neurons are located within the petrous temporal bone and constitute the vestibular ganglion.[5] Axons leave the petrous temporal bone through the internal acoustic meatus adjacent to the cochlear portion of the eighth cranial nerve. Fibers course to the lateral aspect of the rostral medulla and penetrate the brainstem between the caudal cerebellar peduncle and the spinal tract of the trigeminal nerve. The majority of fibers of the eighth cranial nerve terminate in the four vestibular nuclei (rostral, medial, lateral, and caudal) located in the lateral wall of the fourth ventricle of the rostral medulla oblongata.[1] Some of these fibers form the vestibulocerebellar tract and directly enter the caudal cerebellar peduncle to terminate in the fastigial nucleus and flocculonodular lobes of the cerebellum. The afferent supply to the vestibular nucleus is primarily from the maculae, the crista ampullaris, and the cerebellum. These sensory fibers synapse with second-order neurons in the vestibular nuclei which extend fibers to the motor neurons of the spinal cord, the nuclei of the cranial nerves that control eye position, the cerebellum, the autonomic nervous system, the reticular formation, and the cerebral cortex.[2, 5]

The vestibulospinal tract courses in the ipsilateral ventral funiculus and terminates in interneurons of the ventral gray column. Stimulation of the vestibulospinal tract is facilitatory to alpha and gamma motor neurons of the ipsilateral extensor muscles, inhibitory to the alpha motor neurons of the ipsilateral flexor muscles, and inhibitory to contralateral extensor muscles.[2] The net result is ipsilateral extensor tonus and contralateral flexor tonus which act as an adaptive mechanism against gravity by catching the body and preventing a fall in the direction of vestibular stimulation.[6]

Axons from the medial vestibular nucleus project through the medial longitudinal fasciculus. The ascending portions of the medial longitudinal fasciculus course to the motor nuclei of the third, fourth, and sixth cranial nerves (oculomotor, trochlear, and abducens).[4, 9] These fibers coordinate conjugate eye movement with changes in head position. This pathway, in conjunction with cerebellar input, controls physiologic (vestibular) nystagmus.[2] Physiologic nystagmus is a normal reflex which allows the eyes to remain fixed on a stationary object while the head is moving.[5] Nystagmus is characterized by involuntary, conjugate, rhythmic eyeball oscillations with a fast and slow phase. The direction of nystagmus is defined by the direction of the fast phase and is induced by rapid movements of the head. Rapid dorsiflexion of the neck results in vertical nystagmus, whereas side-to-side movement of the head induces horizontal nystagmus. Turning the head to the left results in a horizontal nystagmus with the fast phase to the left. The accompanying slow phase is in a direction opposite to body motion and allows the eyes to fix on a stationary image. The fast phase is initiated when the eyeball reaches the lateral limit of ocular movement and allows the eyeballs to jump forward and focus on a new image.[5, 6] The slow phase is controlled by vestibular input and the fast phase is a function of the brainstem.[2] Physiologic nystagmus induced by rapid manipulation of the head is called the oculocephalic reflex. This reflex occurs independent of vision.[10] Descending portions of the medial longitudinal fasciculus travel in the ventral funiculus of the cervical and cranial thoracic spinal cord segments and control the position and activity of the limbs and trunk in coordination with head position.[2, 5]

Fibers from the vestibular nuclei that project to the reticular formation provide afferents to the vomit center, which is the pathway for the development of motion sickness. Reticulospinal tracts also aid in the maintenance of extensor tone to support the body against gravity.[2, 5]

Vestibular impulses enter the cerebellum via the caudal cerebellar peduncles. Fibers of the vestibulocerebellar tracts terminate primarily in the flocculonodular lobe and fastigial nucleus.[2] The flocculonodular lobe appears to be closely linked to the semicircular canals in the control of dynamic equilibrium.[5] The cerebellum functions to coordinate protagonistic, antagonistic, and synergistic muscle groups for controlled responses to gravity. The vestibular apparatus provides information to the cerebellum dictating the relative degree of contraction necessary to maintain equilibrium.[5]

Vestibular signals travel through to the contralateral medial geniculate nuclei of the thalamus to the cerebral cortex. In addition to proprioceptive information from other parts of the body, the cerebral cortex facilitates conscious perception of orientation.[2]

The vestibular system is capable only of detecting movement and orientation of the head in relationship to the rest of the body. Afferent pathways from the neck allow the head to be cognizant of the orientation of the rest of the body.[5, 8] Proprioceptive receptors in the joints of the neck that transmit signals to the reticular formation are essential to the righting reflex.[7, 8] Exteroceptor receptors of the skin and proprioceptive receptors in other joints are also integrated in the cerebellum and reticular formation to aid in the maintenance of equilibrium. These signals allow the vestibular system to know if the body remains in an appropriate position with respect to gravity while the head is bent. Visual images can help to maintain balance by visual detection of the upright stance. In addition, slight linear or angular movement of the head shifts the image on the retina which relays directional information to equilibrium centers. Visual compensation may be capable of maintaining balance in the face of complete vestibular destruction, if the eyes are open and motions are performed relatively slowly.[5]

The seventh cranial nerve (the facial nerve) emerges from the lateral medulla ventral to the vestibulocochlear nerve at the level of the trapezoid body. The two nerves are both closely associated with the petrous temporal bone and enter the internal auditory meatus together.[11] Within the internal auditory meatus, the facial nerve separates from the vestibular nerve and courses through the facial canal of the petrosal bone. The facial nerve exits the cranium from the stylomastoid foramen located immediately caudal to the external auditory meatus.[12] It is common for both nerves to be affected simultaneously by a single disease process owing to the proximity of the facial and vestibular nerves.[12]

Sympathetic innervation to the eye is also anatomically associated with the petrous temporal bone. Damage to this nerve (Horner's syndrome), in conjunction with vestibular and facial nerve deficits, frequently occurs with petrous temporal bone trauma and otitis media in small animals.[10] The association of Horner's syndrome, facial nerve paralysis, and vestibular disease is rarely documented in the horse.[2]

CLINICAL SIGNS

Knowledge of the anatomy and function of structures related to the peripheral and central vestibular system aids in neuroanatomical localization of the lesion.[10] Differentiation of central vs. peripheral vestibular disease is important for establishing a list of differential diagnoses, initiating therapy, and formulating a prognosis. A thorough physical and neurologic examination of a horse with vestibular disease may identify nonvestibular neurologic signs, lending significant insight into the location of the lesion. Historical information, including duration of condition, rate of onset, and disease progression, may also aid in differentiation of central from peripheral vestibular disease.

Signs of acute peripheral vestibular system dysfunction include head tilt, nystagmus, falling, circling, reluctance to move, and asymmetric ataxia with preservation of strength.[2, 4, 8, 10, 12, 13] Horses affected with peracute vestibular disease are often violent owing to disorientation.[1] A true head tilt is a consistent sign of vestibular disease and is characterized by ventral deviation of the poll of the head toward the affected side[4, 14] (Fig. 9–26). The horse will prefer to lie on the side of the lesion and may lean on the wall toward the affected side when standing. When forced to move, the horse will take short, uncoordinated steps in a circle toward the direction of the lesion. The body may be flexed laterally with a concavity toward the lesion.[4, 6] Extensor hypotonia ipsilateral to the lesion and mild hypertonia and hyper-reflexia of the extensor muscles of the contralateral side result in asymmetric ataxia.[15] Extensor hypotonia occurs due to loss of facilitatory neurons of the vestibulospinal tract to ipsilateral extensor muscles. Contralateral extensor hyperto-

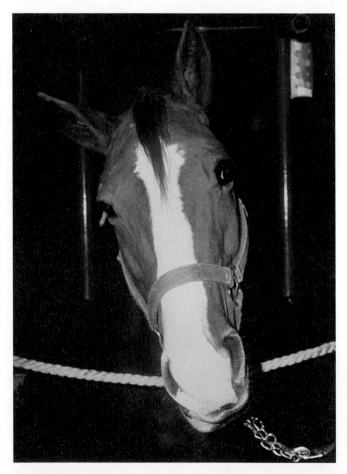

Figure 9–26. Thoroughbred with right-sided peripheral vestibular disease due to a pathologic fracture of the petrous temporal bone secondary to otitis media-interna. The head tilt, dropped pinna, and eyelid droop occur on the affected side, whereas the muzzle is pulled toward the contralateral side.

nia occurs due to loss of inhibitory neurons and unopposed extensor tone of the contralateral vestibulospinal tract.[2, 6, 14] Central vestibular disease will present with similar clinical signs, but general proprioceptive deficits, weakness, and multiple cranial nerve deficits may also be present resulting from damage to the surrounding neurologic structures. The onset of vestibular signs in a horse with an expanding space-occupying central lesion will not be as dramatic as peripheral nerve damage; adjustments by compensatory mechanisms occur during slow development of the lesion. These lesions, however, are not likely to show significant clinical improvement after the onset of clinical signs, as may occur with peripheral vestibular lesions.

Pathologic nystagmus is involuntary, rhythmic oscillations of the eyes occurring while the head is in a normal position and is indicative of a lesion in either the vestibular system or cerebellum.[12] As in physiologic nystagmus, a fast and slow phase are identified. The direction of nystagmus is defined by the direction of the fast phase.[2, 5, 12] Pathologic nystagmus may be spontaneous, occurring with the head in the resting position, or positional, which is induced by elevation or lateral flexion of the head.[2] Nystagmus usually appears with the onset of other peripheral vestibular signs, but may last only 2 to 3 days because of central compensation.[4, 15] Concomitant blinking of the eyelid may hinder detection of nystagmus.[2]

Peripheral vestibular dysfunction may result in either horizontal or rotary nystagmus. The fast phase of nystagmus is directed away from the lesion and will not change with changing head position.[2, 3, 6] The direction of rotary nystagmus is defined by the direction the limbus moves from the 12 o'clock position during the fast phase.[2] Horizontal, rotary, or vertical nystagmus can result from a central vestibular lesion. In addition, the type of nystagmus observed may change with changing head position in a patient with central vestibular disease.[1, 12, 14] Often the fast phase is directed away from the central lesion, but this is not a consistent finding.[2]

In the healthy animal, a constant stream of electrical stimulation arises in each vestibular end-organ and transmits signals which control ocular position via the medial longitudinal fasciculus. These signals normally drive the eyes toward the opposite direction. The eyes are maintained centrally, however, because vestibulo-ocular pathways are opposed in an equal and opposite manner. Unilateral vestibular disease upsets this balance resulting in slow deviation of both eyes toward the lesion. Rapid eye movements return the eyes to midposition. Individuals that are blind at birth or have been blind for an extended time may exhibit irregular eyeball oscillation with no slow or fast component.[16]

Ataxia and dysmetria are often severe with peripheral vestibular disease; however, strength is maintained. Postural reactions will remain normal with the exception of the righting reflex. The motor system is unable to accurately control movement and identify the location of different parts of the body at a given time. Therefore, an exaggerated response will be made toward the side of the lesion as the horse attempts to stand.[2]

Loss of hearing is a common finding with peripheral vestibular disease owing to the proximity of the cochlea to the vestibular receptor organs. In the central nervous system diffuse pathways control auditory signals and extensive central disease would be necessary to cause hearing loss.[14]

If vestibular signs are accompanied by depression, weakness, or conscious proprioceptive deficits, a central vestibular system lesion is likely. With a central lesion, abnormal conscious proprioception occurs due to damage, within the brainstem, of the descending upper motor neuron tracts to the limbs.[2] Damage to the spinocerebellar tracts or caudal cerebellar peduncles will result in abnormal unconscious proprioception and hypermetria.[1] The nuclei of the trigeminal (fifth cranial nerve) and the abducens nerves (sixth cranial nerve) are in anatomical proximity to the vestibular nuclei and are readily damaged in a common disease process. Trigeminal nerve paralysis creates a loss of sensation to the head and atrophy of the muscles of mastication. Trochlear nerve damage results in medial strabismus.[10]

Destructive space-occupying lesions in the cerebellopontine angle or flocculonodular lobe may result in paradoxical central vestibular disease.[1, 17] This syndrome is manifested by vestibular ataxia and a head tilt contralateral to the side demonstrating general proprioceptive ataxia and postural reaction deficits. When this unusual combination of neurologic signs is present, localization of the lesion is defined by the side of general proprioceptive deficits.[2, 10]

Central or peripheral vestibular disease may produce strabismus. Ventrolateral strabismus is observed ipsilateral to the vestibular lesion with elevation of the head and extension of the neck.[2, 10] Mild ventral deviation of the eyes is observed in normal horses when the head is elevated, but it is a symmetric finding. Ventrolateral strabismus of vestibular disease is not a sign of a cranial nerve deficit of the extraocular muscles.[2] It is a reflection of abnormal upper motor neuron influences on the oculomotor nucleus from the ipsilateral vestibular nucleus via the medial longitudinal fasciculus. If the strabismus is purely vestibular in origin, normal ocular mobility will be seen with manipulation of the head.[14]

Signs of vestibular disease may rapidly improve 2 to 3 weeks after onset owing to visual and central accommodation.[2, 13] Central vestibular lesions are slower to compensate than peripheral vestibular lesions; signs may even progress if the central lesion is an expanding space-occupying mass.[14] Humans compensate satisfactorily for unilateral disease, but are not required to be coordinated athletes performing at high speed.[4] Blindfolding a horse with compensated disease will result in ataxia and a head tilt (Romberg's test). Blindfolding eliminates visual and limb proprioceptive orientation; the body is forced to rely on the impaired vestibular system for equilibrium.[2, 10, 11] This test is unreliable for localizing the side of the lesion.[3] Horses may decompensate dramatically when the blindfold is placed over the eyes, resulting in anxiety, disorientation, and falling.[2] The test should be performed with caution on a padded surface with good footing.

Horses affected with bilateral peripheral disease demonstrate no head tilt, circling, or pathologic nystagmus, and physiologic nystagmus cannot be induced by rapid manipulation of the head (the oculocephalic reflex) or by caloric testing. The head may sway with wide excursions from side to side.[4] As with all peripheral vestibular disease, strength is preserved.[2] Clinically, horses affected with bilateral vestibular disease will exhibit more symmetric ataxia very similar to generalized cerebellar disease.[1]

Facial nerve (seventh cranial nerve) paralysis frequently occurs concurrently with peripheral vestibular disease because of its proximity to the vestibular nerve within the petrous temporal bone. Facial nerve paralysis worsens the long-term prognosis and complicates the management of vestibular disease patients. The facial nerve innervates the muscles of facial expression and damage to this nerve results in muzzle deviation away from the affected side, lack of menace and palpebral response, ear droop, decreased nostril flare impeding air flow, and buccal impaction of feed.[4, 11, 12] Keratitis and corneal ulceration are common owing to inability to blink and decreased tear production.[4, 18] Decreased tear production results from damage to parasympathetic fibers to the lacrimal gland. Preganglionic fibers travel with the facial nerve through the internal auditory meatus and separate in the facial canal proximal to the geniculate nucleus.[12] The fibers split from the facial nerve to join the superior petrosal nerve which carries fibers to the sphenopalatine ganglion. Postganglionic fibers join the sympathetic fibers to the eye and travel with the vasculature to the lacrimal gland.[2, 12] Corneal ulcerations occur in the inferior portion of the cornea, and are slow to heal owing to ongoing exposure.[11] Lack of tear production aids in localization of the lesion, indicating the damage is within the petrous temporal bone, proximal to the geniculate nucleus.[2, 12] Clinical signs of facial nerve paralysis may not appear for several days after the onset of vestibular disease, because damage to the nerve may be the result of hematoma, callus, or an extension of inflammation and secondary neuritis.[4] Owing to the proximity of the nuclei of the facial and vestibular nerves, extensive lesions of the medulla may involve both nerves. If no improvement of facial nerve deficits occurs within 3 to 4 months after the onset of disease, a poor prognosis is given for recovery of these signs. If even mild improvement is noted in the first 4 months, facial nerve function may return.[4] Horses may learn to retract the globe, allowing the eyelid and nictitating membrane to slide across the surface of the cornea, distributing lubrication and protecting the eye from trauma.[11] Careful observation is necessary to differentiate this adaptation from improvement of lid function.

PERIPHERAL VESTIBULAR DISEASE

Acute onset of peripheral vestibular disease and facial nerve paralysis is not a rare occurrence in the horse.[15, 19] Damage to the temporal bone is the most likely anatomical location when these nerves are affected concurrently. Otitis media-interna and traumatic skull fractures are the most common causes of these signs in large animals.[1]

Otitis Media

Otitis media-interna is less common in the horse when compared with other species.[4] It is a disease of adult horses with no breed or sex predilection. Rupture of the tympanic membrane and drainage of exudate from the external meatus can occur in the horse, but is uncommon.[11, 15] Instead, as in lambs, the infectious process migrates ventrally, creating chronic inflammation of the tympanic bulla and proximal stylohyoid bone.[20] Inflammation induces bony proliferation of these bones with loss of the joint space and fusion of the temporohyoid joint. The hyoid apparatus is linked in series to the tongue and larynx; fusion of the temporohyoid joint results in impaired flexibility of the unit. A stress fracture of the petrous temporal bone, the stylohyoid bone, or both may result from eating or vocalization with normal tongue movement.[6, 15] Petrous temporal bone fracture is most common. The fracture line extends into the cranial vault at the level of the internal auditory meatus, resulting in direct neural tissue trauma and hemorrhage into the middle and inner ear.[1, 15] No neurologic signs are apparent during the formation of proliferative osteitis and temporohyoid joint fusion. The onset of neurologic signs corresponds with the occurrence of the stress fracture. Occasionally, the fracture extends to the foramen lacerum, caudal to the petrous temporal bone, where the glossopharyngeal and vagus nerves exit the skull. Trauma to these nerves by the fracture may result in dysphagia for several days, in addition to acute vestibular disease.[11]

As a result of extension of the inflammation through the internal acoustic meatus, focal suppurative meningitis may occur at the level of the pons, resulting in fever and depression.[21] Secondary meningitis complicates the treatment and management and worsens the prognosis for recovery.[15]

The origin of the infectious process of otitis media is presently unknown. Extension from otitis externa and tympanic membrane rupture is very unlikely.[21] Hematogenous spread of bacteria to the inner ear and ascending infection from the eustachian tube are both highly suspected.[4, 11, 15, 21] Acute vestibular disease as the result of extension of an aspergillosis guttural pouch infection to the stylohyoid and petrous temporal bone has been documented.[22] However, otitis media is rarely associated with concurrent guttural pouch infection. In addition, microorganisms isolated from the guttural pouch did not correlate to microorganisms obtained from the middle ear of normal horses.[1, 18] Pathogenic organisms isolated from the middle ear of horses include *Actinobacillus, Salmonella, Enterobacter, Pseudomonas, Streptococcus, Staphylococcus,* and *Aspergillus.*[1, 18]

Radiographic examination of the skull is necessary for establishing the diagnosis of osteitis. Dorsoventral radiographs are most valuable in identifying the characteristic periosteal proliferation and sclerosis of the stylohyoid bone and petrous temporal bone[4, 11, 18] (Fig. 9–27). The fracture line is difficult to identify owing to minimal displacement of the fracture fragments, and lateral oblique radiographs at varying angles may aid in localization of a petrous temporal bone fracture. Several acute-onset cases of otitis media did not initially demonstrate characteristic radiographic evidence of disease. Moderate bony proliferation may not occur for several weeks and must be present to diagnose the condition radiographically.[18] Bone scintigraphy is a noninvasive technique that may allow for an immediate identification of early lesions of the petrous temporal bone. Radiography can only identify structural abnormalities of bone. Bone scintigraphy is capable of detecting dynamic characteristics of bone. Increased metabolic activity and blood supply to the bone, due to infection or fracture, will result in increased uptake of the radiolabeled compound (technetium 99m–labeled phosphate) prior to radiographic evidence of bony proliferation.[23–25]

Otoscopy is difficult in the horse owing to the long, bony, narrow, horizontal ear canal. The accumulation of ceruminous debris also impedes visualization.[12, 18] Anesthesia

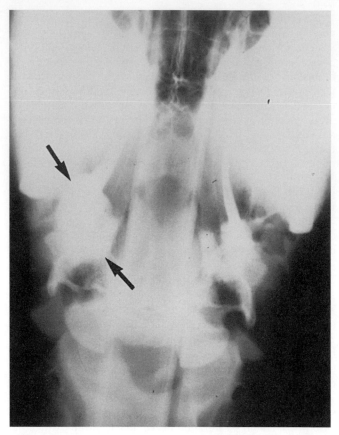

Figure 9–27. Ventrodorsal skull radiograph demonstrating bony proliferation of the proximal left stylohyoid and petrous temporal bones *(arrows)* secondary to chronic otitis interna-media.

allows for complete cleaning of the external auditory canal and is likely to be necessary for a thorough otoscopic examination given the uncooperative nature of the awake horse. Even with a thorough examination, it is difficult to detect subtle changes of the tympanic membrane. Transtympanic lavage may aid in the diagnosis of otitis media. Sterile saline (0.5 mL) is infused via a myringotomy with immediate withdrawal of fluid. A cloudy or yellow tap is a positive finding. Fluid is submitted for cytology, protein evaluation, and culture. Anaerobic and aerobic culture and sensitivity may allow for identification of the pathogenic organism and aid in appropriate antibiotic selection.[18]

Cerebrospinal fluid analysis should be performed in all cases of acute vestibular disease.[1, 2] In the case of otitis media, cerebrospinal fluid analysis, culture, and sensitivity will help to reveal the presence of secondary bacterial meningitis, identify the causative organism, and direct the selection of an appropriate antibiotic.[15]

Endoscopy of the pharynx and guttural pouch is generally diagnostic in horses with proliferative osteitis of the stylohyoid bone. This noninvasive procedure should be performed on every suspected case, because bony proliferation of the proximal stylohyoid bone can often be identified within the guttural pouch[1, 22] (Fig. 9–28).

Treatment should include long-term administration (30 days) of broad-spectrum antibiotics. Potentiated sulfa, ampi-

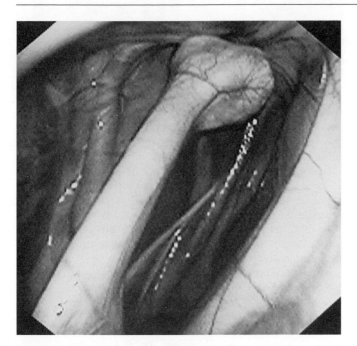

Figure 9–28. Endoscopic view of the right guttural pouch of a horse with acute onset of right-sided vestibular disease and facial nerve paralysis. Bony proliferation of the proximal stylohyoid bone is consistent with chronic osteitis due to otitis interna-media.

cillin 2 mg/kg IM b.i.d. or t.i.d., and chloramphenicol 15–25 mg/kg PO q.i.d. have been recommended when culture and sensitivity cannot be obtained.[11, 15] Phenylbutazone 2 to 4 mg/kg PO b.i.d. will help alleviate inflammation.[1] If central nervous system involvement is identified, dimethyl sulfoxide 1 g/kg IV in 10% solution is recommended to reduce brain inflammation and edema.[1] Corticosteroid therapy should be avoided if an infectious process is suspected. Intensive supportive care and topical therapy for corneal ulceration may also be necessary.

Diagnosis prior to acute neurologic signs is difficult because most horses may exhibit no clinical signs. Some horses may demonstrate early signs of otitis media, including ear-rubbing, head-tossing, chomping movements, and ear sensitivity prior to the onset of neurologic signs. Affected horses may exhibit signs of pain on palpation at the base of the ear. Head-tossing is a common problem in the horse, with multiple causes; the primary problem is rarely identified.[18] Ventrodorsal radiographs of the skull and endoscopy of the guttural pouches should be performed on the headshaking horse to identify an early case of otitis media. Surgical removal of a 2-cm segment of the stylohyoid bone has been attempted on several headshaking horses with bony proliferation of the petrous temporal bone, in an attempt to prevent secondary stress fracture and neurologic signs. A fibrous non-union of the stylohyoid bone should interrupt the transmission of hyoid forces to the temporohyoid joint. Long-term success of the surgery has not yet been established.[18]

Head Trauma

Traumatic fractures of the petrous temporal bone result in damage to the vestibular and facial nerves. Profuse aural hemorrhage or loss of cerebrospinal fluid from the external ear canal is frequently observed. Bleeding from the nose occurs if the fracture extends to the cribriform plate.[4] Clinical signs usually appear immediately following trauma and include vestibular disease, facial nerve paralysis, recumbency, or coma. Damage to nervous tissue may be caused by hematoma, callus formation, or displacement of fracture fragments resulting in delayed onset of clinical signs. Signs from brainstem contusion or concussion may be more severe than vestibular dysfunction. If blindness is present, the prognosis worsens due to the loss of visual compensation of vestibular disease in the future. If the oculocephalic reflex (physiologic nystagmus) cannot be elicited, damage to the medial longitudinal fasciculus is suspected, indicating extensive brainstem damage; a poor prognosis is indicated.[2] Recall that bilateral peripheral vestibular disease will also result in loss of the oculocephalic reflex; this, however, is an unlikely scenario for trauma.

Fractures of the basioccipital and basisphenoid bones occur most frequently in horses that rear over backward and hit on the poll of the head. This fracture is not the result of referred impact from the poll. It is thought to be an avulsion fracture from the pull of the powerful ventral straight muscle of the neck (rectus capitis ventralis) on its insertion on the basioccipital bone.[26] Basioccipital fractures result in neurologic signs associated with damage to the brainstem; signs of vestibular disease are common.

Petrous temporal bone fractures are difficult to identify radiographically; tympanosclerosis appears as early as 20 days post trauma and will obscure the fracture line.[4] Basioccipital fractures are often easily identified, but can be confused for the suture lines in the base of the skull.[26]

Treatment of vestibular signs secondary to head trauma is similar to that of otitis media. Anti-inflammatory drugs such as phenylbutazone and dimethyl sulfoxide are indicated to reduce swelling and edema. Broad-spectrum antibiotics are required to prevent secondary bacterial infection. Dexamethasone 0.1 to 0.2 mg/kg IM q.4–6h. for 1 to 4 days should be administered if brain concussion or contusion is suspected.[1] Acepromazine maleate will lower the seizure threshold and is contraindicated in cases of head trauma.[27] Xylazine may potentiate an active bleeding process due to transient hypertension and should be avoided in the early period following head trauma.[28]

Drug toxicities can result in unilateral or bilateral peripheral vestibular disease and deafness. Degeneration of the hair cells within the peripheral receptor organs of the auditory and vestibular system occurs with prolonged administration of aminoglycoside antibiotics. Severely affected animals also develop neural degeneration.[3] A more common manifestation of aminoglycoside toxicity is renal failure. As renal clearance of the aminoglycoside decreases, the ototoxic effects of the antibiotics are potentiated.[1, 10, 21] Clinical signs of vestibular disease appear prior to deafness. Early vestibular disease may be reversible or centrally compensated, but loss of auditory function is permanent.[2, 10, 21] Streptomycin preferentially affects the vestibular system, whereas dihydrostreptomycin, kanamycin, gentamicin, neomycin, and vancomycin are more toxic to the auditory system.[2, 15] Vincristine, a vinca alkaloid, can cause bilateral cochlear nerve damage in humans. Auditory function improves several months after discontinuation of the drug.[3] This antimitotic drug is a common component of multiagent chemotherapy protocols in the treatment of lymphosarcoma in the horse.[29] Vincristine is also used for immunosuppression and stimulation of platelet function in refractory cases of immune-mediated thrombocytopenia.[30] Auditory function should be carefully monitored when this drug is employed.

Sudden loud noises can result in degeneration and necrosis of the sensory hair cells of the inner ear.[21] A lightning strike, although usually fatal, is reported to cause acute onset of unilateral vestibular disease in the horse. Facial nerve paralysis may or may not accompany the vestibular signs. Documentation of histopathologic findings in one case revealed hemorrhage and necrosis of the temporal bone, vestibular nerve, and adjacent tissue. Whether the mechanism of damage is electrocution or noise trauma is unknown.[31]

CENTRAL VESTIBULAR DISEASE

The vestibular nuclei and related tracts may be damaged by any inflammatory disease or space-occupying mass of the central nervous system. Clinical signs vary with the type and extent of the disease process. A central nervous system disease should be suspected if abnormal mentation, seizures, blindness, or multiple cranial nerve abnormalities with general proprioceptive deficits are present. An electroencephalogram (EEG) should be performed to detect the location and extent of the central nervous system lesion. The EEG can detect only cerebral damage and cannot identify lesions of the brainstem. Inflammatory, parasitic, and neoplastic diseases have been implicated in central vestibular disease of the horse.

Inflammatory disease affecting the central nervous system includes bacterial abscess, equine protozoal myelitis, polyneuritis equi, and viral encephalitis. Cerebrospinal fluid analysis should be performed to identify the inflammatory process. In the case of brain abscessation, a culture of the cerebrospinal fluid may identify the causative organism; *Streptococcus equi* is a common causative agent.[32, 33] Equine protozoal myeloencephalitis is a common neurologic disease in the United States and Canada and should be suspected if multifocal disease is present.[1] It is not uncommon for polyneuritis equi to present with vestibular dysfunction, but the signs of cauda equina neuritis will predominate.[2] Rabies may present as either an encephalitis or spinal cord disease and should be considered in the differential diagnosis of any horse with neurologic disease. Spinal ataxia is the primary neurologic deficit observed in horses affected with equine herpesvirus myelitis, but the presence of concurrent vestibular disease is reported.[34] The major clinical signs observed with a togavirus (eastern, western, and Venezuelan equine encephalitis) infection are depression and seizure, although cranial nerve deficits are observed.[6, 33]

Aberrant parasite migration of the central nervous system in horses results in acute onset of neurologic signs. Clinical signs vary, but progression of clinical signs occurs in most instances. Neurologic signs are generally asymmetric owing to the random nature of migration. The parasites most frequently identified are *Hypoderma, Habronema, Strongylus,* and *Setaria* species. *Strongylus vulgaris* is most common and may also produce parasitic thromboembolism to the brain.[31, 33] Migration of *Micronema deletrix* and *Setaria* may produce severe, diffuse brain and spinal cord disease.[35] Cerebrospinal fluid analysis may reveal eosinophilic or neutrophilic leukocytosis with evidence of hemorrhage. *Micronema* may be identified in the cerebrospinal fluid and urine.[31] Treatment includes anti-inflammatory (flunixin meglumine, phenylbutazone, dexamethasone) and antiparasitic drugs (ivermectin 200 mg/kg; fenbendazole 50 mg/kg/day for 1 to 3 days; thiabendazole 440 mg/kg s.i.d. for 2 days). Recovery may be dramatic.[31] Fungal granulomas caused by *Aspergillus* and *Cryptococcus neoformans* have been reported as space-occupying masses within the cranium of a horse.[31, 36] Cholesteatoma (cholesterol granuloma) could involve the vestibular system by extending from the choroid plexus of the fourth ventricle of the brain.[1] Neoplastic diseases of the central nervous system are rare in the horse. Any tumor affecting the cerebellomedullary angle could result in vestibular signs.[2] Lymphosarcoma, ependymoma, meningeal melanoma, and melanotic hamartoma have been reported to affect the central nervous system of the horse.[2, 37]

ANCILLARY DIAGNOSTIC TESTS
Caloric Testing

The caloric test is a diagnostic aid that may be helpful in differentiation of central from peripheral vestibular disease. The test is able to assess each peripheral vestibular sensory organ separately. In the normal animal, irrigation of ice-cold water (12°F) into the external auditory canal for 3 to 5 minutes will induce a horizontal nystagmus with the fast phase away from the tested labyrinth.[2, 3, 5, 6] Endolymph closest to the tympanic membrane is cooled, increasing its density. A density gradient is created within the semicircular canal and the cooled endolymph will sink, causing displacement of the hair cells. Warm water (45°F) irrigation of the external auditory canal results in horizontal nystagmus with a fast phase toward the tested labyrinth. The warm water test is less reliable.[10, 16] In a nonfunctional labyrinth, no nystagmus is induced. Animals may resist the procedure, making the test difficult to interpret, and in some animals, no nystagmus can be induced. If an asymmetric response is obtained, the depressed reaction indicates the abnormal labyrinth.[2] The test is difficult to perform and not entirely reliable, although it may be a helpful diagnostic aid in the anesthetized or comatose horse.[6]

Brainstem Auditory Evoked Response

The cochlea will be damaged by trauma or inflammation of the peripheral vestibular receptor organs and detection of hearing loss may help to differentiate central from peripheral vestibular disease. Unilateral hearing loss is difficult to assess subjectively in the horse. Brainstem auditory evoked response (BAER) is a method of objective assessment of auditory function in the horse. This noninvasive, electrodiagnostic test stimulates the auditory system with a series of clicks. Far-field potentials of the brainstem auditory components are recorded via cutaneous electrodes and a signal averaging system.[6, 38] The response is a series of evoked potentials occurring within 10 ms after the stimulus. In the horse, the evoked potentials appear on the oscilloscope as a series of five waveforms.[39] In humans, five to seven waveforms are present and each corresponds to a specific neurologic structure.[38, 39] Abnormalities of the specific waveforms can identify a lesion of the corresponding neurologic structure. In the horse, functional loss of the cochlea or eighth cranial nerve results in the loss of the entire waveform on the side of injury and the presence or absence of the waveform can differentiate a central from a peripheral vestibular lesion.[38] The test is reliable with sedation and general anesthesia. General anesthesia is not necessary to perform the test, but sedation is recommended.[38]

REFERENCES

1. Mayhew IG: *Large Animal Neurology: A Handbook for Veterinary Clinicians.* Philadelphia, Lea & Febiger, 1989, p 179.
2. deLahunta A: Vestibular system—special proprioception. In deLahunta A, ed: *Veterinary Neuroanatomy and Clinical Neurology.* Philadelphia, WB Saunders, 1983, p 238.
3. Luxon L: Diseases of the eighth cranial nerve. In Dyke P, Thomas P, Lambert E, eds: *Peripheral Neuropathy.* Philadelphia, WB Saunders, 1975, p 1301.
4. Firth E: Vestibular disease and its relationship to facial paralysis in the horse: A clinical study of 7 cases. *Aust Vet J* 53:560, 1977.
5. Guyton A: Motor functions of the brainstem and basal ganglia—reticular formation, vestibular apparatus, equilibrium and brainstem reflexes. In Guyton A, ed: *Organ Physiology: Structure and Function of the Nervous System.* Philadelphia, WB Saunders, 1976, pp 140–155.
6. Watrous B: Head tilt in horses. *Vet Clin North Am Equine Pract* 3:353, 1987.
7. Ganong W: Control of posture and movement. In Ganong W, ed: *The Nervous System.* Los Altos, Calif, Lange, 1979, p 135.
8. Kuffler S, Nicholls J, Martin A: Integrative mechanisms in the cns for the control of movement. In Kuffler S, Nicholls J, Martin A, eds: *From Neuron to Brain.* Sunderland, Mass, Sinauer Associates, 1984, p 446.
9. Breazile JE: Regulation of motor activity. In Swenson MJ, Reece WO, eds: *Duke's Physiology of Domestic Animals,* ed 11. Ithaca, NY, Comstock, 1993, p 836.
10. Chrisman C: Disorders of the vestibular system. *Compend Contin Educ Pract Vet* 1:744, 1979.
11. Power H, Watrous B, deLahunta A: Facial and vestibulocochlear nerve disease in six horses. *J Am Vet Med Assoc* 183:1076, 1983.
12. Geiser D, Henton J, Held J: Tympanic bulla, petrous temporal bone, and hyoid apparatus disease in horses. *Compend Contin Educ Pract Vet* 10:740, 1988.
13. Palmer A: Pathogenesis and pathology of the cerebello-vestibular syndrome. *J Small Anim Pract* 11:167, 1970.
14. Greene C, Oliver J: Neurologic examination. In Ettinger S, ed: *Textbook of Veterinary Internal Medicine.* Philadelphia, WB Saunders, 1983, p 419.
15. Blythe L, Watrous B, Schmitz J, et al: Vestibular syndrome associated with temporohyoid joint fusion and temporal bone fracture in three horses. *J Am Vet Med Assoc* 185:775, 1984.
16. Palmer A: Nystagmus and its focal causes. In Palmer A, ed: *Introduction to Animal Neurology.* Oxford, Blackwell, 1976, p 59.
17. Raphel C: Brain abscess in three horses. *J Am Vet Med Assoc* 180:874, 1982.
18. Blythe L: Otitis media and interna in the horse: Its relationship to head tossing and skull fractures. In Pidgeon G (ed): *Proceedings of the Seventh American College of Veterinary Internal Medicine Forum.* Madison, WI, OmniPress, 1989, p 1015.
19. Montgomery T: Otitis media in a thoroughbred. *Vet Med Small Anim Clin* 76:722, 1981.
20. Jensen R, Pierson R, Weibel J: Middle ear infection in feedlot lambs. *J Am Vet Med Assoc* 181:805, 1982.
21. Jubb K, Kennedy P, Palmer N: The ear. In Jubb K, Kennedy P, Palmer N, eds: *Pathology of Domestic Animals.* Orlando, Fla, Academic Press, 1985, p 393.
22. Cook W: Disease of the ear, nose and throat of the horse. Part 1: The ear. In Grunsell O, ed: *The Veterinary Annual.* Bristol, England, John Wright & Sons, 1971, p 12.
23. Ueltschi G: Bone and joint imaging with 99m Tc labelled phosphates as a new diagnostic aid in veterinary orthopedics. *J Am Vet Radiol Soc* 18:80, 1977.
24. Lamb C, Koblik P: Scintigraphic evaluation of skeletal disease and its application to the horse. *Vet Radiol* 29:16, 1988.
25. Devous M, Twardock R: Techniques and applications of nuclear medicine in the diagnosis of equine lameness. *J Am Vet Med Assoc* 3:318, 1984.
26. Cook W: Skeletal radiology of the equine head. *J Am Vet Radiol Soc* 11:35, 1970.
27. Clement S: Convulsive and allied syndromes of the neonatal foal. *Vet Clin North Am Equine Pract* 3:333, 1987.
28. Booth N: Non-narcotic analgesics. In Booth N, McDonald LE, eds: *Veterinary Pharmacology and Therapeutics.* Ames, Iowa State University Press, 1982, p 311.
29. Couto, G. Personal communication, 1992.
30. Morris D: Immune-mediated thrombocytopenia. In Robinson E, ed: *Current Therapy in Equine Medicine.* Philadelphia, WB Saunders, 1987, p 310.
31. Mayhew IG: *Large Animal Neurology: A Handbook for Veterinary Clinicians.* Philadelphia, Lea & Febiger, 1989, p 90.
32. Ford J, Lokai M: Complications of *Streptococcus equi* infections. *Equine Pract* 2:41, 1980.
33. Mittel L: Seizures in the horse. *Vet Clin North Am Equine Pract* 3:323, 1987.
34. Kohn CW: Equine herpes myeloencephalitis. *Vet Clin North Am Equine Pract* 3:405, 1987.
35. Jubb K, Kennedy P, Palmer N: Parasitic infestations. In Jubb K, Kennedy P, Palmer N, eds: *Pathology of Domestic Animals.* Orlando, Fla, Academic Press, 1985, p 311.
36. Teuscher E, Vrins A, Lemaire T: A vestibular syndrome associated with *Cryptococcus neoformans* in a horse. *Zentralbl Veterinarmed* [A] 31:132, 1984.
37. Mair T, Pearson G: Melanotic hamartoma of the hind brain in a riding horse. *J Comp Pathol* 102:239, 1990.
38. Marshall A, Byars T, Whitlock R, et al: Brainstem auditory evoked response in the diagnosis of inner ear injury in the horse. *J Am Vet Med Assoc* 178:282, 1981.
39. Rolf S, Reed S, Melnick W, et al: Auditory brainstem response testing in anesthetized horses. *Am J Vet Res* 48:910, 1987.

9.7

Diseases of the Cerebellum

Barbara A. Byrne, DVM

Cerebellar abnormalities have been reported in horses and are primarily confined to a small number of breeds. The cerebellum is essential for the coordination of movement.

Afferent information arises from the general and special (vestibular) proprioceptive systems and the special somatic (auditory and visual) systems. It is responsible for the regulation of the rate, range, and strength of movement, as well as integration and coordination for balance and posture. Cerebellar abnormalities in horses are unusual; however, when present, they can have a profound impact on gait and posture.

STRUCTURE AND FUNCTION

Knowledge of the structure and development of the cerebellum is important for understanding cerebellar function in health and disease. The cerebellum is located in the metencephalon dorsal to the pons. It is attached to the pons via three cerebellar peduncles[1] (Fig. 9–29). The caudal peduncle is composed primarily of afferent fibers arising from the medulla, the vestibular nuclei via the vestibulocerebellar tracts, and the spinal cord via the spinocerebellar tracts. The middle cerebellar peduncle contains only afferent fibers to the cerebellum which arise from the transverse fibers of the pons. The rostral cerebellar peduncle is the primary connection to the mesencephalon and carries the majority of cerebellar efferent fibers, although a few afferent fibers arise from the spinocerebellar tracts. The cerebellum consists of two hemispheres and a central region known as the vermis.[1] The extensive convolutions of the cerebellar cortex are termed *folia*. The cortex covers the surface of the cerebellum. On cut section, the cerebellar medulla is identified as a central region of white matter with multiple projections, called arbor vitae. These branches extend to the cerebellar cortex and form the white matter portion adjacent to the cerebellar cortex.

There are three nuclei in the cerebellar medulla: the fastigial, interpositional and lateral nuclei from medial to lateral on each side of the cerebellum. The cerebellum can also be divided into three bilateral longitudinal regions in association with these nuclei.[1, 2] The medial zone, containing the vermis and the fastigial nucleus, primarily regulates the tone, posture, and equilibrium of the body in general. The intermediate zones contain the interpositional nucleus and cortex adjacent to the vermis and adjust the orientation of limbs in space, maintaining balance, posture, and muscle tone during complex movements. The lateral zones, consisting of the lateral nuclei and lateral portions of the cerebral hemispheres, have a similar function, but do not influence posture or muscle tone directly.[2]

The cerebellum arises from the alar plate region of the metencephalon. It originates initially as a proliferation of cells in the rhombic lip which extend dorsally and medially to form the dorsal portion of the metencephalon.[1] Germinal cells proliferating in the rhombic lip eventually migrate into the cerebellum and differentiate to form the specialized neurons of the cerebellar cortex. There are three layers of the cerebellar cortex: the outer molecular, the middle Purkinje, and the inner granular (Fig. 9–30). The molecular layer is relatively acellular and consists primarily of the dendritic zones of the Purkinje cells and axons of the granular cells.[1] The Purkinje layer is only one cell thick and consists of Purkinje neurons. The granular layer is densely cellular with granular neurons. It is important for normal function that all layers be present and aligned in proper orientation.

Organization of the specialized structure of the cerebellar cortex allows integration and coordination of movement. The cerebellum primarily provides regulation of skeletal movement, allowing coordinated movement; it does not initiate muscular activity. Afferent information regarding movement and balance arising from the mesencephalon, the brainstem, and the spinal cord enters the cerebellum via the cerebellar peduncles and regulation of movement is coordinated by the inhibitory influence of Purkinje neurons on the cerebellar nuclei. Information enters the cerebellum via the cerebellar peduncles and is carried on two major afferents termed *mossy fibers* and *climbing fibers*.[1] Mossy fibers originate from the brainstem and spinal cord. They send collateral fibers to synapse with the cerebellar nuclei; they terminate by synapsing with granule neurons in the cerebellar cortex. These fibers are facilitory at these synapses. The axons that granule neurons send to the molecular layer course transversely through this layer to synapse with the dendritic zone of multiple Purkinje cells and also provide facilitory influence at these synapses. Climbing fibers originate in the olivary nucleus which provides most of the extrapyramidal projections to the cerebellum. Similar to mossy fibers, climbing fibers send collaterals to synapse on neurons in the cerebellar nuclei; however, the axon continues through the cerebellar cortex to synapse with the dendritic zone of the Purkinje neurons in the molecular layer. As with mossy fibers, climbing fibers provide a facilitative influence at the synapses.

Purkinje neurons provide the sole efferent fibers from the cerebellar cortex.[1] The majority of Purkinje cell axons terminate on neurons in the cerebellar nuclei, although there are direct projections from these neurons to the vestibular

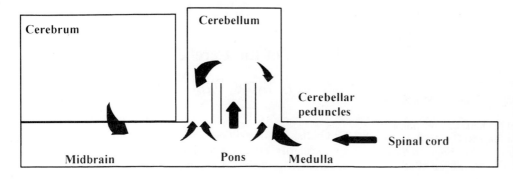

Figure 9–29. Schematic diagram of cerebellar efferent and afferent information pathways via the cerebellar peduncles. The arrow size reflects the relative contribution of each pathway. See text for details.

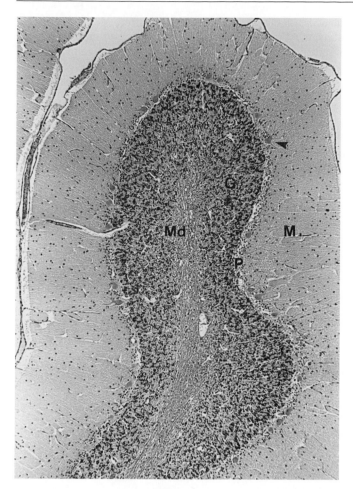

Figure 9–30. Photomicrograph of a normal cerebellum. *M,* molecular layer; *P,* Purkinje layer; *G,* granular layer; *Md,* medulla. The *arrowhead* indicates a Purkinje neuron. ×55, hematoxylin-eosin. (Courtesy of the Washington Animal Disease Diagnostic Laboratory, Pullman, WA.)

nuclei via the caudal cerebellar peduncle. Purkinje neurons are inhibitory and utilize the neurotransmitter γ-aminobutyric acid.[1] Efferents from the cerebellum are primarily from the cerebellar nuclei which facilitate activity of upper motor neurons originating in the brainstem.

Thus, much of the influence of the cerebellum on skeletal muscle activity is to modulate the upper motor neuron. Information regarding movement and balance enters the cerebellar cortex via the cerebellar peduncles. This afferent activity stimulates inhibitory Purkinje neurons by climbing or mossy fibers. Purkinje neurons in turn modulate the activity of the cerebellar nuclei in order to regulate movement and muscular tone. Purkinje neurons also provide direct inhibitory input to the vestibular nuclei.

CLINICAL SIGNS

Clinical signs associated with cerebellar disease generally reflect the loss of coordination. Mentation is normal in horses with cerebellar disease provided that other regions of the brain are unaffected and metabolic disturbances such as

septicemia or endotoxemia are not present. Cerebellar disturbances result in ataxia and inability to regulate the rate, range, and force of movement.[1] Dysmetria refers to alterations in the range of gait. Hypermetria is an exaggerated range of movement. When moving, the limb will have a higher or longer flight when compared to normal. Hypometria is a diminished movement; for example, the arc of flight of a limb in motion may be lower. Horses showing hypometria tend to hit objects with the limb when stepping over them and may fail to extend the limb far enough to set the foot down on a step. Initiation of movement may be jerky and awkward and the trunk may sway from side to side when the horse moves. Spasticity is caused by hypertonia and results in a jerky stiff gait. Paresis is not a feature of cerebellar disease since the cerebellum does not initiate voluntary motion, although a horse that is unable to regulate rate and range of motion may sometimes appear weak and drag its toes. Diffuse cerebellar disease results in bilateral signs. In general, unilateral lesions result in signs ipsilateral to the lesion.

Intention tremor is another prominent sign of diffuse severe cerebellar disease. Tremor is most obvious as vertical or horizontal head motions and can be readily observed as a horse approaches feed or attempts to nurse. The tremor is present only when a movement is initiated and tends to become more exaggerated as the horse approaches an object.

Cerebellar disease may also cause loss of the blink reflex and vestibular abnormalities. The horse may fail to blink in response to an ocular menace. The exact mechanism for this deficiency is unknown; however, it is likely that a portion of the visual pathway from the visual cortex to the facial nucleus (which initiates the blink) travels through the cerebellum.[1] Disruption of the flocculonodular lobe, located in the ventral cerebellum, or the fastigial nucleus may result in vestibular signs characterized by disequilibrium, a variable nystagmus, which may be positional, and positioning difficulties.[1] Unilateral lesions may result in a head and body tilt toward the side of the lesion and nystagmus with the fast phase away from the lesion. Paradoxical vestibular syndrome characterized by a head tilt away from the lesion and nystagmus with the fast phase toward the lesion can be seen with unilateral lesions involving the cerebellar peduncle.[1, 2]

DISEASES OF THE CEREBELLUM
Cerebellar Abiotrophy and Degeneration

Cerebellar abiotrophy is the most commonly reported cerebellar disease in horses.[3–10] Abiotrophy in the nervous system refers to premature degeneration of neurons due to some intrinsic abnormality in their structure or metabolism.[11] Cerebellar abiotrophy has been reported in Arabian, Gotland pony, and Oldenburg horse breeds. Degenerative cerebellar lesions have been observed in one Thoroughbred and two Paso Fino newborn foals.[12] Arabian and part-Arabian horses are most frequently affected in North America.[3–6, 8–10] The incidence in some Arabian horse herds has been reported to be as high as 8%.[5] In one report, colts were more frequently affected than fillies, although subsequent reports have not substantiated this finding.[5] The cerebellar abiotrophy that occurs in Oldenburg horses is progressive and fatal with atypical histologic lesions compared with the syndrome that occurs in Arabian foals.[13]

Cerebellar abiotrophy generally affects foals less than 1 year of age and occurs most frequently in 1- to 6-month-old foals. Adult-onset cerebellar abiotrophy has been reported in other species such as the dog and has been observed in two equine cases.[1] Many foals are born with no abnormalities and later develop disease; however, occasionally they are affected at or shortly following birth.[5, 6, 9]

Clinical signs associated with cerebellar abiotrophy include intentional head tremor, ataxia, wide-based stance and gait, dysmetria, and spasticity.[3-10] The most frequently reported initial signs noted by owners are an intentional head tremor, either vertical or horizontal, or a very hypermetric forelimb gait.[3, 9] The neurologic examination reveals that there is no change in mentation. Nystagmus is almost never observed and has been reported in only one case of abiotrophy in a Gotland pony.[7] A menace reflex is frequently absent or diminished.[6, 9] This finding must be interpreted with caution as normal foals may lack or have a depressed menace reflex until at least 2 weeks of age.[14]

Stance and gait abnormalities seen with cerebellar abiotrophy generally consist of a wide-based stance or gait and ataxia.[6, 8, 9] The foal may move stiffly and have a high "goose-stepping" gait. There may be protraction of the limb when walking, resulting in slamming the foot to the ground. Movement may be spastic and circumduction may be observed. Gait abnormalities are exacerbated by walking on an incline, when the foal is asked to step over obstacles, or when blindfolded. Generally, gait abnormalities are symmetric although in a Welsh cob–Arabian cross foal the initial signs were characterized by a stiff motion in the left front limb. Signs in this foal progressed to severe ataxia.[4] Foals affected at birth may have difficulty rising.[5-7] Despite this finding, weakness is not a feature of the clinical signs associated with cerebellar abiotrophy. Spinal reflexes are usually normal. Some affected animals will fall when startled or when the head is raised. Signs are generally progressive for several months following diagnosis. Once the animal has reached maturity the condition becomes static, although mild improvement has been observed.[10]

Ancillary testing is of limited value in diagnosing cerebellar abiotrophy; however, it can be helpful to rule out other causes of ataxia. The complete blood count and serum biochemistry profile are normal in affected foals. Abnormalities in cerebrospinal fluid (CSF) can be detected. In one study, three of four foals had an elevated CSF creatine kinase activity.[9] Values in affected foals ranged from 6.6 to 62 IU/μL (normal range, 0–8 IU/μL).[9] CSF creatine kinase elevations are generally associated with neural necrosis or degeneration, although they are not specifically associated with a particular disease.[15-17]

In addition, CSF total protein may be elevated. In the study cited above, three foals had elevated total protein with an average of 226 mg/dL (normal, 0–100 mg/dL) in all foals with cerebellar abiotrophy.[9] As with creatine kinase, total protein elevations are not specific for abiotrophy and may occur with disruption of the blood-brain barrier or with central nervous system inflammation or degeneration. Many foals with cerebellar abiotrophy will have normal CSF analysis. Electroencephalographic abnormalities, including increased synchrony and increased number of abrupt frequency

changes, may also be detected in affected foals.[9] In this study, these abnormalities were not observed in normal foals anesthetized under similar conditions. Skull and cervical radiographs are unremarkable. However, since mentation is normal in foals with cerebellar abiotrophy, electroencephalographic examination is not necessary to make a diagnosis and is primarily useful to exclude seizure disorders as a cause of the tremors observed.

Antemortem diagnosis of cerebellar abiotrophy is made on the basis of a typical history and the clinical signs of intention tremor, lack of menace, and failure to blink to bright light, and ataxia in Arabian or part-Arabian foals or Gotland pony foals. The differential diagnoses for cerebellar abiotrophy include cranial malformations; congenital spinal malformations, including atlanto-axial malformations and stenotic myelopathy; inflammation or infection of the cerebellum; and trauma. These conditions can be ruled out on the basis of the neurologic examination, CSF analysis, and radiography. The signs of characteristic ataxia and head tremor without weakness in the appropriate breed is nearly pathognomonic.

Postmortem examination provides a definitive diagnosis of this disorder. Generally, there are no gross abnormalities noted; however, careful examination of the cerebellum may reveal an increased lobular pattern with prominent folia. In the Gotland pony, the weight ratio of the cerebellum to the cerebrum is significantly reduced in foals with cerebellar abiotrophy.[7] Normal foals had a ratio of 13% and affected foals had a 10% ratio. In the degenerative cerebellar condition seen in the Paso Fino and Thoroughbred foals, there was a decrease in the cerebellar-to-whole brain weight ratio.[12] This ratio in normal foals was 8%, and was 6% in affected foals.

Histologic abnormalities are consistent in cases of cerebellar abiotrophy. The most prominent finding is the widespread loss of Purkinje neurons[3-10] (Fig. 9–31). Degenerative changes, such as shrunken and angular neurons with hyperchromasia and dispersion of Nissl substance, can be seen. Occasional "baskets" or clear spaces where the Purkinje

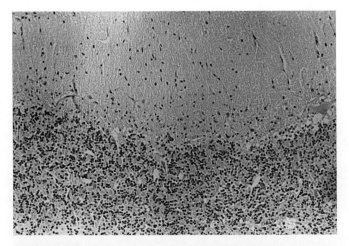

Figure 9–31. Photomicrograph of the cerebellum from a 9-month-old foal with cerebellar abiotrophy. Note the decreased number of Purkinje neurons. ×139, hematoxylin-eosin. (Courtesy of the Washington Animal Disease Diagnostic Laboratory, Pullman, WA.)

neuron is lost may be observed. There is thinning of the molecular layer with gliosis. The granular layer is also thin with a loss of cellularity. Similar histologic findings were found in Thoroughbred and Paso Fino foals with vacuolation and proliferation of Bergmann's glia in the Purkinje cell layer.[12]

The pathogenesis of cerebellar abiotrophy is unknown. Viral, toxic, and genetic causes have been suggested.[3, 5, 6, 9] To date there has been no evidence to support an infectious cause. No virus has been isolated from the CSF or brain of affected foals and no viral inclusions have been observed on histologic examination. No toxin has been consistently associated with cerebellar abiotrophy of Arabian foals. A genetic cause may be present. Pedigree analysis of affected Arabian foals has shown a high degree of inbreeding of affected foals, although this breed is generally inbred.[5] Interestingly, in this study three of six foals from one mare suffered from cerebellar ataxia; all affected foals had different sires. A similar pedigree analysis was performed in the Gotland pony in which an autosomal recessive mode of inheritance was suggested.[7] Similar to Arabian foals, a high degree of inbreeding was noted, making a highly significant conclusion difficult. Attempts to breed affected individuals in this study were unsuccessful. Although a definitive mode of inheritance has not been demonstrated in either breed, a familial tendency is suggested.

There is no treatment for cerebellar abiotrophy. As noted above, signs may be progressive until the foal reaches maturity. Signs may stabilize or improve slightly with time.

Gomen Disease

Gomen disease is a degenerative cerebellar condition recognized in the northwest part of New Caledonia.[18] It is a progressive cerebellar disease which causes mild to severe ataxia. Horses that are indigenous or introduced to the region may be affected. The disease is seen only in horses that are allowed to roam free and signs may take 1 to 2 years to develop once a horse is introduced into an endemic area. Horses that are confined generally are unaffected. Clinical signs consist of ataxia, which is most prominent in the hindlimbs; toe-dragging; and a wide-based stance. As the disease progresses, weakness becomes prominent and horses may have difficulty rising. The signs are primarily referable to involvement of the cerebellum; however, weakness is likely due to brainstem or spinal cord involvement. Nystagmus is not observed. Ataxia is progressive over 3 to 4 years until the horse dies or is euthanized.

Mild cerebellar atrophy may be apparent on gross examination of the brain. Histologically, there is severe depletion of Purkinje neurons throughout the cerebellum.[19] Purkinje neurons may contain lipofuscin pigment and vacuoles. One horse examined had moderate loss of granule cells. There is moderate-to-severe lipofuscin pigmentation of neuron cell bodies throughout the brain and spinal cord. Although lipofuscin accumulation may be considered a normal variation seen with aging, the degree of pigment accumulation is far more severe than that seen in horses of similar age.

The pathogenesis of this disease is unknown. Pedigree analysis has not revealed any genetic component for susceptibility to development of disease.[18] There is a condition of

neuronal lipofuscinosis in dogs which has some similarities to this disease.[19] The accumulation of lipofuscin pigment and association with free-ranging horses is suggestive of a metabolic disorder, perhaps resulting from toxicity.[18, 19]

Developmental Abnormalities

Dandy-Walker syndrome is characterized by a midline defect of the cerebellum and cystic dilatation of the fourth ventricle, which separates the cerebral hemispheres.[20] Frequently, all or portions of the cerebellar vermis fail to form and the corpus callosum may be absent. This is a rare condition in horses and has been observed in Thoroughbred and Arabian foals.[21, 22] Foals with this syndrome may be neurologically abnormal from birth, with difficulty rising, seizures, and absence of the suckle reflex.[21] The forehead may be excessively domed. Ataxia, nystagmus, aggression, and difficulty in training may persist as the foal ages.[21, 22] Diagnosis is generally made at postmortem examination; however, one case was diagnosed antemortem using computed tomography.[21]

Several individual cases of equine developmental cerebellar abnormalities have been described. Cerebellar hypoplasia has been described in a Thoroughbred foal which had difficulty rising and developed seizures shortly after birth.[23] This report did not describe the histologic findings of cerebellar hypoplasia in detail; thus, the relationship between this finding and cerebellar abiotrophy or degeneration seen in Arabian foals is unknown. Bilateral focal cerebellar cortical hypoplasia has been reported in a 6-year-old Thoroughbred gelding.[24] No gait abnormalities were detected in this horse, although it had fallen over repeatedly prior to euthanasia. The relationship between falling and the cerebellar abnormality is unclear. It is possible that the abnormality in this adult horse was the result of a secondary problem, such as vascular injury, rather than a developmental defect.[13]

A single case of cerebellar dysplasia has been described in a 4-year-old Thoroughbred horse.[25] This horse had a 7-month history of circling and collapsing to the left side. In this case, there was hyperplasia of the right side of the cerebellum with no associated central white matter. Histologically, there was thinning of the granule layer, increased thickness of the molecular layer, and cavitation of the white matter.

Additional reported developmental disorders include cerebellar hypoplasia with internal hydrocephalus and cerebellar aplasia with hydranencephaly in two fetuses from Haflinger mares with hydrops allantois.[26] Mild cerebellar degenerative changes consisting of Purkinje neuron granularity has been noted in a standardbred filly with a chromosomal abnormality.[27] This abnormality was accompanied by mild spongiotic degeneration of the cerebrum. Abnormal neurologic signs in this filly included difficulty standing at birth, mental dullness, and a head tilt. These signs were accompanied by growth retardation, small inactive ovaries, and a consistently wrinkled muzzle.

Infectious Conditions

Unlike the case in many other large animals, there are no infectious agents that have the cerebellum as their primary target; however, a number of agents may affect the cerebellum. Any agent that targets the central nervous system, especially those that have a multifocal distribution, may also involve the cerebellum.

Equine protozoal myelitis is a protozoal disease caused by *Sarcocystis neurona*. This agent causes multifocal inflammation and necrosis of the central nervous system. The most common signs associated with *S. neurona* infection are spinal ataxia, weakness, and muscle atrophy, although this agent can also affect the cerebellum. Clinical signs associated with cerebellar involvement may reflect diffuse or focal involvement. A head tilt or asymmetric ataxia without weakness or lower motor neuron signs may be associated with focal disease. Diagnosis can be made on the basis of multifocal neurologic disease and the presence of antibody to *S. neurona* in the CSF. Additional information regarding this disease may be found in Chapter 9.10.

Equine herpesvirus type 1 causes multifocal meningoencephalitis due to vasculitis, vascular thrombosis, and ischemia of nervous tissue. Although the primary signs associated with this agent include spinal ataxia, cranial nerve abnormalities, and signs associated with involvement of the cauda equina, this agent may also affect the cerebellum. As with equine protozoal myelitis, involvement may be focal, multifocal, or diffuse.

Occasionally, disseminated *Streptococcus equi* infection ("bastard strangles") may result in a cerebellar abscess.[28] Neurologic abnormalities in one reported case included proprioceptive deficits in the right forelimb, nystagmus, and a head tilt. Meningitis contributed to other central nervous signs such as depression, blindness, and recumbency. Diagnosis of this condition can be based on a history of previous *S. equi* infection, evidence of severe suppurative inflammation in the CSF, and culture of *S. equi* from the CSF. Treatment consists of penicillin. The prognosis is guarded; however, successful surgical drainage of a cerebral *S. equi* abscess has been reported.[29]

Focal involvement of the cerebellum has been associated with aberrant parasite migration in the horse.[4, 30] In a 6-year-old pony, infection with *Halicephalobus deletrix* resulted in severe ataxia.[30] Histologic study showed lesions scattered throughout the cerebellum, brainstem, thalamus, and pituitary gland, and nematodes were observed throughout the lesions. A second case involving a 1-year-old Thoroughbred colt had a sudden onset of severe ataxia.[4] Multifocal malacia with numerous eosinophils was observed throughout the cerebellar white matter. No nematode was detected, although parasitic involvement was suspected based on the eosinophilic inflammation.

Miscellaneous Conditions

A familial neurologic condition in newborn Thoroughbred foals has been reported.[31] A thoroughbred mare had three of five foals affected by this syndrome. The foals were normal at birth and developed signs of severe incoordination, a wide-based stance, and recumbency at 2 to 5 days of age. The condition appeared more severe when the foals became excited or struggled; consequently they were treated symptomatically with diazepam. The signs would improve with this treatment and return as the sedation wore off. These foals improved with stall rest over 7 to 10 days. The cause of the clinical signs in these foals is unknown; however, the authors suggested possible viral or toxic causes.

Cerebellar ataxia in two Thoroughbred fillies has been associated with hematoma in the fourth ventricle.[32] These two horses demonstrated fever, dysmetria, spasticity, and weakness. Clinical signs most likely resulted from compression of the adjacent cerebellum. CSF analyses in these cases revealed xanthochromia, elevated red and white blood cell counts, and elevated total protein concentrations. The cause of the hematomas was not identified; damage to regional small vessels and a vascular anomaly were suspected.

Chronic methylmercurial poisoning in horses can cause a number of clinical abnormalities, including cerebellar ataxia.[33] Severe poisoning can result in incoordination, dysmetria, and gross head-nodding in the experimental setting. Associated clinical signs include lethargy, anorexia, exudative dermatitis, and laminitis. Lesions in the cerebellum consisted of focal atrophy and cellular depletion in the granular layer with little-to-no involvement of Purkinje cells. Additional abnormalities included neuronal necrosis and gliosis in the cerebrum, lymphocytic perivascular cuffing, and swollen axons in the spinal cord. Preferential accumulation of inorganic mercury in the brain and resulting cell injury most likely led to the neurologic signs observed. Diagnosis of methylmercurial poisoning can be based on clinical signs and measurement of mercury in the liver and kidney (see Chapter 19).

REFERENCES

1. deLahunta A: *Veterinary Neuroanatomy and Clinical Neurology.* Philadelphia, WB Saunders, 1983, p 225.
2. Holliday TA: Clinical signs of acute and chronic experimental lesions of the cerebellum. *Vet Sci Commun* 3:259, 1979.
3. Dungworth DL, Fowler ME: Cerebellar hypoplasia and degeneration in a foal. *Cornell Vet* 55:17, 1966.
4. Fraser H: Two dissimilar types of cerebellar disorder in the horse. *Vet Rec* 78:608, 1966.
5. Sponseller ML: Equine cerebellar hypoplasia and degeneration. *Proc Am Assoc Equine Pract* 13:123, 1967.
6. Palmer AC, Blakemore WF, Cook WR, et al: Cerebellar hypoplasia and degeneration in the young Arab horse: Clinical and neuropathological features. *Vet Rec* 93:62, 1973.
7. Bjork G, Everz KE, Hansen HJ, et al: Congenital cerebellar ataxia in the Gotland pony breed. *Zentralbl Veterinarmed [A]* 20:341, 1973.
8. Baird JD, MacKenzie CD: Cerebellar hypoplasia and degeneration in part-Arab horses. *Aust Vet J* 50:25–28, 1974.
9. Turner-Beatty MT, Leipold HW, Cash W, et al: Cerebellar disease in Arabian horses. *Proc Am Assoc Equine Pract* 31:241, 1985.
10. DeBowes RM, Leipold HW, Turner-Beatty M: Cerebellar abiotrophy. *Vet Clin North Am Equine Pract* 3:345, 1987.
11. deLahunta A: Abiotrophy in domestic animals: A review. *Can J Vet Res* 54:65, 1990.
12. Mayhew IG: Neurological and neuropathological observations on the equine neonate *Equine Vet J* (suppl)5:28, 1988.
13. Innes JRM, Saunders LZ: *Comparative Neuropathology.* New York, Academic Press, 1962, p 303.
14. Adams R, Mayhew IG: Neurological examination of newborn foals. *Equine Vet J* 16:306, 1984.
15. Sherwin AL, Norris JW, Bulcke JA: Spinal fluid creatine kinase in neurologic disease. *Neurology* 19:993, 1969.

16. Furr MO, Tyler RD: Cerebrospinal fluid creatine kinase activity in horses with central nervous system disease: 69 cases (1984–1989). *J Am Vet Med Assoc* 197:245, 1990.
17. Culebras-Fernandez A, Richards NG: Glutamic oxaloacetic transaminase, lactic dehydrogenase, and creatine phosphokinase content in cerebrospinal fluid. *Clev Clin Q* 38:113, 1971.
18. LeGonidec G, Kuberski T, Daynes P, et al: A neurologic disease of horses in New Caledonia. *Aust Vet J* 57:194, 1981.
19. Hartley WJ, Kuberski T, LeGonidec G, et al: The pathology of Gomen disease: A cerebellar disorder of horses in New Caledonia. *Vet Pathol* 19:399, 1982.
20. Jubb KVF, Kennedy P, Palmer N: *Pathology of Domestic Animals.* San Diego, Academic Press, 1993, p 275.
21. Cudd TA, Mayhew IG, Cottrill CM: Agenesis of the corpus callosum with cerebellar vermian hypoplasia in a foal resembling the Dandy-Walker syndrome: Pre-mortem diagnosis by clinical evaluation and CT scanning. *Equine Vet J* 21:378, 1989.
22. Oaks GL: Personal communication, 1994.
23. Oliver RE: Cerebellar hypoplasia in a thoroughbred foal. *N Z Vet J* 23:15, 1975.
24. Wheat JD, Kennedy PC: Cerebellar hypoplasia and its sequela in a horse. *J Am Vet Med Assoc* 131:291, 1957.
25. Poss M, Young S: Dysplastic disease of the cerebellum of an adult horse. *Acta Neuropathol* 75:209, 1987.
26. Waelchli RO, Ehrensperger F: Two related cases of cerebellar abnormality in equine fetuses associated with hydrops of fetal membranes. *Vet Rec* 123:513, 1988.
27. Makela O, Gustavsson I, Hollmen T: A 64,X,i(Xq) karyotype in a Standardbred filly. *Equine Vet J* 26:251, 1994.
28. Bell RJ, Smart ME: An unusual complication of strangles in a pony. *Can Vet J* 33:400, 1992.
29. Allen JR, Barbee DD, Boulten CR, et al: Brain abscess in a horse: Diagnosis by computed tomography and successful surgical treatment. *Equine Vet J* 19:552, 1987.
30. Blunden AS, Khalil LF, Webbon PM: *Halicephalobus deletrix* infection in a horse. *Equine Vet J* 19:255, 1987.
31. Mayhew IG, Schneiders DH: An unusual familial neurological syndrome in newborn thoroughbred foals. *Vet Rec* 133:447, 1993.
32. Miller LM, Reed SM, Gallina AM, et al: Ataxia and weakness associated with fourth ventricle vascular anomalies in two horses. *J Am Vet Med Assoc* 186:601, 1985.
33. Seawright AA, Costigan P: Chronic methylmercurialism in a horse. *Vet Hum Toxicol* 20:6, 1978.

9.8

Cervical Vertebral Stenotic Myelopathy

Randolph H. Stewart, DVM, MS
Bonnie Rush Moore, DVM, MS

Cervical stenotic myelopathy (CSM) is a developmental disease of the cervical vertebrae characterized by stenosis of the cervical vertebral canal resulting in intermittent or continuous compression of the spinal cord.[1–3] There are two general manifestations of this syndrome: cervical vertebral instability (CVI) and cervical static stenosis (CSS).[1,2] CVI is a dynamic condition in which spinal cord compression is intermittent, and occurs when the cervical vertebrae are in the ventroflexed position.[4,5] The intervertebral sites most commonly involved in CVI-affected horses are C3–4 and C4–5.[6,7] In horses with CSS, spinal cord compression is continuous regardless of cervical position, and occurs predominantly in the caudal cervical region, C5–6 and C6–7.[2,7]

CSM occurs most frequently in rapidly growing, young male horses.[4,8–10] Although CSM has been reported in most light and draft breeds, it occurs more commonly in Thoroughbreds and quarter horses.[2,4,5,9] Early reports of CSM suggested that cranial and middle cervical lesions occurred in young horses (6–30 months) and caudal lesions in older horses (>5 years).[5] Subsequent studies, however, have not supported this observation. A retrospective study of 306 myelograms involving mostly Thoroughbreds reported 1- to 2-year-old horses to be most frequently affected and showed C3–4 to be the most commonly affected intervertebral site.[7] In most instances, there is no difference in site distribution of lesions between horses less than or equal to 2 years of age and those greater than 2 years of age.[7]

CLINICAL SIGNS

Cervical vertebral stenotic myelopathy is characterized by symmetric ataxia, paresis, and spasticity, which are usually worse in the rearlimbs than forelimbs.[4,9,10] At rest, affected horses will often assume a wide-based stance and demonstrate delayed responses to proprioceptive positioning. Stumbling, toe-dragging, circumduction of the hindlimbs, and truncal sway are observed at a walk. These signs are accentuated by manipulation during neurologic examination using circles, hills, obstacles, and elevation of the head.[4,5,9] The laryngeal adductor response test may be abnormal. Clinical signs of ataxia often progress for a short period of time and then stabilize.[4,5] A history of a traumatic incident is often associated with the onset of CSM; however, ataxia was likely present prior to the traumatic incident. In many cases the fall is a result of mild neurologic deficits and the traumatic incident exacerbates the clinical signs of spinal cord compression.

Infrequently, there is evidence of gray matter and spinal nerve root damage such as cervical pain, atrophy of the cervical musculature, or cutaneous hypalgesia adjacent to the affected cervical vertebrae.[8,9,11] These signs are more commonly observed in horses over 4 years of age with significant arthropathy of the caudal cervical vertebrae (C5–7).

Clinical signs of concurrent developmental orthopedic disease of the appendicular skeleton, such as physeal enlargement of the long bones, joint effusion secondary to osteochondrosis, and flexural limb deformities, are often present in young horses with CSM.[4,5,12]

PATHOGENESIS AND PATHOLOGIC FINDINGS

One of the most consistent pathologic changes observed in horses with CSM is narrowing of the vertebral canal as evidenced by decreased minimum sagittal diameter (MSD).[8, 11, 13, 14] The MSD can be determined for each cervical vertebra by taking the smallest sagittal diameter of the vertebral canal via radiographic or postmortem examination.[8] Horses affected with CSM have a narrowed MSD at C3–6, regardless of the site of spinal cord compression.[8, 11, 13, 14] In cases of CSS, narrowing of the canal diameter is exacerbated by thickening of the dorsal lamina, enlargement of the ligamentum flavum, and degenerative articular processes with thickened joint capsules.[2, 12] Abnormalities of the dorsal lamina and ligamentum flavum are not observed in young CSM-affected Thoroughbreds[13] and appear to be more common in the older CSM-affected horses.[2] In some cases of CSS, flexion of the neck will stretch the thickened ligamentum flavum and relieve spinal cord compression, whereas hyperextension exacerbates compression.[6, 8] Pathologic changes of the cervical vertebrae most commonly observed in horses with CVI are instability and subluxation of adjacent vertebrae, malformation of the caudal vertebral physis or epiphysis (caudal epiphyseal flare), and malformation or malarticulation of the articular processes.[1, 8] Histopathologic examination of the spinal cord reveals wallerian degeneration, malacia, and fibrosis at the sites of spinal cord compression and demyelination in the ascending and descending white matter tracts within adjacent segments of the spinal cord proximal and distal to the site of spinal cord compression.[8, 9]

Many studies have identified an association between CSM and developmental orthopedic disease in horses, although no causal relationship has been established.[1, 2, 12, 13] Osteochondrotic lesions are more severe in the articular processes of the cervical vertebrae and are more frequent and severe in the appendicular skeleton in horses affected with CSM than in clinically normal horses.[13] Instability between adjacent vertebrae, caused by osteochondrosis and subsequent degenerative joint disease of the articular processes, may lead to generation of excessive or inappropriate biomechanical forces on the ligamentum flavum, joint capsule, and dorsal lamina.[2] Thickening and fibrosis of these structures contribute to narrowing of the vertebral canal in horses with CSS. Osteochondrosis of the articular processes is not always present at the site of spinal cord compression in horses with CVI.[8, 13] Physeal osteochondrosis may produce caudal epiphyseal malformation and vertebral instability in cases of spinal cord compression wherein osteochondrosis of the articular processes is not present. Conversely, CSM and osteochondrosis may be two separate manifestations of developmental orthopedic disease characterized by an underlying inability to form normal cartilage and bone, and the occurrence of CSM may result from generalized failure of vertebral canal development rather than from osteochondrosis.[13] Nonetheless, the association between osteochondrosis and CSM indicates that the cause and pathophysiology of these two conditions are similar.

The cause of CSM appears to be multifactorial involving genetic and environmental influences. There is no evidence that CSM is directly heritable by simple mendelian dominant or recessive patterns.[15] Rather, the mode of inheritance may involve multiple alleles and variable penetrance determining a genetic predisposition to CSM. Nutrition, rapid growth, trauma, and abnormal biomechanical forces likely contribute

to the development of CSM in genetically predisposed individuals.[1, 16–19]

Dietary factors investigated in the pathogenesis of osteochondrosis and CSM include dietary copper, zinc, protein, and carbohydrate. Low dietary copper and high zinc concentrations produce severe osteochondrotic lesions in foals.[20, 21] Additionally, diets containing 15 ppm copper produce three times as many osteochondrotic lesions of the appendicular and axial skeleton compared to diets containing 55 ppm copper.[16–18, 22] Correction of trace mineral balance including zinc, calcium, and phosphorus, in conjunction with copper supplementation, decreases the incidence of developmental orthopedic disease in foals.[16, 17, 22] Copper supplementation does not completely eliminate developmental orthopedic disease, suggesting other etiologic factors must exist. Excessive carbohydrate in the diet is hypothesized to contribute to the pathogenesis of osteochondrosis through endocrine imbalance.[19, 23–26] A high carbohydrate meal (130% of the National Research Council [NRC] recommendation) results in postprandial elevation of serum insulin concentration and depression of serum thyroxine concentration.[23] Insulin stimulates the zone of chondrocyte proliferation and thyroxine stimulates the zone of chondrocyte maturation at the growth plate.[25, 26] High insulin and low thyroxine concentrations are suspected to promote cartilage proliferation and retention without promoting maturation. Cartilage retention and failure of maturation are consistent with the histopathologic appearance of osteochondrosis. Endocrine alterations associated with a high carbohydrate diet are the basis for the "paced diet" program for prevention and treatment of CSM.[27, 28] A correlation between dietary protein concentrations and the incidence of osteochondrosis and CSM has not been identified.[16–18]

DIAGNOSIS

The differential diagnosis of CSM includes neurologic diseases that produce tetraparesis and incoordination, such as equine herpesvirus type 1 myeloencephalitis, equine protozoal myeloencephalitis, equine degenerative myeloencephalopathy, occipitoatlantoaxial malformation, spinal cord trauma, vertebral fracture or luxation, vertebral abscessation, and verminous myelitis.[4] Neurologic examination, cerebrospinal fluid (CSF) analysis, and radiographic procedures are indicated in horses with symmetric tetraparesis and ataxia.[29]

Lateral radiographic views of the cervical vertebrae are examined to obtain objective determination of vertebral canal diameter and subjective assessment of vertebral malformation. Characteristic malformations of the cervical vertebrae in horses with CSM include flare of the caudal epiphysis of the vertebral body, abnormal ossification patterns of the articular processes, subluxation between adjacent vertebrae, extension of the dorsal laminae, and degenerative joint disease (DJD) of the articular processes.[27, 28] DJD of the articular processes is the most frequent and severe malformation observed in CSM-affected horses.[14] However, DJD of the articular processes occurs in 10% to 50% of nonataxic horses,[8, 14, 30] and subjective evaluation of DJD of the articular processes in the caudal cervical spine results in the false-positive diagnosis of CSM.[7] Although the presence of characteristic vertebral malformations supports the diagnosis of CSM, subjective evaluation of bony malformation from radiographs of the cervical vertebrae does not reliably discriminate between CSM-affected and unaffected horses.[7, 14]

Objective assessment of the vertebral canal diameter is more accurate than subjective evaluation of bony malformation for identification of horses with CSM.[14] The most reliable objective determination of vertebral canal diameter from standing radiographs of the cervical vertebrae is the sagittal ratio technique. The sagittal ratio is calculated by dividing the MSD by the width of the vertebral body.[14] The vertebral body width is measured perpendicular to the vertebral canal at the widest point of the cranial aspect of the vertebral body (Fig. 9–32). This technique eliminates variability in absolute MSD values due to magnification. The vertebral body is located within the same anatomical plane as the vertebral canal; therefore, the proportion of these two objects will be the same regardless of the degree of radiographic magnification.[31] The sagittal ratio technique has a sensitivity and specificity equal to or greater than 89% for vertebral sites C4–7, and should be used to determine the likelihood of the presence of CSM in an individual with spinal ataxia.[14] If the sagittal ratio at a particular vertebral site is below the reference value for that site, myelographic examination should be performed to confirm the diagnosis of CSM. If the sagittal ratio is above the reference value, myelographic examination should be avoided or postponed until diagnostic tests focused on alternative causes of spinal ataxia are performed. The reference values for sagittal ratio measurements of the cervical vertebrae are 52% at C4–6, and 56% at C7. Accurate measurement of the sagittal ratio value requires a precise, lateral radiograph of the cervical vertebrae. Obliquity of the cervical vertebrae results in indistinct margins of the ventral aspect of the vertebral canal, producing erroneous values for MSD and vertebral body width.

A semiquantitative scoring system for assessment of cervical radiographs has been developed for identification of

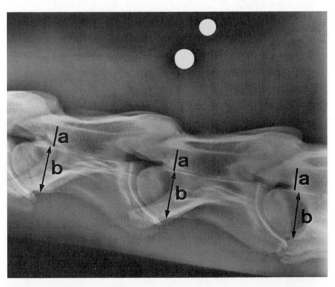

Figure 9–32. Lateral radiographic view of the fourth, fifth, and sixth cervical vertebrae. The sagittal ratio is determined at each vertebral site by dividing the minimum sagittal diameter *(a)* by the width of the cranial aspect of the vertebral body *(b)* at its widest point.

CSM in Thoroughbred foals up to 1 year of age.[27, 28, 32] The semiquantitative scoring system incorporates objective determination of vertebral canal stenosis and subjective evaluation of vertebral malformation. The maximum total score is 35 points and a total score of 12 or higher constitutes a radiographic diagnosis of CSM. Stenosis of the vertebral canal is assessed by determination of the inter- and intravertebral MSD; the maximum score designated for vertebral canal stenosis is 10 points. The inter- and intravertebral MSDs are corrected for radiographic magnification by dividing the MSD by the length of the vertebral body. Malformation of the cervical vertebrae is determined by subjective assessment of each of the following five categories: (1) enlargement of the caudal physis of the vertebral body, (2) caudal extension of the dorsal lamina, (3) angulation between adjacent vertebrae, (4) delayed ossification of bone, and (5) degenerative joint disease of the articular process. The maximum score allotted for each category of bony malformation is 5 points. This semiquantitative scoring system is a noninvasive method for predicting and diagnosing the presence of CSM in Thoroughbred foals up to 1 year of age.[32]

Myelographic examination is required for definitive diagnosis of CSM.[6, 33] Use of the sagittal ratio method for determination of specific sites of spinal cord compression will overestimate the number of sites of spinal cord compression within the CSM-affected population.[8, 11, 13] In addition, subjective evaluation of bony malformation will result in inaccurate diagnosis of the sites of spinal cord compression. The severity of vertebral abnormalities does not necessarily correspond to the site of spinal cord compression, and spinal cord compression can occur from stenosis of the vertebral canal at vertebral sites that lack bony malformation.[7, 8, 13] Therefore, radiographs of the cervical vertebrae cannot replace myelographic examination for identification of the location, number of affected sites, and classification of spinal cord compressive lesions in horses with CSM.[29]

Definitive diagnosis of CSM is determined by 50% or greater decrease in the sagittal diameter of the dorsal and ventral dye columns at diametrically opposed sites.[6, 33] This decrease is quantified by comparing it with the midvertebral site cranial or caudal to the compressed site. The ventral column is often totally obliterated at the intervertebral sites in normal studies, particularly in the flexed position; therefore, 50% or greater decrease in opposing dorsal and ventral columns must be present for diagnosis of CSM. In horses with obvious sites of spinal cord compression identified on myelographic views with the cervical vertebrae in the neutral position, excessive manipulation of the neck should be avoided so as to obtain flexed and extended myelographic views to prevent exacerbation of spinal cord injury.

Although myelographic examination has been shown to be a relatively safe procedure,[6, 7] it is not without risk. The contrast agent metrizamide may produce depression, increased ataxia, fever, seizures, meningitis, and muscle fasciculations.[34–36] Nonionic, water-soluble contrast agents, such as iopamidol and iohexol, provide superior radiographic contrast with fewer adverse effects than metrizamide.[33, 37] Regardless of the contrast agent used, myelographic examination should be reserved for use in those cases in which the risk and the cost are justified. Indications for myelographic examination include confirmation of a definitive diagnosis of CSM at the owner's request, insurance purposes, prior to euthanasia, and identification of the exact site(s) of spinal cord compression prior to surgical intervention.

Analysis of CSF shows it is often within reference ranges in horses with CSM.[4, 9, 29] In instances when CSF is abnormal in horses with CSM, the alterations are consistent with acute spinal cord compression, such as mild xanthochromia or mild increases in protein concentrations.[9]

TREATMENT

Surgical intervention is the most widely reported treatment for CSM.[38–44] Stall rest, glucocorticoids, dimethyl sulfoxide, and other anti-inflammatory drugs may provide transient improvement in clinical signs, but effective treatment must be directed at preventing further spinal cord injury.[5] The goals of surgical intervention in horses with CSM are stabilization of the cervical vertebrae and decompression of the spinal cord. Cervical vertebral interbody fusion provides intervertebral stability for horses with dynamic spinal cord compression (CVI). Affected cervical vertebrae are fused in the extended position to provide immediate relief of spinal cord compression and prevent repetitive spinal cord trauma.[39, 40, 42, 43]

Immediate decompression of the spinal cord in cases of CSS is achieved by subtotal dorsal laminectomy in which portions of the dorsal lamina, ligamentum flavum, and joint capsule overlying the compressed site are removed.[5, 41, 45, 46] This procedure effectively decompresses the spinal cord, but is associated with significant postoperative risk.[40] Interbody fusion of caudal cervical vertebrae in horses with CSS produces remodeling and atrophy of the articular processes resulting in delayed decompression of the spinal cord over a period of weeks to months.[38, 39] Decompression is immediate with dorsal laminectomy; however, because of its relative safety, interbody fusion is selected by some surgeons as the technique of choice for CSS and CVI.[40]

Cervical vertebral interbody fusion results in improvement in neurologic status in 44% to 90% of horses with CVI and CSS, and 12% to 62% of horses return to athletic function.[5, 39, 40, 42, 44] Subtotal dorsal laminectomy results in improvement in neurologic status in 40% to 75% of horses with CSS.[40, 41] Both subtotal dorsal laminectomy and cervical vertebral interbody fusion for CSS of the caudal cervical vertebrae are associated with fatal postoperative complications, including vertebral body fracture, spinal cord edema, and implant failure.[40] The most important patient factor for determination of postoperative prognosis is duration of clinical signs prior to surgical intervention; horses with clinical signs for less than 1 month prior to surgery are more likely to return to athletic function than are horses with clinical signs of greater than 3 months' duration.[40] The number of spinal cord compressive sites and patient age do not affect the long-term surgical outcome of cervical vertebral interbody fusion.

The duration of convalescence and rehabilitation following cervical vertebral interbody fusion is approximately 6 to 12 months.[39, 40] An individualized exercise program, dependent on capability, projected use, and neurologic status of the horse, should be designed for promotion of muscular strength. Extended exercise at slow speed, including ponying and lunging on inclines, is recommended during the rehabili-

tation process. The point at which the horse is competent to return to athletic function following interbody fusion should be determined by neurologic examination. It is unlikely that significant improvement in neurologic status will occur beyond the 1-year postoperative time period.

Successful conservative management of CSM has been achieved using the paced diet program in foals less than 1 year of age. The goal of this dietary program is to retard bone growth, enhance bone metabolism, and allow the vertebral canal diameter to enlarge to relieve compression of the spinal cord.[27, 28] This dietary program is restricted in protein and energy (65%–75% of NRC recommendations), but maintains balanced vitamin and mineral intake (at least 100% of NRC recommendations). Vitamins A and E are provided at three times the NRC recommendations and selenium is supplemented to 0.3 ppm. Roughage is provided by grass of low-quality (6%–9% crude protein) timothy hay. Individual dietary plans are specially formulated according to the age and weight of the foal. Solitary stall confinement is recommended to reduce the risk of spinal cord compression due to dynamic instability. This program of dietary management and restricted exercise has been successful in prevention of the development of neurologic signs in foals with radiographic evidence of CSM and in treatment of foals demonstrating clinical signs of CSM.

REFERENCES

1. Reed S, Newbery J, Norton K: Pathogenesis of cervical vertebral malformation. *Proc Am Assoc Equine Pract* 31:37–42, 1985.
2. Powers BE, Stashak TS, Nixon AJ, et al: Pathology of the vertebral column of horses with cervical static stenosis. *Vet Pathol* 23:392–399, 1986.
3. Rooney J: Disorders of the nervous system. In Rooney J, ed: *Biomechanics in Lameness.* Baltimore, Williams & Wilkins, 1969, pp 219–233.
4. Reed S, Bayly W, Traub J: Ataxia and paresis in horses. Part I: Differential diagnosis. *Compend Contin Educ Pract Vet* 3:S88–S99, 1981.
5. Wagner PC, Grant BD, Reed SM: Cervical vertebral malformations. *Vet Clin North Am Equine Pract* 3:385–396, 1987.
6. Rantanen N, Gavin P: Ataxia and paresis in horses. Part II: Radiographic and myelographic examination of the cervical vertebral column. *Compend Contin Educ Pract Vet* 3:S161–171, 1981.
7. Papageorges M, Gavin P, Sande R, et al: Radiographic and myelographic examination of the cervical vertebral column in 306 ataxic horses. *Vet Radiol* 28:53–59, 1987.
8. Mayhew I, deLahunta A, Whitlock R: Spinal cord disease in the horse. *Cornell Vet* 68(suppl 6):44–105, 1978.
9. Mayhew IG: *Large Animal Neurology. A Handbook for Veterinary Clinicians.* Philadelphia, Lea & Febiger, 1989, pp 243–335.
10. Rooney JR: Equine incoordination I. Gross morphology. *Cornell Vet* 53:411–421, 1963.
11. Moore B, Holbrook T, Reed S, et al: Contrast-enhanced computed tomography in six horses with cervical stenotic myelopathy. *Equine Vet J* 24:197–202, 1992.
12. Mayhew IG, Krook L, Whitlock RH, et al: Nutrition, bones and bone pathology. *Cornell Vet* 68(suppl 6):71–102, 1978.
13. Stewart R, Reed S, Weisbrode S: The frequency and severity of osteochondrosis in cervical stenotic myelopathy in horses. *Am J Vet Res* 52:873–879, 1991.

14. Moore BR, Reed SM, Biller DS, et al: Assessment of vertebral canal diameter and bony malformations of the cervical part of the spine in horses with cervical stenotic myelopathy. *Am J Vet Res* 55:5–13, 1994.

15. Wagner PC, Grant BD, Watrous BS, et al: A study of the heritability of cervical vertebral malformation in horses. *Proc Am Assoc Equine Pract* 33:43–50, 1957.

16. Gabel A, Knight D, Reed S, et al: Comparison of incidence and severity of developmental orthopedic disease on 17 farms before and after adjustment of ration. *Proc Am Assoc Equine Pract* 33:163, 1987.

17. Knight D, Reed S, Weisbrode S, et al: Correlation of dietary mineral to the incidence and severity of osteochondrosis in cervical vertebral malformation of horses. *Proceedings of the Eighth American College of Veterinary Internal Medicine Forum.* Blacksburg, Va, ACVIM, 1990, pp 989–991.

18. Knight D, Weisbrode S, Schmall L, et al: The effects of copper supplementation on the prevalence of cartilage lesions in foals. *Equine Vet J* 22:426–432, 1990.

19. Glade M: The role of endocrine factors in developmental orthopedic disease. *Proc Am Assoc Equine Pract* 33:171, 1987.

20. Bridges C, Harris E: Experimentally induced cartilaginous fractures in foals fed low-copper diets. *J Am Vet Med Assoc* 193:215–221, 1988.

21. Bridges C, Moffitt P: Influence of variable content of dietary zinc on copper metabolism of weanling foals. *Am J Vet Res* 51:275–280, 1990.

22. Knight D: Copper supplementation and cartilage lesions in foals. *Proc Am Assoc Equine Pract* 33:191, 1987.

23. Glade M, Reimers T: Effects of dietary energy supply on serum thyroxine, triiodothyronine and insulin concentrations in young horses. *J Endocrinol* 104:93, 1985.

24. Glade M, Belling T: A dietary etiology for osteochondritic cartilage. *Equine Vet Sci* 6:151–155, 1985.

25. Kronfeld D: Dietary aspects of developmental orthopedic disease. *Vet Clin North Am Equine Pract* 451–466, 1990.

26. Kronfeld D, Donoghue S: Metabolic convergence in developmental orthopedic disease. *Proc Am Assoc Equine Pract* 33:195, 1987.

27. Donawick W, Mayhew I, Galligan D, et al: Early diagnosis of cervical vertebral malformation in young thoroughbred horses and successful treatment with restricted, paced diet and confinement. *Proc Am Assoc Equine Pract* 35:525–528, 1989.

28. Donawick W, Mayhew I, Galligan D, et al: Recognition and non-surgical management of cervical vertebral malformation in foals. In *Proceedings of the 20th Annual Surgical Forum,* 1992, pp 103–105.

29. Moore BR, Granstom DE, Reed SM: Diagnosis of equine protozoal myelitis and cervical stenotic myelopathy. *Compend Contin Educ Pract Vet* 17:419–426, 1995.

30. Whitwell KE, Dyson S: Interpreting radiographs. 8: Equine cervical vertebrae. *Equine Vet J* 19:8–14, 1987.

31. Pavlov H, Torg J, Robie B: Cervical spinal stenosis: Determination with vertebral body ratio method. *Radiology* 164:771–775, 1987.

32. Mayhew I, Donawick W, Green S, et al: Diagnosis and prediction of cervical vertebral malformation in Thoroughbred foals based on semi-quantitative radiographic indicators. *Equine Vet J* 25:435–440, 1993.

33. Neuwirth L: Equine myelography. *Compend Contin Educ Pract Vet* 14:72–79, 1992.

34. Nyland T, Blythe L, Pool R, et al: Metrizamide myelography in the horse: Clinical, radiographic and pathologic changes. *Am J Vet Res* 41:204–211, 1980.

35. Hubbell J, Reed S, Myer C, et al: Sequelae of myelography in the horse. *Equine Vet J* 20:438–440, 1988.

36. Beech J. Metrizamide myelography in the horse. *J Am Vet Rad Soc* 20:22–32, 1979.

37. May SA, Wyn-Jones G, Church S: Iopamidol myelography in the horse. *Equine Vet J* 18:199–203, 1986.

38. DeBowes RM, Grant BD, Bagby GW, et al: Cervical vertebral interbody fusion in the horse: A comparative study of bovine xenografts and autografts supported by stainless steel baskets. *Am J Vet Res* 45:191–199, 1984.

39. Grant B, Barbee D, Wagner P: Long term results of surgery for equine cervical vertebral malformation. *Proc Am Assoc Equine Pract* 31:91–96, 1985.

40. Moore B, Reed S, Robertson J: Surgical treatment of cervical stenotic myelopathy in horses: 73 cases (1983–1992). *J Am Vet Med Assoc* 203:108–112, 1993.

41. Nixon A, Stashak T, Ingram J: Dorsal laminectomy in the horse. III. Results in horses with cervical vertebral malformation. *Vet Surg* 12:184–188, 1983.

42. Wagner P, Grant B, Bagby G: Evaluation of cervical spinal fusion as a treatment in the equine "wobbler" syndrome. *Vet Surg* 8:84–88, 1979.

43. Wagner P: Surgical stabilization of the equine cervical spine. *Vet Surg* 3:7–12, 1979.

44. Wagner PC, Grant BD, Gallina AM: Ataxia and paresis in horses. Part III. Surgical treatment of cervical spinal cord compression. *Compend Contin Educ Pract Vet* 3:S192–202, 1981.

45. Nixon A, Stashak T, Ingram J: Dorsal laminectomy in the horse. I. Review of the literature and description of a new procedure. *Vet Surg* 12:172–176, 1983.

46. Nixon A, Stashak T, Ingram J: Dorsal laminectomy in the horse. II. Evaluation in the normal horse. *Vet Surg* 12:177–183, 1983.

9.9

Equine Degenerative Myeloencephalopathy

Hilary K. Matthews, DVM

Equine degenerative myeloencephalopathy (EDM) is a noncompressive, diffuse, symmetric, degenerative neurologic disease characterized by ataxia, weakness, and spasticity (hypometria) in young horses of many breeds and both sexes.[1–3] A similar syndrome has been observed in Mongolian wild horses (*Equus przewalski*)[4] and Grant's zebras.[2, 5] The disease has been diagnosed in England and North America and is reported to occur more frequently in the northeastern United States.[6] A familial tendency has been observed in the Paso Fino,[7] Arabian,[2] appaloosa,[8, 9] and Thoroughbred breeds and in Grant's zebras.[7] Neuroaxonal dystrophy (NAD), a similar but less diffuse disease of Morgan horses, also appears to have a familial occurrence.[10, 11] No pattern of inheritance for EDM or NAD has been proved.

CLINICAL SIGNS

The age of onset of clinical signs varies from less than 1 month to several years. Most horses manifest signs at less than 6 months of age with the mean age of onset being 0.4 year.[1, 3] However, in one study of 128 horses with EDM, age of onset ranged from 1 month to 20 years, with 16% of the horses showing signs at greater than 28 months of age.[11]

Onset of signs may be abrupt or insidious.[1, 2, 6] Signs are referable to upper motor neuron and general proprioceptive deficits and include symmetric ataxia, weakness, and spasticity of all four limbs, often worse in the pelvic limbs.[1–3] Signs may begin in the pelvic limbs and progress to the thoracic limbs. The gait is characterized by dysmetria and stabbing of the ground with the limbs.[2, 6] Often, hindlimb interference and dragging or scuffing of the toes are present.[2, 6] When backed, the horse may resist or rock back on the pelvic limbs and "dog-sit."[2, 6] Postural placing reactions may show conscious proprioceptive deficits. When circled, affected horses often pivot on the inside hindlimb and circumduct the outside limb.[6] Affected horses may have trouble stopping and it is not unusual for them to fall while running in the pasture or being worked.[3, 6] Cranial nerve involvement, muscle atrophy, or changes in skin sensation or tail tone are absent in EDM.[1, 2] Hyporeflexia over the neck and trunk with diminished-to-absent cervical, cervicofacial, cutaneous trunci, and laryngeal adductor reflexes may be found, especially in severe and longstanding cases.[12]

Neuroaxonal dystrophy in Morgan horses has similar clinical signs, but even in very severely affected horses only pelvic limb deficits may be seen. Pelvic limb dysmetria, asynchrony, and ataxia are generally less severe than in EDM.[9]

PATHOLOGY

Gross necropsy findings in EDM are unremarkable.[1, 2] Classic histologic changes are evident in the caudal brainstem nuclei (medulla oblongata) and especially the spinal cord and include diffuse neuronal fiber degeneration (dystrophy) of the white matter.[1, 2] Generally, the lateral and medial cuneate nuclei, gracile nucleus, lateral cervical and thoracic nuclei, and lumbosacral and cervical intermediate gray columns are affected.[1, 2] Astrocytosis, astrogliosis, vacuolization, myelin loss, spheroid formation, and lipofuscin-like pigment accumulation are present in these areas.[1, 2] With chronicity, the dorsal and ventral spinocerebellar tracts and the medial part of the ventral funiculi of the thoracic segments are more severely affected.[1, 2] Neurochemical studies of the spinal cord show a significant loss of myelin and component lipids.[1] Demyelination occurs to a greater extent than axon loss.[1]

Histologic changes in NAD of Morgan horses lack the diffuse nature of the changes seen in EDM. In NAD, histologic changes may be confined to the accessory cuneate nuclei.[10]

PATHOPHYSIOLOGY

The pathogenesis of EDM is unknown. However, it is most likely due to a complex interaction of many factors. Degenerative myelopathy in other species, which bears clinical and histopathologic similarities to EDM, has been linked to vitamin E and copper deficiencies, hereditary factors, and toxic insults. Possibly, one or more of these factors with environmental and management stress factors may play a role in the pathogenesis of EDM.

Vitamin E deficiency has received much attention as a possible cause of EDM. This association is based on the presence of degenerative myelopathy in rats,[13, 14] monkeys,[15] humans,[16–18] and captive Przewalski's horses[4] with low serum vitamin E concentrations. One study reported a high incidence of EDM on two breeding farms in which low serum vitamin E concentrations were found. Vitamin E supplementation decreased the incidence from 40% to less than 10%. However, affected and unaffected horses on both farms were found to be vitamin E–deficient.[7] Another study measured serum vitamin E and blood glutathione peroxidase concentrations in 40 horses with histologically confirmed EDM and in 49 normal age-matched control horses. This study found no significant differences in serum vitamin E and blood glutathione peroxidase concentrations between the two groups.[19] The role of vitamin E or glutathione peroxidase in the development of EDM remains unclear.

A recent study documented significantly lower vitamin E concentrations and clinical signs compatible with EDM in eight of nine foals sired by an EDM-affected stallion.[20] Age-matched control foals raised in the same environment had normal serum vitamin E concentrations, and no signs of EDM.[20] Oral vitamin E absorption tests were performed on both groups, and no significant differences were found between the groups.[20] Thus, an inability to absorb vitamin E from the gastrointestinal tract does not appear to be a factor in the low serum vitamin E concentrations in EDM-affected horses.[20]

Similar histologic changes and clinical signs have been observed in copper-deficient sheep,[21, 22] goats,[23] guinea pigs,[24] young pigs,[25] calves,[26] and rats.[27] In one study plasma and liver copper concentrations were measured in 25 horses with histologically confirmed EDM and compared with values in 35 normal age-matched control horses. This study found no significant differences in plasma and liver copper concentrations between the two groups.[28] Thus, the role of copper in EDM remains unclear.

Recently, a study on affected and normal horses was done to identify risk factors associated with the development of EDM. Comparison of affected (56 horses) and control (179 horses) groups identified three risk factors: (1) use of insecticides, (2) exposure to wood preservatives, and (3) spending frequent time on a dirt lot.[29] Spending time on green pastures was found to be a protective factor. Additionally, a foal was 25 times more likely to develop EDM if its dam had any other foals diagnosed with EDM.[12] These factors alone probably do not cause EDM, but may interact with other factors to produce disease. Also, these factors should be considered in preventing or minimizing the risk of developing EDM.

Hereditary factors must also be considered in the pathogenesis of EDM and NAD in horses, as the diseases have been observed in familial clusters.[9] Heterofamilial neuroaxonal dystrophy has been shown to occur in kittens[1, 30] and Suffolk sheep[1, 31] and is inherited as an autosomal recessive trait. However, the mode of inheritance has not been identified in EDM- or NAD-affected horses.

Toxic compounds such as organophosphates,[1, 32, 33] diethyldithiocarbamate,[1, 34] and cycad palm[35] have been reported to cause histologic changes and clinical signs similar to NAD in horses of several species. Their effect is due to the neurotoxic properties of the compounds. No direct association of toxic compounds with EDM or NAD in horses has been shown.

DIAGNOSIS

Definitive diagnosis of EDM can be made only with histopathologic examination of the spinal cord and brainstem. Antemortem diagnosis is based on clinical signs and ruling out other neurologic diseases (especially cervical vertebral malformation and equine protozoal myeloencephalitis). In EDM, cerebrospinal fluid (CSF) analysis and cervical spinal radiographs are usually within normal limits, although increased CSF creatine phosphokinase (CPK) levels have been found in horses affected with EDM.[1] Serum vitamin E levels of less than 1 mg/mL in horses showing clinical signs of EDM may help support a diagnosis.[3] The normal reference range for serum vitamin E concentration does vary, but is usually greater than 1.5 mg/mL.[3] It should be noted that a single serum vitamin E sample may not adequately reflect the true vitamin E status of the horse, as up to 12% variation in concentrations can occur normally.[36]

TREATMENT AND PREVENTION

There is no specific treatment for EDM in horses. Affected horses may benefit from oral vitamin E supplementation coupled with monitoring of serum vitamin E concentrations. The earlier vitamin E treatment is instituted, the better the chance for a response. Horses with clinical signs of EDM may benefit from very large doses of vitamin E (6,000 IU/ day) for an extended period of time.[37] Horses with very low serum vitamin E concentration may also benefit from 1,000 (foals and yearlings) to 2,000 (adults) IU of vitamin E in oil given intramuscularly every 10 days. Dietary vitamin E levels should be maintained at 500 to 1,000 IU/kg dry weight.[3] Heat-treated pellets, stored oats, and sun-baked forages have marginal vitamin E concentrations (0–5 IU/kg dry weight).[3, 7] Horses fed a diet of these should have frequent access to fresh green forage or vitamin E supplementation at 600 to 1,800 mg or tocopheryl acetate 1.5 to 4.4 mg/kg/ day to meet their reported needs.[38] To date, vitamin E toxicity associated with supplementation has not been reported. Also, farms with a high incidence of EDM may benefit from prophylactic vitamin E supplementation.[7]

PROGNOSIS

Equine degenerative myeloencephalopathy is generally progressive, necessitating euthanasia. Once clinical signs are evident, no improvement or remission occurs. However, signs may plateau.[3, 7] Generally, horses with EDM do not progress to a state of recumbency.[1, 3] Severely affected horses usually have an earlier age of onset and rapid disease progression.[6] Mildly affected horses usually have a later age of onset, and the disease has a less rapid course.[6]

REFERENCES

1. Mayhew IG, deLahunta A, Whitlock RH, et al: Spinal cord disease in the horse. *Cornell Vet* 68(suppl 6):11, 1978.
2. Mayhew IG, deLahunta A, Whitlock RH: Equine degenerative myeloencephalopathy. *J Am Vet Med Assoc* 170:195, 1977.
3. Mayhew IG: *Large Animal Neurology. A Handbook for Veterinary Clinicians.* Philadelphia, Lea & Febiger, 1989, p 294.
4. Liu S-K, Dolensek EP, Adams CR, et al: Myelopathy and vitamin E deficiency in six Mongolian wild horses. *J Am Vet Med Assoc* 183:1266, 1983.
5. Montali RJ, Bush M, Sauer RM, et al: Spinal ataxia in zebras: Comparison with the wobbler syndrome of horses. *Vet Pathol* 11:68, 1974.
6. Beech J: Equine degenerative myeloencephalopathy. In Reed SM, ed. *Veterinary Clinics of North America.* Philadelphia, WB Saunders, 1987, p 379.
7. Mayhew IG, Brown CM, Stowe HD, et al: Equine degenerative myeloencephalopathy: A vitamin E deficiency that may be familial. *J Vet Intern Med* 1:45, 1987.
8. Blythe LL: Can wobbler disease be a family affair? In *Proceedings of Eastern States Veterinary Conference.* Abstract No. 160, 1986.
9. Blythe LL, Hultgren BD, Craig AM, et al: Clinical, viral, and genetic evaluation of equine degenerative mycloencephalopathy in a family of Appaloosas. *J Am Vet Med Assoc* 198: 1005, 1991.
10. Beech J: Neuroaxonal dystrophy of the accessory cuneate nucleus in horses. *Vet Pathol* 21:384, 1984.
11. Beech J, Haskins M: Genetic studies of neuraxonal dystrophy in the Morgan. *Am J Vet Res* 48:109, 1987.
12. Mayhew IG, Brown C, Trapp A: Equine degenerative myeloencephalopathy. In *Proceedings of the Fourth Annual Veterinary Medical Forum.* 2:11, 1986.
13. Pentschew A, Schwarz K: Systemic axonal dystrophy in vitamin E deficient adult rats with implications in human neuropathology. *Acta Neuropathol* 1:313, 1962.
14. Towfighi J: Effects of chronic vitamin E deficiency on the nervous system of the rat. *Acta Neuropathol* 54:261, 1981.
15. Nelson JS, Fitch CD, Fischer VW, et al: Progressive neuropathologic lesions in vitamin E–deficient rhesus monkeys. *J Neuropathol Exp Neurol* 40:166, 1981.
16. Sokol RJ, Guggenheim MA, Iannaccone ST, et al: Improved neurologic function after long-term correction of vitamin E deficiency in children with chronic cholestasis. *N Engl J Med* 313:1580, 1985.
17. Elias E, Muller DPR, Scott J: Association of spinocerebellar disorders with cystic fibrosis or chronic childhood cholestasis and very low serum vitamin E. *Lancet* 2:1319, 1981.
18. Harding AE, Muller DPR, Thomas PK, et al: Spinocerebellar degeneration secondary to chronic intestinal malabsorption: A vitamin E deficiency syndrome. *Ann Neurol* 15:419, 1982.
19. Dill SG, Kallfelz FA, deLahunta A, et al: Serum vitamin E and blood glutathione peroxidase values of horses with degenerative myeloencephalopathy. *Am J Vet Res* 50:166, 1989.
20. Blythe LL, Craig AM, Lassen ED, et al: Serially determined plasma α-tocopherol concentrations and results of the oral vitamin E absorption test in clinically normal horses and in horses with degenerative myeloencephalopathy. *Am J Vet Res* 52:908, 1991.
21. Cancilla PA, Barlow RM: Structural changes of the central nervous system in swayback (enzootic ataxia) of lambs. *Acta Neuropathol* 12:307, 1969.
22. Innes JRM, Shearer GD: "Swayback": A demyelinating disease of lambs with affinities to Schilder's encephalitis in man. *J Comp Pathol Ther* 43:1, 1940.
23. Owen ED, Prodfoot R, Robert JM, et al: Pathological and

biochemical studies of an outbreak of swayback in goats. *J Comp Pathol* 75:241, 1965.

24. Everson GJ, Tsai H-CC, Wang T-I: Copper deficiency in the guinea pig. *J Nutr* 93:533, 1968.

25. McGavin MD, Ranby RD, Tammemsgi L: Demyelination associated with low liver copper levels in pigs. *Aust Vet J* 38:8, 1962.

26. Sanders DE, Koestner A: Bovine neonatal ataxia associated with hypocupremia in pregnant cows. *J Am Vet Med Assoc* 176:728, 1980.

27. Carlton WW, Kelly WA: Neural lesions in the offspring of female rats fed a copper-deficient diet. *J Nutr* 97:42, 1969.

28. Dill SG, Hintz HF, deLahunta A, et al: Plasma and liver copper values in horses with equine degenerative myeloencephalopathy. *Can J Vet Res* 53:29, 1989.

29. Dill SG, Correa MT, Erb HN, et al: Factors associated with the development of equine degenerative myeloencephalopathy. *Am J Vet Res* 51:1300, 1990.

30. Woodard JC, Collins GH, Hessler JR: Feline hereditary neuroaxonal dystrophy. *Am J Pathol* 74:551, 1974.

31. Cordy DR, Richards WPC, Bradford GE: Systemic neuroaxonal dystrophy in Suffolk sheep. *Acta Neuropathol* 8:133, 1967.

32. Stubbings DP, Gilbert FR, Giles N, et al: An organophosphate worming compound and paraplegia in pigs. *Vet Rec* 99:127, 1976.

33. Beck BE, Wood CD, Whenhan GR: Triaryl phosphate poisoning in cattle. *Vet Pathol* 14:128, 1977.

34. Howell LJM, Ishmael J, Ewbank R, et al: Changes in the central nervous system of lambs following administration of sodium diethyldithiocarbamate. *Acta Neuropathol* 15:197, 1970.

35. Hooper PT, Best SM, Campbell A: Axonal dystrophy in the spinal cords of cattle consuming cycad palm, *Cycas media. Aust Vet J* 50:146, 1974.

36. Craig AM, Blythe LL, Lassen ED, et al: Variations of serum vitamin E, cholesterol, and total serum lipid concentrations in horses during a 72-hour period. *Am J Vet Res* 50:1527, 1989.

37. Blythe LL, Craig AM, Lassen ED: Vitamin E in the horse and its relationship to equine degenerative myeloencephalopathy. In *Proceedings of the Seventh Annual Veterinary Medical Forum.* 1:1007, 1989.

38. Roncus BO, Hakkarainen RV, Lindholm CA, et al: Vitamin E requirements of adult Standardbred horses evaluated by tissue depletion and repletion. *Equine Vet J* 18:50, 1986.

9.10

Equine Protozoal Myeloencephalitis

David E. Granstrom, DVM, PhD
William J. Saville, DVM

HISTORY

Equine protozoal myeloencephalitis (EPM) was initially identified as segmental myelitis by J.R. Rooney at the University of Kentucky in 1964.[1] The first cases were recognized among standardbreds returning to Kentucky from racetracks in the northeastern United States. Subsequent cases have been reported among native horses in most of the United States as well as in Canada, Panama, and Brazil.[2-5] The disease was called segmental myelitis because discrete lesions were found distributed randomly throughout the spinal cord. As more cases were examined, it became apparent that the brain was frequently involved, resulting in the name focal myelitis-encephalitis. The lesions of EPM include multifocal areas of necrosis and hemorrhage along with nonsuppurative inflammation of the white and gray matter. Ten years later, a "*Toxoplasma*-like" protozoan was recognized in histopathologic sections and the disease gradually became known as equine protozoal myeloencephalitis.[6-8]

Dubey, in a 1976 review of sarcocystosis in domestic animals, was the first to suggest that EPM was caused by a member of the genus *Sarcocystis*.[9] It was another 15 years before he was able to culture the organism from the spinal cord of an affected horse.[10] He named the organism *Sarcocystis neurona* because it often develops within neurons. Until recently, little information was available regarding the life cycle of the organism. and only asexual stages of the parasite were known. Sporocysts of *S. falcatula* from the opossum were tested by an *S. neurona*–specific polymerase chain reaction (PCR) assay and found to be positive. Subsequent sequence analysis demonstrated 99.89% sequence homology between the 18S small subunit ribosomal DNA sequences of *S. neurona* and *S. falcatula*.[11]

EPIDEMIOLOGY

A majority of the information known about EPM was gathered from naturally occurring infections. Regional epidemiologic studies of EPM have yielded dissimilar results.[12, 13] Although regional differences probably occur, the most reliable general information for North America was provided by an EPM workshop convened at the Veterinary Medical Forum of the American College of Veterinary Internal Medicine in 1988.[14] It was based on 364 histologically confirmed cases from California, Florida, Illinois, Kentucky, New York, Ohio, Oklahoma, Pennsylvania, Texas, and Ontario, Canada. Data were compiled from histologically confirmed cases from animal diagnostic centers in each state or province. The average period reported was 6 years with a range of 4 to 12 years. In descending order of frequency, Thoroughbreds, standardbreds, and quarter horses were most often affected, although many other breeds and ponies were represented. Usually only one animal in a herd or location was affected. The age of affected horses ranged from 2 months to 19 years, but over 60% were 4 years old or less. No geographic or seasonal predilection could be established.

Affected horses often have a history of recent stress, that is, shipment, heavy training or racing, foaling, and so on. Many affected horses have been moved frequently, making it difficult to determine where exposure occurred. If the onset of clinical signs is stress-related, the incubation period and seasonal occurrence would be highly variable. Clinical signs are confined to the central nervous system (CNS) and may include seizures and cranial nerve or spinal cord signs. Affected horses may stumble and fall or show weakness, ataxia, and spasticity in one or more limbs.

Preliminary seroprevalence data have been collected using immunoblot testing to detect antibodies to *S. neurona*–

specific proteins in equine serum samples (Granstrom, unpublished). Initial testing in Kentucky and Ohio detected an average exposure rate above 20% among clinically normal horses. Recent investigations conducted at the University of Kentucky laboratory on serum samples collected from horses in Ohio, Kentucky, and Pennsylvania have demonstrated an exposure rate above 40% among clinically normal horses. Exposure rates on individual farms ranged from approximately 0% to 100%. In 1978, the New York State Veterinary College at Cornell University, Ithaca, reported that 25% of all their equine neurologic disease accessions were due to EPM.[13] The number of cases diagnosed at the Livestock Disease Diagnostic Center at the University of Kentucky, Lexington, has been 8% to 9% of all neurologic accessions over the last few years. A recent report from the Ohio State University Veterinary Hospital, Columbus, revealed a 25% incidence of EPM in all horses presented with spinal ataxia from December 1991 to March 1994 based on Western blot analysis of serum and cerebrospinal fluid (CSF).[15] It is difficult to determine whether the increase is real or due to heightened awareness caused by the availability of immunoblot testing of serum and CSF. Horses that actually reach the postmortem room represent a small portion of the total number affected annually. Samples processed for immunoblot testing at the Gluck Equine Research Center, Lexington, suggest that several thousand cases occur in the United States each year. Recent evidence suggests that *Neospora* spp may also be a cause of EPM. However, *Neospora* Spp have a worldwide distribution but can be reported to be a disease of the Americas.[15a] The role of this organism in EPM is likely limited.

ETIOLOGY AND LIFE CYCLE

Sarcocystis neurona has been cultured from CNS lesions of eight horses from several different locations: New York,[10] California (three cases),[16, 17] Panama,[4] and Kentucky (three cases).[18] Preliminary morphologic, immunologic, and DNA comparisons have detected only minor differences among isolates.[4, 18] Cultured organisms multiply asexually by a type of merogony (or schizogony) known as endopolygeny, whereby many merozoites (or tachyzoites) are formed from a single nucleus.[10] This is in contrast to endodyogeny, the method of merogony that produces merozoites of *Toxoplasma gondii*. As the term implies, each individual *Toxoplasma* merozoite divides to form two new merozoites. The term *meront* (or *schizont*) refers to the small intracellular body of rapidly budding merozoites seen in histopathologic sections and in cell culture. Cultured merozoites contain a conoid, numerous micronemes, and a central nucleus, but no rhoptries.[4] This stage of *Sarcocystis* species is not known to be transmissible to other animals. Cultured merozoites have been injected epidurally, intramuscularly, intravenously, and subcutaneously without producing clinical signs in horses (Granstrom, unpublished). Transplacental infection has not been reported but cannot be ruled out.

Many normal foals have been produced by EPM-suspect mares. Recently, one of the mares was euthanized and a diagnosis of EPM was confirmed histologically. Her foal, taken at euthanasia, died of pneumonia at 8 weeks of age without neurologic signs. No lesions were present in the CNS. Although the mare was immunoblot-positive in serum and CSF, the foal was immunoblot-negative. The earliest EPM case reported occurred in a 2-month-old foal.[14] If transplacental transmission does not occur, the minimum incubation period may be 8 weeks. However, a recent case suggests the incubation period may be much shorter. Serum and CSF collected 4 days after onset of clinical signs were both negative for antibodies to *S. neurona*. Serum and CSF collected 3½ weeks later were both positive. This indicates that the parasite was ingested and caused clinical signs in the 10 to 12 days required to produce a detectable antibody response.

Sarcocystis belongs to the phylum Apicomplexa which includes several genera of coccidia that utilize an obligatory, predator-prey or scavenger-carrion life cycle.[3, 19] The host range for an individual species of *Sarcocystis* is usually narrow. *Sarcocystis* species produce sporulated oocysts by sexual reproduction (gametogony) in the gut wall of the appropriate predator or definitive host. However, the oocyst wall is very fragile and usually ruptures before being passed in the feces. Infective sporocysts are introduced into the food and water supply of the prey animal or intermediate host by fecal contamination from the predator. Birds and insects may serve as transport hosts to further disseminate sporocysts. Once ingested by the intermediate host, sporocysts excyst, releasing four sporozoites which penetrate the gut and enter arterial endothelial cells in various organs. Meronts develop rapidly and eventually rupture the host cell releasing merozoites into the bloodstream. This is usually followed by a second round of merogony in capillary endothelial cells throughout the body. Second-generation merozoites are released into the bloodstream and usually enter skeletal muscle cells where they develop into specialized meronts known as sarcocysts. Mature sarcocysts contain bradyzoites which are only able to complete the life cycle when ingested by the appropriate predator or scavenger. *Sarcocystis fayeri* uses this general method to cycle between horses and canids and is not very pathogenic in either host.[3] The prevalence of *S. fayeri* in North America has been estimated at approximately 30%, increasing with age.[20]

Sarcocysts of *S. neurona* have not been found in affected horses, precluding transmission of the parasite to the definitive host.[3, 20] The horse is an aberrant, dead-end host.[19, 20] *Sarcocystis falcatula* cycles normally between the opossum and various avian species. Sarcocysts are found in the muscles of infected birds. Opossums shed sporocysts in their feces following ingestion of the infected muscle.

It seems likely that *S. neurona* sporozoites penetrate the horse's intestinal tract, enter vascular endothelial cells, and complete at least one merogonous generation. Ultimately, merozoites must pass through the vascular endothelium of the blood-brain barrier to reach the CNS. *Sarcocystis neurona* only rarely has been observed in vascular endothelium or in leukocytes attached to endothelial lining.[19] It is uncertain whether merozoites pass through the blood-brain barrier within leukocytes or cross directly through the cytoplasm of endothelial cells. It should be possible to determine their mode of entry once large numbers of sporozoites can be introduced simultaneously by experimental infection.

The clinical severity of experimental sarcocystosis, in appropriate intermediate hosts studied, is directly related to the number of sporocysts fed.[21] It appears that the ability of any individual to resist infection is related to the size of the infective dose, immunocompetence, environmental stress, and the species of *Sarcocystis*. Some individuals may be inherently more susceptible to infection, which may have variable heritability. It seems premature to speculate about this possibility until more is learned about the pathogenesis of clinical infection.

CLINICAL SIGNS

The clinical signs of *S. neurona* infection can be quite variable. Variability of clinical signs is a reflection of the focal, multifocal, or diffuse nature of the lesions, which occur randomly in the gray and white matter of the brain, brainstem, or spinal cord. Usually the physical examination is within normal limits and the horse appears bright and alert, although focal muscle atrophy may be observed. The onset of clinical signs may be gradual, but more typically there are mild signs acutely with sometimes very rapid progression.[22–24] The neurologic examination often reveals ataxia and incoordination in all four limbs, which sometimes show lateralization, or there may be gait abnormalities with only one limb involved.[22–24] Infection with *S. neurona* can result in brainstem as well as spinal cord signs and often causes damage to the lower motor neuron of spinal cord or cranial nerves, leading to muscle atrophy. The muscle atrophy is most common in the quadriceps and gluteal regions in the hindlimbs, but also may mimic sweeney, radial paralysis, or polyneuritis equi.[23, 24] If the brainstem is involved, atrophy of the temporal-masseter muscles and occasionally the tongue may be evident along with head tilt, facial nerve paralysis, and difficulty swallowing.[22–24] It is important to carefully examine for signs of muscle wasting as well as loss of sensation along the face, neck, or body.

A frequent complaint is obscure lameness which can progress to ataxia, spasticity, and incoordination of the limbs. Poor coordination and weakness are worsened by walking with the head elevated or walking up or down a slope. The asymmetry of clinical signs is important to recognize as this can be an early indication of EPM. Horses with brainstem involvement often have head tilt, facial paralysis, loss of sensation of the cornea and internal nares, as well as dysphagia, circling, and acute recumbency.[13, 25] Some horses have a tendency to lean toward the side of the lesion and will use the wall of the stall to balance themselves. At least three horses have been observed with seizures as the only clinical signs.[26]

PATHOLOGY

Sarcocystis neurona probably causes few pathologic changes in the appropriate intermediate host. However, CNS lesions in the horse are often extensive.[6–8, 13] Multifocal areas of hemorrhage to light discoloration of the brain or spinal cord may be visible on gross examination. Lesions may be microscopic to several centimeters wide. The brainstem and spinal cord are affected most often. Microscopically, lesions are characterized by focal-to-diffuse areas of nonsuppurative inflammation and necrosis with perivascular infiltration of mononuclear cells, including lymphocytes, macrophages, and plasma cells. Giant cells, eosinophils, and gitter cells also are present in inflammatory infiltrates. Gray or white matter, or both, are affected. Organisms have been found in neurons, leukocytes, and vascular endothelium, although they tend to develop most often in neurons.[6, 7, 10, 13, 16, 22, 27–29]

IMMUNODIAGNOSIS

Immunoblot analysis of serum and CSF provides antemortem information about exposure to *S. neurona*.[30] The test utilizes cultured merozoites to detect antibodies directed against proteins that are unique to *S. neurona*. Antibodies produced to proteins shared with *S. fayeri* or other organisms can be differentiated. Unfortunately, other immunoassays are confounded by cross-reactivity with *S. fayeri* or other organisms that share antigens with *S. neurona*. Immunoblot testing of CSF has demonstrated greater than 90% specificity and sensitivity among approximately 150 neurologic cases that received postmortem examination. One half of the cases were histologically confirmed as EPM. Positive serum (specific antibody present) indicates exposure only. However, greater than 90% of histologically confirmed cases have tested seropositive.

Positive CSF indicates that parasites have penetrated the blood-brain barrier and stimulated a local immune response. If the integrity of the blood-brain barrier is compromised, circulating antibodies may leak across and produce a false-positive test result. It is especially important to determine total IgG and albumin in both serum and CSF in such cases. If the ratio of total IgG in CSF and serum is normal (IgG index) with an increase in blood-brain permeability (designated by the albumin quotient, AQ), leakage may have occurred.[31] However, if the AQ is normal or increased, along with an increase in the IgG index, intrathecal antibody production has occurred, which may be due to the presence of parasites in the CNS.[31] False-negative results have been rare, but may occur. Some horses may simply fail to respond to the *S. neurona*–specific proteins identified.

The possible causes of false-negative responses are important to consider so that affected horses are not misdiagnosed. Horses that initially tested positive have become negative after several weeks of treatment and are apparently recovered. Chronically affected horses may test negative and still be infected or the horse may still exhibit neurologic signs. We speculate that this may be due to permanent CNS damage and that parasites are either no longer present or antibody production is below test sensitivity. The use of polymerase chain reaction (PCR) testing aids in parasite detection when the antibody level is low. Acute cases that test negative should be retested in 2 to 3 weeks. However, the incubation period appears to be sufficiently long to allow production of detectable amounts of IgG before the onset of clinical signs in most cases. As was discussed before, one exception with a very short incubation period has been observed. Additional positive reactions were not observed when the immunoblot assay was modified for the detection of IgM.

DIFFERENTIAL DIAGNOSIS

Differential diagnosis for horses suspected to have *S. neurona* infection may be any disease affecting the CNS, although, depending upon the neuroanatomical localization, certain problems may be more probable. That is to say, in a horse with weakness, ataxia, and spasticity of all four limbs, with no muscle atrophy or cranial nerve deficits, the horse may have cervical vertebral stenotic myelopathy (CVM) or equine degenerative myeloencephalopathy.[13, 22, 25, 32] Both affect young horses (1–3 years of age), but CVM occurs more often in males.[13, 22, 32] The clinical signs are often symmetric with the hindlimbs usually a grade worse than the forelimbs.[13, 22, 32] The signs may be exaggerated by flexing or hyperextending the neck.[13, 24, 32]

Equine herpesvirus (EHV-1) myeloencephalitis often has an acute onset following an episode of fever, cough, and nasal discharge or following one or more abortions on a farm. This condition often affects more than one horse on a farm. Herpesvirus has a rapid onset and often results in severe hindlimb weakness and ataxia along with bladder dysfunction. Urine dribbling may sometimes occur. The ataxia and weakness is usually symmetric and may result in recumbency. Occasionally, the horses will dog-sit. Cranial nerve involvement is not common.[33–36]

Another disease that must be considered in the differential for EPM is polyneuritis equi. This disease can occur both acutely and insidiously. It is more common in mature horses and usually starts with hyperesthesia progressing to anesthesia. There is progressive paralysis of the tail, rectum, bladder, and urethra, leading to urine dribbling. Rearlimb ataxia with gluteal atrophy may be present. Asymmetric cranial nerve deficits with involvement of cranial nerves V, VII, and VIII have been reported in 50% of the cases.[37–40]

Verminous myeloencephalitis should also be considered, as the signs are extremely variable depending on the parasite's migratory pathway. Diffuse or multifocal brain and spinal cord lesions have been reported. The onset is usually sudden with rapid deterioration and death. The incidence of this disease is very low, perhaps owing to more intense parasite control.[41–43]

TREATMENT

Several regimens have been described previously for the treatment of EPM.[22–24, 44, 45] EPM has been described as successfully treated in 55% to 60% of the cases.[44] In the proceedings of the American Association of Equine Practitioners (AAEP) in 1994, 101 cases of EPM were diagnosed by clinical signs, Western blot analysis, and 22 postmortem examinations. It could be speculated that the 79 (approximately 78%) that did not die responded to therapy. The treatment has involved the combination of potentiated sulfonamides (trimethoprim-sulfas) and pyrimethamine. This combination causes a sequential blockade of folate metabolism in apicomplexan protozoa. A synergistic effect by this drug combination against *Toxoplasma* in other animal species has led to the current therapy.[45] Many veterinarians currently recommend a dosage of pyrimethamine of 0.25 to 0.5 mg/kg PO b.i.d. for 3 days, followed by the same dose once a day[44, 45] or 0.25 mg/kg body weight PO s.i.d.[23] We believe this dose is not adequate. Based on a recent pharmacokinetic study of pyrimethamine in horses, the dose required to reach the minimum inhibitory concentration (MIC) for *Toxoplasma gondii* in CSF is 1.0 mg/kg.[20, 46] The success rate of treated cases appears to be greater than 65%, or close to 80%, with no complaints of anemia or thrombocytopenia.

Still others recommend pyrimethamine at a dose of 1 to 2 mg/kg s.i.d. for 96 to 120 days; however, the increased dosage for the full term may result in anemia. Previous work using the 1-mg/kg dose of pyrimethamine once a day did

not result in anemia, but that dose was only administered for 10 days.[46] Owing to the synergistic effect of the pyrimethamine–trimethoprim-sulfa combination on the parasites, perhaps the dose of pyrimethamine could be reduced and subsequently the incidence of anemia lowered. The trimethoprim-sulfa combinations have been previously recommended at a dose of 15 to 20 mg/kg PO b.i.d. or 15 mg/kg PO t.i.d.[23, 44, 45] We recommend sulfadiazine at a dose of 20 mg/kg PO t.i.d. for the full treatment period. Most of the treatments are administered for at least 6 weeks, but must sometimes be extended to 12 weeks or more. After the initial therapy has been completed, some clinicians recommend periodic treatments when animals undergo some unusual stress. Other therapies, such as once every 2 to 4 weeks or the first week of every month, also have been used.[23, 45] However, careful controlled studies to determine the efficacy of these strategies have not been performed. Periodic treatment may lead to parasite resistance in that particular horse, resulting in the need for ever-increasing doses.

When the horse has an acute onset of EPM that results in dramatic and progressive clinical signs, the use of anti-inflammatory medications has been recommended.[23, 24, 44, 45] The use of flunixin meglumine or phenylbutazone may be helpful. The usual dose of flunixin meglumine is 1.1 mg/kg b.i.d. parenterally; intravenous administration of medical-grade dimethyl sulfoxide (Domoso, Syntex Animal Health, West Des Moines, Iowa) at a dose of 1.0 mL/kg (approximately 1 g/kg) in a 10% solution once-daily for 3 days in a row; and although not uniformly recommended, some clinicians use dexamethasone parenterally in severely affected horses at a dose rate of 0.05 mg/kg b.i.d. or sometimes empirically at 50 mg b.i.d.[23, 45] However, we believe corticosteroids should be used judiciously. The exacerbation of signs in stressed patients and reports of horses with EPM showing a worsening of signs following the use of these medications suggest immunosuppression should be avoided.[22, 25] Ancillary treatments may include padded helmets, slings, good supportive care, and a deeply bedded stall.

Many horses appear to relapse days, weeks, or months after treatment has stopped.[19, 23] Some apicomplexans have latent stages, most notably *Toxoplasma* pseudocysts and *Plasmodium* hypnozoites. *Sarcocystis* species are not known to form pseudocysts or hypnozoites. However, *Sarcocystis faculata* encephalitis in birds may persist for several months without reinfection. This phenomenon may simply represent a low-level infection and not the development of a true latent parasitic stage. *Eimeria tenella* has been shown to develop latent stages in leukocytes which reactivate after stress. A great deal concerning the life cycle of coccidia remains unknown. The ability to produce experimental infections will help determine whether *S. neurona* forms a latent stage or maintains a persistent, low-level focus of infection. Reinfection may also be responsible in some cases. The efficacy of preventive therapies is open to debate.

Because of the suspicion that protozoal infections occur more commonly in immunocompromised patients, immunomodulators or other therapies that may have a nonspecific enhancement of the immune system may be helpful. One clinician includes levamisole as part of the treatment regimen for her cases of EPM. Studies have shown that levamisole is a nonspecific immunomodulator which affects T cell–mediated immunity, including delayed-type hypersensitivity, and increases the phagocytic activity of macrophages.[47, 48] Reaction to other *Sarcocystis* species in domestic animals appears to be a delayed-type hypersensitivity reaction involving mononuclear cell infiltration.[3] The use of these products may have merit, but further investigation is necessary. It is possible that these drugs may also enhance the immunopathologic effects associated with CNS infection.

Prolonged therapy with antifolate medications should be monitored for signs of bone marrow suppression with resultant anemia, thrombocytopenia, or neutropenia.[23, 24, 45] We sometimes recommend supplementation with folic acid at a rate of 20 to 40 mg/day PO. Commercially available products are available. Folic Acid & Vitamin E Pak (Buckeye Feed Mills Inc., Dalton, Ohio), which includes vitamin E, thiamine, niacin, folic acid, and choline, is an excellent supplement. Antifolate medications may also cause reduced spermatogenesis in stallions and may be teratogenic to the fetus in mares.[23, 24, 45] Pregnant mares should routinely receive folic acid supplementation during treatment with antifolates. Acute colitis has also been associated with use of trimethoprim-sulfa combinations.

REFERENCES

1. Prickett ME: Equine spinal ataxia. *Proc Am Assoc Equine Pract* 14:147–158, 1968.
2. deBarros CSL, de Barros SS, Dos Santos MN: Equine protozoal myeloencephalitis in southern Brazil. *Vet Rec* 117:283–284, 1986.
3. Dubey JP, Speer CA, Fayer R: *Sarcocystosis of Animals and Man.* Boca Raton, Fla, CRC Press, 1989, pp 1–215.
4. Granstrom DE, Alvarez JO, Dubey JP, et al: Equine protozoal myelitis in Panamanian horses and isolation of *Sarcocystis neurona. J Parasitol* 78:909–912, 1992.
5. Masri MD, Lopez de Alda J, Dubey JP: *Sarcocystis neurona*–associated ataxia in horses in Brazil. *Vet Parasitol* 44:311–314, 1992.
6. Beech J, Dodd DC: Toxoplasma-like encephalomyelitis in the horse. *Vet Pathol* 11:87–96, 1974.
7. Cusick PK, Sells DM, Hamilton DP, et al: Toxoplasmosis in two horses. *J Am Vet Med Assoc* 164:77–80, 1974.
8. Dubey JP, Davis GW, Koestner A, et al: Equine encephalomyelitis due to a protozoan parasite resembling *Toxoplasma gondii. J Am Vet Med Assoc* 165:249–255, 1974.
9. Dubey JP: A review of *Sarcocystis* of domestic animals and other coccidia of cats and dogs. *J Am Vet Med Assoc* 169:1061–1078, 1976.
10. Dubey JP, Davis SW, Speer CA, et al: *Sarcocystis neurona* n. sp. (Protozoa: Apicomplexa), the etiologic agent of equine protozoal myeloencephalitis. *J Parasitol* 77:212–218, 1991.
11. Fenger CK, Granstrom DE, Langemeir JL, et al: Identification of the opossum *(Didelphus virginiana)* as the definitive host of *Sarcocystis neurona. J Parasitol* 81:916–919, 1995.
12. Boy MG, Galligan DT, Divers TJ: Protozoal encephalomyelitis in horses: 82 cases (1972–1986). *J Am Vet Med Assoc* 196:632–634, 1990.
13. Mayhew IG, de Lahunta A, Whitlock RH, et al: Spinal cord disease in the horse. *Cornell Vet* 68(suppl 6):1–20, 1978.
14. Fayer R, Mayhew IG, Baird JD, et al: Epidemiology of equine protozoal myeloencephalitis in North America based on histologically confirmed cases. *J Vet Intern Med* 4:54–57, 1990.
15. Reed SM, Granstrom D, Rivas LJ, et al: Results of cerebrospinal fluid analysis in 119 horses testing positive to the Western blot test on both serum and CSF to equine protozoal encephalomyelitis. *Proc Am Assoc Equine Pract* 40:199, 1994.
15a. Marsh AE, Barr BC, Madigan J, et al: Neosporosis as a cause of equine protozoal myeloencephalitis. *J Am Vet Med Assoc* 209(11):1907–1913, 1996.
16. Davis SW, Daft BN, Dubey JP: *Sarcocystis neurona* cultured in vitro from a horse with equine protozoal myelitis. *Equine Vet J* 23:315–317, 1991.
17. Davis SW, Speer CA, Dubey JP: In vitro cultivation of *Sarcocystis neurona* from the spinal cord of a horse with equine protozoal myelitis. *J Parasitol* 77:789–792, 1991.
18. Granstrom DE, MacPherson JM, Gajadhar AA, et al: Differentiation of *Sarcocystis neurona* from eight related coccidia by random amplified polymorphic DNA assay. *J Mol Cell Probes* 8:353–356, 1994.
19. Fayer R, Dubey JP: Comparative epidemiology of coccidia: Clues to the etiology of equine protozoal myeloencephalitis. *Int J Parasitol* 17:615–620, 1987.
20. Granstrom DE, Dubey JP, Giles RC, et al: Equine protozoal myeloencephalitis: Biology and epidemiology. In Nakajima H, Plowright W: Refereed Proceedings. R & W Publications (Newmarket) Ltd, 1994.
21. Cawthorn RJ, Speer CA: *Sarcocystis:* Infection and disease of humans, livestock, wildlife and other hosts. In Long PL, ed: *Coccidiosis of Man and Animals.* Boca Raton, Fla, CRC Press, 1990, pp 91–120.
22. Madigan JE, Higgins RJ: Neurologic disease: Equine protozoal myeloencephalitis. *Vet Clin North Am Equine Pract* 3:397–403, 1987.
23. MacKay RJ, Davis SW, Dubey JP: Equine protozoal myeloencephalitis. *Compend Contin Educ Pract Vet* 14:1359–1366, 1992.
24. Cox JH, Murray RC, DeBowes RM: Diseases of the spinal cord. In Kobluk CN, Ames TR, Geor RJ, eds: *The Horse Diseases and Clinical Management.* Philadelphia, WB Saunders, 1995, pp 443–472.
25. Mayhew IG, deLahunta A, Whitlock RH, et al: Equine protozoal myeloencephalitis. *Proc Am Assoc Equine Pract* 22:107–114, 1976.
26. Dunigan CE, Oglesbee MJ, Mitten LA, et al: Seizure activity associated with equine protozoal myeloencephalitis. *Prog Vet Neurol* 6(2):50–54, 1995.
27. Clark EG, Townsend HGG, McKenzie NT: Equine protozoal myeloencephalitis: A report of two cases from western Canada. *Can Vet J* 22:140–144, 1981.
28. Dorr TE, Higgins RJ, Dangler CA, et al: Protozoal myeloencephalitis in horses in California. *J Am Vet Med Assoc* 185:801–802, 1984.
29. Bowman DD: Equine protozoal myeloencephalitis: History and recent developments. *Equine Pract* 13:28–33, 1991.
30. Granstrom DE, Dubey JP, Davis SW, et al: Equine protozoal myeloencephalitis: Antigen analysis of cultured *Sarcocystis neurona* merozoites. *J Vet Diagn Invest* 5:88–90, 1993.
31. Andrews FM, Maddux JM, Faulk D: Total protein, albumin quotient, IgG and IgG index determinations for horse cerebrospinal fluid. *Prog Vet Neurol* 1:197–204, 1991.
32. Nixon AJ, Stashak TS, Ingram JT: Diagnosis of cervical vertebral malformation in the horse. *Proc Am Assoc Equine Pract* 28:253–266, 1982.
33. Jackson T, Kendrick JW: Paralysis of horses associated with equine herpesvirus 1 infection. *J Am Vet Med Assoc* 158:1351–1357, 1971.
34. Ostlund EN, Powell D, Bryans JT: Equine herpesvirus 1: A review. *Proc Am Assoc Equine Pract* 36:387–395, 1990.
35. Ostlund EN: The equine herpesviruses. *Vet Clin North Am Equine Pract* 9:283–294, 1993.
36. Wilson JH, Erickson DM: Neurological syndrome of rhinopneumonitis. *Proc Am Coll Vet Intern Med Forum* 9:419–421, 1991.

37. Beech J: Neuritis of the cauda equina. *Proc Am Assoc Equine Pract* 22:75–76, 1976.

38. Greenwood AG, Barker J, McLeish I: Neuritis of the cauda equina in a horse. *Equine Vet J* 5:111–115, 1973.

39. Rousseaux CG, Futcher KG, Clark EG, et al: Cauda equina neuritis: A chronic idiopathic polyneuritis in two horses. *Can Vet J* 25:214–218, 1984.

40. White PL, Genetzky RM, Pohlenz JFL: Neuritis of the cauda equina in a horse. *Compend Contin Educ Pract Vet* 6:S217–S224, 1984.

41. Blunden AS, Khalil LF, Webbon PM: *Halicephalobus deletrix* infection in a horse. *Equine Vet J* 19:255, 1987.

42. Lester G: Parasitic encephalomyelitis in horses. *Compend Contin Educ Pract Vet* 14:1624–1630, 1992.

43. Mayhew IG, Brewer BD, Reinhard MK, et al: Verminous (*Strongylus vulgaris*) myelitis in a donkey. *Cornell Vet* 74:30–37, 1984.

44. Reed SM, Granstrom DE: Equine protozoal encephalomyelitis. *Proc Am Coll Vet Intern Med Forum* 11:591–592, 1993.

45. Welsch BB: Update on equine therapeutics: Treatment of equine protozoal myeloencephalitis. *Compend Contin Educ Pract Vet* 13:1599–1602, 1991.

46. Clarke CR, MacAllister CG, Burrows GE, et al: Pharmacokinetics, penetration into cerebrospinal fluid, and hematologic effects after multiple oral administrations of pyrimethamine to horses. *Am J Vet Res* 53:2296–2299, 1992.

47. Hoebeke J, Franchi G: Influence of tetramisole and its optical isomers on the mononuclear phagocytic system: effect of carbon clearance in mice. *J Reticuloendothel Soc* 14:317–323, 1973.

48. Renoux G, Renoux M, Teller MN, et al: Potentiation of T cell–mediated immunity by levamisole. *Clin Exp Immunol* 75:288–296, 1976.

9.11

Equine Herpesvirus 1 Myeloencephalopathy

W. David Wilson, BVMS, MS

A diffuse multifocal hemorrhagic myeloencephalopathy with leptomeningeal vasculitis occurs in a small proportion of horses infected with equine herpesvirus type 1 (EHV-1), one of four distinct herpesviruses known to cause disease in horses.[1–4] The classification of these viruses, designated EHV-1 (equine abortion virus), EHV-2 (equine cytomegalovirus), EHV-3 (equine coital exanthema virus), and EHV-4 (equine rhinopneumonitis virus), reflects differences between them with regard to their pathogenicity, epidemiology, antigenicity, genetic composition, and other features.[2, 4, 5] Until recently, EHV-1 and EHV-4 were thought to be a single virus (EHV-1) capable of causing respiratory disease, abortion, early neonatal death, and neurologic disease in horses. However, major antigenic differences corresponding to the site of isolation (fetal or respiratory) of EHV-1 strains have been observed for many years.[6, 7] Restriction endonuclease fingerprint analysis of viral DNA and serologic testing subse-quently confirmed the existence of two distinct viruses with less than 20% homology of their DNA sequences and substantial differences in two of the six major antigenic sites.[5, 8–13] Although these alphaherpesviruses, initially designated EHV-1, subtype 1 (EHV-1) and EHV-1, subtype 2 (EHV-4), can now be readily differentiated by cultural characteristics and serologic testing using specific monoclonal antibodies, as well as by analysis of viral DNA,[2, 5, 8–10, 13–16] these tests are not routinely performed in many diagnostic laboratories. While EHV-1 can cause abortion, neonatal disease, myeloencephalopathy, and respiratory disease, EHV-4 rarely causes abortion or neonatal disease and there is only one report of its isolation from a horse with neurologic disease.[5, 11–13, 17] In contrast, EHV-4 is an important respiratory pathogen and a more common cause of respiratory disease in young horses than is EHV-1.[5, 11, 13]

Restriction endonuclease fingerprinting of DNA has permitted further subclassification of EHV-1 into two electropherogram genotypes, 1P and 1B.[12, 18] The majority of EHV-1 abortions in the United States prior to 1981 were caused by subtype 1P, whereas subtype 1B has been responsible for the majority of abortions investigated since that time, although both subtypes continue to be active in the horse population.[5, 12, 18] It is likely that both subtypes 1P and 1B are capable of causing neurologic disease, although this has not been documented.

EPIDEMIOLOGY

The first definitive association between EHV-1 and myeloencephalopathy was made in 1966 in Norway with the isolation of the virus from the brain and spinal cord of a horse that showed signs of severe neurologic dysfunction.[19] However, descriptions of a clinical syndrome resembling EHV-1 myeloencephalopathy first appeared in the late nineteenth century.[20] The myeloencephalopathic form of EHV-1 infection is now considered to have a worldwide distribution, having been recognized in Denmark,[21, 22] Germany,[23] Sweden,[24] Austria,[25] Britain,[26–28] Ireland,[29] Australia,[30] India,[31] the United States,[3, 32–37] and Canada.[38–42]

In view of the ubiquitous occurrence of EHV-1 infection in horse populations, outbreaks of EHV-1 myeloencephalopathy are rare. The special circumstances that predispose to their occurrence are at present undefined.[37, 43] In many instances, cases of neurologic EHV-1 infection occur in association with outbreaks of abortion or respiratory disease, although some outbreaks occur in the absence of other manifestations of EHV-1 infection and without the introduction of new horses into the group. Recrudescence of latent infection or contact with inapparently infected horses may be the source of infection under these circumstances.[5, 43–45] Virus may be shed by clinically affected and inapparently infected horses for up to 2 weeks in infected aerosols, ocular and nasal secretions, saliva, and feces, in addition to the products of EHV-1 abortions.[46] Disease spread is by direct horse-to-horse contact, inhalation of aerosols of virus-containing secretions, contact with contaminated equipment and clothing, and trafficking of horses on the farm and between one property and another.[5, 46] EHV-1 may remain infective in the environment for up to 14 days and on horse hair for 35 to 42 days.[47]

The myeloencephalopathic form of EHV-1 infection may occur as sporadic individual cases or, more often, as outbreaks involving multiple individuals over a period of several weeks on a single farm, stable, or racetrack, or on several premises within a limited geographical region.[19, 21–28, 31, 35–42, 48] Secondary or tertiary waves of clinical disease may occur as previously unexposed horses become infected from a common source over a short period of time.[5, 26] Morbidity rates ranging from less than 1% to almost 90% of exposed individuals, and mortality rates ranging from 0.5% to 40% of in-contact horses have been reported.[3, 22, 24, 27, 35–40, 42, 48] Neurologic EHV-1 infection can occur at any time of year, but the highest incidence is in late winter, spring, and early summer, perhaps reflecting the seasonal occurrence of abortigenic EHV-1 infections during the same months.[37]

Experimentally, the neurologic form of EHV-1 infection is most readily induced in pregnant mares, and some field studies suggest that pregnant mares may be at increased risk.[26, 27, 32, 33] Pregnancy is not, however, a prerequisite for infection of the central nervous system (CNS) and field cases have been observed in nonpregnant mares, geldings, stallions, and foals,[3, 5, 19, 23, 26, 27, 30, 34–39, 42] although foals appear to be affected less often and less severely than mature horses.[26] In experimental studies of pregnant mares, the stage of gestation appears to be important in determining the outcome of infection.[32, 33] Mares infected during the first two trimesters of gestation are more likely to develop neurologic signs without abortion, whereas mares infected during the last trimester are likely to abort without showing neurologic signs.[33] Similarly, in field outbreaks, it is not common to see neurologic signs in mares that also abort, although this has been recorded.[5, 23, 27, 41, 49]

All breeds of horses appear to be susceptible to the neurologic form of EHV-1 infection and other equids may also be affected. EHV-1 was the suspected cause of myeloencephalopathy which developed in a zebra 1 week after an in-contact onager (*Equus hemionus* subsp. *onager*) aborted an EHV-1-infected fetus.[50] I am unaware of reports of neurologic EHV-1 affecting donkeys and mules, although donkeys and mules have shown seroconversion indicating infection with EHV-1 while in contact with affected horses during outbreaks.[35, 36, 48] Indeed, donkeys and mules returning from a show were thought to be responsible for dissemination of EHV-1 and propagation of multiple outbreaks of neurologic EHV-1 infection in Southern California in 1984.[48] It is not known whether a donkey-adapted variant of EHV-1 with an increased neuropathogenicity in horses plays a role in outbreaks of EHV-1 myeloencephalopathy. However, the isolation from donkeys of an alphaherpesvirus, designated asinine herpesvirus 3 (AHV-3), closely related to EHV-1, has led to the hypothesis that EHV-1 may be recently derived from a donkey virus and that donkeys may remain an alternative host for EHV-1, serving as a reservoir to infect horses.[2]

Severe neurologic EHV-1 was reported in two geldings and one pregnant mare 8 to 11 days after administration of a modified live EHV-1 vaccine of monkey cell line origin.[34] This vaccine was subsequently shown to be associated with neurologic disease in 486 of 60,000 recipients, prompting its withdrawal from the market in 1977.[9] There are no reports of EHV-1 myeloencephalopathy associated with recent use of the modified live vaccine currently approved for horses.

PATHOGENESIS

The acute onset of clinical signs of EHV-1 myeloencephalopathy is the result of vasculitis of arterioles in the brain and especially the spinal cord. This causes functional impairment of blood flow and metabolic exchange and, in severe cases, hypoxic degeneration and necrosis with hemorrhage into adjacent neural tissue of the white and, to a lesser extent, gray matter.[5, 32, 33, 40, 41, 43, 51]

Acquisition of EHV-1 infection is followed by attachment of the virus to, and replication in, the epithelium of the nose, pharynx, trachea, and bronchi.[5] From these sites it is disseminated to lymphoid follicles of the pharynx and regional lymph nodes of the respiratory tract.[5] Extension of infection beyond the respiratory tract mucosa and draining lymph nodes occurs through infection of local inflammatory cells and entry of virus-infected monocytes and lymphocytes into the bloodstream to establish a viremia associated with buffy coat cells, particularly T lymphocytes.[5, 13, 52] The intracellular site appears to be immunologically privileged since virus can be recovered from buffy coat cells in the presence of high levels of neutralizing antibody.[53] Like other herpesviruses, EHV-1 is capable of spreading directly from one infected cell to contiguous cells without an extracellular phase.[5] Replication of virus in vascular endothelium is important for systemic dissemination of EHV-1 and appears to be the mechanism by which EHV-1 reaches secondary target organs from the circulating intraleukocytic location in the presence of neutralizing antibody.[33, 54, 55] In experimental infections, the endothelium of arterioles appears to be the initial site of infection within the CNS.[33, 54] Viremia can occur during primary and all successive infections with EHV-1, even when no clinical signs are apparent; thus all EHV-1 infections pose a threat of inducing neurologic disease or abortion.[13]

There is no satisfactory explanation as to why some outbreaks of EHV-1 infection are associated with a high incidence of neurologic disease, while others are not, or why, during outbreaks, different horses show different clinical manifestations of EHV-1 infection.[28] In contrast to the observation by Studdert and coworkers[30] that those strains of EHV-1 which show a propensity to induce neurologic disease may be differentiated from other EHV-1 strains by restriction endonuclease analysis, other workers have been unable to demonstrate definitive biological or genetic markers for neuropathogenicity.[25, 56]

Encephalitic herpesvirus infections, such as herpes simplex in humans, infectious bovine rhinotracheitis (IBR) in cattle, and pseudorabies in pigs, demonstrate a primary neurotropism with viral replication and inclusion bodies in neurons, and neurophagia.[37] In contrast, EHV-1 did not appear to be neurotropic, even after direct inoculation into the equine brain,[33, 57] whereas subcutaneous inoculation of the same strain (Army 183) resulted in a paralytic syndrome characterized by severe vasculitis.[32, 33] Intracerebral inoculation studies in suckling mice, and the application of sensitive immunoperoxidase staining techniques to tissues from clinical cases, further indicate that the propensity of certain EHV-1 isolates to induce myeloencephalopathy does not reflect specific neurotropism, but, rather, a marked endotheliotropism.[28, 32, 33, 54–56, 58] Unlike the inflammation observed in EHV-1-infected tissues elsewhere in the body, where parenchymal cells are directly involved and inclusion bodies are present, axonal swelling and malacic foci in the CNS appear to develop secondary to ischemia resulting from vasculitis and thrombosis of small vessels.[21, 28, 32, 33, 40, 43, 54, 55]

The nature and extent of lesions resulting from EHV-1 infection likely also reflect the age and immune status of the horse, the amount of challenge, and perhaps the route of infection.[28] Endothelial cell infection and perivascular cuffing within the CNS appeared to be at least as pronounced in foals that died during an EHV-1 outbreak without showing neurologic signs, as in two severely paretic mares that died or were destroyed during the same outbreak.[28] Despite the presence of viral antigen in small veins and arterioles of the gray matter, white matter, and meninges of the cerebrum, medulla, and spinal cord of the foals, parenchymal CNS lesions were minimal and clinical signs of neurologic disease were absent.[28] It is likely that the majority of EHV-1 infections that cause neurologic signs represent reinfection rather than a new infection.[22, 24, 59] Neurologic EHV-1 infection has been observed in regularly vaccinated horses.[3, 36, 37, 42] Myeloencephalopathy was readily induced in mares with significant preexisting serum levels of neutralizing antibody and those mares that developed the most severe clinical signs were also the ones that showed the most rapid increase in titer after infection.[32, 33]

In addition, the characteristic vascular lesions seen in neural tissues of affected horses are typical of type III (Arthus) hypersensitivity reactions, suggesting that the myeloencephalopathic form of EHV-1 may be the result of immune-complex vasculitis rather than of direct viral infection of neural tissues.[5, 24, 32, 33, 44, 59] The presence of circulating immune complexes has been demonstrated at the onset of clinical signs of neurologic disease and corresponds to high serum levels of complement-fixing (CF) and neutralizing antibody to EHV-1.[54] An immune-mediated mechanism is further supported by the difficulty experienced in isolating the virus from neural tissues of affected horses compared with the relative ease with which it can be isolated from the respiratory tract and from aborted fetuses in other forms of EHV-1 infection.[28, 39, 43] In addition, assessment of risk factors during outbreaks of neurologic EHV-1 infection in Southern California in 1984 revealed that horses vaccinated with either killed or modified live EHV-1 vaccine within the previous year were significantly (9–14 times) more likely to develop neurologic manifestations of infection than were non-vaccinated horses.[48]

An alternative immune-mediated mechanism was investigated by Klingeborn and coworkers[59] who documented the presence of circulating antibodies to the neuritogenic myelin protein P2 in the serum of horses that died from EHV-1 myeloencephalopathy but not in horses that recovered. At this time, it is not known whether this antibody plays a role in the pathogenesis of neurologic EHV-1 infection or whether it represents leakage of neuritogenic myelin protein P2 after damage induced by another mechanism.

Evidence for an immune-mediated pathogenesis for EHV-1 myeloencephalopathy is by no means conclusive. In experimental EHV-1 infections in which the onset of neurologic signs correlated with a peak in the level of circulating immune complexes, vasculitis was not present in vessels in which endothelial cells did not support viral replication, nor in organs such as the kidney that would be expected to trap circulating immune complexes.[54] In addition, the onset of neurologic signs 8 to 9 days post infection was correlated with an increase in circulating CF antibody and a return toward normal of platelet counts which had become markedly depressed 2 days after experimental infection, presumably as a result of consumption in thrombi secondary to endothelial damage. These findings suggest that the neuropathologic changes are initiated before circulating immune complexes peak and that the action of immune complexes is secondary and localized.[54] Failure to isolate the virus from the CNS may be attributable to high levels of circulating antibody and to the endotheliotropism of the virus.[54]

PATHOLOGY

Lesions are frequently not confined to the CNS of horses with EHV-1 myeloencephalopathy. Widespread hemorrhagic and inflammatory changes of mild-to-moderate degree may be seen in the nasal passages, guttural pouches, posterior trachea, and pulmonary parenchyma, with draining lymph nodes showing edema or hemorrhage.[28, 32, 33, 43, 58] Vasculitis and well-demarcated areas of necrosis may be present in the endometrium of affected pregnant mares, even those that do not abort.[33] Subcutaneous congestion and hemorrhage resulting from self-inflicted trauma or recumbency are also common findings.[28, 33, 43] In horses that die from EHV-1 myeloencephalopathy, pulmonary congestion, pneumonia, bowel atony, impaction, intussusception, cystitis, and rupture of the urinary bladder are frequent findings.[5]

Gross pathologic lesions in the CNS are frequently not observed in horses that die or are euthanized because of EHV-1 myeloencephalopathy.[5, 28, 33, 41, 43] In others, small (2–6 mm) focal areas of hemorrhage are distributed randomly throughout the meninges and parenchyma of the brain and spinal cord.[5, 33, 41–43] More diffuse dural hemorrhage is noted in some cases and may extend to spinal nerve roots and the cauda equina.[32, 33, 43] Small plum-colored areas of degeneration and hemorrhage are sometimes grossly visible in fresh tissue at various levels of the spinal cord, and malacic foci may be seen macroscopically in sliced fixed sections of brain.[32, 33, 41–43]

The gross and histologic lesions in the CNS reflect vasculitis, congestion, and secondary degeneration of nervous tissue.[28, 32, 33, 41, 43] While vasculitis is a consistent finding, degeneration of nervous tissue is evident chiefly in those horses with clinical evidence of severe neurologic disease.[28, 33] The vasculitis is often severe and has a widespread, random, multifocal distribution, which may involve the cerebrum and cerebellum, although the most severe lesions are usually seen in the brainstem and spinal cord.[28, 32, 33, 43] In some instances, sheaths of nerve roots and nerves, and capsules of ganglia are also involved.[28, 32, 33, 43] Trigeminal ganglionitis may be present but is usually not manifest clinically.[40]

The orientation of affected blood vessels and resulting lesions is rather consistent, both in the brain and spinal cord.[33] In the brain, the meningeal and penetrating or radiating vessels in gray matter are the major sites of vascular involvement. Thus foci of axonal swelling and malacia develop in the gray and white matter, particularly adjacent to the meningeal surface and in the deep cortex adjacent to the white matter.[32, 33, 43] In the spinal cord, a similar orientation to meningeal vessels results in degeneration of white matter within ovoid, linear, or wedge-shaped foci affecting predominantly the lateral and the ventral white columns.[33] The axes of these foci extend toward the central canal and the base of the wedge-shaped lesions is oriented toward the meningeal surface.[33] Less commonly, small foci of malacia are found in spinal gray matter.[33]

Early changes in affected blood vessels include proliferation of endothelial cells, some of which may appear multinucleate, followed by endothelial cell necrosis and inflammatory cell infiltration involving the endothelium, subendothelium, tunica intima, and tunica media.[33] The cellular response to endothelial necrosis initially involves neutrophils, but later lymphocytes become the predominant cell type.[33] Necrosis of the tunica intima and media in more severely affected arteries leads to disruption of vessel walls of focal or segmental extent and may be accompanied by thrombosis as dense aggregates of leukocytes, erythrocytes, and platelets accumulate as cellular thrombi adjacent to damaged endothelium.[32, 33, 43] Necrosis of vessel walls leads to hemorrhage and extravasation of plasma protein into the perivascular spaces and consequent congestion.[33, 43] In lesions of longer standing, thrombosis and necrosis become much less prominent and are succeeded by progressive segmental accumulation of lymphocytes, macrophages, and plasma cells in the adventitia as large dense cellular cuffs around meningeal and surface-oriented vessels, especially the arteries.[28, 33]

In experimental infections, malacic foci are first visible 7 days after infection as neuropil vacuolation and cellular necrosis with few macrophages present initially.[33] Reactive changes in and around malacic foci tend to correlate with the duration of severe paralysis, although foci of differing ages may be observed in the same brain, as can variation in the extent of vessel wall necrosis and thrombosis compared with perivascular cuffing.[33, 43] In horses that have shown signs for several days to a week or more prior to death, malacic foci may be invaded and lined by macrophages containing abundant phagocytosed lipid materials, accompanied by occasional plasma cells, with swelling and degeneration evident in oligodendroglia in local white matter and early gliosis in some cases.[32, 33, 43] Involvement of neurons is minimal and no neurophagia is present.[32, 43] Arterial thrombosis, while a common feature, is not a prerequisite for the development of foci of malacia since such foci have been seen in association with perivascular cuffing in the absence of thrombosis.[28] It is possible that partial or complete occlusion of thin-walled vessels might result from compression caused by perivascular cellular infiltration.[28]

Ocular lesions, including uveal vasculitis with perivascular mononuclear cell cuffing in the ciliary body and optic nerve, and extensive retinal degeneration, have been observed in field and experimental EHV-1 infections.[28, 33, 43, 60] EHV-1-induced uveal vasculitis may have been responsible for the clinical signs of bilateral hypopyon and iritis observed in three foals during an outbreak of paresis.[26] In addition, EHV-1 was likely the cause of severe visual impairment and chorioretinopathy, without anterior segment involvement, which developed following resolution of clinical signs of respiratory disease 28 days after experimental infection of a 3-month-old foal with EHV-1.[60] The presence of similar lesions in other experimentally infected foals has led to the suggestion that EHV-1 may produce ocular and neural damage in the absence of gross signs of neurologic or visual impairment.[60] During paralytic infections, secondary viral replication occurs in blood vessels of the testis and epididymis in addition to the CNS, and may be responsible for reported signs of scrotal edema and loss of libido in affected stallions.[26, 61]

CLINICAL SIGNS

In experimental infections, neurologic signs appear 6 to 10 days after infection by the intranasal or subcutaneous routes.[32, 33, 38, 54, 55, 58, 62] The incubation period appears to be of similar length in field cases and is slightly shorter than that required for EHV-1 abortion, perhaps reflecting the more rapid manifestation of signs of anoxia in the CNS as compared to the endometrium and fetus.[55] The onset of neurologic signs may be preceded or accompanied by signs of upper respiratory disease, fever, inappetence, or hindlimb edema within the previous 2 weeks, although in many instances no antecedent disease is noted.[3, 26, 27, 37, 41, 63, 64] There is, however, frequently a herd or stable history of current or recent cases of respiratory tract infection, fever, inappetence, distal limb edema, abortion, neonatal death, foal diarrhea, or neurologic disease.[26, 27, 35, 37]

Affected horses are occasionally febrile at the onset of neurologic disease, although most are normothermic and some are hypothermic.[26, 27, 51, 63–65] Neurologic signs are generally of acute or peracute onset, after which they tend to stabilize rapidly and generally do not progress after the first 1 or 2 days.[1, 3, 22, 26, 27, 37, 49, 66] Clinical signs are highly variable, reflecting the location and severity of lesions.[5, 37] However, clinical signs in most horses predominantly reflect involvement of the spinal white matter.[37] Ataxia and paresis of the limbs are the predominant signs, with hypotonia of the tail and anus, tail elevation, and urinary incontinence being common but not invariable findings.[22, 27, 37, 49, 64] Clinical signs are usually bilaterally symmetric or only mildly asymmetric, although hemiparesis, or sudden onset of unilateral hind- or forelimb lameness progressing to unilateral or more generalized ataxia, paresis, and recumbency, have been reported.[1, 37, 40, 51] Lesions in peripheral nerves, as well as the spinal cord, were observed in some of these cases.[40]

The hindlimbs are generally affected more severely and earlier in the disease course than the front limbs.[1, 3, 37, 49, 51, 65] In mildly affected horses, transient ataxia and stiffness of the pelvic limbs or dribbling of urine secondary to overflow from a distended atonic bladder may be the only signs noted.[27, 37] Conscious proprioceptive deficits in these cases may be noted as reluctance to move, clumsiness, toe-dragging, knuckling, stumbling, pivoting, and circumduction in one or more limbs on circling, with spasticity evident in some cases.[26, 37, 65] These signs may be very subtle and it is likely that they go unnoticed in some cases. More severely affected horses show more profound limb weakness and swaying of the hindquarters, and a small proportion show complete paralysis of affected limbs, manifest as paraplegia and dog-sitting, complete recumbency, or tetraplegia.[5, 37, 65] Affected stallions and geldings may develop penile flaccidity and paraphimosis or repeated erections, while vulvar flaccidity may be noted in mares.[5, 22, 26, 49, 64, 65] In addition, stallions may experience reduced libido and swelling of the testes.[28] Edema of the scrotum may accompany hindlimb edema at the onset of neurologic signs in some cases.[26–28, 41, 49] Distention of the urinary bladder is common and may cause signs of colic or dribbling of urine which frequently results in scalding of the perineum, legs, and other areas.[36] Cystitis is a frequent complication, particularly when repeated catheterization is necessary to relieve bladder distention.[66]

Sensory deficits are uncommon, but perineal hypalgia or analgesia has been noted[22, 27, 65] and analgesia of the caudal half of the body was observed in one affected horse.[37] Consistent with predominant involvement of the white matter of the spinal cord, flexor reflexes are normal and perineal reflexes are preserved.[37] In recumbent horses, spinal tendon reflexes can be tested and may be increased.[37] Atrophy is rarely seen, even in the later stages of the disease.[37]

Affected horses usually remain alert and have a good appetite, even when recumbent, although some show modest depression and inappetence.[26, 64] Severe depression, when it occurs, is more often due to secondary complications than to primary brain involvement.[64] Unequivocal signs of brain disease are rare, although infarction of the brainstem may lead to depressed sensorium, altered behavior, and cranial nerve damage resulting in vestibular signs and in lingual, mandibular, and pharyngeal paresis, which may manifest as dysphagia.[1, 23, 42, 49, 63, 64] Strabismus, nystagmus, circling, and head tilt have been observed on occasion.[23, 37, 42, 65] Signs of cerebellar disease are rare because the cerebellum is relatively spared in EHV-1 myeloencephalopathy.[28]

Affected horses show variable progression of clinical signs. Those that are mildly affected frequently stabilize rapidly over a period of hours to a few days as edema and hemorrhage resolve, and generally recover completely over a period of days to several weeks.[22, 26, 65] If recumbency occurs, it generally does so during the first 24 hours, with some horses showing such complete motor paralysis that they are unable to lift their heads.[40] Severely affected horses may show progression of signs during the first few days and may die in coma or convulsion or be euthanized because of secondary complications.[65]

DIAGNOSIS

The multifocal distribution of lesions in EHV-1 myeloencephalopathy results in variability of clinical presentation, necessitating the inclusion of a number of conditions in the differential diagnosis. These include equine protozoal myeloencephalitis, cervical stenotic myelopathy and cervical vertebral instability (wobbler syndrome), cervical vertebral fracture or other CNS trauma, neuritis of the cauda equina, fibrocartilaginous infarction, aberrant parasite migration, degenerative myelopathy, rabies, botulism, togaviral encephalitis, CNS abscess, and a variety of plant and chemical intoxications.[3, 37]

Sudden onset and early stabilization of neurologic signs, including ataxia, paresis, and urinary incontinence; involvement of multiple horses on the premises; and a recent history of fever, abortion, or viral respiratory disease in the affected horse or its herdmates is sufficient to make a tentative diagnosis of EHV-1 myeloencephalopathy.[3] Antemortem diagnosis is further supported by the ruling out of other conditions; demonstration of xanthochromia and elevated protein concentration in cerebrospinal fluid (CSF); isolation of EHV-1 from the respiratory tract, buffy coat, or CSF; and demonstration of a fourfold increase in serum-neutralizing (SN) or CF antibodies in acute and convalescent serum samples collected 7 to 21 days apart.[67] However, antemortem confirmation of a diagnosis of EHV-1 myeloencephalitis is frequently not possible, particularly when an individual horse is affected, because the above tests do not yield consistent results in all cases.

Xanthochromia and an increased protein concentration (100–500 mg/dL) in CSF are anticipated but not invariable findings, reflecting vasculitis and protein leakage into CSF.[1, 28, 32, 33, 37, 43, 51, 66] The white blood cell count in CSF is usually normal (0–5 cells per deciliter), but is occasionally increased.[1, 28, 32, 33, 37, 43, 51, 66] Abnormalities in CSF are not present at the onset of clinical signs in some horses and changes resolve rather quickly; thus the CSF may be normal within 2 weeks of onset of clinical signs.[33, 37, 66] Fewer than half (11/24) of the horses with EHV-1 myeloencephalopathy reviewed in one university study had elevated CSF protein concentrations, and of these, none had abnormal cell counts.[37]

Antibodies to EHV-1 are absent from the CSF of normal horses, even in the presence of high serum titers following vaccination with a modified live EHV-1 vaccine.[67] In experimentally induced EHV-1 myeloencephalopathy, neutralizing antibody titers in CSF were consistently increased, ranging from 2.4 to 23.0 within 6 to 15 days following experimental inoculation.[33] While the finding of antibodies to EHV-1 in the CSF of field cases is strongly suggestive of a diagnosis of EHV-1 myeloencephalopathy, such antibodies are absent in many cases.[3, 23, 33, 37, 59] The presence of EHV-1 antibodies in the CSF likely reflects leakage across a damaged blood-brain or blood-CSF barrier secondary to vasculitis rather than local antibody production within the CNS.[59, 68] Since the ratio of CSF albumin to serum albumin is elevated in these horses, neutralizing antibodies are more likely to be present in the CSF of affected horses with concomitantly high serum titers.[33, 37, 59]

Blood contamination during collection of CSF and other diseases that cause an increase in the permeability of the blood-brain barrier, or bleeding into the subarachnoid space, may falsely elevate CSF antibody titers if serum titers are also high. Such a situation was observed in a horse with a fractured petrous temporal bone and evidence of hemorrhage into the CSF.[67] Caution should therefore be exercised in the interpretation of EHV-1 neutralizing antibody titers in CSF, and both the serum titer and CSF albumin concentration should be taken into account. It has been suggested, based on a study of four horses (one of which had viral encephalitis) with low EHV-1 neutralizing antibody titers detectable in CSF, that a positive CSF antibody titer may have increased diagnostic significance when the ratio of serum titer to CSF titer is less than 96.[68] This observation remains to be confirmed by comparison of the results from a large number of affected and unaffected horses.

Isolation of EHV-1 from the CSF of affected horses would confirm a diagnosis, but is rarely successful.[36, 37, 59] Similarly, isolation of EHV-1 from nasopharyngeal swabs or buffy coat samples is strongly supportive of a diagnosis of EHV-1 myeloencephalitis and should be attempted by submission of nasopharyngeal swabs and citrated or heparinized blood.[3, 13, 37, 69] However, the results may be negative because the peak of virus shedding has usually passed by the time neurologic signs appear.[69] Thus, the likelihood of isolating EHV-1 during outbreaks of neurologic disease is increased by monitoring in-contact horses and collecting nasal swab and buffy coat samples during the prodromal febrile phase before neurologic signs develop.[26] Even so, interpretation of positive culture results can be confused by the fact that both EHV-1 and EHV-4 have been isolated from the respiratory tract of normal horses.[46] In addition, EHV-4 is not distinguished from EHV-1 using routine procedures employed by many diagnostic laboratories.

The polymerase chain reaction (PCR) technique has been shown to be more sensitive than virus isolation for detecting viral antigen in nasopharyngeal swabs collected from horses with respiratory tract disease caused by EHV-1 or EHV-4.[70] Application of this technique, or immunodiagnostic techniques such as indirect immunoperoxidase staining, to nasopharyngeal, buffy coat, or CSF samples collected from horses with suspected EHV-1 myeloencephalopathy shows great promise for improving the sensitivity of antemortem diagnosis.

Demonstration of a fourfold or greater increase in serum antibody titer, using SN or CF tests on acute and convalescent samples collected 7 to 21 days apart, provides presumptive evidence of infection.[3, 5, 22, 35, 42, 64, 69] However, many affected horses do not show a fourfold rise in SN titer and some actually show a decline. Of 22 horses on which paired samples were tested during investigation of an outbreak of suspected EHV-1 myeloencephalopathy in southern California, only 3 affected horses showed a fourfold or greater increase in SN titer, while 8 showed increases ranging from one- to threefold, 5 showed no titer change, and 4 showed decreases in titer ranging from one- to threefold.[36] More than half of the affected horses retained low titers (1:32 or less) in convalescent samples.[36] This may be explained by the finding that, when antibody titers rise, they do so rapidly, within 6 to 10 days of infection, so that they may have already peaked by the time neurologic signs appear.[32, 33, 35, 62, 69] While serologic SN testing has limitations in confirming a diagnosis of EHV-1 myeloencephalopathy in an individual horse, testing of paired serum samples from in-contact horses is recommended because a significant proportion of both affected and unaffected in-contact horses will seroconvert, providing indirect evidence that EHV-1 is the etiologic agent.[3, 35, 36, 42]

When horses with suspected EHV-1 myeloencephalopathy die or are euthanized, the whole carcass or the head, spine, spleen, thyroid, and lung should be submitted for postmortem examination.[46] Whereas widespread multifocal vasculitis with thrombosis and secondary ischemic degeneration of neural tissue is typically found and is considered diagnostic for EHV-1 infection, the virus is infrequently isolated from the CNS of affected horses.[5, 23, 28, 30, 37, 40–42, 54, 62] Thus attempts should be made to isolate the virus from other sites to support the diagnosis. Those sites most likely to yield virus or to contain viral antigen include the turbinates and nasal passages; lymph nodes draining the upper respiratory tract; lung; thyroid; spleen; and endometrium in addition to the brain.[28, 37, 62] For virus isolation, tissue homogenates are usually inoculated onto rabbit or equine kidney cell and equine embryonic lung monolayers and examined for cytopathic effect for up to 8 days.[28, 62]

The difficulty experienced in isolating EHV-1 from tissues of affected horses has prompted investigation of other tests to identify viral antigen. Immunofluorescent antibody (IFA) testing of brain and spinal cord sections is considered to be more sensitive than virus isolation, but false-negative results have been observed.[28, 37, 39] Recently an indirect immunoperoxidase (IP) method using orthodox light microscopy was described and was shown to be highly sensitive for identifying individual antigen-containing cells in the CNS and other areas of the body, even at sites where there were few, or no, lesions or inclusion bodies and virus could not be detected by IFA or virus isolation.[28] This technique and PCR show great promise for routine application to samples collected antemortem or at necropsy from affected horses.[28, 55, 70]

TREATMENT

Because EHV-1 is a contagious and potentially devastating infection, horses suspected of being affected should be promptly and strictly isolated until EHV-1 is ruled out by confirmation of an alternative diagnosis.[64] Since no specific treatment is available, management of horses with EHV-1 myeloencephalopathy is directed toward supportive nursing and nutritional care, and reduction of CNS inflammation.[3] Horses that are not recumbent should be encouraged to remain standing and protected from self-inflicted trauma by the provision of good footing, removal of obstacles, placement of food and water at a convenient height above ground level, and other measures, such as the use of padded hoods. Maintenance of hydration is important and provision of a laxative diet or the administration of laxatives such as bran mashes, mineral oil, or psyllium may be necessary to reduce intestinal impaction. Administration of enemas or manual emptying of the rectum may also be necessary to promote defecation and improve patient comfort.[3]

If affected horses are unable to stand and posture to urinate or if bladder function is significantly impaired, manual evacuation of the bladder by application of pressure per rectum may be necessary. If these measures are unsuccessful, judicious urinary catheterization is indicated and should be performed aseptically with the collection tubing attached to a sterile closed bag to minimize the risk of inducing urinary tract infection.[3, 64, 65] Cystitis is, however, a frequent complication, particularly in recumbent horses with distended urinary bladders, and can lead to bladder wall necrosis, bladder rupture, and systemic sepsis. Urine scalding can become a major problem, particularly in mares that are dribbling urine. Prevention involves regular washing of the perineum, tail, and hindlegs with water, application of water-repellent ointments, and braiding or wrapping the tail to simplify cleaning.[3]

Patients that become recumbent should be maintained in a sternal position on a thick cushion of dry absorbent bedding and should be rolled frequently (at least every 2–4 hours) to reduce the risk of developing myonecrosis and decubital ulcers. Whenever possible, they should be lifted to, and supported in, the standing position, using an appropriately fitted sling. Slings are most beneficial for moderately affected horses that are too weak to rise but able to maintain a standing position with minimal assistance. Slings are less useful for paraplegic or tetraplegic horses, which are unable to support their own weight. These horses tend to hang in the sling and experience problems related to pressure and constriction from the limited area of support provided by most slings if left hanging for periods of more than a few minutes.

Affected horses usually maintain a good appetite, even when recumbent, and should be provided with accessible food and water freely. Hand-feeding may be necessary to encourage some horses to eat. The caloric and water needs of anorectic patients can usually be met by feeding gruels of alfalfa-based or similar pelleted feeds in water or a balanced electrolyte solution via nasogastric tube. If oral intake is insufficient to meet the daily water needs of 60 to 80 mL/kg body weight per day, hydration can be maintained by intravenous administration of balanced electrolyte solutions.[37] Partial or total parenteral nutrition can also be used to meet the caloric needs of anorectic recumbent horses.

Because vasculitis, hemorrhage, and edema are prominent early lesions and may have an immune basis, treatment with corticosteroids early in the disease course is indicated and appears to be beneficial in some cases.[26, 37, 64] A short course of treatment with prednisolone acetate 1 to 2 mg/kg/day or dexamethasone 0.05 to 0.25 mg/kg parenterally twice-daily for 2 to 3 days, with reduced doses over a further 1 to 3 days, is recommended.[3, 37, 49, 57, 65] Dimethyl sulfoxide (DMSO) at a dose of 0.5 to 1.0 g/kg IV as a 10% to 20% solution in normal saline or 5% dextrose once-daily for up to 3 days is commonly used to treat horses with suspected CNS trauma or inflammatory disease, such as EHV-1 infection.[3, 49] At this time, no objective data are available to determine whether DMSO used alone or in combination with corticosteroids is superior to corticosteroids alone, or no anti-inflammatory treatment, in the management of EHV-1 myeloencephalopathy.

Because of the high risk of development of cystitis and other secondary bacterial infections in recumbent horses subjected to repeated catheterization of the bladder, it is advisable to administer broad-spectrum antibiotics such as potentiated sulfonamides, alone or in combination with penicillin G, particularly when corticosteroids are being given.[3, 37] The choice of antibiotics for treating established secondary bacterial infections of the urinary tract, respiratory tract, or other areas should be based on the results of culture and susceptibility testing.

PROGNOSIS

Affected horses that remain standing have a good prognosis and improvement is generally seen within a few days, although a period of several weeks to more than a year may be required before horses with severe deficits show complete recovery.[1, 22, 26, 35, 37, 49, 65, 66] In these instances control of urination frequently returns before gait abnormalities resolve completely.[64] Some horses may be left with residual neurologic deficits.[35-37] Horses that become recumbent, in addition to having more severe neurologic involvement, have a greatly increased likelihood of developing complications such as myonecrosis, urinary tract infection, decubital ulcers, respiratory tract infection, gastrointestinal obstruction and ulceration, injuries, and complications of dehydration and malnutrition. Their prognosis for recovery is therefore poor, particularly if they are unable to stand after being lifted with a sling, and these horses may die or require euthanasia. However, there are reports of horses standing again and recovering completely to race successfully after being recumbent for several days to 3 weeks.[26, 40, 41] Thus euthanasia should not be elected prematurely in valuable horses. Recurrence or exacerbation of neurologic signs in horses that have recovered completely has not been documented.[37] Recovered cases do have the potential to remain latently infected and show recrudescence of viral shedding if immunosuppressed by stress or glucocorticoid administration.[5, 45, 64]

PREVENTION

During outbreaks of EHV-1 infection, control measures are aimed at reducing spread by infected aerosols, direct contact, and fomites, and at reducing stress-induced recrudescence of latent EHV-1 infection. If abortions, early neonatal deaths, respiratory disease, or neurologic disease suggestive of EHV-1 infection occurs, affected animals should be promptly and completely isolated in a well-ventilated airspace separate from the remainder of the herd, and in-contact horses should be isolated as one or more small groups.[4, 5, 13, 26, 63] Aborted fetuses and fetal membranes should be collected at the site where they are found and placed in leakproof containers such as heavy-gauge plastic bags for submission for diagnostic evaluation or for disposal by burning.[13] Similarly, bedding and dirt contaminated with fetal fluids should be disposed of or burned and stalls or other areas occupied by infected horses should be thoroughly cleaned, disinfected with an iodophor or phenolic product, and left empty for several weeks.[5] Equipment used to handle, groom, feed, water, muck out, or transport affected horses should also be cleaned and disinfected or disposed of. Thereafter, separate equipment and personnel should be used for affected and unaffected horses, or at least caretakers should handle affected horses last and wear disposable gloves and protective clothing when doing so.[5, 49] Traffic of horses and people on the premises should be minimized and movement of horses onto and off the infected premises should be suspended until at least 3 weeks after resolution of acute signs in the last clinical case.[3-5, 13, 49] These measures aimed at reducing transmission of infection to susceptible horses may not stop the outbreak completely, since transmission of infection before control measures are implemented may result in a secondary wave of disease 1 to 2 weeks later.[5, 26]

There is no known method to reliably prevent the neurologic form of EHV-1 infection because the virus survives by inducing latent infections and by productively infecting immunologically experienced horses as well as immunologically naive introductions to horse herds.[5] However, routine management practices aimed at reducing the chances of introducing and disseminating infection are logical.[4, 5, 51, 71] New arrivals should be isolated for at least 3 weeks before joining the herd, distinct herd groups should be maintained based on the age and use of the horses, and care should be taken to minimize or eliminate commingling of resident horses with visiting or transient horses. In particular, pregnant broodmares should be maintained in groups separate from the remaining farm population. In addition, it is judicious to minimize stress associated with overcrowding and handling procedures in an attempt to reduce recrudescence of latent EHV-1 infection.[5, 45, 51, 71]

Appropriate repetitive administration of currently available EHV-1 vaccines appears to induce some immunity to respiratory disease and reduce the incidence of abortion, although it does not block infection with EHV-1 or eliminate the possibility of abortion, myeloencephalopathy, or establishment of the carrier state.[5, 13, 42, 71–74] None of the EHV-1 or EHV-4 vaccines currently available carry a claim that they prevent EHV-1 myeloencephalopathy and the disease has been observed in horses vaccinated regularly at 3- to 4-month intervals with inactivated and modified live vaccines.[3, 36, 37, 42] Indeed, previous vaccination appeared to constitute a risk factor in one outbreak.[48] However, it is logical to maintain appropriate vaccination procedures in an attempt to reduce the incidence of other manifestations of EHV-1 infection and reduce virus shedding within the population. This may indirectly help prevent EHV-1 myeloencephalopathy.[37] It is common practice to give booster vaccinations to exposed pregnant mares during outbreaks of abortigenic EHV-1 infection.[5, 13] However, vaccination of exposed horses during outbreaks of EHV-1 myeloencephalopathy has not been investigated and cannot be recommended at this time because of the possibility of an immune-mediated pathogenesis for this disease.[49] Booster vaccination of as yet unexposed horses has been recommended and may limit spread of the virus and associated morbidity.[3, 5, 49]

REFERENCES

1. deLahunta A: *Veterinary Neuroanatomy and Clinical Neurology.* Philadelphia, WB Saunders, 1983, p 227.
2. Browning GF, Ficorilli N, Studdert MJ: Asinine herpesvirus genomes: Comparison with those of the equine herpesviruses. *Arch Virol* 101:183, 1988.
3. Wilson JH: Neurologic syndrome of rhinopneumonitis. In *Proceedings of the Ninth American College of Veterinary Internal Medicine Forum,* 1991, p 419.
4. Powell DG: Viral respiratory disease. In Robinson NE, ed: *Current Therapy in Equine Medicine,* ed 3. Philadelphia, WB Saunders, 1992, p 581.
5. Allen GP, Bryans JT: Molecular epizootiology, pathogenesis, and prophylaxis of equine herpesvirus-1 infections. *Prog Vet Microbiol Immunol* 2:78, 1986.
6. Shimizu T, Ishizaki R, Ishii S, et al: Isolation of equine abortion virus from natural cases of equine abortion in horse kidney cell culture. *Jpn J Exp Med* 29:643, 1959.
7. Burrows R, Goodridge D: In vivo and in vitro studies of equine rhinopneumonitis strains. In Bryans JT, Gerber H, eds: *Equine Infectious Diseases III (Proceedings of the Third International Conference on Equine Infectious Diseases).* Basel, Karger, 1972, p 306.
8. Sabine M, Robertson GR, Whalley JM: Differentiation of subtypes of equine herpesvirus 1 by restriction endonuclease analysis. *Aust Vet J* 57:148, 1981.
9. Studdert MJ, Simpson T, Roizman B: Differentiation of respiratory and abortigenic isolates of equine herpesvirus 1 by restriction endonucleases. *Science* 214:562, 1981.

10. Turtinen LW, Allen GP, Darlington RW, et al: Serologic and molecular comparisons of several equine herpesvirus type 1 strains. *Am J Vet Res* 42:2099, 1981.
11. Studdert MJ: Restriction endonuclease DNA fingerprinting of respiratory, foetal, and perinatal foal isolates of equine herpes type 1. *Arch Virol* 77:249, 1983.
12. Allen GP, Yeargan MR, Turtinen LW, et al: Molecular epizootiologic studies of equine herpesvirus-1 infections by restriction endonuclease fingerprinting of viral DNA. *Am J Vet Res* 44:263, 1983.
13. Ostlund EN, Powell D, Bryans JT: Equine herpesvirus 1: A review. *Proc Am Assoc Equine Pract* 36:387, 1990.
14. Studdert MJ, Blackney MH: Equine herpesviruses: On the differentiation of respiratory and foetal strains of type 1. *Aust Vet J* 55:488, 1979.
15. Fitzpatrick DR, Studdert MJ: Immunologic relationships between equine herpesvirus type 1 (equine abortion virus), and type 4 (equine rhinopneumonitis virus). *Am J Vet Res* 45:1947, 1984.
16. Yeargan MR, Allen GP, Bryans JT: Rapid subtyping of equine herpesvirus 1 with monoclonal antibodies. *J Clin Microbiol* 21:694, 1985.
17. Meyer H, Thein P, Hübert P: Characterization of two equine herpesvirus (EHV) isolates associated with neurological disorders in horses. *J Vet Med B* 34:545, 1987.
18. Allen GP, Yeargan MR, Turtinen LW, et al: A new field strain of equine abortion virus (equine herpesvirus-1) among Kentucky horses. *Am J Vet Res* 46:138, 1985.
19. Saxegaard F: Isolation and identification of equine rhinopneumonitis virus (equine abortion virus) from cases of abortion and paralysis. *Nord Vet Med* 18:504, 1966.
20. Comény M: De la paraplégie infectieuse du cheval. *Rec Med Vet* 5:288, 1888.
21. Dalsgaard H: Enzootic paresis as a consequence of outbreaks of rhinopneumonitis (virus abortion). *Dan Dyrlaegeforen* 53:71, 1970.
22. Bitsch V, Dam A: Nervous disturbances in horses in relation to infection with equine rhinopneumonitis virus. *Acta Vet Scand* 12:134, 1971.
23. Thein P: Infection of the central nervous system of horses with equine herpesvirus serotype 1. *J S Afr Vet Assoc* 52:239, 1981.
24. Dinter Z, Klingeborn B: Serological study of an outbreak of paresis due to equid herpesvirus 1 (EHV-1). *Vet Rec* 99:10, 1976.
25. Chowdhury SI, Kubin G, Ludwig H: Equine herpesvirus type 1 (EHV-1) induced abortions and paralysis in a Lipizzaner stud: A contribution to the classification of equine herpesviruses. *Arch Virol* 90:273, 1986.
26. Greenwood RES, Simson ARB: Clinical report of a paralytic syndrome affecting stallions, mares and foals on a Thoroughbred studfarm. *Equine Vet J* 12:113, 1980.
27. Crowhurst FA, Dickinson G, Burrows R: An outbreak of paresis in mares and geldings associated with equid herpesvirus 1. *Vet Rec* 109:527, 1981.
28. Whitwell KE, Blunden AS: Pathological findings in horses dying during an outbreak of the paralytic form of equid herpesvirus type 1 (EHV-1) infection. *Equine Vet J* 24:13, 1992.
29. Collins JD: Virus abortion outbreak in Ireland. *Vet Rec* 91:129, 1972.
30. Studdert MJ, Fitzpatrick DR, Horner GW, et al: Molecular epidemiology and pathogenesis of some equine herpesvirus type 1 (equine abortion virus) and type 4 (equine rhinopneumonitis virus) isolates. *Aust Vet J* 61:345, 1984.
31. Batra SK, Jain NC, Tiwari SC: Isolation and characterization of 'EHV-1' herpesvirus associated with paralysis in equines. *Indian J Anim Sci* 52:671, 1982.
32. Jackson T, Kendrick JW: Paralysis of horses associated with

equine herpesvirus 1 infection. *J Am Vet Med Assoc* 158:1351, 1971.

33. Jackson TA, Osburn BI, Cordy DR, et al: Equine herpesvirus 1 infection of horses: Studies on the experimentally induced neurologic disease. *Am J Vet Res* 38:709, 1977.

34. Liu IKM, Castleman W: Equine posterior paresis associated with equine herpesvirus 1 vaccine in California: A preliminary report. *J Equine Med Surg* 1:397, 1977.

35. Pursell AR, Sangster LT, Byars TD, et al: Neurologic disease induced by equine herpesvirus 1. *J Am Vet Med Assoc* 175:473, 1979.

36. Franklin TE, Daft BM, Silverman VJ, et al: Serological titers and clinical observations in equines suspected of being infected with EHV-1. *Calif Vet* 39:22, 1985.

37. Kohn CW, Fenner WR: Equine herpes myeloencephalopathy. *Vet Clin North Am Equine Pract* 3:405, 1987.

38. Little PB, Thorsen J, Moran K: Virus involvement in equine paresis. *Vet Rec* 95:575, 1974.

39. Thorsen J, Little PB: Isolation of equine herpesvirus type 1 from a horse with an acute paralytic disease. *Can J Comp Med* 39:358, 1975.

40. Little PB, Thorsen J: Disseminated necrotizing myeloencephalitis: A herpes-associated neurological disease of horses. *Vet Pathol* 13:161, 1976.

41. Charlton KM, Mitchell D, Girard A, et al: Meningoencephalomyelitis in horses associated with equine herpesvirus 1 infection. *Vet Pathol* 13:59, 1976.

42. Thomson GW, McCready R, Sanford E, et al: An outbreak of herpesvirus myeloencephalitis in vaccinated horses. *Can Vet J* 20:22, 1979.

43. Platt H, Singh H, Whitwell KE: Pathological observations on an outbreak of paralysis in broodmares. *Equine Vet J* 12:118, 1980.

44. Bryans JT, Allen GP: Equine viral rhinopneumonitis. *Rev Sci Tech Off Int Epizootiology* 5:837, 1986.

45. Edington N, Bridges CG, Huckle A: Experimental reactivation of equid herpesvirus 1 (EHV 1) following the administration of corticosteroids. *Equine Vet J* 17:369, 1985.

46. EHV-1: A recurrent problem. *Vet Rec* 124:443, 1989.

47. Campbell TM, Studdert MJ: Equine herpesvirus type 1 (EHV 1). *Vet Bull* 53:135, 1983.

48. Hughes PE, Ryan CP, Carlson G, et al: An epizootic of equine herpes virus-1 myeloencephalitis. Unpublished observations, 1987.

49. Kortz G: Equine herpes myeloencephalopathy. In Robinson NE, ed: *Current Therapy in Equine Medicine,* ed 3. Philadelphia, WB Saunders, 1992, p 550.

50. Montali RJ, Allen GP, Bryans JT, et al: Equine herpesvirus type 1 abortion in an onager and suspected herpesvirus myelitis in a zebra. *J Am Vet Med Assoc* 187:1248, 1985.

51. Mayhew IG: *Large Animal Neurology.* Philadelphia, Lea & Febiger, 1989, p 272.

52. Scott JC, Dutta SK, Myrup AC: In vivo harboring of equine herpesvirus-1 in leukocyte populations and subpopulations and their quantitation from experimentally infected ponies. *Am J Vet Res* 44:1344, 1983.

53. Bryans JT: On immunity to disease caused by equine herpesvirus 1. *J Am Vet Med Assoc* 155:294, 1969.

54. Edington N, Bridges CG, Patel JR: Endothelial cell infection and thrombosis in paralysis caused by equid herpesvirus-1: Equine stroke. *Arch Virol* 90:111, 1986.

55. Edington N, Smyth B, Griffiths L: The role of endothelial cell infection in the endometrium, placenta and foetus of equid herpesvirus 1 (EHV-1) abortions. *J Comp Pathol* 104:379, 1991.

56. Nowotny N, Burtscher H, Bürki F: Neuropathogenicity for suckling mice of equine herpesvirus 1 from the Lipizzan outbreak in 1983 and of selected other EHV 1 strains. *J Vet Med B* 34:441, 1987.

57. Prickett ME, Bryans JT: Contribution to discussion on equine herpesvirus. In Bryans JT, Gerber H, eds: *Equine Infectious Diseases II (Proceedings of the Second International Conference on Equine Infectious Diseases).* Basel, Karger, 1970, p 60.

58. Patel JR, Edington N, Mumford JA: Variation in cellular tropism between isolates of equine herpesvirus-1 in foals. *Arch Virol* 74:41, 1982.

59. Klingeborn B, Dinter Z, Hughes RAC: Antibody to neuritogenic myelin protein P2 in equine paresis due to equine herpesvirus 1. *Zentralblatt Veterinar Med [B]* 30:137, 1983.

60. Slater JD, Gibson JS, Barnett KC, et al: Chorioretinopathy associated with neuropathology following infection with equine herpesvirus-1. *Vet Rec* 131:237, 1992.

61. Smith KC, Tearle JP, Whitwell KE, et al: EHV-1 pathogenesis. *Animal Health Trust Scientific Report* 1990–1991, p 1.

62. Mumford JA, Edington N: EHV1 and equine paresis. *Vet Rec* 106:277, 1980.

63. Roberts RS: A paralytic syndrome in horses. *Vet Rec* 77:404, 1965.

64. MacKay RJ, Mayhew IG: Equine herpesvirus myeloencephalitis. In Colahan PT, Mayhew IG, Merritt AM, eds: *Equine Medicine and Surgery,* ed 4. Goleta, Calif, American Veterinary, 1991, p 751.

65. George LW: Equine herpesvirus 1 myeloencephalitis (rhinopneumonitis myelitis). In Smith BP, ed: *Large Animal Internal Medicine.* St Louis, Mosby–Year Book, 1990, p 913.

66. Braund KG, Brewer BD, Mayhew IG: Equine herpesvirus type 1 infection. In Oliver JE, Hoerlein BF, Mayhew IG, eds: *Veterinary Neurology.* Philadelphia, WB Saunders, 1987, p 223.

67. Blythe LL, Mattson DE, Lassen ED, et al: Antibodies against equine herpesvirus 1 in the cerebrospinal fluid in the horse. *Can Vet J* 26:218, 1985.

68. Keane DP, Little PB, Wilkie BN, et al: Agents of equine viral encephalomyelitis: Correlation of serum and cerebrospinal fluid antibodies. *Can J Vet Res* 52:229, 1988.

69. Mumford JA: The development of diagnostic techniques for equine viral diseases. *Vet Annu* 24:182, 1984.

70. Sharma PC, Cullinane AA, Onions DE, Nicolson L: Diagnosis of equid herpesviruses-1 and -4 by polymerase chain reaction. *Equine Vet J* 24:20, 1992.

71. Mumford JA: Equid herpesvirus 1 (EHV 1) latency: More questions than answers. *Equine Vet J* 17:340, 1985.

72. Eaglesome MD, Henry JNR, McKnight JD: Equine herpesvirus 1 infection in mares vaccinated with a live-virus rhinopneumonitis vaccine attenuated in cell culture. *Can Vet J* 20:145, 1979.

73. Burrows R, Goodridge D, Denyer MS: Trials of an inactivated equid herpesvirus 1 vaccine: Challenge with subtype 1 virus. *Vet Rec* 114:369, 1984.

74. Bürki F, Rossmanith W, Nowotny N, et al: Viraemia and abortions are not prevented by two commercial equine herpesvirus-1 vaccines after experimental challenge of horses. *Vet Q* 12:80, 1990.

9.12

Polyneuritis Equi

William J. Saville, DVM

Polyneuritis equi (PNE) is an uncommon neurologic disease of all equine species that is characterized by tail and anal sphincter paralysis, often accompanied by cranial and peripheral nerve damage.[1-13] Previous reports referred to the disease as neuritis of the cauda equina because of the susceptibility of this region, but frequent involvement of the cranial and peripheral nerves led to the term *polyneuritis equi*.[2] Although the disease has been more readily recognized in Europe where it was first reported by Dexler in 1897, cases have now been reported from Great Britain, Canada, and the United States.[3, 4, 6, 14] There does not appear to be a breed, sex, or age predilection, but the youngest horse affected was 17 months of age.[2, 5, 6, 13-15]

The cause of this disease is unknown. Primary immune reaction and viral inflammatory disease have been suggested, although very possibly one may be a consequence of the other.[2] Several infectious agents have been suggested, such as equine herpesvirus type 1 (EHV-1), equine adenovirus, and streptococcal bacteria.[10, 12, 16] The pathologic lesions resemble those of Guillain-Barré syndrome in humans and the disease is also similar to experimental allergic neuritis (EAN) in rats.[10, 13] There is evidence to suggest that the immune system is involved, as horses with PNE have circulating antibodies to P2 myelin protein, which is present in rats with EAN.[10, 17] The significance of this is that PNE may be both an inflammatory and an immune-mediated disease.

CLINICAL SIGNS

The disease will often manifest itself in two forms: (1) the acute signs include hyperesthesia of the perineal or head region, or both; (2) in the chronic form horses show paralysis of the tail, anus, rectum, and bladder. This is often accompanied by fecal and urinary retention, urinary scalding of the hindlimbs, and in male horses, penile paralysis.[1-3, 6, 8, 9, 12, 13, 15]

The hindlimb signs in affected horses are often symmetric, whereas the head signs are often asymmetric.[6, 13, 15] Muscle atrophy in the gluteal region is sometimes present along with mild degrees of ataxia.[2, 3, 5, 6, 9] Muscle atrophy associated with cranial nerve involvement may occur in the head region. Damage to peripheral motor nerves may result in gait deficits and abnormal use of fore- or hindlimbs.[1, 12, 13, 15]

Although cranial nerve involvement is primarily reported to affect cranial nerves V, VII, and VIII, any of cranial nerves II, III, IV, VI, IX, X, and XII may also be involved.[2, 4, 5, 8, 13] The horses may have trouble with mastication and swallowing.[12] A head tilt, ear droop, lip droop, and ptosis are common signs.[8, 12, 13] There has been one report of a horse with brachial neuritis along with involvement of cranial nerves V, VII, and XII.[2] The horse also exhibited mild ataxia and weakness in all four limbs.[2] The hopping test was performed poorly on the right thoracic limb and the horse resented palpation in the right caudal cervical and prescapular region.[2]

Colic due to fecal retention may be the primary sign when initially examining horses with PNE. Fecal retention leads to an impaction due to the flaccid anal sphincter, often accompanied by an atonic, distended bladder.[1] If presented in the acute or hyperesthetic form, this usually progresses to the chronic form of hypalgesia or anesthesia. The area of anesthesia may be surrounded by an area of hyperesthesia.[1, 2, 8]

DIAGNOSIS

The definitive diagnostic test is a postmortem examination. The peripheral white blood cell (WBC) count usually reveals a mature neutrophilia with hyperfibrinogenemia, mild-to-moderate anemia, and an increased total protein, all indications of a chronic inflammatory process.[3, 5, 13, 15] Examination of the cerebrospinal fluid (CSF) may reveal an elevated protein (70–300 mg/dL) along with an elevated WBC count. The WBC count indicates a mononuclear inflammatory reaction, although CSF cytology may be normal, particularly in the acute stage of the disease.[2, 3, 5, 6, 8, 11, 13]

Radiography may be required to rule out trauma to the tail head or cranial nerve involvement such as a fractured petrous temporal bone.[2, 8]

Some horses with clinical signs exhibit the presence of circulating P2 myelin antibody in the serum.[10, 17] However, the presence of this antibody is only supportive of the diagnosis; the same antibody has been detected in horses with EHV-1 and equine adenovirus infections.[1, 2, 10, 13, 16, 18]

Classically, the primary pathologic lesions involve the extradural nerve roots, but the intradural nerve roots may also be involved.[2, 3, 5, 12, 13] The lesions are granulomatous with various degrees of inflammation and infiltration of lymphocytes, eosinophils, macrophages, giant cells, and plasma cells. This inflammation leads to myelin degeneration, subsequent axonal degeneration, and thickening of the epineurium, endoneurium, and perineurium with proliferation, which causes obliteration of the neural architecture by the fibrous tissue.[1, 2, 9, 13] The most severe lesions are in the cauda equina, but swelling, edema, and hemorrhage of cranial nerves may be seen. The fibrous tissue formation may lead to adhesions between the meninges and the periosteum of the vertebral bodies.[13] There are reports of involvement of the autonomic nervous system, but no changes in clinical signs have been reported (postmortem only).[2, 4]

The polyneuritis lesions are typical of the Guillain-Barré syndrome in humans, EAN in rats, and coonhound paralysis in dogs.[2, 5, 11-13] This may indicate a combination of inflammatory and immune-mediated mechanisms in the pathophysiology of PNE.

DIFFERENTIAL DIAGNOSIS

The most important differential disease is trauma to the sacrococcygeal area of the spinal canal. This can be differentiated by radiography of the area looking for fractures or displacements.[2, 6, 8]

Equine protozoal myeloencephalitis (EPM) is the second most common disease in the differential of PNE. The usual signs of EPM include asymmetric damage in the limbs and brain and brainstem lesions causing cranial nerve deficits with alterations in attitude, whereas the cranial nerve deficits of PNE are peripheral, with no change in attitude.[6] This disease may be differentiated from PNE by Western blot analysis of the CSF.[19]

Equine herpesvirus (EHV-1) myeloencephalitis often has an acute onset following an episode of fever, cough, and nasal discharge or following one or more abortions on a farm. This condition often affects more than one horse on a farm. Herpesvirus has a rapid onset and often results in severe hindlimb weakness and ataxia along with bladder dysfunction. Urinary dribbling may sometimes occur. The ataxia and weakness is usually symmetric and may result in recumbency. Occasionally the horses will dog-sit. Cranial nerve involvement is not common.[20–23]

Verminous myeloencephalitis should be considered; the signs are extremely variable and depend on the parasite's migratory pathway. Diffuse or multifocal brain and spinal cord lesions have been reported. The onset is usually sudden with rapid deterioration and death. The incidence of this disease is very low, perhaps owing to more intense parasite control.[24–26]

Equine motor neuron disease should be considered in the differential diagnosis. Horses with motor neuron disease have symmetric muscle wasting or atrophy and weight loss with marked weakness, sweating, and muscle fasciculations.[27] However, these horses are not ataxic and their unique clinical feature is that they walk better than they stand.[27] This disease is a denervation atrophy of type I muscle fibers only and may be diagnosed by a spinal accessory nerve biopsy or sacrodorsalis caudalis muscle biopsy.[27]

TREATMENT

The primary therapy is palliative. There is no known treatment for the disease. Removing feces from the rectum, and bladder evacuation are usually necessary. If there is a cystitis due to bladder distention, systemic antibiotics may be indicated. Some attempts have been made at treating the inflammation with corticosteroids, but the effects have been short-lived. The prognosis is usually poor, but the progression of the disease is slow. Some animals may be maintained for many months.[2, 4–6, 8, 12, 13, 15]

REFERENCES

1. Reed SM: Neuritis of the cauda equina: Polyneuritis equi in the horse. *Proc J D Stewart Memorial Refresher Course for Veterinarians* 183:385–386, 1992.
2. Vatistas NJ, Mayhew IG, Whitwell KE, et al: Polyneuritis equi: A clinical review incorporating a case report of a horse displaying unconventional signs. *Prog Vet Neurol* 2:67–72, 1991.
3. Rousseaux CG, Futcher KG, Clark EG, et al: Cauda equina neuritis: A chronic idiopathic polyneuritis in two horses. *Can Vet J* 25:214–218, 1984.
4. Wright JA, Fordyce P, Edington N: Neuritis of the cauda equina in the horse. *J Comp Pathol* 97:667–675, 1987.
5. White PL, Genetzsky RM, Pohlenz JFI, et al: Neuritis of the cauda equina in a horse. *Compend Contin Educ Pract Vet* 6:S217–S224, 1984.
6. Scarratt WK, Jortner BS: Neuritis of the cauda equina in a yearling filly. *Compend Contin Educ Pract Vet* 7:S197–S202, 1985.
7. Milne FJ, Carbonell PL: Neuritis of the cauda equina of horses: a case report. *Equine Vet J* 2:179–182, 1970.
8. Mayhew IG: *Large Animal Neurology.* Philadelphia, Lea & Febiger, 1989, pp 349–357.
9. Greenwood AG, Barker J: Neuritis of the cauda equina in a horse. *Equine Vet J* 5:111–115, 1973.
10. Fordyce PS, Edington N, Bridges GC, et al: Use of an ELISA in the differential diagnosis of cauda equina neuritis and other equine neuropathies. *Equine Vet J* 19:55–59, 1987.
11. Cummings JF, deLahunta A, Timoney JF: Neuritis of the cauda equina, a chronic polyradiculoneuritis in the horse. *Acta Neuropathol* 46:17–24, 1979.
12. Beech J: Neuritis of the cauda equina. *Proc Am Assoc Equine Pract* 21:75–76, 1976.
13. Yvorchuk K: Polyneuritis equi. In Robinson NE, ed: *Current Therapy in Equine Medicine,* ed 3. Philadelphia, WB Saunders, 1992, pp 569–570.
14. Yvorchuk-St Jean K: Neuritis of the cauda equina. *Vet Clin North Am Equine Pract* 421–427, 1987.
15. Cox JH, Murray RC, DeBowes RM: Disease of the spinal cord. In Kobluk CN, Ames TR, Geor RJ, eds: *The Horse: Diseases and Clinical Management.* Philadelphia, WB Saunders, 1995, pp 443–472.
16. Edington N, Wright JA, Patel JR, et al: Equine adenovirus 1 isolated from cauda equina neuritis. *Res Vet Sci* 37:252–254, 1984.
17. Kadlubowski M, Ingram PL: Circulating antibodies to the neuritogenic protein, P2, in neuritis of the cauda equina of the horse. *Nature* 293:299–300, 1981.
18. Klingeborn B, Dinter Z, Hughes RAC: Antibody to neuritogenic myelin protein P2 in equine paresis due to equine herpesvirus 1. *Zentralbl Veterinarmed* 30:137–140, 1983.
19. Granstrom DE, Dubey JP, Giles RC, et al: Equine protozoal myeloencephalitis: Biology and epidemiology. In Nakajima H, Plowright W: Refereed Proceedings. R & W Publications (Newmarket) Ltd, 1994.
20. Jackson T, Kendrick JW: Paralysis of horses associated with equine herpesvirus 1 infection. *J Am Vet Med Assoc* 158:1351–1357, 1971.
21. Ostlund EN, Powell D, Bryans JT: Equine herpesvirus 1: A review. *Proc Am Assoc Equine Pract* 36:387–395, 1990.
22. Ostlund EN: The equine herpesviruses. *Vet Clin North Am Equine Pract* 9:283–294, 1993.
23. Wilson JH, Erickson DM: Neurological syndrome of rhinopneumonitis. *Proc Am Coll Vet Intern Med* 9:419–421, 1991.
24. Blunden AS, Khalil LF, Webbon PM: *Halicephalobus deletrix* infection in a horse. *Equine Vet J* 19:255, 1987.
25. Lester G: Parasitic encephalomyelitis in horses. *Compend Contin Educ Pract Vet* 14:1624–1630, 1992.
26. Mayhew IG, Brewer BD, Reinhard MK, et al: Verminous (*Strongylus vulgaris*) myelitis in a donkey. *Cornell Vet* 74:30–37, 1984.
27. Divers TJ, Cummings JF, Mohammed HO, et al: Equine motor neuron disease. *Proc Am Coll Vet Intern Med* 13:918–921, 1995.

9.13

Togaviral Encephalitis

Joseph J. Bertone, DVM, MS, Dip ACVIM

Togaviridae are small, lipid- and protein-enveloped RNA viruses. Several insect-borne viruses (arboviruses) of the genera *Alphavirus* and *Flavivirus* have been associated with encephalitis in horses. The structure of the viruses and associated clinical presentations are similar among the viruses, but the epizootiology and antigenicity are distinct. *Alphavirus* species (formerly arbovirus group A) tend to be more infectious and are more often associated with epidemics compared with *Flavivirus* species (formerly arbovirus group B). *Flavivirus* species tend to be associated with sporadic outbreaks. In the Togaviridae, equine arteritis virus, a *Rubivirus* species, has been associated with some neurologic deficits and central nervous system edema.[1] This is discussed elsewhere.

In general, birds, rodents, and reptiles act as reservoirs. Often, mosquitoes play a role in transmitting the disease among these species. Mosquitoes and, less commonly, other insects feed on sylvatic hosts and subsequently transmit the disease to horses and humans.

ALPHAVIRUS ENCEPHALITIDES: EASTERN, WESTERN, AND VENEZUELAN EQUINE ENCEPHALOMYELITIS

The predominant togaviral encephalitides in the Western Hemisphere are associated with eastern (EEE), western (WEE), and Venezuelan (VEE) equine encephalitis (Table 9–9).

Etiology

EEE and WEE are specific and discrete togaviral particles. There are North and South American antigenic variants of EEE. WEE variants include eastern, western, and Highlands J strains. The various strains have equivocal differences in antigenic properties and biological behavior, and extensive geographical overlap occurs.[2] The molecular basis for the antigenic variation between EEE and WEE has been described.[3] There are four subtypes of VEE virus. Type I, variants A, B, and C are associated with disease and epidemics. Type I, variants D, E, and F, and types II, III, and IV are endemic and usually not associated with clinical disease.[4-7]

Epizootiology

Encephalitis similar to the viral encephalitides has been reported in the United States for many years with high morbidity and mortality rates.[8, 9] Evidence that an eastern and western virus exist and are antigenically distinct was first reported in 1933.[10] Horses immunized with strains of virus isolated from infected horses from the East or West were differentially protected when vaccinated with attenuated virus from one location and exposed to virus from the other.[10-12]

Distribution. In general, disease associated with EEE, WEE, and VEE is restricted to the Western Hemisphere and ranges from temperate to desert climates. Each virus and incidence of associated equine disease has a characteristic distribution. The range of positive serology for the viruses is often far greater than the range of clinical disease[13-39] (Fig. 9–33). For example, clinical disease associated with VEE was identified in southern Texas in 1971. However, asymptomatic horses with significant titers for VEE (type II) are often identified in Florida where the disease syndrome has not been evident.[16] The WEE virus is recognized in reservoir avian hosts in the eastern United States; however, clinical disease is rarely identified there. Geographical variation in viral virulence may be an explanation. Some importance of the vector in eliciting a more virulent virus lies in the fact that the vector for WEE in the East is *Culiseta melanura*, which is the common vector for EEE. This mosquito may not be able to generate the virulent state of WEE, since clinical disease in that region is rare. Equine disease associated with WEE is rare on the eastern seaboard of the United States, but is recognized.[40] Outside of the Western Hemisphere, EEE has been identified in the Philippines,[41] and there is some indication it may be seen in Europe.[42]

Epidemic. There are several requirements for epidemics associated with EEE, WEE, or VEE to develop. Long lapses can occur between outbreaks if all of these conditions are not met. These prerequisites include adequate and adjacent numbers of reservoir animals, sufficient quantities of virulent viruses, infected intermediate hosts, insect vectors, and susceptible horse and human populations.[43, 44] Prediction of outbreaks has been attempted but without success.[36, 45, 46] This indicates that other, unknown factors may exist.

Reservoirs. With minor exceptions, Togaviridae persist by

Table 9–9. A Summary of the Major Togaviral Equine Encephalitides*

Virus†	Major Disease Vector	Zoonotic Potential	Amplification from Horses	Disease Spread	Viremia	Equine Mortality	Human Mortality
EEE	*Aedes* spp.	Unlikely	Unlikely	Vector	Low	75%–100%	50%–75%
WEE	*Culex tarsalis*	Unlikely	Unlikely	Vector ± secretions	Low	20%–50%	5%–15%
VEE	*Culex melanoconium,* *Aedes* spp. *Phosphora* spp.	Occurs	Occurs	Vector ± secretions	High	40%–80%	1%

*The statements made are generalities and some degree of variation occurs.
†EEE, WEE, and VEE are eastern, western, and Venezuelan equine encephalitis, respectively.

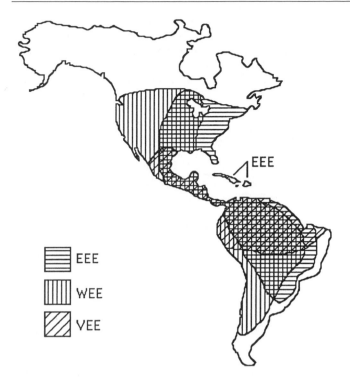

Figure 9–33. Predominant distribution of *Alphavirus* spp.–associated equine encephalitis in the Western Hemisphere. This figure represents the disease distribution. Positive serology for the diseases is more widespread. *EEE, WEE,* and *VEE* denote eastern, western, and Venezuelan equine encephalitis virus, respectively.

asymptomatically infecting wild animals (sylvatic hosts), such as birds, small mammals, and reptiles, by unknown mechanisms.[47] The viruses survive during the winter or non-vector season in sylvatic populations.[46, 48]

Vectors. There is specificity of the viruses for particular vectors. Vector distribution, to a large degree, explains viral distribution. The vectors for EEE include *C. melanura* and *Aedes* species.[13, 29, 49, 50] *Culiseta melanura* is, for the most part, confined to freshwater swamps, feeds primarily on swamp birds, and is rarely found in areas of increased horse populations.[13] In general, *C. melanura* serves as the vector for the enzootic cycle, which involves swamp birds. *Aedes* species appear to be more important in epizootics and epidemics.

In Florida, WEE persists continuously in *C. melanura* (see above).[13] Important WEE vectors include *Culex tarsalis, Dermacentor andersoni,*[51, 52] and *Triatoma sanguisuga* (assassin bug).[53, 54] The cliff swallow bug (*Oeciacus vicarius*) may be an overwintering reservoir[51, 55] (see below).

The vectors for VEE include *Culex melanoconium,* and *Mansonia, Aedes,* and *Phosphora* species.[16, 17, 23, 24]

Virulence Induction. Some puzzles exist in light of some mosquitoes' and other insects' ability to carry two or three viruses, but the inability of these viruses to induce disease. Some form of virulence induction specific to the viruses may occur. The existence or mechanism of virulent mutation

is controversial. The intermediate host may play a key role in this process, but that is speculative.

Vector Ecology. Vector transmission is the most important way infection is spread. WEE and VEE may be spread by nasal secretions, but this is less likely.[16, 17, 54, 56]

Vectors transmit viral particles between sylvatic hosts when taking a blood meal. If the virus is able to penetrate the vector's gut, it may pass through the hemolymph to oral glands, multiply, and subsequently be shed in saliva and other oral secretions. If the blood meal contains adequate numbers of viral particles, multiplication may not be required for transmission. In most instances and judiciously assumed, the mosquito remains infected for life.[50, 57]

Seasonal Incidence. In most instances, the diseases occur during the height of the vector season. In temperate climates the highest number of cases occur between June and November. In warm climates, where the vector season is longer, the disease problem lasts longer.[23, 27, 30, 31, 50, 54, 57]

Zoonology. Clinical infection in humans usually involves very old or very young persons. Signs, symptoms, morbidity, and mortality rates are virus-specific.[58]

Circulating virus concentrations are often too low for transmission of EEE from infected horses to humans, mosquitoes, and other animals. Human disease is most likely associated with insect vector contact and often coincides with, or is preceded by, equine epizootics.[45] In the acute stages of equine disease a transient, substantial viremia occurs. Therefore, if vector density is increased, an acutely infected horse could be a transient amplifier of EEE. Spread from horse to horse is possible.[49] Clinical signs in humans include acute fulminant encephalitis, headache, altered consciousness, and seizures. The mortality rate is approximately 50% to 75%.[58]

Both humans and horses are terminal hosts for WEE. Human cases of WEE occur yearly, but fatality and incomplete recovery are rare. These cases are associated with vector contact. Environmental conditions that decrease exposure to insects decrease the incidence of disease.[59] Increased numbers of animals with clinical equine disease are an indication of heavy sylvatic concentrations of virus and are not a potential source of infection for humans. Generally, increased numbers of horse cases precede cases in humans by 2 to 5 weeks.[60] Thus, horses are sentinels for humans in a given area. Clinical signs in humans include fever, headache, confusion, stupor, and seizures, with a 5% to 15% mortality rate.[58]

Horses with VEE have sufficient circulating viral concentrations that they act as amplifiers of disease.[23, 61] Ocular and nasal secretions from infected horses contain high concentrations of VEE.[16, 17] Infection via entry through the respiratory tract may occur by direct contact with infected animals. Equine and human survivors of VEE infection and clinical disease may develop chronic relapsing viremias and serve as chronic disease amplifiers.[61] Clinical signs in humans include fever, headache, myalgia, and pharyngitis. There is a 1% mortality rate.[58]

With any of the alphaviral equine encephalitides, sufficient viral particles for infection may be present in central nervous and other tissues and precautions should be taken when performing a necropsy examination on suspect cases. Strict mosquito control and vaccination can prevent both human and equine cases and all equine cases should be reported to state health officials.[45, 61]

Other Domestic Species. Calves may be affected naturally and experimentally with EEE.[62, 63] Pigs may be affected by EEE[64] and VEE.[65] The signs of disease in these species are similar, but are milder than disease in horses for the respective viruses. Burros and mules may contract all three diseases and the disease is as severe as that identified in horses.[66]

Pathogenesis

After viruses are inoculated, they multiply in muscle, enter the lymphatic circulation, and localize in lymph nodes. Viruses replicate in macrophages and neutrophils and subsequently are shed in small numbers. Many of the viral particles are cleared at this time. If clearance mechanisms are successful, no further clinical signs develop. Neutralizing antibodies will still be produced. Several mechanisms of viral immunologic avoidance exist and include erythrocyte and leukocyte absorption. If viral elimination is not complete, the remaining viruses infect endothelial cells and concentrate in highly vascular organs, such as liver and spleen. Viral replication in these tissues is subsequently associated with circulating virus. The second viremic period is often associated with early clinical signs of disease. Infection of the central nervous system occurs within 3 to 5 days.[6, 17, 67, 68]

Clinical Signs

Clinical signs are more profound in unvaccinated animals.[60, 69] Acute clinical signs of EEE and WEE are nonspecific and include mild fever to severe pyrexia, anorexia, and stiffness. Viremia occurs during this period. After an experimental dose of EEE and WEE there is a 1- to 3-week incubation period. The incubation period is often shorter with EEE than WEE. Early signs of the diseases include fever and mild depression. This stage is transient and, presumably, often undetected because of lack of overt clinical signs. The acute signs may last for up to 5 days after they are first manifest. Many cases of WEE do not progress beyond this point. With EEE, progression is more common. Once nervous signs develop, the viremia is past and it is unlikely that the animals can amplify the disease. In progressive cases the fever may rise and fall sporadically. Cerebral signs may develop at any time, but often occur a few days after infection. Acute signs often range from propulsive walking, depression, and somnolence to hyperesthesia, aggression, and excitability. Some horses may become frenzied after any sensory stimulation. Often conscious proprioceptive deficits are evident in the early stages. With progression, signs become less disparate and more consistent between EEE and WEE. The later signs are evidence of the dynamic nature of these conditions and increased severity of cerebral cortical and cranial nerve dysfunction. These signs include head-pressing, propulsive walking, blindness, circling, head tilt, and facial and appendicular muscle fasciculations. Paralysis of the pharynx, larynx, and tongue is com-

mon. Death is often preceded by recumbency for 1 to 7 days. Animals that are comatose rarely survive. If animals are to survive they show gradual improvement of function over weeks to months.[69–72]

VEE may have similar or different clinical presentations as compared with WEE and EEE. This is most likely due to the difference in strain pathogenicity.[16, 68] The pyrexia in cases of VEE peaks early and remains increased through the course of the disease. In experimental disease, endemic strains are associated with mild fever and leukopenia. Epidemic strains are associated with severe pyrexia and leukopenia.[6, 68] Diarrhea, severe depression, recumbency, and death may be prominent before neurologic deficits are evident. Neurologic signs occur at approximately 4 days following infection. Other associated signs include abortion, oral ulceration, pulmonary hemorrhage, and epistaxis.[16, 17]

Diagnosis

The presumptive diagnosis is based upon findings at clinical presentation and the presence of associated epidemiologic features. Serologic and necropsy evaluation will provide a definitive determination.

Clinical Immunology and Virology. Viral infections are usually identified by complement fixation, hemagglutination inhibition, and cross-serum neutralization assays. A combination of these techniques increases the likelihood of a positive diagnosis.[73] A fourfold rise in antibody titer in convalescent sera is commonly recommended for diagnosis. However, it is possible that a rise in titer may not be detected. Viral antibodies are commonly present within 24 hours after the initial viremia and their presence often precedes clinical encephalitis.[42] The concentration of antibodies increases rapidly and then decreases over 6 months.[74] An initial sample is often taken when encephalitic signs are present. This may be after peak titers have been reached. Therefore, it is possible that a second sample may have a decreased titer compared with the initial sample. If increased titers exist for hemagglutination inhibition, complement fixation, and neutralizing antibody, then a presumptive diagnosis can be made on a single sample.[73] In the case of suspected VEE, an enzyme-linked immunosorbent assay (ELISA) can detect viral-specific IgM antibodies to surface glycoprotein by 3 days after the onset of clinical signs. These antibodies are not produced in response to vaccine. The antibodies disappear by 21 days following infection.[74] This test should be used for confirmation of acute VEE infection when convalescent serum samples cannot be collected. It is unlikely that viral cultures will be fruitful, except in the case of acute VEE. The virus may be isolated from cerebrospinal fluid of horses with acute infections.[17] The usefulness of cerebrospinal fluid viral titers in light of a negative viral isolation is questioned. Fluorescent antibody, ELISA, and viral isolation are useful in identifying virus in brain tissue.[75, 76]

Colostral antibodies may interfere with diagnosis in foals. The antibody titers to VEE, WEE, and EEE viruses in the sera of 2- to 8-day-old foals are similar to those of dams. The serum half-life of maternal antibodies in foals is approximately 20 days.[77]

Clinical Pathology. The cerebrospinal fluid changes associated with togaviral infections are similar to those of other viral encephalitides and include increased cellularity (50–400 mononuclear cells per microliter) and protein concentration (100–200 mg/dL).

Necropsy Findings. Animals that die or are euthanized should be necropsied and a gross and histologic examination performed with special reference to the central nervous system. The brain and spinal cord often have a normal gross appearance. In some cases vascular congestion and discoloration of the central nervous system is found. Histologic findings include nonseptic mononuclear cell and neutrophilic inflammation of the entire brain.[16, 78–80] Severe lesions are found in the cerebral cortex, thalamus, and hypothalamus. Specific lesions include marked perivascular cuffing with mononuclear and neutrophil cell infiltration, gliosis, neuronal degeneration, and mononuclear cell meningeal inflammation. With VEE, liquefactive necrosis and hemorrhage of the cerebral cortex, atrophy of the pancreatic acinar cells, and hyperplasia of the pancreatic duct cells are commonly seen.[79]

Differential Diagnosis. The differential diagnosis for EEE, WEE, and VEE should include other conditions that are associated with diffuse or multifocal neurologic deficits. These include other togaviral encephalitides, trauma, hepatoencephalopathy, rabies, leukoencephalomalacia, bacterial meningoencephalitis, equine protozoal myeloencephalitis, and verminous encephalitis.

Treatment

There is no known effective, specific treatment of the viral encephalitides. Treatment is primarily supportive. Nonsteroidal anti-inflammatory drugs (phenylbutazone 4 mg/kg q.12h.; flunixin meglumine 1 mg/kg q.12–24h.) are used to control pyrexia, inflammation, and discomfort. Dimethyl sulfoxide 1 g/kg IV in 20% solution may be useful in controlling inflammation and provides some analgesia and mild sedation. The use of corticosteroids is controversial since beneficial effects are short term and there is increased risk of developing secondary bacterial infections. Convulsions may be controlled by the use of pentobarbital, diazepam 0.05 to 2.2 mg/kg IV, phenobarbital 2 mg/kg PO, or phenytoin 0.2 to 1.0 mg/kg IV. If horses develop secondary bacterial infections, appropriate antibiotic therapy should be employed. Hydration should be monitored and balanced fluid solutions administered orally or intravenously, as needed. Other supportive care should include dietary supplementation. Laxatives should be administered to minimize the risk of gastrointestinal impaction. If anorexia persists for more than 48 hours, enteral or parenteral supplementation should be employed. Commercial formulations can be used. For the short term, pelleted feeds may be put into suspension and administered orally. Protection from self-induced trauma may employ protective leg wraps and head protection. If the horse is recumbent, attempts should be made to provide support in a sling. All animals should be bedded heavily.

Prognosis

Complete recoveries from the neurologic deficits associated with these viruses are reported, but they are rare.[81] Animals that have recovered from EEE often have residual neurologic deficits that commonly include ataxia, depression, and abnormal behavior. Neurologic sequelae are similar, but less common in horses that recover from WEE. For horses that develop neurologic disease the mortality rate for EEE is 75% to 100%; for WEE, 20% to 50%; and for VEE, 40% to 80%.[16, 42] If horses recover from any of the diseases, they seem to be variably protected for up to 2 years after infection. It is wise to assume that no protection is afforded by infection.

Prevention

Prevention of these diseases should aim at reduction of the concentration of insect vectors and implementation of vaccination programs.[33–35, 82–84] Most vaccines are killed (formalin-inactivated) viruses of chick tissue culture origin. Significant increases in antibody titer occur at 3 days after vaccination.[16, 17, 85–88] Vaccination of susceptible horse populations with monovalent, divalent, or trivalent vaccines containing EEE, WEE, or VEE should be employed. There is increased specific antibody production to all viruses when trivalent vaccines are administered. There is some cross-protection between EEE and WEE and between EEE and VEE, but none between WEE and VEE.[77, 89, 90] If VEE vaccine is to be given, it is recommended that all three be administered simultaneously.[91, 92] The response to VEE vaccination alone is poorer in horses previously vaccinated against WEE and EEE.[87, 88, 92, 93] VEE vaccination does not seem to interfere with responses to EEE or WEE vaccination.[94] Annual vaccination should be completed in late spring or several months prior to the beginning of the encephalitis season. Adequate titers appear to last for 6 to 8 months. In areas where the mosquito problem is prolonged or continuous, biannual or triannual vaccination is suggested. Vaccination of susceptible horses in the face of an outbreak is recommended. If vaccinated horses develop disease the affected individuals are often very young or old. Vaccination of mares 1 month prior to foaling will enhance colostral antibody concentrations.[77] Antibody concentrations in foals born to immunized mares appear by 3 hours after colostrum is fed and persist for 6 to 7 months.[77] Vaccination may begin at any age, but if vaccinated early, foals should be revaccinated at 6 months and 1 year to ensure adequate protection. Foals will respond to vaccination with VEE in utero.[95]

Insecticides and repellents should be used when possible and practical. Standing water should be eliminated. In endemic areas or during an outbreak, environmental insecticide application and screened stalls may be implemented. Horses with VEE can be persistently viremic and are quarantined for 3 weeks after complete recovery. Cases of VEE must be reported in the United States. Other measures of disease control may be instituted by public health officials.

FLAVIVIRUS ENCEPHALITIS

Flavivirus species are sporadically associated with encephalitis in the United States and abroad. Seroconversion is often evident, but clinical disease is rare.

Japanese B Encephalitis

Sporadic cases of equine encephalitis have been observed and serum neutralization tests have indicated the presence of Japanese encephalitis in affected horses.[96–102] In most instances, Japanese B encephalitis is a disease of humans and humans are the source of infection for animals.

The disease is widely distributed throughout the eastern pacific rim. As in the case of most togaviral encephalitides, mosquitoes are the natural vectors. The mosquitoes *Culex tritaeniorhyncus* and *Culex pipiens* are the principal vectors. The virus may overwinter in these mosquitoes.[103] In general, horses are dead-end hosts, but horse-to-horse transmission by mosquitoes is reported.[104] A cycle that involves humans, mosquitoes, and pigs maintains the infection throughout the year. Wading birds, such as egrets, are the major sylvatic hosts.[105] In pigs, which are a major reservoir, the disease is associated with abortion and nonsuppurative encephalitis in animals less than 6 months of age.[106] Subclinical infection occurs in cattle, sheep, and goats.[107]

Clinical signs of the disease in horses vary widely in presentation and severity. Mild signs are pyrexia, depression, and icterus for a few days. More severe signs include severe pyrexia and depression, icterus, and petechiation of mucosal surfaces. Dysphagia and ataxia are common. Transient signs may include radial paralysis, blindness, hyperexcitability, profuse sweating, and muscle tremor. These severe signs are uncommon, but when present, often precede death. In most cases, complete recovery occurs in 5 to 10 days. The disease is differentiated from other virus-associated encephalitides of horses by serologic and virus isolation tests.[104]

Formalin-attenuated vaccines protect against natural and experimental encephalitis in pigs and horses.[108]

Borna Disease

Borna disease, first identified in Germany, and Near Eastern equine encephalomyelitis, found in the Middle East, are indistinguishable structurally and antigenically. The virus has a strict tropism for neural tissues where it can persist indefinitely. The method of viral transmission is unknown, but thought to be by inhalation,[109] ingestion, or tick (*Hyalomma anatolicum*) transmission.[110] Other vectors may exist. The infection of horses is often accidental and outside an apparent tick and wild bird cycle. Morbidity is low, but mortality is high. Borna disease in Germany may be associated with transfer of virus from the Near East to Europe by migratory birds.

The signs of disease are similar to other equine encephalitides. The incubation period is unusually long and can range from 4 weeks to 6 months. The long incubation is due to the time required for transport of the virus in dendrite and axonal processes from the site of inoculation to the hippocampus. Necropsy findings are similar to other viral encephalitides, but there are characteristic intranuclear inclusion bodies in nerve cells of the hippocampus and olfactory lobes of the cerebral cortex.[109, 111]

The disease has zoonotic potential.[110, 112, 113] A vaccine is available that appears to be protective for horses.[110, 114]

Other Togaviridae

The viruses discussed below have been classified as *Flavivirus* species. Some have been classified into other groups of viruses from time to time.

California encephalitis is caused by a group of closely related viruses. California serogroup viruses are often classified as Bunyaviridae, as well. The important vectors seem to be *Aedes dorsalis, Aedes triseratus,* and *Culex tarsalis.* They can be associated with encephalitis in horses (snowshoe hare virus).[115] Seroconversion without clinical disease is widespread.[43, 60, 87, 116–121] In the rare instance when horses develop clinical disease, they often recover completely within 7 to 10 days. Pyrexia and depression appear to be common signs.[116, 120–122]

St. Louis virus is most commonly associated with encephalitis in humans. It may be involved in equine disease. Experimental inoculation in horses produces viremia, but no clinical signs. Neutralizing antibody is often present. *Culex pipiens* and *Culex tarsalis* are the major vectors. Wild birds seem to be the primary reservoir.[26, 123–125]

West Nile virus meningoencephalitis occurs in horses in the French Mediterranean. Seroconversion without evidence of disease occurs in humans, sheep, pigs, and birds. *Culex modestus* appears to be the important vector.[126–128]

Powassan virus has been associated with nonsuppurative, focal necrotizing meningoencephalitis in horses. Antibodies for Powassan virus are commonly identified in Ontario and the eastern United States. *Ixodes cookei, Ixodes marxi,* and *Dermacentor andersoni* appear to be important vectors, with snowshoe hares and striped skunks as major reservoirs. Zoonoses occur after bites by infected ticks. Approximately 13% of horses sampled across Ontario in 1983 were serologically positive for the virus.[129] Experimental infection with Powassan virus strain M794 in horses was associated with neurologic deficits within 8 days. A nonsuppurative encephalomyelitis, neuronal necrosis, and focal parenchymal necrosis occur. Signs include tremors of the head and neck, ptyalism, myalgia, ataxia, and recumbency. No clinical signs were identified in inoculated rabbits, but widespread encephalitis characterized by lymphoid perivascular cuffing, lymphocytic meningitis, and lymphocytic choroiditis occurred.[43, 129]

Main Drain virus was isolated from the brain of a horse with encephalitis in Sacramento County, California. Signs included incoordination, ataxia, stiffness of the neck, headpressing, dysphagia, pyrexia, and tachycardia. The major vector is *Culicoides varipennis,* which transmits the virus from infected rabbits and rodents.[122]

Horses have been identified with titers for *Ross River* and *Murray Valley viruses.* Experimental infection with either virus produced transient pyrexia, myalgia, and ataxia. Horses are unlikely to be efficient amplifiers of either virus or important pathogens.[130–133] In Australia, significant titers for Murray Valley encephalitis virus are identified. This is more commonly a disease of humans. An epidemic in humans was associated with significant titers in horses. Some horses with clinical signs, significant titers, and histologic evidence of viral encephalitis were identified.[130, 133]

In Michigan, evidence of *Cache Valley* and *Jamestown Canyon virus* were identified in clinically normal horses.[125] Other viruses, identified in areas around the world, that have been implicated in equine encephalitis or that are associated with encephalitis in other species and for which significant titers have been identified in horses include the *louping ill*,[134, 135] *Maguari*,[26, 117, 136] *Ross River*,[133] *Aura*,[26, 136] *Una*,[26, 136, 137] *Highlands J*,[48, 125, 138] *Semliki forest*,[139] and *getah viruses*.[102]

REFERENCES

1. Jones TC, Doll ER, Bryans JT: The lesions of equine arteritis. *Cornell Vet* 47:3–68, 1957.
2. Casal J: Antigenic variants of equine encephalitis virus. *J Exp Med* 119:547–565, 1964.
3. Trent DW, Grant JA: A comparison of new world alphaviruses in the western equine encephalomyelitis complex by immunochemical and oligonucleotide fingerprint techniques. *J Gen Virol* 47:261–282, 1980.
4. Calisher CH, Kinney RM, de Souza Lopes O, et al: Identification of a new Venezuelan equine encephalitis virus from Brazil. *Am J Trop Med Hyg* 31:1260–1272, 1982.
5. Martin DH, Dietz WH, Alvarez OJ, et al: Epidemiological significance of Venezuelan equine encephalomyelitis virus in vitro markers. *Am J Trop Med Hyg* 31:561–568, 1982.
6. Walton TE, Alvarez O, Buckwalter RM, et al: Experimental infection of horses with enzootic and epizootic strains of Venezuelan equine encephalomyelitis virus. *J Infect Dis* 128:271–282, 1973.
7. Dietz WH, Alvarez O, Martin DH, et al: Enzootic and epizootic Venezuelan equine encephalomyelitis virus in horses infected by peripheral and intrathecal routes. *J Infect Dis* 137:227–237, 1978.
8. Udall DH: A report on the outbreak of "cerebro-spinal meningitis" (encephalitis) in horses in Kansas and Nebraska. *Cornell Vet* 3:17–43, 1913.
9. Meyer KF, Haring CM, Howitt B: Newer knowledge of neurotropic virus infections of horses. *JAMA* 79:376–389, 1931.
10. TenBroeck C, Merrill MH: A serological difference between eastern and western equine encephalomyelitis virus. *Proc Soc Exp Biol Med* 31:217–220, 1933.
11. Records E, Vawter LR: Equine encephalomyelitis cross-immunity in horses between western and eastern strains of virus. *J Am Vet Med Assoc* 85:89–95, 1934.
12. Records E, Vawter LR: Equine encephalomyelitis cross-immunity in horses between western and eastern strains of virus. Supplemental report. *J Am Vet Med Assoc* 86:764–772, 1935.
13. Hoff GL, Bigler WJ, Buff EE, et al: Occurrence and distribution of western equine encephalomyelitis in Florida. *J Am Vet Med Assoc* 172:351–352, 1978.
14. Goldfield M: Arbovirus infection of animals in New Jersey. *J Am Vet Med Assoc* 153:1780–1787, 1968.
15. Shahan MS, Giltner LT: A review of the epizootiology of equine encephalomyelitis in the United States. *J Am Vet Med Assoc* 197:279–287, 1945.
16. Kissling RE, Chamberlain RW: Venezuelan equine encephalitis. *Adv Vet Sci Comp Med* 11:65–84, 1967.
17. Kissling RE, Chamberlain RW, Nelson DB, et al: Venezuelan equine encephalomyelitis in horses. *Am J Hyg* 63:274–287, 1956.
18. Gilyard RT: A clinical study of Venezuelan virus equine encephalomyelitis in Trinidad, BWI. *J Am Vet Med Assoc* 106:267–277, 1945.
19. Young NA, Johnson KM: Antigenic variants of Venezuelan equine encephalitis virus: Their geographic distribution and epidemiologic significance. *Am J Epidemiol* 89:286–307, 1969.
20. Scherer WF, Anderson K, Pancake BA, et al: Search for epizootic-like Venezuelan encephalitis virus at enzootic habitats in Guatemala during 1969–1971. *Am J Epidemiol* 103:576–588, 1976.
21. Scherer WF, Madalengoitia J, Flores W, et al: Ecologic studies of Venezuelan encephalitis virus in Peru during 1970–1971. *Am J Epidemiol* 101:347–355, 1975.
22. Sudia WD, Fernandez L, Newhouse VF, et al: Arbovirus vector ecology studies in Mexico during the 1972 Venezuelan equine encephalitis outbreak. *Am J Epidemiol* 101:51–58, 1975.
23. Sudia WD, Newhouse VF: Epidemic Venezuelan equine encephalitis in North America: A summary of virus-vector-host relationships. *Am J Epidemiol* 101:1–13, 1975.
24. Sudia WD, Newhouse VF, Beadle ID, et al: Epidemic Venezuelan equine encephalitis in North America in 1971: Vector studies. *Am J Epidemiol* 101:17–35, 1975.
25. Sudia WD, McLean RG, Newhouse VF, et al: Epidemic Venezuelan equine encephalitis in North America in 1971: Vertebrate field studies. *Am J Epidemiol* 101:36–50, 1975.
26. Monath TP, Sabattini MS, Pauli R, et al: Arbovirus investigations in Argentina, 1977–1980. IV. Serologic surveys and sentinel equine program. *Am J Trop Med Hyg* 34:966–975, 1985.
27. Dietz WHJ, Galindo P, Johnson KM: Eastern equine encephalomyelitis in Panama: The epidemiology of the 1973 epizootic. *Am J Trop Med Hyg* 29:133–140, 1980.
28. Srihongse S, Grayson MA, Morris CD, et al: Eastern equine encephalomyelitis in upstate New York: Studies of a 1976 epizootic by modified serologic technique, hemagglutination reduction, for rapid detection of virus infections. *Am J Trop Med Hyg* 27:1240–1245, 1978.
29. Bigler WJ, Lassing EB, Buff EE, et al: Endemic eastern equine encephalomyelitis in Florida: A twenty-year analysis, 1955–1974. *Am J Trop Med Hyg* 25:884–890, 1976.
30. Bast TF, Whitney E, Benach JL: Considerations on the ecology of several arboviruses in eastern Long Island. *Am J Trop Med Hyg* 22:109–115, 1973.
31. Bryant ES, Anderson CR, Van der Heide L: An epizootic of eastern equine encephalomyelitis in Connecticut. *Avian Dis* 17:861–867, 1973.
32. Morgante O, Vance HN, Shemanchuk JA, et al: Epizootic of western encephalomyelitis virus infection in equines in Alberta in 1965. *Can J Comp Med* 32:403–408, 1968.
33. Ellis RA: Emergency measures and mosquito control during the 1975 western encephalomyelitis outbreak in Manitoba. *Can J Public Health* 67(suppl 1):59–60, 1976.
34. Donogh NR: Public information on western encephalomyelitis and emergency mosquito control in Manitoba—1975. *Can J Public Health* 67(suppl 1):61–62, 1976.
35. Lillie LE, Wong FC, Drysdale RA: Equine epizootic of western encephalomyelitis in Manitoba—1975. *Can J Public Health* 67(suppl 1):21–27, 1976.
36. Potter ME, Currier RW, Pearson JE, et al: Western equine encephalomyelitis in horses in the northern Red River Valley. *J Am Vet Med Assoc* 170:1396–1399, 1977.
37. Morier L, Cantelar N, Soler M: Infection of a poikilothermic cell line (XL-2) with eastern equine encephalitis and western equine encephalitis viruses. *J Med Virol* 21:277–281, 1987.
38. Carneiro V, Cunha R: Equine encephalomyelitis in Brazil. *Arch Inst Biol* 14:157–194, 1943.
39. Meyer KF, Wood F, Haring CM: Susceptibility of non-immune hyperimmunized horses and goats to eastern, western and Argentine virus of equine encephalomyelitis. *Proc Soc Exp Biol Med* 32:56–58, 1934.
40. Holden P: Recovery of western equine encephalomyelitis virus from naturally infected English sparrows of New Jersey. *Proc Soc Exp Biol Med* 88:490–492, 1955.
41. Livesay HR: Isolation of eastern equine encephalitis virus

from naturally infected monkey (*Macacus philippensis*). *J Infect Dis* 84:306–309, 1949.

42. Gibbs EPJ: Equine viral encephalitis. *Equine Vet J* 8:66–71, 1976.

43. Keane DP, Little PB, Wilkie BN, et al: Agents of equine viral encephalomyelitis: Correlation of serum and cerebrospinal fluid antibodies. *Can J Vet Res* 52:229–235, 1988.

44. Sellers RF: Weather, host and vector—their interplay in the spread of insect-borne animal virus diseases. *J Hyg (Lond)* 85:65–102, 1980.

45. Grady GF, Maxfield HK, Hildreth SW, et al: Eastern equine encephalitis in Massachusetts, 1957–1976. A prospective study centered upon analysis of mosquitos. *Am J Epidemiol* 107:170–178, 1978.

46. Shahan MS, Giltner LT: Equine encephalomyelitis studies: I, Cross-immunity tests between eastern and western types of virus. *J Am Vet Med Assoc* 86:7664–7672, 1935.

47. Smart DL, Trainer DO: Serologic evidence of Venezuelan equine encephalitis in some wild and domestic populations of southern Texas. *J Wildl Dis* 11:195–200, 1975.

48. McLean RG, Frier G, Parham GL, et al: Investigations of the vertebrate hosts of eastern equine encephalitis during an epizootic in Michigan, 1980. *Am J Trop Med Hyg* 34:1190–1202, 1985.

49. Sudia WD, Stamm DD, Chamberlain RW, et al: Transmission of eastern equine encephalomyelitis to horses by *Aedes sollicitans* mosquitos. *Am J Trop Med Hyg* 5:802–808, 1956.

50. Crans WJ, McNelly J, Schulze TL, et al: Isolation of eastern equine encephalitis virus from *Aedes sollicitans* during an epizootic in southern New Jersey. *J Am Mosquito Control Assoc* 2:68–72, 1986.

51. Hayes RO, Wallis RC: An ecology of western equine encephalomyelitis in the eastern United States. *Adv Virus Res* 21:37–83, 1977.

52. Syverton JT, Berry GP: The tick as a vector for the virus disease equine encephalomyelitis. *J Bacteriol* 33:60, 1937.

53. Kitselman CH, Grundman AW: Equine encephalomyelitis virus isolated from naturally infected *Triatoma sanguisuga*. *Kans Agricultural Exp Station Tech Bull* 50:15, 1940.

54. Hardy JL: The ecology of western equine encephalomyelitis virus in the central valley of California, 1945–1985. *Am J Trop Med Hyg* 37(suppl 3):18s–32s, 1987.

55. Hayes RO, Francy DB, Lazuick JS: Role of the cliff swallow bug (*Oaeciacus vicarius*) in the natural cycle of a western equine encephalitis–related alphavirus. *J Entomol* 14:257–262, 1977.

56. Vawter LR, Records E: Respiratory infection in equine encephalomyelitis. *Science* 78:41–42, 1933.

57. Chamberlain RW: Vector relationships of the arthropod-borne encephalitides in North America. *Ann N Y Acad Sci* 70:312–319, 1958.

58. Whitley RJ: Viral encephalitis. *N Engl J Med* 323:242–250, 1990.

59. Gahlinger PM, Reeves WC, Milby MM: Air conditioning and television as protective factors in arboviral encephalitis risk. *Am J Trop Med Hyg* 35:601–610, 1986.

60. McLintock J: The arbovirus problem in Canada. *Can J Public Health* 67(suppl 1):8–12, 1980.

61. Parker RL, Dean PB, Zehmer RB: Public health aspects of Venezuelan equine encephalitis. *J Am Vet Med Assoc* 162:777–778, 1973.

62. Pursell AR, Mitchell FE, Seibold HR: Naturally occurring and experimentally induced eastern encephalomyelitis in calves. *J Am Vet Med Assoc* 169:1101–1103, 1976.

63. Giltner LT, Shahan MS: Transmission of infectious equine encephalomyelitis in mammals and birds. *Science* 78:63–64, 1933.

64. Karsted L, Hanson RP: Natural and experimental infections

in swine with the virus of eastern equine encephalomyelitis. *J Infect Dis* 105:293–296, 1959.

65. Pursell AR, Peckham JC, Cole JR, et al: Naturally occurring and artificially induced eastern encephalomyelitis in pigs. *J Am Vet Med Assoc* 161:1143–1146, 1972.

66. Byrne RH, French GR, Yancy FS, et al: Clinical and immunologic interrelationship among Venezuelan, eastern, and western equine encephalomyelitis viruses in burros. *Am J Vet Res* 25:24–31, 1964.

67. Binn LN, Sponseller ML, Wooding WL, et al: Efficacy of an attenuated western encephalitis vaccine in equine animals. *Am J Vet Res* 27:1599–1604, 1966.

68. Henderson BE, Chappell WA, Johnston JG, et al: Experimental infection of horses with three strains of Venezuelan equine encephalomyelitis. *Am J Epidemiol* 93:194–205, 1971.

69. Wilson JH, Rubin HL, Lane TJ, et al: A survey of eastern equine encephalomyelitis in Florida horses: Prevalence, economic impact, and management practices, 1982–1983. *Prev Vet Med* 4:261–271, 1986.

70. Doby PB, Schnurrenberger PR, Martin RJ, et al: Western encephalitis in Illinois horses and ponies. *J Am Vet Med Assoc* 148:422–427, 1966.

71. Sponseller ML, Binn LN, Wooding WL, et al: Field strains of western encephalitis virus in ponies: Virologic, clinical, and pathologic observations. *Am J Vet Res* 27:1591–1598, 1966.

72. Cox HR, Philip CB, Marsh H, et al: Observations incident to an outbreak of equine encephalomyelitis in the Bitterroot Valley of western Montana. *J Am Vet Med Assoc* 94:225–232, 1938.

73. Calisher CH, Emerson JK, Muth DJ, et al: Serodiagnosis of western equine encephalitis virus infections: Relationships of antibody titer and test to observed onset of clinical illness. *J Am Vet Med Assoc* 183:438–440, 1983.

74. Calisher CH, Mahmud MI, el Kafrawi AO, et al: Rapid and specific serodiagnosis of western equine encephalitis virus infection in horses. *Am J Vet Res* 47:1296–1299, 1986.

75. Scott TW, Olson JG, All BP, et al: Detection of eastern equine encephalomyelitis virus antigen in equine brain tissue by enzyme-linked immunosorbent assay. *Am J Vet Res* 49:1716–1718, 1988.

76. Monath TP, McLean RG, Cropp CB, et al: Diagnosis of eastern equine encephalomyelitis by immunofluorescent staining of brain tissue. *Am J Vet Res* 42:1418–1421, 1981.

77. Ferguson JA, Reeves WC, Hardy JL: Studies on immunity to alphaviruses in foals. *Am J Vet Res* 40:5–10, 1979.

78. Roberts ED, Sanmartin C, Payan J: Neuropathologic changes in 15 horses with naturally occurring Venezuelan equine encephalomyelitis. *Am J Vet Res* 31:1224–1229, 1970.

79. Monlux WS, Luedke AJ: Brain and spinal cord lesions in horses inoculated with Venezuelan equine encephalomyelitis virus (epidemic American and Trinidad strains). *Am J Vet Res* 34:465–473, 1973.

80. Hurst EW: The histology of equine encephalomyelitis. *J Exp Med* 59:529–542, 1934.

81. Devine EH, Byrne RJ: A laboratory confirmed case of viral encephalitis (equine type) in a horse in which the animal completely recovered from the disease. *Cornell Vet* 50:494–497, 1960.

82. Eldridge BF: Strategies for surveillance, prevention, and control of arbovirus diseases in western North America. *Am J Trop Med Hyg* 37(suppl):77S–86S, 1987.

83. Spertzel RO, Kahn DE: Safety and efficacy of an attenuated Venezuelan equine encephalomyelitis vaccine for use in equidae. *J Am Vet Med Assoc* 20:128–130, 1971.

84. Byrne RJ: The control of eastern and western arboviral encephalomyelitis of horses. In *Proceedings of the Third Conference on Equine Infectious Diseases*, 1972, pp 115–123.

85. Gochenour WS, Berge TO, Gleiser CA, et al: Immunization of burros with living Venezuelan equine encephalomyelitis virus. *Am J Hyg* 75:351–362, 1962.

86. Berge T, Banks IS, Tigertt WD: Attenuation of Venezuelan equine encephalomyelitis virus by in vitro cultivation in guinea-pig heart cells. *Am J Hyg* 73:209–218, 1961.

87. Ferguson JA, Reeves WC, Milby MM, et al: Study of homologous and heterologous antibody responses in California horses vaccinated with attenuated Venezuelan equine encephalomyelitis vaccine (strain TC-83). *Am J Vet Res* 39:371–376, 1978.

88. Baker EF, Sasso DR, Maness K: Venezuelan equine encephalomyelitis vaccine (strain TC-83): a field study. *Am J Vet Res* 39:1627–1631, 1978.

89. Walton TE, Jochim MM, Barber TL, et al: Cross-protective immunity between equine encephalomyelitis viruses in equids. *Am J Vet Res* 50:1442–1446, 1989.

90. Jochim MM, Barber TL: Immune response of horses after simultaneous or sequential vaccination against eastern, western, and Venezuelan equine encephalomyelitis. *J Am Vet Med Assoc* 165:621–625, 1974.

91. Barber TL, Walton TE, Lewis KJ: Efficacy of trivalent inactivated encephalomyelitis virus vaccine in horses. *Am J Vet Res* 39:621–625, 1978.

92. Vanderwangen LC, Pearson JL, Franti CE, et al: A field study of persistence of antibodies in California horses vaccinated against western, eastern and Venezuelan equine encephalomyelitis. *Am J Vet Res* 36:1567–1571, 1975.

93. Calisher CH, Sasso DR, Sather GE: Possible evidence for interference with Venezuelan equine encephalitis virus vaccination of equines by pre-existing antibody to eastern or western equine encephalitis virus, or both. *Appl Microbiol* 26:485–488, 1973.

94. Ferguson JA, Reeves WC, Hardy JL: Antibody studies in ponies vaccinated with Venezuelan equine encephalomyelitis (strain TC-83) and other alphavirus vaccines. *Am J Vet Res* 38:425–430, 1977.

95. Morgan DO, Bryans JT, Mock RE: Immunoglobulins produced by the antigenized equine fetus. *J Reprod Fertil Suppl* 23:735–738, 1975.

96. Hale JH, Witherington DH: Encephalitis in race horses in Malaya. *J Comp Pathol* 63:195–198, 1953.

97. Patterson PY, Ley HL, Wisseman DL, et al: Japanese encephalitis in Malaya. I. Isolation of virus and serological evidence of human and equine infections. *Am J Hyg* 56:320–333, 1952.

98. Rosen L: The natural history of Japanese encephalitis virus. *Annu Rev Microbiol* 40:395–414, 1986.

99. Chong SK, Teoh KC, Marchette NJ, et al: Japanese B encephalitis in a horse. *Aust Vet J* 44:23–25, 1968.

100. Yamada T, Rojanasuphot S, Takagi M, et al: Studies on an epidemic of Japanese encephalitis in the northern region of Thailand in 1969 and 1970. *Biken J* 14:267–296, 1971.

101. Nakamura H: Japanese encephalitis in horses in Japan. *Equine Vet J* 4:155–156, 1974.

102. Matsumura T, Goto H, Shimizu K, et al: Prevalence and distribution of antibodies to getah and Japanese encephalitis viruses in horses raised in Hokkaido. *Nippon Juigaku Zasshi* 44:967–970, 1982.

103. Fukimi H, Hayashi K, Mifune K, et al: Ecology of Japanese encephalitis virus in Japan. 1. Mosquito and pig infection with the virus in relation to human incidences. *Trop Med* 17:97–110, 1975.

104. Gould DJ, Byrne RJ, Hayes DE: Experimental infection of horses with Japanese encephalitis virus by mosquito bite. *Am J Trop Med Hyg* 13:742–746, 1964.

105. Scherer WF: Ecologic studies of Japanese encephalitis virus in Japan. Swine infection. *Am J Trop Med Hyg* 8:698, 1959.

106. Kheng CS, Chee TK, Marchette NJ, et al: Japanese encephalitis in a horse. *Aust Vet J* 44:23–25, 1968.

107. Spradbow P: Arbovirus infections of domestic animals. *Vet Bull* 36:53–61, 1966.

108. Goto H: Efficacy of Japanese encephalitis vaccine in horses. *Equine Vet J* 8:126–127, 1976.

109. Carbone KM, Duchala CS, Griffin JW, et al: Pathogenesis of borna disease in rats: Evidence that intra-axonal spread is the major route for virus dissemination and the determinant for disease incubation. *J Virol* 61:3431–3440, 1987.

110. Daubney R, Mahalu EA: Viral encephalomyelitis of equines and domestic ruminants in the Near East—part 1. *Res Vet Sci* 8:375–397, 1967.

111. Blinzinger K, Anzil AP: Large granular nuclear bodies (karyosphaeridia) in experimental borna virus infection. *J Comp Pathol* 83:589–596, 1973.

112. Rott R, Herzog S, Richt J, et al: Immune-mediated pathogenesis of borna disease. *Zentralbl Bakteriol Mikrobiol Hyg [A]* 270:295–301, 1988.

113. Rott R, Herzog S, Fleischer B, et al: Detection of serum antibodies to borna disease virus in patients with psychiatric disorders. *Science* 228:755–756, 1985.

114. Ludwig H, Thein P: Demonstration of specific antibodies in the central nervous system of horses naturally injected with borna disease virus. *Med Microbiol Immunol (Berl)* 163:215–226, 1977.

115. Parkin WE: The occurrence and effects of the local strains of the California encephalitis group of viruses in domestic mammals of Florida. *Am J Trop Med Hyg* 22:788–795, 1973.

116. Artsob H, Wright R, Shipp L, et al: California encephalitis virus activity in mosquitoes and horses in southern Ontario, 1975. *Can J Microbiol* 24:1544–1547, 1978.

117. Calisher CH, Monath TP, Sabattini MS, et al: A newly recognized vesiculovirus, calchaqui virus, and subtypes of melao and maguari viruses from Argentina, with serologic evidence for infections of humans and horses. *Am J Trop Med Hyg* 36:114–119, 1987.

118. Campbell GL, Reeves WC, Hardy JL, et al: Distribution of neutralizing antibodies to California and Bunyamwera serogroup viruses in horses and rodents in California. *Am J Trop Med Hyg* 42:282–290, 1990.

119. Clark GG, Crabbs CL, Bailey CL, et al: Identification of *Aedes campestris* from New Mexico: With notes on the isolation of western equine encephalitis and other arboviruses. *J Am Mosquito Control Assoc* 2:529–534, 1986.

120. Lynch JA, Binnington BD, Artsob H: California serogroup virus infection in a horse with encephalitis. *J Am Vet Med Assoc* 186:389, 1985.

121. McFarlane BL, Embree JE, Embil JA, et al: Antibodies to snowshoe hare virus of the California group in the snowshoe hare (*Lepus americanus*) and domestic animal populations of Prince Edward Island. *Can J Microbiol* 27:1224–1227, 1981.

122. Emmons RW, Woodie JD, Laub RL, et al: Main Drain virus as a cause of equine encephalomyelitis. *J Am Vet Med Assoc* 183:555–558, 1983.

123. Kokernot RH, Hayes J, Will RL, et al: Arbovirus studies in the Ohio-Mississippi basin, 1964–1967. II. St. Louis encephalitis virus. *Am J Trop Med Hyg* 18:750–761, 1969.

124. Bailey CL, Eldridge BF, Hayes DE, et al: Isolation of St. Louis encephalitis virus from overwintering *Culex pipiens* mosquitos. *Science* 199:1346–1349, 1978.

125. McLean RG, Calisher CH, Parham GL: Isolation of Cache Valley virus and detection of antibody for selected arboviruses in Michigan horses in 1980. *Am J Vet Res* 48:1039–1041, 1987.

126. Guillon JC, Oudar J, Joubert L, et al: Histological lesions of the nervous system in West Nile virus infection in horses [in French]. *Ann Inst Pasteur (Paris)* 114:539–550, 1968.

127. Joubert L, Oudar J, Hannoun C, et al: Experimental reproduction of meningoencephalomyelitis of horses with West Nile arbovirus. 3. Relations between virology, serology, and anatomo-clinical evolution. Epidemiological and prophylactic consequences [in French]. *Bull Acad Vet Fr* 44:159–167, 1971.

128. Oudar J, Joubert L, Lapras M, et al: Experimental reproduction of meningoencephalomyelitis of horses with West Nile arbovirus. II. Anatomo-clinical study [in French]. *Bull Acad Vet Fr* 44:147–158, 1971.

129. Little PB, Thorsen J, Moore W, et al: Powassan viral encephalitis: A review and experimental studies in the horse and rabbit. *Vet Pathol* 22:500–507, 1985.

130. Campbell J, Hore DE: Isolation of Murray Valley encephalitis virus from sentinel chickens. *Aust Vet J* 51:1–3, 1975.

131. Kay BH, Young PL, Hall RA, et al: Experimental infection with Murray Valley encephalitis—pigs, cattle, sheep, dogs, rabbits, chickens, and macropods. *Aust J Exp Biol Med Sci* 63:109–126, 1985.

132. Kay BH, Pollitt CC, Fanning ID, et al: The experimental infection of horses with Murray Valley encephalitis and Ross River viruses. *Aust Vet J* 64:52–55, 1987.

133. Gard GP: Association of Australian arboviruses with nervous disease in horses. *Aust Vet J* 53:61–66, 1977.

134. Timoney PJ, Donnelly WJC, Clements LO, et al: Encephalitis caused by louping ill virus in a group of horses in Ireland. *Equine Vet J* 8:113–117, 1976.

135. Timoney PJ: Susceptibility of the horse to experimental inoculation with louping ill virus. *J Comp Pathol* 90:73–86, 1980.

136. Sabattini MS, Monath TP, Mitchell CJ, et al: Arbovirus investigations in Argentina, 1977–1980. I. Historical aspects and description of study sites. *Am J Trop Med Hyg* 34:937–944, 1985.

137. Narayan O, Herzog S, Frese K, et al: Pathogenesis of borna disease in rats: Immune-mediated viral ophthalmoencephalopathy causing blindness and behavioral abnormalities. *J Infect Dis* 148:305–315, 1983.

138. Karabatsos N, Lewis AL, Calisher CH, et al: Identification of Highlands J virus from a Florida horse. *Am J Trop Med Hyg* 40:228–231, 1989.

139. Robin Y, Bourdin P, Le Gonidec E, et al: Semliki forest virus encephalomyelitis in Senegal [in French]. *Ann Microbiol (Inst Pasteur)* 125A:235–241, 1974.

9.14

Rabies

Carla S. Sommardahl, DVM, Dip ACVIM

EPIDEMIOLOGY AND PATHOGENESIS

Rabies is an uncommon disease in the equine, but because of its zoonotic potential, should be considered in the differential diagnosis in horses showing neurologic signs of less than 10 days' duration. In the United States during 1993, 606 cases of rabies were reported in domestic animals, with 0.5% of these being in horses and mules.[1]

The rabies virus is a large, cylindrical, bullet-shaped neurotropic rhabdovirus (genus *Lyssavirus,* family Rhabdoviridae).[2] Rhabdoviruses are enveloped with single-stranded RNA. They are heat-labile, and susceptible to degradation by radiation, strong acids, alkalis, most disinfectants, lipid solvents, and anionic solvents.[2, 4] Rabies virus is transmitted by saliva-contaminated wounds. In the horse, the most common method of infection is a bite wound from a wild carnivore or insectivorous bat carrying the virus.[5] The most common reservoir hosts in the United States are skunks, raccoons, and the red fox.[2] However, domestic dogs, cats, and other horses may transmit rabies to horses by bite wounds. Furthermore, rabies virus can be transmitted by droplet inhalation, orally, or transplacentally. Droplet transmission has been reported to have occurred in foxes, coyotes, opossums, and raccoons in a bat cave in Texas.[3] In that report, the virus was isolated from the air in the cave.[3] Also, aerosolization of the virus caused an outbreak of rabies in a laboratory.[2] Transplacental transmission of virus has occurred in naturally infected cattle and experimentally infected mice and bats.[2]

Rabies virus infects and replicates in myocytes at the inoculation site and may remain undetectable for weeks or months before moving centrally. The virus infects peripheral nerves by traversing neuromuscular and neurotendinous spindles. Progression along the nerve is thought to occur in the tissue spaces of the nerve fasciculus.[3] After progressing centripetally up the peripheral nerve by axoplasmic flow, the virus replicates in spinal and dorsal root ganglia of the corresponding peripheral nerve. Once the virus reaches the central nervous system (CNS), spread occurs rapidly through multiplication in neurons of the brain, spinal cord, sympathetic trunk, and glial cells. Also, spread of rabies virus can occur through passive transport within cerebrospinal fluid or blood.[2, 4, 5] Finally, tissues outside the CNS are reached via centrifugal movement of the virus along nerve axons.[2, 4]

The incubation period for rabies varies from 9 days to 1 year in horses. The incubation period can be affected by the virus strain, host species, inoculum size, and proximity of the inoculation site to the CNS.[2, 5] Retention of virus in myocytes at the inoculation site may be a mechanism for variation in the incubation period.[2] Also, a shorter incubation period may be explained by the virus entering peripheral nerves soon after exposure and rapidly migrating centripetally to the CNS without replication in non-neural tissue.[2]

CLINICAL SIGNS

There are no pathognomonic signs for rabies infection in horses. Clinical signs on presentation are variable and range from lameness to sudden death.[6–9] Hyperesthesia, ataxia, behavior change, anorexia, paralysis or paresis, and colic have been reported as initial clinical signs.[6–11] A bite wound is rarely found and the horse may or may not be febrile. The site of inoculation and its proximity to the CNS influence what clinical signs are seen.[2, 7, 8] The neurologic signs exhibited in rabies-infected horses can be classified into three forms depending on the neuroanatomical location in the CNS infected by the virus. First, in the cerebral or furious form, aggressive behavior, photophobia, hydrophobia, hyperesthesia, straining, muscular tremors, and convulsions may be seen.[12] Second, in the brainstem or dumb form, signs commonly seen are depression, anorexia, head tilt, circling, ataxia, dementia, excess salivation, facial and pharyngeal paralysis, blindness, flaccid tail and anus, urinary incontinence, and self-mutilation.[10, 12, 13] Finally, in the paralytic or spinal form, progressing ascending paralysis, ataxia, or shifting lameness with hyperesthesia, and self-mutilation of an extremity may be seen.[11–14] Most affected animals with the paralytic form become recumbent in 3 to 5 days with normal eating and drinking often remaining.[13] The neurologic signs may vary as the virus spreads to other portions of the CNS. Thus, horses may present with clinical signs of two or all three forms of rabies. Disease progresses rapidly and death is usually inevitable regardless of the clinical manifestation. Anti-inflammatory therapy can delay virus progression.[12] But death usually occurs within 5 to 10 days after onset of clinical signs.[9, 13]

DIAGNOSIS

Antemortem diagnosis of rabies is difficult, but the disease should be considered in horses showing rapidly progressing or diffuse neurologic signs. Other diseases that should be considered include hepatoencephalopathy, togaviral encephalitis, protozoal encephalomyelitis, nigropallidal encephalomalacia, botulism, lead poisoning, cauda equina neuritis, meningitis, space-occupying mass, trauma to the brain or spinal cord, and esophageal obstruction.[4, 5, 13] Clinical laboratory data of body fluids are nonspecific. Cerebrospinal fluid may be within normal reference range or may show a moderate increase in total protein concentration (60–200 mg/dL) and a pleocytosis (5–200/dL).[4, 5, 13] Fluorescent antibody of tactile hair follicles of facial skin taken on biopsy or corneal epithelium may be done to help diagnose rabies antemortem. The fluorescent antibody technique detects the rabies virus antigen in these tissues. Unfortunately, a negative test does not exclude rabies as a differential diagnosis.[9] Definitive postmortem diagnosis can be achieved by submitting half the brain in 10% formaldehyde for histologic examination, and the other half frozen to a public health diagnostic laboratory for immunofluorescent antibody tests, mouse inoculation, and monoclonal antibody techniques. The whole brain may be shipped unfrozen on ice for further rabies evaluation and testing. The rest of the carcass should be examined only with careful precautions against transmission of the virus, if present, by wearing gloves, caps, and masks until a negative rabies diagnosis is made.

Common histopathologic changes are a mild nonsuppurative encephalomyelitis, perivascular cuffing by mononuclear cells, gliosis, glial nodules, and neuronal degeneration.[4, 13] These lesions are most commonly seen in the hippocampus, brainstem, cerebellum, and gray matter of the spinal cord. Large intracytoplasmic eosinophilic inclusions within neurons and ganglion cells, known as Negri bodies, are pathognomonic for rabies.[2, 4, 13] However, in 15% to 30% of confirmed rabies cases, Negri bodies are not present in histopathologic sections, especially if the animal died or was euthanized early in the disease process.[2] The most commonly used and fastest diagnostic test for rabies is the fluorescent antibody test. This technique may identify 98% of infected brain specimens.[2, 4] The mouse inoculation test is the most

accurate method for diagnosing rabies virus infection, but requires 5 to 6 days to complete. The mouse inoculation test involves the injection of suspect brain or salivary gland tissue homogenates intracerebrally in mice and observation of clinical and neurologic signs or death.[2, 4] The monoclonal antibody test (MCAT) has most recently been employed for rabies diagnosis in horses. The MCAT can differentiate specific street, fixed, or vaccinal strains of rabies virus by their glycoprotein or nucleocapsid antigens.[2] The importance of this is in postexposure vaccination of humans and animals when it is important to use the specific strain of virus.

TREATMENT AND PREVENTION

There is no specific treatment for rabies in horses. Symptomatic treatment and supportive care may help prolong the disease course to complete diagnostics and to rule out other diseases with similar signs. This, however, creates a risk of exposure to handlers and other animals. Therefore, any animal suspected of having rabies should be isolated and handled as little as possible. Horses that are known to have been exposed to rabies should have all wounds cleaned and lavaged with iodine or quaternary ammonium disinfectant, and rabies antiserum, if available, infiltrated around the bite wound.[4, 13] There is no postexposure protocol for unvaccinated or vaccinated horses. However, exposed horses should be quarantined for 6 months and observed for the occurrence of neurologic signs.[5] Unvaccinated horses should not receive postexposure prophylaxis until after the 6 months of quarantine.[5] There are two inactivated diploid vaccines (Imrab-1, Pitman-Moore, Inc., Terre Haute, Ind., and Rabguard, Norden Laboratories Inc., Lincoln, Neb.) approved for use in horses. These are recommended annually in high-risk areas to be given to horses over 3 months of age.[12, 13] The dosage is 2 mL administered in the semimembranosus or semitendinosus muscle group. The manufacturer does not recommend administration into the neck muscles.[5]

There are several ongoing arguments concerning vaccination of horses against rabies. The potential for a rare vaccine reaction, illness with neurologic signs following the use of a modified live virus (SAD strain) rabies vaccine, has been reported in the United States.[6] There is also the risk that vaccinated horses that are bitten by a rabid animal will have a silent or attenuated form of the disease and will shed the virus.[12] This, however, is not a proven theory. Public concern and safety outweigh the potential risks of vaccinating horses. Therefore, recommendations to vaccinate in endemic areas should be followed. Any animal positively diagnosed with rabies should be reported to public health officials.

REFERENCES

1. Krebs JW, Strine TW, Smith JS, et al: Rabies surveillance in the United States during 1993. *J Am Vet Med Assoc* 205: 1695, 1994.
2. Martin ML, Sedmak PA: Rabies. Part I. Epidemiology, pathogenesis, and diagnosis. *Compend Contin Educ Pract Vet* 5: 521, 1983.
3. Baer GM: Pathogenesis to the central nervous system. In Baer GM, ed: *The Natural History of Rabies,* vol. 1. New York, Academic Press, 1975, p 181.

4. Mayhew IG, Mackay RJ: Rabies. In Mansmann RA, McAllister ES, Pratt PW, eds: *Equine Medicine and Surgery,* ed 3. Santa Barbara, Calif, American Veterinary Publications, 1982, p 1192.

5. Kent Lloyd KC: Rabies. In Robinson NE, ed: *Current Therapy in Equine Medicine,* ed 2. Philadelphia, WB Saunders, 1987, p 364.

6. West GP: Equine rabies. *Equine Vet J* 17:280, 1985.

7. Striegel P, Genetzky RM: Signs of rabies in horses: A clinical review. *Mod Vet Pract* 64:983, 1983.

8. Joyce JR, Russell LH: Clinical signs of rabies in horses. *Compend Contin Educ Pract Vet* 3:S56, 1981.

9. Smith JM, Cox JH: Central nervous system disease in adult horses. Part III. Differential diagnosis and comparison of common disorders. *Compend Contin Educ Pract Vet* 9:1042, 1987.

10. Sommardahl CS, Henton JE, Peterson MG: Rabies in a horse. *Equine Pract* 12:11, 1990.

11. Siger L, Green SL, Merritt AM: Equine rabies with a prolonged course. *Equine Pract* 11:6, 1989.

12. Mayhew IG: *Large Animal Neurology.* Philadelphia, Lea & Febiger, 1989, p 82.

13. George LW: Diseases of the nervous system. In Smith BP, ed: *Large Animal Internal Medicine.* St Louis, Mosby–Year Book, 1990, p 922.

14. Meyer EE, Morris PG, Elcock LH, et al: Hindlimb hyperesthesia associated with rabies in two horses. *J Am Vet Med Assoc* 188:629, 1986.

Chapter 10

Diseases of the Skin

Karen A. Moriello, DVM ∎ Douglas J. DeBoer, DVM ∎
Susan D. Semrad, DVM, PhD

BASIC STRUCTURE AND FUNCTION OF THE SKIN

General Functions

The most important functions of the skin are protection from external injury and prevention of excess loss of water, electrolytes, and other macromolecules. Other functions of the skin include temperature regulation, blood pressure control, immunoregulation, production of adnexa, secretion and excretion, sensory perception, protection from solar damage via pigmentation, acting as an indicator of general health, and storage of water, electrolytes, fat, vitamins, protein, and other materials.[1]

Gross Anatomy

The skin is the largest organ in the body. At each body orifice it is continuous with mucous membranes. Skin thickness varies from 1 mm to 5 mm depending upon the body region. In general, skin thickness decreases from the dorsum to the ventrum and from proximal to distal on the limbs.[2, 3] In horses, the skin is thickest on the forehead, dorsal neck, dorsal thorax, and base of the tail. The skin is thinnest on the ears and in the axillary, inguinal, and perianal areas.[3]

The sebaceous and sweat glands of the horse are larger and more numerous than in other large animals.[3] The sebaceous glands are particularly well developed on the lips, prepuce, mammary glands, perineum, and labia of the vulva. Apocrine sweat glands are present over the entire body, but are most numerous in the flank, lateral wing of the nostril, mammary glands, and penis.

The ergot is a small mass of cornified tissue located in a tuft of hair on the flexor surface of the fetlock. It is a vestige of the second and fourth digits of extinct Equidae. The chestnut refers to a mass of horny tissue on the medial surface of the radius. It is believed to be a vestige of the first digit. The hoof is the horny covering over the distal end of the third digit.

The coat consists of simple primary hairs. Hair replacement occurs in a mosaic pattern and is influenced most by the photoperiod and ambient temperature. Hair cycle and coat are unaffected by castration, but are accelerated by thyroid hormones and suppressed by excessive glucocorticoids.[4] The texture of the hair coat varies with ambient temperature. In warm ambient temperatures it is composed of thick medullated hairs. Piloerection of hairs allows for maximum cooling. In contrast, in cold ambient temperatures the coat is composed of longer, finer, and poorly medullated fibers. This allows for greater insulation from cold. The hairs of the fetlock, mane, and tail are not shed in cycles. Figure 10–1 summarizes a normal hair growth cycle in a mammal.

EXAMINATION OF THE PATIENT

The diagnosis of equine skin diseases is dependent upon the practitioner's history-taking skills, visual acumen, and the judicious choice of diagnostic tests. The major goals of the physical examination are (1) to determine the type and configuration of the lesions present, (2) to determine the distribution of the lesions, and (3) to evaluate the overall health of the horse. It is important to perform a complete physical examination because some skin diseases are manifestations of systemic illnesses.

History

The medical history of a patient with skin disease should be pursued with the same amount of care as a patient with any other medical or surgical problem. Unfortunately, the history is often the most neglected part of the diagnostic evaluation. Standardized forms should be used to collect the history (Fig. 10–2). Key points in the history are age, breed, familial occurrence of similar disease, seasonal or environmental influence, evidence of contagion or zoonosis, previous skin diseases, response to past and current therapy (including ivermectin), initial skin lesions and a description of lesion progression, and the presence or absence of pruritus.

Physical Examination

The skin is one of the easiest body organs to examine because the gross pathologic lesions are visible to the veterinarian. Unfortunately, many examinations of the skin are performed too rapidly and under poor circumstances. Horses with skin disease are best examined outdoors in strong sunlight. It is often necessary to clip the coat to visualize the lesions. In addition, a handheld magnifying lens should

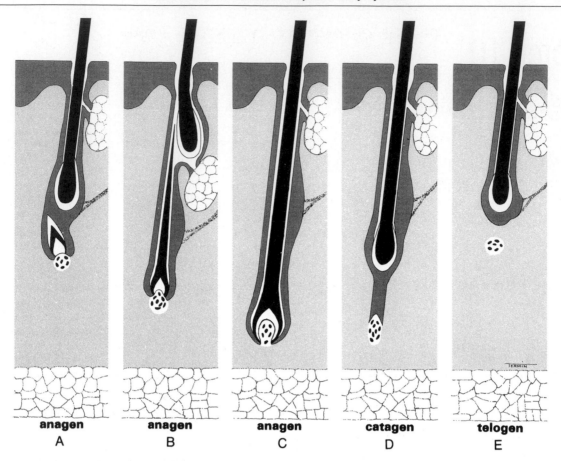

anagen   **anagen**   **anagen**   **catagen**   **telogen**
A   B   C   D   E

Figure 10–1. Phases in the life cycle of a hair. *A,* Anagen begins with the renewal of the intimate relationship between the papilla and the undifferentiated cells that partially enclose it. *B,* As anagen proceeds, matrix cells generate a new hair that pushes upward toward the surface and in the process dislodges the old club hair. *C,* Mature anagen hair follicle consists of infundibular, isthmus, and inferior segments. *D,* During catagen, the entire inferior segment of the follicle shrivels upward as a thin cord of epithelial cells and is followed upward by the papilla. *E,* During telogen, the club hair rests in its cornified sac at the level of the hair erector muscle. (From Moschella SL, Herley HJ: Dermatology, ed 3. Philadelphia, WB Saunders, 1992, p. 61.)

be available. Specific lesions and patterns of distribution of the important skin diseases of horses are discussed below.

COMMON CAUSES OF PRURITIC DERMATOSES

Pruritus may be defined as the sensation that elicits the desire to scratch, or in more general terms, an uneasy sensation in the skin.[5] Typically, horses will rub or bite at their skin when pruritic. Clinical evidence of pruritus includes broken hairs, excoriations, hemorrhagic crusts, alopecia, and postinflammatory hyperpigmentation.

Although simplistic, it is helpful to categorize skin diseases into pruritic and nonpruritic (Fig. 10–3). In general, this is a useful approach, but it is important to remember that some skin diseases are variable with respect to pruritus: bacterial infections, dermatophytosis, and seborrhea. In addition, some patients with classically nonpruritic skin diseases may be pruritic because of secondary inflammation or infection. The reader may find the algorithms in Figures 10–4 and 10–5 useful for the diagnosis of equine pruritus.

Parasitic Skin Diseases
Lice (Pediculosis)

Lice are the most common ectoparasites of horses. The sucking louse of horses, *Haematopinus asini,* is most commonly found in the mane and tail, and in the hairs behind the fetlock and pastern. The biting louse, *Damalinia equi,* tends to concentrate on the dorsolateral trunk. Biting lice feed on epidermal debris, while sucking lice feed on blood and lymph.

Lice are host-specific and complete their entire life cycle on the host, and females attach their eggs to hairs. In cool moist environments, lice can live for 2 to 3 weeks in the environment; otherwise they can only live for several days off the host. Lice infestations are transmitted by direct or indirect contact. It is important to remember that contaminated brushes, combs, and tack are sources of fomite transmission. Adult horses may act as asymptomatic reservoirs of infection.

Lice infestations occur year-round; however clinical signs tend to be more evident in the winter in northern climates. There are several reasons for this. First, the longer winter hair coat is more hospitable to lice. Secondly, horses tend to

EQUINE DERMATOLOGY HISTORY FORM

Date _____

Age when purchased _____

What is this horse's use? _____

What is your complaint about the horse's skin? _____

Age of horse? _____ Age when skin problem started? _____

Where on the body did the problem start? _____

What did the skin problem look like initially? _____

_____

How has it spread or changed? _____

Is the problem continual or intermittent? _____

What season did the problem start? _____

Is the problem seasonal or year-round? _____

If seasonal, what seasons is the disease present? _____

_____

Does the horse itch? _____ If so, where? _____

_____

Do any horses in contact with the affected horse have skin problems? _____

If so, are they similar or different from this horse's problem? _____

Do any people in contact with the horse have skin problems? _____

Do you use insect control? _____ If so, describe. _____

_____

Do any relatives of this horse have skin problems? _____ If yes, explain. _____

_____

Please list any injectable, oral, or topical medications that have been used to treat the problem (veterinary or "home remedies"): _____

_____

Did any help the condition? _____ If yes, which ones? _____

Did any aggravate the condition? _____ If yes, which ones? _____

Describe the environment where the horse is kept: Indoors _____

_____ Outdoors _____

What is the horse fed? _____

What feed additives do you use? _____

What is your deworming schedule? _____

Did the horse receive ivermectin? _____ If so, when? _____

List any other major medical problems or drugs that the horse received: _____

_____

List any additional information you feel is relevant to the skin disease: _____

_____

Figure 10–2. Sample equine history form.

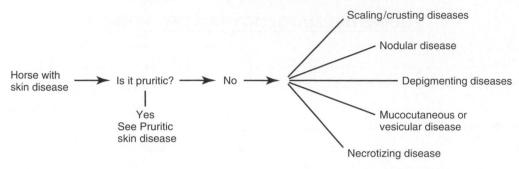

Figure 10–3. Simplified guide to equine skin disease.

congregate more closely, increasing the chances of transmission. Finally, the life cycle of the louse is affected by temperature, and biting lice do not propagate when skin temperature exceeds 38°C which can easily occur in the summer.[6] The cooler skin and hair coat temperatures of horses in the winter are most favorable for development of eggs within the female, oviposition, and egg development. Heavy louse populations may develop. The skin temperatures on the legs, with the possible exception of draft horses, are too cold for louse development.

There is no documented breed, sex, or age predilection for lice infestations. Anecdotal reports and clinical observations suggest that foals and draft horses may be predisposed. However, management practices in individual stables may greatly influence these observations. Infested horses may be restless or have a poor appetite. Affected animals will have a dry, dull hair coat with patchy areas of hair loss and excoriations. The coat may appear moist and have a sour or "mousy" odor. Skin fasciculations may be the only evidence of early infestations in foals. Some horses may also be asymptomatic carriers and are only detected when foals or other susceptible animals become infested. Heavy infestations of sucking lice may cause anemia or severe debilitation.

Lice infestations are diagnosed by demonstration of the adult or eggs attached to hairs. This is not always easy to do and is best done by careful examination of the hair coat in direct sunlight. Combing the hair coat with a fine-toothed metal comb or household scrub brush, collecting the debris in a flat pan, and examining the material under a microscope is very useful when lice are suspected, but cannot be found. Skin biopsy reveals varying degrees of superficial perivascular eosinophilic dermatitis. Microscopic intraepidermal microabscesses may also be present.[7]

Elimination of lice requires treatment of all horses on the premises. Ivermectin 200 μg/kg PO every 2 weeks for three treatments is very effective, but is not approved for this use in horses. The efficacy of ivermectin in the treatment of biting lice may be questionable and concurrent use of a topical sponge-on dip or spray is recommended. Topical treatment alone may be very effective, but only if the parasiticide is thoroughly applied to the entire body. Household vinegar diluted 1:1 with water and used as a rinse prior to using a sponge-on will help loosen lice and nits attached to hairs. Pyrethrin, pyrethroid, lime sulfur, and organophosphate sponge-on dips applied weekly for six to eight treatments are effective. It is, however, advisable to avoid products containing organophosphates because of the potential

for toxicity. Although few owners are receptive to the suggestion, clipping the long winter hair coat, or the long shaggy hairs on the fetlock of draft horses, will speed recovery and limit contagion. The environment should be decontaminated using a commercial premise spray licensed to kill fleas since adult lice may survive for days to weeks in the environment and nits attached to hairs are sources of contagion and reinfestation. Tack, blankets, and other fomites also should be decontaminated with a parasiticidal premise flea spray. Reinfestation is difficult to prevent, but animals returning from shows, breeding farms, or from training should be treated prophylactically.

Acariasis (Mange)

The important mites of horses are *Sarcoptes scabiei* var. *equi* (scabies, head mange), *Chorioptes equi* (leg mange), *Psoroptes equi* (body mange), *Pyemotes tritici* (straw itch mite), and *Trombicula* and *Eutrombicula* species (chiggers). Pruritus is caused by a combination of mechanical irritation and hypersensitivity to the mite and mite byproducts (e.g., feces).[8, 9] The primary lesion of acariasis is a maculopapular eruption, but these lesions may be difficult to find on horses with longstanding infestations.

In the United States, *S. scabiei* infestations in horses are reportable to the United States Department of Agriculture (USDA). This mite is highly contagious and will infest horses and may transiently affect people in contact with parasitized horses. Scabies mites burrow in the superficial epidermis where they lay eggs. In early infestations, mites are found in highest concentration around the head and neck. As the disease progresses, mites will spread over the entire body. Affected horses usually have intense pruritus, generalized scaling, and crusting with excoriations and lichenification. An "itch" reflex may be elicited by scratching the horse over the withers, causing the horse to tuck its nose close to its chest and make smacking noises and exaggerated movements with its lips. This reflex, however, may also be elicited from normal horses.[10]

Chorioptes equi mites are host-specific and do not parasitize people. This mite spends its entire life cycle on the host. The mite prefers to infest the distal limbs and perineum of horses and causes extreme pruritus. Affected horses will stamp their limbs, scratch at their legs, and rub their perineum. Infestations are most common in draft horses and other breeds with feathered fetlocks. This mite is a com-

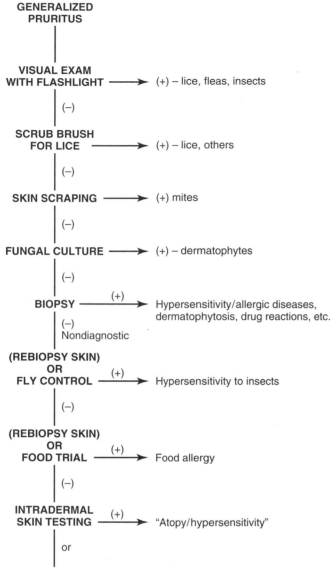

GENERALIZED
PRURITUS
|
VISUAL EXAM
WITH FLASHLIGHT ⟶ (+) – lice, fleas, insects
|
(–)
|
SCRUB BRUSH
FOR LICE ⟶ (+) – lice, others
|
(–)
|
SKIN SCRAPING ⟶ (+) mites
|
(–)
|
FUNGAL CULTURE ⟶ (+) – dermatophytes
|
(–)
|
BIOPSY —(+)⟶ Hypersensitivity/allergic diseases,
dermatophytosis, drug reactions, etc.
(–)
Nondiagnostic
|
(REBIOPSY SKIN)
OR
FLY CONTROL —(+)⟶ Hypersensitivity to insects
|
(–)
|
(REBIOPSY SKIN)
OR
FOOD TRIAL —(+)⟶ Food allergy
|
(–)
|
INTRADERMAL
SKIN TESTING —(+)⟶ "Atopy/hypersensitivity"
|
or
|
Corticosteroid therapy or hydroxyzine therapy,
200 to 400 mg b.i.d. or t.i.d.

Figure 10–4. Flowchart for diagnosis of equine pruritic skin diseases.

monly overlooked cause of pastern dermatitis (Fig. 10–6) (scratches, grease heal).

In the United States, *Psoroptes* mite infestations in horses are reportable to the USDA. *Psoroptes* also is highly contagious but does not parasitize people. Mite infestations usually begin on the mane and tail and spread to the trunk, but may also infest the ear canal causing otitis externa.[7] Affected horses may present with headshaking or rubbing. The intensity of the pruritus is variable, ranging from none to marked.

Trombiculidiasis is caused by infestation with the larvae of free-living adult mites of the genus *Eutrombicula* or *Trombicula*. Larvae are most prevalent in grasses, forests, or swamps in late summer and fall. Skin lesions consist of wheals and papules with small brightly colored orange, red, or yellow dots (trombiculid larvae) in the center. Lesions are most commonly found on the face, muzzle, distal limbs,

ventral thorax, and abdomen. This disease is self-limiting, but severely affected animals may require one treatment of a topical insecticide (lime sulfur or pyrethrin) and prednisolone or prednisone 0.5 mg/kg PO for 3 to 5 days. Pruritus varies from none to marked.

Pyemotes tritici (straw itch mite) normally parasitizes the larvae of grain insects, but infestations of horses and people have been reported.[11] Horses are infested from contaminated hay fed from overhead racks. This mite causes a maculopapular crusted eruption on the head, neck, and trunk that is predominantly nonpruritic. The disease is self-limiting and contaminated forage should be removed or horses should be fed from the ground until all the contaminated forage has been used. Infestations from fomites or hay fed on the ground have not been reported.

Definitive diagnosis of acariasis is made by finding mites or eggs on skin scrapings. The best sites to scrape are nontraumatized areas adjacent to newly developing lesions. Mineral oil should be liberally painted on the skin, and wide deep skin scrapings performed. Histologic examination of tissue will reveal nondiagnostic superficial perivascular eosinophilic dermatitis; it is rare to find a mite on histologic examination of skin. Complete blood counts may show an eosinophilia.

Ivermectin 200 μg/kg PO repeated two to three times at 2-week intervals is very effective in the eradication of *Sarcoptes*, *Chorioptes*, and *Psoroptes* species infestations. Alternatively, topical therapy is effective, and is enhanced, if the animals are aggressively brushed and washed to remove contaminated crusts prior to the application of topical parasiticidal agents. The following topical treatments are effective: six weekly treatments of lime sulfur (Lym Dyp, DVM Miami, Florida) (2%–5%), or two treatments of malathion (0.5%) or methoxychlor (0.5%) at 2-week intervals.[7]

Chorioptes infestations in draft horses are difficult to treat even with systemic ivermectin therapy. We have found the concurrent use of a topical sponge-on pyrethrin dip to be very beneficial. Clipping of the hair will greatly enhance penetration of the dip, if the owner will comply. Alternatively, the lower legs can be soaked in buckets of pyrethrin or lime sulfur dip for 4 to 5 minutes every 5 days during the treatment period. Amitraz should not be used in horses because of the adverse side effects. Horses sprayed with 0.025% amitraz developed depression, ataxia, weakness, and progressive large intestinal impactions within 24 to 48 hours of treatment.[12]

The environment should be decontaminated because these mites can live for days to weeks off the host in cool moist environments.[13, 14] Commercial premise sprays formulated for eradicating fleas are effective and convenient to use. One to two applications are recommended. In addition, blankets, tack, combs, etc. should be washed and thoroughly sprayed with an insecticide.

Fleas

Fleas occasionally infest horses. Infestations tend to occur in the summer and fall when populations are at their highest. *Tunga penetrans* (chigoe, jigger, sand flea) and *Echidnophaga gallinacea* (sticktight flea) are the most common species of fleas found on horses.[7]

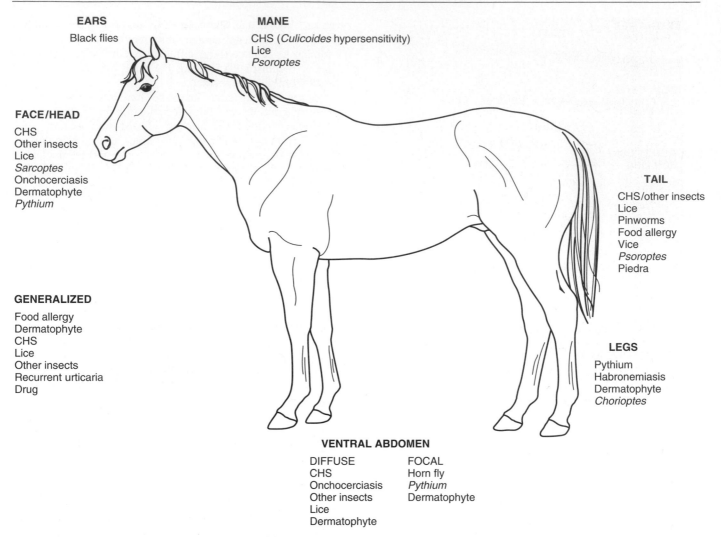

EARS

Black flies

MANE

CHS (*Culicoides* hypersensitivity)
Lice
Psoroptes

FACE/HEAD

CHS
Other insects
Lice
Sarcoptes
Onchocerciasis
Dermatophyte
Pythium

TAIL

CHS/other insects
Lice
Pinworms
Food allergy
Vice
Psoroptes
Piedra

GENERALIZED

Food allergy
Dermatophyte
CHS
Lice
Other insects
Recurrent urticaria
Drug

LEGS

Pythium
Habronemiasis
Dermatophyte
Chorioptes

VENTRAL ABDOMEN

DIFFUSE	FOCAL
CHS	Horn fly
Onchocerciasis	*Pythium*
Other insects	Dermatophyte
Lice	
Dermatophyte	

Figure 10–5. Regional pruritus: Differential diagnosis of pruritic skin diseases.

The clinical signs include generalized pruritus, excoriations, papules, crusting, and secondary hair loss. *Tunga penetrans* fleas are found in the southern United States. The adult female flea burrows into the skin and swells to the size of a pea and causes a painful ulcer. Necrosis, gangrene, and tetanus are possible sequelae to infestation. *Tunga penetrans* infestations are commonly confused with chigger bites. Diagnosis is made by clinical signs and finding fleas or flea excreta.

Successful eradication of flea infestations requires treatment of both the horse and the environment. For the horse, residual action pyrethrin or pyrethroid insecticidal sprays are recommended. *Tunga penetrans* fleas may require mechanical removal with forceps or mosquito hemostats. Control of fleas in the environment is difficult and efforts should be directed at the stable and paddock. It is impractical to attempt to eliminate fleas from the pasture area. Bedding should be removed, burned, and the environment thoroughly sprayed with a commercial parasiticide diluted and used according to the manufacturer's instructions. However, the flea burden can be greatly decreased if attention is directed at cool, moist, shaded areas; fleas cannot live and reproduce in areas with direct sunlight. Organic material should be removed and insecticide sprinkled under shady protected areas. Outdoor insecticides are available at most garden supply stores.

Ticks

Ticks are members of the spider family and are an important ectoparasite of horses. Ticks cause disease by sucking blood, causing tick paralysis, creating wounds that predispose the horse to secondary bacterial infection or myiasis, and by the transmission of a variety of viral, protozoal, rickettsial, and bacterial infections. Tick infestations are most common in spring and summer.

Argasid ticks lay their eggs in cracks and crevices in the environment and immature ticks infect hosts after hatching. Larvae and nymphs suck blood and lymph and then drop off to develop into adults. These ticks infest barns, sheds, and other areas where animals are found. In horses, *Otobius megnini* (spinose ear tick) tends to infest the ears and ear canal. Clinical signs of infestation include otitis externa,

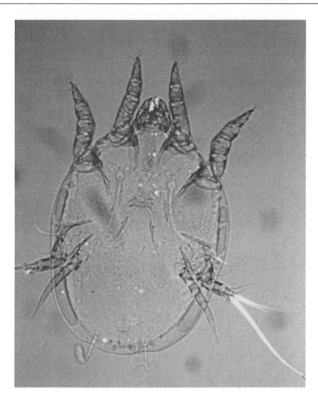

Figure 10–6. *Chorioptes* mite.

head tilt, headshaking, ear rubbing, and occasionally aural hematomas.

Dermacentor, Ixodes, and *Amblyomma* species are the most common ixodid ticks of horses. These ticks are found outdoors, have complicated life cycles, and all stages of the life cycle are parasitic. The severity of clinical signs depends upon the density of the infestation and whether or not the horse develops a hypersensitivity reaction to the bites. Ears, face, neck, groin, distal limbs, and tail are most commonly infested. Early lesions consist of papular to pustular eruptions which rapidly develop into crusts, erosions, ulcers, and hair loss. Hypersensitivity reactions can be localized or generalized. Local responses appear as nodules that develop at the site of the tick bite. Although the pathogenesis is unknown, cutaneous basophil hypersensitivity is believed to be involved.[15] Systemic reactions are characterized by whole-body urticaria or multifocal urticarial plaques. In Australia, a hypersensitivity reaction to *Boophilus microplus* has been observed in sensitized horses.[16] Intense pruritus, papules, and wheals develop as soon as 30 minutes after ticks begin to feed.

Definitive diagnosis is made by finding ticks attached to the horse or in the ear canal. Treatment is directed at killing the ticks on the horse. Pyrethrin or pyrethroid sponge-on dips should be applied to the horse's body. Extra care should be taken to soak skinfold areas. Usually only one treatment is necessary unless reinfestation is occurring. Resistance to insecticides can occur rapidly and knowledge of the local resistance patterns is important. Infestations of *O. megnini* require mechanical removal of as many ticks as possible. One part rotenone and three parts mineral oil applied twice-weekly is an effective otic parasiticide for horses.[17] Ivermectin 200 μg/kg PO is also effective.

Onchocerciasis

Onchocerciasis is a nonseasonal skin disease of horses caused by *Onchocerca cervicalis*. This nematode lives in the ligamentum nuchae and produces microfilaria which migrate to the skin and are ingested by the intermediate host, *Culicoides* species gnats. Microfilariae populations in the skin are variable and the highest concentrations are found in the dermis of face, neck, and ventral midline, especially at the umbilicus[18] (Fig. 10–7). Microfilariae populations vary seasonally and are highest in the spring, which, interestingly, is the peak season for the *Culicoides* vector.[19] In addition, microfilaria also are more superficial in the dermis during the spring and summer months. Clinical signs of onchocerciasis are believed to be due to an idiosyncratic hypersensitivity reaction to microfilarial antigen(s) because many horses that have circulating microfilariae do not have any gross skin or ocular lesions.[20] It is unknown if the reaction is directed only at dying or dead microfilariae.

Onchocerciasis has no breed or sex predilection and usually affects horses age 4 years and older. Clinical signs are nonseasonal, but may be worse in the spring and summer, most likely due to the added irritation from the vector. Lesions may be seen on the face and neck, on the ventral chest and abdomen, or in all these areas.[21, 22] Early lesions begin as thinning of the hair coat. As the disease progresses, lesions may vary from focal to generalized areas of alopecia, scaling, crusting, and plaques. Affected areas may be severely excoriated, ulcerated, oozing, and lichenified. Annular lesions in the center of the forehead are believed to be suggestive of the disease (Fig. 10–8). Leukoderma usually develops at the site of lesions and is irreversible. Ocular lesions include sclerosing keratitis, vitiligo of the bulbar conjunctiva, white nodules in the pigmented conjunctiva, uveitis, and a crescent-shaped patch of depigmentation bordering the optic disk.[23]

A presumptive diagnosis of onchocerciasis may be made by demonstrating the microfilariae in the skin of animals with compatible historical and clinical findings. Skin scrapings and direct blood smears are often negative. Microfilaria are most reliably demonstrated with a mince preparation or via histologic examination of skin from a biopsy

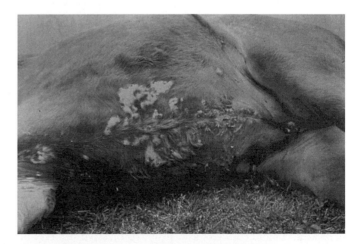

Figure 10–7. Ventral midline dermatitis due to onchocerciasis.

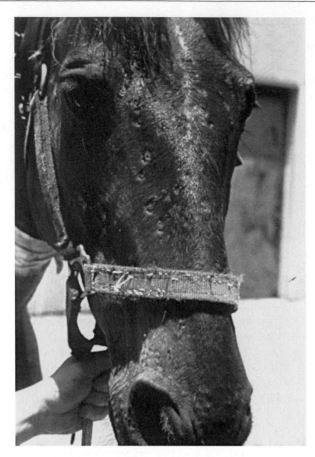

Figure 10–8. Equine onchocercosis.

and fever. It is important to remember that none of the current anthelmintics will kill the adult worms in the ligamentum nuchae and affected individuals will need periodic retreatment with ivermectin when reexacerbations occur. The prevalence of cutaneous onchocerciasis has decreased significantly because of the advent of routine dewormings with ivermectin.

Fly Bite Dermatitis

Fly bite dermatitis is a very common cause of skin disease in horses. Mosquitoes and species of *Culicoides* (gnats, biting midges, sandflies, "no-see-ums," "sweet itch"), *Simulium* (black flies), *Tabanus* (horse flies), *Chrysops* (deer flies), *Haematopota* (breeze flies), *Stomoxys calcitrans* (stable flies), *Haematobia* (horn flies), *Musca, Gasterophilus,* bees, and wasps have all been observed to cause skin lesions in horses.[7]

Bites or strikes from these flying insects cause disease in several ways. Firstly, the bite itself may cause a wound in the skin large enough to ooze serum and predispose the horse to a secondary bacterial infection or myiasis. Secondly, the bites of the larger flies, for example, *Tabanus* and *Chrysops* species, cause painful wheals or nodules which are very irritating to the horse. Thirdly, many of these flying insects are vectors for viral, bacterial, and protozoal diseases. Finally, many flying insects have been incriminated as a cause of insect hypersensitivity in horses. The most common is *Culicoides,* but *Simulium, Stomoxys calcitrans,* and *Haematobia* species also are involved.[7, 19, 22] Insect hypersensitivity reactions represent type I and type IV hypersensitivity reactions to salivary antigens or injected toxins.[25]

Insect Hypersensitivity

Insect hypersensitivity is one of the most common pruritic skin diseases of horses. This disease is seasonal in colder climates and nonseasonal in warmer climates. Any age, sex, or breed may be affected and there is some suggestion that there may be a heritable component. The distribution of the disease is variable and it may be dorsal, ventral, or dorsal and ventral.[7, 19, 22, 26, 27] Face, ears, dorsal trunk, and tail head are most commonly affected in dorsal insect hypersensitivity (Fig. 10–9). Severe self-trauma of the mane and tail may result in almost total hair loss. Horses are intensely pruritic and will bite and rub, creating hair loss, excoriations, and lichenification. Often a generalized papular-crusted eruption is present. Ventral insect hypersensitivity is usually characterized by pruritus and a papular-crusted eruption on the ventral midline, groin, axilla, thorax, and intermandibular area. The intense pruritus and irritation caused by insect hypersensitivity may affect the horse's temperament.

The diagnosis of insect hypersensitivity is based on a compatible history, physical findings, and the elimination of other causes of pruritus in the horse. Skin scrapings are usually not helpful. Histologic examination of a skin biopsy specimen is the most useful routine diagnostic test. A superficial or deep perivascular eosinophilic dermatitis with epidermal spongiosis (intercellular edema of the epidermis), necrosis, and collagen degeneration is very suggestive of insect hypersensitivity if other causes of pruritus have been

specimen.[22] Mince preparations are easy to perform and require a 4- to 6-mm punch specimen of tissue taken from the ventral abdomen. The tissue specimen is placed in a Petri dish with a small amount of physiologic saline, minced with a scalpel blade or razor, and incubated at room temperature for 30 to 60 minutes. The specimen is then examined under a microscope for the rapid motion of the microfilariae. Skin biopsies will reveal superficial perivascular eosinophilic dermatitis. Often microfilariae will be seen in the superficial dermis.[7]

Ivermectin 200 μg/kg PO has rapidly become the drug of choice for the treatment of equine onchocerciasis.[7, 21, 24] A single dose often produces remission of clinical signs within 2 to 3 weeks, but some horses may require two to three monthly treatments before clinical signs resolve. About 25% of horses have an adverse reaction, such as ventral midline edema or pruritus, which occurs 1 to 10 days after treatment. In rare cases, severe umbilical and eyelid edema and fever may occur. In confirmed cases of onchocerciasis, a thorough ocular examination should be performed to look for any signs of eye disease associated with onchocerciasis. Anecdotal reports suggest treatment may precipitate an episode of uveitis.

Prednisolone or prednisone 0.5 mg/kg PO may be necessary in the first week of treatment to prevent exacerbation of skin and ocular lesions as a result of massive destruction of microfilariae, but is not needed routinely. Indications include the development of ventral midline edema, pruritus, eliminated. Occasionally, a V-shaped area of necrosis is observed, suggesting a previous insect bite in the area.[27] Intradermal skin testing with dilutions of insect antigen (Greer, Lenoir, N.C.) may be very helpful in making a diagnosis of insect hypersensitivity.[27] Unfortunately, the cost of the antigens and their intermittent availability from manufacturing companies may limit the usefulness of this diagnostic test. Identification of the exact offending insect is often impossible. Fortunately, therapy and environmental control measures are similar for most biting and flying insects, and therefore, it is not crucial to confirm the diagnosis via intradermal skin testing.

The treatment of fly bite dermatitis involves insect control and the judicious use of glucocorticoids.[27] Recommendations are summarized in Tables 10–1, 10–2, and 10–3. Ideally, horses should be stabled during the target insect's peak feeding period. The windows should be screened with a small-mesh screen (32 × 32) and sprayed with a residual parasiticide. If possible, breeding areas for flies should be eliminated, that is, standing water, manure, etc. Horses should be sprayed with residual insecticides, for example, pyrethrins or pyrethroids. Frequency of application varies with the product and environmental conditions. Label recommendations should be followed initially and then therapeutic changes made appropriately. Cattle tags impregnated with insecticide may be helpful if attached to manes, tails, or halters. Commercial bath oils diluted 1:1 with water (Skin-So-Soft bath oil, Avon Products, Inc., New York, N.Y.) may be helpful as a repellant but should be used with care because this preparation can cause contact reactions.

Anecdotal reports suggest that it is important that repellents and insecticide sprays be applied to the horse when the skin is cool and dry. This may minimize the development of sensitivity reactions to these products by limiting the percutaneous absorption of the substance. Many horses have a sensitivity to petroleum-based products and will develop erythematous skin and hair loss in the area where insecticide, fly wipe, or bath oil has been applied to the skin. If a horse has a history of this, it is advisable to perform an open patch test with any new product before applying the spray to the entire body. An open patch test is performed by applying a small amount of the test substance to an area of skin and

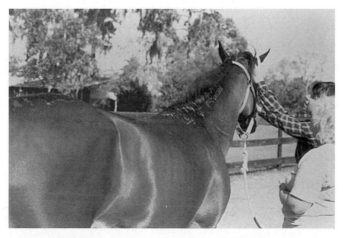

Figure 10–9. Two-year-old horse with *Culicoides* hypersensitivity.

Table 10–1. Primary Management Strategies for Common Equine Pests*

1. Stabling
   Tabanids: Diurnal and crepuscular periods
   Black flies: Diurnal and crepuscular periods
   Biting midges: Under fans, nocturnal and crepuscular periods
2. Exclusion devices
   Black flies: Ear nets
   House flies: Face masks
   Face flies: Face masks
3. Hay and manure management
   Stable flies: Particularly hay in pastures
   House flies: General sanitation
4. Cattle management
   Horn flies: Control pest on natural host
   Face flies: Undisturbed cattle manure requisite for larval development
5. Water management
   Mosquitoes: Only certain species
   Biting midges: Only certain species
6. Source identification and removal
   Straw itch: Normally infested hay
   Blister beetle: Normally products containing alfalfa
7. Restricted grazing or movement
   Chiggers: Erratic distribution in spring or fall
   Ticks: Mowing and understory control also helpful
   Tabanids: Allow horses to escape from wooded areas
   Poultry pests (sticktight and lice): Separate horses from poultry

*From Foil L, Foil C: Control of ectoparasites. In Robinson NE, ed: *Current Therapy in Equine Medicine*, Vol 3. Philadelphia, WB Saunders, 1992, p 689.

observing the site for 72 hours for signs of erythema, swelling, and hair loss.

In many cases, insect control is not sufficient to alleviate discomfort and clinical signs. Hydroxyzine HCl may be beneficial in some horses with insect hypersensitivity when administered orally at a dosage of 200 to 400 mg b.i.d. or t.i.d.[29] Additionally, this drug has been very helpful in managing insect-induced urticaria and the only observed side effect has been transient sedation for several days. If there is no response to hydroxyzine HCl, systemic glucocorticoids are the next drug of choice. Prednisolone 1 mg/kg PO is administered daily until the pruritus is relieved. The dose is then tapered to the smallest alternate-day therapy that is effective. Daily bathing of affected animals not only removes crusts and scales but decreases pruritus. A double-blind study on the efficacy of immunotherapy in the treatment of *Culicoides* hypersensitivity showed that this therapy was ineffective when compared with untreated controls.[30]

Allergic Skin Diseases

Insect Hypersensitivity

The reader is referred to this section under Parasitic Skin Diseases.

Table 10–2. Pesticides Recommended for External Parasite Control on Horses*†

Residual Insecticides	Other Compounds
Pyrethroids	Repellents
Cypermethrin	MGK 326 *di-n-propyl isocinchomeronate*
Fenvalerate	Stabilene: butoxypolypropylene glycol
Permethrin	Botanicals
Resmethrin	Pyrethrins (also insecticidal)
Tetramethrin	Synergists
S-Bioallethrin	Piperonyl butoxide *5-[[2-(2-butoxyethoxy) ethoxy]methyl]-6-propyl-1,3-benzodioxole*
Sumethrin	MGK 264 *N-octyl bicycloheptene dicarboximide*
Organophosphates	
Coumaphos	
Dichlorvos	
Malathion	
Tetrachlorvinphos	
Organochlorines	
Lindane	
Methoxychlor	

*From Foil L, Foil C: Control of ectoparasites. In Robinson NE, ed: *Current Therapy in Equine Medicine*, Vol 3. Philadelphia, WB Saunders, 1992, p 689.
†Categories may overlap: e.g., some pyrethrins are also insecticidal, and some pyrethroids are repellent. William B. Warner and Roger O. Drummond assisted in compiling this list.

Food Allergy

Documented cases of feed-related hypersensitivities are rare in horses and most of the information on this condition is based on anecdotal reports. Food hypersensitivity refers to an immune-mediated adverse reaction to a feedstuff unrelated to any physiologic effect of the feed. The pathomechanism of dietary hypersensitivity in horses is unknown, but it is believed to involve type I, type III, and type IV hypersensitivity reactions. The skin, respiratory tract, and gastrointestinal tract may be affected. The most commonly incriminated foods include potatoes, malt, beet pulp, buckwheat, fishmeal, wheat, alfalfa, red and white clover, Saint Johnswort, chicory, glucose, barley, bran, oats, and tonics.[31]

Dermatologic manifestations of food allergy include generalized pruritus with or without papules, urticaria, and pruritus ani. Flatulence, loose stools, heaves, or asthma may accompany skin lesions.

Diagnosis is made by eliminating more common causes of pruritus in horses and by positive response to a food elimination trial (see Fig. 10–4). Hypoallergenic diets are individualized for each patient and it is critical to obtain a very thorough dietary history from the owner. It is important to identify any change in the diet (vitamin supplements, grains, hays) to optimize chances of success. It is practical to start by eliminating any supplements and concentrates from the diet. Dusty feedstuffs should not be fed during the trial because some horses can develop inhalant allergy to feedstuffs. Feed the horse oats, grass, or alfalfa hay for 4 to 8 weeks and note whether or not a decrease in the pruritus occurs. If the animal is notably less pruritic, reinstitute the previous diet to confirm that the pruritus is due to a food allergy and that improvement was not coincidental. If the food allergy is present, the pruritus will return and the hypoallergenic diet should be reinstituted until clinical signs subside. The offending substance is identified by reintroducing one dietary item to the special diet per week and observing the horse for the reappearance of clinical signs.

Table 10–3. General Insecticide Types Used for Equine Pests*†

Insecticides	Insecticides and repellents
Face flies	Biting midges
Facultative myiasis	Black flies
Horn flies	Chiggers
House flies	Facultative myiasis
Lice	Mosquitoes
Mosquitoes	Stable flies
Sticktight flea	Ticks
Poultry lice	Premise treatment
Ticks	House flies
Repellents	Mosquitoes
Black flies	Stable flies
Biting midges	
Chiggers	
Horseflies	

*Modified from Foil L, Foil C: Control of ectoparasites. In Robinson NE, ed: *Current Therapy in Equine Medicine*, Vol 3. Philadelphia, WB Saunders, 1992, p 689.
†Categories may overlap, owing to differences in management systems or life cycles of different species.

Contact Allergy

True contact allergies are rare in horses perhaps in part because the hair coat acts as a protective barrier. Irritant contact reactions are much more common (see below). These allergies, when they occur, are type IV hypersensitivity reactions. Potential allergens are usually small molecules that penetrate the skin, bind to dermal collagen or carrier proteins, and are then presented to antigen-presenting cells (Langerhans cells) in the dermis. Upon subsequent reexposure, an inflammatory response occurs that results in skin disease. Development of allergic contact reactions usually takes months to years.

Contact reactions are most likely due to pasture plants, changes in bedding material, insect repellents, topical medications, and tack items.[32] Parasiticides and bath oils applied as insect repellents are the most commonly identified causes of contact allergy in our experience. Repeated application of chemicals to the coat of sweating horses may predispose them to the development of a contact allergy because the protective barrier of the skin is compromised.

The clinical signs of contact allergy are variable and depend upon how long the allergic reaction has been present. Early in the course of the reaction, erythema, swelling, oozing, pain, or pruritus, singly or severally, develop within 2 to 3 days after application of the offending substance. This often progresses over a period of weeks or months to alopecia, lichenification, and crusting, if left untreated. The distribution of the lesions may suggest the cause: legs (plants, bedding), face and muzzle (plants, bedding), face and trunk (tack), face, ears, neck, trunk (insect repellents).[32]

Definitive diagnosis is made by either provocative exposure or patch testing. Provocative exposure involves avoiding the suspect substance for 10 days or until lesions resolve, reexposing the horse to the substance, and noting the recurrence of the lesions or clinical signs over the next 7 to 10 days.[32] Provocative testing will not distinguish between an irritant reaction and an allergic reaction, but it will identify the offending substance. Patch testing involves the application of the suspect substance to an area of the skin for 48 to 72 hours. Plant, bedding or other particulate matter will not adhere well to the skin and are best tested under an occlusive dressing (closed patch test). A 3-cm² area of hair is clipped on the thorax or dorsum for each test item. A small amount of the suspect substance is applied to the skin and the site is covered with a gauze sponge and bandaged for 48 to 72 hours. A control site should also be bandaged. When the bandages are removed, the area is assessed for erythema, swelling, induration, pain, and exudation. A biopsy of the control and the test site(s) should be obtained and the tissue examined histologically to confirm the diagnosis. Liquid substances can be applied to the skin daily and do not require an occlusive bandage.

Successful treatment involves accurate identification of the offending substance and avoidance. If that is not possible, short-term systemic glucocorticoids and mild cleansing shampoos should be prescribed.

Cutaneous Drug Reactions

Cutaneous drug reactions in horses are rare and can mimic any known skin disease. Drug reactions are believed to involve type I, II, III, or IV hypersensitivity reaction. Any therapeutic agent administered by any route may cause a drug reaction. The most commonly incriminated drugs are penicillin, streptomycin, oxytetracycline, neomycin, chloramphenicol, sulfonamides, phenothiazines, phenylbutazone, guaifenesin, aspirin, and glucocorticoids. Clinical signs are variable and pruritus may or may not be present. Urticaria is a commonly observed skin reaction. Less commonly, mucocutaneous ulceration or vesiculation may be present.

The diagnosis of a drug reaction is dependent upon an accurate medication history. Skin biopsies may be helpful in supporting a clinical diagnosis and the most commonly reported patterns of inflammation are a perivascular dermatitis, interface or lichenoid (band of cellular infiltrate at or beneath the basement membrane zone) dermatitis, and intraepidermal or subepidermal vesicular dermatitis.[32] The diagnosis can be definitively confirmed by provocative challenge but this may lead to anaphylaxis or death and, therefore, this is not recommended.

Treatment requires removal of the offending drug, symptomatic therapy, and avoiding related compounds. Drug reactions, in general, do not respond well to glucocorticoids. A drug reaction usually subsides within 2 to 3 weeks, but may last for months.

Atopy

Atopy is defined as pruritic dermatitis due to inhaled allergens. This disease has only recently been recognized in horses[33] and is a classic example of a type I hypersensitivity disorder and occurs in genetically predisposed animals. Reaginic (IgE) antibody binds to dermal mast cells. When an allergen binds to allergen-specific antibody on a mast cell, degranulation occurs and vasoactive chemicals and inflammatory mediators are released. Trees, grasses, and weed pollens and molds are the most common allergens involved in equine atopy in our experience.

Atopy in horses is manifest by seasonal or nonseasonal pruritic skin disease. Urticaria and concurrent "heaves" or asthma are common clinical presentations. Atopy can mimic any of the pruritic dermatoses of horses and may occur concurrently with insect hypersensitivity.

A tentative diagnosis can be made after other causes of pruritus have been eliminated and upon positive response to exogenous glucocorticoids. Diagnosis is confirmed via intradermal skin testing. Treatment is individualized and may include any combination of the following: avoidance of the offending substances (often not practical), hydroxyzine 200 to 400 mg/kg PO t.i.d., hyposensitization, or oral prednisolone 0.5 mg/kg PO s.i.d. or q.o.d.

Infectious Causes of Pruritus

Dermatophytosis and bacterial skin infections can cause pruritus in horses. They are more commonly recognized in the field as crusting or exfoliative dermatoses and are discussed next.

COMMON CAUSES OF SCALING AND CRUSTING DERMATOSES

Exfoliative dermatoses in horses have a wide range of causes. Again, the historical and physical findings are ex-

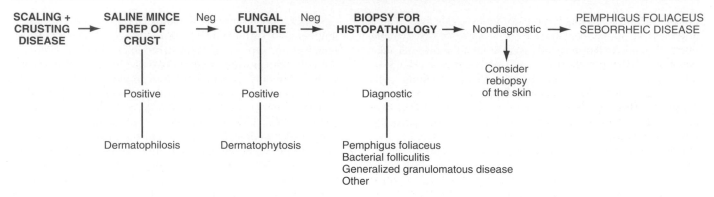

Figure 10–10. Flowchart for diagnosis of equine scaling and crusting diseases.

tremely important in differentiating these diseases. Skin scrapings, fungal cultures, bacterial cultures, mince preparations of crusts for cytologic examination for dermatophilosis, and skin biopsies may all be required to make a diagnosis in difficult cases. If cost constraints are present, the most useful diagnostic test is a carefully obtained skin biopsy. It is critical *not* to scrub or prepare the skin in any way prior to obtaining the skin biopsy specimen. In addition, extreme care should be taken to collect the crust when obtaining a skin biopsy from a horse with an exfoliative skin disease. We routinely submit extra crust specimens for processing. In many instances, the causative agent or evidence of a definitive diagnosis is obtained from histopathologic examination of the crust. A simplified approach to the diagnosis of exfoliative dermatoses is shown in Figure 10–10.

Infectious Causes of Exfoliation

Dermatophilosis (Rain Scald)

Dermatophilosis is a bacterial skin disease of horses and other large animals caused by the gram-positive, facultative anaerobic actinomycete *Dermatophilus congolensis*. The normal habitat of the organism is unknown, but it is thought that it exists in a quiescent state on carrier animals until conditions are optimal for proliferation.[34] It is unknown if these carrier animals act as reservoirs of infection for other animals.

The development of lesions is dependent upon chronic moisture and skin damage.[34, 35] The organism cannot penetrate intact healthy skin and moisture is required to cause the release of the zoospores. The skin can be damaged from chronic maceration due to moisture, biting flies, vegetation, or underlying pruritic skin diseases. Chronic moisture is more conducive to the organism's growth than intermittent but heavy rainfall. Once these two prerequisites (moisture and trauma) are met, the organism can multiply. Moisture induces the release of infective, motile, flagellated zoospores. These organisms are attracted to low concentrations of carbon dioxide and repelled by high concentrations of carbon dioxide. As the organism multiplies and inflammatory cells migrate into the area, the carbon dioxide concentration in the skin rises and the zoospores migrate toward the surface of the skin in search of a more suitable environment. The organism again multiplies and their numbers increase. There is a concurrent influx of inflammatory cells and both factors

result in an increase in the concentration of carbon dioxide. The zoospores again migrate toward the skin surface seeking a low carbon dioxide concentration and this cycle is repeated over and over again resulting in layered, crusting, and matting of the hair coat. Zoospores can remain viable in crusts at ambient temperatures of 28° to 31°C for up to 42 months.[34]

Clinical signs of dermatophilosis can develop within 24 hours. The disease has a follicular orientation and appears as crusted, moist, mats of hair which can resemble small "paintbrushes." Under fresh crusts, the skin is moist, exudative, and yellow-tinged. Exudative crusted lesions tend to be found on the back, gluteal area, on the face and neck, and on the distal extremities (Fig. 10–11). Lesions on the limbs may cause pain, swelling, and erythema, especially in white or lightly pigmented areas. Racehorses or horses in training commonly develop abrasions on the cranial surface of the

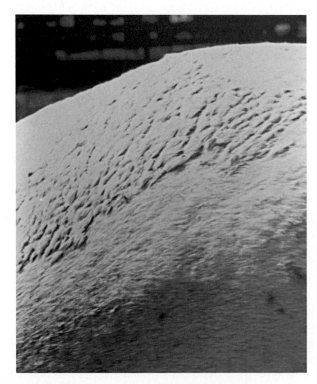

Figure 10–11. Horse with matting of coat due to dermatophilosis.

hind legs. These lesions are prime sites for infection. Some lesions are isolated to the cranial aspect of the cannon bone or muzzle. Severely affected horses may be febrile, depressed, lethargic, anorectic, and have regional lymphadenopathy.

Dermatophilosis is diagnosed by demonstration of the organism. This can be done by cytologic examination of a crust or by histologic examination of a skin biopsy specimen. "Dermatophilosis preps" can be made from dried or fresh crusts or from direct smears of the exudate. Dried crusts are finely minced in a few drops of sterile saline, allowed to dry for 45 minutes, and stained. Direct smears or dried mince preparations may be stained with a fast Giemsa, Diff Quik, or Gram's stain. The organism is best visualized under $\times 1,000$ oil immersion and appears as fine-branching multiseptate hyphae with transverse and longitudinally arranged cocci (railroad track appearance) (Fig. 10–12). When collecting a skin biopsy from a horse with suspected dermatophilosis, it is very important to submit a specimen with the crust attached to the skin or hairs. Key histologic findings include folliculitis, intraepidermal pustules, intracellular edema, and alternating layers of parakeratotic (epidermal cells with retained nuclei) and orthokeratotic (keratinized epidermal cells without nuclei) hyperkeratosis with leukocyte debris.[33] The organism is often found only in crusts.

Horses with mild infections may be treated with topical therapy alone. Crusts should be gently soaked and removed using a mild antibacterial shampoo such as chlorhexidine or benzoyl peroxide. Sedation may be required in some horses where this is difficult or painful. The animal should be towel-dried and a topical antibacterial sponge-on dip applied (chlorhexidine 1:32 dilution of 2% stock solution, or lime sulfur 1:32 dilution of stock solution). This should be done daily for 5 to 7 days until healing is evident, then twice-weekly until all of the lesions have resolved. Horses with lesions on the muzzle may benefit from a topical antibiotic cream with or without corticosteroids. Severely affected animals may benefit greatly from systemic antibiotics, for example, procaine penicillin 22,000 IU/kg IM b.i.d. for 5 days. In either case, exposure to excessive moisture and skin trauma should be eliminated.

Dermatophytosis (Ringworm)

Dermatophytosis is the most common contagious skin disease of horses. *Trichophyton equinum, Trichophyton mentagrophytes, Microsporum gypseum,* and *Microsporum canis* are the most frequent isolates.[36] The infection is self-limiting but can seriously affect the function of the horse and is of zoonotic importance.

Dermatophytosis is transmitted by direct contact with an infected host or by indirect contact via contaminated fomites or the environment. Illness, poor nutrition, overcrowding, age (young or old immunosuppressed individuals), and stressful environments predispose horses to infection. In addition, chronic moisture from sweating or the environment damages the skin's protective barrier, enhancing the opportunity for infection. When fungal spores contact the hair coat, infection may or may not occur. The spores may be mechanically removed, they may be unable to compete with the normal flora of the skin, or they may remain on the coat in a dormant state until conditions are optimal for infection. Dermatophytes invade the keratin of the epidermis and hair with the aid of enzymes that are allergenic to the host. Dermatophytosis is considered a biological contact dermatitis.[37] The incubation period is usually several weeks. During this time, fungi are invading the epidermal keratin, hair follicles, and the hair shaft itself. The epidermis responds to the intruder by increasing epidermal cell turnover in an effort to mechanically remove the fungi. Clinically, this is represented as scaling. Hair shaft integrity is compromised and hairs either fall out or are easily fractured, accounting for the hair loss associated with this disease. The infection is eliminated from a particular hair when it is shed, enters the telogen stage, or if the dermatophyte elicits an inflammatory response.

The clinical signs of dermatophytosis, including pain and pruritus, are variable. The infection is follicular in distribution and early lesions often begin as a papular eruption with erect hairs (Fig. 10–13). This may be preceded by an urticarial eruption 24 to 72 hours prior to the owner noticing the papules.[38] Lesions rapidly progress to crusted papules that spread circumferentially. The classic lesion is a circular patch of alopecia with stubbly hairs on the margin and variable amounts of scaling (Fig. 10–14). Erythema and hyperpigmentation may be present. In rare instances, dermatophytosis may present as generalized scaling without significant hair loss.[38] If the dermatophyte causes follicular

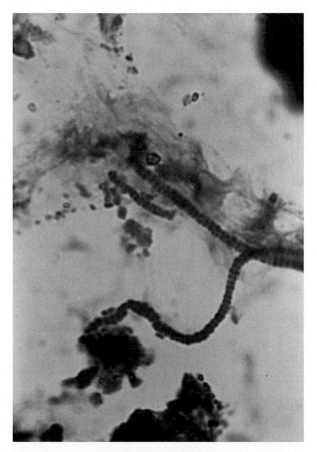

Figure 10–12. Microscopic appearance of *Dermatophilus congolensis.*

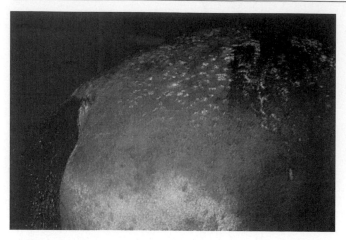

Figure 10–13. Dermatophytosis. Note the papular eruption on the advancing edge of lesions.

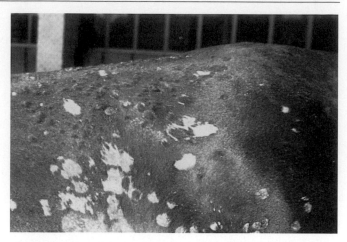

Figure 10–14. Classic signs of dermatophytosis (ringworm).

rupture, nodules, ulcers, or a kerion reaction (inflammatory dermatophyte infection that may resemble an abscess) may develop. Lesions are most common in areas where tack contacts the skin, but may be limited to the posterior pastern.

Diagnosis is made by demonstration and identification of the organism. Wood's lamp examinations are not particularly useful in the field for logistical reasons and, more important, because few cases of equine dermatophytosis are caused by *M. canis*. Direct examination of hair and scale is useful, but requires special training. The most reliable tests are fungal culture and skin biopsy. The details of superficial fungal culture techniques have been reviewed elsewhere.[36, 39] It is important to note that hairs collected for culture should be collected from the periphery of a newly developing lesion. It is critical to avoid areas that the owner may have treated. Additionally, the area should be gently wiped with an alcohol swab prior to collecting hair samples as this will minimize the growth of contaminants. Hairs should be plucked in the direction of growth and transported to the laboratory or clinic in a paper envelope for inoculation on dermatophyte test medium (DTM). Sab-Duets plates (Bacti-Labs, Mountain View, Calif.) are our preferred commercial fungal culture media. Each plate contains Sabouraud's glucose medium and DTM. Using both media plates greatly enhances the

culturing of suspect organisms. *Trichophyton* species isolation will be improved if a few drops of B vitamin complex are added to the surface of the media and the plate incubated at 37°C. Skin biopsy sites should be selected with care. Do not scrub or wipe the area prior to sampling. Again, early lesions with crusts are ideal. Histologic findings include folliculitis, perifolliculitis, and furunculosis; superficial perivascular dermatitis with ortho- or parakeratosis; and intraepidermal vesicular or pustular dermatitis. Septate fungal hyphae and oval spores may be present in the superficial keratin or hair follicle.[36]

Dermatophytosis is a self-limiting disease and most cases heal spontaneously within 1 to 6 months. Treatment is strongly advised to minimize contagion to other animals and people. In horses, antifungal sponge-on dips are the treatment of choice. The more commonly used preparations are listed in Table 10–4. Recent research on the efficacy of topical antifungal preparations has shown that many commonly used topical antifungal therapies do not alter the course of infection. Chlorhexidine, Captan, and povidine-iodine are not effective and should not be used (K.A. Moriello, D.J. DeBoer, University of Wisconsin, Madison, unpublished data, 1993). Systemic antifungal drugs, such as griseofulvin (50 mg/kg PO once daily) or itraconazole (5–10

Table 10–4. Topical Antifungal Preparations for Equine Dermatophytosis

Product	Brand Name	Recommended Administration	Comments
Lime sulfur	Lym Dyp (DVM)	4 oz to 8 oz/gal water applied as a dip every 3–5 days	Strong sulfur odor; may cause yellow discoloration of white hair coats; concentrations >4 oz/gal may cause irritant reaction
Enilconazole	Imaverol (Janssen Animal Health, Belgium)	1:50 dilution used as a dip every 3 days for 4 treatments	Excellent therapy; not available in United States

mg/kg PO once daily) are effective, but expensive. In instances where it is necessary or desirable to treat an infected herd, itraconazole 5 to 10 mg/kg PO once-daily for 15 days will abort the infection. Concurrent topical therapy with lime sulfur is necessary.

Elimination of dermatophytosis from single or multiple horse barns requires elimination of the organism from infected hosts and decontamination of the environment. Table 10–5 summarizes one approach to treatment. Commercial antifungal vaccines for equine dermatophytosis are not available in the United States. Autogenous vaccines are not recommended at this time because of lack of information on their efficacy and the potential for serious side effects, including sterile abscesses, hypersensitivity reactions, generalized anaphylaxis, and death.

Bacterial Infections

Bacterial folliculitis in horses is caused by *Staphylococcus* and, less commonly, *Streptococcus* species. Infections are most frequent in the summer when heat, moisture, increased insect populations, and increased use of the horse act in concert as predisposing factors.

The pathogenesis of bacterial folliculitis in the horse is similar to that of other animals. The causative agents are normally found on the host and when the skin's natural protective barrier is compromised, bacteria invade and multiply within hair follicles. This results in inflammation, destruction of the hair follicle, and shedding of the hair. As the infection spreads, lesions enlarge. If hair follicles rupture, furunculosis and deep pyoderma may occur.

Clinically, bacterial folliculitis may be indistinguishable from dermatophytosis. One differentiating factor is that bacterial lesions are much more likely to be painful and are only rarely pruritic. Infection is most common in the saddle and tack area, but bacterial folliculitis may be limited to the pastern area. Deep pyoderma of the tail base also occurs.

Definitive diagnosis is best made by cytology, bacterial culture, and skin biopsy. It is very important to differentiate bacterial folliculitis from dermatophytosis. Skin biopsy reveals varying degrees of folliculitis, intraepidermal pustules, and perivascular inflammation. Neutrophils are the primary inflammatory cell. Keratinocytes often show intracellular edema, parakeratosis and orthokeratosis are common in the crust. Special stains often show bacteria within crusts and hair follicles.

Treatment depends upon the severity of the clinical signs. Mild infections may be self-limiting, but benefit from topical therapy. Severe cases require daily topical antibacterial shampoos with benzoyl peroxide or chlorhexidine and oral antimicrobials. Systemic antimicrobial therapy should be based upon culture and sensitivity but, in general, procaine penicillin 22,000 IU/kg IM b.i.d. daily until resolution of clinical signs is usually effective.[39] A minimum of 10 to 14 days is recommended.

Table 10–5. Topical Antifungal Preparations for Equine Dermatophytosis (Ringworm, Fungus) of Multiple Horses*

In the treatment of ringworm or superficial fungal infections of the skin, it is important to accomplish three things:
  1. Kill the fungus on the animal to stop progression of the disease.
  2. Kill the fungus on the animal to prevent spread to other animals, people, and the environment.
  3. Decontaminate the environment.
The following suggestions have been helpful when treating outbreaks in the multiple horse barn. It should be kept in mind that fungal infections may take *6–8 weeks* to heal completely.
  1. *Isolate* all affected horses from normal horses.
  2. Treat the barn by cleaning out all bedding and spraying stalls and exposed surfaces with 1:10 dilution of household bleach.
  3. Treat all affected horses daily with lime sulfur sponge-on (4 oz/gal) for 7 days, then once weekly. It is vital to treat the horse's *entire body,* not just the affected areas. Sponge-on preparations should be allowed to dry on the horse and horses should not be bathed between treatments.
  4. Use individual brushes and tack for each horse. Disinfect brushes and tack frequently. Do not transfer equipment between horses.
  5. Blankets used with household bleach should be disinfected twice weekly or more often. It is best *not* to use blankets or sheets as this may enhance the spread of the lesions.
  6. Ideally, the people who handle affected horses should not handle normal horses. If this is not possible, normal horses should be handled first, then affected horses. It is important to wash *well* between animals with a chlorhexidine scrub.
  7. Ringworm is contagious to other animals and people; handlers should be careful to wash well and report the development of any lesions. If possible, gloves should be worn when handling affected horses.
  8. Ideally, horses affected with ringworm should be rested from training or riding until lesions are gone. Continued riding or training may contribute to skin microtrauma, and spread of infection.

---

*Adapted from client education handouts used at the College of Veterinary Medicine, University of Florida, and the School of Veterinary Medicine, University of Wisconsin.

Parasitic Causes of Exfoliation

Insect hypersensitivities (discussed earlier) are the most common parasitic cause of exfoliation in horses. The major differentiating feature is the presence of pruritus, lack of circumferentially spreading lesions, and the absence of pain. Skin biopsy findings of superficial or deep eosinophilic perivascular dermatitis with or without collagen degeneration are very suggestive of insect hypersensitivity.

Nutritional Causes of Exfoliation

True nutritional deficiencies are rare in horses and much of the information has been extrapolated from work done with other species or experimentally induced deficiencies.

Protein

Protein deficiency may occur in foals or horses with fever, dysphagia, burns, proteinuria, liver disease, horses with gastrointestinal diseases, or any disease in which metabolic demand increases and production of protein decreases. The skin uses 25% to 30% of the daily protein intake for hair production and maintenance of the epidermis.[40] This requirement may increase fivefold in disease states. In experimental deficiencies created in ruminants and laboratory animals, protein-deficient animals developed dry, dull, brittle, thin hair. Prolonged shedding was also reported.[41] Presumably, horses with protein-deficient diets would manifest similar clinical signs.

Zinc

Naturally occurring zinc deficiencies have not been reported in horses. Classically, this deficiency appears as crusting skin disease. Experimentally induced zinc deficiencies in foals resulted in alopecia, dense scaling on the lower limb that progressed to the trunk, inappetence, decreased growth rate, and low tissue and serum zinc concentrations.[41] Definitive diagnosis is made by finding histologic lesions compatible with zinc deficiency: diffuse epidermal and follicular parakeratosis and response to oral supplementation with zinc sulfate 10 mg/kg PO s.i.d. A marked response is usually seen within 2 to 3 weeks and therapy may or may not be lifelong.

Iodine

Suspected iodism caused by excessive supplementation therapeutically or in feeds has been reported in horses.[42] Noncutaneous signs included cough, lacrimation, nasal discharge, and joint pain. Severe dry seborrhea with or without dorsal alopecia was also present. No treatment was necessary and

the horses recovered spontaneously once the source of excessive iodine was removed.

Immunologic Causes of Exfoliation

Pemphigus Foliaceus

Pemphigus foliaceus is a rare autoimmune skin disease that causes severe crusting and matting of the hair coat. This disease is caused by an autoantibody against the glycocalyx of keratinocytes. The antibody binds to the glycocalyx which results in the release and activation of keratinocyte proteolytic enzymes into the intercellular space. The glycocalyx is hydrolyzed and intercellular cohesion is lost, leading to acantholysis.[43]

There is no age or sex predilection, but Appaloosa horses may be predisposed.[44] Lesions usually begin on the face and limbs and may take weeks or months before becoming generalized. In some horses only the coronary band is affected.[44] The primary lesion, a subcorneal pustule, is rarely observed because of the horse's hair coat. The most common clinical presentation is severe matting and crusting of the coat with oozing of serum from the skin (Fig. 10–15). Most horses are depressed and show signs of systemic illness. Swelling and pain of the distal extremities, in addition to lameness, are common. Pruritus and pain on the trunk, ventral edema, and regional or generalized lymphadenopathy are variable.

Definitive diagnosis is made by routine histologic examination of a skin biopsy specimen. It is critical to submit a

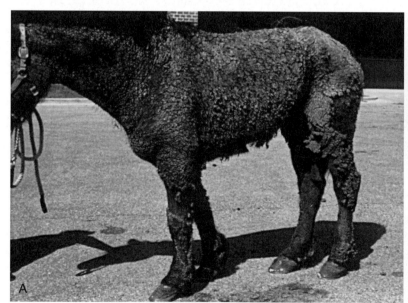
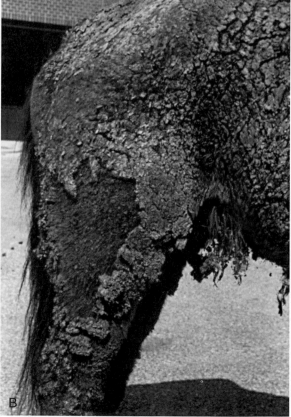

Figure 10–15. A, Pemphigus foliaceus in a horse. **B,** Note the marked crusting of the skin.

skin biopsy with intact crusts attached to the underlying skin or hairs. Histologically, pemphigus foliaceus is characterized by intragranular to subcorneal acantholysis. Often, layered rafts of acantholytic cells are observed within the crusts interspersed among neutrophils.[44] Direct immunofluorescence is unreliable but when positive shows diffuse intercellular fluorescence. A tentative diagnosis of pemphigus foliaceus may be made based on impression smears of the content of intact pustules or the underside of exudative crusts (Fig. 10–16). Rafts of deeply basophilic acantholytic cells and nondegenerate neutrophils are highly suggestive of this disease.

Pemphigus foliaceus in horses less than 1 year of age is usually self-limiting.[45] Spontaneous remission is common in foals and they often do not require long-term therapy. In adults, treatment is difficult and often unrewarding, thus many owners elect euthanasia. Remission and control of the disease is induced using large doses of prednisone or prednisolone 1 mg/kg PO b.i.d. until no new lesions develop. This usually occurs within 7 to 10 days, at which point alternate-day therapy is instituted at the same dose.[46] It is difficult to maintain clinical normalcy with prednisolone therapy alone and adjuvant immunosuppressive agents may have to be added to the treatment program. Even in cases where prednisolone therapy is effective, the potential for laminitis and immunosuppression warrants the use of other agents. Chrysotherapy (gold salts) has been used in horses, even though it is expensive.[46] Two test doses of aurothioglucose (Solganal, Schering Corp., Kenilworth, N.J.) 1 week apart are administered IM, 20 and 40 mg, respectively. If no adverse effects (stomatitis, urticaria, sloughing of skin, blood dyscrasia) are observed, weekly therapy is begun at 1 mg/kg IM until the disease responds (6–12 weeks). Treatment is then tailored to the individual animal, for example, biweekly or monthly therapy. Complete remission of clinical signs may not be possible to achieve even with combination therapy. The most common side effects of aurothioglucose therapy in people, dogs, and cats are an immune-mediated thrombocytopenia and proteinuria. Presumably, this could occur in the horse. It is recommended that a complete blood count and urinalysis be performed weekly for the first month and then monthly if no abnormalities develop.

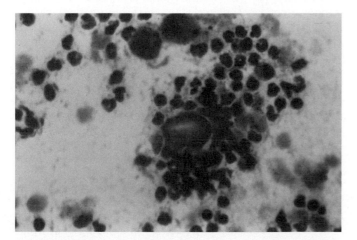

Figure 10–16. Cytologic appearance of a touch preparation from a lesion of pemphigus. Note rounded cells (acanthocytes).

Irritant Contact Dermatitis

Irritant contact dermatoses are fairly common in horses. This reaction differs from allergic contact dermatitis because the offending substance invariably causes a reaction if left in contact with the skin; prior sensitization is not needed.

The mechanism of irritant contact reactions depends upon the causative chemical, but moisture and tissue maceration are important predisposing factors. Common irritating substances include feces, urine, wound secretions, caustic substances, crude oil, diesel oil, turpentine, "blisters," leg sweats, improperly used insecticides, fly wipes, concentrated disinfectants, irritating plants, and soiled bedding.[47]

There is no age, sex, or breed predilection.[47–49] Direct contact with the offending substance is required for irritant reactions to occur. Acute lesions are often erythematous, vesiculated, erosive or ulcerated, and painful. As the condition continues, necrosis, crusting, scaling, and hair loss occur. Leukoderma and leukotrichia are common and may be permanent. Pruritus and pain are variable.

Diagnosis is made from the history, clinical signs, and inspection of the horse's environment. Provocative testing is very useful in identifying and confirming the causative agent as long as there is minimal risk to the horse. Histologic examination of skin reveals necrosis, spongiotic vesicles, and ulceration.

Treatment requires identification and removal of the offending substance. Affected areas should be washed daily with copious amounts of water and topical 0.5% chlorhexidine soaks applied. Astringent topical solutions, for example, aluminum acetate (Domeboro, available as an over-the-counter preparation) may be beneficial, but often cause pain or delay wound healing. Healing may be promoted by topical antimicrobial creams free of corticosteroids. Healing is usually rapid once the irritant is removed.

Allergic Contact Dermatitis

Allergic contact dermatitis has been discussed earlier. It is important to note that it may cause scaling and crusting in addition to pruritus. Lesions are usually distributed in a pattern that reflects contact with the offending substance.

Photodermatitis

Photodermatitis can be caused directly by sunburn, or indirectly by photoallergy or photosensitization.

Sunburn

Sunburn is a phototoxic reaction caused by excessive exposure to ultraviolet B light. Horses with white or light skin or hair are at risk. The affected area becomes erythematous and scaly. If severe, necrosis and exudation may occur. Diagnosis is based on history and clinical signs. Topical glucocorticoid creams will alleviate pain, but, excessive use has the potential to cause minor side effects (depigmentation, failure, slowing of hair regrowth) or possibly serious side effects (laminitis) because these drugs are absorbed systemically. Stabling horses during periods of intense sunlight and application of water-repellent sunscreens may be helpful.

Photoallergy

Photoallergy is believed to be caused by contact with a chemical or plant (species unknown) and ultraviolet light. This is most commonly observed on white muzzles and extremities of horses housed on pasture containing clover, particularly alsike clover.[38] Erythema, vesicles, and crusts develop. Diagnosis is made by clinical findings. If the offending substance cannot be identified and removed from the environment, then horses should be stabled during daylight, if possible, to minimize exposure to the offending substance.

Photosensitization

Photosensitization may develop as a result of hepatogenous photosensitization, aberrant pigmentation formation, or a primary photodynamic agent that has been ingested, injected, or applied to the skin. In many cases the cause is not identified.

Regardless of the source of the photodynamic agent, the pathophysiology of skin disease is similar.[47, 50] Photodynamic agents are deposited in the skin and absorb energy when exposed to sunlight. These molecules are elevated to a high energy state and, in the presence of oxygen, produce free radicals which damage cell membranes. Lysosomes and other organelles release hydrolytic enzymes and other mediators of inflammation.

Lesions are most common in white or lightly pigmented areas, but have been observed to extend into dark-colored areas.[38, 47] Eyelids, lips, face, perineum, and coronary bands are commonly affected. There is usually an acute onset of erythema, edema, pruritus, and pain. Vesicles and bullae may develop (Fig. 10–17). Necrosis, ulceration, and crusting often occur.

Diagnosis is made by clinical signs, history, and laboratory tests. Liver function tests should always be performed regardless of whether or not the horse is showing clinical signs of hepatic disease.

Treatment requires identification of the underlying cause. Prognosis is variable in horses with liver disease. One of us (S.S.) treated several horses with photosensitization due to

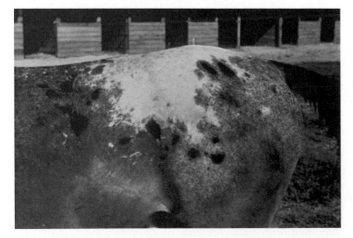

Figure 10–17. Horse with photosensitization.

acute hepatitis that recovered and did well. Therapy requires removal of the offending substance, avoidance of sunlight, and topical or systemic glucocorticoids.[38]

Seborrhea and Localized Disorders of Keratinization as Causes of Scaling and Crusting

Seborrhea

Seborrhea is a clinically descriptive term for excessive scaling and crusting. It may or may not be the result of excessive sebum production. Most seborrheic skin conditions are secondary, resulting from dermatophytosis, dermatophilosis, or parasitic or bacterial skin diseases. The skin's natural response to insult is proliferation, either as a mechanism by which to remove an offending organism or as a result of inflammation. Primary seborrhea is a disorder of keratinization in which epidermal cell turnover time and basal cell proliferation are increased. Genetic factors may be involved in the control of these mechanisms. Secondary seborrhea, the most common form of seborrhea, can occur in any inflammatory, infectious, or parasitic skin disease (see above).

Idiopathic or primary seborrhea in horses may be generalized or localized to the tail and mane. There is no age, sex, or breed predilection. Generalized seborrhea appears clinically as diffuse matting of the coat. The coat's texture may be oily and thick adherent crusts may be easily removed. Oily or dry adherent scales are present at the base of the hairs. Lesions are usually generalized and involve the face and legs (Fig. 10–18). The animal is odoriferous and is not usually pruritic. Seborrhea of the mane and tail is very common and presents as crusts or scales attached to the base of hairs. Pain and inflammation are generally absent.

Primary seborrhea is a diagnosis of exclusion. Therefore, it is very important to rule out other causes of scaling. Severe generalized seborrhea must be differentiated from pemphigus foliaceus. Skin scrapings, fungal cultures, dermatophilosis preparations, and skin biopsies should be performed on all suspected cases. Skin biopsies may help in determining if primary or secondary seborrhea is present.[51] In early cases of generalized equine seborrhea where there is little secondary inflammation, skin biopsy findings are strongly suggestive of a primary disorder of keratinization. The noncornified epidermis is not hyperplastic (thickened), but there is marked orthokeratotic hyperkeratosis attached to an epidermis of normal thickness. The superficial dermis shows only a mild perivascular to diffuse cellular infiltrate of neutrophils. The "mismatch" in the thickness of the noncornified epidermis vs. the cornified epidermis suggests a keratinization defect. In cases in which there is secondary inflammation or the seborrheic condition has been more longstanding, the biopsy findings may not be as easily interpreted. The cornified epidermis is acanthotic (thickened) and there is marked orthokeratotic or parakeratotic hyperkeratosis. Superficial perivascular inflammation often is present in the superficial dermis.

Secondary seborrhea is treated by eliminating the predisposing cause. Primary seborrhea is usually incurable and is managed symptomatically with topical therapy. Seborrheic conditions can usually be managed quite satisfactorily with

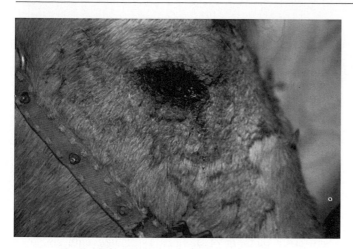

Figure 10–18. Horse with primary seborrhea.

antiseborrheic shampoos. The horse should be washed with a cleansing shampoo just prior to using a medicated shampoo. This removes excess dirt and scale, improves the efficacy of the medicated shampoo, and decreases the amount of medicated shampoo that the owner needs to use, minimizing the potential for a contact reaction to develop. As with people, horses are individuals and several brands of shampoos may need to be used before a suitable shampoo is found. In general, dry seborrhea responds best to sulfur-based shampoos and oily seborrhea to tar-based shampoos. Benzoyl peroxide–based shampoos also work well in cases of oily seborrhea. Antiseborrheic shampoos formulated for small animals work well in horses, but may be expensive. Human shampoos should be avoided because these products are often more expensive than veterinary products and they lather excessively, making rinsing difficult. Owners should allow the antiseborrheic shampoo to contact the coat for 10 to 15 minutes before rinsing the shampoo from the hair. It is very important to thoroughly rinse the horse, especially in the axillary and inguinal region, because shampoo residues are irritating to the skin. Initially, owners may need to shampoo the horse daily for 1 to 2 weeks. After the horse's coat is normal, shampooing can be decreased to twice a week; owners must realize therapy is lifelong. If shampoo therapy dries the coat and worsens dry seborrhea, a moisturizing lotion or spray can be used.

Cannon Keratosis

Cannon keratosis ("stud crud") is an idiopathic skin disease characterized by the presence of hyperkeratotic plaques and patches on the cranial aspect of the rear cannon bones.[52, 53] This disorder of keratinization is uncommon and does not appear to have any recognized age, breed, or sex predilection. Clinically, well-circumscribed plaques of tightly adherent crusts and scales with or without alopecia develop over the cranial surface of the rear cannon bones. The lesions are not pruritic.

Diagnosis is usually made by clinical examination and can be confirmed by skin biopsy. It is important to differentiate cannon keratosis from dermatophilosis and dermatophytosis. Treatment consists of antiseborrheic shampoos.

Topical glucocorticoids may be useful. Finally, topical vitamin A cream (tretenoin, Retin-A cream 0.1%, Ortho Pharmaceutical Corp., Raritan, N.J.) may be beneficial in removing crusts and plaques.

Linear Keratosis

Linear keratosis is an uncommon idiopathic disorder of keratinization.[52, 53] The disease appears to be heritable, especially in quarter horses. There is no age or sex predilection.

Lesions develop between 1 and 5 years of age. One or more painless, nonpruritic unilateral, vertically oriented bands of alopecia and hyperkeratosis develop on the neck or lateral thorax. Lesions are of variable size ranging from 0.25 to 3.5 cm in width to 5 to 70 cm in length.[52] Early lesions may begin as coalescing groups of papules. Lesions are not painful or pruritic.

Diagnosis is usually made by clinical signs alone. Skin biopsy findings include regular, irregular, or papillated epidermal hyperplasia with marked compact orthokeratotic hyperkeratosis.[51] Superficial perivascular dermatitis may or may not be present. If the linear keratosis does not interfere with the function of the horse, no treatment is necessary; otherwise, surgical excision of small lesions may be curative. Topical vitamin A cream or salicylic acid cream may be useful in nonsurgical cases. These agents are keratolytic and may decrease the height, width, or thickness of the keratosis, allowing the horse to be used. Affected animals should not be bred.

Idiopathic Causes of Scaling and Crusting

Equine Exfoliative Eosinophilic Dermatitis and Stomatitis

This is an idiopathic disease of horses characterized by ulcerative stomatitis, severe wasting, marked exfoliation, and eosinophil infiltration of the skin.[32, 54–56] There is no age, sex, or breed predilection, but lesions tend to occur more commonly in the winter.

Early lesions begin as scaling, crusting, exudation, and fissuring at the coronary band. Oral ulcers are usually present at this stage. Over a period of several weeks, a generalized exfoliative dermatosis develops. Hairs are easily epilated and alopecia with multifocal areas of ulceration and exudation develops. The horse may be pruritic. Affected horses without ulcerative stomatitis have a good appetite and may even be ravenous, but soon begin to develop severe weight loss. Some horses may have a protein-losing enteropathy or concurrent malabsorption syndrome, or both.

Definitive diagnosis is made on the basis of the history, physical examination, and skin biopsy. It is critical to rule out pemphigus foliaceus and bullous pemphigoid in the differential diagnosis. The chronic wasting nature of the disease and the multisystemic signs are key to making a diagnosis. Laboratory features include hypoalbuminemia, hypoproteinemia, impaired small intestinal carbohydrate absorption, and elevated γ-glutamyltransferase (GGT), serum alkaline phosphatase (SAP), and bile duct isoenzymes. A superficial and deep eosinophilic and lymphoplasmacytic dermatitis with marked irregular epidermal hyperplasia is present.[54, 55] Exocytosis of eosinophils and lymphocytes and necrosis of keratinocytes are noted.[32, 54, 55] Perivascular collagen degeneration, lymphoid nodules, and a lichenoid inflammatory infiltrate may be present. Eosinophilic infiltrates of the pancreas, salivary glands, oral cavity, and gastrointestinal tract are common. Peripheral eosinophilia is usually absent.

Two horses have responded to dexamethasone 0.2 mg/kg IM for the first 5 days, followed by prednisolone 0.5 mg/kg PO b.i.d. for 7 days, and then 1.0 mg/kg s.i.d. for a week, followed by alternate-day therapy.[32, 54, 55] However, most horses respond poorly to systemic glucocorticoids and the prognosis is grave. Recently, however, there was one report of a single horse with this disease that showed partial response to hydroxyurea and dexamethasone.[57]

Generalized Granulomatous Dermatitis

Generalized granulomatous disease is a rare idiopathic skin disease characterized by exfoliation, severe wasting, and granulomatous inflammation of multiple organ systems.[58] This disease has also been called "equine sarcoidosis" because it resembles sarcoidosis of humans. The use of this term should be avoided because of possible confusion with sarcoid tumors. The cause of this disease is unknown. The disease may be an abnormal host reaction to an infectious or allergenic agent[59] or a nonmalignant neoplastic proliferation of cells.

There is no recognized breed, age, or sex predilection. The skin disease begins as scaling, crusting, and alopecia on the face, limbs, and trunk (Fig. 10–19). The clinical signs rapidly become generalized. Occasionally the disease is focal or multifocal in distribution.[58] Peripheral lymphadenopathy may develop concurrent with weight loss, muscle wasting, anorexia, exercise intolerance, and fever.

Definitive diagnosis is made by skin biopsy.[58] Perifollicular and mid-dermal noncaseating granulomatous dermatitis is seen with frequent multinucleated giant cells. Neutrophils, lymphocytes, and plasma cells are present in small numbers. The granulomas are present in the superficial portion of the

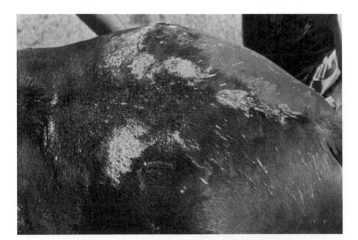

Figure 10–19. Horse with generalized granulomatous dermatitis. (Courtesy of A.A. Stannard, University of California at Davis.)

dermis. Granulomatous infiltrates are also seen in other organs, including the lymph nodes, lung, gastrointestinal organs, liver, and spleen. A complete blood count reveals leukocytosis, increased fibrinogen, and hyperglobulinemia. Anemia secondary to chronic infection may be present.

The prognosis is grave and there is no treatment. Horses are usually euthanized within several months. Large doses of prednisolone 2 mg/kg PO s.i.d. may be beneficial in the early stage of the disease. Occasionally, spontaneous remission may occur.

DISEASES CHARACTERIZED BY PAPULES AND NODULES

There are a plethora of diseases associated with single or multiple nodules in the skin of horses. It is almost impossible to make a definitive diagnosis based upon history and clinical signs alone. The most useful and cost-effective diagnostic test is a skin biopsy. Figure 10–20 is a diagnostic algorithm for equine nodular skin disease.

Infectious Causes of Nodules

Bacterial Granulomas (Botryomycosis)

Bacterial granulomas may be caused by a wide variety of organisms, but most commonly staphylococci are isolated.

They begin as traumatic injuries to the skin during which an infectious organism is inoculated into the dermis. The granulomatous reaction develops because the organism is capable of eliciting a response from the host, but the host is only able to contain the infection and not eradicate it. Bacterial granulomas develop in areas of previous trauma and are common on the limbs and scrotum.[60] The lesions are poorly circumscribed, firm, draining lesions that may or may not be painful. The center of the lesion may be ulcerated. In some cases, variable numbers of white to yellow pieces of particulate matter resembling grains of sand (tissue grains) may be present in the exudate.[60]

Diagnosis is confirmed by skin biopsy and the causative organism is identified by bacterial or fungal culture. Histologic examination of a skin biopsy shows nodular to diffuse pyogranulomatous inflammation with or without tissue grains. Bacteria may be seen in the sections.

Surgical drainage or antimicrobial therapy rarely is indicated individually or in combination.[60] Surgical excision or radical debulking followed by long-term antimicrobial therapy based upon culture and sensitivity has been most successful.[39, 60] Organisms may be difficult to isolate from biopsy tissue samples and submission of large wedges of tissue obtained at the time of surgery is recommended. If possible, tissue submitted for culture should be obtained from the deepest portion of the lesion to increase the likelihood of isolating an infective agent. Tissue should be submitted for aerobic, anaerobic, and deep fungal cultures.

Corynebacterial Infections

Corynebacteria are gram-positive pleomorphic rods and cause two clinical syndromes in the horse—abscesses and ulcerative lymphangitis.[35, 39, 61]

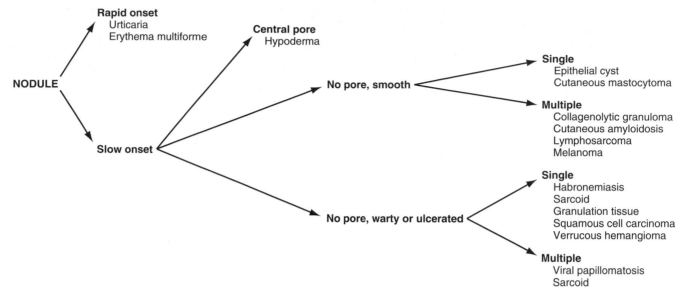

Figure 10–20. Flowchart for equine nodular dermatitis.

Abscesses

Corynebacterial abscesses are frequently seen in horses in the western United States. Lesions tend to be seasonal, occurring most commonly during the summer and fall concurrent with peak fly season, especially in dry dusty conditions. The organism is believed to be transmitted by flies, particularly horn flies. For unknown reasons, fly bites are very susceptible to infection.

Lesions develop slowly and may be single or multiple.[35] The pectoral and ventral abdominal areas are most commonly affected. These abscesses drain a creamy to caseous material that may be whitish to greenish in color. Pitting edema, ventral midline dermatitis, depression, fever, and lameness may be present.[61] The course of the disease may be chronic and recurrent internal abscesses are frequent.

Diagnosis is suspected based upon the season and the appearance of the abscess and exudate. As it may be difficult to identify the organism on cytologic examination of exudate, culture is always recommended.

Treatment is protracted and is complicated by the limited response of the organism to systemic antimicrobials. The abscess should be allowed to mature ("come to a head"), surgically incised, and drained.[39] Systemic antimicrobial use before abscess rupture may be followed by recurrence of the abscess when the drug is discontinued. If drainage cannot be accomplished, large doses of procaine penicillin (50,000 IU/kg IM b.i.d.) for up to 6 months may be curative.[35, 39, 60, 61] Toxoids and bacterins have not been useful.

Ulcerative Lymphangitis

Ulcerative lymphangitis is an infection of the cutaneous lymphatics caused most commonly by *C. pseudotuberculosis*. Infection is believed to begin by wound contamination. The disease is infrequently seen today.

There is no age, sex, or breed predilection. Lesions usually develop on the hindlimbs, especially at the fetlock.[35] Hard to fluctuant chains of nodules which abscess, ulcerate, and drain are most commonly seen. Old lesions heal within 1 to 2 weeks, but new lesions develop.[35] The affected limb may be swollen and painful, and the horse may be depressed. Regional lymphatics appear corded. In chronic cases, permanent thickening of the tissue surrounding the regional lymphatics is common.

Diagnosis is made based upon the appearance of the lesion and identification of the organism. Direct smears of exudate stained with either a fast Giemsa or Gram's stain and a culture and sensitivity usually confirm the diagnosis.

Treatment must be initiated rapidly to prevent permanent debilitation and disfigurement. In early cases, hydrotherapy, exercise, surgical drainage, and large doses of procaine penicillin 20,000 to 80,000 IU/kg IM b.i.d. for at least 30 days post clinical normalcy may be curative.[60] Nonsteroidal anti-inflammatory drugs may be beneficial. If the area has begun to become fibrotic and motion of the joint is restricted, there is little chance for a cure.

Mycetomas

Mycetomas (Table 10–6) are chronic subcutaneous infections characterized by swelling, draining tracts, and tissue granules. Mycetomas may be caused by either filamentous bacteria or eumycetic fungi (fungi that inhabit the soil or vegetation). These organisms gain entrance to the body through traumatic inoculation. As with other granulomatous reactions, the body is able to recognize the intruder and isolate it, but not eliminate it.

Single or multiple nodules of varying sizes can occur almost anywhere on the horse's body. The nodules are often pigmented and ulcerated and may discharge tissue grains (small sandlike particles). The tissue grains are believed to be masses of hyphae from the organism. Gross examination of the cut surface often reveals dark-brown pigment or granules scattered in yellow to pink tissue.

It is impossible clinically to distinguish among bacterial

Table 10–6. Fungal Diseases of Horses

Disease	Common Etiologic Agents	Clinical Signs
Superficial Infections		
Dermatophytosis	*Microsporum* and *Tricophyton* spp.	Circular patches or hair loss, crusting and scaling, urticaria, papules
Piedra	*Piedra* spp. or *Trichosporon beigelii*	Black or white flamentous nodules on hair shaft
Intermediate Infections		
Sporotrichosis	*Sporothrix schenckii*	Papules and nodules that occur along lymphatics; nodules may ulcerate, become thickened, and drain a thick brown-to-red-colored exudate
Phaeohyphomycosis (chronic, subcutaneous fungal infection caused by pigmented opportunistic fungi)	*Hormodendrum, Drechslera, Phialophora, Curvuluria, Cladiosporium*	Single or multiple nodules; lesions may be grossly or microscopically pigmented, nonpruritic, nonpainful, cool to the touch
Mycetoma (chronic subcutaneous infection)	Two causes of filamentous bacterial organisms; opportunistic fungi	Single or multiple, nodular lesions; ulcerated, draining tracts are common; mycetomas discharge tissue grains in contrast to phaeohyphomycosis which does not

or fungal mycetomas or any number of other causes of lumps in the skin. Definitive diagnosis requires an excisional or wedge biopsy of a lesion. Histologic examination shows diffuse to nodular pyogranulomatous to granulomatous inflammation surrounding septate branching hyphae. Tissue grains are often visible microscopically. The hyphae contained in tissue grains or tissue may be pigmented or nonpigmented. Fungi are best cultured from tissue grains and, occasionally, exudate. If it can be performed, surgical excision is curative.[39] Antimicrobial therapy is usually ineffective, especially for fungal mycetomas.

Phaeohyphomycosis

Phaeohyphomycosis (see Table 10–6), sometimes referred to as chromomycosis, is a chronic subcutaneous, and occasionally systemic infection caused by pigmented opportunistic fungi, for example, *Hormodendrum, Drechslera, Phialophora, Curvularia,* and *Cladosporium* species. Many of the organisms that cause fungal mycetomas can cause phaeohyphomycosis. The distinguishing difference is the lack of tissue grains.

Pigmented fungi (dematiaceous fungi) causing this disease are soil and vegetative saprophytes that gain entrance into the body via a wound or abrasion. The body is not able to eliminate the organism and it proliferates in tissues. Immunosuppression may be a predisposing factor.

Lesions appear anywhere on the body and may be single or multiple. Some lesions are deeply pigmented on gross examination or pigmentation is only a microscopic feature. Nodules vary in size and are cool, nonpainful, and nonpruritic. Regional granulomatous dermatitis may be present.

Definitive diagnosis is made by histologic examination

of an excised nodule. Skin biopsy reveals suppurative to granulomatous dermatitis, with pigmented septate hyphae. Observation of pigmental septate hyphae in the skin indicates opportunistic invasion of the tissue. Fungal culture of tissue samples is necessary to identify the organism. It is important to note that growth of these organisms is very slow, often requiring weeks, and is best done by a reference laboratory.

Excision is the only effective treatment, but this may be impractical when numerous lesions are present. These organisms are not susceptible to currently available systemic or topical antifungal agents.

Sporotrichosis

Sporotrichosis (see Table 10–6) is a fungal disease caused by *Sporothrix schenckii,* a dimorphic aerobic fungus. The organism is a soil and plant saprophyte that lives in decaying vegetation. It gains entrance via traumatic inoculation, especially from puncture wounds.

In horses, the cutaneous lymphatic form is most common.[62, 63] Early lesions begin as papules that may exude a seropurulent material. Nodules are most common on the thigh or proximal foreleg and chest. If the organism is not eliminated by the immune system, hard subcutaneous nodules develop along the lymphatics draining the area. The lymphatics become corded and drain thick, brown-to-red-colored exudate. Regional lymph nodes are not involved. Occasionally, only a solitary nodule develops. Rarely, the disease becomes systemic.

Definitive diagnosis can be made by demonstration of the organism via cytologic examination of exudate, culturing of tissue or exudate, or skin biopsy. The organism appears as a cigar-shaped yeast in macrophages and neutrophils on

Giemsa-stained smears. Histologic examination of tissue shows nodular to diffuse, suppurative to granulomatous dermatitis. Intraepidermal microabscesses may be seen. The yeast is rarely seen in tissue sections. The number of organisms present in the tissue may be variable and repeat cultures are often necessary.

Sodium iodide (20% solution) has been very successful in treating sporotrichosis in horses.[63, 64] A loading dose of 20 to 40 mg/kg IV for 2 to 5 days is used. This is followed by once-daily oral therapy (20–40 mg/kg) until all clinical lesions are gone; therapy should be administered for at least 3 weeks after lesions disappear. Sodium iodide may be given orally via syringe or mixed in sweet feed. Topical hot packs of 20% sodium iodide may be used on open wounds. Iodism (see above) may develop and may require temporary discontinuation of therapy. Iodines cause abortion and should not be used in pregnant mares.[64]

Pythiosis (Phycomycosis, Florida Leeches, Gulf Coast Fungus, Swamp Cancer)

Pythiosis is caused by an aquatic fungus, *Pythium insidiosum,* common in the Gulf Coast region of the United States, South America, and Australia.[65] This organism is a plant parasite and normally lives on aquatic vegetation or organic debris. Damaged animal tissue is chemotactic for the organism and most probably the fungus gains entrance into animal tissue via wounds in prolonged contact with contaminated water.[65]

Typically, ventral body areas, including legs, abdomen, and chest, are affected (Fig. 10–21). Nasal tissue can also be

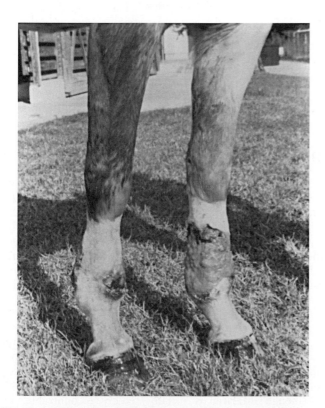

Figure 10–21. Horse with bilateral pythiosis on the legs.

involved. Wire cuts, puncture wounds, and ventral midline dermatitis caused by horn flies or *Culicoides* gnats are prime locations. Early signs of fungal invasion are single or multiple minute foci of necrosis that progress very rapidly and develop into circular, ulcerative, granulomatous masses with serosanguinous discharges.[63–65] These masses are intensely pruritic and are often hemorrhagic from self-trauma. Thick, sticky, material exudes from the wound. This discharge often contains a classic hallmark of this disease, "kunkers," which are hard, gritty, white to yellow masses that develop in tissue tracts. These granules branch macroscopically, which distinguishes them from granules seen in other skin diseases. Kunkers are composed of fungal hyphae, host exudate, and protein. Lameness, regional lymph node involvement, anemia, and hypoproteinemia are common noncutaneous findings. Anemia and hypoproteinemia develop secondarily to the loss of blood and serum from the mass. Occasionally, the disease may become systemic. This disease is not a known zoonosis, but, protective latex gloves should be worn when examining patients.

Pythiosis is difficult to differentiate from habronemiasis, exuberant granulation tissue, bacterial granulomas, and invasive squamous cell carcinoma. Definitive diagnosis requires biopsy, culture, and cytologic examination of exudate and kunkers. Both tissue specimens and kunkers should be submitted for histologic examination. Common findings include pyogranulomatous inflammation with large numbers of eosinophils. If hyphae are seen, they are 2.6 to 6.4 μm in diameter, thick-walled, and irregular in size.[66] Pythiosis can be grown on fungal culture medium, requires incubation in a vegetable extract agar, and a laboratory familiar with appropriate isolation techniques. Kunkers should be collected, washed in sterile saline, and deeply embedded in the media. This disease occasionally can be diagnosed by cytologic inspection of the kunkers. Small kunkers are macerated and minced with a scalpel, the material placed on a glass microscope slide, and incubated overnight in a 1:1 mixture of 10% potassium hydroxide and India ink. Hyphae stain black and appear as broad, thick-walled branching structures.

The prognosis is poor as treatment is very difficult. If the disease is diagnosed early, surgical excision may be possible. Relapses are common, however, and repeated excision is required. Surgery sites should be monitored closely for evidence of recurrence: focal areas of edema with dark hemorrhagic patches 1 to 5 mm in diameter with serosanguinous discharge in the granulation tissue.

Systemic antifungal drugs are not particularly effective in the treatment of this disease.[65, 67] Systemic amphotericin B (Fungizone IV, Bristol-Myers, Squibb, New Brunswick, N.J.), combined with topical amphotericin B, may be curative in *rare* isolated cases. Amphotericin B is administered 0.3 mg/kg in 5% dextrose IV daily until a total dose of 350 mg has been administered. This dose is then administered on alternate days until the horse is cured. In addition, the lesions are treated topically with gauze dressings soaked in an amphotericin B and dimethyl sulfoxide (DMSO) solution (50 mg amphotericin B, 10 mL sterile water and 10 mL DMSO). Amphotericin B also may be injected into lesions. Amphotericin B is nephrotoxic and serum creatinine and serum urea nitrogen concentrations and hydration should be monitored daily. Immunotherapy with a phenolized, ultrasonicated preparation from fungal culture is reportedly curative if administered early in the course of the disease.[67, 68] In a small number of cases, vaccine administration resulted in a decrease in the size of the lesion. This therapy may be of benefit if used preoperatively to enhance complete removal of infected tissue. Unfortunately, the vaccine is not commercially available. Because of the cost of medical or surgical therapy, the risks of treatment, and the high probability that excision is incomplete, euthanasia is often elected.

Parasitic Causes of Nodules
Habronemiasis

Cutaneous habronemiasis is caused when infective larvae of *Habronema muscae, Habronema majus,* or *Draschia megastoma* are deposited by their intermediate host (*Musca* and *Stomoxys* species) into wounds.[7, 22, 38] This occurs when the intermediate host feeds on serum, blood, or moist areas on the horse's body. Larvae are also capable of penetrating intact skin.

The exact pathogenesis of the disease is unknown, but it is believed to involve a hypersensitivity reaction to the presence of dead or dying larvae.[38] The disease is seasonal and lesions spontaneously resolve in the winter. The occurrence is sporadic within a group of horses, but certain individuals may be genetically predisposed to yearly recurrences. There is no age, sex, or breed predilection.[7, 22, 38] The disease usually begins in the spring with the rise in fly populations.

Lesions are most commonly seen on the legs, ventrum, medial canthus of the eye, prepuce, urethral process, or at the site of a wound. They develop rapidly from a papule to a nodule and may be solitary or multiple. Ulceration, exudation, intermittent hemorrhage, and pruritus are common. Wounds often contain very small calcified granules (1 mm). Anecdotal reports suggest that reactions in donkeys are much more severe than in horses. The reason for this is unknown.[38]

Diagnosis is often made solely on the basis of the history and clinical signs and the location of lesions. Skin scrapings are unreliable diagnostic aids because they are not consistently positive and fly larvae other than *Habronema* and *Draschia* species may be found. Biopsy is the test of choice. Histologic findings include nodular to diffuse eosinophilic dermatitis.[51] Multifocal areas of discrete coagulation necrosis with or without degenerating nematode larvae in the center are characteristic of this disease. The lesion must be differentiated from sarcoids and excessive granulation tissue. Occasionally, squamous cell carcinomas, pythiosis, and excessive granulation tissue will be secondarily infected with habronemiasis.

Treatment is aimed at reducing the size of the lesion(s), reducing the inflammation, and preventing reinfestation. Massive lesions often require surgical excision. Intralesional or sublesional injections of 4 to 5 mg per site of triamcinolone acetate (<20 mg per horse total) every 14 days works well to reduce smaller lesions. Prednisone or prednisolone 1 mg/kg/day PO for 7 to 14 days followed by 0.5 mg/kg/day of prednisone for an additional 10 to 14 days is recommended for large lesions and results in a dramatic reduction in the size of the mass. The use of organophosphates to kill larvae are of little value because the pathogenesis of this disease is centered on dead and dying larvae. Ivermectin works over a 2- to 3-week period to kill larvae as they enter the skin, but probably does little to decrease the size of the original lesion.[37, 38, 69] Strict fly control and wound care is mandatory to prevent recurrences.

Warbles (Hypodermiasis, Grubs)

Warbles occasionally occur in horses. They are caused by a larval stage of *Hypoderma bovis* and *Hypoderma linateum.*[7] In horses, larvae do not usually complete their life cycle.[22] Horses that develop infestations are usually pastured or housed with cattle. Adult flies lay eggs on the hairs and larvae migrate toward the skin surface and eventually penetrate the skin. Once in the host's body, the larvae migrate to reach the subcutaneous tissues of the neck and trunk. A swelling develops at the site of the larvae development which eventually becomes perforated as a breathing pore is formed. Nodules are seen most commonly over the withers and almost all develop a breathing pore. The nodules are often painful. Spontaneous rupture may cause anaphylaxis.[22] Occasionally, aberrant migrations cause neurologic signs.

The presence of dorsal swelling or a nodule with a breathing pore is diagnostic. The major differential consideration is collagenolytic granuloma; however, these nodules lack a breathing pore. Hypodermiasis is treated by gently enlarging the breathing pore surgically and removing the grub, removing the entire nodule surgically, or allowing the grub to fall out spontaneously.[22] In areas of high occurrence, pour-on insecticides may be used as a preventive.[70] Horses should be treated at the same time of the year as affected cattle in the area would be.

Ticks

Tick bites can result in a hypersensitivity reaction characterized by nodules (see Parasitic Skin Diseases). These lesions are usually less than 0.5 cm in diameter.

Urticaria

Urticaria is a nodular skin disease of horses characterized by wheals, edema, and often pruritus. It is most commonly caused by a type I hypersensitivity reaction. However, urticaria can also result from nonimmunologic factors such as pressure, sunlight, heat, exercise, stress, and drugs. Pre-race stress, insect or arthropod bites, bacterial infections, topical parasiticides, systemic drugs (penicillin, phenylbutazone, aspirin, guaifenesin, phenothiazine, quinidine, streptomycin, oxytetracycline), feedstuffs, soaps, leather conditioners, vaccines, snake bites, inhalants, and plants can cause urticaria in horses.[32] In our experience, urticaria is a common manifestation of atopy and insect hypersensitivity. Mosquito swarmings commonly result in urticaria.

There is no age, sex, or breed predilection for urticaria. Lesions may develop rapidly or slowly and may be localized or generalized. Lesions are raised, cool to the touch, pit when depressed, and may or may not exude serum or blood. Pruritus is variable. In rare instances, lesions may coalesce to form bizarre patterns.

Although urticaria is usually readily recognizable, its causes can be very difficult to identify. The cause of an acute urticaria episode (<6 weeks in duration) is much more likely to be identified than the cause of a chronic episode (>6 weeks). A detailed history is critical to finding the cause. Important questions to answer are:[33]

1. Is this a corticosteroid-responsive urticaria? This suggests an allergic cause such as atopy, insect hypersensitivity, or food allergy.

2. Does the development of the lesion correlate with the administration of systemic drugs or the application of topical medications? This would suggest a drug reaction.

3. Does the application of fly repellents aggravate or alleviate the urticaria? Worsening of the urticaria suggests an allergic contact reaction, whereas alleviation suggests an insect hypersensitivity.

4. Do lesions resolve with stabling the horse for 24 to 48 hours or moving to a new environment? If so, this would suggest an environmental cause of the urticaria (molds, inhaled dust from bedding, hay, feedstuffs, feathers from roosting birds).

5. Do lesions improve if the horse is moved off pasture? A positive answer would suggest plant antigen as a cause of the urticaria.

6. Do the lesions improve if the feed is changed? Improvement in clinical signs suggests an ingestant allergy or inhaled allergy to feedstuffs. A lack of improvement rules out an ingestant allergy, but not an inhalant allergy to pollens or molds.

In cases where lesions are bizarre in appearance, chronic, or exudative, a skin biopsy should be performed to rule out other causes of nodular disease. Typical histologic findings for urticaria show vasodilation, edema in the dermis, and mild to moderate eosinophilic perivascular inflammation. Complete blood cell counts and serum chemistry profiles are rarely useful. Before beginning expensive or involved diagnostic testing, be sure to eliminate allergic reactions to shampoos, tack cleaners, soaps, and so forth. All horses with chronic urticaria should undergo a food trial, be moved to a new environment for 5 to 7 days, and undergo a program of insect control before being referred for intradermal skin testing. Intradermal skin testing is the best method for identifying the cause of allergic inhalant dermatitis. Horses should not receive antihistamines or tranquilizers for 1 week, or corticosteroids for 4 weeks, prior to intradermal skin testing.

Treatment is directed at eliminating the underlying cause, if possible. Hydroxyzine 200 to 400 mg PO t.i.d. is very effective in eliminating urticarial swellings in most cases of acute or chronic urticaria.[29] Transient sedation of several days' duration may be seen with this drug. If the horse is nonresponsive to hydroxyzine, prednisone 1 mg/kg PO, IV or IM may be beneficial on a short-term (<1 week) basis.

Idiopathic Inflammatory Causes of Nodules

Eosinophilic Granuloma with Collagen Degeneration (Nodular Collagenolytic Granuloma, Nodular Necrobiosis)

Eosinophilic granulomas are a frequent cause of nodules in the skin of horses.[38] The exact cause of these lesions is unknown, but they may be due to a hypersensitivity reaction

to insect bites.[38] Lesions, however, have been reported to develop spontaneously or as a result of trauma, suggesting multiple causes.[71] Regional variability in the occurrence of lesions has been noted by us.

These lesions have no sex, breed, or age predilection, but tend to be most common in warmer months. They may be single or multiple and vary greatly in size (0.5–10 cm in diameter). The nodules may occur anywhere on the body but are most common on the neck, withers, and dorsal trunk (Fig. 10–22). Individual lesions are rounded, well circumscribed, firm, haired, nonpainful, and nonpruritic. Owners of horses with seasonal problems have reported that early lesions are often soft and fluctuant and develop into firm masses over weeks to months. If lesions are under the saddle, the horse may exhibit pain.

Definitive diagnosis is made by skin biopsy. Histologic examination of tissue reveals multifocal areas of collagen degeneration surrounded by granulomatous eosinophilic inflammation. Chronic lesions may have marked dystrophic mineralization.[51]

Solitary lesions that do not cause the horse discomfort require no treatment. Problem lesions respond to excision or sublesional injections of triamcinolone acetonide (3–5 mg per lesion) or methylprednisolone acetate (5–10 mg per lesion).[38] No more than 20 mg per horse of triamcinolone acetonide should be injected because of the danger of laminitis. Horses with multiple lesions may be treated with oral prednisolone 1 mg/kg PO s.i.d. for 2 to 3 weeks.[38] Once

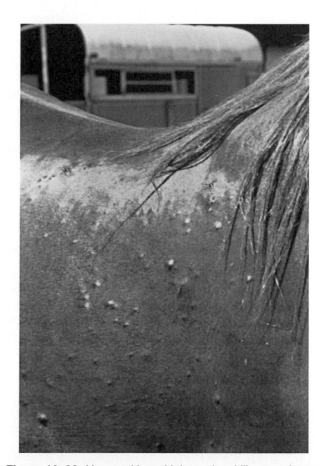

Figure 10–22. Horse with multiple eosinophilic granulomas.

lesions have resolved, the dose of prednisolone should be tapered and discontinued over a 5- to 10-day period. Horses with seasonal recurrences in which insect hypersensitivity is involved and documented via intradermal skin testing might benefit from hyposensitization to insects.

Equine Axillary Nodular Necrosis

This is a very rare idiopathic skin disease of horses. The disease is similar to equine eosinophilic granuloma with collagen degeneration, except that the lesions are localized to the axillary region.[72]

There is no known age, sex, or breed predilection. Clinically, single or multiple nodules develop unilaterally in the axillae. The nodules are painless, nonpruritic, haired, well-circumscribed firm masses which vary in size from 0.5 cm to 4.0 cm or greater in diameter. Horses with multiple lesions tend to have them arranged in a row.

Skin biopsy is diagnostic. Biopsy findings include pyogranulomatous, eosinophilic dermatitis with foci of coagulation necrosis. Collagen degeneration is not a common finding.

Treatment is the same as for equine eosinophilic granuloma. Corticosteroids often do not work well, and surgical excision may be necessary. Lesions tend to recur.

Equine Unilateral Papular Dermatosis

Equine unilateral papular dermatosis is another rare idiopathic skin disorder of horses.[72] This disease has been seen in several breeds of horses but may be more common in quarter horses. Lesions develop in the warm months and are characterized by the unilateral development of multiple (30–300) papules and nodules on the trunk (Fig. 10–23). Lesions are firm, well circumscribed, nonpainful, and nonpruritic.

Diagnosis is by skin biopsy. Histologic examination of tissue shows eosinophilic folliculitis and furunculosis.

Spontaneous remission may occur, otherwise prednisone 1 mg/kg PO s.i.d. for 2 to 3 weeks is recommended until nodules resolve. Relapses the same or next year may occur.

Neoplastic Causes of Nodules

It is beyond the scope of this chapter to review all of the neoplastic skin conditions of horses. Only the skin tumors of horses that commonly masquerade as nodules are discussed: sarcoids, melanomas, mast cell tumors, and cutaneous lymphoma. Some cutaneous neoplasms can be diagnosed via exfoliative cytology, but biopsy is the diagnostic test of choice. The reader is referred to several excellent reviews for information on other neoplastic skin diseases of horses.[73–75]

Sarcoids

Sarcoids account for up to one third of all reported tumors of horses. Sarcoids are locally invasive fibroblastic neoplasms.[76–81]

The etiology is controversial and currently papovavirus is believed to be involved in the development of lesions.[73, 77, 78] Polymerase chain reaction nucleotide sequences strongly

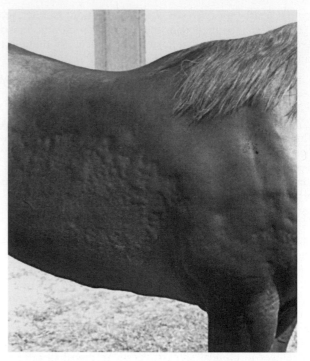

Figure 10–23. Horse with unilateral papular dermatitis. (Courtesy of V. Fadock, University of Florida.)

suggest that equine sarcoids are caused by bovine papillomavirus types 1 and 2.[79] Evidence for this includes the clinical observations that lesions often develop in areas of previous trauma, lesions may spread to other areas on the same horse or to other horses, epizootics of equine sarcoid have been described, and autotransmission is possible under experimental conditions. Finally, equine sarcoids were produced in donkeys inoculated with bovine papillomavirus. A predisposition or susceptibility also appears to play a part in the pathogenesis. Certain genetically related horses have a higher frequency of occurrence of sarcoids, suggesting a genetic susceptibility.[78]

There is no sex or breed predilection, but over 70% of sarcoids develop in horses less than 4 years of age. They may arise spontaneously or at a site of previous trauma and may occur anywhere on the body. However, there is a predilection for the head, ears, and limbs. One third of affected horses have multiple lesions. There are four clinical presentations of sarcoids: (1) flat (occult), (2) verrucous (warty), (3) fibroblastic (proliferative), or (4) or a combination of verrucous and fibroblastic (mixed) (Fig. 10–24 and 10–25). Flat sarcoids appear grossly as annular rings of hair loss with scaling and crusting. However, they may extend deeply into the dermis and subcutaneous tissue. They may be grossly indistinguishable from dermatophytosis, dermatophilosis, or bacterial folliculitis; however, one distinguishing characteristic is that flat sarcoids do not rapidly change or spread, unlike infectious causes of hair loss and scaling. Verrucous sarcoids are warty in appearance, rarely greater than 6 cm in diameter, and may be grossly indistinguishable from papillomas. Fibroblastic sarcoids are clinically similar to squamous cell carcinomas, exuberant granulation tissue, pythiosis, bacterial and fungal granulomas, and habronemiasis. They appear as nodules or large, ulcerated masses.

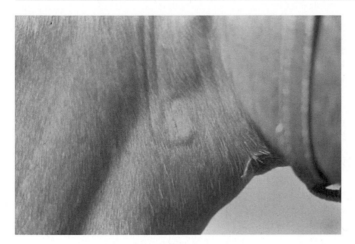

Figure 10–24. Flat sarcoid.

Skin biopsy is required to confirm the diagnosis. Fibroblastic proliferation of the dermis with concurrent epidermal hyperplasia is classic.[51] The collagen in the dermis shows a whorled, tangled, or herringbone pattern. Individual cells are spindle-shaped, fusiform to stellate, and may be atypical. Fibroblasts at the dermal-epidermal junction may be perpendicular to the basement membrane. The epidermis is hyperplastic and hyperkeratotic.

These tumors do not metastasize but do wax and wane, complicating treatment. Flat sarcoids usually remain static unless traumatized and present a clinical challenge because the trauma from skin biopsy may induce a dramatic change in behavior to that of a fibroblastic nature. If a solitary nonchanging lesion is present and no evidence of a bacterial or fungal infection is found, "watchful neglect" may be the best therapeutic option. If biopsy is elected, it should be by wide excision.

Sarcoids have been treated with radioactive isotope implants, excision and immediate split-thickness skin grafts, radiation-induced hyperthermia, cryosurgery, and intralesional bacille Calmette-Guérin (BCG) and other immunostimulants. Cryosurgery and intralesional BCG are the most commonly used therapies available.[80, 81] Cryosurgery is very successful for treating sarcoids, especially after large tumors have been excised. Lesions should be frozen two to three times to at least $-20\,^{\circ}$C. Tissue should be allowed to thaw completely before being refrozen, and the use of cryoprobes to monitor tissue temperature is highly recommended. Time for complete healing may take more than 8 weeks and owners should be warned of the odor and exudate from necrotic tissue. Spontaneous regression of multiple sarcoids postcryosurgery has been reported. In addition, single untreated lesions may spontaneously regress.

Immunotherapy with BCG is an alternative treatment.[81] Live BCG vaccine (BCG Vaccine, Organon, Inc, West Orange, N.J.) is available. Occasionally, acute fatal anaphylactic reactions occur following its use. However, killed purified protein derivative vaccines are currently used and commercially available. Patients should be selected carefully and the diagnosis confirmed by biopsy. The best candidates are horses with single or multiple nodular sarcoids less than 0.5 cm in diameter. The anatomical site of the sarcoid is an important consideration when considering immunotherapy with BCG. Tumors in the inguinal or axillary region are hard to inject without anesthesia. BCG therapy is particularly suited for tumors located in critical areas that may be damaged by scarring, secondary to cryosurgery. Large or multiple tumors are difficult to treat with BCG because of possible vaccine reactions.

Pretreatment with flunixin meglumine 1.0 mg/kg IV and antihistamines intramuscularly is recommended.[81] Tetanus prophylaxis should be current. Large proliferative tumors should be debulked by sharp dissection to the skin level, if necessary. Using an 18-gauge needle, approximately 1.0 mL of BCG per 1.0 to 2.0 cc of tumor is injected into the tumor and intradermally adjacent to the sarcoid's base. The total volume of BCG should not exceed 6.0 cc per tumor.[81] BCG is very difficult to inject because of the viscous nature of the product and the dense connective tissue of the sarcoid. Edema, inflammation, and swelling occur within 24 to 48 hours of treatment. If the sarcoid begins to regress or slough within 14 days, one treatment will suffice. In most cases, two to five treatments are needed. Postinjection reactions are mildest with the first treatment, and intensify with each subsequent treatment. Wounds should be cleaned daily and monitored closely for myiasis.

Melanomas

Melanomas may arise from dermal melanocytes or melanoblasts and may be benign or malignant. These tumors are most commonly seen in older horses of the Arabian and

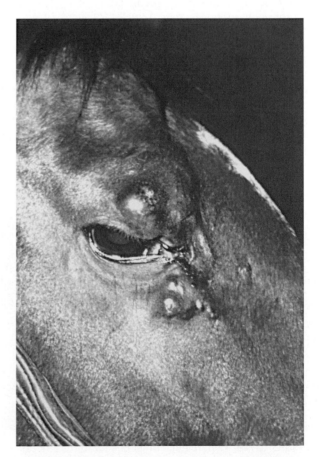

Figure 10–25. Fibroblastic (proliferative) sarcoid.

Percheron horse breeds.[82] There is also a widely recognized relationship between the development of melanomas and gray coat color.[82] Melanomas appear to occur exclusively in horses that are gray or become dapple-gray with age. It has been estimated that up to 80% of gray horses over 15 years of age have melanomas.[83]

Lesions may be solitary or multiple and occur most commonly on the perineum or ventral surface of the tail. Tumors are usually firm, nodular, and may be hairless and ulcerated. They are almost always black. Vitiligo may precede the development of the lesions.[82] Three growth patterns have been described: (1) slow growth without metastasis, (2) slow growth with sudden metastasis, and (3) rapid growth and malignancy from the onset.[83]

Diagnosis is usually based upon clinical signs. Biopsy is usually not needed to confirm the diagnosis unless the lesion is bizarre in appearance.

No treatment is needed unless the melanoma is interfering with function, for example, defecation; early radical excision does not guarantee the melanoma will not recur. Recently, cimetidine (Tagamet) 2.5 mg/kg t.i.d. has been reported to cause partial to complete regression of tumors. The number and size of the melanomas decreases by 50% to 90% in horses treated for 3 months. Once the tumors have regressed, daily maintenance therapy at 1.6 mg/kg PO once-daily is recommended.[84]

Mastocytoma

Mast cell tumors are uncommon in horses. Equine mast cell tumors show a definitive sex predilection, being five times more common in males than females.[85] There is no age predilection, but there is a breed predilection in that tumors are very rare in Thoroughbreds, but much more common in Arabian horses.[38]

There are two distinct types of mast cell tumors in horses: a hyperplastic type and a neoplastic type. Most equine mast cell tumors are hyperplastic rather than neoplastic. Clinically, there are two forms of equine mastocytomas that have been reported.[38] The most common form is a single cutaneous nodule, most frequently located on the head (Fig. 10–26). Nodules range in size from 2 to 20 cm in diameter. The

surface of the nodule may be normal, hairless, or ulcerated. The second form consists of a diffuse swelling on a lower extremity, usually below the carpus or hock. The swelling is firm and the overlying skin is normal in appearance.[38] Radiographs of the limb commonly show multifocal areas of soft tissue mineralization.

Diagnosis is made by biopsy. Diffuse to nodular proliferations of mast cells are seen in the dermis. Tumor cells may be well differentiated or more atypical. Tissue eosinophilia, collagen degeneration, and dystrophic mineralization are commonly seen in horses.[51]

Solitary tumors can be treated by excision, sublesional triamcinolone acetate 5 to 10 mg per lesion or with cryosurgery.[73, 74] Spontaneous remission may occur following incomplete excision or in young horses.[83, 86, 87] Metastasis has not been reported.

Lymphoma

Cutaneous lymphoma is rare in horses.[71, 73] There is no recognized age, sex, or breed predilection. Most affected animals have another concurrent systemic disease and weight loss, anorexia, anemia, and lymphadenopathy are commonly present.[73, 88] Lesions develop slowly or rapidly. They may occur anywhere on the body, but the trunk and neck are most commonly affected. Individual lesions may be firm or fluctuant, resembling urticaria. The overlying skin is usually normal. Involvement of internal organs may occur.

Definitive diagnosis is made by histologic examination of a skin biopsy. Several representative sample tissues should be submitted for examination. Histologically, lymphosarcoma is characterized by diffuse dermal and subcutaneous infiltration of malignant lymphocytes.[89] If the owners want to pursue treatment, there are several treatment options. Prednisolone 1 mg/kg PO s.i.d. for 7 days and then every other day has been used successfully. In addition, PEG-L-asparaginase 10,000 IU/m^2 once-weekly may be beneficial, although expensive. Recently, low-dose cyclophosphamide and immunization with vaccinia virus–infected autologous tumor cells was successful in inducing a 19-month remission in a 13-year-old horse[90]; however, this therapy is experimental.

Pseudolymphoma

Pseudolymphomas are relatively common in horses compared to lymphomas.[38] It is very important to differentiate the two diseases as the prognosis for pseudolymphoma is excellent.

Pseudolymphomas are nodular to papular lesions that develop in the skin as a result of chronic antigenic stimulation. It is believed that the most common antigenic stimuli are insect bites and drug reactions. Lesions occur most commonly in late summer and fall and are usually solitary, but may be multiple.[38, 73] Pseudolymphomas usually occur on the head and trunk. Individual lesions are firm, raised, and haired.

Definitive diagnosis is by skin biopsy. Histologic examination of tissue shows dense dermal and subcutaneous infiltration of lymphocytes, histiocytes, plasma cells, and eosinophils. Lymphoid nodules and eosinophils are present and are

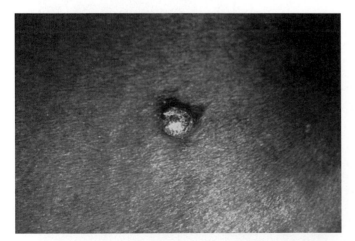

Figure 10–26. Hyperplastic mast cell tumor in a horse.

an important aid in the differentiation of pseudolymphoma from lymphoma.[51, 73]

Pseudolymphomas often spontaneously regress, but may be surgically excised or injected sublesionally with triamcinolone acetonide 3 to 5 mg per lesion).[73]

Congenital Causes of Nodules

Dermoid Cysts

A *dermoid cyst* is defined as a tumor of developmental origin consisting of a wall of fibrous tissue lined with stratified epithelium containing hair follicles, sweat glands, sebaceous glands, nerves, or teeth, or any combination of these. They may be congenital or hereditary.

Dermoid cysts have been reported in horses 6 months to 9 years of age and are common in Thoroughbreds.[91] They occur frequently on the dorsal midline between the rump and withers. The cysts appear as soft, fluctuant swellings with normal overlying skin. Diagnosis is made by histologic examination after excision.

Atheroma (False Nostril Cyst)

An atheroma is a cyst in the false nostril.[87] They are believed to develop from hair follicle retention cysts or from displaced germ material.[87] Atheromas are present at birth, usually unilateral, and enlarge with time. They are not usually noticed until they enlarge to greater than 2 cm. The tumor is firm on palpation but is rarely painful.

Diagnosis is by clinical signs. Treatment is not necessary unless breathing is compromised or the owner is disturbed by the lesion mass. Surgical excision is the treatment of choice, but, care must be taken to remove the entire cyst, lest recurrence or chronic drainage occur.[87]

DISORDERS OF PIGMENTATION

Skin and hair color are dependent upon melanin production in the skin.[92] Pigment is produced within melanocytes which are found at the dermal-epidermal junction and in the outer root sheath of the hair follicle. There is one melanocyte for every 10 to 20 keratinocytes. Melanin pigments have a wide range of colors including black-brown eumelanins, yellow-red pheomelanins, and a range of intermediate pigments. Melanin pigment is produced in special tyrosinase-rich organelles called melanosomes found in the cytoplasm of melanocytes.[92] Tyrosine is converted to dopa which is oxidized to dopaquinone.[92] Both reactions are catalyzed by the copper-containing enzyme tyrosinase.[92] Subsequent intermediate products polymerize, eventually forming melanin. Melanocytes secrete or inject melanosomes into adjacent keratinocytes. The production of melanin is controlled by genetics, hormones, local keratinocytes, and Langerhans' cells.[92] Ultraviolet light, inflammation, byproducts of the arachidonic acid cycle, androgens, estrogens, glucocorticoids, and thyroid hormones can also influence pigmentation.[92]

Skin and hair color are determined by the number, size, type, and distribution of melanosomes. Melanosomes are responsible for coat color, photoprotection, free radical scavenging, and heat conservation.

Causes of Hyperpigmentation

Hyperpigmentation is almost always an acquired change. Both the skin and the hair can become hyperpigmented. The usual cause of localized or patchy hyperpigmentation is chronic inflammation or irritation. Macular patches of noninflammatory hyperpigmentation, called lentigo, can occur in horses. Lentigo is most frequently seen at mucocutaneous junctions. The most important differential diagnosis for lentigo is cutaneous melanoma. A skin biopsy of the affected area is the most useful diagnostic test. Generalized hyperpigmentation of the coat or skin has not been reported; however, it would suggest a hormonal cause.

Causes of Hypopigmentation

Hypopigmentation describes a decrease in normal melanin pigmentation. Depigmentation specifically refers to a loss of preexisting melanin. *Leukoderma* and *leukotrichia* are clinical terms used to describe the loss of color in skin and hair, respectively. Amelanosis is a total lack of melanin.

Albinism and Lethal White Foal Disease

Albinism is rare in horses and is transmitted by an autosomal dominant gene. Affected animals have white skin and hair, hypopigmented irides, and photophobia. Lethal white foal disease has two forms. One is caused by an autosomal dominant gene characterized by early embryonic death in the homozygous state.[93] The second form results from the breeding of two Overo paint horses and is an autosomal recessive disorder.[94] Affected foals are characterized by albinism and congenital defects of the intestinal tract.

Leukoderma

Leukoderma develops in areas of previous trauma or inflammation and may be temporary or permanent. Affected areas appear normal but depigmented leukoderma occurs commonly in horses with onchocerciasis, lupus erythematosus, pressure sores, ventral midline dermatitis, viral skin diseases, freezing, burns, or sun damage (Fig. 10–27). Leu-

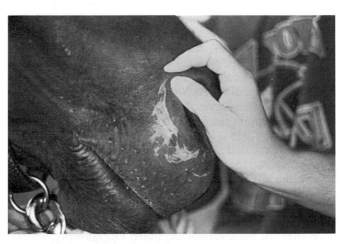

Figure 10–27. Idiopathic leukoderma in a horse.

Black and White Follicle Dystrophy

Affected horses (juvenile and adult) have abnormal hairs growing in either patches of white- or black-haired areas. These hairs are short, brittle, and dull. Affected areas may be hypotrichotic. There is no known treatment.[102]

Curly Coat

This a hereditary condition of Percherons, Missouri fox trotting, and Bashkin horse breeds.[102] It is inherited as an autosomal recessive trait. Clinically affected animals have unusually curly coats.

Endocrine Causes of Hair Abnormalities

Hyperadrenocorticism

Equine hyperadrenocorticism is most commonly the result of an adenoma of the pars intermedia of the hypophysis.[103] These adenomas secrete adrenocorticotropic hormone (ACTH), α- and β-melanocyte-stimulating hormone (MSH), corticotropin-like intermediate lobe peptides, and β-endorphins. For reasons unknown, secretion of these peptides is resistant to glucocorticoid administration, making the dexamethasone suppression test of little diagnostic use in horses.

Hyperadrenocorticism is most common in older mares.[103, 104] The first clinical sign noted by the owner is a rapid regrowth of long hair after a shedding season or a failure to shed the coat. The coat becomes very shaggy and body hairs can reach lengths of 10 to 12 cm. Interestingly, the mane, tail, and fetlock hairs are unaffected. Secondary seborrhea may develop. Affected horses may be predisposed to dermatophytosis, dermatophilosis, or secondary bacterial pyoderma. Nondermatologic signs include polydipsia, polyuria, muscle wasting, lethargy, weight loss, pendulous abdomen, and flaccid muscles. Neurologic disorders and blindness may develop.

Diagnosis is based upon clinical signs and laboratory tests. Complete blood counts will show a neutrophilia, lymphopenia, and eosinopenia. Urinalysis shows a low specific gravity and occasionally glucosuria. Serum chemistry panel may show any combination of the following: hyperglycemia, hypercholesterolemia, and lipemia.[103] The diagnostic tests available are the ACTH response test and measurement of endogenous ACTH plasma levels.[104] The ACTH response test may be performed using either IM (1 IU/kg ACTH gel) or IV ACTH (100 IU aqueous ACTH). Basal serum samples are collected before ACTH administration and post-ACTH serum samples are collected at either 2 hours (IV protocol) or 8 hours (IM protocol). Although horses with hyperadrenocorticism reportedly show a greatly exaggerated response to ACTH exogenously administered,[104] caution must be used in interpreting ACTH response tests, as there is evidence that the test does not adequately distinguish between normal and abnormal horses. Plasma ACTH concentrations in horses with hyperadrenocorticism will be markedly elevated (>400 pg/mL; normal, 32 ±5 pg/mL).[104] This is a better test, but more difficult and expensive to perform. Dexamethasone suppression tests are not completely reliable in the horse, but are widely used because of their ease of administration and the lack of a better alternative.

The prognosis for treatment of these animals is poor. Horses do not respond well to mitotane. Cyproheptadine and pergolide have been used on a few horses with some success.[104] Details of therapy are discussed elsewhere; see Chapter 17.

Hypothyroidism

Hypothyroidism in the horse is rare and much of the information on this endocrinopathy is anecdotal. Horses with naturally occurring hypothyroidism reportedly present with a wide range of clinical signs including loss of mane and tail hairs, muscle weakness, hyperpigmentation, seborrhea, lethargy, poor performance, infertility, agalactia, myxedema, and dry, dull, brittle hair. Juvenile hypothyroidism was reported in a Thoroughbred foal with skeletal lesions, delayed appearance of ossification centers, delayed bone development in cartilage models, delayed closure of epiphyseal plates, bone cysts, osteochondrosis dissecans, and transverse trabeculation in metaphyses.[105, 106]

Definitive diagnosis is made by measuring thyroid hormone concentrations. The test of choice is a function test, either a thyroid-stimulating hormone (TSH) response test or a thyrotropin-releasing hormone (TRH) response test.[107] The major advantage of using a function test is avoidance of the difficulties encountered in evaluating basal thyroid hormone concentrations. Basal thyroid hormones may be spuriously low due to exogenous drugs (glucocorticoids, phenylbutazone), illness, frequent hard training and racing, and individual variation in euthyroid horses. The disadvantages of function tests are cost, limited availability of the testing hormones, and time commitment. The TSH response test can be performed using either an intramuscular or intravenous protocol after a basal serum sample is collected. If used intramuscularly, 5 IU TSH is injected and a second serum sample is collected between 6 and 12 hours after TSH administration.[103] If used intravenously, 5 IU TSH is injected and a second serum sample is collected 4 hours after drug administration.[103] Euthyroid horses will show at least a twofold increase in the basal thyroxine (T_4) hormone concentration. If TRH is used, 0.5 to 1.0 mg is administered IV after a basal serum sample is collected.[107] A second sample is collected 4 hours after TRH administration. Euthyroid horses will show a two- to threefold increase in basal thyroid hormone concentrations.

Treatment regimens are anecdotal because of the paucity of clinical case material. Sodium levothyroxine is the treatment of choice in other species, and there is no reason to suspect that the horse is different. Dosage recommendations for the horse vary, but 10 mg orally once daily is most commonly recommended.[107]

Miscellaneous Disorders Affecting the Hair Coat

Anagen Defluxion and Telogen Effluvium

Anagen defluxion refers to a condition in which a disease or drug interferes with anagen hair growth. This results in abnormal hairs or hair shaft abnormalities or both. Hair loss occurs within days of the insult or drug. This is most commonly seen in horses with high fevers, systemic illnesses, or malnutrition[108] (Fig. 10–29). Typically, the mane and tail are not affected.

Telogen effluvium refers to a condition in which a stressful situation causes the sudden cessation of anagen hair growth and the sudden synchrony of many hair follicles in the telogen hair cycle stage.[108] Two to 3 months later there is a sudden shedding and a wave of new hair growth.

These conditions cannot be distinguished clinically. Diagnosis is based upon examining the hair shaft of easily epilated hairs. Anagen defluxion is characterized by dysplastic hairs, the shaft may be weak or narrow, and the root end contains a root sheath. Telogen effluvium is characterized by uniform hairs with no shaft abnormalities and a nonpigmented root end lacking a root sheath. Both conditions resolve spontaneously when the animal recovers from the predisposing condition.

Trichorrhexis Nodosa

Trichorrhexis nodosa is an acquired hair shaft disorder of horses caused by physical or chemical trauma.[96] Overzealous grooming, shampoos, pesticides, alcohol, or solvents are the most common causes. The lesions are visible without magnification and appear as small white to gray nodules on the hair shaft. The hair shaft is easily fractured and broken at these sites. Under the microscope, the affected hairs have the appearance of two brooms shoved together. Therapy consists of eliminating the trauma.

Piedra

Piedra is a rare superficial fungal disease of horses which causes nodules on the hair shaft.[64] Black or white filamentous

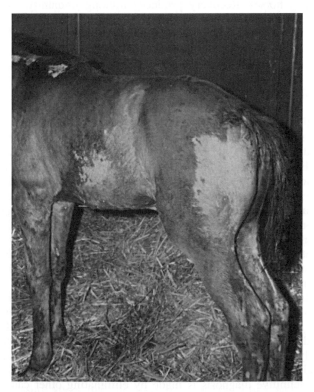

Figure 10–29. Foal with telogen effluvium after illness.

nodules consisting of tightly packed hyphae are most commonly seen on the mane or tail. Affected hairs break at the site of infection. Definitive diagnosis is made by fungal culture and microscopic identification of the agent, *Piedra* sp. or *Trichosporon beigelii*. Affected animals are treated by clipping the hair and the application of topical fungicides (see Table 10–4).

Abnormal Shedding

Shedding is controlled by photoperiod and temperature. Most horses will have a spring and fall shed. Abnormal shedding in horses may result in large areas of alopecia.[96] Large areas of hair loss may develop on the face, shoulders, or even over the entire body. The pathogenesis is unknown. Skin biopsy is recommended to eliminate infectious or parasitic causes of hair loss. Skin biopsy is normal and shows normal hair follicles in various stages of development. Horses spontaneously recover in up to 3 months.[96]

Alopecia Areata

Alopecia areata is a rare idiopathic skin disease of horses characterized by focal areas of alopecia.[95] Lesions may be single or multiple and the underlying skin is otherwise normal. If and when hair regrows, it may be of a different color. Diagnosis is made by biopsy. Classically, in early lesions skin biopsy shows an accumulation of lymphoid cells around the proximal end of the anagen hair follicles.[96] This change is diagnostic, but it may require numerous biopsies before it can be seen. The prognosis is uncertain. In humans, alopecia areata may resolve spontaneously in 3 to 5 years. It is unknown if this will occur in horses.

MUCOCUTANEOUS VESICULAR DISEASES

A vesicle is an elevated fluctuant fluid-filled lesion of less than 1 cm in size. A vesicular eruption suggests a viral, autoimmune, or irritant etiology. In horses, vesicles are very transient because the epidermis is thin and these lesions rupture very easily. Erosions or ulcerations are often the first clue that a vesicle-producing disease is present. Additionally, vesicular diseases may masquerade as pustular eruptions. Vesicles in horses rapidly fill with inflammatory cells making them indistinguishable from frank pustules. In rare instances, horses may develop bullae (>1 cm in diameter) which are very large vesicles. Occasionally, bullae may fill with blood and are red-purple in color.

Viral Causes of Vesicular Eruptions

Equine Herpes Coital Exanthema

Coital exanthema is a rare contagious venereal disease of horses caused by equine herpesvirus type 3 (EHV-3), which occurs worldwide. It is transmitted via coitus, insects, fomites, and inhalation. Early lesions begin as papules which rapidly progress to vesicles or bullae or pustules on the vulva or perineum of mares and the penis and prepuce of rope burns, counterirritants, or radiation. The majority of burns occurring in horses are the result of barn fires.

Large thermal injuries in horses are very difficult to manage.[112–115] The large surface area of the burn dramatically increases the potential for the loss of fluids, electrolytes, and caloric losses. Burns on 50% or more of the body are usually fatal, but this does depend on the depth of the burn.[112, 115] Massive wound contamination is almost impossible to prevent because of the impossibility of maintaining a sterile environment.[112, 115] Long-term restraint is required to prevent continued trauma; wounds are often pruritic and self-mutilation is common.[113] Burned horses are frequently disfigured, preventing them from returning to full function.

Burns are classified by the depth of the injury.[112–115] First-degree burns involve only the most superficial layers of the epidermis. These burns are characterized by erythema, edema, desquamation of superficial layers of the skin, and pain. The germinal layer of the epidermis is spared and these burns heal without complication.[114] Second-degree burns involve the entire epidermis and can be superficial or deep. Superficial second-degree burns involve the stratum corneum, stratum granulosum, and a few cells of the basal layer. Deep second-degree burns involve all layers of the epidermis. Clinically, these burns are characterized by erythema, edema at the epidermal-dermal junction, necrosis of the epidermis, accumulation of white blood cells at the basal layer of the burn, eschar (slough produced by a thermal burn) formation, and minimal pain. The only germinal cells spared are those within the ducts of sweat glands and hair follicles. Second-degree burns heal well with good wound care.[114] Third-degree burns are characterized by loss of the epidermal and dermal components. There is fluid loss and a marked cellular response at the margins and deeper tissue, eschar formation, lack of pain, shock, wound infection, and possible bacteremia and septicemia. Healing is by contraction and epithelialization occurs only from the wound margins. These burns are frequently complicated by infection and problems with wound healing.[114] Fourth-degree burns involve all of the skin and underlying muscle, bone, and ligaments.

Burns cause both local and systemic effects.[113–116] Local tissue damage results from massive protein coagulation and cellular death. In the immediate area of the burn, arteries and venules constrict and capillary beds dilate. Capillary wall permeability is increased in response to vasoactive amines released as a result of tissue damage and inflammation.[116] These vascular responses result in fluid, protein, and inflammatory cells accumulating in the wound. There is vascular sludging, thrombosis, and dermal ischemia, resulting in further tissue damage. The tissue ischemia continues for 24 to 48 hours after the injury and is believed to be due to the local release of thromboxane A_2.[115, 116] Lipid layers in the skin are destroyed and there is a fourfold increase in the loss of fluid. Fluid losses result in increased heat loss from evaporation and an increased metabolic rate. It is important to note that the full extent and depth of the burn may not be evident for several days. Neutrophil function and chemotaxis are markedly decreased, predisposing the wound to local infection, bacteremia, and septicemia. Burns are frequently colonized by *Pseudomonas aeruginosa*, *Staphylococcus*, *Escherichia coli*, *Klebsiella*, nonhemolytic *Streptococcus*, *Proteus*, *Clostridium*, and *Candida* species.[112–115]

Systemic effects are life-threatening and include hypovolemia, fluid and electrolyte losses, protein loss, pulmonary edema, anemia, increased basal metabolic rate, increased caloric needs, and depressed cell-mediated and humoral immune responses. A decrease in cardiac output secondary to a circulating myocardial depressant factor is exacerbated by hypovolemia.[116]

First-degree burns and superficial second-degree burns should be treated immediately with ice or cold water to prevent further tissue necrosis.[112, 115] Aloe vera cream or a water-soluble antibacterial cream should be applied to the wound to prevent infection. In addition, nonsteroidal analgesics should be administered to alleviate pain and to help reduce dermal ischemia via their antiprostaglandin effects. Aspirin 10 to 20 mg/kg PO s.i.d. or b.i.d. decreases thromboxane production and may also halt further dermal ischemia and may be the initial drug of choice.[115]

Deep second-degree burns are managed initially as described above; however, these burns tend to form blisters which should be left intact as long as possible because the vesicular fluid is a good medium for reepithelialization.[112, 113, 115] Ruptured blisters should be trimmed and the area cleaned with copious amounts of water. The wound should be covered with an antibacterial dressing, xenograft, or an eschar should be allowed to form.[112–115] The bandage should allow drainage and be changed daily or more often.

Full-thickness burns (third and fourth degree) can be managed by occlusive dressings (closed technique), eschar production (exposure technique), continuous wet dressings (semiopen technique), or excision and grafting techniques.[115] The most practical therapy for large burns in horses is the semiopen method-leaving the eschar intact with continuous application of moist bandages and antibacterial agents.[115] The moist dressings help prevent heat and moisture loss from the eschar, provide protection of the eschar, and help prevent bacterial invasion of the wound.[112–115]

Routine use of systemic antibiotics is not recommended in burn patients. Short-term systemic antibiotics may be useful in the initial 3 to 5 days after the burn to minimize bacterial colonization of burns and systemic sepsis.[115] In the absence of sepsis, systemic antibiotics are contraindicated. Extensive use of antibiotics may cause altered microbial flora in the gut and in mucous membranes. This may predispose the patient to infections from antibiotic-resistant gram-negative bacteria or from fungi.[112] Topical medications should be water-based, easily applied and removed, not interfere with wound healing, and be readily excreted or metabolized. Silver sulfadiazine and aloe vera are very effective. Silver sulfadiazine is effective against gram-negative bacteria, causes no discomfort to the horse, penetrates eschar, and has a duration of action of 24 hours.[112–115] Aloe vera is reported to relieve pain, decrease inflammation, stimulate cell growth, and kill bacteria and fungi.[117] Aloe vera is most useful in the early treatment of wounds.[117] The reader is referred to several excellent references for further information on the long-term medical and surgical management of horses with large thermal burns.[112, 114, 115]

Frostbite

Frostbite occurs when tissue is exposed to extreme cold. Sick, debilitated, and neonatal animals are more at risk.

Cold temperatures inhibit cell metabolism and cause tissue dehydration, cell disruption by ice crystals, ischemia, and vascular damage. The most commonly affected areas are the glans penis, ear tips, coronary bands, and heels.[47] The initial lesion of frostbite is paleness of the skin. Erythema, scaling, and hair loss follow. Pigment loss may occur. In severe cases necrosis and dry gangrene occur.

Mild cases of frostbite do not require treatment. More severe cases require rapid thawing in warm water (41°–44 °C).[47] After rewarming, nonsteroidal antibiotic ointments should be applied to the area. In very severe cases with necrosis and sloughing, topical wet soaks and symptomatic therapy with antibiotics may be needed to prevent sepsis. Surgical debridement should not be attempted until an obvious demarcation is present between viable and nonviable tissue. Previously frostbitten areas may be more susceptible to cold injury.

Chemical Toxicoses
Selenium Toxicosis

In addition to causing disorders of the hair coat, selenosis may result in necrosis and sloughing of the hoof. (See Chemical and Plant Causes of Coat Abnormalities.)

Stachybotryotoxicosis

Stachybotryotoxicosis is a mycotoxicosis caused by the toxins of the fungus *Stachybotrys atra*.[47] This fungus grows on hay and straw and produces toxins referred to as macrocytic trichothecenes. These toxins cause bone marrow suppression, profound neutropenia and thrombocytopenia, and necrotic-ulcerative lesions of the skin and mucous membranes.

Commonly, lesions begin at the mucocutaneous junction as focal areas of necrosis and ulceration. Petechiae, ulcers, large areas of necrosis, catarrhal rhinitis, suppurative rhinopharyngitis, and laryngitis follow. Skin lesions occur as early as 24 hours after ingestion of the toxin. Systemic signs include lethargy, anorexia, weight loss, hyperactivity, proprioceptive deficits, colic, muscular stiffness, and second-degree atrioventricular block. Affected animals develop hemorrhagic diathesis, hemorrhagic enteritis, septicemia, and then die.

Diagnosis is based upon history, clinical signs, and finding the toxin in the feed. If recognized early in the course of the disease, withdrawal of affected feed has resulted in resolution of the signs. Animals with extensive lesions and chronic exposure have a poor prognosis.

Bites and Stings of Venomous Insects, Spiders, and Reptiles

Many species of snakes, spiders, and insects have venomous bites and stings. Except for snake bites, these animals lack sufficient quantity of venom to cause more than transient pain or local inflammation. Venoms contain a wide variety of substances, including enzymes, peptides, polypeptides, amines, and glycosides, which act locally by causing tissue necrosis, vascular thrombosis, and hemorrhage, or systemically by causing widespread hemolysis and neurotoxicity.

Snake Bite

Of the poisonous snakes in the United States, rattlesnake, water moccasin, and copperhead bites occur most commonly in horses.[118] The venom from these snakes is mainly hemotoxic and proteolytic and produces extreme local swelling with marked tissue and red blood cell destruction.

Most of the bites occur in the spring and summer. Horses are most commonly bitten on the nose, head, neck, and legs. Snake bites may or may not involve envenomation and may be either "dry" or "wet." Bites in which no venom is injected swell minimally and are only slightly painful (dry bite). When envenomation occurs (wet bite), rapid swelling, pain, and local hemorrhage develop, usually within 60 minutes of the bite. Fang marks are often very difficult to find because of the tissue swelling. Edema, erythema, and tissue necrosis develop over days and the skin may slough (Fig. 10–30). Bites occurring on the face or head are serious because of the risk of respiratory distress due to upper respiratory and nasal edema. If respiratory distress is severe, a tracheotomy may be needed.

Snake bites are treated symptomatically. The wound should be cleaned and hydrotherapy with cool water instituted to minimize swelling. If swelling is already present, warm hydrotherapy may stimulate circulation and removal of tissue edema. It is unknown, however, if this increases the absorption of venom in the early stages of a bite. Broad-spectrum systemic antibiotics are indicated to prevent secondary infection. The use of glucocorticoids is controversial but they may be beneficial in decreasing inflammation and pain. Nonsteroidal anti-inflammatory agents may also be beneficial. Surgical debridement and wound closure may be necessary if severe necrosis and sloughing occur. Although specific antivenoms are available, they are of limited use. Maximum benefit is attained only when they are administered within hours of the bite. Additionally, the volume of antivenom necessary to treat snake bites in horses is cost-prohibitive.

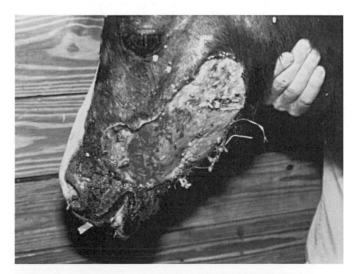

Figure 10–30. Face of a horse after being bitten by an Eastern diamondback rattlesnake.

Fire Ant Bites

Fire ants, *Solenopsis* species, are common in the southern United States. Single or small numbers of stings are acutely painful and rapidly develop into a pustule or crust. Horses tend to be bitten commonly on the legs, nose, and ventrum, but massive exposure can occur if the horse rolls on an anthill and is bitten by hundreds or thousands of ants. Complications of massive exposure include infection, anaphylactic shock, bronchospasms, and sloughing of the epidermis. Single or small numbers of solitary stings usually require little or no treatment. It is prudent to apply an antibiotic ointment to minimize the chance of myiasis, but otherwise wounds heal without complication. If massive exposure has occurred, systemic antibiotics, and nonsteroidal, anti-inflammatory drugs may be needed to decrease pain and swelling.

Spider Bites

Black, brown, and red widow spiders (*Latrodectus* species) and the brown recluse (*Loxosceles reclusa*) spider are common in America. In Australia, the black house spider (*Ixeuticus*) causes painful bites.[74] Spider bites are characterized by hot, edematous painful swellings in the area of the bite. The brown recluse spider has a dermal necrotoxin that can cause severe dermal necrosis, but this has not been reported in horses.

Treatment is symptomatic. Cold ice packs applied to the area and systemic glucocorticoids or antihistamines, or both, may be helpful. It is very important to spray the horse's environment with a parasiticide, for example, a premise spray formulated for flea control. Discarded furniture, newspapers, old cloths, and trash should be removed from the premises as these are favorite living areas for venomous spiders.

Vasculitis and Purpura Hemorrhagica

Vasculitis is a rare inflammatory reaction occurring in the wall of the blood vessel. Vasculitides are classified by inflammatory cell type. Neutrophilic vasculitides are further subdivided into leukocytoclastic (neutrophils undergoing karyorrhexis) or nonleukocytoclastic.

The immunologic mechanisms involved are believed to be type I and type III reactions.[46] Equine viral arteritis, equine influenza, *Corynebacterium pseudotuberculosis*, and *Streptococcus* species (especially *S. equi*) infections may result in a vasculitis.[32] Vasculitis also may result secondary to *Rhodococcus equi* pneumonia, bronchopneumonia, and cholangiohepatitis and some antimicrobial treatments. Often, however, the underlying cause is never identified.

Idiopathic vasculitis has no known breed, sex, or age predilection. The most common location for lesions is on the distal limbs, ears, lips, and periocular areas.[32] Oral ulcers and bullae may be present. Skin lesions consist of purpura, edema, and erythema (Fig. 10–31). Systemic signs may include pyrexia, depression, anorexia, weight loss, and lameness.

Purpura hemorrhagica is an acute noncontagious disease of horses characterized by extensive edema and hemorrhage

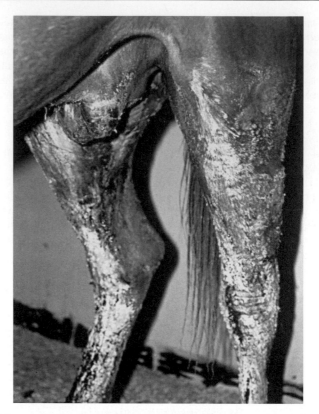

Figure 10–31. Horse with vasculitis secondary to strangles.

of the subcutaneous tissue. Hemorrhage in the mucosae and viscera are common. Most cases are secondary to strangles or equine influenza.[32, 119] Clinical signs usually develop within 2 to 4 weeks of the respiratory infection. Urticaria followed by pitting edema of the distal limbs, head, and ventral abdomen is common. Severe edema of the head may compromise breathing.[16] Tissue exudation and sloughing may occur. Pain and pruritus are rare. Affected horses are usually depressed, reluctant to move, and often anorectic.

Vasculitis is diagnosed by skin biopsy. It is important to obtain skin biopsy specimens from lesions 8 to 24 hours old because these lesions tend to have the most diagnostic changes. Lesions older than 24 hours may be nondiagnostic because of intense secondary cellular infiltrates or necrosis. Skin biopsy reveals neutrophilic, eosinophilic, lymphocytic, or mixed cellular infiltrates in the vessel wall.[51] Fibrinoid degeneration and hemorrhage are common.[51] Direct immunofluorescence testing is occasionally useful as an adjuvant diagnostic aid.

Success of treatment is unpredictable. It is important to identify and treat the underlying cause, if possible. Idiopathic vasculitis may respond to large doses of prednisone 1 mg/kg PO b.i.d. for 5 to 7 days followed by alternate-day therapy. Treatment should continue for several weeks after clinical cure. Equine purpura hemorrhagica requires early recognition and institution of therapy to enhance the prognosis. Horses may die from secondary bacterial infections or renal failure. Penicillin is the antimicrobial of choice. Because of the slight possibility that prior penicillin treatment may be the source (e.g., for streptococcal infections) of the vasculitis, extra care should be taken when first administering this agent. Penicillin K 22,000 IU/kg IV q.i.d. is administered in the early stages of severe disease. This is followed by penicillin G 22,000 IU/kg IM s.i.d. for at least 1 week post remission.[119] Prednisone 1 mg/kg PO or IM b.i.d. should be administered until remission is induced. In addition, hydrotherapy and exercise are beneficial.

Panniculitis and Fat Necrosis

Panniculitis refers to inflammation of the subcutaneous fat. This condition is rare in horses and results from widespread death of lipocytes. Fat cells are very vulnerable to trauma, ischemia, and neighboring inflammation. When lipocytes are damaged, lipid is released which undergoes hydrolysis into glycerol and fatty acids. Fatty acids are potent inflammatory agents that elicit further inflammatory reactions.

Panniculitis may be precipitated by a wide range of causes including trauma, infections, autoimmune diseases, pancreatic disease, glucocorticoid therapy, vasculitis, vitamin E deficiency, and, of course, idiopathic causes. In the horse, few cases have been reported and the causes of those were obscure. Vitamin E deficiency was suspected in a few cases.[72, 120]

Clinically, horses with panniculitis present with deep-seated nodules and plaques.[120] The lesions may be single or multiple and vary in size. Nodules may be very hard and well defined or soft and ill defined. Initially, lesions are not fixed to the overlying skin, but as the disease progresses nodules become cystic and rupture onto the skin surface. The ulcerating nodules drain a yellow to brown to bloody oily material. Pain is variable. Healed lesions may leave depressed scars. Affected animals may be febrile, depressed, lethargic, and anorectic.

Definitive diagnosis is made by skin biopsy. Tissue for histopathologic study must be collected by deep excisional biopsy using a scalpel blade. Skin biopsy punches will not obtain sufficiently deep samples to be diagnostic. Special stains (e.g., positive acid-Schiff, Gomori's methamine silver, Brown and Benn's) for etiologic agents should be requested. Skin biopsy reveals lobular to diffuse pyogranulomatous inflammation in the panniculus.

Underlying causes should be investigated and treated appropriately. Idiopathic panniculitis may respond well to prednisolone 1 to 2 mg/kg PO s.i.d. for 7 to 14 days[72, 120] or to a single treatment of dexamethasone 20 to 30 mg IM. Clinical improvement is usually seen within 7 to 14 days. Relapses may occur and lifelong therapy may be required.

DERMATOSES OF THE LOWER LIMB

Skin diseases of the lower limbs of horses are common dermatologic problems. These diseases may be extensions of generalized dermatoses or unique clinical syndromes.

Infectious Diseases of the Lower Limb
Bacterial Pastern Folliculitis

Bacterial folliculitis of the pastern is a rare disease of horses caused by *Staphylococcus aureus, Staphylococcus hyicus,* or a beta-hemolytic streptococcus.[74, 87] This disease is considered a primary pyoderma, but the mechanism by which these organisms initiate the disease is unknown.

Lesions are limited to the posterior aspect of the pastern and fetlock region. Single or multiple limbs may be involved. The initial lesion consists of papules and pustules that eventually coalesce and produce large areas of ulceration and suppuration. The disease is not associated with systemic signs.

Diagnosis is made by clinical signs, skin scraping, cytologic examination of the exudate, Gram's stain, and bacterial culture and sensitivity. Cytologic examination of pustule contents usually reveals large numbers of neutrophils engulfing bacteria.

Sedation may be necessary for the initial treatment, as these lesions are very painful.[74] The hair from affected areas should be clipped and the area washed daily in an antimicrobial scrub or shampoo, for example, chlorhexidine shampoo or scrub. An appropriate antimicrobial ointment without corticosteroids should be applied twice daily. Systemic antimicrobial therapy is not usually necessary.

Ulcerative Lymphangitis

Ulcerative lymphangitis is a bacterial infection of the cutaneous lymphatics of horses. The organisms most commonly isolated from affected horses are *Corynebacterium pseudotuberculosis,* and *Staphylococcus* and *Streptococcus* species, with *Pseudomonas aeurigonosa* and *Rhodococcus equi* being less commonly isolated.[121]

There is no age, breed, or sex predilection. Lameness is a common complaint. Lesions are most common on the hind legs, especially distal to the hock. These consist of hard to fluctuant nodules which abscess, ulcerate, and drain pus. Individual nodules may heal, but new lesions develop. Cording of the regional lymphatics is common. Edema and fibrosis are common. The regional lymph nodes are not usually involved.

Definitive diagnosis is made by direct smears, Gram's stain, and culture of a nodule. Skin biopsy reveals superficial and deep perivascular dermatitis that may be suppurative or pyogranulomatous. Special stains (Brown and Brenn's and Gram's) may reveal the organism.

If the disease is treated early, therapy may be effective and permanent disfigurement and debilitation prevented. The drug of choice pending culture and sensitivity is procaine penicillin 20,000 to 80,000 IU/kg IM b.i.d. for 30 days or longer. Adjunct hydrotherapy may be beneficial. Once fibrosis occurs, there is little chance for cure.[74, 121] The affected area should be cleaned daily with copious amounts of water and washed with an antimicrobial scrub, for example, chlorhexidine.

Viral Papillomatosis

Equine viral papillomatosis is caused by a DNA papovavirus.[111] Viral papillomatosis is common in horses and occurs most frequently in horses less than 3 years of age. There is no sex or breed predilection. Transmission appears to be by direct contact because groups of young horses are often more frequently affected than horses of the same age but housed individually. Lesions are most common on the muzzle, genitalia, and distal legs. They are usually multiple and resemble papillomatosis of other species.

Definitive diagnosis is by skin biopsy. Epithelial proliferation without connective tissue proliferation is typical.

These lesions are best treated by "watchful neglect" because spontaneous remission almost always occurs. Surgical removal should only be considered when the lesion interferes with function. Anecdotal reports that surgical removal or damage to part of the lesion will induce remission of the lesion are unproven.[73] In fact, controlled studies suggested that the duration of the lesions may be increased by such intervention.[73, 74] Finally, autogenous vaccines are unproven.

Sporotrichosis

Sporotrichosis is caused by the dimorphic fungus *Sporothrix schenckii* and was discussed in detail under Infectious Causes of Nodules.

One form of sporotrichosis is a cutaneous lymphatic form that may localize to the distal extremities of horses. The lymphatics become corded and large nodules ulcerate and drain a thick brown-red discharge. Regional lymph nodes are not involved. Edema production is rare. Diagnosis and treatment already have been discussed.

Parasitic Diseases of the Lower Limb

The common parasitic diseases of horses have been discussed previously (see Parasitic Skin Diseases). Lice, *Chorioptes,* and chiggers are the most common parasitic dermatoses that cause lower limb pruritus.

Neoplastic and Non-Neoplastic Proliferative Diseases of the Lower Limb
Keloids

A keloid is a non-neoplastic fibroblastic response that occurs on the pastern of horses. Clinically it resembles a cluster of grapes. This condition is not seen as commonly as it once was, now that "soring" practices are illegal. Definitive diagnosis is made by biopsy. These lesions do not respond to surgical excision and may, in fact, be exacerbated by surgery.[74] Keloids are treated best by the intralesional injection of triamcinolone acetonide (do not exceed 20 mg per horse). Unfortunately, most lesions are so massive that response to therapy is poor.

Hemangiomas

Hemangiomas are benign tumors of the endothelial cells of blood vessels. These lesions are most commonly seen in horses less than 1 year of age and some horses are born with them.[73] Hemangiomas tend to be solitary tumors occurring on the distal limbs. The clinical appearance varies and may be circumscribed, nodular, firm to fluctuant, blue to black in color, dermal or subcutaneous, hyperkeratotic, and verrucous. Ulceration and bleeding are common.

Diagnosis is by skin biopsy, which reveals proliferation of blood-filled vascular spaces lined by single layers of well-differentiated endothelial cells.[50, 73] Equine hemangiomas are characterized by a multinodular capillary hemangioma with hyperplasia and hyperkeratosis of the overlying epidermis.[51, 73]

Surgical excision is the treatment of choice. Equine verrucous hemangioma is difficult to excise and cryosurgery may be beneficial. Recurrence is common.

Autoimmune Diseases of the Lower Limbs
Pemphigus Foliaceus

Pemphigus foliaceus was discussed under Immunologic Causes of Exfoliation. It is important to remember that in some horses only the coronary band is affected.[38] The coronary band of all four limbs will be crumbly, degenerating, and exudative. Pain, lameness, and edema of the lower limb may occur.

Systemic Lupus Erythematosus

This is a multisystemic autoimmune disease that is extremely rare in horses. Profound lymphedema of the lower limbs may be the only clinical sign observed. The disease is treated with immunosuppressive doses of prednisone 2 mg/kg PO b.i.d. The prognosis is grave.

Vasculitis

Vasculitis was discussed earlier under Vasculitis and Purpura Hemorrhagica. In some horses, cutaneous vasculitis has been restricted to the white skin of the pasterns and face of horses in the summer.[38] The characteristic lesions are erythema, swelling, pain, and exudation and may resemble photodermatitis. This suggests a photo-induced etiology. Edema of the pastern and face is marked.

Pastern Dermatitis (Grease-Heel, Scratches)

Skin disease of the lower limbs is a common and frustrating problem in horses. "Pastern dermatitis", "scratches", "grease-heel", and "mud fever" are all colloquial terms for a moist exudative dermatitis of the caudal heel and pastern area. It is important to remember that these terms are nonspecific and only describe a variety of inflammatory skin conditions of the lower leg of horses.

The pathogenesis of the syndrome is not completely understood. The initial lesion may be due to a primary infection or may be due to a bacterial infection secondary to a predisposing cause, for example, pemphigus foliaceus, mites. Horses with long fetlock hair or horses kept in muddy paddocks, unsanitary conditions, or rough stubbly pasture are most at risk for developing pastern dermatitis. The problem also is common in horses worked on tracks consisting of grit particles, which can cause microtrauma to the skin.

The clinical signs depend greatly upon whether or not the condition is acute or chronic, and whether or not the owner has treated the lesions. Many horse owners often do not recognize the acute development of skin disease, thus minimizing the opportunity to identify the underlying cause. To

Table 10–7. Skin Diseases with Systemic Manifestations

Disease	Cutaneous Signs	Systemic Signs
Environmental		
Gangrene	Wet: moist swelling, discoloration, malodorous, tissue decomposition Dry: dry, discolored, leathery skin	Depends upon underlying cause, fever
Burns	Superficial: erythema, edema, pain, vesicles Deep: necrosis, ulceration, anesthesia, scarring	Shock, respiratory compromise
Selenosis	Painful coronary band, sloughing and necrosis of hoof, rough hair coat, progressive loss of long hairs of mane and tail	Lameness, weight loss
Arsenic poisoning	Severe seborrhea, ulcer, nonhealing wounds, hypertrichosis	Gastroenteritis, emaciation, variable appetite
Mercury poisoning	Progressive alopecia	Gastroenteritis, lameness, emaciation
Iodism	Severe dry seborrhea with or without hair loss	Cough, variable appetite, joint pain, seromucoid nasal discharge, lacrimation
Hepatogenous photosensitization	Erythema, edema, pruritus, pain, in white or light-skinned area; vesicles and bullae may progress to oozing, necrosis, and sloughing	Acute: hepatic encephalopathy, icterus, depression, decreased appetite Chronic: weight loss, depression neurologic signs
Ergotism	Swelling of coronary band, necrosis of feet, sloughing of ears, tail, feet	Lameness of hind legs, fever, weight loss, poor appetite
Leucaenosis	Hoof dystrophies, shedding of hair	Laminitis, lameness
Hairy vetch toxicosis	Cutaneous plaques and papules that ooze yellow pus; pruritus, hair loss	Conjunctivitis, anorexia, pyrexia, weight loss
Bacterial Diseases		
Strangles	Limb edema, edema of lips, eyelids; petechial hemorrhages of mucous membranes and sclera	History of acute contagious upper respiratory infection; pyrexia, mucopurulent nasal discharge, abscesses in the mandibular or retropharyngeal lymph nodes
Corynebacterium pseudotuberculosis abscesses	Single or multiple deep abscesses that develop slowly or rapidly; 50% occur in the pectoral or ventral abdominal area; ventral midline edema	Pitting edema, depression, fever, lameness, internal abscess, prolonged fever, abortion
Dermatophilosis	Exudative crusted lesions on dorsal trunk, face, pastern, or coronets	Depression, fever, lethargy, poor appetite, weight loss, fever, lymphadenopathy; lesions on legs may cause edema, pain, and lameness
Actinobacillosis	Thick-walled abscess of soft tissue	In newborn foals disease is a highly fatal septicemic disease and skin lesions are rare
Clostridial infections	Malignant edema—swelling at site of infection, pitting edema, local erythema; skin may become hot to touch, painful, or slough; crepitus Blackleg—hot, painful, swelling which progresses to a cold painful swelling with edema and subcutaneous emphysema	High fever, anorexia, muscle tremors, acute death possible within 24–48 hr
Glanders (farcy) *Pseudomonas mallei* (not in United States)	Subcutaneous nodules begin most commonly on medial aspect of hock; lesions rapidly ulcerate and drain a honey-colored material; lymphadenopathy and cording of lymphatitis is common	Respiratory infection that rapidly leads to death
Fungal Disease		
Histoplasmosa farciminosus (epizootic lymphangitis)	Unilateral nodules on face, head, neck and occasionally trunk; nodules initially are firm but rupture and exude light-green blood-tinged exudate; large ulcer may form and lesions may spread bilaterally	Lacrimation, conjunctivitis, and respiratory signs may occur
Parasites		
Lice	Pruritus, scaling, alopecia	Anemia in severe infestations with sucking lice
Black flies	Painful papules, and wheals which may become vesicular, hemorrhagic, and necrotic; lesion may be localized to ears or intermandibular areas	Toxin in bite can cause increased capillary permeability; depression, weakness, staggers, tachypnea, tachycardia, weak pulse, shock, and possible death

Table continued on following page

Table 10–7. Skin Diseases with Systemic Manifestations (Continued)

Disease	Cutaneous Signs	Systemic Signs
Immune-Mediated Diseases		
Atopy	Chronic pruritic urticaria, excoriations, alopecia, lichenification	Respiratory difficulty, especially on expiration
Pemphigus foliaceus	Crusts, scales, oozing, annular eruption, matting of the coat; lesions may be limited to coronary band	Depression, weight loss, poor appetite, pyrexia
Bullous pemphigoid	Vesicles and bullae in mouth, groin, and axilla; crusts, ulcers, and epidermal crusts	Anorexia, depression, fever
Systemic lupus erythematosus	Lymphedema, panniculitis, alopecia, leukoderma; scaling of face, neck, and trunk	Polyarthritis, thrombocytopenia, proteinuria, fever, depression, weight loss
Transfusion reactions and graft-versus-host disease (may occur in horse post unmatched blood transfusion)	Exfoliative to ulcerative dermatitis, ulcerative stomatitis	Diarrhea, increased heart and respiratory rates, lacrimation, muscle fasciculation
Erythema multiforme	Symmetric maculopapular lesions, urticaria that results in annular arciform or polycyle shapes; wheals do not disappear	Occurs secondary to pregnancy, drugs, neoplasia, connective tissue disease, infections, and idiopathic
Vasculitis	Purpura, edema, erythema, necrosis, crusts; purpura hemorrhagica causes edema, hemorrhagic swelling in tissue, mucosa, and viscera	May occur secondary to strangles or influenza; depression, fever, reluctance to move, colic, diarrhea
Equine exfoliative eosinophilic dermatitis and stomatitis	Scaling and crusting that progress to generalized exfoliation, alopecia, ulceration, and exudation; pruritus variable	Severe progressive weight loss; no diarrhea, ravenous appetite
Equine cutaneous amyloidosis	Papules, nodules, and plaque over the head and neck that develop rapidly	Diffuse nodules in upper respiratory tract may cause severe dyspnea
Endocrine Disease		
Hypothyroidism	Dull rough hair coat, delayed shedding of coat, edema of face and limb	Anecdotal reports of laminitis, infertility, anhidrosis, anemia, myopathy; weight gain and decreased food intake; skeletal limb disorders have been reported in foals
Hyperadrenocorticism	Long shaggy hair that fails to shed; mane and tail unaffected	Polydipsia, polyuria, muscle wasting, weight loss, lethargy, swayback appearance, pendulous abdomen, blindness, chronic infections, neurologic disorders or signs
Sweat Gland Disorders		
Anhidrosis	Acute episode—none	Acute—labored breathing, fever, flared nostrils, lack of sweating, collapse, death
	Chronic—dry hair coat, excessive scaling, partial alopecia, pruritus	Chronic—polydipsia, polyuria, poor appetite, loss of body condition
Miscellaneous Diseases		
Panniculitis	Firm to fluctuant nodules most commonly found on trunk in subcutaneous tissue that ruptures and drains an oily yellow-brown to bloody discharge	Anorexia, depression, lethargy, pyrexia
Neoplastic Diseases		
Hemangioma and hemangiosarcoma	Two types: (1) well-circumscribed nodules that are blue-black in appearance; (2) dark hyperkeratotic and verrucous lesions that bleed easily	Anemia
Lymphosarcoma	Single or multiple dermal-to-subcutaneous nodule, especially on trunk	Internal organ involvement, usually fatal

complicate matters further, many owners treat these lesions before seeking veterinary care. Many common over-the-counter medicaments can induce irritant or allergic reactions making it almost impossible to distinguish between these reactions and the original skin disease. Then it is critical to know what the owners have applied to the affected skin.

Regardless of the cause, the clinical signs are similar[74] (Fig. 10–32). Acute lesions usually begin at the heel. Pain, swelling, moist exudation, and hair loss are common. As the disease process continues, lesions spread proximally and anteriorly. Matting of the hair occurs and the horse is often noticeably lame. Crusting is common. If the underlying disease process involves a vasculitis, ulceration may be present. If left untreated, a foul odor develops. Because of the constant flexion in the area, fissures often develop. In draft horses, vegetative granulomatous growths commonly result. Lesions may occur on one or multiple limbs or just on extremities with white markings.

Definitive diagnosis requires a complete medical history. Liver function tests are mandatory in any horse in which the lesions are limited to the unpigmented areas of the skin. Dermatophilus preparations, fungal cultures, and skin scrapings should be performed in all cases. In horses with long hairs on the fetlocks, the hair should be thoroughly combed with a fine-toothed metal comb. This often is the only successful method for finding lice. In difficult cases, tissue should be submitted for bacterial and fungal culture.

Correct therapy requires identifying the underlying cause. Specific therapy for most of the diseases can be found elsewhere in this chapter or in the references. In all cases, the long hairs of the fetlock area should be clipped. The affected areas should be thoroughly washed in an antimicrobial scrub, for example, 2% chlorhexidine. Iodine preparations are best avoided as they can be irritating. All crusts and exudation should be removed, daily if necessary. In all cases, exposure to moisture and irritants should be avoided. It is critical to avoid the use of "home remedy" concoctions, which may be irritating. Cases of idiopathic grease-heal often respond very well to cleaning of the area, improved hygiene of the stall, and systemic corticosteroid therapy, assuming a bacterial cause is not present. Large doses of prednisolone 1 mg/kg PO s.i.d. may be needed to induce remission of clinical signs. It is important not to decrease the dose of glucocorticoids too rapidly or relapse may occur. If oral prednisolone does not induce remission, dexamethasone 0.2 mg/kg PO s.i.d. for 3 to 5 days may be effective.

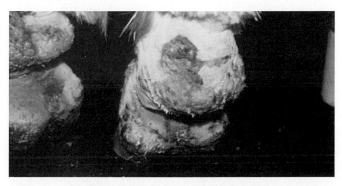

Figure 10–32. Pastern dermatitis.

SYSTEMIC DISEASES WITH CUTANEOUS MANIFESTATIONS

It is beyond the scope of this chapter to review all the skin diseases that may or do present with systemic clinical signs. An effort has been made to include the most common systemic findings in this chapter. Table 10–7 is a brief summary.

REFERENCES

1. Scott DW: *Large Animal Dermatology.* Philadelphia, WB Saunders, 1988, p 1.
2. Talukdar AH, et al.: Microscopic anatomy of the skin of the horse. *Am J Vet Res* 33:2365, 1972.
3. Sisson S, Grossman JD: *Anatomy of Domestic Animals.* Philadelphia, WB Saunders, 1975, p 728.
4. Ebling FJ: Comparative and evolutionary aspects of hair replacement. In Rook AJ, Walton GS, eds: *Comparative Physiology and Pathology of the Skin.* Oxford, Blackwell, 1965, p 507.
5. Irke P: Pruritus. In Ettinger SJ, ed: *Textbook of Veterinary Internal Medicine.* Philadelphia, WB Saunders, 1983, p 115.
6. Murray MD: Influence of skin temperature on populations of *Linognathus pedalis. Aust J Zool* 8:357, 1960.
7. Scott DW: *Large Animal Dermatology.* Philadelphia, WB Saunders, 1988, p 207.
8. Martineua GP: Pathophysiology of sarcoptic mange in swine—pt 1. *Compend Cont Educ Pract Vet* 9:F51, 1987.
9. Martineua GP: Pathophysiology of sarcoptic mange in swine—pt 2. *Compend Cont Educ Pract Vet* 9:F93, 1987.
10. Smythe R: In Hayes MH, ed: *Veterinary Notes for Horse Owners.* New York, ARCO, 1968, p 169.
11. Kunkle GA, Greiner EC: Dermatitis in horses and man caused by the straw itch mite. *Am J Vet Med Assoc* 181:467, 1982.
12. Roberts MC, Argenzio A: Amitraz induced large intestinal impaction in the horse. *Aust Vet J* 55:553, 1979.
13. Arlian LG, Runyan RA, Sorlie BS, et al.: Host seeking behavior of *Sarcoptes scabie. J Am Acad Dermatol* 11:594, 1987.
14. Arlian LG, Runyan RA, Archars J, et al.: Survival and infestivity of *Sarcoptes scabie var. canis and var. hominis. J Am Acad Dermatol* 11:210, 1984.
15. Dvorak HF: Cutaneous basophil hypersensitivity. *J Allergy Clin Immunol* 58:229, 1976.
16. Pascoe RR: The nature and treatment of skin conditions observed in horses in Queensland. *Aust Vet J* 49:35, 1979.
17. Ackerman LJ: *Practical Equine Dermatology.* Goleta, Calif, American Veterinary Publications, 1989, p 42.
18. Rabalasis FC, Votava CL: Cutaneous distribution of *Onchocerca cervicalis* in horses. *Am J Vet Res* 35:1369, 1974.
19. Foil L, Foil C: Parasitic skin diseases. *Vet Clin North Am Equine Pract* 5:529, 1983.
20. Stannard AA, Cello RM: Onchocera cervicalis infection in horses from the western United States. *Am J Vet Res* 36:1029, 1975.
21. Foil CS: Cutaneous onchocerciasis. In Robinson NE, ed: *Current Therapy in Equine Medicine,* vol 2. Philadelphia, WB Saunders, 1987, p 627.
22. Fadok VA, Mullowney PC: Dermatologic diseases of horses. Pt 1: Parasitic dermatoses of the horse. *Compend Cont Educ Pract Vet* 5:S615, 1983.
23. Lavach JD: *Large Animal Ophthalmology.* St Louis, Mosby–Year Book, 1989, p 257.
24. Anderson RR: The use of ivermectin in horses: Research and

clinical observations. *Compend Cont Educ Pract Vet* 6:S516, 1984.

25. Baker KP: The pathogenesis of insect hypersensitivity. *Vet Dermatol News* 8:11, 1983.
26. Baker KP, Quinn PJ: A report on the clinical aspects and histopathology of sweet itch. *Equine Vet J* 10:243, 1973.
27. Fadok VA: Culicoides hypersensitivity. In Robinson NE, ed: *Current Therapy in Equine Medicine,* vol 2. Philadelphia, WB Saunders, 1987, p 624.
28. Foil, L, Foil C: Control of ectoparasites. In Robinson NE, ed *Current Therapy in Equine Medicine,* vol 3. Philadelphia, WB Saunders, 1992, p 688.
29. Rosenkrantz W, Griffin C: Treatment of equine urticaria and pruritus with hyposensitization and antihistamines. In *Proceedings of the Annual Meeting of the American Academy of Veterinary Dermatology and the American College of Veterinary Dermatology,* New Orleans, Spring, 1986.
30. Barbet JL, Bevier D, Greiner EC. Specific immunotherapy in the treatment of *Culicoides* hypersensitive horses: A double-blind study. *Equine Vet J* 22:232, 1990.
31. Ackerman LJ: *Practical Equine Dermatology.* Goleta, Calif, American Veterinary, 1989, p 107.
32. Scott DW: *Large Animal Dermatology.* Philadelphia, WB Saunders, 1988, p 284.
33. Evans A: Recurrent urticaria due to inhaled allergens. In Robinson NE, ed: *Current Therapy in Equine Medicine,* vol 2. Philadelphia, WB Saunders, 1987, p 619.
34. Lloyd DH, Sellers KC: *Dermatophilosis Infection in Domestic Animals and Man.* New York, Academic Press, 1976.
35. Scott DW: *Large Animal Dermatology.* Philadelphia, WB Saunders, 1988, p 120.
36. Scott DW: *Large Animal Dermatology.* Philadelphia, WB Saunders, 1988, p 168.
37. Hay RJ: Fungal infection. In Mackie RM, ed: *Current Perspectives in Immunodermatology.* Edinburgh, Churchill Livingston, 1984 p 208.
38. Stannard A, Fadok VA: Equine dermatology. *Proc Mod Vet Pract Semin* 1984.
39. Barbet JL, Baxter GM, McMullan WC: Diseases of the Skin. In Colahan PT, Mayhew IG, Merritt AM, et al. eds: *Equine Medicine and Surgery.* Goleta, Calif, American Veterinary Publications, 1991, p 1569.
40. Buffington CAT: Nutrition and the skin. In *Proceedings of the 11th Annual Kal Kan Symposium,* the Ohio State University, Columbus, Ohio, 1987, p 11.
41. Scott DW: *Large Animal Dermatology.* Philadelphia, WB Saunders, 1988, p 358.
42. Fadok VA, Wild S: Suspected cutaneous iodism in a horse. *J Am Vet Med Assoc* 183:1104, 1983.
43. Halliwell REW, Gorman NTL *Veterinary Clinical Immunology.* Philadelphia, WB Saunders, 1989, p 285.
44. Scott DW, Walton DK, Slater MR: Immune-mediated dermatoses in domestic animals: Ten years after: Pt 2. *Compend Cont Educ Pract Vet* 9:S39, 1987.
45. Manning T, Sweeney C: Immune-mediated equine skin diseases. *Compendium Continuing Educ Pract Vet* 12:979, 1986.
46. Manning TO: Pemphigus foliaceus. In Robinson NE, ed: *Current Therapy In Equine Medicine.* Philadelphia, WB Saunders, 1983, p 541.
47. Scott DW: *Large Animal Dermatology.* Philadelphia, WB Saunders, 1988, p 65.
48. Irke PJ: Contact dermatitis. In Robinson NE, ed: *Current Therapy in Equine Medicine.* Philadelphia, WB Saunders, 1983, p 547.
49. Mullowney PC: Dermatologic diseases of horses. Pt 4. Environmental, congenital, and neoplastic diseases. *Compend Cont Educ Pract Med* 7:S22:1985.
50. Honigsman H, Wolff K, Fitzpatrick TB, et al.: Oral photochemotherapy with psoralens: Principles and practice. In Fitzpatrick TM, Eisen AZ, Wolff K, et al, eds: *Dermatology in General Medicine,* ed 3. New York, McGraw-Hill, 1987, p 1533.
51. Yager JA, Scott DW: The skin and appendages. In Jubb KV, Kennedy J, eds: *Pathology of Domestic Animals,* ed 3, vol 1. New York, Academic Press, 1985, p 407.
52. Scott DW: *Large Animal Dermatology.* Philadelphia, WB Saunders, 1988, p 411.
53. Ihrke PJ: Diseases of abnormal keratinization (seborrhea). In Robinson NE, ed: *Current Therapy in Equine Medicine.* Philadelphia, WB Saunders, 1983, p 546.
54. Wilkie JSN, Yager JA, Nation PN: Chronic eosinophilic dermatitis: A manifestation of a multisystemic, eosinophilic, epitheliotrophic disease in five horses. *Vet Pathol* 22:297, 1985.
55. Lindberg R: Clinical and pathophysiological features of granulomatous enteritis and eosinophilic granulomatosis in the horse. *Zentralbl Vet Med Assoc* 32:526, 1985.
56. Roberts MC: Chronic eosinophilic dermatitis. In Robinson NC, ed: *Current Therapy in Equine Medicine.* Philadelphia, WB Saunders, 1992, p 688.
57. Hillyer MH, Mair TS: Multisystemic eosinophilic epitheliotrophic disease in a horse: Attempted treatment with hydroxyurea and dexamethasone. *Vet Rec* 130:392, 1992.
58. Stannard AA: Generalized granulomatous disease. In Robinson NE, ed: *Current Therapy In Equine Medicine,* vol 2. Philadelphia, WB Saunders, 1987, p 645.
59. Kerdel FA, Moschella S: Sarcoidosis. An updated review. *J Am Acad Dermatol* 11:1, 1984.
60. Mullowney PC, Fadok VA: Dermatologic diseases of horses—Pt 2: Bacterial and viral skin diseases. *Compend Cont Educ Pract Vet* 6:S16, 1984.
61. Miers KC, Ley WB: *Corynebacterium pseudotuberculosis* infection in the horse: Study of 117 clinical cases and consideration of etiopathogenesis. *J Am Vet Med Assoc* 117:250, 1980.
62. Blackford J: Superficial and deep mycoses in horses. *Clin Vet North Am Large Anim Pract* 6:47, 1984.
63. Morris P: Sporotrichosis. In Robinson NE, ed: *Current Therapy in Equine Medicine.* Philadelphia, WB Saunders, 1983, p 555.
64. Mullowney PC, Fadok VA: Dermatologic diseases of horses—Pt 3: Fungal skin diseases. *Compend Cont Educ Pract Vet* 6:S324, 1984.
65. Scott DW: *Large Animal Dermatology.* Philadelphia, WB Saunders, 1988, p 168.
66. Miller RI, Campbell RSF: The comparative pathology of equine cutaneous phycomycosis. *Vet Pathol* 21:325, 1984.
67. Miller RI: Equine phycomycosis. *Compend Cont Educ Pract Vet* 5:S472, 1983.
68. Miller RI: Treatment of equine phycomycosis by immunotherapy and surgery. *Aust Vet J* 57:377, 1981.
69. Herd RP, Donham JC: Efficacy of ivermectin against cutaneous *Draschia* and *Habronema* infection (summer sores) in horses. *Am J Vet Res* 42:1953, 1981.
70. Scharff DK: Control of cattle grubs in horses. *Vet Med Small Anim Pract* 68:791, 1973.
71. Thomsett LR: Noninfectious skin diseases of horses. *Vet Clin North Am Large Anim Pract* 6:57, 1984.
72. Scott DW: Nodular skin disease in the horse. In Robinson NE, ed: *Current Therapy in Equine Medicine,* vol 2. Philadelphia, WB Saunders, 1987, p 634.
73. Scott DW: *Large Animal Dermatology.* Philadelphia, WB Saunders, 1988, p 419.
74. Barbet JL, Baxter GM, McMullan WC: Diseases of the skin. In Colahan PT, Mayhew IG, Merritt AM, et al, eds: *Equine Medicine and Surgery.* Goleta, Calif, American Veterinary Publications, 1991, p 1569.

75. Theilen GH, Madewell BR: *Veterinary Cancer Medicine.* Philadelphia, Lea & Febiger, 1987.

76. Barbet JL, Baxter GM, McMullan WC: Diseases of the skin. In Colahan PT, Mayhew IG, Merritt AM, et al, eds: *Equine Medicine and Surgery.* Goleta, Calif, American Veterinary Publications, 1991, p 1657.

77. Sullins KE: Equine sarcoid. *Equine Pract* 8:21, 1986.

78. Lazary S: Equine leukocyte antigens in sarcoid affected horses. *Equine Vet J* 17:283, 1985.

79. Otten N, Tscharner C von, Lazary S, et al.: DNA of bovine papillomavirus type 1 and 2 in equine sarcoids: PCR detection and direct sequencing. *Arch Virol* 132:121, 1993.

80. Barbet JL, Baxter GM, McMullan WC: Diseases of the skin. In Colahan PT, Mayhew IG, Merritt AM, et al, eds: *Equine Medicine and Surgery.* Goleta, Calif, American Veterinary Publications, 1991, p 1635.

81. Rebhun WC: Immunotherapy for sarcoids. In Robinson NE, ed: *Current Therapy in Equine Medicine,* vol 2. Philadelphia, WB Saunders, 1981, p 637.

82. Tuthill RE: Equine melanotic disease: A unique animal model for human dermal melanocytic disease (abstract). *Lab Invest* 46:85A, 1982.

83. Stannard AA, Pulley LT: Tumors of the skin and soft tissue. In Moulton JE, ed: *Tumors in Domestic Animals,* vol 2. Berkeley, University of California Press, 1978, p 16.

84. Goetz TE: Cimetidine for treatment of melanoma in three horses. *J Am Vet Med Assoc* 196:449, 1990.

85. Doran RE: Mastocytoma in a horse. *Equine Vet J* 18:500, 1986.

86. Prasse KW: Generalized mastocytosis in a foal resembling urticaria pigmentosa of man. *J Am Vet Med Assoc* 166:68, 1975.

87. Pascoe RR: *Equine Dermatoses: The Post Graduate Foundation in Veterinary Science.* Sydney, Australia, University of Sydney 1981, no. 22.

88. Neufeld TL: Lymphosarcoma in a mare and a review of cases at Ontario Veterinary College. *Can Vet J* 14:149, 1973.

89. Sheahan BJ: Histiolymphocytic lymphosarcoma in the subcutis of two horses. *Vet Pathol* 17:123, 1980.

90. Gallagher RD, Ziola B, Chelack BJ: Immunotherapy of equine cutaneous lymphosarcoma using low dose cyclophosphamide and autologous tumor cells infected with vaccinia virus. *Can Vet J* 34:371, 1993.

91. Pascoe RR, Summers RM: Clinical survey of tumors and tumor-like lesions in horses in southeast Queensland. *Equine Vet J* 13:235, 1981.

92. Wick MM, Hearing VJ, Rorsman J: Biochemistry of melanization. In Fitzpatrick TM, Eisen AZ, Wolff K, et al, eds: *Dermatology in General Medicine,* ed 3. New York, McGraw-Hill 1987, p 251.

93. Pulos WL, Hutt FB: Lethal dominant white horses. *J Hered* 60:59, 1969.

94. Schneider JE, Leipold HW: Recessive lethal white in two foals. *J Equine Med Surg* 2:479, 1978.

95. Mullowney PC: Dermatologic disease of horse. Part V: Allergic, immune-mediated, and miscellaneous skin disorders. *Compend Cont Educ Pract Vet* 7:S217, 1985.

96. Scott DW: *Large Animal Dermatology.* Philadelphia, WB Saunders, 1988, p 387.

97. Stannard AA: Hyperesthetic leukotrichia, In Robinson NE, ed: *Current Therapy in Equine Medicine,* vol 2. Philadelphia, WB Saunders, 1987, p 647.

98. Oehme, FW: Selenium. In Robinson NE, ed: *Current Therapy in Equine Medicine,* vol 2. Philadelphia, WB Saunders, 1987, p 670.

99. Oehme, FW: Arsenic. In Robinson NE, ed: *Current Therapy in Equine Medicine,* vol 2. Philadelphia, WB Saunders, 1987, p 668.

100. Schmitz DG: Toxic Nephropathies. In Robinson NE, ed: *Current Therapy in Equine Medicine,* vol 2. Philadelphia, WB Saunders, 1987, p 704.

101. Jones, RJ: Toxicity of *Leucaena leucocophala. Aust Vet J.* 54:387, 1978.

102. Scott DW: *Large Animal Dermatology.* Philadelphia, WB Saunders, 1988, p 334.

103. Scott DW: *Large Animal Dermatology.* Philadelphia, WB Saunders, 1988, p 374.

104. Beech J: Tumors of the pituitary gland (pars intermedia). In Robinson NE, ed: *Current Therapy in Equine Medicine,* vol 2. Philadelphia, WB Saunders, 1987, p 182.

105. Shauer JR, Fretz P, Doige CE, et al.: Skeletal manifestations of a suspected hypothyroidism in two foals. *J Equine Med Surg* 3:269, 1979.

106. Vivrette SL. Skeletal disease in a hypothyroid foal. *Cornell Vet* 74:373, 1984.

107. Chen DCL, Li OWI: Hypothyroidism. In Robinson NE, ed: *Current Therapy in Equine Medicine,* vol 2. Philadelphia, WB Saunders, 1987, p 188.

108. Bertolino AP, Freedberg IM: Hair, In Fitzpatrick TM, Eisen AZ, Wolff K, Freedberg IM, Austen KF, eds: *Dermatology in General Medicine* (ed. 3). New York: McGraw Hill Book Co., 1987, p 627.

109. Bowen JM. Veneral diseases of Stallions. In Robinson NE, ed: *Current Therapy in Equine Medicine II.* Philadelphia: WB Saunders, 1987, p 567.

110. Sorensen DK: Vesicular stomatitis. In Howard JC, ed: *Current Veterinary Therapy:* Food Animal Practice. Philadelphia: WB Saunders, 1981, p 576.

111. Gillespie JH, Timoney JF: *Hagen and Bruner's Infectious Diseases of Domestic Animals.* Ithaca: Cornell University Press, 1981, p 532.

112. Geiser DR, Walker RD: Management of large animal thermal injuries. *Compend Cont Ed Pract Vet* 7:S69, 1985.

113. Fubini SL: Burns. In Robinson NE, ed: *Current Therapy in Equine Medicine.* Philadelphia: WB Saunders, 1987, p 639.

114. Fox SML Management of a large thermal lesion in a horse. *Compend Cont Ed Pract Vet* 10:88, 1988.

115. Baxter GM: Management of burns. In Colahan PT, Mayhew IG, Merritt AM, Moore JN, eds: *Equine Medicine and Surgery,* (ed. 4). Goleta: American Veterinary Publications, Inc. 1991, p 1625.

116. Asch MJ: Systemic and pulmonary hemodynamic changes accompanying thermal injuries. *Ann Surg* 178:218, 1973.

117. Swaim SF: Topical wound medications: A review. *J Am Vet Med Assoc* 190:1588, 1988.

118. Oehme FW: Snake bite. In Robinson NE, ed: *Current Therapy in Equine Medicine II.* Philadelphia: WB Saunders, 1987, p 663.

119. Sonea IM: Strangles. In Robinson NE, ed: *Current Therapy in Equine Medicine II.* Philadelphia: WB Saunders, 1987, p 590.

120. Scott DW: *Large Animal Dermatology.* Philadelphia: WB Saunders, 1988, p 399.

121. Abu-Samra MT: Ulcerated lymphangitis in a horse. *Equine Vet J* 12:149, 1980.

Chapter 11

Diseases of the Hemolymphatic System

Debra Deem Morris, DVM, MS, Dip ACVIM

HEMATOLOGIC DISORDERS

Normal Hematopoiesis

In order to fully understand diseases affecting the cellular components of blood, a basic knowledge of normal blood production, or hematopoiesis, is necessary. During postnatal life, most hematopoiesis occurs in the bone marrow. Although all marrow is initially hematopoietically active, maturation is attended by hematopoiesis receding from the shafts of the long bones and the replacement of red marrow by resting yellow marrow. Active hematopoiesis continues throughout life in the epiphyses of long bones as well as in flat bones such as the skull, vertebrae, sternum, ribs, and pelvis. Transition from yellow to red marrow occurs in response to increasing demand for erythrocytes via the glycoprotein hormone erythropoietin.[1]

The bone marrow consists of the various differentiated blood cells and their recognizable precursors, undifferentiated progenitor cells, reticular cells and fibers, endothelial-lined sinusoids, and adipocytes. The hematopoietic cells are found in the intrasinusoidal spaces. All blood cells originate from a population of lymphoid-appearing cells, called pluripotent stem cells, that give rise to committed progenitors of the lymphoid and myeloid systems.[1] Pluripotent stem cells are capable of slow but definite self-renewal, whereas the committed progenitor cells disappear through differentiation and their numbers depend upon the influx from the stem cell pool. The first myeloid cell progenitor is a trilineage stem cell, also called spleen colony-forming unit (CFU), which gives rise to the committed progenitors for megakaryocytes and erythrocytes, phagocytic cells, and eosinophils (Fig. 11–1). Megakaryoblast stem cells and erythroid blast-forming units may arise from a common precursor, and the stem cells for granulocytes and monocytes arise from yet another. The erythroid blast-forming unit undergoes one more maturation process to the erythroid CFU (CFU-E), which is the immediate progenitor for the first morphologically recognizable erythroid cell, the rubriblast.[2]

A number of hormones regulate the amplification and differentiation of the hematopoietic progenitors. The colony-stimulating factors are polypeptide growth factors produced by endothelial cells, macrophages, fibroblasts, and T lymphocytes that stimulate the formation of neutrophils, eosinophils, basophils, and monocytes, and platelets from progenitor cells within the bone marrow.[3] Currently, four human colony-stimulating factors have been identified and charac-

terized as cloned gene products that have considerable overlap in their actions and wide-reaching effects on mature leukocytes as well as stem cells.[4] Granulocyte-macrophage colony-stimulating factor is produced by activated T cells, macrophages, fibroblasts, and endothelial cells,[5] then interacts with bone marrow progenitor cells to increase production of neutrophils, monocytes, eosinophils, and platelets.[6] Granulocyte colony-stimulating factor and macrophage colony-stimulating factor are produced by macrophages, fibroblasts, and endothelial cells and induce the maturation of neutrophils and monocytes, respectively.[7] Interleukin-3 (IL-3) is produced exclusively by T lymphocytes and stimulates production of neutrophils, monocytes, eosinophils, basophils, and platelets.[8] Molecules with similar action are likely present in horses.

The proliferation and differentiation of erythroid-committed stem cells appears to be under control of burst-promoting activity as well as erythropoietin.[2] Mononuclear phagocytes, certain T lymphocytes, and IL-1-stimulated endothelial cells and fibroblasts produce burst-promoting activity, which promotes the differentiation of spleen CFU to the erythroid stem cell as well as stimulating its proliferation.[9, 10] There is strong evidence that burst-promoting activity and IL-3 activities may be shared by a single molecule produced by IL-2-stimulated T cells.[11] Other T lymphocytes produce material (probably interferon-γ) that inhibits erythroid blast-forming unit development.[12] Factors with less well-characterized effects on erythropoiesis include hemin, leukotrienes, and prostaglandin E.[2]

Erythropoietin, the most important erythropoietic growth factor, is produced almost exclusively by the kidneys in adult mammals. Committed erythroid stem cells become progressively more sensitive to erythropoietin stimulation as they mature. The mitotic activity of the erythroid blast-forming unit can be stimulated by high concentrations of erythropoietin, whereas very low concentrations of erythropoietin will stimulate the proliferation of CFU-E. Erythropoietin is essential as a differentiation factor triggering the transformation of CFU-E into rubriblasts and shortens marrow transit time for erythrocyte precursors.[2] The production of erythropoietin is stimulated by tissue hypoxia. Low oxygen content of the blood can result from low partial pressure of blood oxygen (PO_2), anemia, methemoglobinemia, and increased hemoglobin affinity for oxygen.

Under homeostatic conditions, production of blood cells by the marrow proceeds at a rate that precisely approximates

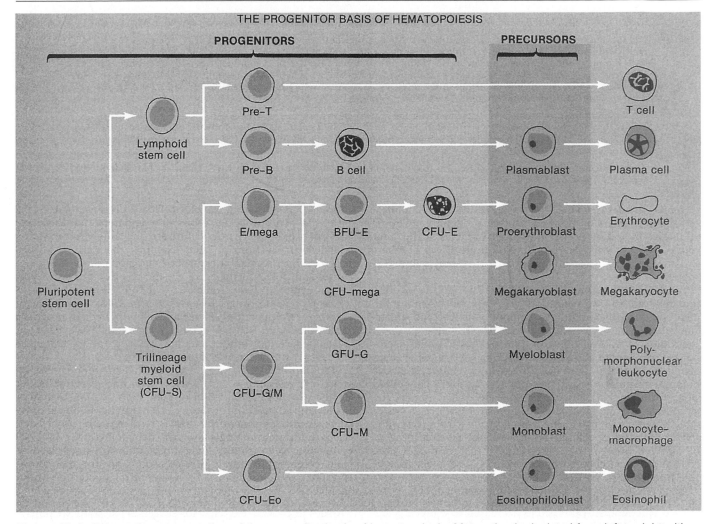

Figure 11–1. Schematic representation of the progenitor basis of hematopoiesis. Maturation is depicted from left to right with circulating blood cells as the final product on the far right of the drawing. Progressive amplification of progenitors and precursors as they mature and differentiate is not shown. *CFU-S*, colony-forming unit–spleen; *CFU-6M*, CFU–granulocyte macrophage; *CFU-eo*, CFU-eosinophil; *BFU-E*, burst-forming unit, erythroid; *CFU-mega*, CFU-megakaryocyte; *CFU-E*, CFU-erythrocyte. (From Nathan DG: Hematologic diseases. In Wyngaarden JB, Smith LH, eds: *Cecil Textbook of Medicine*, ed 18. Philadelphia, WB Saunders, 1988, p 875.)

the rate of destruction. The life spans of equine erythrocytes and platelets are approximately 155 days and 7 days, respectively.[13] Granulocytes have a half-life of disappearance from the peripheral blood of about 10½ hours.[14] Increased use or peripheral loss of one or more of the marrow-derived blood cells results in production amplification of the necessary component(s). Complete marrow failure causes clinical signs referable to the life span and turnover of peripheral blood cells. Initially, there is enhanced susceptibility to infection owing to the loss of granulocytes. Petechial hemorrhages and tendency to bleed secondary to thrombocytopenia follow, and finally pallor and signs of anemia occur.

Lymphocyte precursor maturation and differentiation are considerably more complex than that of the other hematopoietic cells.[1] Lymphoid precursors of B cells arise in the bone marrow, spleen, and lymph nodes where maturation and differentiation continue. The thymus influences the commitment of marrow-derived lymphoid progenitor cells to differentiate into subsets of T lymphocytes. They are then ex-

ported to the spleen, lymph nodes, and marrow to establish final residence and perform many of their functions. Circulating lymphocytes, most of which are T cells, represent only a small fraction of the total lymphocyte pool. Many of these cells are in transit to and from the secondary lymphoid organs where the majority of cellular interactions with antigenic challenge occur. In addition to lymph nodes, lymphoid accumulations occur in great abundance associated with the mucosal surfaces.[15] Throughout postnatal life, the spleen constitutes the largest single mass of lymphocytes in the body[16] and plays a major role in cellular and humoral immune defense. The spleen functions only briefly in hematopoiesis during fetal life, but retains this potential into adult life and actively produces erythrocytes, granulocytes, and megakaryocytes, when necessary.

The unique architecture of the spleen with its network of fixed phagocytic cells bestows the important function of filtering aged or damaged cells, particulate debris, and microorganisms from the blood. As erythrocytes slowly traverse the tortuous microcirculation of the spleen, they are subjected to adverse anatomical and metabolic conditions (e.g., hypoxia, low pH) that result in stress of senescent or damaged cells, and their retention within the red pulp and destruction by macrophages.[17] Hemoglobin is degraded and iron is stored within phagocytes until it is subsequently released into the plasma for reutilization during erythropoiesis. Splenic macrophages also perform a "pitting function" by removing inclusions such as Heinz bodies (denatured hemoglobin) or intraerythrocytic parasites from erythrocytes. Damaged leukocytes and platelets are also removed by the spleen.

Another splenic function that is extraordinarily important in horses is serving as a reservoir for erythrocytes. Owing to the large amount of epinephrine-responsive smooth muscle in the equine splenic capsule, the packed cell volume of horses can increase by as much as 40% during exercise or with excitement, and similarly, can decrease subsequent to sedation.[18, 19] Horses that are physically fit seem to exhibit a more profound change, and normalization of red blood cell values after a period of marked excitement or exhaustive exercise may require up to 1 hour. Thus, ascertaining the actual normal resting packed cell volume of horses may not be possible when they are apprehensive or excited. The spleen also serves as a reservoir of platelets that are in dynamic exchange with those circulating in the blood. At any time, up to one third of the total available platelets are retained in the spleen.[16] In rare instances, splenomegaly may cause mild thrombocytopenia due to the enlarged space for available platelets.

Anemia

Anemia is functionally defined as decreased oxygen-carrying capacity of the blood. The diagnosis of anemia is most accurately based on reduction of the packed cell volume below that considered normal for the horse's age, breed, and use (Tables 11–1 and 11–2). The total red blood cell count and hemoglobin concentration should also be reduced. The packed cell volume and other red blood cell values must always be interpreted in light of the patient's hydration status and the level of excitement.

Anemia accompanies a number of different disease processes in horses, and develops due to one of three basic pathophysiologic mechanisms: (1) blood loss; (2) increased erythrocyte destruction (hemolysis); and (3) decreased erythrocyte production, or any combination of these.[20, 21] In the first two situations, the bone marrow responds to the loss of red blood cells by increased erythropoiesis and the anemia is said to be regenerative. In the last instance, the bone marrow does not replace senescent erythrocytes at a normal rate and a nonregenerative anemia ensues. The classification of anemia by etiology and pathogenesis is more difficult in horses than in other species because reticulocytes are rarely released into the peripheral blood despite intense erythropoiesis.[2, 16] Therefore, the useful indications of regenerative anemia in other species, such as reticulocytosis, polychromasia, macrocytosis, and metarubricytosis, are not commonly observed in horses. A bone marrow examination is necessary to accurately characterize the anemia as regenerative or nonregenerative.[20]

History and Clinical Signs

History of any current or past illness, drug administration, deworming rate, vaccinations, diet, housing conditions, recent travel, and Coggins test status are all important in determining the cause of anemia. The clinical signs of anemia are due to reduced tissue oxygenation and are determined by its severity and rate of development. Signs are manifest at a higher red blood cell mass when anemia develops acutely. Anemia with a gradual onset allows physiologic compensation for the reduced oxygenation of body tissues. Reduced exercise tolerance, depression, weakness, tachycardia, tachypnea, and mucosal pallor are the more common signs of anemia in horses. A low-grade systolic murmur is sometimes auscultable when the packed cell volume drops below 15% to 18%. Other clinical signs may help determine the pathophysiologic mechanism and associated underlying disease process. Fever, icterus, or pigmenturia,

Table 11–1. Influence of Age on Normal Erythron Values (Mean ± 1SD) of Hot-Blooded Horses*†

	Age								
	1 day	2–7 days	8–14 days	21–30 days	1–3 mo	8–18 mo	2 yr	3–4 yr	≥5 yr
RBC (× 10⁶/μL)	10.5 ± 1.4	9.5 ± 0.8	9.0 ± 0.8	11.2 ± 1.3	11.9 ± 1.3	8.6 ± 0.6	9.9 ± 1.3	9.1 ± 1.2	8.6 ± 1.0
Hgb (g/dL)	14.2 ± 1.3	12.7 ± 0.9	11.8 ± 1.2	13.1 ± 1.1	13.4 ± 1.6	14.7 ± 1.6	14.7 ± 1.6	14.3 ± 1.4	14.4 ± 1.6
PCV (%)	41.7 ± 3.6	37.1 ± 3.7	34.9 ± 3.3	38.3 ± 4.1	34.5 ± 3.8	41.4 ± 4.2	40.8 ± 4.3	40.8 ± 4.3	40.8 ± 4.1
MCV (fL)	40.1 ± 3.8	39.2 ± 2.8	39.1 ± 2.2	34.0 ± 2.4	32.4 ± 1.9	40.1 ± 2.9	42.7 ± 2.8	44.8 ± 3.4	47.8 ± 4.0
MCH (pg)	13.6 ± 1.2	13.4 ± 1.0	13.1 ± 0.8	11.8 ± 0.8	11.2 ± 0.6	13.7 ± 1.3	14.9 ± 1.1	15.7 ± 1.2	16.8 ± 1.3
MCHC (%)	33.9 ± 1.6	34.2 ± 1.2	33.6 ± 0.9	34.5 ± 1.0	34.9 ± 1.2	34.1 ± 1.4	34.9 ± 1.3	35.2 ± 1.5	35.4 ± 1.4

*From Morris DD: Review of anemia in horses, pt 1: Clinical signs, laboratory findings and diagnosis. *Equine Pract* 11:27–34, 1989; adapted from Jain NC, ed: *Schalm's Veterinary Hematology*, ed 4. Philadelphia, Lea & Febiger, 1986.

†Abbreviations: RBC red blood cells; Hgb, hemoglobin; PCV, packed cell volume; MCV, mean corpuscular volume; MCH, mean corpuscular hemoglobin; MCHC, mean corpuscular hemoglobin concentration.

Table 11–2. Influence of Breed on Normal Erythron Values (Mean ± SD) in Adult Horses*†

Breed	RBC (× 10⁶/µL)	Hgb (g/dL)	PVC (%)	MCV (fL)	MCH (pg)	MCHC (%)
Thoroughbred	9.35 ± 1.05	14.8 ± 1.3	41.7 ± 3.8	44.7 ± 3.4	15.9 ± 1.4	35.8 ± 1.4
Standardbred	8.37 ± 1.02	13.6 ± 1.6	38.3 ± 3.5	46.1 ± 4.0	16.3 ± 1.4	35.5 ± 1.6
Quarter horse	8.26 ± 1.02	13.3 ± 1.6	38.0 ± 4.0	46.2 ± 3.9	16.1 ± 1.7	34.9 ± 1.6
Appaloosa	8.60 ± 1.11	13.3 ± 1.6	38.4 ± 4.7	44.8 ± 4.4	15.5 ± 1.3	34.5 ± 0.8
Arabian	8.41 ± 1.21	13.8 ± 2.1	39.3 ± 5.0	46.9 ± 1.9	16.4 ± 0.9	34.9 ± 1.0
Clydesdale	7.30 ± 0.87	12.4 ± 1.1	33.0 ± 3.0	44.6	—	38.1
Percheron	7.39 ± 1.08	11.7 ± 1.4	—	—	—	—
Mixed cold-blooded	7.76 ± 1.23		33.0 ± 7.0	42.3	—	—

*From Morris DD: Review of anemia in horses, pt 1: Clinical signs, laboratory findings and diagnosis. *Equine Pract* 11:27–34, 1989; adapted from Jain NC, ed: *Schalm's Veterinary Hematology*, ed 4. Philadelphia, Lea & Febiger, 1986.

†For abbreviations, see footnote, Table 11–1.

individually or together, often occur when there is ongoing hemolytic disease. Epistaxis, hematuria, or melena may signal a source of chronic blood loss. Anorexia, lethargy, and weight loss suggest an underlying chronic disease process.

Laboratory Evaluation

The laboratory assessment of anemia should initially include a complete blood count (CBC), total plasma protein (TPP), and plasma fibrinogen concentration.[20] The presence of clinical icterus warrants quantitation of total and direct serum bilirubin concentrations. Unique features of the equine erythron must be kept in mind during evaluation of the CBC. The erythrocyte reservoir function of the equine spleen precludes accurate assessment of a horse's packed cell volume after exercise or excitement and during disease states that produce endotoxemia.[22, 23] Since the packed cell volume of at least one blood sample must be less than 30% before an individual horse can be assessed as anemic, splenic contraction can mask the presence and severity of this abnormality. The response of the spleen to acute hemorrhage, with subsequently increased packed cell volume, and red blood cell and hemoglobin concentrations precludes estimation of the magnitude of blood loss for 12 to 24 hours.[24]

Small nuclear remnants called Howell-Jolly bodies may be found in a small number of erythrocytes in normal horses and are not indicative of increased erythropoiesis, as in other species.[25] Although mild anisocytosis and a modest increase in mean corpuscular volume (MCV) may occur during intensified erythropoiesis, characterization of an anemia as regenerative or nonregenerative in a horse is most accurately done by *bone marrow examination*.[20, 21] Aspirates for cytology are adequate to characterize marrow erythropoiesis and these are most easily obtained from the sternum using a 3½-in., 18-gauge disposable spinal needle. Thin smears should be prepared rapidly, air-dried, then stained with Wright's or another modified Romanowsky's stain. The normal myeloid-erythroid ratio (M/E), based on counting 500 cells, usually ranges from 0.5 to 1.5 in horses, thus an M/E ratio of less than 0.5 classifies an anemia as regenerative.

The small size of equine erythrocytes (5–6 µm) and their tendency to adhere to one another to form a "stack," like coins (rouleau), further complicate peripheral blood assessment. Marked rouleaux may be confused with autoagglutination, sometimes seen during immune-mediated hemolysis. This tendency for natural aggregation of equine erythrocytes leads to their rapid separation from plasma, necessitating thorough mixing of blood samples before erythron data are measured.

Finally, equine plasma is normally quite yellow compared with that of other animals, owing to the combined effects of blood carotenoids from green feed and the greater concentration of bilirubin.[16, 26] Fasting causes a marked increase in equine serum bilirubin concentration that peaks after 2 to 3 days and can result in clinical icterus in some horses with values of up to 8 mg/dL occasionally being measured.[27] This fasting hyperbilirubinemia is due to reduced hepatic uptake, conjugation, and secretion of bilirubin; thus the increase in bilirubin consists of the unconjugated form. There is no definitive explanation for fasting-induced unconjugated hyperbilirubinemia in horses, but a net decrease in competition for intracellular binding proteins (particularly ligandin) has been proposed.[27–29] This has to be taken into account when considering hemolytic disease, which also results in clinical icterus due to increased serum unconjugated bilirubin.

Red blood cell morphology should always be evaluated as a routine part of the equine CBC. Precipitates of oxidized hemoglobin (Heinz bodies), parasites, spherocytosis, and schistocytes may be seen, which would aid in defining the cause of anemia. Since peripheral erythrocytes are nearly always mature and iron deficiency states are extremely rare in horses, the red blood cell indices are not highly useful. Hemolysis, in vivo or in vitro, causes an increased mean corpuscular hemoglobin (MCH) due to the presence of free plasma hemoglobin.

The leukogram and plasma fibrinogen concentrations are used to detect chronic inflammatory disease which may be associated with the cause of anemia. The ability of adult horses to increase circulating neutrophils in response to disease is limited and chronic inflammation may be attended by a normal or only mildly elevated white blood cell (WBC) count. Alternatively, during an intense erythropoietic response to anemia, neutrophilia with a mild left shift may occur.[16] Hyperfibrinogenemia may be more indicative of the presence and severity of inflammatory disease than the WBC count in up to 50% of affected horses;[29] however, in these cases a normal WBC count is often attended by a left shift. Foals older than 7 days and up to 1 year of age seem to be exceptions, and often present with neutrophilic leukocytosis in inflammatory or infectious disease.

The TPP is useful as a guide to evaluation of hydration status, as well as a clue to the pathophysiologic cause of anemia. Reduced packed cell volume in the presence of increased TPP suggests that the horse may be hemoconcentrated and that the anemia is actually more severe than the packed cell volume indicates. Mild anemia may be masked by dehydration in addition to splenic contraction in horses. An increase in TPP sometimes occurs due to the hypergammaglobulinemia that accompanies chronic infection. Reduction of both the TPP and the packed cell volume is suggestive of chronic blood loss.

Generally, the history, thorough physical examination, and baseline laboratory data allow the clinician to categorize the anemia into one of the three broad pathophysiologic classifications—blood loss, hemolysis, or inadequate erythropoiesis. Additional laboratory tests can then be performed to specifically address the suspected cause of anemia. In complicated cases where there is more than one mechanism of anemia operative, a bone marrow examination is necessary to determine the presence or absence of erythroid regeneration. This may also have prognostic as well as diagnostic significance.

Treatment

Identification and elimination of the primary cause, provision of nursing care, ensuring adequate tissue perfusion, and minimizing stress are the hallmarks of therapy for anemia in horses. Blood transfusion should always be reserved for those instances in which oxygen delivery to the tissues is inadequate to support life.[31, 32] The proper procedures for transfusion are covered in the section on blood and plasma therapy (p. 591).

Blood Loss Anemia

Blood loss may be acute or chronic and occur externally or internally.[32] The clinical and laboratory findings are largely determined by these factors.

Acute blood loss generally follows trauma, surgery, or rupture of a major blood vessel. The most common causes of acute blood loss in horses include postcastration hemorrhage, rupture of a uterine artery post partum, or erosion of the carotid artery by guttural pouch mycosis. Acute massive hemorrhage induces hypovolemic shock characterized by tachycardia, tachypnea, hypothermia, pale and dry mucous membranes, prolonged capillary refill time, cold extremities, and muscle weakness. Signs of shock generally develop when blood volume is reduced by more than 30%.[16] Compensatory mechanisms are triggered immediately in an attempt to maintain circulating blood volume. Catecholamines induce vasoconstriction and increased cardiac output, while antidiuretic hormone causes water and sodium resorption into the bloodstream. Plasma volume is expanded by withdrawal of fluid from the interstitium, increased resorption of

water in the renal tubules, and absorption of fluid from the gastrointestinal tract. The intitial fall in capillary pressure due to blood loss followed by arteriolar constriction allows movement of protein-free fluid from the interstitial space to the capillaries. This first phase of plasma volume regulation begins as early as 30 minutes after blood loss and continues for up to 6 hours.[33] It was estimated that horses restore as much as 2 L of lost plasma volume before the end of an experimental bleeding period carried out over 2 hours.

Splenic contraction in response to massive hemorrhage injects a concentrated mass of stored erythrocytes into the circulation almost immediately, thereby masking the extent of the loss during the first several hours post hemorrhage. In the intact horse, fluid movement into the bloodstream to compensate for plasma loss is also overshadowed by the massive splenic injection of erythrocytes[24] which may be as great as 30% of the original blood volume.[20] The second phase of plasma volume expansion follows the central nervous system release of multiple hormones, including cortisol, that increase extracellular osmolality.[34] Intracellular fluid is drawn into the interstitium, increasing interstitial fluid volume and pressure, which is followed by return of interstitial albumin through lymphatics and a restoration of plasma volume. Fluid movement into the vascular system continues at a decreasing rate for up to 72 hours.[35] The first hematologic evidence of acute blood loss in a horse is decline in the TPP within 4 to 6 hours of the insult. A reduction in packed cell volume and other red blood cell parameters is usually not appreciated until 12 to 24 hours post hemorrhage when plasma volume has expanded to exceed the immediate compensatory effort of the spleen to increase circulating red blood cells.

Diagnosis of acute blood loss is based on clinical signs, evidence of recent hemorrhage, and, depending upon the interval since hemorrhage, anemia accompanied by hypoproteinemia. External blood loss from wounds or body openings is obvious, but hemothorax or hemoperitoneum must be documented by paracentesis. Platelet-free bloody fluid in a body cavity and cytologic evidence of erythrophagocytosis support the presence of internal hemorrhage rather than peripheral blood contamination.

Therapy of acute blood loss should be aimed at stopping the source of hemorrhage and maintaining circulatory blood volume. Pressure wraps and packing or ligatures may minimize external hemorrhage; however, it is rarely possible to control internal hemorrhage since the source is difficult to find and the patient is a poor risk for general anesthesia. The rapid intravenous administration of large volumes (40–80 mL/kg) of sodium-containing crystalloid solution is necessary to control hypovolemic shock. Colloids such as plasma, albumin, or dextran may be more beneficial but are usually cost-prohibitive in horses. Dogs with experimental hemorrhagic shock required at least four times higher volumes of crystalloids than colloids to maintain central hemodynamics at preshock levels.[36] The clinical response to fluid administration, evaluated concomitantly with ongoing losses, is used to gauge the necessary replacement volume. Preliminary data in horses suggest that small volumes of hypertonic saline (4–5 mL/kg 7.5% sodium chloride) may effectively reduce the pathophysiologic sequelae of experimental hemorrhagic shock.[37] Although positive results have been reported in other species, clinical studies are necessary to fully evaluate this therapy in horses.[38, 39]

Blood transfusion should be reserved for those instances in which the erythrocyte mass is insufficient to maintain adequate tissue oxygenation. The more rapidly an anemia develops, the higher the packed cell volume at which grave signs occur. The slow loss of blood provides time for plasma volume replacement, which maintains venous return, and for physiologic adaptations to occur, which prevent tissue hypoxia. A packed cell volume of less than 20% suggests that all erythrocyte reserves have been depleted. As long as the packed cell volume stabilizes at 12% or greater and the horse is not stressed, blood transfusion is usually unnecessary. Renal hypoxia causes erythropoietin production which subsequently causes marrow proliferation of erythrocyte progenitor cells, which begins to replenish erythrocytes within 4 to 6 days. Depending upon the severity of blood loss, the anemia generally resolves within 4 to 12 weeks.[13, 39, 40] Prerequisites for an optimal marrow response include adequate iron, protein, copper, cobalt, and B vitamins. The normal equine diet includes an excess of all necessary nutrients. The exception is a milk diet, which may contain insufficient iron. Iron-deficient states are extremely uncommon in horses and are generally associated with chronic blood loss.

Chronic blood loss of small quantities causes a slowly developing anemia because the bone marrow has a chance to regenerate erythrocytes as they are lost. Anemia develops only when the bone marrow's rate of erythropoiesis is exceeded by the rate of blood loss. Chronic external blood loss may be complicated by iron deficiency, which causes a maturation arrest within marrow erythroid precursors.[16] Gradually developing tissue hypoxia allows physiologic adaptation; thus clinical signs of anemia are generally masked until the packed cell volume drops below 15%. The gastrointestinal tract is the usual source of chronic hemorrhage in horses, although blood loss may occur from any external orifice or within body cavities.

Causes of gastrointestinal blood loss include parasitism (particularly large strongylosis); gastric or duodenal ulcers (usually in foals); nonsteroidal anti-inflammatory drug (NSAID) toxicosis; and neoplasia, particularly gastric squamous cell carcinoma.[32] The hemorrhage is usually occult and rarely results in frank melena. Because chemical tests for fecal occult blood are excessively sensitive but not highly specific, the diagnosis of chronic gastrointestinal hemorrhage should be supported by a high index of clinical suspicion and ruling out other sources of hemorrhage. Swallowed blood from the respiratory tract or bleeding induced by rectal examination may induce a positive test for fecal occult blood. Blood loss from the upper respiratory tract is usually identified by the presence of constant or intermittent epistaxis. Guttural pouch mycosis, ethmoidal hematoma, and fungal rhinitis are the more common causes of upper respiratory tract blood loss. Hemorrhage from the lower respiratory tract subsequent to severe pneumonia, lung abscesses, pulmonary neoplasia, or exercise may be manifested by epistaxis; however, pulmonary bleeding is often occult and only recognized by finding hemosiderin-laden macrophages on cytology of a tracheal aspirate or bronchial lavage specimen.

Chronic blood loss anemia due to urogenital lesions is rare but may be caused by hemorrhagic or erosive cystitis, urogenital neoplasia, or vascular anomalies. Grossly normal urine cannot exclude urinary blood loss since chronic microscopic hematuria can induce anemia. The presence of intact red blood cells in urine sediment differentiates hematuria from other causes of pigmenturia or positive urine occult blood.

Hemostatic dysfunction may result in chronic blood loss anemia. Severe coagulation factor deficiencies, such as warfarin toxicosis,[41] moldy sweet clover toxicosis,[43] hemophilia A,[44] and other heritable coagulopathies,[45–47] generally induce clinically recognizable hemorrhage into joints or other body cavities, or external bleeding following trauma or surgery. Anemia may be acute or chronic depending upon the inciting cause. Thrombocytopenia (e.g., immune-mediated thrombocytopenia) or more complex coagulation disorders, such as disseminated intravascular coagulation (DIC), are usually associated with mucosal petechial and ecchymotic hemorrhages, epistaxis, and occult blood loss from the bowel and urinary tract.[48] Anemia develops slowly unless there is trauma or surgery, which incites severe acute blood loss.

Therapy of chronic blood loss anemia is directed at identification and treatment of the primary disease process. Chronic external blood loss may lead to iron deficiency (discussed later), especially in foals, which have comparatively low body iron stores.[49]

Hemolytic Anemia

Hemolytic anemia ensues when the rate of erythrocyte destruction exceeds the bone marrow's erythropoietic capacity. Although intravascular hemolysis occurs in some disease processes, most causes of hemolytic anemia result in an accelerated rate of extravascular erythrocyte destruction and shortened intravascular life span. Members of this class of anemias would more accurately be termed "anemia associated with increased erythrocyte destruction."[40]

Clinical manifestations of hemolysis vary with the rate of erythrocyte destruction, the degree of anemia, and the underlying disease process. Icterus is characteristic of hemolytic anemia, although in some low-grade hemolytic processes the liver may be able to excrete bilirubin at a rate sufficient to avoid clinical icterus. Other causes of icterus must be ruled out and clear hematologic evidence of anemia should exist if icterus is caused by a hemolytic process. Acute intravascular hemolysis produces hemoglobinemia and hemoglobinuria, manifest as pink plasma and reddish-brown urine, respectively. Constant or intermittent fever due to underlying infections or active erythrocyte destruction is not uncommon.

There are numerous causes of hemolytic anemia (Table 11–3) and the mechanisms responsible for enhanced erythrocyte destruction vary widely. Hemolysis results in a regenerative anemia without reduction in TPP. Intensified erythropoiesis is often associated with a neutrophilia and regenerative left shift. Total and indirect bilirubin concentrations are generally elevated. Other laboratory findings are determined by the cause of the anemia (see Table 11–3). In addition to a CBC, TPP, and serum bilirubin determination, the diagnostic evaluation of suspected hemolytic anemia should include a thorough blood smear examination, urinalysis, Coombs' test, and Coggins test. The adequacy of regeneration can only be evaluated by bone marrow examination.

Table 11–3. Hemolytic Anemia in Horses

Causes	Diagnosis
Immune-mediated	
Neonatal isoerythrolysis	Hemolytic crossmatch
Equine infectious anemia	Coggins test
Autoimmune hemolytic anemia	Coombs test
Secondary immune-mediated anemia (drugs, infection, neoplasia)	History, signs, Coombs test
Incompatible blood transfusion	History, crossmatch
Oxidant-induced	
Phenothiazine toxicosis	History, Heinz bodies on blood smear
Onion toxicosis	History, odor, Heinz bodies on blood smear
Red maple leaf toxicosis	History, methemoglobinemia, Heinz bodies on blood smear
Parasitic	
Babesiosis (equine piroplasmosis)	Complement fixation test
Microangiopathic	
Disseminated intravascular coagulation	Thrombocytopenia, and prolonged prothrombin time or activated partial thromboplastin time
Acute hepatic failure?	Liver enzymes, biopsy

From Morris DD: Review of anemia in horses, pt 2: Pathophysiologic mechanisms, specific diseases and treatment. *Equine Pract* 11:34–46, 1989.

Treatment of hemolytic anemia is aimed at the primary disease process whenever possible. Acute, severe hemolysis that results in life-threatening tissue hypoxia warrants blood or packed cell transfusion; however, in cases of immune-mediated anemia, identification of compatible donors is exceedingly difficult.

Immune-Mediated Hemolytic Anemia

Hemolysis occurs when antibodies combine with antigens on the erythrocyte membrane. Erythrocytes coated with immunoglobulins or immune complexes are generally removed from circulation by tissue-fixed macrophages in the spleen, liver, and bone marrow (mononuclear phagocyte system, MPS). When sensitizing antibodies are IgM or complement-activating IgG, complement-mediated intravascular hemolysis occurs. Immune-mediated hemolysis may be a primary process, such as neonatal isoerythrolysis, transfusion reactions, or idiopathic autoimmune hemolytic anemia, wherein antibodies are directed against antigens on the erythrocyte membrane.[40] More commonly, however, immune-mediated erythrocyte destruction is a secondary problem in association with viral, bacterial, or protozoal infections; neoplasia, particularly lymphosarcoma; and exposure to certain drugs.[32]

Neonatal Isoerythrolysis

NI is a hemolytic syndrome in newborn foals caused by a blood group incompatibility between the foal and dam, and mediated by maternal antibodies against foal erythrocytes (alloantibodies) absorbed from the colostrum (see Chapter 1).[50–52] The disease most often affects foals of multiparous dams since sensitization usually occurs late in gestation or during the birth of a previous incompatible foal. A primiparous mare can produce a foal with NI if she has received a prior sensitizing blood transfusion or developed placental abnormalities in early gestation which allowed leakage of fetal red blood cells into her circulation.

Clinical Signs and Laboratory Findings. Foals with NI are born clinically normal, then become depressed, weak, and have a reduced suckle response within 12 to 72 hours of birth. The rapidity of onset and severity of disease are determined by the quantity and activity of absorbed alloantibodies. Affected foals have tachycardia, tachypnea, and dyspnea. The oral mucosa is initially pale, then becomes icteric in foals that survive 24 to 48 hours. Hemoglobinuria may rarely occur. Seizures due to cerebral hypoxia are a preterminal event.

The salient laboratory findings are anemia and hyperbilirubinemia. Most of the elevated bilirubin is unconjugated, although the absolute concentration of conjugated bilirubin generally is elevated well above normal (>0.4 mg/dL). Urine may be red to brown in color and positive for occult blood.

Etiology and Pathogenesis. There are several prerequisites for the natural development of NI. First, the foal must inherit from the sire and express an erythrocyte antigen (alloantigen) that is not possessed by the mare. Blood group incompatibility between the foal and dam is not particularly uncommon, but most blood group factors are not strongly antigenic under the conditions of exposure through previous parturition or placental leakage. Factor Aa of the A system and factor Qa of the Q system are, however, highly immunogenic and nearly all cases of NI are caused by antibodies to these alloantigens.[53–55] Mares that are negative for Aa or Qa, or both, are considered to be at risk for producing a foal with NI. This would involve approximately 19% and 17% of Thoroughbred and standardbred mares, respectively.[53] Second, and perhaps most important, the mare must become sensitized to the incompatible alloantigen and produce antibodies to it. The mechanism for this is not known in many instances, but is generally believed to result from transplacental hemorrhage during a previous pregnancy involving a foal with the same incompatible blood factor.[51, 52]

Sensitization via transplacental contamination with fetal erythrocytes earlier in the current pregnancy is possible, but an anamnestic response is generally necessary to induce a pathogenic quantity of alloantibodies.[50] Ten percent of Thoroughbred mares and 20% of standardbred mares have antibodies to the Ca blood group antigen without known exposure to erythrocytes.[53] It is postulated that some common environmental antigen may lead to production of anti-Ca antibodies.[56] Data suggest that these "natural" antibodies may suppress an immune response to other blood group antigens because mares negative for Aa and that have anti-Ca antibodies often do not produce antibodies to Aa of their foal's erythrocyte that also contain Ca antigen.[56] This antibody-mediated immunosuppression is thought to result from the destruction of fetal cells before the dam mounts an immune response to other cell surface antigens.[57] Natural alloantibodies have not been associated with NI in horses.

After the mare becomes sensitized to her foal's erythrocytes, alloantibodies are concentrated in the colostrum during the last month of gestation. Unlike the human neonate, which acquires alloantibodies in utero and thus is born with hemolytic disease, the foal is protected from these antibodies prior to birth by the complex epitheliochorial placentation of the mare. Thus the final criterion for foal development of NI is ingestion in the first 24 hours of life of colostrum-containing alloantibodies specific for foal alloantigens. Immunoglobulin-coated foal erythrocytes are prematurely removed from circulation by the MPS or lysed intravascularly via complement. The rapidity of development and severity of clinical signs are determined by the amount of alloantibodies that were absorbed and their innate activity. Alloantibodies against Aa are potent hemolysins and are generally associated with a more severe clinical syndrome than antibodies against Qa or other alloantigens.[50, 52] Highest alloantibody titers are likely to be produced by mares that were sensitized in a previous pregnancy, then subsequently reexposed to the same erythrocyte antigen during the last trimester of the current pregnancy. Prior sensitization of a mare by blood transfusion or other exposure to equine blood products may predispose to NI.[50]

Diagnosis. A tentative diagnosis of NI can be made in any foal that has lethargy, anemia, and icterus during the first 4 days of life. Blood loss anemia due to birth trauma is attended by pallor. Icterus due to sepsis or liver dysfunction would not be associated with anemia. The definitive diagnosis of NI must be based upon demonstration of alloantibodies in the dam's serum or colostrum that are directed against foal erythrocytes. The most reliable serodiagnostic test for NI is the hemolytic crossmatch using washed foal erythrocytes, mare serum, and an exogenous source of absorbed complement (usually from rabbits).[52, 58] Although this test is impractical in a practice setting, there are a number of qualified laboratories that routinely perform this diagnostic service (Table 11–4). The direct antiglobulin test (Coombs'[3] test) may demonstrate the presence of antibodies on foal

Table 11–4. Veterinary Hematology Laboratories That Perform Equine Hemolytic Crossmatch*

†Serology Laboratory
Department of Veterinary Reproduction
University of California
Davis, CA 95616

†Stormont Laboratory, Inc.
1237 East Beamer Street, Suite D
Woodland, CA 95695

†Shelterwood Equine Laboratory Inc.
Box 215
Carthage, TX 75633

Rood and Riddle Equine Hospital
2150 Georgetown Road
Lexington, KY 40511

Hagyard-Davidson-McGee Associates
848V Nandini Blvd.
Lexington, KY 40511

Equine Immunogenetics Laboratory
School of Veterinary Medicine
Louisiana State University
Baton Rouge, LA 70803

George D. Widener Hospital
New Bolton Center
University of Pennsylvania
382 West Street Road
Kennett Square, PA 19348

*Serum and acid-citrate-dextrose (ACD)–anticoagulated blood are required from donor and recipient.
†These laboratories also provide blood-typing services.

erythrocytes; however, there are many false-negatives. Routine saline agglutination crossmatch between mare serum and foal cells can be performed by most human or veterinary hematology laboratories. Because some equine alloantibodies act only as hemolysins, agglutination tests may be falsely negative. Most field screening tests of colostrum have not proved to be reliable enough for practical use.[54, 58]

Treatment. If NI is recognized when the foal is less than 24 hours old, the dam's milk must be withheld and the foal should be fed an alternative source of milk during the first day of life. This can be accomplished by muzzling the foal and feeding it via nasogastric tube. The minimum necessary amount of milk is 1% of body weight every 2 hours (e.g., a 50-kg foal should receive 500 mL or 1 pt of mare's milk or milk replacer every 2 hours). The mare's udder should be stripped regularly (at least every 4 hours) and the milk discarded. In most instances, clinical signs are not apparent until after the foal is 24 hours old when colostral antibodies have been depleted or the absorptive capacity of the foal's intestine for immunoglobulin has diminished. Withholding milk at this point is of minimal benefit.

Supportive care to ensure adequate warmth and hydration is paramount. The foals should not be stressed and exercise must be restricted. It is best to confine the mare and foal to a box stall. Intravenous fluids are indicated to promote and minimize the nephrotoxic effects of hemoglobin as well as to correct any fluid deficits and electrolyte and acid-base imbalances. Antimicrobials may be necessary to prevent secondary infections.

Foals should be carefully monitored for the necessity of blood transfusion, although transfusion should be used only as a lifesaving measure. When the packed cell volume drops below 12%, blood transfusion is warranted to prevent life-threatening cerebral hypoxia. Erythrocytes from the dam are perfect in terms of nonreactivity with the foal's blood; however, the fluid portion of the dam's blood has to be completely removed from the cells to prevent administration of additional harmful alloantibodies to the foal. Dam erythrocytes from blood collected in acid-citrate-dextrose solution can be pelleted by centrifugation or gravity, and then the plasma aseptically drawn off by suction apparatus or syringe and replaced by sterile isotonic (0.9%) saline. The cells are thoroughly mixed with the saline, then centrifugation or sedimentation is repeated, followed by aspiration and discarding of saline. This washing process should be performed at least three times. The packed erythrocytes can then be suspended in an equal volume of isotonic saline for administration. Erythrocyte washing by centrifugation is more desirable than gravity sedimentation because antibody removal is more complete and packed cell preparations can be prepared more quickly (each gravity sedimentation requires 1–2 hours). Packed red blood cells are advantageous in overcoming the problem of volume overload.

When equipment or conditions do not allow the safe utilization of dam erythrocytes, an alternative donor is necessary. Since the alloantibodies absorbed by the foal are generally directed against Aa or Qa, and the latter are highly prevalent among most breeds of horses, a compatible blood donor is very difficult to identify. The odds of finding a donor without Aa or Qa are higher in quarter horses, Morgans, and standardbreds than in Thoroughbreds and Arabians.[59] Previously blood-typed individuals negative for Aa and Qa and free of alloantibodies are optimal. Two to 4 L of blood or 1 to 2 L of packed erythrocytes should be given over a 2- to 4-hour period. These allogeneic cells have a very short life span and represent a large burden to the neonatal MPS which may cause increased susceptibility to infection. In addition, these cells sensitize the foal to future transfusion reactions. All potential harm must be measured against the benefit in each particular situation.

Client Education. The prognosis for NI in foals depends on the quantity and activity of absorbed antibodies and is indirectly proportional to the rate of onset of signs. Peracute cases may die before the problem is recognized, while foals with slowly progressive signs often live with appropriate supportive care.

Like most diseases, NI is much more effectively prevented than treated. Any mare that has produced a foal with NI should be suspect for the production of another affected foal; thus all subsequent foals should be provided with an alternative colostrum source and the dam's colostrum discarded unless she is bred to a stallion with known blood type compatibility. Mares negative for Aa and Qa alloantigens are most at risk of producing affected foals, thus they should be identified by blood-typing. Subsequently, breeding of these mares may be restricted to Aa- and Qa-negative

stallions, thus eliminating the possibility of producing an affected foal.[54] In breeds with a high prevalence of Aa or Qa alloantigens (e.g., Thoroughbreds, Arabians), a stallion negative for these and suitable on the basis of other criteria may be difficult to identify. It is often more reasonable to breed these "at-risk" mares as desired than to screen their serum in the last month of pregnancy for the presence of erythrocyte alloantibodies[53] (see Table 11–3). Mares with low or equivocal titers must be retested closer to the time of parturition. If alloantibodies are detected, the dam's colostrum should be withheld and their foals must then be provided with an alternative colostrum source. Maternal alloantibodies to Ca do not appear to mediate NI in foals and may actually be preventive by removing potentially sensitizing cells from the circulation;[56] therefore, foals from mares possessing anti-Ca antibodies should not be deprived of dam colostrum, even when Ca is present on their erythrocytes. Rarely, the antigens De, Ua, Pa, and Ab have been associated with NI in foals;[51] however, it is not practical to consider mares without these alloantigens to be at risk for NI.

Immune-Mediated Hemolytic Disease

IMHD is composed of autoimmune hemolytic anemia and secondary immune-mediated hemolytic anemia, which are frequently clinically indistinguishable.[60] Autoimmune hemolytic anemia generally arises as an idiopathic process wherein an individual's own erythrocytes are not recognized as "self" and antibodies are produced and directed against an alloantigen.[61] Secondary immune-mediated hemolytic anemia is associated with infections, drugs, or neoplasia that causes antibodies or complement components to bind to erythrocytes either specifically or nonspecifically. Extravascular destruction of erythrocytes in the MPS ensues and may also be accompanied by intravascular hemolysis. Prior sensitization by drugs or infection is not always easy to exclude; thus many cases of primary IMHD may actually be secondary to an underlying unidentified process.[40] The occurrence of this IMHD is uncommon, but affected individuals can be any age, sex, or breed.

Clinical Signs and Laboratory Findings. The clinical signs of IMHD are referable to reduced oxygenation of tissues and signs of any underlying disease. Affected horses have variable exercise intolerance, depression, weakness, or dyspnea, or any combination of these. Tachypnea and tachycardia are generally present at rest and worsen with exercise. Fever may be present depending upon the severity and rate of hemolysis as well as any concomitant disease. Mucous membranes and sclerae are usually moderately icteric, although chronic IMHD cannot be ruled out by the absence of icterus. Pigmenturia is uncommon.

In rare cases of IMHD, blood shows gross erythrocyte agglutination. This finding must be interpreted cautiously since severe inflammatory states can result in erythrocyte clumping, which may resemble autoagglutination. Immune-mediated erythrocyte aggregation persists when the anticoagulated blood is diluted 1:2 in isotonic saline, whereas false autoagglutination is easily dispersed.[62] Spherocytosis is rare owing to the small size of the equine erythrocyte.[20] In addition to anemia, there may be neutrophilic leukocytosis subsequent to general bone marrow regeneration. An increase in

MCH suggests the presence of intravascular hemolysis, which also causes pink plasma. Hyperbilirubinemia due to elevated indirect bilirubin is common. When pigmenturia is present, urine is occult blood–positive without microscopic hematuria. Cytologic examination of a bone marrow aspirate usually reveals an orderly regenerative erythron (M/E ratio <0.5).

Etiology and Pathogenesis. True autoimmunity results when beta-cell clones become abnormally reactive and fail to recognize self.[63] Dysfunction of suppressor T cells or increased activity of helper T cells may have a role. A weak antigenic determinant may escape T-cell suppression when placed in close association with a strong determinant such as a viral antigen. Thus, even true autoimmune hemolysis may occur secondarily.

Secondary IMHD is often caused by immune complexes that bind to erythrocyte membranes and mediate extravascular red blood cell destruction ("innocent bystander effect"). In other situations the erythrocyte membrane is altered by the primary disease process, and then elicits an abnormal immune response because it is no longer recognized as self. Finally, stimulation of the immune system by another antigen may result in the production of antibodies with cross-reactivity to the patient's normal erythrocytes. Partial phagocytosis of immunoglobulin-coated cells in the MPS may result in spherocyte formation. Secondary IMHD in horses has been described in association with equine infectious anemia (EIA),[64] *Clostridium perfringens* infection,[65] injection site abscesses,[66] lymphosarcoma,[66–68] other internal neoplasias,[66] protein-losing enteropathy,[69] purpura hemorrhagica,[67] and penicillin therapy.[70]

Diagnosis. Definitive diagnosis of IMHD is based upon demonstration of patient antibodies that react with their erythrocytes. If true autoagglutination is not evident, diagnosis is most accurately made with the direct antiglobulin (Coombs') test, performed by incubating washed patient erythrocytes with antiserum to equine IgG, IgM and complement components.[62] Positive results are indicated by gross or microscopic agglutination. The Coombs' test reliably detects erythrocyte membrane-bound immunoglobulin or complement provided a purified antiserum is used in appropriate dilutions with controls. Since the test endpoint is agglutination, autoagglutinated blood cannot be evaluated. The latter is evidence enough of IMHD, provided false agglutination is excluded. A false-negative Coombs' test may occur immediately following a hemolytic crisis, when corticosteroid therapy has been initiated, or when the Coombs' antiserum is inappropriately diluted. The Coombs' test may be positive in the absence of IMHD if a disease process results in immunoglobulin or complement coating of erythrocytes; therefore, the diagnosis of IMHD must be made by combining clinical and laboratory evidence of hemolytic anemia along with autoagglutination or a positive Coombs' test.

The indirect antiglobulin (indirect Coombs') test is used in humans to detect the presence of circulating nonagglutinating autoantibodies through utilization of normal erythrocytes of the same blood group.[62] Because the most active antibodies are already bound to the patient's erythrocytes and there are numerous equine blood groups, the indirect

Coombs' test yields many false-negatives and has not been widely adopted for veterinary use.

The osmotic fragility test is a screening test for IMHD since erythrocytes bound by antibody are less resistent to osmotic stress and will lyse more easily than normal erythrocytes when subjected to various concentrations of saline solution.[20] Often two populations of cells are evident in IMHD: (1) the osmotically less resistant cells that are bound by immunoglobulin and (2) a population of erythrocytes that are more resistant to hypotonic lysis, comprising younger erythrocytes that have been released in the regenerative response to hemolysis. Advantages of this test include ease of performance and lack of necessity for specialized reagents; however, positive results are not specific for IMHD and may occur in other diseases that compromise erythrocyte membrane function (e.g., oxidative insult).

Horses with IMHD should have a thorough diagnostic workup in search of neoplasia because of the common association between these two disease processes. Also, the Coggins test for EIA should not be overlooked.

Treatment. Any current medication should be immediately discontinued in an attempt to exclude the possibility of drug-associated IMHD. Antimicrobials used for confirmed sepsis should be replaced by the most chemically dissimilar substitute (e.g., penicillin should be replaced by erythromycin or perhaps trimethoprim rather than ampicillin).

After samples have been drawn for diagnostic testing, horses with rapidly developing or severe anemia due to IMHD often require corticosteroid therapy. Since corticosteroids may worsen a primary infectious process and cause recrudescence of viremia in horses with chronic EIA, the Coggins test should be negative prior to their use. Although the beneficial actions of corticosteroids in IMHD are not entirely known, they will reduce erythrocyte clearance by the MPS and impair autoantibody production.[71, 72] Dexamethasone 0.05 to 0.2 mg/kg IV or IM once-daily seems to be more effective than prednisolone in therapy of equine IMHD.[60] The packed cell volume should be carefully monitored, and the dose rate of dexamethasone increased to twice-daily if the packed cell volume does not stabilize within 24 to 48 hours. The full effect of corticosteroid therapy often requires 4 to 7 days and blood transfusion may be necessary if life-threatening anemia develops in the interim.

Once the packed cell volume stabilizes at a concentration of 20% or greater, the dose of dexamethasone can be decreased by 10% every 24 to 48 hours while carefully monitoring for a relapse. When the dose of necessary dexamethasone is 20 mg/day or less, therapy can usually safely be given orally. Dexamethasone can be discontinued when the packed cell volume remains stable during therapy with 0.01 mg/kg every 24 to 48 hours. At any point during therapy, prednisolone or prednisone can be used in place of dexamethasone at a dose approximately seven times greater given every 12 hours (e.g., the immunosuppression provided by 20 mg dexamethasone every 24 hours would be approximated by 135 mg prednisone every 12 hours). Corticosteroids should be tapered as soon as possible to the lowest necessary dose and given on alternate days for 1 week before discontinuation; however, some cases of IMHD require treatment for several weeks.

Client Education. Horses believed to have idiopathic IMHD requiring constant corticosteroid therapy are often found to have incurable underlying disease (e.g., lymphosarcoma). The prognosis for horses with secondary IMHD depends upon that of the underlying disease process.

Equine Infectious Anemia

This is a multisystemic retroviral disease of Equidae, characterized by hemolytic anemia that is immune-mediated.[64] All ages and breeds of horses are affected, but the disease is most prevalent in the southeastern United States.[73] Because of its importance, EIA is briefly considered separately from other causes of equine IMHD.

Clinical Signs and Laboratory Findings. The clinical manifestations of EIA depend upon the dose and virulence of the virus, host resistance, and concomitant stress factors. Three forms of clinical disease have been described: (1) acute, (2) subacute to chronic, and (3) chronic inapparent.[64, 74] Clinical signs of acute EIA seen within 7 to 30 days after first exposure to the virus include fever, depression, anorexia, and mucosal petechial hemorrhages. Anemia is not seen at this stage.[64] The more classic clinical signs of EIA occur in horses that have been infected greater than 30 days and these include weight loss, anemia, icterus, edema of the limbs and ventral abdomen, and intermittent fever spikes. Less common clinical signs are colic, ataxia, abortion, and infertility, which result from viral-induced inflammatory changes in all body systems.[64, 75, 76] Any deaths usually occur during this subacute to chronic form of the disease. Most horses recover, but periodic flare-ups of clinical disease at unpredictable time intervals may occur, most frequently within the first year of infection. Severe environmental or managemental stresses and treatment with corticosteroids are known to induce recrudescence of EIA.[77] A large number of horses infected with the EIA virus do not show clinical illness. Although these animals remain virus carriers, are seropositive, and are a potential source of infection to other horses, many would go undetected unless subjected to serologic testing.

During acute EIA, thrombocytopenia is the first and most consistent laboratory finding.[78] Leukopenia is often present with mild lymphocytosis and monocytosis. During the subacute to chronic stages of disease, the packed cell volume, red blood cell count, and hemoglobin are reduced and there are other laboratory indications of hemolysis. The Coombs' test is often positive during periods of active hemolysis. Hypergammaglobulinemia, increased liver enzymes, and proteinuria may develop. Chronic inapparent carriers are hematologically normal, as are chronically infected horses between clinical flare-ups.

Etiology and Pathogenesis. The virus that causes equine infectious anemia is a nononcogenic member of the retrovirus family in the genus *Lentivirus*.[79] This high-molecular weight RNA virus is enveloped and possesses an RNA-directed DNA polymerase that allows incorporation within the genome of host macrophages throughout the body. In infected horses, viremia is maintained persistently throughout life, despite a detectable immune response.

Infection by the EIA virus usually occurs by transmission of blood between infected and uninfected horses, although other body secretions may contain virus and could serve as a source of infection.[76] Natural transmission of the virus generally occurs through the interrupted feeding of hematophagous arthropods; horseflies (*Tabanus* species) and deer flies (*Chrysops* species) are most incriminated.[64, 80, 81] Horses that are febrile and show other clinical signs of EIA have a higher titer of viremia and are much more likely to serve as a source of disease transmission than are inapparent carriers.[80] The virus titer of infected horses is greatly reduced between clinical episodes, at which time their propensity for disease transmission is reduced. The EIA virus can cross the placenta and in utero transmission has been reported.[82]

Once the virus gains access to the blood, it multiplies in macrophages throughout the body, elaborating viral proteins that stimulate strong humoral and cell-mediated immunologic responses. Acute disease is thought to be associated with massive virus replication in, and destruction of, infected macrophages.[64] Most horses develop a detectable serologic response within 16 to 42 days[64] from infection with the EIA virus. This response persists indefinitely owing to the continual virus production, resulting in lymphoreticular hyperplasia and hypergammaglobulinemia in chronically infected horses.[83]

The clinical signs of subacute-chronic EIA result from viral-induced immunologically mediated damage to a variety of body tissues.[83] The IMHD during EIA is likely secondary to immune complex attachment to erythrocytes via the viral hemagglutinin.[84, 85] There also appears to be decreased bone marrow erythrocyte production.[86] The periodic flare-ups of disease in some horses may be due to antigenic drift in the EIA virus and stimulation of a new wave of immunologic responses.

Diagnosis. The easiest and most sensitive and specific assay for the diagnosis of EIA is the Coggins test, an agar gel immunodiffusion procedure for the detection of serum antibodies directed against the EIA virus.[64, 73, 78] As with any serologic procedure, the Coggins test may be falsely negative during acute EIA prior to the production of measurable antibodies, and false-positives occur in foals that have absorbed colostrum from infected dams. Both drawbacks can be overcome by repeated testing: most infected horses have a measurable antibody titer by 45 days (usually after 10–14 days) and foals' maternally derived antibodies are gone by 6 months of age. The accuracy of the Coggins test is due to the fact that horses are persistently infected with the EIA virus and the constant antigenic stimulation maintains antibody production. Other serologic tests and fluorescent antibody for EIA virus are more sensitive but less specific than the Coggins test.[64]

Treatment. No treatment eliminates EIA virus from the body. Supportive care such as rest, fluid therapy, and blood transfusion may aid clinical recovery; however, the horse is always subject to clinical episodes of EIA and remains a source of infection to other horses.

Client Education. The prognosis of EIA is currently hopeless. Even horses that never show signs of EIA have pathologic lesions,[76, 80] and thus their athletic capacity and overall performance may be reduced. Because of their potential to infect other horses, it is my opinion that any horse with a positive Coggins test should be humanely destroyed, unless it can be strictly separated from all other Equidae. Although the chance of virus transmission by these horses is low,[80, 87] horses with chronic inapparent EIA can effectively transmit the disease under natural conditions,[88] even when the suggested 200-yd quarantine is enforced.[81] Also, a horse with inapparent EIA may eventually develop the subacute form.[76] Before introducing new horses to a herd, they should be tested seronegative for EIA twice, separated by 30 days.

Oxidant-Induced Hemolytic Anemia

Exposure to a variety of oxidizing agents causes oxidative denaturation of hemoglobin through disulfide bond formation between sulfhydryl groups. This oxidized hemoglobin subsequently precipitates onto erythrocyte membranes as small aggregates termed *Heinz bodies*. Erythrocytes containing Heinz bodies are less deformable, more prone to osmotic lysis, and readily removed by the MPS.[89] Certain types of oxidants also result in methemoglobin formation wherein iron in hemoglobin is transformed from the ferrous (Fe^{2+}) to the ferric (Fe^{3+}) state, which does not accommodate oxygen transport. The causes of Heinz body hemolytic anemia in horses are discussed here because of their marked clinical similarities. There is generally a history of relevant exposure and any type of horse may be affected. The administration of phenothiazine and the ingestion of onions, wilted red maple leaves, or agents rich in indole have been associated with Heinz body hemolytic anemia in horses.

Clinical Signs and Laboratory Findings. Typical clinical signs of depression, weakness, anorexia, tachycardia, and tachypnea are present. Sometimes the first manifestation is pigmenturia due to the presence of hemoglobin. Affected horses are not usually febrile and mucous membranes are generally icteric. Horses with red maple leaf toxicosis often have a brownish discoloration of membranes due to the presence of concomitant methemoglobinemia.[90, 91]

In addition to the reduced packed cell volume and red blood cell count, hematologic study often shows an increase in MCH due to hemoglobinemia. Heinz bodies may be obvious on routinely stained peripheral blood smears as pale areas within, or bleblike projections from, erythrocyte membranes; however, they are best visualized with new methylene blue stain of a wet-mount preparation of blood. Urine is usually positive for blood and protein, and plasma creatinine is often elevated subsequent to hemoglobinuric nephrosis.[91, 92] As with all cases of hemolysis, there is indirect hyperbilirubinemia. Horses with red maple leaf toxicosis may have methemoglobinemia causing a marked brownish color of the blood and urine and elevated hepatic enzymes.

Etiology and Pathogenesis. Horses given larger than recommended doses of *phenothiazine* may develop Heinz body hemolytic anemia due to the oxidant metabolite phenothiazine disulfide.[32, 93] Some horses appear to have an idiosyncratic sensitivity. Hemolysis ensues within 1 week of phenothiazine exposure. Phenothiazine toxicosis is very uncommon owing to the low rate of current phenothiazine

usage in horses; however, cases still occur in horses with access to ruminant supplements or salt blocks that contain phenothiazine.

Consumption of wild or domestic *onions* can cause Heinz body hemolytic anemia in horses,[94] but more commonly in cattle, sheep, and dogs.[95] Allyl propyl disulfide (closely related to di-n-propyl disulfide) is considered the constituent of onion oil responsible for oxidative erythrocyte damage. The amount of onions required to produce toxicosis is unlikely to be voluntarily ingested by horses, and would result in a distinct onion odor of breath, urine, and feces.

The most common cause of Heinz body hemolytic anemia in horses is *red maple leaf toxicosis*.[90–92] Horses and ponies grazing areas inhabited by red maple trees *(Acer rubrum)* during the summer and fall in the eastern United States are affected. Although the erythrotoxic oxidant has not been definitively isolated, this syndrome can be reproduced by administration of dried red maple leaves.[90, 96] The viable vegetation appears not to produce the syndrome. Many affected horses develop a marked methemoglobinemia that results in chocolate-brown blood, brown urine, and a brownish discoloration of the mucous membranes, in addition to other signs of acute hemolytic anemia.

Hemoglobin is normally oxidized at a slow rate by the oxygen it carries, but this process is reversed by an intracellular reducing system composed of metabolically generated NADPH and glutathione.[16] The ingestion of exogenous oxidant can overwhelm this natural protective mechanism. There seems to be a variation among species in the intraerythrocytic reductive capacity and this potential is relatively poor in horses.[89] It is not entirely clear why some oxidative insults produce primarily methemoglobin, some cause Heinz body hemolytic anemia, and others result in both methemoglobinemia and Heinz body hemolytic anemia. When both oxidative insults are manifest, the clinical disease is much more severe because both are additive in terms of reduced oxygenation of the tissues. Neurologic signs due to central nervous system hypoxia and death are common in horses with red maple leaf toxicosis.[91, 92]

Acute renal failure is associated with hemoglobinuria, although the exact mechanism is unknown. Tubular obstruction by pigment precipitation, direct toxic injury to renal tubular epithelial cells causing altered glomerular permeability, increased filtrate reabsorption, and reflex afferent arteriolar vasoconstriction have all been proposed and may work in concert.[97, 98] Hemodynamic renal ischemia is known to result from pigmenturia, and renal failure rapidly ensues. In cases of mild to moderate hemolysis, the associated renal failure is often the limiting factor to recovery.

Diagnosis. The diagnosis of Heinz body hemolytic anemia is based upon an appropriate history of exposure to an erythrotoxic oxidant, typical clinical signs, and the presence of Heinz bodies in the peripheral blood. Since Heinz bodies may be difficult to identify on a routine Romanowsky's-stained blood smear, new methylene blue or another vital stain (e.g., crystal violet) should be used to evaluate a wet-mount blood film. One drop of new methylene blue can be mixed with one drop of blood on a glass slide, and the blood evaluated under a microscope after applying a coverslip. Heinz bodies appear as bluish-green, oval-to-serrated refractile granules located near the red blood cell margin or protruding from the cell. An attempt should always be made to rule out other causes of hemolytic anemia. The Coggins and Coombs' tests are negative in Heinz body hemolytic anemia; however, the osmotic fragility of erythrocytes may be increased. Chocolate-brown blood and brownish mucous membranes strongly suggest the diagnosis of red maple leaf toxicosis. The concentration of methemoglobin as a percentage of total hemoglobin can be estimated by comparing the hemoglobin concentration measured by the cyan-methemoglobin method (all hemoglobin) and that by the oxyhemoglobin method.[40] Abnormal values exceed 3%.

Treatment. Treatment of Heinz body hemolytic anemia is largely supportive and aimed at minimizing hemoglobin-induced nephrotoxicosis. The horse should be removed from access to the oxidant as soon as it is identified and housed to minimize stress and exercise. The packed cell volume must be monitored closely for development of life-threatening anemia. Clinical signs of red maple leaf toxicosis are typically more severe than would be suggested by the erythron data, owing to the inability of methemoglobin to transport oxygen. Intravenous therapy with isotonic balanced crystalloid solutions (80–100 mL/kg/24 hrs) is paramount to insure hydration and promote diuresis. The serum electrolyte and acid-base status should be monitored closely and corrected as needed. Other appropriate measures to treat renal failure may be warranted such as dopamine, furosemide, or mannitol, singly or combined. Methylene blue or other reductive therapy is not used since these agents are relatively ineffective in accelerating methemoglobin reduction in equine erythrocytes and may even enhance Heinz body formation.[99]

Client Education. The prognosis for Heinz body hemolytic anemia is determined by the amount of oxidant ingested and its innate activity. Red maple leaf toxicosis carries a poor prognosis, especially when methemoglobinuria is present.[92] Prevention is based on limiting access to excess phenothiazine, onions, or wilted red maple leaves.

Parasite-Induced Hemolytic Anemia

Babesiosis (Equine Piroplasmosis)

Babesiosis is caused by tick-borne protozoan parasites of the genus *Babesia*;[100] it is the only intraerythrocytic parasitic disease that affects horses. It is widely distributed throughout tropical and subtropical areas and to a less extent in temperate regions, corresponding to the habitat of natural tick vectors. All equids are susceptible and older animals are more severely affected. Affected horses generally have recently traveled to endemic areas, which include parts of Florida, Texas, Mexico, Cuba, and Central and South America.

Clinical Signs and Laboratory Findings. Clinical disease generally develops 5 to 28 days after susceptible horses are placed with infected horses in an endemic area. Signs include fever, depression, anorexia, weakness, ataxia, lacrimation, mucoid nasal discharge, chemosis, icterus, and hemoglobinuria.[100, 101] Death may occur within 48 hours or chronic disease (fever and anemia) may persist for months. Horses raised in endemic areas often carry *Babesia* without showing clinical signs.

Laboratory data are consistent with hemolytic anemia. Parasitized erythrocytes may be easily seen on routine blood smears during the febrile period but are often absent in the hemolytic crisis. *Babesia* species appear as pyriform bodies in groups of two to four with their pointed ends meeting at an acute angle.[16] Severe cases are attended by intravascular hemolysis which results in pink plasma and pigmenturia. Pigment nephropathy may ensue.

Etiology and Pathogenesis. Horses are susceptible to infection with *Babesia caballi* and *Babesia equi*, although only *B. caballi* is considered endemic to the United States.[101] Both species cause equine disease in parts of Europe, Asia, Africa, the Middle East, and Russia.[100] The organisms divide by binary fission and *B. caballi* appears as a pair of 3×2-µm pyriform bodies in parasitized erythrocytes. *Babesia equi* is much smaller (1–2 µm) and usually appears as ovoid structures in groups of four to form a Maltese cross.[100] Natural transmission of *Babesia* species occurs via ticks, although they may be transmitted by contaminated instruments or needles. *Dermacentor nitens*, permanently established in areas where the temperature remains above 16° C (60° F), is the primary vector for *B. caballi* in the United States. *Babesia caballi* is passed vertically (transovarially) from one tick generation to the next. *Babesia equi* is transmitted horizontally (transstadially) by species of *Dermacentor, Hyalomma,* and *Rhipicephalus*, which can rarely serve as vectors for *B. caballi* as well.[100]

Once they gain access to the host, *Babesia* species multiply and develop within erythrocytes. Many parasitized erythrocytes are removed via the MPS; however, intravascular hemolysis can occur. Clinical disease associated with *B. equi* infection is much more severe than that caused by *B. caballi* and the mortality rate is higher. Horses that survive clinical babesiosis remain inapparent carriers for an indeterminable period of time, unless treated. Foals born in endemic areas are believed to experience subclinical infection as maternal immunity is waning and develop strong active immunity dependent upon the constant presence of the organism (premunition). Stress such as training, transportation, inclement weather, or pregnancy can induce clinical disease in carrier horses.

Diagnosis. Definitive diagnosis of babesiosis relies upon demonstration of parasitized erythrocytes on Giemsa-stained blood smears or by positive serology. Since parasitemia is brief and usually precludes hemolysis, diagnosis is most often made serologically. Antibodies to *Babesia* species are detectable within 14 days of infection by a complement fixation or indirect fluorescent antibody test.[100, 101] Horses imported to the United States must have a negative complement fixation test for both *B. caballi* and *B. equi*.

Treatment. Imidocarb diprionate can effectively depress parasitemia and usually eradicates *B. caballi* infection when given at an appropriate dose and rate (2.2 mg/kg q.24h. × 2). *Babesia equi* is much more resistant and imidocarb therapy (4 mg/kg q.72h. × 4) is only 50% to 60% effective in eliminating infection, particularly of eastern European origin.[103] Imidocarb may cause colic, hypersalivation, diarrhea, and death. Donkeys appear to be particularly sensitive and often die if given imidocarb at the rate to eliminate *B. equi*.[104] Supportive care should include rest, intravenous fluids, and NSAIDs.

Client Education. The prognosis for *B. caballi* infection is fair to good with imidocarb treatment. The prognosis for *B. equi* infection is variable. There are currently no vaccines for prevention of equine babesiosis. Disease transmission can be minimized by tick control and sanitary veterinary practices in endemic areas. All attempts should be made to quarantine carrier horses until they are effectively treated with imidocarb.

Microangiopathic Hemolysis

Thrombosis or fibrinoid change within the lumen of small blood vessels, can result in damage and subsequent lysis of erythrocytes.[105] This microangiopathic hemolytic disease is a characteristic of chronic DIC and has been reported in horses.[106] Usually hemolysis is mild and any anemia is due to blood loss.

A fulminant intravascular hemolytic syndrome has been reported in horses with terminal *liver failure*.[107] Acute hemolysis and intense icterus are attended by marked hemoglobinuria.[40] Most affected horses die. Lesions at necropsy resemble those described for DIC.[108] Alterations in exchangeable red blood cell membrane lipoproteins and the effect of bile acids on erythrocyte metabolism during liver failure have been suggested in the pathogenesis.[40]

Anemia Due to Inadequate Erythropoiesis

When the rate of erythropoiesis is inadequate to replenish aged erythrocytes removed by the MPS, anemia ensues. This type of depression anemia is termed *nonregenerative* and can be caused by (1) deficiency in substances essential for erythrocyte production, (2) systemic disease processes that interfere with erythropoiesis, or (3) conditions that damage or displace normal bone marrow elements. Anemia that is solely due to inadequate erythropoiesis develops slowly because of the normally long life span of equine erythrocytes. Depressed erythropoiesis associated with blood loss or hemolysis can produce a rapidly progressive and life-threatening anemia. Definitive classification of anemia as nonregenerative requires cytologic or histologic evaluation of the bone marrow.

Iron deficiency anemia is extremely rare in horses since they have constant access to dirt, which has a high iron content, as do legumes. Iron deficiency only develops when the rate of iron loss from the body exceeds the absorption of iron from the diet. Milk is a particularly poor source of iron; thus foals are more susceptible to iron deficiency than adults.[49] After the absorption of dietary iron from the intestinal tract, it is transported in the blood to body tissues by the carrier protein, transferrin. Iron is stored in various body tissues (especially liver and spleen) as either a soluble, mobile fraction in ferritin, or as insoluble aggregated deposits of hemosiderin. The amount of storage iron determines its relative distribution between ferritin and hemosiderin, with the latter increasing with storage iron concentration. Iron necessary for hematopoiesis is delivered to the bone marrow via transferrin and may come directly from the intestinal tract or from the storage pool. Since circulating erythrocytes account for greater than 65% of the total iron stores in the body, iron deficiency is often associated with chronic external blood loss.

Clinical Signs and Laboratory Findings. Iron deficiency develops gradually and clinical signs do not differ from those of chronic blood loss (see p. 563). Initially, the anemia is normocytic and normochromic with decreased marrow iron.[32] As blood loss continues, serum iron and percent saturation of transferrin decrease while the total iron binding capacity (TIBC) increases.[49] The TIBC is a measure of serum transferrin, being derived from the iron content of serum after total iron saturation of its carrier protein. Since transferrin can bind more iron than is normally present, the TIBC is greater than the serum iron concentration. Serum iron may be expressed as a percentage of TIBC or as the percent saturation. Hypoproteinemia is commonly associated with chronic blood loss, and moderate to severe iron deficiency eventually induces a reduction in erythrocyte size and color, and microcytic hypochromic anemia.

Etiology and Pathogenesis. Severe ulcerative gastrointestinal lesions such as gastroduodenal ulcers, NSAID toxicosis, and neoplasia, which result in chronic external blood loss, are common causes of iron deficiency. Anemia due to iron deficiency is particularly prevalent in horses with gastric squamous cell carcinoma. Coagulopathies and severe external or intestinal parasitism are other potential causes. Iron deficiency results in an erythrocyte maturation arrest in the bone marrow due to delayed hemoglobin synthesis.[16] Late rubricytes awaiting hemoglobin synthesis may undergo cell division, producing a few erythrocytes that are smaller than normal and deficient in hemoglobin. These poorly structured erythrocytes have reduced deformability and a modestly shortened life span.

Diagnosis. Iron deficiency should not be diagnosed solely on the basis of decreased serum iron concentration,[109] since serum iron declines in response to acute phase inflammatory reactions, renal disease, and chronic inflammation,[110] in addition to iron deficiency. The TIBC may help differentiate true iron deficiency from other disease processes, because it is usually normal in iron deficiency and tends to be low in association with inflammation. Serum ferritin has been shown to be a much better indicator of total body iron content than serum iron and serum ferritin less than 45 ng/mL is suggestive of iron deficiency in horses.[111] Unfortunately, ferritin is also an acute phase protein and may be falsely increased by inflammation. The assay is species-specific and tests for equine ferritin are not routinely available. The presence of bone marrow iron (detected by examination of Prussian blue–stained slides) specifically eliminates iron deficiency as the cause of anemia. Iron deficiency bone marrow cytology is characterized by a predominance of rubricytes and metarubricytes with scanty irregularly stained cellular boundaries.

Treatment. Therapy should be aimed at identification and correction of the primary disease process. Since parenteral iron solutions can cause anaphylactoid reactions, only oral iron supplementation is safe. Supplements are unnecessary if chronic blood loss is stopped.

Client Education. The prognosis depends upon that for the cause of chronic blood loss. Iron deficiency anemia is reversible.

Anemia of Inflammatory Disease

Also known as the anemia of chronic disease, this is the most common form of anemia in horses.[32, 40] Clinical signs are usually ascribed to the primary disease process and anemia tends to be mild, slowly progressive, and of little clinical consequence. Hematologic features include a mild nonresponsive anemia (packed cell volume, 23%–30%) with other data that suggest a chronic inflammatory response (neutrophilic leukocytosis, hyperfibrinogenemia, and hypergammaglobulinemia). Serum iron is usually decreased and TIBC is normal or slightly low, but serum ferritin in increased.[109, 110]

Chronic disease processes such as pneumonia, pleuritis, peritonitis, abscessation (e.g., bastard strangles), and neoplasia are the most common underlying disorders. Kinetic data indicate that the anemia of inflammatory disease develops because the bone marrow fails to compensate for a modest decrease in circulating erythrocyte life span.[112] The latter may be secondary to red blood cell damage while passing through inflamed tissues or destruction by the hyperplastic MPS. Impaired erythropoiesis is due to altered iron metabolism and sequestration by cells of the MPS.[112] This decrease in iron availability may be a protective response against bacteria that require iron for multiplication. IL-1, tumor necrosis factor (TNF), and other cytokines released in the "acute phase" response to infection may have a role in inhibition of erythropoiesis.

The presence of nonresponsive anemia in the face of clinical and laboratory evidence of chronic underlying disease is generally suggestive of anemia of chronic disease. Marrow iron stores are normal to increased, as are serum ferritin concentrations. Therapeutic efforts should be aimed at the underlying disease.

Anemia associated with renal disease is due to inadequate erythropoiesis. Although failure of normal erythropoietin production has been proposed, there is no evidence that serum erythropoietin is actually decreased.[113] It is more likely that defective marrow response to erythropoietin in combination with reduced erythrocyte longevity accounts for the anemia of renal disease.[16] Therapy must be aimed at the renal disease; the prognosis is poor.

Myelophthisic anemia is due to destruction of the normal marrow habitat by neoplastic or inflammatory tissue, and the net result is peripheral pancytopenia. Because of the shorter half-life of granulocytes and platelets, clinical signs of bleeding diathesis and localized or generalized infections generally precede those associated with anemia. Blood loss generally hastens anemia development, which is exemplified by lethargy, anorexia, and mucosal pallor. Hematologic study reveals severe neutropenia and thrombocytopenia in addition to nonresponsive anemia.

Myelophthisic anemia has been described in horses with several types of myeloid neoplasia (see p. 575).[114–117] In these myeloproliferative disorders, a marrow-derived blood cell proliferates at the expense of all others. Myelophthisic disease could also result from metastasis of neoplasia to the bone marrow, although this is exceedingly rare in horses.

Myelophthisis is confirmed by bone marrow examination, which reveals replacement of normal marrow elements by the proliferation of atypical cells. Occasionally, abnormal cells are found in the peripheral blood.[115] Blood transfusions are only palliative. Hematopoietic neoplasia is considered fatal in horses.

Bone Marrow Aplasia (Aplastic Anemia)

This is caused by failure of stem cells to undergo differentiation, either due to intrinsic damage, or interruption of their interactions with supporting cells that constitute the microenvironment.[118] There is no evidence of a primary disease infiltrating or suppressing hematopoietic tissue. The net result is marrow hypoplasia associated with peripheral pancytopenia. Aplastic anemia is very uncommon in horses and generally is an acquired disorder. Idiopathic hypoplastic anemia has been reported,[119–121] and rare cases have been associated with phenylbutazone use.[122, 123]

Clinical Signs and Laboratory Findings. The clinical features of aplastic anemia are similar to those accompanying myelophthisic disease and relate to inadequate numbers of functional peripheral blood cells. Disease onset is insidious, characterized by vague historical complaints of poor performance,[122] weight loss,[119] and intermittent fever.[121, 123] Neutropenia causes increased susceptibility to infections, especially arising from bacterial invasion of the gastrointestinal and respiratory tracts. Hemorrhagic diathesis secondary to thrombocytopenia is often the first indication of disease,[120, 123] manifest by epistaxis, gingival bleeding, mucosal petechial hemorrhages, hematomas, or prolonged hemorrhage following injections, trauma or surgical procedures. As aplasia progresses, other signs of anemia develop.

Hematologic findings depend upon the stage of disease. Neutropenia, monocytopenia, and thrombocytopenia occur first, followed by severe anemia. Blood loss often hastens the development of anemia and some cases may have a positive Coombs' test. The production of lymphocytes is reportedly not impaired; however, absolute lymphopenia is not uncommon.[124] The circulating lymphocytes are occasionally highly reactive, confusing the diagnosis with neoplasia or a preleukemic syndrome.[123] Plasma proteins may be low, normal, or reflect chronic antigenic stimulation; however, changes are neither consistent nor specific.

Etiology and Pathogenesis. In humans, marrow aplasia can be categorized into one of two general processes: (1) an intrinsic or acquired defect in primitive stem cells that renders them unable to differentiate, or (2) an immunologically mediated disorder that causes an inappropriate cellular or microenvironmental milieu for stem cell maturation.[124] The cause cannot be proved in most instances. Exposure to a diverse array of chemicals; drugs such as alkylating agents, antimetabolites, antimicrobials, and sedatives; ionizing radiation; viral infections; bacterial toxins; neoplasia; or immune-mediated diseases have been implicated. These associations make it unlikely that a single pathogenic mechanism can explain all cases of aplastic anemia. Approximately 50% of human cases are termed *idiopathic* and there is no apparent clinical difference between these and secondary forms of the disease.

Regardless of the exact cause, aplastic anemia results from failure of pluripotential stem cell development.[124] The vulnerability of some individuals may be caused by a genetic or acquired defect in drug detoxification or stem cell sensitivity. Immunologic rejection of stem cells probably plays a role in both idiopathic[125] as well as secondary forms of aplastic anemia[124] and interferon from activated suppressor lymphocytes may be pathogenetically important.[126]

Diagnosis. The diagnosis of aplastic anemia is based upon peripheral pancytopenia and fatty replacement of normal bone marrow elements. Because the erythrocyte life span in horses is approximately 140 days,[2] clinically significant anemia due to marrow failure requires a substantial developmental period, although blood loss may hasten its development. Neutropenia, with no left shift, and thrombocytopenia are the early and most consistent hematologic manifestations.

Because sternal bone marrow aspirates are frequently contaminated by peripheral blood, a core marrow biopsy from the rib or ileal wing should be examined histologically. The key diagnostic feature for aplastic anemia is a fatty marrow with essentially empty stroma.[118] Nucleated red blood cells usually are the most numerous cell type, accompanied by lymphocytoid cells, reticulum cells, mast cells, and plasma cells. Benign lymphoid nodules create confusion with lymphosarcoma. Because of the unavoidable heterogeneity of a large organ, biopsies from at least two sites are necessary to definitively substantiate marrow failure.

Treatment. The major thrust of therapy is to remove the horse from suspected causative drugs, chemicals, or environmental toxins and to provide supportive care until spontaneous remission occurs. Immunosuppressive or myelostimulatory drugs have produced discouraging results in adult humans with marrow aplasia and are largely unproven in horses. The treatment of choice for human aplastic anemia is bone marrow transplantation.[118, 125] This is an unlikely treatment option in horses, because of the necessity of absolute leukocyte antigen compatibility between donor and recipient to prevent fatal graft-versus-host disease.[127, 128] Blood or platelet transfusions only provide temporary relief and should be reserved for life-threatening anemia (packed cell volume <10%), or actual bleeding episodes (see discussion of idiopathic thrombocytopenia under Coagulation Dysfunction). Early, intense broad-spectrum antimicrobial therapy should be instituted after appropriate samples have been taken for culture and sensitivity. Serial blood cultures to identify the potential pathogen are indicated when there is fever without localizing signs.

Testosterone and orally active synthetic androgens (such as oxymetholone) stimulate erythropoiesis in certain circumstances and have been used to treat human aplastic anemia. The toxicity of androgens is high and their potential usefulness is subject to debate, since granulocyte and platelet responses are much less common than a rise in packed cell volume. Experience with androgens in horses with severe bone marrow aplasia is limited.

Client Education. Too few horses with aplastic anemia have been studied to give a clear indication of prognosis. Human aplastic anemia may be a severe disease, with mortality within 6 months, or a milder syndrome that is protracted and may smoulder for many years.

Erythrocytosis (Polycythemia)

Erythrocytosis is defined as an elevation of packed cell volume, red blood cell count, and hemoglobin concentration above those considered normal for the species.[129] Early in the evaluation of the erythrocytosis, it must be determined whether there is an increase in total red blood cell mass (absolute erythrocytosis) or a decrease in plasma volume (relative erythrocytosis). Relative erythrocytosis is common in horses, whereas absolute erythrocytosis is exceptionally rare.

Relative Erythrocytosis

A relative increase in the packed cell volume, red blood cell count, and hemoglobin concentration is usually due to a reduction in plasma volume (dehydration). Relative erythrocytosis may also occur subsequent to a red blood cell mass at the upper end of normal, combined with a low normal plasma volume. Splenic contraction due to excitement, exercise, or endotoxemia generally underlies this form of relative erythrocytosis.

Clinical signs of relative erythrocytosis are associated with the primary disease process. Clinical evidence of dehydration such as tacky mucous membranes and reduced skin pliability make the diagnosis obvious. Endotoxemia or other forms of shock would be manifested by tachycardia, cool extremities, and mucosal congestion or pallor.

Any disease condition that prevents adequate oral fluid intake or causes loss of body water in excess of that absorbed from the gastrointestinal tract will produce relative erythrocytosis. These include the causes of dysphagia, diarrhea, overexertion and heat stress, proximal enteritis, and other diseases that cause adynamic ileus. Endotoxemia generally arises from gastrointestinal diseases that cause colic or diarrhea, but may also be associated with severe gram-negative pleuropneumonia and postpartum metritis.

The diagnosis of relative erythrocytosis is easily made by resolution of the condition following intravenous fluid therapy to replace plasma volume. Treatment is aimed at fluid administration necessary to maintain hydration and whatever is indicated for the primary disease process.

Absolute Erythrocytosis

Absolute erythrocytosis refers to an increased circulating red blood cell mass without any change in plasma volume. Primary absolute erythrocytosis results from autonomous proliferation of erythroid progenitor cells. Excessive stimulation of an otherwise normal bone marrow by erythropoietin causes secondary absolute erythrocytosis.

Irrespective of the underlying cause, absolute erythrocytosis causes certain common clinical manifestations due to expanded blood volume and increased blood viscosity. Generalized vascular expansion and venous engorgement cause the characteristic "muddy" hyperemia of mucous membranes. A marked decrease in cardiac output accompanies blood hyperviscosity and ultimately impairs tissue oxygenation, producing the vague signs of lethargy and weight loss. Epistaxis and gastrointestinal bleeding or an increase in thrombotic complications such as laminitis and renal failure may occur. Laboratory findings in addition to the increased packed cell volume, red blood cell count, and hemoglobin concentration usually include increased unconjugated bilirubin concentration.

Primary erythrocytosis may occur as a single cell disorder or as a component of polycythemia vera. Both are idiopathic myeloproliferative disorders characterized by excessive autonomous proliferation of erythroid elements that results in an absolute increase in red blood cell mass. In polycythemia vera, there is also abnormal proliferation of myeloid cells and megakaryocytes resulting in elevated granulocyte and platelet counts.[129] It has been suggested that primary erythrocytosis arises in the committed erythroid stem cell compartment, rather than the pluripotent stem cell affected by polycythemia vera. The diagnosis of polycythemia vera is based on demonstration of increased erythrocyte mass that is not associated with excessive erythropoietin production, as well as increased bone marrow production of granulocytes and platelets. Affected patients have erythrocytosis that is not responsive to intravenous fluid therapy, as well as leukocytosis, thrombocytosis, and a normal arterial oxygen concentration. When hematologic and bone marrow abnormalities are restricted to proliferation of the erythroid series, the diagnosis of primary erythrocytosis would be made. A case of erythrocytosis has been described in a horse with no identifiable cause of secondary erythrocytosis and without an elevated concentration of plasma erythropoietin.[130] This may have represented primary erythrocytosis. Although bone marrow examination is indicated in the evaluation of all cases of erythrocytosis, the marrow may appear normal and erythroid hyperplasia is not specific for primary or secondary erythrocytosis.

Treatment. The initial therapy of primary erythrocytosis must include phlebotomy to keep the packed cell volume less than 50% to minimize the complications of hypervolemia and blood hyperviscosity. Initially, 10 mL/kg body weight of blood should be removed every 2 to 3 days until a normal packed cell volume is attained. Phlebotomies are then performed as needed. As iron deficiency supervenes, the frequency of phlebotomy can be greatly reduced. Although alkylating agents and radioactive phosphorus reliably produce myelosuppression in humans, these modalities are associated with many side effects such as cytopenia and malignant transformation.[129] Hydroxyurea causes reversible bone marrow suppression and has been used successfully in humans[129] and dogs[131] with primary erythrocytosis. Side effects are much fewer than occur with other myelosuppressive drugs. The dose of hydroxyurea must be individualized, but 30 mg/kg/day PO for 7 to 10 days, followed by 15 mg/kg/day, has been suggested for dogs.[131] There is no experience with the use of hydroxyurea in horses.

Secondary erythrocytosis. Increased concentrations of erythropoietin or other erythroid stimulatory substances result in secondary erythrocytosis. Causes can further be subdivided into conditions in which increased erythropoietin production represents a physiologically appropriate response to arterial hypoxemia and poor tissue oxygenation and disorders characterized by excessive autonomous production of erythropoietic stimulatory substances.

Physiologically appropriate erythrocytosis is the most common form of absolute erythrocytosis in domestic animals. Chronic tissue hypoxia that attends residence at high altitude, congenital heart defects that produce right-to-left shunting, and some forms of chronic pulmonary disease induce a compensatory increase in plasma erythropoietin that results in absolute secondary erythrocytosis.

To insure adequate offloading of oxygen to tissues, the Po_2 in capillaries must be maintained close to 40 mm Hg. Erythropoietin production in response to hypoxia causes erythrocytosis in an attempt to increase the oxygen-carrying capacity of circulating blood. At elevated altitudes, diminished atmospheric Po_2 produces a much smaller alveolar:capillary Po_2 gradient and an inadequate driving force for tissue oxygenation. Of the domestic animals, cattle are most susceptible to the effects of high altitude and some develop erythrocytosis at 1,800 m above sea level.[132] Horses develop an increased erythrocyte mass above 2,200 m, especially when in training.

Congenital cardiac disorders that produce right-to-left shunting of blood away from the lungs cause absolute erythrocytosis in horses. Tetralogy of Fallot is the most common defect to cause a right-to-left shunt, although a number of other defects, including ventricular septal defect, may eventually result in right-to-left shunting and secondary erythrocytosis.[133] Chronic impairment of alveolar ventilation may eventually cause erythrocytosis, although most chronic pulmonary diseases in horses are not associated with significant hypoxemia. Chronic obstructive pulmonary disease may produce enough ventilation:perfusion mismatching to reduce the arterial Po_2 below normal; however, the degree of resultant hypoxemia is insufficient to induce erythrocytosis.

Physiologically appropriate erythrocytosis can be diagnosed by documenting low arterial Po_2. Thoracic radiographs, transtracheal aspiration, and echocardiology may more thoroughly delineate cardiorespiratory function. In spite of the need for increased oxygen-carrying capacity of the blood, the beneficial effect of expanded red blood cell mass is ultimately offset by the detrimental effect of increased blood viscosity on cardiac output, systemic oxygen transport, and tissue oxygen delivery. Oxygen delivery is impaired when the packed cell volume exceeds 60%, thus phlebotomy is indicated when the packed cell volume is greater than 60%. The optimal packed cell volume for patients living at high altitudes or those with right-to-left cardiac shunts must be determined by trial and error.

Physiologically inappropriate erythrocytosis may rarely accompany renal, hepatic, or endocrine disorders that result in inappropriate elaboration of erythropoietin. Carcinomas of the liver, kidney, adrenal gland, and ovary have been reported in humans to produce erythropoietin, although the proportion of tumors that cause erythrocytosis is highly variable. Secondary erythrocytosis may accompany nonmalignant renal disorders such as cystic disease and hydronephrosis in which local intrarenal ischemia is believed to mediate increased erythropoietin production. Rarely, erythrocytosis may be caused by androgenic steroids, administered therapeutically or produced during adrenal disorders. Increased plasma erythropoietin and secondary erythrocytosis have been identified in one horse with hepatocellular carcinoma and interstitial nephritis.[134] Erythrocytosis may rarely accompany chronic hepatic disease in horses.

The diagnosis of inappropriate secondary erythrocytosis is based upon elevated serum erythropoietin in the absence of hypoxemia. It may not be possible to demonstrate the elevation of erythropoietin since equine erythropoietin must be determined by bioassay. Renal, hepatic, and adrenal function can be explored by appropriate laboratory testing.

Client Education. Congenital cardiac defects, neoplastic diseases, and chronic organ insufficiency carry a guarded prognosis. Primary erythrocytosis may be managed by phlebotomy, although there are no long-term follow-ups for horses with these disorders.

Myeloid Neoplasia

Myeloid neoplasia is characterized by the unregulated proliferation of a bone marrow–derived blood cell line. The eventual outcome is severe myelophthisis with loss of normal marrow elements. Forms of myeloid neoplasia described in horses, include granulocytic leukemia,[116] myelomonocytic leukemia,[117, 135–137] monocytic leukemia,[114] and eosinophilic myeloproliferative disorder.[115]

There appears to be no age predilection for equine myeloid neoplasia, as affected cases have ranged from 10 months[115] to 9 years of age.[116] Predominant clinical signs include depression, weight loss, edema, anemia, and mucosal petechial hemorrhages. Fever,[115, 117, 135, 137] peripheral lymphadenopathy,[117, 137] hemorrhagic diathesis,[115] and oral ulcers[136, 137] were identified in some of the horses. Severe destruction of normal marrow architecture by the neoplastic cell line results in myelophthisic disease characterized by inadequate production of erythrocytes, platelets, and normal leukocytes. Most horses are anemic and have thrombocytopenia. The total WBC count of affected horses may be elevated, normal, or reduced, but abnormal leukocytes have been invariably found in the peripheral blood. Bone marrow aspirates were dominated by abnormal leukocytes.

The cause of myeloid neoplasia remains undefined. Clinical signs are due to the loss of normal blood cells which predisposes to hemorrhagic diathesis, infections, and inadequate oxygenation of tissues. The diagnosis in all reported cases was based on abnormal morphology of the circulating neoplastic leukocytes; the type of cell was delineated by cytochemistry or special stains. Treatment was attempted with cytotoxic agents in one case of acute myelomonocytic leukemia but was unsuccessful.[117] All horses died or were humanely destroyed as a result of the effects of myelophthisic disease. At postmortem examination, abnormal leukocytes were found in various organs in addition to the bone marrow, most commonly in the lymph nodes, spleen, and liver.

Lymphoid Neoplasia

Lymphosarcoma

The most common type of neoplasia to involve the equine hemolymphatic system is lymphosarcoma.[138] Four anatomical forms have been described (generalized, intestinal, mediastinal, cutaneous) based upon the major site of tumor involvement;[138–140] however, the forms overlap substantially, both clinically and pathologically. The typical age of onset is between 5 and 10 years,[141] although lymphosarcoma has been documented in horses ranging in age from birth through 25 years.[142–144] There is no sex predilection.[145] The incidence of lymphosarcoma is unknown, but the reported prevalence of affected horses at postmortem examination is 2% to 5%.[146, 147]

Clinical Signs and Laboratory Findings. The most common clinical signs of lymphosarcoma are chronic weight loss, ventral subcutaneous edema, and regional lymphadenopathy.[145, 148, 149] Although peripheral lymphadenopathy is common, this finding is not consistently present. Clinical manifestations are highly variable depending upon the organs involved and the duration of the disease process. Lymphosarcoma involving the thoracic cavity may cause tachypnea, dyspnea, cough, and pleural effusion.[143, 150] In addition to weight loss, signs of gastrointestinal involvement may include colic or diarrhea.[151–153] Although skin or eye masses may be the only manifestation of lymphosarcoma,[139] concomitant internal organ involvement is not unusual.[138, 154, 155] The regional or generalized occurrence of multiple subcutaneous nodules 1 to 20 cm in diameter, unassociated with other lesions of lymphosarcoma, has been reported in horses.[139] Nodules may appear suddenly, grow slowly, remain static or regress, and recur at a later time. Tumor masses in localized areas may result in dysphagia, unresponsive nasal discharge, chemosis, ataxia, and jugular venous distention.[148, 150, 154, 156–161] Pseudohyperparathyroidism, resulting in hypercalcemic nephropathy and polyuria or polydypsia, has been reported in a horse with splenic lymphosarcoma.[162] Splenic enlargement, internal lymphadenopathy, or abdominal masses may be palpated on rectal examination. Most clinical signs are progressive over weeks or months, although they may have a sudden onset.

The laboratory findings are highly variable. Hematologic indications of chronic inflammatory disease are common, including neutrophilic leukocytosis, nonresponsive anemia, hyperfibrinogenemia, and hypergammaglobulinemia.[149, 150] Lymphocytic leukemia with peripheral lymphocytosis and large numbers of circulating neoplastic lymphocytes is rare and usually associated with bone marrow involvement.[152, 163–166] Although the lymphocyte count is usually normal or reduced, the presence of atypical or obviously neoplastic lymphocytes on a peripheral blood smear occurs in 30% to 50% of cases.[145, 149, 166–170] The TPP may be low, normal, or elevated, but the albumin-globulin ratio is often reduced, particularly when there is gastrointestinal involvement.[153, 171] Polyclonal gammopathy is not unusual and monoclonal gammopathy associated with serum hyperviscosity and a hemorrhagic diathesis has been described.[172] In some patients, Coombs'-positive immune-mediated hemolytic anemia or thrombocytopenia, or both, may occur.[170, 173, 174] A mild elevation in liver-derived serum enzymes may occur subsequent to hepatic involvement. Hyperbilirubinemia is usually due to anorexia or hemolysis. Hypercalcemia can occur in association with pseudohyperparathyroidism.

Etiology and Pathogenesis. A viral etiology has not been documented in the development of equine lymphosarcoma;[158, 175] however, there is one report describing virus-like particles in the lymph node of a foal with lymphosarcoma that died shortly after birth.[144] Clinical signs and laboratory changes of lymphosarcoma are generally due to loss of normal organ and tissue function subsequent to infiltration by lymphocytes or physical obstruction by tumor masses or the excessive generation of tumor cell products. Some neoplastic lymphocytes appear to be of the T-lymphocyte lineage[166, 169] and may have suppressor effects, since decreased serum concentrations of IgM and other indications of immunosuppression have been noted in horses with lymphosarcoma.[176] Other neoplastic lymphocytes may arise from autoreactive B-cell clones that produce antibodies responsible for gammopathies and immune-mediated cytopenias. Neoplastic proliferation of large granular lymphocytes that had natural killer cell activity was described in one case.[177] Extensive intestinal infiltration by neoplastic lymphocytes typically produces intestinal malabsorption, which contributes to hypoalbuminemia and weight loss.

Diagnosis. The diagnosis of lymphosarcoma is made by demonstration of neoplastic lymphocytes in affected tissue. Histologic examination of a biopsy from a tumor mass or affected lymph node is the most reliable method, and excisional biopsies are much preferred over needle biopsies or aspirates. Without lymph nodes or other masses accessible for biopsy, antemortem diagnosis is often difficult.[143, 160, 170, 178] Diagnosis is only rarely possible on a peripheral blood smear[164, 166] and generally requires careful cytologic evaluation of bone marrow, pleural effusion, or peritoneal fluid.[150, 179, 180] Neoplastic lymphocytes may rarely be found by transcutaneous liver biopsy[168] and laparoscopy has been used to better envision a mass for biopsy.[143] Radiography and ultrasonography may be useful in locating and perhaps enabling biopsies of masses in the thorax or abdomen. Often, diagnosis of lymphosarcoma is possible only by exploratory laparotomy or postmortem examination.[151, 160, 170, 178]

The morphology of neoplastic lymphocytes in horses is highly variable.[142] On cytologic preparations, they often appear as large lymphoid cells with a variable nucleus-cytoplasm ratio, multiple nucleoli, nuclear chromatic clumping, cytoplasmic basophilia, and vacuolation. Mitotic figures and binucleate cells may be seen. The cytologic diagnosis of lymphosarcoma is best left to those experienced in evaluation of equine fluid specimens, since normal "reactive" lymphocytes and mesothelial cells may be difficult to distinguish from well-differentiated neoplastic cells. Histologically, the neoplastic cellular morphology is also variable, but destruction of normal tissue architecture by a population of lymphoid cells aids the diagnosis.

Treatment. There is limited experience in treating horses with lymphosarcoma. They are generally markedly debilitated by the time diagnosis is made. Transient improvement in generalized forms has occurred following use of cytotoxic drugs, immunomodulators, and corticosteroids;[148, 178] however, the long-term response is poor. The localized cutaneous form of lymphosarcoma may be responsive to corticosteroid therapy, but often recurs in a more pathogenic form when treatment is stopped.[139]

Client Education. The prognosis for equine lymphosarcoma is grave. Most horses die or are humanely destroyed within 6 months of the onset of signs. Rarely, survival for a number of years occurs.

Plasma Cell Myeloma

Plasma cell myeloma (multiple myeloma), characterized by proliferation of neoplastic plasma cells in the bone marrow, spleen, liver, and lymph nodes, is very rare in horses. Clinical signs include weight loss, weakness, recurrent fever, ventral edema, hemorrhage, lameness, and posterior paralysis.[181-184] Renal failure and infections are not uncommon. In humans and dogs, skeletal pain and pathologic fractures result from neoplastic invasion of bone that causes osteolytic "punched-out" lesions;[185, 186] osteolysis, however, does not consistently occur in horses.

Laboratory findings include anemia, hypercalcemia, azotemia, and hyperproteinemia with monoclonal gammopathy. Light-chain proteinuria (Bence Jones proteins) is variable. Criteria for diagnosis of plasma cell myeloma include plasmacytosis in the bone marrow or a soft tissue lesion, evidence of invasiveness, and the presence of monoclonal gammopathy or light-chain proteinuria.[185] Because of the overlap in histologic and clinicopathologic findings with some cases of lymphosarcoma, definitive diagnosis of plasma cell myeloma can be difficult.[172, 187] Treatment of plasma cell myeloma in horses has not been attempted.

HEMOSTATIC DISORDERS
Physiology of Normal Hemostasis

A thorough knowledge of normal hemostasis is the basis for the diagnosis and treatment of disorders that produce hemostatic dysfunction in horses.[108] The mechanism of hemostasis has been much more extensively studied in laboratory animals and humans than in horses. Thus, much of our current understanding is based upon extrapolation from data in other species. Hemostasis is a complex series of events that function to arrest bleeding from damaged blood vessels and maintain nutrient blood flow to all body tissues.[188] Hemostasis is composed of two interrelated components, namely, coagulation and fibrinolysis, both with their respective inhibitors.

Coagulation

The cooperation of platelets and blood procoagulant proteins with the blood vessel wall constitutes the basis for coagulation, which culminates in the formation of fibrin. The *vasculature*, a frequently neglected component of hemostasis, is now known to be important in the regulation of both coagulation and fibrinolysis.[189] Immediately after injury, reflex vasoconstriction limits blood loss and the vessel wall provides a scaffold for fibrin clot formation. More important, endothelial cells release a number of substances that activate or inhibit the other components of coagulation and fibrinolysis, to be discussed subsequently. These compounds include platelet activating factor (PAF), tissue factor (TF) or thromboplastin, von Willebrand's factor (vWF), prostacyclin, thrombomodulin, protein S, heparin-like glycosaminoglycans, tissue plasminogen activator (t-PA), and plasminogen activator inhibitor (PAI).

The interaction of *platelets* with a discontinuous vascular surface forms a plug that provides primary hemostasis. Platelets adhere to subendothelial collagen via factor VIII:vWF, then undergo activation, aggregation, and the release reaction.[190] Platelet spheration centralizes granules in preparation for subsequent secretion and pseudopods are necessary for aggregation (platelets adhering to one another). Primary platelet aggregation is reversible and occurs without a release reaction, whereas secondary aggregation is irreversible and associated with granule secretion. An initial platelet release of adenosine 5'-diphosphate (ADP) into the extracellular environment in response to adhesion promotes primary aggregation.[191] Platelet aggregation requires the exposure of fibrinogen receptors to which fibrinogen binds in the presence of divalent cations. Secondary irreversible aggregation is a consequence of thromboxane A_2 (TXA_2) formation and secretion of platelet granule constituents, which include adenosine triphosphate (ATP), ADP, divalent cations, fibrinogen, vWF, thrombomodulin, factor V, platelet factor 4, and lysosomal hydrolases. The liberated TXA_2 and ADP bind specific platelet surface receptors and stimulate hydrolysis of inositol phosphate, Ca^{2+} mobilization, and protein phosphorylation to amplify platelet responses via enhancing cytosolic Ca^{2+}.

The synergistic activity of TXA_2 and ADP produce positive feedback loops that culminate in maximal platelet contraction and secretion of granular contents. Platelet factor 3 provides the phospholipid (PL) necessary at numerous steps during the subsequent interaction of coagulant proteins. The

platelet plug is limited to the site of vascular damage by the release of ectoenzymes that inactivate ADP and by the secretion of prostacyclin by healthy endothelial cells.[188] During and after platelet plug formation, an insoluble fibrin meshwork forms at the site of injury by blood procoagulants. The platelet surface protects coagulant proteins from plasma anticoagulants and localizes clot formation to the hemostatic plug. Although the mechanism remains obscure, platelets prevent spontaneous hemorrhage into the skin and mucous membranes by maintaining "vascular integrity."

Coagulation proteins (or coagulation factors) circulate in the peripheral blood as inactive enzymes (zymogens) that must be altered to become active. With the exception of factor XIII, all enzymes of the coagulation system are serine proteases that are converted to the active form through cleavage of a portion of the molecule to expose an "active site" serine. Coagulation has been referred to as a "cascade" because it is a self-amplifying series of linked proteolytic events in which a zymogen is transformed to a proteinase that effects the subsequent zymogen-proteinase transition.[192] There are numerous links between what have classically been considered the extrinsic and intrinsic pathways, although the initiating mechanisms remain fairly distinct. These pathways join at the point of activated factor X, then coagulation proceeds through thrombin and fibrin formation via a single common path (Fig. 11–2).

In the extrinsic pathway, factor Xa is formed via the action of TF, which complexes with factor VII in the presence of Ca^{2+}. The lipoprotein TF is not normally present in the blood, but is widely distributed throughout tissues and thus accesses the circulation when vasculature is disrupted by inflammation or tissue necrosis.[193] Pericytes and fibroblasts in the blood vessel adventitia express surface TF constitutively, while vascular endothelial cells, tissue macrophages, and blood monocytes are activated to produce TF by agonists such as endotoxin, TNF, and IL-1.[189] When blood contacts fluid or cells with TF activity, factor VII is activated, and the complex initiates coagulation. The mechanism by which

Figure 11–2. Schematic representation of blood coagulation showing the numerous interactions between coagulation factors in the classic extrinsic and intrinsic pathways. *Arrow*, primary action; *dashed arrow*, actions of secondary importance; *a*, activated form; *HMWK*, high-molecular-weight kininogen; *TF*, tissue factor; *PL*, phospholipid; *Prekal*, prekallikrein. (From Morris DD: Recognition and management of disseminated intravascular coagulation in horses. Vet Clin North Am Equine Pract 4:115–143, 1988.)

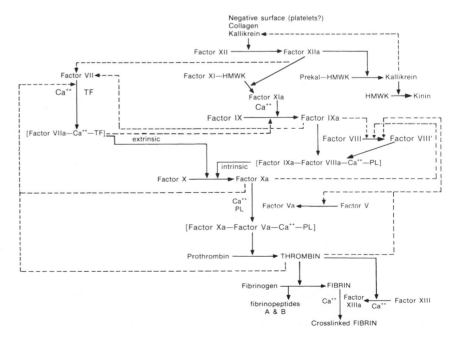

factor VII is initially activated remains unresolved. Factor Xa is an efficient activator of factor VII, and once generated, factor Xa preferentially activates factor VII complexed to TF,[194] which causes its continued production. The TF:VII complex may possess some minimal proteolytic activity for factor X[193] or there may be trace amounts of plasma factor VIIa that complex with TF to cause activation of factor Xa.[195]

The intrinsic pathway to factor Xa formation is initiated when blood is exposed to a negatively charged surface such as the platelet plug or subendothelial collagen.[196] Through association of the plasma protein factor XII (Hageman factor), prekallikrein, and high-molecular-weight kininogen (HMWK), factor XIIa is formed, which converts factor XI to XIa to perpetuate the intrinsic cascade. The activation of factor XII remains ill-defined: reciprocal proteolytic activation between factor XII and prekallikrein may occur or factor XII may autoactivate. Prekallikrein and factor XI circulate bound to HMWK, which serves as a nonenzymatic cofactor in contact interactions. Once generated, factor XIa activates factor IX in the presence of Ca^{2+}. Factor IXa finally becomes bound with PL, Ca^{2+}, and factor VIIIa, and this complex activates factor X. Factor VIII generally circulates bound to vWF in an inactive form, but acquires procoagulant cofactor properties through limited proteolysis by thrombin or factor Xa on a PL surface.[197] Because there is reciprocal activation between factor XII and prekallikrein, the intrinsic coagulation pathway stimulates the formation of kinins, complement, and other inflammatory mediators.

Once factor Xa is generated, it forms a prothrombinase complex with factor Va, PL and Ca^{2+}, which cleaves prothrombin to thrombin. Factor V is similar to factor VIII in requiring activation by thrombin or factor Xa.[197] The mechanism by which factors V and VIII are initially activated remains unclear; nascent forms may have trace cofactor activity. Since factor V is stored in platelet alpha granules, the local concentrations of factor V at sites of platelet aggregation are much higher than in the plasma.[198] Newly formed thrombin dissociates from the PL surface and cleaves fibrinogen to yield fibrin monomers, which spontaneously polymerize. Thrombin activates factor VII, which cross-links the fibrin, increasing the clot's mechanical strength and resistance to fibrinolysis.[188] In addition to its direct actions in fibrin formation and clot stabilization, thrombin induces platelet aggregation, enhances the cofactor activity of factors V and VIII, and activates protein C (see below).

There are a number of plasma *anticoagulant proteins* that localize the coagulation process to the site of injury and thereby protect against generalized thromboses. One major anticoagulant mechanism involves a group of proteins (serpins) that irreversibly inhibit the serine proteases.[199] The two most important serpins are antithrombin III (AT-III) and heparin cofactor II, which account for approximately 75% and 20%, respectively, of thrombin-inhibiting activity in plasma. Although AT-III is the main thrombin inhibitor, it also can neutralize factors Xa, IXa, XIa, and XIIa, as well as kallikrein and plasmin.[192] Heparin produces a conformational change in AT-III that results in a 2,000-fold acceleration of the latter's inhibitory action. The luminal surface of endothelial cells expresses heparin sulfate proteoglycan, which also serves this function.[189] Heparin has no innate anticoagulant effect other than enhancing the action of other anticoagulant proteins. Heparin cofactor II functions similarly to AT-III and its actions are likewise accelerated by optimal heparin concentrations. Another endothelial glycosaminoglycan, dermaton sulfate, strongly accelerates inhibition of thrombin by heparin cofactor II, but not by AT-III.[200]

The second major plasma anticoagulant mechanism is provided by the protein C system.[201] Protein C, a liver-derived vitamin K–dependent protein, circulates as a serine protease zymogen. When thrombin is complexed to a protein on the luminal surface of endothelial cells called thrombomodulin, it activates protein C rather than its other substrates.[202, 203] The clotting of fibrinogen and activation of platelets, as well as factors V, VIII, and XIII, are all inhibited by binding of thrombin to thrombomodulin in a 1:1 complex. The subsequent activated protein C (APC) cleaves and inactivates factors Va and VIIIa in the presence of Ca^{2+} and PL. Thus, the formation of APC by thrombin-thrombomodulin is a powerful anticoagulant event, just as thrombin-induced activation of factors V and VIII is a powerful procoagulant event. The inhibition of factors Va and VIIIa by APC requires another vitamin K–dependent cofactor, protein S, which increases its affinity for PL surfaces and reverses the species-specificity of APC.[204] The fibrinolytic actions of APC are discussed below. Two different serpins, which form covalent complexes with and thus inactivate APC, have been isolated from human plasma, although their physiologic significance remains uncharacterized.[205]

The catalytic activity of the TF–factor VIIa complex for factor Xa is inhibited by a newly discovered protein called extrinsic pathway inhibitor (EPI).[195] Apparently EPI is first bound by factor Xa, and then EPI:Xa forms a complex with TF:VIIa that causes the latter to become nonfunctional. In this way, the concentration of factor Xa can modulate its own formation via the extrinsic pathway.

Fibrinolysis

The fibrinolytic system is activated simultaneously with coagulation and functions to prevent tissue ischemia which would result from the continued presence of fibrin clots.[206, 207] Fibrinolysis limits extension of the fibrin clot as well as providing a mechanism for fibrin removal.

The key *fibrinolytic protein*, plasmin, is formed from the circulating zymogen, plasminogen, by the action of several plasminogen activators (Fig. 11–3). Plasmin is a general proteolytic serine protease that hydrolyzes fibrinogen and fibrin with equal affinity and destroys factors V, VII, IX, XI, and XIIa. Plasmin is also capable of complement activation and generation of kinins.[207] For a number of reasons discussed later, physiologic plasmin activity is limited to its effect on fibrin.

The most physiologically relevant activator of plasminogen is t-PA, which is synthesized primarily by endothelial cells.[208] Both t-PA and plasminogen have a high avidity for fibrin, and the presence of fibrin strikingly enhances the activation rate of plasminogen by t-PA. This is mainly due to an increased affinity of fibrin-bound t-PA for plasminogen, resulting in formation of a ternary complex.[208] The cofactor activity of fibrin in the reaction between t-PA and plasminogen results in clot lysis primarily from within and largely avoids systemic generation of plasmin and widespread fibrinolysis, complement activation, and kinin generation. Stasis

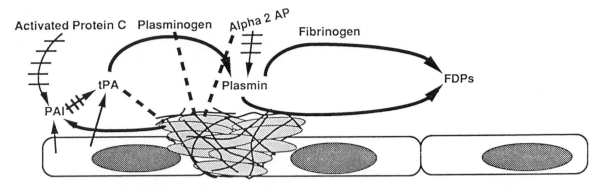

Figure 11–3. Plasmin is the key fibrinolytic protein, formed from plasminogen by tissue plasminogen activator *(t-PA)*. The actions of t-PA are controlled by plasminogen activator inhibitor *(PAI)*. Plasmin is inactivated by α_2-antiplasmin *(Alpha 2 AP)*. *Arrow*, primary pathway; *hatched arrow*, inhibition; *black dashed line*, bound for physiologic activity; FDPs = fibrin/fibrinogen degradation products.

upstream from an occluded vessel is the primary stimulus for t-PA release and the additional uptake of t-PA by the clot tips the balance of hemostasis toward fibrinolysis.[206] Effective in vivo thrombus dissolution requires continuous replacement of consumed plasmin by new plasminogen at the fibrin surface. Other enzymes capable of plasminogen activation do not have an affinity for fibrin and thus are not physiologically significant during fibrinolysis. The most notable of these is urokinase, present in normal urine and other tissues, which may be important for pericellular proteolysis involved in tissue remodeling and inflammatory processes. Although previously used as a thrombolytic agent in humans, streptokinase (a product of group C β-hemolytic streptococci) does not activate equine plasminogen.[209]

To insure localization of plasmin generation and subsequent activities to the fibrin clot, there is an efficient array of *antifibrinolytic proteins.* The plasma contains small amounts of a specific PAI that rapidly binds and inactivates physiologic concentrations of t-PA and urokinase.[210] Endothelial cells are the primary source of this type 1 PAI (PAI-1) in plasma, although the release of PAI-1 from platelet alpha granules during coagulation may play an important role in prevention of premature clot lysis. Another type of PAI (PAI-2) arises from the uterus and certain other cell types, but its significance during physiologic fibrinolysis remains unproven.[211]

The inhibition of plasmin activity in the blood is solely and instantaneously carried out by the serpin α_2-antiplasmin (AP).[192, 208] During coagulation, AP competes with plasminogen for binding to fibrin; thus a normal clot does not lyse spontaneously, despite fixation of some t-PA. With fixation of additional t-PA, as noted, plasmin formation proceeds at a rate that exceeds the inhibitory capacity of bound AP, allowing fibrinolysis to occur. Plasmin formed on the fibrin surface has its active site bound, thus is only slowly inactivated by plasma AP.[208] In physiologic states, fibrinolysis remains in dynamic equilibrium with blood coagulation to maintain an intact, patent vascular system. Numerous diseases are associated with dysfunction of normal hemostasis.

Vasculitis

Definition

Vasculitis is a general pathologic term that refers to inflammation of blood vessels of any type, in any location, regardless of cause.[212, 213] Vasculitis may be the primary process, or a component of some underlying disease. The category of diseases characterized by vasculitis is composed of heterogeneous syndromes with overlapping clinical and pathologic features. In human medicine, numerous classification schemes for vasculitic syndromes have emerged based upon clinical and pathologic findings as well as proposed etiology.[213, 214] Vasculitis in horses generally develops as a secondary manifestation of a primary infectious, toxic or neoplastic process and has characteristics of hypersensitivity vasculitis in humans.

Although the antigenic stimuli associated with this group of disorders vary, hypersensitivity vasculitides are characterized by predominant involvement of small blood vessels in the skin. In most cases the postcapillary venules are involved, although some syndromes (e.g., equine viral arteritis) affect the arterioles. The most common inflammatory pattern is *leukocytoclasis*, defined by the presence of neutrophilic nuclear debris in and around the involved vessels. Vessel wall necrosis and fibrinoid changes occur.

Clinical Signs and Laboratory Findings

In horses, vasculitis is characterized by well-demarcated areas of cutaneous edema that may involve any portion of the body.[215] The distal extremities and ventral body wall are most commonly affected and the edematous area is often hot and painful. Affected horses are generally depressed and reluctant to move. Hyperemia, petechial and ecchymotic hemorrhages, and ulcerations are commonly present on mucous membranes of the mouth, nose, vulva, etc. A host of other signs may reflect edema, hemorrhage, and infarction in other body systems. Lameness, colic, diarrhea, dyspnea, or ataxia can result from involvement of vessels in joints, muscles, gastrointestinal tract, respiratory tract, and central nervous system. Subclinical renal disease may occur. Secondary complications such as laminitis, thrombophlebitis, and localized infections are common. Affected skin often weeps serum and eventually sloughs.

Hematologic and serum biochemical findings in vasculitis are usually determined by the underlying disease, length of illness, other organ involvement, and secondary complications; none are characteristic. Chronic inflammation is usually attended by neutrophilia, mild anemia, hyperglobulinemia, and hyperfibrinogenemia. The platelet count is generally normal unless there is concomitant consumptive coagulopathy or immune-mediated thrombocytopenia. With renal involvement, serum creatinine may be elevated or urinalysis may reveal hematuria or proteinuria, or both.

Etiology and Pathogenesis

Equine diseases characterized by hypersensitivity vasculitis with predominant cutaneous involvement include equine purpura hemorrhagica (EPH), equine viral arteritis (EVA), equine infectious anemia (EIA), and equine ehrlichiosis (EE).[216] In addition, vasculitic syndromes for which the cause and clinical course are poorly defined occur in horses.[217, 218] The antigenic stimulus of hypersensitivity vasculitis is usually a microbe, drug, toxin, or foreign or endogenous protein[213] and vessel wall damage results from immunopathogenic mechanisms.[219] The deposition of circulating immune complexes with subsequent vessel wall damage is widely accepted as the major event in the pathogenesis of vasculitic syndromes.[212, 213, 221] Soluble immune complexes, formed in moderate antigen excess, become deposited in blood vessel walls in areas of increased permeability. The release of vasoactive amines from platelets or IgE-complexed mast cells has been suggested to cause areas of vessel wall permeability. PAF may also have a role. Deposited immune complexes activate complement with resultant formation of C5a, which is a potent chemotactic factor for neutrophils. Infiltrating neutrophils release lysosomal and other cytoplasmic enzymes, such as elastase and collagenase, that directly damage vessel walls. The net effect is vessel wall leakage and luminal compromise, which result in edema, hemorrhage, thrombosis, and ischemic changes in supplied tissues.

Aside from vessel wall necrosis, vasculitis results in vascular dysfunction characterized by a net increase in vasoconstriction and platelet aggregation, which contribute to tissue ischemia.[220] The diseased endothelium releases endothelin, a polypeptide that causes contraction of underlying smooth muscle,[222] and produces less dilator substances like endothelial-derived relaxing factor.[223] Injury to the vessel wall also results in diminished prostacyclin production, which usually serves to maintain vasodilation and platelet nonreactivity.[213] Thus, endothelial dysfunction contributes to ultimate vessel failure subsequent to vasculitis.

The factors that determine which individuals develop hypersensitivity vasculitis remain undefined. Genetic predisposition, altered immunoregulatory mechanisms, and the amount, relative size, and type of complement components in circulating immune complexes are very important in determining the potential risk of developing vasculitis, since these factors determine how quickly immune complexes are cleared by the MPS.[224] Maybe even more significant in this potential risk are genetic and acquired differences in the number and activity of receptors for complement and IgG on erythrocytes and macrophages. This can markedly affect immune complex handling and distribution.[221, 225] Receptors for complement and the Fc of IgG mediate immune complex transport to, and removal by, the macrophages of the MPS. Physical factors such as turbulence of blood flow, hydrostatic pressure within vessels, and previous endothelial damage likely determine the size, type, and location of blood vessels involved in vasculitis.[213] The propensity for lesion formation in skin of dependent body portions is likely due to the hydrostatic pressure in affected postcapillary venules in these areas.[213]

Diagnosis

The diagnosis of vasculitis rests on demonstration of typical histologic changes (e.g., leukocytoclasis, fibrinoid necrosis) in involved vessels. Full-thickness punch biopsies (≥ 6 mm in diameter) of skin in an affected area should be obtained and preserved in 10% formalin for histopathologic study. Samples saved in Michel's transport medium can subsequently be processed for immunofluorescence analysis to detect immune complexes.[226] Multiple biopsies from various sites are optimal in reaching a diagnosis since distribution of histologic lesions and immune complexes is patchy; however, affected skin is often on the distal limbs where there is increased risk of cellulitis or exuberant granulation tissue. The irregular distribution of histologic lesions, coupled with difficulty in obtaining biopsies, makes the definitive diagnosis of vasculitis difficult. Often vasculitis is diagnosed on clinical grounds based on history, signs, and response to therapy.

Specific Equine Vasculitic Syndromes

Equine purpura hemorrhagica is believed to be an allergic response to streptococci or antigens of the equine influenza virus. This vasculitic syndrome typically follows clinical signs of *Streptococcus equi* (strangles) infection by 2 to 4 weeks.[227] Sometimes EPH occurs without prior signs in a previously sensitized horse exposed to infected horses. Rarely, EPH may follow infections with *Streptococcus zooepidemicus* or influenza. Immune complexes containing IgA and the M protein of *S. equi* have been demonstrated in the serum of horses with EPH;[228] however, the disease is difficult to reproduce experimentally[229] and immunofluorescence studies have been performed in few natural cases.[230]

Classic signs of EPH are demarcated areas of edema on the limbs, ventral abdomen, head, and trunk, with mucosal petechial hemorrhages. Edema and hemorrhage of other tissues occasionally causes dysphagia, dyspnea, colic, lameness, or renal disease.[229–231] Hematologic study generally reflects chronic inflammation, as stated above. Some horses with EPH develop moderate anemia (packed cell volume, 20%–25%) which may be due to fluid shifts or increased erythrocyte destruction.[227] The diagnosis of EPH is based on appropriate history and clinical signs. Documentation of *leukocytoclastic* venulitis in the dermis and subcutaneous tissue supports the diagnosis. Although most horses with EPH respond to appropriate therapy (see below), some cases seem refractory. Deaths are usually secondary to laminitis or septic complications.

Equine viral arteritis is caused by a nonarthropod-borne togavirus classified in 1985 as the sole member of the genus *Arterivirus*.[232] Although there is only one serotype of the EVA virus, the pathogenicity of strains varies considerably. The virus is classically transmitted via inhalation of aerosolized secretions from an infected horse and widespread lateral transmission can occur between closely associated horses.[233] Subsequent to an epizootic of EVA in Kentucky in 1984, it became apparent that venereal transmission may play a significant role in EVA dissemination.[234] Infected stallions can remain carriers and shed virus in their semen from several weeks to several years.[235]

Exposure to the EVA virus may result in clinical disease of variable severity or an inapparent infection.[236, 237] The virus multiplies in macrophages and endothelial cells throughout the body and seems to have a predilection for the media of small muscular arteries. Although necrosis of arteries with a well-developed muscular coat is a unique lesion for EVA, inflammation of thin-walled vessels such as capillaries, veins, and lymphatics is more important in producing the clinical syndrome.[238] Clinical signs develop after an incubation period of 3 to 5 days and include any of the following: fever up to 41 °C, depression and anorexia, periorbital and palpebral edema with conjunctivitis, petechial hemorrhages, ocular and nasal discharge, edema of the legs and ventral abdomen, and respiratory distress.[237, 239] Host factors such as age and immunity and dose and pathogenicity of the virus account for the variation in severity of clinical manifestations. Pregnant mares seem to be most severely affected and up to 90% in the last trimester abort 3 to 8 weeks' post infection.[240] Abortions usually occur from 5 to 30 days after the mare's febrile response and may or may not be associated with other clinical signs.[239–241] Autolytic changes in the aborted fetuses are not consistently present. Other less common clinical signs of EVA include corneal opacity, coughing, diarrhea, icterus, ataxia, and dermatitis.[234, 236, 241] Leukopenia, primarily due to lymphopenia, usually accompanies the early febrile response.

The diagnosis of EVA is based on viral isolation or seroconversion. Appropriate samples for virus isolation include nasopharyngeal and conjunctival swabs, citrated blood samples, semen, and placental or fetal fluids. Samples should be collected early in the course of disease and transported on ice to an appropriate diagnostic facility. Serum antibodies to EVA are usually assayed using a complement-enhanced microtitration procedure.[237] A fourfold increase in titer in two samples collected 10 to 14 days apart is considered evidence of infection. A number of state diagnostic laboratories perform these tests. Affected horses usually make an uneventful recovery with only supportive care within 3 weeks. Infected stallions can remain persistent carriers and shedders of virus for an unpredictable period of time. Infection can be prevented by immunization of susceptible horses with a modified live vaccine at least 3 weeks prior to exposure to the virus.[236]

Infections with the *equine infectious anemia* virus often causes necrotizing vasculitis that affects the skin as well as a variety of other organ systems.[64, 76] The classic signs of EIA include fever, icterus, mucosal petechiae, ventral edema, anemia, and weight loss. A complete discussion of EIA can be found on p. 568. Diagnosis of equine infectious anemia is confirmed by an agar gel immunodiffusion (Coggins) test for serum antibodies to the EIA virus. Horses remain viremic for life.

Equine ehrlichiosis, caused by infection with the rickettsial agent *Ehrlichia equi*, is a vasculitic syndrome usually seen in horses from northern California.[242] Individual cases have been reported in other states, so the disease is not absolutely geographically restricted.[243] Clinical signs are more severe in horses over 3 years of age and characterized by fever, depression, anorexia, mucosal petechial hemorrhages, icterus, edema of the distal extremities, weakness, ataxia, and reluctance to move.[242] Hematologic examination often reveals mild-to-moderate leukopenia, thrombocytopenia, and anemia. Although not proven, ticks are the proposed vector for *E. equi*, which is antigenically distinct from the etiologic agent for Potomac horse fever (equine ehrlichial colitis), *Ehrlichia risticii*. The disease is often regionally distributed, but does not appear to be contagious since most cases are sporadic. Infection generally confers immunity for up to 2 years; this is not associated with the development of a carrier state. Diagnosis of EE is based on demonstration of typical pleomorphic inclusion bodies in the cytoplasm of circulating neutrophils and eosinophils. The inclusions stain bluish-gray on Giemsa-stained blood smears. Affected horses generally recover within 2 weeks with supportive care alone. Oxytetracycline 7 mg/kg IV once daily for 5 days often causes a prompt remission of clinical signs within 1 to 2 days of starting therapy and may be useful in aiding a clinical diagnosis.

Idiopathic vasculitic syndromes with an uncharacterized pathogenesis and unpredictable clinical course have been described in horses.[217, 218, 230] Clinical signs may include fever, weight loss, lameness, alopecia, hyperkeratosis, and hypopigmentation of the skin, with or without edema and hemorrhages in various parts of the body. Positive serology for rheumatoid factor or antinuclear antibody may indicate significant involvement of organ systems other than the skin. It is speculated that these idiopathic syndromes represent diseases similar to systemic necrotizing vasculitis in humans.[214, 220]

Treatment

The aims in the therapy of equine vasculitic syndromes are to (1) remove the antigenic stimulus if possible, (2) reduce vessel wall inflammation, (3) normalize the immune response, and (4) provide supportive care. Regardless of the cause, vasculitis in horses generally warrants aggressive nursing care, which should be instituted immediately. Edema can be minimized by hydrotherapy, and pressure wraps are useful on the limbs. Animals that become severely depressed and fail to drink or those with dysphagia due to pharyngeal edema require fluids, intravenously or via nasogastric tube. A tracheostomy may be necessary in horses with stridor and dyspnea secondary to edema of the upper respiratory tract. Phenylbutazone, flunixin meglumine, or other NSAIDs are indicated to reduce vascular inflammation and provide analgesia. Corticosteroid administration may also be warranted (see below). Antimicrobial therapy may reduce the incidence or severity of cellulitis or other septic sequelae.

Since no treatment effectively eliminates the viruses of EIA from the body, neither disease warrants specific therapy. Although EE will spontaneously resolve, elimination of the organism by oxytetracycline therapy considerably shortens the clinical course of disease.

When the cause is conjectural, vasculitis can be difficult to treat because the antigenic stimulus remains undefined and may not be easily eliminated. Any drug being used at the time that signs occur should be discontinued. A thorough search for an underlying infection or neoplasia is warranted. Horses with a recent history of strangles or that have been exposed to the disease should receive procaine penicillin G 22,000 units/kg, IM, q.12h. or potassium penicillin G IV q.6h. for at least 2 weeks. Accessible abscesses should be drained. Even though the sensitizing infection has usually resolved by the time there are signs of EPH, ongoing sepsis and antigen production will prolong the allergic vasculitis. The use of corticosteroids (mentioned above) for the treatment of hypersensitivity vasculitis remains controversial;[213] however, clinical experience suggests that horses with EPH or idiopathic vasculitic syndromes respond favorably to corticosteroid therapy.[227, 230]

Mild cases may resolve without immunosuppressive therapy, but life-threatening edema involving the upper respiratory tract or causing organ system dysfunction necessitates early aggressive corticosteroid treatment. Dexamethasone 0.05 to 0.2 mg/kg IV or IM q.12–24h. should be given at the dose and rate necessary to effect reduction in edema. Prednisolone 0.5 to 1.0 mg/kg IM q.12h. may be substituted for dexamethasone, but is often not as effective. Once edema and hemorrhages start to resolve, the corticosteroid dose can be gradually reduced (by 10%–15%, q.24–48h.) while the horse is carefully monitored for a relapse. It is not uncommon for horses with EPH to require corticosteroid therapy for a period of 4 to 6 weeks before edema permanently resolves.

Occasionally horses suffer disease flare-ups that require the corticosteroid dose to be increased over the previously efficacious level. In these instances, flunixin meglumine may enhance steroid efficacy. Once the dose of dexamethasone has been reduced to less than 0.05 mg/kg/day, it can usually be safely replaced by oral prednisone of an equivalent dose. Dexamethasone is approximately seven times more potent and has a half-life twice as long as prednisolone and prednisone (e.g., a dose of dexamethasone 20 mg, q.24h. is equivalent to 140 mg prednisone q.12h.). Antimicrobials are indicated throughout the period of systemic corticosteroid administration to reduce the incidence and severity of secondary sepsis.

Prognosis

The prognosis for vasculitis depends upon the initiating disease process. With early aggressive therapy and supportive care, most horses recover from EPH within 4 weeks, although numerous sequelae may prolong the convalescence. Dermal infarction in the distal limbs often leads to skin sloughing followed by exuberant granulation tissue. This may require excision followed by skin grafting. Laminitis and various infections such as cellulitis, pneumonia, colitis, and thrombophlebitis are common and may be complications of long-term corticosteroid therapy.

As stated above EVA and EE carry a good prognosis and disease confers some immunity to reinfection. Horses with EIA are persistently infected and may suffer recurrent clinical relapses. Horses with idiopathic vasculitic syndromes have an unpredictable response to therapy and some have a poor prognosis. Inadequate resolution of hypersensitivity

vasculitis in humans is usually due to failure to identify the antigenic stimulus or completely eliminate it from the body.[213] Although most cases undergo spontaneous remission, some have debilitating cutaneous disease or develop systemic necrotizing vasculitis with a poor prognosis.

Coagulation Dysfunction

Inability to form a stable fibrin clot that prevents loss of blood from the vasculature constitutes the basis for coagulation dysfunction. Disorders that produce coagulopathy are characterized by hemorrhagic diatheses of variable severity or the tendency for thrombus formation. The latter may be manifested clinically as organ failure or edema of tissue proximal to the obstruction, depending upon the type, size, and location of the occluded vessels.

Specific Diseases

Idiopathic Thrombocytopenia Purpura

ITP is an uncommon coagulation disorder characterized by an insufficient number of circulating platelets in the absence of other recognizable hemostatic dysfunction.[174, 244, 245] ITP is thought to be due to immune-mediated destruction of platelets in the MPS. Any age, sex, or breed of horse may be affected, although the syndrome seems to be more prevalent among young adult Thoroughbreds.

Clinical Signs and Laboratory Findings. Thrombocytopenia results in diffuse bleeding from small blood vessels and is characterized by petechial hemorrhages on the oral, nasal or vaginal (preputial) mucous membranes, and the nictitans or sclerae. Epistaxis, hyphema, occult melena, and hematuria are not uncommon. Spontaneous profuse hemorrhage is rare, but prolonged bleeding from injections or wounds and hematomas following minor trauma occurs when the platelet count drops below 20,000/μL.[244, 246] Other clinical signs are determined by the presence and nature of any underlying disease process. Horses with primary ITP are generally bright and appear clinically normal, often not manifesting overt hemorrhage despite severely reduced platelet numbers. Alternatively, horses with ITP secondary to sepsis or neoplasia seem particularly susceptible to hemorrhage.[170, 174]

Laboratory findings consistent with ITP include severe thrombocytopenia (<40,000/μL), prolonged bleeding time, and abnormal clot retraction. The prothrombin time (PT), activated partial thromboplastin time (APTT), and thrombin time (TT) are normal. The concentration of plasma fibrinogen is not reduced and may be increased owing to another disease process. Serum concentrations of fibrin or fibrinogen degradation products may be mildly increased (10–40 μg/mL). If the condition is chronic, anemia and hypoproteinemia may occur. Feces and urine are often positive for occult blood.

Etiology and Pathogenesis. The clinical course and therapeutic response of ITP in horses resembles similar syndromes in humans[247, 248] and dogs,[249–251] wherein antibodies coat the platelet surface and mediate the phagocytic destruction of platelets by cells of the MPS. The platelet-associated immunoglobulin in primary ITP is usually complement-fixing IgG, produced principally in the spleen and directed against a platelet membrane antigen.[248] These IgG- and complement-coated platelets are removed prematurely from the circulation by mononuclear phagocytes via the Fc and C3 receptors. Platelets heavily coated with antibodies are cleared primarily by the liver, whereas lightly coated platelets are destroyed in the spleen, and complement-coated platelets may be removed by both.[252] The mean half-life of circulating platelets and the platelet count are inversely proportional to the quantity of platelet-associated IgG and complement components. Macrophages activated by infection or neoplasia have an increased number and avidity of receptors for Fc of IgG and C3, which results in an increased rate of platelet destruction. The spleen seems to be the major site of platelet phagocytosis since 30% of the platelet mass is normally present in the spleen, antiplatelet antibody is secreted locally, and the stagnant splenic blood flow allows sensitized platelets to pass slowly through a dense network of phagocytic cells.[245, 248] Less commonly in humans, ITP may be associated with platelet-directed IgM, and the subsequent binding of complement by IgM may initiate platelet clearance by the MPS.[247, 253, 254]

Despite the fact that megakaryocyte numbers generally increase as a compensatory response to ITP, there is evidence in humans that autoantibodies may cause decreased platelet production in addition to increased destruction.[255] ITP and decreased megakaryocyte numbers have been reported in horses.[256] Antibodies may cause megakaryocyte destruction or prevent newly formed platelets from entering the circulation. The potential mechanisms for autoantibody production include suppressor T-cell dysfunction, increased self-reactive inducer T-cell activity, abnormal response of B cells to T-cell regulation, and stimulation of autoreactive B-cell clones by infectious or inflammatory states.[257]

Secondary ITP results from nonspecific binding of immune complexes to the platelet surface via platelet Fc receptors. Antigenic stimuli for secondary ITP include bacterial infections, viral diseases, other systemic immune-mediated disorders, neoplasia, or the administration of certain drugs.[174] Thrombocytopenia has been reported in horses secondary to EIA,[64] lymphosarcoma,[150, 170] and autoimmune hemolytic anemia.[174] Drugs implicated in the pathogenesis of human ITP that are commonly used in horses include phenylbutazone, aspirin, heparin, quinidine, digoxin, rifampin, penicillin, erythromycin, sulfa drugs, tetracycline, and gold salts.[245] The foreign antigen that perpetuates ITP is either being constantly replenished or is difficult to excrete. Drug-induced ITP generally abates within days after the offending agent is discontinued, unless the thrombocytopenia is secondary to systemic gold therapy. Whether due to the slow release of tissue-bound gold or induction of true autoimmunity, ITP associated with chrysotherapy may persist weeks to years after drug withdrawal.[249]

The bleeding diathesis posed by thrombocytopenia is caused by insufficiency of numerous hemostatic functions provided by platelets (see p. 577).

Diagnosis. Clinical evidence of small blood vessel hemorrhage and severe thrombocytopenia in a horse with normal coagulation times (PT, APTT) and neutrophil count are sufficient for the presumptive diagnosis of ITP. Response to corticosteroid therapy (see Treatment) adds support to the diagnosis. Definitive diagnosis of immune-mediated thrombocytopenia requires demonstration of increased platelet-associated Ig or C3; however, methods used to detect antibody and complement on platelet membranes[250, 255, 258] have not been developed for horses. The platelet factor 3 immunoinjury technique has been used in horses as an indirect indicator of plasma antiplatelet antibodies,[259] but results of this test have a very poor correlation with clinical evidence of equine ITP.[246] This test is not used in humans because of its low sensitivity. The bone marrow in horses with ITP generally shows evidence of hyperplasma,[174, 246] although lack of marrow megakaryocytes has been reported.[256]

Profound thrombocytopenia in a horse with minimal evidence of hemorrhage should be reevaluated. Spuriously low platelet counts can result from improper blood collection, inadequate volume of anticoagulant, or platelet clumping in ethylenediaminetetraacetic acid (EDTA).[260–263] The mechanism of platelet agglutination in EDTA is unknown, but in humans the phenomenon seems to be mediated by a blood protein fraction, somehow related to fibrinogen.[263] In some cases, this protein appears to be IgM or IgG against unidentified platelet antigens that is maximally reactive at lower temperatures in the presence of reduced calcium concentrations or EDTA.[260, 262] EDTA-induced platelet clumping is reported to be most prevalent in patients with prolonged severe illness.[261, 263] When pseudothrombocytopenia is suspected, the platelet count should be determined on two blood samples collected at the same time, one anticoagulated with EDTA and the other with 3.8% sodium citrate. If the platelet count on the sample prepared with citrate (corrected for dilution) is considerably higher than that from the test tube with EDTA, pseudothrombocytopenia is likely. A smear prepared from the EDTA-anticoagulated blood should demonstrate platelet clumping.[261]

Treatment. The approach to, and rationale of, initial treatment for ITP are very similar to those outlined for IMHA (see p. 565). Any medication should be stopped or replaced by the chemically most dissimilar substitute. Most cases of drug-induced ITP rapidly improve in the absence of the sensitizing agent. In the unlikely event of life-threatening hemorrhage, a transfusion of fresh whole blood (8–16 mL/kg body weight), platelet-rich plasma, or platelet concentrate should be administered (see Blood and Plasma Therapy). Platelet-rich plasma can be manually produced by centrifugation of fresh blood collected in acid-citrate-dextrose solution 3 to 5 minutes at 250 × g.[174] Any contact of blood with glass should be minimized to prevent platelet adhesion and activation. Platelet-rich blood components may also be produced by continuous flow centrifugation thrombocytopheresis using a continuous flow blood cell separator.[264] Approximately 8×10^{11} platelets are contained in 300 mL of normal equine platelet-rich plasma, which could theoretically raise the platelet count of a 500-kg horse by approximately 30,000/μL, sufficient to normalize hemostasis. Blood and plasma components should always be held at 4° C, but storage for longer than 6 hours is attended by a rapid loss of hemostatic activity.

Horses with suspected ITP generally respond favorably to corticosteroids, used as prescribed for IMHA. In addition to their effects on the immune response and MPS clearance, corticosteroids improve capillary integrity and increase thrombocytopoiesis.[245] Dexamethasone 0.05 to 0.2 mg/kg IM or IV daily usually results in an increase in the platelet count within 4 to 7 days, although full benefit may not be evident for 1 to 3 weeks. Once the platelet count is greater than 100,000/μL, the dosage of dexamethasone can be decreased by 0.01 mg/kg/day while monitoring the platelet count closely for a relapse. Prednisolone (initial dose 1 mg/kg IM q12h.) may be used in lieu of dexamethasone; however, some horses appear only to be sensitive to the immunosuppressive effects of dexamethasone.[174, 216] Corticosteroids should not be discontinued until the platelet count has been normal for at least 5 days. If the period of necessary glucocorticoid administration has extended beyond 2 weeks, alternate-morning low-dose therapy (dexamethasone 0.01 mg/kg or prednisolone 0.07 mg/kg) should be continued for 10 more days to prevent iatrogenic hypoadrenocorticism.

Alternative methods of treating ITP in horses are largely unproven since so few cases are refractory to corticosteroids. Splenectomy to remove the major site of platelet destruction, as well as a large source of antiplatelet antibodies, is successful in some people[245, 265] and dogs[266, 267] with ITP. Splenectomy has been used to treat ITP in horses, but the long-term outcome remains to be documented. Postsplenectomy sepsis is a large potential drawback to this procedure.

Cytotoxic drugs are moderately successful for treating ITP in humans[245] and dogs[267, 268] refractory to corticosteroids and splenectomy. The vinca alkaloids (vincristine and vinblastine) appear to increase platelet production as well as induce immunosuppression. Vincristine[2] 0.01–0.025 mg/kg IV every 7 days, combined with glucocorticoids, has been successfully used in horses that were refractory to corticosteroids alone.[244] There are no data regarding the effect of azathioprine and cyclophosphamide in equine ITP. Cytotoxic drugs can induce severe bone marrow suppression and increase susceptibility to sepsis; therefore, they should be used with extreme caution in horses, and only after 10 days of non-response to corticosteroids.

Remission (both short-term and complete) of ITP has been reported in humans given concentrated gammaglobulin 200–1,000 mg/kg/day IV for 2–5 days.[269, 270] The large dose of immunoglobulins may block Fc receptor-mediated phagocytosis, sterically hinder antibody binding, enhance suppressor T-cell function, and reduce B-cell function. Although this high-dose immunoglobulin therapy carries much less risk than splenectomy or cytotoxic drugs, at least 80 L of plasma would be necessary to achieve the total Ig dose for a 500-kg horse. This expense is obviously prohibitive for most equine patients.

Client Education. Most horses with ITP recover within 3 to 4 weeks if treated appropriately. This suggests that many cases are secondary, yet the initiating cause is rarely found. Horses with EIA[64] or underlying neoplasia[170] obviously have a poor prognosis since the primary disease is incurable. Chronic, recurrent primary ITP, requiring prolonged corticosteroid therapy, has been reported in horses.[246]

Disseminated Intravascular Coagulation

Also called consumption coagulopathy, defibrination syndrome, or intravascular coagulation or fibrinolysis, DIC is the most common form of hemostatic dysfunction in horses.[108] DIC is defined as a pathologic activation of coagulation that causes microvasculature clotting and may lead to a hemorrhagic diathesis subsequent to consumption of procoagulants or the action of fibrinolytic byproducts.[271–274] Practically, DIC may be regarded as a state of intermittent or continuous activation of coagulation, the duration and manifestations of which are dependent upon the strength of the initial stimulus.[275] Never a primary disorder, DIC represents an intermediary mechanism of some underlying disease. Disease processes in horses known to be associated with DIC include localized or systemic sepsis,[276] systemic neoplasia,[276] hemolytic anemia,[69] enteritis and colitis,[69, 277] and numerous other gastrointestinal disorders that cause colic.[278–281]

Clinical Signs and Laboratory Findings. Because of the heterogeneity of initiating diseases and the dynamic nature of DIC, clinical manifestations range from diffuse thrombosis and ischemic organ failure to a severe hemorrhagic diathesis. Clinical syndromes associated with DIC have been termed "consumptive thrombohemorrhagic disorders."[282] In horses, DIC is manifest more as a thrombotic disorder than one causing massive hemorrhage.[108]

Clinical manifestations depend upon the organ involved and the degree of hypoperfusion. Renal afferent arteriolar obstruction produces ischemic cortical necrosis leading to azotemia. Clinical signs of renal dysfunction include oliguria and polyuria, depression, and ileus. Acute renal failure poses a serious threat to life and contributes greatly to the morbidity and mortality of the primary disease process. Gastrointestinal microthrombosis during DIC may induce colic, complicating the clinical picture in horses with primary gastrointestinal disease. Any gastrointestinal hemorrhage is usually occult and rarely causes melena. Digital microthrombosis with ischemia frequently accompanies DIC in horses and may play a key role in the development of acute laminitis.[283] Laboratory evidence of DIC has been documented during the developmental phase of laminitis[284, 285] and the prevalence of laminitis among horses with endotoxemia or sepsis,[283] along with histopathologic evidence of digital microvascular thrombosis,[286] implicates coagulation dysfunction in the pathogenesis.

The tendency for thrombosis of peripheral veins is another prominent manifestation of coagulation dysfunction in horses.[108] Sometimes a jugular vein will undergo complete thrombosis within hours of a routine blood sampling procedure. Spontaneous thrombosis of smaller cutaneous vessels also occurs. Pulmonary microthrombosis may rarely cause tachypnea and hypoxemia. Altered consciousness, delirium, convulsions, or coma may follow cerebral microvascular thrombosis, although these signs are not specific nor are they highly indicative of DIC in horses. Because DIC is so frequently initiated by conditions that cause colic, and horses may display abnormal behavior in response to pain, the incidence of cerebral dysfunction in horses with DIC is difficult to estimate. Although reported, microangiopathic hemolysis, hemoglobinemia, and hemoglobinuria are rare in horses with DIC.[106]

Depending upon the rate of DIC, platelet and clotting factor depletion and the generation of fibrinolytic byproducts cause the tendency for hemorrhage. Petechial or ecchymotic hemorrhage on mucous membranes and sclerae and the tendency to bleed following venipuncture or minor trauma are the principal signs. Spontaneous epistaxis, hyphema, and melena occur less commonly. Life-threatening hemorrhage is rare in horses with DIC, unless there is initiating trauma (e.g., nasogastric intubation).

Numerous tests of hemostasis may be abnormal during DIC, reflecting generalized activation of the coagulation mechanism. Unfortunately, none constituently nor specifically indicate the presence of DIC.[108, 207, 278, 287–292] Excessive coagulation causes reduced plasma concentrations of platelets, coagulation proteins, and anticoagulants, while secondary increased fibrinolysis results in elevated fibrin degradation products (FDPs) and reduced concentrations of fibrinolytic and antifibrinolytic proteins. Laboratory changes of DIC include thrombocytopenia and prolonged PT, APTT, TT, and activated coagulation time (ACT); reduced plasma concentrations of fibrinogen, factor V, factor VIII, AT-III, plasminogen, and α_2-antiplasmin; and increased serum concentrations of FDPs and soluble fibrin monomer. None of these changes are consistently present or uniquely specific for DIC, since the latter is a heterogeneous dynamic process and blood concentrations of cells and proteins that are directly or indirectly measured by these hemostatic function tests are also influenced by the rate of synthesis, catabolism, and loss by other routes. One consistent feature of DIC is the presence of multiple hemostatic abnormalities. Serial analyses of hemostatic data should reveal reduced platelet numbers and a trend toward prolongation of the PT, APTT, TT, and ACT.

Etiology and Pathogenesis. Disease processes that trigger DIC either generate excessive procoagulant activity within the blood or cause abnormal surfaces to contact blood. Procoagulant substances released or generated by diseases that initiate DIC include TF, PLs, ADP, leukocyte procoagulant activity (PCA), PAF, and tumor products that directly activate clotting factors. Endothelial disruption by certain diseases (e.g., vasculitis) exposes collagen, which may directly activate platelets and the intrinsic coagulation pathway. Substantial vascular compromise allows TF to enter the blood. Diseases may act by multiple mechanisms to induce the overwhelming stimulus needed to trigger DIC. The nature and intensity of the procoagulant force, the concentration of natural coagulation inhibitors, and the functional capacity of the MPS, all play vital roles in determining whether an individual with a given disease process develops DIC.

The most common disorders associated with DIC in horses are gastrointestinal diseases that cause colic[277–280] and bacterial sepsis.[108, 276] Endotoxemia is the pathophysiologic mechanism common to both. Endotoxins, the lipopolysaccharide (LPS) portion of gram-negative bacterial cell walls, are released by death or rapid proliferation of the bacteria and initiate severe morbidity and mortality if they gain access to the blood. The equine gastrointestinal tract normally contains a large quantity of luminal endotoxins, only a small amount of which are absorbed into the portal blood and then removed by the liver. Conditions that cause intestinal ischemia, mucosal edema, and endothelial disruption result in increased endotoxin absorption, which overcomes Kupffer cell clearance capacity and allows LPS to access the

peripheral circulation. Intestinal strangulating obstruction, thromboembolic infarction, and severe colitis are commonly associated with endotoxemia.[293, 294] The proliferation of gram-negative bacteria within tissues and the blood is also accompanied by endotoxemia, and gram-negative sepsis is a frequent initiator of DIC in both humans[292, 295] and animals.[296, 297]

Endotoxins induce hemostatic dysfunction by numerous mechanisms,[189, 298, 299] which, if they remain unchecked, culminate in DIC (Fig. 11–4).[294, 295, 300–302] Endotoxins can directly activate factor XII[303] and cause extensive endothelial cell damage exposing collagen, which activates the intrinsic pathway. Endothelial cell damage can also release TF, which initiates the extrinsic pathway.[189] Activated neutrophils, complement components and macrophage products, IL-1, and TNF are all involved in endotoxin-induced endothelial perturbation.[189] Platelets are stimulated to release TXA_2, which promotes platelet aggregation.[188]

Probably the most important mediators of endotoxin-induced coagulopathy are released from stimulated leukocytes and macrophages. A PCA that functions identically to TF is produced by monocytes and macrophages in response to endotoxins,[304–306] and this PCA has been characterized in equine monocytes.[307] Endotoxin-stimulated granulocytes and macrophages release a PAF which augments the numerous contributions of platelets to coagulation.[308] Equine platelets are highly sensitive to PAF, further substantiating its role in equine coagulopathy.[309] Other macrophage products, particularly IL-1[310] and TNF,[311] amplify the procoagulant actions of LPS. Endothelial cells, perturbed by LPS or macrophage mediators, do not express the same amount of heparin-like activity of thrombomodulin as do normal cells, causing the anticoagulant actions of AT-III and protein C to be reduced.[189] Finally, endotoxemia causes an overall inhibition of fibrinolysis associated with increased production and plasma concentrations of PAI,[210, 312–314] and downregulation of protein C.[189, 201]

Endotoxemia is not the only mechanism by which sepsis triggers DIC.[277, 290, 315] Circulating antigen-antibody complexes during any infectious disease can cause endothelial damage as well as directly activate factor XII. Tissue destruction during the inflammatory process may result in TF release or PCA production by activated leukocytes. Any triggering mechanism for DIC produces the systemic generation of excess thrombin and plasmin. The major role of thrombin in hemostasis is the proteolytic cleavage of fibrinogen to fibrin monomers that subsequently polymerize to form the fibrin clot. However, thrombin also activates factor XIII to render fibrin more resistant to fibrinolysis, enhances the cofactor activity of factors Va and VIIIa, induces platelet aggregation, and enhances the exposure of platelet PL.[192] The results of exaggerated thrombin formation are widespread fibrin deposition in the microcirculation, circulatory obstruction, and organ hypoperfusion, which may lead to ischemic necrosis and failure.

AT-III and the protein C system inhibit the actions of thrombin; however, they may become depleted during acute DIC.[288, 289, 316] Fibrinopeptides A and B, liberated by the action of thrombin on fibrinogen, induce systemic vasoconstriction, which compounds hypoperfusion and eventual organ failure. Polymerized fibrin entraps platelets, enhancing their consumption, and damages red blood cells. Microangio-

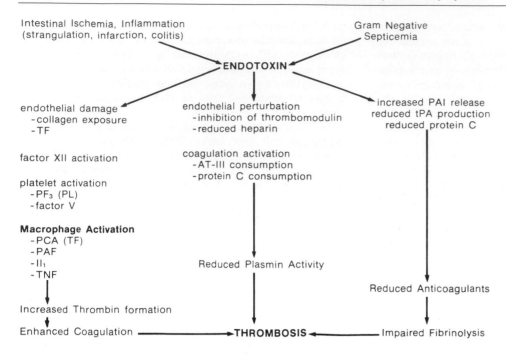

Figure 11–4. This figure depicts the various means by which endotoxin induces hemostatic dysfunction. The net effect is procoagulant producing the tendency for thrombosis. *AT III*, antithrombin III; *II₁*, interleukin-1; *PAF*, platelet activating factor; *PCA*, procoagulant activity; *PF₃*, platelet factor 3; *PL*, phospholipid; *TF*, tissue factor; *t-PA*, tissue plasminogen activator; *TNF*, tumor necrosis factor; *PAI*, plasminogen activator inhibitor. (From Morris DD: Thrombophlebitis in horses: The contribution of hemostatic dysfunction to pathogenesis. *Compendium Continuing Educ Pract Vet* 11:1386–1395, 1989.)

pathic hemolysis provides ADP and PL to continue the process of DIC.

Excessive thrombin generation is linked to the systemic generation of plasmin via t-PA release from underperfused tissues and interaction between factor XIIa and prekallikrein. The resultant FDPs have antithrombin activity, interfere with fibrin monomer polymerization, and cause platelet dysfunction,[317] thereby predisposing to hemorrhage. Paradoxically, the combination of clotting factor consumption and fibrinolysis potentiates bleeding at the same time that disseminated thromboses occur.

Hemostasis is intimately related to other plasma protein enzyme systems that contribute to the pathophysiologic manifestations of DIC. Factor XIIa is responsible for the generation of kallikrein, which not only converts plasminogen to plasmin but produces kinins from kininogen. Kinins cause pain and hypotension and increase vascular permeability, contributing to shock and reduced organ perfusion. Plasmin activates the C1 and C3, which are capable of mediating cytolysis, and multiple immunologic phenomena. The MPS has a vital, often overlooked role in the pathogenesis of DIC. The tissue-fixed macrophages of the spleen and liver normally remove activated clotting factors and FDPs from the peripheral circulation, and the latter are increased only when their rate of formation exceeds the ability of the MPS to clear them. Shock and hypoperfusion of the liver and spleen, or diseases associated with excessive tissue debris (e.g., sepsis, metastatic neoplasia), will reduce the function of the MPS and predispose to, or perpetuate, DIC. The thrombotic events of DIC may eventually cause MPS failure and a positive feedback "circular pathophysiology."

Diagnosis. Numerous tests of hemostatic function may be abnormal during the genesis of coagulopathy, but no one test result consistently or specifically indicates the presence of DIC. Laboratory criteria for the diagnosis of DIC are extremely arbitrary and must always be interpreted in light of

the patient's underlying disease process.[273] For example, plasma fibrinogen and factor VIII are rarely decreased in horses with DIC since the chronic infectious or inflammatory processes that predispose to coagulopathy usually cause increased synthesis of these acute phase reactants.[108] Clinical signs and specific situations suggest the possibility of DIC, and laboratory data only provide support.

The combination of thrombocytopenia with prolongation of the PT and APTT strongly suggests the presence of DIC in horses. Thrombocytopenia is a sensitive indicator of severe DIC in most species,[296] but patients with chronic compensated coagulopathy may have normal platelet numbers.[282, 289] Thrombocytopenia is not specific for DIC since it may also occur with ITP, bone marrow aplasia, or myelophthisic disease. These latter conditions are not associated with other abnormalities of hemostatic function (e.g., PT, APTT). PT is a crude measure of the extrinsic and common coagulation pathways, becoming prolonged in humans when factors V, VII, or X are less than 50% of normal values.[272] This test is less sensitive to defects of prothrombin and fibrinogen.[318] APTT assesses the function of the intrinsic and common pathways, becoming prolonged when factors VIII, IX, XI, XII, or prekallikrein are 30% of normal or less. APTT may be falsely prolonged by inhibitors such as FDPs or heparin, which can be documented by correction of the abnormality by diluting one part of the patient's plasma with one part of normal control plasma.[319] TT becomes prolonged with severe hypofibrinogenemia, dysfibrinogenemia, and in the presence of thrombin inhibitors such as FDPs and heparin. TT is often prolonged in horses with DIC, despite normal or high plasma fibrinogen.[278] This is probably due to the inhibitory effects of FDPs or soluble fibrin monomers.[319] Clotting times are very insensitive to coagulation factor deficiencies, and thus are usually only prolonged late in the genesis of hemostatic dysfunction.

Unlike humans, adult horses with DIC rarely develop

hypofibrinogenemia.[108, 276, 278, 281, 319] Because infection or inflammation generally initiates coagulopathy in horses, the acute phase hepatic response to increased fibrinogen synthesis probably compensates for consumptive loss.[276, 282] The metabolic events that constitute the acute phase response are elicited by products of activated macrophages, particularly IL-1,[320] TNF,[321] and IL-6.[322] Endotoxins are potent macrophage inducers,[323] so hemostatic dysfunction secondary to endotoxemia is often associated with hyperfibrinogenemia.[108, 281, 319, 324] Hypofibrinogenemia has only been reported in horses with fulminant hepatic failure.[107]

Increased serum FDPs reflect the proteolytic action of plasmin on fibrin (locally) or fibrinogen (systemically) at a rate that exceeds FDP clearance by the MPS.[207] The commercially available test kit[3] does not distinguish the lytic byproducts of fibrin from those of fibrinogen; therefore, fibrinolysis localized to the microcirculation cannot be differentiated from systemic fibrinolysis. Hyperfibrinolysis with FDPs greater than 40 μg/mL usually indicates DIC,[282] but the absence of FDPs does not rule out a coagulopathy since there may be MPS compensation or degradation of FDPs to undetectable forms. An elevation in FDPs is a late manifestation of DIC in horses. FDPs are often not increased during the initial activation of hemostasis.[278, 279] Severe inflammation, localized intravascular coagulation, or other hemorrhagic disorders, like ITP, can increase serum FDPs, although the concentrations in these conditions rarely exceed 40 μg/mL.[174, 325]

Since the aforementioned tests have low sensitivity or specificity for detecting subclinical coagulopathy in horses, a number of other hemostatic system components have been evaluated.[108, 278, 307, 324] Factor assays rarely provide significantly more information than the clotting times. Factors V and VIII are reported to be most reduced during DIC in humans[207, 274] because they are rendered unstable by thrombin[272] and digested by plasmin,[207] in addition to being consumed during coagulation. This is not a consistent finding,[282, 303] as clotting factor concentrations may be normal, decreased, or even increased during DIC, depending upon its rate and severity as well as the adequacy of compensatory mechanisms. Factor VIII is another acute phase reactant that may be increased by inflammatory states like endotoxemia. Ponies developed significantly increased plasma factor VIII during chronic activation of hemostasis by colitis.[324] Reduced plasma AT-III seems to be a sensitive indicator of DIC in humans;[214, 289, 326] however, it is also reduced by liver disease, protein-losing diseases, protein catabolic states, and certain drugs.[289, 326] Although correlated with activation of hemostasis in adult horses, reduced plasma AT-III activity seems not to be as sensitive in the early identification of coagulopathy as in other species.[278, 327] Horses with liver disease often have increased plasma AT-III activity, suggesting that it may behave as an acute phase reactant in adult horses.[328]

Hyperfibrinolysis, secondary to hemostatic activation, may result in reduced plasma concentrations of plasminogen and antiplasmin.[192, 289] These changes are not specific for DIC since they have been identified in humans with severe liver disease or during thrombolytic therapy.[329] Alternatively, their increased consumption may be masked by accelerated synthesis during neoplasia, chronic inflammation, or thrombotic disease.[329, 330] Adult horses normally have lower plasma plasminogen concentrations than do other species,[331] but plasminogen actually rose during a chronic procoagulant stimulus in ponies,[324] suggesting that plasminogen may function as an acute phase reactant. On the other hand, antiplasmin was significantly reduced in these ponies, suggesting that it may be utilized in excess of synthesis during chronic coagulopathy in horses.[324]

Reduced plasma concentrations of protein C have been associated with liver disease, DIC, respiratory distress syndrome, and postsurgical states in humans.[201] Assays have been developed for equine protein C and normal values for adult horses have been generated.[332, 333] Research is currently under way to evaluate the significance of protein C in adult horses with hemostatic dysfunction.[333] Since DIC is a dynamic process, serial monitoring of hemostatic data may enable its earlier diagnosis and differentiation from disease processes not characterized by multiple abnormalities of hemostasis such as ITP and warfarin toxicosis.

Treatment. Therapy of DIC is highly controversial, and the only widely accepted modalities are those directed at identification and treatment of the primary disorder, along with general supportive measures to combat shock and maintain tissue perfusion.[108, 188, 272, 282] Intravenous fluid administration helps to prevent organ dysfunction subsequent to microvascular thrombosis and can correct existing acid-base or electrolyte imbalances. Septic conditions require appropriate antimicrobial therapy. Necrotic tissue and purulent exudate should be removed whenever possible. Strangulating intestinal obstruction necessitates immediate surgical intervention to resect nonviable bowel. Because endotoxemia commonly promotes DIC in horses, treatment to alleviate the deleterious effects of LPS is indicated. Flunixin meglumine reduces eicosanoid generation during endotoxemia at a dosage (0.25 mg/kg IV q.8h.) that has minimal analgesic action, thus not masking clinical signs.[334] Corticosteroids are not indicated and may even worsen DIC[274] since they (1) reduce the phagocytic action of the MPS, which allows FDPs and activated clotting factors to accumulate in the circulation, and (2) potentiate the vasoconstrictor effects of catecholamines.

Once specific or supportive measures have been taken to treat the primary disorder, a clinical judgment must be made to determine whether these will sustain the patient and allow time for spontaneous resolution of DIC. Fresh plasma administration (15–30 mL/kg) to replace utilized coagulant, anticoagulant, or fibrinolytic proteins has been suggested if there is life-threatening hemorrhage.[188, 273, 335] The argument has been advanced, however, that plasma therapy may "fuel" the coagulation process and cause additional organ impairment.[336] Consequently, some authors have suggested concomitant heparin administration to prevent further thromboses.[188, 301] In humans, the consequences of continued hemorrhage outweigh the chance of additional fibrin deposition. Controlled studies have not been performed in horses of any age. There are reports of significant side effects of heparin use in horses.[337–340] Encouraging results have been obtained using concentrates of AT-III to treat DIC in humans.[341] Because AT-III is often depleted in humans with DIC, and heparin's anticoagulant activity depends upon the presence of AT-III, supplementation of AT-III may be valuable to prevent thromboses.[301] Pretreatment of rats solely with AT-III prior to development of septic shock significantly ameliorated DIC and dramatically increased survival.[342] In a similar study, AT-III caused a significant improvement in endotoxin-induced coagulopathy in dogs.[343]

Since plasma concentration of protein C is reduced in some individuals with DIC,[316, 344] it seems reasonable to administer protein C therapeutically. In a baboon model of septicemia, infusion of exogenous protein C at the same time as a lethal dose of *Escherichia coli* prevented coagulopathic, hepatotoxic, and lethal effects of the bacteria.[345] Because the clinical manifestations of coagulopathy in horses are more often due to disseminated thrombosis than to hemorrhage,[108] concentrates of AT-III and protein C may be useful in DIC. At this point these plasma components are not commercially available. Experience with horses suggests that aggressive therapy of the primary disease is the most effective treatment for DIC.[108] Since DIC is a dynamic process, serial monitoring of hemostatic data may enable its earlier diagnosis and differentiation from disease processes not characterized by multiple abnormalities of hemostasis, such as ITP and warfarin toxicosis.

Client Education. The prognosis for DIC in horses depends upon the nature and severity of the primary disease process and how early and effectively the latter is treated. Mild cases of DIC associated with gastrointestinal-induced endotoxemia generally resolve. However, debilitating sequelae such as laminitis or renal failure may result in the horse's ultimate demise. Once DIC has progressed to the stage at which blood incoagulability predominates, the prognosis is generally grave.

Warfarin Toxicosis

Horses may rarely develop coagulation dysfunction subsequent to *warfarin toxicosis.* This coumarin derivative anticoagulant is used therapeutically in some horses to treat navicular disease[346] and is a rodenticide in grains and other feedstuffs to which horses may be exposed.[41]

Clinical Signs and Laboratory Findings. Warfarin-induced coagulopathy is usually manifested by mucosal ecchymotic hemorrhages, hematomas, epistaxis, melena, and anemia.[41] Petechial hemorrhages do not occur. Owing to the short half-life of factor VII, the earliest laboratory indication of warfarin toxicosis is prolongation of PT. As the disease progresses, APTT becomes prolonged and horses develop anemia and hypoproteinemia due to chronic blood loss.

Etiology and Pathogenesis. Therapeutic amounts of warfarin may become toxic by a cumulative effect if there is concurrent use of highly protein-bound drugs or there is a dietary alteration that contains less vitamin K. Warfarin, as well as other coumarin derivatives, acts as an antagonist of the enzyme responsible for regeneration of the active form of vitamin K, which is necessary for liver production of clotting factors II, VII, IX, and X.[42, 48] Without vitamin K, hepatic γ-glutamyl carboxylase is unable to incorporate the necessary γ-carboxyglutamic acid into factors II, VII, IX, and X.[347, 348] Subsequently, functional prothrombinase cannot be produced and hemostasis is impaired. Factors VII, IX, X, and XI have increasingly greater half-lives; therefore, factor VII of the extrinsic system is the first to become depleted by warfarin toxicosis, causing prolongation of PT within 36 hours of toxicosis. Over the next 2 to 3 days, factors II, IX, and X become deficient.

Warfarin is rapidly absorbed from the gastrointestinal tract,[349] then highly bound to plasma proteins. This protein-bound portion of warfarin is pharmacologically inactive, but acts as a reservoir for the free drug. Drugs that are normally protein-bound, most notably phenylbutazone and chloral hydrate, can greatly enhance the toxicity of warfarin by allowing a greater proportion to be circulating in the unbound form. Similarly, hypoalbuminemia can increase the propensity for warfarin toxicosis. Hormones such as T_4 and corticosteroids lower the necessary therapeutic dose of warfarin by enhancing receptor affinity, as well as increasing clotting factor catabolism. Rapid withdrawal of drugs that induce hepatic microsomal enzyme metabolism, such as rifampin, chloramphenicol, and barbiturates, without altering the administered dose of warfarin can also potentiate toxicosis because warfarin metabolism is enhanced by these drugs. Finally, any hepatic dysfunction or reduced content of dietary vitamin K (e.g., good- to poor-quality roughage) can precipitate warfarin toxicosis. The concomitant use of heparin and aspirin may be synergistic in promoting hemorrhage.

Diagnosis. Warfarin toxicosis is diagnosed by history of exposure, a hemorrhagic tendency that does not result in petechiae, and a prolonged PT with or without a prolonged APTT, with no other hemostatic abnormalities. Occasionally hemorrhage precedes abnormal laboratory data; thus warfarin toxicosis should not be ruled out when the history and clinical findings are supportive. Within 24 hours, the PT should become prolonged.

Treatment. The administration of, or access to, warfarin must be stopped. Vitamin K_1 should be administered at a rate of 1 mg/kg subcutaneously every 6 hours until clinical signs have abated and the PT is normal for at least 2 days. Treatment may be necessary for several days because of continued absorption of warfarin from the gastrointestinal tract and the necessary period for clotting factor production. Warfarin is eliminated rapidly; however, some potentiated coumarins used as rodenticides have a prolonged half-life. Vitamin K_3 should be avoided because of its poor therapeutic benefit and the potential for nephrotoxicosis.[350] Life-threatening hemorrhage can be controlled by transfusion of fresh plasma (4–20 mL/kg) to replenish clotting factors. Fresh plasma is essential since clotting factor degradation occurs under normal storage conditions. Life-threatening anemia can be treated with whole blood (see p. 593).

Client Education. Prevention is based on limiting access of horses to rodenticides and carefully monitoring the therapeutic use of warfarin. The benefits of warfarin in horses are highly controversial and many question whether the advantages outweigh the risks. Both owner and veterinarian should consider warfarin therapy potentially dangerous. A history or clinical or laboratory evidence of hepatic disease or hemostatic dysfunction is a strong contraindication to warfarin use. The administration of other drugs (particularly phenylbutazone) should be limited during warfarin therapy and the dose of the latter reevaluated if the dose or rate of other medications is changed. The potential for trauma must be minimized, particularly during the initial warfarin dose adjustment period. The PT should be monitored daily and the dose of warfarin adjusted as needed to achieve an increase no greater than twofold. During warfarin therapy, the PT should be checked at least twice-weekly and more often if there is a change in diet, concurrent disease, or other medication.

Sweet Clover Toxicosis

This toxicosis, caused by ingestion of moldy sweet clover (*Melilotus*) hay, is reported in all herbivores but is most commonly seen in cattle in the northern Great Plains states.[43]

Clinical Signs and Laboratory Findings. Initially, there may be epistaxis and melena, with the development of subcutaneous hematomas and periarticular swellings as the disease progresses. Visible swellings are often at points of trauma such as the tuber coxae, hocks, or carpi and are not hot or painful, although they may cause stiffness and disinclination to move. Accidental and surgical wounds can precipitate fatal blood loss anemia.

Laboratory data are similar to that described for warfarin toxicosis, with prolonged PT being the earliest abnormality. As the disease progresses, the APTT becomes prolonged and blood loss anemia develops. The platelet count remains normal.

Etiology and Pathogenesis. White sweet clover (*Melilotus albus*) and yellow sweet clover (*Melilotus officinalis*) commonly grow along roadsides in the United States and are sometimes planted for use as fresh forage, silage, and hay. The plants contain coumarin, a nontoxic substance that imparts a bitter taste and vanilla fragrance. When sweet clover hay is improperly cured, a medium for growth of numerous fungi (*Penicillium, Mucor*, etc.) is produced, and the fungi convert coumarin to 4-hydroxycoumarin which condenses to dicumarol.[351] Animals that ingest the moldy hay develop a syndrome identical to warfarin toxicosis, in that dicumarol acts as a competitive inhibitor of vitamin K and interferes with hepatic synthesis of clotting factors II, VII, IX, and X. Affected animals develop severe coagulation dysfunction within 2 to 7 days after ingesting the moldy hay and are subject to internal and external hemorrhage.[352] Continued ingestion of mold-infested hay generally results in a lethal hemorrhagic crisis.

The succulent nature of sweet clover creates a high incidence of molding in hay prepared from it. Grazing the crop is not dangerous. The dicumarol concentration is highest in small bales, presumably because of exposure to more moisture and oxygen that are necessary for fungal growth. Concentrations of dicumarol toxic to cattle are in excess of 10 mg/kg feed.[353]

Diagnosis. History of access to moldy sweet clover hay, with the signs and laboratory changes described for warfarin toxicosis, provides the diagnosis.

Treatment. The sweet clover forage should obviously be removed from the ration and replaced by good-quality al-falfa. The suspect hay should be disposed of since toxic concentrations of dicumarol may remain in sweet clover for up to 4 years.[351] Therapy with vitamin K_1, as described for warfarin toxicosis, is paramount. Blood transfusion and supportive care should be performed as indicated.

Client Education. Horses are rarely affected by this disease; however, it is safest not to use sweet clover hay as their forage source. Affected forage is not visibly moldy because fungi grow within the stems.

Inherited Coagulation Disorders

Inherited coagulation disorders that have been reported in horses include deficiencies of factor VIII (hemophilia A),[44, 354] factors IX and XI,[46] prekallikrein,[45, 47] and the contact phase of intrinsic coagulation.[355] *Hemophilia A* is by far the most common of these and has been reported in Thoroughbreds,[44, 356, 357] standardbreds,[358] and quarter horses.[359, 360] This disease is transmitted as a sex-linked recessive trait and only the hemizygous male is clinically affected.

Clinical Signs and Laboratory Findings. Clinical signs are usually manifest within the first few weeks of life. Subcutaneous or intramuscular hematomas and joint swellings due to hemarthroses are the most common complaints, although any form of excessive hemorrhage may be seen. Affected joints are not hot or painful to palpation, but foals may have a recurrent shifting lameness. Signs of abdominal pain, depression, or dyspnea may occur subsequent to hemorrhage into body cavities. There is an increased tendency to bleed following minor trauma and surgical procedures, which may rarely lead to fatal hemorrhage. Petechial hemorrhages are noticeably absent and epistaxis is rare. The most prominent laboratory abnormality is prolongation of the APTT. Other hemostatic data are normal.

Etiology and Pathogenesis. The basic defect in hemophilia A is an inability to form functional factor VIII. In the blood, procoagulant factor VIII (factor VIII:C) generally circulates in a complex with a large-molecular-weight protein, von Willebrand's factor (vWF), part of which is immunologically active and called factor VIII–related antigen (VIII:RA).[354, 361] The synthesis and secretion of factor VIII:C is decreased in most patients with hemophilia A, although it is suspected that a defective form of factor VIII:C molecule is synthesized in some. Plasma and endothelial concentrations of vWF are normal and VIII:RA levels may even be increased. Deficiency of factor VIII:C causes a compromised intrinsic coagulation pathway that results in a hemorrhagic diathesis, the severity of which is inversely correlated with the plasma concentration of factor VIII:C. Severe hemophilic bleeding occurs when factor VIII:C activity is less than 1% of normal; a moderate defect is associated with levels between 1% and 5%, while a mild syndrome accompanies coagulant activity between 5% and 20%.

Diagnosis. The diagnosis of hemophilia A must be based on hemostatic data. The APTT is prolonged to at least two times normal, while the PT, TT, plasma fibrinogen concentration, and platelet count are near normal. The abnormal APTT can be corrected by mixing patient plasma 1:1 with normal horse plasma. Definitive diagnosis of hemophilia A is based on a factor VIII:C activity that is less than 20% of normal, as determined by a specific assay for factor VIII.[362] Carrier mares generally have factor VIII:C between 30% and 60% of normal and a ratio of VIII:R/factor VIII:C of greater than 2; however overlap with normal values can occur.[360, 363] Since factor VIII:C greater than 50% of normal is necessary to prevent hemorrhage after surgery or major trauma,[354] some of these carrier mares may be at risk for bleeding in these situations.

Treatment. The only effective treatment for hemophilia is repeated transfusion with fresh plasma (15–20 mL/kg IV) to maintain normal hemostasis. The half-life of transfused factor VIII:C is only 8 to 12 hours, necessitating transfusions on at least a daily basis. Cryoprecipitate or factor VIII concentrates, used to treat human hemophilia A, are not available for horses. Whole blood can be administered as needed if there is severe blood loss. Affected horses should be rested in a safe enclosure so that the chances of trauma are minimized.

Client Education. The long-term prognosis for hemophilia A in horses is poor. There is no cure for the disease and therapy is only palliative and highly impractical. Most affected foals die or are humanely destroyed because of progressive debilitation by 6 months of age, although a mildly affected Thoroughbred was described at 3 years of age.[356] The latter case seems to be unusual as the disease in horses is usually severe.

Carrier mares serve to perpetuate the disease, and their removal from the breeding population is the basis for prevention of affected foals. Definitive diagnosis of hemophilia A in a colt documents the mare as a carrier. She should not be used for breeding since 50% of the male progeny will be hemophiliacs and 50% of the female progeny will be carriers. Carriers have plasma factor VIII:C that is 30% to 60% normal; however, since factor VIII:C may be elevated from the last trimester through 60 days post partum, suspect mares should not be rebred until factor VIII:C can be accurately determined.[360] Available tests do not always confirm the carrier state.[361]

Thrombophlebitis

Thrombophlebitis is venous thrombosis accompanied by vessel wall inflammation.[364] Hemostatic dysfunction characterized by enhanced activity of thrombin or impaired activity of plasmin results in thrombus formation, and the mere presence of thrombosis induces vessel wall inflammation. Jugular thrombophlebitis is common in horses with severe gastrointestinal diseases accompanied by endotoxemia.

Clinical Signs and Laboratory Findings. The initial sign of jugular thrombophlebitis is edema of the head and hyperemia of the oral mucosa. Bilateral jugular thrombosis can lead to dysphagia and dyspnea subsequent to lingual, pharyngeal, and laryngeal edema. Collateral circulation develops rapidly, and is manifest as superficial arborizing vessels on the patient's neck and face. The thrombosed vein is firm and may be accompanied by heat, swelling, and signs of pain, which strongly suggests sepsis. Septic thrombophlebitis is

further indicated if the horse is febrile or resists manipulation of the neck. Depression, anorexia, toxemia, hemoconcentration, and shock occur in the unlikely event of systemic sepsis. Endocarditis, pneumonia, or pulmonary abscess formation may result from embolization.

There are no characteristic laboratory changes in thrombophlebitis. Hemostatic data consistent with DIC may occur. Neutrophilic leukocytosis and hyperfibrinogenemia generally attend septic thrombophlebitis, although these may also arise from the primary disease process.

Etiology and Pathogenesis. Stasis of blood flow, injury to the vessel wall, and a hypercoagulable state predispose to thrombophlebitis.[364, 365] Thrombosis may be considered as an inappropriate form of hemostasis or "hemostasis in the wrong place"[365, 366] when the action of thrombin is enhanced relative to that of plasmin.[367] The combined effects of endogenous heparin–antithrombin III and the protein C system physiologically oppose the action of thrombin. Insufficient anticoagulant mechanisms can predispose patients to thrombosis.[368]

The most common mechanism by which excess thrombin is generated in the blood is DIC.[282, 296] In horses, DIC is generally caused by conditions that induce endotoxemia[108, 279, 280] and the latter are also accompanied by a high rate of thrombophlebitis.[369] Not only is there a tendency for excess generation of thrombin but endotoxemia produces an overall inhibition of fibrinolysis and anticoagulant mechanisms associated with increased plasma PAI and the downregulation of protein C, respectively.[189, 210]

A hypercoagulable state that predisposes to thrombosis may also be induced by profound loss of anticoagulants.[370] Owing to the small size of AT-III, protein-losing states can induce a deficiency of AT-III that correlates with the degree of hypoalbuminemia. Horses with chronic glomerulonephritis[371] or protein-losing enteropathy[69, 152] have a propensity for venous thrombosis. Vessel wall trauma likely plays a large role in the development of equine thrombophlebitis. Frequency of venipuncture, the thrombogenicity of the catheter materials, blood flow turbulence at the catheter tip, and the physical characteristics of infused solutions are all important.

Diagnosis. Thrombophlebitis of the jugular vein or other peripheral veins is usually clinically obvious. Ultrasonography aids detection of an occult thrombus and characterizes the extent and severity of known thrombosis.

Treatment. At the first clinical indication of thrombophlebitis, catheters should be aseptically removed and cultured. Venipuncture of the involved vein is contraindicated. Hydrotherapy increases blood supply and reduces local inflammation. Topical anti-inflammatory agents, such as 50% DMSO or antiphlogistic salves are sometimes useful. Systemic nonsteroidal anti-inflammatory therapy might be indicated, but the intravenous use of phenylbutazone should be avoided because of the drug's tendency to cause severe intimal irritation. Intravenous therapy should be kept to a minimum. Heparin and warfarin may reduce the incidence of thromboembolism, but have no mechanism for resolving existing thrombi. Since the incidence of thromboembolism in horses is low and anticoagulant therapy is attended by numerous potential complications,[339, 340, 348, 372] the risk and expense of the latter outweigh marginal benefits.[369] Although used in humans,[208] safe and affordable thrombolytic therapy is not available for horses.

Systemic antimicrobial therapy is indicated for septic thrombophlebitis. The choice of drugs should be based on the results of bacterial culture and sensitivity performed on the removed catheter, on exudate from the thrombosed vein, or blood. If a sample cannot be obtained for culture, broad-spectrum antimicrobial therapy should be continued for at least 10 days or until signs of local and systemic sepsis have abated. Mild, localized sepsis usually resolves with conservative therapy. Perivascular tissue necrosis and abscess formation might necessitate surgical drainage of the area. Surgical removal of the infected vessel is indicated by intermittent fever, leukocytosis, and pain in the region of the vein for longer than 2 weeks after initiation of systemic antimicrobial therapy.

Client Education. Nonseptic thrombophlebitis has a good prognosis. Resolution of thrombophlebitis changes the vessel into a firm cord of fibrous tissue, but large vessels such as the jugular vein may eventually become patent again. Venipuncture of thrombosed vessels should be avoided because intimal irritation in a region of resolving inflammation can reinitiate or worsen thrombosis and bacterial contamination of a thrombus can result in sepsis. The prognosis for septic thrombophlebitis depends upon the extent of vein involvement, pathogenicity of the involved microorganisms, rapidity of diagnosis, and appropriateness of treatment. Most cases resolve with long-term antimicrobial therapy; however, surgical extirpation of the vein may be necessary.

The incidence of serious thrombophlebitis in horses can be reduced by therapy to mitigate the effects of endotoxemia and shock and measures taken to minimize trauma and bacterial contamination of veins. Irritating solutions should be diluted prior to intravenous administration. Catheters are required for large volumes of medication and for treating uncooperative patients. Measures to minimize catheter-induced thrombophlebitis should be strictly adhered to.[369, 373, 374] Repeated venipuncture of large vessels should be avoided.

Fibrinolytic Dysfunction

The main function of fibrinolysis is to remove fibrin clots that have served their function to arrest blood loss from a damaged vessel. An imbalance between the actions of thrombin and of plasmin on fibrin leads to a thrombotic diathesis.[366] Failure of fibrinolysis to remove occlusive arterial thrombi causes tissue ischemia and organ failure. Fibrinolytic dysfunction can also contribute to the development and persistence of venous thrombosis. Patients with fibrinolytic dysfunction are clinically in a hypercoagulable state.[365]

Pathogenesis

Decreased fibrinolysis results from inadequate release of t-PA, increased plasma concentrations of PAI, or both.[375–377] The exact mechanisms for this are very poorly characterized. In studies performed thus far in humans, PAI has been measured in assays based on titration of PAI with t-PA.

Therefore, increased PAI activity can be caused either by increased PAI or decreased t-PA.[210] Poor release of t-PA may represent inadequate response to certain stimuli or decreased t-PA reserved in the endothelial cells.[365, 378] In blood, PAI behaves as an acute phase reactant protein.[210, 379] Plasma PAI activity is also induced by endotoxin[312, 380] and this effect is enhanced by concomitant downregulation of protein C.[381]

Disease States

Owing to lack of established assays for equine t-PA and PAI, there are no data that document the association of fibrinolytic dysfunction with any recognized disease process. Reduced fibrinolytic activity has been shown in human patients with deep vein thrombosis,[380, 382] coronary vascular disease,[312] acute myocardial infarction,[382] and gram-negative bacterial sepsis.[383–385] The changes in the fibrinolytic system during sepsis are related to circulating levels of endotoxin[383] and the concentration of PAI may be inversely related to prognosis.[383–385] One may extrapolate from these studies in humans that altered function of the fibrinolytic mechanism contributes to development of the coagulopathy that accompanies endotoxemia in horses[108] and likely predisposes to thrombophlebitis.[309]

BLOOD AND PLASMA THERAPY

The objective of whole-blood administration is to improve oxygen delivery to the tissues during anemia; however, it should be viewed only as a temporary lifesaving procedure. There are two important reasons why blood transfusion should be used only as needed. Allogeneic equine erythrocytes, even when crossmatch-compatible, are removed from the circulation by the MPS within 4 days of administration.[386] Thus, the benefit derived from improved oxygen-carrying capacity is transient and the increased load of cellular debris that must be processed by the MPS has the potential to immunocompromise the patient. Secondly, blood transfusion impedes the bone marrow response to anemia by blunting renal production of erythropoietin. Since transfused erythrocytes remain in the circulation less than 5 days, a bone marrow response in the interim is highly important to ultimate recovery from anemia.

Plasma has an integral role in primary or supportive care of many equine diseases by providing immunoglobulins, clotting factors, enzymes, and transport proteins, as well as helping to maintain vascular oncotic pressure. Applications of plasma therapy include its use in failure of passive transfer of maternal antibodies in foals, and in diseases that cause hypoproteinemia, such as protein-losing enteropathy or nephropathy. Horses with TPP of less than 4 g/dL, hemoconcentration, or associated peripheral edema, as well as those with a TPP of less than 3 g/dL, regardless of signs, probably warrant a plasma transfusion to restore plasma oncotic pressure. In addition, plasma may be useful in management of selected patients with DIC, septicemia or endotoxemia, or ITP.

Donor Selection and Management

The selection of an appropriate blood donor is highly important to prevent potentially fatal transfusion reactions as well as to maximize in vivo survival of transfused erythrocytes. The short life span of transfused cells is likely due to minor antigenic incompatibilities that are only identified through blood-typing. Compatibility testing to identify the presence of antibodies to allogeneic erythrocytes (alloantibodies) in the donor or recipient is suggested prior to transfusion; however, donor identification is complicated by the high degree of blood group polymorphism in horses.[59, 387] Over 30 different erythrocyte antigens (alloantigens) constituting eight blood groups have been identified in horses, accounting for more than 400,000 phenotypes.[387] Although identification of a donor with completely compatible alloantigen and alloantibody profiles as the recipient is nearly impossible, compatibility testing can help avert severe transfusion reactions by identifying existing alloantibodies. Following first exposure to a foreign alloantigen, alloantibodies are produced within 5 to 7 days and memory cells are committed. Subsequent exposure to the same alloantigens results in a rapid anamnestic response with alloantibody-mediated erythrocyte destruction. Thus, each transfusion from the same or different donors must be preceded by compatibility testing.

Alloantigens Aa of the A system and Qa of the Q system are the most immunogenic of equine alloantigens and are highly prevalent among light horse breeds.[53, 388] Transfusion of blood containing one or both of these alloantigens to horses that lack them results in a high titer of alloantibodies that mediate severe hemolysis upon subsequent exposure. In addition to transfusion, horses can become sensitized by previous pregnancy,[52] plasma, or other blood component therapy that contains contaminating erythrocytes[50] or by immunization with an equine-origin biological.[389]

Routine compatibility testing generally involves the saline agglutination crossmatch procedure. This test is performed by incubating washed erythrocytes from donor (major) and recipient (minor) with serum from the other, followed by gross and microscopic examination for clumping. Unfortunately, the routine crossmatch only demonstrates agglutinins and many equine alloantibodies act primarily as hemolysins.[52, 387] The latter can only be reliably detected by adding exogenous complement to the reaction mixture,[50, 52] which is usually provided by absorbed rabbit serum.[5] Although agglutination tests can be performed by most veterinary practices and human hospitals, the need for special handling and storage of rabbit serum limits hemolysin testing to a number of specialized veterinary hematology laboratories (see Table 11–4). In an emergency setting, the agglutination crossmatch is recommended as a general screening test for donor-recipient incompatibility, but one must realize that test results may not always predict a serious transfusion reaction.[386] The first transfusion to a recipient that has not received prior blood component therapy or had an incompatible pregnancy is generally well tolerated because natural equine alloantibodies are rare and weakly reactive;[31] however, accurate history of prior sensitization may be unavailable. In lieu of testing in a life-threatening situation, a 1- or 2-year-old horse of either sex with no history of blood or plasma therapy is the best potential donor. After transfusion, alloantibodies to incompatible erythrocyte antigens may develop within days, making subsequent transfusions from the same or a different donor hazardous.[32]

The safest and easiest approach to donor identification is

through prior blood-typing. Since most serious transfusion reactions involve alloantibodies to Aa or Qa, horses that lack alloantigens Aa and Qa as well as serum alloantibodies are generally safe blood or plasma donors for any horse.[31, 387, 388] Such horses can be identified by sending samples of serum and blood, anticoagulated with acid-citrate-dextrose, from a number of potential donors to a laboratory experienced with equine blood-typing procedures (see Table 11–4). Suitable donors are most easily found among quarter horses and standardbreds since both breeds have a lower prevalence of Aa than other light horses,[59] and standardbreds rarely possess Qa. Multiparous mares should not be considered. Identified donors should be retested annually, after any major illness or after pregnancy, to insure that they have not acquired serum alloantibodies.

Plasma donor selection is similar to that for whole blood, but only alloantibodies in the donor serum for recipient erythrocytes (minor crossmatch) must be considered. Donors lacking alloantibodies for Aa and Qa usually are adequate, although the best donor would lack all erythrocyte alloantibodies. Plasma harvested manually (by aspirating or squeezing the plasma from the top of a container of centrifuged or sedimented erythrocytes) is usually contaminated with a small number of erythrocytes, which may be sufficient for recipient sensitization. Subsequent blood transfusions may be incompatible, and a recipient filly's foal would be predisposed to neonatal isoerythrolysis.[389] Thus, plasma donors would optimally lack alloantigens Aa and possibly Qa, as these are the most immunogenic.

Blood Collection

Blood for transfusion should be aseptically collected into sterile bottles or bags containing a volume of acid-citrate-dextrose solution to provide a ratio of 1:9 with blood. Sterile intravenous solution bags in 1- to 3-L sizes are commercially available,[6] to which acid-citrate-dextrose can be added prior to blood collection. The acid-citrate-dextrose solution can be made by mixing 11 g dextrose, 9.9 g sodium citrate, 3.3 g citric acid, and enough distilled water to total 300 mL, then autoclaved.[390] Most adult horses can safely donate 8 to 10 L of blood, which represents 20% to 25% of their total blood volume, every 30 days.[31] This amount is more than needed for a foal and is usually therapeutic for severe anemia in the adult since replacing 20% to 40% of the lost erythrocytes is generally sufficient to maintain life until the bone marrow can respond.[391] Accurate data regarding safe storage life of equine blood are not available; thus blood for transfusion should be used immediately or stored upright in a refrigerator (4 °C) for less than 24 hours.

Plasma Preparation

Plasma can be produced by collecting the liquid portion of whole blood that has been centrifuged or allowed to sit at room temperature for 1 to 2 hours. This manual technique is simple and fast, but fraught with the risk of bacterial contamination and recipient sensitization. Apheresis using centrifugation or membrane filtration blood fractionation equipment[7] is the optimal method of plasma production. The donor is included as part of a closed loop, whereby whole blood is withdrawn and separated into its component parts (plasma, erythrocytes, granulocytes, platelets), plasma is collected, and the remaining blood components are returned. This technique produces cell-free sterile plasma.[264] These devices are used to produce commercially available frozen plasma from donors that lack Aa and Qa alloantigens and serum alloantibodies (numerous sources). Usually this commercial plasma can be administered safely without the need for prior compatibility testing. Immunoglobulins are preserved for longer than a year in frozen plasma, but hemostatic proteins may deteriorate.

Blood Components

Concentrates of specific equine plasma components could provide more focused therapy and in a lower necessary volume.[335] Concentrated immunoglobulins could be used to treat failure of passive transfer, other humoral immunodeficiencies, and possibly ITP. Cryoprecipitate, which is a combination of factor VIII:C, fibrinogen, and fibronectin, would be useful for foals with hemophilia A. Purified fibronectin may be indicated in treating selected cases of DIC or endotoxemia that accompany neonatal septicemia, acute colitis, intestinal strangulation, obstruction, and pleuropneumonia. Concentrates of the anticoagulant proteins AT-III and protein C may reduce the incidence of thrombotic disease in horses that have been depleted of these proteins during DIC or through gastrointestinal or renal loss.

Centrifugation apheresis allows collection of granulocyte, platelet, and erythrocyte concentrates. Granulocyte transfusion may improve survival in neonatal foal septicemia, as has been shown in human neonates.[392] Platelets and erythrocytes are useful in the treatment of life-threatening thrombocytopenia or anemia.

Transfusion Technique

After warming to 37 °C in a water bath, any blood product should be administered intravenously through a size 0.22 μM in-line filter to remove clots or debris. The vital signs of the recipient are recorded prior to transfusion, then blood or plasma 0.1 mL/kg body weight should be slowly administered (10 minutes). If temperament and vital signs do not change, the transfusion is continued at a rate of 5 to 20 mL/kg/hr. In the absence of hypovolemia (e.g., hemolytic anemia, hypoproteinemia), slower flow rates may be necessary to prevent volume overload, especially in foals. Slower administration is also safer since it allows detection of delayed adverse reactions prior to excessive blood delivery. Horses should be monitored continuously during transfusion and the transfusion stopped if the recipient has any change in demeanor.

The necessary dose of whole blood for a severely anemic horse can only be estimated. In most instances, replacing 20% to 40% of the calculated blood loss is sufficient to maintain life until the bone marrow can respond. Assuming the 500-kg horse has 40 L of blood (8% of body weight), a drop in the packed cell volume from 36% to 12% would represent a loss of about 27 L. In this instance, 6 to 8 L of blood should be therapeutic. Using the estimated values for plasma volume and extravascular protein distribution, a rule

of thumb for plasma therapy is that intravenous infusion of 7 L of plasma containing protein at 7 g/dL in a 500-kg horse raises the TPP by about 1 g/dL. Ongoing losses must be considered.

Potential Complications

More common signs of "transfusion reactions" include restlessness, tachypnea, dyspnea, tachycardia, piloerection, sweating, defecation, and muscle fasciculations. These signs are nonspecific and may indicate a number of potential complications. Immunologic sequelae such as hemolysis or anaphylaxis are mediated by recipient antibodies to donor blood components. Endotoxemia or recipient complement activation may be caused by blood that has been improperly obtained or contaminated during handling or administration. Rarely, citrate in the acid-citrate-dextrose solution may result in hypocalcemia. Since it is not possible to immediately determine the cause of a transfusion reaction, blood component administration should be stopped immediately and replaced by isotonic crystalloid solution. Flunixin meglumine may be indicated and calcium gluconate should be given if hypocalcemia is identified. Collapse or profound dyspnea is highly suggestive of anaphylaxis and should be treated with epinephrine 0.01 to 0.02 mL/kg of 1:1,000 solution IM. Another blood or plasma donor should be identified unless the cause of the adverse reaction is known not to be immunologically mediated. Extreme care must be taken to ensure sterile procurement and handling of all blood components for therapy.

REFERENCES

1. Nathan DG: Hematologic diseases. In Wyngaarden JB, Smith LH, eds: *Cecil Textbook of Medicine*, ed 18. Philadelphia, WB Saunders, 1988, p 873.
2. Harvey JW: Erythrocyte metabolism. In Kaneko JJ, ed: *Clinical Biochemistry of Domestic Animals*, ed 4. New York, Academic Press, 1989, p 185.
3. Clark SC, Kamer R: The human hematopoietic colony-stimulating factors. *Science* 236:1229, 1987.
4. Weisbart RH: Colony-stimulating factors and host defense. *Ann Intern Med.* 110:297, 1989.
5. Chan JY, Slamon DJ, Nimer SD, et al: Regulation of expression of human granulocyte-macrophage colony-stimulating factor (GM-CSF). *Proc Natl Acad Sci U S A* 83:8669, 1986.
6. Tomonaga M, Golde DW, Gasson JC: Biosynthetic (recombinant) human granulocyte-macrophage colony-stimulating factor: Effect on normal bone marrow and leukemia cell lines. *Blood* 67:31, 1986.
7. Hammond WP IV, Price TH, Souza LN, et al: Treatment of cyclic neutropenia with granulocyte colony-stimulating factor. *N Engl J Med* 320:1306, 1989.
8. Yang YC, Ciaretta AB, Temple PA, et al: Human Il-3 (Multi-CSF): Identification by expression cloning of a novel hematopoietic growth factor related to murine Il-3. *Cell* 47:3, 1986.
9. Rich IN: A role for the macrophage in normal hemopoiesis. I. Functional capacity of bone-marrow-derived macrophages to release hemopoietic growth factors. *Exp Hematol* 14:738, 1986.
10. Zucali JR, Broxmeyer HE, Dinarello CA, et al: Regulation of early human hematopoietic (BFU-E and CFU-GEMM)

progenitor cells *in vitro* by interleukin 1-induced fibroblast-conditioned medium. *Blood* 69:33, 1987.

11. Stanley ER, Jubinsky PT: Factors affecting the growth and differentiation of haematopoietic cells in culture. *Clin Haematol* 13:329, 1984.

12. Burdach SEG, Levitt LJ: Receptor-specific inhibition of bone marrow erythropoiesis by recombinant DNA-derived interleukin-2. *Blood* 69:1368, 1987.

13. Valli VE, Lumsden JN, Carter EI, et al: The kinetics of hematopoiesis in the normal light horse: The life span of peripheral blood cells and plasma proteins. In Kitchen H, Krehbiel JD, eds: *Proceedings of the First International Symposium of Equine Hematology.* Golden, Colo, American Association of Equine Practitioners, 1976, p 91.

14. Carakostas MC, Moore WE, Smith JE: Intravascular neutrophilic granulocyte kinetics in horses. *Am J Vet Res* 42:623, 1981.

15. Stokes C, Bourne JF: Mucosal Immunity. In Halliwell REW, Gorman NT, eds: *Veterinary Clinical Immunology*, Philadelphia, WB Saunders, 1989, p 164.

16. Jain NC: *Schalm's Veterinary Hematology*, ed 4. Philadelphia, Lea & Febiger, 1986, p 350.

17. Weiss L, Tavassoli M: Anatomical hazards to the passage of erythrocytes through the spleen. *Semin Hematol* 7:372, 1970.

18. Meagher DM, Tasker JB: Effects of excitement and tranquilization on the equine hemogram. *Mod Vet Pract* 53:41, 1972.

19. Persson SGB, Ekman L, Lydin G, et al: Circulating effects of splenectomy in the horse. 1. Effect on red-cell distribution and variability in the horse. *Zentralbl Veterinar med*, 20:441, 1973.

20. Bloom JC, Roby KAW: Evaluation of the erythron. In Robinson NE, ed: *Current Therapy in Equine Medicine*, Vol 2. Philadelphia, WB Saunders, 1987, p 291.

21. Morris DD: Review of anemia in horses, Part I: Clinical signs, laboratory findings and diagnosis. *Equine Pract* 11:27, 1989.

22. Burrows GE: Equine *E. coli* endotoxemia: Comparison of intravenous and intraperitoneal endotoxin administration. *Am J Vet Res* 40:991, 1979.

23. Morris DD, Whitlock RH, Corbeil LB: Endotoxemia in horses: Protection provided by antiserum to core lipopolysaccharide. *Am J Vet Res* 47:544, 1986.

24. Torten M, Schalm OW: Influence of the equine spleen on rapid changes in the concentration of erythrocytes in peripheral blood. *Am J Vet Res* 25:500, 1964.

25. Sonoda M: Clinical and experimental studies on the erythrocytes which include Jolly's bodies in horses. *Jpn J Vet Res* 8:1, 1960.

26. Tennant B, Baldwin BH, Silverman SL, et al: Clinical significance of hyperbilirubinemia in the race horse. In Kitchen H, Krehbiel JD, eds: *Proceedings of the First International Symposium of Equine Hematology.* Golden, Colo, American Association of Equine Practitioners, 1975, p 246.

27. Naylor J, Kronfeld DS, Johnson K: Fasting hyperbilirubinemia and its relationship to free fatty acids and triglycerides in the horse. *Proc Soc Exp Biol Med* 165:86, 1980.

28. Engelking LR, Anwer S, Lofstedt J: Hepatobiliary transport of indocyanine green and sulfobromophthalein in fed and fasted horses. *Am J Vet Res* 46:2278, 1985.

29. Grownwall R, Engelking LR, Noonan N: Direct measurement of biliary bilirubin excretion in ponies during fasting. *Am J Vet Res* 41:125, 1980.

30. Schalm OW: Equine hematology III. Significance of plasma fibrinogen concentration in clinical disorders in horses. *Equine Pract* 1:24, 1979.

31. Becht JL, Gordon BJ: Blood and plasma therapy. In Robinson NE, ed: *Current Therapy in Equine Medicine*, Vol 2. Philadelphia, WB Saunders, 1987, p 317.

32. Morris DD: Review of anemia in horses, Part II: Pathophysiologic mechanisms, specific diseases and treatment. *Equine Pract* 11:34, 1989.

33. Gann DS: Endocrine control of plasma protein and volume. *Surg Clin North Am* 56:1135, 1976.

34. Gann DS: Pirkle JC: Role of cortisol in the restitution of blood volume after hemorrhage. *Am J Surg* 130:565, 1975.

35. Elman R, Lischer C, Davey HW: Plasma proteins (albumin and globulin) and red cell volume following a single severe non-fatal hemorrhage. *Am J Physiol* 138:569, 1943.

36. Hein LG, Albrecht M, Dworsehak M, et al: Long-term observation following traumatic hemorrhage shock in the dog: A comparison of crystalloidal vs. colloidal fluids. *Circ Shock* 26:353, 1988.

37. Schmall LM, Muir WW, Robertson JT: Haemodynamic effects of small volume hypertonic saline in experimentally induced haemorrhagic shock. *Equine Vet J* 22:273, 1990.

38. Rocha-E-Silva M, Negraes GA, Soares AM, et al: Hypertonic resuscitation from severe hemorrhagic shock: Patterns of regional circulation. *Circ Shock* 19:165, 1986.

39. Mazzoni MC, Borgstrom P, Arfors KE, et al: Dynamic fluid redistribution in hyperosmotic resuscitation of hypovolemic hemorrhage. *Am J Physiol* 255:H629, 1988.

40. Carlson GP: Diseases associated with increased erythrocyte destruction (hemolytic anemia). In Smith BP, ed: *Large Animal Internal Medicine*. St Louis, Mosby–Year Book, 1990, p 1084.

41. Byers TD: Warfarin toxicosis. In Robinson NE, ed: *Current Therapy in Equine Medicine*, Vol 2. Philadelphia, WB Saunders, 1987, p 305.

42. Vrins A, Carlson G, Feldman B: Warfarin: A review with emphasis on its use in the horse. *Can Vet J* 24:211, 1983.

43. Blood DC, Radostits OM, Arundel JH et al: *Veterinary Medicine*, ed 7. Philadelphia, Bailliere Tindall, 1989, p 1332.

44. Archer RK, Allen BV: True hemophilia in horses. *Vet Rec* 91:655, 1972.

45. Geor RJ, Jackson ML, Lewis KD, et al: Prekallikrein deficiency in a family of Belgian horses. *J Am Vet Med Assoc* 197:741, 1990.

46. Hinton M, Jones DRE, Lewis IM, et al: A clotting factor defect in an Arab colt foal. *Equine Vet J* 9:1, 1977.

47. Turrentine MA, Sculley PW, Green EM, et al: Prekallikrein deficiency in a family of miniature horses. *Am J Vet Res* 47:2464, 1986.

48. Morris DD: Diseases associated with blood loss or hemostatic dysfunction. In Smith BP, ed: *Large Animal Internal Medicine*, St Louis, Mosby–Year Book, 1990, p 1068.

49. Harvey JW, Asquith RL: Serum ferritin, serum iron and erythrocyte values in foals. *Am J Vet Res* 48:1348, 1987.

50. Becht JL: Neonatal isoerythrolysis in the foal. Part 1. Background, blood group antigens and pathogenesis. *Compendium Continuing Educ Pract Vet* 5:S591, 1983.

51. Scott AM, Jeffcott LB: Haemolytic disease of the newborn foal. *Vet Rec* 103:71, 1978.

52. Stormont C: Neonatal isoerythrolysis in domestic animals: A comparative review. *Adv Vet Sci Comp Med* 19:23, 1975.

53. Bailey E: Prevalence of anti-red blood cell antibodies in the serum and colostrum of mares and its relationship to neonatal isoerythrolysis. *Am J Vet Res* 43:1917, 1982.

54. McClure JJ: Immunologic disorders. In Smith BP, ed: *Large Animal Internal Medicine*. St Louis, Mosby–Year Book, 1990, p 1598.

55. Morris DD: Immunologic disease of foals. *Compendium Continuing Educ Pract Vet* 8:S139, 1986.

56. Bailey E, Albright DG, Henney PJ: Equine neonatal isoerythrolysis: Evidence for prevention by maternal antibodies to the Ca blood group antigen. *Am J Vet Res* 49:1218, 1988.

57. Pollack W, Gorman JG, Freda VJ: Rh immune suppression: Past, present and future. In Frigoletti FD Jr, Jewett JF, Konu-

gres AA, eds: *Rh Hemolytic Disease: New Strategy for Eradication*. Boston, GK Hall, 1982, pp 9–70.

58. Becht JL, Semrad SD: Hematology, blood typing and immunology of the neonatal foal. *Vet Clin North Am Equine Pract* 1:91, 1985.

59. Bowling AT, Clark RS: Blood group and protein polymorphism gene frequencies for seven breeds of horses in the United States. *Anim Blood Groups Biochem Genet* 16:93, 1985.

60. Morris DD: Immune-mediated hematologic disorders in horses. In *Proceedings of the Fourth Annual Forum of the American College of Veterinary Internal Medicine*, Washington, DC, 1986, pp 7–9.

61. Beck BJ: A case of primary autoimmune haemolytic anaemia in a pony. *Equine Vet J* 22:292, 1990.

62. Halliwell REW, Gorman NT: Autoimmune blood diseases. In Halliwell REW, Gorman NT, eds: *Veterinary Clinical Immunology*, Philadelphia, WB Saunders, 1989, p 308.

63. Rose NR: Pathogenic mechanisms in autoimmune diseases. *Clin Immunol Immunopathol* 53:57, 1989.

64. Clabough DL: The immunopathogenesis and control of equine infectious anemia. *Vet Med*, 1020, 1990.

65. Reef V: *Clostridium perfringens* cellulitis and immune-mediated hemolytic anemia in a horse. *J Am Vet Med Assoc* 182:251, 1983.

66. Mair TS, Taylor FGR, Hillyer MH: Autoimmune haemolytic anaemia in eight horses. *Vet Rec* 126:51, 1990.

67. Farrelly BT, Collins JD, Collins SM: Autoimmune haemolytic anemia (AHA) in the horse. *Ir Vet J* 20:42, 1966.

68. Reef V, Dyson SS, Beech J: Lymphosarcoma and associated immune-mediated hemolytic anemia and thrombocytopenia in horses. *J Am Vet Med Assoc* 184:313, 1984.

69. Morris DD, Vaala WE, Sartin E: Protein-losing enteropathy in a yearling filly with subclinical DIC and autoimmune hemolytic disease. *Compendium Continuing Educ Pract Vet* 4:S542, 1982.

70. Blue JT, Dinsmore RP, Anderson KL: Immune-mediated hemolytic anemia induced by penicillin in horses. *Cornell Vet* 77:263, 1987.

71. Beck JS, Browning MCK: Immunosuppression with glucocorticoid—a possible explanation for interpatient variation in sensitivity. *J R Soc Med* 76:473, 1983.

72. Fries LF, Brickman CM, Frank MM: Monocyte receptors for the Fc portion of IgG increase in number in autoimmune hemolytic anemia and other hemolytic states and are decreased by glucocorticoid therapy. *J Immunol* 131:1240, 1983.

73. Pearson JE, Knowles RC: Standardization of the equine infectious anemia immunodiffusion test and its application to the control of the disease in the United States. *J Am Vet Med Assoc* 184:298, 1984.

74. Roberts DH, Lucas MH: Equine infectious anaemia. *Vet Annu* 27:147, 1987.

75. McClure JJ, Lindsay WA, Taylor W, et al: Ataxia in four horses with equine infectious anemia. *J Am Vet Med Assoc* 180:279, 1982.

76. Tashjian RJ: Transmission and clinical evaluation of an equine infectious anemia herd and their offspring over a 13-year period. *J Am Vet Med Assoc* 184:282, 1984.

77. Kono Y, Hirasawa K, Fukanaga Y, et al: Recrudescence of equine infectious anemia by treatment with immunosuppressive drugs. *Natl Inst Anim Health Q (Tokyo)* 16:8, 1976.

78. Coggins L, Norcross NL, Nusbaum SR: Diagnosis of equine infectious anemia by immunodiffusion test. *Am J Vet Res* 33:11, 1972.

79. Gonda MA, Charman HP, Walker JL, et al: Scanning and transmission electron microscopic study of equine infectious anemia virus. *Am J Vet Res* 39:731, 1978.

80. Issel CJ, Adams WV, Meek L, et al: Transmission of equine infectious anemia virus from horses without clinical signs of disease. *J Am Vet Med Assoc* 180:272, 1982.

81. Issel CJ, Foil LD: Studies on equine infectious anemia virus transmission by insects. *J Am Vet Med Assoc* 184:293, 1984.

82. Kemen MJ Jr, Coggins L: Equine infectious anemia: transmission from infected mares to foals. *J Am Vet Med Assoc* 161:496, 1972.

83. Henson JB, McGuire TC: Immunopathology of equine infectious anemia. *Am J Clin Pathol* 56:306, 1971.

84. Perryman LE, McGuire TC, Banks KL, et al: Decreased C_3 levels in a chronic virus infection: EIA. *J Immunol* 106:1074, 1971.

85. Sentsui H, Kono Y: Hemagglutination by equine infectious anemia virus. *Infect Immun* 14:325, 1976.

86. McGuire TC, Henson JB, Quist SE: Impaired bone marrow response in EIA. *Am J Vet Res* 30:2091, 1969.

87. Coggins L: Carriers of equine infectious anemia virus. *J Am Vet Med Assoc* 184:279, 1984.

88. Hall RF, Pursell AR, Cole JR, et al: A propagating epizootic of equine infectious anemia on a horse farm. *J Am Vet Med Assoc* 193:1082, 1988.

89. Harvey JW, Kaneko JJ: Mammalian erythrocyte metabolism and oxidant drugs. *Toxicol Appl Pharmacol* 42:253, 1977.

90. Divers TJ, George LW, George JW: Hemolytic anemia in horses after the ingestion of red maple leaves. *J Am Vet Med Assoc* 180:300, 1982.

91. Warner AE: Methemoglobinemia and hemolytic anemia in a horse with acute renal failure. *Compendium Continuing Educ Pract Vet* 6:S465, 1984.

92. Tennant B, Dill SB, Glickman LT, et al: Acute hemolytic anemia, methemoglobinemia and Heinz body formation associated with ingestion of red maple leaves by horses. *J Am Vet Med Assoc* 179:143, 1981.

93. McSherry BJ, Roe CK, Milne FJ: The hematology of phenothiazine poisoning in horses. *Can Vet J* 7:3, 1966.

94. Pierce KR, Joyce JR, England RB et al: Acute hemolytic anemia caused by wild onion poisoning in horses. *J Am Vet Med Assoc* 160:323, 1972.

95. Harvey JW, Rackear D: Experimental onion-induced hemolytic anemia in dogs. *Vet Pathol* 22:387, 1985.

96. George LW, Divers TJ, Mahaffey EA, et al: Heinz body hemolytic anemia and methemoglobinemia in ponies given red maple (*Acer rubrum*) leaves. *Vet Pathol* 19:521, 1982.

97. Allen TA, Fettman MJ: Comparative aspects of nonoliguric acute renal failure. *Compendium Continuing Educ Pract Vet* 9:293, 1987.

98. Divers TJ, Whitlock RH, Byars TD, et al: Acute renal failure in six horses resulting from haemodynamic causes. *Equine Vet J* 19:178, 1987.

99. Keitt AS, Leibach JR, Kitchens CS: Aniline induced methemoglobinemia: Hazards of methylene blue and ascorbate (abstract). *Clin Res* 26:795A, 1978.

100. Zaugg JL: Babesiosis. In Smith BP, ed: *Large Animal Internal Medicine*, St Louis, Mosby–Year Book, 1990, p 1088.

101. Knowles RC: Equine piroplasmosis. *Equine Pract* 2:10, 1980.

102. Schein D, Rehbein G, Voigt WP, et al: *Babesia equi* 1. Development in horses and in lymphocyte culture. *Tropenmed Parasitol* 32:223, 1981.

103. Kutler KL, Zaugg JL, Gipson GA: Imidocarb and paravaquone in the treatment of piroplasmosis (*Babesia equi*) in equids. *Am J Vet Res* 48:1613, 1987.

104. Frerichs MW, Allen PC, Holbrook AA: Equine piroplasmosis (*B. equi*): Therapeutic trials of imidocarb dihydrochloride in horses and donkeys. *Vet Rec* 93:73, 1973.

105. Marder VJ, Martin SE, Francis CW, et al: Consumptive thrombohemorrhagic disorders. In Colman RW, Hirsch J, Marder VJ, et al, eds: *Hemostasis and Thrombosis: Basic*

Principles and Clinical Practice, ed 2. Philadelphia, JB Lippincott, 1987, p 975.

106. MacLachlan NJ, Divers TJ: Hemolytic anemia and fibrinoid change of renal vessels in a horse. *J Am Vet Med Assoc* 181:716, 1982.

107. Tennant BC, Evans CD, Kaneko JJ, et al: Intravascular hemolysis associated with hepatic failure in the horse. *Calif Vet* 27:15, 1972.

108. Morris DD: Recognition and management of disseminated intravascular coagulation in horses. *Vet Clin North Am Equine Pract* 4:115, 1988.

109. Stone MS, Freden GO: Differentiation of anemia of inflammatory disease from anemia of iron deficiency. *Compendium Continuing Educ Equine Pract* 12:963, 1990.

110. Smith JE, Cipriano JE, DeBowes R, et al: Iron deficiency and pseudo-iron deficiency in hospitalized horses. *J Am Vet Med Assoc* 188:285, 1986.

111. Smith JE, Moore K, Cipriano JE, et al: Serum ferritin as measure of stored iron in horses. *J Nutr* 114:677, 1984.

112. Feldman BF, Kaneko JJ, Farver TB, et al: The anemia of inflammatory disease in the dog: Clinical characterization. *Am J Vet Res* 42:1109, 1981.

113. Radtke HW, Clausner A: Serum erythropoietin concentrations in chronic renal failure: relationship of degree of anemia and excretory renal function. *Blood* 54:877, 1979.

114. Burkhardt E, Saldern FV, Huskamp B: Monocytic leukemia in a horse. *Vet Pathol* 21:394, 1984.

115. Morris DD, Bloom JC, Roby KAW, et al: Eosinophilic myeloproliferative disorder in a horse. *J Am Vet Med Assoc* 185:993, 1984.

116. Searcy GP, Orr JP: Chronic granulocytic leukemia in a horse. *Can Vet* 22:148, 1981.

117. Spier SJ, Madewell BR, Zinkl JG, et al: Acute myelomonocytic leukemia in a horse. *J Am Vet Med Assoc* 188:861, 1986.

118. Keitt AS: Anemia due to bone marrow failure. In Wyngaarden JB, Smith LH, eds: *Cecil Textbook of Medicine*, ed 18. Philadelphia, WB Saunders, 1988, p 884.

119. Archer RK, Miller WC: A case of idiopathic hypoplastic anaemia in a two-year-old thoroughbred filly. *Vet Rec* 77:538, 1965.

120. Berggren PC: Aplastic anemia in a horse. *J Am Vet Med Assoc* 179:1400, 1981.

121. Ward MV, Mountain PC, Dodds WJ: Severe idiopathic refractory anemia and leukopenia in a horse. *Calif Vet* 34:19, 1980.

122. Dunavant ML, Murry ES: Clinical evidence of phenylbutazone induced hypoplastic anemia. In Kitchen H, Krehbiel JD, eds: *Proceedings of the First International Symposium of Equine Hematology*. Golden, Colo, American Association of Equine Practitioners, 1975, p 383.

123. Lavoie JP, Morris DD, Zinkl J, et al: Pancytopenia caused by bone marrow aplasia in a horse. *J Am Vet Med Assoc* 191:1462, 1987.

124. Erslev AJ: Hemopoietic stem cell disorders—Aplastic anemia. In Williams WJ, Beutler E, Erslev AJ, et al, eds: *Hematology*, ed 3. New York, McGraw-Hill, 1983, p 151.

125. Thomas ED, Storb R: Acquired severe aplastic anemia: Progress and perplexity. *Blood* 64:325, 1984.

126. Zoumbos NC, Gascon P, Djeu JY, et al: Circulating activated suppressor T lymphocytes in aplastic anemia. *N Engl J Med* 312:257, 1985.

127. Bue CM, Davis WC, Magnuson NS, et al: Correction of equine severe combined immunodeficiency by bone marrow transplantation. *Transplant* 42:14, 1986.

128. Krantz SB: Special Features: New therapies for aplastic anemia. *Am J Med Sci* 291:371, 1986.

129. Berk PD: Erythrocytosis and polycythemia. In Wyngaarden JB, Smith LH, eds: *Cecil Textbook of Medicine*, ed 18. Philadelphia, WB Saunders, 1988, p 975.

130. Beech J, Bloom JC, Hodge TG: Erythrocytosis in a horse. *J Am Vet Med Assoc* 150:1493, 1984.

131. Campbell KL: Diagnosis and management of polycythemia in dogs. *Compendium Continuing Educ Pract Vet* 12:543, 1990.

132. Blood DC, Radostits OM, Henderson JA eds: *Veterinary Medicine*, ed 7. London, Bailliere Tindall, 1989, p 1231.

133. Bayly WM, Reed SM, Leathers CW, et al: Multiple congenital heart anomalies in five Arabian foals. *J Am Vet Med Assoc* 181:684, 1982.

134. Roby KAW, Beech J, Bloom JC, et al: Hepatocellular carcinoma associated with erythrocytosis and hypoglycemia in a yearling filly. *J Am Vet Med Assoc* 196:465, 1990.

135. Blue J, Perdrizet J, Brown E: Pulmonary aspergillosis in a horse with myelomonocytic leukemia. *J Am Vet Med Assoc* 190:1562, 1987.

136. Boudreaux MK, Blue JT, Durham SK, et al: Intravascular leukostasis in a horse with myelomonocytic leukemia. *Vet Pathol* 21:544, 1984.

137. Brumbaugh GW, Stitzel KA, Zinkl JG, et al: Myelomonocytic myeloproliferative disease in a horse. *J Am Vet Med Assoc* 180:313, 1982.

138. Theilen GH, Madewell BR: *Veterinary Cancer Medicine*. Philadelphia, Lea & Febiger, 1979, pp 204–288.

139. Carlson GP: Lymphosarcoma in horses. In Smith BP, ed: *Large Animal Internal Medicine*. St Louis, Mosby–Year Book, 1990, p 112.

140. VanDenHoven R, Franken P: Clinical aspects of lymphosarcoma in the horse. *Equine Vet J* 15:49, 1983.

141. Neufeld JL: Lymphosarcoma in the horse: A review. *Can Vet J* 14:129, 1973.

142. Haley PJ, Spraker T: Lymphosarcoma in an aborted equine fetus. *Vet Pathol* 20:647, 1983.

143. Mackey VS, Wheat JD: Reflections on the diagnostic approach to multicentric lymphosarcoma in an aged Arabian mare. *Equine Vet J* 17:467, 1985.

144. Tomlinson MJ, Doster AR, Wright ER: Lymphosarcoma with virus-like particles in a neonatal foal. *Vet Pathol* 16:629, 1983.

145. Morris DD: Diseases of the hemolymphatic system. In Colahan P, Mayhew IG, Merritt A, et al, eds: *Equine Medicine and Surgery*, ed 4. Goleta, Calif, American Veterinary Publications, 1991, pp 1753–1859.

146. Baker J, Ellis C: A survey of postmortem findings in 480 horses, 1958–1980, (1) Causes of death. *Equine Vet J* 13:43, 1985.

147. Kerr KM, Alden CL: Equine neoplasia: A ten-year survey. In *Proceedings of the 17th Annual Meeting of the American Association of Veterinary Laboratory Diagnosticians*, Roanoke, Va, 1974, pp 183–187.

148. Rebhun WC, Bertone AL: Equine lymphosarcoma. *J Am Vet Assoc* 184:720–721, 1984.

149. Schalm OW: Lymphosarcoma in the horse. *Equine Pract* 3:23, 1981.

150. Mair TS, Lane JG, Laucke VM: Clinicopathological features of lymphosarcoma involving the thoracic cavity in the horse. *Equine Vet J* 17:428, 1985.

151. Bertone AL, Yovich JV, McIlwraith CW: Surgical resection of intestinal lymphosarcoma in a mare. *Compendium Continuing Educ Pract Vet* 7:S506–S511, 1985.

152. Traub-Dargatz JL, Bayly WM, Reed SM, et al: Intraabdominal neoplasia as a cause of chronic weight loss in the horse. *Compendium Continuing Educ Pract Vet* 5:S526–S536, 1983.

153. Wiseman A, Petrie L, Murray M: Diarrhea in the horse as a result of alimentary lymphosarcoma. *Vet Rec* 95:454–457, 1974.

154. Lane PC: Palatine lymphosarcoma in two horses. *Equine Vet J* 17:465, 1985.

155. Sheahan BJ, Atkins GJ, Russell RJ, et al: Histiolymphocytic

lymphosarcoma in the subcutis of two horses. *Vet Pathol* 17:123, 1980.

156. Adams R, Calderwood-Mays MB, Peyton LC: Malignant lymphoma in three horses with ulcerative pharyngitis. *J Am Vet Assoc* 193:674, 1988.

157. Esplin DJ, Taylor JL: Hypercalcemia in a horse with lymphosarcoma. *J Am Vet Med Assoc* 170:180, 1977.

158. Kannegieter NJ, Alley MR: Ataxia due to lymphosarcoma in a young horse. *Aust Vet J* 64:377, 1987.

159. Murphy CJ, Lavoie JP, Groff J, et al: Bilateral eyelid swelling attributable to lymphosarcoma in the horse. *J Am Vet Med Assoc* 194:939, 1989.

160. Rousseaux CG, Doige CE, Tuddenham TJ: Epidural lymphosarcoma with myelomalacia in a seven-year-old Arabian gelding. *Can Vet J* 30:751, 1989.

161. Shamis LB, Everitt JI, Baker GJ: Lymphosarcoma as the cause of ataxia in a horse. *J Am Vet Assoc* 184:1517, 1984.

162. Marr CM, Love S, Pirie HM: Clinical, ultrasonographic and pathological findings in a horse with splenic lymphosarcoma and psdudohyperparathyroidism. *Equine Vet J* 21:221, 1989.

163. Roberts MC: A case of primary lymphoid leukaemia in a horse. *Equine Vet J* 9:216, 1977.

164. Bernard WV, Sweeney CR, Morris CR, et al: Primary lymphocytic leukemia in a horse. *Equine Pract* 10:24, 1988.

165. Green PD, Donovan LA: Lymphosarcoma in a horse. *Can Vet J* 18:257, 1977.

166. Madewell BR, Carlson GP, MacLachlan NJ, et al: Lymphosarcoma with leukemia in a horse. *Am J Vet Res* 43:807, 1982.

167. Allen BV, Wannop CC, Wright IM: Multicentric lymphosarcoma with lymphoblastic leukemia in a young horse. *Vet Rec* 115:130, 1984.

168. Hambright MB, Meuten DJ, Scrutchfield WL: Equine lymphosarcoma. *Compendium Continuing Educ Pract Vet* 5:S53, 1983.

169. Perryman LE, Wyatt CR, Magnuson NS: Biochemical and functional characterization of lymphocytes from a horse with lymphosarcoma and IgM deficiency. *Comp Immunol Microbiol Infect Dis* 7:53, 1984.

170. Reef VB, Dyson SS, Beech J: Lymphosarcoma in associated immune-mediated hemolytic anemia and thrombocytopenia in horses. *J Am Vet Med Assoc* 184:313, 1984.

171. Roberts MC, Pinsent PJN: Malabsorption in the horse associated with alimentary lymphosarcoma. *Equine Vet J* 7:166–172, 1975.

172. Jacobs RM, Kociba GJ, Ruoff WW: Monoclonal gammopathy in a horse with defective hemostasis. *Vet Pathol* 20:643, 1983.

173. Farrelly BT, Collins JD, Collins SM: Autoimmune hemolytic anemia in the horse. *Ir Vet J* 20:42–45, 1966.

174. Morris DD. Immune-mediated thrombocytopenia In Robinson NE, ed: *Current Therapy in Equine Medicine*, vol 2. Philadelphia, WB Saunders, 1987, pp 310–312.

175. Marayama K, Swearingen GR, Dmochowsku L, et al: Herpes type virus and type C particles in spontaneous equine lymphoma. In *Proceedings of the 28th Annual Meeting of the Electron Microscope Society of America*, 1970, pp 162–163.

176. Dopson LC, Reed SM, Roth JA, et al: Immunosuppression associated with lymphosarcoma in 2 horses. *J Am Vet Med Assoc* 182:1239, 1983.

177. Grinden CB, Roberts MC, McEntee MF, et al: Large granular lymphocyte tumour in a horse. *Vet Pathol* 26:86, 1989.

178. McConnel S, Katada M, Fiske RA, et al: Equine lymphosarcoma diagnosed as equine infectious anemia in a young horse. *Equine Vet J* 14:160, 1982.

179. Lock PF, Macy DW: Equine ovarian lymphosarcoma. *J Am Vet Med Assoc* 175:72, 1979.

180. Thatcher CD, Roussel AJ, Chickering WR, et al: Pleural effusion with thoracic lymphosarcoma in a mare. *Compendium Continuing Educ Pract Vet* 7:S726, 1985.

181. Cornelius CE, Goodbary RF, Kennedy PC: Plasma cell myelomatosis in a horse. *Cornell Vet* 49:478, 1959.

182. Drew RA, Greatorex JC: Vertebral plasma cell myeloma causing posterior paralysis in a horse. *Equine Vet J* 6:131, 1974.

183. MacAllister C, Qualls C, Ryler L, et al: Multiple myeloma in a horse. *J Am Vet Med Assoc* 191:337, 1987.

184. Markel MD, Dorr TE: Multiple myeloma in a horse. *J Am Vet Med Assoc* 188:621, 1986.

185. Salmon SE: Plasma cell disorders In Wyngaarden JB, Smith LH, eds: *Cecil Textbook of Medicine*, ed 18. Philadelphia, WB Saunders, 1988, pp 1026.

186. Seide RK, Jacobs RM, Dobblestein TN, et al: Characterization of a homogenous paraprotein from a horse with spontaneous multiple myeloma syndrome. *Vet Immunol Immunopathol* 17:69, 1987.

187. Thrall MA: Lymphoproliferative disorders: Lymphocytic leukemia and plasma cell myeloma. *Vet Clin North Am* 11:321, 1981.

188. Mosher DF: Disorders of blood coagulation. In Wyngaarden JB, Smith LH, eds: *Cecil Textbook of Medicine*, ed 18. Philadelphia, WB Saunders, 1988, p 1060.

189. Muller-Berghaus G: Septicemia and the vessel wall. In Verstraete M, Vermylen J, Lijnen R, et al, eds: *Thrombosis and Hemostasis: 1987*. Leuven, Belgium, Leuven University Press, 1987, p 619.

190. Seiss W: Molecular mechanisms of platelet activation. *Physiol Rev* 69:58, 1989.

191. Haslam RJ: Signal Transduction in Platelet Activation. In Verstraete M, Vermylen J, Lijnen R, et al, eds: *Thrombosis and Hemostasis: 1987*. Leuven, Belgium, Leuven University Press, 1987, p 147.

192. Lammle B, Griffin JH: Formation of the fibrin clot: The balance of procoagulant and inhibitory factors. *Clin Haematol* 145:281, 1985.

193. Nemerson Y: Tissue factor and hemostasis. *Blood* 71:1, 1988.

194. Rao LVM, Rapaport SE: Activation of factor VII bound to tissue factor: a key early step in the tissue factor pathway of coagulation. *Proc Natl Acad Sci U S A* 85:6687, 1988.

195. Rapaport SE: Inhibition of Factor VIIa/Tissue Factor–induced blood coagulation: with particular emphasis upon a factor Xa-dependent inhibitory mechanism. *Blood* 73:359, 1989.

196. Kaplan AP, Silverberg M: The coagulation-kinin pathway of human plasma. *Blood* 70:1, 1987.

197. Kane WH, Davie EW: Blood coagulation factors V and VIII: Structural and functional similarities and their relationship to hemorrhagic and thrombotic disorders. *Blood* 71:539, 1988.

198. Tracy PB, Eide LL, Bowie EJW, Mann KG: Radioimmunoassay of factor V in human plasma and platelets. *Blood* 60:59, 1982.

199. Carroll RW, Christey PB, Boswell DR: Serpins: antithrombin and other inhibitors of coagulation and fibrinolysis: Evidence from amino acid sequences. In Verstraete M, Vermylen J, Lijnen R, et al, eds: *Thrombosis and Hemostasis: 1987*. Leuven, Belgium, Leuven University Press, 1987, p 1.

200. Tollefson DM, Pestka CA, Monafo WJ: Activation of heparin cofactor II by dermatan sulfate. *J Biol Chem* 258:6731, 1983.

201. Clouse LH, Camp PC: The regulation of hemostasis: The protein C system. *N Engl J Med* 314:1298, 1986.

202. Dittman WA, Majerus PW: Structure and function of thrombomodulin: A natural anticoagulant. *Blood* 75:329, 1990.

203. Esmon CT: The roles of protein C and thrombomodulin in the regulation of blood coagulation. *J Biol Chem* 264:4743, 1983.

204. Esmon CT: Protein-C: Biochemistry, physiology and clinical implications. *Blood* 62:1155, 1983.

205. Heeb MJ, Epaña F, Griffin JH: Inhibition and complexation of activated protein C by 2 major inhibitors in plasma. *Blood* 73:446, 1989.

206. Bachman F: Fibrinolysis. In Verstraete M, Vermylen J, Lijnen

R et al, eds: *Thrombosis and Hemostasis: 1987.* Leuven, Belgium, Leuven University Press, 1987, p 1.

207. Bick RL: The clinical significance of fibrinogen degradation products. *Semin Thromb Hemost* 8:302, 1982.

208. Verstraete M, Collen D: Thrombolytic therapy in the eighties. *Blood* 67:1529, 1986.

209. Wohl RC, Sinio L, Summario L, et al: Comparative activation kinetics of mammalian plasminogens. *Biochem Biophys Acta* 745:20, 1983.

210. Sprenger ED, Kluft C: Plasminogen activator inhibitors. *Blood* 69:381, 1987.

211. Brandtzaeg P, Joo GB, Brusletto B, et al: Plasminogen activator inhibitor 1 and 2, alpha-2-antiplasmin, plasminogen, and endotoxin levels in systemic meningococcal disease. *Thromb Res* 57:271, 1990.

212. Cupps TR, Fauci AS: The vasculitides. In Smith LH, ed: *Major Problems in Internal Medicine.* Philadelphia, WB Saunders, 1981, p 1.

213. Wolff SM: The vasculitic syndromes. In Wyngaarden JB, Smith LH, eds.: *Cecil Textbook of Medicine,* ed 18. Philadelphia, WB Saunders, 1988, p 2025.

214. Bacon PA: Vasculitis—clinical aspects and therapy. *Acta Med Scand Suppl* 715:157, 1989.

215. Morris DD: Vasculitis in horses. In *Proceedings of the Fourth Scientific Forum of the American College of Veterinary Internal Medicine,* Washington, DC, 1986, pp 3–7.

216. Morris DD: Diseases associated with blood loss and hemostatic dysfunction. In Smith BP, ed: *Large Animal Internal Medicine.* St Louis, Mosby–Year Book, 1990, p 1068.

217. Morris DD, Miller WH Jr, Goldschmidt MH, et al: Chronic necrotizing vasculitis in a horse. *J Am Vet Med Assoc* 183:579, 1983.

218. Werner LL, Gross TL, Hillidge CJ: Acute necrotizing vasculitis and thrombocytopenia in a horse. *J Am Vet Med Assoc* 185:87, 1984.

219. Kingston ME, Mackey D: Skin clues in the diagnosis of life-threatening infections. *Rev Infect Dis* B:1, 1986.

220. Conn DT: Update on systemic necrotizing vasculitis. *Mayo Clin Proc* 64:535, 1989.

221. Smiley JD, Moore SE: Southwestern Internal Medicine Conference: Immune-complex vasculitis: Role of complement and IgG-Fc receptor functions. *Am J Med Sci* 298:257, 1989.

222. Yanagisawa M, Kurihara H, Kimura S, et al: A novel potent vasoconstrictor peptide produced by vascular endothelial cells. *Nature* 332:411, 1988.

223. Vanhoutte PM: The endothelium-modulator of vascular smooth-muscle tone (editorial). *N Engl J Med* 319:512, 1988.

224. Schifferli JA, Ng YC, Peters DK. The role of complement and its receptor in the elimination of immune complexes. *N Engl J Med* 315:488, 1986.

225. Fearon DT: Complement, C receptors, and immune complex disease. *Hosp Pract* 23:63, 1988.

226. Caciolo PL, Hurvitz AI, Nesbitt GH. Michel's medium as a preservative for immunofluorescent staining of cutaneous biopsy specimen in dogs and cats. *Am J Vet Res* 45:128, 1984.

227. Schalm OW, Carlson GP. The blood and blood-forming organs. In Mannsman RA, McAllister ES, Pratt PW, eds. *Equine Medicine and Surgery,* ed 3. Santa Barbara, Calif, American Veterinary, 1982, p 410.

228. Galan JE, Timoney JR. *Streptococcus equi* associated immune complexes in the sera of horses with purpura haemorrhagica. Presented at Conference on Research Work on Animal Diseases, Chicago, 1984, abstr 98.

229. Gunson DE, Rooney JR: Anaphylactoid purpura in a horse. *Vet Pathol* 14:324–331, 1977.

230. Morris DD: Cutaneous vasculitis in horses: 19 cases. *J Am Vet Med Assoc* 191:460, 1987.

231. Roberts MC, Kelly WR: Renal dysfunction in a case of purpura haemorrhagica in a horse. *Vet Rec* 110:144, 1982.

232. Westaway EG, Brinton MA, Gaidamovich SY, et al: Togaviridae. *Intervirology* 24:125, 1985.

233. McCollum WH, Prickett ME, Bryans JT: Temporal distribution of equine arteritis virus in respiratory mucosa, tissues and body fluids of horses infected by inhalation. *Res Vet Sci* 2:459, 1971.

234. Timoney PJ, McCollum WH, Roberts AW, et al: Status of equine viral arteritis in Kentucky, 1985. *J Am Vet Med Assoc* 191:36, 1987.

235. Timoney PJ, McCallum WH, Roberts AW, et al: Demonstration of the carrier state in naturally acquired equine arteritis virus infection in the stallion. *Res Vet Sci* 4:279, 1986.

236. Timoney PJ, McCollum WH: Equine viral arteritis. *Can Vet J* 28:693, 1987.

237. Traub-Dargatz JL, Ralston SL, Colins JK, et al: Equine viral arteritis. *Compendium Continuing Educ Pract Vet* 7:S490, 1985.

238. Crawford TB, Henson JB: Immunoflourescent, light microscopic and immunologic studies of equine viral arteritis. In *Proceedings of the Third International Conference on Equine Infectious Diseases.* Basel, S. Karger, 1973, p 282.

239. Jones TC: Clinical and pathologic features of equine viral arteritis. *J Am Vet Med Assoc* 155:315, 1969.

240. Cole JR, Hall RF, Gosser HS, et al: Transmissibility and abortigenic effect of equine viral arteritis in mares. *J Am Vet Med Assoc* 189:769, 1986.

241. Doll ER, Knappenberger RE, Bryans JT: An outbreak of abortion caused by the equine arteritis virus. *Cornel Vet* 47:69, 1957.

242. Madigan JE, Gribble D: Equine ehrlichiosis in northern California: 49 cases (1968–1981). *J Am Vet Med Assoc* 190:445, 1987.

243. Carlson GP: Equine ehrlichiosis. In Smith BP, ed: *Large Animal Internal Medicine.* St Louis, Mosby–Year Book, 1990, p 1115.

244. Byars TD, Greene CE: Idiopathic thrombocytopenic purpura in the horse. *J Am Vet Med Assoc* 180:1422–1424, 1982.

245. Marcus AJ: Hemorrhagic disorders: abnormalities of platelet and vascular function. In Wyngaarden JB, Smith LH, eds.: *Cecil Textbook of Medicine,* ed 18. Philadelphia, WB Saunders, 1988, p 1042.

246. Morris DD, Whitlock RH: Relapsing idiopathic thrombocytopenia in a horse. *Equine Vet J* 15:73, 1983.

247. Hegde UM, Ball S, Zuiable A, et al: Platelet associated immunoglobulins (PAIgG and PAIgM) in autoimmune thrombocytopenia. *Br J Haemotol* 59:221, 1985.

248. Karpatkin S: Autoimmune thrombocytopenic purpura. *Blood* 56:329, 1980.

249. Bloom JC, Blockmer SA, Bugelski PJ, et al: Gold-induced thrombocytopenia in the dog. *Vet Pathol* 22:492, 1985.

250. Campbell KL, George JW, Greene CE: Application of the enzyme-linked immunosorbent assay for the detection of platelet antibodies in dogs. *Vet Med* 45:2561–2564, 1984.

251. Shebani OI, Jain NC: Mechanisms of platelet destruction in immune-mediated thrombocytopenia: in vitro studies with canine platelets exposed to heterologous and isologous antiplatelet antibodies. *Res Vet Sci* 47:288, 1989.

252. Kernoff LM, Malan E: Complement (C_3) binding to platelets in autoimmune thrombocytopenia. *Clin Lab Haematol* 5:1, 1983.

253. Cines DB, Wilson SB, Tomaski A, et al: Platelet antibodies of the IgM class in immune thrombocytopenic purpura. *J Clin Invest* 75:1183, 1985.

254. Lehman HA, Lehman LO, Rustagi PK, et al: Complement-mediated autoimmune thrombocytopenia. *N Engl J Med* 316:194, 1987.

255. Ballem PJ, Segal GM, Stratton JR, et al: Mechanisms of thrombocytopenia in chronic autoimmune thrombocytopenic purpura. *J Clin Invest* 80:33, 1987.

256. Sockett DC, Traub-Dargatz J, Weiser MG: Immune-mediated hemolytic anemia and thrombocytopenia in a foal. *J Am Vet Med Assoc* 190:308, 1987.

257. Rose NR: Pathogenic mechanisms in autoimmune diseases. *Clin Immunol Immunopathol* 53:S7, 1989.

258. Arnott J, Horsewood P, Kelton JG: Measurement of platelet-associated IgG in animal models of immune and nonimmune thrombocytopenia. *Blood* 69:1294, 1987.

259. Dodds WJ, Wilkins RJ: Immune-mediated thrombocytopenia, autoimmune thrombocytopenia, idiopathic thrombocytopenic purpura. *Am J Pathol* 86:489, 1977.

260. Onder O, Weinstein A, Hoyer LW: Pseudothrombocytopenia caused by platelet agglutinins that are reactive in blood anticoagulated with chelating agents. *Blood* 56:177, 1980.

261. Payne BA, Pierre RV: Pseudothrombocytopenia: A laboratory artifact with potentially serious consequences. *Mayo Clin Proc* 59:123, 1984.

262. Pegels JG, Bruynes ECE, Engelfriet CP, et al: Pseudothrombocytopenia: An immunologic study on platelet antibodies dependent on ethylene diamine tetra-acetate. *Blood* 59:157, 1982.

263. Savage RA: Pseudoleukocytosis due to EDTA-induced platelet clumping. *Am J Clin Pathol* 81:317, 1984.

264. Gordon BJ, Latimer KS, Murray CM, et al: Evaluation of leukapheresis and thrombocytapheresis in the horse. *Am J Vet Res* 47:997, 1986.

265. Coon WW: Splenectomy for idiopathic thrombocytopenic purpura. *Surg Gynecol Obstet* 164:225, 1987.

266. Feldman BF, Handagama P, Lubberink AAME: Splenectomy as adjunctive therapy for immune-mediated thrombocytopenia and hemolytic anemia in the dog. *J Am Vet Med Assoc* 187:617, 1985.

267. Jans HE, Armstrong J, Price GS: Therapy of immune-mediated thrombocytopenia: a retrospective study of 15 dogs. *J Vet Intern Med* 4:4, 1990.

268. Greene CE, Scoggin J, Thomas JE, et al: Vincristine in the treatment of thrombocytopenia in five dogs. *J Am Vet Med Assoc* 180:140, 1982.

269. Bussel JB, Pham LC, Aedort L, et al.: Maintenance treatment of adults with chronic refractory immune thrombocytopenic purpura using repeated intravenous infusions of gammaglobulin. *Blood* 72:121, 1988.

270. Gernsheimer T, Stratton J, Ballem PJ, et al: Mechanisms of response to treatment in autoimmune thrombocytopenia purpura. *N Engl J Med* 320:974, 1989.

271. Corrigan JJ: Disseminated intravascular coagulopathy. *Pediatr Rev* 1:37, 1979.

272. Colman RW, Marder VJ: Disseminated intravascular coagulation (DIC): Pathogenesis, pathophysiology, and laboratory abnormalities. In Colman RW, Hirsh J, Marder VJ, et al, eds: *Hemostasis and Thrombosis: Basic Principles and Clinical Practice.* Philadelphia, JB Lippincott, 1982, p 654.

273. Feinstein DI: Diagnosis and management of disseminated intravascular coagulation: The role of heparin therapy. *Blood* 60:284, 1982.

274. Moore DJ: Disseminated intravascular coagulation: A review of its pathogenesis, manifestations and treatment. *J S Afr Vet Assoc* 50:259, 1979.

275. Nyman D: To the discussion on the definition of DIC and its treatment. *Scand J Clin Lab Invest* 45:31, 1985.

276. Morris DD, Beech J: Disseminated intravascular coagulation in six horses. *J Am Vet Med Assoc* 183:1067, 1983.

277. Johnstone IB, Blackwell T: Disseminated intravascular coagulation in a horse with postpartum ulcerative colitis and laminitis. *Can Vet J* 25:195, 1984.

278. Johnstone IB, Crane S: Hemostatic abnormalities in equine colic. *Am J Vet Res* 47:356, 1986.

279. Johnstone IB, McAndrew KH, Baird JD: Early detection and successful reversal of DIC in a Thoroughbred mare presented with a history of diarrhea and colic. *Equine Vet J* 18:337, 1986.

280. Meyers K, Reed S, Keck M, et al: Circulating endotoxin-like substance(s) and altered hemostasis in horses with gastrointestinal disorders: An interim report. *Am J Vet Res* 43:2233, 1982.

281. Pablo LS, Purohit RC, Teer PA, et al: Disseminated intravascular coagulation in experimental intestinal strangulation obstruction in ponies. *Am J Vet Res* 44:2115, 1983.

282. Marder VJ: Consumptive thrombohemorrhagic disorders. In Buetler E, Erslev AJ, Lichtman, eds: *Hematology.* New York, McGraw-Hill, 1983, p 1433.

283. Baxter GM: Equine laminitis caused by distal displacement of the distal phalanx: 12 cases (1976–1985). *J Am Vet Med Assoc* 189:326, 1986.

284. Hood DM, Gremmel SM, Amoss MS, et al: Equine laminitis III. Coagulation dysfunction in the developmental and acute disease. *Equine Med Surg* 3:355, 1979.

285. McClure JR, McClure JJ: Intravascular coagulopathies associated with alimentary-induced acute laminitis in the pony. In *Proceedings of the First Equine Endotoxemia-Laminitis Symposium.* Golden, Colo, American Association of Equine Practitioners, 1982, p 124.

286. Sprouse RF, Garner HE: The Schwartzman reaction in horses and ponies with endotoxin and alimentary-induced laminitis. In *Proceedings of the First Equine Endotoxemia-Laminitis Symposium.* Golden, Colo, American Association of Equine Practitioners, 1982, p 119.

287. Bick RL: Clinical implications of molecular markers of hemostasis and thrombosis. *Semin Thromb Hemost* 10:290, 1984.

288. Bick RL, Bick MD, Fekete LJ: Antithrombin III patterns in disseminated intravascular coagulation. *Am J Clin Pathol* 73:577, 1980.

289. Cembrowski GS, Griffin JH, Mosher DF: Diagnostic efficacy of six plasma proteins in evaluating consumptive coagulopathies. *Arch Intern Med* 146:1997, 1986.

290. Colman RW, Robboy SJ, Minna JD: Disseminated intravascular coagulation: a reappraisal. *Annu Rev Med* 30:359, 1986.

291. Feldman BF, Madewell BR, O'Neill S: Disseminated intravascular coagulation: Antithrombin, plasminogen, and coagulation abnormalities in 41 dogs. *J Am Vet Med Assoc* 179:151, 1981.

292. Spero JA, Lewis JH, Hasiba A: Disseminated intravascular coagulation: Findings in 346 patients. *Thromb Haemost* 43:28, 1980.

293. King JN, Gerring EL: Detection of endotoxemia in cases of equine colic. *Vet Rec* 123:269, 1988.

294. Moore JN: Recognition and treatment of endotoxemia. *Vet Clin North Am* 4:105, 1988.

295. Ziegler EJ. Extraintestinal infections caused by enteric bacteria. In Wyngaarden JB, Smith LH eds: *Cecil Textbook of Medicine,* ed 18. Philadelphia, WB Saunders, 1988, p 1658.

296. Feldman BF: Disseminated intravascular coagulation. *Compendium Continuing Educ Pract Vet* 3:46, 1981.

297. Wig DA, Yamada T, Havley JB, et al: Model for disseminated intravascular coagulation: Bacterial sepsis in rhesus monkeys. *J Lab Clin Med* 92:239, 1978.

298. Morrison DC, Ryan JL: Endotoxins and disease mechanisms. *Annu Rev Med* 38:417, 1987.

299. Francis GL, Read LC, Ballard FJ, et al: Purification and partial sequence analysis of insulin-like growth factor-1 from bovine colostrum. *Biochem J* 233:207, 1986.

300. Muller-Berghaus G. Interference of endotoxin with blood co-

agulation. In Eaker D, Wadstrom T, eds: *Natural Toxins*. New York, Pergamon Press, 1980, p 139.

301. Fruchtman S, Aledort LM: Disseminated intravascular coagulation. *J Am Coll Cardiol* 8:159B, 1986.
302. Karakusis PH: Considerations in the therapy of septic shock. *Med Clin North Am* 70:933, 1986.
303. Morrison DC, Cochrane CG: Direct evidence for Hageman factor (factor XII) activation by bacterial lipopolysaccharides (endotoxins). *J Exp Med* 140:797, 1974.
304. Edwards RL, Rickles FR: Macrophage procoagulants. *Prog Hemost Thromb* 7:183, 1984.
305. Lyberg T: Clinical significance of increased thromboplastin activity on the monocyte surface—a brief review. *Haemostasis* 14:430, 1984.
306. Maier RV, Hahnel GB: Potential for endotoxin-activated Kupffer cells to induce microvascular thrombosis. *Arch Surg* 119:62, 1984.
307. Henry MM, Moore JN: Endotoxin-induced procoagulant activity in equine peripheral blood monocytes. *Circ Shock* 26:297, 1988.
308. Handley DA, Van Valen RG, Melden MK, et al: Inhibition and reversal of endotoxin-aggregated IgG and PAF-induced hypotension in the rat by SRI 63-072, a PAF receptor antagonist. *Immunopharmacology* 12:11, 1986.
309. Carrick JB, Moore JN, Morris DD: Inhibition of PAF-induced aggregation of equine platelets by a PAF-receptor antagonist (SR 63–441). In Handley DA, Saunders RN, Houlihan WJ, et al, eds: *Platelet Activating Factor in Endotoxin and Immune Diseases*. New York, Marcel Dekker, 1989, p 77.
310. Newton RC: Human monocyte production of interleukin-1: Parameters of the induction of IL-1 secretion by lipopolysaccharides. *J Leukoc Biol* 39:299, 1986.
311. Männel DN, Northoff, Bauss F, et al: Tumor necrosis factor: A cytokine involved in toxic effects of endotoxin. *Rev Infect Dis* 9:S602, 1987.
312. Paramo JA, Fernandez Diaz FJ, Rocha E: Plasminogen activator inhibitor activity in bacterial infection. *Thromb Haemost* 59:451, 1988.
313. Schwartz BS, Monroe MC, Levin EG: Increased release of plasminogen activator inhibitor type 2 accompanies the human mononuclear cell tissue factor response to LPS. *Blood* 71:734, 1988.
314. Suffredini AF, Harpel PC, Parrillo JE: Promotion and subsequent inhibition of plasminogen activation after administration of intravenous endotoxin to normal subjects. *N Engl J Med* 320:1165, 1989.
315. Wigton DH, Kociba GJ, Hoover EQ: Infectious canine hepatitis: Animal model for viral-induced disseminated intravascular coagulation. *Blood* 47:287, 1976.
316. Marlar RA, Brooks JE, Miller C: Serial studies of protein C and its plasma inhibitor in patients with disseminated intravascular coagulation. *Blood* 66:59, 1985.
317. Martinez-Brotons F, Oncins JR, Mestres J, et al: Plasma kallikrein-kinin system in patients with uncomplicated sepsis and septic shock—comparison with cardiogenic shock. *Thromb Haemost* 58:709, 1987.
318. Giddings C, Peake R: Laboratory support in the diagnosis of coagulation disorders. *Clin Haematol* 14:571, 1985.
319. Meyers K, Menard M, Wardrop KJ: Equine hemostasis: description, evaluation and alteration. *Vet Clin North Am Equine Pract* 3:485, 1987.
320. Dinarello CA. An update on human interleukin-1: from molecular biology to clinical relevance. *J Clin Immunol* 5:287, 1985.
321. Perlmutter DH, Dinarello CA, Punsal PI, et al: Cachectin/tumor necrosis factor regulates hepatic acute-phase gene expression. *J Clin Invest* 78:1349, 1986.
322. Le J, Vilcek J. Interleukin 6: A multifunctional cytokine regulating immune reactions and the acute phase protein response. *Lab Invest* 61:588, 1989.
323. McCuskey RS, McCuskey PA, Urbascheck R, et al: Species differences in Kupffer cells and endotoxin sensitivity. *Infect Immun* 45:278, 1984.
324. Morris DD, Messick J, Whitlock RH, et al: Effects of equine ehrlichial colitis on the hemostatic system in ponies. *Am J Vet Res* 49:1030, 1988.
325. Garcia Frade LJ, Landin L, Avello AG, et al: Changes in fibrinolysis in the intensive care patient. *Thromb Res* 47:593, 1987.
326. Bick RL: Clinical relevance of antithrombin III. *Semin Thromb Hemost* 8:276, 1982.
327. Morris DD: Hemostatic function tests in horses: current and future trends. In Milne FJ, ed: *Proceedings of the 33rd Annual Convention of the American Association of Equine Practitioners,* Golden, Colo, 1987, p 331.
328. Johnstone IB, Petersen D, Crane S: Antithrombin III (AT III) activity in plasma from normal and diseased horses, and in normal canine, bovine, and human plasma. *Vet Clin Pathol* 16:14, 1987.
329. Friberger P. Chromogenic peptide substrates: Their use for the assay of factors in the fibrinolytic and the plasma kallikrein-kinin systems. *Scand J Clin Lab Invest Supp* 42 (162):1, 1982.
330. Wehrmacher WH: Molecular markers of hemostasis: introduction and overview. *Semin Thromb Hemost* 10:215, 1984.
331. Morris DD, Ward MV, Whitlock RH. Plasma plasminogen concentrations in clinically normal horses: the effect of age, sex and pregnancy. *Equine Vet J* 21:119, 1989.
332. Welles EG, Prasse KW, Moore JN: Use of a newly developed assay for protein C and plasminogen in horses with signs of colic. *Am J Vet Res* 52:345–351, 1991.
333. Prasse KW, Allen D, Moore JN, et al: Evaluation of coagulation and fibrinolysis during the prodromal stage of experimental equine acute laminits and reference values in normal horses. *Am J Vet Res* 51:1950–1955, 1990.
334. Semrad SD, Hardee GE, Hardee MM, et al: Flunixin meglumine given in small doses: Prostaglandin inhibition in healthy horses. *Am J Vet Res* 46:2474, 1985.
335. Morris DD: Blood products in large animal medicine: A comparative account of current and future technology. *Equine Vet J* 19:272, 1987.
336. Bick RL: DIC and related syndromes: Etiology, pathophysiology, diagnosis and management. *Am J Hematol* 5:265, 1978.
337. Stick JA: Laminitis. In Robinson NE, ed: *Current Therapy in Equine Medicine*, vol 2. Philadelphia, WB Saunders, 1987, p 277.
338. Silver D, Kapsch D, Tsoi E: Heparin-induced thrombocytopenia, thrombosis and hemorrhage. *Ann Surg* 198:301, 1983.
339. Duncan SG, Meyers KM, Reed SM: Reduction of the red blood cell mass of horses: Toxic effect of heparin anticoagulant therapy. *Am J Vet Res* 44:2271, 1983.
340. Moore JN, Mahaffey EA, Zboran M: Heparin-induced agglutination of erythrocytes in horses. *Am J Vet Res* 48:68, 1987.
341. Sakata Y, Yoshida N, Matsuda M, et al: Treatment of DIC with AT-III concentrates. *Bibl Haematologica* 49:307, 1983.
342. Emerson TE, Fournel MA, Leach WJ, et al: Protection against DIC and death by AT-III in the *E. coli* endotoxemic rat. *Circ Shock* 21:1, 1987.
343. Hauptman JG, Hassouna NI, Bell TG, et al: Efficacy of AT-III in endotoxin-induced DIC. *Circ Shock* 25:111, 1988.
344. Heeb MJ, Mosher D, Griffin JH: Activation and complexation of protein C and cleavage and decrease of protein S in plasma of patients with DIC. *Blood* 73:455, 1989.
345. Taylor FB, Chang A, Esmon CT, et al: Protein C prevents the coagulopathic and lethal effects of *E. coli* infusion in the baboon. *J Clin Invest* 79:918, 1987.
346. Colles CM: Anticoagulant therapy for navicular disease. *Vet Rec* 108:107, 1981.
347. Esmon CT, Sadowsky JI, Suttie JW: A new carboxylation

reaction. The vitamin K-dependent incorporation of $H^{14}CO_3^-$ into prothrombin. *J Biol Chem* 250:4744, 1975.

348. Stenflo J, Fernland P, Egan W, et al: Vitamin K dependent modification of glutamic acid residues in prothrombin. *Proc Natl Acad Sci U S A* 71:2730, 1974.

349. Scott EA, Byars TD, Lamar AM: Warfarin: Effects of anticoagulant, hematologic and blood enzyme values in normal ponies. *Am J Vet Res* 40:142, 1979.

350. Rebhun WC, Tennant BC, Dill SG, et al: Vitamin K_3-induced renal toxicosis in the horse. *J Am Vet Med Assoc* 184:1237, 1984.

351. Burrows GE, Tyrl RJ: Plants causing sudden death in livestock. *Vet Clin North Am Food Anim Pract* 5:263, 1989.

352. Osweiler GD, Rurh LP: Plants affecting blood coagulation. In Howard JS, ed: *Current Veterinary Therapy Food Animal Practice*, vol 2. Philadelphia, WB Saunders, 1986, p 404.

353. Casper HH, Benson ME, Kunerth W: Spectrophotometric determination of dicoumarol in sweet clover. *J Assoc Anal Chem* 64:689, 1981.

354. Feldman BF, Carroll EJ, Jain NC: Coagulation and its disorders. In Jain NC, ed: *Schalm's Veterinary Hematology*, ed 4. Philadelphia, Lea & Febiger, 1986, p 388.

355. Ainsworth DM, Dodds WJ, Brown CM: Deficiency of the contact phase of intrinsic coagulation in a horse. *J Am Vet Med Assoc* 187:71, 1985.

356. Mills JN, Bolton JR: Haemophilia A in a 3-year-old Thoroughbred horse. *Aust Vet J* 60:60, 1983.

357. Nossel HL, Archer RK, Macfarlane RG: Equine haemophilia: report of a case and its response to multiple infusions of heterospecific AHG. *Br J Haematol* 8:335, 1962.

358. Hutchins DR, Lepherd EE, Crook IG: A case of equine hacmophilia. *Aust Vet J* 43:83, 1967.

359. Feldman BF, Giacopuzzi RL: Hemophilia A (Factor VIII) deficiency in a colt. *Equine Pract* 4:24, 1982.

360. Henninger RW: Hemophilia in two related Quarter Horse colts. *J Am Vet Med Assoc* 193:91–94, 1988.

361. Hoyer LW: The factor VIII complex: structure and function. *Blood* 58:1, 1981.

362. Littlewood JD, Bevan SA, Corke MJ: Hemophilia A (classic hemophilia, factor VIII deficiency) in a Thoroughbred foal. *Equine Vet J* 23:70, 1991.

363. Veltkamp JJ: Diagnosis of carriers of hemophilia A. In Brinkhous KM, Hemker HC, eds: *Handbook of Hemophilia*. Amsterdam, Excerpta Medica, 1975, pp 277–281.

364. Knotos HA: Vascular diseases of the limbs. In Wyngaarden JB, Smith LH, eds: *Cecil Textbook of Medicine*, ed 18. Philadelphia, WB Saunders, 1988, p 375.

365. Schafer AI: The hypercoagulable state. *Ann Intern Med* 102:814, 1985.

366. Bauer KA, Rosenberg RD: The pathophysiology of the prethrombotic state in humans: Insights gained from studies using markers of hemostatic system activation. *Blood* 70:343, 1987.

367. Owen J, Kvam D, Nossel HL, et al: Thrombin and plasmin activity and platelet activation in the development of venous thrombosis. *Blood* 61:476–482, 1983.

368. Thaler E, Lechner K: Antithrombin III deficiency and thromboembolism. In Prentice CRM, ed: *Clinics in Haematology*, vol 10. London, WB Saunders, 1981, p 369.

369. Morris DD: Thrombophlebitis in horses: The contribution of hemostatic dysfunction to its pathogenesis. *Compendium Continuing Educ Pract Vet* 11:1386, 1989.

370. Green RA: Clinical implications of antithrombin III deficiency in animal disease. *Compendium Continuing Educ Pract Vet* 6:537, 1984.

371. Morris DD: Glomerulonephritis. In Robinson WE, ed: *Current Therapy in Equine Medicine*, ed 2. Philadelphia, WB Saunders, 1987, p 310.

372. Mahaffey EA, Moore JN: Erythrocyte agglutination associated with heparin treatment in three horses. *J Am Vet Med Assoc* 181:1478, 1986.

373. Bayly WM, Vale BH: Intravenous catheterization and associated problems in the horse. *Compendium Continuing Educ Pract Vet* 4:S227, 1982.

374. Deem DA: Complications associated with the use of intravenous catheters in large animals. *Calif Vet* 6:19, 1981.

375. Nilsson IM, Ljungner H, Tengborn L: Two different mechanisms in patients with venous thrombosis and defective fibrinolysis: Low concentration of plasminogen activator or increased concentration of plasminogen activator inhibitor. *Br Med J* 290:1453, 1985.

376. Sloan IG, Firkin BG: Impaired fibrinolysis in patients with thrombotic or haemostatic defects. *Thromb Res* 55:559, 1989.

377. Kluft C, Verheijen JH, Jie AFH, et al: The postoperative fibrinolytic shutdown: A rapidly reverting acute phase pattern for the fast-acting inhibition of tissue-type plasminogen activator after trauma. *Scand J Clin Lab Invest* 45:605, 1985.

378. Wiman B, Ljungberg B, Chmielewski J, et al: The role of the fibrinolytic system in deep vein thrombosis. *J Clin Lab Med* 105:265, 1985.

379. Kluft C, Verheijen JH, Jie AFH, et al: The postoperative fibrinolytic shutdown: a rapidly reverting acute phase pattern for the fast-acting inhibitor of tissue-type plasminogen activator after trauma. *Scand J Clin Lab Invest* 45:605, 1985.

380. Suffredini AF, Harpel PC, Parillo JE: Promotion and subsequent inhibition of plasminogen activation after administration of intravenous endotoxin to normal subjects. *N Engl J Med* 320:1165, 1989.

381. Van Hinsbergh VWH, Bertina RM, Van Wijngaarden A, et al: Activated protein C decreases plasminogen activator-inhibitor activity in endothelial cell-conditioned medium. *Blood* 65:444, 1985.

382. Almer L-O, Ohlin H: Elevated levels of the rapid inhibitor of plasminogen activator (t-PAI) in acute myocardial infarction. *Thromb Res* 47:335, 1987.

383. Brandtzaeg P, Joo GB, Brusletto B, et al: Plasminogen activator inhibitor 1 and 2, alpha-2-antiplasmin, plasminogen, and endotoxin levels in systemic meningococcal disease. *Thromb Res* 57:271, 1990.

384. Engebretsen LF, Kierulf P, Brandtzeg P: Extreme plasminogen activator inhibitor and endotoxin values in patients with meningococcal disease. *Thromb Res* 42:713, 1986.

385. Pralong G, Colandra T, Glauser MP, et al: Plasminogen activator inhibitor 1: a new prognostic marker in septic shock. *Thromb Haemost* 61:459, 1989.

386. Kallfelz FA, Whitlock RH, Schultz RD: Survival of ^{59}Fe-labeled erythrocytes in cross-transfused equine blood. *Am J Vet Res* 39:617, 1978.

387. Stormont CJ: Blood groups in animals. *J Am Vet Med Assoc* 181:1120, 1982.

388. Wong PL, Nickel LS, Bowling AT, et al: Clinical survey of antibodies against red blood cells in horses after homologous blood transfusion. *Am J Vet Res* 47:2566, 1986.

389. Doll ER, Richards MG, Wallace ME, et al: The influence of equine fetal tissue vaccine upon hemagglutination activity of mare serums: Its relation to hemolytic icterus of newborn foals. *Cornell Vet* 42:495, 1952.

390. Schmotzer WB, Riebold TW, Porter SL, et al: Time-saving techniques for the collection, storage and administration of equine blood and plasma. *Vet Med* 89, 1985.

391. Morris PG: Blood transfusion. In Robinson NE, ed: *Current Therapy in Equine Medicine*. Philadelphia, WB Saunders, 1983, p 325.

392. Morris DD, Bruce J, Gaulin G, et al: Evaluation of granulocyte transfusion therapy in healthy neonatal foals. *Am J Vet Res* 48:1187, 1987.

Chapter 12

Gastrointestinal Disease

Problems Involving the Mouth

Gordon J. Baker, BVSc, PhD, MRCUS, Dip ACVS

The word *mouth* is used commonly to signify either the first part of the alimentary canal or the entrance to it.[1] It is bounded laterally by the cheeks, dorsally by the palate, and ventrally by the body of the mandible and by the mylohyoideus muscles. The caudal margin is the soft palate. The horse's mouth is long and cylindrical and when the lips are closed the contained structures almost fill the cavity. A small space remains between the root of the tongue and the epiglottis and is termed the *oropharynx*. The cavity of the mouth is subdivided into sections by the teeth. The space external to the teeth and enclosed by the lips is termed the *vesicle of the mouth* and, in the resting state, the lateral margins of the vesicle, that is, the buccal mucosa, are in close contact with the cheek teeth. Caudally, it communicates with the pharynx through the aditus pharyngis. The mucous membrane of the mouth is continuous at the margin of the lips with the skin and during life it is chiefly pink in color but can be more or less pigmented, depending on the skin color and the breed type.

MORPHOLOGY AND FUNCTION

The lips are two muscular membranous folds that unite at angles close to the first cheek teeth. Each lip presents an outer and an inner surface, and the upper lip has a shallow median furrow (philtrum). The lower lip has a rounded prominence or chin (mentum). The internal surface is covered with a thick mucous membrane that contains small pitted surfaces which are the openings of the ducts of the labial glands. There are small folds of the mucous membrane that pass from the lips to the gum, the frenula labii. The free border of the lip is dense and bears short stiff hairs. The arteries of the mouth are derived from the maxillary, mandibular, labial, and sphenopalatine artery of the major palatine artery. The veins drain chiefly to the lingual facial vein. Sensory nerves originate from the trigeminal nerve (cranial nerve V) and the motor nerves from the facial nerve (VII). The cheeks spread back from the lips and form both sides of the mouth. They are attached to the alveolar borders of the bones of the jaws. They are comprised of skin and a muscular and glandular layer and then the internal mucous membrane. The skin is thin and pliable. The oral mucous membrane, by contrast, is dense and in many areas of the oral cavity is firmly attached to the periosteum so that construction of oral mucosal flaps can only be achieved by horizontal division of the periosteal attachment. Such a feature is important in reconstructive techniques applied to the oral cavity. The blood supply to the cheeks comes from the facial and buccal arteries, sensory nerves from the trigeminal, and motor nerves from the facial nerve.

The hard palate (palatum durum) is bounded rostrally and laterally by the alveolar arches and is continuous with the soft palate caudally. It has a central raphe which divides the surface into two equal portions. From the line of the rostral cheek tooth, the hard palate is markedly concave to the line of the caudal cheek tooth. Paired transverse ridges (about 18) traverse the concavity and have their free edges directed caudally. The incisive duct is a small tube of mucous membrane which extends obliquely through the palatine fissure. The dorsal component communicates by a slitlike opening in the rostral portion of the ventral nasal meatus. Its palatine end is blind and lies in the submucosa of the palate. When stallions display their flehmen response, watery secretions enter the nose from the glands of the vomeronasal duct. It is not yet known to what extent these secretions aid in pheromone reception.[2]

That portion of the palatine mucosa immediately behind the incisor teeth is frequently swollen (lumpas) during eruption of the permanent teeth. This swelling is physiologic and not pathologic.

The tongue is situated on the floor of the mouth between the bodies of the mandible and is supported by the sling formed by the mylohyoideus muscles. The root of the tongue is attached to the hyoid bone, soft palate, and pharynx. The upper surface and the rostral portion of the tongue are free; the body of the tongue has three surfaces. The apex of the tongue is spatulate and has a rounded border. The mucous membrane adheres intimately to the adjacent structure and on the dorsum it is very dense and thick. From the lower surface of the free part of the tongue, a fold of mucous membrane passes to the floor of the mouth forming the lingual frenulum. Caudally, a fold passes on each side of the dorsum to join the soft palate, forming the palatoglossal arch. Dorsally from the soft palate, the palatopharyngeal arch attaches and circumvents the aditus laryngis and attaches to the roof of the nasopharynx. The mucous membrane of the tongue presents four kinds of papillae. (1) Filiform papillae are fine threadlike projections across the dorsum of the tongue. They are absent on the root of the tongue, and are small on the rostral portion of the tongue. (2) The fungiform papillae are larger and easily seen at the rounded free end. They occur principally on the lateral portion of the tongue. (3) Vallate papillae are usually two or three in number and are found on the caudal portion of the dorsum of the tongue. The free surface bears numerous small, round secondary papillae. (4) Foliate papillae are situated rostral to the palatoglossal arches of the soft palate where they form a rounded eminence about 2 or 3 cm in length marked by transverse fissures. Foliate, vallate, and fungiform papillae are covered with taste buds and secondary papillae.

The lingual and sublingual arteries supply the tongue from the linguofacial trunk and matching veins. The linguofacial trunk drains into the linguofacial vein. The lingual muscles are innervated by the hypoglossal nerve (XII) and the sensory supply is from the lingual and glossopharyngeal (IX) nerves.

EQUINE DENTITION

The formula for the deciduous teeth of the horse is I$\frac{3}{3}$ C$\frac{0}{0}$ P$\frac{3}{3}$ × 2 = 24. The permanent dental formula is I$\frac{3}{3}$ C$\frac{1}{1}$ P$\frac{3}{3}$ or P$\frac{4}{3}$ M$\frac{3}{3}$ × 2 = 40 or 42. In the mare, the canine teeth are usually very small or do not erupt, hence reducing the number to 36 or 38. The first premolar tooth (wolf tooth) is often absent and has been reported as occurring in only 20% of the upper dentition of Thoroughbred horses.[3] The teeth of the horse are complex in shape and are compounded of different materials (dentine, cementum, and enamel). They function as grinding blades to masticate and macerate cellulose food in the important first stage of the digestive process. Study of the cheek teeth in the horse is a well-documented feature of the evolution of *Equus caballus*.

Eruption Times

Deciduous Teeth. The first incisor is present at birth or the first week of life; the second incisor, at 4 to 6 weeks of age; the third incisor, at 6 to 9 months of age; the first and second premolars, birth to 2 weeks of age; the third premolar, 3 months of age.

Permanent Teeth. The eruption times are first incisor, 2½ years of age; second incisor, 3½ years of age; third incisor, 4½ years of age; the canine tooth, 4 to 5 years of age; the first premolar (wolf tooth), 5 to 6 months of age; the second premolar, 2½ years of age; the third premolar, 3 years of age; the fourth premolar, 4 years of age; the first molar, 10 to 12 months of age; the second molar, 2 years of age; the third molar, 3½ to 4 years of age. It is clear from this eruption sequence that the eruption of the second and third permanent premolar teeth give the potential for dental impaction.

The modern horse has six incisor teeth in each jaw that are placed close together so that the labile edges form a semicircle. The occlusal surface has a deep enamel invagination (infundibulum) which is only partially filled with cementum. As the incisor teeth are worn, a characteristic pattern forms in which the infundibulum is surrounded by rings of enamel, dentine, enamel, and crown cementum in a concentric pattern. Each incisor tooth tapers from a broad crown to a narrow root so that as the midportion of the incisor is exposed to wear, the cross-sectional diameters are about equal, that is, at 14 years of age, the central incisor tooth of the horse has an occlusal surface that is an equilateral triangle. Observations on the state of eruption, the angles of incidence of the incisor teeth, and the pattern of the occlusal surfaces are used as guides for aging of horses. The canine teeth are simple teeth without complex crowns and are curved. The crown is compressed and is smooth on its labial aspect, but carries two ridges on its lingual aspect. No occlusal contact is made between the upper and lower canine teeth.

When erupted, the six cheek teeth of the horse function as a single unit in the mastication of food. Each arcade consists of three premolar and three molar teeth. The maxillary arcade is slightly curved and the teeth have a square occlusal surface. The occlusal surfaces of the mandibular teeth are more oblong in appearance, and each arcade is straighter. The horse is anisognathic, that is, the distance between the mandibular teeth is narrower (one-third) than the distance between the upper cheek teeth. This anatomical arrangement affects the inclination of the dental arcade as the jaws slide across each other in the food preparation process. The unworn upper cheek tooth presents a surface in which there are two undulating and narrow ridges, one of which is lateral and the other medial. On the rostral and lingual side of the medial style, there is an extra hillock. The central portion of these surfaces is indented by two depressions that are comparable to, but much deeper than, the infundibula of the incisor teeth. When the teeth have been subjected to wear, the enamel that closed the ridges is worn through and the underlying dentine appears on the surface. The result is that after a time the chewing surface displays a complicated pattern that may be likened to the outline of an ornate letter *B*, the upright stroke of the *B* being on the lingual aspect. Dentine supports the enamel internally, cementum supports the enamel lakes, and the peripheral cementum fills in the spaces between the teeth so that all six teeth may function as a single unit, that is, the dental arcade. Each tooth is crossed by transverse ridges so that the whole maxillary arcade seems to consist of a serrated edge. The serrations are formed so that a valley is present at the area of contact with adjacent teeth. These serrations are matched by fitting serrations on the mandibular arcade.

The true roots of the cheek teeth are short when compared with the total length of the tooth. There are three roots—two small lateral roots and one large medial root. It is customary to refer to that portion of the crown that is embedded within the dental alveolus as the reserve crown and to confine the term *root* to that area of the tooth that is comparatively short and enamel-free. As the tooth wears away, the reserve crown is gradually exposed, and the roots lengthen. In an adult 1,000-lb horse, the maxillary cheek teeth are between 8.0 and 8.5 cm in length. Dental wear accounts for erosion and loss of tooth substance at a rate of 2 mm/yr.

The pulp chambers of the horse's teeth are also complex. The incisors and canines have a single pulp chamber. The mandibular cheek teeth have two roots and two separate pulp chambers. The maxillary cheek teeth, although they have three roots, have, in fact, five pulp chambers. As occlusal wear proceeds, the pulp chambers are protected by the deposition of secondary dentine within the pulp chambers (e.g., the dental star, medial to the infundibulum on the incisor teeth).

In the mandibular cheek teeth, the transverse folding of the enamel anlage (during morphogenesis of the tooth) does not take place, and the occlusal surface is a simple surface of central dentine surrounded by enamel. Each tooth is then conformed to a single arcade by the presence of peripheral crown cementum.

SALIVARY GLANDS

Saliva is important for lubrication and softening of food material. The horse has paired parotid, mandibular, and polystomatic sublingual salivary glands. The parotid gland is the largest of the salivary glands in the horse. It is situated in the space between the ramus of the mandible and the wing of the atlas. The parotid duct is formed at the ventral part of the gland near the facial crest by the union of three or four smaller ducts. It leaves the gland above the linguofacial vein, crosses the tendon of the sternocephalicus muscle, and enters the mouth obliquely in the cheek opposite the third upper cheek tooth. Its orifice is small, but there is some dilatation of the duct and a circular mucous fold (the parotid papillae) at this point. The mandibular gland is smaller than the parotid gland and extends from the atlantal fossa to the basihyoid bone. For the most part, it is covered by the parotid gland and by the lower jaw. The mandibular duct is formed by union of a number of small duct radicles which emerge along the concave edge of the gland and run rostral to the border of the mouth opposite the canine tooth. The orifice is at the end of a sublingual caruncle. The mandibular gland possesses serous, mucous, and mixed alveolar glandular components. The parotid gland is a compound alveolar serous gland.

The parotid salivary gland can secrete saliva to yield minute rates of 50 mL/min, and a total daily parotid secretion can be as much as 12 L in a 500-kg horse. Parotid secretion only occurs during mastication, and its secretion can be blocked by atropine or anesthesia of the oral mucosa. Parotid saliva is hypotonic compared with plasma, but at high rates of flow there are increases in sodium, chloride, and bicarbonate ions. There is a high concentration of calcium in parotid saliva in the horse, and occasionally calculus deposition will form within the duct radicles of the parotid salivary gland.

The lips of the horse are extremely mobile and prehensile. In many ways they function like the tip of the elephant's trunk in that they test, manipulate, and sample the environment for potential nutritive value. Consequently, loss of motor function (e.g., facial palsy) will affect the efficiency of the prehensile system. Food is grasped by the lips in grazing or browsing, and sectioned by the incisor teeth. After mastication and lubrication with saliva, the bolus of food is formed and is manipulated from side to side across the mouth assisted by the tight cheeks of the horse and the palatine ridges. Swallowing is initiated by the food bolus contacting the base of the tongue and the pharyngeal walls. During swallowing there is elevation of the soft palate to close the nasopharynx, elevation of the base of the tongue, and rostral movement of the hyoid bone and the larynx secondary to contraction of the hyoid muscles. During this process, the rima glottidis is closed and the epiglottis tilts dorsally and caudally to protect the airway so that food is swept through lateral food channels around the sides of the larynx into the laryngoesophagus. In fluoroscopic studies in nursing foals in the dorsoventral view, it was shown that there is contact between the lateral food channels in the midline so that in outline the food bolus achieves a bow tie shape.[4]

MOUTH DISEASES

The oral cavity and oropharynx are subject to a wide variety of diseases. However, many conditions affecting the first portion of the alimentary system produce the same clinical signs regardless of their cause. The clinical signs may include inappetence or reluctance to eat, pain on eating or swallowing, oral swelling, oral discharge, and a fetid breath. Affected animals may show some interest in food but hesitate to eat it. There may be excessive salivation, which may be contaminated with purulent exudate or blood. The occurrence of bruxism (i.e., grinding of teeth) can be an indication of discomfort in other areas of the alimentary tract, for example, bruxism and frothing oral saliva is a characteristic feature of gastric ulceration in the horse.

The clinician needs to be aware that considerable weight loss can occur rapidly with inability to feed and swallow. Diseases that result in denervation of the pharynx and inappropriate swallowing can have the complication of inhalation pneumonia.

Examination and Clinical Signs

After a complete physical examination and ascertaining the history as to time of onset, and so forth, a systematic approach should be used in all cases. A considerable portion of the mouth and teeth can be examined from the outside by palpation of the structures through the folds of the cheek. Most horses allow an oral examination without sedation or the use of an oral speculum. In many cases, however, the dental detailed oral examination is best achieved by sedation and the use of an oral speculum and a light source. The mouth should be irrigated to wash out retained food material, so that the lips, cheeks, teeth, and gums can be inspected as well as palpated.

The classic signs of dental disease in the horse include difficulty and slowness in feeding, together with a progressive unthriftiness and loss of body condition. In some instances, the horse may quid, that is, it may drop poorly masticated food boluses from the mouth, and halitosis may be obvious. Additional problems reported by owners include biting and riding problems and headshaking or head shyness. There may be facial or mandibular swelling. Nasal discharge can result from dental disease that is associated with maxillary sinus empyema. Mandibular fistulas are frequently caused by lower cheek tooth apical infections. Some correlation can be achieved between the animal's age and clinical signs (Table 12–1).

Ancillary Diagnostic Techniques

Ancillary aids for a complete examination of the oral cavity of the horse may include radiology, endoscopic examination,

Table 12–1. Correlation Between Dental Disease and Dental Therapy*

Age	Examine for	Necessary Dentistry
2–3 yr	1. 1st premolar vestige (wolf teeth)	1. Remove wolf teeth if present
	2. 1st deciduous premolar (upper and lower)	2. Remove deciduous teeth if ready; if not, file off corners and points of premolars
	3. Hard swelling on ventral surface of mandible beneath 1st premolar	3. Obtain x-ray film; extract retained temporary premolar if present
	4. Cuts or abrasions on inside of cheek in region of the 2nd premolars and molars	4. Lightly float or dress all molars and premolars if necessary
	5. Sharp protuberances on all premolars and molars	5. Rasp protuberances down to level of other teeth in arcade
3–4 yrs	1. (1), (2), (4), and (5) above	1. (1), (2), (4), and (5) above
	2. 2nd deciduous premolar (upper and lower)	2. Remove if present and ready
4–5 yrs	1. (1), (4), and (5) above	1. (1), (4), and (5) above
	2. 3rd deciduous premolar	2. Remove if present and ready
5 yrs and older	1. (1), (4), and (5) above	1. (1), (4), and (5) above
	2. Uneven growth and "wavy" arcade	2. Straighten if interfering with mastication
	3. Unusually long molars and premolars	3. Unusually long molars and premolars may have to be cut if they cannot be filed down

*From Baker GJ: Diseases of the teeth. In Colohan PT, Mayhew IG, Merritt AM, et al, eds: *Equine Medicine and Surgery,* ed 4, vol 1. Goleta, Calif, American Veterinary Publications, 1991, p 550.

fluoroscopy, biopsy, and culture. Care should always be taken if endoscopic evaluation of the oral cavity is made using a flexible endoscope. I recommend sedation and the use of an oral speculum to prevent inadvertent mastication of the endoscope. If general anesthesia is to be used as part of the diagnostic workup, then endoscopic evaluation of the oral cavity is made much easier.

Congenital and Developmental Abnormalities

Cleft Palate. Palatine clefts may be the result of an inherited defect and are caused by failure of the transverse palatal folds to fuse in the oral cavity. Very few palatine clefts in the horse are accompanied by harelip. The degree of palatine clefting depends on the stage at which interruption in the fusion of the palatopalatal folds occurs. Toxic or teratogenic effects are documented in other species, but little data are available in the horse.

In recent years, treatment for repair of uncomplicated palatine defects has been recommended but is generally poor because of the considerable nursing care required and the incidence of surgical failures. Emphasis should be placed on early surgery and the use of mandibular symphysiotomy in affording surgical exposure. The combination of mandibular symphysiotomy and transhyoid pharyngotomy to approach the caudal margins of the soft palate affords surgical access, and mucosal flaps can be constructed to repair the defects. There is, however, a high incidence of surgical breakdown and healing by first intention is the exception rather the rule. A recent surgical report documented the successful closure of a median cleft of the lower lip and mandible in a donkey.[5]

Campylorhinus Lateralis. Foals that are born with a se-verely deviated premaxilla and palate present with a wry nose. Surgical correction of the deviated premaxilla can be achieved by submucosal division of the premaxilla across the nose at the line of the first cheek tooth. There is circumstantial evidence that such a defect has a genetic cause and it has been seen most frequently in the Arabian breed.

Cysts. Other developmental abnormalities are subepiglottic cysts as a result of cystic distortion of remnants of the thyroglossal duct which may cause dyspnea and choking in foals. Surgical removal of these cysts results in normal function.

Parrot Mouth. The most significant developmental defect of dental origin is the circumstance in which the maxilla is relatively longer than the mandible, that is, the horse is parrot-mouthed. An overbite of some 2 cm in the incisor arcade may be present in a horse with a mismatch of less than 1 cm between the first upper and lower cheek teeth. Both parrot mouth and monkey or sow mouth are thought to be inherited conditions. Some correction of minor incisor malocclusion will occur up to 5 years of age.

Recognition and detection of parrot mouth are important in the examination of potential breeding stock. Surgical attempts to inhibit overgrowth of the premaxilla by wiring or by the application of dental bite plate procedures have been documented in recent years.[6]

Oral Wounds

As has been indicated, the horse is, by nature, a curious animal and uses its lips as a means of exploring a variety of objects. It is therefore not uncommon to find that wounds of the lips, incisive bone, and the mandibular incisor area occur commonly in the horse. These usually occur as a result of the horse getting the lips, jaw, or teeth caught in feeding buckets, in fence posts, in halters, or having a segment of tongue encircled with hair in tail chewing. As the horse panics and pulls away from its oral entrapment, considerable trauma can occur to the lips, teeth, and gums.

Most wounds repair satisfactorily provided they are seen early and the basic principles of wound hygiene, excision of necrotic tissue, and wound closure are observed. It is important to insure that oral mucosal defects are closed and effective oral seals are made before external wounds are closed. In some cases it may be necessary to offer specially constructed diets or even to feed the horse by nasogastric tube or esophagostomy during the healing processes.

Oral Neoplasia

Oral and pharyngeal neoplasias are not common in the horse, with the exception of viral papillomas on the lips and muzzle.[7, 8] Perhaps the commonest oral malignancy is squamous cell carcinoma of the oral or pharyngeal mucosa. Lesions have been seen as ulcerated granulating masses of the hard palate, on the tongue, on the gingiva, and on the larynx. Malignant melanoma occurs as a primary tumor within the parotid salivary gland. Another form is multiple infiltrating lesions of the lips and buccal mucosa. Such tumors occur more frequently in gray horses. The management of malignant melanoma is problematic. Many cases progress extremely slowly. Consequently, the response to therapy may be difficult to assess. Local excision or cryotherapy and the use of histamine blockers[9] or combinations of such therapies have all been reported as being successful.

Foreign Bodies

Foreign body penetration has been reported in grazing and browsing horses and in particular in horses that have certain hay sources that contain desiccated barley awns or yellow "bristle" grass.[10] Ulcerative stomatitis is also seen as a consequence of the toxicity of phenylbutazone therapy.[11] Exposure and ingestion of the fungus *Rhizoctonia leguminicola* (slaframine intoxication slobbers) in the horse has been reported (see Chapter 19). Affected red clover and alfalfa, if ingested by horses, will result in excess salivation. There is no effective treatment for this problem other than removal of the horse from the affected clover or alfalfa pastures. Horses may be returned to the pasture if plant regrowth is free of the fungus.[12]

Actinobacillosis

Actinobacillus lignieresii, the causative agent of actinobacillosis, has been isolated and identified from ulcers on the free border of the soft palate and oral and laryngeal granulomas. It was also reported in a sublingual caruncle in a horse with a greatly swollen tongue.[13] Therapy with 150 mL of 20% sodium iodide and 5 g of ampicillin b.i.d. or t.i.d. affected a clinical cure.

Dental Diseases

Eruption Disorders. The normal eruption times of the teeth have been listed. Tooth eruption is a complex phenomenon involving the interplay of dental morphogenesis and those vascular forces that are responsible for creating the eruption pathway. These changes are responsible for osteitis and bone remodeling within the maxilla and mandible. Young horses frequently show symmetric, bony swelling as a result of these "eruption cysts." In some cases, additional clinical signs of nasal obstruction with respiratory stridor or nasal discharges may be seen.

Pathologic problems associated with maleruption include a variety of dental diseases. Oral trauma can displace or damage erupting teeth or the permanent tooth buds. As a result, teeth may be displaced and erupt in abnormal positions or may have abnormal shapes. Supernumerary teeth, both incisors and molars, can develop as well as palatal displacement of impacted teeth (maxillary P3-3, or third cheek tooth). In almost all of these conditions some form of surgical treatment is necessary.

There is significant evidence from the location of apical osteitis diseased teeth (Table 12–2) that confirms that dental impaction is a major cause of dental disease in the horse. In a series of 142 extracted teeth, 63 were P3-3 or P4-4 (cheek tooth 2 or 3, respectively).[14] Early observations had indicated that the first molar (M1, or cheek tooth 4) was the most commonly diseased tooth, and it has been suggested that an "open infundibulum" in this tooth was the cause.[15] Studies on cementogenesis of the maxillary cheek teeth have shown, however, that in fact most maxillary cheek teeth have a greater or lesser degree of hypoplasia of cementum within the enamel lakes and that it is rare for this "lesion" to expand into the pulp. The central infundibular hole is the site of its vascular supply to the unerupted cement lake. On those occasions in which caries of cementum occurs, that is, secondary inflammatory disease and acid necrosis of the cementum, there may develop apical osteitis.

Dental Decay. Pulpitis is key to the pathogenesis of dental decay in the horse. The initiation of inflammatory pulp changes may be a sequela to dental impaction, dental caries, or it may result from fracture of a tooth. If the onset of the inflammatory process is slow, then the pulp and the tooth may be protected by the formation of secondary dentine within the pulp chambers. This arises from stimulation of odontoblasts within the pulp chamber. Such changes are the normal process of protection during dental wear and attrition as crown substances are worn away and the reserve crown comes into wear. In acute disease, however, this defense mechanism is ineffective, and the changes that are seen and that are sequelae to pulpitis reflect the location of each individual affected tooth. For example, pulpitis and apical osteitis of the third mandibular cheek tooth will, most commonly, result in the development of a mandibular dental fistula. Pulpitis of the third maxillary cheek tooth will, however, result in an inflammatory disease within the rostral maxillary sinus and to development of chronic maxillary sinus empyema (Fig. 12–1).

The diagnosis of dental decay is greatly assisted by oblique radiographs to demonstrate sinus track formation, sequestration of bone, mandibular osteitis, hyperplasia of

Table 12–2. Sites of Apical Infections in Diseased Cheek Teeth in the Horse*

	Cheek Tooth†												Number Affected
	1		2		3		4		5		6		
	R	*C*	*R*	*C*	*R*	*C*	*R*	*C*	*R*	*C*	*R*	*C*	
Maxillary	2	7	9	9	10	11	7	8	0	0	0	0	
Total	9		18		21		15		0		0		63
Mandibular	0	4	18	22	13	10	5	3	3	1	0	0	
Total	4		40		23		8		4		0		79
													142

*From Baker GJ: Diseases of the teeth. In Colohan PT, Mayhew IG, Merritt AM, et al, eds: *Equine Medicine and Surgery,* ed 4, vol 1. Goleta, Calif, American Veterinary Publications, 1991, p 550.

†R, rostral root; C, caudal root.

cementum, and new bone formation (so-called alveolar periosteitis).[16]

The management of dental decay in the horse usually involves surgical extraction of the diseased tooth. In limited cases, apicoectomy and retrograde endodontic techniques can be used to save the diseased tooth. Care needs to be taken, however, in selection of patients. Most cases of apical osteitis in the horse that result from dental impaction have very immature root structures so that achieving an apical seal of the exposed pulp is not easy.

Periodontal Disease

Gingival hyperemia and inflammation occur during the eruption of the permanent teeth and are a common cause of a sore mouth in young horses (particularly 3-year-olds as the first dental caps loosen). Such periodontal changes usually resolve as the permanent dental arcade is established. During normal mastication, the shearing forces generated by the occlusal contact of the cheek teeth essentially clean the teeth of plaque and effectively inhibit deposition of dental calculus. Wherever there is ineffective occlusal contact, periodontal changes and calculus buildup occur; for example, it is common to see the deposition of calculus on the canine teeth of mature geldings and stallions. Routine dental prophylaxis forms an important component of the maintenance of normal occlusal contact, and it is for this reason that arcade irregularities that result in enamel point formation on the buccal edges of the maxillary cheek teeth and the lingual edges of the mandibular cheek teeth should be removed. These edges need to be removed annually in horses that are at grass and twice yearly in young horses, aged horses, and stabled horses. It has been shown that horses at grass have a greater range of occlusal contact and, therefore, better periodontal hygiene than stabled horses. In stabled horses the range of occlusal contact is narrower and the formation of enamel points occurs more frequently with subsequent buccal ulceration and the initiation of a cycle of altered occlusal contact and hence irregular arcade formation. It is this process that leads to severe forms of periodontal disease and wave mouth formation.

Periodontal disease occurs when there is abnormal occlusal contact and the cycle of irregular wear and abnormal contact is initiated. Such changes progress to loss of alveolar bone, gross peridontal sepsis, and loss of support for the tooth. In this sense it is truly the scourge of the horse's mouth and results in tooth loss.[17]

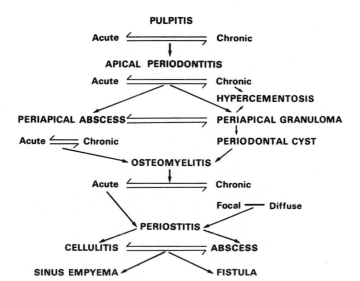

Figure 12–1. Possible sequelae of pulpitis in the horse. (From Baker GJ: Diseases of the teeth. In Colohan PT, Mayhew IG, Merritt AM, et al, eds: *Equine Medicine and Surgery,* ed 4, vol 1. Goleta, Calif, American Veterinary Publications, 1991, p 569.)

REFERENCES

1. Sisson S: Equine digestive system. In Getty G, ed: *Sisson and Grossman's the Anatomy of the Domestic Animal,* ed 5, vol 1. Philadelphia, WB Saunders, 1975, p 454.
2. Lindsay FEF, Burton FL: Observational studies of "urine testing" in the horse and donkey stallion. *Equine Vet J* 15:330, 1983.
3. Baker GJ: Oral examination and diagnosis: Management of oral disease. In Harvey CE, ed: *Veterinary Dentistry.* Philadelphia, WB Saunders, 1985, p 217.

4. Baker GJ: Fluoroscopic investigations of swallowing in the horse. *Vet Radiol* 23:84, 1982.

5. Farmand M, Stohler T: The median cleft of the lower lip and mandible and its surgical correction in a donkey. *Equine Vet J* 22:298, 1990.

6. DeBowes RM: Brachygnathia. In White NA, Moore JN, eds: *Current Practice of Equine Surgery*. Philadelphia, JB Lippincott, 1990, p 469.

7. Cotchin E: A general survey of tumours in the horse. *Equine Vet J* 9:16, 1977.

8. Leyland A, Baker JR: Lesions of the nasal and paranasal sinuses causing dyspnoea. *Br Vet J* 131:339, 1975.

9. Goetz TE, Ogilvie GK, Keegan KG, et al: Cimetidine for treatment of melanomas in three horses. *J Am Vet Med Assoc* 196:449, 1990.

10. Bankowski RA, Wichmann RW, Stuart EE: Stomatitis of cattle and horses due to yellow bristle grass (*Setaria lutescens*). *Am Vet Med Assoc* 129:149, 1956.

11. Snow DH, Bogan JA, Douglas TA, et al: Phenylbutazone toxicity in ponies. *Vet Res* 105:26, 1979.

12. Sockett DC, Baker JC, Stowe CM: Slaframine (*Rhizoctonia leguminicola*) intoxication in horses. *J Am Vet Med Assoc* 181:606, 1979.

13. Baum KH, Shin SJ, Rebhun WC, et al: Isolation of *Actinobacillus lignieresii* from enlarged tongue of a horse. *J Am Vet Med Assoc* 185:792, 1984.

14. Baker GJ: Diseases of the teeth. In Colohan PT, Mayhew IG, Merritt AM, et al, eds: *Equine Medicine and Surgery*, ed 4, vol 1. Goleta, Calif, American Veterinary, 1991, p 550.

15. Hofmeyr CFB: Comparative dental pathology (with particular reference to caries and paradental disease in the horse and the dog). *J S Afr Vet Med Assoc* 29:471, 1960.

16. Baker GJ: Some aspects of dental radiology. *Equine Vet J* 3:46, 1971.

17. Baker GJ: Some aspects of equine dental decay. *Equine Vet J* 6:127, 1974.

12.2

The Esophagus

Michael J. Murray, DVM, MS

ANATOMY

The esophagus is a musculomembranous tube that originates from the pharynx dorsal to the larynx and terminates at the cardia of the stomach.[1] In adult Thoroughbred horses the esophagus is approximately 120 cm long, with the cervical portion being approximately 70 cm long, the thoracic portion approximately 50 cm long, and the very short abdominal portion only approximately 2 cm long. The cervical esophagus lies dorsal and to the left of the trachea, and once the esophagus passes through the thoracic inlet it lies dorsal to the trachea. Within the mediastinum, the thoracic esophagus crosses to the right of the aortic arch and dorsal to the heart base.

The esophagus has no digestive or absorptive functions.

It serves as a conduit of feed, water, and salivary secretions to the stomach and lower digestive tract. The esophagus is lined by keratinized stratified squamous epithelial mucosa.[1] The submucosa contains elastic fibers that contribute to the longitudinal folds of the esophagus. In the proximal two thirds of the equine esophagus, the tunica muscularis is composed of striated skeletal muscle, whereas in the distal third the muscular layer is smooth muscle. In the proximal esophagus the skeletal muscle layers spiral across one another at angles. Within the smooth muscle layers of the distal esophagus the outer layer becomes more longitudinal while the inner layer thickens and becomes circular. The wall of the terminal esophagus can be 1 to 2 cm thick. Deep cervical fascia, pleura, and peritoneum contribute externally to the thin fibrous adventitia of the esophagus. Only the abdominal portion of the esophagus has a serosal covering.

Motor innervation to the striated skeletal muscle of the esophagus includes the pharyngeal and esophageal branches of the vagus nerve, which originate in the nucleus ambiguus of the medulla.[2] Parasympathetic fibers of the vagus nerve supply the smooth muscle of the distal esophagus and originate in the medulla. There is minimal sympathetic innervation of the esophagus.

FUNCTION

Passage of ingesta through the esophagus can be considered as part of the process of swallowing, which consists of oral, pharyngeal, and esophageal stages.[3] The oral stage is voluntary and involves transport of the food bolus from the mouth into the oropharynx. During the involuntary pharyngeal stage, the food bolus is forced through the momentarily relaxed upper esophageal sphincter by simultaneous contractions of the pharyngeal muscles. In the esophageal phase of swallowing the upper esophageal sphincter closes immediately, the lower esophageal sphincter opens, and esophageal peristalsis propels the bolus into the stomach.[4] Owing to gravitational forces, liquids can reach the lower esophageal sphincter independent of the peristaltic wave.

The upper esophageal sphincter prevents esophagopharyngeal reflux, with subsequent tracheobronchial aspiration, and hindrance of air distention of the esophagus during inspiration. Upper esophageal pressure increases secondary to increased intraluminal acidity or increased intraluminal pressure.[5]

The lower esophageal sphincter (LES) is functional smooth muscle located at the gastroesophageal junction.[5] The LES restricts gastroesophageal reflux and permits passage of ingested material from the esophagus to the stomach during relaxation. Normally, the LES remains closed due to intrinsic myogenic tone and gastric distention with ingesta. Distention of the stomach with ingesta results in tight constriction of the LES. Also, increased intragastric pressure causes further constriction of the LES by a vagal reflex, a safety mechanism against gastroesophageal reflux. Along with the absence of a vomiting reflex in the horse, these mechanisms prevent spontaneous decompression of excessive gastric fluid, which can result in gastric rupture.

CLINICAL SIGNS AND SIGNALMENT

Most esophageal disorders in foals and horses are obstructive, result from complications secondary to obstruction, or are secondary to failure of the LES to prevent gastroesophageal reflux. The predominant sign in horses with esophageal disorders is dysphagia.[6-8] Characteristic signs of dysphagia in the horse include frequent, ineffectual attempts to swallow, stretching of the neck, and retching. Coughing during swallowing, ptyalism, and nasal regurgitation of feed mixed with saliva also are observed in horses with esophageal disease.[7, 8] Enlargement of the cervical esophagus is palpable in some cases of esophageal obstruction. Esophageal perforation is suggested by cervical cellulitis, cervical subcutaneous emphysema, and fistulous tracts, which may drain more copiously following ingestion of feed. With a chronic disorder, such as esophageal stricture, weight loss may occur. Dehydration and electrolyte and acid-base imbalances may also accompany obstructive esophageal disorders.

The age of the animal is often relevant to the cause of dysphagia. In foals, dysmaturity, septicemia, botulism, and congenital disorders can cause dysphagia. In young horses, esophageal impaction secondary to improper mastication during dental eruption should be considered. Neoplasia and improper mastication are considerations for esophagcal disease in the aged horse. Feeding and management practices should be ascertained, since esophageal obstruction by feed material or foreign objects often results from deficiencies in management. Individual animal temperament also is an important consideration, particularly with regard to recommending methods of avoiding future esophageal obstruction.

The onset of clinical signs can relate to the cause of dysphagia. With acute mechanical obstruction, clinical signs develop rapidly, whereas with chronic or slowly developing disorders, such as neoplasia, luminal stricture, or external compression, clinical signs may occur gradually.

An important consideration when cataloguing the clinical signs exhibited by a patient is to ascertain whether these signs reflect a primary problem, or whether dysphagia is secondary to another disorder, and, in fact, whether the signs actually represent dysphagia. For instance, the bilateral nasal discharge that results from esophageal obstruction can be an unmistakable mixture of saliva and grass or hay, or it may be a fetid, mucoid discharge. The latter may represent chronic esophageal obstruction, but may also occur with guttural pouch empyema, pharyngeal abscessation, severe pneumonia, or pulmonary edema. Ptyalism in foals is characteristically attributed to gastroduodenal ulceration, and often results from gastroesophageal reflux. Ptyalism may also occur with botulism or sepsis, and has been observed secondary to pharyngeal trauma from administering improper boluses of medication.

DIAGNOSTIC PROCEDURES

The objectives of diagnostic procedures for esophageal disorders are to determine whether the cause of the observed clinical signs is related to the esophagus, whether the disorder is obstructive, and if it is, the location of the obstruction, whether it is intra- or extraluminal, and to play the most appropriate course of treatment. These procedures include gentle passage of the nasogastric tube, endoscopy, radiography, and ultrasonography. In foals and at appropriate referral centers, computed tomography (CT) scans of the thoracic esophagus can be performed.

When passing a nasogastric tube into a suspected obstructed esophagus, care should be taken not to damage the mucosa. A Silastic tube is relatively compliant, and less likely to traumatize the esophagus than a stiff tube. A nasogastric tube sometimes can be passed beyond an obstruction and enter the stomach, giving the false impression that either an obstruction did not exist or had been relieved.

Esophagoscopy should be done if the proper equipment is available. The proximal esophagus can be examined with endoscopes of 1 m working length. A length of 170 to 190 cm is required to examine the entire esophagus of adult horses. The normal esophageal mucosa is whitish-tan to slightly pink in color and glistening in appearance. In the normally collapsed esophagus, longitudinal and transient transverse folds can be seen (Fig. 12–2). In the thoracic esophagus, changes in intrapleural pressure may produce visible expansion and collapse of the esophageal lumen. The esophagus normally relaxes and then contracts in peristaltic waves. It is often easiest to examine the mucosa and advance the endoscope as the esophagus relaxes. At the gastroesophageal junction the LES is usually closed, but it may open in response to a peristaltic wave. If possible, gastroscopy should be performed, since ulceration of the stomach at the cardia may result in esophageal dysfunction. In some cases, the esophageal mucosa is better observed as the endoscope is withdrawn and air is insufflated.

Useful radiographic procedures for diagnosis of esophageal disorders include survey radiographs, and single and

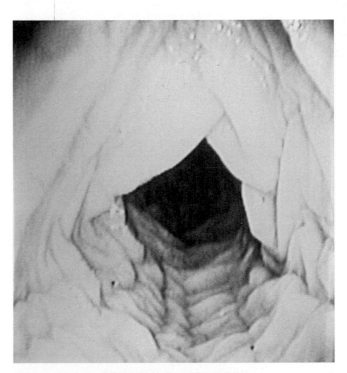

Figure 12–2. Endoscopic view of the cervical esophagus of an adult horse. Both longitudinal and transverse folds are seen during relaxation of the esophagus.

double contrast esophagraphy.[8–10] Survey radiographs usually do not delineate the esophagus unless there is excessive air, gas, or foreign material. Impacted feed material often appears as a granular density within the esophageal lumen. Benign accumulations of air may accompany aerophagia due to excitement or general anesthesia, but are transient. Repeated films will help determine whether air densities pass with peristalsis or are stationary. Subcutaneous emphysema may be evident with perforations of the cervical esophagus. Radiographs of the thorax may reveal air accumulation in the esophagus or pneumomediastinum, or displacement of the esophagus.

Preferably, radiography of the esophagus should be done in the standing, untranquilized animal. If tranquilization is required for completion of the procedure, acepromazine can be used with minimal effect on swallowing. Xylazine can impair the swallowing reflex and cause esophageal relaxation. The latter may result in an artifactual dilatation or air accumulation within the esophageal lumen. This can be advantageous when performing a double contrast esophagram, in which the esophageal lumen is distended with air. In foals, the pharynx; the cervical, thoracic, and abdominal esophagus; and the stomach can be studied using portable radiographic equipment and rare earth screens. In most adult horses, only the pharynx and cervical esophagus are readily studied with portable equipment.

Various contrast materials can be used to optimize the detection of different esophageal disorders. Fifty to 100 mL of a 40% barium sulfate suspension can be given via a catheter tip syringe or by tube at a rate that allows adequate swallowing.[4] Standing lateral radiographs are taken immediately after swallowing. Initially, the smaller volume of barium suspension should be given, since this may outline an obstruction or constriction, and will not be likely to reflux into the pharynx and be aspirated. Larger volumes of barium suspension, up to 500 mL, can be administered through a cuffed nasogastric tube (Bivona Inc., Gary, Ind.).[7] Barium paste can be given at a dose of 30 to 100 mL.

The esophagus is usually collapsed when coated with the barium suspension or paste, allowing visualization of the smooth, longitudinal esophageal folds. Esophageal disorders that can be diagnosed using this technique include complete intraluminal obstruction, mural neoplasms, extensive esophageal compression, and some strictures. Up to 500 mL of a 40% barium suspension, followed by an equal volume of air, can be administered through a cuffed nasogastric tube to demonstrate circumferential lesions, such as esophageal rings, strictures, and megaesophagus[4] (Fig. 12–3). If an esophageal perforation is suspected, barium should be avoided because it is a tissue irritant, and a soluble iodinated contrast medium used.

Ultrasonography is useful when there is cervical swelling. Pockets of fluid, gas accumulation, and foreign bodies may be appreciated with ultrasonography. Thoracic ultrasonography can be used to examine the cranial mediastinum and to detect the presence of pleural effusion or pulmonary consolidation, as might occur secondary to severe aspiration pneumonia.

ESOPHAGEAL DISORDERS
Obstruction (Choke)

Obstruction is the most frequently diagnosed esophageal disorder in the horse and is usually due to an intraluminal

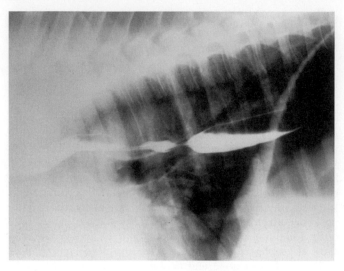

Figure 12–3. Double contrast esophagram in a horse with circumferential esophageal stricture following esophageal luminal obstruction. Note the narrowing of the barium column in the esophagus, and the pre- and poststenotic dilatation of the esophagus.

impaction.[2, 7, 8] Esophageal obstruction should be considered an emergency, because prolonged pressure on the esophageal mucosa by the obstructing material can result in extensive tissue damage, with resultant scar tissue formation and stricture, or lead to esophageal perforation.

Many substances have been identified as causing esophageal obstruction, including grain, hay, pelleted feeds, corncobs, pieces of fruit or vegetable, wood shavings, and medicinal boluses.[2, 7, 8, 11–13] In many cases there is a predisposing factor, such as improper mastication in older horses with poor dentition or in young horses with erupting teeth, recovery from general anesthesia, or exhaustion. Horses that have a stricture, diverticulum, megaesophagus, or compression on the esophagus will experience recurrent obstruction at the affected site.[7, 11]

Most obstructions occur proximally in the cervical esophagus (high choke). Obstructions also occur at the thoracic inlet (low choke) because the distensibility of the esophagus is restricted at that site. Intrathoracic obstruction is less common, which is fortunate since these are most difficult to resolve. Passage of a nasogastric tube or palpation of the neck may help to identify the site of obstruction. Endoscopy, if available, will pinpoint the site of obstruction.

Although some cases of esophageal obstruction resolve spontaneously, once a diagnosis is made treatment should be given immediately. The most conservative approach is to administer acepromazine 10 to 15 mg/500 kg. In cases with mild obstruction, this may offer sufficient muscle relaxation to allow the obstruction to pass. A nasogastric tube can be used cautiously in alleviating many cases of esophageal impaction. The obstruction may pass into the stomach with gentle pressure by the tube. Vigorous pressure should be avoided. Administration of xylazine hydrochloride 1.1 mg/kg IV will provide proper sedation, muscle relaxation, and lowering of the head. With the head lowered, saliva and other fluids trapped proximal to the obstruction are less likely to be aspirated. Gentle lavage of the esophagus can

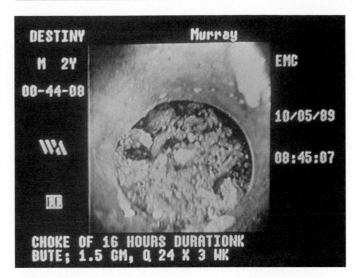

DESTINY   Murray

M 2Y   EMC

00-44-08

                10/05/89

WA

                08:45:07

f.f.

CHOKE OF 16 HOURS DURATIONK
BUTE; 1.5 GM, Q 24 X 3 WK

Figure 12–4. Endoscopic view of a feed impaction causing obstruction in the cervical esophagus, as seen through a cuffed nasotracheal tube placed in the esophagus. The tube was used to vigorously lavage the impaction. This was done several times, and after each lavage the mass and esophageal mucosa were inspected endoscopically.

be done with warm water or, preferably, a 0.9% sodium chloride solution. A soft, flexible nasogastric tube can be gently advanced as the obstruction diminishes in size, while pumping is continued, until the impaction is relieved.

Vigorous esophageal lavage should only be done using a cuffed nasoesophageal tube and with appropriate sedation (Fig. 12–4). This is necessary to prevent aspiration of fluid and material within the esophagus subsequent to lavage. If the impaction is not relieved, lavage can be done intermittently. The horse can be sedated and muzzled, crosstied, or put into an unbedded stall between attempts, during which time spontaneous recovery may occur. The use of lubricating agents, such as mineral oil, or softening agents, such as docusate sodium (D-S-S), is contraindicated because these might be aspirated.

In most cases, these procedures will relieve the esophageal obstruction. If initial attempts are not successful and the patient's condition is stable, a general anesthetic may be administered, the horse placed in lateral recumbency with the head lowered, and intubated with an endotracheal tube. Continued lavage through a nasoesophageal tube will be enhanced by the additional muscle relaxation accompanying anesthesia.

Removal of a foreign body often is more difficult than an aggregate of feed. Foreign body removal may be attempted with the horse sedated, but general anesthesia often is preferred, since there is better esophageal relaxation and procedures can be performed with greater efficiency. Proximally lodged foreign bodies can occasionally be retrieved manually with the horse anesthetized. There are several endoscopic accessories that can be used to retract or section foreign bodies.[13] If numerous intubations are necessary to remove multiple objects, the endoscope can be repeatedly passed through a preplaced large tube, which also protects the esophageal mucosa from lacerations by sharp objects.

Aspiration of saliva and feed frequently occurs in horses with esophageal obstruction. In some cases this can lead to severe aspiration pneumonia. If a horse develops a fever following resolution of the esophageal impaction, aspiration pneumonia should be considered and broad-spectrum antimicrobial agents given. A transtracheal aspirate will help characterize the severity of inflammation and identify pathogenic organisms, with corresponding antimicrobial sensitivity patterns.

Medical therapy in cases of esophageal obstruction is aimed at correcting dehydration and electrolyte disturbances, minimizing esophageal inflammation, and treating aspiration pneumonia. Intravenous polyionic fluids should be given if dehydration is present and in cases in which water consumption is restricted. Some horses with excessive salivary loss have been noted to have hypochloremic metabolic alkalosis.[7] In such cases, 0.9% sodium chloride IV is the fluid of choice. Oral fluid therapy should be utilized only after the obstruction has been relieved and the pharyngeal or esophageal inflammation has subsided.

Anti-inflammatory drugs are used to control pain and inflammation. Nonsteroidal anti-inflammatory drugs, such as flunixin meglumine (Banamine, Schering Corp., Kenilworth, N.J.) and phenylbutazone, are preferred. Broad-spectrum antimicrobials are indicated if aspiration pneumonia occurs, and should be targeted against enteric organisms and anaerobic bacteria. Initially, antimicrobial drugs should be administered parenterally, since oral administration may exacerbate the esophageal disorder.

After the obstruction has been relieved, the esophageal mucosa should be evaluated endoscopically to determine whether mucosal or submucosal damage occurred, the extent of injury, and appropriate management of the patient. If the impaction was transient and there is minimal mucosal damage, the horse can be fed handfuls of hay or grazed within a few hours. In horses with esophageal irritation or mild to moderate ulceration, small amounts of hay or grass may be provided within 24 hours, but other feed should be withheld for 24 to 72 hours. The hay may be soaked in water to soften it. Eating small amounts of presoftened hay or grass may be beneficial by mechanically debriding damaged mucosa. Another potential benefit is the exposure of the damaged mucosa to salivary epidermal growth factor, a polypeptide that stimulates reepithelialization.[14] Subsequently, nonirritating, moist feed substances should be provided, such as a slurry of pelleted feed, with or without the addition of mineral oil. With severe esophageal damage, parenteral feeding should be considered. The damaged esophageal tissue requires time to heal and may require careful debridement via endoscopy to facilitate the healing process. Oral feedings of any type should be prohibited as long as any evidence of dysphagia persists.

Esophageal Stricture

Esophageal stricture is a sequela to damage to the esophageal submucosa secondary to obstruction, corrosion, or trauma. Fortunately, esophageal stricture occurs in the minority of cases with obstruction. Tissue damage limited to the mucosa results in a mild, transient esophageal narrowing attributable to the acute inflammatory response.[15]

With injury to the submucosa or muscularis, fibroplasia results in scar tissue formation. With longitudinal defects, the resultant scar tissue causes minimal interference to passage of feed. However, with circumferential lesions, scar tissue formation and contraction result in diminution of the luminal diameter.[16] In one study, the esophageal luminal diameter gradually diminished between 21 and 30 days after the original insult, with maximum luminal reduction by 30 days.[17] Subsequently, the luminal diameter began to increase, reaching a maximum increase at 60 days post injury. It is therefore advisable that in cases in which significant mucosal injury is evident, esophagrams or endoscopy be done regularly for up to 8 weeks post obstruction.

The classic clinical sign of esophageal stricture is recurrent esophageal feed impaction.[2, 7, 8] Dysphagia is observed most frequently after ingesting solid feed. With chronicity, the esophagus dilates proximal to the stricture and can accommodate considerable amounts of ingested feed, in which case dysphagia may be delayed for some period after eating. Eventually, weight loss may be apparent. A history of previous esophageal injury is likely. The diagnosis of esophageal stricture is confirmed by a contrast esophagram or endoscopy. A double contrast esophagram will clearly define the stricture not evident in the collapsed esophagus, as will a barium and feed mixture.[4, 7]

Dietary management is important in horses with esophageal stricture. The principle of feeding is to provide soft feed materials in small amounts at frequent intervals. Types of feeds that may be employed in the dietary program include grass, preformented softened hay, alfalfa leaves, and pellet or grain slurries. When formulating a diet for a horse with an esophageal stricture, consideration must be given to the nutritional balance of the diet and the potential effects on the large colon.

Bougienage is a safe, nonsurgical method of dilating the stenotic region.[18] Bougienage is the passage of a bougie, a slender cylinder, through a tubular organ with the purpose of increasing the diameter of the lumen by distending it at the site of the stricture.[4] The procedure is performed repeatedly in a patient, resulting in progressive breakdown of scar tissue. Since developing scar tissue is more easily disrupted by bougienage than mature scar tissue, the procedure is best applied at the earliest signs of stricture formation. Human instrumentation in use today includes mercury-filled rubber dilators (23F–60F), and metal olive dilators (16F–45F).[18]

Green and MacFadden[4] describe a procedure for bougienage in the sedated horse following withholding feed. After passage of a guidewire into the esophagus, a lubricated dilator is attached to a dilator shaft and passed over the guidewire through the strictured area. If necessary, three progressively sized dilators can be passed during one session. Daily sessions can be continued, if necessary. A cuffed nasogastric tube also can be used to reverse early stricture development following deep, circumferential esophageal injury from luminal obstruction. Reports of failures of bougienage in the horse may be related to the stage of stricture maturation at which the procedure is attempted, although I have seen the technique applied successfully in a horse with a stricture of at least 90 days' duration.

In some cases, surgery is required. Esophageal resection, esophagomyotomy, esophagoplasty, and patch grafting techniques have been reported.[19–23]

Table 12–3. Esophageal Disorders in Foals and Horses

Foals
Gastroesophageal reflux
 Esophagitis
 Esophageal ulceration
 Acquired megaesophagus
Congenital megaesophagus
Extrinsic compression
 Retropharyngeal abscess
 Mediastinal abscess
 Hilar lymph node abscess
 Persistent right aortic arch
Esophageal cyst
Esophageal stricture

Horses
Esophageal luminal impaction (choke)
Esophageal luminal constriction
Extrinsic esophageal compression
 Retropharyngeal abscess
 Cervical cellulitis
 Mediastinal mass
 Diaphragmatic hernia
Esophageal perforation
Esophagitis
 Gastroesophageal reflux
 Iatrogenic (medicinal bolus)
Esophageal diverticulum
 Congenital
 Acquired
Neoplasia
 Squamous cell carcinoma
 Melanoma
 Fibroma
Megaesophagus
 Secondary to obstruction/stricture
 Neuromuscular disease (botulism, myasthenia gravis)
 Central neurologic disorder (equine protozoal myelitis, equine herpesvirus)

Extrinsic Esophageal Compression

Extrinsic compression of the esophagus is less common than intraluminal obstruction. Typical causes of compression of the esophagus are listed in Table 12–3. The diagnosis of extrinsic compression is made on the basis of the findings of a physical examination, endoscopy, and radiography. Treatment is for the primary problem.

Esophagitis

Esophagitis is a very common disorder in humans, but has been diagnosed infrequently in horses. The incidence probably is greatest in foals, as a sequela to gastroduodenal ulceration, but it occurs occasionally in adult horses.

The most common cause of esophagitis is reflux of gastric acid into the distal esophagus. Chemicals administered orally have the potential to induce esophagitis, particularly some antihelminthics no longer in frequent use. Reflux esophagitis effects the distal esophagus, and in humans the condition can be very painful, even without endoscopic evidence of mucosal damage. Normally, the cardia in the horse restricts gastroesophageal reflux, but with gastroduodenal ulceration, particularly when the ulceration involves the lesser curvature of the stomach or cardia, the sphincter function of the cardia is impaired. Endoscopically, this can be seen as a partial, persistent opening of the cardia, rather than the closed slit that appears normally (Fig. 12–5).

Clinical signs of esophagitis can be subtle and difficult to pinpoint. Esophageal inflammation produces pain, with or without esophageal ulceration. In foals, esophagitis is associated with ptyalism and anorexia. Bruxism could relate to esophageal discomfort as much as to gastric or duodenal pain. In adult horses, esophagitis produces signs that mimic colic or esophageal obstruction.

Esophagitis is diagnosed by endoscopy. The presence of mucosal erosion or ulceration confirms the diagnosis (Fig. 12–6), although this may be absent in many cases. With an incompetent LES, gastroesophageal reflux may be seen in the thoracic esophagus. If the cardia appears open and remains open, gastroesophageal reflux should be presumed. If the stomach can be examined, this should be done, since most foals and horses with reflux esophagitis will have gastric lesions.

Lower esophageal inflammation leads to reduced LES pressure; consequently, esophagitis can become self-perpetuating. Continued inflammation results in motility disturbances, and esophageal dilatation. In severe cases, the LES can remain dilated due to chronic inflammation and fibrosis, resulting in persistent esophageal dilatation.[24]

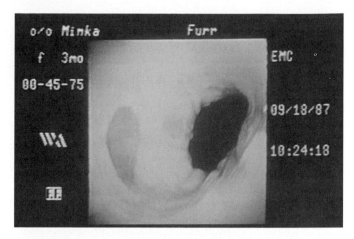

Figure 12–6. Endoscopic view of the distal esophagus of a 7-month-old foal with duodenal obstruction, which resulted in delayed gastric emptying and reflux esophagitis. There are several ulcerative lesions in the distal esophagus and generalized hyperkeratosis of the esophageal mucosa. The foal also had megaesophagus secondary to chronic gastroesophageal reflux.

Treatment of reflux esophagitis is based on treating confirmed or presumed gastroduodenal ulceration and enhancing lower esophageal motility, LES tone, and gastric emptying. Use of a histamine type 2 receptor (H_2) antagonist is recommended to decrease gastric acidity. This is effective in healing gastroduodenal ulceration and in healing esophageal mucosal injury. Even severe esophageal mucosal lesions can heal completely within less than 5 days if gastric acidity is suppressed. Recommended treatments include cimetidine (Tagamet, SmithKline & French, Carolina, P.R.) 10 to 15 mg/kg every 6 to 8 hours, or ranitidine (Zantac, Glaxo Inc., Research Triangle Park, N.C.) 6.6 mg/kg every 6 to 8 hours. Mild acid-induced esophagitis can be effectively treated with antacids. As an example, Maalox (Rorer Pharmaceutical Corp., Fort Washington, Pa.) 8 to 10 oz PO six times daily has been effective in such cases.

Prokinetic drugs that stimulate lower esophageal and gastric motility should be used. Metoclopramide (Reglan, A.H. Robins, Richmond, Va.) and bethanechol (Urecholine, Merck & Co., Rahway, N.J.) have been effective. Metoclopramide is a dopamine antagonist that also sensitizes the muscularis to acetylcholine.[25] Bethanechol is a cholinergic agent. These drugs increase the strength of esophageal contractions, increase LES pressure, and promote coordination of gastric and small intestinal motility.[26]

Adverse neurologic side effects occur with metoclopramide when used at effective dosages (0.25 mg/kg) in the horse, and for that reason this drug may not be preferable. Bethanechol has appeared to be as effective, with few side effects. Bethanechol can be given subcutaneously at 0.025 to 0.030 mg/kg every 4 hours for 24 hours in animals that cannot be medicated orally. The oral dosage of bethanechol is 0.35 to 0.45 mg/kg every 6 to 8 hours. At higher dosages diarrhea can occur. Cisapride, a drug that also affects dopamine-receptor interaction, has beneficial prokinetic properties, but is currently only under investigation in the United States.

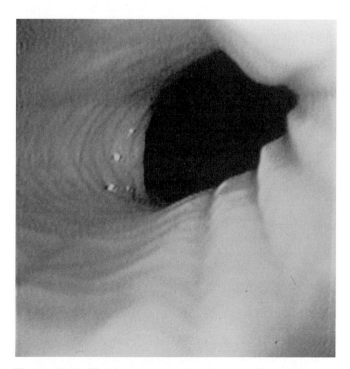

Figure 12–5. Distal esophagus in a horse with severe gastric ulceration and distal esophagitis that presented with a history of intermittent colic of 30 days' duration. The lower esophageal sphincter is open, and when observed for 2 minutes, it remained open. This abnormality resulted in reflux of gastric contents into the distal esophagus.

Dietary management should be considered in some cases. Soft pelleted slurries and grass should be fed in small quantities at frequent intervals. With severe ulceration, all solid feed should be withheld until the lesions have healed. In some patients, total parenteral nutrition may be indicated.

Esophageal Perforation

Esophageal perforation can result from laceration or occur secondary to mural pressure necrosis from chronic obstruction.[27, 28] Iatrogenic perforation during attempts to alleviate an intraluminal obstruction using a nasogastric tube is an important consideration (Fig. 12–7).

With perforation that originates luminally, saliva, esophageal secretions, and swallowed feed material leak subcutaneously and cause severe cellulitis, with swelling and subcutaneous emphysema. The cellulitis can become progressive and dissect along fascial planes, and can lead to sloughing of overlying skin, mediastinitis, and pleuritis.

Open wounds result from penetrating objects or from necrosis and sloughing of skin overlying a previously closed esophageal wound. The wound discharge consists of saliva and feed material. The diagnosis of esophageal wounds is based upon clinical signs with confirmation by esophagraphy and esophagoscopy. If esophageal perforation is suspected, a water-soluble iodine-based contrast material should be used instead of barium.

Esophageal perforations are allowed to heal by secondary intention. Surgical intervention is usually limited to debridement and establishment of adequate drainage, by creating or enlarging a skin wound.

Acutely, excessive salivary loss through the perforation can result in metabolic acidosis, but after just a few days pronounced hyponatremia, hypochloremia, and metabolic alkalosis can occur.[29] If the wound is large, the horse can be fed through an esophagotomy tube while the wound con-

tracts. When small enough to permit only minimal leakage of feed, oral feeding can be resumed. Complete healing requires several weeks. The prognosis is guarded, but return to normal function is possible if diligent care is maintained. Possible complications of esophageal perforation include chronic weight loss, esophageal traction diverticulum formation, esophageal stricture, chronic esophagocutaneous fistula, laryngeal hemiplegia, and Horner's syndrome.[4]

Esophageal Diverticula

Esophageal diverticula are occasionally seen in horses. These represent herniation of the mucosa through a defect in the muscular layers of the esophagus.[30] Diverticula may be congenital or acquired, the latter being more common in the horse. Acquired diverticula are classified as pulsion or traction diverticula.

A pulsion diverticulum results when increased intraluminal pressure occurs near a site of obstruction or stenosis, forcing the mucosal layer between the muscular layers. Injury to the muscular layer also can precipitate a pulsion diverticulum. Traction diverticula develop during the healing process following esophageal injury. The diverticulum results from distortion of the wall of the esophagus as scar tissue contracts around the wall of the esophagus. The result is an outpouching. Unlike pulsion diverticula, the traction diverticula consist of all four histologic layers of the esophagus (mucosa, submucosa, muscularis, and adventitia).

While small pulsion diverticula can be asymptomatic, larger diverticula can permit accumulation of feed and postprandial enlargement of the neck. Diagnosis is made by radiography and endoscopy. On an esophagram, contrast material may partially or completely outline the fundus of the diverticulum. In some cases a barium-feed mixture best outlines the diverticular pouch.[4] Treatment of diverticula is usually conservative, involving dietary management. Large diverticula may require surgical correction.[30, 31]

Congenital Disorders

Congenital disorders of the esophagus are rarely reported in horses. They have included ectasia (dilatation),[32] persistent right aortic arch,[8] and esophageal cysts.[33, 34] The clinical signs are those of dysphagia and diagnosis is by endoscopy and radiography.

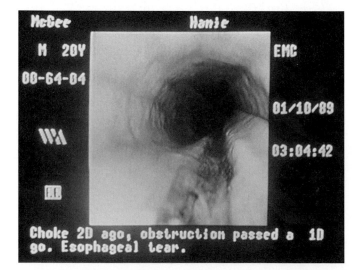

Figure 12–7. Endoscopic view of the cervical esophagus of a horse that had repeated passages of a stiff nasogastric tube during attempts to relieve an esophageal obstruction. There is a deep, linear lesion within the esophageal mucosa that appears to extend into the submucosa.

REFERENCES

1. The alimentary canal. In Schummer A, Nickel R, Sack WO, eds: *The Viscera of the Domestic Mammals.* New York, Springer-Verlag, 1979, p 99.
2. O'Brien JA, Harvey CE, Brodey RS: The esophagus. In Anderson NV, ed: *Veterinary Gastroenterology.* Philadelphia, Lea & Febiger, 1980, p 372.
3. Meyer GW, Castell DO: Anatomy and physiology of the esophageal body. In Castell DO, Johnson LF, eds: *Esophageal Function in Health and Disease.* New York, Elsevier Science, 1983, p 1.
4. Green EM, MacFadden KE: Disorders of the esophagus. In Smith BP, ed: *Large Animal Internal Medicine.* St Louis, Mosby–Year Book, 1990, p 636.

5. Gerhardt DC, Castell DO: Anatomy and physiology of the esophageal sphincters. In Castell DO, Johnson LF, eds: *Esophageal Function in Health and Disease.* New York, Elsevier Science, 1983, p 17.

6. Cattau EL, Castell DO: Symptoms of esophageal dysfunction. In Castell DO, Johnson LF, eds: *Esophageal Function in Health and Disease.* New York, Elsevier Science, 1983, p 31.

7. Stick JA: Esophageal disease. In Robinson NE, ed: *Current Therapy in Equine Medicine.* Philadelphia, WB Saunders, 1987, p 12.

8. Freeman DE: The esophagus. In Mansmann RA, McAllister ES, Pratt PW, eds: *Equine Medicine and Surgery.* Santa Barbara, Calif, American Veterinary, 1982, p 476.

9. Alexander JE: Radiologic findings in equine choke. *J Am Vet Med Assoc* 151:47, 1967.

10. Greet TRC: Observations on the potential role of oesophageal radiography in the horse. *Equine Vet J* 14:73, 1982.

11. DeBowes RM, Grant BD, Sande RD: Esophageal obstruction by antibiotic boluses in a Thoroughbred filly: A case report. *Equine Vet Sci* 23, 1982.

12. MacDonald MH, Richardson DW, Morse CC: Esophageal phytobezoar in a horse. *J Am Vet Med Assoc* 191:1455, 1987.

13. Monnier P, Savary M: New endoscopic techniques. In *International Trends in General Thoracic Surgery—Benign Esophageal Disease.* St Louis, Mosby–Year Book, 1987, p 61.

14. Gysin B, Muller RKM, Otten U, et al: Epidermal growth factor is increased in rats with experimentally induced gastric lesions. *Scand J Gastroenterol* 23:665, 1988.

15. Kikendall JW, Johnson LF: Esophageal injury: Caustics and pills. In Castell DO, Johnson LF, eds: *Esophageal Function in Health and Disease.* New York, Elsevier Science, 1983, p 255.

16. Eastwood GL: Esophagitis and its consequences. In Castell DO, Johnson LF, eds: *Esophageal Function in Health and Disease.* New York, Elsevier Science, 1983, p 175.

17. Todhunter RJ, Stick JA, Trotter GW, et al: Medical management of esophageal stricture in seven horses. *J Am Vet Med Assoc* 185:784, 1984.

18. Peura DA, Johnson LF: Treatment of esophageal obstruction. In Castell DO, Johnson LF, eds: *Esophageal Function in Health and Disease.* New York, Elsevier Science, 1983, p 305.

19. Derksen FJ, Stick JA: Resection and anastomosis of esophageal stricture in a foal. *Equine Pract* 5:17, 1983.

20. Fretz PB: Repair of esophageal stricture in a horse. *Mod Vet Pract* 53:31, 1972.

21. Gideon L: Esophageal anastomosis in two foals: *J Am Vet Med Assoc* 184:1146, 1984.

22. Nixon AJ, Aanes WA, Nelson AW, et al: Esophagomyotomy for relief of an intrathoracic esophageal stricture in a horse. *J Am Vet Med Assoc* 183:794, 1983.

23. Suann CJ: Oesophageal resection and anastomosis as a treatment for oesophageal stricture in the horse. *Equine Vet J* 14:163, 1982.

24. Murray MJ, Ball MM, Parker GA: Megaesophagus and aspiration pneumonia secondary to gastric ulceration in a foal. *J Am Vet Med Assoc* 192:381, 1988.

25. Albibi R, McCallum RW: Metoclopramide: Pharmacology and clinical application. *Ann Intern Med* 98:86, 1983.

26. Hunt JM, Gerring EL: Effects of propanolol, yohimbine, bethanecol, and metoclopramide in an equine model of postoperative ileus. In *Proceedings of Equine Colic Research Symposium,* vol 2, Athens, Ga, October 5, 1986, pp 89–94.

27. DeMoor A, Wouters L, Mouens Y, et al: Surgical treatment of a traumatic oesophageal rupture in a foal. *Equine Vet J* 11:265, 1979.

28. Raker CW, Sayers A: Esophageal rupture in a Standardbred mare. *J Am Vet Med Assoc* 185:371, 1958.

29. Stick JA, Robinson NE, Krehbiel JD: Acid-base and electrolyte alterations associated with salivary loss in the pony. *Am J Vet Res* 42:733, 1981.

30. Diverticula and diverticulosis. In Enterline H, Thompson J, eds: *Pathology of the Esophagus.* New York, Springer-Verlag, 1984, p 43.

31. Fraunfelder HC, Adams SB: Esophageal diverticulectomy in a horse. *J Am Vet Med Assoc* 180:771, 1982.

32. Rohrbach BW, Rooney JR: Congenital esophageal ectasia in a Thoroughbred foal. *J Am Vet Med Assoc* 177:65, 1980.

33. Scott EA, Snoy P, Prasse KW, et al: Intramural esophageal cyst in a horse. *J Am Vet Med Assoc* 171:652, 1977.

34. Orsini JA, Sepesy L, Donawick WJ, et al: Esophageal duplication cyst as a cause of choke in the horse. *J Am Vet Med Assoc* 193:474, 1988.

12.3

Gastroduodenal Ulceration

Michael J. Murray, DVM, MS

Disorders of the stomach of foals and horses are being diagnosed with increasing frequency because the means for making antemortem diagnoses are available in a greater number of hospitals. The use of endoscopy, in particular, has enhanced the recognition of several syndromes of gastric ulceration in both foals and adult horses.

Just as the term "colic" describes a clinical presentation, and encompasses a large number of disorders, the terms "gastric" and "gastroduodenal ulceration" describe a clinical finding, the cause of which is likely to be multifactorial and different from case to case. The equine stomach is lined by a stratified squamous epithelial mucosa dorsally and a glandular epithelial mucosa ventrally, and different clinical syndromes and pathophysiologic processes apply to the different types of tissue lining the stomach of the horse. Under the umbrella term "gastroduodenal ulceration" are included focal or multifocal ulceration, generalized gastritis, gastric emptying disorders, focal duodenal ulceration, duodenal erosions, and duodenitis. Gastric ulceration can occur in conjunction with, and often secondary to, duodenal ulceration in foals. In recent years, the prevalence of gastric and duodenal ulceration in foals and adult horses has been characterized, but the causes of these disorders remain largely undetermined. Recognition of animals at risk and clinical signs, both overt and subtle, referable to gastric and duodenal lesions will facilitate proper treatment and prevention of gastroduodenal disease.

PATHOPHYSIOLOGY

The term "peptic ulceration" is used in human medicine as a catchall for disorders associated with ulceration or inflammation of the stomach and duodenum. There are several discrete clinical syndromes under the umbrella of peptic ulceration, some of which are associated with acid hypersecretion,[1] acid hyposecretion,[1] infection with *Helicobacter pylori*,[2] ingestion of nonsteroidal anti-inflammatory agents (NSAIDs),[3] and severe physiologic stress.[4] There are several risk factors in humans, such as smoking and ingestion of alcohol, for developing peptic ulceration that are irrelevant to horses. An important concept that is applicable to the understanding of equine gastroduodenal ulcer syndromes is one of imbalance between aggressive and protective factors that influence the microenvironment of the gastric and duodenal mucosa.

The predominant aggressive factors are hydrochloric acid and pepsin, an enzyme that initiates protein digestion. Hydrochloric acid is secreted by parietal cells in the gastric glands. Secretion of acid is via an H^+, K^+ = ATPase (adenosine triphosphatase) pump on the luminal side of the parietal cell.[5]

Several peptides can stimulate or inhibit the secretion of acid by the parietal cell (Table 12–4). The predominant stimuli to hydrochloric acid secretion are gastrin, histamine, and acetylcholine via the vagus nerve.[1] Gastrin is released by G cells within the gastric glands, while histamine is released by mast cells and enterochromaffin-like (ECL) cells in the gastric gland. Histamine, in effect, increases parietal cell cyclic adenosine monophosphate (cAMP), which results in phosphorylation of enzymes that "activate" the proton pump. Gastrin and acetylcholine stimulate another enzyme system that also activates the proton pump. Other stimuli to acid secretion include gastrin-releasing peptide (GRP) which has an overall effect of stimulating gastric secretion (acid and pepsin),[6] and brain peptides, which mediate gastric secretion through the vagus nerve.[7]

Gastric acid secretion by parietal cells is primarily inhibited by somatostatin, released by fundic and antral D cells. Somatostatin release increases with decreased luminal pH (increased acidity), and decreases when luminal pH increases.[8] The inhibitory effect of somatostatin is primarily paracrine, or cell to cell, but plasma levels of somatostatin increase with increased gastric luminal acidity, and vice versa. Parietal cell acid secretion also is inhibited by epidermal growth factor (EGF), a peptide produced in saliva.[9]

Significant gastric acid secretion occurs as early as 2 days of age in foals, since pH measurements of the glandular mucosal surface and gastric contents revealed a highly acidic pH.[10] This contrasts somewhat with other species, particularly the rat, in which gastric acid secretion is negligible until approximately 20 days of age.[11] In rats, the initiation of gastric acid secretion is associated with increased serum cortisol, and can be induced precociously by administration of exogenous corticosteroid.[12] In contrast, serum cortisol levels are greatest at birth in foals,[13] and plasma gastrin levels in neonatal foals are similar to those of adult horses.[13, 14] Plasma somatostatin levels are relatively low in foals at birth, but increase twofold by 4 days of age.[13] These findings suggest a precocious development of gastric secretory function in foals.

The horse secretes acid in a continuously variable pattern, such that acid secretion occurs in the absence of ingestion of feed.[15] Acid output, acid concentration, and gastric fluid volume approximately doubled in response to pentagastrin administration in fasted young horses.[16] On a body weight basis the horse has a greater basal acid output, but a similar stimulated acid output, compared to humans.

Eating affects the acidity of the stomach of horses. Horses with free access to hay had greater median 24-hour gastric pH (less acidity) than did horses withheld from feed for 24 hours (3.1 vs. 1.6).[17] Ingestion of feed should actually stimulate acid secretion, but the acid is largely neutralized by the buffering capacity of feed and by bicarbonate-rich salivary secretions that are stimulated by feed.[18] There is a circadian pattern to basal gastric acid secretion in humans,[19] and gastric acidity is greatest during the late night hours.[20] A circadian pattern of gastric acidity has not been reported in horses, and in the study of Murray and Schusser[17] no such pattern was detected.

Pepsin is released from the chief cells in the gastric gland as proenzyme pepsinogen, which itself has minimal proteolytic activity. Pepsinogen must be enzymatically cleaved to pepsin, which only occurs at a pH of less than 3.0.[21] Pepsin secretion is stimulated by acetylcholine, secretin, GRP, and vasoactive intestinal peptide, among other stimuli.[22]

There are many mucosal factors that protect the lining of the stomach from digestion by hydrochloric acid and pepsin. It is important to recognize that the gastric squamous epithelium is intrinsically more sensitive to acid-pepsin injury than the glandular epithelium, because the former mucosa has less advanced mucosal protective properties. Principal among these are the mucus-bicarbonate layer that covers the glandular mucosal surface, prostaglandin E_2, mucosal blood flow, cellular restitution, and probably EGF. The mucus-bicarbonate layer that covers the gastric mucosa (glandular mucosa of the horse) is approximately 200 μm thick, but creates a lumen-to-mucosa gradient in pH from 1.5 to 6.5.[23] This represents a 100,000-fold attenuation in acidity from the lumen to the mucosal surface! Mucus-secreting cells are present on the luminal surface of the mucosa and within the gastric glands. Prostaglandin E_2 enhances the secretion of bicarbonate-rich mucus, promotes mucosal blood flow, and suppresses hydrochloric acid secretion.[3, 24] Mucosal capillary perfusion is an integral component of mucosal protection,

Table 12–4. Mediators of Gastric Acid Secretion That Have Paracrine, Endocrine, or a Central Effect Within the Brain

Stimulatory		Inhibitory	
Paracrine or Endocrine	Central	Paracrine or Endocrine	Central
Gastrin	Thyrotropin-releasing hormone	Somatostatin	Gastrin-releasing peptide
Histamine	Cholecystokinin	Prostaglandin E_2	Opiates
Acetylcholine	Somatostatin	Secretin	Corticotropin-releasing factor
Gastrin-releasing peptide	Oxytocin		

since disruption of mucosal perfusion readily produces ulceration. Cellular restitution refers to the regeneration of surface epithelial cells in response to an irritating substance. This involves migration of cells from within the gastric gland to the surface, a phenomenon that requires several minutes to a few hours to be completed.[25]

Unlike the mucosal protective factors that are intrinsic to the stomach, EGF is produced in the salivary glands.[26] It is a relatively large peptide (53 amino acids) and can pass to the lower digestive tract with its activity intact. EGF promotes cellular DNA synthesis, and thus growth of gastrointestinal mucosa, and when administered parenterally it inhibits secretion of hydrochloric acid by parietal cells.[27] EGF is produced at other sites, notably in Brunner's glands of the duodenum and the kidney, although salivary EGF seems more important in protection against duodenal ulceration than duodenal EGF.[28] Interestingly, experimental creation of gastric ulcers in rats stimulated salivary EGF synthesis.[26]

The equine gastric stratified squamous mucosal epithelium does not benefit from mucus-bicarbonate secretion. Additionally, such secretions originating in the glandular portion of the stomach do not adhere to the squamous mucosa. Mechanisms that have been postulated to afford protection of gastrointestinal squamous epithelium from acid-pepsin injury include intercellular mucopolysaccharide glycoconjugates, intercellular tight junctions, intercellular buffering of hydrogen ions by bicarbonate, and intracellular buffering of H^+.[29–31] Orlando et al.,[31] in 1992, postulated that intercellular mucopolysaccharides in the superficial epithelial layers provide a diffusion barrier to H^+. If, however, H^+ penetrates this diffusion barrier, cells in the stratum spinosum of the epithelium will concentrate H^+ and epithelial necrosis will subsequently occur. I have observed an increase in intraepithelial mucosubstances in mucosa adjacent to gastric squamous epithelial ulcers compared with normal mucosa from horses. The significance of this finding has not been established, however.

In rats, the development of gastric glandular mucosal resistance to ulceration by hydrochloric acid occurs coincident with the development of gastric acid secretion.[32] Also, resistance to ulceration, as well as acid secretion, can be induced precociously by administration of exogenous corticosteroid. Thus, the development of both acid secretory capability and mucosal protective processes coincide. However, the balance of these aggressive and protective factors may not be highly fine-tuned in the neonate, which may make the young foal more susceptible than adult horses to ulceration in the glandular mucosa of the stomach.

Few specific causes of gastric ulceration in foals and adult horses have been determined. Excessive administration of NSAIDs results in ulceration of both glandular and squamous mucosal linings in foals and adult horses.[33, 34] Through inhibition of prostaglandin E_2 synthesis, NSAIDs promote acid secretion and diminished blood flow in the glandular mucosa. A direct effect on the squamous mucosa has not been determined, but increased acid secretion may account for the ulceration seen secondary to NSAID administration in this tissue in foals and horses.

Stress has been implicated as contributing to, or even causing, gastroduodenal ulcers in foals. Stress is difficult to quantify, but a clinical disorder is likely to represent stress to a foal, and foals with clinical disorders have a greater prevalence of glandular mucosal lesions than normal age-matched foals.[35, 36] Different stress models have been used in laboratory animals in an effort to reproduce and characterize stress-related gastric lesions. Application of different stressors resulted in ulceration of the glandular mucosa, which appeared to have been a result of focal decreased mucosal capillary perfusion that occurred secondary to high-amplitude, low-velocity muscular contractions of the stomach.[37] Such contractions could literally squeeze the blood out of the capillaries, and when sustained, limit perfusion for enough time that acid injury could occur.

Helicobacter (formerly *Campylobacter*) *pylori* is highly prevalent in people with peptic ulcer disease, and is considered by many investigators to be a primary pathogenic agent.[2] To date, there have been no reports that this organism has been identified in any equine species. Bacteria can be found in association with gastric ulcers in foals,[38] but because so many types of bacteria have been associated with the lesions, none has appeared to be of primary pathogenicity. *Candida* has been reported to be associated with gastric lesions in foals,[39] but, again, it was not determined whether the organism was primary or secondary.

Two apparently important factors contributing to gastric squamous mucosal ulceration in horses are the level of training and eating behavior. Repeat gastroscopy in 2-year-old Thoroughbred horses revealed normal mucosa at the beginning of training, but often severe ulceration after the horses had raced just once or were ready to race (M.J. Murray, unpublished data, 1992). Eating behavior may be important since horses that are not eating have significantly higher gastric acidity than horses that are eating,[17] and this degree of acidity (pH <2.0) should be sufficient to cause gastric squamous mucosal ulceration.

PREVALENCE

The overall prevalence of gastric ulcers in foals has been reported to be as high as 25% to 50%, depending on location within the stomach, the presence of a clinical disorder, and age.[35, 40–42] Duodenal ulceration was found in 28 of 511 (5%) foals necropsied at a veterinary teaching hospital[43] (Table 12–5), but the relative difficulty of performing duodenoscopy in foals has precluded a definitive antemortem prevalence from being determined.

Gastric ulcers occur in yearling and adult horses as well as foals. In a report of horses necropsied in Hong Kong, 66% of 195 mature horses had gastric ulcers.[44] Of 100 apparently normal horses examined by gastroendoscopy, 52 had ulcers in the gastric squamous mucosa, while 80 of 87 horses with poor appetite, poor bodily condition, or signs and history of abdominal discomfort had ulcers.[45] Also, horses with clinical signs suggestive of gastric ulceration had significantly greater severity of ulceration than asymptomatic horses. In the same study, 67 of 74 race horses had ulcers in the squamous mucosa of the stomach. In another endoscopic survey, 33 of 33 (100%) racing Thoroughbred horses had ulcers, which in most cases worsened as they continued to race (M.J. Murray, unpublished data, 1992). Also, horses actively racing had a higher prevalence and greater severity of ulcers than did horses at the racetrack, but not in intense training.

Table 12–5. Prevalence of Gastric Lesions in Foals and Horses

Age	Site of Lesion in Stomach	Prevalence	References
2–50 days	Squamous mucosa adjacent to margo plicatus along greater curvature	50%	40–42
2–90 days	Glandular mucosa	4–40%	35, 40–42
90–270 days	Squamous mucosa adjacent to margo along lesser curvature	10–30%	35
2 days–1 yr	Duodenum	≤5%	43
Yearling	Squamous mucosa	<10%*	
Adult, racing	Squamous mucosa	80%–90%	44, 45
Adult, nonracing	Squamous mucosa	30%	44, 45

*Based on observations from 20 normal yearlings examined by the author using endoscopy.

It is apparent that gastric ulceration is a widespread phenomenon, affecting a large number of foals and horses. The adverse health effects in the majority of foals and horses with gastric lesions remain undetermined, although recent experience suggests that the effects of gastric ulceration on condition and performance are much greater than has been recognized.

CLINICAL SYNDROMES

Foals

Gastric Ulceration

The clinical signs that typically are associated with gastric ulcers in foals include bruxism, dorsal recumbency (Fig. 12–8), salivation, interrupted nursing, and colic. These signs, though, are observed in the minority of foals with ulcers, and usually reflect the presence of lesions in the gastric glandular mucosa or duodenum. It is important to recognize that by the time the classic clinical signs of gastroduodenal ulceration are observed in foals, the disorder usually has progressed to a severe stage. This is particularly true if signs of salivation are noted, since this often indicates that

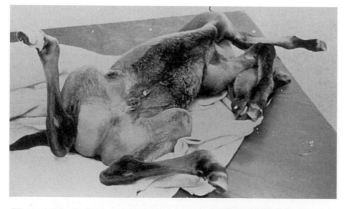

Figure 12–8. Ten-day-old foal with omphalitis and septic physitis. The foal remained in dorsal recumbency, as depicted in this photograph, and on endoscopic examination was found to have a deep ulcer in the gastric glandular mucosa.

gastroesophageal reflux is occurring. Gastric perforation occurs infrequently, but is almost always fatal. Many foals with gastric perforation appeared normal, with no signs suggestive of gastric ulceration until perforation occurred. Thus, although most foals with gastric lesions do not develop clinical disease as a result, one cannot predict in which foals the lesions will be benign and in which more serious consequences might develop.

As mentioned, stress has been associated with gastric ulceration in foals. Retrospectively, 14 (23%) of 61 foals up to 85 days of age with a clinical disorder were found to have lesions in the glandular mucosa of the stomach,[35] and prospectively 8 (40%) of 20 foals up to 30 days of age with a clinical disorder had glandular ulceration.[36] By contrast, only 4% to 9% of foals examined in endoscopic surveys[40–42] had lesions observed in the gastric glandular mucosa. Thus, stress ulceration appears to be an important ulcer syndrome in foals.

The majority of foals with gastric ulcers do not have lesions in the glandular mucosa or duodenum, but they have them in the squamous mucosa.[35, 40–42] The distribution of lesions in the squamous mucosa varies with the age of the foal. In foals less than 50 days old, lesions typically originate in the squamous mucosa adjacent to the margo plicatus along the greater curvature (Fig. 12–9). Such lesions can be seen in foals as young as 2 days of age and have been observed in 50% of foals less than 50 days old. Histologic examination of these lesions has revealed disruption of the epithelial layers of the mucosa and a neutrophilic infiltration.

Another phenomenon that occurs in young foals is the shedding, or desquamation, of squamous epithelium, which appears as flakes or sheets of epithelium. Desquamation occurs without ulceration in up to 80% of foals less than 35 days of age. Desquamation can occur without ulceration, but in many cases is associated with ulceration or erosion and a neutrophilic infiltration.

Some of the erosive or ulcerative lesions adjacent to the margo plicatus in young foals can coalesce into larger, or deeper, areas of ulceration. At this point, there may be hemorrhage associated with the lesions. In the majority of foals, though, the squamous mucosal lesions resolve without treatment and without causing a clinical problem.[36] If clinical signs do occur, diarrhea and poor appetite are those most frequently observed. Diarrhea is the most frequent sign in

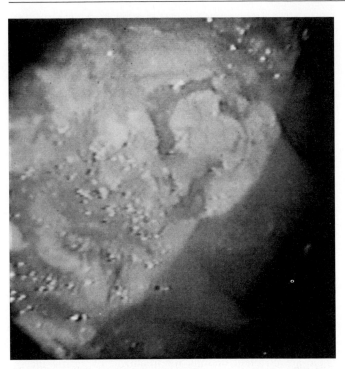

Figure 12–9. Endoscopic view of the stomach of a 23-day-old foal. There is a focal ulcer in the squamous mucosa adjacent to the margo plicatus along the greater curvature of the stomach.

symptomatic foals with squamous mucosal lesions, and is associated with more diffuse erosion or ulceration of the squamous mucosa than occurs in asymptomatic foals. In some foals, poor growth, rough hair coat, or a "potbelly" appearance, or all of those, occur in conjunction with moderate to severe squamous mucosal ulceration. In cases with severe or diffuse squamous ulceration, bruxism or colic may occur.

In older foals, lesions become more prevalent in the squamous mucosa surrounding the cardia, and along the lesser curvature between the cardia and pylorus.[36] Lesions also are found in the squamous mucosa of the fundus and adjacent to the margo plicatus. These lesions can be very severe, and are often associated with clinical signs such as diarrhea, poor appetite, and poor growth and bodily condition. In some cases, lesions surrounding the cardia have occured in association with anatomical or functional obstruction to gastric emptying. When gastric emptying is impaired, gastroesophageal reflux may also occur, and ulceration of the distal esophagus will be present.

Duodenal Ulceration

The signs of duodenal ulceration are the same as described for gastric ulceration (bruxism, colic, salivation, diarrhea), but the consequences of duodenal ulceration are often more severe. Lesions occur primarily in the proximal duodenum, and range from diffuse inflammation to focal bleeding and perforating ulcers. Foals with duodenal ulceration often have delayed gastric emptying and may have gastroesophageal reflux. Complications can include duodenal rupture, duode-

nal stricture, ascending cholangitis, severe gastric ulceration, and aspiration pneumonia secondary to gastroesophageal reflux.[46–48]

The causes of duodenal ulceration in foals are poorly understood. In humans, duodenal ulceration is associated with increased gastric acid secretion.[1] The age distribution of the disease in foals and the rarity of the disease in adult horses suggest that immature regulation of acid secretion and mucosal protection may be an important factor in the development of duodenal lesions in foals, but this is speculative at this time. Gastric ulceration that occurs secondary to duodenal ulceration tends to be severe, and is frequently associated with gastroesophageal reflux and esophagitis. Gastric ulcers may occur during the active phase of duodenal inflammation or as a result of impaired gastric emptying due to sequelae of duodenal ulceration.

Duodenal ulceration can be difficult to confirm. Duodenoscopy is the most specific means of diagnosis, although the procedure is more difficult than gastroscopy. Additionally, an endoscope at least 200 cm in length is needed for foals up to 5 to 7 months old, and a longer endoscope usually is required for older animals.

Excessive enterogastric reflux of bile through the pylorus suggests duodenal dysfunction. Also, ulceration at the pylorus or pyloric antrum is suggestive of duodenal ulceration. If gastroendoscopy, but not duodenoscopy, can be performed, the severity of lesions, particularly in the glandular mucosa and in the squamous mucosa of the lesser curvature dorsal to the pyloric antrum, will usually be severe when duodenal ulcers are present. Also, histamine H_2 receptor antagonist therapy may be less effective in resolving gastric lesions than in cases of primary gastric ulceration.

Yearlings and Adult Horses

In yearlings and mature horses lesions occur predominantly in the squamous mucosa, particularly adjacent to the margo plicatus. In more severe cases, lesions extend dorsally into the squamous fundus. Endoscopy has revealed that in normal yearlings and 2-year-old horses in training for racing there can be mild multifocal lesions in the squamous mucosa. These lesions typically are very small, and seem to be inconsequential. Clinically relevant lesions typically affect a greater portion of the squamous mucosa and can be deep enough to cause bleeding (Fig. 12–10). However, bleeding from ulcers in the gastric squamous mucosa is typically *not* associated with anemia or hypoproteinemia, and if these abnormalities are present, another cause must be determined.

When lesions are observed in the glandular mucosa, NSAID administration should be suspected. The low prevalence of spontaneous glandular lesions in adult horses compared with foals suggests that adult horses have a more mature mucosal protective capability.

The clinical signs associated with gastric ulcers in adult horses include acute or recurrent colic, poor bodily condition, poor appetite, poor performance, and attitude changes (Table 12–6). In contrast to foals, diarrhea is not associated with gastric ulcers in adult horses, although ulcers can occur concurrent with a disorder causing diarrhea. Of 87 horses with these clinical signs examined by gastroendoscopy, 81 (93%) had gastric ulcers, compared with 52 of 100 asymp-

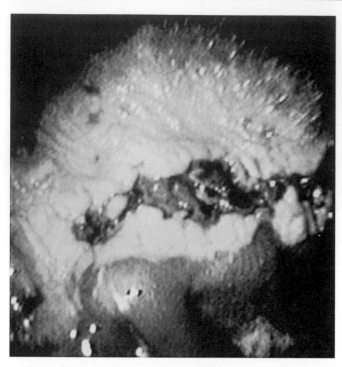

Figure 12–10. Endoscopic view of the right side of the stomach of a horse with recurrent colic and poor appetite. There is a large area of ulceration of the squamous mucosa adjacent to the margo plicatus.

tomatic horses.[45] Lesions were significantly more severe in the symptomatic horses. Horses in active training for racing, including Thoroughbreds trained for flat-racing and steeplechase racing, and standardbreds trained for trotting or pacing, were at greater risk of having gastric ulcers than horses not in training. Of 37 reportedly asymptomatic horses in training, 29 (78%) had ulcers compared with 23 of 63 (36%) reportedly asymptomatic horses not in training.

Gastric ulcers can cause colic and can occur secondary to other intestinal disorders that cause colic.[49] The severity of pain associated with ulcers can vary from mild to severe. Some horses with gastric ulcers develop recurrent colic with colonic gas distention that resolves when the ulcers are treated. A few horses have had such severe pain that exploratory surgery was done. No intestinal lesions were found, but severe ulcers were seen by endoscopy. In other horses, ulcers caused colic after a primary problem, such as a large colon impaction, was resolved. Yet in some other horses, ulcers occurred secondary to ileocecal intussusception, enteritis, and colitis. Determination of ulcers as the cause of colic can best be made by endoscopic confirmation of ulcers, ruling out other possible causes of colic, clinical response to treatment, and endoscopic evidence of ulcer healing.

Given the high prevalence of gastric ulcers in adult horses, particularly those in racing, it is important for the practitioner to consider this disorder in the differential diagnosis of a horse with a poor appetite, mild to moderate weight loss, poor bodily condition, and colic for which another cause has not been determined.

DIAGNOSIS

Diagnosis of gastric ulceration is based on the presence of age-related clinical signs, endoscopic findings, and response to treatment. The diagnosis of gastric ulceration in the majority of foals and horses can be definitively determined only by gastroendoscopic examination. The procedures and equipment required for endoscopic examination of the stomach of foals and adult horses have been described.[50] An endoscopic diagnosis of gastric ulceration allows the examiner to determine that ulcers are present, the location of the lesions, the severity of the lesions, and the response to therapy. The presence of clinical signs, and the results of diagnostic tests, such as fecal occult blood and contrast radiography, can be unreliable indicators of the presence of gastric ulcers. Testing for fecal occult blood is of value only in young foals, since the colonic microflora thoroughly digest hemoglobin. In my experience, the test has been negative in horses with actively bleeding gastric lesions.

TREATMENT

There are different options for treatment of gastric ulcers, and the decision as to which agent(s) to use should be based on the location and severity of lesions as determined by endoscopy, severity of clinical signs, and expense of treatment (Table 12–7). Of these considerations, the location of the ulcer is most important, since lesions in the squamous mucosa and those in the glandular mucosa will not be treated identically.

If gastroendoscopy is unavailable, some guidelines to therapy can be employed, but the efficacy of the treatment will be based on clinical signs, which are often vague or nonspecific. Signs of colic or diarrhea that result from gastric ulcers often resolve within 48 hours. Improvements in appetite, bodily condition, and attitude can be noted within 1 to 3 weeks. If improvement in clinical signs is not observed, either treatment has not been effective or gastric ulceration was not the primary problem.

The principal therapeutic agents available for ulcer treatment are the H_2 antagonists cimetidine, ranitidine (Zantac, Glaxo, Inc., Research Triangle Park, N.C.), famotidine (Pep-

Table 12–6. Signs of Gastric Ulcers in Adult Horses

Signs of Colic	Signs of Poor Appetite or Condition	Attitude Changes
Mild discomfort after eating	Does not finish feed	Nervous
Mild discomfort after training	Slow to finish feed	Sluggish
Moderate abdominal pain, acute or recurrent	50–75 kg underweight	Difficult to handle
Severe acute pain		Poor training, racing

Table 12–7. Therapeutic Agents and Recommended Dosages for Treating Gastric and Duodenal Ulcers in Foals and Horses

Classification	Drug	Dosage
Histamine H_2 receptor antagonist	Cimetidine	50 mg/kg/day PO divided t.i.d. or q.i.d.
		26 mg/kg/day IV divided q.i.d.
	Ranitidine	20 mg/kg/day PO divided t.i.d.
		4.5 mg/kg/day IV divided t.i.d.
	Famotidine	10–15 mg/kg/day divided b.i.d. or t.i.d.
Mucosal adherent	Sucralfate	10–20 mg/kg PO q.6–8h.
Antacid	Aluminum/ magnesium hydroxide	40–50 mL/100 kg PO 4–6 times daily
H^+, K^+-ATPase blocker	Omeprazole	.7–1 mg/kg* PO once-daily

*Prilosec enteric-coated granules administered by nasogastric tube.

cid, Merck & Co., Inc., Rahway, N.J.), nizatidine (Axid, Eli Lilly & Co., Indianapolis, Ind.), the mucosal adherent sucralfate (Carafate, Marion Merrill Dow, Kansas City, Kans.), the proton pump blocker omeprazole (Prilosec, Merck & Co., Inc., Rahway, N.J.), and antacids. The H_2 antagonists suppress hydrochloric acid secretion through competitive inhibition of the parietal cell histamine receptor. This inhibition can be partially overcome with agents such as exogenous pentagastrin. Use of H_2 antagonists has been successful in resolving gastric lesions and the presenting problem in both foals and adult horses.[47, 49, 51]

Omeprazole blocks secretion of H^+ at the parietal cell membrane by irreversibly binding to the H^+, K^+-ATPase proton pump of the cell.[52] The effect of the drug, therefore, is to completely suppress acid secretion, and depending on the dose administered, the effect can last 24 hours. Omeprazole has been evaluated experimentally in the horse and it effectively suppressed acid secretion.[53–55] The drug has not been thoroughly clinically evaluated in horses, and its biggest drawback at this time is effective oral delivery.

Clinical experience and the results of research[56, 57] have demonstrated that the lower the dosage of an H_2 antagonist, the greater the individual variability in response. Some horses respond relatively poorly to higher doses of drug (6.6 mg/kg ranitidine, 3.3 mg/kg famotidine), and not at all to lower doses (4.4 mg/kg ranitidine, 1.0 mg/kg famotidine). Similar dose-related variability has been noted in humans taking omeprazole.[58] Thus, the goal in treating horses with acid-suppressive agents is to administer a dose that is *effective* in the greatest number of patients. Lower doses are less expensive, but if they are ineffective they will not have been cost-effective.

Cimetidine should be given at a dosage of 60 to 90 mg/kg/day, and ranitidine at 20 mg/kg/day. Famotidine probably should be given at 10 to 15 mg/kg/day. My preferred dosage

schedule is ranitidine at 6.6 mg/kg every 8 hours. Lower dosages, such as 2.2 mg/kg, have seemed effective in alleviating clinical signs of gastric ulcers (diarrhea, inappetance, etc.), but gastroscopic examination revealed that significant ulceration was still present. This suggests that the degree of suppression of acid secretion required to heal lesions is greater than that required to provide relief from discomfort. A relationship between dosage and alleviation of symptoms has been difficult to establish in humans, because even though people are able to articulate symptoms of dyspepsia, there is often poor correlation between these symptoms and the presence of ulcers![59] On the other hand, a positive correlation between dosages of H_2 antagonists and ulcer healing has been determined for humans.[56]

The H_2 antagonist therapy should continue for 14 to 21 days to ensure complete healing. In many cases, complete healing will occur within this time, but in others it may take 30 to 40 days. It has become apparent from treating horses in training for racing that if the horse is kept in training while being treated, clinical signs resolve but the lesions do not. Once the medication is discontinued, clinical signs often return. Thus, for healing of the ulcers to be achieved, treatment with an H_2 antagonist should be accompanied by refraining from athletic activity.

Currently, cimetidine and ranitidine are available in injectable, tablet, and liquid forms. Famotidine and nizatidine are available in tablets.

The use of antacids in the treatment of gastric ulcers has not been critically examined in the horse. In people, antacids must be taken frequently, 6 to 10 times daily, to have a significant effect on the healing of peptic ulcers.[60] There also may be a rebound secretion of acid in response to the increase in gastric pH following antacid administration. The duration of acid suppression of antacid (180 mL Maalox, Rorer Pharmaceutical Corp., Fort Washington, Pa.) in horses was only 30 to 45 minutes.[57] Thus, antacids may be effective in treating equine gastric ulcers, but large volumes will have to be administered every 2 to 3 hours. Antacids have appeared useful in mature horses in alleviating clinical signs of gastric ulcers, particularly poor appetite. Antacids have not been critically evaluated as a maintenance therapy.

Sucralfate, sucrose octasulfate (SOS), and aluminum hydroxide are effective in the treatment of peptic ulcers in humans.[61] The mechanism of action likely involves adherence to ulcerated mucosa, stimulation of mucus secretion, enhanced prostaglandin E synthesis, and concentration of growth factor at the site of ulceration. These are all factors relevant to glandular mucosa, and the efficacy of sucralfate in treating ulcers in the equine gastric squamous mucosa remains undetermined, but in this regard it is unlikely to be of important benefit. Consequently, sucralfate should not be used as the single therapeutic agent in treatment of gastric ulcers unless gastroscopy has revealed lesions confined to the glandular mucosa. It is advisable to utilize sucralfate as an adjunct to H_2 antagonist therapy. Sucralfate may be effective in prevention of stress-induced ulcers in young foals, since these occur in the glandular mucosa, although no clinical evidence directly supports this concept. Sucralfate should be given at a dosage of 10 to 20 mg/kg every 6 to 8 hours.

Because of evidence that sucralfate adheres to gastric

mucosa in an acidic environment, it has been advised to administer sucralfate 1 to 2 hours prior to administering an H_2 antagonist. However, this is probably unnecessary since more recent evidence suggests that sucralfate will adhere to gastric mucosa at pH levels greater than 5.[62] Also, it is likely that at the time of administration of an H_2 antagonist the gastric pH will have returned to a relatively acidic pH since the last dosage, and it will remain so for approximately 60 minutes after administration of an H_2 antagonist, certainly enough time for binding of sucralfate to the glandular mucosa. Thus, I recommend concurrent administration of sucralfate and H_2 antagonist.

The use of synthetic prostaglandin E_1 analogs has been effective in the treatment of gastric and duodenal ulcers in humans, and the proposed mechanism of action involves both inhibition of gastric acid secretion and mucosal cytoprotection.[63] Misoprostil (Cytotec, The Upjohn Co., Kalamazoo, Mich.) effectively heals duodenal ulcers,[64] but frequently reported adverse effects include intestinal cramping and diarrhea. These adverse effects would be unacceptable in an equine patient, and thus the use of misoprostil to treat ulcers in horses has not been reported.

Prokinetic drugs should be considered in foals with duodenal disease, gastroesophageal reflux, and when delayed gastric emptying is suspected. Metoclopramide (Reglan, A.H. Robins Co., Inc., Richmond, Va.) has been used in selected cases to prevent gastroesophageal reflux and enhance gastric emptying. The effect on gastrointestinal smooth muscle is mediated principally by antagonism of dopamine at dopamine receptors. Reported experience with metacloramide in the horse is limited.[65, 66] Dosages ranging from 0.10 to 0.25 mg/kg PO or SC three to four times daily are used clinically.

Several adverse reactions to metoclopramide occur in up to 20% of human patients, most frequently drowsiness and lassitude. Extrapyramidal effects and dyskinesias, resulting from the central dopamine inhibitory effects of metoclopramide, also occur.[67] In the horse, sudden neurologic excitation has been reported[65, 66] and observed on several occasions by me. Excitation, with violent outbursts, may occur with a variety of dosages, and thus it is advisable to administer a test dose, at the desired dosage, as an intravenous drip over a 60-minute period. In one foal that I treated, chronic administration of metoclopramide resulted in tachycardia, bilateral facial sweating, miosis, and enophthalmos. These signs resolved when the drug was discontinued.

In my experience, the cholinergic drug bethanechol (Urecholine, Merck & Co., Inc., Rahway, N.J.) has effectively enhanced gastric emptying or minimized gastroesophageal reflux in foals, with fewer adverse effects than observed with metoclopramide. In cases of acute gastric atony, bethanechol 0.025 to 0.030 mg/kg, SC every 3 to 4 hours has been effective in promoting gastric motility and emptying, followed by oral maintenance dosages of 0.35 to 0.45 mg/kg three to four times daily. Adverse effects can include diarrhea, inappetance, salivation, and colic, but at the dosages stated, adverse effects have been infrequent and mild.

REFERENCES

1. McGuigan JE: Peptic ulcer disease. In Braunwald E, Isselbacher KJ, eds: *Harrison's Principles of Internal Medicine.* New York, McGraw-Hill, 1983, p 1697.

2. Graham DY: *Campylobacter pylori* and peptic ulcer disease. *Gastroenterology* 96:615, 1989.

3. Richardson CT: Pathogenic factors in peptic ulcer disease. *Am J Med* 79(suppl 2c):1, 1985.

4. Glotzer DJ: Stress ulcer control in critically ill patients. *J Crit Illness* 3:S59, 1988.

5. Smolka A, Sachs G, Lorentzen P: Cell-free synthesis of rat and rabbit gastric proton pump. *Gastroentrology* 97:873, 1989.

6. Hirschowitz BI, Molina E: Relation of gastric acid and pepsin secretion to serum gastrin levels in dogs given bombesin and gastrin-17. *Am J Physiol* 244:G546, 1983.

7. Tache Y: Central nervous system action of neuropeptides to influence or prevent experimental gastroduodenal ulceration. In Szabo S, Pfeiffer CJ, eds: *Ulcer Disease: New Aspects of Pathogenesis and Pharmacology.* Boca Raton, Fla, CRC Press, 1989, p 179.

8. Schubert ML, Edwards NF, Makhlouf GM: Regulation of gastric somatostatin secretion in the mouse by luminal acidity: A local feedback mechanism. *Gastroenterology* 94:317, 1988.

9. Lewis JJ, Goldenring JR, Asher VA, et al: Effects of epidermal growth factor on signal transduction in rabbit parietal cells. *Am J Physiol* 258:G476, 1990.

10. Murray MJ, Grodinsky C: Regional gastric pH measurements in horses and foals. *Equine Vet J* 7(suppl):73, 1989.

11. Takeuchi K, Peitsch W, Johnson LR: Mucosal gastrin receptor. V. Development in newborn rats. *Am J Physiol* 240:G163, 1981.

12. Peitsch W, Yakeuchi K, Johnson LR: Mucosal gastrin receptor. VI. Induction by corticosterone in newborn rats. *Am J Physiol* 240:G442, 1981.

13. Murray MJ, Luba NK: Plasma gastrin, somatostatin, and serum thyroxine (T_4), triiodothyronine (T_3), reverse triiodothyronine (rT_3), and cortisol in foals from birth to 28 days of age. *Equine Vet J* 25:237, 1993.

14. Brown CM, Sonea I, Nachreiner RF, et al: Serum immunoreactive gastrin activity in horses: Basal and postprandial values. *Vet Res Commun* 11:497, 1987.

15. Campbell-Thompson ML, Merritt AM: Effect of ranitidine on gastric acid secretion in young male horses. *Am J Vet Res* 48:1511–1515, 1987.

16. Campbell-Thompson ML, Merritt AM: Basal and pentagastrin-stimulated gastric secretion in young horses. *Am J Physiol* 259:R1259–R1266, 1990.

17. Murray MJ, Schusser G: Application of gastric pH-metry in horses: Measurement of 24 hour gastric pH in horses fed, fasted, and treated with ranitidine. *Equine Vet J* 25:417–421, 1993.

18. Alexander F, Hickson JCD: The salivary and pancreatic secretions of the horse. In Phillipson AT, ed: *Physiology of Digestion and Metabolism in the Ruminant.* Oriel, London, 1970, pp 375–389.

19. Moore JG: Circadian dynamics of gastric acid secretion and pharmacodynamics of H_2 receptor blockade. *Ann N Y Acad Sci* 618:150, 1990.

20. Merki HS, Witzel L, Kaufman D, et al: Assessment of intragastric acidity in man: Modern aspects, reproducibility of intragastric pH-monitoring, and pharmacodynamic results obtained with H_2-receptor antagonists. *Scand J Gastroenterol Suppl* 23(146):142, 1988.

21. Piper DW, Fenton BW: pH stability and activity curves of pepsin with special reference to their clinical importance. *Gut* 6:506, 1965.

22. Sutliff VE, Raufman JP, Jensen RT, et al: Actions of vasoactive intestinal peptide and secretin on chief cells prepared from guinea pig stomach. *Am J Physiol* 251:G96, 1986.

23. Ross IN, Bahari HMM, Turneberg LA: The pH gradient across mucus adherent to rat fundic mucosa in vivo and the effect of potential damaging agents. *Gastroenterology* 81:713, 1981.

24. Kauffman G: The role of prostaglandins in the regulation of gastric mucosal blood flow. *Prostaglandins* 21:33, 1981.

25. Gronbech JE, Varhaug JE, Svanes K: Restituted gastric mucosa: Tolerance against low luminal pH and restricted mucosal blood flow in the cat. *Gastroenterology* 96:50, 1989.
26. Gysin B, Muller RKM, Otten U, et al: Epidermal growth factor is increased in rats with experimentally induced gastric lesions. *Scand J Gastroenterol* 23:665, 1988.
27. Hatt JF, Manson PJ: Inhibition of gastric acid secretion by epidermal growth factor. *Biochem J* 25:789, 1988.
28. Konturek SJ, Dembinski A, Warzecha Z, et al: Role of epidermal growth factor in healing chronic gastroduodenal ulcers in rats. *Gastroenterology* 94:1300, 1988.
29. Orlando RC: Esophageal epithelial defense against acid injury. *J Clin Gastroenterol* 13(suppl 2):S1, 1991.
30. Tobey NA, Orlando RC: Mechanisms of acid injury to rabbit esophageal epithelium. *Gastroenterology* 101:1220, 1991.
31. Orlando RC, Lacy ER, Tobey NA, et al: Barriers to paracellular permeability in rabbit esophageal epithelium. *Gastroenterology* 102:910, 1992.
32. Dial EJ, Lichtenberger LM: Development of gastric mucosal protection against acid in the rat. *Gastroenterology* 91:318, 1986.
33. Traub JL, Gallina AM, Grant BD, et al: Phenylbutazone toxicosis in the foal. *Am J Vet Res* 44:1410, 1983.
34. Murray MJ: Phenylbutazone toxicosis in a horse. *Compendium Continuing Educ Pract Vet* 7:S389, 1985.
35. Murray MJ: Gastroendoscopic appearance of gastric lesions in foals: 94 cases (1987–1988). *J Am Vet Med Assoc* 195:1135, 1989.
36. Furr MO, Murray MJ: The effects of stress on gastric ulceration and serum T_3, T_4, and cortisol in neonatal foals. *Equine Vet J* 24:37–40, 1992.
37. Garrick T, Bauck S, Minor TR, et al: Predictable and unpredictable shock stimulates gastric contractility and causes mucosal injury in rats. *Behav Neurosci* 103:124, 1989.
38. Collobert-Laugier C, Vaissaire J, Jacquet A, et al: Bacterial species in gastroduodenal ulcerations in foals. *Equine Vet J* 7(suppl):139, 1989.
39. Gross TL, Mayhew IG: Gastroesophageal ulceration and candidiasis in foals. *J Am Vet Med Assoc* 182:1370, 1983.
40. Murray MJ, Hart J, Parker GA: Equine gastric ulcer syndrome: Prevalence of gastric lesions in asymptomatic foals. In *Proceedings of the American Association of Equine Practitioners,* 1987, New Orleans, p 769.
41. Murray MJ, Murray CM, Sweeney HJ, et al: The prevalence of gastric ulcers in foals in Ireland and England: An endoscopic survey. *Equine Vet J* 22:6, 1990.
42. Murray MJ, Grodinsky C, Cowles RR, et al: The progression of gastric lesions in young Thoroughbred foals: An endoscopic study. *J Am Vet Med Assoc* 196:1623, 1990.
43. Wilson JH: Gastric and duodenal ulcers in foals: A retrospective study. In *Proceedings of the Second Equine Colic Research Symposium,* October, 1985. Lawrenceville, NJ, Vet Learning System, 1986, p 126.
44. Hammond CJ, Mason DK, Watkins KL: Gastric ulceration in mature Thoroughbred horses. *Equine Vet J* 18:284, 1986.
45. Murray MJ, Grodinsky C, Anderson CW, et al: Gastric ulcers in horses: A comparison of endoscopic findings in horses with and without clinical signs. *Equine Vet J* 7(suppl):68, 1989.
46. Murray MJ, Ball MM: Megaesophagus and aspiration pneumonia secondary to gastric ulceration in a foal. *J Am Vet Med Assoc* 192:381, 1988.
47. Becht JL, Byars TD: Gastroduodenal ulcers in foals. *Equine Vet J* 18:307, 1986.
48. Orsini JA, Donawick WJ: Surgical treatment of gastroduodenal obstructions in foals. *Vet Surg* 15:205, 1986.
49. Murray MJ: Gastric ulceration in horses with colic: 91 cases (1987–1990). *J Am Vet Med Assoc* 102:117, 1992.
50. Adamson P, Murray MJ: Stomach. In Brown CM, Traub-Dargatz JL, eds: *Equine Endoscopy.* St Louis, Mosby–Year Book, 1990, p 119.
51. Furr MO, Murray MJ: Treatment of gastric ulcers in horses with histamine type 2 receptor antagonists. *Equine Vet J* 7(suppl):77, 1989.
52. Larsson H, Mattsson H, Carlsson E: Gastric acid antisecretory effect of two different dosage forms of omeprazole during prolonged oral treatment in the gastric fistula dog. *Scand J Gastroenterol* 23:1013, 1988.
53. Andrews F, Jenkins C, Frazier D, et al: Effect of oral omeprazole on basal and pentagastrin-stimulated gastric secretion in young female horses. *Equine Vet J* 13(suppl):80, 1992.
54. Jenkins C, Andrews F, Frazier D, et al: Pharmacokinetics and antisecretory effects of intravenous omeprazole in horses. *Equine Vet J* 13(suppl):84, 1992.
55. Jenkins C, Blackford J, Andrews F, et al: Duration of antisecretory effects of oral omeprazole in horses with chronic gastric cannulae. *Equine Vet J* 13(suppl):89, 1992.
56. Burget DW, Chiverton SG, Hunt RH: Is there an optimal degree of acid suppression for healing of duodenal ulcers? *Gastroenterology* 99:345, 1990.
57. Murray MJ, Grodinsky C: The effects of famotidine, ranitidine, and magnesium hydroxide/aluminum hydroxide on gastric fluid pH in adult horses. *Equine Vet J* 11(suppl):52, 1992.
58. Sharma BK, Walt RP, Pounder RE, et al: Optimal dose of oral omeprazole for maximum 24 hour decrease in intragastric acidity. *Gut* 25:957, 1984.
59. Bates S, Sjoden P-O, Fellenius J, et al: Blocked and nonblocked acid secretion and reported pain in ulcer, nonulcer dyspepsia, and normal subjects. *Gastroenterology* 97:376, 1989.
60. Peterson WL, Sturdevant RAL, Frankl HD, et al: Healing of duodenal ulcer with an antacid regime. *N Engl J Med* 297:341, 1975.
61. Van Deventer GM, Schneidman D, Walsh JH: Sucralfate and cimetidine as single agents and in combination for treatment of active duodenal ulcers. *Am J Med* 79(suppl 2C):39, 1985.
62. Danesh BJZ, Duncan A, Russell RI, et al: Effect of intragastric pH on mucosal protective action of sucralfate. *Gut* 29:1379, 1988.
63. Mahachai V, Walker K, Sevelius H, et al: Antisecretory and serum gastrin lowering effect of enprostil in patients with duodenal ulcer disease. *Gastroenterology* 89:555, 1985.
64. Birnie GG, Watkinson G, Shroff NE, et al: Double-blind comparison of two dosage regimens of misoprostol in the treatment of duodenal ulceration. *Dig Dis Sci* 33:1269, 1988.
65. Gerring EEL, Hunt JM: Pathophysiology of equine postoperative ileus: Effect of adrenergic blockade, parasympathetic stimulation and metoclopramide in an experimental model. *Equine Vet J* 18:249, 1986.
66. Kritchevsky JE, Adams SB, Lamar CH: Metoclopramide in the horse: Dosage and effects on gastrointestinal motility. In *Proceedings of Conference of Research Workers in Animal Diseases,* Chicago, November, 1984, p 49.
67. Albibi R, McCallum RW: Metoclopramide: Pharmacology and clinical application. *Ann Intern Med* 98:86, 1983.

12.4

Duodenitis–Proximal Jejunitis

Michael J. Murray, DVM, MS

Duodenitis–proximal jejunitis (DPJ) describes a clinical syndrome that is characterized by inflammation of the small intestine, resulting in excessive fluid and electrolyte secretion by the small intestine and, consequently, large volumes of enterogastric reflux. The disorder also has been referred to as anterior enteritis and proximal enteritis. The syndrome was first described in 1982[1] and was more fully characterized in 1987.[2] A subsequent report[3] described clinical and clinicopathologic findings in horses with DPJ that differed somewhat from the cases initially reported,[1] suggesting that either the cases were of similar pathogenesis but of different severity, or of different pathogenesis with the only similarity being the segment of bowel affected.

The events that led to the recognition of DPJ as a clinical entity reflect the evolution of the approach to the treatment of the horse with acute abdominal pain. Horses later recognized as having DPJ were routinely taken to surgery because they presented with current or recent acute abdominal pain, had large volumes of fluid recovered from nasogastric intubation, and had evidence of distended small intestine on rectal examination. These signs were indicative of small intestinal obstruction, but at surgery no obstruction was found. Rather, the duodenum or proximal small intestine, or both, had extensive serosal hyperemia and hemorrhage, was sometimes thickened, and contained large volumes of fluid. Despite evacuating the fluid into the colon at surgery, postoperatively these horses continued to produce copious volumes of enterogastric reflux, were difficult to maintain metabolically, and frequently died.

Once DPJ was recognized as a clinical syndrome, it appeared that the survival rate for those that had surgery was worse than for horses treated medically. Recent retrospective reports revealed that, indeed, the survival rate for horses with DPJ that had surgery (3/18, or 17%)[2] was poor compared with that of horses treated medically (30/32 or 94%).[3] This great difference in survival rates has been attributed to the stress of general anesthesia and surgery on horses already compromised metabolically. However, another important factor may be the severity of the disease in the groups of horses in different reports.[2, 3] For instance, horses diagnosed with DPJ that I treated and observed while at the University of Georgia by and large had more severe signs in terms of volume and duration of enterogastric reflux and incidence of complications (laminitis) than the horses with DPJ I have subsequently treated and observed in Virginia. There was little difference in the intensity of intravenous fluid administration or other supportive treatment. Others have noted apparent geographically related differences in incidence and severity of the syndrome, with more cases seen in the southeastern United States.

CLINICAL SIGNS

Because of the experience that horses with DPJ that had surgery tended to have a worse survival rate than those treated with medical therapy only, it was important to develop diagnostic criteria that distinguished horses with DPJ from those with small intestinal obstruction. Johnston and Morris[3] reported that horses diagnosed as having DPJ that were admitted to the University of Pennsylvania veterinary hospital were older, had greater severity of depression, had less severe abdominal pain, had lower heart rates, and produced greater volumes of nasogastric reflux than horses with small intestinal obstruction. These results were generated from 34 horses with small intestinal obstruction and 34 horses diagnosed *by clinical signs* as having DPJ.

Certainly, when the veterinarian is confronted with a horse with colic that has enterogastric reflux and small bowel distention on rectal examination, the differentiation between DPJ and obstruction can be very difficult. Horses with DPJ frequently present with a history of an acute onset of moderate to severe abdominal pain. At the time of examination the horse may still exhibit abdominal discomfort, or may no longer be in pain but rather, appear depressed. Other clinical signs accompanying DPJ include large volumes (6–20 L with each decompressive effort) of nasogastric reflux that is often orange-brown–colored with a fetid odor, moderate to severe small intestinal distention palpated on rectal examination, fever of 38.6° to 39.1°C (101.5°–102.5 °F), dehydration, injected mucous membranes, depressed or absent borborygmi, prolonged capillary refill time, tachycardia (> 60/min), and tachypnea. Although the signs of abdominal pain usually resolve after gastric decompression, most horses remain severely depressed. If the fluid that accumulates in the proximal intestinal tract is not removed periodically, signs of abdominal pain recur. Horses with DPJ often require gastric decompression at 2-hour intervals, with 2 to 10 L of fluid recovered each time.

CLINICOPATHOLOGIC FINDINGS

Typical clinical laboratory findings include an increased packed cell volume and total plasma protein reflective of hemoconcentration, a metabolic acidosis in longstanding or severe cases, an increased peritoneal fluid protein concentration (often > 3.5 g/dL), and a mild to moderate elevation of the peritoneal white blood cell count, although the count usually is less than 10,000 cells per microliter.[3, 4] The peritoneal fluid is usually yellow and turbid, but in severe cases diapedesis occurs, resulting in a serosanguinous color. The white blood cell count in the peripheral blood may be normal or increased. In addition, hyponatremia, hypochloremia, hypokalemia, and acid-base alterations can develop. The loss of enteric bicarbonate through evacuation of enterogastric reflux and poor tissue perfusion from hypovolemia can lead to metabolic acidosis.

A definitive diagnosis of DPJ can be made in most cases by gross examination of the duodenum and proximal jejunum at surgery or at necropsy. In horses with DPJ, lesions are always found in the duodenum, but the severity and frequency of lesions in the jejunum are variable. Occasionally, lesions are found in the pyloric portion of the stomach. The lesions of DPJ are typically transmural with the serosal surface appearing smooth and containing bright-red to dark-red petechial and ecchymotic hemorrhages.[2] Inflammation and edema may cause thickening of the proximal small intestinal wall. The mucosa appears a deep-red color and the proximal small intestinal contents can be similarly discolored depending on the amount of mucosal damage. While the stomach and proximal small intestine are moderately distended with fluid, the distal jejunum and ileum are usually flaccid. Lesions are rarely found in the distal jejunum, ileum, and large intestine.[1, 2]

The histologic lesions in the duodenum and proximal jejunum vary in severity from case to case but are consis-

Table 12–8. Physical and Laboratory Examination Findings in Horses with Duodenitis–Proximal Jejunitis (DPJ), and an Operable Small Intestinal Lesion*

Examination	DPJ	Strangulating Obstruction	Nonstrangulating Obstruction
Abdominal Pain	Acute onset	Acute onset	Acute onset
Attitude	*Depressed, painful*	*Painful*	*Painful*
Heart rate (beats/min)	40–80	≥80	40–80
Respiratory rate (breaths/min)	16–28	24–40	15–35
Rectal temperature (°F)	*101.5–102.5*	*≤101*	*99–101*
Capillary refill time	>3 sec	≥3 sec	1.5–3.0 sec
Intestinal sounds	Mildly to markedly depressed	Markedly depressed to absent	Mildly depressed to absent
Nasogastric reflux	3–4 gal orange-brown	2–4 gal, ±malodorous	2–3 gal with ingesta character, ±malodorous
Rectal examination	Dilated to moderately distended	Moderately to markedly distended	Mild to moderately distended, ±ileal impaction
Response to nasogastric decompression	*Depressed, quiet*	*Temporary to no pain relief*	*Temporary to no pain relief*
Complete blood count	±Increased WBC, mature neutrophilia	±Increased WBC, slight neutrophilia	Normal to increased WBC
Peritoneal fluid protein	>3.0 g/dL and may be >4.5 g/dL	2.5–4.5 g/dL	2.5–3.5 g/dL
Peritoneal fluid nucleated cell count	*≤5,000/μL*	*3,000–>20,000/μL*	*3,000/1–12,000/μL*

*Findings in which differences between DPJ and obstructive disorders are often present are italicized.

tently more severe from proximal to distal in individual cases. Lesions include hyperemia and edema of the mucosa and submucosa progressing to villus epithelial degeneration and mucosal necrosis, epithelial cell sloughing, marked neutrophil infiltration, hemorrhages in the muscular layers, and fibrinopurulent exudation onto the serosal surface. Thus, the term *hemorrhagic fibrinonecrotic duodenitis-proximal jejunitis* has been suggested as a more descriptive name for this syndrome.[2] Similar lesions have been reported in humans and neonatal pigs with *Clostridium perfringens* infection.

PATHOGENESIS

An etiologic agent or agents that cause DPJ have not been identified, although *Salmonella* and *Clostridium* species have been recovered from enterogastric reflux and the contents of the small intestine of affected horses. Inoculation of horses with species of *Salmonella* or *Clostridium* has not reproduced the disease, however. Nevertheless, an infectious agent seems most plausible as the cause of the disorder, since the lesions are not typical of those resulting from a primary vascular insult. Also, the volume of fluid produced by the small bowel is typical of an active secretory process, rather than passive secretion resulting from a vascular insult.

Active secretion can be stimulated by increased levels of mucosal membrane adenylate or guanylate cyclase activity, increased mucosal cellular prostaglandin E₂, or increased mucosal cell membrane calcium permeability and influx.

The net effect is increased movement of chloride and sodium into the mucosal cell from the interstitium, with secretion of chloride and sodium into the bowel lumen. Water follows the directional flux of chloride and sodium through highly permeable intercellular spaces. Several bacterial toxins and endogenous mediators (Table 12–8) can cause active secretion.

Passive secretion of protein-rich fluid into the lumen undoubtedly also occurs, secondary to damage to the mucosal epithelium and capillary endothelium and submucosal inflammation in the proximal small intestine. The clinically relevant events that result from the active and passive fluid secretion are proximal small intestinal distention and nasogastric reflux, dehydration, and circulatory shock.

Although an accelerated transmucosal fluid movement is the primary cause of the intestinal distention and nasogastric reflux in horses with DPJ, adynamic ileus of the small intestine is probably another contributing factor. Irritation and inflammation of the seromuscularis inhibits intestinal motility. It is reasonable to conclude, therefore, that adynamic ileus could result from the intramuscular hemorrhage and fibrinopurulent exudate on the serosa of the proximal small intestine of horses with DPJ.[5] Allen and Clark[5] postulated that changes in serosal microvascular hemodynamics and endothelial permeability that result from inflammation of the small intestinal serosa result in exudation of protein-rich fluid from the serosal capillaries and into the peritoneal fluid. The peritoneal fluid protein concentration increases as a result of the inflammatory processes affecting the visceral peritoneum. Capillary endothelial barriers become more permeable to protein and with continued microvascular damage and tissue inflammation, white blood cells begin to migrate through this vascular barrier. The leukotactic response to serositis may also contribute to the mild elevations in the peritoneal fluid nucleated cell count. Furthermore, horses severely affected with DPJ may have sufficient mural damage to allow toxins to enter the peritoneal cavity and elicit granulocyte invasion. As stated previously, however, the peritoneal fluid nucleated cell counts in horses with DPJ are highly variable and should be used in conjunction with other laboratory test and clinical findings in differentiating DPJ from small intestinal obstruction.

TREATMENT

Because the etiologic agent(s) for DPJ is unknown, treatment remains empirical and consists of aggressive supportive therapy. The continuous production of enterogastric reflux requires frequent gastric decompression (every 1–2 hours) to relieve pain and to prevent gastric rupture. Affected horses should receive nothing by mouth until small intestinal function has returned, recognized clinically by cessation or reduction of the nasogastric reflux concurrent with improved borborygmi. The duration of increased transmucosal fluid movement and intestinal ileus that result in gastrointestinal reflux varies with the severity of the intestinal lesion and usually is 3 to 7 days. Repeated rectal examinations after the first day of therapy may or may not reveal distended loops of small intestine, depending on the frequency of removal of the reflux and the severity of the initial lesion.

Intravenous administration of a balanced electrolyte solution is necessary to treat hypovolemia, electrolyte imbalances, and maintain renal filtration. Continuous administration of large volumes of fluid are usually required and in large horses this may necessitate administration of fluid via both jugular veins. Horses will typically require 50 to 100 L of intravenous fluid daily in the acute stages of the disorder. If long-term intravenous fluid therapy is required, attention should be paid to serum concentrations of ionized calcium and magnesium. Commercial balanced polyionic fluids do not provide sufficient calcium and magnesium for long-term administration, and supplementation often is required.

Ironically, the intravenous fluid therapy itself may accelerate the flux of fluid from the vasculature into the intestinal lumen because of a reduction in intravascular oncotic pressure and an increased capillary perfusion pressure. This can result in an increased volume of gastrointestinal reflux. However, one should not consider reducing the volume of intravenous fluid therapy because excessive fluid losses continue to occur. One should monitor plasma protein concentration, the overall hydration of the patient, and the volume of reflux, and then determine the rate of intravenous fluid administration. During the initial hours of therapy, even aggressive intravenous fluid administration will result in only moderate clinical improvement. The clinical response, as evidenced by improved hydration status, decreased nasogastric reflux, improved attitude, and improvement in values reflecting kidney function (decreased blood urea nitrogen and creatinine), will correlate with improvement of the intestinal damage.

Because horses with DPJ can go several days without eating and are often in a hypermetabolic state, parenteral nutritional support should be considered. Parenterally administered solutions containing glucose, balanced amino acid solutions, lipid emulsions, balanced electrolyte and trace minerals, and vitamins have been administered to adult horses with small intestinal ileus or colitis. Based on a small number of horses, this therapy has proved promising in terms of minimizing protein losses and decreasing the duration of illness. Providing for part of the horse's nutritional requirements (8,000–12,000 kcal/day) is possible with glucose–amino acid solutions, which are of moderate cost. It is reasonable to suppose that providing nutritional support to an anorectic, severely ill horse will facilitate the healing process and even shorten the duration of illness. Thus, the overall cost of providing nutritional supplementation, enteral or parenteral, to horses with DPJ may well be offset by quicker recovery and diminished requirements for other, expensive treatments.

Nonsteroidal anti-inflammatory agents should be used, albeit judiciously. A dosage of flunixin meglumine (Banamine, Schering Corp., Kenilworth, N.J.) of 0.25 to 0.50 mg/kg four times daily can be used to reduce the untoward effects of arachidonic acid metabolites, especially thromboxane.

Because *Clostridium* species are suspected as an etiologic agent, penicillin is usually administered. However, broad-spectrum antimicrobial coverage should be considered in horses with DPJ. An aminoglycoside (gentamicin, amikacin) or third-generation cephalosporin (ceftiofur [Naxcel], Upjohn Co., Kalamazoo, Mich.) can be added to the penicillin therapy.

Medical therapy is sufficient in most cases of DPJ, but in those cases that continue to produce copious enterogastric reflux, surgery should be considered as an option. Surgery may be elected to determine the extent of the lesions and intestinal dysfunction and to perform intestinal bypass so that enterogastric reflux is directed toward the cecum and colon, where the fluid can be reabsorbed. Allen and Clark[5] have described two approaches for surgical therapy in such cases. A standing right flank laparotomy with resection of the last rib has been used to approach the duodenum and cecal base. Using this approach, a small stoma can be made between the duodenum and cecum using a handsewn 1.0- to 1.5-cm side-to-side anastomosis. The stoma may act as a shunt to decompress the proximal small intestine and deliver the small intestinal fluid to the cecum for reabsorption. Following recovery, the stoma will likely close.

The preferred method described by Allen and Clark for evaluating and decompressing the small intestine in horses with DPJ is via a ventral midline celiotomy. Although potentially more stressful to the patient than a standing flank laparotomy, this approach permits a more complete evaluation of the gastrointestinal tract and facilitates development of a more physiologic intestinal shunt. Upon entrance into the abdominal cavity, dilated small intestine is immediately apparent. After the extent of the diseased intestine is determined, a segment of normal distal jejunum is laid side to side to the proximal diseased intestine in an isoperistaltic fashion, as far proximal on the affected bowel as possible without extending to bowel that cannot be removed from the abdominal cavity. A small 1.0- to 1.5-cm handsewn anastomosis can then be made between the two segments of intestine. This provides an adequate stoma for direct intestinal decompression while minimally compromising the digestive and absorptive capacity of the small intestine. Potential complications of this procedure include development of an intestinal incarceration through the loop that is formed and the development of small intestinal adhesions.

Complications of DPJ include peritonitis, adhesions of the proximal small intestine, and laminitis. Approximately 95% of horses with DPJ will survive the primary intestinal insult with appropriate management.[3] Death or functional losses from this disease are more commonly related to the secondary complications such as laminitis and intraabdominal adhesions.

Because laminitis is commonly encountered as a complication of DPJ, therapy directed toward prevention is routinely incorporated into the medical therapy. Unfortunately, no definitive preventive therapies have been universally effective, but there are treatments that clinicians have considered to be of help.

Nonsteroidal anti-inflammatory drugs are indicated, with flunixin meglumine preferred because of its effects on blocking synthesis of vasoconstrictive prostaglandins. Some clinicians have used sodium heparin 40 to 60 IU/kg SC two to three times daily.[6, 7] A concern with heparin is that it forms microaggregates of red blood cells that could exacerbate capillary stasis. Dimethyl sulfoxide (DMSO) administered IV at a wide range of dosages (20 mg/kg up to 1 g/kg) one to two times daily, diluted in isotonic electrolyte solution (10%–20% DMSO), has been used because it scavenges hydroxyl radicals that result from inflammatory processes and that can severely disrupt the integrity of cell walls and the interstitial matrix.[8] Acepromazine 10 to 20 mg/500 kg SC two to three times daily has been used for its possible vasodilating effects on the pedal vasculature. Pentoxyfylline, a pharmacologic relative of theophylline, has been used because it enhances the deformability of red blood cells and possibly preserves pedal capillary blood flow.

Routine foot care is indicated and where practical, horses should be stalled in deep wood shavings or in a sand stall to provide sole and frog support. Otherwise, the sole and frog area can be supported somewhat using gauze sponges or a roll of gauze held in place with an adhesive elastic bandage or frog pads.

Intraabdominal adhesions are infrequently encountered after DPJ, except in cases in which surgical manipulation of affected small intestine has occurred. Specific treatments to prevent abdominal adhesions are unavailable at the present time, but the supportive measures and therapies used in treating the initial disease process, including the complications of peritonitis and laminitis, may help to minimize the development of adhesions.[9] Broad-spectrum antimicrobial therapy, and possibly heparin therapy at 80 to 100 IU/kg SC two to three times daily may have a role in adhesion prevention.

CONCLUSION

A practitioner confronted with a horse that has exhibited abdominal discomfort, has rectally palpable small intestinal distention, and has greater than 2 L of gastric reflux should recommend referral of the horse to a facility that is capable of performing abdominal surgery. The chance that such a horse has an intestinal obstruction is too great to decide to treat it as if it may have DPJ. Indeed, it is not unusual for surgery to be performed on such horses, even though DPJ is considered, to rule out an obstruction. At present, the survival of horses with DPJ that undergo surgery is much greater than previously, and certainly greater than that of horses with small intestinal obstruction that do not have surgery! Thus, we have in a sense come full circle. With improvement in the quality and intensity of postoperative aftercare during the past decade, the survival rate of horses with DPJ that have surgery is much improved since the days when the disorder was first encountered.

REFERENCES

1. Blackwell RB, White NA: Duodenitis–proximal jejunitis in the horse. In *Proceedings of Equine Colic Research Symposium* 1982, p 106.
2. White NA, Tyler DE, Blackwell RB, et al: Hemorrhagic fibrinonecrotic duodenitis–proximal jejunitis in horses: 20 cases (1977–1984). *J Am Vet Med Assoc* 190:311–316, 1987.
3. Johnston JK, Morris DD: Comparison of duodenitis–proximal jejunitis and small intestinal obstruction in horses: 68 cases: (1977–1985). *J Am Vet Med Assoc* 191:849–854, 1987.
4. Morris DD, Johnston JK: Peritoneal fluid constituents in horse with colic due to small intestinal disease. In Moore JN, White NA, Becht JL, eds: *Proceedings of the Second Equine Colic Research Symposium.* Lawrenceville, NJ, Veterinary Learning Symposium, 1986, pp 197–199.
5. Allen D, Clark ES: Duodenitis-proximal jejunitis. In Smith BP, ed: *Large Animal Internal Medicine.* St Louis, Mosby–Year Book, 1989.
6. Moore JN, Allen D, Clark ES: The pathophysiology of colic. In Gordon BJ, Allen D, eds: *Colic Management in the Horse.* Lanexa, Veterinary Medicine, 1988.
7. Morris DD: Medical therapy of colic. In Gordon BJ, Allen D, eds: *Colic Management in the Horse.* Lanexa, Veterinary Medicine, 1988.
8. Doran R: Postoperative care and management of colic patients. In Gordon BJ, Allen D, eds: *Colic Management in the Horse.* Lanexa, KS, Veterinary Medicine, 1988.
9. Baxter GM: Surgical colic: Postoperative complications and treatment. In Gordon BJ, Allen D, eds: *Colic Management in the Horse.* Lanexa, Veterinary Medicine, 1988.

12.5

Diseases of the Small Intestine

Jonathan H. Foreman, DVM, MS, Dip ACVIM

PHYSIOLOGY OF DIGESTION AND ABSORPTION

Much of what is known about the physiology of digestion and absorption of feedstuffs in horses is borrowed or extrapolated from better scientific data in other species. It is logical, however, that the absorption of simple carbohydrates, amino acids and small peptides, and lipids should be essentially the same in most mammalian species. Horses are almost unique in that they are herbivores, not ruminants, even though they have an organ, the cecum, which provides many of the functions of the rumen in the animal species that chew the cud.

The small intestine is uniquely adapted for digestion and absorption. Morphologically, the mucosal surface has numerous folds, each of which contains villi with innumerable microvilli, all designed to maximize the absorptive surface area. These various levels of folding and infolding are not unlike those of the primary, secondary, and tertiary laminae which make up the sensitive and insensitive laminae within the horse's hoof. At the base of the villi are the intestinal crypts (crypts of Lieberkühn), where rapidly dividing mucosal cells give rise, by simple mitosis, to the epithelial cells on the outer surface of each villus.[1] New cells migrate up the villus and reach the tip within 3 to 6 days. As they migrate, they mature in function so that the majority of intestinal absorption is performed at the tips of the villi by mature epithelial cells, while the majority of secretory function is performed by the immature crypt cells. Diseases that cause a sloughing of small intestinal villi (e.g., viral enteritis) produce their malabsorptive effects by the loss of absorptive mucosal cells at the tips of the villi, as well as by the loss of considerable absorptive surface area.

Mastication combined with the action of gastric-origin digestive agents such as hydrochloric acid and pepsin (activated from pepsinogen by gastric HCl) causes a semidigested slurry to be presented to the duodenum through the pylorus. The consistency of the ingesta is primarily a function of the type of diet, in that the greater the amount of fiber ingested, the thicker the consistency of the ingesta. Immediately upon presentation to the upper small intestine, a number of secretions are added to the slurry via the pancreatic duct, the bile duct, and the epithelial cells to further enhance digestion. There are multiple digestive and absorptive processes going on in the small intestine at three interrelated levels at all times: (1) within the lumen of the intestine, (2) at the epithelial surface (brush border), and (3) intracellularly. The goal of the digestive process within the small intestine is the absorption of the single or bimolecular basic building blocks of proteins, carbohydrates (starch), and lipids.

Endocrine cells distributed throughout the stomach, small intestine, and pancreas are called the amine precursor uptake and decarboxylation (APUD) cells.[2] These cells are stimulated by chemical changes, such as alterations in luminal pH. In response to such chemical stimuli, APUD cells release small polypeptide hormones to stimulate local actions within the gastrointestinal tract. For example, presentation of acidic ingesta to the pyloric antrum stimulates the cholinergic-mediated release of gastrin, a small polypeptide responsible for numerous gastric and postgastric digestive effects.[2] Gastrin's effects include the stimulation of increased pancreatic enzyme secretion, the volume of which has been measured in 70-kg ponies to be as high as 10 mL/min,[3] a rate that is three to five times higher than that measured in dogs.[4]

Secretin is another small polypeptide released by the small intestine itself in response to acidic ingesta being presented to the duodenum.[2] Secretin stimulates the release of pancreatic bicarbonate and water, which are crucial to the neutral-

ization of acidic ingesta. This effect is less important in the horse than in other monogastric species, since the abundance of bicarbonate in equine saliva buffers the gastric pH to a range of 4.0 to 6.0 upon presentation to the duodenum.[5] Cholecystokinin-pancreozymin (CCK-PZ) is released by the duodenum upon presentation of fat and protein ingesta and stimulates the release of pancreatic digestive enzymes along with gastrin.[2] These enzymes include trypsinogen (activated to trypsin), chymotrypsinogen (activated to chymotrypsin), and carboxypeptidase A and B (activated by trypsin).

Pancreatic α-amylase is secreted in its active form, while pancreatic lipase seems to require some degree of activation from bile acids.[5] Secretion can also be stimulated by cholinergic nerve fibers, but the equine pancreas is unique in that only a limited amount of increased pancreatic enzyme secretion can be attributed to direct cholinergic stimulation (e.g., only about 5% of the level of the swine pancreas).[3, 5]

The regulation of the release of these local hormones is poorly studied in the horse and other domestic species. Negative feedback for most gastrointestinal peptides has not been well documented. Another small polypeptide hormone, vasoactive intestinal peptide (VIP), has been shown in the dog to have competitive inhibitory effects against secretin by competing for the same receptor sites.[6] The rates of salivary, gastric, pancreatic, small intestinal, and colonic secretions are also regulated by changes in concentrations of cyclic adenosine monophosphate (cAMP) and cyclic guanosine monophosphate (cGMP) within the enterocytes.[7, 8] Infectious diarrheal agents (e.g., enteropathogenic *Escherichia coli*) can cause enough inflammatory infiltrate to result in increased local levels of prostaglandins and leukotrienes. These eicosanoid mediators stimulate increased adenyl cyclase activity, resulting in increased intracellular concentrations of cAMP or cGMP. These mediators cause increased enterocyte secretion and a net fluid loss into the lumen of the intestine (secretory diarrhea).[7, 8]

Only soluble carbohydrates (starches) with α-glucose bonds are digested in the small intestine (i.e., not cellulose).[5] Pancreatic α-amylase enzymatically hydrolyzes these α-bonds in the small intestinal lumen. In monogastric species other than the horse, the vast volumes of pancreatic α-amylase cause complete digestion of starches by the time the ingesta reach the distal duodenum.[9] This process seems to take longer in the horse, owing in part to lower concentrations of pancreatic α-amylase.[5] The final luminal products of carbohydrate digestion are maltose (two glucose molecules bound together), maltotriose (three glucose molecules combined), and several glucose molecules combined into α-dextrins. Dietary lactose and sucrose are not affected by pancreatic α-amylase.

Further carbohydrate breakdown occurs in the brush border of the upper jejunum. Oligosaccharidases (α-dextrinase, maltase) hydrolyze the multiple glucose polymers into monosaccharide glucose molecules for active transport (adenosine triphosphate [ATP]–dependent) into the epithelial cells. Lactose and sucrose are enzymatically cleaved into their component monosaccharides (glucose, galactose, fructose), which are then actively transported across the epithelial cell membrane.[10] In the case of glucose and galactose, this transport requires the presence of sodium.[10] Some glucose is utilized in the transport of these monosaccharides into the cell. Lactase activity decreases in most species as individuals grow older[5] and become no longer solely dependent upon milk for their diet.

Protein digestion begins with gastric pepsin's hydrolytic action on ingested proteins. Pancreatic trypsinogen is activated to trypsin by the action of enterokinase in the mucosal brush border of the small intestine.[11] Trypsin then activates chymotrypsinogen and carboxypeptidase A and B, as well as additional trypsinogen. These enzymes cleave proteins into smaller-component oligopeptides and single amino acids. At the brush border, single amino acids (about 20% of ingested proteins) and di- and tripeptides (about 80%) are then absorbed across the epithelial cell membrane into the cytosol. This absorption is active in nature, requiring various different active transport systems located within the cell membrane.[11] As with glucose and galactose absorption, these processes also require the presence of Na^+.[11]

Once inside the cell, about 90% of the remaining di- and tripeptides that were not previously cleaved into single amino acids are completely hydrolyzed by intracellular peptidases.[5] Some amino acids are utilized by intestinal cells for production of intestinal proteins. The remainder are transported outside the cell for synthesis into proteins elsewhere in the body, particularly in the liver and muscle. A fraction of the absorbed amino acids and small peptides are deaminated within the intestinal mucosal cells and their carbon framework is utilized for energy production through the tricarboxylic acid (TCA) cycle.[11]

Owing to the predominantly low fat content of the typical equine diet, fat digestion is the least important component of digestion in the horse. However, several recent investigations have focused on the use of increased dietary fat (primarily in the form of oils added to the diet) for greater available energy and for glycogen-sparing effects in exercising horses.[12–14] Both pancreatic lipase and bile salts are needed for luminal lipolysis.[15] Most dietary fat is presented to the small intestine as small collections of triglycerides. Pancreatic lipase acts on these fat emulsions to cleave off one monoglyceride and two free fatty acids from each triglyceride molecule.[15] These individual components are made more water-soluble by the detergent action of bile acids, which bring the insoluble portions together into a polar multimolecular mass called a micelle.[16]

The epithelial membrane is typically lipid in constitution. A thin layer of water overlying the epithelium is the primary barrier to lipid absorption. This barrier is overcome by organizing the lipid molecules into the polar micelles which then passively diffuse through the polar water layer.[16] The lipid molecules then dissociate from the micelle and diffuse freely and passively through the lipid membrane into the cytosol of the epithelial cells.[16] Once inside the cells, the free fatty acids are recombined into triglycerides which are subsequently combined with proteins and phospholipids into lipoproteins and chylomicrons.[15] These fat-soluble aggregates are analogous to the micelle in that they facilitate passive transport of the absorbed lipid molecules through the opposite side of the mucosal cell membrane into the lymphatic system, in which they travel through the thoracic duct and then are deposited into the normal circulation.

Aqueous pores within the lipid epithelial lining of the villi allow for the absorption of other water-soluble solutes and water.[17] The pore radius is small (<200 Å) and diminishes as the tract progresses aborally.[17] Thus, the majority of the absorption of larger molecules, such as many orally administered medications, occurs in the upper small intestine. Absorption of drugs is also affected by the pH of the ingesta, which is approximately 6.5 in the duodenum and rises to 8.0 in the lower small intestine. The luminal pH in relation to the dissociation constant (pK_a) of the drug determines where, and to what extent, the drug is absorbed,[18] since most drugs are absorbed across the lipid cell membrane as electrically neutral lipid-soluble salts in their nondissociated form. Those drugs that have enterohepatic cycles also have their blood levels affected by the kinetics of small intestinal absorption, biliary excretion, and small intestinal reabsorption.

PATHOPHYSIOLOGY OF MALDIGESTION AND MALABSORPTION

Maldigestion syndromes are uncommon in the horse compared with other domestic species (e.g., dogs with pancreatic exocrine insufficiency). Lactose intolerance in suckling foals is due to a deficiency of small intestinal lactase,[19] the hydrolytic enzyme responsible for cleaving lactose into its absorbable monosaccharide components (glucose and galactose). Two forms of lactase have been identified in the equine brush border: neutral β-galactosidase (digestive) and acidic β-galactosidase (lysozomal).[20] Lactase activity in the horse is highest during the initial period of lactose ingestion as a neonate and drops to negligible levels by 3 years of age.[20]

Primary lactase deficiencies are rare in horses, but secondary or acquired lactase deficiencies are common in any enteritis that results in the loss of some or all of the crypt cells responsible for lactase secretion.[20] Any condition, such as viral enteritis, that results in sloughing of small intestinal epithelial cells will then result in some degree of lactase deficiency. An inability to digest lactose in the pediatric diet will then result in an osmotic diarrhea since the disaccharide lactose molecules are osmotically active particles, causing excessive amounts of water and electrolytes to remain within the small intestinal lumen.

Clinical signs of lactase deficiency are indistinguishable from those of the original disease (e.g., viral enteritis) which resulted in the loss of villous tips containing the lactase-secreting epithelial cells. Diarrhea, dehydration, acidosis, and hypoglycemia are all interrelated problems in these foals. A presumptive diagnosis may be made in a suckling foal with a prolonged course of diarrhea, especially one in which the foal initially seemed to recover but then relapsed. Definitive diagnosis can be made with an oral lactose tolerance test performed by administering 1 g/kg of a 20% lactose solution via nasogastric tube after a minimum 4-hour fast.[21] Blood glucose levels should peak within 60 to 90 minutes of lactose administration in normal foals, with peak levels reaching a level of at least 35 mg/dL over baseline values.[21]

Oral administration of fluids or glucose may not be helpful and may actually be dangerous since such therapies may not be absorbed well and may, in fact, contribute to the osmotic diarrhea. Dietary rest, particularly in the form of withholding the mare's milk, is often corrective. Separating the mare and foal but continuing to milk the mare by hand is indicated. Muzzling the foal will prevent it from nursing but, in its frustration to nurse, the foal may aggravate the mare by continually bumping its head into her udder to stimulate milk letdown. Continued lactose intolerance may require early weaning or dietary supplementation with a soy-based, non-lactose-containing milk replacer.[20]

Pancreatic exocrine insufficiencies are common causes of maldigestion in other species but are very rare in the horse. A limited number of cases were reviewed by Carlson[22] and were reported to be ponies (n = 2) and draft horses (n = 5). Presenting complaints usually centered on chronic weight loss and intermittent colic. Horses progressively deteriorated, but the definitive diagnosis of chronic pancreatic necrosis was made only at necropsy. The two ponies had clinicopathologic evidence of secondary diabetes mellitus. While little to no laboratory analysis was performed in these cases, their rarity underscores the reasoning behind the infrequent use of serum and peritoneal fluid amylase and lipase determinations as a matter of routine in biochemical panels or profiles in the horse. (Normal values are shown in Table 12–9.) Acute pancreatitis is also rare in the horse and, when seen, presents as an acute gastritis with voluminous reflux and uncontrollable abdominal pain.[23] Definitive diagnosis is made at necropsy, and little in the way of antemortem therapy can be offered in the event a diagnosis is made via documentation of elevated serum amylase or lipase levels.

Diseases of malabsorption are much more common in the horse than are diseases of maldigestion. Any abnormality of the normal absorptive mechanisms in the small intestine will contribute to a malabsorption syndrome. Horses suffering from malabsorption routinely present with client complaints of chronic weight loss, depression, and lethargy, sometimes despite aggressive appetites. Diarrhea is a common component in such presentations, but a horse need not have diarrhea in order to have a malabsorptive problem.

Insufficient absorptive surface area is clearly a cause of malabsorption in horses. After extensive small intestinal resection due to severe strangulation-obstruction, horses may have trouble gaining and maintaining body weight and condition.[24, 25] The greater the amount of small intestine resected, the more likely a malabsorption problem. Small sections of resected bowel will have no untoward long-term effects, but extensive resections may result in the horse becoming a "digestive cripple." Such horses may benefit

from being fed highly digestible feeds. Feeds with high-quality fiber content may also contribute to body weight gain in that they may be more extensively converted from cellulose to volatile free fatty acids in the cecum.[25] Feeding more frequent meals in smaller amounts may also aid in better digestion and absorption.

Another example of malabsorption is the horse with chronic weight loss after a bout of viral enteritis. With sufficient sloughing of villous tips, the absorptive surface area may be compromised and the horse may simply not have enough epithelial cells to absorb normal amounts of nutrients from the intestinal lumen. In foals, this may also result in lactase deficiency if the villous sloughing goes deeply enough into the intestinal crypts to affect secretory cells responsible for lactase production.[20] In either event, little can be done until the intestinal epithelium recovers sufficiently to produce new villous cells with sufficient maturity to absorb normally. This maturation and healing process may take weeks, or even months in severe cases.

Infiltration of the small intestinal wall by inflammatory cells can also contribute to malabsorption. Such infiltrates may occur with simple viral enteritis, or may occur with more permanent consequences in horses with noninfectious inflammatory bowel disease. Such noninfectious diseases have been variously classified as *granulomatous enteritis*[26, 27] or *eosinophilic gastroenteritis*[28, 29] (or enterocolitis),[30] depending upon the predominant cellular infiltrate. Villous atrophy is common[26] and contributes to malabsorption due to loss of absorptive surface area and loss of absorptive epithelial cells at the tips of the villi. Inflammation of the intestinal wall may cause enlargement of the junctional pores between mucosal cells. These pores are normally responsible for absorption of larger molecules, but when enlarged, may actually contribute to a net loss of fluid and protein into the lumen. Mucosal ulcerations caused by inflammatory infiltrates[26] may also cause fluid and protein transudation into the lumen.

The cause of granulomatous enteritis remains unproven. Uncontrolled immunologic reactions (delayed hypersensitivity) to various dietary or infectious antigens have been proposed.[27] Standardbreds have been reported to be overrepresented,[27] but no case-control epidemiologic studies have been undertaken to prove this apparent breed predisposition. The pathologic lesions resemble those of Johne's disease in cattle and sheep and Crohn's disease in humans.[26, 27] Both the small and large intestines are usually involved, as are mesenteric lymph nodes.[26] Histologically, the lamina propria is infiltrated by mononuclear cells (lymphocytes, macrophages, epithelioid cells, plasma cells, and rare multinucleated giant cells).[26] The ileum is most affected while the large colon is least affected.[26] Severe villous atrophy of the small intestine is commonly observed. Eosinophilic dermatitis has also been reported in subjects with eosinophilic gastrointestinal infiltrates.[29, 30] Therapy is unproven and generally ineffective, although cases with eosinophilic infiltrates have been reported to be inconsistently corticosteroid-responsive.[30] The prognosis, however, remains guarded to poor, since the necessity for steroid therapy may continue throughout the horse's life.

Enteric neoplasms may also cause chronic weight loss[31] and malabsorption.[32] Neoplastic infiltration of bowel wall interferes with normal cellular absorptive mechanisms.[32]

Table 12–9. Normal Serum and Peritoneal Fluid Values Determined in Fifteen Thoroughbred and Two Arabian Horses (N = 17)*

	Serum	Peritoneal Fluid
Glucose (mmol/L)	4.0–5.6	4.9–6.4
Lactate (mmol/L)	0.7–1.7	0.4–1.2
Amylase (units/L)	14–35	0.0–14
Lipase (units/L)	23–87	0.0–36
γ-Glutamyltransferase (units/L)	9–29	0.0–6.0

*Modified from Parry BW, Crisman MV: Serum and peritoneal fluid amylase and lipase reference values in horses. *Equine Vet J* 23:390–391, 1991.

Neoplasms may also cause obstruction of normal mural lymphatics, resulting in lymphangiectasia, transudative fluid loss into the bowel lumen (resulting in diarrhea), and failure to transport chylomicrons and lipoproteins into the normal circulation. Mucosal neoplastic lesions may also manifest as ulcers, which exacerbate luminal fluid and protein losses. Such ulcers may even result in bleeding into the lumen.[33] Luminal bleeding results in a blood loss anemia in addition to the typical anemia of chronic inflammation or neoplasia caused by the tumor. The most common intestinal mural neoplasm resulting in chronic weight loss in the horse is lymphosarcoma.[32, 33] Other reported equine abdominal tumors resulting in weight loss rarely involve the small intestine (e.g., squamous cell carcinoma,[34] adenocarcinoma[35]). Leiomyoma and leiomyosarcoma are most commonly reported in horses in the small intestine, but are usually presented for chronic or intermittent to acute colic pain, not weight loss.[36–38]

Infectious granulomatous enterocolitis has been rarely reported in horses associated with enteric tuberculosis[27, 39] or paratuberculosis.[40] There are also rare reports of enteric fungal infections due to *Aspergillus fumigatus*[41, 42] or *Histoplasma capsulatum*.[41–43] It has been stated that these fungal infections are manifested in horses undergoing chronic antibiotic[41, 42] or corticosteroid therapy.[42] This sterilizing of the gut and chronic immunosuppression with steroids is thought to promote the growth of enteric fungal infections. In reality, enteric manifestations of fungal infections are probably only one of several sites affected in horses with systemic fungal infections,[42] particularly in the arid southwestern portion of the United States. Therapy is with systemic antifungals (amphotericin B, miconazole) and is generally unrewarding.

Parasitism may be the only treatable cause of intestinal malabsorption in the adult horse (i.e., excluding lactase deficiencies in suckling foals). While chronic gastrointestinal parasitism is usually associated primarily with its large colon effects, a complete and simple separation of small intestinal and large intestinal effects is difficult. Horses with profound large colon burdens of parasites may have sufficient small intestinal burdens to result in malabsorptive disorders. Diagnosis via glucose or xylose tolerance testing followed by larvacidal dewormings with ivermectin or high-dose benzimidazoles may be corrective.

Diagnosis

Diagnosis of malabsorption in the horse is made by performing a glucose[44] or xylose[45–47] absorption test. Xylose, a 5-carbon molecule, is the preferred test compound since glucose is a naturally occurring 6-carbon molecule that is subject to metabolism by the subject during the test, thus clouding interpretation of the peak values obtained. D-Xylose 0.5 g/kg in a 10% solution is administered via nasogastric tube in a horse which has been fasted overnight. Heparinized venous blood samples are taken before administration of the xylose and at 30-minute intervals afterward for up to 2½ to 3½ hours. Most reports of D-xylose responses in normal horses document peaks of plasma xylose at 60 to 90 minutes after administration[45–47] (Fig. 12–11). Peak values vary between reports and between laboratories, but most investiga-

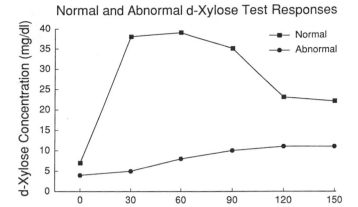

Normal and Abnormal d-Xylose Test Responses

Figure 12–11. Normal D-xylose test response from a male yearling mule with chronic weight loss due to chronic diarrhea. This mule had large colon abnormalities at postmortem, but a normal small intestine. Abnormal D-xylose response from a male yearling standardbred with chronic weight loss. This standardbred had lymphohistiocytic (granulomatous) enteritis, with a normal large colon, confirmed at postmortem. Both yearlings received 0.5 g/kg D-xylose in a 10% solution via nasogastric tube, after a 12-hour fast, at time 0 on the curves.

tors agree that the curve should be bell-shaped after administration and that a definitive peak should be achieved. Peak absolute plasma values reported are routinely 15 mg/dL greater than baseline values in normal horses.[45–47] Xylose or glucose absorption can be increased in younger horses[47] and by feeding high carbohydrate diets,[45] and can be decreased by delayed gastric emptying and enteritis. It must be remembered that an abnormal xylose or glucose absorption test proves only an inability to absorb simple sugars; it is presumed that the documented abnormality of monosaccharide malabsorption is reflective of a larger inability to absorb the primary constituents of proteins and lipids.

Protein-Losing Enteropathy

Many horses with maldigestive or malabsorptive conditions develop hypoproteinemia. This condition is due to a failure to absorb sufficient dietary protein, often combined with a protein-losing enteropathy. Enteric protein loss can be due to a number of mechanisms, including mucosal ulcers, mural inflammatory cell infiltrates, and lymphangiectasia. Sufficiently low serum protein levels (<4 g/dL), especially if due to low albumin concentrations (<2 g/dL), cause a decrease in the colloid osmotic pressure of the plasma. The end result is the development of increased interstitial fluid manifested as pitting peripheral edema of the distal limbs, ventral midline, pectoral region, and prepuce.

Diagnosis of protein-losing enteropathy is difficult in most clinical situations, and thus is also usually presumptive. The definitive diagnosis is made by administering radioactively labeled albumin parenterally and observing the feces for subsequent increased levels of radioactivity. Since this method is generally impractical, a presumptive diagnosis is usually based upon clinical presentation, dietary history, and by ruling out other mechanisms for development of hypoproteinemia. Malabsorption, hepatic failure to produce circulating proteins, and other routes of excessive protein loss, including renal, abdominal, and thoracic, must be investigated. Protein-losing enteropathy can, however, occur in the presence or in the absence of a malabsorptive disorder (i.e., neither excludes the other).

PATHOPHYSIOLOGY OF DIARRHEA

Most investigators agree that, for diarrhea to develop in the adult horse, the large colon must be primarily involved.[48] An extensive review of the pathogenesis of large colon diarrhea is presented in Chapter 12.10. However, viral and protozoal (coccidial) enteritis are diarrheal conditions unique to the small intestine, particularly in younger foals.

Viral Enteritis

Viral intestinal infections produce their effects by invading epithelial cells lining intestinal villi, causing epithelial cell death, sloughing, and blunting of villi. Maldigestion results from loss of the normal small intestinal brush border enzymes. Malabsorption also results from the loss of villous tip enterocytes as well as from the loss of considerable absorptive surface area. With failure of normal digestion and absorption, there are increased numbers of osmotic particles within the lumen of the intestine, resulting in a net flow of fluid and electrolytes out of the small intestine rather than being absorbed. As immature crypt cells divide and migrate out onto the blunted villous tips, they may actually contribute to a worsening of the diarrhea by adding a secretory component not previously present.

Rotavirus infection is the most commonly implicated virus in young foals with profuse watery diarrhea at approximately 1 to 4 weeks of age.[49, 50] Coronavirus and adenovirus (in Arabian foals with severe combined immunodeficiency) have also been implicated.[50] Affected foals are often febrile, but leukocyte shifts may be more reflective of secondary bacterial flora changes than of simple viral infection. Foal heat diarrhea must be considered as a differential diagnosis, but rotavirus foals are often somewhat older than the typical foal heat diarrhea age of 4 to 10 days old.

Rotavirus is a common environmental pathogen on many breeding farms.[51] If found on electron microscopic or commercial ELISA (enzyme-linked immunosorbent assay) examination of diarrheal feces from an affected foal, rotavirus should be considered as the likely pathogen. Outbreaks involving several foals on a given farm are common, frustrating, and time-consuming for the practitioner. Therapy is directed at volume replacement and maintenance, balancing the electrolyte and acid-base status, and controlling abdominal pain, if present. Broad-spectrum antibiotics are indicated if secondary bacterial sepsis is of concern. Plasma from donors hyperimmunized against equine rotavirus is commercially available.

Most foals recover in a few days if the diarrhea remains uncomplicated. The development of secondary bacterial sepsis is a poor prognostic sign. Development of severe villous atrophy and blunting may result in longer-term soft-to-diarrheal stools until the villi regenerate and develop full absorptive capabilities again. Prevention should be directed at good hygiene between foaling mares and between affected foals and other horses. New arrivals should be isolated for 2 to 4 weeks whenever practical. Stalls that have housed a rotavirus-positive foal should be disinfected with phenolic compounds,[51] since rotavirus is resistant to killing by the more commonly used chlorine bleach disinfectants. A vaccine to be used in pregnant mares is being investigated and is currently available under limited licensure (Fort Dodge, Iowa).

Protozoal Enteritis

Oocysts of the coccidium *Eimeria leukarti* have been identified in the feces of numerous normal horses as well as in those of horses with chronic diarrhea.[52] The pathogenicity of *Eimeria* in horses is unclear, but is thought to be low. Clinical enteritis has been associated with its presence, but the feces in such cases are not hemorrhagic as in the coccidial infections of other domestic species.[53] If pathogenic, its effect in causing diarrhea is probably related to its local intracellular invasion of enterocytes, resulting in cell death, villous sloughing, and maldigestion and malabsorption. It may also stimulate increased enteric secretion, thus contributing to the diarrhea. However, most investigators agree that it is usually not pathogenic.

Diagnosis is difficult, since simple fecal flotation may not sufficiently concentrate the oocysts to allow visualization in large numbers. Use of a saturated sodium nitrate solution has been suggested.[53] However, in most cases, definitive diagnosis is based on visualization of the affected segment of small intestine and the microscopic examination of biopsies of these areas. The exact life cycle is unknown, making control of transmission difficult.[53] Treatment with oral sulfa antibiotics may be indicated, as in other coccidial diseases, if *Eimeria* infection were suspected as the cause of diarrhea in a group of horses.

Cryptosporidium species have conventionally been thought to be pathogenic only in immunosuppressed foals (i.e., Arabian foals with severe combined immunodeficiency).[54] Recent data, however, suggest that these coccidia may be pathogenic in immunocompetent foals as well as calves.[55, 56] Unlike other coccidia, *Cryptosporidium* species attach to the epithelial surface at the brush border rather than entering the cytoplasm of enterocytes. No intermediate host is required for infectivity or transmission, which is by the fecal-oral route. The incubation period is 3 to 7 days, with signs of diarrhea lasting for 5 to 16 days. Clinically apparent infection is more common in experimental foals separated from their dams and hand-reared within the first 30 days of life.[56] These data implicate dietary changes and stress as contributory factors, and raise concern about the susceptibility of hand-reared orphaned foals to *Cryptosporidium* infections.[56]

Diagnosis is by detection of fecal oocysts. This technique is frustrating because of difficulties in identifying the smaller cryptosporidial oocysts (4–6 μm) and in concentrating them in sufficient numbers for identification. Dimethyl sulfoxide–modified, acid-fast stain has been reported to be useful in aiding in oocyst identification.[56, 57] Auramine O fluorochrome dye has also been used to stain direct fecal smears.[58] Postmortem diagnosis is based upon identification of routinely stained fresh enteric tissue.

Most affected foals recover with only moderate to intensive supportive care including intravenous fluids and electrolytes.[56] No specific coccidiostats have been shown to be efficacious in treating equine cryptosporidiosis. Prevention should be aimed at better hygiene, including minimizing contact between younger suckling or orphaned foals and other species more commonly infected with *Cryptosporidium* (e.g., calves). Like other coccidia, these oocysts are resistant to disinfectants and are rendered noninfective only by 10% formalin, 5% ammonia,[59] and sodium hypochlorite (common chlorine bleach).[56] It must be emphasized that *Cryptosporidium* species are not species-specific and that there is always a possibility for zoonotic transmission to the client and veterinarian.

MEDICAL COLIC OF SMALL INTESTINAL ORIGIN
Spasmodic Colic

Spasmodic colic is probably the most common cause of abdominal pain in the horse. It is thought to occur from spasms or abnormal and uncontrolled contractions of the muscular portion of the intestinal wall. These dysfunctional contractions do not contribute to aboral movement of ingesta through the intestinal tract, but still result in considerable pain to the horse due to the stimulation of mural stretch receptors. Numerous causes have been proposed, but none have been proved.[60] This lack of etiologic knowledge of the condition is due to the transient nature of the abdominal pain, resulting in an inability to reproduce the condition routinely for accurate experimental study. Proposed mechanisms include verminous migration through the bowel wall or vessels; moldy feed or excessive grain or insufficient fiber resulting in excessive gas production and subsequent bowel wall distention; and other environmental influences such as the natural excitability of an individual horse and excitement or fatigue due to exercise.

Horses with spasmodic colic often have acute bouts of pain which resolve with minimal or no therapy. They are probably the most usual cause of the "false-alarm" colics common in typical field practice, in which the horse's colic pain is often resolved by the time the practitioner arrives at the farm. After an initial bout of pain and a period of quiescence, the pain may recur without warning. Auscultation is often the key to diagnosis since one or more of the various quadrants will yield increased or hypermotile bowel sounds which may even be so loud as to be audible to the practitioner without a stethoscope. Rectal examination, nasogastric intubation, and abdominocentesis are routinely normal.

Many horses respond to no treatment. However, if still painful upon presentation, some form of analgesic relief should be provided. This condition may be the one good indication for the use of dipyrone, which is labeled as an antispasmodic agent. Xylazine, detomidine, and nonsteroidal anti-inflammatories (flunixin meglumine, phenylbutazone) are also often used. The additional analgesia provided by narcotics (morphine, meperidine) and narcotic-like agents (butorphanol) are not usually necessary to control the pain

of horses with spasmodic colic. Oral therapies (mineral oil, or surface-acting agents such as docusate sodium) are often administered since the practitioner cannot be certain that the horse does not have a cranial impaction that is beyond the reach of rectal palpation.[61] The prognosis for recovery is good provided there is no subsequent or associated malpositioning of the bowel resulting in a more severe strangulating displacement or obstruction.

Ileal Hypertrophy

Muscular hypertrophy of the ileum is an uncommon cause of ileal impaction and obstruction.[62–64] The cause is unknown. Proposed mechanisms include primary lesions caused by chronically deranged parasympathetic nervous dysfunction resulting in chronically increased muscle tone and subsequent hypertrophy of the muscular layers of the ileal wall. Another proposed pathogenesis is that neurogenically induced chronic hypertonicity of the ileocecal valve leads to chronic ileal muscular hypertonicity, which leads to muscular hypertrophy. Secondary causes may include verminous migration.[62]

Clinical signs are generally those of mild colic, but may be more severe if a moderate-to-severe ileal impaction results from the decreased diameter of the intestinal lumen. Therapy is aimed at control of abdominal pain with xylazine, detomidine, or nonsteroidal anti-inflammatories such as flunixin meglumine or phenylbutazone. Severe presentations require surgery. Exploratory laparotomy allows definitive diagnosis and corrective ileal resection, ileocecal bypass, or ileal myotomy.

Ileal Impaction and Obstruction

Ileal impaction resulting in ileal obstruction is a poorly understood phenomenon seen more commonly in the southeastern part of the United States.[65, 66] Embertson et al.[55] proposed that the common local management practice of feeding Bermuda grass hay resulted in more frequent cases of ileal impaction in Florida.[65] Nonstrangulating infarction of the ileum has also been proposed as a mechanism for deranged motility resulting in ileal impaction.

Clinical findings are those of a simple small intestinal obstruction without displacement or strangulation. Mild-to-moderate pain, gradually worsening gastric reflux, and normal abdominal fluid are common findings. When reflux becomes more apparent, mild-to-moderate small intestinal distention will also become more apparent rectally. Abdominal fluid white blood cell counts and total protein levels will increase as the degree of small intestinal distention increases.

In the early stages of the disease, mild pain may be responsive to analgesic therapy such as xylazine or nonsteroidal anti-inflammatories. In the later stages, however, horses may present with severe pain, which is uncontrollable with conventional analgesic therapy. Such cases present as surgical candidates, with uncontrollable pain, reflux, rectally palpable small intestinal distention, and moderately abnormal abdominal fluid. Surgical correction should include ileal resection and subsequent jejunocecostomy if there is any degree of ileal muscular hypertrophy at all.[66] Cases in which simple surgical massage of the impaction results in initial relief are often presented again at a later date for a recurrence of the problem, resulting eventually in a second surgery and ileal resection.

The prognosis for an early and easily massaged impaction should be fair, but the prognosis for horses with recurring ileal impactions is poor without ileal resection. Ileal resection was originally thought to cause a loss of some intestinal functions, particularly the absorption of vitamin B_{12} and bile acids, and the transmural exchange of bicarbonate and chloride.[5] The cell membrane–bound carriers for facilitating absorption of these compounds are generally located only in the ileum.[17] This concern has subsequently been abandoned owing to the overwhelming empirical clinical data which indicate that horses surviving ileal resection do not have problems gaining weight or performing up to expectations following recovery from surgery. It is now believed that the cecum and large intestine probably acquire the ability to absorb those compounds originally thought to be restricted solely to the ileum.

Nonstrangulating Infarction (Thromboembolic Colic)

Nonstrangulating infarction of the small intestine, cecum, or large intestine has been associated with verminous arteritis caused by the vascular migratory stages of *Strongylus vulgaris*.[67] It has traditionally been termed *thromboembolic colic*. Conventionally, it was taught that the verminous arteritis lesions within the aorta and cranial mesenteric artery give rise to emboli which lodge downstream and obstruct the blood supply to a portion of the intestinal tract. This traditional mechanism is, however, inaccurate, in that emboli have not been demonstrated in most horses with gross postmortem lesions characteristic of nonstrangulating infarction.[67]

Other proposed mechanisms include the release of vasoactive mediators from the thrombi into the artery, resulting in vasospasm and subsequent infarction downstream from the cranial mesenteric thrombus.[68] The irritation of vessel walls caused by larval migration may result in endothelial activation resulting in platelet aggregation, thrombus formation, and production of thromboxane, a potent vasoconstrictive eicosanoid related to prostaglandin. The thrombus itself may cause obstruction and subsequent low flow problems resulting in more gradual intestinal infarction. Strongyle larvae, through their traditional migratory patterns, may affect the blood supply in smaller vessels. Some thrombi are large enough to occlude the cranial mesenteric artery without the actual embolization process.

This disease has been made infrequent or even rare with the widespread use of ivermectin. This first-generation derivative of the avermectin family was the first commercially available dewormer to kill the offending migratory stages of *S. vulgaris*.[69] This unique characteristic has resulted in a phenomenal decrease in the frequency of cranial mesenteric thrombi once seen routinely at necropsy, a sign of the efficacy of the compound. As a result of fewer thrombi in all horses, there has been a concomitant decline in the frequency of clinically apparent nonstrangulating intestinal infarction.

Affected horses present with significant pain, which may not be controllable with conventional analgesic therapy. Serosanguinous abdominal fluid is common in such cases because of the infarction of the bowel wall. Free or phagocytosed bacteria may be evident later in the disease process as the bowel wall becomes thinner and more fragile. Small intestinal distention may be rectally palpable, but is not usually as severe as in small intestinal displacement and strangulation. If the small intestinal tract is affected for long, reflux via a nasogastric tube will be obtained as part of the routine examination.

The presence of uncontrollable pain, serosanguinous abdominal fluid, rectally palpable small intestinal distention, or gastric reflux often leads to the conclusion that the horse has a surgical lesion. Upon exploratory laparotomy, however, the nonstrangulating infarct-like nature of the condition is readily apparent. Intestinal resection is usually impractical given the amount of bowel involved. With or without exploration, therapy is aimed at controlling the patient's pain and impending peritonitis. Broad-spectrum antibiotics such as penicillin combined with an aminoglycoside (gentamicin or amikacin) are frequently used. Nonsteroidal anti-inflammatories are used for their analgesic and anti-endotoxic effects.[70] Anticoagulant therapy such as heparin is sometimes used for the infarct-like nature of the condition as well as for its anti-endotoxic effects.[71] Supportive care, such as large-volume fluid replacement, is a mainstay of therapy and may be the most important reason for the timely referral of such cases, since large-volume fluid administration is often impractical for the field practitioner. The prognosis for any nonstrangulating infarction must remain guarded, especially if the amount of bowel involved is large or if peritonitis develops.

REFERENCES

1. Banks WJ: *Applied Veterinary Histology*, ed 2. Baltimore, Williams & Wilkins, 1986, p 409.
2. Makhlouf GM: The neuroendocrine design of the gut. *Gastroenterology* 67:159, 1974.
3. Alexander F, Hickson JCD: The salivary and pancreatic secretions of the horse. In Phillipson AT, ed: *Physiology of Digestion and Metabolism in the Ruminant*. Newcastle upon Tyne, England, Oriel, 1970, p 375.
4. Jankowitz HD: Pancreatic secretion of fluid and electrolytes. In *Handbook of Physiology: Alimentary Canal*. Washington, DC, American Physiology Society, 1968, p 925.
5. Argenzio RA: Comparative physiology of the gastrointestinal system. In Anderson NV, ed: *Veterinary Gastroenterology*. Philadelphia, Lea & Febiger, 1980, p 172.
6. Konteruk SJ, Thor P, Dembinski A, et al: Comparison of secretin and vasoactive intestinal peptide on pancreatic secretion in dogs. *Gastroenterology* 68:1527, 1975.
7. Kimberg DV: Cyclic nucleotides and their role in gastrointestinal secretion. *Gastroenterology* 67:1023, 1974.
8. O'Loughlin EV, Scott RB, Gall DG: Pathophysiology of infectious diarrhea: Changes in intestinal structure and function. *J Pediatr Gastroenterol Nutr* 12:5, 1991.
9. Gray GM: Mechanisms of digestion and absorption of foods. In Sleisenger MH, Fordtran JS, eds: *Gastrointestinal Disease*. Philadelphia, WB Saunders, 1973, p 250.
10. Nervi FO: Normal mechanisms of carbohydrate absorption. In Dietschy JM, ed: *Disorders of the Gastrointestinal Tract: Disorders of the Liver: Nutritional Disorders*. New York, Grune & Stratton, 1976, p 35.
11. Nervi FO: Normal mechanisms of protein absorption. In

Dietschy JM, ed: *Disorders of the Gastrointestinal Tract: Disorders of the Liver: Nutritional Disorders.* New York, Grune & Stratton, 1976, p 36.

12. Hintz HF, Ross MW, Lesser FR, et al: The value of dietary fat for working horses. *J Equine Med Surg* 2:483, 1978.

13. Hambleton PL, Slade LM, Hamar DW, et al: Dietary fat and exercise conditioning effect on metabolic parameters in the horse. *J Anim Sci* 51:1330, 1980.

14. Pagan JD, Essen-Gustavsson B, Lindholm A, et al: The effect of dietary energy source on exercise performance in Standardbred horses. In Gillespie JR, Robinson NE, eds: *Equine Exercise Physiology,* vol 2. Davis, Calif, SpICCEP, 1987, p 686.

15. Johnston JM: Mechanisms of fat absorption. In *Handbook of Physiology: Alimentary Canal.* Washington, DC, American Physiology Society, 1968, p 1323.

16. Westergaard H: Normal mechanisms of lipid absorption. In Dietschy JM, ed: *Disorders of the Gastrointestinal Tract: Disorders of the Liver: Nutritional Disorders.* New York, Grune & Stratton, 1976, p 38.

17. Fordtran JS: Diarrhea. In Sleisenger MH, Fordtran JS, eds: *Gastrointestinal Disease.* Philadelphia, WB Saunders, 1973, p 291.

18. Curran PF, Schultz SG: Transport across membranes: General principles. In *Handbook of Physiology: Alimentary Canal.* Washington, DC, American Physiology Society, 1968, p 1217.

19. Martens RJ, Scrutchfield WL: Foal diarrhea: Pathogenesis, etiology and therapy. *Compendium Continuing Educ Pract Vet* 4:S175, 1982.

20. Roberts MC, Kidder FD, Hill FW: Small intestinal beta-galactosidase activity in the horse. *Gut* 14:535, 1973.

21. Martens RJ, Malone PS, Brust DM: Oral lactose tolerance test in foals: Technique and normal values. *Am J Vet Res* 46:2163, 1986.

22. Carlson GP: The exocrine pancreas. In Mansmann RA, McAllister ES, Pratt PW, eds: *Equine Medicine and Surgery,* ed 3. Santa Barbara, Calif, American Veterinary, 1982, p 643.

23. Lilley CW, Beeman GM: Gastric dilatation associated with acute necrotizing pancreatitis. *Equine Pract* 3:8, 1981.

24. Tate LP, Ralston SL, Kock CM, et al: Effects of extensive resection of the small intestine in the pony. *Am J Vet Res* 44:1187, 1983.

25. Sojka JE: Malabsorption. In Colahan PT, Mayhew IG, Merrit AM, et al, eds: *Equine Medicine and Surgery,* ed 4. Goleta, Calif, American Veterinary, 1991, p 607.

26. Cimprich RE: Equine granulomatous enteritis. *Vet Pathol* 11:535, 1974.

27. Merrit AM, Cimprich RE, Beech J: Granulomatous enteritis in nine horses. *J Am Vet Med Assoc* 169:603, 1976.

28. Pass DA, Bolton JR: Chronic eosinophilic gastroenteritis in the horse. *Vet Pathol* 19:486, 1982.

29. Nimmo Wilke JS, Yager JA, Nation PN, et al: Chronic eosinophilic dermatitis: A manifestation of a multisystemic, eosinophilic, epitheliotropic disease in five horses. *Vet Pathol* 22:297, 1985.

30. Gibson KT, Alders RC: Eosinophilic enterocolitis and dermatitis in two horses. *Equine Vet J* 19:247, 1987.

31. Traub JL, Bayly WM, Reed SM, et al: Intraabdominal neoplasia as a cause of chronic weight loss in the horse. *Compendium Continuing Educ Pract Vet* 5:S526, 1983.

32. Roberts MC, Pinsent PJN: Malabsorption in the horse associated with alimentary lymphosarcoma. *Equine Vet J* 7:166, 1975.

33. Platt H: Alimentary lymphomas in the horse. *J Comp Pathol* 97:1, 1987.

34. Sendberg JP, Bunstein T, Page EH, et al: Neoplasms of equidae. *J Am Vet Med Assoc* 170:150, 1977.

35. Honnas CM, Snyder JR, Olander HJ, Wheat JD: Small intestinal adenocarcinoma in a horse. *J Am Vet Med Assoc* 191:845, 1987.

36. Collier MA, Trent AM: Jejunal intussusception associated with leiomyoma in an aged horse. *J Am Vet Med Assoc* 182:810, 1982.

37. Hanes GE, Robertson JT: Leiomyoma of the small intestine in a horse. *J Am Vet Med Assoc* 182:1398, 1983.

38. Livesey MA, Hulland TJ, Yovich JV: Colic in two horses associated with smooth muscle intestinal tumors. *Equine Vet J* 18:334, 1986.

39. Platt H: Chronic inflammatory and lymphoproliferative lesions of the equine small intestine. *J Comp Pathol* 96:671, 1986.

40. Larsen AB, Moon HW, Merkal RS: Susceptibility of horses to *Mycobacterium paratuberculosis. Am J Vet Res* 33:2185, 1972.

41. Kohn CW: Acute diarrhea. In Mansmann RA, McAllister ES, Pratt PW, eds: *Equine Medicine and Surgery,* ed 3. Santa Barbara, Calif, American Veterinary, 1982, p 528.

42. McCullough C: Mycotic diseases. In Robinson NE, ed: *Current Therapy in Equine Medicine,* vol 1. Philadelphia, WB Saunders, 1983, p 32.

43. Goetz TE, Coffman JR: Ulcerative colitis and protein losing enteropathy associated with intestinal salmonellosis and histoplasmosis in a horse. *Equine Vet J* 16:439, 1984.

44. Roberts MC, Hill FWG: The oral glucose tolerance test in the horse. *Equine Vet J* 5:171, 1973.

45. Bolton JR, Merritt AM, Cimprich RE, et al: Normal and abnormal xylose absorption in the horse. *Cornell Vet* 66:183, 1976.

46. Jacobs KA, Norman P: Effect of diet on the oral D-xylose absorption test in the horse. *Am J Vet Res* 43:1856, 1982.

47. Merritt T, Mallonee PG, Merrit AM: D-Xylose absorption in growing foals. *Equine Vet J* 18:298, 1986.

48. Merritt AM: Pathophysiology of diarrhea. In Colahan PT, Mayhew IG, Merrit AM, et al, eds: *Equine Medicine and Surgery,* ed 4. Goleta, Calif, American Veterinary, 1991, p 498.

49. Conner ME, Darlington RW: Rotavirus infection in foals. *Am J Vet Res* 41:1699, 1980.

50. Palmer JE: Gastrointestinal diseases of foals. *Vet Clin North Am Equine Pract* 3:101, 1987.

51. Dwyer RM: Methods of environmental disinfection and sanitation during foal diarrhea outbreaks (a case report). In Royer MG, ed: *Proceedings of the 36th Convention of the American Association of Equine Practitioners.* 1991, San Francisco, p 692.

52. McQueary CA, Worley DE, Catlin JE: Observations on the life cycle and prevalence of *Eimeria leuckarti* in horses in Montana. *Am J Vet Res* 38:1673, 1977.

53. Mayhew IG, Griener EC: Protozoal diseases. *Vet Clin North Am Equine Pract* 2:439, 1986.

54. Snyder SP, England JJ, McChesney AE: Cryptosporidiosis in immunodeficient Arabian foals. *Vet Pathol* 15:12, 1978.

55. Klei TR: Other parasites: Recent advances. *Vet Clin North Am Equine Pract* 2:329, 1986.

56. Austin SM, DiPietro JA, Foreman JH: *Cryptosporidium* sp.: A cause of diarrhea in immunocompetent foals. *Equine Pract* 12:10, 1990.

57. Bronsdon MA: Rapid dimethyl sulfoxide–modified acid-fast stain of *Cryptosporidium* oocysts in stool specimens. *J Clin Microbiol* 19:952, 1984.

58. Heuschele WP, Oosterhuis J, Janssen D, et al: Cryptosporidial infections in captive wild animals. *J Wild Dis* 22:493, 1986.

59. Campbell I, Tzipori S, Hutchison G, et al: Effect of disinfectants on survival of *Cryptosporidium* oocysts. *Vet Rec* 111:414, 1982.

60. Soyka JE, Adams SB: Diseases affecting multiple sites. In Colahan PT, Mayhew IG, Merrit AM, et al, eds: *Equine Medicine and Surgery,* ed 4. Goleta, Calif, American Veterinary, 1991, p 532.

61. Foreman JH, White NA: Incidence of equine colic in the University of Georgia ambulatory practice. In Moore JN, White NA, Becht JL, eds: *Proceedings of the Second Equine Colic Research Symposium.* Lawrenceville, NJ, Veterinary Learning Systems, 1986, p 30.

62. Rooney JR, Jeffcott LB: Muscular hypertrophy of the ileum in a horse. *Vet Rec* 83:217, 1968.

63. Schneider JE, Kennedy GA, Leipold WH: Muscular hypertrophy of the small intestine in a horse. *J Equine Med Surg* 3:226, 1977.

64. Lindsay WA, Confer AW, Ochoa R: Ileal smooth muscle hypertrophy and rupture in a horse. *Equine Vet J* 13:66, 1981.

65. Embertson RM, Colahan PT, Brown MP, et al: Ileal impaction in the horse. *J Am Vet Med Assoc* 186:570, 1985.

66. Doran RE, White NA, Allen D: Clinical aspects of ileal impaction in the horse. In Moore JN, White NA, Becht JL, eds: *Proceedings of the Second Equine Colic Research Symposium.* Lawrenceville, NJ, Veterinary Learning Systems, 1986, p 182.

67. Wright AI: Verminous arteritis as a cause of colic in the horse. *Equine Vet J* 4:169, 1972.

68. White NA: Thromboembolic colic in horses. *Compendium Continuing Educ Pract Vet* 7:S156, 1985.

69. Klei TR, Torbert BJ, Chapman MR, et al: Efficacy of ivermectin in injectable and oral paste formulations against 8-week old *Strongylus vulgaris* larvae in ponies. *Am J Vet Res* 45:183, 1984.

70. Semrad SD, Hardee GE, Hardee MM, et al: Low dose flunixin meglumine: Effect on eicosanoid production and clinical signs induced by experimental endotoxaemia in horses. *Equine Vet J* 19:201, 1987.

71. Meyers K, Reed SM, Keck M, et al: Circulating endotoxin-like substances and altered hemostasis in equine patients with gastrointestinal disorders: An interim report. *Am J Vet Res* 43:2233, 1982.

12.6

Pathophysiology of Intestinal Injury

Samuel L. Jones, MS, DVM
Jack R. Snyder, DVM, PhD, Dip ACVS
Sharon J. Spier, DVM, PhD, Dip ACVIM

INTESTINAL EDEMA

Net fluid movement between the vascular and interstitial compartments is described by Starling's hypothesis of fluid exchange. The balance between capillary and interstitial oncotic and hydrostatic pressures prevents the accumulation of interstitial fluid. If capillary hydrostatic pressure increases or plasma oncotic pressure decreases, fluid moves from the vascular space into the interstitium.[1] As the volume of fluid in the interstitial space increases, the interstitial oncotic pressure decreases and the hydrostatic pressure increases, resulting in a new equilibrium resisting further movement of fluid into the interstitium.[1] Lymph flow increases, draining accumulated fluid from the interstitial space; however, lymph

drainage plays a minor role in preventing the formation of interstitial edema.[1] The homeostatic mechanisms preventing edema formation are effective, at least in the small intestine, over a range of pressures as high as 15 mm Hg.[1] However, once the pressure exceeds a critical point, interstitial edema can form.

The severe intestinal edema often present in natural intestinal injury probably develops from the gradual strangulation that obstructs the more pliable venous vessels. Owing to the venous obstruction, the capillary hydrostatic pressure increases above a critical point, resulting in the formation of interstitial edema.[1, 2] Endotoxin, oxygen radicals, histamine, kinins, and hypoxemia increase capillary permeability and potentiate the formation of edema fluid.[3–5] Not only does a larger volume of fluid move into the interstitium but the fluid has a higher oncotic pressure since large molecules such as albumin are able to permeate the capillary barrier. The oncotic pressure of the interstitial fluid increases, further increasing the movement of fluid into the interstitium.

LUMINAL DISTENTION

Obstruction of the large intestine often produces distention from the accumulation of gas, fluid, or ingesta. Colonic obstruction initiates a series of events that result in the accumulation of fluid above the site of obstruction. As luminal pressure increases, a reversal of net absorption to net secretion of isotonic fluid into the lumen occurs. Increased movement of sodium from the plasma to the lumen with a concomitant movement of water into the lumen is the primary reason for the increase in net secretion; however, the transmission of the luminal pressure across the mucosa to the interstitium increases the interstitial hydrostatic pressure and may result in the diffusion of fluid into the lumen or across the serosa.[6] Net secretion continues even after the obstruction is relieved.

It is unlikely that luminal distention plays an important role in the pathogenesis of intestinal damage. Pressures much higher than those measured in natural cases of intestinal obstruction in horses are required to affect blood flow to the tissues. Intraluminal pressures above 35 cm H_2O are required to reduce intestinal blood flow in cats.[7] Intraluminal pressures up to 25 cm H_2O did not produce intestinal hemodynamic changes in dogs.[8] Intraluminal pressures in horses with intestinal obstruction ranged from 4.5 to 21 cm H_2O.[9] In experimental studies of small intestinal distention, intraluminal pressures of 9 and 18 cm H_2O for 4 hours resulted in the formation of interstitial edema and separation of individual cells; however, the cells and the basement membrane remained intact.[10] These minor morphologic changes can be accounted for by the movement of fluid out of the capillaries into the interstitium as a result of an increase in the hydrostatic pressure. The capillary hydrostatic pressure increases as the venous vessels collapse under the pressure exerted from the lumen. The morphologic damage to the intestine observed in natural cases of intestinal obstruction may not be fully explained by luminal distention; however, the effects of increased intraluminal pressure may act in concert with other factors to culminate in significant pathologic changes to the intestine.

ISCHEMIA

The reversibility of cellular damage resulting from ischemia and reperfusion depends largely on the severity of the ischemia.[11] Experimental models of nonocclusive ischemia have shown that the small intestinal circulation is capable of regulating blood flow during periods of low perfusion pressure.[2, 12, 13] As the perfusion pressure falls, the blood flow to the tissues eventually decreases, but the efficiency of oxygen uptake by the intestinal tissue increases.[13] As blood flow falls below a critical level, regulatory systems are no longer effective and oxygen uptake by the tissues decreases, eventually resulting in tissue damage. The equine colonic tissue is more resistant to ischemic damage than the small intestinal tissue. The duration required to produce severe morphologic damage to the equine colon is approximately 25% longer than the small intestine (240 vs. 180 min).[14, 15] Tissue hypoxia is thought to be the primary mechanism of tissue injury in the colon, and the mucosa is the layer most susceptible to ischemic damage. The villus tip is the most susceptible region affected by hypoxia in the equine small intestine, largely due to the countercurrent exchange mechanism of blood flow in the small intestinal villus.[11] The base of the villus receives a larger concentration of oxygen than the tip, rendering the tip relatively more hypoxic than the base, and more sensitive to changes in blood oxygen concentration.[11] The mucosa of the equine colon has a markedly different pattern of blood supply.[11, 14] The mucosal layer of the colon may not have significant differences in oxygenation among regions, at least partially explaining the resistance to ischemic damage relative to the small intestine.

The first biochemical event to occur during hypoxia is a loss of oxidative phosphorylation.[16] The generation of adenosine triphosphate (ATP) slows down or stops. The diminished ATP concentration causes failure of the energy-dependent Na^+, K^+-ATPase resulting in accumulation of sodium, and subsequently intracellular water. Cell swelling occurs, as osmotically active sodium, lactic acid, and other metabolites accumulate.[16] The pH of the cytosol drops as lactic acid and inorganic phosphates accumulate from anaerobic glycolysis.[16] The falling pH damages cell membranes, including lysosomal membranes, resulting in the release and activation of lysosomal enzymes into the cytosol, further damaging cellular membranes. Damage to the cell membrane allows the accumulation of high concentrations of calcium in the cytosol, which activates calcium-dependent degradative enzymes.

Ultrastructural alterations observed using transmission electron microscopy occur much earlier during ischemia than can be detected by light microscopy.[17] Damage to the mitochondria, rough endoplasmic reticulum, nuclear membrane, and basement membrane are detectable within 10 minutes of complete ischemia in the dog small intestine. Subepithelial accumulations of vacuoles containing organelles of enterocyte origin enclosed by a single membrane are seen in the equine small intestine and colon. The extrusion of fluid from the cell in these vacuoles is thought to occur to remove excess cellular water and sodium accumulating intracellularly as the Na^+, K^+-pump becomes de-energized.[18] The function of cellular organelles also changes during short periods of ischemia. Oxygen consumption and high-energy phosphate (ATP) concentrations decrease 25%

and 50% respectively after 30 minutes of ischemia.[19] Based on morphologic studies in the small intestine and colon, however, the physical separation of intestinal cells by the buildup of subepithelial fluid probably occurs before irreversible biochemical damage, and is likely responsible for permanent damage to the cells.[15, 17–19]

The early morphologic changes observed in the equine large colon during total ischemia are different from those described in the equine small intestine.[15] In the colon, small groups of superficial luminal cells are affected first, developing signs of necrosis, and breaking away from the basement membrane and surrounding cells.[14] Subepithelial blebs (vacuoles) form, separating the cells from the basement membrane.[20] Edema, hemorrhage, and mucosal sloughing progress over time.[20] The degree of morphologic alteration of the colonic tissue is based on the degree of hemorrhage and edema in the mucosa and submucosa, the percentage of superficial and crypt cellular damage, and the interstitial:crypt ratio.[14] The interstitial:crypt ratio compares the space occupied by connective tissue relative to the space occupied by the crypts in the lamina propria, and is thought to reflect mucosal pressure.[14]

REPERFUSION INJURY

Tissue damage has been shown to continue in ischemic small intestine and colon in the horse once the circulation has been reestablished to the ischemic tissues.[11, 20, 21] Biochemical evidence of reperfusion injury in the equine colon includes decreased superoxide dismutase activity and formation of lipid peroxides in reperfused colonic tissue.[21] The formation of oxygen metabolites and oxygen radicals and subsequent oxidant injury when the tissue is oxygenated is considered to be a major cause of reperfusion injury. Superoxide and hydroxyl radicals, singlet oxygen, and hydrogen peroxide are formed during reperfusion of ischemic tissue.[22–24] During hypoxia, cellular xanthine dehydrogenase, which reduces cellular NAD^+, is converted to xanthine oxidase within intestinal epithelial and endothelial cells, a process dependent on the accumulation of intracellular calcium during ischemia.[25–27] Xanthine dehydrogenase is found in low concentrations in the equine large colon tissue, but is found in high concentrations in equine blood.[25] In addition, adenyl dehydrogenase is found in high concentrations in colonic tissue, and is converted to adenyl oxidase during hypoxia.[28] Also during the hypoxic period, ATP is converted to adenosine diphosphate (ADP), and finally to hypoxanthine.

Once oxygen returns during reperfusion, radicals form. Xanthine oxidase generates superoxides by transferring electrons from hypoxanthine to oxygen. In the colon, adenyl oxidase transfers electrons from adenyl compounds to oxygen. Superoxide dismutase converts superoxides to hydrogen peroxide, which is converted to water by catalase. Hydroxyl radicals can be generated from superoxides and hydrogen peroxide via the Haber-Weiss reaction, or by interaction of hydrogen peroxide with transitional metals such as ferrous (reduced) iron.[16] Superoxides, hydrogen peroxide, and hydroxyl radicals are also produced and liberated by neutrophils through oxidative metabolism. Hydroxyl radicals appear to be the most potent of the oxygen metabolites formed.[25] Myeloperoxidase released from neutrophils catalyzes a two-electron oxidation of chloride by hydrogen peroxide, producing hypochlorous acid and chloramines, both potent cytotoxic agents.[29] Tissue damage attributable to oxygen radicals includes lipid peroxidation of cellular and mitochondrial membranes, denaturation of proteins, and damage to interstitial matrix leading to alterations in membrane permeability and enzyme activation.[23] Oxidant injury severely disrupts cellular integrity and homeostasis, often resulting in cell death.

The severity of reperfusion injury in intestinal tissue is enhanced by the presence of neutrophils.[29–31] Large numbers of neutrophils are present in reperfused tissue, including the equine colon.[20] When oxygen radical scavengers are used to prevent reperfusion injury experimentally, neutrophilic influx is also blocked, suggesting that oxygen radicals are involved in the attraction of neutrophils. In addition, damage to endothelium resulting in the release of chemotactic factors such as leukotrienes (LTB$_4$) and the activation of complement (C5a, C3a) stimulate the influx of neutrophils. Blocking adherence of neutrophils to vascular endothelium effectively blocks neutrophil-induced tissue damage during reperfusion.[30] Activated neutrophils migrating into an ischemic area are an important source of oxygen radicals during reperfusion, and may block the perfusion of ischemic tissue (no reflow phenomenon) by becoming less pliable and plugging capillaries.[11] Experimental studies in ponies have shown that large numbers of platelets are also present in the microvasculature, progressively occluding the vessels.[20] These platelets were degranulated, suggesting that the release of platelet factors plays a role in reperfusion injury in the horse.

Mammalian cells have adapted mechanisms for blocking and preventing cellular injury by oxygen radicals using endogenous antioxidants and free-radical scavenging molecules.[16, 32] Enzymes that reduce hydrogen peroxide to water and oxygen are glutathione peroxidase and catalase. Superoxide dismutase reduces superoxides to hydrogen peroxide. Ascorbate (vitamin C) and α-tocopherol (vitamin E) and sulfhydryl-containing compounds (cysteine and glutathione) scavenge free radicals. Transferrin is thought to act as an antioxidant by binding ferrous iron.[16] Under normal conditions, these systems prevent damage to cellular constituents by free radicals. However, during intestinal ischemia and reperfusion, these systems are overwhelmed, rendering the cell susceptible to injury from free radicals.[29]

REFERENCES

1. Granger DN, Barrowman JA: Microcirculation of the alimentary tract: I. Physiology of transcapillary fluid and solute exchange. *Gastroenterology* 84:846–868, 1983.
2. Folkow B, Lungren O, Wallentin I: Studies on the relationship between flow resistance capillary filtration coefficient, and regional blood volume in the intestine of the cat. *Acta Physiol Scand* 57:270–283, 1963.
3. Granger DN, Taylor AE: Permeability of intestinal capillaries to endogenous macromolecules. *Am J Physiol* 238:H457–H464, 1983.
4. Mortillara NA, Granger DN, Kvietys PR, et al: Effects of histamine and histamine antagonists on capillary permeability. *Am J Physiol* 240:G381–G386, 1982.
5. Parks DA, Bulkley GB, Granger DN: Role of oxygen-derived

6. Bury KD, McClure RL, Wright HK: Reversal of colonic net absorption to net secretion with increased intraluminal pressure. *Arch Surg* 108:854–857, 1974.
7. Granger DN, Kvietys PR, Mortillara NA, et al: Effects of luminal distention on transcapillary fluid exchange. *Am J Physiol* 239:G516–G523, 1980.
8. Hanson KM: Hemodynamic effects of distention of the dog small intestine. *Am J Physiol* 225:456–460, 1973.
9. Allen D, White NA, Tyler DE: Factors for prognostic use in equine obstructive intestinal disease. *J Am Vet Med Assoc* 189:777–780, 1986.
10. Allen D, White NA, Tyler DE: Morphologic effects of experimental distention of equine small intestine. *Vet Surg* 17:10–14, 1988.
11. Snyder JR: The pathophysiology of intestinal damage: Effects of luminal distention and ischemia. *Vet Clin North Am Equine Pract* 5:247–270, 1989.
12. Bulkley GB, Kvietys PR, Parks DA, et al: Relationship of blood flow and oxygen consumption to ischemic injury of the canine small intestine. *Gastroenterology* 89:852–857, 1986.
13. Shepherd AP, Granger DN: Metabolic regulation of intestinal circulation. In Shepherd AP, Granger DN, eds: *Physiology of Intestinal Circulation*. New York, Raven Press, 1984, pp 33–47.
14. Snyder JR, Olander NJ, Pascoe JR, et al: Morphologic alterations observed during experimental ischemia of the equine large colon. *Am J Vet Res* 49:801–809, 1988.
15. White NA, Moore JN, Trim CM: Mucosal alterations in experimentally induced small intestinal strangulating obstruction in ponies. *Am J Vet Res* 41:193–198, 1980.
16. Cotran RS, Kumar V, Robbins SL: Cellular injury and adaptation. In Cotran RS, Kumar V, Robbins SL, eds: *Pathologic Basis of Disease*. Philadelphia, WB Saunders, 1989, pp 1–38.
17. Brown RA, Chin CJ, Scott HJ, et al: Ultrastructural changes in canine ileal mucosal cell after mesenteric arterial occlusion. *Arch Surg* 101:290–297, 1970.
18. Wagner R, Gabbert H, Hohn P: The mechanism of epithelial shedding after ischemic damage to the small intestinal mucosa. *Virchows Arch [B]* 30:25–31, 1929.
19. Chiu CJ, McArdle AH, Brown R, et al: Intestinal mucosal lesions in low flow states. I: A morphologic, hemodynamic, and metabolic reappraisal. *Arch Surg* 101:478–483, 1920.
20. Meschter CL, Craig D, Hackett R: Histopathological and ultrastructural changes in simulated large colonic torsion and reperfusion in ponies. *Equine Vet J* 23(6):426–433, 1991.
21. Dabreiner RM, Snyder JR, Sullivan KE, et al: Evolution of the microcirculation of the equine jejunum and ascending colon after ischemia and reperfusion. *Am J Vet Res* 54:1683–1692, 1983.
22. Granger DN, Rutili G, McCord JM: Superoxide radicals in feline intestinal ischemia. *Gastroenterology* 81:22–29, 1981.
23. McCord JM: Oxygen-derived free radicals in post-ischemic tissue injury. *N Engl J Med* 312:159–163, 1985.
24. Parko DA, Granger DN: Contributions of ischemia and reperfusion to mucosal lesion formation. *Am J Physiol* 250:G749–G753, 1986.
25. Rochat MC: An introduction to reperfusion injury. *Compendium Continuing Educ Pract Vet* 13:923–929, 1991.
26. Hernandez LA, Grisham MB, Ritter C von, et al: Biochemical localization of xanthine oxidase in the cat small intestine. *Gastroenterology* 92:1433–1438, 1987.
27. Javaseh ED, Bruder G, Heid HM: Significance of xanthine oxidase in capillary endothelial cells. *Acta Physiol Scand Suppl* 548:39–43, 1986.
28. Parks DA, Bulkley GB, Granger DN: Role of oxygen-derived

free radicals in digestive tract diseases. *Surgery* 94:415–422, 1983.

free radicals in digestive tract diseases. *Surgery* 94:415–422, 1983.

29. Grisham MB, Hernandez AL, Granger WD: Xanthine oxidase and neutrophil infiltration in intestinal ischemia. *Am J Physiol* 251:G567–G574, 1986.

30. Engler RL, Dahlgren MD, Peterson MA, et al: Accumulation of polymorphonuclear leukocytes during 3-hour experimental myocardial ischemia. *Am J Physiol* 251:H93–H100, 1986.

31. Hernandez LA, Grisham MB, Twohig B, et al: Role of neutrophils in ischemia-reperfusion induced microvascular injury. *Am J Physiol* 253:H699–H703, 1987.

32. Simpson PJ, Mickelson JK, Lucchesi RB: Free-radical scavengers in myocardial ischemia. *Am Soc Exp Biol* 46:2413–2421, 1987.

12.7

Endotoxemia

Bruce Kuesis, DVM

Sharon J. Spier, DVM, PhD, Dip ACVIM

Endotoxemia (gram-negative sepsis, endotoxic shock) is a systemic disorder that originates from the host response to gram-negative bacteria. Endotoxin or lipopolysaccharide (LPS) is the outer cell wall structural glycolipid that is central to this process. Endotoxemia frequently accompanies pathologic processes when gram-negative bacteria or endotoxin gains access to the systemic circulation. The LPS molecule is a potent inflammatory stimulant capable of both direct and indirect induction of multiple host inflammatory and immunologic processes. Endotoxemia is associated with the activation of host cellular populations and the liberation of inflammatory peptides, arachidonic acid metabolites, complement, kinins, and reactive oxygen radicals. Once the inflammatory cascades are initiated, alterations in homeostatic mechanisms governing endothelial integrity, hemodynamics, hemostasis, and metabolism may lead to tissue ischemia and organ failure. Clinical signs of endotoxemia include depression, fever, tachycardia, tachypnea, abdominal pain, altered fecal consistency, and evidence of perfusion deficits.

The horse is particularly prone to gram-negative sepsis secondary to gastrointestinal disorders and neonatal septicemia.[1–3] Toxic metritis and gram-negative pneumonia and pleuropneumonia are other disease processes associated with high mortality and remain leading causes of death and debilitation among equines. Despite recent advances in the understanding of molecular and cellular pathophysiology, many of the processes leading to septic shock remain undefined. Treatment of endotoxin-associated conditions remains difficult owing to rapid widespread activation of host inflammatory and immunologic processes. Therapeutic goals are aimed at eliminating the primary source of gram-negative sepsis, providing general support to the patient, and curtailing the host's inflammatory response.

STRUCTURE OF LIPOPOLYSACCHARIDE

All gram-negative bacteria share a similar outer cell wall structure consisting of two main components: an inner mucopolysaccharide-peptidoglycan layer, and an outer LPS layer. Endotoxin is an aggregation of LPS combined with cell wall capsular polysaccharide and proteins. The basic LPS structure has been phylogenetically conserved among gram-negative bacterial species. In addition to activating various cellular populations of the host, the LPS moiety also serves as a virulence factor in that it inhibits the bactericidal actions of serum complement and intracellular phagocytic killing.[4] LPS is an amphipathic molecule containing both hydrophobic and hydrophilic regions. Most of the toxic effects of LPS are attributable to the hydrophobic region termed *lipid A.* The hydrophilic region consists of the O-specific chain (also called O-specific antigens or O-somatic antigens) and the core polysaccharide which are responsible for most of the antigenic properties of LPS (Fig. 12–12).

The O-specific chain consists of repeating oligosaccharide units that contain up to six sugar residues. Among differing gram-negative species, there is tremendous variation in the structure, composition, and arrangement of these oligosaccharide constituents. O-antigens are specific for the gram-negative organism from which they are derived and are important for determining specific serologic identity. This region of the LPS molecule is highly antigenic and gram-negative sepsis models have demonstrated the protective effects of O-specific antisera against homologous endotoxin challenge.[5] However, the strain-specificity of the O-chain and diversity of possible gram-negative pathogens preclude the clinical usefulness of O-specific antisera in most circumstances.

The core polysaccharide consists of two main regions, an outer core region that lies in close association with the O-specific side chains, and a lipid A proximal inner core. In contrast to the O-specific chain, constituents of the inner core region tend to be antigenically conserved among gram-negative bacteria. Hence, different gram-negative organisms share common core antigens. Antigenic similarity appears most evident in the 2-keto-3-deoxyoctonic acid (KDO)–containing inner core region. The recognition of cross-anti-

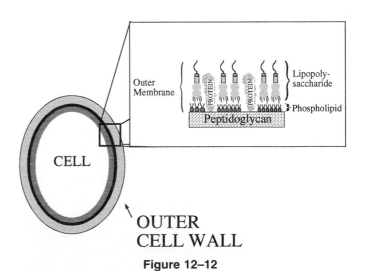

Figure 12–12

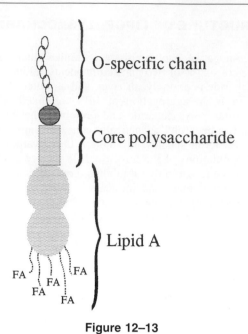

O-specific chain

Core polysaccharide

Lipid A

Figure 12–13

genicity of core antigens has prompted investigation into the clinical use of antisera directed at core epitopes in humans and various animal species. Passive and active immunotherapy is discussed further under Treatment (Fig. 12–13).

The bioactive properties of endotoxin (herein called endotoxic activity) are largely mediated through the lipid A constituent of the LPS molecule. Administration of lipid A appears to exert the same biological effect as endotoxin infusion.[6] The toxic effects of lipid A are largely mediated through interaction, and activation of various inflammatory and immunologic cell populations of the host. The KDO protion of the core polysaccharide may contribute to some extent by upregulating the endotoxic effects of lipid A.[7] Endotoxic activity associated with lipid A appears to require mandatory molecular structures including a biphosphorylated B(1–6)–linked disaccharide and associated fatty acid chains. This structure is well conserved in gram-negative organisms.[8] Deviation in the disaccharide region or in the number or structure of fatty acid chains results in diminished endotoxic activity and in some circumstances the ability to antagonize endotoxin-mediated cellular events. This concept has served as the basis for investigation of lipid A analogs that may attenuate the endotoxic activity of LPS.[9]

ETIOLOGY

Lipopolysaccharide is liberated from gram-negative bacteria following rapid multiplication or bacteriolysis. In the horse, endotoxemia commonly occurs in association with various gastrointestinal disorders, peritonitis, pneumonia and pleuritis, toxic metritis, and neonatal septicemia. Intact epithelium offers the first line of defense against invading microorganisms. Host phagocytic cells, lymphocytes, and humoral factors, including immunoglobulins, complement, and acute phase reactants, constitute the essential secondary host defense mechanisms. Functional deficiencies of these protec-

tive barriers facilitate bacterial invasion and proliferation. Hospitalized patients are at risk of acquiring infections from pathogenic gram-negative organisms displaying antimicrobial resistance patterns. Stresses of hospitalization, and concurrent antimicrobial therapy contribute to nosocomial infections. Contaminated intravenous solutions may also serve as a source of gram-negative infections. In human patients endotoxemia is associated with gram-negative infections involving the meninges, urinary tract, and burns.

Gastrointestinal disorders, particularly those causing mucosal damage to the intestinal tract, are the main source of endotoxemia in adult horses. Concentrations as high as 80 μg of endotoxin per milliliter of cecal contents have been measured in clinically normal horses.[10] The normally functioning mucosal barrier allows only minute quantities of endotoxin access into the portal circulation or peritoneal cavity. Binding of endotoxin by bile salts within the intestinal lumen serves as an additional deterrent to systemic absorption of endotoxin.[11] Severe mucosal inflammation, enterocyte necrosis, and loss of the epithelial barrier may occur secondary to various gastrointestinal insults. Invasive enteric pathogens, including *Salmonella* and *Clostridium* species, are capable of causing direct mucosal damage. Strangulating and nonstrangulating obstructions may result in intestinal ischemia, reperfusion injury, and mucosal necrosis.[12] Toxicosis resulting from the ingestion of cantharidin from blister beetles (*Epicauta* species), oak, or heavy metals can also lead to severe mucosal inflammation and subsequent endotoxin absorption. Nonsteroidal anti-inflammatory drugs (NSAIDs), including phenylbutazone, flunixin meglumine, and ketoprofen inhibit prostaglandin synthesis, and can threaten mucosal integrity at toxic doses. Prostaglandins E_1 and E_2 (PGE$_1$, PGE$_2$) are important for the maintenance of mucosal blood flow, epithelialization, and the mucus-bicarbonate barrier.[13] Toxicity associated with these NSAIDs has resulted in clinical signs of endotoxemia secondary to severe ulcerative lesions distributed throughout the gastrointestinal tract.[14–16]

Normal resident gastrointestinal microbes are important contributors to the luminal environment. Commensal organisms reduce the risk of virulent bacterial overgrowth by competing for limiting substrates, binding sites, and through the release of metabolic byproducts that inhibit the growth of competing bacteria. A number of frequently encountered clinical situations pose considerable threat to the normal flora. Rapid dietary changes to rations containing easily fermentable carbohydrates with minimal roughage can alter the luminal environment, allowing pathogenic organisms to flourish. Experimentally induced carbohydrate overload results in decreased cecal pH and elevated endotoxin and lactate concentrations.[10] Enteral and parenteral antimicrobial agents, including lincomycin, clindamycin, erythromycin, rifampin, metronidazole, trimethoprim-sulfas, tetracyclines, and various β-lactam antibiotics, have been associated with enterocolitis. Antimicrobial administration may selectively inhibit anaerobic or gram-positive populations, allowing for overgrowth of coliforms. Additionally, antimicrobial agents such as erythromycin may affect normal motility patterns and alter the luminal environment. Surgical enterotomy and evacuation of the colon, as necessitated by various gastrointestinal disorders, may also significantly deplete resident flora. Probiotic agents aimed at replacing normal gastrointestinal flora are commercially available for the horse. Although the use of probiotic agents has been associated with a decreased incidence of gastrointestinal disorders and improved feed efficiency in other species, critical studies in the horse have not been reported.

The neonatal foal is predisposed to severe bacterial infections. This may be attributable to the foal's obligatory requirement for colostral immunoglobulins, decreased complement activity, and immature cell-mediated immune response.[17-19] Exposure to gram-negative bacteria may occur in utero or in the early postfoaling environment. Neonatal bacterial infections are commonly acquired through enteric, respiratory, and umbilical routes. On the basis of blood culture, gram-negative organisms, especially *Escherichia coli, Klebsiella pneumoniae,* and *Actinobacillus* and *Salmonella* species, remain the most commonly isolated bacteria in neonatal septicemia. Two retrospective studies have incriminated gram-negative organisms in the majority of positive blood cultures obtained from septic neonatal foals presented to intensive care units.[20, 21] A contributory role for endotoxemia associated with neonatal sepsis is supported by the relevant clinical signs, hematologic alterations, and the recent identification of tumor necrosis factor (TNF) in septic foals.[9, 22]

PATHOGENESIS

Upon gaining access to the systemic circulation, LPS initially complexes with high- and low-density lipoproteins, LPS-binding protein, and other plasma constituents. These complexes may play an important role in the kinetics, transport, and cellular interactions of systemically absorbed endotoxin.[23, 24] LPS exerts deleterious effects upon the host by direct and indirect induction of an overzealous inflammatory response. Directly, LPS activates the complement, coagulation, and fibrinolytic cascades via activation of Hageman factor (factor XII).[25] Host cell populations, including lymphocytes, neutrophils, endothelial cells, platelets, and, most important, mononuclear cells, are activated via specific and nonspecific LPS interactions. The exact nature of the LPS-cellular interaction and coupled response remains unclear. Nonspecific intercalation of lipid A into the plasma membrane may occur.[26] However, recent evidence supports the presence of specific membrane-associated proteins that act as receptors for lipid A or lipid A–protein complexes.[27] Binding of the specific receptor triggers intracellular events leading to cell activation and the release of inflammatory and proinflammatory mediators. These processes have been highly conserved through evolution and represent vital host responses aimed at eliminating microorganisms. When the host response progresses in an unattenuated fashion, widespread endothelial inflammation, coagulopathy, and cardiovascular dysfunction result.[14]

The mononuclear phagocytic system (MPS) is comprised of circulating monocytes, tissue-residing macrophages, and bone marrow stem cells. Kupffer cells of the liver, pulmonary intravascular macrophages (PIMs), and alveolar macrophages of the lung make up a large proportion of the fixed macrophages in the horse. These cells are important in removing bloodborne particles, including LPS, from the portal and systemic circulation. Mononuclear cells are pivotal in

the pathogenesis of gram-negative sepsis. Endotoxin-active mononuclear cells liberate peptide mediators (cytokines), most notably TNF, interleukin-1 (IL-1), and interleukin-6 (IL-6). Endotoxin triggers monocytic phospholipase A_2 and phospholipase C activity which results in the production of arachidonic acid mediators (eicosanoids) and platelet activating factor (PAF). Through the early release of these peptide and lipid mediators, monocytes activate host leukocytes, endothelial cells, and platelets, thus initiating the inflammatory response.

Endotoxin, cytokines, lipid mediators, and complement induce functional alterations in host neutrophils. Activated neutrophils contribute to the inflammatory response through the release of proteolytic enzymes and reactive oxygen radicals. Endotoxin and TNF stimulate neutrophil migration and endothelial adhesion. The expression of adhesion proteins expressed by neutrophils and endothelial cells leads to margination of neutrophils in vessels.[28, 29] Following activation of complement, neutrophils demonstrate decreased deformability, which favors additional sequestration in the microvasculature.[30] Adherence to endothelium, interactions with LPS, and the presence of complement enhance the oxidative capacity of neutrophils.[31] Release of reactive oxygen radicals and lysomal enzymes results in local endothelial and tissue damage.

Endothelial cells contribute to derangement of host inflammatory and coagulation processes during gram-negative sepsis. Endothelial damage inflicted from LPS and activated neutrophils results in the release of thromboplastin and the exposure of subendothelial collagen which activate the extrinsic and intrinsic coagulation cascades, respectively. Endothelial cells activated by LPS and cytokines contribute to alterations in coagulation through the production of tissue factor-like procoagulant activity, tissue plasminogen activator, and plasminogen activator inhibitor.[32] Endothelial cells contribute to the propagation of inflammatory and hemodynamic derangements through the production and release of IL-1, PAF, and prostacyclin (PGI_2).

Cytokines

Cytokines are a diverse group of peptide mediators that are derived from activated host cell populations. These cellular messengers are capable of inducing multiple activities in local or distant host cells. Cytokines are essential to the modulation of host inflammatory and immunologic processes. Research efforts have demonstrated the important role of various peptide mediators in the pathogenesis of septic shock attributable to endotoxemia. Although multiple cytokines have been demonstrated to be operant during clinical endotoxemia, this chapter focuses on TNF, IL-1, and IL-6. The contributory role of these three cytokines in the pathogenesis of septic shock is an area of active investigation. The bioactivity of the various cytokines is complex owing to their overlapping and interrelated functions.

Tumor Necrosis Factor (TNF, Cachectin). TNF, a small polypeptide molecule, is produced in relatively large quantities from LPS-activated macrophages. TNF appears to be distributed preferentially to the liver, skin, kidneys, and gastrointestinal tract where it interacts with specific cellular receptors.[33] The clinical manifestations of gram-negative sepsis are mediated through TNF via activation of host cell populations, including neutrophils, lymphocytes, mononuclear cells, and endothelial cells which act to amplify the inflammatory response.[34-37] Induction of phospholipase activity by TNF results in the liberation of membrane-derived lipid mediators, including prostaglandins, thromboxane, leukotrienes, and PAF. Neutrophils are activated by TNF, demonstrating increased respiratory burst activity, increased liberation of lysosomal enzymes and oxygen radicals, increased antibody-dependent cell-mediated cytotoxicity, and endothelial adhesion.[38-40] Vascular endothelial cells demonstrate expression of procoagulant activity and depressed thrombomodulin activity, which contribute to the hypercoagulable state of endotoxemia. The metabolic effects of TNF include increased circulating systemic cortisol, glucagon, insulin, increased gluconeogenesis, and inhibition of adipocyte lipoprotein lipase. Fever is induced by TNF via direct hypothalamic PGE production and indirectly through the induction of IL-1 and IL-6. TNF also functions in the regulation and activation of host T lymphocytes.[41]

The important role of TNF in the pathogenesis of endotoxemia has been documented in many species, including the horse. In rats, mice, and dogs, intravenous infusion of TNF produces the same clinical and pathologic sequelae as endotoxin infusion.[42-44] The manifestations of TNF in these studies included hypotension, hypermetabolism, metabolic acidosis, elevated cortisol production, hemorrhagic or ischemic necrosis of the gastrointestinal tract, renal tubular necrosis, and pulmonary parenchymal hemorrhage and leukocyte accumulation. Additional credence for TNF as a central mediator of endotoxic shock is provided by passive immunization studies performed in mice and baboons. In these studies, passively acquired anti-TNF antibodies provided protection against intravenous challenge with both endotoxin and *E. coli*.[45, 46] Elevated TNF activity has been identified and associated with poor outcome in human patients with meningococcal septicemia, in horses with strangulating obstructive and inflammatory gastrointestinal disorders, and in septic neonatal foals.[22, 47-49] TNF activity recently has been documented in adult horses and foals following intravenous LPS administration.[28] Adult horses receiving a low-dose continuous infusion of *E. coli* endotoxin demonstrated TNF activity within the first hour of LPS infusion. Activity peaked at approximately 2 hours following initiation of endotoxin and then rapidly diminished.

Interleukin-1 (IL-1, Endogenous Pyrogen, Lymphocyte Activating Factor). IL-1 is a polypeptide cytokine that is important in mediating normal host inflammatory and immunologic responses. IL-1 is produced by antigen-activated macrophages during antigen processing, and functions to activate T lymphocytes, and stimulate B-lymphocyte antibody synthesis. Other sources of IL-1 include endothelial cells, synovial cells, gingival and corneal epithelial cells, astrocytes, and renal mesangial cells.[50] The majority of IL-1 produced during endotoxemia is derived from macrophages in response to LPS, TNF, or leukotrienes.[51-54] During endotoxemia, IL-1 functions to activate host cell populations, and shares overlapping bioactivity with, and potentiates the effect of, TNF.[55, 56] IL-1 participates with other cytokines in the induction of fever, the acute phase response, phospholipase

activation, muscle catabolism, hematologic alterations, lymphocyte activation, and endothelial derangements. The severity of septic shock has been associated with increased IL-1 activity in human patients.[55, 57]

Interleukin-6 (IL-6). IL-6 is a polypeptide cytokine that was first recognized to be important in the final differentiation of lymphocytes into functional antibody-producing cells.[58] IL-6 subsequently has been shown to participate in many aspects of host immunologic and inflammatory function, including the acute phase response, T-cell activation and proliferation, cytotoxic T-cell differentiation, multilineage blast cell stimulation, and adrenocorticotropic hormone production.[58, 59] IL-6 is the predominant cytokine responsible for induction of the acute phase response. The acute phase response is an important nonspecific host inflammatory response that includes fever, leukocytosis, and increased hepatic production of a number of acute phase proteins, including fibrinogen, ceruloplasmin, amyloid A, and C-reactive protein. In this regard, IL-6 may serve as an early hematologic marker of inflammation.[60] Many cells are capable of producing IL-6, including monocytes, macrophages, endothelial cells, and fibroblasts. Endotoxin, TNF, and IL-1 are among substances known to induce IL-6 production.[61, 62] The role of IL-6 in septic shock is not fully understood. Elevated IL-6 activity has been identified in combination with other cytokines from clinically septic human patients and equine patients with experimental endotoxemia.[60, 63-65] In mice, pretreatment with antibodies to IL-6 provided protection when challenged with LPS and TNF.[66]

Lipid Mediators

Platelet Activating Factor (PAF). PAF is a phosphoglycerol mediator produced from activated leukocytes, endothelial cells, platelets, and other cell populations. Tissue hypoxia, endotoxin, and TNF result in increased phospholipase activity and the hydrolytic liberation of arachidonic acid from cell membrane phospholipids. The remaining membrane lysophospholipid is converted to PAF through the action of acetyltransferase. PAF functions in normal physiologic processes as well as inflammatory processes. PAF induces hypotension by decreasing vascular tone and through its negative inotropic properties. In addition, PAF increases vascular permeability, induces pulmonary and bronchial edema, and ischemic bowel necrosis.[67] Equine peritoneal macrophages produce the vasoactive eicosanoids prostacyclin and thromboxane in response to PAF.[68] Elevated circulating PAF is observed following administration of LPS, and infusion of PAF results in some of the same clinical signs observed during endotoxemia.[69, 70] Additionally, PAF antagonists lessen the severity of endotoxin-induced hypotension and hyperglycemia, and improve survivability.[71]

Eicosanoids. Eicosanoids are a group of lipid mediators including prostaglandins, thromboxanes, and leukotrienes. Like PAF, the eicosanoids are derived from cell membrane phospholipids, and participate in normal physiologic and inflammatory processes. During endotoxemia, arachidonic acid serves as a precursor to the eicosanoids. Arachidonic acid may be converted to prostaglandins and thromboxanes

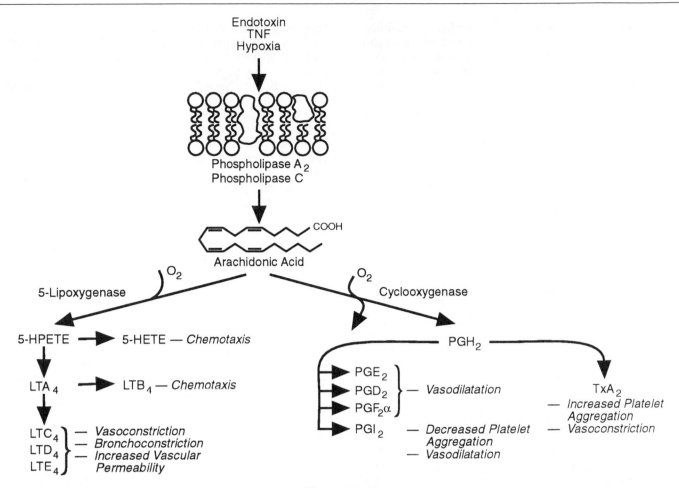

Figure 12–14

through the action of the enzyme cyclooxygenase, or leukotrienes may be produced through the enzymatic conversion of arachidonic acid by lipoxygenase. Eicosanoids are produced from many cells, including neutrophils, macrophages, vascular endothelial cells, platelets, and smooth muscle cells.[72] These mediators are operant in both local and generalized inflammatory processes.[73]

Prostaglandins and thromboxanes collectively possess diverse physiologic function. Thromboxane A_2 (TXA$_2$) is responsible for vasoconstriction, platelet aggregation, and bronchoconstriction. This contributes to early endotoxin-induced hemodynamic and microvasculature alterations that lead to tissue ischemia.[72–74] PGI$_2$ appears later during septic shock and antagonizes many of the activities of thromboxane. PGI$_2$ inhibits platelet aggregation, induces vasodilation, and contributes to systemic hypotension.[72–74] PGE derangements affect regional blood flow, thermoregulatory function, gastrointestinal motility, and immune function.[73] PGF$_{2\alpha}$ has vasoconstrictive properties and causes lysis of the corpus luteum.

The role of the various leukotrienes in septic shock is not well defined. Several areas of research support the importance of leukotrienes in the pathophysiology of septic shock.[75–79] Administration of leukotrienes results in many of the same clinical signs of endotoxemia. Endotoxin challenge is associated with increased leukotriene production and sig-

nificant reduction in hepatobiliary clearance.[80, 81] In mice, the administration of a lipoxygenase inhibitor and leukotriene receptor antagonist provides protection in lethal endotoxemia. Leukotriene B$_4$ (LTB$_4$) induces alterations in neutrophil function, including increased chemotactic activity, lysosomal degranulation, and production of reactive oxygen species. The sulfpeptidyl leukotrienes comprise LTC$_4$, LTD$_4$, and LTE$_4$, previously known as slow reacting substance of anaphylaxis. Major biological effects of the sulfpeptidyl leukotrienes include vasoconstriction, bronchoconstriction, increased vascular permeability, and smooth muscle contraction of the stomach and ileum[82] (Fig. 12–14).

Reactive Oxygen Radicals

Free radicals are molecular species that are highly unstable and reactive due to an unpaired electron. Hypoxia, eicosanoid metabolism, and the respiratory burst of leukocytes contribute to the formation of oxygen-derived free radicals including the superoxide radical (O^{2-}), hydroxyl radical (HO·), hydrogen peroxide (H$_2$O$_2$), and leukocyte-derived hypochlorous acid. These molecules induce oxidative damage to surrounding tissue. Damage to cellular membrane phospholipids referred to as lipid peroxidation results in loss of membrane fluidity, membrane protein damage, and disruption of membrane electrical and ionic gradients.[83] Additionally, membrane damage leads to increased phospholipase activity and the production of arachidonic acid metabolites.[84]

Numerous additional mediators contribute to cardiovascular collapse and tissue damage that ensue with septic shock. Complement components, catecholamines, endorphins, histamine, and serotonin are examples of such. The contributions of these substances are addressed as they pertain to the clinical manifestations of septic shock.

CLINICAL MANIFESTATIONS

Prompt recognition of the clinical signs accompanying different stages of endotoxemia allows early therapeutic intervention. The clinical manifestations of sepsis depend upon the route and dose of endotoxin or gram-negative organisms, the duration of sepsis, and a number of individual host factors. The clinical manifestations may be further confounded by physiologic alterations resulting from the underlying disorder. Based on clinical criteria, human physicians have defined the terms *sepsis, septic syndrome,* and *septic shock* to facilitate staging of the septic process.[85] Likewise, a *sepsis score* based on clinical and laboratory findings has proved useful in the evaluation of neonatal foals.[86] Clinical signs frequently demonstrated by endotoxic horses include hyperthermia, depression, tachycardia, tachypnea or labored respiratory effort, mucous membrane alterations, poor peripheral perfusion, abdominal pain, diarrhea, laminitis, and abortion. The manifestations of gram-negative sepsis in neonates may initially appear subtle, such as depression, interrupted suckling, and weakness. Frequently, progressive clinical deterioration follows these observations. (See Chapter 12.14 for further discussion of the clinical manifestations of sepsis in foals.)

Fever and depression are early clinical signs associated with endotoxemia. Fever usually occurs early and is associated with cytokine-induced (TNF, IL-1, IL-6) elevations of PGE$_2$ at the hypothalamic thermoregulatory center. Temperature increases may be marked, exceeding 40.5 °C (105 °F). With progression, hypothermia may result from peripheral circulatory alterations. Neonatal foals fail to consistently demonstrate a fever, and normothermia or hypothermia in a foal does not exclude the possibility of sepsis. The febrile "masking" effects of NSAIDs, including flunixin meglumine, phenylbutazone, and ketoprofen, should be considered.

Numerous models of equine endotoxemia have demonstrated significant hemodynamic derangements.[87-95] The alterations observed are dependent on the LPS dose and route of administration. Relatively high doses of LPS result in early pulmonary hypertension and systemic vasoconstriction followed by systemic hypotension. Cerebral and myocardial blood flow decrease while gastrointestinal perfusion and splanchnic pooling of blood occur.[92, 93] Hypoxemia occurs in both adult horses and foals following moderate to high LPS challenge.[94, 95] Horses given lower doses of LPS experience decreased cecal blood flow and transient pulmonary hypertension without systemic hypotension. The complex hemodynamic changes are attributable to a number of mediators, including thromboxanes, prostaglandins, leukotrienes, PAF, and catecholamines. The vasoconstrictive properties of thromboxane and the hypotensive role of prostacyclin have

been well documented in equine endotoxin models.[87, 92] Initial vasoconstriction is represented clinically by pale, blanched-appearing mucous membranes. Loss of vascular tone follows, with the mucous membranes appearing dark, congested, and "toxic." Capillary refill time is frequently prolonged at this time.

Horses demonstrating clinical signs of endotoxemia are prone to derangements in fluid and electrolyte balance. Splanchnic vascular pooling results in a decreased effective circulating plasma volume. Additionally, widespread microvascular damage results in increased permeability and loss of circulating volume. Plasma volume in horses has been estimated to decrease by approximately 15% following a single intravenous dose of endotoxin.[96] The primary underlying disorder also may contribute to functional volume deficits. Profuse diarrhea associated with enterocolitis, gastric reflux secondary to duodenitis–proximal jejunitis, and third-compartment sequestration of fluids, as occurs with volvulus of the ascending colon, are relevant examples.

Pulmonary alterations secondary to endotoxemia have been described in a number of species. Human patients suffering from gram-negative sepsis are at risk of developing severe pulmonary damage referred to as the adult respiratory distress syndrome (ARDS). High mortality despite intensive supportive care results from widespread pulmonary damage, noncardiogenic pulmonary edema, decreased lung compliance, and hypoxemia. Pulmonary alterations similar to those occurring in ARDS have recently been described in the veterinary literature.[97] Pulmonary hypertension and hypoxemia appear to be the most consistent alterations observed experimentally.[19, 88-91] Horses subject to experimental *E. coli* septicemia suffered profound pulmonary damage that shared similarities with that of ARDS.[98] Interstitial hemorrhage progressing to septal and intra-alveolar accumulation of neutrophils and fluid were observed histopathologically. Horses suffering from endotoxemia demonstrate histopathologic evidence of pulmonary vascular damage.[99] Vasoactive and bronchoconstrictive mediators, including thromboxane, prostaglandins, leukotrienes, and PAF, may contribute to ventilation:perfusion ($\dot{V}/\dot{Q}$) mismatch and hypoxemia associated with ARDS. These alterations account for the tachypnea and labored respiratory effort demonstrated by some horses with gram-negative sepsis.

Cardiac output is frequently depressed during septic shock. Systemic and pulmonary circulatory alterations and fluid loss secondary to increased vascular permeability result in decreased venous return. Reduction in cardiac output occurs secondary to diminished preload. Direct myocardial contractility may be affected by the release of myocardial depressant factors, leukocyte-induced cellular damage, myocardial edema, and alterations of cell membrane and contractile apparatus function.[100] Studies have demonstrated that myocardial depression associated with LPS administration is dose-dependent.[101, 102] In septic human patients, maintenance of a high cardiac output is associated with improved survival.[103]

Circulatory compromise is further exacerbated by disruption of host coagulation and fibrinolysis. Disseminated activation of the extrinsic and intrinsic coagulation systems occurs under the direction of LPS and derived mediators. LPS initiates the intrinsic cascade through the exposure of subendothelial collagen and activation of factor XII. Extensive endothelial damage results in the release of thromboplastin (tissue factor) and activation of the extrinsic cascade. Platelets are activated to aggregate, contract, and degranulate with exposure to subendothelial collagen. TNF downregulates the natural anticoagulant system through decreased activity of thrombomodulin and protein C, and increased expression of plasminogen activator inhibitor (PAI). Equine monocytes contribute to the hypercoagulable state through the endotoxin-induced expression of procoagulant activity.[104, 105] Progression of the hypercoagulable state leads to depletion of antithrombin III (AT-III), an essential circulating anticoagulant protein. Disseminated intravascular coagulation (DIC) ensues with microvasculature thrombosis, and hemorrhage secondary to consumption of coagulation factors. This may be manifest by excessive hemorrhage associated with abdominal surgery, venipuncture, or intravenous catheterization. Petechial and ecchymotic hemorrhages involving the scleral and mucous membranes are also commonly observed in horses with DIC.[32, 106]

Complex circulatory derangements and increased cellular oxygen requirements during sepsis promote cellular hypoxia and death. Cell populations of the cerebrum, renal tubules, liver, lungs, and gastrointestinal mucosa are particularly susceptible owing to their high metabolic requirements. Cerebral hypoxia may lead to lethargy and alterations in mentation.[93] Renal failure appears to occur frequently with endotoxin-associated coagulopathy.[107] Diarrhea, abdominal pain, bowel edema, and ileus have been observed following experimental endotoxemia.[1, 88, 91, 92]

Abortion in mares has been known to occur following conditions associated with endotoxemia. Multiple pathophysiologic mechanisms may be responsible for abortion associated with sepsis. These include profound hemodynamic alterations induced by various inflammatory mediators. $PGF_{2\alpha}$ release during endotoxemia is an important cause of abortion in the first 2 months of gestation.[108, 109] $PGF_{2\alpha}$ results in lysis of the corpus luteum. Since the corpus luteum is responsible for the maintenance of plasma progesterone during early pregnancy, lysis results in a significant decline in plasma progesterone. Experimental endotoxemia induced in mares 21 to 44 days pregnant resulted in a high rate of abortion. Supplementation with altrenogest (Rebumate, Hoechst-Roussel Pharmaceuticals, Inc., Agri-Vet, Somerville, N.J.), a synthetic progestogen, following experimental endotoxemia through day 70 of gestation prevented endotoxin-induced abortion.[109] The administration of flunixin meglumine prevents endotoxin-induced abortion by inhibiting $PGF_{2\alpha}$ production.[108] Flunixin appeared effective only if administered prior to or early in the course of endotoxin challenge.

Hematologic Alterations

During the initial stages of gram-negative sepsis, neutropenia occurs due to vascular margination. This is a consistent response, and peripheral neutrophil counts may be less than $1,000/\mu L$. Mononuclear-derived factors including TNF, IL-1, and granulocyte and granulocyte-macrophage colony-stimulating factors (G-CSF and GM-CSF, respectively) enhance myeloid proliferation within the bone marrow. This is usually evidenced by neutrophilia, which accompanies the latter stages of gram-negative sepsis. Toxic changes consisting of cytoplasmic vacuolation and toxic granules and immature band neutrophils are often present. Increases in red blood cell count, packed cell volume (PCV), and hemoglobin and plasma protein concentration are noted secondary to extravascular fluid loss. Total plasma protein concentration remains a more reliable indicator of fluid deficits since red blood cell parameters are frequently increased secondary to catecholamine-mediated splenic contraction.

Hyperproteinemia occurs early during endotoxemia, but protein levels may decrease significantly with intestinal losses. Severe enterocolitis commonly leads to protein loss from the damaged bowel and strangulating obstructions may result in protein loss from the bowel or into the peritoneal cavity. Total protein and IgG levels are frequently depressed (IgG <800 mg/dL) in the neonatal foal with failure of passive transfer. The clinician should use discretion when interpreting these values as they may be falsely elevated in foals that are hypovolemic. Decreased peripheral circulation and hypoxemia result in peripheral anaerobic metabolism evidenced by metabolic acidosis and increased serum lactate and anion gap. Elevations of creatine and blood urea nitrogen (BUN) are associated with renal or prerenal azotemia. Further assessment of renal function by urinalysis, including urine specific gravity determination, will differentiate renal from prerenal azotemia. Repeat creatinine and BUN determinations following plasma expansion also assist the clinician in assessing fluid therapy. Hyperglycemia secondary to increased hepatic glycogenolysis occurs in the early stages of sepsis. This is followed by hypoglycemia secondary to decreased gluconeogenesis and increased peripheral glucose utilization. Hyperlipidemia may be noted secondary to endotoxin-induced inhibition of lipoprotein lipase activity. In the young foal, this may be difficult to differentiate from serum chylomicrons obtained from suckling.

Derangements in the clotting panel reflect the state of hemostatic dysfunction. Increases in prothrombin time (PT) and activated partial thromboplastin time (APTT) are common but may not reflect early factor consumption. Elevated fibrin degradation products (FDPs) and depressed plasma fibrinogen are associated with increased fibrinolysis. Depression of AT-III activity is a consistent indicator of coagulopathy in horses with colic and may serve as a negative prognostic indicator.[106, 110]

DIAGNOSIS

Endotoxemia should be suspected based upon the aforementioned clinical and laboratory findings. The detection of serum endotoxin and endotoxin-derived mediators requires controlled assays, which at the present time are used mainly as a research tool. Bacteriologic culture remains important in establishing an etiologic diagnosis and determining antimicrobial sensitivity. Blood cultures should be routinely performed on any foal with presumptive septicemia. Blood culture is indicated in adult horses at risk of bacteremia, especially those displaying fever of unknown origin. Previous antimicrobial administration, transient bacteremia, or low-level bacteremia may result in false-negative blood cultures. Bacteriologic culture and cytology should be performed on specimens that may be associated with the septic process. This may include analysis of peritoneal, pleural, joint, and cerebrospinal fluid. When possible, evaluation of septic foals should include abdominal ultrasonography. Ultrasonography has proved especially useful in identifying infected umbilical structures and various gastrointestinal disorders in foals.

TREATMENT

Treatment of conditions associated with endotoxemia should be expeditious once a presumptive diagnosis has been reached. Treatment is aimed at stabilizing the patient, resolving the source of gram-negative sepsis, controlling the inflammatory response, and providing supportive care. Immediate patient stabilization, and, if necessary, resuscitation are the first priority. These should precede emergency surgical procedures if possible. Arterial blood gas determinations should be performed on horses displaying respiratory distress or cyanosis. Oxygen therapy should be provided to hypoxic patients, and ventilatory support may be required in foals that demonstrate hypoventilation.

The restoration of circulating volume is the most important factor in reestablishing peripheral perfusion. Clinical assessment of the patient will allow estimation of plasma volume deficits. Signs of decreased functional plasma volume in horses with sepsis include elevated heart rate, poor pulse pressure, dry mucous membranes with poor refill, decreased jugular vein distensibility, and cool extremities. Plasma protein and packed cell volume determinations are easily obtained, and allow a more objective assessment of plasma volume.

Intravenous fluid replacement is important in reestablishing functional circulating volume in horses that are significantly volume-depleted. Balanced polyionic solutions such as lactated Ringer's solution (LRS) or 0.9% sodium chloride are the initial fluids of choice. Since hypoglycemia is common in septic foals, 1 L of 5% dextrose or isotonic electrolyte solution supplemented with 2.5% glucose should be administered in foals that appear weak or recumbent. The need for additional glucose supplementation should be based on the blood glucose determination. Fluid rates vary according to the condition of the patient. Fluids can be administered at rates of 10 to 20 mL/kg/hr (5–10 L/500 kg/hr) in horses that are severely compromised. Because of microvascular alterations that may exist with sepsis, overhydration and increased hydrostatic pressure may lead to the development of pulmonary edema. Foals and patients with low plasma protein (colloid oncotic pressure) are particularly susceptible. Clinical signs in these patients include shallow, rapid respiratory effort, the development of auscultable crackles or wheezes, and radiographic evidence of pulmonary edema.

Intravenous administration of small volumes of hypertonic saline (4 mL/kg of 7.5% NcCl) may provide a means of rapid volume expansion. Numerous clinical and experimental studies have shown that hypertonic saline administration results in rapid increases in plasma volume and improved cardiac performance in hemorrhagic shock.[111–115] Similar results have been observed in experimental endotoxemia in horses and dogs.[116, 117] Increased intravascular solute concentration results in extravascular-to-intravascular fluid shifts and subsequent plasma volume expansion. Further research will help define the role of hypertonic saline as a means of rapid volume expansion during endotoxemia.

Horses with pronounced fluid deficits and related tissue hypoperfusion may suffer from metabolic acidosis. In most instances, establishing normal peripheral perfusion through volume expansion results in correction of the base deficit. Severe cases of acidosis may require intravenous alkali therapy with sodium bicarbonate. This is usually reserved for cases with a base balance of less than 10 mEq/L. The total carbon dioxide concentration can be used to calculate base balance since it approximates the bicarbonate concentration. Intravenous and oral potassium chloride will aid in preventing hypokalemia, which can occur with the correction of metabolic acidosis.

Plasma protein levels may be severely depressed as a result of protein catabolism or protein loss through damaged intestinal mucosa. Administration of colloid solutions to provide oncotic pressure should be considered in patients with plasma protein values less than 4 g/dL. Colloid solutions include plasma obtained from a commercial source or harvested from an appropriate donor (horses negative for Aa and Qa isoantibodies). Commercially available high-molecular-weight dextran solutions may provide an alternative for an emergency situation such as general anesthesia. Five liters of plasma or more is usually required in adult horses to significantly elevate plasma protein values. Foals with IgG levels less than 800 mg/dL should receive 1 to 2 L of plasma. Frequent monitoring of plasma protein and IgG is necessary since protein levels may fall rapidly with continued protein loss or catabolism.

Inotropic agents may prove beneficial in horses that are hypotensive or are experiencing anuria despite correction of fluid deficits. Consideration should be given to horses that demonstrate mean arterial pressures of less than 60 mm Hg. Mean arterial pressure can be measured easily through tail cuff manometry. Dopamine hydrochloride and dobutamine (Dobutrex, Eli Lilly Industries, San Juan, P.R.) are agents that have demonstrated positive cardiovascular responses in horses.[118–120] These agents have a short serum half-life necessitating continuous intravenous administration. Dobutamine improves myocardial contractility, peripheral perfusion, and oxygen delivery. Dobutamine can be administered at a rate of 2 to 5 μg/kg/min IV. Horses demonstrating anuria or profound hypotension may benefit from dopamine at a rate of 1 to 5 μg/kg/min IV. This dose results in increased cerebral and renal blood flow through selective vasodilation. The lower end of the dose should be administered initially and gradually increased to effect. Frequent monitoring of heart rate, rhythm, and mean arterial pressure should be performed.

Elimination of the septic focus relies upon the removal of infected or devitalized tissue, and the rational use of antimicrobial agents. Abdominal surgery may be required to remove necrotic intestinal segments and infected umbilical structures. Drainage of septic exudates involving the pleural and peritoneal cavity should be performed. Mares appearing septic following parturition should be examined carefully for retained placenta or uterine tears.

The rational use of antimicrobials remains an important aspect in treating horses that have clinical signs of sepsis. This involves administering an antimicrobial agent or agents at a dosage that will be effective against the offending organism(s) in the particular environment in which they exist. Broad-spectrum antimicrobials should be administered immediately following the collection of specimens for bacteriologic culture and sensitivity.

The aminoglycosides, third-generation cephalosporins, potentiated sulfonamides, and expanded-spectrum penicillins are antimicrobials that demonstrate moderate to good activity against gram-negative bacteria. Effective antibiotic combinations used in treating septic equine patients include penicillin or ampicillin used in combination with an aminoglycoside or a third-generation cephalosporin. Drugs that are effective against gram-positive organisms are also indicated since mixed bacterial infections are common. The profound neutropenia that frequently accompanies gram-negative species may also predispose patients to gram-positive infections. The use of therapeutic monitoring is indicated when using the aminoglycoside antimicrobials. Administration of gentamicin at recommended doses to septic horses resulted in significant variability in optimal plasma concentration and rate of elimination.[121] Likewise, septic neonatal foals with azotemia or hypoxemia treated with amikacin demonstrated significant variability in serum amikacin peak, trough, and clearance values.[122] Individualizing dosage regimens through therapeutic monitoring provides a means of establishing effective drug concentrations while minimizing toxic effects.[122, 123]

Since host inflammation is the major factor responsible for hemodynamic derangement, coagulopathy, and tissue damage during gram-negative sepsis, a major goal of therapy focuses on attenuation of inflammation. Agents such as corticosteroids, NSAIDs, and free radical scavengers are aimed at limiting the inflammatory response by reducing inflammatory mediators. Immunotherapy, passive or active, focuses on reducing LPS activity through decreased release, increased clearance, or decreased host cellular interactions. Because of the rapid initiation of multiple inflammatory cascades, efforts to control the inflammatory response are most efficacious when initiated early in the course of sepsis.

Corticosteroids

The use of corticosteroids in the treatment of septic shock remains an area of dispute. Corticosteroids mediate multiple anti-inflammatory effects through alterations in gene transcription and translation. Corticosteroids significantly decrease the synthesis of TNF, which results in significant downregulation of the inflammatory response.[85] Corticosteroids increase the synthesis of lipocortin, a protein that inhibits phospholipase A_2 activity and the formation of arachidonic acid–derived eicosanoids. The early release of TNF and eicosanoids supports studies which demonstrate that glucocorticoids are only effective if administered prophylactically, or early in the course of sepsis. There are many potential disadvantages associated with the use of corticosteroids for the treatment of sepsis. Profound immunosuppression results from decreased neutrophil chemotaxis, antigen-antibody complexing, and opsonization, thus leading to refractory or even secondary infections. Corticosteroid administration is known to induce laminitis in some horses by potentiating catecholamine-induced digital vasoconstriction.[124] This may be particularly important in septic patients that are already at risk of developing laminitis. Studies investigating the application of corticosteroids in equine endotoxemia have failed to show any therapeutic benefit.[125, 126]

Nonsteroidal Anti-Inflammatory Drugs

Cyclooxygenase-inhibiting drugs used in the treatment of equine endotoxemia have traditionally included the NSAIDs flunixin meglumine, phenylbutazone, and aspirin. Ketoprofen, a new NSAID approved for use in horses, may also prove beneficial in treating endotoxemia. Inhibition of cyclooxygenase by the NSAIDs results in decreased synthesis of prostaglandins and thromboxanes. Numerous studies have demonstrated the NSAIDs to be beneficial in the treatment of equine endotoxemia. Of this group, flunixin meglumine appears to provide the most potent anti-endotoxic effects. Administration of flunixin meglumine has been shown to improve hemodynamic derangement, gastrointestinal motility, and long-term survival in endotoxic horses.[92, 93] Beneficial effects of flunixin have been observed at a dosage of 1.1 mg/kg every 8 to 12 hours or 0.25 mg/kg every 6 to 8 hours.[127] In addition to inhibiting cyclooxygenase, aspirin opposes thrombus formation by altering platelet function. NSAIDs cause significant alterations to local blood flow through inhibition of vasodilator prostaglandins. Clinically, this is important as administration of NSAIDs may predispose patients to gastrointestinal ulceration and renal ischemia. Avoidance of NSAID-associated toxicity relies on careful patient monitoring, the maintenance of adequate hydration, and administering the lowest effective dose.

The leukotrienes contribute to hemodynamic, hematologic, and pulmonary manifestations of septic shock. The beneficial effects of lipoxygenase-inhibiting drugs and leukotriene receptor antagonists have been demonstrated in other species. The leukotrienes are labile and difficult to assay. This has resulted in relatively few clinical studies when compared to prostaglandins and thromboxanes. To our knowledge, there are no clinical trials investigating the use of specific lipoxygenase-inhibiting drugs and leukotriene antagonists in the horse.

Ketoprofen is an NSAID that has recently been licensed for use in horses. There is some evidence that ketoprofen possesses antilipoxygenase activity, but this has not been uniformly accepted. Diethylcarbamazine (DEC) is an antifilarial agent that demonstrates lipoxygenase-inhibiting activity. DEC has been used in the horse to treat onchocerciasis and parasitic arteritis caused by *Strongylus vulgaris*. In mice, DEC used in combination with a leukotriene receptor antagonist provided 100% survival in a lethal endotoxemia model. The therapeutic use of ketoprofen and DEC in equine septic shock has not been reported to date.

IMMUNOTHERAPY

The use of antibodies aimed against LPS core antigens forms the basis of immunologic therapy. Antibodies to common core polysaccharide antigens are cross-protective since different gram-negative organisms share these structures. Rough or R-mutant gram-negative organisms, which lack the genome for synthesis of outer O-specific antigens, are used for the production of core-specific antibodies. R-mutants are categorized by the subscript a, b, c, d, or e based on the length of core structure that is present. *Escherichia coli* 0111:B4 (J5) and *Salmonella minnesota* (R_e 595) are rough mutants that have been used as bacterins for active

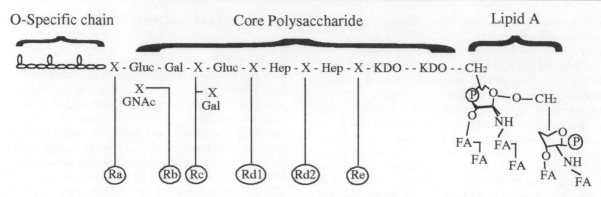

Figure 12–15 Schematic representation of lipopolysaccharide used to stimulate anti-polysaccharide antibody formation depicting position of R mutant organisms (Ra, Rb, Rc, Rd1, Rd2, Re).

immunization, or for the production of hyperimmune sera to treat horses and foals with endotoxemia (Fig. 12–15).

Passive immunotherapy involves the administration of hyperimmune antisera to horses or foals that are at high risk of endotoxemia. Antibodies aimed at the LPS core region may promote opsonization and reticuloendothelial clearance of gram-negative organisms and LPS.[128, 129] Additionally, anti-core polysaccharide antibodies may sterically inhibit biological interaction of the LPS molecule.[130] In humans and animals, a number of studies have shown beneficial effects derived from the use of anti-core LPS immunoglobulins.[128, 131-133] The use of core-LPS immunoglobulins in equine studies has shown mixed results in experimental endotoxemia models and clinical trials.[131-135] In a double blind randomized clinical trial, administration of J5 hyperimmune plasma (4.4 ml/kg body weight) to horses with clinicopathologic evidence of endotoxic shock (horses with strangulating intestinal obstruction or enterocolitis) resulted in improved clinical appearance, survival, and decreased hospitalization time compared with horses receiving control plasma.[132] Like other treatment modalities, the use of LPS-core antisera would be expected to provide the greatest benefit when initiated early in the septic process.

Effective active immunoglobulin production through the use of bacterins derived from R-mutant gram-negative organisms has proved beneficial in the treatment of gram-negative infections in various animal species.[133] In horses subject to carbohydrate overload, the use of R-mutant bacterins has been shown to decrease the incidence of laminitis and delay the onset of clinical signs of endotoxemia.[131] Although the benefits of active immunization to core-LPS antigens appear promising, additional investigation is required to assess the beneficial effects of this form of therapy.

SUMMARY

Endotoxin is absorbed systemically from gram-negative bacterial invasion or as free endotoxin from damaged epithelial surfaces. Systemic LPS is a potent stimulus of host inflammation. The host responds to LPS through the activation of various defense mechanisms which initiate a series of inflammatory processes aimed at halting bacterial infection. This response may remain attenuated and localized with few systemic effects, or escalate to a state of generalized immune-inflammatory activation. Once initiated, propagation of the host response may occur in the presence or absence

of widespread gram-negative infection. Thus, the overzealous host response to bacterial endotoxin is the key feature that leads to the clinical manifestations observed during gram-negative sepsis. Clinical manifestations of endotoxemia in the horse include fever, tachycardia, hypotension, coagulopathy, vascular damage, and perfusion defects, which lead to vital organ damage. Because of the multiple abnormalities that exist, treatment of endotoxin-related conditions remains difficult and frequently expensive. The focus of treatment is based upon establishing tissue perfusion, controlling the inflammatory response, eliminating the source of endotoxin, and providing general patient support.

REFERENCES

1. Burrows GE: Endotoxemia in the horse. *Equine Vet J* 13:88–94, 1981.
2. Moore JN: Recognition and treatment of endotoxemia. *Vet Clin North Am Equine Pract* 4:105–113, 1988.
3. Morris DD: Endotoxemia in horses. A review of cellular and humoral mediators involved in its pathogenesis. *J Vet Intern Med* 5:167–181, 1991.
4. Makela PH, Hovi M, Saxen H, et al: Role of LPS in the pathogenesis of salmonellosis. In Nowotny A, ed: *Cellular and Molecular Aspects of Endotoxin Reactions. Endotoxin Research Series,* vol 1. Amsterdan, Elsevier Science, 1990, p 537.
5. Pennington GE, Menkes E: Type specific vs. cross protective vaccination for gram-negative bacterial pneumonia. *J Infect Dis* 144:599–603, 1982.
6. Galanos C, Luderitz O, Reitschel ET, et al: Synthetic and natural free lipid A expresses identical endotoxic activities. *Eur J Biochem* 148:1, 1985.
7. Haeffner-Cavaillon N, Caroff M, Cavaillon JM: Interleukin-1 induction by lipopolysaccharide: Structural requirement of the 3-deoxy-*d*-manno-2-octulosonic acid (KDO). *Mol Immunol* 26:485, 1989.
8. Rietschel ETH, Seydell U, Zahringer U, et al: Bacterial endotoxin: Molecular relationship between structure and activity. *Infect Dis Clin North Am* 5:753–779, 1991.
9. Stutz P, Liehl E: Lipid A analogs aimed at preventing the detrimental effects of endotoxin. *Infect Dis Clin North Am* 5:847–873, 1991.
10. Moore JN, Garner HE, Berg JN, et al: Intracecal endotoxin and lactate during the onset of equine laminitis: A preliminary report. *Am J Vet Res* 40:722, 1979.
11. Cahill CJ, Pain JA, Bailey ME: Bile salts, endotoxin and renal function in obstructive jaundice. *Surg Gynecol Obstet* 165:519–522, 1987.

12. Snyder JR: The pathophysiology of intestinal damage: Effects of luminal distension and ischemia, advances in equine abdominal surgery. *Vet Clin North Am* 249–270, 1989.

13. Murray MJ: Nonsteroidal antiinflammatory drug toxicity. In Smith BP, ed: *Large Animal Internal Medicine.* St. Louis, Mosby–Year Book, 1990, p 665.

14. Lees P, Creed RFS, Gerring EEL, et al: Biochemical and hematological effects of phenylbutazone in horses. *Equine Vet J* 15:158–167, 1983.

15. Traub JL, Gallina AM, Grant BD, et al: Phenylbutazone toxicosis in the foal. *Am J Vet Res* 44:1410–1418, 1983.

16. Karcher LF, Dill SG, Anderson WI, et al: Right dorsal colitis. *J Vet Intern Med* 4:247–253, 1990.

17. Hietala SK, Ardans AA: Neutrophil phagocytic and serum opsonic response of foals to *Corynebacterium equi. Vet Immunol Immunopathol* 14:279–294, 1987.

18. Rernoco M, Liu IKM, Wuest-Ehlert CJ, et al: Chemotactic and phagocytic function of peripheral blood polymorphonuclear leucocytes in newborn foals. *J Reprod Fertil* 35(suppl): 599–605, 1987.

19. Lavoie JP, Madigan JE, Cullor JS, et al: Haemodynamic, pathological, haematological and behavioural changes during endotoxin infusion in equine neonates. *Equine Vet J* 22:23–29, 1990.

20. Koterba AM, Brewer BD, Tarplee FA: Clinical and clinicopathological characteristics of the septicaemic neonatal foal: Review of 38 cases. *Equine Vet J* 16:376–383, 1984.

21. Wilson WD, Madigan JE: Comparison of bacteriologic culture of blood and necropsy specimens for determining the cause of foal septicemia: 47 cases 1978–1987. *J Am Vet Med Assoc* 195:1759–1763, 1989.

22. Morris DD, Moore JN: Tumor necrosis activity in serum from neonatal foals with presumed septicemia. *J Am Vet Med Assoc* 199:1584–1589, 1991.

23. Schumann RR, Leong SR, Flaggs GW, et al: Structure and function of lipopolysaccharide binding protein. *Science* 249:1429, 1990.

24. Wright SD, Ramos RA, Tobias PS, et al: CD14, a receptor for complexes of lipopolysaccharide and LPS binding protein. *Science* 249:1431, 1990.

25. Sable CA, Wispelwey B: Pharmacologic interventions aimed at preventing the biologic effects of endotoxin. *Infect Dis Clin North Am* 5:883–898, 1991.

26. Shands JW Jr: Affinity of endotoxin for membranes. *J Infect Dis* 128:189, 1973.

27. Morrison DC: The case for specific lipopolysaccharide receptors expressed on mammalian cells. *Microb Pathog* 7:389, 1989.

28. Old LJ: Tumor necrosis factor. *Sci Am* 258:59–75, 1988.

29. Gamble JR, Harlan JM, Klebanoff SJ, et al: Stimulation of the adherence of neutrophils to the umbilical vein endothelium by human recombinant tumor necrosis factor. *Proc Natl Acad Sci U S A* 82:8667–8671, 1985.

30. Worthen G, Schwab B, Elson E, et al: Mechanics of stimulated neutrophils: Cell stiffening induces retention in capillaries. *Science* 245:183–186, 1989.

31. Wilson ME: Effects of bacterial endotoxins on neutrophil function. *Rev Infect Dis* 7:404–418, 1985.

32. Morris DD: Endotoxemia in horses. A review of cellular and humoral mediators involved in its pathogenesis. *J Vet Intern Med* 199:167–181, 1991.

33. Beutler B, Milsark IW, Cerami A: Cachectin/tumor necrosis factor: Production, distribution, and metabolic fate in vivo. *J Immunol* 135:3972–3977, 1985.

34. Beutler B, Cerami A: The endogenous mediator of endotoxic shock. *Clin Res* 35:192–197, 1987.

35. Camussi G, Bussolino F, Salvidio G, et al: Tumor necrosis factor/cachectin stimulates peritoneal macrophages, polymorphonuclear neutrophils and vascular endothelial cells to synthesize and release platelet-activating factor. *J Exp Med* 166:1390–1404, 1987.

36. Meyrick B, Jesmok G, Brigham KL: Human recombinant tumor necrosis factor alpha (TNF) causes cytotoxicity and prostanoid release from large and small lung vessel endothelial cells in culture. *Am Rev Respir Dis* 137:362, 1988.

37. Beutler B, Cerami A: The biology of cachectin/TNF, a primary mediator of the host response. *Annu Rev Immunol* 7:625–655, 1989.

38. Shalaby M, Aggarwal B, Rinderknecht E, et al: Activation of human polymorphonuclear neutrophil functions by interferon-gamma and tumor necrosis factors. *J Immunol* 135:2069–2063, 1986.

39. Klebanoff S, Vadas MA, Harlan JM, et al: Stimulation of neutrophils by tumor necrosis factor. *J Immunol* 136:4220–4225, 1986.

40. Grunfeld C, Palladino MA: Tumor necrosis factor. Immunologic, antitumor, metabolic, and cardiovascular activities. *Adv Intern Med* 35:45–72, 1990.

41. Scheurich P, Thoma B, Ucer U, et al: Immunoregulatory activity of recombinant human tumor necrosis factor (TNF)-alpha: Induction of TNF receptors on human T cells and TNF-gamma mediated enhancement of T cell response. *J Immunol* 138:1786–1790, 1987.

42. Tracey KJ, Beutler B, Lowry SL, et al: Shock and tissue injury induced by recombinant human cachectin. *Science* 234:470–474, 1986.

43. Remick DG, Kunkek RG, Larrick JW, et al: Acute in vivo effects of human recombinant tumor necrosis factor. *Lab Invest* 56:583–590, 1987.

44. Tracey KJ, Lowry SF, Fahey TJ III, et al: Cachectin/tumor necrosis factor induces lethal shock and stress hormone responses in the dog. *Surg Gynecol Obstet* 164:415–422, 1987.

45. Beutler B, Milsark IW, Cerami AC: Passive immunization against cachectin/tumor necrosis factor protects mice from lethal effect of endotoxin. *Science* 229:869–871, 1985.

46. Tracey KJ, Fong Y, Hesse DG, et al: Anti-cachectin/TNF monoclonal antibodies prevent septic shock during lethal bacteraemia. *Nature* 330:662–664, 1987.

47. Waage A, Halstensen A, Epsevik T: Association between tumor necrosis factor in serum and fatal outcome in patients with meningococcal disease. *Lancet* 1:1355–1357, 1987.

48. Morris DD, Moore JN, Crowe N: Serum tumor necrosis factor activity in horses with colic attributable to gastrointestinal tract disease. *Am J Vet Res* 52:1565–1569, 1991.

49. MacKay RJ, Merritt AM, Zertuche JM, et al: Tumor necrosis factor activity in the circulation of horses given endotoxin. *Am J Vet Res* 52:533–538, 1991.

50. Dinarello CA: Interleukin-1. *Rev Infect Dis* 6:51–84, 1984.

51. Newton RC: Human monocyte production of IL-1: Parameters of the induction of IL-1 secretion by LPS. *J Leukoc Biol* 39:299–311, 1986.

52. Rola-Pleszcynski M, Lemaire I: Leukotrienes augment interleukin-1 production by human monocytes. *J Immunol* 135:3958–3961, 1985.

53. Dinarello CA, Cannon JG, Wolff SM, et al: Tumor necrosis factor (cachectin) is an endogenous pyrogen and induces interleukin-1. *J Exp Med* 163:1433–1450, 1986.

54. Samuelson B: Leukotrienes: A new class of mediators of immediate hypersensitivity reactions and inflammation. *Adv Prostaglandin Thromboxane Leukotriene Res* 11:1–13, 1983.

55. Le J, Vilcek J: Biology of disease: Tumor necrosis factor and interleukin-1: Cytokines with multiple overlapping biological activities. *Lab Invest* 56:234, 1987.

56. Tracey KJ, Beutler B, Lowry SF, et al: Shock and tissue injury induced by recombinant human cachectin. *Science* 234:470, 1986.

57. Calandra T, Baumgartner JD, Grau GE, et al: Prognostic values of tumor necrosis factor/cachectin, interleukin-1, interferon-alpha and interferon-gamma in the serum of patients with septic shock. *J Infect Dis* 161:982, 1990.

58. Kishimoto T: The biology of interleukin-6. *Blood* 74:1–10, 1989.

59. Helle M, Brakenhoff JPJ, De Groot ER, et al: Interleukin 6 is involved in interleukin 1 induced activities. *Eur J Immunol* 18:957, 1988.

60. Macay RJ, Lester GD: Induction of the acute-phase cytokine, hepatocyte stimulating factor/interleukin 6, in the circulation of horses treated with endotoxin. *Am J Vet Res* 53:1285–1289, 1992.

61. Jablons GM, Mule JJ, MacIntosh JK, et al: Interleukin-6/interferon-beta-2 as a circulating hormone, induction by cytokine administration in humans. *J Immunol* 142:1542–1547, 1985.

62. Helfgoit PC, Tatter SB, Santhanam U, et al: Multiple forms of interferon-beta-2/interleukin-6 in serum and body fluids during acute bacterial infection. *J Immunol* 142:948–953, 1989.

63. Waage A, Brandtzaeg, Halstensen A, et al: The complex pattern of cytokines in serum from patients with meningococcal septic shock. *J Exp Med* 169:333, 1989.

64. Morris DD: Interleukin 6: A novel cytokine with possible significance in equine endotoxemia. In *Proceedings of the Ninth Annual Meeting of the American College of Veterinary Internal Medicine,* New Orleans, 1991, pp 393–395.

65. Robinson JA, Allen GK, Green EM: Equine neonatal endotoxemia: Involvement of interleukin-6. In *Proceedings of the 10th Annual Meeting of the American College of Veterinary Internal Medicine,* San Diego, 1992, pp 309–311.

66. Starnes HF, Pearce MK, Tewari A, et al: Anti-IL-6 monoclonal antibodies protect against lethal *Escherichia coli* infection and lethal tumor necrosis factor-alpha challenge in mice. *J Immunol* 145:4185, 1990.

67. Hanahan DJ: Platelet activating factor: A biologically active phosphoglyceride. *Annu Rev Biochem* 55:483–509, 1986.

68. Morris DD, Moore JN: Equine peritoneal macrophage production of thromboxane and prostacyclin in response to platelet activating factor and its receptor antagonist SRI 63-441. *Circ Shock* 28:149–158, 1989.

69. Hosford D, Braquet P: The potential role of platelet-activating factor in shock and ischemia. *J Crit Care* 5:115–136, 1990.

70. Lefer AM: Induction of tissue injury and altered cardiovascular performance by platelet-activating factor: Relevance to multiple systems organ failure. *Crit Care Clin* 5:331–351.

71. Terashita Z, Imura Y, Nishikawa K, et al: Is platelet activating factor (PAF) a mediator of endotoxic shock? *Eur J Pharmacol* 109:257–261, 1985.

72. Bottoms GD, Johnson M, Ward D, et al: Release of eicosanoid from white blood cells, platelets, smooth muscle cells and endothelial cells in response to endotoxin and A 23187. *Circ Shock* 20:25–34, 1986.

73. Bottoms GD, Adams RH: Involvement of prostaglandins and leukotrienes in the pathogenesis of endotoxemia and sepsis. *J Am Vet Med Assoc* 200:1842–1848, 1992.

74. Temple GE, Strong JW, Wise WC, et al: The role of eicosanoids in mediating blood flow alterations in endotoxin shock. In Passman JC, Reichard SM, eds: *Perspectives in Shock Research: Metabolism, Immunology, Mediators, and Models.* New York, Alan R Liss, 1989, pp 33–43.

75. Feverstein G, Hallenbeck JM: Prostaglandins, leukotrienes and platelet-activating factor in shock. *Annu Rev Pharmacol Toxicol* 27:301–313, 1987.

76. Cook JA, Wise WC, Haluska PV: Protective effect of a selective leukotriene antagonist in endotoxemia in the rat. *J Pharmacol Exp Ther* 235:470–474, 1985.

77. Pacitti N, Bryson SE, McKechnie K, et al: Leukotriene antagonist FPL 57231 prevents the acute pumonary effects of *Escherichia coli* endotoxin in cats. *Circ Shock* 21:155–168, 1987.

78. Keppler D, Hagmann W, Rapp S: Role of leukotrienes in endotoxin action in vivo. *Rev Infect Dis* 5(suppl):S580–584, 1987.

79. Keppler D, Hagmann W, Denzlinger C: Leukotrienes as mediators in endotoxin shock and tissue trauma. *Prog Clin Biol Res* 236a:301–309, 1987.

80. Hagmann W, Denslinger C, Keppler D: Role of peptide leukotrienes and their hepatobiliary elimination in endotoxin action. *Circ Shock* 14:223–235, 1984.

81. Pfeifer CA, Bottoms GD, Johnson MA, et al: Leukotriene C4 disposition and metabolism in the anesthetized and endotoxemic dog. *Circ Shock* 33:68–83, 1990.

82. Hardie EM, Kruse-Elliot K: Endotoxic shock. Part 1: A review of causes. *J Vet Intern Med* 4:258–266, 1990.

83. Hess ML, Manson NG: Molecular oxygen. Friend or foe. Part 1. *Mol Cell Cardiol* 16:969–985, 1984.

84. Brown SA, Hall ED: Role of oxygen derived free radicals in the pathogenesis of shock and trauma, with focus on central nervous system injuries. *J Am Vet Med Assoc* 200:1849–1859, 1992.

85. Bone RC: Sepsis syndrome: New insights into its pathogenesis and treatment. *Infect Dis Clin North Am* 5:793–806, 1991.

86. Brewer BD, Koterba AM: Development of a scoring system for the early diagnosis of equine neonatal sepsis. *Equine Vet J* 20:18–22, 1988.

87. Bottoms GD, Templeton CB, Fessler JF, et al: Thromboxane, prostaglandin I_2 (epoprostenol), and the hemodynamic changes in equine endotoxin shock. *Am J Vet Res* 43:999–1002, 1982.

88. Burrows GE: Hemodynamic alterations induced by rapid intravenous injection of *Escherichia coli* in anesthetized ponies. *Am J Vet Res* 31:1976–1973, 1970.

89. Burrows GE: Hemodynamic alterations in the anesthetized pony produced by slow intravenous administration of *Escherichia coli* endotoxin. *Am J Vet Res* 46:1975–1982, 1970.

90. Olson N: Effects of endotoxin on lung water, hemodynamics and gas exchange in anesthetized ponies. *Am J Vet Res* 46:2288–2293, 1985.

91. Clark ES, Gantley B, Moore JN: Effects of slow infusion of a low dosage of endotoxin on systemic haemodynamics in conscious horses. *Equine Vet J* 23:18–21, 1991.

92. Bottoms GD, Fessler JF, Roesel OF, et al: Endotoxin-induced hemodynamic changes in ponies: Effects of flunixin meglumine. *Am J Vet Res* 42:1514–1518, 1981.

93. Templeton CB, Bottoms GD, Fessler JF, et al: Effects of repeated endotoxin injections on prostanoids, hemodynamics, endothelial cells and survival in ponies. *Circ Shock* 16:253–264, 1985.

94. King JN, Gerring EL: The action of low dose endotoxin on equine bowel motility. *Equine Vet J* 23:11–17, 1991.

95. Moore JN, Garner HE, Shapland JE, et al: Lactic acidosis and arterial hypoxemia during sublethal endotoxemia in conscious ponies. *Am J Vet Res* 41:1696–1698, 1980.

96. Spurlock GH, Landry SL, Sams R, et al: Effect of endotoxin administration on body fluid compartments in the horse. *Am J Vet Res* 46:1117–1200, 1985.

97. Frevert CW, Warner AE: Respiratory distress resulting from acute lung injury in the veterinary patient. *J Vet Intern Med* 6:154–165, 1992.

98. Sembrat R, Di Stazio J, Reese J, et al: Acute pulmonary failure in the conscious pony with *Escherichia coli* septicemia. *Am J Vet Res* 39:1147–1153, 1978.

99. Schaub RG, Moore JN, Garner HE, et al: Pulmonary vascular damage in the pony induced by endotoxin: Effects of lido-

caine. In *Proceedings of Equine Endotoxemia and Laminitis Symposium,* 1981, pp 87–96.

100. Vincent JL: Cardiovascular management of septic shock. *Infect Dis Clin North Am* 5:807–816, 1991.

101. Abel FL: Myocardial function in sepsis and endotoxin shock. *Am J Physiol* 257:1265–1281, 1989.

102. McDonough KH, Brumfield BA, Lang CH: In vitro myocardial performance after lethal and nonlethal dose of endotoxin. *Am J Physiol* 250:240–246, 1986.

103. Siegel JH: Relations between circulatory and metabolic changes in sepsis. *Ann Rev Med* 32:175–194, 1981.

104. Henry MM, Moore JN: Endotoxin-induced procoagulant activity in equine peripheral blood monocytes. *Circ Shock* 26:297–309, 1988.

105. Henry MM, Moore JN: Clinical relevance of monocyte procoagulant activity in horse with colic. *J Am Vet Med Assoc* 198:843–848, 1991.

106. Welch RD, Watkins JP, Taylor TS, et al: Disseminated intravascular coagulation associated with colic in 23 horses. *J Vet Intern Med* 6:29–35, 1992.

107. Morris DD: Recognition and management of disseminated intravascular coagulation in horses. *Vet Clin North Am Equine Pract* 4:115–143, 1988.

108. Daels PF, Stabenfeldt GH, Hughs JP, et al: Effects of flunixin meglumine on endotoxin-induced prostaglandin F_2 alpha secretion during early pregnancy in mares. *Am J Vet Res* 52:276–282, 1991.

109. Daels PF, Stabenfeldt GH, Hughes JP, et al: Evaluation of progesterone deficiency as a cause of fetal death in mares with experimentally induced endotoxemia. *Am J Vet Res* 52:282–288, 1991.

110. Darien BJ, Potempa J, Moore JN, et al: Antithrombin III activity in horses with colic: An analysis of 46 cases. *Equine Vet J* 23:211–214, 1991.

111. Maier RV, Carrico CJ: Developments in the resuscitation of the critically ill surgical patient. *Adv Surg* 19:271–329, 1986.

112. Kramer GC, Perron PR, Lindsey DC, et al: Small-volume resuscitation with hypertonic saline dextran solution. *Surgery* 100:239–247, 1986.

113. Defillippe J, Timoner J, Velasco IT, et al: Treatment of refractory hypovolemic shock by 7.5% sodium chloride injections. *Lancet* 2:1002–1004, 1980.

114. Schmall LM, Muir WW, Robertson JT: Haemodynamic effects of small volume hypertonic saline in experimentally induced haemorrhagic shock. *Equine Vet J* 22:273–277, 1990.

115. Schmall LM, Muir WW, Robertson JT: Haematological, serum electrolyte and blood gas effects of small volume hypertonic saline in experimentally induced haemorrhagic shock. *Equine Vet J* 22:278–283, 1990.

116. Bertone JJ: New perspectives in septic shock: metabolism and intravenous hypertonic saline solution. In *Proceedings of the 12th Annual Equine Seminar, Louisiana Veterinary Medicine Equine Association,* Bossier City, September 1989.

117. Mullins RJ, Hudgens RW: Hypertonic saline resuscitates dogs in endotoxic shock. *J Surg Res* 43:37–44, 1987.

118. Swanson CR, Muir WW, Bednarski RM, et al: Hemodynamic responses in halothane-anesthetized horses given infusions of dopamine or dobutamine. *Am J Vet Res* 46:365–370, 1986.

119. Trim CM, Moore JN, White NA: Cardiopulmonary effects of dopamine hydrochloride in anaesthetized horses. *Equine Vet J* 17:41–44, 1985.

120. Donaldson LL: Retrospective assessment of dobutamine therapy for hypotension in anesthetized horses. *Vet Surg* 17:53–57, 1988.

121. Sojka JE, Brown SA: Pharmocokinetic adjustment of gentamicin dosing in horses with sepsis. *J Am Vet Med Assoc* 189:784–789, 1986.

122. Green SL, Conlon PD, Mama K, et al: Effects of hypoxia and azotemia on the pharmacokinetics of amikacin in neonatal foals. *Equine Vet J* 24:475–479, 1992.

123. Koritz GD: Practical aspects of pharmacokinetics for the large animal practitioner. *Compendium Continuing Educ Pract Vet* 11:201–204, 1989.

124. Eyre P, Elmes PJ: Corticosteroid-potentiated vascular responses of the equine digit: A possible pharmacologic basis for laminitis. *Am J Vet Res* 40:135–138, 1979.

125. Moore JN: Equine endotoxemia: Characterization and treatment. *Diss Abstr Int B* 42:4315, 1982.

126. Green EM, Garner HE, Sprouse RF: Laminitis/endotoxemia: Pathophysiology and therapeutic strategy. In *Proceedings of the Sixth Annual Veterinary Medical Forum of the American College of Veterinary Internal Medicine,* 1988, pp 323–327.

127. Semrad SD, Hardee GE, Hardee MM, et al: Low dose flunixin meglumine: Effects on eicosanoid production and clinical signs induced by experimental endotoxemia in horses. *Equine Vet J* 19:201–206, 1987.

128. Ziegler EJ, McCutchan JA, Fierer J, et al: Treatment of gram-negative bacteremia and shock with human antiserum to a mutant *Escherichia coli. N Engl J Med* 307:1225–1230, 1982.

129. Fenwick BW, Cullor JS, Osburn BI, et al: Mechanisms involved in the protection provided by immunization against core lipopolysaccharides of *Escherichia coli* J5 from lethal hemophilus pleuropneumonia infections in swine. *Infect Immun* 53:298–304, 1986.

130. Braude AI, Zeigler EJ, Douglas H, et al: Antibody to cell wall glycolipid of gram-negative bacteria: Induction of immunity to bacteremia and endotoxemia. *J Infect Dis* 136(suppl):S167–173, 1977.

131. Garner HE, Sprouse RF, Green EM: Active and passive immunization for blockade of endotoxemia. *Proc Am Assoc Equine Pract* 31:525–532, 1985.

132. Spier SJ, Lavoie JP, Cullor JS, et al: Protection against clinical endotoxemia in horses by using plasma containing antibody to an Rc mutant *E. coli* (J5). *Circ Shock* 28:235–248, 1989.

133. Tyler JW, Cullor JS, Spier SJ, et al: Immunity targeting common core antigens of gram-negative bacteria. *J Vet Intern Med* 4:17–25, 1990.

134. Morris DD, Whitlock RH, Corbeil LB: Endotoxemia in horses: Protection provided by antiserum to core lipopolysaccharide. *Am J Vet Res* 41:1696–1698, 1980.

135. Morris DD, Whitlock RH: Therapy of suspected septicemia in neonatal foals using plasma containing antibodies to core lipopolysaccharide (LPS). *J Vet Intern Med* 1:175–182, 1987.

12.8

Physiology of the Large Intestine

Samuel L. Jones, MS, DVM

Jack R. Snyder, DVM, PhD, Dip ACVS

Sharon J. Spier, DVM, PhD, Dip ACVIM

ANATOMY

The large intestine includes all sections distal to the ileocecal orifice, the cecum, and the ascending colon (both the right and left ventral colon and the right and left dorsal colon). The cecum has an average length of 1 m with an average capacity of 33 L. The body of the cecum has four longitudinal bands of the ascending and descending colons. The lateral band can be traced to the point at which it joins the cecocolic fold; the dorsal band joins the ileocecal fold, and the lateral and ventral bands join each other at the apex of the cecum. The ascending mesocolon attaches the cecum to the body wall on the right side of the mesenteric root.

The ascending colon is 3 to 4 m in length and has a capacity of as much as 130 L. The ascending colon originates from the cecocolic orifice as the right ventral colon (RVC), which is attached to the lateral band of the cecum by the cecocolic fold. The ascending colon travels cranially to the sternal flexure (SF), continues caudally as the left ventral colon (LVC), decreases in diameter, and turns 180 degrees at the pelvic inlet to form the pelvic flexure (PF). The PF may vary in location, but is usually left of midline at the pelvic inlet. The ascending colon continues cranially from the pelvic flexure as the larger-sized left dorsal colon (LDC), and forms the diaphragmatic flexure dorsal to the SF. The ascending colon then turns 180 degrees, continuing caudodorsally to the right as the right dorsal colon (RDC). At the root of the mesentery, the RDC decreases sharply in diameter and turns medially to form the transverse colon (TC), which passes from right to left cranial to the cranial mesenteric artery (CMA). The ascending colon is attached to the body wall at the most proximal and distal aspects only (right ventral and dorsal colons). The LVC has distinct wide bands confluent with the adjacent intestinal wall, and well-formed haustra. The PF has one band that is located along the mesenteric border. The LDC has three bands, which are similar to those found on the ventral colon, but no haustra. The ascending colon gives rise to the descending colon at the TC. The descending colon reaches a length of 2.5 to 4.0 m and continues to the rectum on the left side of the abdomen. The descending colon has two wide bands which are raised above the rest of the surface.[1]

The vascular supply to the large colon originates from the CMA, whereas in most other species the large colon is supplied by both the CMA and caudal mesenteric artery. The dorsal colon is supplied by the right colic artery, a branch of the CMA. The CMA becomes the ileocolic artery and gives off the colic branch artery, which supplies the ventral colon. Both colic vessels are located on the mesenteric border of the colon, and anastomose at the PF. The terminal branches of the ileocolic artery supply the cecum, with a small vessel supplying the antimesenteric border of the ileum. The descending colon is supplied by the caudal mesenteric artery and the middle colic artery, a branch of the CMA.

The colonic tissue is supplied through numerous arterial branches from the mesenteric vessels. These initial branches form a vascular rete that surrounds the mesenteric vein before progressing to the serosal surface toward the antimesenteric border. These subserosal vessels travel approximately 3 to 4 cm, penetrate the muscle layers, and continue into the submucosa, forming a vascular network that supplies all layers of the intestinal wall.[2] The mucosal vessels form a plexus around the colonic glands, continue toward the lumen, form a subluminal anastomotic plexus, and drain into the submucosal veins.[2]

DIGESTION, SECRETION, ABSORPTION

The large intestine plays a vital role in digestion and water balance in the horse. The large intestine secretes and recovers a volume of fluid equal to the extracellular fluid volume every 24 hours.[3] Up to 75% of the energy requirements in the horse are met by products of microbial fermentation of carbohydrates in the cecum and colon.[4] The importance of maintaining a stable environment for the microbial population is manifested by the devastating sequelae of profound changes in the flora produced by grain overload or administration of certain antimicrobials. The large intestine must absorb the products of fermentation, resorb large volumes of fluid, and maintain optimal conditions for microbial fermentation (primarily pH, osmolarity, and hydration).[4]

The microorganisms that populate the equine large intestine have not been intensively studied. Ciliated protozoa and strict anaerobic bacteria have received the most attention and make up the largest proportion of the population.[5, 6] Bacteria from the family Enterobacteriaceae are present in relatively small numbers.[5] The important cellulolytic bacteria found in the equine large intestine appear to be similar to those found in the rumen of cud-chewing species.[4, 7] The conditions for fermentation (pH, osmolarity, anaerobiasis, hydration) also appear to be similar to the rumen.[4] The pH of the large intestinal contents normally fluctuates within a narrow range (6.0–6.8) and the osmolarity remains relatively stable at approximately 300 mOsm/L.[4, 8, 9]

Fermentation of soluble and insoluble carbohydrates yields volatile fatty acids (primarily acetic, propionic, and butyric acid) carbon dioxide, methane, and small amounts of lactate. Volatile fatty acids (VFAs) are passively absorbed through the mucosa into the blood, where they are transported to the liver to be metabolized. Acetic acid is produced in the greatest proportion, but the ratio of acetic:propionic acid decreases as the ratio of soluble:insoluble carbohydrate increases.[10] The amount of soluble carbohydrate reaching the large intestine varies with the diet and may be as high as 50% of the amount ingested.[4] When ponies are fed a pelleted diet every 12 hours, the production of VFAs fluctuates between periods of high production (0–8 hours after feeding) and periods of low production (8–12 hours after feeding).[8, 10] The period of high VFA production is associated with a rapid increase in fluid volume of the large intestine, production of large quantities of osmotically active organic acids, and gas formation.[3, 10]

Homeostatic mechanisms in the large intestine which buffer formed organic acids include transport of bicarbonate-rich fluid from the small intestine, secretion of bicarbonate by the large intestinal mucosa, and rapid absorption of VFAs. Bicarbonate entering the large intestine from the ileum is rapidly depleted by reacting with acids in the cecum.[4] Bicarbonate is secreted by the mucosa of the ascending colon during periods of VFA production. Accumulation of bicarbonate in the luminal fluid is linked to acetate absorption. The amount of bicarbonate appearing in the luminal fluid during acetate absorption is one half to one third of the amount of VFAs absorbed.[11] The remainder of the bicarbonate is titrated by hydrogen ions in the luminal fluid. An independent Na^+, H^+-transport mechanism secretes H^+ in exchange for sodium ions.[11] The experimental removal of Na^+ from the luminal fluid results in the appearance of bicarbonate in the luminal fluid equivalent to the amount of acetate absorbed.[11]

Ninety-nine percent of the VFAs are dissociated (ionized) at the average pH of the large intestine.[12] The ionized form of VFA is poorly absorbed as compared with the lipid-soluble un-ionized (undissociated) form. During periods of rapid VFA production, the pH drops and a higher percentage of VFAs is un-ionized. The absorption of acetate is three times as great at pH 6.3 as at 7.2.[11, 12] It appears that the hydration of carbon dioxide to carbonic acid, which then dissociates to bicarbonate and H^+, provides a source of H^+ to form more readily absorbable undissociated VFAs.[11] As the lipid-soluble un-ionized VFAs are absorbed, bicarbonate accumulates in the luminal fluid. Large volumes of water and Na^+ are also secreted during the period of VFA production. The Na^+, H^+-transport system is partially responsible for resorbing Na^+. Resorption of Na^+ by this mechanism seems to be partially under local control by prostaglandins.[13] Aldosterone also appears to play an important role in Na^+ transport.[14, 15] The H^+ that are exchanged for Na^+ combine with VFAs to form undissociated acid, which can be absorbed, or titrated by bicarbonate.[11, 16] Phosphate found in the luminal fluid in high concentrations also serves as an important buffer for H^+, especially in the distal colon.[4] The osmolarity of the luminal content remains relatively stable in spite of the formation of organic acids, owing to the secretion of water. Water is absorbed by the ascending and descending colons, resulting in a net absorption of 90% to 95% of the luminal water.[3]

Undigested protein entering the large intestine is digested by the microbial flora to ammonia. The ammonia can then be recycled to synthesize amino acids and microbial protein.[4, 17] Soluble carbohydrates are required for synthesis of amino acids and protein by the microbes. The capability of the large intestine to absorb amino acids is controversial; however, the amount absorbed is probably small compared with that absorbed by the small intestine.[18, 19] The majority of the protein degraded in the large intestine is lost in the feces or utilized by the horse as ammonia.[4] The ammonia produced by microbial flora is absorbed into the blood and transported to the liver to be converted to urea.

LARGE INTESTINAL MOTILITY

The function of the large intestine as the primary site of digestion in the horse requires that the motor activity accomplish the task of retention and mixing of ingesta to allow microbial fermentation of insoluble carbohydrates (cellulose). The large intestine can be *functionally* divided into four compartments: cecum, ventral ascending colon, dorsal ascending colon, and descending colon. The cecocolic valve, PF, and TC act as barriers for aboral movement of ingesta.[3] Ingesta is retained and mixed in the first three compartments for long periods. Movement of liquid markers through the cecum can take up to 5 hours, and movement through the ascending colon can take up to 50 hours.[3] The movement of particles of ingesta is even slower and the rate appears to be indirectly proportional to particle size.[4] Thorough mixing of the large volume of ingesta for 48 to 72 hours is necessary to allow sufficient contact between the microflora and the ingesta, buffering of organic acids, and hydration of the material to promote fermentation and allow absorption of VFAs and other microbial byproducts. The motor activity of the large intestine can be divided into three phases: mixing, propulsion, and retropulsion.

Mixing activity is accomplished by local contractions oc-

curring in the cecum and colon.[20] These contractions are characterized by rapid, short spike bursts of electrical activity lasting only seconds which generate frequent (3–5/min) low-amplitude contractions involving adjacent haustra.[20, 21] Strong propulsive contractions in the cecum and large colon are progressive and move ingesta aborally. Propulsive contractions are characterized by long spike bursts of electrical activity and occur every 4 minutes in the cecum. They originate from an apparent pacemaker in the body of the cecum and are propagated to the cranial base of the cecum, through the cecocolic orifice, into the RVC.[20, 21] Similar contraction patterns originate every 2 to 3 minutes at the pacemaker site in the PF and move into the LDC.[21, 22] The relative frequency of short spike bursts and long spike bursts determines the amount of mixing vs. aboral movement of ingesta.[20]

Retropulsive contractions that are electrically and mechanically similar to propulsive events are occasionally propagated from the pacemaker site in the PF into the LVC and through the RVC to the cecocolic orifice.[23, 24] Retropulsive contractions also occur in the cecum, propagating from the body of the cecum to the caudal base of the cecum, or vice versa. The dorsal plica of the base of the cecum prevents ingesta from moving through the cecocolic orifice.[21, 24] Retropulsive contractions appear to delay transit of ingesta which tends to keep the ascending colon and cecum filled. The end result is to retain the ingesta to allow microbial fermentation.[24]

Control of the motor activity of the large intestine is complex. The smooth muscle of the intestinal wall has intrinsic contractility. Extrinsic factors serve to modify the contractility of the smooth muscle and can be divided into autonomic and endocrine mechanisms.[20] Autonomic innervation of the large intestine includes parasympathetic and sympathetic contributions. Parasympathetic nerves originate from the brain (vagus nerve) and the spinal cord (pelvic nerve) to supply the proximal (cecum and ascending colon) and distal (descending colon) large intestine, respectively. Preganglionic parasympathetic fibers of the vagus and pelvic nerves terminate in the intramural ganglia of the myenteric plexus. Postganglionic fibers arising from the intramural ganglia synapse at the myoneural junction of the intestinal smooth muscle. Stimulation of the preganglionic fibers results in release of acetylcholine (ACh) at the ganglionic synapse, which stimulates postganglionic fibers to release ACh at the myoneural junction, stimulating contraction of the smooth muscle. Parenteral administration of parasympathomimetic drugs may stimulate nicotinic (ganglionic) or muscarinic (myoneural) receptors, or both. Bethanechol, for example, stimulates both nicotinic and muscarinic receptors, which causes contraction of the intestinal smooth muscle. Neostigmine inhibits acetylcholinesterase, resulting in ACh accumulation at nicotinic and muscarinic sites, also stimulating contraction. Atropine, a parasympatholytic drug, antagonizes ACh at muscarinic but not nicotinic receptors, inhibiting contraction.[25]

The sympathetic innervation of the large intestine consists of preganglionic nerves arising in the spinal cord which synapse in the superior and inferior mesenteric ganglia. Postganglionic adrenergic fibers terminate on cholinergic neurons in the intramural ganglia. Norepinephrine released by the postganglionic sympathetic fibers generally inhibits cholinergic fibers of the intramural ganglia via α_2-receptors, resulting in decreased motility.[20] Xylazine, a selective α_2-adrenergic agonist, inhibits contractile activity in the cecum and ventral colon in ponies, presumably via α_2-receptors.[25, 26] The inhibitory effect of xylazine on large intestinal motility can be antagonized by α_2-antagonists, such as tolazoline and yohimbine.[26, 27]

Reflexive control of motility plays an important regulatory role in the large intestine. Intestinal receptors give rise to impulses that enter the spinal cord and brainstem, which in turn can modify the efferent outflow to the viscera. Local reflexes are also important in regulating contractile activity.[28] Chemoreceptors and mechanoreceptors in the mucosa respond to changes in pH, osmotic pressure, VFA concentration, and the presence of ingesta in the lumen.[20, 28] Increasing VFA concentration has been shown to stimulate short spike activity and mixing contractions in the large intestine.[20] Stretch receptors in the muscle layers and serosa respond to distention. Fullness of the colon or distention of the large intestinal wall initiates an increase in long spike burst activity which initiates a complex of contractile activity resulting in enhanced propulsion of ingesta.[20] The distention reflex appears to be a local reflex; however, distention of proximal visceral segments also will cause an increase in large intestinal contractility, a phenomenon called the "colic motor complex."[20, 29] Feeding also stimulates large intestinal motility. The feeding reflex can be divided into two phases: an early phase that is neurally mediated, and a later phase that appears to be independent of enervation and may be hormonally mediated.[20, 28]

The role of the endocrine system in controlling large intestinal motility is unclear. Serotonin, substance P, prostaglandins, enkephalins, insulin, glucagon, and other hormones serve a regulatory role in gastrointestinal motility, but, only serotonin, substance P, and prostaglandins (PGE_1 and $PGF_{2\alpha}$) have been investigated in regard to motility in the equine large colon. Serotonin and substance P appear to stimulate motility in the equine large colon.[27] Substance P also increases colonic blood flow.[27] PGE_1 on the other hand, was found to *inhibit* motility in the ascending and descending colons in a dose-dependent manner.[30] The mechanism of action of these mediators is speculative at this time.

Pharmacologic manipulation of intestinal motility has revealed evidence of β-adrenergic, opiate, and dopaminergic influence on the contractility of the intestine. α-Adrenergic mechanisms appear to be more important than β-adrenergic mechanisms in the equine large intestine.[28] Opiate agonists have well-documented effects mediated by opiate receptors which increase segmental contraction and decrease propulsive movement of ingesta.[25, 31, 32] Opiate agonists have similar effects on the equine colon, but, at pharmacologic doses, opiate agonists can also cause transient relaxation of the large intestine that is not blocked by opiate antagonists, suggesting that mechanisms other than opiate receptor–mediated mechanisms, such as inhibition of ACh or substance P release or stimulation of α_2-adrenergic receptors, may play a role at these doses.[28] Naloxone, an opiate antagonist, stimulates propulsive activity of the equine large colon.[31] Metaclopramide has variable effects on equine large intestinal motility, and cholinergic mechanisms as well as antagonism of dopamine may be involved.[28] The physiologic role of opiate, dopaminergic, and β-adrenergic receptors in equine large intestinal motility remains unclear.

REFERENCES

1. Nickel R, Schummes A, Seiferle E: The alimentary canal. In Schummes A, Nickel K, Sack WO, eds: *The Viscera of the Domestic Animal,* ed 2. New York, Springer-Verlag, 1979, pp 180–197.
2. Snyder JR, Tyler WS, Pascoe JR, et al: Microvasculature of the equine colon, a correlative study of the pelvic flexure using scanning electron microscopy of vascular replicas, microangiography, and light microscopy. *Am J Vet Res* 50:2075–1083, 1989.
3. Argenzio RA, Lowe JE, Pickard DW, et al: Digesta passage and water exchange in the equine large intestine. *Am J Physiol* 226:1035–1042, 1974.
4. Argenzio RA: Functions of the equine large intestine and their interrelationship to disease. *Cornell Vet* 65:303–327, 1975.
5. Mackie RI, Wilkins CA: Enumeration of anaerobic bacterial microflora of the equine gastrointestinal tract. *Appl Environ Microbiol* 54:2155–2160, 1988.
6. Kern DL, Shytes LL, Leffel EC, et al: Ponies vs steers: Microbial and chemical characteristics of intestinal ingesta. *J Anim Sci* 38:559–564, 1974.
7. Russell JB, Bruckner GG: Microbial ecology of the normal animal: Intestinal tract. In Woolcock JB, ed: *Microbiology of Animals and Animal Products.* New York, Elsevier Science, 1991, pp 1–18.
8. Argenzio RA, Stevens CE: Cyclic changes in ionic composition of digesta in the equine intestinal tract. *Am J Physiol* 228:1224–1230, 1975.
9. Murray MJ: Digestive physiology of the large intestine in adult horses: Part I. Mechanisms of fluid, ions, and volatile fatty acid transport. *Compendium Continuing Educ Pract Vet* 10:1204–1210, 1988.
10. Argenzio RA, Southworth M, Stevens CE: Sites of organic acid production and absorption in the equine gastrointestinal tract. *Am J Physiol* 226(5):1043–1050, 1974.
11. Argenzio RA, Southworth M, Lowe JE, et al: Interrelationship of Na, HCO_3, and volatile fatty acid transport by equine large intestine. *Am J Physiol* 233:E469–E478, 1977.
12. Argenzio RA: Transport of electrolytes and water by equine large colon. In *Proceedings of the First Equine Colic Research Symposium.* 1982, pp 44–52.
13. Clarke LL, Argenzio RA: NaCl transport across equine proximal colon and the effect of endogenous prosteroids. *Am J Physiol* 259:G62–G69, 1990.
14. Clarke LL, Ganjam VK, Fichtenbaum B, et al: Effect of feeding on renin-angiotensin-aldosterone system in the horse. *Am J Physiol* 254:R524–R530, 1988.
15. Argenzio RA, Clarke LL: Electrolyte and water absorption in the hind gut of herbivores. *Acta Vet Scand Suppl* 86:29–33, 1989.
16. Argenzio RA: Physiology of digestive, secretory, and absorptive processes. In White NA, ed: *The Equine Acute Abdomen.* Philadelphia, Lea & Febiger, 1990, pp 25–35.
17. Wootton JF, Argenzio RA: Nitrogen utilization within equine large colon. *Am J Physiol* 229:1062–1067, 1975.
18. Tisserand JL: Microbial digestion in the large intestine in relation to monogastric and polygastric herbivores. *Acta Vet Scand Suppl* 86:83–91, 1989.
19. Freeman DE, Donawick WJ: *In vitro* transport of cycloleucine by equine cecal mucosa. *Am J Vet Res* 52:539–542, 1991.
20. Ruckebusch Y: Motor functions of the intestine. *Adv Vet Sci Comp Med* 25:345–369, 1981.

21. Sellers AF, Lowe JE, Rendano VT: Equine colonic motility: Interactions among wall motion, propulsion, and fluid flow. *Am J Vet Res* 45:357–360, 1984.
22. Sellers AF, Lowe JE, Brondum J: Motor events in equine large colon. *Am J Physiol* 237:E457–E464, 1979.
23. Ross MW, Donawick WJ, Sellers AF, et al: Normal motility of the cecum and right ventral colon in ponies. *Am J Vet Res* 47:1756–1762, 1986.
24. Sellers AF, Lowe JE, Drost CJ, et al: Retropulsion—propulsion in equine large colon. *Am J Vet Res* 43:390–396, 1982.
25. Adams SB: Equine intestinal motility: An overview of normal activity, changes in disease, and effects of drug administration. *Proc Am Assoc Equine Pract* 33:539–555, 1987.
26. Roger T, Ruckebusch Y: Colonic α_2-adrenoreceptor-mediated responses in the pony. *J Vet Pharmacol Ther* 10:310–318, 1987.
27. Sellers AF, Lowe JE, Cummings JF: Trials of serotonin, substance P, and α_2-adrenergic receptor effects on the equine large colon. *Cornell Vet* 75:319–323, 1985.
28. Clark ES: Intestinal Motility. In White NA, ed: *The Equine Acute Abdomen*. Philadelphia, Lea & Febiger, 1990, pp 36–48.
29. King JN, Gerring EL: Observations on the colic motor complex in a pony with a small intestinal obstruction. *Equine Vet J* 7(suppl):43–45, 1986.
30. Hunt JM, Gerring EL: The effect of prostaglandin E_1 on motility of the equine gut. *J Vet Pharmacol Ther* 8:165–173, 1985.
31. Kohn CW, Muir WW: Selected aspects of the clinical pharmacology of visceral analgesics and gut motility modifying drugs in the horse. *J Vet Intern Med* 2:85–91, 1988.
32. Roger TH, Bardon TH, Ruckebusch Y: Colonic motor responses in the pony: Relevance of colonic stimulation by opiate antagonists. *Am J Vet Res* 46:31–35, 1985.

12.9

Examination for Disorders of the Large Intestine

Samuel L. Jones, MS, DVM

Jack R. Snyder, DVM, PhD, Dip ACVS

Sharon J. Spier, DVM, PhD, Dip ACVIM

PHYSICAL EXAMINATION

Examination of patients with disease of the large intestine must include evaluation of the metabolic and cardiovascular status of the patient, since acute conditions of the large intestine have the potential to lead to endotoxemia and sepsis. Examination of the cardiovascular system (heart, peripheral pulse, and mucous membranes), lungs, and abdomen is essential to detect clinical signs of endotoxemia, coagulation disorders, metabolic acidosis, ileus, shock, and other systemic manifestations of sepsis resulting from injury to the large intestine. Clinical signs of endotoxemia and sepsis are covered in detail in Chapter 12.7.

Physical examination of the large intestine is accomplished primarily by abdominal auscultation, transabdominal ballottement, and transrectal palpation. Abdominal distention often is an indication of distention of the large intestine; however, small intestinal distention can also cause visible abdominal distention if a large proportion of the small intestine is severely distended. Abdominal palpation can be done in neonatal foals; after several weeks of age, however, the abdominal wall is too rigid to allow effective palpation of intraabdominal structures.

Abdominal auscultation is particularly useful when assessing the motility of the large intestine. Progressive motility of the small intestine, conversely, is difficult to distinguish from nonprogressive motility by auscultation. The distinct character of the borborygmi produced during propulsive contractions of the cecum and ascending colon allow evaluation of the frequency and strength of retropulsion and propulsion. Propulsive contractions of the cecum and ventral colon occur every 3 to 4 minutes and give rise to prolonged rushing sounds heard over long segments of intestine.[1] Retropulsive sounds presumably sound similar to propulsive sounds, but they occur less frequently. The distinction of propulsion from retropulsion is not important clinically since both types of contractions signify normal motility. Inter- and intrahaustral mixing contractions produce nonspecific sounds of fluid and ingesta movement that are difficult to distinguish from other borborygmi, such as small intestinal contractions or spasmodic contractions.[1]

Auscultation over the right flank, and proceeding along the caudal edge of the costal margin toward the xiphoid, allows evaluation of the cecal borborygmi. Auscultation over a similar area on the left side allows evaluation of the pelvic flexure and ascending colon. Typical progressive borborygmi heard every 3 to 4 minutes on both sides of the abdomen indicate normal motility of the cecum and ascending colon. Less frequent progressive sounds may indicate a pathologic condition of the large intestine or may result from anorexia, nervousness (sympathetic tone), or pharmacologic inhibition of motility (i.e., α_2-adrenergic agonists such as xylazine).[2, 3] Absolute absence of any auscultable borborygmi suggests abnormal motility and indicates ileus resulting from a serious pathologic condition, but is not specific to the large intestine.[3, 4] If borborygmi are heard, but progressive sounds are not detected, it is difficult to determine whether a significant abnormality exists.[4]

Borborygmi heard more frequently than normal may result from increased motility following feeding, from excessive stimulation from irritation, distention, inflammation, or after administration of parasympathomimetic drugs such as neostigmine. Large intestinal motility increases in the early stages of intestinal distention regardless of the site.[5] Mild inflammation or irritation of the large intestinal mucosa also can stimulate motility.[3] Parasympathomimetic drugs stimulate contractions and auscultable borborygmi in the large intestine; however, an increase in parasympathetic tone may result in segmental contractions, which actually inhibit progressive motility.[2]

Sand or gravel in the large intestinal ingesta can be detected by auscultation behind the xiphoid process. Sand or gravel particles can be heard grinding together during progressive contractions of the ascending colon.[6] The presence of sand in the ingesta becomes clinically detectable by auscultation or fecal sedimentation before the amount of sand is enough to produce clinical signs of pain or irritation (diarrhea).[7] If progressive contractions are heard without hearing sand sounds, it is unlikely that clinically important quantities of sand are present. If the frequency of progressive contractions is low or absent, the detection of sand by auscultation is difficult.

Percussion of the abdomen during auscultation can reveal gas in the large intestine. The characteristic ping produced by simultaneous digital percussion and auscultation over a gas-filled viscus often is associated with abnormal accumulation of gas under pressure. This technique is particularly useful in foals, ponies, and miniature horses because of the limitations of palpation per rectum.

Transabdominal ballottement can be used to detect large, firm masses, or an abnormal volume of peritoneal fluid. The usefulness of this technique is usually limited to animals too small to palpate per rectum. Soft tissue masses or fetuses can be detected by bumping the structures with a hand or fist. If excessive peritoneal fluid is present, a fluid wave can be generated by ballottement; however, this technique is not as useful in horses older than 4 weeks because the abdominal wall is rigid.

Transrectal palpation is the most specific physical examination technique for investigation of large intestinal disease, and is particularly valuable when evaluating obstructive diseases.[8] The primary objective of transrectal palpation is to assess the size, consistency, and position of the segments of the large intestine. Evaluation of the wall thickness and texture and the mesenteric structures (blood and lymphatic vessels, and lymph nodes) also may aid in the diagnosis of large intestinal disease. The interpretation of transrectal palpation findings in light of clinical signs and laboratory results is an important diagnostic aid for development of appropriate treatment strategies for large intestinal diseases manifested by abdominal pain.

Enlargement of one or more segments of large intestine detected by transrectal palpation provides evidence of obstruction at or distal to the enlarged segment. By systematically evaluating each segment, the site of obstruction may be elucidated. Obstruction of the pelvic flexure, for instance, results in enlargement of the pelvic flexure and ventral colon, but the dorsal and descending colons are of normal size. Enlargement of a segment of the large intestine is usually accompanied by abnormal consistency of the contents. Accumulation of gas, fluid, or ingesta may be distinguished, and foreign bodies in palpable segments may be detected. Accumulation of gas and fluid infers complete and acute obstruction, while accumulation of ingesta infers chronic and incomplete obstruction. Accumulation of fluid usually indicates ileus. The consistency of the contents must be evaluated in light of the size of the segment; ingesta in the ventral colon of a dehydrated patient may be firm, but the size of the ventral colon will be normal. Conversely, if the ingesta is firm because of a distal obstruction, the ventral colon will be enlarged.

Displacement of a segment of the large intestine may create an obstruction which can be detected by enlargement of the segment and accumulation of gas and fluid, even if the site of obstruction is not palpable. Torsion of the ascending colon at the sternal and diaphragmatic flexures results in acute accumulation of gas and fluid proximal to the torsion, causing distention of the left dorsal and ventral colons. Depending on the degree of torsion, the position of the ventral and dorsal colons may not be markedly abnormal. Often, displacement of a segment of large intestine results in incomplete obstruction, and the diagnosis relies solely on detection of the displaced segment in an abnormal position. The position of the displaced segment may not be palpable, and the diagnosis then relies on the inability to find the segment in a normal position. Care must be taken to insure that the segment that appears to be displaced is not in a normal position, but has become too small to palpate from a decrease in the volume of ingesta. The cecum, right dorsal and ventral colons, pelvic flexure, and descending colon can be palpated in most horses.

Evaluation of the wall thickness and mesenteric vessels can reveal venous congestion (mural edema and enlarged blood and lymphatic vessels) or inflammation (mural edema with normal vessels). Disruption of arterial blood flow will not cause venous congestion, but the arterial pulse will not be detected. Mesenteric tears may not be palpable, but the entrapped ischemic intestinal segment may be thickened with edema. Acute or chronic inflammation with cellular infiltration of the intestinal wall may be detected as thickening of the wall without edema. Enlargement of mesenteric lymph nodes may also be noted. Abnormalities in the wall or vessels should be interpreted in light of the size, consistency, and position of the segment of intestine and the clinical signs.

Rectal tears can be detected and carefully evaluated by palpation. Mural masses can be detected in palpable segments of intestine or mesentery; however, if a mass is causing obstruction, the result of the obstruction can be detected in proximal segments of intestine even if the mass is unreachable. Palpation of the mesenteric vessels may reveal thickening and thrombosis, which can lead to ischemia or infarction.

Visual inspection of the mucosa of the rectum and descending colon can be accomplished with a speculum or flexible endoscope. Rectal tears or perforations can be evaluated using these techniques, and mural masses, strictures, or mucosal inflammation can be evaluated. Guided biopsy can also be accomplished. The obvious limitations are the amount of fecal material interfering with the examination and the distance of the lesion of interest from the anus. These techniques offer little advantage over palpation in many cases unless the patient is too small to palpate.

CLINICAL PATHOLOGY

Evaluation of the hemogram is essential when assessing conditions of the large intestine. However, hematologic alterations associated with diseases of the large intestine are often nonspecific, reflecting systemic response to inflammation, endotoxemia, or sepsis. Neutrophilic leukocytosis and normochromic normocytic anemia, with or without hyperfibrinogenemia, are commonly associated with chronic inflammatory conditions of the large intestine. Anemia of chronic blood loss is seen infrequently; usually anemia is secondary to inflammation, as are alterations in the leukon and plasma fibrinogen concentrations. Plasma protein concentrations vary depending on gastrointestinal losses of albumin and globulin, and elevation of globulin concentration from antigenic stimulation. Immunoglobulin quantification can be useful in selected cases; immunosuppression with low IgM concentration has been shown to occur in some cases of lymphosarcoma.[9] Parasitic infections, especially strongylosis, may be characterized by elevated serum IgG(T) concentrations.[10]

Acute disease of the large intestine is not accompanied by significant alterations of the hemogram unless severe inflammation, dehydration, endotoxemia, or sepsis is present. During the early stages of endotoxemia, elevations in circulating concentrations of inflammatory mediators, epinephrine, and cortisol produce characteristic changes in the hemogram. Leukopenia, with neutropenia and a left shift, toxic changes in the neutrophilic cytoplasm, and lymphopenia are seen.[11] Hemoconcentration and hyperfibrinogenemia are also common. Thrombocytopenia, coagulopathies, and disseminated intravascular coagulation (DIC) are also features of endotoxemia. Indeed, thrombocytopenia may be the earliest indicator of sepsis.[12] Endotoxemia and circulating mediators of inflammation activate the coagulation cascade, first causing a hypercoagulable state that can lead to consumption of coagulation factors and coagulation defects, manifested as elevated prothrombin time, partial thromboplastin time, fibrin degradation products, and bleeding time, and reduced activity of antithrombin III.[13–15] During the later stages of endotoxemia, neutrophilic leukocytosis is seen.[13]

The most common serum biochemical abnormalities with diseases of the large intestine are electrolyte imbalances. Serum calcium concentrations are often low, with strangulating obstructions and acute inflammatory diseases of the large intestine.[16] Inflammation of the mucosa can severely disrupt electrolyte fluxes and when diarrhea occurs, sodium, potassium, calcium, and bicarbonate may be lost. Ischemia of the large intestine causing hypoxia and cellular damage may be reflected by an elevated serum phosphate concentration resulting from phosphate leakage from damaged cells.[17] Ischemia and cellular hypoxia also cause a shift in energy metabolism to anaerobic glycolysis, resulting in increased production of lactate and elevated serum lactate concentration.[18, 19] Reduced perfusion of peripheral tissues from hypotensive shock, as well as intestinal ischemia, can cause elevations in serum lactate. However, obstruction of the large intestine during ischemia may result in absorption of lactate from the lumen.[18, 19] Anion gap is an indirect measurement of organic acid production during states of tissue hypoxia, and is a reasonable estimate of serum lactate concentration.[19] Metabolic acidosis may accompany lactic acidemia, but an inconsistent association exists between the two, especially when mixed acid-base imbalances are present.[19, 20]

Hemoconcentration, increases in the circulating red blood cell (RBC) mass (splenic contraction), and changes in RBC deformability from hypoxia or hypocalcemia may increase blood viscosity.[21] Blood viscosity has been shown to increase in patients with acute obstructive disease.[21] Hyperviscosity reduces perfusion of capillary beds, thereby exacerbating ischemia and tissue hypoxia.[21] Hyperviscosity is one manifestation (along with lactic acidemia, coagulopathies, and clinical signs of shock) of the pathophysiologic events that take place during acute inflammatory or vascular injury to the large intestine. Laboratory tests designed to reflect the systemic effects of endotoxemia, ischemia, sepsis, and shock are important to design therapeutic strategies, and monitor response to therapy.

Examination of Peritoneal Fluid. Abdominocentesis and analysis of peritoneal fluid (PF) is a diagnostic technique performed on many patients with disease of the large intestine. Cytologic examination and quantification of peritoneal fluid, white blood cell (WBC) and RBC counts, protein, fibrinogen, lactate, phosphate, and glucose concentration, lactate dehydrogenase (LDH), creatine kinase (CK), and alkaline phosphatase (AP) activity, and pH can be done. The results of PF analysis may help establish a specific diagnosis, but more important, may reflect inflammatory, vascular, or ischemic injury to the large intestine requiring surgical intervention.

A sequence of events takes place during acute vascular injury to the large intestine that is reflected in the PF. First, the PF protein concentration increases, followed by increases in the RBC count and fibrinogen.[22, 23] A transudative process resulting from vascular congestion and increased endothelial permeability allows small molecules (albumin) to escape into the PF, followed by larger molecules (globulin and fibrinogen), and finally diapedesis of cells (RBCs, then WBCs).[22, 23] If ischemic inflammation of the intestine and visceral peritonitis occur, an exudative process ensues. Severe inflammation of the intestine and visceral peritoneum causes large quantities of protein and WBCs, primarily neutrophils, to escape into the PF.[23] As damage to the bowel progresses, the protein concentration and RBC and WBC counts continue to rise. As the degree of irreversible damage to the intestine increases, the PF characteristics become more exudative.[22, 23] Eventually, bacteria begin to translocate across the intestinal wall and appear in the PF as the mucosal barrier breaks down.[22] Neutrophils predominate, and the cytoplasm becomes granulated and Döhle's bodies can be seen. If perforation occurs, bacteria and particles of ingesta appear in the PF, and the neutrophils become degenerate, that is, pyknotic, with karyorrhexis, karyolysis, and smudge cells.[22]

Elevated PF protein concentration is a sensitive indicator of early inflammation, while elevated RBC counts in the presence of normal WBC counts suggest vascular damage without marked tissue ischemia.[23] Elevation of the WBC count usually indicates severe tissue inflammation or intestinal injury.[24] The gross color of the PF can be helpful in detecting injury and necrosis of the intestine. A serosanguinous appearance indicates vascular injury, while an orange or brown-red color indicates necrosis with the release of pigments such as hemosiderin. Serial samples of PF are most useful in determining the nature and extent of damage to the intestine, but in many cases of ischemia, by the time PF abnormalities are seen, irreversible tissue damage has occurred.

Tissue hypoxia and ischemia cause a rapid elevation of peritoneal fluid LDH, CK, and AP activity, and lactate concentration.[18, 19, 25] Phosphate concentration will increase when cellular disruption occurs.[17] Peritoneal fluid enzyme activities, phosphate, and lactate concentration increase faster and higher than serum activities.[17–19, 25] Peritoneal fluid pH and glucose concentration tend to decrease during intestinal ischemia.[26] Although biochemical alterations may provide early indicators of intestinal ischemia and necrosis, they are nonspecific, and offer no advantage over conventional methods of PF analysis in many cases. Peritoneal fluid AP has been shown to arise predominantly from degenerating WBCs, and elevations of other enzyme activities may occur with many inflammatory diseases.[25] Peritoneal fluid pH and glucose concentration may also decrease if infectious peritonitis is present.[26] However, in selected cases where conventional PF analysis and physical examination do not provide sufficient information to develop a treatment plan, biochemical analysis of the PF may be useful.

Chronic inflammatory conditions of the large intestine may be reflected in the cells of the PF examined cytologically, especially eosinophilic or lymphocytic processes.[27] Infectious and inflammatory conditions often cause increases in the neutrophil count, and may be indistinguishable unless bacteria are seen. Neoplastic diseases of the large intestine, other than lymphosarcoma, are rarely detectable by PF examination. Chronic infection and inflammation may be associated with elevated PF protein and fibrinogen concentration. Culture of PF is required to distinguish bacterial infections from noninfectious inflammation unless bacteria can be seen cytologically. However, culture of PF is often unrewarding because factors that are found in inflammatory PF inhibit bacterial growth, and many bacteria in the PF are phagocytosed by leukocytes.[28]

FECAL EXAMINATION

Gross examination of the feces can provide information about digestion and transit time in the large intestine. Large fiber particles in the feces represent poor mastication or poor digestion in the large intestine. Small, mucus-covered, hard fecal balls indicate prolonged transit through the descending colon, whereas increased fluidity implies decreased transit time. Feces containing sand or gravel are not necessarily abnormal. However, a significant amount of sand implies that large quantities are present in the colon. Frank blood indicates substantial bleeding into the distal colon from mucosal damage.

Laboratory analysis of the feces is performed frequently in cases of diarrhea. Fecal cytology and tests for occult blood are used to detect mucosal inflammation, erosion, or ulceration. Severe inflammatory diseases in humans, invasive bacterial infections in particular, have been shown to increase the shedding of leukocytes in the feces.[29] A higher percentage of horses with salmonellosis and diarrhea have fecal leukocyte counts greater than 10 cells per high power field than horses with negative fecal cultures for Salmonella.[29] These results suggest that high fecal leukocyte counts indicate salmonellosis in horses with diarrhea. However, additional work needs to be done to characterize the fecal leukocyte counts in a larger number of horses with known diarrheal disease other than salmonellosis. Low fecal leukocyte counts do not rule out salmonellosis.[29] Fecal occult blood tests are used to detect blood in the feces, presumably from erosion or ulceration of the mucosa. This test does not distinguish the source of the blood. Large volumes of blood (1–2 L) given by nasogastric tube were required to produce a positive test for occult blood in the feces, but the amount of blood originating from the large intestine required to produce a positive test is unknown.[30] A positive test implies significant hemorrhage into the gastrointestinal tract. Newer, more sensitive tests not only detect occult blood but also degraded blood, and may be useful to determine the site and

quantity of blood loss.[30] A positive test implies significant hemorrhage into the gastrointestinal tract.

Bacteriologic examination of the fecal flora has been used to quantitate specific bacterial species in the feces of horses with diarrhea. Quantitation of clostridial species may be beneficial in diagnosing clostridial infection of the large intestine.[31] Tests to detect clostridial toxins in intestinal contents or feces are important to determine whether clostridia cultured from the feces are causing disease. By far, the most common bacterial pathogen isolated from the feces of horses is Salmonella. The number of Salmonella organisms isolated from the feces of horses with clinical salmonellosis is usually higher than from horses with asymptomatic infections. However, the volume of feces in many cases of acute diarrhea is high, and the concentration of Salmonella organisms may be lower than would be expected, accounting for many false-negative fecal cultures. The sensitivity of fecal cultures for detection of Salmonella infection may be as low as 20%.[32] Culture of five consecutive daily fecal samples is recommended to increase the sensitivity of the test. Because salmonella is an intracellular organism, culture of rectal scrapings or a rectal biopsy sample, along with fecal material, may increase the sensitivity of culture for detecting Salmonella infection to 50%.[32]

Qualitative fecal examination is a technique used to detect nematode and cestode ova, protozoan oocysts, parasitic larvae, and protozoan trophozoites. A direct smear of fecal material is a rapid method to screen feces for ova and oocysts and to detect parasite larvae and trophozoites, and to observe motility of ciliates and parasite larvae.[33] Fecal flotation is a more sensitive technique for isolating and detecting ova and oocysts because the eggs are concentrated from the sample. Zinc sulfate and sucrose solutions are often used to concentrate less dense ova and oocysts. Zinc sulfate produces less distortion of trophozoites and larvae than sucrose solutions. Fecal sedimentation is particularly appropriate for ciliates, Giardia, and trichomonads. Quantitative techniques such as the Cornell-McMaster method allow the number of eggs per gram of feces to be estimated, and are most appropriate in monitoring parasite control programs.[33]

RADIOGRAPHY OF THE EQUINE ABDOMEN

Radiography of the adult equine abdomen is an effective technique in detecting radiodense material in the large intestine, such as enteroliths, sand, and metallic objects.[34, 35] The large size and density of the adult abdomen precludes evaluation of soft tissue structures because the detail and contrast of the radiographs are usually poor. Small ponies and miniature horses can be radiographed with a better chance of producing diagnostically useful films. Accumulation of gas can be seen on radiographs of adult horses, but it is often difficult to distinguish normal intestinal gas from obstruction. Horses should be fasted for 24 to 48 hours to reduce the amount of ingesta in the large intestine prior to radiography.

Abdominal radiography is more useful in foals than adult horses. Radiographs are more detailed, and contrast can be good. Radiographic evidence of gas distention in the large intestine may indicate large intestinal obstruction, and radiographic signs of displacement are often diagnostic.[36, 37] Impactions, intussusceptions, foreign bodies and other diseases may be diagnosed with the aid of radiography. Functional ileus may be difficult to distinguish from mechanical obstruction.[36, 37]

HISTOPATHOLOGIC EXAMINATION

Histopathologic examination of tissues from the large intestine is often required to diagnose chronic inflammatory, infiltrative, or neoplastic conditions, and can be useful in evaluating the extent of injury after obstruction or ischemia. Rectal mucosal biopsies are easy to collect with few complications. However, to collect a full-thickness biopsy of the large intestine requires a surgical approach (flank or ventral midline approach). Laparoscopy offers a safer technique to observe the large intestine and abdominal structures.[38] Biopsies of masses, lymph nodes, mesentery, or intestinal serosa can be obtained via laparoscopy.

REFERENCES

1. Sellers AS, Lowe JE: Visualization of auscultation sounds of the large intestine. *Proc Am Assoc Equine Pract* 29:359–363, 1983.
2. Argengio RA: Functions of the large intestine and their interrelationship with disease. *Cornell Vet* 65:303–327, 1975.
3. Adams SB: Equine intestinal motility: An overview of normal activity, changes in disease, and effects of drug administration. *Proc Am Assoc Equine Pract* 33:539–553, 1987.
4. Parry BW, Anderson GA, Gay CC: Prognosis in equine colic: A study of individual variables used in case assessment. *Equine Vet J* 15:337–344, 1983.
5. Kin JN, Gerring EL: Observation on the colic motor complex in a pony with a small intestinal obstruction. *Equine Vet J* 7(suppl):42–43, 1986.
6. Ragle CA, Meagher DM: Abdominal auscultation as an aid to diagnosis of sand colic. *Proc Am Assoc Equine Pract* 33:521–523, 1987.
7. Ragle CA, Meagher DM, Schrader JL, et al: Abdominal auscultation in the detection of experimentally induced gastrointestinal sand accumulation. *J Vet Intern Med* 3:12–14, 1984.
8. Adams SB, McIlwraith CW: Abdominal crisis in the horse: A comparison of presurgical evaluation with surgical findings and results. *Vet Surg* 7:63–69, 1978.
9. Dopson LC, Reed SM, Roth JA, et al: Immunosuppression associated with lymphosarcoma in two horses. *J Am Vet Med Assoc* 182:1239–1241, 1983.
10. Patton S, Mock RE, Drudge JH, et al: Increase of immunoglobulin T concentrations in ponies as a response to experimental infection with the nematode *Strongyles vulgaris. Am J Vet Res* 39:19–22, 1978.
11. Feldman RG: The hemogram: A key to seeing beyond the signs of colic. *Vet Med* 12:935–938, 1988.
12. Porkitt TR, Porkitt PK: Thrombocytopenia of sepsis: The role of circulating IgG-containing immune complexes. *Ann Intern Med* 145:891–894, 1985.
13. Duncan SG, Meyers KM, Reed SM, et al: Alterations in coagulation and hemograms of horses given endotoxin for 24 hours via hepatic portal infusions. *Am J Vet Res* 46:1287–1293, 1985.
14. Johnstone IB: Coagulation abnormalities in cases of equine colic. In Moore JN, White NA, Becht JL, eds: *Proceedings of the Second Equine Colic Research Symposium.* Lawrenceville, NJ, Veterinary Learning Systems, 1986, pp 163–165.
15. Holland M, Kelly AB, Snyder JR, et al: Antithrombin III activities in horses with large colon torsions. *Am J Vet Res* 47:897–899, 1986.
16. Dart AJ, Snyder JR, Spier SJ, et al: Ionized calcium concentrations in horses with surgically managed gastrointestinal disease: 147 cases (1988–1990). *J Am Vet Med Assoc* 201:1244–1248, 1992.
17. Arden WA, Stick JA: Serum and peritoneal fluid phosphate concentrations as predictors of major intestinal injury associated with equine colic. *J Am Vet Med Assoc* 193:927–931, 1988.
18. Moore JN, Owen RR, Lumsden JH: Clinical evaluation of blood lactate levels in equine colic. *Equine Vet J* 8:49–54, 1976.
19. Gosset KA, Cleghorn B, Martin GS: Correlation between anion gap, blood lactate concentrations and survival in horses. *Equine Vet J* 19:29–30, 1987.
20. Gossett KA, French DD, Cleghorn B: Laboratory evaluation of metabolic acidosis. In Moore JN, White NA, Becht JL, eds: *Proceedings of the Second Equine Colic Research Symposium.* Lawrenceville, NJ, Veterinary Learning Systems, 1986, pp 161–167.
21. Andrews FM, Hamlin RL, Stalnaker PS: Blood viscosity in horses with colic. *J Vet Intern Med* 4:183–186, 1990.
22. Morris DD, Johnstone JK: Peritoneal fluid constituents in horses with colic due to small intestinal disease. In Moore JN, White NA, Becht JL, eds: *Proceedings of the Second Equine Colic Research Symposium.* Lawrenceville, NJ, Veterinary Learning Systems, 1986, pp 134–141.
23. Hunt E, Tennant BC, Whitlock RH: Interpretation of peritoneal fluid erythrocyte counts in horses with abdominal disease. In Moore JN, White NA, Becht JL, eds: *Proceedings of the Second Equine Colic Research Symposium.* Lawrenceville, NJ, Veterinary Learning Systems, 1986, pp 134–141.
24. Moore JN, White NA: Acute abdominal disease: Pathophysiology and preoperative management. *Vet Clin North Am Large Animal Pract* 4:61–78, 1982.
25. Turner AS, McIlwraith CW, Trotter GW, et al: Biochemical analysis of serum and peritoneal fluid in experimental colonic infarction in horses. In *Proceedings of the First Equine Colic Research Symposium.* 1982, pp 79–87.
26. Parry BW: Use of clinical pathology in evaluation of horses with colic. *Vet Clin North Am Equine Pract* 3:529–542, 1987.
27. Bach CG, Ricketts SW: Paracentesis as an aid to diagnosis of abdominal disease in the horse. *Equine Vet J* 6:116–121, 1974.
28. Rumbaugh GE, Smith BP, Carlson GP: Internal abdominal abscesses in the horse: A study of 25 cases. *J Am Vet Med Assoc* 172:304–309, 1978.
29. Morris DD, Whitlock RH, Palmer JE: Fecal leukocytes and epithelial cells in horses with diarrhea. *Cornell Vet* 73:265–274, 1983.
30. Pearson EG, Smith BB, McKim JM: Fecal blood determinations and interpretation. *Proc Am Assoc Equine Pract* 33:77–81, 1987.
31. Wierup M, DiPietro JA: Bacteriologic examination of equine fecal flora as a diagnostic tool for equine intestinal clostridiosis. *Am J Vet Res* 42:2167–2619, 1981.
32. Palmer JE, Whitlock RH, Benson CE, et al: Comparison of rectal mucosal cultures and fecal cultures in detecting *Salmonella* infection in horses and cattle. *Am J Vet Res* 46:697–698, 1985.
33. Georgi JR: Antemortem diagnosis. In Georgi JR, ed: *Parasitology for Veterinarians.* Philadelphia, WB Saunders, 1985, pp 228–265.
34. Rose JA, Rose EM, Sande RD: Radiography in the diagnosis of equine enterolithiasis. *Proc Am Assoc Equine Pract* 26:211–220, 1980.

35. Rose JA, Rose EM: Colonic obstruction in the horse. Radiographic and surgical considerations. *Proc Am Assoc Equine Pract* 33:95–101, 1987.
36. Cudd TA, Toal RL, Embertson RM: The use of clinical findings, abdominocentesis, and abdominal radiographs in assessing surgical versus non-surgical abdominal disease in the foal. *Proc Am Assoc Equine Pract* 33:41–33, 1987.
37. Fischer AT, Kerr LY, O'Brien TR: Radiographic diagnosis of gastrointestinal disorders in the foal. *Vet Radiol* 28:42–48, 1987.
38. Fischer AT, Lloyd KCK, Carlson GP, et al: Diagnostic laparoscopy in the horse. *J Am Vet Med Assoc* 189:289–292, 1986.

12.10

Pathophysiology of Colonic Inflammation and Diarrhea

Samuel L. Jones, MS, DVM

Sharon J. Spier, DVM, PhD, Dip ACVIM

Colitis in the horse is a common and often devastating condition that can lead to massive fluid and electrolyte loss, endotoxemia, sepsis, shock, and death.[1] Many causes of colitis are known in other species, but, few causes of colitis have been documented in horses. The pathophysiology of colitis and diarrhea has not been studied extensively in horses. Many pathophysiologic principles of colonic inflammation and diarrhea in horses are extrapolated from work done in other species. However, the basic principles of inflammatory processes in colonic tissue and mechanisms of diarrhea appear to apply to many species, including horses.

INFLAMMATION

The inflammatory process appears to play a central role in the pathogenesis of acute diarrhea from colitis.[2] The colonic mucosa, like other epithelial barriers, is rich in inflammatory and immune cells capable of mounting a rapid and significant inflammatory response to stimulation by antigens or by tissue damage. Secretory diarrhea without inflammation can occur in some species from infection with organisms such as *Vibrio cholerae* or *Escherichia coli* by stimulation of secretory processes in the mucosa by enterotoxins. These events, however, are generally specific to the small intestine.[3] Most organisms that infect the colon and cause diarrhea are invasive, and inflammation of the colon is an important event leading to altered secretion, absorption, and motility in the colon.[4] Noninfectious causes of colitis also appear to initiate diarrhea through inflammatory mechanisms.[5]

Inflammation in the colon can be stimulated by a variety of organisms or toxins. The lamina propria seems to be an important regulatory site of inflammation. Immune and inflammatory cells in the lamina propria have been shown

to be the primary site of production of several inflammatory mediators.[6] Neutrophils have been extensively studied and clearly are responsible for many aspects of the inflammatory reaction in several species.[6-8] Depletion of neutrophils from colonic tissue infected with *Salmonella* prevents the elaboration of some mediators of inflammation, such as prostaglandins.[7] The release of vasoactive lipids (prostaglandins and leukotrienes), as well as proteolytic enzymes, reactive oxygen metabolites, and other mediators, perpetuates the inflammatory reaction, and induces cellular and tissue damage. Activation of the complement cascade has been shown to be an important constituent of inflammation in the colon, primarily by enhancing chemotaxis of neutrophils by components C3a and C5a.[2] Kinins, bacterial products, and leukotriene B_4 are also important constituents of colonic inflammation and have potent chemotactic activity toward neutrophils.[2,4] Mast cells, macrophages, lymphocytes, platelets, and even endothelial cells have important but less clearly defined roles in colonic inflammation.

Upon stimulation of the immune and inflammatory cells of the lamina propria by bacteria or their toxins, mediators of inflammation are released that initiate a cascade of events that may result in diarrhea if not controlled. Prostaglandins, leukotrienes, kinins, histamine, serotonin, platelet activating factor, reactive oxygen metabolites, and other products have been shown not only to be involved in inflammation of the colon but to affect secretion, absorption, and motility as well.[2,3,8-11] Many of the cytokines produced by inflammatory cells appear to affect colonic function through mechanisms mediated by vasoactive lipids, such as prostaglandins E and F (PGE, PGF).[8-10] PGE and PGF have been intensively studied and they are clearly involved in the regulation of secretory activity of colonic mucosal cells in many species, including horses.[3,12,13] Prostaglandin infusion not only increases secretion of water and chloride by colonic mucosa but also increases protein efflux into lymphatics of the colon and across the colonic mucosa.[14] Elevated PGE_1 concentrations have been found in colonic tissue from animals with experimentally produced colitis and from humans with inflammatory bowel disease.[2,14,15] Alterations in chloride and fluid secretion and sodium chloride absorption are blocked by cyclooxygenase inhibitors such as indomethacin and aspirin in several models of colitis, including chemical colitis and infection with some species of *Salmonella*.[3,16]

Histamine and kinins such as bradykinin are released by neutrophils and mast cells during inflammation. Experimental studies have shown that these products are able to affect secretion and absorption in colonic mucosa, and that these effects are in part mediated by prostaglandins.[9,10,17] Histamine also has H_1 receptor–mediated effects on colonic secretion.[17] Kinins can be potent chemotactic factors for neutrophils, stimulating the influx of neutrophils into colonic tissue, potentiating the inflammatory rection. Serotonin has a less clearly defined role in colonic inflammation. Histamine and, to a lesser extent, kinins and serotonin not only play a role in infectious and toxic colitis but are also important in producing colonic secretion and diarrhea during type I hypersensitivity responses, and anaphylaxis.[10,18]

Phagocytic leukocytes, such as neutrophils, produce reactive oxygen metabolites during the respiratory burst via the hexose-monophosphate shunt and the NADPH oxidase enzyme complex.[8] Hydrogen peroxide, superoxides, hypochlorite, hydroxyl radicals, and chloramines are produced.[8] During active inflammation, the ability of the colon to degrade and inactivate these metabolites may be overwhelmed. Reactive oxygen metabolites have been implicated in the production of cellular injury in colonic mucosa and disruption of the interstitial matrix during inflammation.[2, 8] Phagocytes from the colon of human patients with inflammatory bowel disease have elevated reactive oxygen metabolism.[8, 19] Many reactive oxygen metabolites, hydroxyl radicals, hypochlorite, and chloramines in particular, have potent cytotoxic activity by peroxidation of lipid membranes and other mechanisms.[8] In addition, oxygen radicals may play a role in damaging the interstitial matrix by potentiating the activity of proteolytic enzymes released by phagocytic cells during the inflammatory process, and inhibiting antiproteases naturally found in the colonic mucosa that normally prevent protease-induced damage.[8] These mechanisms contribute to the formation of erosions and ulcers during colonic inflammation.[8] Hydrogen peroxide and other oxidants also stimulate secretion via prostaglandin-mediated mechanisms in colonic mucosa.[8] Antioxidants such as 5-aminosalicylic acid, a metabolite of sulfasalazine, are effective in preventing the effects of oxygen radicals on colonic mucosa in experimental models of colitis in laboratory animals.[8]

SECRETION

Secretion by the inflamed colon contributes a large part of the volume of fluid lost in the feces.[20] Both active and passive secretion play a role in the loss of fluid through the mucosa.[2] Active secretion is an energy-dependent process that results in the secretion of electrolytes and consequently water through the mucosal cell, whereas passive secretion is the movement of fluid, solutes, and macromolecules from the vascular compartment to the mucosa and into the lumen by energy-independent processes. Active and passive secretory processes work in concert to effect net secretion in the colon.[21]

The pathophysiology of active electrolyte and water secretion during inflammation and in response to enterotoxins has been extensively studied in the small intestine in many species, but the mechanisms of secretion are less clear in the colon, especially the equine colon. Abnormal secretion of chloride ions seems to be the singular event that governs the loss of fluid and other electrolytes by the colonic mucosa, resulting in the loss of electrolytes and water.[3, 20] Extracellular signals controlling chloride secretion are transduced primarily through two pathways, via the activation of adenyl cyclase and the increase of intracellular cyclic adenosine monophosphate (cAMP) concentrations, or by the activation of calcium channels and the increase of intracellular calcium concentrations.[22] These pathways are not exclusive; in fact they may act synergistically.[23] The role of cyclic guanosine monophosphate (cGMP) in the control of secretion in the small intestine is important, but the role in the colon is less clear. cAMP and calcium activate specific secretory activities, such as calcium-dependent chloride channels, when the intracellular concentrations increase.[2, 22] Chloride secretion increases, which increases the secretion of water directly and by decreasing the absorption of sodium.

Evidence from equine studies and studies in other species

suggests that eicosanoids play an important role in the regulation of active secretion in the colon, primarily by activating adenyl cyclase, but in some instances by increasing intracellular calcium concentration.[6, 12, 13, 15] Acute inflammation of the colon appears to increase secretion by mucosal cells in large part through mechanisms mediated by prostaglandins, especially PGE and PGF, and, to a lesser extent by leukotrienes.[2, 3, 6] Many of the mediators of inflammation increase intracellular concentrations of cAMP and calcium, and therefore secretion, by stimulating the release of arachidonic acid, and the synthesis of prostaglandins. PGE has been shown to increase intracellular cAMP in colonic mucosal cells and secretion of chloride in many species, including horses.[3, 13, 14] Histamine, kinins, reactive oxygen metabolites, platelet activating factor, and other mediators appear to enhance prostaglandin production, primarily by the inflammatory cells of the lamina propria, but also by mucosal cells.[6, 8–11, 17, 19] Prostaglandins also modify neural activity, which exerts some control on secretion by the colonic mucosa, resulting in increased secretion.[6] Lastly, prostaglandins can alter passive secretory activity, discussed later.

Other active mechanisms exist that increase secretion. For example, bacterial enterotoxins are capable of stimulating adenyl cyclase activity directly. The classic example is cholera toxin, but *Salmonella* and *E. coli* produce enterotoxins that interact directly with membrane receptors.[3] Mediators that have been shown to stimulate secretion via prostaglandin production have other effects acting in concert. Histamine can increase secretion by directly stimulating H_1 receptors.[10, 17] Platelet activating factor has been shown to increase colonic secretion by prostaglandin-dependent and prostaglandin-independent mechanisms.[11] Kinins can potentiate the effects of other mediators, and directly modify neural activity, controlling secretion.[9] Clearly, the pathophysiologic mechanisms governing active mucosal secretion of chloride and water causing fluid loss are interwoven and complex. But many of these processes have common themes, and seem to exert their effects on cellular events through similar signal transduction pathways.

The vascular space is the source of the fluid secreted by the colonic mucosa during acute colitis. Passive secretion of fluid in the colon is dependent on the hydraulic conductance of the vascular bed (capillary filtration coefficient), and hydrostatic and oncotic pressures of the interstitium and vascular space as described by Starling's law.[21] Changes in the characteristics of the interstitium and vascular endothelium can profoundly affect the exchange of fluid and solutes from the vascular space and into the interstitial space.[21] The mucosal barrier is also important in that the colonic mucosa is relatively impermeable to electrolytes and water compared to the small intestine, a property dependent on the tight junctions between epithelial cells.[24] Injury to the colonic mucosa or increased active secretion by the mucosal cells, coexisting with increased passive secretory activity originating from the vascular and interstitial tissues, can cause large increases in the rate of fluid and solute secretion into the colonic lumen.[21]

The vascular endothelium has a variety of structural and functional features that render the barrier relatively permeable to water, solutes, and macromolecules. Endothelial fenestrae, endothelial membrane pores, pinocytotic vesicles, the density of intercellular junctions, and transendothelial channels all contribute to the regulation of fluid and macromolecules across the vascular endothelium.[21] Fluid exchange across the endothelium is determined by the capillary filtration coefficient, dependent on the number of perfused capillaries and the number of pores in each capillary, the hydrostatic pressure, and the oncotic pressure in the capillary.[21] These properties can be markedly influenced by colonic inflammation. Inflammatory mediators, such as PGE, kinins, and histamine, not only affect blood pressure and ultimately hydrostatic pressure in the colonic capillaries but also can increase the number of perfused capillaries and increase the permeability of the endothelium.[14, 21] PGE has been shown to increase the passive secretion of fluid, and also of macromolecules such as proteins (albumin).[14] Loss of protein (albumin) during acute colitis can contribute to fluid exchange across the endothelium by decreasing the vascular oncotic pressure and potentiating passive secretory activity.[2]

With a vascular bed as permeable as that found in the colon, it becomes evident that the interstitial matrix is an important regulator of fluid and macromolecule exchange. The interstitial matrix, a gel formed by collagen and mucopolysaccharides (primarily hyaluronic acid), immobilizes interstitial fluid.[21] The hydraulic conductance across the matrix is normally very low. However, the hydraulic conductance is inversely related to the hydration of the matrix (interstitial edema).[21] In addition, the conductance of macromolecules such as albumin is inversely related to the hydration of the matrix.[21] Normally, small fluctuations in Starling's forces do not cause interstitial edema because of factors that resist expansion of the matrix (edema safety factors).[21] However, if these factors are overcome, as in acute colitis, expansion of the matrix greatly increases water and macromolecule flow through the interstitium to the mucosa, ultimately to be secreted into the lumen. Damage to the interstitium during inflammation by proteases, reactive oxygen metabolites, collagenases and other substances released by immune cells (phagocytes), by enzymes and toxins released by invasive bacteria, and by cellular constituents leaking from injured mucosal cells act to disrupt the interstitial matrix, contributing to expansion of the matrix and causing interstitial edema.[3, 7, 8, 21] Interstitial edema is a pathologic feature of many forms of acute colitis that plays an important role in the secretion of fluid and macromolecules, causing diarrhea.

ABSORPTION

The absorptive capacity of the colon is remarkably large. The large intestine of the horse secretes and resorbs a volume of fluid equal to the daily plasma volume, the efficiency of which is dependent on an intact mucosa and tight junctions.[20, 24] Because of the absorptive capacity of the colon, increased secretion of fluid can be compensated for by increased absorption. However, colonic injury is often associated with decreased absorptive capacity by the colonic mucosa, primarily by disruption of the absorptive cells of the mucosa and the tight junctions.[3, 5, 20] Not only is the absorptive activity of the cells altered but the ability of the mucosa to retain absorbed fluid is lost when the tight junctions are disrupted.[20, 24] In fact, the absorptive (apical) cells may be the cells most susceptible to injury by toxins and bacteria.[3, 5] Therefore, even the normal secretory activity of the secretory (crypt) cells of the mucosa overwhelms the

absorptive capacity, and increased secretory activity can lead to massive fluid loss.[24] In addition, mediators of inflammation, such as histamine, and bacterial toxins, such as *Salmonella* enterotoxin and cytotoxin, can inhibit the absorptive ability of the mucosal cells by prostaglandin and non-prostaglandin-mediated mechanisms.[10, 16] Sodium chloride absorption is inhibited by PGE in many species, including horses.[3, 14] Other mediators of inflammation may inhibit absorption in the colon by stimulating the synthesis of prostaglandins by inflammatory and epithelial cells.

MOTILITY

Disturbances in motility patterns occur during inflammatory diseases of the colon, but the role of motility alterations in the pathogenesis of diarrhea remains unclear. Invasive bacteria cause characteristic motor patterns in the colon consisting of rapid bursts of motor activity that appear to decrease transit time through the large intestine.[3] As a result, the clearance of bacteria from the large intestine is reduced, which may contribute to the virulence of the organism.[3] Absorption of endotoxin and the release of inflammatory mediators such as prostaglandins disrupts the motility patterns of the large intestine, resulting in less coordinated contractions, and may contribute to the alterations in motility seen with invasive bacteria.[25] Although the effect of endotoxin and prostaglandins on transit time is not profound, the disruption of coordinated activity may play a role in causing diarrhea.[25] Thorough mixing and prolonged retention time of ingesta are important not only in microbial digestion of nutrients but also in absorption of microbial byproducts and fluid.[20, 26] The ingesta is viscous and therefore must be mixed to bring luminal ingesta in contact with the mucosa for absorption.[26] In addition, poor mixing increases the thickness of the unstirred layer, decreasing contact of ingesta with the mucosa, and decreasing absorption.[20, 26]

Progressive motility must be present, however, if a diarrheal state is to occur.[3, 26] Ileus may be accompanied by increased fluid in the lumen of the large intestine, but without progressive motility the fluid is not passed. Frequently, acute colitis causes a period of ileus that is characterized by scant stool. Diarrhea is only seen when motility returns and the ingesta is passed. Increased progressive motility has been suggested to cause diarrhea by decreasing transit time, and is thought to play a role in irritant catharsis and in the mechanism of action of some laxatives.[27] Irritation and distention increase motility and may well decrease transit time, but increased secretion is also thought to contribute to diarrhea caused by these substances.[24]

REFERENCES

1. Palmer JE, Whitlock RH: Inflammation, infectious, and immune diseases. In Colahan PT, Mayhew IG, Merritt AM, et al, eds: *Equine Medicine and Surgery,* ed 4. Santa Barbara, Calif, American Scientific, 1991, pp 642–656.
2. Murray MJ: Digestive physiology of the large intestine in adult horses. Part II: Pathophysiology of colitis. *Compendium Continuing Educ Pract Vet* 10:1309–1316, 1988.
3. O'Loughlin EV, Scott RB, Gall DG: Pathophysiology of infectious diarrhea: Changes in intestinal structure and function. *J Pediatr Gastroenterol Nutr* 12:5–20, 1991.

4. Gianella RA: Pathogenesis of acute bacterial diarrheal disorders. *Annu Rev Med* 32:341–357, 1981.

5. Roberts MC, Clarke LL, Johnson CM: Castor-oil induced diarrhea in ponies: A model for acute colitis. *Equine Vet J* 7(suppl):60–67, 1986.

6. Bern MJ, Sturbaum CW, Karaylacin SS, et al: Immune system control of rat and rabbit colonic electrolyte transport: Role of prostaglandins and enteric nervous system. *J Clin Invest* 83:1810–1820, 1989.

7. Gianella RA: Importance of the intestinal inflammatory reaction in *Salmonella*-mediated intestinal secretion. *Infect Immun* 23:140–145, 1979.

8. Yamada T, Grisham MB: Role of neutrophil-derived oxidants in the pathogenesis of intestinal inflammation. *Klin Wochenschr* 69:988–994, 1991.

9. Gaginella TS, Kachur JF: Kinins as mediators of intestinal secretion. *Am J Physiol* 256:G1–G15, 1989.

10. Wang YZ, Cooke HJ, Su HC, et al: Histamine augments colonic secretion in guinea pig distal colon. *Am J Physiol* 258:G432–G439, 1990.

11. Buckley TL, Hoult JRS: Platelet activating factor is a potent colonic secretagogue with actions independent of specific PAF receptors. *Eur J Pharmacol* 163:275–283, 1989.

12. Clarke LL, Argenzio RA: NaCl transport across equine proximal colon and the effect of endogenous prostaglandins. *Am J Physiol* 259:G62–G69, 1990.

13. Rachmilewitz D: Prostaglandins and diarrhea. *Dig Dis Sci* 25:897–899, 1980.

14. Granger DN, Shackleford JS, Taylor AE: PGE-induced intestinal secretion: Mechanism of enhanced transmucosal protein efflux. *Am J Physiol* 5:E788–E796, 1979.

15. Racusen LC, Binder HJ: Effect of prostaglandin on ion transport across isolated colonic mucosa. *Dig Dis Sci* 25:900–903, 1980.

16. Gianella RA, Gots RE, Charney AN, et al: Pathogenesis of *Salmonella*-mediated intestinal fluid secretion: Activation of adenylate cyclase and inhibition by indomathacin. *Gastroenterology* 69:1238–1245, 1975.

17. Hardcastle J, Hardcastle PT: Involvement of prostaglandin in histamine-induced fluid and electrolyte secretion by rat colon. *J Pharm Pharmacol* 40:106–110, 1988.

18. Castro GA, Harari Y, Russell D: Mediators of anaphylaxis-induced ion transport changes in small intestine. *Am J Physiol* 253:G176–G183, 1985.

19. Karayalcin SS, Sturbaum CW, Wacksman JT, et al: Hydrogen peroxide stimulates rat colonic prostaglandin production and alters electrolyte transport. *J Clin Invest* 86:60–68, 1990.

20. Argenzio RA: Physiology of diarrhea—Large intestine. *J Am Vet Med Assoc* 173:667–672, 1978.

21. Granger DN, Barrowman JA: Microcirculation of the alimentary tract. I: Physiology of transcapillary fluid and solute exchange. *Gastroenterology* 84:846–868, 1983.

22. Böhme M, Diener M, Rummel W: Calcium and cyclic AMP–mediated responses in isolated colonic crypts. *Pflugers Arch* 419:144–151, 1991.

23. Cartwright CA, McRoberts JA, Mandel KG, et al: Synergistic action of cyclic AMP and calcium mediated chloride secretion in a colonic cell line. *J Clin Invest* 76:1837–1843, 1985.

24. Ewe K: Intestinal transport in constipation and diarrhoea. *Pharmacology* 36:73–84, 1988.

25. King JN, Gerring EL: The action of low dose endotoxin on equine bowel motility. *Equine Vet J* 23:11–17, 1991.

26. Read NW: Colon: Relationship between epithelial transport and motility. *Pharmacology* 36(suppl 1):120–125, 1988.

27. Adams SB: Equine intestinal motility: An overview of normal activity, changes in disease, and effects of drug administration. *Proc Am Assoc Equine Pract* 33:539–553, 1987.

12.11

Inflammatory Diseases of the Large Intestine Causing Diarrhea

Samuel L. Jones, MS, DVM
Sharon J. Spier, DVM, PhD, Dip ACVIM

INFECTIOUS DISEASES

Salmonellosis

Pathogenesis

Salmonella is a genus of gram-negative facultatively anaerobic bacteria that is a common gastrointestinal pathogen in horses. Many serotypes of *Salmonella* have been reported to infect horses, but those classified in group B appear to be more commonly associated with disease than those in other groups. Group B includes *Salmonella typhimurium* and *Salmonella agona,* two of the species most frequently isolated from horses.[1–3] *Salmonella typhimurium* is the most pathogenic serotype in horses, and is associated with a higher case fatality rate than other species of *Salmonella.*[1] Approximately 10% to 20% of horses are inapparently infected with and actively shed *Salmonella,* and are a potential source of infection to susceptible horses.[1, 4] The virulence of the bacteria varies with serotype and even among strains of the same serotype. Host susceptibility plays an important role in the pathogenicity of particular organisms. The infective dose is generally on the order of millions of organisms inoculated orally, but various environmental and host factors can reduce the infective dose to a few thousand or even hundreds of organisms.[5–7] Environmental factors or stresses are not well defined, but it is known that high ambient temperature, for example, can greatly increase the prevalence of *Salmonella* infections in horses.[6, 7] In fact, the peak incidence of salmonellosis in horses occurs in late summer and fall.[6, 7] Other environmental and host factors that affect susceptibility to infection include transportation, antibiotic administration, gastrointestinal surgery, general anesthesia, preexisting diseases, and immunosuppression.[1, 7]

Host factors that restrict gastrointestinal colonization and invasion by pathogens include gastric pH, normal gastrointestinal flora, gastrointestinal motility, and immunity.[1, 8] Acidic pH in the stomach is important in preventing live organisms from reaching the intestine.[8] Altering the gastric pH, with histamine H_2 receptor antagonists, for example, may increase susceptibility to infection. Gastrointestinal flora inhibit the proliferation and colonization of *Salmonella* by secreting bacteriocins, short-chain fatty acids, and other substances that are toxic to *Salmonella.*[8] In addition, the normal flora compete for nutrients and space, especially on the mucosa.[8] Being predominantly anaerobic, the normal flora maintain a low oxidation-reduction potential in the environment of the large intestine, which inhibits the growth of many bacterial pathogens.[10] The importance of normal host gastrointestinal ecology is illustrated by the fact that disturbances of the colonic flora with antibiotics, changes in feed, or underlying gastrointestinal disease markedly increases the susceptibility of the host to infection by *Salmonella,* often resulting in serious disease. Peristaltic activity tends to control the population of pathogens by mechanically removing them from the colon.

The immune status of the host may be one of the most important factors determining not only the susceptibility to *Salmonella* infections but also the degree of invasion and subsequent outcome of the infection. Local immunity, such as antibody secretion, prevents colonization of the mucosa.[8, 11] Opsonizing antibodies and activation of the complement cascade are important in fighting systemic invasion by *Salmonella* by increasing the efficiency of phagocytosis and by direct bactericidal activity. Humoral immunity, however, is often ineffective in preventing disease and dissemination once invasion occurs. *Salmonella* possesses protective mechanisms that enable the organism to escape many host immune functions, such as phagocytosis, lysosomal killing, and complement binding.[8–11] In addition, *Salmonella* is capable of surviving and multiplying within cells, rendering humoral (noncellular) immune systems ineffective.[12] Specific cellular immunity may be the most effective defense mechanism in the host arsenal against systemic infections by *Salmonella.*[11, 12] Protective immunity in horses and calves may be induced by oral inoculation with small numbers of virulent organisms, but the duration of the immunity is not known.[13, 14] Oral and parenteral vaccines using killed or attenuated organisms and bacterial products have been promising, but are effective only against homologous organisms, and are usually not cross-protective among different serogroups.[13, 14]

Bacteria that infect the large intestine are generally invasive.[8] In horses, *Salmonella* primarily infects the cecum and proximal colon. The pathogenicity of *Salmonella* is dependent upon the ability of the bacteria to invade the gastrointestinal mucosa.[8, 9] The virulence factors that determine pathogenicity are not well defined, but several factors have been identified. First the bacteria must migrate to and adhere to colonic mucosa. The mucosa releases factors that are chemotactic to *Salmonella,* increasing the number of organisms on the surface of the mucosa.[8] Enzymes produced by the bacteria that break down the mucosal barrier have been suggested to enhance colonization.[8] Adherence of *Salmonella* to the mucosal cells is accomplished by interaction between certain protein structures, such as pili and fimbrae, and receptors on the mucosal cell surface.[8, 9] Pili have been shown to bind to the carbohydrate moiety of glycoprotein receptors on mucosal cells.[9] Receptor proteins must be present and available on mucosal cell membranes for adherence to occur. Absence of receptors may render individuals or species resistant to infection by certain gastrointestinal pathogens, such as enterotoxigenic *Escherichia coli.*[8] Lipopolysaccharide and inflammatory mediators elaborated during invasion of the mucosa disrupt motility patterns of the large intestine, decreasing the clearance of bacteria from the luminal contents.[15, 16]

Invasion of the mucosa occurs by penetration of the apical membrane of the mucosal cell, transcytosis across the cell, and penetration through the basolateral membrane.[9] Infection of epithelial cells, as well as macrophages and other cells of the lamina propria, occurs.[9] Invasion is facilitated by toxins produced by *Salmonella.* Lipopolysaccharide (endotoxin) is an important virulence factor that has been shown to increase, but is not required for, invasion of the mucosa.[8–10] *Salmonella* produces at least two exotoxins. One is a cytotoxin that inhibits protein synthesis in mucosal cells, causing morphologic damage and increased permeability of mucosal cells.[17] Presumably, this toxin directly affects the ability of the organism to invade by injuring mucosal cells. *Salmonella* also produces an enterotoxin that is similar to the heat-labile (LT) toxin produced by *E. coli.*[18, 19] The enterotoxin has been shown to increase secretion of chloride and water, and decrease absorption of sodium chloride by colonic mucosal cells in many species, including horses, by increasing intracellular cAMP concentration.[18–20] Direct stimulation of membrane receptors by the *Salmonella* enterotoxin may occur, as with LT toxin. However, evidence suggests that *Salmonella* enterotoxin stimulates the release of prostaglandins which in turn stimulate cAMP synthesis in the mucosal cells.[19, 21] The effects of both exotoxins contribute to mucosal damage and fluid loss in the feces.

Once *Salmonella* has invaded the mucosa, dissemination to other tissues occurs via the reticuloendothelial system.[9] Cytotoxin may aid in dissemination by allowing spread through the tissues of the colon.[8, 17] Motility of the bacteria may also contribute to the ability to disseminate, since flagella are an established virulence factor.[8–10] Dissemination may be local, to the mesenteric lymph nodes, or systemic, to the blood, spleen, liver, etc. Survival in the host is enhanced by the ability of *Salmonella* to resist digestion by phagocytes, resist binding of complement and antibodies in serum, mobilize iron stores, and survive intracellularly.[8, 9, 13] Both the O-specific side chains of cell wall endotoxin and capsular proteins are important in mediating resistance to host immunity.[8–10, 13]

Some virulence factors are encoded by chromosomal genes, but others are encoded by plasmids. Plasmid virulence factors can easily be spread to other *Salmonella* species of the same or different serotypes, and even to other gram-negative bacteria. Antibiotic resistance is well documented to be encoded by plasmids, but virulence plasmids have been identified that encode the ability to invade beyond the intestine, and encode serum resistance.[9, 22, 23]

The virulence of *Salmonella,* as mentioned previously, is related to invasiveness, but the ability to stimulate an inflammatory response plays a central role in the pathogenesis of diarrhea.[24] Invasive species of *Salmonella* have been shown to increase secretion most effectively in vitro when inflammation of the colonic mucosa is produced.[24] In addition, the presence of neutrophils is important in order to stimulate secretion by colonic mucosal cells.[24] Inflammatory mediators, such as prostaglandins, leukotrienes, reactive oxygen metabolites, and histamine, are potent stimulators of chloride secretion in the colon of many species.[8, 16, 25] Macrophages, in response to bacterial toxins (exotoxin and endotoxin) and other bacterial products, produce a variety of cytokines that activate the immune and inflammatory systems. Activation of neutrophils and other inflammatory cells by cytokines released by macrophages and lymphocytes results in the release of many of the mediators of inflammation that produce both morphologic and physiologic alterations.

Most of the inflammatory mediators studied stimulate colonic secretion by prostaglandin-dependent mechanisms, resulting in either increased intracellular cAMP or calcium concentrations, or both, in mucosal cells.[16] In addition, these mediators may stimulate active and passive secretion by prostaglandin-independent mechanisms, inhibit sodium and water absorption, cause motility disturbances, and potentiate tissue injury, all of which enhance the pathogenicity and dissemination of *Salmonella,* and contribute to the pathogenesis of diarrhea.[16, 25] Potentially massive losses of electrolytes, water, and protein can occur. Systemic metabolic disturbances, such as endotoxemia and septicemia, may result from systemic invasion of the bacteria.

Clinical Signs and Diagnosis

Four clinical syndromes of *Salmonella* infection have been documented clinically and reproduced experimentally: (1) inapparent infections with latent or active carrier states; (2) depression, fever, anorexia, and neutropenia without diarrhea or colic; (3) fulminant or peracute enterocolitis with diarrhea; and (4) septicemia.[21, 26] Septicemia and enterocolitis may occur concurrently. Inapparent infections can be activated in compromised horses, such as horses with colic or horses being treated with antibiotics, causing mild-to-severe enterocolitis. In addition, latent infections (nonshedding) can become active infections (shedding) under certain conditions, such as transportation stress and antibiotic treatment. Horses with depression, anorexia, fever, and neutropenia without diarrhea generally have a good prognosis, and recover in several days without specific treatment.[26] The focus of this discussion is on acute enterocolitis.

Acute enterocolitis is characterized by severe fibrinonecrotic typhlocolitis, with interstitial edema and intramural vascular thrombosis.[1] Severe ulceration of the large intestinal mucosa may occur, with serosal ecchymoses and congestion. The earliest signs of enterocolitis are usually fever and anorexia.[1, 7] Signs of colic may be seen early in the course of the disease, especially if ileus is present. Clinical signs of endotoxemia are common, and range from fever, elevated heart and respiratory rates, poor peripheral perfusion, and ileus, to fulminant and rapidly progressive signs of endotoxemic shock. Oral mucous membranes are often pale with a dark gingival margin, but may be brick-red or reddish-blue, with prolonged capillary refill time. Weakness, muscle fasciculations, cold extremities, and other signs suggestive of sepsis and shock; synchronous diaphragmatic flutter; abdominal pain; and marked metabolic and electrolyte abnormalities may be noted in severe cases of enterocolitis. Signs of mild-to-moderate dehydration may be noted before diarrhea is seen; however, once diarrheal feces are evident, dehydration may become rapidly severe. Occasionally, horses die peracutely, without developing diarrhea.

Diarrhea may not be seen for several days, but usually occurs by 24 to 48 hours after the fever is noted.[1, 7] The duration of the diarrhea may be days to weeks. The character of the first diarrheal feces is usually watery with particles of roughage, but may rapidly become fluid without solid material. Finding frank blood and fibrin in the feces is unusual. The volume of feces is often large, with frequent defecation. Straining or signs of colic may be noted when the patient is defecating, and rectal prolapse may occasionally occur. Abdominal borborygmi are often absent early in the course

of the disease because of ileus, but become evident later, usually when diarrhea begins. Fluid and gas sounds are commonly heard, but normal progressive motility is less frequently heard than normally. Transrectal palpation may reveal edematous rectal mucosa and colon and fluid-filled colon and cecum. Gastric reflux may be obtained, especially early in the course when ileus is evident.

Hematologic abnormalities early in the course of the disease include moderate-to-severe neutropenia, lymphopenia, and leukopenia, a mild-to-moderate left shift, and toxic changes in the neutrophils.[1] Thrombocytopenia, moderate-to-severe hemoconcentration, and hyperfibrinogenemia are also common. Neutropenia is an early but nonspecific indicator of salmonellosis, often occurring concurrently with the onset of fever.[1] Later in the course of disease, neutrophilic leukocytosis may be seen, indicating recovery. A degenerating left shift, with metamyelocytes and myelocytes seen in the peripheral blood, is a poor prognostic sign.

Serum biochemical analysis may reveal azotemia, elevations in serum sorbitol dehydrogenase and γ-glutamine aminotransferase activity, and elevated serum lactic acid concentration. Azotemia is often prerenal, but acute renal failure may be seen in severely dehydrated, endotoxemic, or septicemic patients, especially patients receiving nephrotoxic drugs. Hyponatremia may also contribute to prerenal azotemia. Elevations in hepatocellular enzymes are usually mild, and reflect damage to the hepatocytes from such absorbed toxins as endotoxin. Lactic acidemia is usually a result of poor perfusion. Plasma protein rapidly drops, as protein is lost in the gastrointestinal tract, causing moderate-to-severe hypoalbuminemia and hypoglobulinemia. Hypokalemia, hyponatremia, hypochlorinemia, and hypocalcemia are common electrolyte abnormalities in patients with enterocolitis. Metabolic acidosis is also common. Coagulopathies, such as decreased antithrombin III activity and disseminated intravascular coagulation (DIC), may be noted. Urinalysis may reveal isosthenuria, proteinuria, hematuria, cylindruria, and glucosuria if renal disease is present. The number of leukocytes in the feces is usually elevated, and occult blood may be detected. Peritoneal fluid is usually normal except when severe mural inflammation or colonic infarction occurs.

Diagnosis of salmonellosis is routinely accomplished by frequent culture of large samples (10–30 g) of feces using enrichment techniques.[1, 27] However, the sensitivity of fecal culture can be as low as 30% to 50%, even if several fecal samples collected daily are cultured.[27] Concurrent culture of rectal biopsy specimens and feces increases the sensitivity of culture techniques to 60% to 75%.[27] Culture of peripheral blood may allow isolation of the organism if bacteremia or septicemia is present, but is less sensitive than culture of feces. Young animals and foals are more likely to become septicemic, but culture of blood is recommended in all cases with signs suggestive of septicemia. Increased numbers of fecal leukocytes suggest an invasive process in the colon, but are not specific for salmonellosis.

Early in the course of the disease, dehydration, electrolyte and acid-base imbalances, endotoxemia, and sepsis may be life-threatening. Aggressive treatment during the acute stages to replace fluids lost in the diarrhea and to control sepsis and endotoxemia is often effective in controlling the primary disease. Weight loss and hypoproteinemia are often severe. Complications such as laminitis, acute renal failure, venous thrombosis and septic phlebitis, peripheral edema accumulation, irreversible protein-losing enteropathy or chronic malabsorption, pulmonary aspergillosis, and gastrointestinal infarction can occur. In many instances, horses recover from acute salmonellosis with aggressive treatment, only to succumb to complications of the disease, partially explaining the high fatality rate of equine salmonellosis compared to human salmonellosis. Chronic, mild-to-moderate diarrhea is occasionally seen in horses after a bout of severe salmonellosis, usually with protein-losing enteropathy. If the chronic diarrhea persists beyond 4 to 5 weeks after the onset of signs, the prognosis for recovery is poor.[7]

Treatment

The principles of therapy for salmonellosis include replacement of fluid and electrolyte losses, control of colonic inflammation and reduction of fluid secretion, control of endotoxemia and sepsis, and reestablishment of normal flora. Prompt treatment is essential to prevent life-threatening metabolic disturbances and to minimize complications, and aggressive treatment may be required.

Replacement of fluid and electrolyte losses is of primary concern in treating horses with salmonellosis. Depending on the severity of the disease, fluid losses may be minimal or massive. Fluid and electrolytes can be administered by two routes, orally or intravenously. Some horses with mild-to-moderate diarrhea may maintain hydration and electrolyte balance by consuming water and electrolytes voluntarily. Fresh water and water containing electrolytes should be available in all cases. In many instances, periodic nasogastric intubation and administration of water and electrolytes via the tube may be sufficient to maintain hydration. In more severe cases, indwelling nasogastric tubes can be maintained, and up to 4 to 8 L of fluid can be administered by the tube every 20 to 30 minutes, if ileus is not evident. However, intravenous administration of fluids is preferred in most cases, requiring significant quantities of fluid to replace and maintain hydration and electrolyte balance. It is not unusual for patients with severe diarrhea to require large volumes (50–100 L/day) of intravenous fluids to maintain hydration. Frequent monitoring of packed cell volume, serum electrolyte concentration, venous blood gases or total serum carbon dioxide, blood urea nitrogen (BUN) and creatinine, urine cytology and biochemistry, and body weight is important to monitor hydration, electrolyte and acid-base balance, and kidney function.

Isotonic sodium chloride or lactated Ringer's solution is frequently used to restore and maintain fluid and electrolyte balance. Potassium chloride can be added to the fluids and administered at a rate up to 0.5 to 1.0 mEq/kg/hr. Generally, a rate of less than 0.5 mEq/kg/hr is used. Hypertonic NaCl solutions (1–2 L of 3%–5% NaCl) have been used in horses that are severely hyponatremic (<120 mEq/dL). Hypertonic solutions should not be administered to severely dehydrated horses, but have been used clinically without complication and with considerable beneficial effect in hemoconcentrated patients showing signs suggestive of endotoxemia. The beneficial effects of hypertonic NaCl are short-lived (30–60 minutes). Isotonic solutions should be administered concurrently, or immediately following administration of hyper-

tonic NaCl solutions. Isotonic (1.3%) or hypertonic (5.0%) sodium bicarbonate solutions are used to correct metabolic acidosis. Prolonged administration of sodium-containing fluids may promote diuresis and renal water loss or accumulation of peripheral edema, and should be used conservatively when a relative free water loss is noted. Administration of isotonic dextrose (5%) solution may be beneficial when free water loss (relative sodium excess) is evident.

Control of colonic inflammation and secretion is a difficult and poorly studied aspect of salmonellosis. The role of inflammation and mediators such as prostaglandins and leukotrienes as a cause of fluid loss is well known during *Salmonella* infection. Cyclooxygenase inhibitors (nonsteroidal anti-inflammatory drugs, NSAIDs) and lipoxygenase inhibitors have antisecretory effects when studied using models of salmonellosis, and the clinical benefits of using such drugs have been speculated on.[8, 18–21, 24] In fact, NSAIDs are commonly administered to horses with salmonellosis. However, NSAIDs have been shown to exacerbate colonic inflammation in humans with inflammatory colitis, and have well-documented detrimental effects on colonic mucosa in horses.[28, 29] Gastric ulceration is not unusual in horses with enterocolitis, and may be related to treatment with NSAIDs. No work has been done to study the effect of NSAIDs on colonic mucosa during enterocolitis in horses. Prostaglandins such as prostaglandin E (PGE) are cytoprotective to gastrointestinal mucosa, and the doses of NSAIDs used pharmacologically to inhibit colonic inflammation and secretion may in fact be detrimental if not used judiciously. Shunting of arachidonic acid metabolism toward the lipoxygenase pathway and increased synthesis of leukotrienes has been suggested to contribute to mucosal damage from NSAIDs.[30]

Specific lipoxygenase inhibitors are not available for clinical use; however, calcium channel blockers have been used to inhibit leukotriene synthesis, since calcium is required for lipoxygenase activity. Verapamil, for instance, significantly reduced tissue concentrations of leukotriene B_4 (LTB_4), improved fluid absorption, and decreased ulceration in experimentally produced models of colonic inflammation in rats, without affecting secretion.[30] Development of treatment strategies that inhibit leukotriene synthesis in horses with colitis may prove to be beneficial in reducing inflammation and fluid loss, and preventing some of the detrimental effects of NSAIDs.

In light of the role of reactive oxygen metabolites in colonic inflammation, free radical scavengers have been advocated to reduce the effects of these molecules. Sulfasalazine metabolites have been shown to reduce reactive oxygen metabolite–induced colonic inflammation in other species, and sulfasalazine has been used to treat chronic inflammatory disease in horses, but has not been used to treat acute inflammation. The only practical free radical scavenger used in horses is dimethyl sulfoxide (DMSO). DMSO 0.1 to 1.0 g/kg IV q.12–24h. in a 10% solution has been used in clinical cases of colitis, but its efficacy has not been established. Bismuth subsalicylate solutions administered orally are often used to decrease inflammation and secretion in the colon. In adult horses, the volume of solution necessary to be beneficial is large (3–4 L, q.4–6h.). Often, the solution is administered twice daily instead of four to six times daily. If a beneficial effect is not achieved within 3 to 4 days of treatment, administration of bismuth subsalicylate solution is discontinued. More frequent administration can be accomplished in foals, and clinical improvement is more often seen in foals than in adult horses.

Endotoxemia frequently occurs in patients with salmonellosis. Oral administration of activated charcoal and mineral oil is commonly used to reduce absorption of endotoxin. Low doses of NSAIDs such as flunixin meglumine 0.1 to 0.25 mg/kg IV q.6–8h. inhibit eicosanoid synthesis induced by endotoxin. Flunixin meglumine has been shown to inhibit eicosanoid production and reduce the severity of clinical signs of endotoxemia at these doses when administered prior to endotoxin.[31] In addition, NSAIDs are administered to prevent laminitis from endotoxemia, a devastating complication of salmonellosis. It is clear that the benefits of NSAIDs outweigh the risks of gastrointestinal damage, but judicious use is recommended.

Treatment with plasma harvested from donor horses immunized with rough mutants of *E. coli* (J5) or *S. typhimurium* has been used to prevent systemic effects of endotoxin, and has been shown to be beneficial in horses with clinical endotoxemia from gastrointestinal disease.[32] In addition, plasma provides an important source of protein for hypoproteinemic patients, and may provide an important source of other proteins, such as antithrombin III. Large volumes (6–8 L/day) may be required to significantly increase and maintain plasma protein concentration. Both oral and intravenous routes have been used to administer plasma to horses with enterocolitis, but the intravenous route is preferred.

Treatment with antibiotics is controversial in horses with salmonellosis. Treatment with antibiotics is not thought to alter the course of the enterocolitis. However, in neutropenic patients, or patients with signs of septicemia, administration of broad-spectrum antibiotics is recommended. Neutropenia is associated with an increased risk of septicemia and septic complications, such as septic phlebitis and infection of surgical sites.[1] Septicemia is a potential life-threatening complication of enterocolitis, and may be caused by *Salmonella* or by other enteric bacteria that invade the injured colon. Lipid-soluble antibiotics are ideally suited for *Salmonella* infections, since the bacteria can live intracellularly. Potentiated sulfa drugs, such as trimethoprim-sulfadiazine and chloramphenicol, have been advocated for this reason. Additionally, third-generation cephalosporins or combinations of penicillin and aminoglycosides are useful in neutropenic patients to prevent bacteremia and septic complications.

Heparin has been suggested to prevent laminitis in equine models of endotoxemia, and is commonly administered to horses with enterocolitis for this reason.[33] In addition, hypercoagulability is a common complication of enterocolitis, presumably from endotoxemia. Administration of heparin 20 to 80 IU/kg SQ or IV q.6–12h. may prevent thrombosis in these patients, provided antithrombin III concentrations are adequate in the plasma. Concentrated sources of antithrombin III are not available for use in horses, but whole plasma may provide an important source. Treatment with heparin is thought to decrease thrombosis, especially of the jugular vein, a serious complication of salmonellosis. Low-dose aspirin treatment (15 mg/kg PO q.24–48h.) in conjunction with heparin treatment may provide added benefit by irreversibly inhibiting platelet function.[34] Heparin may also enhance the phagocytotic activity of the reticuloendothelial system by enhancing the efficiency of opsonins such as fibronectin

and immunoglobulin, thereby stimulating phagocytosis of products of coagulation and possibly other particles, including bacteria.[35, 36]

Maintenance of the bacterial flora and antagonism of pathogenic bacteria such as *Salmonella* in the gastrointestinal tract is an important defense mechanism preventing colonization by pathogenic bacteria. The use of probiotic preparations containing beneficial bacteria has been shown to prevent colonization of pathogenic bacteria, including *Salmonella,* in poultry.[37] Little work has been done to investigate the efficacy of these products in preventing salmonellosis in horses, but ongoing studies may provide important information in this regard. Probiotic and other preparations designed to restore normal flora to the gastrointestinal tract, such as fecal suspensions, sour milk, and yogurt, have been used clinically to shorten the course of salmonellosis, with variable results. Therefore, prevention of infection by using probiotic agents and other means is important. Exposure of susceptible horses to *Salmonella* should be avoided, but is a difficult task, especially since asymptomatic infections are common and the bacteria are ubiquitous in the environment. Prophylactic use of probiotic preparations, judicious use of antibiotics in susceptible horses, control of environmental conditions such as temperature, and minimalization of exposure to pathogenic bacteria are important in control of salmonellosis.

Good nursing care and adequate nutrition are vital to the treatment of horses with salmonellosis. Salmonellosis is a severely catabolic disease, increasing caloric requirements greatly. Normal intake of roughage to provide energy may be inadequate; however, feeding of grains must be done carefully to prevent carbohydrate overload. Enteral and parenteral nutrition (total and partial) have been used successfully to provide calories to anorectic horses. Catheter care and strictly aseptic drug and fluid administration must be the rule. Grooming, exercise, and foot care provide immeasurable benefits in patient attitude and well-being that are frequently overlooked.

Potomac Horse Fever

Pathogenesis

Potomac horse fever (equine monocytic ehrlichiosis) is caused by the obligate intracellular rickettsial organism *Ehrlichia risticci.*[38–40] The disease is most common from late summer to early fall, with a peak incidence in July and August.[38] The disease was first described in the Northeast, but has since been discovered in most areas of the continental United States, with a particularly high prevalence in the Northeast and Midwest. The geographical distribution is characterized by a significantly higher percentage of cases found along waterways and rivers.[38] The disease occurs sporadically, both temporally and geographically, and can affect any age group of horses. The epidemiologic data, the fact that many other rickettsial diseases are transmitted by insect vectors, and the finding that the disease can be transmitted via whole blood have implicated insects such as ticks and biting flies as vectors, but the mode of transmission is as yet unknown.[38] Attempts to transmit the disease experimentally with ticks (*Dermacentor variablis*) or biting flies (*Stomoxys calcitrans*) have been unsuccessful.[41, 42] Oral transmission has not been ruled out.

The pathogenesis of *E. risticci* has not been extensively studied. Experimental transmission has been produced by inoculation of infected whole blood and cultured cell lines via parenteral and oral routes.[39, 43] However, it is not known how natural infection occurs. The organism can be found in blood monocytes during natural infections, but the sequence of events resulting in enterocolitis remains speculative. The organism appears to first infect blood monocytes, which may be the vehicle of organ infection.[39, 44] The target organ is the gastrointestinal mucosa, with the most severe lesions found in the large intestine.[44, 45] Infection of human colonic cells in vitro does not cause major cytopathologic effects for several days.[46] Disruption of the microvilli in the region of the plasma membrane where sodium chloride channels are located has been observed in human colonic cell cultures.[46] Infection in horses is associated with variable degrees of morphologic damage.[44, 45] Mild morphologic damage and mononuclear cell infiltration of the lamina propria occur early during the infection, but fibrinous, necrotizing typhlocolitis with severe mucosal ulceration and inflammation of the lamina propria may occur later in the disease. Vasculitis and intravascular coagulation are consistent features in the large intestine, with perivascular edema.[45] *Ehrlichia risticci* can be observed in mucosal cells and macrophages and mast cells of the lamina propria.[44, 45] Evidence suggests that the organism can survive and multiply in macrophages by avoiding lysosomal digestion by inhibiting phagosome-lysosome fusion.[47] Oxytetracycline appears to prevent the mechanism by which *E. risticci* inhibits lysosomal fusion in vitro.[47]

Evidence of impaired sodium chloride absorption in the colon has been suggested to contribute to diarrhea in infected horses, and may be related to destruction of the membrane structure in the region of sodium chloride channels.[46, 48] Direct injury to the mucosa by *E. risticci* and colonic inflammation are likely to be prominent features leading to diarrhea, especially later in the disease.[45] Fluid, protein, and electrolyte loss is likely to be due to increased passive and active fluid secretion. Effects of inflammatory mediators on the vascular system, interstitium, and mucosa are well known to increase passive and active secretion and decrease active absorption. Vasculitis, along with increased vascular permeability induced by inflammatory mediators, causes interstitial edema, which disrupts the interstitial matrix, potentiating passive secretion and fluid and protein loss. Altered mucosal permeability from cellular injury and ulceration results in reduced absorption of fluid and sodium. In addition, inflammation of the large intestine may well disrupt motility, contributing to the diarrhea. Injury to the intestinal mucosa, particularly in the large intestine, results in the absorption of bacterial products, such as endotoxin, and translocation of bacteria. Endotoxemia and septicemia are potential complications of *E. risticci* infections, and contribute to the clinical signs seen during the disease.

Clinical Signs

Ehrlichia risticci infection is clinically similar to other forms of enterocolitis, and is characterized by anorexia, depression, and fever.[43, 49] Experimental infections produce a biphasic

fever occurring 6 to 7 days apart.[43, 49] Decreased gastrointestinal motility, manifested as reduced borborygmi, occurs during the early stages, before the onset of diarrhea. Diarrhea is seen in 75% of cases, and occurs 2 days after the second fever episode during experimental infections.[42a, 43, 49] The diarrhea can be moderate to severe and dehydrating. Ileus can develop at any stage of the disease, and can cause signs of moderate-to-severe colic. Systemic signs of endotoxemia and shock are common, and are similar to those described for salmonellosis. Laminitis is a complication of 20% to 30% of naturally occurring cases, and is often severe.[38] Complications such as protein-losing enteropathy, renal failure, and others, as described for salmonellosis, can occur. The fatality rate has been reported to be as high as 30%.

Hematologic abnormalities reflect endotoxemia, dehydration, and sepsis, and are essentially identical to those described for salmonellosis. Neutropenia with a left shift is a consistent feature and occurs concurrently with or soon after the onset of diarrhea.[43] Thrombocytopenia is common and often severe.[43] Neutrophilic leukocytosis occurs later in the course of the disease. Hyperfibrinogenemia is usually more pronounced than that seen with salmonellosis. Serum electrolyte, acid-base, and biochemical abnormalities are also similar to those described for salmonellosis. Coagulopathies are commonly seen during *E. risticci* infection, and reflect activation of coagulatory pathways. DIC is not uncommon, and may be the cause of the high frequency of laminitis associated with *E. risticci* infection.[50]

Diagnosis of *E. risticci* infection cannot be based on clinical signs since the disease is clinically similar to other forms of enterocolitis. Serologic evidence of infection, such as rising antibody titers to *E. risticci* detected by indirect immunofluorescence in paired serum samples, is considered diagnostic, but single samples are meaningless since many horses in endemic areas have positive titers.[38] Isolation of the organism from blood is possible, but is difficult, and is useful only in the research laboratory. Recent development of a polymerase chain reaction test for *E. risticci* DNA holds promise of a highly sensitive and specific test for *E. risticci* infection.[51]

Treatment

Principles of therapy are similar to those for other causes of enterocolitis and diarrhea described earlier. Maintenance of hydration and electrolyte and acid-base balance is of primary concern, and often requires intravenous fluid administration. Treatment of colonic inflammation and secretion with NSAIDs is indicated, but low doses of NSAIDs are often used to reduce injury to gastrointestinal mucosa and avoid renal toxicity. NSAIDs are also important to prevent laminitis. Bismuth subsalicylate solutions administered orally are used to reduce colonic secretion and inflammation. Plasma containing antibodies to the core regions of endotoxin is often administered to reduce the systemic effects of endotoxin, and provide a source of plasma protein. Mineral oil and activated charcoal administered orally may reduce the absorption of endotoxin. The use of probiotic preparations to compete with potentially pathogenic bacteria in the large intestine may be beneficial. Heparin 20 to 40 IU IV or SQ q.6–8h. and aspirin may be of particular benefit in light of the hypercoagulability and intravascular coagulation that appear to be a consistent feature of *E. risticci* infections.

As with other causes of enterocolitis, the use of antibiotics is controversial. Fear of inducing salmonellosis or other forms of antibiotic-induced diarrhea and the difficulty of diagnosing the disease early have caused most authors to recommend judicious use of antibiotics.[38] Lipid-soluble drugs are desirable, since the organism can live within cells. Oxytetracycline 6.6 mg/kg IV q.24h., trimethoprim-sulfadiazine (5 mg/kg trimethoprim PO or IV q.8–12h.; 25 mg/kg sulfadiazine q.8–12h.), or erythromycin-rifampin 30 mg/kg PO q.12h. and 5 mg/kg PO q.12h., respectively, has been used effectively to treat clinical cases.[38, 52] Oxytetracycline may be the most effective and inexpensive antibiotic available. Treatment is most successful if initiated before the onset of diarrhea.[38] In patients with a high suspicion of *E. risticci* infection, treatment with antibiotics is indicated. In addition, severely neutropenic patients are susceptible to sepsis, and broad-spectrum antibiotics are indicated.

Prevention of the disease by reducing exposure to the etiologic organism is difficult since the mode of transmission is not known. However, a killed vaccine has been developed that is relatively effective in preventing clinical illness other than fever in 80% of challenged horses.[53] Anecdotal evidence of the vaccine's efficacy in the field has been satisfactory, but controlled field trials have not been done. Prior inoculation with *Ehrlichia sennetsu* has been shown to prevent clinical signs of Potomac horse fever in horses challenged with *E. risticci*.[54] Passive transfer of protective immunity in naive mice challenged with *E. risticci* has been documented using serum and purified IgG from infected mice.[55] This evidence suggests that humoral immunity is important in preventing clinical signs of disease from *E. risticci* infection, and provides information that may be useful in developing a more effective vaccine.

Equine Intestinal Clostridiosis

Pathogenesis

Clostridial infections are an important cause of enterocolitis in foals; however, the pathogenicity of *Clostridium* species in adult horses is controversial. *Clostridium perfringens* type A has been suggested to cause acute colitis in adult horses.[56] In a clinical study comparing a group of normal horses with a group of horses with gastrointestinal disease, horses with acute diarrhea and signs of toxemia were found to have elevated numbers of *C. perfringens* type A colony-forming units (CFU) in the feces in the absence of other known gastrointestinal pathogens.[56] In the same study, normal horses and horses with diarrhea without systemic signs had very low numbers of *C. perfringens* type A CFU in the feces. In other studies, horses with diarrhea induced by oxytetracycline were found to have increased numbers of fecal *C. perfringens* type A.[56] Oral administration of broth cultures of *C. perfringens* type A has been shown to induce signs of mild enterocolitis in horses.[56] Intravenous administration of virulent *C. perfringens* type A bacteria induced signs of systemic shock, colic, and hemorrhagic gastroenteritis in ponies.[57] However, the isolation of *C. perfringens* type A enterotoxin from diarrheal feces or intestinal fluid has not been done to support the role of *C. perfringens* type A as a

gastrointestinal pathogen in adult horses. Quantitative culture of *C. perfringens* type A from feces is used to screen for infection in elderly human patients with diarrhea, but definitive diagnosis requires isolation of the enterotoxin from the feces.[58]

Dietary factors are known to affect the numbers of *Clostridium* species shed in the feces of horses. Feeding dietary protein supplements containing lysine and methionine has been shown to increase the number of fecal *C. perfringens* type A CFU without causing diarrhea.[56] In addition, experimental induction of colic has been shown to increase fecal shedding of *Clostridium* species in the absence of diarrhea.[59] As mentioned previously, induction of diarrhea in ponies with oxytetracycline increases fecal shedding of *C. perfringens* type A. Antibiotic-associated *C. perfringens* type A infection is well documented in elderly human patients.[58] Clearly, disruption of gastrointestinal flora can increase the shedding of *Clostridium* species of bacteria in the feces; however, the role of *C. perfringens* type A as a gastrointestinal pathogen is as yet unclear. It is likely that overgrowth of *C. perfringens* type A and possibly other *Clostridium* species is an important component in the pathogenesis of enterocolitis in horses with altered gastrointestinal flora.

Clostridium perfringens types B and C are known to cause enterocolitis in foals, lambs, and calves.[60] *Clostridium difficile* has been shown to cause acute enterocolitis in foals and pseudomembranous colitis in humans.[61] *Clostridium cadaveris* has been isolated from feces of ponies with clindamycin- and lincomycin-induced diarrhea and has been suggested to be a cause of acute enterocolitis in horses.[62] However, the causal relationship between *Clostridium* species and enterocolitis in adult horses has yet to be established.

The pathogenicity of *Clostridium* depends on the production of enterotoxins.[60] *Clostridium* organisms inhabiting the gastrointestinal tract are normally found in very low numbers, and do not produce enterotoxin. In some circumstances, such as during antibiotic treatment, the numbers of clostridia increase in the large intestine. The conditions resulting in enterotoxin production are not fully understood; however, only certain serotypes are enterotoxigenic. Large intestinal disease attributed to *C. perfringens* type A infection in horses is manifested by hemorrhagic to necrotizing typhlocolitis.[56] Enterotoxigenic *C. perfringens* type A produces α-toxin (phospholipase C), which interferes with glucose uptake, energy production, and synthetic pathways in mucosal cells.[60] Oral administration of α-toxin does not cause tissue necrosis, but causes increased secretion by small intestinal mucosal cells in humans.[58, 60] However, the effects of the toxin during infection of equine or human large intestine are less well characterized.

Clinical Signs and Diagnosis

Equine intestinal clostridiosis is clinically similar to other forms of acute enterocolitis in horses. Fever, anorexia, and depression may be noted prior to the onset of gastrointestinal signs, but more commonly no prodromal signs are seen.[56] Acute signs of colic and severe, dehydrating diarrhea may be accompanied by signs of endotoxemia and shock.[56] Diarrhea may not be profuse, but is usually dark and foul-smelling.[56] Hematologic and serum biochemical abnormalities are also similar to those associated with other forms of enterocolitis, and reflect fluid, protein, and electrolyte loss and endotoxemia. Neutropenia, leukopenia, and hemoconcentration are common. Hypoproteinemia may be profound. Hyponatremia, hypokalemia, hypochloremia, hypocalcemia, and azotemia are often noted, as well as metabolic acidosis and coagulopathies. Serum concentrations of hepatocellular enzymes, such as sorbitol dehydrogenase, are characteristically elevated, and liver function is reduced, as demonstrated by increases in bromosulfophthalein retention time.[56] The clinical course may be acute or peracute with rapid death. Occasionally, a milder, more prolonged clinical course is seen.

Diagnosis of equine intestinal clostridiosis is based on the isolation of greater than 100 CFU of *C. perfringens* type A per gram of feces from patients with diarrhea and signs suggestive of toxemia.[56, 63] Similar criteria are used to screen human patients for *C. perfringens* type A infection.[58] Normal horses shed fewer than 100 CFU/g of feces and usually horses with intestinal clostridiosis shed greater than 10^6 CFU/g.[56, 64] However, identification of increased numbers of *Clostridium* organisms in the feces does not prove infection. Detection of *C. perfringens* type A enterotoxin in feces or intestinal contents in horses with increased numbers of fecal CFU is conclusive evidence of enterotoxigenic infection.

Treatment

The principles of therapy for equine intestinal clostridiosis are similar to those for other forms of acute enterocolitis. Maintenance of hydration and electrolyte and acid-base balance with intravenous fluid administration is of primary importance. Prevention of systemic effects of endotoxin absorbed across the damaged mucosa with NSAIDs and plasma containing antibody to rough mutants of *E. coli* or *S. typhimurium* is also important. Plasma provides an important source of plasma protein as well. Gastrointestinal protectants such as bismuth subsalicylate solutions are beneficial in reducing inflammation and secretion. Anticoagulants such as heparin, and antiplatelet drugs such as aspirin, may be used to prevent thrombosis. Broad-spectrum antibiotics, such as third-generation cephalosporins, or penicillin-aminoglycoside combinations, are beneficial if neutropenia or sepsis is present. Oral administration of metronidazole is used to treat humans with *C. difficile* and *C. perfringens* type A enterocolitis.[58, 64] The use of metronidazole to treat horses with suspected intestinal clostridiosis has not been investigated.

Since altered large intestinal flora appears to play an important role in the pathogenesis of equine intestinal clostridiosis, probiotic preparations have been advocated to treat affected horses.[56] Sour milk, a product containing lactose-producing *Streptococcus* species, appears to markedly improve the clinical course in horses suspected of having *C. perfringens* type A infection.[56] Sour milk may benefit the patient by altering the flora and antagonizing enterotoxigenic *C. perfringens* type A, but also is reported to be bactericidal against *C. perfringens* type A.[56] Other probiotic preparations may be equally beneficial.

Strongylosis

Pathogenesis

Strongyle infections in horses are caused by two groups of nematodes: large and small strongyles (see Cyathostomiasis). Large strongyles that are pathogenic in horses include *Strongylus vulgaris*, *Strongylus edentatus*, and *Strongylus equinus*. Of these species, *S. vulgaris* is by far the most important cause of disease in the large intestine, and in fact is the most pathogenic parasitic infection in horses.[65] *Strongylus vulgaris* infection in horses is manifested clinically by two forms, causing acute and chronic disease.[65] The age and resistance of the host, the infective dose, and the size and function of the affected arteries influence the type and degree of disease that occurs.[65] Sudden ingestion of large numbers of infective larvae by a naive host causes acute strongylosis, whereas ingestion of fewer infective larvae over a long period of time by an older, more resistant host causes chronic strongylosis. Acute strongylosis is more likely to cause colic than diarrhea, and may be rapidly fatal. Chronic strongylosis tends to cause debilitation and signs of colic, but may also cause diarrhea.

Diarrhea associated with acute strongylosis occurs within several days of infection, and is likely to be caused by migration of the larvae through the intestinal wall. Fourth-stage larvae migrate through the mucosa and submucosa into the arterioles of the intestine, causing mural edema, hemorrhage, and infiltration with inflammatory cells into the intestinal wall.[65, 66] Increased secretion and decreased absorption of fluid and electrolytes, stimulated by inflammatory mediators such as prostaglandins and histamine, may play a role in the diarrhea induced by *S. vulgaris*. Interstitial edema and damage to the interstitial matrix may occur as a result of inflammation and migration of the parasites, causing increased passive secretion of fluid and albumin. Abnormal gastrointestinal motility may also play a role in the development of diarrhea. Migration of larvae through the intestinal wall early in the course of infection affects myoelectrical activity and motility in the large intestine and may affect retention of ingesta and absorption of fluid.[67, 68] Migration of nematode larvae in murine intestine has been shown to decrease transit time, resulting in decreased absorption of fluid.[16] The cause of death in acute strongylosis has not been addressed, but may be related to massive migration through the vasculature, causing ischemia and infarction of the intestine.

Chronic strongylosis causes typical verminous arteritis and is more commonly associated with natural infections in horses than acute strongylosis.[65] Lesions of the large intestinal vasculature caused by migration of larvae through the intima are characterized by thrombus formation, narrowing of the arterial lumen, fibrosis, and thickening of the arterial wall.[65, 66] Embolization may occur, causing acute segmental infarction of the large intestine, but more commonly reduced blood flow without embolization causes ischemia and occasionally infarction.[66, 69] Postmortem examination of horses with colonic infarction failed to reveal embolization as the cause in the majority of cases.[69] Reduced blood flow in the tissues of the intestine usually results from narrowing of the arterial lumen by the thrombus and formation of microthrombi at sites independent of the parasites. Release of vasoconstrictive inflammatory mediators, such as leukotrienes, from platelets, neutrophils, and eosinophils, as well as elaboration of parasitic antigens or toxins, may cause vasoconstriction and ischemia.[70] Horses with experimental strongylosis were found to have a 50% reduction of blood flow in the colonic vasculature.[71]

Clearly, reduced blood flow is an important effect of chronic strongylosis, but the relationship between blood flow and diarrhea is unclear. Disrupted motility resulting from ischemia may lead to diarrhea by reducing the retention of ingesta and absorption of fluid. Acute infarction and mucosal ulceration have been found to cause severe, chronic diarrhea in naturally infected horses.[72] Release of inflammatory mediators, such as prostaglandins, histamine, and kinins, from inflammatory cells associated with thrombi and inflamed intestine may also affect secretion, absorption, and motility, leading to diarrhea.

Clinical Signs and Diagnosis

The clinical signs of acute strongylosis caused by *S. vulgaris* infection are characterized by depression, moderate-to-severe colic, and fever. Diarrhea is less often a feature of acute strongylosis than colic.[65] Most cases of acute strongylosis occur in young naive horses that are introduced to an infested environment or are inoculated experimentally with infective larvae. This form of strongylosis is not often recognized naturally. Chronic strongylosis, however, is most commonly observed as a natural syndrome. Weight loss or poor weight gain; chronic, intermittent colic; fever; poor appetite; and diarrhea are frequently observed.[65, 66] Diarrhea may be profuse and watery, or the feces may be soft but of normal volume. Transrectal palpation may reveal thickening and fremitus in the cranial mesenteric artery. Young horses are most commonly affected, but older horses may also be affected. Horses with acute infarction or large intestinal ulceration secondary to chronic strongylosis may have signs of severe abdominal pain, sepsis, and endotoxemia, and profuse, watery diarrhea is common.

Hematologic abnormalities associated with strongylosis include neutrophilic leukocytosis and eosinophilia.[73, 74] Neutrophilia appears to be an early event during the course of the disease, and eosinophilia tends to appear later.[73, 74] Hyperfibrinogenemia may also be seen, especially later in the course of the disease. Serum α- and β-globulin and IgG(T) concentrations are characteristically elevated.[73–75] Horses with chronic ulcerative colitis secondary to strongylosis may exhibit severe hypoalbuminemia.[72] Peritoneal fluid analysis may reveal an elevated protein concentration and eosinophilia.[73, 74] Tentative diagnosis is based on clinical signs, hematologic abnormalities, and peritoneal fluid analysis. Elevated serum α- and β-globulin concentrations and IgG(T) concentration support the diagnosis.[75] Fecal analysis may reveal strongyle eggs, but often fecal egg counts are unreliable since the disease is caused by nonpatent larvae.

Treatment

Treatment of *S. vulgaris* infection requires treatment of the migrating parasite larvae and the lesions produced by the parasite. Thiabendazole 440 mg/kg PO q.24h. for 2 days, fenbendazole 50 mg/kg PO q.24h. for 3 days or 10 mg/kg PO q.24h. for 5 days, and ivermectin 200 mg/kg PO have been found to be effective in killing fourth-stage larvae.[65] Other anthelmintics may also be effective when given at higher doses than those required to kill adult worms. The efficacy of these anthelmintics against larvae within thrombi is not known.

Thrombolytic and antithrombotic therapy designed to reduce the thrombi induced by the larvae has been advocated.[65, 72] Heparin 20 to 80 IU IV or SQ q.6–12h. is often administered as an anticoagulant. Aspirin 15 to 30 mg/kg PO q.12–48h. is usually combined with heparin to inhibit platelet function by irreversibly inhibiting cyclooxygenase. Aspirin may also inhibit release of platelet products, such as thromboxane, that affect the motility of the large intestine. Low-molecular-weight dextrans have been advocated as anticoagulants that act by inhibiting platelet function.[72] The clinical efficacy of dextran administration appears to be good, but no controlled studies have been performed.

Additional supportive care may be required if severe diarrhea or colic is present. Intravenous fluid administration, analgesic therapy, and broad-spectrum antibiotics may be indicated if severe diarrhea, colic, or sepsis is a complication of the primary disease. Gastrointestinal protectants, such as bismuth subsalicylate, may be beneficial in reducing secretion by the large intestine. Appropriate preventive measures are important in controlling this disease, including such management procedures as preventing overcrowding and reducing exposure of susceptible individuals, and instituting proper deworming schedules. Monitoring fecal egg counts as a means of evaluating the efficacy of parasite control measures is recommended.

Cyathostomiasis
Pathogenesis

Infection with small strongyles (cyathostomiasis) is less recognized as a cause of diarrhea and large intestinal disease in horses than large strongyle infection. However, clinical evidence of cyathostome infection associated with chronic diarrhea and hypoalbuminemia in horses clearly implicates cyathostome infection as an important cause of disease of the large intestine.[76–78] The cyathostome life cycle requires migration by fourth-stage larvae through the mucosa of the large intestine, and may include a period of hypobiosis, during which the larvae remain encysted within the mucosal layer of the large intestine.[79]

After a period of hypobiosis, the larvae emerge in response to a largely unknown stimulus.[79] In temperate zones of the Northern Hemisphere, hypobiosis occurs over winter, and emergence occurs during the late winter and spring.[79] Emergence of hypobiotic larvae is thought to be the cause of diarrhea and other clinical signs in horses with cyathostomiasis.[77–79] Most cases occur when larval emergence takes place, classically in the late winter and spring in the northern temperate zones. However, migration of the larvae through the mucosa affects motility patterns causing increased and disorganized motility associated with diarrhea.[67] Chronic, eosinophilic, granulomatous colitis and diarrhea with histopathologic evidence of hypobiotic cyathostome larvae in the large intestine has been reported in two horses during a period in which emergence of larvae would not be expected to occur (early winter).[78] Clearly, the pathogenesis of diarrhea resulting from cyathostome infection is not well understood.

Emergence of cyathostome larvae causes shedding and ulceration of the large intestinal mucosa, which may even result in bleeding into the lumen.[66] Mild-to-moderate eosinophilic and mononuclear inflammation of the lamina propria is seen.[66] Moderate-to-severe interstitial edema is frequently observed.[66] Colonic inflammation and interstitial edema may contribute to the diarrhea, in conjunction with the loss of the mucosal barrier, by causing increased active and passive secretion of fluid, electrolytes, and protein. Protein loss is often significant, resulting in profound hypoalbuminemia. Chronic, granulomatous colitis has been reported to occur in response to encysted larvae, and may cause diarrhea by increased secretion secondary to granulomatous inflammation or disruption of the interstitium by granulomatous infiltration.

Clinical Signs and Diagnosis

Clinical signs of cyathostomiasis are characterized by moderate-to-severe weight loss or poor weight gain, ventral edema, intermittent fever, and intermittent, mild colic.[66, 76–78] Diarrhea is typically profuse and watery, but may be mild and the consistency of bovine feces.[76–78] Appetite is usually normal, but occasionally affected horses will have a ravenous appetite.[76–78] Transrectal palpation usually does not reveal any abnormalities. Any age of horse may be affected, and clinical signs are more common during periods of emergence of larvae, corresponding to late winter and spring in northern temperate zones. The deworming history may appear to be adequate.

Neutrophilic leukocytosis is typically evident, but the white blood cell count may be normal.[76–78] Profound hypoalbuminemia is a characteristic feature of cyathostomiasis, manifested clinically by ventral edema.[76–78] Plasma α- and β-globulin concentrations are often elevated, which may result in a normal total plasma protein concentration in spite of hypoalbuminemia.[76–78] The serum IgG(T) concentration, however, has been reported to be normal, which may help distinguish cyathostomiasis from S. vulgaris infection.[77, 78] In addition, peritoneal fluid analysis does not usually reveal any abnormalities, in contrast to horses with S. vulgaris infection. Fecal analysis may be unrewarding since the infection is often not patent when clinical signs are apparent. Rectal scrapings or rectal mucosal biopsies may reveal evidence of cyathostome larvae.[78] Definitive diagnosis may require microscopic examination of biopsy specimens of the large intestine, usually the cecum and ascending colon.[77, 78] Collection of biopsy specimens from the small intestine is recommended to rule out other causes of weight loss and diarrhea. Appropriate diagnostic tests, such as culture of feces for pathogenic bacteria, should be included in the workup to further rule out other causes.

Treatment

Anthelmintic administration is usually the only treatment necessary for mild-to-moderate cases of cyathostomiasis treated early in the course of the disease (within 1–3 weeks of onset). Fenbendazole 50 mg/kg PO q.24h. for 3 days or ivermectin 200 mg/kg PO has been advocated as effective larvacidal anthelmintics.[79] Anti-inflammatory therapy may also be beneficial, especially in severe or refractory cases. NSAID administration may have limited value, but dexamethasone appears to be efficacious in refractory cases when used in conjunction with larvacidal anthelmintics.[78] Presumably, dexamethasone reduces inflammation in the colon by suppressing the response of immune and inflammatory effector cells. In fact, some authors have suggested that an immune-mediated mechanism may be a component of the disease, especially when emergence of the larvae does not appear to be contributing to the pathophysiology.[78] Bismuth subsalicylate is often administered orally as an antisecretory agent. Supportive care may be necessary in severe cases. Intravenous fluid administration is occasionally required. Proper nutritional support is also important. Preventive measures, as described for S. vulgaris, are also appropriate.

TOXICOLOGIC DISEASES

Antibiotic-Associated Diarrhea

Pathogenesis

Antibiotic-associated diarrhea has been reported in many species, including horses.[80] Certain antibiotics, such as tetracyclines, clindamycin, and lincomycin, are associated with well-characterized enterocolitis syndromes in horses that have been induced experimentally.[62, 80, 81] Other antibiotics, such as trimethoprim-sulfonamide combinations, penicillins, erythromycin, rifampin, and metronidazole, have been anecdotally linked to enterocolitis in horses. In some cases, such as those seen with trimethoprim-sulfonamide combinations, the geographical incidence of antibiotic-associated diarrhea appears to differ markedly.

The most common mechanism by which antibiotics cause diarrhea is by disrupting the gastrointestinal flora. The normal large intestinal flora, comprised of mainly obligate anaerobes and streptococci, protects the host from colonization by pathogenic bacteria by colonization resistance.[10] Ecologic factors play an important role in colonization resistance. For example, surface bacteria in the large intestine interact with receptors on the mucosal cells, facilitating adherence to the mucosa.[8, 10] In doing so, the normal organisms compete more successfully for an important ecologic niche. Competition for space and nutrients is an important means of preventing colonization and proliferation of pathogenic bacteria.[8, 10] In addition, anaerobic bacteria produce short-chain fatty acids and other metabolites that are toxic to facultative anaerobic bacteria, especially in the conditions of the large intestine.[8, 10] Organisms of the normal flora also produce bacteriocins that inhibit growth of potential pathogens.[10]

Antibiotics that deplete the population of obligate anaerobes and streptococci efficiently decrease colonization resistance.[10] Production of fatty acids is diminished, and competition for space and nutrients is reduced. As a result, the gram-negative enteric bacteria, such as Salmonella, are able to proliferate. In addition, pathogenic anaerobes normally found in low numbers can proliferate. Tetracycline administration has been shown to be associated with an increase in the numbers of gram-negative enteric bacteria and Clostridium perfringens in the feces of horses as well as reactivation of salmonellosis and prolongation of fecal shedding of *Salmonella*.[56, 82] Antibiotic-resistant strains of bacteria, especially gram-negative enteric bacteria, may be selected by antibiotic administration, allowing proliferation of pathogenic bacteria resistant to many antibiotics.[83]

Decreased carbohydrate fermentation and production of short-chain fatty acids by depleted anaerobic bacterial populations also contributes to the pathogenesis of antibiotic-associated diarrhea by decreasing absorption of sodium and water by the colonic mucosa.[84] Ampicillin has been shown to decrease colonic fermentation of carbohydrates in humans.[85] Human patients with antibiotic-associated diarrhea were found to have markedly impaired colonic fermentation, resulting in very low production of short-chain fatty acids.[86] Erythromycin, ampicillin, or metronidazole treatment was associated with decreased production of short-chain fatty acids in patients with and without diarrhea.[86] Absorption of sodium and water is known to be stimulated by absorption of short-chain fatty acids in the equine colon.[84]

Broad-spectrum antibiotics exert a more profound effect on the gastrointestinal flora than narrow-spectrum antibiotics.[87] Antibiotics administered orally, especially those that are poorly absorbed, are more likely to cause diarrhea than parenterally administered antibiotics.[87] For instance, doxycycline administered intravenously is less likely to cause diarrhea in humans than tetracycline administered orally. Similarly, clindamycin in humans is less likely to cause diarrhea when administered intravenously than when administered orally.[87] Antibiotics with extensive enterohepatic circulation, such as tetracyclines and erythromycin, are excreted in high concentrations in the bile, and are more commonly associated with diarrhea than antibiotics that do not undergo enterohepatic circulation.[87]

Antibiotics may cause diarrhea by other means than by disrupting the normal flora. Direct toxic effects may play a role in producing irritation, increasing secretion, and disrupting motility patterns. Tetracyclines are irritating to the gastrointestinal mucosa, and may cause inflammation and increase secretion.[87] Erythromycin has been shown to interact with smooth muscle cells, affecting gastrointestinal motility.[87] Normal peristalsis plays an important role in regulating the population size of potentially pathogenic bacteria.[8, 10] Bacteria that are prevented from adhering to the mucosa by colonization resistance are swept aborally by peristalsis, and excreted in the feces. Disruption of normal motility patterns may prevent clearance of pathogenic bacteria, contributing to the colonization of mucosal surfaces.

Clinical Signs and Diagnosis

Diarrhea induced by antibiotics can occur during antibiotic administration, or can occur several days after cessation of antibiotic treatment. The clinical syndrome of antibiotic-associated diarrhea can vary from mild diarrhea to fulminant enterocolitis with severe diarrhea. Mild cases of diarrhea are common, especially in foals receiving erythromycin, trimethoprim-sulfa combinations, or rifampin.[88] Mild cases of diarrhea are usually not clinically significant. However, acute, severe enterocolitis can occur in all ages of horses receiving antibiotics, and can be life-threatening.[62, 80] Clinical signs are identical to other causes of acute enterocolitis. In fact, antibiotic administration may induce salmonellosis or clostridiosis, as discussed earlier. Severe, dehydrating diarrhea, endotoxemia, sepsis, and shock may occur. Hemoconcentration, neutropenia, hypoproteinemia, and electrolyte and acid-base imbalances are common. Severe hyponatremia may occur in foals with antibiotic-associated diarrhea, especially if trimethoprim-sulfa and rifampin combinations are the cause.[88] More detailed descriptions of the clinical and laboratory findings were given earlier. Diagnosis is presumptive since definitive diagnosis of antibiotic-associated diarrhea is impossible. Fecal examination may reveal *Salmonella* or *Clostridium* infection.

Treatment

The principles of therapy are similar to those for other causes of acute enterocolitis. Maintenance of fluid, electrolyte, and acid-base balance is imperative. Patients with mild diarrhea may maintain hydration by oral consumption of water and electrolyte solutions, and may not require intravenous fluids. More severe cases require intravenous administration of fluids and plasma. In most cases, discontinuation of all antibiotics is desirable. In cases of mild diarrhea, reduction of the dose of the antibiotic may alleviate the signs. In cases with severe neutropenia or septicemia, continuation of antibiotic treatment with a different antibiotic regimen using as narrow a spectrum of antibiotic as possible, and a drug that does not undergo enterohepatic circulation, administered parenterally, will reduce the effects of the antibiotic on the gastrointestinal flora. Metronidazole 15 to 25 mg/kg PO q.6–12h. may be beneficial if clostridiosis is suspected. Treatment of colonic inflammation, endotoxemia, sepsis, coagulopathies, and complications from the enterocolitis is accomplished as with other forms of acute enterocolitis. NSAIDs and oral gastrointestinal protectants, such as bismuth subsalicylate, are important components of therapy.

Oral probiotic preparations may provide a means of reestablishing normal gastrointestinal flora. Preparations of lactic acid–producing bacteria and other bacteria are administered orally or by enema to provide nonpathogenic organisms to compete with pathogenic bacteria and increase colonization resistance.[37] Lactic acid–producing bacteria (lactobacilli and enterococci) administered orally to human patients receiving antibiotics such as erythromycin were shown to decrease the incidence of diarrhea.[89] In addition, administration of lactic acid–producing enterococci significantly reduced the severity, and was associated with faster resolution, of diarrhea in patients with acute antibiotic-associated enteritis.[90] Fecal organisms from adult chickens fed to newly hatched chicks prevented the colonization of *Salmonella*.[37] Clearly, probiotic preparations are beneficial in some species, especially when preventing antibiotic-associated diarrhea caused by colonization of pathogenic bacteria in the large intestine, but their efficacy in horses has not been established.

Nonsteroidal Anti-Inflammatory Drug Toxicity

Pathogenesis

Toxicity resulting from NSAID administration has been well documented in several species, including horses.[91–93] In horses and humans, NSAID toxicity is manifested by renal and gastrointestinal disease.[91–93] Elderly human patients are more susceptible to NSAID toxicity, but the effects of age on NSAID toxicity in horses are less well defined.[93, 94] Foals are considered to be more susceptible than adult horses to gastrointestinal disease secondary to NSAID administration, and ponies may be more susceptible than horses. All NSAIDs are capable of inducing gastrointestinal and renal damage at toxic concentrations and the relative toxicity is not significantly different among products. However, aspirin has been suggested to be more toxic than other NSAIDs since aspirin irreversibly inactivates cyclooxygenase by acetylation, whereas other NSAIDs reversibly inhibit cyclooxygenase.[91, 94] Phenylbutazone is the drug most commonly reported to cause toxicity in horses, but this is likely to be due to its widespread usage by veterinarians and horse owners. The focus of this discussion is on the toxic effects of NSAIDs on the large intestine, but necessarily includes elements of upper gastrointestinal and renal disease.

Horses with large intestinal disease resulting from NSAID toxicity generally have received inappropriately large doses. The dosage regimen recommended for phenylbutazone (4.4 mg/kg b.i.d. for 1 day, then 2.2 mg/kg b.i.d.) is considered to be safe. Experimental studies in horses, however, have shown toxicity to occur when less than the recommended dosage (6.6 mg/kg/day) is administered for several days.[93] Administration of phenylbutazone at the recommended dosage has been reported to cause a significant decrease in plasma protein concentration.[95, 96] Dehydration, sepsis, and endotoxemia exacerbate the renal and gastrointestinal toxicity of NSAIDs. Clearly, the margin of safety is quite narrow for phenylbutazone, and probably for other NSAIDs used in horses as well.

Gastrointestinal disease induced by NSAIDs is manifested by mucosal ulceration, bleeding, and protein-losing enteropathy.[29, 94, 96] NSAID administration has been shown to cause an acute relapse of preexisting colonic inflammatory disease and worsen colonic inflammation in humans.[28, 92, 94] The mechanism by which NSAIDs induce mucosal damage is probably multifactorial. Direct irritation may play a role in oral and gastric irritation and ulceration; however, parenteral administration of NSAIDs produces oral and gastric ulceration as well.[30] Inhibition of prostaglandin synthesis by cyclooxygenase inhibition is likely to be the most important mechanism of mucosal injury.[30, 91, 94, 96] PGE and PGF predominate in the gastrointestinal mucosa of all species studied, and have been found to be important in the colonic mucosa in horses.[94, 97] PGE and PGF have different physiologic roles in the alimentary tract, but both are considered to be mucosal-protective.[91, 94] PGE has been shown to increase mucosal blood flow; increase secretion of mucus, water, and bicarbonate; increase mucosal cell turnover rate and migration; stimulate adenyl cyclase activity; and exert other protective effects in the gastric mucosa of several species.[91, 94] The role of prostaglandins in mucosal protection in the colon is less well defined. PGE has been shown to prevent chemical injury in the colonic mucosa in several species.[94] Protection from chemical injury has been shown to occur in the stomach and small intestine as well.[94] In addition, administration of PGE prevents many of the morphologic effects of NSAID toxicity on gastrointestinal mucosa in humans and horses.[94, 96]

Other mechanisms may play a role in NSAID-induced injury to gastrointestinal mucosa. Shunting arachidonic acid metabolism to the lipoxygenase pathway by inhibiting cyclooxygenase may result in an increase in leukotriene production.[30, 91, 94] Leukotrienes are vasoconstrictive, and may cause injury to gastrointestinal mucosa by causing ischemia or by other means.[91, 94] Prostaglandins may also have other, less well-defined functions on cellular metabolism that have adverse effects at high concentrations.[94] In addition, NSAID-induced vascular injury has been suggested to cause mural edema and mucosal ischemia and injury in horses.[29]

Clinical Signs and Diagnosis

Nonsteroidal anti-inflammatory toxicity is characterized by gastrointestinal ulceration, mural vascular thrombosis and edema, protein-losing enteropathy, and mucosal hemorrhage.[28, 96] Microulceration of the colonic mucosa may be evident.[28, 96, 97] The colon may be more severely affected than the proximal gastrointestinal tract. Recently, a syndrome of NSAID toxicity has been recognized that is characterized by right dorsal colitis with ulceration and severe inflammation in the absence of lesions in the rest of the gastrointestinal tract.[98]

Clinical signs of NSAID toxicity may vary from mild diarrhea with no systemic signs to severe dehydrating diarrhea with anorexia, fever, depression, peripheral edema, and intermittent colic.[28, 93, 96] Oral and gastric ulceration may be seen. Endotoxemia and sepsis may occur, manifested as poor peripheral perfusion, tachycardia, and tachypnea. Cyanotic oral mucous membranes are commonly observed.[28, 93, 96] Hematuria or oliguria may be observed if renal involvement is present. Exacerbation of a preexisting enterocolitis may occur when inclusion of NSAIDs in the treatment regimen is associated with worsening of the patient's condition. Complications associated with other forms of severe enterocolitis, such as laminitis, thrombophlebitis, and severe weight loss, may occur.

Hematologic abnormalities are nonspecific, and include neutropenia with a left shift or leukocytosis, and hemoconcentration. Serum biochemical analysis is characterized by profound hypoproteinemia, hyponatremia, and metabolic acidosis.[93, 95] Hypocalcemia, hypokalemia, hypochloremia, and elevated hepatocellular enzyme activities may also be seen. Hypoproteinemia may occur without signs of diarrhea. Azotemia may occur secondary to dehydration, but is frequently associated with renal disease. Urinalysis frequently reveals hematuria, proteinuria, cylindruria and isosthenuria. Fecal occult blood is frequently detected.

Diagnosis is presumptive, with a history of overdose of NSAIDs being strong evidence of NSAID toxicity, but as discussed earlier, toxicity may occur with dosage regimens that are not considered inappropriate. Gastrointestinal ulceration, profound metabolic acidosis, hypoproteinemia, and hyponatremia are highly suggestive but not specific for NSAID toxicity. Other causes of enterocolitis, such as salmonellosis, Potomac horse fever, and antibiotic-associated diarrhea, must be ruled out.

Treatment

Principles of therapy for horses with NSAID toxicity include cessation of NSAID administration, maintenance of hydration and electrolyte and acid-base balance, replacement of plasma protein, and gastrointestinal mucosal protection. Intravenous administration of fluids and plasma is often required. Profound hyponatremia and metabolic acidosis may require administration of hypertonic solutions of sodium chloride and bicarbonate. Sucralfate 20 to 40 mg/kg PO q.6h. and H$_2$-receptor blockers, such as cimetidine 4.4 mg/kg PO q.6–8h., are effective in treating ulceration of the upper gastrointestinal tract, but not the large intestine.[94] Bismuth subsalicylate solution 5 to 10 mL/kg PO q.6–8h. is administered to control colonic mucosal inflammation, but has the potential to worsen the effects of NSAIDs on the alimentary mucosa.

Synthetic PGE, such as misoprostol, is effective in preventing and treating NSAID-induced mucosal injury in humans, and may be equally beneficial in horses, especially foals.[94, 96] The beneficial effects of PGE have been characterized in the upper gastrointestinal tract in humans, and have been shown to protect the colonic mucosa against chemical injury.[94] Since shunting of arachidonic acid metabolism toward the lipoxygenase pathway may occur, inhibition of leukotriene synthesis may be effective in reducing the effects of NSAIDs on the colonic mucosa. Specific lipoxygenase inhibitors are not available clinically; however, calcium channel blockers inhibit leukotriene synthesis by limiting intracellular calcium concentration.[29] Verapamil has been shown to decrease macroscopic ulceration and increase the rate of healing in chemically induced models of colitis in rats.[29]

Treatment of endotoxemia is best accomplished with intravenous administration of fluids and plasma containing antibodies against rough mutants of gram-negative bacteria, such as *E. coli* (J5). Administration of NSAIDs, even at low doses, should be avoided. If laminitis occurs, judicious administration of NSAIDs may be required, but control of pain can be achieved with opiates and local nerve anesthesia. Heparin 20 to 80 IU SQ or IV q.6–8h. is often administered to prevent laminitis and vascular thrombosis. Horses with severe neutropenia or signs suggestive of septicemia require broad-spectrum antibiotic administration. Aminoglycosides should be avoided since they may potentiate NSAID-induced renal toxicity. Cephalosporins, ampicillin, and trimethoprim-sulfa combinations are commonly used. Treatment of concurrent renal disease may be required, and is described in Chapter 16.

Recovery from NSAID toxicity is often prolonged, with persistent diarrhea, hyponatremia, and hypoproteinemia being common. Medical treatment of right dorsal colitis is frequently unsuccessful, and surgical bypass or resection of the ulcerated segment may be required for definitive treatment.

Cantharidin Toxicity

Cantharidin is the toxic principle found in beetles of the genus *Epicauta,* commonly known as blister beetles.[99] Ingestion of the beetles by horses eating contaminated hay causes release of the toxin from the tissues of the beetle, and absorption through the gastrointestinal tract. Transcutaneous absorption may occur, but appears to be rare in horses.[100] Blister beetles feed on the flowers of alfalfa, and may be incorporated into processed alfalfa hay if the hay is cut and

processed simultaneously, as by crimping.[99] The beetles often swarm, and large numbers of beetles may be found in relatively small portions of hay.[99] The lethal dose of cantharidin is less than 1 mg/kg, but the concentration of cantharidin varies from species to species of blister beetles, and between sexes.[99, 100] As many as 100 to as few as six to eight beetles may be lethal. Usually, only one or a few horses fed contaminated hay will ingest beetles since the beetles are concentrated in a small portion of the hay. However, outbreaks involving many horses on a farm have occurred. Most cases occur in Texas and Oklahoma, but horses in other states may be affected as well, especially if hay is imported from states where blister beetles are common.

Cantharidin is a potent irritant, causing acantholysis and vesicle formation when applied topically.[99, 101] Cantharidin is absorbed from the gastrointestinal tract and excreted via the kidney. The chemical is thought to disrupt oxidative metabolism in the mitochondria, causing mitochondrial swelling, plasma membrane damage, and changes in membrane permeability.[99] Cell swelling and necrosis occur, resulting in acantholysis and mucosal ulceration.[99] The mucosa of the gastrointestinal tract is most commonly affected in horses since they ingest the toxin. Oral, esophageal, gastric, and small and large intestinal ulceration have been observed in natural and experimental canthariasis.[101] Severe fibrinous to pseudomembranous inflammation and submucosal edema of the intestine have also been reported.[101] Diarrhea probably results from the severe ulceration and inflammation of the large intestine, causing increased secretion of water, electrolytes, and protein, and decreased absorption of fluid. Large volumes of fluid and protein are lost in the gastrointestinal tract, causing hemoconcentration and profound hypoalbuminemia in some cases.[99, 101]

Cystitis and myocarditis occur in natural and experimentally produced cases of cantharidin toxicity.[99, 101] Cystitis occurs from the high concentration of cantharidin in the urine, since the toxin is excreted via the kidneys. Occasionally, hemorrhagic cystitis may occur, resulting in hematuria or frank hemorrhage into the bladder.[99] The cause of the myocarditis and myocardial necrosis is unknown, but may also be a direct effect of the toxin on the myocardium. Elevated plasma creatine kinase activity is often observed, and has been postulated to arise from the damaged myocardium.[99, 100] Horses have a characteristically stiff gait, but histopathologic evidence of skeletal muscle injury that explains the elevated plasma creatine kinase activity has not been observed.[99] The kidneys are often pale, swollen, and moist, with occasional infarcts.[101]

Hypocalcemia and hypomagnesemia are biochemical features of cantharidin toxicity in horses that have not been explained.[99, 100] Hypocalcemia may occur from hypoalbuminemia, but the ionized calcium concentration is often decreased along with the total calcium concentration, indicating that hypoalbuminemia is not responsible for the hypocalcemia.[100] In addition, clinical signs of hypocalcemia, such as synchronous diaphragmatic flutter, are often associated with hypocalcemia from cantharidin toxicity. Hypocalcemia associated with hypoalbuminemia alone does not produce clinical signs.

Clinical Signs and Diagnosis

Cantharidin toxicity can cause a range of clinical signs, from mild depression and abdominal discomfort to fulminant signs of toxemia and rapid death, depending on the ingested dose of toxin.[99, 100] Most commonly, clinical signs include depression, abdominal pain, elevated heart and respiratory rates, fever, and profuse diarrhea. Blood is rarely seen in the feces. Affected horses frequently posture to urinate. Stranguria and pollakiuria are characteristic of cantharidin toxicity.[99] Signs of hypocalcemia include synchronous diaphragmatic flutter and tremors. A stiff and stilted gait may be evident. Signs of endotoxemia may be seen in severe cases. Some horses develop severe depression and toxemia, and may die within hours after ingestion of cantharidin without developing diarrhea.[99]

Hematologic abnormalities include hemoconcentration and neutrophilic leukocytosis.[99, 100] Occasionally, neutropenia and leukopenia may accompany endotoxemia. Serum biochemical analysis usually reveals elevated creatine kinase activity, hypocalcemia, and hypoalbuminemia.[100] The ionized calcium concentration is usually correlated with the serum total calcium concentration.[100] A mildly elevated BUN may be observed, but the serum creatinine concentration is usually normal. Urine specific gravity is characteristically in the hyposthenuric range.[99, 100] Microscopic hematuria and mild proteinuria may be evident. Fecal occult blood is often present, but hematochezia is unusual.

Tentative diagnosis can be made based on clinical signs and the finding of blister beetles in the hay. Determining the species of the insects may be necessary to estimate the amount of cantharidin ingested. All species of *Epicauta* contain cantharidin, but some have small amounts. Definitive diagnosis requires the measurement of the cantharidin concentration in gastric contents and urine.[99, 102] Measurement of cantharidin concentration in the beetles is often done, but is not necessary.

Treatment

Mild cases of cantharidin toxicity may resolve without treatment. However, most cases require treatment. Supportive care is the most important principle of therapy for cantharidin toxicity. Intravenous fluid administration, maintenance of electrolyte balance, especially calcium, and prevention of further renal and urinary tract damage is important. Diuresis by intravenous fluid administration is often sufficient to prevent renal failure. Furosemide is often administered after rehydration of the patient to further promote diuresis, to decrease the concentration of the toxin in the urine, which may ameliorate some of the effects on the urinary tract mucosa.[99] Diuresis may also increase clearance of the toxin, but no evidence for this has been found. Judicious use of NSAIDs may be necessary to control abdominal pain, but should be reserved until the patient is rehydrated. Cantharidin is lipid-soluble; therefore oral administration of mineral oil may prevent further absorption of the toxin.[99] Activated charcoal is often administered with the mineral oil. Prognosis is guarded, but if the patient survives several days, recovery is probable.

Arsenic Toxicosis
Pathogenesis

Arsenic toxicosis is an unusual cause of diarrhea in horses, resulting from ingestion of arsenic-containing herbicides,

insecticides, and other pest control products contaminating water or roughage used as a food source.[103] The toxicity of arsenic depends on the valence of the element.[103, 104] Arsenate may be reduced to arsenite in mammalian systems.[104] Arsenite is thought to be more toxic than arsenate, and less rapidly excreted in urine.[104] Arsenate and arsenite uncouple oxidative phosphorylation, leading to breakdown of energy metabolism in the cells of many tissues.[104] Widespread cellular injury and death occur rapidly during acute arsenic toxicosis. Multiorgan failure is usually the result. In fact, cardiomyopathy and pulmonary disease are common causes of death in humans.[105] Damage to the large intestine is probably due in part to direct cellular toxicity and corrosion by the compound. However, vasculitis is a hallmark of the disease in humans and horses, and is thought to be the most important mechanism of large intestinal disease in humans.[103, 106] Acute hemorrhagic colitis is a feature of arsenic toxicosis, with severe mural edema and mucosal ulceration.[103] Profuse, hemorrhagic diarrhea and abdominal pain result. Chronic arsenic toxicity can occur, but appears to be rare in horses.

Clinical Signs and Diagnosis

Acute depression, weakness, abdominal pain, hemorrhagic diarrhea, and shock are characteristic of acute arsenic toxicosis in horses.[103] Death may occur before diarrhea is evident. Initial clinical signs may be difficult to distinguish from other peracute forms of colitis, and are related to endotoxic shock, metabolic disturbances, and dehydration. Later, cardiac arrhythmias, pulmonary edema, acute renal failure, and neurologic deficits (ataxia and stupor) may develop.[103] Anuria or polyuria may be observed. Hemolytic anemia due to preferential binding of arsenic compounds to red blood cells is a feature of arsenic poisoning in humans.[105] Hematologic abnormalities may be seen after the peracute stages from injury to bone marrow cells and ongoing hemolysis. Leukopenia and thrombocytopenia have been described in human patients.[105] Serum biochemical analysis may reveal azotemia, hepatocellular enzyme activities higher than generally attributed to endotoxemia, and elevated creatine kinase activity.[103] Urine specific gravity may be in the isosthenuric range, with hematuria, cylindruria, and proteinuria evident by urinalysis.

Diagnosis may be possible by measuring blood and urine arsenic concentration, but these tests may not be diagnostic. Postmortem diagnosis is made by measuring the arsenic concentration in liver and kidney samples.[103] History of exposure and clinical signs remain the primary means of diagnosis.

Treatment

Reduction of arsenic absorption by administration of cathartics such as mineral oil and magnesium sulfate slurries and activated charcoal by nasogastric tube should be initiated immediately.[103] Chelation therapy with sodium thiosulfate 20 to 30 g in 300 mL of water PO and dimercaprol (BAL) 3 mg/kg IM q.4h. is indicated.[103] Dimercaprol is a specific antidote for trivalent arsenicals, but its efficacy in horses is questionable. Intravenous fluid administration may help treat shock, replace fluid lost in feces, and promote diuresis, but should be monitored carefully since pulmonary edema is a frequent complication. More specific treatment of renal, cardiac, pulmonary, or neurologic disease may be required. The prognosis is poor.

MISCELLANEOUS DISORDERS OF THE LARGE INTESTINE

Colitis X

Pathogenesis

Colitis X is a syndrome in horses characterized by peracute, rapidly fatal colitis and toxemia of unknown cause.[107-109] The pathogenesis is difficult to describe without a clear conception of the cause. The syndrome is clinically and pathologically similar to known causes of colitis, such as salmonellosis and antibiotic-associated diarrhea.[80, 81, 108] *Clostridium cadaveris, Clostridium difficile,* and *Clostridium perfringens* type A have been implicated as causes.[56, 62] Experimental fatal endotoxemia closely mimics the clinical signs of colitis X. In addition, experimental anaphylaxis may elicit gastrointestinal signs and pathologic features similar to colitis X.[109, 110] These observations suggest that severe type I hypersensitivity in conjunction with severe endotoxemia or other forms of toxemia may produce a colitis X-like syndrome. The large intestine appears to be a shock organ in horses, and colitis X may well result from a combination of acute type I hypersensitivity localized to the gastrointestinal tract associated with an underlying disorder of the large intestine. Some authors have suggested that stress usually precedes the onset of colitis X, but this is not universally true.[109] Exhaustion of host resistance has been implicated as a predisposing factor, resulting from a preexisting disease, with stress or other environmental factors superimposed. However, this hypothesis has not been investigated experimentally.

Colitis X has been classically described as a peracute, fulminant colitis and toxemia that is often fatal.[107-109] Severe intramural edema and hemorrhagic inflammation of the large intestine is characteristic, often producing submucosal thickening on the order of many centimeters. Vascular thrombosis may be widespread with mucosal and serosal petechiae and ecchymoses.[108, 109] Diarrhea results in part from intestinal inflammation, and may also result from other factors, such as type I hypersensitivity. Many of the mediators of type I hypersensitivity, such as histamine, have well-documented stimulatory effects on mucosal secretory activity, and intramural edema may increase passive secretion of fluid. Endotoxemic and septic shock may be overwhelming. Infarction of intestinal segments and other organs may occur from intravascular coagulation. Ileus, abdominal distention, and moderate-to-severe abdominal pain may result from metabolic disturbances and infarction of the large intestine.

Clinical Signs and Diagnosis

The clinical signs are similar to those described for other forms of peracute colitis. Characteristically, severe shock, signs of endotoxemia and sepsis, and severe metabolic disturbances are observed.[107-109] Heart and respiratory rates may be markedly elevated, with other signs of cardiovascular collapse. Endotoxic shock produces weak and thready peripheral pulses, with peripheral vasoconstriction. However, peripheral vasodilation may be seen later in the course of disease. Dark-red, muddy, or cyanotic mucous membranes with a prolonged capillary refill time signify septic physiology. Borborygmi are usually absent and abdominal tympany may be heard on percussion, secondary to ileus. Moderate-to-severe colic may accompany ileus. Severe diarrhea may occur, but death may occur before diarrhea is evident. Multiorgan failure from DIC is not unusual. Rapid onset of weakness, staggering, and trembling commonly precedes death. The syndrome may cause death in 4 to 24 hours.

Hematologic abnormalities include severe neutropenia and leukopenia, thrombocytopenia, and hemoconcentration.[108] Serum biochemical alterations include hyponatremia, hypokalemia, hypocalcemia, and severe metabolic acidosis.[108] BUN and creatinine may be elevated from prerenal or renal azotemia. If acute renal failure accompanies the colitis, hyperkalemia may result. Hepatocellular enzyme activity may be elevated in the serum from endotoxemia. Severe coagulopathies are common, resulting in prolonged coagulation times, elevated fibrinogen, decreased antithrombin III activity, and elevated plasma concentration of fibrin degradation products. Analysis of peritoneal fluid may be valuable since infarction of the large intestine is not unusual. Protein concentration and the white blood cell count may be elevated. Red blood cell counts are less likely to be elevated, since infarction and not strangulation of the intestine occurs.

Diagnosis is based on clinical signs, postmortem findings, and exclusion of other causes. Cultures and toxicologic analysis of fecal samples and gastrointestinal tissues fail to demonstrate a clear cause. Other diagnostic tests are also inconclusive.

Treatment

Treatment of colitis X, in principle similar to other forms of colitis, is often unsuccessful, owing to the rapidly progressive nature of the syndrome.[107-109] Supportive care may necessitate administration of large volumes of intravenous fluids, along with calcium, potassium, and sodium bicarbonate solutions. Inclusion of heparin in the intravenous fluids (20–80 IU/kg IV q.8–12h.) may help prevent vascular thrombosis. Administration of hypertonic saline solutions may prove to be useful during initial periods of endotoxic shock. Administration of large volumes (2–4 L) of plasma containing antibody against rough mutants of gram-negative bacteria is indicated. Early treatment with shock doses of prednisolone succinate 10 to 20 mg/kg IV or dexamethasone 0.1 to 1.0 mg/kg IV may be essential for successful treatment, especially if type I hypersensitivity is suspected.[108] Administration of low doses of NSAIDs (0.1–0.25 mg/kg IV q.6–8h.) is indicated to reduce the systemic effects of endotoxin, reduce inflammation, and help control abdominal pain. Additional analgesics, such as xylazine, butorphanol, combinations of the two drugs, or other narcotics, may be required. Broad-spectrum antibiotic treatment may be indicated, especially if neutropenia is present. Oral administration of mineral oil and activated charcoal followed by bismuth subsalicylate may reduce absorption of bacterial toxins and moderate intestinal inflammation.

Carbohydrate Overload

Pathogenesis

Overeating of soluble carbohydrates, especially so-called hot grains such as corn, overwhelms the digestive capability of the small intestine, resulting in a high percentage of the soluble carbohydrates entering the large intestine. The amount of soluble carbohydrates that will produce diarrhea varies according to the previous dietary history of the individual. Horses fed diets higher in soluble carbohydrates are more resistant to the deleterious effects of carbohydrate overload. Gradual accommodation to a diet high in carbohydrates can be accomplished over several weeks. However, horses fed an unusually large amount of grains or other form of soluble carbohydrates often develop diarrhea, and may, depending on the amount ingested, develop severe colitis, endotoxemia, metabolic acidosis, and laminitis.[111–114]

The pathogenesis of colitis from carbohydrate overload is mediated primarily by the microbial flora in the large intestine.[112] A sudden influx of soluble carbohydrates into the large intestine is rapidly fermented by gram-positive lactic acid–producing bacteria, causing a sudden increase in organic acid production.[113] The cecal pH rapidly decreases and the lactic acid concentration rapidly increases.[113] Rapid organic acid production overwhelms the buffering capacity of the large intestine, not only by directly depleting the buffers found in the contents but also by reducing the efficiency of buffer secretion. Bicarbonate secretion is linked to absorption of volatile fatty acids, which are produced in low amounts by fermentation of soluble carbohydrates. The contents of the large intestine become profoundly acidic, resulting in unfavorable conditions for the microbial flora. Lactic acid–producing bacteria flourish, while the gram-negative bacteria, especially the Enterobacteriaceae, are killed in large numbers by the acids. Large quantities of endotoxin are released from the dying bacteria.[113]

The osmotic load from the lactic acid produced in the large intestine is an important factor in the development of diarrhea since organic acids such as lactic acid are poorly absorbed. Mild cases of carbohydrate overload may result purely from osmotic diarrhea. In more severe cases, the acidic contents of the large intestine are caustic to the mucosa, causing necrosis of the mucosal tissues, similar to that seen in ruminal acidosis. Diarrhea in this case is partially osmotic, but intestinal inflammation also contributes. Mucosal ulceration allows absorption of large quantities of endotoxin and lactic acid, normally poorly absorbed by intact mucosa.[114] Systemic endotoxemia and sepsis may be overwhelming, and profound metabolic acidosis may occur. Secretory diarrhea, with loss of bicarbonate, worsens the acidosis. Rapid and severe dehydration occurs secondary to the diarrhea. Endotoxemia, along with intestinal inflammation, adversely affects intestinal motility, and ileus develops. Ileus and gas production from fermentation of the carbohydrates may cause severe distention of the large intestine and signs of abdominal pain. Laminitis is a frequent complication of endotoxemia and lactic acidosis. In fact, carbohydrate overload is used to induce laminitis as an experimental model because of the consistency of the laminitis produced.[112–114]

Clinical Signs and Diagnosis

Clinical signs of colitis from carbohydrate overload can vary according to the amount of carbohydrate ingested and accommodation of the flora to a high carbohydrate diet. Mild cases may result in a transient osmotic diarrhea, with no systemic effects. More severe cases are characterized by signs similar to those described for other forms of colitis, including abdominal pain, moderate-to-severe diarrhea, and dehydration. Signs of endotoxemia and sepsis are frequently present in severe cases. Elevated heart and respiratory rates are common, with peripheral vasoconstriction early in the disease, followed by peripheral vasodilation as the disease progresses. Depression may be profound from metabolic acidosis and endotoxemia. Abdominal auscultation and percussion may reveal ileus and intestinal tympany. Nasogastric intubation may yield significant gastric acidic reflux. Particles of grain may be noted in the gastric reflux and the feces, if grain overload is the source of the carbohydrate overload. Laminitis may complicate both mild and severe cases of carbohydrate overload, especially if the animal has had previous bouts of laminitis.

Hematologic abnormalities include neutropenia and leukopenia. Severe dehydration may result in profound hemoconcentration. Protein loss later in the course of disease may result in hypoproteinemia. Serum biochemical abnormalities include azotemia, elevated hepatocellular enzyme activity, hyponatremia, and hypokalemia. Severe hypocalcemia and metabolic acidosis are characteristic of the disease. Serum lactate concentrations are elevated in the absence of evidence of intestinal strangulation or infarction. Peritoneal fluid analysis often reveals no abnormalities.

Treatment

Mild cases of carbohydrate overload may not require treatment other than exclusion of grains from the diet for several days to weeks, and gradual reintroduction of grain into the diet later if extra energy is needed. Patients showing signs of colic or diarrhea without other systemic signs may benefit from administration of mineral oil, charcoal, and fluids via nasogastric tube. Flushing of residual carbohydrate from the stomach may also be accomplished with the nasogastric tube. Often, NSAIDs such as phenylbutazone 2.2 to 4.4 mg/kg/day PO or IV or flunixin meglumine 0.1 to 0.25 mg/kg IV or PO q.6–8h. or 1 mg/kg PO or IV q.12h. are administered to prevent laminitis. Phenoxybenzamine and heparin given before the onset of laminitis may decrease or ablate the degree of laminitis produced.[34, 115]

More severe cases with dehydrating diarrhea, systemic signs of endotoxemia, or metabolic acidosis require intravenous fluid support to maintain water, electrolyte, and acid-base balance in addition to the previously mentioned treatments. Large amounts of bicarbonate-containing solutions may be required. Care should be taken when administering hypertonic bicarbonate solutions, since many patients are already hyperosmotic from lactic acidemia. Isotonic sodium bicarbonate 1.3% may be useful in the hyperosmotic patient. Careful attention to calcium balance is also important, since severe hypocalcemia may occur. Intravenous administration of plasma containing antibodies against rough mutants of gram-negative bacteria may be beneficial, especially in endotoxic patients. Intravenous broad-spectrum antibiotics are administered to combat bacteremia and septicemia, which frequently complicate carbohydrate overload–induced colitis.

In extreme cases, especially if the patient has ingested a very large quantity of grain, surgical removal of the grain from the large intestine may be indicated, especially before the onset of severe clinical signs. However, administration of oral cathartics, such as magnesium sulfate slurries or mineral oil, or a combination of these, is sufficient to clear the carbohydrate from the large intestine before fermentation, mucosal damage, and absorption of endotoxins and lactic acid occur. Oral administration of activated charcoal may prevent absorption of endotoxins by binding the molecules in the lumen of the bowel. In any case, feeding of the source of the soluble carbohydrate, such as grains, should be discontinued. Low carbohydrate and protein roughages such as grass or oat hays should be fed until the microbial flora recovers. Oral administration of probiotic preparations containing lactobacillus is contraindicated; however, other sources of normal equine large intestinal microbial flora, such as fecal extracts from normal feces, may be useful to reintroduce appropriate microorganisms. Complications from laminitis and sepsis are common, and often cause death.

Infiltrative Diseases

Chronic infiltrative diseases of the gastrointestinal tract include lymphosarcoma, granulomatous enterocolitis, and eosinophilic enterocolitis. These diseases primarily affect the small intestine, and the clinical signs usually reflect protein-losing enteropathy and malabsorption rather than diarrhea.[116–119] However, the large intestine may also be involved, especially in the case of eosinophilic enterocolitis causing chronic diarrhea. The pathogenesis of these diseases is largely unknown, but may involve immune-mediated mechanisms in the case of eosinophilic and granulomatous enterocolitis.[117, 119] Granulomatous enterocolitis in horses has been associated with mycobacterial and fungal infections and hairy vetch poisoning, but is usually idiopathic.[116–118] Food allergy and parasites have been suggested as causes of eosinophilic enterocolitis, since the eosinophil is the primary inflammatory cell involved.[119] However, very little data are available regarding the pathogenesis.

Since infiltrative diseases primarily affect the small intestine and only rarely cause clinical signs attributed solely to large intestinal disease, they are more appropriately covered under the heading of diseases of the small intestine. However, with regard to the pathophysiology of the diarrhea observed when the large intestine is involved, chronic inflammation of the intestine is a likely cause of secretion of fluid, and may account for the diarrhea to a large degree. Inflammation causes fluid secretion by infiltration of the submucosa and lamina propria with inflammatory cells, disruption of the interstitium, and release of inflammatory mediators. Infiltration of the interstitium disrupts normal fluid forces governing passive secretion, and may result in a net secretion of fluid into the lumen. In addition, reduced absorption of fluid may result from infiltration of the intestinal wall. Inflammatory mediators have well-described effects on the secretory activity of the mucosa.

Since clinical signs, diagnosis, and treatment relate primarily to small intestinal disease, these details are described elsewhere.

Sand Enteropathy

Sand enteropathy is described in more detail under the heading of obstructive diseases, since acute obstruction is often associated with abnormally large amounts of sand in the large intestine. However, chronic colitis is a distinct syndrome that can occur at any age from abnormal accumulation of sand in the large intestine.[120, 121] Chronic diarrhea and signs of colic may be seen without obstruction. The pathogenesis of sand accumulation in individual horses, other than simple ingestion of large quantities, is unclear, as described in Chapter 12.12. Presumably the sand causes irritation, and may disrupt motility, leading to diarrhea. The diarrhea is usually not severe and dehydrating, and may be intermittent. Weight loss is characteristic, and can be severe in some cases.[120] Complications may occur, such as peritonitis and acute obstruction.[120]

Diagnosis is based on finding abnormal amounts of sand in the feces and auscultation of characteristic sand sounds in the ventral abdomen. Occasionally, radiography may be required to diagnose the disease.[120] Treatment requires removal of the sand from the gastrointestinal tract as described in Chapter 12.12, using psyllium products and magnesium sulfate slurries administered orally. Analgesics may be required initially to relieve pain and stimulate appetite. A diet high in roughage often stimulates further passage of sand. Treatment may require several weeks to remove as much sand as possible. Prevention of the disease is important, and recurrence is not unusual.

REFERENCES

1. Smith BP: *Salmonella* infection in horses. *Compendium Continuing Educ Pract Vet* 3:S4–S17, 1981.
2. Smith BP, Reina-Guerra M, Hardy AJ: Prevalence and epizootiology of equine salmonellosis. *J Am Vet Med Assoc* 172:353–356, 1978.
3. Donahue JM: Emergence of antibiotic resistant *Salmonella agona* in horses in Kentucky. *J Am Vet Med Assoc* 188:592–595, 1986.
4. Traub-Dargatz JL, Salman MD, Jones RL: Epidemiologic study of *Salmonella* shedding in the feces of horses and the potential risk factors for development of the infection in hospitalized horses. *J Am Vet Med Assoc* 196:1617–1622, 1990.
5. Smith BP: Understanding the role of endotoxins in gram-negative sepsis. *Vet Med* 12:1148–1161, 1986.
6. Carter JD, Hird DW, Farver TB, et al: Salmonellosis in hospitalized horses: Seasonality and case fatality rates. *J Am Vet Med Assoc* 188:163–164, 1986.
7. Morse EV, Duncan MA, Page EA, et al: Salmonellosis in equidae: A study of 23 cases. *Cornell Vet* 66:198–213, 1976.
8. Gianella RA: Pathogenesis of acute bacterial diarrheal disorders. *Annu Rev Med* 32:341–357, 1981.
9. Finlay BB, Falkow S: Virulence factors associated with *Salmonella* species. *Microbiol Sci* 5:324–328, 1988.
10. Hirsch DC: The alimentary canal as a microbial habitat. In Biberstein EL, Zee YC, eds: *Review of Veterinary Microbiology.* Boston, Blackwell Scientific, 1990, pp 93–97.
11. Hirsch DC: *Salmonella.* In Biberstein EL, Zee YC, eds: *Review of Veterinary Microbiology.* Boston, Blackwell Scientific, 1990, pp 110–113.
12. Clarke RC, Gyles CL: *Salmonella.* In Gyles CL, Thoen CO,

eds: *Pathogenesis of Bacterial Infections in Animals.* Ames, Iowa State University Press, 1986, pp 95–109.

13. Smith BP, Hardy AJ, Reina-Guerra M: A preliminary evaluation of some preparations of *Salmonella typhimurium* as vaccines in horses. In Moore JN, White NA, Becht JL, eds: *Proceedings of the First Equine Colic Symposium.* Lawrenceville, NJ, Veterinary Learning Systems, 1982, pp 211–215.

14. Smith BP, Reina-Guerra M, Hoiseth SK, et al: Aromatic dependent *Salmonella typhimurium* as modified live vaccines for calves. *Am J Vet Res* 45:59–66, 1984.

15. King JN, Gerring EL: The action of low dose endotoxin on equine bowel motility. *Equine Vet J* 23:11–17, 1991.

16. O'Loughlin EV, Scott RB, Gall DG: Pathophysiology of infectious diarrhea: Changes in intestinal structure and function. *J Pediatr Gastroenterol Nutr* 12:5–20, 1991.

17. Koo FC, Peterson JW, Houston CW, et al: Pathogenesis of experimental salmonellosis: Inhibitors of protein synthesis by cytotoxin. *Infect Immun* 43:93–100, 1984.

18. Gianella RA, Gots RE, Charney AN, et al: Pathogenesis of *Salmonella*-mediated intestinal fluid secretion: Activation of adenylate cyclase and inhibition by indomethacin. *Gastroenterology* 69:1238–1245, 1975.

19. Peterson JW, Molina NC, Houston CW, et al: Elevated cAMP in intestinal epithelial cells during experimental cholera and salmonellosis. *Toxicon* 21:761–775, 1983.

20. Murray MJ: Enterotoxin activity of a *Salmonella typhimurium* of equine origin in vivo in rabbits and the effect of *Salmonella* culture lysates and cholera toxin on equine colonic mucosa in vitro. *Am J Vet Res* 47:769–773, 1986.

21. Duebbert IE, Peterson JW: Enterotoxin-induced fluid accumulation during experimental salmonellosis and cholera: Involvement of prostaglandin synthesis by intestinal cells. *Toxicon* 23:157–172, 1985.

22. Rumschlag HS, Boyce JR: Plasmid profile analysis of *Salmonellae* in a large-animal hospital. *Vet Microbiol* 13:301–311, 1987.

23. Gulig PA: Virulence plasmids of *Salmonella typhimurium* and other *Salmonellae*. *Microb Pathog* 8:3–11, 1990.

24. Gianella RA: Importance of the intestinal inflammatory reaction in *Salmonella*-mediated intestinal secretion. *Infect Immun* 23:140–145, 1979.

25. Murray MJ: Digestive physiology of the large intestine in adult horses. Part II: Pathophysiology of colitis. *Compendium Continuing Educ Pract Vet* 10:1309–1316, 1988.

26. Smith BP, Reina-Guerra M, Hardy AJ, et al: Equine salmonellosis: Experimental production of four syndromes. *Am J Vet Res* 40:1072–1077, 1979.

27. Palmer JE, Whitlock RH, Benson CE, et al: Comparison of rectal mucosal cultures and fecal cultures in detecting *Salmonella* infection in horses and cattle. *Am J Vet Res* 46:697–698, 1985.

28. Kaufmann HJ, Taubin HL: Nonsteroidal anti-inflammatory drugs activate quiescent inflammatory bowel disease. *Ann Intern Med* 107:513–516, 1987.

29. Meschter CL, Krook MG, Maylin G, et al: The effects of phenylbutazone on the intestinal mucosa of the horse: A morphologic, ultrastructural, and biochemical study. *Equine Vet J* 22:255–263, 1990.

30. Fedorak RN, Empey LR, Walker K: Verapamil alters eicosanoid synthesis and accelerates healing in experimental colitis in rats. *Gastroenterology* 102:1229–1235, 1992.

31. Semrad SD, Hardee GE, Hardee MM, et al: Low dose flunixin meglumine: Effects on eicosanoid production and clinical signs induced by experimental endotoxemia in horses. *Equine Vet J* 19:201–206, 1987.

32. Tyler JW, Cullor JS, Spier SJ, et al: Immunity targeting common core antigens of gram-negative bacteria. *J Vet Intern Med* 4:17–25, 1990.

33. Belknap JK, Moore JN: Evaluation of heparin for prophylaxis of equine laminitis: 71 cases (1980–1986). *J Am Vet Med Assoc* 195:505–507, 1989.

34. Cambridge H, Lees P, Hooke RE, et al: Anti-thrombotic action of aspirin in the horse. *Equine Vet J* 23:123–127, 1991.

35. Van de Water L, Schroeder S, Crenshaw EB, et al: Phagocytosis of gelatin-latex particles by a murine macrophage line is dependent on fibronectin and heparin. *J Cell Biol* 90:32–34, 1981.

36. Doran JE, Mansberger AR, Edmondson HT, et al: Cold insoluble globulin and heparin interactions in phagocytosis by macrophage monolayers: Mechanism of heparin enhancement. *J Reticuloendothelial Soc* 29:285–294, 1981.

37. Fuller R: Probiotics in man and animals. *J Appl Bacteriol* 66:365–378, 1989.

38. Mulville P: Equine monocytic ehrlichiosis (Potomac horse fever): A review. *Equine Vet J* 23:400–404, 1991.

39. Dutta SK, Myrup AC, Rice RM, et al: Experimental reproduction of Potomac horse fever in horses with a newly isolated *Ehrlichia* organism. *J Clin Microbiol* 22:265–269, 1985.

40. Rikihisa Y, Perry BD: Causative ehrlichial organism in Potomac horse fever. *Infect Immun* 49:513–517, 1985.

41. Levine JF, Levy MG, Nicholson WL, et al: Attempted *Ehrlichia risticci* transmission with *Dermacentor variabilis* (Acaridae:Ixodidae). *J Med Entomol* 27:931–933, 1990.

42. Burg GJ, Roberts AW, Williams NM, et al: Attempted transmission of *Ehrlichia risticci* (Rickettsiaceae) with *Stomoxys calcitrans* (Diptera:Muscidae). *J Med Entomol* 27:874–877, 1990.

43. Ziemer EL, Whitlock RH, Palmer JE, et al: Clinical and hematologic variables in ponies with experimentally induced equine ehrlichial colitis (Potomac horse fever). *Am J Vet Res* 48:63–67, 1987.

44. Rikihisa Y, Perry BD, Cordes DO: Ultrastructural study of ehrlichial organisms in the large colons of ponies infected with Potomac horse fever. *Infect Immun* 49:505–512, 1985.

45. Cordes DO, Perry BD, Rikihisa Y, et al: Enterocolitis caused by *Ehrlichia* sp in the horse (Potomac horse fever). *Vet Pathol* 23:471–477, 1986.

46. Rikihisa Y: Growth of *Ehrlichia risticci* in human colonic epithelial cells. *Ann N Y Acad Sci* 590:104–110, 1989.

47. Wells MY, Rikihisa Y: Lack of lysosomal fusion with phagosomes containing *Ehrlichia risticci* in P388D cells: Abrogation of inhibition with oxytetracycline. *Infect Immun* 56:3209–3215, 1988.

48. Rikihisa Y, Johnson GC, Cooke HJ, et al: Pathophysiologic changes of large colon of horses infected with *Ehrlichia risticci* (abstract). In Moore JN, White S, Morris DD, eds: *Proceedings of the Third Equine Colic Symposium.* Lawrenceville, NJ, Veterinary Learning Systems, 1988.

48a. Rikihisa Y, Johnson GC, Wang Y-Z, et al: Loss of absorptive capacity for sodium and chloride in the colon causes diarrhea in Potomac horse fever. *Res Vet Sci* 52:353–362, 1992.

49. Dutta SK, Penney BE, Myrup AC, et al: Disease features in horses with induced equine monocytic ehrlichiosis (Potomac horse fever). *Am J Vet Res* 49:1747–1751, 1988.

50. Morris DD, Messick J, Whitlock RH, et al: Effects of equine ehrlichial colitis on the hemostatic system in ponies. *Am J Vet Res* 49:1030–1036, 1988.

51. Biswar B, Mukherjee D, Mattingly-Napier BL, et al: Diagnostic application of polymerase chain reaction for detection of *Ehrlichia risticci* in equine monocytic ehrlichiosis (Potomac horse fever). *J Clin Microbiol* 29:2228–2233, 1991.

52. White G, Prior SD: Comparative effects of oral administration of trimethoprim-sulphadiazine or oxytetracycline on the fecal flora of horses. *Vet Rec* 111:316–318, 1982.

53. Ristic M, Holland CJ, Goetz TE: Evaluation of a vaccine for equine monocytic ehrlichiosis. In *Proceedings of Symposium on Potomac Horse Fever,* 1988, pp 89–100.

54. Rikihisa Y, Pretzman CI, Johnson GC, et al: Clinical, histopathological, and immunological response of ponies to *Ehrlichia sennetsu* and subsequent *Ehrlichia risticci* challenge. *Infect Immun* 56:2960–2966, 1988.

55. Kaylor PS, Crawford TB, McElwain TF, et al: Passive transfer of antibody to *Ehrlichia risticci* protects mice from ehrlichiosis. *Infect Immun* 591:2058–2062, 1991.

56. Weirup MO: Equine intestinal clostridiosis. An acute disease in horses associated with high intestinal counts of *Clostridium perfringens* type A. *Acta Vet Scand Suppl* 62:1–182, 1977.

57. Ochoa R, Kern SR: The effects of *Clostridium perfringens* type A enterotoxin in Shetland ponies—clinical, morphological, and clinicopathological changes. *Vet Pathol* 17:738–747, 1980.

58. Samuel SC, Hancock P, Leigh DA: An investigation into *Clostridium perfringens* enterotoxin–associated diarrhoea. *J Hosp Infect* 18:219–230, 1991.

59. Linerode PA, Goode RL: The effect of colic on the microbial activity of the equine large intestine. *Proc Am Assoc Equine Pract* 16:321–341, 1970.

60. Niilo L: Enterotoxemic *Clostridium perfringens.* In Gyles CL, Toen CO, eds: *Pathogenesis of Bacterial Infections in Animals.* Ames, Iowa State University Press, 1986, pp 80–86.

61. Jones RL, Adney WS, Alexander AF, et al: Hemorrhagic necrotizing enterocolitis associated with *Clostridium difficile* infection in four foals. *J Am Vet Med Assoc* 193:76–79, 1988.

62. Prescott JF, Staempeli HR, Barker IK, et al: A method for reproducing fatal idiopathic colitis (colitis X) in ponies and isolation of a *Clostridium* as a possible agent. *Equine Vet J* 20:417–420, 1988.

63. Wierup M, DiPietro JA: Bacteriologic examination of equine fecal flora as a diagnostic tool for equine intestinal clostridiosis. *Am J Vet Res* 42:2167–2169, 1981.

64. Smilack JD, Wilson WR, Cockerill FR: Tetracyclines, chloramphenicol, erythromycin, and metronidazole. *Mayo Clin Proc* 66:1270–1280, 1991.

65. Drudge JH: Clinical aspects of *Strongylus vulgaris* infection in the horse. *Vet Clin North Am Equine Pract* 1:251–265, 1979.

66. Owen J, Slocombe D: Pathogenesis of helminths in equines. *Vet Parasitol* 18:139–153, 1985.

67. Bueno L, Ruckebusch Y, Dorchies P: Disturbances of digestive motility in horses associated with strongyle infection. *Vet Parasitol* 5:253–260, 1979.

68. Lester GD, Bolton JR, Cambridge H, et al: The effect of *Strongylus vulgaris* larvae on equine intestinal myoelectrical activity. *Equine Vet J* 7(suppl):8–13, 1986.

69. White NA: Intestinal infarction associated with mesenteric vascular thrombotic disease in the horse. *J Am Vet Med Assoc* 178:259–262, 1981.

70. Becht JL: The role of parasites in colic. *Proc Am Assoc Equine Pract* 33:301–309, 1987.

71. Sellers AF, Lowe JE, Drost OJ, et al: Retropulsion-propulsion in the equine large colon. *Am J Vet Res* 43:390–395, 1982.

72. Greatorex JC: Diarrhea in horses associated with ulceration of the colon and caecum from *Strongylus vulgaris* larval migration. *Vet Rec* 97:221–225, 1975.

73. Amborski GF, Bello TR, Torbert BJ: Host response to experimentally induced infections of *Strongylus vulgaris* in parasite-free ponies and naturally infected ponies. *Am J Vet Res* 35:1181–1188, 1974.

74. Klei TR, Torbert BJ, Ochoa R, et al: Morphologic and clinico-pathologic changes following *Strongylus vulgaris* infections of immune and nonimmune ponies. *Am J Vet Res* 43:1300–1307, 1982.

75. Patton S, Mock RE, Drudge JH, et al: Increased immunoglobulin T concentration in ponies as a response to experimental infection with the nematode *Strongylus vulgaris. Am J Vet Res* 39:19–22, 1978.

76. Chiejina SN, Macon JA: Immature stages of *Trichonema* spp as a cause of diarrhea in adult horses in spring. *Vet Rec* 100:360–361, 1977.

77. Giles CJ, Urquhart KA, Longstaffe JA: Larval cyathostomiasis (immature *Trichonema*-induced enteropathy): A report of 15 clinical cases. *Equine Vet J* 17:196–201, 1985.

78. Church S, Kelly DF, Obriolo MJ: Diagnosis and successful treatment of diarrhea in horses caused by immature small strongyles apparently insusceptible to anthelmintics. *Equine Vet J* 18:401–403, 1986.

79. Uhlinger CA: Equine small strongyles: Epidemiology pathology, and control. *Compendium Continuing Educ Pract Vet* 13:863–869, 1991.

80. Andersson G, Ehman L, Manson I, et al: Lethal complications following administration of oxytetracycline in the horse. *Nord Vet Med* 23:9–22, 1971.

81. Raisbeck MF, Holt GR, Osweiler GD: Lincomycin-associated colitis in horses. *J Am Vet Med Assoc* 179:362–363, 1981.

82. Owen RR, Fullerton J, Barnum DA: Effects of transportation, surgery, and antibiotic therapy in ponies infected with *Salmonella. Am J Vet Res* 44:46–50, 1983.

83. Knothe H: The effects of trimethoprim-sulphonamide, trimethoprim, and sulphonamide on the occurrence of resistant Enterobacteriaceae in human intestinal flora. *Infection* 7(suppl 4):S321–S323, 1979.

84. Argenzio RA: Physiology of diarrhea—Large intestine. *J Am Vet Med Assoc* 173:667–672, 1978.

85. Rao SCC, Edwards CA, Austen CJ, et al: Impaired colonic fermentation of carbohydrate after ampicillin. *Gastroenterology* 94:928–932, 1988.

86. Clausen MR, Bonnen H, Tvede M, et al: Colonic fermentation to short-chain fatty acids is decreased in antibiotic-associated diarrhea. *Gastroenterology* 101:1492–1504, 1991.

87. Grossman RF: The relationship of absorption characteristics and gastrointestinal side effects of oral antimicrobial agents. *Clin Ther* 13:189–193, 1991.

88. Lakritz J, Madigan J, Carlson GP: Hypovolemic hyponatremia and signs of neurologic disease associated with diarrhea in a foal. *J Am Vet Med Assoc* 200:1114–1116, 1992.

89. Wunderlich PF, Braun C, Fumagalli I, et al: Double blind report of the efficacy of lactic acid–producing enterococcus SF68 in the prevention of antibiotic-associated diarrhoea and the treatment of acute diarrhoea. *J Int Med Res* 17:333–338, 1989.

90. Siitonen S, Vapaatalo H, Salminen S, et al: Effect of *Lactobacillus* GG yoghurt in prevention of antibiotic-associated diarroea. *Ann Med* 22:57–59, 1990.

91. Kore A: Toxicology of non-steroidal antiinflammatory drugs. *Vet Clin North Am Small Anim Pract* 20:419–430, 1990.

92. Gilson GR, Whiteacre EB, Ricotti GA: Colitis induced by nonsteroidal antiinflammatory drugs: Report of four cases and review of the literature. *Arch Intern Med* 152:625–632, 1992.

93. Murray MJ: Phenylbutazone toxicity in a horse. *Compendium Continuing Educ Pract Vet* 7:S389–S394, 1985.

94. Semble EL, Wu WL: Prostaglandins in the gut and their relationship to nonsteroidal antiinflammatory drugs. *Baillieres Clin Rheumatol* 3:247–269, 1989.

95. Lees P, Creed RFS, Gerring EEL, et al: Biochemical and hematological effects of phenylbutazone in horses. *Equine Vet J* 15:158–167, 1983.

96. Collins LG, Tyler DE: Experimentally induced phenylbutazone toxicosis in ponies: Description of the syndrome and its prevention with synthetic prostaglandin E_2. *Am J Vet Res* 46:1605–1615, 1985.

97. Clarke LL, Argenzio RA: NaCl transport across equine proximal colon and the effect of endogenous prostaglandin. *Am J Physiol* 259:G62–G69, 1990.

98. Karcher LF, Dill SG, Anderson WI, et al: Right dorsal colitis. *Vet Intern Med* 4:247–253, 1990.

99. Scmitz DG: Cantharidin toxicosis in horses. *J Vet Intern Med* 3:208–215, 1989.

100. Shawley RV, Rolf LL: Experimental cantharidiasis in the horse. *Am J Vet Res* 45:2261–2266, 1984.

101. Scoeb TR, Panciera RJ: Pathology of blister beetle (*Epicauta*) poisoning in horses. *Vet Pathol* 16:18–31, 1979.

102. Ray AC, Kyle ALG, Murphy MJ, et al: Etiologic agents, incidence, and improved diagnostic methods of cantharidin toxicosis in horses. *Am J Vet Res* 50:187–191, 1989.

103. Osweiler GD, Carron JL, Buck WB, et al: *Clinical and Diagnostic Veterinary Toxicology,* ed 3. Dubuque, Iowa, Kendal/Hunt, 1985, pp 253–266.

104. Tamaki S, Frankenberger WT: Environmental biochemistry of arsenic. *Rev Environ Contam Toxicol* 124:79–108, 1992.

105. Louria DB: Trace metal poisoning. In Wyngaarden JB, Smith LH, eds: *Cecil Textbook of Medicine,* 18th ed. Philadelphia, WB Saunders, 1988, pp 2385–2393.

106. Mack RB: Arsenic intoxication. *N C Med J* 44:753–755, 1983.

107. Dunkin TE: Colitis X. *Proc Am Assoc Equine Pract* 15:371–376, 1969.

108. Olson NE: Acute diarrheal disease in the horse. *J Am Vet Med Assoc* 148:418–421, 1966.

109. Rooney JR, Bryans JT, Prickett ME, et al: Exhaustion shock in the horse. *Cornell Vet* 56:220–235, 1966.

110. Mansmann RA: Equine anaphylaxis (abstract). *Fed Proc* 31:661, 1972.

111. Garner HE, Hutcheson DP, Coffman JR, et al: Lactic acidosis: A factor associated with equine laminitis. *J Anim Sci* 45:1037–1041, 1977.

112. Garner HE, Moore JN, Johnson JH, et al: Changes in the caecal flora associated with the onset of laminitis. *Equine Vet J* 10:249–252, 1978.

113. Moore JN, Garner HE, Berg JN, et al: Intracecal endotoxin and lactate during the onset of equine laminitis: A preliminary report. *Am J Vet Res* 6:722–723, 1979.

114. Sprouse RF, Garner HE, Green EM: Plasma endotoxin levels in horses subjected to carbohydrate-induced laminitis. *Equine Vet J* 19:25–28, 1987.

115. Hood DM, Stephen KA, Amoss MS: The use of alpha and beta adrenergic blockade as a preventive in the carbohydrate model of laminitis: A preliminary report. In *Proceedings of the First Equine Endotoxin Laminitis Symposium,* 1982, pp 141–150.

116. Platt H: Chronic inflammatory and lymphoproliferative lesions of the equine small intestine. *J Comp Pathol* 96:671–684, 1986.

117. Merritt M, Cimprich RE, Beech J: Granulomatous enteritis in nine horses. *J Am Vet Med Assoc* 169:603–609, 1976.

118. Dade AW, Lichfeldt WE, McAllister HA: Granulomatous colitis in a horse with histoplasmosis. *Vet Med Small Anim Clin* 3:279–281, 1973.

119. Pass DA, Bolten JR: Chronic eosinophilic gastroenteritis in the horse. *Vet Pathol* 19:486–496, 1982.

120. Bertone JJ, Traub-Dargatz JL, Wrigley RW, et al: Diarrhea associated with sand in the gastrointestinal tract of horses. *J Am Vet Med Assoc* 193:1409–1412, 1988.

121. Ramey DW, Reinertson EL: Sand-induced diarrhea in a foal. *J Am Vet Med Assoc* 185:537–538, 1984.

12.12

Obstructive Conditions of the Large Intestine

Samuel L. Jones, MS, DVM
Jack R. Snyder, DVM, PhD, Dip ACVS
Sharon J. Spier, DVM, PhD, Dip ACVIM

NONSTRANGULATING DISPLACEMENT OF THE ASCENDING COLON

Pathogenesis

Displacement of the ascending colon is a common cause of large intestinal obstruction.[1, 2] The ascending colon is freely movable except for the right dorsal and ventral colons. Contact with adjacent viscera and the abdominal wall tends to inhibit movement of the ascending colon from a normal position; however, accumulation of gas and fluid or ingesta may cause the colon to migrate.[3] Feeding behavior is thought to play a role in normal function of the large intestine.[4] Feeding large meals at infrequent intervals encourages the rapid consumption of large amounts of food. Ingestion of large meals high in concentrates has been shown to disrupt normal motility patterns throughout the intestinal tract.[4] The rate of passage of the ingesta is increased, allowing a greater percentage of soluble carbohydrates to reach the large intestine.[4] The rate of fermentation is enhanced, and the amount of gas and volatile fatty acids increases rapidly. The production of large amounts of volatile fatty acids stimulates the secretion of large volumes of fluid into the colon.[5] Displacements of the ascending colon seem to be more prevalent in horses fed a high-concentrate, low-roughage diet.[6] Rapid changes in gas and fluid volume of the colon may well play a part in the migration of the ascending colon from a normal position.

Abnormal motility patterns of the ascending colon have also been suggested to contribute to the development of colonic displacement.[2] Feeding stimulates colonic motility via the gastrocolic reflex, but large meals may disrupt normal motility patterns and concurrently allow rapid accumulation of gas and fluid from fermentation. Feeding large meals is more likely to affect normal motility patterns than feeding small frequent meals.[4] Distention associated with gas and fluid and the production of volatile fatty acids (VFAs) have been shown to increase colon motility.[7] Further, obstruction with distention of the small intestine also increases the motility of the ascending colon (colic motor complex).[8] Displacements of the large colon have been associated with naturally occurring small intestinal obstruction, such as epiploic foramen entrapment and ileal impaction.[9, 10] Migration of parasite larvae (strongyles) through the intestinal wall or in the vasculature has been suggested to disrupt motility patterns directly or secondarily by causing intermittent ischemia.[11] Other experimental studies have also shown that *Strongylus vulgaris* infection results in reduced blood flow to segments of the large intestine without necessarily causing infarction.[12] Electrical activity of the colon and cecocolic junction increases after infection with *S. vulgaris* and cyathostome larvae, probably reflecting a direct effect of migration through the intestine and an early response to reduced blood flow.[13, 14]

Displacements of the ascending colon are generally divided into three types: left dorsal displacement, right dorsal displacement, and retroflexion.[3] Left dorsal displacement is characterized by entrapment of the ascending colon in the renosplenic space. The colon is often twisted 180 degrees such that the left ventral colon is situated in a dorsal position relative to the left dorsal colon. The entrapped portion may only be the pelvic flexure, or may involve a large portion of the ascending colon, with the pelvic flexure situated near the diaphragm. The colon may become entrapped by migrating dorsally between the left abdominal wall and the spleen, or may migrate in a caudodorsal direction over the renosplenic fold.[3, 15] Occasionally, the ascending colon can be palpated between the spleen and abdominal wall, lending support to the first mechanism of displacement. Gastric distention is thought to predispose horses to left dorsal displacement of the ascending colon by displacing the spleen medially, allowing the colon room to migrate along the abdominal wall.[15]

Right dorsal displacement begins by movement of the colon cranially, then either medial (medial flexion) or lateral (lateral flexion) to the cecum. The proportion of right dorsal displacements with medial vs. lateral flexion is approximately 1:15.[15] In either case, the pelvic flexure ends up adjacent to the diaphragm. Retroflexion of the ascending colon occurs by movement of the pelvic flexure cranially without movement of the sternal or diaphragmatic flexures.

Displacement of the ascending colon partially obstructs the lumen, resulting in accumulation of gas or ingesta, causing distention. The distention may be exacerbated by the secretion of fluid in response to the distention.[16] Tension and stretch of the visceral wall is an important source of the pain associated with colonic displacement. Tension on mesenteric attachments and the root of the mesentery by the enlarged colon may also cause pain.[1] Ischemia is rarely associated with nonstrangulating displacement of the colon. However, vascular congestion and edema are often seen in the displaced segments of colon, resulting from increased hydrostatic pressure from reduced venous outflow. Morphologic damage to the tissues is usually minor.

Clinical Signs and Diagnosis

Displacement of the ascending colon is characterized by intermittent signs of mild to moderate abdominal pain of acute onset, but, an insidious onset of colic is not unusual.[3, 15] Mild-to-moderate dehydration may be noted if the duration of the displacement is sufficient. The heart rate may be elevated during periods of abdominal pain, but is often normal. Abdominal distention may be present if the colon is enlarged by gas, fluid, or ingesta. Fecal production is reduced and abdominal borborygmi are heard less frequently than normal, and progressive motility of the large intestine is absent. Percussion may reveal evidence of gas distention of the colon.

Left dorsal displacements are often diagnosed by transrectal examination. The left ventral colon can be felt in a dorsal position, and is often gas-filled. The ascending colon can be traced to the renosplenic space, and the spleen may be displaced medially. Right dorsal displacements are characterized by the presence of the distended ventral colon running across the pelvic inlet, and may be felt between the cecum and the body wall if a lateral flexion is present. The pelvic flexure is usually not palpable. Retroflexion of the ascending colon may produce a palpable kink in the colon. If the displaced colons are not distended by gas in the instance of right dorsal displacement and retroflexion, the ascending colon may not be palpable and is conspicuous by its absence from a normal position.

Peritoneal fluid may be increased in amount, but the color, clarity, and white blood cell count are usually normal. The protein concentration may be elevated from inflammation of the serosa of the displaced segment. The displaced segment is often edematous, and fluid leaking through the serosa into the peritoneal fluid increases the protein concentration.

Treatment

Surgical correction of colon displacement is the most effective means of resolving this disorder. Delay in surgical intervention may lead to disastrous results such as ischemic injury or rupture of the colon. Left dorsal displacements have been corrected using a technique of rolling the horse under general anesthesia.[10] This technique is effective in many cases if the colon is not distended.[10] Distention of the colon not only increases the difficulty of reducing the displacement by rolling but increases the likelihood of rupture. Furthermore, other obstructive disorders, such as torsion of the ascending colon, may coexist with the displacement, necessitating surgical treatment after reducing the left dorsal displacement conservatively.[1, 3, 10] The majority of cases of ascending colon displacements corrected surgically recover well. Most horses begin eating a roughage diet soon (within 24 hours) after surgery. Left dorsal displacements have a higher rate of recurrence than right dorsal displacements.

Strict withdrawal of food in combination with supportive care may lead to resolution of the displacement. Intravenous administration of polyionic fluids and analgesic drugs are important. Flunixin meglumine 0.25 to 0.5 mg/kg t.i.d. or q.i.d. or 1.1 mg/kg b.i.d. provides good analgesia while reducing inflammation of the colon. During periods of severe pain, more potent analgesic drugs such as xylazine 0.3 to 1.0 mg/kg or butorphanol 0.01 to 1.0 mg/kg, or a combination of the two drugs, provides very effective short-term analgesia. Administration of analgesic drugs should be done cautiously if surgical correction of the displacement is an option so that signs of deteriorating condition are not masked. Intravenous fluid administration should be done conservatively at a maintenance rate. Overzealous intravenous fluid administration may contribute to fluid accumulation in the displaced colon.

STRANGULATING OBSTRUCTION OF THE LARGE INTESTINE
Pathogenesis

Strangulating obstruction of the large intestine occurs when the vasculature of the affected segment is disrupted. Volvulus or torsion of the ascending colon is the most frequent cause of strangulating displacement of the large intestine.[3, 17] Torsion of the ascending colon occurs at the sternal and diaphragmatic flexures, while volvulus of the ascending colon usually occurs at the mesenteric attachment, but may include the cecum.[17] Torsion or entrapment of the descending colon also occurs, but is unusual.[3] Strangulating obstruction of the ascending colon was found in 11% to 17% of adult horses undergoing surgical exploration for colic.[18, 19] Periparturient mares are thought to be predisposed to torsion or volvulus of the ascending colon, but the condition is also seen in males and in mares independent of parturition.[17, 20] Development of torsion or volvulus of the ascending colon may be associated with the same factors as found in nonstrangulating displacements, such as gas or ingesta accumulation in the colon, or altered motility.[3] Patients with torsion of the ascending colon often have ingesta in the dorsal colon, with a gas-distended ventral colon.[17] Whether the accumulation of ingesta in the dorsal colon and gas in the ventral colon led to the development of a torsion or occurred after the torsion developed is unknown. The reason for the high incidence in periparturient mares is unknown, but may be related to an increase in the volume of the abdomen during pregnancy.

Torsion or volvulus greater than 270 degrees results in strangulation of the vasculature at the site of the twist. Rotation of the ascending colon greater than 360 degrees is associated with a poor prognosis for survival, presumably owing to the extreme strangulation of the colonic tissue and vessels.[17, 20] Torsion or volvulus of the ascending colon can occur in a dorsomedial or dorsolateral direction. Dorsolateral rotation is more common, possibly because the cecocolic ligament resists dorsomedial rotation.[20] Strangulating obstruction of the descending colon may result from torsion, but is more commonly associated with entrapment in a mesenteric rent, or strangulation by a lipoma.[3] Strangulating obstruction of the large intestine causes complete obstruction of the lumen, resulting in rapid and severe distention of the displaced segment. Severe distention and intestinal ischemia contribute to the pain seen clinically.

Strangulating obstruction of the large intestine may be classified as hemorrhagic or ischemic strangulation.[17] Hemorrhagic strangulation occurs when the venous outflow from the segment is obstructed, while the arterial supply is intact. The serosa appears dark red to purple, and the mucosa becomes black with time. Marked hemorrhage and edema of the intestinal wall are seen grossly and microscopically. Ischemic strangulation occurs when the arterial blood flow is obstructed before significant venous obstruction occurs. The serosa and mucosa appear gray, with less edema than seen with hemorrhagic strangulation.[17] Hemorrhagic strangulation represents a syndrome characterized experimentally as a low flow state, whereas ischemic strangulation is referred to as a no flow state.[21] The pathogenesis of intestinal injury is similar in either case: ischemia leading to cellular death and necrosis of mucosal cells, followed by the muscular and serosal layers.[21] Morphologic and biochemical evidence of reperfusion injury during experimental ischemia and reperfusion of the equine colon have been reported, and may explain the failure of the mucosal layer to recover in some cases of strangulating obstruction.[21–23] A no flow state leads to irreversible morphologic and biochemical damage more readily than a low flow state, and may be more prone to develop reperfusion injury.[21]

Thrombosis of the vessels supplying the mucosa has been seen histologically in biopsy samples from natural cases of ascending colon torsion.[24] This thrombosis is thought to occur from the aggregation and activation of platelets in areas of injured epithelium, with activation of the coagulation cascade by vascular injury, platelet products, endotoxin, and inflammatory mediators.[24] Coagulopathies, decreased antithrombin III activity, and disseminated intravascular coagulation (DIC) have been documented in horses with endotoxemia, and strangulating obstruction of the ascending colon.[25–27] Thrombosis of the vessels supplying the mucosa may be in part responsible for the continued deterioration of the colonic mucosa after the blood supply has been restored to the affected segment of colon.[24]

Ischemic injury to the mucosa and loss of mucosal cells disrupts the barrier preventing the absorption of endotoxins and the translocation of bacteria. Normal fluxes of electrolytes and water are also severely affected. As a result, endotoxemia, septicemia, electrolyte and acid-base imbalances, dehydration, and shock are common clinical features of torsion or volvulus of the ascending colon.[17, 20] Diarrhea, which may be life-threatening, commonly occurs after surgical correction of strangulating obstruction of the ascending colon.[20] The duration and degree (i.e., low flow vs. no flow state) of strangulation dictate the severity of complicating factors associated with mucosal injury. The percentage of cellular necrosis of the mucosa seen histopathologically correlates with survival, largely owing to the complications associated with the loss of the mucosal barrier. The percentage of crypts that undergo necrosis correlates with survival also, since the crypt cells are the only source of cells capable of regenerating and reepithelializing the colonic mucosa.[17]

Clinical Signs and Diagnosis

Strangulating obstruction of the ascending colon or cecum is characterized clinically by acute, moderate-to-severe abdominal pain.[17, 20] Abdominal distention develops rapidly and may be severe enough to compromise respiration and venous return from compression of the diaphragm and caudal vena cava. The heart rate is often markedly elevated, but not in all cases.[17] Shock may be a feature, manifested as tachycardia, poor pulse quality, slow capillary refill time, cool extremities, and pale mucous membranes. The respiratory rate is often elevated with shallow respirations, especially if abdominal distention is severe. Mild to moderate dehydration may be noted. If intestinal ischemia has caused significant mucosal injury, signs of endotoxemia and sepsis may be seen, most notably endotoxemic shock.

Feces production is decreased and abdominal borborygmi are usually absent. Abdominal percussion may reveal tympanic resonance over gas-distended viscus. Transrectal palpation is often diagnostic when strangulating obstruction of the ascending colon is present.[17, 20] Severe gas distention of the ascending colon or cecum or both, may be felt. The strangulated segment of ascending intestine will be markedly edematous, and congestion of the mesenteric vasculature may be palpable. Often, the degree of distention of the colon precludes accurate evaluation of the position of the segments of colon; however, the left ventral colon is most prominent, and may be situated in a dorsal position at the pelvic inlet. Strangulating obstruction of the descending colon causes severe gas distention of the descending colon. The strangulated segment of descending colon becomes edematous, as with the ascending colon.

Hematologic and serum biochemical abnormalities are often not evident early in the course of a strangulating displacement. Later, hemoconcentration and metabolic acidosis may be seen.[20] The serum calcium concentration may be abnormally low. The serum and peritoneal fluid phosphate and lactate concentrations and serum anion gap may be elevated from tissue ischemia and cellular necrosis. Peritoneal fluid may be normal in color and clarity. The protein concentration is usually elevated (>2.0 g/dL).[20] The red and white blood cell counts rise as vascular and tissue damage progresses. The color of the fluid becomes serosanguinous, orange, or red-brown. Glucose concentration and pH decrease from ischemia of the tissues. Biochemical or cellular abnormalities signify advanced ischemia of the intestine, but, normal peritoneal fluid does not rule out significant damage. Severe metabolic abnormalities signify a poor prognosis.[20]

Treatment

Strangulating displacements of the large intestine require timely surgical treatment. The duration of the strangulation directly affects the prognosis. Correction of acid-base imbalances, electrolyte abnormalities, and dehydration should be done as rapidly as possible before surgery. Intravenous administration of large volumes of polyionic fluids is often required to treat shock and dehydration. Hypertonic saline (5% NaCl) and colloids are useful for treating many forms of shock, and their usefulness for treating horses with strangulating obstruction is being evaluated.[28] Hypertonic saline solutions in conjunction with colloids (dextrans) provide a means of rapid intravascular volume expansion.

Potent analgesic drugs are necessary for controlling pain. Relatively high doses of xylazine 0.25 to 1.1 mg/kg IV, butorphanol 0.01 to 0.1 mg/kg IV, or a combination of these drugs is often required to provide adequate short-term analgesia. Nonsteroidal anti-inflammatory drugs are ineffective as analgesic drugs in most cases. Nonsteroidal anti-inflammatory drugs such as flunixin meglumine 0.25 to 1.1 mg/kg IV are, however, effective in preventing the cardiovascular and metabolic effects of endotoxemia and as anti-inflammatory drugs, and are routinely administered prior to surgery.[29, 30] Intravenous administration of broad-spectrum antibiotics is also valuable prior to surgery since enterotomy of the colon is routinely done, and sepsis is a frequent complication of intestinal ischemia. Plasma or serum harvested from equine donors vaccinated with a bacterin made with rough mutants of *Escherichia coli* or *Salmonella typhimurium* has been shown to reduce many of the effects of endotoxemia experimentally and in clinical cases of colic when administered intravenously.[31, 32] These products are ideally given prior to surgery, but may be given during or after surgery. Specific treatment of endotoxemia and endotoxic shock is discussed in Chapter 12.7.

The viability of the strangulated segment of large intestine must be evaluated carefully during surgery to assess the need for resection. The color of the serosa, and the return of an arterial pulse after the strangulation has been relieved is not an effective means of assessing viability of the colon, especially the mucosa. Surface oximetry, tissue temperature, fluorescein dye perfusion, and histopathologic examination of frozen sections of colonic tissue are more accurate means of assessing tissue viability.[17] If questionable tissue is not removed, further deterioration of the segment may occur from reperfusion injury or thrombosis of mesenteric and intramural blood vessels.

Anti-inflammatory drugs are an important component of therapy in situations where ischemic tissue is not removed. The inflammatory response is responsible for the majority of injuries occurring during and after ischemia.[21] Agents that block lipoxygenase activity, and therefore leukotriene formation, are useful to prevent inflammation and neutrophil chemotaxis, but, few lipoxygenase inhibitors are clinically available.[21] Ibuprofen has been shown to decrease myocardial infarct size in dogs.[33] The mechanism is unclear, but appears to be a direct effect on the neutrophil, by preventing chemotaxis or release of neutrophil products. Other nonsteroidal anti-inflammatory drugs, such as flunixin meglumine, may also be useful as anti-inflammatory drugs.

Free radical scavengers such as allopurinol, dimethyl sulfoxide, and superoxide dismutase have been advocated to prevent reperfusion injury and have been investigated using experimental ischemia of the equine large intestine.[34–37] Allopurinol blocks the conversion of xanthine dehydrogenase to xanthine oxidase.[21] Since little xanthine dehydrogenase is found in the equine colon, this drug may be of little value when used to prevent reperfusion injury in the large intestine. Dimethyl sulfoxide acts as a hydroxyl radical scavenger.[21] Superoxide dismutase catalyzes the conversion of superoxides to hydrogen peroxide.[21] The efficacy of these agents in preventing reperfusion injury in the equine large intestine is controversial, and no clear experimental evidence exists supporting their use.

The administration of intravenous fluids is important to maintain adequate perfusion pressure once the strangulated segment is corrected. Heparin 20 to 100 IU/kg IV, then SC, b.i.d. to q.i.d. has been used effectively as an anticoagulant to prevent the formation of intravascular thrombi in strangulated segments of large intestine.[21, 38] Heparin requires antithrombin III as a cofactor to exert an effect on coagulation. Antithrombin III activity has been found to be reduced in cases of strangulating displacement of the ascending colon.[26] The replacement of antithrombin III with plasma may be required for heparin therapy to be effective, and has been shown to be useful in treating DIC in dogs.[39] However, a concentrated source of equine antithrombin III is not clinically available, and the effect of administering normal plasma to antithrombin III–deficient horses has not been evaluated.

Aspirin 12 mg/kg PO every other day is used to prevent and treat intravascular thrombosis and as an antithrombotic and thrombolytic agent.[40] Aspirin is a potent and irreversible inhibitor of platelet cyclooxygenase by acetylation of the enzyme.[40] Oral administration of low doses of aspirin (12 mg/kg) have been shown to increase bleeding time for 48 hours.[40] Inhibition of platelet function prevents intravascular thrombosis by blocking the synthesis of vasoactive lipids such as thromboxane, which stimulate platelet adhesion and activation.[40] The use of aspirin in combination with recombinant tissue plasminogen activator (t-PA) as thrombolytic agents has been advocated for treatment of human myocardial infarction.[41] t-PA activates plasminogen to plasmin, which is a potent fibrinolytic enzyme. Recombinant t-PA is cost-prohibitive for systemic use in the horse, but local infusion via mesenteric vessels would reduce the quantity required and may allow the agent to be used clinically. The beneficial effects of heparin, aspirin, and other anticoagulants should be weighed against the detrimental effects, such as bleeding and agglutination of red blood cells. The partial thromboplastin time should be carefully monitored when instituting anticoagulant therapy, and should not exceed two times normal.

Postoperative management of patients with strangulating obstruction consists of careful monitoring of clinical signs, acid-base and electrolyte balance, and hydration. Sepsis and endotoxemia are frequent postoperative complications of strangulating obstruction of the large intestine, especially if bowel with questionable viability is not removed. Treatment with broad-spectrum antibiotics, nonsteroidal anti-inflammatory drugs, anti-endotoxin plasma or serum, and intravenous fluids is required for variable periods after surgery. Functional ileus and colitis may also occur after surgery, and may require treatment discussed elsewhere in this book.

PRIMARY IMPACTION OF THE LARGE INTESTINE

Pathogenesis

Primary impaction is one of the most common causes of obstruction of the large intestine.[42] Impaction frequently occurs in the ascending colon at the pelvic flexure, but can occur in other segments of the ascending colon, the cecum, or the descending colon.[43] Primary impaction of the ascending colon occurs in all breeds and age groups, but impaction of the descending colon appears to be more common in ponies and miniature horses.[3, 44]

The pathogenesis of impaction remains unclear. Impaction of the ascending colon can be induced by the drug amitraz, an acaricide associated with clinical cases of colon impaction.[45] Amitraz causes a dissociation of mechanical events of the ascending colon.[45] The pacemaker located at the pelvic flexure appears to be modified, resulting in uncoordinated motility patterns between the left ventral and left dorsal colon. Since the pelvic flexure is an important site regulating the aboral movement of ingesta, disruption of motility in this area increases the retention time of ingesta in the left ventral colon. Absorption of water from the ingesta increases with retention time, dehydrating the contents of the colon, resulting in impaction. Impacted ingesta extends as far orad as the cecum, and may extend aborally to the transverse colon, suggesting that the drug affects other areas of the colon as well, either directly or indirectly, by modifying the activity at the pelvic flexure.[45] Clearly, factors affecting progressive motility patterns contribute to formation of impactions, but the initiating cause is unknown in the majority of natural cases of large intestinal impaction.

Migrating *S. vulgaris* larvae causing arteritis, thrombosis, and intermittent ischemia of the colon have been incriminated as being a cause of impaction by altering the motility of the colon, and have been shown to decrease blood flow to the colon.[11, 12] Migration of cyathostome larvae through the mucosa and submucosa of the large intestine may also disrupt motility by a direct effect.[13] Feeding patterns (i.e., large, infrequent meals), limited exercise, poor dentition, coarse roughage, dehydration, or motility-altering drugs also appear to contribute to the formation of impactions of the colon.[3] Horses housed in confinement and fed dry roughage are thought to be predisposed to impaction of the colon. Water deprivation and dehydration are also associated with impaction formation. The development of cecal impactions has been observed in horses recovering from general anesthesia.[46]

Distention of the large intestine causes much of the pain associated with impaction. Distention of the wall causes reflex contraction of the impacted segments of intestine as well as other segments, which can also be quite painful. Obstruction is not complete, and the distention is not severe, resulting in mild-to-moderate abdominal pain. Ischemia rarely occurs with primary impaction, but progressive distention weakens the wall in some cases, resulting in eventual rupture.

Clinical Signs and Diagnosis

Primary impaction of the large intestine is characterized by mild-to-moderate, intermittent abdominal pain of insidious onset.[3] Partial to complete anorexia develops over a period of hours, to days in some cases. Fecal production is reduced, and the feces are often hard, dry, and mucus-covered. The heart rate may be mildly elevated during episodes of pain, but is often normal. Abdominal borborygmi are reduced in frequency, and progressive motility is often absent. Signs of dehydration appear after long periods of anorexia.

Hematologic evaluation may reveal hemoconcentration, but other parameters are usually normal. The diagnosis of impaction usually relies on transrectal palpation.[3] The enlarged impacted segment is often easily felt per rectum. However, differentiation of primary vs. secondary impaction is often difficult. Abdominal radiography can be used to confirm impaction of the large intestine in small ponies, miniature horses, and foals. Foreign bodies causing secondary impaction may be evident on the radiograph, but cannot be ruled out if not seen. Peritoneal fluid is usually normal with uncomplicated primary impaction.

Treatment

Many cases of primary impaction of the ascending colon can be managed with medical treatment. If the impaction persists for greater than 48 hours of medical treatment, or if evidence suggesting damage to the intestine is seen (i.e., increasing pain, abnormal peritoneal fluid, or signs of sepsis), surgical treatment is indicated. Impaction of the cecum and descending colon is notoriously refractive to medical treatment, possibly because the impaction is secondary to underlying motility disorders.[46, 47] Cecal impactions are prone to perforation, and may recur after resolution of the original impaction.[46] For these reasons, surgical treatment of impactions of the cecum or descending colon is often required for a successful outcome.[46, 47]

Medical treatment of primary impaction consists of management of pain, administration of laxatives and cathartics, and hydration. Nonsteroidal anti-inflammatory agents such as flunixin meglumine 0.25 to 0.5 mg/kg t.i.d. or q.i.d. are effective at controlling abdominal pain when used judiciously. Cases requiring more potent analgesics may be better treated with surgery. Administration of oral water and laxatives such as mineral oil 2 to 4 L by nasogastric tube q.12–24 h. and the anionic surfactant docusate sodium (D-S-S) 6 to 12 g/500 kg diluted in 2 to 4 L of water by nasogastric tube q.12–24 h. are commonly used to soften the impaction.[3] Saline cathartics, such as magnesium sulfate 0.1 mg/kg in 2 to 4 L by nasogastric tube, are useful if the impaction is primary.[3] The use of saline cathartics in cases of secondary impaction is contraindicated. Fluids must be administered intravenously concurrently with saline cathartics to prevent dehydration. Overhydration is effective to rehydrate and break up the impacted ingesta. Administration of polyionic fluids at two to five times maintenance rates (4–10 mL/kg/hr) for 24 to 48 hours has been quite successful in refractory cases. Xylazine has been used to inhibit contraction of the colon to allow hydration of the impacted material and provide analgesia. Prolonged use of xylazine may affect the motility of the colon to a degree that, as the impaction softens, the colon cannot break up the mass.

LUMINAL OBSTRUCTION OF THE LARGE INTESTINE

Enteroliths

Pathogenesis

Enteroliths are intestinal calculi found in the large intestine. They are composed of magnesium ammonium phosphate (struvite).[48] All breeds are affected by enteroliths, but Arabians appear to have the highest incidence. Most horses with enteroliths are between the ages of 5 and 10 years, and rarely under 4 years old.[49] Individual farms may have a higher incidence of enterolithiasis than other farms. The occurrence of enteroliths has been reported over a wide geographical area, but the highest prevalence appears to be on the West Coast (California), and in the Southeast (Florida).[49]

The calculi appear to form by depositing layers of struvite around a dense nidus. Nidi include hair, metal, or other foreign objects, and, perhaps most commonly, silicon dioxide, a flintlike stone.[48] The pathogenesis is unclear, but elevated dietary intake of magnesium and protein may play a role.[48, 49] Many horses that develop enteroliths are fed a diet consisting mainly of alfalfa hay. Analysis of California hay revealed a concentration of magnesium approximately six times the daily requirements of the horse, and California water samples also have elevated concentrations of magnesium.[49] The high protein concentration in alfalfa hay may contribute to calculi formation by increasing the ammonia nitrogen load to the large intestine.[3] Most horses fed a diet of alfalfa hay do not develop enteroliths, indicating that the pathogenesis is multifactorial.[3] Increased colonic pH may cause a precipitation of the minerals, leading to calculi formation.[50] Colonic contents from patients with enterolithi-

asis had a pH greater than 7.0. A pH of less than 6.6 appeared to reduce the weight of experimentally implanted enteroliths.[50] The presence of a nidus may facilitate the formation of organized calculi. Alfalfa hay may buffer the colonic contents, resulting in an alkaline pH. Feeding diets higher in soluble carbohydrates (grains) tended to reduce the pH of colonic contents.[50] The effect of feeding vinegar to alter the pH of the colonic contents and prevent enterolith formation is being investigated.[50]

Intestinal calculi vary in location within the intestinal tract, but large calculi occur in the right dorsal colon. Smaller calculi may enter the transverse colon and descending colon. Calculi may form singly or in groups of several to hundreds of small calculi. Obstruction occurs when calculi enter a segment of large intestine and lodge, causing variable amounts of distention with gas and ingesta proximal to the stone. Occasionally, multiple small calculi cause pain without causing obstruction, presumably by irritating the colon and by stretching the wall. Pressure necrosis can occur from prolonged obstruction, but is unusual. Rarely, large stones can cause perforation in exercising horses without previous signs of obstruction.

Clinical Signs and Diagnosis

Enterolithiasis is characterized by episodic, mild-to-moderate, intermittent abdominal pain.[49] Progressive anorexia and depression may develop. The amount of pain is dependent on the degree of obstruction and amount of distention. Obstruction of the descending colon is often complete, causing acute, unrelenting abdominal pain with abdominal distention. Partial luminal obstruction allows the passage of scant, pasty feces. Heart rate is variable, and dependent on the degree of pain. Abdominal borborygmi are decreased in frequency, and progressive motility is absent. If large numbers of small calculi are present without luminal obstruction, progressive borborygmi may be heard, and the calculi moving against one another produce a characteristic gravelly sound in the ventral abdomen. Transrectal palpation may reveal distention of the obstructed segment with gas or ingesta. The enterolith may be felt if it is large or located in the descending colon. Palpation with the patient's front feet on a ramp or step facilitates feeling the enterolith by moving it caudally.

Peritoneal fluid is normal unless pressure necrosis of the intestine occurs, which causes the fluid to become exudative. Diagnosis may be made with abdominal radiography. This technique is unrewarding in larger horses, and inability to visualize an enterolith radiographically does not rule out enterolithiasis.

Treatment

Definitive treatment requires surgical removal of the enterolith in most cases, but medical management may resolve the obstruction. Medical management consists of analgesia and administration of large volumes of intravenous fluids similar to managing primary impaction of the large intestine. The possibility of pressure necrosis and perforation accompanies medical treatment, and obstruction is likely to recur without removal of the enterolith. Obstruction of the descending colon rarely responds to medical treatment, and is more likely to cause perforation. Currently, feeding a diet consisting of no more than one-half alfalfa by weight is advocated to prevent formation of enteroliths. Preventive treatment by feeding vinegar is under investigation, but the effectiveness of feeding vinegar to decrease the size of the enterolith in clinical cases appears poor.

Sand Impaction

Pathogenesis

Impaction of the large intestine with sand occurs in all ages of horses, and is most common in horses living in areas with loose sandy soil.[51] Horses may consume sand inadvertently while eating hay off the ground, or grazing grass. Some horses, especially foals, deliberately eat sand. Fine sand accumulates in the ventral colon, while coarse sand may accumulate in the dorsal colon.[3] The pathogenesis of sand impaction is unknown, but may involve similar mechanisms as primary impaction. Sand impaction may be associated with underlying displacement of the ascending colon.[51] Poor motility may cause accumulation of sand before impaction, since some horses can clear consumed sand whereas others cannot. Distention from the impaction itself, or gas proximal to the impaction, as well as reflex spasms of contraction stimulated by the distention, causes abdominal pain.

Clinical Signs and Diagnosis

The clinical signs of sand impaction are often identical to those of primary impaction, except diarrhea may be noticed prior to the episode of obstruction from sand enteritis. Mild-to-moderate, intermittent abdominal pain is evident.[51] Feces may be scant, and sand may be present in the feces in abnormally high amounts. Transrectal palpation may reveal the impacted segment, unless the transverse or right dorsal colon is involved and not a palpable segment. Auscultation of the abdomen reveals decreased frequency of borborygmi and progressive contractions. Without progressive contractions, the characteristic sound of sand grinding in the colon may not be heard, even if large amounts of sand are present. If normal progressive motility is heard without hearing sand sounds, accumulation of abnormal amounts of sand in the colon is unlikely.

Abdominal radiography is helpful in visualizing radiodense sand in the gastrointestinal tract, especially in foals, ponies, and small horses. Abdominal paracentesis is risky when large quantities of sand are present in the ventral colon, because inadvertent perforation of the colon may occur.[51] Peritoneal fluid is often normal, but may have an elevated protein concentration. Feces may contain frank or occult blood.

Treatment

Medical management with an analgesic such as flunixin meglumine 0.25 to 1.1 mg/kg IV or PO, as needed, and administration of oral laxatives, cathartics, and intravenous fluids is similar to management of primary impactions. The laxative of choice for sand impactions, however, is psyllium hydrophilic mucilloid (Metamucil) at a dose of 0.25 to 0.5

kg/500 kg body weight.[3] The psyllium product is mixed with 4 to 8 L of water and the mixture is administered rapidly through a nasogastric tube. A preferable method allows administration through the tube without fear of forming a gel too quickly and obstructing the tube. The powder is mixed with 2 L of mineral oil, which will not form a gel, and can be pumped through a nasogastric tube easily. Two to 4 L of water are then pumped through the tube. The psyllium leaves the oil phase and mixes with the water, forming a gel. Psyllium is thought to act by stimulating motility, or by agglutinating the sand, allowing the sand to be passed.[3] If a severe impaction is present, the psyllium should not be given until the impaction is softened by administrating intravenous or oral fluids, and other laxatives. Perforation is a potential complication because the sand stretches and irritates the intestinal wall, and causes inflammation. Surgical treatment is required in refractory cases, cases with unrelenting pain or displacement of the colon, or if the white blood cell count begins to rise in the peritoneal fluid.

Once clinical signs are relieved, prolonged therapy is often necessary to remove accumulated sand. Dry psyllium, one to two cups per 500 kg, can be fed daily for 2 to 3 weeks. Abdominal auscultation for sand sounds can be done routinely to detect sand still present in the colon. Fecal sand content can be monitored to determine if sand is being passed in response to treatment, and when the sand ceases to be passed. Psyllium can be fed routinely (one to two cups/500 kg) daily for a week, every 4 to 6 weeks, to prevent sand accumulation. Feeding in elevated bins and allowing grazing only in fields with adequate growth to prevent ingestion of sand are vital to avoid this condition.

Foreign Body and Fecalith Obstruction

Pathogenesis, Clinical Signs, and Treatment

Like enterolith obstruction, foreign body obstruction usually occurs in the transverse or descending colon.[52] Foreign indigestible material such as bedding, rope, plastic, fence material, and feedbags can cause obstruction, resulting in impaction with ingesta, resulting in distention of the intestine.[52, 53] Young horses are usually affected.[3] Fecaliths are common in ponies, miniature horses, and foals.[54] Composed of long strands of dense fibrous plant material held together by concretions, fecaliths may form from poor mastication of roughage, or poor digestion.[55] Older horses with poor dentition or foals unable to digest the material may be predisposed to forming fecaliths. Fecaliths commonly cause obstruction in the descending colon, and the clinical features are similar to enterolithiasis of the descending colon.[54, 55] Obstruction of the descending colon by fecaliths is often characterized by tenesmus.[54] Abdominal radiography may be useful in smaller patients to identify the obstruction, especially if gas distention around the foreign body or fecalith provides contrast. Surgical treatment is usually required.

Mural Masses and Strictures

Pathogenesis

Mural masses can cause luminal obstruction and impaction. Mural abscesses, tumors (adenocarcinoma, lymphosarcoma), granulomas, and hematomas are examples of mural masses that can cause obstruction. Older horses are usually affected. Impaction may result from obstruction of the lumen or impaired motility in the segment of intestine with the mass. Abscesses may originate from the lumen of the intestine, or may extend from the mesentery or mesenteric lymph nodes. Intramural hematomas form most commonly in the descending colon, and cause acute abdominal pain.[56, 57] Once the acute pain from the hematoma subsides, impaction proximal to the hematoma develops due to impaired motility through the affected portion of the colon. Trauma, ulceration of the mucosa, and parasitic damage are speculated causes of intramural hematomas.[56, 57] Stricture of the large intestine occurs when fibrous tissue forms in a circular pattern around or within the intestine, reducing the luminal diameter and the ability of the wall to stretch. Strictures may be congenital, or secondary to peritonitis, previous abdominal surgery, or ischemia of the intestine from verminous arteritis or other causes.

Clinical Signs and Diagnosis

Clinical signs vary according to the degree of luminal obstruction. Partial obstruction and impaction tend to produce mild-to-moderate abdominal pain of insidious onset. Mural hematomas tend to produce signs of acute abdominal pain.[56, 57] Transrectal examination may reveal the presence of a mass, or simply the impacted segment without feeling the mass itself. Fever, weight loss, and anorexia may be noted if an abscess or tumor is the cause. An elevated white blood cell count, hyperfibrinogenemia, hyperglubulinemia, or normocytic, normochromic anemia may be seen with abscesses or tumors. Lymphosarcoma has been associated with low concentrations of serum IgM in some cases.[58] Peritoneal fluid may reflect the cause of the mass. Tumor cells may be seen, or inflammatory fluid with bacteria if an abscess or granuloma is the cause. Culture may allow isolation of the organism. Hematomas may cause hemorrhage into the peritoneal fluid. If tissue necrosis occurs, the peritoneal fluid can become quite exudative.[56, 57] Endoscopy and biopsy may be useful if the mass is located in the rectum.

Treatment

Treatment usually requires surgical resection of the mass. Abscesses may be treated with appropriate antibiotics if the impaction can be resolved medically with oral or intravenous analgesics and laxatives. *Streptococcus* species, *Actinomyces pyogenes, Corynebacterium pseudotuberculosis, Rhodococcus equi,* and anaerobic bacteria are commonly involved in abscesses, but gram negative enteric species are not unusual. Laxatives are useful to decrease the tendency to form impactions at the site of the mass or stricture if surgical resection is not an option. Coarse, dry roughages have a higher tendency to become impacted. Fresh grass, and pelleted food and bran mixed with water and mineral oil to form a mash have been used successfully to feed patients with strictures or other forms of mural obstruction.

INTUSSUSCEPTION OF THE LARGE INTESTINE
Pathogenesis

Intussusception of the cecum or colon is a rare condition in the horse.[59] Cecal intussusception may involve either the apex of the cecum (cecocecal), or the ensheathing of the cecum into the right ventral colon (cecocolic).[59, 60] Intussusception of the ascending colon may occur at the pelvic flexure and the left dorsal colon.[3, 61] Younger horses are most commonly affected.[59] Intussusception of the cecum has been associated with *Eimeria leukarti* infection in foals, *Anoplocephala perfoliata* infection, mural abscesses, administration of parasympathomimetic drugs such as organophosphates, and *Strongylus vulgaris* infection.[59, 62, 63] The pathogenesis appears to rely on abnormal motility or hypermotility of particular segments of large intestine, or the presence of a wall defect such as an abscess or tapeworms that allows telescoping of the intestine and intussusception to take place. The intussuscipiens may become strangulated, resulting in ischemic necrosis. Complete obstruction or ischemia may cause severe pain, or incomplete obstruction and maldigestion may occur.

Clinical Signs and Diagnosis

Two syndromes may occur with intussusception of the large intestine. Acute, severe, unrelenting abdominal pain may be seen, or a syndrome of chronic, intermittent abdominal pain and weight loss may be noted.[3] The duration of clinical signs may be hours to days. Secondary impaction of the colon may accompany the intussusception. Strangulation and necrosis of the intussuscipiens may result in perforation. Heart rate and other clinical parameters are variable, depending on the degree of obstruction and duration of signs. Signs of sepsis may be seen if perforation or necrosis of the intestine allows absorption of endotoxin or translocation of bacteria. Transrectal palpation often reveals impaction or gas distention and edema of the colon or cecum, but, palpation of the intussusception may not be possible. The intussusception feels similar to a mural mass on palpation. Hematologic parameters are often normal, but may reflect sepsis. Abdominal fluid is variable depending on whether strangulation of the intussuscipiens occurs, and whether the necrotic portion of intestine communicates with the peritoneal fluid or is walled off. Frank or occult blood may be present in the feces.

Treatment

Surgical treatment is required for reduction of the intussusception, or resection of the strangulated intestine. In some cases, successful surgical treatment is impossible. Peritoneal contamination and septic peritonitis are not unusual.

PERFORATION OF THE LARGE INTESTINE
Pathogenesis

Perforation of the large intestine, unfortunately, is not unusual in horses. Perforation can occur in any segment of the large intestine and results in gross contamination of the peritoneal cavity with bacteria and ingesta, and carries an extremely poor prognosis. Perforation of the distal rectum may contaminate the perirectal tissues, but not the peritoneal cavity, and is not as devastating as other sites of perforation. Perforation most commonly occurs when the intestinal wall is injured from ischemia, usually when the tissue is necrotic. When the intraluminal pressure exceeds the ability of the compromised tissue to hold, the wall will tear. Pressure from enteroliths or impactions, strangulated obstructions, mural hematomas or abscesses, or infarcts cause injury sufficient to render the tissue susceptible to perforation. *Anoplocephala perfoliata* infection has been suggested as a cause of cecal perforation.[64]

Perforation of the cecum and, less commonly, the ascending colon has been reported in postparturient mares.[65–67] The pathogenesis of postparturient perforation is unknown, but may be related to gas distention of the cecum or colon during abdominal contractions putting excessive pressure on the wall of the intestine. The wall of the intestine rarely has gross or histologic evidence of preexisting injury or underlying disease that would weaken the strength of the tissue.[67]

Iatrogenic perforation of the large intestine during abdominocentesis with cannulas or during placement of abdominal drains can cause significant contamination of the peritoneal cavity. Perforation of the large intestine with a needle during abdominocentesis is less likely to cause clinically significant contamination. Iatrogenic perforation of the rectum from trauma during transrectal palpation may also occur. Rectal perforation is the most severe form of rectal tear, the least severe involving the mucosa only.

Perforation of the large intestine results in contamination of the peritoneal cavity of varying degrees, depending on the size of the perforation. Most natural perforations are large since the intestine is often under pressure. Iatrogenic perforation is less likely to cause severe contamination. Septic peritonitis from a variety of microorganisms occurs, predominantly anaerobic and gram-negative aerobic bacteria. Particles of ingesta also contaminate the peritoneal cavity, increasing inflammation, fibrin deposition, and abscessation since they cannot be effectively cleared. Deposits of fibrin allow sequestration of bacteria, and can also lead to adhesion formation. Endotoxin-mediated shock and sepsis develop quickly and in most cases are fatal.

Clinical Signs and Diagnosis

Clinical signs are related to the degree of peritonitis that develops. Severe contamination results in endotoxemia, septicemia, and septic shock. Elevated heart and respiratory rates, sweating, severe depression and anorexia, peripheral vasoconstriction followed by vasodilation, fever, and weakness may be seen. In less severe cases, a fever, depression, anorexia, and tachycardia may only be present. Mild signs of abdominal pain may be evident. If obstructive disease led to the perforation, sudden relief from severe abdominal pain may signify that perforation has occurred, but less dramatic relief than is seen with gastric rupture. Transrectal palpation may reveal free gas in the peritoneal cavity, rough visceral peritoneum, and the site of perforation if it is in the rectum.

Hematologic evidence of sepsis may be noted: leukopenia, neutropenia with a left shift, and toxic neutrophils. Metabolic acidosis is often seen with an elevated anion gap and serum lactate concentration. Hyperfibrinogenemia may be seen if the duration is long enough. Diagnosis is often made by examining peritoneal fluid. An elevated white blood cell count is usually seen, but not exclusively. The presence of intra- and extracellular bacteria of different types is highly suggestive of perforation. Finding particles of plant material in the fluid is nearly pathognomonic for perforation. Inadvertent puncture of the intestine during abdominocentesis may contaminate the sample with bacteria and particles of ingesta. Immediate examination of the fluid for intracellular bacteria can help distinguish a contaminated sample from peritonitis. Definitive diagnosis requires surgical exploration.

Treatment

Treatment of intestinal perforation with massive contamination of the peritoneum is not feasible. Small perforations resulting in minimal or localized contamination may be treated, but the prognosis is extremely guarded. Surgical repair of the perforation must be done in nearly all cases. Celiotomy is required unless the tear is in the distal rectum. During surgery, the abdomen can be flushed with large volumes of sterile electrolyte solutions, and infected or necrotic tissue can be debrided. Abdominal drainage and flushing are vital after surgery. Intermittent lavage and continuous drainage can be done for several days until the fluid characteristics improve. Heparin 20 to 40 IU/kg q.i.d. is often included in the lavage fluid to minimize adhesion formation. Intraabdominal administration of dextrans or methylcellulose to prevent adhesion formation is contraindicated if bacteria are present.

Intravenous administration of broad-spectrum antibiotics is indicated. Culture of the peritoneal fluid will help determine which antibiotics are appropriate. Metronidazole 15 to 25 mg/kg PO b.i.d. to q.i.d. is commonly used in conjunction with a β-lactam antibiotic, and an aminoglycoside. Nearly all anaerobic bacteria are susceptible to the metronidazole; it penetrates tissues well, and it is effective in an anaerobic environment.[68] Nonsteroidal anti-inflammatory drugs such as flunixin meglumine 0.25 to 0.5 mg/kg t.i.d. or q.i.d. or 1.1 mg/kg b.i.d. are effective in reducing inflammation and possibly adhesion formation, and also ameliorate the cardiovascular effects of endotoxin. Anti-endotoxin plasma or serum is also helpful in counteracting the effects of endotoxin. Intravenous fluid administration and maintenance of acid-base and electrolyte balance are vital. Food should be withheld for at least 1 day, and green grass and pelleted mash and mineral oil should be fed to prevent excessive stretch of the repaired perforation. Coarse, dry roughage should be withheld for days to weeks depending on the size of the perforation.

TYMPANY

Pathogenesis

Tympany of the large intestine may be primary or secondary to another obstructive condition.[3] Primary tympany is recognized clinically when the distention is severe, but may account for many cases of undiagnosed cases of colic. Distention of the cecum or ascending colon with gas produced from fermentation causes tympany. Rapid increases in the fermentation rate occur when large meals are fed, especially when soluble carbohydrates make up a high percentage of the diet.[4, 5] Gas may accumulate if progressive motility is impaired, or if the rate of gas production exceeds the ability of the gastrointestinal tract to move the gas through.[3, 68] Parasitic infections, feeding schedules and behavior, lack of exercise, and other factors may disrupt motility patterns.[3, 4, 68] Moderate to severe distention stretches the wall of the intestine, causing pain. Mild to moderate distention may increase the contractility of other segments of the gastrointestinal tract, resulting in spasms that may cause pain, often referred to as spasmotic colic.

Clinical Signs and Diagnosis

Primary tympany is characterized by acute abdominal pain that may be severe.[3, 68] Abdominal distention occurs in severe cases, especially in the right flank when the cecum is distended. Heart and respiratory rates are often elevated if the pain is severe, or if the distention compromises respiratory function and venous return. Abdominal borborygmi may be increased in frequency if the distention is mild or moderate, but with severe distention abdominal borborygmi are absent. Abdominal percussion may reveal areas of auscultable tympanic resonance over the distended viscus. Peritoneal fluid is normal with primary tympany, and hematologic abnormalities are unusual.

Treatment

Potent analgesic drugs such as xylazine 0.3 to 1.0 mg/kg IV, butorphanol 0.01 to 0.1 mg/kg IV, or a combination may be necessary to control abdominal pain. Nonsteroidal anti-inflammatory drugs are useful for controlling pain in less severe cases. Administration of laxatives such as mineral oil 10 to 40 mL/kg PO help increase motility to move gas distally, and may decrease the rate of fermentation and gas production. Severe tympany may require trocarization and decompression with a needle or catheter, especially if respiratory function or venous return is compromised. The cecum can be trocarized easily, but trocarization of the ascending colon has a higher risk. Primary tympany responds rapidly to medical treatment. Unresponsive cases are likely to have tympany secondary to underlying obstructive disease.

NONSTRANGULATING INFARCTION OF THE LARGE INTESTINE
Pathogenesis

The most common cause of nonstrangulating infarction of the equine large intestine is thromboembolic infarction; however, mesenteric tears can also cause infarction of the large intestine.[69, 70] Thromboembolic infarction occurs most frequently after infection with *Strongylus vulgaris,* but can also occur from other forms of thrombotic disease such as DIC secondary to acute gram-negative bacterial sepsis.[69] Systemic shock may also cause ischemia and infarction of the large

intestine.[71] *Strongylus vulgaris* infection and thromboembolic disease are thought to play important roles in many forms of obstructive disorders of the large intestine.[11, 69] Postmortem examination of horses that died of acute intestinal obstructive disease suggests that *S. vulgaris* infection and thromboarteritis are an infrequent cause of death in these horses.[11] However, the incidence of *S. vulgaris* infection in horses with obstructive disease of the large intestine is not known. Intensive parasite control regimens have significantly reduced the incidence of colic on some farms.[11, 72] *Strongylus vulgaris* infection affects the motility of the ascending colon, and decreases blood flow to the ascending colon, which may also affect motility.[1, 2, 13, 14] *Strongylus vulgaris* infection may be an infrequent cause of infarction of the intestine and death of the animal, but may contribute to the pathogenesis of impactions, displacements, and many undiagnosed cases of colic by modifying motility patterns and blood flow.

Young or immunocompromised horses are most susceptible to infection with *S. vulgaris.* The third-stage larvae migrate through the wall of the intestines, and into the arterial vasculature, primarily affecting the cranial mesenteric artery.[69] Migration through the wall of the arteries causes thromboarteritis with inflammation, fibrosis, and thickening of the wall. Dilatation of the artery may occur, but thickening of the wall with thrombus formation at the site of the parasite is most common.[69] The larvae molt within the inflamed tissue to the fifth stage, and then migrate back to the intestine. The inflammation and endothelial and intimal damage in the arterial wall induce thrombus formation which can narrow the luminal diameter as much as 50%.[69] The vessels supplying the ascending colon and cecum are most often affected.[11, 69] The blood flow through individual arteries can be markedly reduced, but extensive collateral circulation exists to the cecum and ascending colon, the segments most affected by thromboarteritis.[69]

No direct evidence of embolism causing infarction of the intestine has been reported. Recent speculation has implicated vasoactive mediators arising from the site of thrombus formation as a cause of vasoconstriction and ischemia of the intestine.[11, 69] Vasoactive lipids such as thromboxane are released from the tissues surrounding the larvae.[69, 71] In addition, the larvae may release antigens that affect blood flow.[11] The resulting alteration in blood flow may be sufficient to cause ischemia to the tissues, resulting in altered motility or infarction. Intestinal ischemia has been shown to increase motility acutely, but to eventually paralyze the intestine.[11] Sufficient ischemia causes irreversible cell injury and necrosis. Obstruction from ileus develops. Distention and tissue ischemia contribute to abdominal pain. In the absence of ileus, abdominal pain may still be evident, from intermittent ischemia or from migration of stage-three or stage-five larvae into the intestinal wall.

Thrombosis from systemic coagulation disorders such as DIC or embolism from thrombi in distant sites may cause infarction of intestinal segments. Coagulation disorders such as DIC are often associated with endotoxemia and sepsis in horses, especially when the large intestine is the source, as in acute colitis.[27] Direct activation of the coagulation cascade, increased procoagulant activity, depletion of antithrombin III, and endothelial injury occur during endotoxemia in horses, and contribute to hypercoagulable states.[27] Thrombosis of the intestinal vasculature or of peripheral sites such as the jugular vein is not unusual. Ischemia from thrombosis or embolism resulting in acute infarction of the intestine is more likely to affect the large intestine than other segments of the gastrointestinal tract. Systemic shock from sepsis or acute hemorrhage may also cause ischemia and infarction of the large intestine without causing thrombosis of the intestinal vasculature.[71] Ischemia and infarction cause a functional or paralytic ileus of affected segments, but ileus from systemic disease may affect other segments. Paralytic ileus results in intestinal distention, which, along with ischemia of the intestine, is manifested by acute signs of abdominal pain.

Mesenteric tears in postpartum mares cause acute segmental infarction and necrosis of the intestine and are most common in the descending colon.[70] The cause is unknown, but may be related to trauma at parturition. Ischemic necrosis of the large intestine first causes damage to the mucosa, allowing systemic absorption of endotoxins and translocation of bacteria. Endotoxemia and sepsis are complicating factors of acute infarctive disease, as is septic peritonitis if perforation of the injured segment occurs.

Clinical Signs and Diagnosis

Acute infarction of the colon from strongylosis, thrombosis, or shock is characterized by moderate to severe signs of abdominal pain and abdominal distention.[69, 71] Signs of septic shock develop rapidly, such as tachycardia, tachypnea, and poor peripheral perfusion. Abdominal borborygmi are often absent because of ileus, and fecal production is markedly reduced. Transrectal palpation often reveals fluid or gas distention of the large intestine. Other clinical signs associated with the inciting cause of the intestinal infarction are variable.

Hematologic abnormalities associated with acute infarction of the large intestine are usually secondary to endotoxemia and sepsis; leukopenia with a neutropenia and a left shift is often noted. The plasma fibrinogen concentration may increase. Plasma lactate and phosphate concentrations and the anion gap increase as the extent of tissue necrosis increases. The characteristics of the peritoneal fluid may change dramatically or subtly depending on the amount of tissue necrosis. The peritoneal fluid protein concentration increases initially, then the red and white blood cell counts increase as the fluid becomes more characteristic of an exudate. The color of the fluid becomes serosanguinous, brown-red, or orange. Peritoneal fluid lactate and phosphate concentrations increase before plasma concentrations. The glucose concentration and pH decrease in the peritoneal fluid during ischemia. Other clinicopathologic abnormalities associated with the primary condition leading to infarction of the large intestine may be seen.

Chronic, intermittent obstruction of the large intestine may be seen with *S. vulgaris* infection.[69] Alterations in blood flow to the large intestine, and intermittent ischemia can disturb motility, causing signs of mild-to-moderate, intermittent, abdominal pain.[69] Migration of parasite larval stages through the wall of the intestine may also cause intermittent signs of abdominal pain.[13, 14] Chronic, intermittent obstruction of the large intestine is accompanied by other signs of chronic strongylosis, such as weight loss, diarrhea, depression, and fever.[69] Hematologic manifestations of chronic

strongylosis include nonregenerative anemia, neutrophilic leukocytosis, and, occasionally, eosinophilia. Peritoneal fluid may reflect chronic inflammation, and the eosinophil count in the peritoneal fluid may be elevated. Serum IgG(T) concentration is often elevated in horses with strongylosis.[73]

Mesenteric tears are characterized by slowly progressive signs of abdominal pain, impaction of the descending colon, and signs of sepsis in advanced cases.[70] Perforation of the descending colon causes signs of acute septic peritonitis. Hematologic and peritoneal fluid abnormalities may reflect sepsis and peritonitis. Peritoneal fluid may become quite exudative as necrosis of the intestine progresses.[70]

Treatment

Surgical resection of infarcted tissue is required in the majority of cases. If ischemia but not infarction occurs, surgery may not be required, but differentiating between infarction and ischemia may be difficult without surgical exploration. Treatment of endotoxemia with nonsteroidal anti-inflammatory drugs such as flunixin meglumine 0.25 to 0.5 mg/kg IV t.i.d. or q.i.d., anti-endotoxin serum or plasma, and intravenous fluid administration may be required. Broad-spectrum antibiotic treatment is necessary if signs of sepsis or peritonitis are seen. Aspirin 30 mg/kg PO b.i.d. to q.o.d. may be combined with heparin 20 to 40 IU SC t.i.d. or q.i.d. as antithrombotic and thrombolytic therapy, especially in cases of chronic strongylosis, DIC, and other thrombotic diseases.[27, 40, 69] Partial thromboplastin time should be carefully monitored when anticoagulant therapy is instituted, and should not exceed two times normal. Systemic treatment with t-PA, a potent thrombolytic agent, is not feasible in the horse because of its cost. Treatment of underlying conditions causing the infarction, such as DIC, shock, and colitis, is discussed specifically elsewhere in this book.

REFERENCES

1. Hackett RP: Nonstrangulated colonic displacement in horses. *J Am Vet Med Assoc* 182:235–240, 1983.
2. Huskamp B, Kopf W: Right dorsal displacement of the large colon in the horse. *Equine Pract* 5:20–29, 1983.
3. Snyder JR, Spier SJ: Diseases of the large intestine associated with acute abdominal pain. In Smith BP, ed: *Large Animal Internal Medicine.* St Louis, Mosby–Year Book, 1990, pp 694–703.
4. Clarke LL, Roberts MC, Argenzio RA: Feeding and digestive problems in horses: Physiologic responses to a concentrated meal. *Vet Clin North Am Equine Pract* 6:433–450, 1990.
5. Argenzio RA: Functions of the equine large intestine and their interrelationship in disease. *Cornell Vet* 65:303–327, 1975.
6. Morris DD, Moore JN, Ward S: Comparisons of age, breed, history and management in 229 horses with colic. *Equine Vet J* 7(suppl):129–133, 1986.
7. Ruckebusch Y: Motor functions of the intestine. *Adv Vet Sci Comp Med* 25:345–369, 1981.
8. King JN, Gerring EL: Observations on the colic motor complex in a pony with small intestinal obstruction. *Equine Vet J* 7(suppl):43–45, 1986.
9. Snyder JR: Personal communication, 1992.
10. Baird AN, Cohen ND, Taylor TS, et al: Renosplenic entrap-

ment of the large colon in horses: 57 cases (1983–1988). *J Am Vet Med Assoc* 198:1423–1427, 1991.

11. Becht JL: The role of parasites in colic. *Proc Am Assoc Equine Pract* 33:301–311, 1987.

12. Sellars AF, Lowe JE, Drost CJ, et al: Retropulsion and propulsion in equine large colon. *Am J Vet Res* 43:390–396, 1982.

13. Bueno D, Ruckebusch Y, Dorchies P: Disturbances of digestive motility in horses associated with strongyle infection. *Vet Parasitol* 5:253–290, 1979.

14. Lester GD, Bolton JR, Cambridge H, et al: The effect of *Strongylus vulgaris* larvae on equine intestinal myoelectrical activity. *Equine Vet J* 7(suppl):8–13, 1986.

15. Huskamp B: Displacement of the large colon. In Robinson NE, ed: *Current Therapy in Equine Medicine,* ed 2. Philadelphia, WB Saunders, 1987, pp 60–65.

16. Bury KD, McClure RL, Wright HK: Reversal of colonic net absorption to net secretion with increased intraluminal pressure. *Arch Surg* 108:854–857, 1974.

17. Snyder JR, Pascoe JR, Olander HJ, et al: Strangulating volvulus of the ascending colon in horses. *J Am Vet Med Assoc* 195:757–764, 1989.

18. Barclay WP, Foerner JJ, Phillips TN: Volvulus of the large colon in the horse. *J Am Vet Med Assoc* 177:629–630, 1980.

19. Huskamp B: The diagnosis and treatment of acute abdominal conditions in the horse: The various types and frequency seen in the animal hospital in Hoochmoor. In *Proceedings of the First Equine Colic Research Symposium,* 1982, pp 261–272.

20. Harrison IW: Equine large intestinal volvulus: A review of 124 cases. *Vet Surg* 17:77–81, 1988.

21. Snyder JR: The pathophysiology of intestinal damage: Effects of luminal distention and ischemia. *Vet Clin North Am Equine Pract* 5:247–270, 1989.

22. Meschter CL, Craig D, Hackett R: Histopathologic and ultrastructural changes in simulated large colonic torsion and reperfusion in ponies. *Equine Vet J* 23:426–433, 1991.

23. Snyder JR: Unpublished results.

24. Snyder JR, Pascoe JR, Olander HJ, et al: Vascular injury associated with naturally-occurring strangulating obstruction of the equine large colon. *Vet Surg* 19:446–455, 1990.

25. Duncan SG, Meyer KM, Reed SM, et al: Alterations in coagulation and hemograms of horses given endotoxin for 24 hours via portal infusion. *Am J Vet Res* 46:1287–1293, 1985.

26. Holland M, Kelly AB, Snyder JR, et al: Antithrombin III activity in horses with large colon torsion. *Am J Vet Res* 47:897–900, 1986.

27. Morris DD: Recognition and management of disseminated intravascular coagulation in horses. *Vet Clin North Am Equine Pract* 4:115–143, 1988.

28. Bertone JJ, Gossett KA, Shoemaker KE, et al: Effect of hypertonic saline vs isotonic saline solution on responses to sublethal *Escherichia coli* endotoxemia in horses. *Am J Vet Res* 51:999–1007, 1990.

29. Semrad SD, Hardee GE, Hardee MM, et al: Low dose flunixin meglumine: Effect on eicosanoid production and clinical signs induced by experimental endotoxemia in horses. *Equine Vet J* 19:201–206, 1987.

30. Ewert KM, Fessler JF, Templeton CB, et al: Endotoxin-induced hematologic and blood chemical changes in ponies: Effects of flunixin meglumine, dexamethasone and prednisolone. *Am J Vet Res* 46:24–30, 1985.

31. Spier SJ, Lavoie JP, Cullor JS, et al: Protection against clinical endotoxemia in horses using plasma containing antibody to an Rc mutant *Escherichia coli* (J-5). *Circ Shock* 28:235–248, 1989.

32. Tyler JW, Cullor JS, Spier SJ, et al: Immunity targeting core antigens of gram-negative bacteria. *J Vet Intern Med* 4:17–25, 1990.

33. Romsun JL, Hook BG, Rigot UH, et al: The effect of ibuprofen

on accumulation of indium III–labeled platelets and leukocytes in experimental myocardial infarction. *Circulation* 66:1002–1011, 1982.

34. Reeves MJ, Van Steenhouse J, Stashak TS, et al: Evaluation of the significance of reperfusion injury following ischemia of the equine large colon (abstract). In *Proceedings of the Third Equine Colic Research Symposium,* 1988, p 39.

35. Arden WA, Stick JA, Parks AH, et al: Effects of ischemia and dimethyl sulfoxide on equine jejunal vascular resistance, oxygen consumption, intraluminal pressure, and potassium loss. *Am J Vet Res* 50:380–387, 1989.

36. Horne MM, Ducharme NG, Pascoe IK, et al: Effects of three treatments on jejunal mucosal viability following venous and arteriovenous occlusion in the pony (abstract). In *Proceedings of the Third Equine Colic Research Symposium,* 1988, p 49.

37. Reeves MJ, Van Steenhouse J, Stashak TS, et al: Failure to demonstrate reperfusion injury following ischemia of the equine large colon using dimethyl sulfoxide. *Equine Vet J* 22:126–132, 1990.

38. Provost PJ, Stick JG, Hauptman JS, et al: Equine colonic torsion: Effects of heparin (abstract). In *Proceedings of the Third Equine Colic Research Symposium,* 1988, p 3.

39. Hauptman JG, Hassouna HI, Bell TG, et al: Efficacy of antithrombin III in endotoxin-induced disseminated intravascular coagulation. *Circ Shock* 25:111–112, 1988.

40. Cambridge H, Lees P, Hooke RE, et al: Antithrombotic action of aspirin in the horse. *Equine Vet J* 23:123–127, 1991.

41. Coller BS: Platelets and thrombolytic therapy. *N Engl J Med* 33:33–42, 1990.

42. Tennant BC: Intestinal obstruction in the horse. *Proc Am Assoc Equine Pract* 21:426–439, 1925.

43. Meagher DM: Obstructive disease of the large intestine of the horse: Diagnosis and treatment. *Proc Am Assoc Equine Pract* 18:269–279, 1972.

44. Ragle CA, Snyder JR, Meagher DM, et al: Surgical treatment of colic in American Miniature Horses: 15 cases (1980–1987). *J Am Vet Med Assoc* 201(2):329–331, 1992.

45. Sellars AF, Lowe JE: Review of large intestinal motility and mechanisms of impaction in the horse. *Equine Vet J* 18:261–263, 1986.

46. Campbell ML, Colahan PC, Brown MP, et al: Cecal impaction in the horse. *J Am Vet Med Assoc* 184:950–952, 1989.

47. Keller LD: Diseases of the equine small colon. *Compendium Continuing Educ Pract Vet* 7:S113–S120, 1985.

48. Blue MG, Wittkopp RW: Clinical and structural features of equine enteroliths. *J Am Vet Med Assoc* 179:79–82, 1981.

49. Lloyd K, Hintz HF, Wheat JD, et al: Enterolithiasis in horses. *Cornell Vet* 77:172–186, 1987.

50. Hintz HF, Lowe JE, Livesay-Wilkins P, et al: Studies on equine enterolithiasis. *Proc Am Assoc Equine Pract* 34:53–59, 1988.

51. Ragle CA, Meagher DM, LaCroix CA, et al: Surgical treatment of sand colic: Results in 40 horses. *Vet Surg* 18:48–51, 1989.

52. Meagher DM: Obstructive disease in the large intestine of the horse: Diagnosis and treatment. *Proc Am Assoc Equine Pract* 18:269–279, 1972.

53. Gay CC, Spiers VC, Christie BA, et al: Foreign body obstruction of the small colon in six horses. *Equine Vet J* 11:60–62, 1979.

54. McClure JJ, Kobluk C, Voller K, et al: Fecalith impaction in four miniature foals. *J Am Vet Med Assoc* 200:205–207, 1992.

55. Meagher DM, Bugreeff SE: Surgical conditions of the small colon and rectum in the horse. *Proc Am Assoc Equine Pract* 35:71–77, 1989.

56. Speirs VC, van Veenendaal JC, Christie BA, et al: Obstruction of the small colon by intramural hematoma in three horses. *Aust Vet J* 57:88–89, 1981.

57. Pearson H, Waterman AE: Submucosal haematoma as a cause

of obstruction of the small colon in the horse: A review of four cases. *Equine Vet J* 18:340–341, 1986.

58. Dopson LC, Reed SM, Roth JA, et al: Immunosuppression associated with lymphosarcoma in two horses. *J Am Vet Med Assoc* 182:1239–1241, 1983.

59. Gaughan EM: Cecocolic intussusception in horses: 11 cases (1979–1989). *J Am Vet Med Assoc* 197:1373–1375, 1990.

60. Semrad SD, Moore JN: Invagination of the cecal apex in a foal. *Equine Vet J* 15:62–63, 1984.

61. Wilson DG, Wilson WD, Reineston EL: Intussusception of the left dorsal colon in a horse. *J Am Vet Med Assoc* 183:464–465, 1983.

62. White MR: Cecocolic intussusception in a foal with *Eimeria leukarti* infection. *Equine Pract* 10:15–18, 1988.

63. Owen RR, Jagger DW, Quan-Taylor R: Caecal intussusception in horses and the significance of *Anoplocephala perfoliata*. *Vet Rec* 124:34–37, 1989.

64. Beroza GA, Barclay WP, Phillips TW, et al: Cecal perforation and peritonitis associated with *Anoplocephala perfoliata* infection in three horses. *J Am Vet Med Assoc* 183:804–806, 1983.

65. Voss JL: Rupture of the cecum and ventral colon of mares during parturition. *J Am Vet Med Assoc* 155:745–747, 1969.

66. Littlejohn A, Ritchie JDS: Rupture of the caecum at parturition. *J S Afr Vet Assoc* 46:87–89, 1975.

67. Ross MW, Martin BB, Donawick WJ: Cecal perforation in the horse. *J Am Vet Med Assoc* 187:249–253, 1985.

68. Rosenblatt JE, Edson RS: Metronidazole. *Mayo Clin Proc* 58:154–157, 1983.

69. Messer WT, Beeman GM: Distention colic. In Robinson NE, ed: *Current Therapy in Equine Medicine,* ed 2. Philadelphia, WB Saunders, 1987, pp 58–59.

70. White NA: Thromboembolic colic in horses. *Compendium Continuing Educ Pract Vet* 7:S156–S161, 1985.

71. Dart AS, Pascoe JR: Mesenteric tears of the descending (small) colon as a postpartum complication in two mares. *J Am Vet Med Assoc* 199:1612–1615, 1991.

72. Snyder JR, Spier SJ: Diseases of the small intestine associated with acute abdominal pain. In Smith BP, ed: *Large Animal Internal Medicine.* St Louis. Mosby–Year Book, 1990, pp 685–694.

73. Patten S, Mock RE, Drudge JH, et al: Increased immunoglobulin T concentration in ponies as a response to experimental infection with the nematode *Strongylus vulgaris. Am J Vet Res* 39:19–22, 1978.

12.13

Management of Adynamic Ileus

Edward D. Murphey, DVM, PhD

The ability to manage abdominal disorders in the horse has improved markedly over the last two decades. Surgical technique and anesthetic management have advanced to the point that the survival of horses after abdominal surgery is becoming primarily dependent on the ability to manage associated disorders, including metabolic disorders, endotoxemia, and postoperative complications. This discussion focuses on the management of adynamic ileus, an uncommon but serious complication after abdominal surgery.

Intestinal ileus is characterized by a decrease in propulsive motility, an increase in fluid and particulate transit time, and distention of intestine. Hypomotile loops of intestine after colic surgery may contribute to the formation of adhesions between bowel segments.[1] Clinically, horses with ileus are often depressed and may show signs of abdominal discomfort or have an elevated heart rate. Horses with small intestinal ileus have ongoing nasogastric reflux and the presence of distended loops of small intestine palpable rectally. Horses with ileus of the large intestine may have a bloated appearance externally. Therapy consists of supportive care and possibly pharmacologic attempts to stimulate intestinal motility. Surgical decompression of intractable cases of ileus has been described.[2, 3]

SUPPORTIVE THERAPY

Ileus can result in the progressive distention of stomach and intestine and sequestration of fluid and electrolytes. Increased intraluminal pressures, elevation of portal venous and lymphatic pressures, ischemia, and endotoxin absorption may occur in the distended bowel. In humans and many animal species, this distention is relieved by the act of emesis. The horse has a peculiar gastroesophageal junction compared with other species that inhibits its ability to vomit.[4] If the intestinal distention progresses, rupture of the stomach or intestine or breakdown of anastomotic sites may occur.

Nasogastric intubation is an effective means of providing decompression for the proximal intestinal tract. The nasogastric tube may be left in place by securing it to the horse's halter, or it may be passed and removed intermittently after siphoning of the stomach contents (reflux). Up to 6 gal of reflux every 3 hours may be removed from a horse with proximal enteritis.[5] Some clinicians are concerned about intake of large amounts of air through a nasogastric tube left in place. This may be avoided by plugging the outside end of the tube. Alternatively, a Heimlich valve can allow reflux of fluid with minimal passage of air into the horse. A simple valve can be made by taping a finger of a latex surgeon's glove onto the outside end of the tube and cutting the tip of the finger off. Merely leaving a nasogastric tube in place does not insure protection against rupture; in a retrospective study of 54 horses suffering gastric rupture, six horses had a nasogastric tube in place at the time of rupture.[6] It is therefore advisable to attempt to actively siphon the tube at regular intervals. It must also be understood that the presence of a nasogastric tube in the stomach may by itself cause some decrease in motility.[7] Therefore it is appropriate to remove the nasogastric tube when the amount of reflux fluid has subsided to 1 to 2 L/hr.

Intravenous fluid therapy is indicated in horses with adynamic ileus to compensate for fluid and electrolyte losses. Polyionic, balanced electrolyte solutions are commercially available for use in the horse. Laboratory evaluation of calcium, potassium, sodium, and chloride concentrations may indicate electrolyte deficits that should be corrected by the addition of calcium gluconate, potassium chloride, or hypertonic saline to the intravenous fluids.

The importance of maintaining a normal electrolyte balance cannot be overemphasized. Hypokalemia and low ionized calcium are frequently found in horses with gastrointestinal disorders.[8, 9] A study in dogs suggested that potassium depletion contributed more to the loss of motility than did sympathetic hypersensitivity.[10] Experimental work in rats showed that potassium deficits resulted in a decrease in tone and rhythmicity of the stomach and small intestine.[11] The importance of potassium may be due to its requirement for acetylcholine synthesis.[12] Calcium is involved in cholinergic transmitter release and is necessary for the excitation-contraction coupling in smooth muscle.[13]

Nonsteroidal anti-inflammatory drugs (NSAIDs) are commonly used for pain relief and an anti-endotoxic effect. In experimental models, infusion of endotoxin has well-documented effects on motility throughout the intestinal tract. Endotoxemia has been shown to decrease gastric contraction amplitude and rate,[14] to decrease cecal and ventral colon contractile activity,[15] and to decrease the spike rate in the small colon.[16] Endotoxemia invokes a host inflammatory cascade that, in part, consists of the release of prostaglandins and thromboxane via the cyclooxygenase pathway.

Prostaglandins have been found at elevated levels in models of intestinal ischemia.[17] Experimentally, infusion of prostaglandin E_2 (PGE$_2$) and to a lesser extent PGI$_2$ resulted in a hypomotility similar to that seen with endotoxemia.[16] Infusion of PGF$_{2\alpha}$ had no effect.

NSAIDs are commonly used for their ability to block the cyclooxygenase pathway of inflammation and the production of prostaglandins and thromboxane. When given before endotoxin infusion, both flunixin meglumine and phenylbutazone were effective in decreasing gastrointestinal and cardiac effects.[20] NSAIDs such as flunixin meglumine or phenylbutazone have no direct effect on intestinal motility.[18] However, in one study, horses with ileus and treated with flunixin meglumine recovered faster than nontreated horses.[19] In another study, phenylbutazone was superior to flunixin in inhibiting endotoxin-induced ileus.[20]

Some clinicians believe that exercise will stimulate intestinal activity and decrease the incidence of postoperative adhesions. Feeding of horses with ileus of the proximal intestinal tract is contraindicated, but may be beneficial for stimulating motility of the large colon, as total myoelectric spike frequency was higher in the pelvic flexure and left dorsal colon after feeding in one study,[21] and a gastrocolonic reflex has been described in horses.[22]

PHARMACOLOGIC STIMULATION OF INTESTINAL MOTILITY

Unfortunately, in equine medicine there is a lack of scientifically derived recommendations concerning the appropriateness, time of initiation, and clinical usefulness of prokinetic drugs. Variability in experimental models of ileus, variability in methods of determining propulsive motility, and virtually no well-controlled clinical trials all contribute to the confusion.

Transient hypomotility (<9 hours) is common in horses after anesthesia.[23] In humans, the severity of postoperative ileus is worse if the peritoneum is entered, but does not correlate with the duration of surgery.[24] True postoperative ileus often resolves in 2 to 3 days with supportive therapy alone. Some clinicians initiate motility stimulant therapy

immediately in the postoperative period when they have reason to believe that ileus will likely be a complication (e.g., after a small intestine resection or anastomosis). It is unknown whether better effect can be achieved by initiating motility stimulants early in the course of ileus.

Gastrointestinal motility is subject to multiple influences. Cholinergic mechanisms in general exert positive effects on motility while sympathetic nervous input causes an inhibition of motility. In addition, there appears to be a noncholinergic, nonadrenergic mechanism with an unknown method of transmission. Adenosine triphosphate (ATP), dopamine-like compounds, and gastrointestinal polypeptides have all been implicated in this function. Most pharmacologic attempts to increase motility traditionally have been attempts to manipulate one or more of these influencing mechanisms.

The intestinal tract has its own intrinsic control as well—the enteric nervous system. Removing the influence of extrinsic innervation by vagotomy and sympathectomy does not cause marked changes in intestinal activity.[25] However, diseases in which intrinsic innervation is absent, such as Hirschsprung's disease in humans or lethal white syndrome (ileocolonic aganglionosis) in horses, are associated with greatly diminished motility. Therapies aimed at restoring normal function of the enteric nervous system will likely have the highest success at restoring coordinated motility.

Clearly, there is no single drug that is a panacea for adynamic ileus in every horse and some cases may not respond to any of the currently available drugs. However, a clinician may improve the odds of successful therapy by selecting a drug based upon its activity in the affected intestinal segment (Table 12–10).

Narcotic Antagonists

The use of a narcotic antagonist is based upon the premise that high levels of endogenous opioids are circulating in response to pain and are interfering with motility. The three major types of opioid receptors in the gastrointestinal tract of the horse are the mu, delta, and kappa receptors.[26] Stimulation of mu and kappa receptors results in ataxia, sedation, and decreases in gastrointestinal transit time.[27] The intestinal segment in which the most positive effect of narcotic antagonism is seen is the large intestine, and is apparently due to coordination of the timing of contractions. Naloxone induced typical migrating spike bursts in the colon associated with cecal contractions in a fasting model in ponies,[28] but did not prevent the inhibitory effects of morphine on defecation in ponies.[29] At high doses, naloxone can result in diarrhea, increased heart rate, and signs of abdominal discomfort.[30]

Butorphanol, a narcotic agonist-antagonist, apparently has no direct effect on large intestinal motility and may decrease small intestinal propulsive motility.[31] The drug had no effect on borborygmi or time to first defecation in ponies.[29] Butorphanol inhibited jejunal myoelectric activity as measured by an increased duration of the migrating myoelectric complex (MMC), due to increased duration between regular spike activity (RSA).[32]

Cholinergic Agonists

Acetylcholine is a neurotransmitter for both the intrinsic and extrinsic nerves of the gastrointestinal tract. The action of

Table 12–10. Drug Activity in Adynamic Ileus

Motility Drug	Dose	Route	Dosing Interval	References	Region of Action	Side Effects
Bethanechol	0.025 mg/kg	SC	?	34	Stomach	Salivation, mild colic
	2.5 mg	SC	3 hr	8		
Carbachol	0.01 mg/kg	IV	3 hr	28	Ileum	Salivation
Cisapride	0.1 mg/kg	IM	8 hr	35, 48, 52	Small intestine, large intestine	Slight tachycardia, mild colic
	0.1 mg/kg	IV	8 hr	28		
Domperidone	0.2 mg/kg	IV	6 hr	55	Stomach, small intestine	?
Erythromycin	0.033 mg/kg	20-min IV infusion	?	59	Entire tract	Diarrhea
	0.1–1.0 mg/kg	IV	4–6 hr	76		
Metoclopramide	0.04 mg/kg/hr	Continuous IV infusion	Continuous	46	Small intestine	CNS effects, extrapyramidal signs
	0.5 mg/kg initially, then 0.25 mg/kg for subsequent infusions	30-min IV infusion	3-hr intervals	8, 47		
Naloxone	0.01 mg/kg	IV	?	29	Large intestine	Diarrhea, colic
	0.05 mg/kg	IV		28		
Neostigmine	0.022 mg/kg	SC, IV	2 hr	18	Large intestine	Delayed gastric emptying, asystole at high doses, mild colic (especially IV route)
Phenoxybenzamine	200 mg	30-min IV infusion	15–24 hr	42	?	Hypotension
Yohimbine	0.125–0.25 mg/kg	IV	3 hr	29	Entire tract	CNS effects
	0.15 mg/kg	IV		8		
	0.075 mg/kg	IV		15		

cholinergic stimulation on intestinal motility is predominantly excitatory. Inhibition of cholinergic transmission in the enteric nervous system interrupts motility.[33] Cholinergic agonists are used in an attempt to directly stimulate smooth muscle of the gastrointestinal tract. Bethanechol has been used to aid gastric emptying in humans and was recently shown to have a similar effect in horses.[34] It increased gastric contractions without any effect on acid secretion.[34] In an earlier study, however, bethanechol produced some propulsive action in trauma-induced models of ileus but did not alter the transit time of particles.[8] In a similar study, carbachol was demonstrated to stimulate activity in the terminal ileum and cecocolonic region.[14] Bethanechol and carbachol are drugs with limited therapeutic value when given by themselves owing to their inability to produce coordinated motility.[35] Bethanechol given in combination with yohimbine did result in increased phase III (RSA) jejunal activity and improved transit time of spheres from stomach to anus when compared with yohimbine alone.[8] D-Panthenol, a precursor of coenzyme A, is purported to increase the formation of acetylcholine. It had no effect on intestinal motility in one study in ponies.[18]

Cholinesterase Inhibitors

As with cholinergic agonists, cholinesterase inhibitors are used to increase the concentration of acetylcholine at smooth muscle receptors. These two classes of drugs should not be used concurrently because of the possibility of additive effects. Neostigmine not only has anticholinesterase activity but may also directly stimulate cholinergic receptors. Neostigmine appears useful for the stimulation of progressive motility in the large intestine of horses.[18] Conflicting results have been demonstrated for the effect neostigmine has on the small intestine.[8, 19] Continuous spiking activity (intestinal spasm) was seen with the use of neostigmine in horses after experimental strangulation and obstruction.[18] In another study, neostigmine resulted in cyclic increases in the amplitude of rhythmic contractions of the small intestine with both normal and increased intraluminal pressures.[36] Overdose of this drug may cause asystole and at least one death has been attributed to its usage in the horse.[27]

α-Adrenergic Antagonists

Increased activity of the sympathetic nervous system has been suspected in the pathophysiology of ileus since the classic experiments of Bayliss and Starling in 1899.[37] They demonstrated that the hypomotility seen in dogs undergoing laparotomy could be partially reversed by cutting the sympathetic innervation.

The use of α-adrenergic blockers in horses with ileus is based upon the premise that high sympathetic tone results from pain and stress. Yohimbine is a specific α_2-antagonist that reversed the inhibition of cecal myoelectric activity caused by xylazine and amitraz in one study.[38] In dogs, yohimbine not only immediately restored colonic myoelectric activity after α_2-agonist inhibition but also resulted in the induction of propagated giant contractions.[39] In a trauma-induced model of ileus in horses, yohimbine significantly improved the coordination of activity between the stomach and small intestine and also significantly improved stomach-to-anus transit time of spheres.[8] Yohimbine had no direct effect on contractility of isolated jejunal muscle strips.[40] It may be a good choice for ileus due to endotoxemia as it significantly attenuated hypomotility in an endotoxin infusion model.[15]

Acepromazine is a nonspecific α-adrenergic blocker that has been stated to decrease intestinal motility.[35] However, transit time of markers in the small intestine was improved 32% in one study with no changes in spiking activity and only a 5% reduction in slow-wave frequency.[41] Acepromazine can cause hypotension due to vasodilation. Phenoxybenzamine is a nonreversible α-adrenergic blocker that reduced the amount of gastric reflux in horses in a noncontrolled clinical trial.[42] It is reported to have cumulative effects with each dose.[42] As with acepromazine, hypotension is a possible side effect.

Benzamides

Benzamides have been purported to have three beneficial actions for the treatment of ileus. First, benzamides have cholinomimetic activity. Second, they have antidopaminergic activity (both centrally and peripherally). Last, it appears that benzamides may influence activity at serotonin receptors (5-hydroxytryptamine [5-HT] receptors).[43] Although the benzamides have antagonistic activity at 5-HT type 3 receptors, selective antagonists of 5-HT type 3 receptors were much less effective than benzamides for stimulating antral and small intestinal myoelectric activity in dogs.[44] Therefore, benzamides may exert their effect on motility primarily by acting as agonists at 5-HT type 4 receptors.[45]

Metoclopramide has been the most commonly used drug in this category in the United States. Although commonly used to promote gastric emptying, this effect has not been clearly demonstrated in the horse. Metoclopramide had weak and nonspecific motor effects on stomach and small intestine in fasted conscious ponies,[28] and had no effect on the MMC in the jejunum in another study.[32] However, small intestinal transit time was restored to near normal with 100% coordination between stomach and jejunal contractions in horses given metoclopramide in a trauma-induced model of ileus.[8] When used empirically after small intestinal resection and anastomosis in a clinical trial, horses had decreased volume and duration of reflux, and decreased hospital stay compared with control horses.[46] Metoclopramide slightly decreased large colon and small colon activity in fasted horses.[47] This drug can have potent central nervous system (CNS) stimulant effects and is avoided by some clinicians. It is advisable to administer metoclopramide as an infusion that can be terminated if CNS signs become apparent (i.e., head-pressing, headshaking, excitation, etc.).

Cisapride has been widely investigated in Europe for its prokinetic effects and is now available in the United States in tablet form. Unlike other benzamides, cisapride does not antagonize dopamine. Therefore this drug has fewer CNS effects than metoclopramide. In a fasting model of ileus, cisapride produced progressive motility throughout the small intestine, cecum, and large colon.[48] Increased total contraction activity in the stomach was coordinated with increased phase II (intermittent spiking activity) of the small intestine.[48] Cisapride had no effect on gastric emptying in a similar study,[49] and did not significantly improve gastric emptying in neonatal pony foals.[50] Cisapride has been shown to induce typical migrating spike bursts in the colon in association with cecal contractions. The activity was best seen at an intermediate dose (0.1 mg/kg).[48] In a clinical study that included no controls, cisapride was credited with lowering the death rate of postoperative ileus from 19% to 5%.[51] In a randomized clinical trial, cisapride appeared to decrease the incidence and duration of postoperative ileus.[52] Cisapride may not be useful for endotoxemia-induced ileus.[53] Administration of this drug with no available parenteral form might be problematic. Some clinicians have administered cisapride orally despite the presence of reflux; others have given the drug intrarectally. The amount of cisapride absorbed after these methods of administration in horses is unknown. A recent clinical trial in humans showed a nonsignificant increase in resolution of ileus after rectally administered cisapride.[54]

Dopamine Antagonists

Dopamine is a precursor of norepinephrine and may also have a direct negative effect on gastrointestinal motility. Domperidone is a specific dopamine-2 receptor antagonist. It is reported to coordinate gastroduodenal motility like metoclopramide. Domperidone was more effective than cisapride in restoring transit time of spheres from stomach to anus after a trauma-induced model of ileus.[55] CNS side effects are minimal since domperidone does not cross the blood-brain barrier.

Motilin Agonists

Motilin is a 22–amino acid gut neuropeptide that has a physiologic role in modulating gastrointestinal motility. Motilin receptors have been found throughout the intestinal tract in other species.[56, 57] In horses, motilin receptors have been described in the small intestine and erythromycin-induced activity on isolated colon segments would imply the presence of receptors in the large intestine as well.[58, 59] During interdigestive periods, motilin is released into the peripheral circulation at regular intervals that coincide with phase III regular spike activity (RSA) of the migrating myoelectric complex (MMC) in the stomach and small intestine, and can initiate this in the dog.[60] Because the plasma peak of motilin occurs when the phase III (RSA) is in the duodenum, it may be involved in the initiation of this phase. There is some evidence that endogenous motilin in the dog is a result, rather than an initiating factor, of phase III (RSA) activity.[61] It seems likely, however, that motilin is necessary for normal phase III (RSA) activity since motilin antisera given intravenously will abolish phase III (RSA) activity.[62] Motilin agonists have been effective accelerators of gastric emptying in diabetic humans with gastroparesis due to generalized autonomic neuropathy.[63] This is because the activity is directly on motilin receptors on the intestinal smooth muscle rather than via the release of acetylcholine at myenteric neurons. Motilin activity on isolated perfused intestine was not affected by atropine (muscarinic receptor blockade), loxiglumide (cholecystokinin receptor blockade), or spantide (substance P receptor blockade).[64] Motilin was investigated in experimental studies in an equine model of strangulation-obstruction of the jejunum and resulted in improved stomach-to-cecum transit time of fluid markers.[65] In that study, motilin administration decreased time to onset of jejunal phase III (RSA) spiking activity, increased the number of jejunal and ileal MMCs, and decreased the duration of jejunal and ileal MMCs.[65] Mean transit time of a fluid marker from stomach to cecum was reduced from over 360 minutes in controls to less than 160 minutes in motilin-treated horses.[65]

Clinically, stimulation of intestinal motility has been through the use of erythromycin lactobionate. This macrolide antibiotic can function as a motilin receptor agonist.[66] Erythromycin stimulated motor activity of isolated perfused segments of rabbit ileum in a dose-dependent manner, possibly through activation of calcium channels because the effect of the drug could be abolished by the calcium blocker verapamil.[67] Neuronal blockade with tetrodotoxin, muscarinic blockade with atropine, and opiate blockade with naloxone did not alter the response to erythromycin.[67] In horses, erythromycin infusion interrupted the regular myoelectric pattern of the colon with propagated spike bursts.[59] Erythromycin has been administered as an infusion, but evidence of receptor downregulation suggests that small intermittent doses may be more effective. Severe diarrhea has been reported as a complication with the use of erythromycin in adult horses.[68]

Miscellaneous

Intravenous infusion of lidocaine for the treatment of ileus in horses is currently being investigated in a multicenter clinical trial.[69] Lidocaine is proposed to work by decreasing sympathetic inhibition and is purported to also have direct stimulatory effects on intestinal smooth muscle.

Octreotide, a somatostatin analog, enhanced particulate transit time in experimental models of ileus in the dog, but delayed gastric emptying at high doses.[70]

Diatrozoate meglumine (Gastrografin), a water-soluble gastrointestinal radiologic contrast agent, has long been associated with rapid transit through the intestinal tract. It is a hyperosmolar solution containing the wetting agent polysorbate 80, which draws fluid into the intestinal lumen. It was recently evaluated in a clinical trial in humans with partial small bowel obstruction and found to speed resolution.[71] Because the high osmolarity of Gastrografin attracts fluid into the intestinal tract, it is probably contraindicated in horses with proximal obstructions. Gastrografin was found to be an effective enema for the treatment of meconium obstructions in human infants, with 54% resolution after one enema and 67% resolution after two enemas.[72]

Paravertebral anesthesia to block the sympathetic input to the gastrointestinal tract has been investigated in sheep to resolve postoperative ileus,[73] but has not been investigated in horses. Electroacupuncture has been described as beneficial for resolving ileus in rabbits and horses.[74, 75]

REFERENCES

1. Ellis H: *Intestinal Obstruction.* New York, Appleton-Century-Crofts, 1982, p 70.
2. Macharg MA, Foerner JJ, Phillips TN, et al: Bypass surgery for the treatment of small intestinal ileus in the horse. *Vet Surg* 17:15, 1988.
3. Huskamp B: Diagnosis of gastroduodenojejunitis and its surgical treatment by a temporary duodenocaecostomy. *Equine Vet J* 17:314, 1985.
4. Freeman DE: The stomach. In Mansmann RA, McAllister ES, Pratt PW, eds: *Equine Medicine and Surgery,* ed 3. Santa Barbara, Calif, American Veterinary, 1982, p 497.
5. White NA: Medical management of the colic patient. In *Proceedings of the American Association of Equine Practitioners 34th Convention,* 1988, p 81.
6. Todhunter RJ, Hollis EN, Roth I: Gastric rupture in horses: A review of 54 cases. *Equine Vet J* 18:288, 1986.
7. Alexander F: Experiments on the horse stomach. *Q J Exp Physiol* 36:139, 1951.
8. Gerring EL, Hunt JM: Pathophysiology of equine post-operative ileus: Effect of adrenergic blockade, parasympathetic stimulation and metoclopramide in an experimental model. *Equine Vet J* 18:249, 1986.
9. Dart AJ, Snyder JR, Spier SJ, et al: Ionized calcium concentration in horses with surgically managed intestinal disease. In *Proceedings of the Fifth Equine Colic Research Symposium,* 1994, p 10.
10. Mishra NK, Apport HE, Howard JM: Studies of paralytic ileus: Effects of intraperitoneal injury motility of the canine small intestine. *Am J Surg* 129:559, 1975.
11. Winters HA, Hoff HE, Dso L: Effect of potassium deficiency upon gastrointestinal motility. *FASEB J* 8:169, 1949.
12. Neely J, Catchpole BN: Ileus—the restoration of alimentary tract motility by pharmacological means. *Br J Surg* 58:21, 1971.
13. Rubin RP: Role of calcium in release of neurotransmitter substances and hormones. *Pharmacol Rev* 82:389, 1970.
14. King JN, Gerring EL: Antagonism of endotoxin-induced disruption of equine gastrointestinal motility with the platelet activating factor antagonist WEB 2086. *J Vet Pharmacol Ther* 13:333, 1990.
15. Eades SC, Moore JN: Blockade of endotoxin-induced cecal hypoperfusion and ileus with an alpha 2 antagonist in horses. *Am J Vet Res* 54:586, 1993.
16. King JN, Gerring EL: The action of low dose endotoxin on equine bowel motility. *Equine Vet J* 23:11, 1991.
17. Beard WL, Moore RM: Effect of enteric evacuation on the systemic absorption of endotoxin and inflammatory mediators in an ischemic small intestine model. In *Proceedings of the Fifth Equine Colic Research Symposium,* 1994, p 13.
18. Adams SB, Lamar CH, Masty J: Motility of the distal portion of the jejunum and pelvic flexure in ponies: Effects of six drugs. *Am J Vet Res* 45:795, 1984.
19. Ehreiser-Schmidt C, Deegen E, Plocki K, et al: Use of the prostaglandin inhibitor, flunixin meglumine, to prevent shock in horses undergoing surgery for colic. *Pferdeheilkunde* 5:275, 1989.
20. King JN, Gerring EL: Antagonism of endotoxin-induced disruption of equine bowel motility by flunixin and phenylbutazone. *Equine Vet J* 7(suppl):38, 1989.
21. Merritt AM, Panzer RB, Lester GD, et al: Equine colonic

myoelectrical activity during fed and fasted states. In *Proceedings of the Fifth Equine Colic Research Symposium*, 1994, p 29.

22. Roger T, Ruckebusch Y: Colonic α2-adrenoceptor-mediated responses in the pony. *J Vet Pharmacol Ther* 10:310, 1987.

23. Lester GD, Bolton JR, Cullen LK, et al: Effects of general anesthesia on myoelectric activity of the intestine in horses. *Am J Vet Res* 53:1553, 1992.

24. Livingston EH, Passaro EP: Postoperative ileus. *Dig Dis Sci* 35:121, 1990.

25. Gershon MD, Erde SM: The nervous system of the gut. *Gastroenterology* 80:1571, 1981.

26. Lester GD: Disorders of equine motility and the use of prokinetic drugs. In *Proceedings of the 12th American College of Veterinary Internal Medicine Forum*, 1994, p 603.

27. Kohn CW, Muir WW: Selected aspects of the clinical pharmacology of visceral analgesics and gut motility modifying drugs in the horse. *J Vet Intern Med* 2:85, 1988.

28. Ruckebusch Y, Roger T: Prokinetic effects of cisapride, naloxone, and parasympathetic stimulation at the equine ileo-caeco-colonic junction. *J Vet Pharmacol Ther* 11:322, 1988.

29. Roberts MC, Argenzio A: Effects of amitraz, several opiate derivatives and anticholinergic agents on intestinal motility in ponies. *Equine Vet J* 18:256, 1986.

30. Kamerling SG, Hamra JG, Bagwell CA: Naloxone-induced abdominal distress in the horse. *Equine Vet J* 22:241, 1990.

31. Sojka J, Adams SB, Bronson SA, et al: The effect of 2 opiate agonist-antagonists on intestinal motility in the pony. In *Proceedings of the Second Equine Colic Research Symposium*, 1986, p 102.

32. Sojka JE, Adams SB, Lamar CH, et al: Effect of butorphanol, pentazocine, meperidine, or metoclopramide on intestinal motility in female ponies. *Am J Vet Res* 49:527, 1988.

33. Kosterlitz HW, Lees GM: Pharmacological analysis of intrinsic intestinal reflexes. *Pharmacol Rev* 16:301, 1964.

34. Thompson LP, Burrow JA, Madison JB, et al: Effect of bethanecol on equine gastric motility and secretion. In *Proceedings of the Fifth Equine Colic Research Symposium*, 1994.

35. Gerring EL: Factors affecting gut motility. *Equine Vet Educ* 3:146, 1991.

36. Parks AH, Stick JA, Arden WA, et al: Effects of distention and neostigmine on jejunal vascular resistance, oxygen uptake, and intraluminal pressure changes in ponies. *Am J Vet Res* 50:54, 1989.

37. Bayliss WM, Starling EH: The movements and innervations of the small intestine. *J Physiol* 24:99, 1899.

38. Mogg TDK, Pass MA: Amitraz-induced cecal stasis in ponies—the role of α2-adrenoceptors. In *Proceedings of the Fourth Equine Colic Research Symposium*, 1991, p 18.

39. Maugeri S, Ferre JP, Intorre L, et al: Effects of medetomidine on intestinal and colonic motility in the dog. *J Vet Pharmacol Ther* 17:148, 1994.

40. Malone ED, Brown DR, Trent AM, et al: Responses of equine jejunal longitudinal smooth muscle to adrenergic and cholinergic agonists in vitro. In *Proceedings of the Fifth Equine Colic Research Symposium*, 1994, p 18.

41. Davies JV, Gerring EL: Effect of spasmolytic analgesic drugs on the motility patterns of the equine small intestine. *Res Vet Sci* 34:334, 1983.

42. Beadle RE, Brooks DE, Martin GS: Phenoxybenzamine as an adjunct in the therapy for ileus in the horse. In *Proceedings of the Second Equine Colic Research Symposium*, 1986, p 112.

43. Talley NJ: 5-Hydroxytryptamine agonists and antagonists in the modulation of gastrointestinal motility and sensation: Clinical implications. *Aliment Pharmacol Ther* 6:273, 1992.

44. Gullikson GW, Loeffler RF, Virina MA: Relationship of serotonin-3 receptor antagonist activity to gastric emptying and mo-

tor-stimulating actions of prokinetic drugs in dogs. *J Pharmacol Exp Ther* 258:103, 1991.

45. Buchheit KH, Buhl T: Prokinetic benzamides stimulate peristaltic activity in the isolated guinea pig ileum by activation of 5-HT4 receptors. *Eur J Pharmacol* 205:203, 1991.

46. Dart AJ, Peauroi JR, Pascoe JR: Evaluation of the use of metoclopramide in horses undergoing resection and anastomosis of the small intestine. In *Proceedings of the Fifth Equine Colic Research Symposium*, 1994, p 39.

47. Hunt JM, Gerring EL: A preliminary study of the effects of metoclopramide on equine gut activity. *J Vet Pharmacol Ther* 9:109, 1986.

48. King JH, Gerring EL: Actions of the novel gastrointestinal prokinetic agent cisapride on equine bowel motility. *J Vet Pharmacol Ther* 11:314, 1988.

49. Levy M, Sojka J: Control of gastric emptying in the horse: Effect of cisapride. In *Proceedings of the Fourth Equine Colic Research Symposium*, 1991, p 17.

50. Baker SJ, Gerring EL: Gastric emptying of four liquid meals in pony foals. *Res Vet Sci* 56:164, 1994.

51. Gerring EL: Does cisapride prevent postoperative ileus: Results of a multicentre trial. In *Proceedings of the Fourth Equine Colic Research Symposium*, 1991, p 18.

52. Velden MA, Klein WR: The effects of cisapride on the restoration of gut motility after surgery of the small intestine in horses: A clinical trial. *Vet Q* 15:175, 1993.

53. Gerring EL, King JN, Edwards GB, et al: A multicentre trial of cisapride in the prophylaxis of equine postoperative ileus. *Equine Vet Educ* 3:143, 1991.

54. Benson MJ, Roberts JP, Wingate DL, et al: Small bowel motility following major intra-abdominal surgery: The effects of opiates and rectal cisapride. *Gastroenterology* 106:924, 1994.

55. Gerring EL, King JN: Cisapride in the prophylaxis of equine postoperative ileus. *Equine Vet J* 7(suppl):52, 1989.

56. Depoortee I, Peeters TL, Vantrappen G: Distribution and characterization of motilin receptors in the cat. *Peptides* 14:1153, 1993.

57. Peeters TL, Bormans V, Vantrappen G: Regional and temporal variation of motilin receptor density in the human and rabbit gastrointestinal tract. *Dig Dis Sci* 787, 1985.

58. Kitamura N, Yamada J, Calingasa NY, et al: Immunocytochemical distribution of endocrime cells in the gastrointestinal tract of the horse. *Equine Vet J* 16:103, 1984.

59. Masri MD, Merritt AM, Burrow JA: Effect of erythromycin on equine colonic motility. In *Proceedings of the Fourth Equine Colic Research Symposium*, 1991, p 47.

60. Itoh Z, Takeudis S, Aizawa I, et al: Changes in plasma motilin concentration and gastrointestinal contractile activity in conscious dogs. *Dig Dis* 23:929, 1978.

61. Sarna S, Chey WY, Condon RE, et al: Cause-and-effect relationship between motilin and migrating myoelectric complexes. *Am J Physiol* 245:277, 1983.

62. Lee KY, Chang TM, Chey WY: Effect of rabbit antimotilin serum on myoelectric activity and plasma motilin concentration in fasting dogs. *Am J Physiol* 245:547, 1983.

63. Urbain JL, Vantrappen G, Janssens J, et al: Intravenous erythromycin dramatically accelerates gastric emptying in gastroparesis diabeticorum in normals and abolishes the emptying discrimination between solids and liquids. *J Nucl Med* 31:1490, 1990.

64. Harada N, Chijiiwa Y, Misawa T, et al: Direct contractile effect of motilin on isolated smooth muscle cells of guinea pig small intestine. *Life Sci* 51:1381, 1992.

65. Coatney RW, Adams SB: The effect of motilin on equine small intestinal motility during experimental postoperative ileus. In *Proceedings of the Third Equine Colic Research Symposium*, 1988, p 12.

66. Behrns KE, Sarr MG: Diagnosis and management of gastric emptying disorders. *Adv Surg* 27:233, 1994.

67. Armstrong DN, Ballantyne GH, Modlin IM: Erythromycin stimulates ileal motility by activation of dihydropyridine-sensitive calcium channels. *J Surg Res* 52:140, 1992.

68. Plumb DC: *Veterinary Drug Handbook.* White Bear Lake, Pharma Vet. 1991, p 513.

69. Malone ED, Turner TA, Wilson JH: Intravenous lidocaine for the treatment of ileus in the horse. In *Proceedings of the Fifth Equine Colic Research Symposium,* 1994, p 39.

70. Cullen JJ, Eagon JC, Dozois EJ, et al: Treatment of acute postoperative ileus with octrotide. *Am J Surg* 165:113, 1993.

71. Assalia A, Schein M, Kopelman D, et al: Therapeutic effect of oral Gastrografin in adhesive, partial small-bowel obstruction: A prospective randomized trial. *Surgery* 115:433, 1994.

72. Caniano DA, Beaver BL: Meconium ileus: A fifteen year experience with forty-two neonates. *Surgery* 102:699, 1987.

73. Bueno L, Fioramonti J, Ruckebusch Y: Postoperative intestinal motility in dogs and sheep. *Dig Dis* 23:682, 1978.

74. Dai JL, Ren ZJ, Fu ZM, et al: Electroacupuncture reversed the inhibition of intestinal peristalsis induced by intrathecal injection of morphine in rabbits. *Chin Med J [Engl]* 106:220, 1993.

75. Bossut D, Page E: Preliminary study of the treatment of paralytic ileus in horses by electrocacupuncture. In *Proceedings of the International Veterinary Acupuncture Society Congress.*

12.14

Peritonitis

Michael J. Murray, DVM, MS

Peritonitis is an inflammation of the peritoneum, which consists of a single layer of mesothelial squamous cells that lines the peritoneal cavity and serosal surfaces of the intraabdominal viscera. This single layer of cells functions as a semipermeable barrier to the diffusion of water and low-molecular-weight solutes between the blood and the abdominal cavity.[1] The peritoneum secretes a serous fluid that lubricates the abdominal cavity, inhibits adhesion formation, and has minor antibacterial properties.[1, 2] Inflammation of the mesothelial lining of the peritoneal cavity is characterized by desquamation and transformation of mesothelial cells, chemotaxis of neutrophils, release of several soluble mediators of inflammation, and exudation of serum, fibrin, and protein into the peritoneal cavity.

Because the peritonitis that results from a perforated intestinal viscus is usually fatal, the diagnosis of peritonitis may be considered by some, particularly laypersons, to offer a hopeless prognosis. With early diagnosis and aggressive therapy, though, many cases of peritonitis can be treated effectively.

PATHOPHYSIOLOGY

Peritonitis usually occurs secondary to bacterial contamination, vascular insults involving the intestinal tract, abdominal trauma, or chemical insults (urine, bile, pancreatic enzymes, and chyme), but also occurs with some neoplastic processes and viral infections, notably influenza, viral arteritis, and African horse sickness virus.[1–4] Peritonitis can be focal or diffuse, the difference depending on the cause of inflammation and the extent of the inflammatory process (Table 12–11).

Most cases of peritonitis in horses involve bacterial contamination. Bacterial contamination of the peritoneum can occur as a result of hematogenous spread of bacteria from a primary site of infection (*Streptococcus equi, Rhodococcus equi*),[5] perforation of an abdominal viscus, devitalization of bowel secondary to strangulation or infarction, primary abscessation, or as a result of iatrogenic intervention (enterotomy, enterocentesis, trocharization). The intestinal tract contains a mixed population of bacteria, but the quantity of bacteria and prevalence of anaerobic species increase in the distal segments.[1, 6] There are approximately 10^9 anaerobic and 10^5 aerobic bacteria per milliliter of cecal and colonic fluid,[6] thus the potential for bacterial contamination of the peritoneum is great. High mortality is associated with contamination from the lower bowel because of the large numbers of bacteria present.[7] Hirsch and Jang[8] reported isolation of an infective agent from equine peritoneal fluid in approximately 25% of attempts. Obligate anaerobic bacteria were cultured most frequently, followed by members of the Enterobacteriaceae family (*Escherichia coli*). Penicillin-resistant *Bacteroides fragilis* was isolated from 10% to 20% of cases.

Intestinal vascular insults that can cause peritonitis include strangulation and obstruction, verminous arteritis, nonstrangulating infarction, or ruptured uterine artery. Low flow or no flow conditions can result in both mucosal and serosal inflammation, with probable release of inflammatory mediators into the peritoneum.[9, 10] With progressive vascular damage, leakage of protein and diapedesis into the abdomen occurs. Margination and migration of white blood cells in response to tissue injury follows the increase in red blood cells. With severe or prolonged vascular occlusion, leakage of endotoxin and bacteria from devitalized bowel can occur.

Biological events resulting from contamination of the abdomen or injury to the mesothelial cells have been described.[3] These include release of catecholamines, histamine, and serotonin from peritoneal mast cells, vasodilation and hyperemia, increase in peritoneal and vascular permeability, secretion of protein-rich fluid into the peritoneum, transformation of mesothelial cells into macrophages, and influx of polymorphonuclear cells, humoral opsonins, natural antibodies, and serum complement into the peritoneal cavity. Additionally, there can be depression of the peritoneal fibrinolytic activity, fibrin deposits on the peritoneal surface, and sympathetic-mediated ileus of the gastrointestinal tract.

These processes benefit the animal by confining contamination and infection, and indeed, with focal peritonitis, as occurs subsequent to enterocentesis or trocharization, this is effective. However, with greater severity of peritoneal contamination or irritation, these processes are magnified and become deleterious, resulting in problems such as hypovolemia, hypoproteinemia, ileus with resultant bowel distention, ischemia of the bowel wall with subsequent absorption of bacteria and toxins, and adhesion and abscess formation.[1, 8] Additionally, systemic responses to bacterial toxins,

Table 12–11. Causes of Peritonitis in Foals and Horses

Foals
Meconium impaction
Ruptured bladder
Urachal infection
Gastric/duodenal ulcer perforation
Septicemia
Enteritis
Intestinal vascular accident
Ascarid impaction
Intussusception
Streptococcus abscess
Rhodococcus equi abscess
Neoplasia

Adults

Iatrogenic
Rectal tear
Enterotomy
Trocharization
Enterocentesis
Castration
Vaginal perforation

Trauma
Foreign body penetration
   Gunshot
   Capture dart
   Fence post

Trauma Continued
Uterine/vaginal perforation during foaling
Vaginal perforation during breeding
Splenic tear

Vascular Accident
Verminous arteritis
Intestinal strangulation
Nonstrangulating infarction
Thromboembolism
Ruptured uterine artery

Bowel Contamination
Rupture of stomach, cecum, or colon
Strangulating intestinal obstruction
Nonstrangulating intestinal obstruction
Foreign body perforation
Anastomosis leakage/dehiscence
Intestinal mural abscess/neoplasia
Perforating colitis

Other
Mesenteric abscess
Pyometra
Cholelithiasis
Pancreatitis
Retroperitoneal abscess
Neoplasia

---

particularly lipopolysaccharide,[11, 12] can further compromise the metabolic condition of the patient. Equine peritoneal macrophages release several mediators when exposed to bacterial lipopolysaccharide,[13] undoubtedly an important component of septic peritonitis.

CLINICAL SIGNS

Clinical signs of peritonitis depend on the primary disease process, the duration of the problem, the extent of peritoneal inflammation, and the cause. Localized peritonitis may present with little or no systemic manifestations, whereas severe localized or generalized peritonitis often will be accompanied by severe toxemia or septicemia, or both. Septic peritonitis usually causes more severe clinical signs because of the inflammatory mediators released in response to bacterial toxins. Most clinical signs are nonspecific and include fever, depression, inappetance, decreased borborygmi, and dehydration. Additional signs, reported in 30 horses (age 2 months to 16 years) with peritonitis, were colic, ileus, weight loss, and diarrhea.[4]

Cases with peracute peritonitis, as occurs with rupture of the bowel or rectal tear, present with severe toxemia, weakness, depression or severe colic, tachycardia, tachypnea, and circulatory failure. Fever may not be present, particularly if the horse has been given a nonsteroidal anti-inflammatory drug (NSAID). Typical clinical findings include sweating, pawing, muscle fasciculations, weak peripheral pulses, red-

to-purple mucous membranes, prolonged capillary refill time, and decreased skin elasticity. Parietal pain, characterized by reluctance to move, splinting of the abdominal wall, and sensitivity to external abdominal pressure occur in some acute cases. It may be painful for the horse to urinate or defecate, and urine and fecal retention may be evident on rectal examination. Palpation of the abdomen externally may elicit flinching, aversion movements, or groaning. With extensive abdominal fecal contamination, rectal examination may reveal a "gritty" feeling of the serosal and parietal surface of the peritoneum due to fibrin deposition and a dry texture of the peritoneum. In cases with more chronic peritonitis, rectal examination findings can include pain on palpation of fibrinous adhesions, intestinal impaction or distention secondary to ileus, an abdominal mass (abscess or neoplasia), or an impression of bowel floating in fluid. In many cases no abnormalities can be detected on rectal examination.

Horses with localized, subacute, or chronic peritonitis may have signs of chronic or intermittent colic, depression, anorexia, weight loss, intermittent fever, ventral edema, exercise intolerance, decreased or absent intestinal sounds, and mild dehydration. Heart rate and respiratory rate may be normal. Fecal output may be normal; however, cases with chronic diarrhea and weight loss have been reported.[4]

Foals with peritonitis usually exhibit signs of colic (acute or chronic), are febrile, often are depressed, and are inappetant. In some foals with primary peritonitis, pleural effusion occurs. In young foals, peritonitis can cause rapid metabolic deterioration, and determination and correction of the primary problem requires immediate attention. In older foals, peritonitis may occur insidiously, as occurs secondary to *S. equi* or *R. equi* infections.

CLINICOPATHOLOGIC FINDINGS
Hematology and Serum Chemistry

Clinicopathologic abnormalities will vary depending on the severity and onset of peritonitis. Horses with acute, septic peritonitis can have leukopenia, hemoconcentration, metabolic acidemia, azotemia, and electrolyte imbalances, reflective of toxemia and hypovolemia. Horses with peritonitis of a few days' duration may have leukocytosis and hyperfibrinogenemia. Plasma protein levels vary, depending on the hydration status, degree of exudation into the peritoneum, and type of underlying problem. In chronic peritonitis, hyperproteinemia with hyperglobulinemia may be present.

In foals with peritonitis, the clinicopathologic changes vary according to age. In neonates, peritonitis often is accompanied by hyponatremia, hypochloremia, and hyperkalemia. This is particularly true with uroperitoneum, but I have observed similar electrolyte abnormalities in neonates with umbilical infection. In older foals, peritonitis is usually either acute with clinicopathologic findings reflective of toxemia, such as a result of gastric or duodenal perforation, or as a result of chronic abscessation, with clinicopathologic findings reflecting chronic inflammation (anemia, hyperfibrinogenemia, hyperglobulinemia).

Peritoneal Fluid

Peritoneal fluid is collected through puncture of the abdomen on the ventral midline. An area should be clipped and prepared aseptically. Usually, the lowest point of the abdomen is identified 5 to 10 cm caudal to the xiphoid for puncture, although in some cases one may perform paracentesis more caudally, particularly when a specific area of sequestered fluid or abscessation is suspected. Also, one may choose a site to the right of midline in an attempt to avoid the spleen. Peritoneal puncture can be done using a 1½-in., 18-gauge needle, or, following local anesthesia and a no. 15 scalpel blade stab incision, a sterile cannula may be used. Fluid is collected by gravity flow. Fluid should be collected in a tube containing anticoagulant, preferably ethylenediaminetetraacetic acid (EDTA), for cytologic examination, and a sterile tube without anticoagulant for visual inspection and, if desired, for culture. The EDTA tube should be filled to half its volume, since with less fluid the EDTA may interfere with a refractometer reading of total protein and give a falsely increased result.

Peritoneal fluid should be routinely evaluated as to color, turbidity, total protein, white blood cell (WBC) count and differential, and the presence of bacteria as determined by Gram's stain. Normal peritoneal fluid is clear and straw-colored and does not coagulate spontaneously. Peritoneal fluid becomes turbid when increased numbers of WBCs and concentration of protein are present. Pink or red fluid is indicative of free hemoglobin or hemorrhage. Blood introduced into the peritoneal fluid iatrogenically may, in some cases, be differentiated from blood from internal hemorrhage on the basis of the presence of platelets and hematocrit. Fluid with iatrogenic blood contamination will contain platelets, whereas fluid with blood secondary to internal hemorrhage or diapedesis often will not have platelets. Large volumes of dark-brown or green fluid with a fetid odor, obtained from several sites, suggest bowel rupture, but cytology should be performed for confirmation.

The distribution of polymorphonuclear (PMN) and mononuclear cells varies widely, and the results of cell counts and differentials should be interpreted as being supportive of a number of disorders rather than a specific diagnosis. Normal equine peritoneal fluid contains fewer than 5,000 nucleated cells per microliter.[14]

Reportedly, WBC counts in acute peritonitis ($>100,000/\mu L$) are higher than those in chronic peritonitis ($20,000–60,000/\mu L$)[4, 15]; however, this is not always the case and the WBC count is most dependent on the cause of the peritonitis. The WBC level does not always correlate with severity of peritonitis or the prognosis. The peritoneal fluid WBC count can be greater than $100,000/\mu L$ subsequent to enterocentesis, with no clinical signs or problem.[16] Conversely, peritoneal WBC counts of less than $100,000/\mu L$ may be found in foals or horses with intraabdominal abscesses.[5] The peritoneal WBC count can increase to greater than $150,000/\mu L$ following celiotomy[17] and can be higher if an enterotomy is done. Postoperatively, the WBC count normally continues to decline and returns to near normal by 5 to 7 days. Failure of the WBC count to decrease suggests peritonitis resulting from a postoperative complication. Finally, peritoneal fluid WBC counts greater than $500,000/\mu L$ are indicative of severe focal or generalized peritoneal sepsis.

The distribution of PMNs and mononuclear cells varies in normal peritoneal fluid,[14] but PMNs usually predominate. With acute peritonitis, PMNs typically increase to a greater degree than mononuclear cells, but this depends on the cause. In horses that have bowel disease accompanied by endotoxemia, the number of peritoneal mononuclear cells increases, as does transformation of mesothelial cells to macrophages. In chronic cases, transforming mesothelial cells may easily be mistaken for neoplastic cells. This can make diagnosis difficult, particularly when the presenting problem is compatible with a neoplastic process. In such cases, consultation with a clinical pathologist regarding cytology is prudent.

Normal peritoneal fluid protein concentration is less than 1.5 g/dL.[14] Protein levels between 1.5 g/dL and 2.5 g/dL can be difficult to interpret, but levels greater than 2.5 g/dL should be considered to be increased. Fibrinogen concentration increases with inflammation and levels greater than 10 mg/dL in the peritoneal fluid suggest that an acute inflammatory process is present.[18] Fibrinogen content will also increase from blood contamination.

The presence of bacteria free or within WBCs indicates abscessation or compromised bowel. Importantly, though, iatrogenic contamination of a sample can result in both free and intracellular bacteria in peritoneal fluid. I have observed phagocytosis of bacteria by neutrophils within 5 minutes of adding bacteria to a sample of normal peritoneal fluid, and bacterial contamination of a sample can easily occur during collection of the sample. If numerous bacteria of mixed types are observed free in the peritoneal fluid, or if plant material is observed, massive bacterial contamination of the

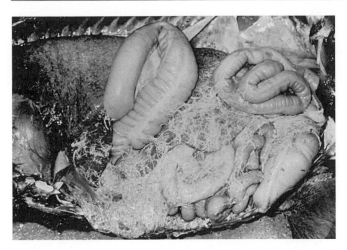

Figure 12–16. The abdomen of a foal that had a perforated gastric ulcer. The peritoneal white blood cell count and protein level were normal, although numerous bacteria were seen. There were extensive fibrinous adhesions associated with the greater omentum.

abdomen following bowel rupture has occurred. To distinguish peritoneal fluid from intestinal contents, look for phagocytosed bacteria within neutrophils, which should be numerous in peritoneal fluid. Fluid acutely contaminated with intestinal contents will contain numerous mixed types of bacteria, plant material, and few WBCs.

In foals, there may be a discrepancy between the peritoneal fluid WBC count and the protein concentration and the observation of bacteria. I have seen cases with severe fibrinous peritonitis secondary to gastric or duodenal ulcer perforation (Fig. 12–16) or ruptured small intestine secondary to ascarid impaction, but the peritoneal fluid WBC count and protein concentration were normal. Large numbers of different types of bacteria were present, indicating bowel rupture. Presumably, the WBCs and protein were sequestered within the extensive fibrinous adhesions. Clearly, when interpreting the results of peritoneal fluid cytology, it is important to correlate all cytologic findings with clinical and clinicopathologic findings.

Increased concentrations of alkaline phosphatase, lactic dehydrogenase, creatine phosphokinase, and aspartate aminotransferase have been measured in the peritoneal fluid of horses with abdominal disorders.[18] Increased lactate concentration is observed with ischemic or inflammatory intestinal disorders.[18, 19] The usefulness of such changes in assisting diagnosis is limited, however.

Peritoneal fluid samples should be submitted in appropriate media for aerobic and anaerobic (Port-A-Cul, Vial BBL Microbiology System) cultures in an attempt to identify a pathogenic organism. Obligate anaerobic bacteria, such as *Bacteroides,* are extremely difficult to culture, because the sample must be collected, transported, and cultured under strict anaerobic conditions. Frequently, bacterial cultures are negative when bacteria are present in peritoneal fluid. In order to enhance recovery of bacteria, peritoneal fluid should be inoculated into blood culture medium (Septi-Chek Columbia, Hoffmann-LaRoche Inc., Nutley, N.J.), and if the horse has received antimicrobial treatment, fluid should first

be passed through an antimicrobial removal device (A.R.D., Becton Dickinson & Co., Cockeysville, Md.).

TREATMENT

Early and aggressive therapy is required if treatment of peritonitis is to be successful. The goals of treatment are to resolve the primary problem, minimize the inflammatory response, and prevent long-term complications. In the acute phase, primary consideration is given to the arrest of endotoxic, septic, or hypovolemic shock; correction of metabolic and electrolyte abnormalities and dehydration; and management of pain. In the absence of blood gas and electrolyte determinations, adequate volumes of a balanced electrolyte solution are required to correct hydration status and support the cardiovascular system. If the horse's plasma protein concentration is less than 3.5 g/dL and peripheral edema develops, administration of plasma should be considered.

Flunixin meglumine (Banamine, Schering Corp., Kenilworth, N.J.) should be administered for its local and systemic anti-inflammatory effects. Dosages vary depending on the severity of peritonitis, degree of toxemia, severity of pain, and hydration status of the horse, and range from 0.25 mg/kg IM or IV every 6 hours, to 1.0 mg/kg IM or IV every 12 hours. The higher dosage provides greater visceral analgesia, whereas the lower dosage was effective in modifying the effects of experimental endotoxemia.[20]

Heparin therapy has been recommended to prevent adhesion formation and to render bacteria more susceptible to cellular and noncellular clearing mechanisms. In experimental models using laboratory animals, heparin therapy was associated with decreased adhesions in septic peritonitis.[21] Heparin has not yet been demonstrated to have similar efficacy in horses, although it may. A dosage range of 40 to 80 IU/kg SC every 8 hours may be considered. It should be noted that heparin induces red blood cell (RBC) aggregation in horses,[22] which may adversely affect capillary blood flow.

Antimicrobial therapy should be initiated once a diagnosis of peritonitis is made and before the results of peritoneal culture are available, since it may take several days to isolate an organism. While the selection of specific antimicrobial drugs will best be determined on the basis of bacteriologic culture and sensitivity results, often the offending organism(s) will not be isolated, or the patient's status may change (fever, depression, leukocytosis, increased fibrinogen), indicating that the initial treatment is not completely effective.

In the majority of cases, peritonitis will have resulted from bowel contamination, and thus a mixed infection with gram-negative aerobic bacteria and gram-positive and gram-negative anaerobic bacteria should be presumed.[9, 22] This should also be presumed in many cases of traumatic peritonitis, as occurs with foreign body puncture, breeding trauma, or foaling trauma. Bacterial synergism can occur, such that infection with one species of bacteria is required for another to become pathogenic.[8]

Intravenous administration of antimicrobials is preferred over oral or intramuscular routes, because more reliable levels of drug are achieved in the tissues and peritoneal fluid than would otherwise be obtained in horses with hypovolemia or decreased intestinal motility.[23] A combination of antimicrobial drugs should be used, since each drug will have a specific spectrum, and generally no one drug will have efficacy against all of the organisms that may be involved in septic peritonitis. An exception may be with abscessation secondary to *Streptococcus* species or *R. equi*, although even with these infections combination therapy is recommended (penicillin or erythromycin plus rifampin).

Aminoglycosides are effective against the majority of gram-negative aerobes but are ineffective against anaerobes. Recommended doses for aminoglycosides vary but currently we use gentamicin at a dosage of 6.6 mg/kg IV once daily or for amikacin we use 15 mg/kg IV every 12 hours. Treatment with amikacin currently is approximately ten times as expensive as with gentamicin, but may be required based on culture and sensitivity results. The potential adverse effects of aminoglycosides are documented,[24] and horses that receive aminoglycosides typically will develop enzymuria (γ-glutamyl transferase:creatinine ratio >30). Also, sick horses will have different disposition of aminoglycosides compared with normal horses,[25] from which pharmacokinetic data and dosage recommendations have been generated.

Thus, therapeutic monitoring of serum levels of aminoglycoside should be considered in patients that will receive the drug for more than a few days. Serum aminoglycoside levels are readily measured by many laboratories. After a patient has received an aminoglycoside for 48 to 72 hours, blood is taken immediately preceding and 30 minutes following administration of a dose. With bolus dosing at the dosages described above, peak levels should be 20 to 25 μg/mL and 35 to 40 μg/mL, respectively, for gentamicin and amikacin.[26] Trough levels should be less than 1.0 μg/mL for gentamicin and less than 2.0 μg/mL for amikacin. Adjustments to dose amount and frequency of administration can be accurately made based on the results of therapeutic monitoring. This can be of tremendous importance in patients that require long-term therapy.

Other antimicrobials that may be considered for treatment of gram-negative infection based on culture and sensitivity results include trimethoprim-sulfa, ticarcillin, ticarcillin-clavulanic acid (Timentin, Beecham Laboratories, Bristol, Tenn.), ceftiofur (Naxcel, Upjohn Co., Kalamazoo, Mich.), and enrofloxacin (Baytril, Haver, Shawnee, Kans.). Enrofloxacin, a quinolone drug, has excellent activity against gram-negative pathogens, is inexpensive, and is an orally administered drug. Unfortunately, it has been shown to cause articular and physeal cartilage damage in animals, sometimes causing severe lameness.[27] Thus, the drug should never be used in an animal with any active physeal growth, and should be used in older horses with caution and only after discussing the potential adverse effects with owners. I have observed the successful use of enrofloxacin in a small number of older horses (>12 years old) without adverse effect, but its use should be considered only if other therapeutic options have been ruled out.

Most gram-positive aerobes and anaerobes are sensitive to penicillin. If abscessation with *Streptococcus* species or *R. equi* is suspected, erythromycin and rifampin may be used in combination. These drugs are lipophilic, and thus penetrate abscesses well, and retain their activity within abscesses.[28] *Bacteroides fragilis* is an anaerobe that frequently is involved in peritonitis secondary to bowel contamination. *Bacteroides* is usually resistant to penicillin, cephalosporins, and erythromycin,[23] but is sensitive to metronidazole or ticarcillin. Metronidazole can be given at 16 mg/kg PO every 6 to 8 hours. Metronidazole may cause adverse effects that include diminished appetite and mild depression, or more severe problems such as paresthesias, bizarre neurologic behavior, and seizure activity.[29] These latter adverse effects are not common in horses, but have occurred.

Drainage or lavage of the peritoneal cavity may be of benefit by removing toxic bacterial byproducts and products of inflammatory cells.[30] High numbers of inflammatory cells and release of their mediators can persist even after the primary stimulus of the inflammatory response has resolved. Infusing large volumes (20–30 L) of isotonic, warmed fluid into the peritoneal cavity also dilutes the inflammatory mediators, possibly reducing their deleterious effects. Most horses will tolerate infusion of up to 30 L of fluid into the abdomen. Abdominal discomfort is usually exhibited when larger volumes of fluid are infused. When successful, peritoneal lavage will result in decreasing the peritoneal fluid WBC count and total protein, reflecting a decrease in diffuse inflammation. Focal inflammation, as from an abscess, a walled-off bowel leakage, or a tumor, may persist. In such cases peritoneal lavage may have to be repeated. In my experience, some cases have benefited from lavage twice daily for up to 7 days, and failure to do so resulted in fever, depression, and increased peritoneal fluid WBCs.

Peritoneal drainage and lavage should be done using a drain of no less than 24F diameter. Foley-type catheters can be used, but "mushroom" drains provide a larger area for fluid to enter the drain. There are two approaches to peritoneal lavage: (1) retrograde irrigation through a ventrally placed ingress-egress drain, and (2) placement of ingress catheter(s) in the paralumbar fossa(e) for infusion of fluids, with a drain placed ventrally for removal of infused fluid. It must be recognized that thorough peritoneal lavage can only be achieved via ventral midline laparotomy. Nonetheless, lavage of the peritoneal cavity as described can be of tremendous benefit in selected cases.

Peritoneal drainage and lavage can be of critical importance in foals with uroperitoneum due to bladder rupture. Peritoneal drainage removes urine that can accumulate to volumes large enough to compress the diaphragm and cause respiratory distress. Peritoneal lavage can assist in restoring more normal electrolyte balance to the extracellular fluid. Concurrent intravenous fluid therapy and eventual surgical correction of the bladder defect are mandatory.

Complications associated with the use of abdominal drains or repeated peritoneal penetration to drain fluid include retrograde infection, local irritation, pneumoperitoneum, and subcutaneous seepage around the drain and resultant cellulitis. If the patient is hypovolemic or hypoproteinemic, volume replacement and administration of plasma should be considered before large quantities of fluid are removed from the abdomen.

In cases of suspected verminous arteritis, larvicidal doses of an anthelmintic should be given once the horse's condition is stabilized. The anthelmintics ivermectin, fenbendazole, and thiabendazole have been recommended for use in larvacidal treatment.

REFERENCES

1. Hosgood G: Peritonitis part I: A review of the pathophysiology and diagnosis. *Aust Vet Pract* 16:184, 1986.

2. Schneider RK: The peritoneum. In Mansmann RA, McAllister ES, Pratt PW, eds: *Equine Medicine and Surgery.* Santa Barbara, Calif, American Veterinary, 1982, p 620.

3. Semrad SE: Peritonitis. In Smith BP, ed: *Large Animal Internal Medicine.* St Louis, Mosby–Year Book, 1990, p 674.

4. Dyson S: Review of 30 cases of peritonitis in the horse. *Equine Vet J* 15:25, 1983.

5. Rumbaugh GE, Smith BP, Carlson GP: Internal abdominal abscesses in the horse: A study of 25 cases. *J Am Vet Med Assoc* 172:304, 1978.

6. Hirsch DC: Microflora, mucosa, and immunity. In Anderson NV, ed: *Veterinary Gastroenterology.* Philadelphia, Lea & Febiger, 1980, p 199.

7. Ahrenholz DH, Simmons RL: In Simmons RL, Howard RJ, eds: *Surgical Infectious Diseases.* New York, Appleton-Century-Crofts, 1982, p 795.

8. Hirsch DC, Jang SS: Antibiotic susceptibility of bacterial pathogens from horses. *Vet Clin North Am* 3:185–186, 1987.

9. Schmid-Schonbein GW: Capillary plugging by granulocytes and the no-reflow phenomenon in the microcirculation. *FASEB J* 46:2397, 1987.

10. Lundin C, Sullins KE, White NA, et al: Induction of peritoneal adhesions with small intestinal ischaemia and distention in the foal. *Equine Vet J* 21:451, 1989.

11. Moore JN: Endotoxemia part II. Biologic reactions to endotoxin. *Compendium Continuing Educ Pract Vet* 3:S392, 1981.

12. Henry MM, Moore JN: Endotoxemia. In Smith BP, ed: *Large Animal Internal Medicine.* St Louis, Mosby–Year Book, 1990, p 668.

13. Henry MM, Moore JN, Feldman EB, et al: Effect of dietary alpha-linoleic acid on equine monocyte procoagulant activity and eicosanoid synthesis. *Circ Shock* 32:173–188, 1990.

14. Brownlow MA, Hutchins DR, Johnston KG: Reference values for equine peritoneal fluid. *Equine Vet J* 13:127, 1981.

15. West JE: Diagnostic cytology in the equine species: Overview of effusions (peritoneal, pleural, and synovial joint) and transtracheal wash. *Proc Am Assoc Equine Pract* 30:169, 1984.

16. Schumacher J, Spano JS, Moll HD: Effects of enterocentesis on peritoneal fluid constituents in the horse. *J Am Vet Med Assoc* 186:1301, 1985.

17. Blackford JT, Schneiter HL, VanSteenehouse JL, et al: Equine peritoneal fluid analysis following celiotomy. In *Proceedings of the Equine Colic Research Symposium,* 1986, p 130.

18. Nelson AW: Analysis of equine peritoneal fluid. *Vet Clin North Am Large Anim Pract* 1:267, 1979.

19. Turner AS, McIlwraith CW, Trotter GW, et al: Biochemical analysis of serum and peritoneal fluid in experimental colonic infarction in horses. In *Proceedings of the Equine Colic Research Symposium.* Athens, University of Georgia, 1982, p 79.

20. Semrad SD, Hardee GE, Hardee MM, et al: Low dose flunixin meglumine: Effects on eicosanoid production and clinical signs induced by experimental endotoxemia in horses. *Equine Vet J* 19:201, 1987.

21. Hau T, Simmons RL: Heparin in the treatment of experimental peritonitis. *Ann Surg* 187:294, 1978.

22. Mahaffey EA, Moore JN: Erythrocyte agglutination associated with heparin treatment in three horses. *J Am Vet Assoc* 189:1478, 1986.

23. Kunesh JP: Therapeutic strategies involving antimicrobial treatment of large animals with peritonitis. *J Am Vet Med Assoc* 10:1222, 1984.

24. Riviere JE, Travers DS, Coppoc DS: Gentamicin toxic nephropathy in horses with disseminated bacterial infection. *J Am Vet Med Assoc* 180:648, 1982.

25. Sojka JE, Brown SA: Pharmacokinetic adjustment of gentamicin dosing in horses with sepsis. *J Am Vet Med Assoc* 189:784, 1986.

26. Aucoin DP: Therapeutic drug monitoring: A tool for rational drug therapy. In *Proceedings of the Seventh American College of Veterinary Internal Medicine,* Forum, 1989, p 450.

27. Neer TM: Clinical pharmacologic features of fluoroquinolone antimicrobial drugs. *J Am Vet Med Assoc* 193:577, 1988.

28. Burrows GE, MacAllister CG, Beckstrom DA, et al: Rifampin in the horse: Comparison of intravenous, intramuscular, and oral administrations. *Am J Vet Res* 46:442, 1985.

29. Snavely SR, Hodges GR: The neurotoxicity of antibacterial agents. *Ann Intern Med* 101:92, 1984.

30. Valdez H, Scrutchfield WL, Taylor TS: Peritoneal lavage in the horse. *J Am Vet Med Assoc* 175:388, 1979.

12.15

Gastrointestinal Neoplasia

Michael J. Murray, DVM, MS

Primary and secondary neoplasia involving the alimentary tract of horses is relatively uncommon,[1] although several cases have been reported. Metastasis of a primary tumor to the alimentary tract is less common than tumors originating from the alimentary tract. The clinical signs of neoplasia are nonspecific and referable to the portion of the alimentary tract that is involved. Typical signs associated with, but not diagnostic for, neoplasia include weight loss and colic. Ascites or edema occur in some cases. If the esophagus is involved, dysphagia will be the predominant sign.[2, 3] Involvement of the stomach with squamous cell carcinoma at the cardia may also result in dysphagia, while involvement at other sites in the stomach may result in signs of obstruction to outflow (colic) or weight loss, or both.[4] Table 12–12 lists the neoplasias affecting the alimentary tract.

When the small or large intestine is affected, the predomi-

Table 12–12. Reported Neoplasias Affecting the Alimentary Tract

Esophagus
Squamous cell carcinoma[2, 3]

Stomach
Squamous cell carcinoma[4]

Small Intestine
Lymphosarcoma[8, 19]
Leiomyosarcoma[15, 16]
Adenocarcinoma[11, 17]
Melanoma[18]
Ganglioneuroma[19]
Intestinal carcinoid[6]

Cecum, Colon, Rectum
Leiomyosarcoma[20]
Lymphosarcoma[8]
Neurofibroma[5]

nant clinical signs are abdominal discomfort (obstruction),[5, 6] chronic weight loss,[7–9] and diarrhea, singly or severally.[8, 10] Septic peritonitis can develop if the neoplasia has eroded through the bowel wall, permitting bacteria to contaminate the peritoneal cavity.

Neoplasia is one of a number of potential conditions to consider when presented with a horse with chronic weight loss, recurrent colic, or chronic diarrhea. The diagnostic evaluation should consist of a complete physical examination, including a rectal examination, routine blood work (complete blood count, serum chemistry panel), urinalysis, and peritoneal fluid analysis. Endoscopy, ultrasonography, laparoscopy, and laparotomy can be used to further evaluate the patient.

Horses with gastrointestinal neoplasia may have anemia, hypo- or hyperproteinemia, and hyperfibrinogenemia. Some blood loss may contribute to the anemia, but probably the majority of the anemia is secondary to chronic inflammation and iron sequestration in bone marrow. Hypoproteinemia can occur secondary to bowel inflammation and protein exudation. Hyperproteinemia can occur secondary to increased serum globulins and will be accompanied by a concomitant decrease in serum albumin. Liver enzymes will be increased with hepatic carcinomas, and serum bile acids will likely be increased with bile duct carcinoma.

Neoplastic cells from a primary gastrointestinal tumor occasionally will be observed in a sample of peritoneal fluid.[11, 12] Carcinomas frequently are exfoliative, and thus neoplastic cells may be observed in peritoneal fluid when the tumor has extended through the serosal surface of intestine into the peritoneal cavity. Mesotheliomas are highly exfoliative, since they arise from the peritoneal lining.[12] Sarcomas are unlikely to be exfoliative. Additionally, evidence of peritonitis can be suggestive of an erosive neoplasm within the bowel.[13]

Endoscopy can be useful, particularly in diagnosing esophageal or gastric squamous cell carcinoma. Ultrasonography can be used to determine whether there is excessive abdominal fluid, to possibly identify a mass, to determine whether there is small bowel thickening, and whether there are any abnormalities within the parenchyma of the liver or spleen. Occasionally, gastric squamous cell carcinoma will metastasize to the spleen, which may be seen by ultrasonography. Neoplasia involving the intestines, mesentery, or peritoneum may be observed by laparoscopy.[11, 14]

Treatment is restricted to those tumors involving a segment of bowel, usually the small intestine, that can be removed surgically. Tumors that may occur as isolated masses in the small intestine include lymphosarcoma,[8] leiomyosarcoma,[15, 16] and adenocarcinoma.[17] When considering surgical removal of a tumor, it is essential to fully explore the abdominal cavity for other neoplastic masses. Additionally, thoracic radiography and ultrasonography should be considered to determine if neoplasia exists at other sites. Any suspicious tissue should be submitted to a pathologist for identification of the mass.

The use of chemotherapy for treatment of abdominal or other visceral neoplasia in the horse is usually not considered because often, by the time a diagnosis is made, the neoplasia is too widespread for medical therapy to be effective. Also, the potential adverse effects of many antineoplastic drugs make them unacceptable for use in the horse. While not reported in the literature, chemotherapy has been applied in a few cases. However, there is limited experience in using antineoplastic chemotherapeutic agents in horses and guidelines for the effective use of such drugs remain to be developed.

REFERENCES

1. Cotchin C: A general survey of tumours in the horse. *Equine Vet J* 9:16, 1977.
2. Moore JN, Kintner LD: Recurrent esophageal obstruction due to squamous cell carcinoma in a horse. *Cornell Vet* 66:589, 1976.
3. Ford TS, Vaala WE, Sweeney CR, et al: Pleuroscopic diagnosis of gastroesophageal squamous cell carcinoma in a horse. *J Am Vet Med Assoc* 190:1556, 1987.
4. Tenant B, Keirn DR, White KK, et al: Six cases of squamous cell carcinoma of the stomach of the horse. *Equine Vet J* 14:238, 1982.
5. Pascoe PJ: Colic in a mare caused by a colonic neurofibroma. *Can Vet J* 23:24, 1982.
6. Orsini JA, Orsini PG, Sepesy L, et al: Intestinal carcinoid in a mare: An etiologic consideration for chronic colic in horses. *J Am Vet Med Assoc* 193:87, 1988.
7. Traub JL, Bayly WM, Reed SM, et al: Intraabdominal neoplasia as a cause of chronic weight loss in the horse. *Compendium Continuing Educ Pract Vet* 5:S526, 1983.
8. Van den Hoven R, Franken P: Clinical aspects of lymphosarcoma in the horse: A clinical report of 16 cases. *Equine Vet J* 15:49, 1983.
9. Roberts MC, Pinsent PJ: Malabsorption in the horse associated with alimentary lymphosarcoma. *Equine Vet J* 7:166, 1975.
10. Wiseman A, Petrie L, Murray M: Diarrhea in the horse as a result of alimentary lymphosarcoma. *Vet Rec* 95:454, 1974.
11. Fulton IC, Brown CM, Yamini B: Adenocarcinoma of intestinal origin in a horse: Diagnosis by abdominocentesis and laparoscopy. *Equine Vet J* 22:447, 1990.
12. Wallace SS, Jayo MJ, Maddux JM, et al: Mesothelioma in a horse. *Compendium Continuing Educ Pract Vet* 9:209, 1987.
13. Edens LM, Taylor DD, Murray MJ, et al: Intestinal myxosarcoma in a Thoroughbred mare. *Cornell Vet* 82:163, 1992.
14. Fischer AT: Diagnostic laparoscopy. In Traub-Dargatz JL, Brown CM, eds: *Equine Endoscopy.* St Louis, Mosby–Year Book, 1990, p 173.
15. Mair TS, Taylor FG, Brown PJ: Leiomyosarcoma of the duodenum in two horses. *J Comp Pathol* 102:119, 1990.
16. Collier MA, Trent AM: Jejunal intussusception associated with leiomyosarcoma in an aged horse. *J Am Vet Med Assoc* 182:819, 1983.
17. Honnas CM, Snyder JR, Olander HJ, et al: Small intestinal adenocarcinoma in a horse. *J Am Vet Med Assoc* 191:845, 1987.
18. Lerner AB, Cage GW: Melanomas in horses. *Yale J Biol Med* 46:646, 1973.
19. Allen D, Swayne D, Belknap JK: Ganglioneuroma as a cause of small intestinal obstruction in the horse. *Cornell Vet* 79:133, 1989.
20. Clem MF, DeBowes RM, Leipold HW: Rectal leiomyosarcoma in a horse. *J Am Vet Med Assoc* 191:229, 1987.

Chapter 13

Diseases of the Liver

Michelle Henry Barton, DVM, PhD
Debra Deem Morris, DVM, MS, Dip ACVIM

THE NORMAL LIVER

Anatomy

The liver is the largest organ in the body, constituting approximately 1% of the body weight in the adult horse.[1] The location of the liver between the gastrointestinal tract and the heart is functionally suited for its metabolic, secretory, excretory, and storage properties. In the normal horse, the liver lies mostly to the right of the median, is completely contained within the rib cage, and does not contact the ventral abdominal floor. The most cranial portion of the liver is located in the ventral third of the sixth to seventh intercostal spaces and extends caudad to the right kidney (fifteenth rib). In disease processes resulting in hepatomegaly, and in the normal equine neonate, the liver may extend beyond the caudal border of the last rib. In older horses, the right liver lobe may be small owing to age-related atrophy.[2]

The equine liver consists of two surfaces, diaphragmatic and visceral, and is divided by fissures into four lobes, right, left, quadrate, and caudate. The visceral surface of the liver in situ is malleable and contains impressions of the organs with which it is in contact. The visceral surface also contains the hilum, or *porta* (door), of the liver, through which blood vessels, lymphatics, and nerves enter, and the hepatic duct exits. In the horse, six ligaments secure the liver in the abdominal cavity.[1] The *coronary ligament* has two laminae, right and left, which attach the diaphragmatic surface of the liver to the caudal vena cava and the abdominal esophagus. The two laminae of the coronary ligament unite ventrally to form the *falciform ligament*. The falciform ligament, a remnant of the fetal ventral mesentery, which extends from the diaphragm to the umbilicus, attaches the quadrate and left lobes to the sternal diaphragm and ventral abdominal floor. The *round ligament,* the remnant of the fetal umbilical vein, is contained within the free border of the falciform ligament. The right and left *triangular ligaments* attach the dorsal right lobe to the right costal diaphragm and the dorsal left lobe to the tendinous center of the diaphragm. The *hepatorenal ligament* connects the caudate process of the quadrate lobe to the right kidney and the base of the cecum.

Histology

At the hilum of the liver, a tree of connective tissue consisting of collagen and fibroblasts enters the hepatic parenchyma. The parenchymal cells, or *hepatocytes,* compose approximately 50% to 60% of the liver's mass and are epithelial cells.[3, 4] The hepatocytes are arranged in rows, or *cords,* at least two cells thick, that anastomose to form blood passageways called *sinusoids* (Fig. 13–1). Hepatic sinusoids are larger than capillaries and are lined with endothelial cells and *Kupffer cells.* Kupffer cells are tissue-fixed macrophages and are estimated to make up 20% of the mass of the liver.[4] The endothelial cells make up approximately 20% of the liver's mass.[4] A cleft, called the *space of Disse,* lies between the hepatocytes and the cells lining the sinusoids. The space of Disse contains fluid similar to the composition of blood, but does not contain erythrocytes.

The afferent hepatic blood vessels, bile ducts, lymphatics, and nerves follow the branching connective tissue tree into the hepatic parenchyma. Two entirely separate sources of

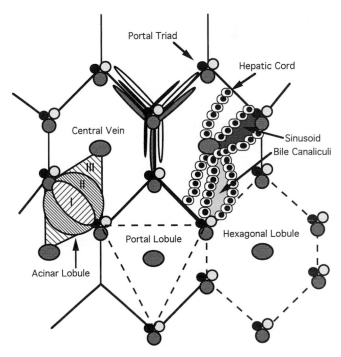

Figure 13–1. Histology of the liver. Roman numerals *I, II,* and *III* represent zones 1, 2, and 3, respectively, of the acinar lobule.

blood supply the liver and empty into the hepatic sinusoids: the *portal vein* and the *hepatic artery.* The portal vein contains poorly oxygenated blood that carries nutrients absorbed from the gastrointestinal tract to the liver for storage, metabolism, transformation, or packaging for export to other tissues. The hepatic artery contains oxygen-rich blood to support the metabolic and energy-generating activities of the liver. The sinusoids drain into *central veins,* which connect with the hepatic vein and caudal vena cava.

The space between contiguous hepatocytes in a cord forms the *bile canaliculus,* through which bile excreted by the hepatocytes drains into bile ductules and ducts. The bile canaliculi are thus formed solely by the cell membranes of the hepatocytes. The bile ductules and ducts are lined with cuboidal and columnar epithelial cells, respectively, that make up approximately 7% of the liver's mass.[4] The bile ducts run in the connective tissue tree, adjacent to branches of the portal vein and hepatic artery, to form a distinct *portal tract, radicle,* or *triad* (see Fig. 13–1). The bile ducts converge at the hilum to form the *hepatic duct,* which drains into the duodenum just distal to the pylorus. Because the horse does not have a gallbladder or a sphincter at the entry site of the hepatic duct into the intestine, the bile is unconcentrated and flows continuously in a direction opposite that of the blood flow in the portal vein and hepatic artery.[1]

The liver can be divided anatomically or functionally into lobules to facilitate histopathologic description of lesions[3] (see Fig. 13–1). The *classic hepatic lobule* in cross section is hexagonal. The corners of the hexagon are defined by three to eight portal tracts with a central vein in the center of the lobule. In contrast, the three corners of the *portal lobule* are defined by central veins, with a portal tract situated in the center. The *acinus lobules* are zones of hepatic parenchyma divided according to the tissue oxygen content. Zone I of the acinus lobule is located immediately adjacent to branching hepatic arteries and portal veins; zone III is located adjacent to central veins; and zone II is situated between zones I and III.

Physiology

The liver is the major organ involved in the regulation of nutrient distribution.[5] The majority of nutrients absorbed from the gastrointestinal tract pass directly to the liver via the portal circulation. The incoming nutrients are metabolized for energy, transformed to other nutrient classes, packaged and exported to peripheral tissues, or stored by the liver. The liver is capable of adjusting to the carbohydrate, protein, and lipid load from the gastrointestinal tract, as well as maintaining consistent blood levels of nutrients between feedings and in response to special needs. In addition to its role in nutrient metabolism and homeostasis, the liver is involved in excretion (bile), detoxification and metabolism of endogenous and exogenous substances, and hematopoiesis.[4]

Protein Metabolism

Amino acids, which are transported to the liver via the portal or hepatic blood, may be used in the biosynthesis of intrinsic hepatocellular proteins, plasma proteins, porphyrins, polyamines, purines, and pyrimidines.[5] The liver synthesizes 90% of the plasma proteins, including albumin, factors involved in coagulation and fibrinolysis (fibrinogen and factors II, V,

VII–XIII, antithrombin III, protein C, plasminogen, plasminogen activator inhibitor, α_2-antiplasmin, α_2-macroglobulin, and α_1-antitrypsin), transport proteins (haptoglobin, transferrin, ceruloplasmin, hormone transport proteins), and acute phase reactant proteins (α- and β-globulins).[4] The liver is the only site of synthesis of albumin and fibrinogen.

The liver is also capable of transamination, or the reversible transfer of an amino group on one amino acid to an α-keto acid, thus forming a new amino acid and a new keto acid. If excess amino acids are presented to the liver, or if carbohydrate is unavailable as an energy source, the amino acids are deaminated by the liver and converted to pyruvate, acetoacetate, and intermediates of the tricarboxylic acid cycle[5] (Fig. 13–2). These intermediates may be oxidized for energy or used as precursors in *gluconeogenesis,* the synthesis of glucose from non-carbohydrate precursors. Both endogenous and exogenous glucocorticoids, glucagon, and thyroid hormone act directly on the liver to increase gluconeogenesis[6–9] (Fig. 13–3) Simultaneously, glucocorticords indirectly influence liver gluconeogenesis by promoting peripheral protein catabolism, thus increasing the availability of amino acids. Insulin inhibits gluconeogenesis in the liver.[7]

In addition to protein synthesis and gluconeogenesis, the liver plays an important role in eliminating the major toxic byproduct of amino acid catabolism, *ammonia.*[10, 11] Ammonia is generated by all tissues and intestinal microflora, and is subsequently released into the circulation. One method by which the liver, as well as certain peripheral tissues, eliminates ammonia is by synthesizing nonessential amino acids from α-keto acids and ammonia in a reversal of deamination. A fundamental reaction in the synthesis of nonessential amino acids is the formation of *glutamate* from α-ketoglutarate and ammonia (Fig. 13–4). Subsequently, glutamate is used in transamination reactions for the formation of other amino acids. Glutamate also participates in the conversion of cytotoxic free ammonia into a nontoxic transport form, *glutamine.* Glutamine may be delivered to the kidney, converted back to free ammonia and excreted, or delivered to the liver for urea synthesis.

The liver has sole responsibility for converting free ammonia or glutamine into *urea,* the principal form of amino group nitrogen excretion by mammals.[4] Urea is formed by the irreversible condensation of two ammonia molecules with carbon dioxide (see Fig. 13–4). The reaction takes place in the hepatocyte mitochondria via the Krebs-Henseleit cycle.[5] The newly formed urea is released from the hepatocyte, secreted into the sinusoidal blood, and transported to the kidney as *blood urea nitrogen (BUN)* for excretion.

Carbohydrate Metabolism

The liver is responsible for the synthesis, storage, and release of glucose.[5] Monosaccharides absorbed from the gastrointestinal tract are delivered via portal blood to the liver. In the hepatocyte, the majority of glucose is phosphorylated to *glucose-6-phosphate* by the enzyme hexokinase (see Fig. 13–2). The remaining glucose is released into the systemic circulation. Other monosaccharides (fructose, galactose) are phosphorylated and converted in the liver to glucose-6-phosphate. The majority of glucose-6-phosphate is converted to glycogen for storage. A small amount of glucose-6-phosphate is oxidized to form adenosine triphosphate (ATP),

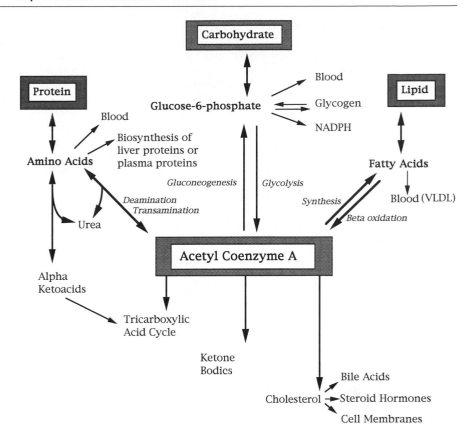

Figure 13–2. Role of the liver in the metabolism of nutrients. *VLDL,* very-low-density lipoprotein; *NADPH,* nicotinamide adenine dinucleotide phosphate.

though the major source of ATP in the liver is amino acid and fatty acid oxidation. Approximately half of the liver glucose enters the phosphogluconate pathway for generation of nicotinamide-adenine dinucleotide phosphate (NADPH), required as a reducing agent in the biosynthesis of fatty acids and cholesterol. Glucocorticoids, catecholamines, glucagon, and thyroid hormone increase gluconeogenesis and glycogenolysis in the liver, while insulin inhibits gluconeogenesis[6-9] (see Fig. 13–3).

Lipid Metabolism

Short-chain fatty acids (fewer than 10 carbon atoms) can be directly absorbed from the gastrointestinal tract, bound to albumin, and delivered to the liver via the portal circulation.[5] However, the majority of short-chain fatty acids are incorporated into phospholipid or triglyceride by the intestinal epithelium and transported to the liver via the portal blood. The remaining fatty acids absorbed from the gastrointestinal tract are transported as triglyceride in *chylomicrons.* After formation in the intestinal epithelial cells and absorption into lymphatics, chylomicrons enter the systemic circulation via the thoracic duct, and subsequently are delivered to the liver. The liver may also take up albumin-bound fatty acids released from adipose tissue.

The fate of fatty acids in the liver depends on the state of energy demand, the rate of fatty acid delivery, and hormonal influences. The primary role of the liver in lipid metabolism is to esterify free fatty acids into triglycerides for export to other tissues[5] (see Fig. 13–3). The triglycerides are packaged with protein, carbohydrate, and cholesterol in the endoplasmic reticulum of the hepatocyte into *very-low-density lipo-*

proteins (VLDLs), which primarily contain triglyceride, and *high-density lipoproteins (HDLs),* which primarily contain protein and phospholipid.[12] The VLDLs and HDLs are released into the hepatic sinusoids. Once in the systemic circulation, the VLDLs are taken up by adipose tissue or their composition is altered by endothelial cell lipases, which remove triglyceride, forming *intermediate-* and *low-density lipoproteins (IDLs, LDLs).*

In addition to exporting plasma lipoprotein, the liver can oxidize free fatty acids for energy to acetyl coenzyme A (acetyl CoA), a fundamental compound in the tricarboxylic acid cycle (see Fig. 13–2). The acetyl CoA thus formed may also be used in the synthesis of other fatty acids, cholesterol, steroids, and ketone bodies, acetoacetate, and β-hydroxybutyrate.[13] Furthermore, through the synthesis of acetyl CoA from glucose and most amino acids, the liver is capable of converting carbohydrate and protein into lipid. Ketone bodies can be exported from the liver and used for energy by peripheral tissues, especially the brain, when glucose is deficient. However, overproduction of ketone bodies can be detrimental, resulting in ketoacidosis.[12]

Lipid metabolism is closely regulated by insulin and glucocorticoids[7, 8] (see Fig. 13–3). Glucocorticoids function primarily to increase fatty acid mobilization from the periphery, while insulin decreases adipose tissue release of fatty acids by activating lipoprotein lipase and inhibiting hormone-sensitive lipase. Insulin acts on the liver to increase fatty acid synthesis from glucose.

Excretion of Bile

Bile consists of several components, including conjugated bilirubin, bile acids, cholesterol, lecithin, water, and electro-

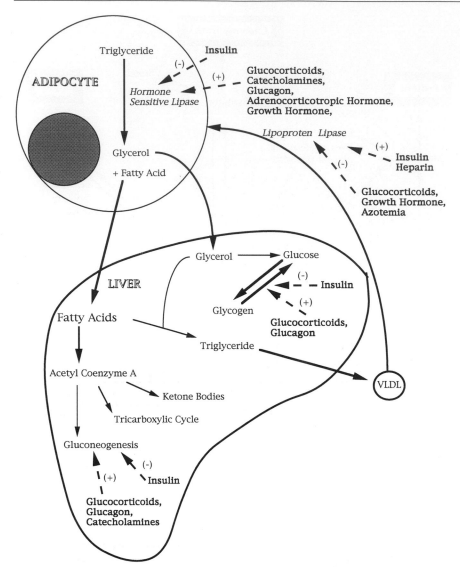

Figure 13–3. Hormonal control of metabolism. (−) represents an inhibitory effect; (+) represents a stimulatory effect.

lytes.[4] Bile is released by hepatocytes into the bile canaliculi where water diffuses passively. Bile is then transported by large bile ducts and the hepatic duct to the intestine. Water and electrolytes exchange takes place between the bile and

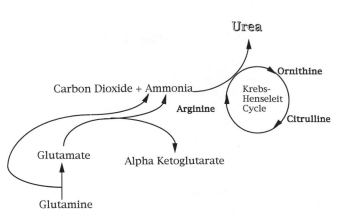

Figure 13–4. The urea cycle.

the bile duct epithelium; however, isotonicity is maintained. Since the horse does not have a gallbladder or a sphincter at the site of entry of the hepatic duct into the duodenum, the bile is unconcentrated and flow is continuous.[1]

Bile acids make up 90% of the organic portion of bile.[14] Bile acids are amphoteric molecules that act as detergents. These detergents facilitate the excretion of cholesterol and phospholipid from the liver into bile and facilitate the absorption of lipids and lipid-soluble compounds (vitamins A, D, E, and K) from the intestinal tract. The principal bile acids in the horse are *cholate* and *chenodeoxycholate*, both of which are conjugated with taurine.[14] More than 95% of the conjugated bile acids excreted in bile and released into the intestinal lumen are reabsorbed by the ileum and returned to the liver via the *enterohepatic circulation.* The bile acids are thus "recycled" between the lumen of the intestinal tract and the liver. It is estimated that the bile acids are recycled at least 38 times a day in healthy ponies.[14]

Bilirubin is the breakdown product of tetrapyroles that function as electron transport pigments.[4] The majority of bilirubin is formed from hemoglobin and myoglobin, but

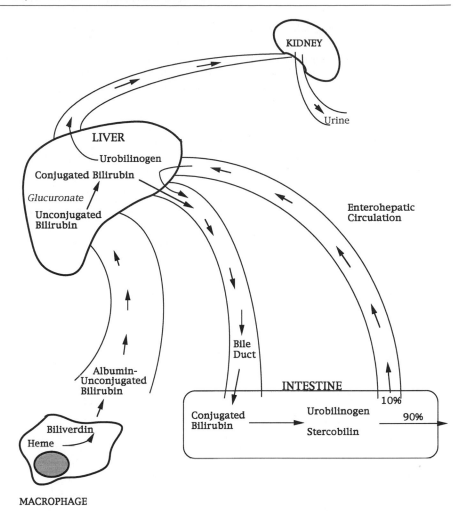

Figure 13–5. Metabolism and excretion of bile.

non-heme pigments, such as the cytochromes, also serve as a source of bilirubin. The pigments are first engulfed by macrophages in the spleen, bone marrow, and liver (Kupffer cells) and are converted to biliverdin (Fig. 13–5). The biliverdin is converted to bilirubin by the macrophage and released from the cell as free, insoluble bilirubin. This form of bilirubin is also referred to as *indirect reacting* or *unconjugated bilirubin.* Unconjugated bilirubin is bound with albumin in the plasma to decrease its hydrophobicity and is delivered to the liver. At the surface of the hepatocyte, the bilirubin is transferred from albumin to *ligandin,* an intrahepatic transport and storage protein.[4, 15] Within the hepatocyte, the bilirubin is conjugated with glucuronide in the endoplasmic reticulum. *Conjugated bilirubin,* also called *direct reacting bilirubin,* is water-soluble, and is excreted into the bile canaliculi. Under normal circumstances, very little conjugated bilirubin escapes into the general circulation.

In the intestinal tract, conjugated bilirubin is reduced by microflora to *urobilinogen* and *stercobilin* (see Fig. 13–5), which impart a yellow-brown color to feces. In herbivores, the presence of chlorophyll pigments in the feces masks the color of urobilinogen.[15] Only in the neonatal herbivore, receiving a milk diet, are the feces yellow. Urobilinogen is absorbed by the intestinal mucosa and transported back to the liver via the enterohepatic circulation. A small amount

of conjugated bilirubin in the intestinal lumen is hydrolyzed to unconjugated bilirubin and is subsequently reabsorbed. The liver extracts the majority of the urobilinogen; however, a small amount spills over into the urine. Urobilinogen is concentrated in the normally alkaline urine of horses and thus is detectable.[16]

Detoxification

The liver is responsible for the *biotransformation* of numerous endogenous and exogenous compounds. Biotransformation involves a series of enzymatic reactions that alter the physical properties or activity of compounds. Biotransformation occurs in two phases.[17] In phase 1, polar groups were added to the compound, or existing polar groups are exposed by oxidation, hydroxylation, deamination, or reduction. In phase 2, the product of phase 1 is conjugated, usually with glucuronate or sulfate. Substrates for detoxification usually are water-insoluble and biotransformation renders them more susceptible to renal or biliary excretion.[4, 18] Examples of endogenous substances biotransformed by the liver include ammonia, bilirubin, and steroid hormones (estrogen, cortisol, aldosterone). There are countless exogenous substances biotransformed by the liver, examples being drugs, plant toxins, insecticides, and mercaptans.

Phase 1 of biotransformation occurs primarily on the enzyme-bound systems of the endoplasmic reticulum, called *microsomes.*[4, 18] The majority of these enzymes are iron-containing enzymes of the P-450 system, thus named because they absorb light at 450 nm. The P-450 enzymes are also called *mixed function oxidases.* Some substrates, referred to as *inducers,* are capable of saturating the enzymes involved in biotransformation. Enzyme saturation and induction causes hypertrophy of the endoplasmic reticulum and all contain enzymes, thus accelerating substance removal rates. Inducers not only accelerate their own removal rate but may also accelerate the biotransformation of other endogenous and exogenous substances. Examples of enzyme inducers are the barbiturates, phenylbutazone, and chlorinated hydrocarbons.[18] Other agents presented for biotransformation may inhibit microsomal enzymes, for example, chloramphenicol, cimetidine, organophosphates, morphine, and quinidine, thus prolonging the effect of other substrates.[18] Hepatic biotransformation sometimes results in the formation of a toxic metabolite from a nontoxic parent compound, examples being aspirin and halothane.[18]

Mononuclear Phagocyte System

Hepatic macrophages, or Kupffer cells, make up a major portion of the mononuclear phagocyte system. Cells of the mononuclear phagocyte system are derived from bone marrow myeloid progenitors and serve two main functions: (1) phagocytosis, and (2) to act as antigen-processing cells for lymphocytes. Kupffer cells are responsive to opsonins and synthesize a vast array of inflammatory mediators, including interleukins, tumor necrosis factor, and eicosanoids. Unlike other macrophages in the mononuclear phagocyte system, Kupffer cells function mainly in phagocytosis and are strategically located along the hepatic sinusoids, where portal blood can be "cleansed," for example, of bacterial endotoxin, prior to exposure to the hepatocytes, and subsequently, the systemic circulation.[19] Kupffer cells also help "cleanse" systemic blood entering via the hepatic artery by removing fibrin degradation products, tissue plasminogen activators, and hemoglobin, as well as microbes, foreign antigens, and other particulate debris.[2, 19]

Miscellaneous Functions

The liver serves as a storage site for several vitamins and trace minerals, including vitamins A, D, and B_{12}, copper, and iron. Vitamin D is first converted in the liver to 25-hydroxycholecalciferol and exported to the kidney, where it is transformed into 1,25-dihydroxycholecalciferol, the active form of the vitamin.[6] In the fetus, the liver is involved in *hematopoiesis.*[4] In the adult, the bone marrow serves as the primary site for hematopoiesis; however, the liver may serve as an extramedullary site of hematopoeisis under intense conditions of erythrocyte regeneration or if a large portion of the bone marrow is destroyed.

HEPATIC INSUFFICIENCY

Definition

Hepatic insufficiency or failure refers to the inability of the liver to properly perform its normal functions. Because the liver is involved in such a diverse array of physiologic activities, any pathologic process may hinder one or several functions without impeding others. Furthermore, most hepatic functions are not impaired until greater than 80% of the hepatic mass is lost.[4, 15, 20] The liver also has the capability to regenerate under certain conditions. If hepatocyte loss is gradual and regeneration parallels destruction, hepatic failure may not necessarily ensue. Thus, hepatic disease may be present without accompanying hepatic failure. Consequently, hepatic disease does not always manifest clinically.

Patterns and Pathology of Hepatic Injury

The severity of the accompanying clinical signs and the course of hepatic disease are variable depending on the pattern, location, rate, and extent of hepatic damage. Hepatic injury may be reversible (fatty degeneration, cloudy swelling), irreversible (necrosis), focal or zonal, generalized, acute, chronic, inflammatory, anatomical, or functional.

Focal Hepatic Injury

Focal hepatic injury occurs when one small area of the liver is uniformly damaged. Examples of focal hepatic injury include hepatic abscesses, solitary infarctions, and neoplastic growths. Because there is adequate hepatic reserve in the unaffected regions, focal hepatic injury rarely is accompanied by clinical signs of hepatic failure, though evidence of hepatic disease may be demonstrable.[17] Hepatic injury may be zonal, that is, certain zones of the liver are uniformly affected throughout the entire organ.[17] The liver often appears pale with an enhanced lobular pattern on the cut surface. The two most common types of zonal hepatic injury are centrolobular and periacinar. In *centrolobular zonal injury,* the area adjacent to the central veins is uniformly affected, whereas in *periacinar zonal injury,* the cells in zones II and III of the acinar lobules are affected (see Fig. 13–1). Hepatocytes in these locations are most susceptible to anoxic damage, since the normal oxygen tension is lowest in these areas. Examples of disease states resulting in centrolobular injury are severe acute anemia, passive congestion due to congestive heart failure, and toxic hepatopathies. Zone I acinar lobular injury may occur with infarction of hepatic vessels, as may occur during verminous arteritis. Similar to focal hepatic injury, hepatic failure infrequently occurs with zonal hepatic injury. However, if widespread zonal injury is present, hepatic disease may be demonstrable and hepatic failure may ensue.

Acute Generalized Hepatic Injury

Acute generalized hepatic injury is often accompanied by clinical signs of hepatic failure, with the extent of damage dictating the severity of the clinical signs.[17] Typically, the liver appears pale and enlarged, and is often friable. Acute generalized hepatic injury may be the result of infection, necrosis, inflammation, or hepatotoxic agents.[4] Bacterial or viral infections, parasitic infestations, or immune disorders may cause acute generalized necrosis or inflammation. Despite its cause, any process that results in an inflammatory response in the hepatic parenchyma is referred to as *hepatitis.* Acute inflammation most commonly accompanies necrosis and is characterized by the presence of neutrophils and lymphocytes in the areas of cell death or surrounding portal triads. Inflammatory processes primarily involving the biliary system are called *cholangitis,* usually the result of ascending infection from the intestinal tract or secondary to cholestasis.

Chronic Generalized Hepatic Injury

Chronic hepatic injury is accompanied by clinical signs of hepatic failure when greater than 80% of the hepatic mass is destroyed or replaced by fibrosis.[4, 20] Fibrosis, the presence of collagen and fibroblasts, occurs when the rate of ongoing necrosis exceeds the rate of regeneration. Typically, the liver appears smaller than normal. Fibrosis commonly follows conditions resulting in chronic hypoxia, chronic inflammation, chronic cholangitis or cholestasis, metastatic neoplasia, trauma, or ingestion of antimitotic agents such as plants containing pyrrolizidine alkaloids. *Cirrhosis,* or an *end-stage liver,* refers to chronic hepatic disease characterized by the presence of widespread fibrosis, nodular regeneration, and biliary hyperplasia.[17] Nodular regeneration, or "islands" of hepatocytes, occurs when the normal architecture and blood supply of the liver are disrupted or destroyed by the presence of fibrosis. The cause of biliary hyperplasia during chronic liver failure is unknown. One form of chronic hepatic disease, called *chronic active hepatitis,* is characterized by the presence of cirrhosis plus an acute inflammatory response.[17]

Anatomical or Functional Injury

Anatomical or functional shunts cause liver injury by anoxic damage. Additionally, if blood habitually bypasses the liver, the liver cannot perform its normal metabolic regulatory or detoxifying functions, thus clinical signs of hepatic failure become imminent. Anatomical shunts can be either congenital or acquired, intrahepatic or extrahepatic.

Clinical Signs of Hepatic Insufficiency

The clinical signs of hepatic insufficiency are highly variable and nonspecific, depending on the extent and duration of hepatic disease. Usually, greater than 80% of the liver mass must be lost before clinical signs become apparent, regardless of the cause of hepatic disease. Thus, despite the duration of hepatic disease, the onset of clinical signs is often abrupt. The most common clinical signs of hepatic insufficiency in horses are hepatic encephalopathy, icterus, and weight loss.[21, 22] Less commonly reported clinical signs include hepatogenic photosensitization, diarrhea, abdominal pain, and hemorrhagic diathesis. Rarely reported clinical signs of hepatic insufficiency in horses are ascites, steatorrhea, pruritus, endotoxic shock, polydipsia, and hemolysis. The appearance of specific clinical signs of hepatic disease often reflects the type of hepatic function(s) that is altered.

Hepatic Encephalopathy

Hepatic encephalopathy (HE) is a complex clinical syndrome characterized by abnormal mental status that accompanies severe hepatic insufficiency.[23–25] Clinical signs are widely variable, but represent manifestations of augmented neuronal inhibition. This syndrome occurs in patients with advanced, decompensated liver disease of all types and may be a feature of acute, subacute, or chronic hepatocellular failure. HE is generally considered to be a potentially reversible metabolic encephalopathy.[24] It is uncertain whether multiple episodes of hepatic encephalopathy could lead to irreversible neuronal damage.

Clinical Signs and Laboratory Findings

There are no specific features of HE that allow this syndrome to be distinguished from other causes of cerebral dysfunction. The earliest phase of HE is probably missed in most equine patients since it represents minimal behavioral changes with subtle impairment of intellect due to bilateral forebrain dysfunction[26] (stage I; Table 13–1). In humans, these early signs are more apparent to close friends and family members than to a physician. As encephalopathy progresses, motor function, intellectual abilities, and consciousness become impaired. This is generally the stage (corresponding to stage II) at which horses become obviously affected. Clinical signs include depression, head-pressing, circling, mild ataxia, aimless walking, persistent yawning, and other manifestations of inappropriate behavior. Next, somnolence develops: the horse is rousable but responds minimally or excessively to the usual stimuli. At this stage (III) the horse often manifests aggressive or violent behavior interspersed with periods of stupor. Finally, consciousness fades, the horse becomes recumbent, and coma ensues. Occasionally seizures occur during the later stages of HE, but in general they are atypical. The severity of encephalopathy corresponds to the degree of hepatic dysfunction; however, neither of these parameters correlates with type or reversibility of the underlying hepatic disease.

Etiology and Pathophysiology

By definition, the cause of HE is insufficient hepatocellular function, irrespective of the cause of the liver disease. It is clear that a normally functioning liver is necessary to maintain normal brain function. The pathogenesis of HE remains

---

Table 13–1. Clinical Stages of Hepatic Encephalopathy*

Stage	Mental Status
I	Mild confusion, decreased attention, slowed ability to perform mental tasks, irritability
II	Drowsiness, lethargy, obvious personality changes, inappropriate behavior, disorientation
III	Somnolent but rousable, marked confusion, amnesia, occasional aggressive uncontrolled behavior
IV	Coma

*Adapted from Gammel SH, Jones EA: Hepatic encephalopathy. *Med Clin North Am* 73:793–813, 1989.

unclear and considering the numerous proposed hypotheses it is almost certain that the cause is multifactorial. The following mechanisms have been suggested for the development of HE and any or all may be involved to greater or lesser degree: (1) gastrointestinal-derived neurotoxins; (2) "false" neurotransmitters subsequent to plasma amino acid imbalance; (3) augmented activity of γ-aminobutyric acid (GABA) in the brain; (4) increased permeability of the blood-brain barrier; and (5) impaired central nervous system (CNS) energy metabolism.

Perhaps the oldest and most "predominant" hypothesis involves the accumulation of toxic materials in the blood, derived from the metabolism of nitrogenous substrates in the gastrointestinal tract, that bypass the liver through functional or anatomical shunts.[23, 27, 28] Accordingly, HE may be due primarily to failure of the liver to adequately remove certain substances in blood that have the direct or indirect ability to modulate function of the CNS. Ammonia, subsequent to the degradation of amino acids, amines, and purines by enteric bacteria, has been widely supported as a major neurotoxin of hepatic disease.[28–30] In patients with liver failure, ammonia is insufficiently metabolized, thus plasma concentrations increase, and ammonia enters the CNS, where it may cause encephalopathy.[28, 31] Ammonia has a toxic effect on cell membrane neurons by inhibition of the Na^+,K^+-dependent ATPase (adenosinetriphosphatase) due to competition with potassium.[30] Hyperammonemia is also associated with a disturbance in CNS energy production caused by alterations in the tricarboxylic acid cycle that result in a decrease in α-ketoglutarate formation and increased glutamine.[32] Whether this disturbance in energy metabolism is the cause or consequence of ammonia-associated encephalopathy remains unresolved.[24, 33] Ammonia can induce encephalopathy experimentally[34] and children with hyperammonemia due to congenital enzyme deficiencies have encephalopathy.[29] Therapy aimed at reducing the absorption of ammonia from the intestine tends to ameliorate hepatic encephalopathy,[26] although these modalities also decrease production and absorption of other putative toxins.[25] Points against ammonia in the pathogenesis of HE are that plasma ammonia concentrations correlate poorly with the severity of HE and ammonia does not induce the electroencephalogram (EEG) changes typical of the encephalopathy of liver disease.[24, 35] Likewise, alterations in brain neurotransmitters during experimental hyperammonemic encephalopathy are different from those occurring in HE (discussed below).[36] Seizures are common in experimental or congenital hyperammonemic syndromes,[29, 34] but are very unusual with HE.[25] Thus, it is clear that the actions of ammonia on the CNS are complex and ammonia is likely involved but not solely responsible for HE.

The synergistic neurotoxins hypothesis for the pathogenesis of HE implicates not only ammonia but other gut-derived neurotoxins, specifically mercaptans, short-chain fatty acids, and phenols.[26, 27] Members of each of these classes of substances are increased in the blood of patients with hepatic failure in concentrations that alone are insufficient to induce encephalopathy. However, the combination of some or all of them is considered to induce encephalopathy by their synergistic actions and by augmenting endogenous metabolic abnormalities.[26, 27] The actions of these and most neurotoxins include inhibition of brain Na^+,K^+-ATPase with subse-

quently impaired neurotransmission.[24] Points in favor of the synergistic toxins hypothesis are that plasma concentrations of these substances increase during hepatic disease and they can alone, or in various combinations, induce experimental encephalopathy.[26, 27] However, blood and brain concentrations of mercaptans, like ammonia, correlate poorly with the stage of HE.[37] Again, these compounds commonly induce seizures.

A separate hypothesis holds that during liver failure the content of true neurotransmitters in the CNS, such as norepinephrine and dopamine, become depleted and that false neurotransmitters, especially octopamine and phenylethanolamine, increase.[25, 38] The net neurophysiologic effect of such changes is reduced neuronal excitation and increased neural inhibition. The mechanism of this effect is related to the increased serum concentrations of aromatic amino acids (AAAs: phenylalanine, tyrosine, tryptophan) and decreased concentrations of branched-chain amino acids (BCAAs: valine, leucine, isoleucine) that occur in liver failure.[39, 40] Serum glucagon is increased in hepatic failure, leading to muscle catabolism and release of amino acids. However, hepatic metabolism of AAAs is reduced, and since BCAAs are metabolized by muscle and adipose tissue, there is a relative increase in AAAs and a decrease in BCAAs. The decreased plasma BCAA/AAA ratio during liver failure and increased brain glutamine concentration (presumably a consequence of ammonia retention) are considered to promote an influx of AAA into the brain and efflux of glutamine from the brain by exchange transport processes at the blood-brain barrier.[24] Phenylalanine can compete with tyrosine for tyrosine hydroxylase, resulting in decreased production of dopamine[40] (Fig. 13–6). The displaced tyrosine may be decarboxylated to tyramine, then converted to the false neurotransmitter, octopamine. Accumulated tyrosine also competes for dopamine β-oxidase and reduces the formation of norepinephrine. Phenylalanine and tryptophan in the CNS are ultimately converted to phenylethanolamine and serotonin, a false neurotransmitter and a neuroinhibitor, respectively.

Consistent with this theory are the observations of increased serum concentrations of AAAs accompanied by increased cerebrospinal fluid (CSF) concentrations of octopamine, serotonin, and phenylethanolamine in patients with HE.[38] Additionally, there seems to be a relationship between plasma or urine octopamine and the stage of encephalopathy.[38] However, the intraventricular administration of large doses of octopamine to rats failed to reduce consciousness in spite of markedly reduced norepinephrine levels.[41] Thus octopamine alone cannot induce encephalopathy. The plasma BCAA/AAA ratio correlates poorly with HE in humans[42] and controlled clinical trials of oral or intravenous BCAA therapy do not indicate consistent amelioration of signs of HE.[40] Implicit in this hypothesis is the notion that dopaminergic neurotransmission is impaired; however, dopaminergic drugs have not been found useful in treatment,[43] nor have functional changes in dopamine receptors been found in patients with HE.[44]

A recently popular theory regarding the pathogenesis of HE involves augmented activity of GABA, the principal inhibitory neurotransmitter of the vertebrate brain.[24, 25, 36] When released from presynaptic neurons, GABA binds to specific receptors on postsynaptic neurons, resulting in increased chloride ion conductance across the postsynaptic

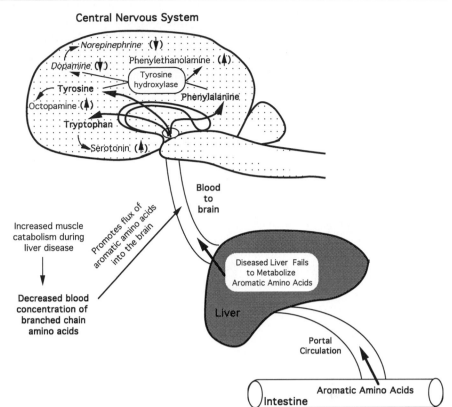

Figure 13–6. Role of aromatic amino acids in the brain in hepatic encephalopathy. Aromatic amino acids (tryptophan, tyrosine, phenylalanine) enter the central nervous system, where they are metabolized, altering the balance of neurotransmitters. True neurotransmitters (dopamine, norepinephrine) decrease *(arrow down)*, while "false" neurotransmitters (octopamine, phenylethanolamine) increase *(arrow up)*. The net effect is increased neuronal inhibition and reduced neuronal excitation.

neural membrane, membrane hyperpolarization, and generation of an inhibitory postsynaptic potential.[36] The GABA receptor is a chloride ionophore supramolecular complex that has interactive binding sites for three classes of synergistic ligands: GABA and agonists, benzodiazepines, and barbiturates.[24, 45] The binding of benzodiazepine or a barbiturate on its binding site of the GABA receptor potentiates GABA-induced sedation. The GABA hypothesis of HE was originally based on a series of observations using a model of HE in rabbits in which increased GABA-like activity was identified in the serum and CSF and there was an increased density of GABA receptors.[36] Since then, at least three possible mechanisms for augmented GABAergic neurotransmission in liver failure have been proposed: (1) increased availability of GABA receptor agonists; (2) increased density or affinity of GABA receptors; and (3) allosteric potentiation of the action of GABA due to the presence of agonist ligands for benzodiazepines or barbiturate binding sites.[24]

Increased plasma GABA has been documented in humans with liver failure[46] and the major source is considered to be the gut.[25] Nonspecific enhanced permeability of the blood-brain barrier during hepatic insufficiency allows plasma GABA to enter the CNS and increase GABAergic neurotransmission.[47] Increased density of the GABA and benzodiazepine receptors in the CNS has been reported in rabbits with hepatic failure[48]; however, this could not be substantiated using a rat experimental model.[49]

The GABA receptor is an oligomeric glycoprotein complex which has been pharmacologically subdivided into a GABA receptor unit, a benzodiazepine receptor unit, and a chloride ionophore that contains receptors for barbiturates.[24] Activation of the GABA receptor opens the chloride iono-

phore and increases membrane permeability to chloride.[50] Entrance of chloride causes neuronal membrane hyperpolarization. Agonists of benzodiazepine increase the frequency of GABA-induced chloride channel openings and barbiturates lengthen the average time that channels are open.[51] Results of studies using electrophysiologic and in vitro techniques to study an animal model of HE provide strong evidence for a functional increase in GABAergic tone that is mediated allosterically through the benzodiazepine receptor by an endogenous diazepam-like substance.[52, 53] Support for this suggestion was provided by clinical studies that showed improved consciousness and reduced EEG changes of HE in patients treated with the benzodiazepine receptor antagonist flumazenil.[44]

Diagnosis

The diagnosis of HE is based upon the presence of neurologic signs of cerebral dysfunction in a horse with physical examination and laboratory findings compatible with liver disease (see Diagnosis and Laboratory Findings of Hepatic Insufficiency). Other possible causes for the neurologic signs should be excluded because there are no specific features of HE that enable this syndrome to be definitively distinguished from other encephalopathies. A partial list of conditions to be ruled out includes eastern, western, and Venezuelan encephalomyelitis; rabies; moldy corn toxicity (leukoencephalomalacia); brain abscess; equine protozoal myeloencephalitis; parasite larval migrans; blister beetle toxicosis; organophosphate toxicity; nigropallidal encephalomalacia; botulism; fluphenazine or other sedative overdose; and heavy metal toxicosis. Many of these conditions have other characteristic clinical signs, the absence of which would exclude them from the differential diagnosis. Access to potential toxins or drugs should be carefully gleaned from the history.

Serum electrolytes, including calcium; creatinine values; and a complete blood count should be performed to aid in ruling out other encephalopathies. Serology for the viral encephalitides and toxicologic screening for organophosphates and heavy metals may be appropriate. A lumbar spinal tap for CSF analysis may be indicated if other causes of encephalopathy are highly suspect. The CSF is normal in horses with HE. In humans, EEG changes of symmetric generalized slowing of cerebral electrical activity are sensitive indicators of HE, but are not specific for this disorder since other metabolic encephalopathies can cause similar abnormalities.[23, 25] Visual evoked potentials (VEPs) are superior to conventional EEGs in terms of specificity and ease of quantitation.[48] An average VEP reflects the pattern and magnitude of postsynaptic neuronal activity evoked by a visual afferent stimulus. Hepatoencephalopathy in humans is attended by a distinctively abnormal VEP trace; however, this testing would be technically difficult in horses and has not been explored. As a general rule, the brain shows no definite light or electron microscopic structural changes. Some human patients with hepatic cirrhosis and portosystemic shunts have an increase in the number and size of astrocytes (Alzheimer type II) in the gray matter of the cerebrum and cerebellum.[24, 26] These changes appear to be reversible and specific for portosystemic shunting of blood. The relevance of these changes, if any, to behavioral dysfunction of hepatic encephalopathy is unknown.

Icterus

Icterus, or *jaundice,* is caused by *hyperbilirubinemia* with subsequent deposition of the pigment in tissues, causing yellow discoloration. Icterus is most apparent in nonpigmented skin; mucous membranes, especially the vulvar mucosa; and the sclerae. Approximately 10% to 15% of horses normally have slightly yellow sclerae.[21] Disease states that result in hyperbilirubinemia can be categorized as follows: increased production of bilirubin, impaired hepatic uptake or conjugation of bilirubin, and impaired excretion of bilirubin.[20] Increased production of bilirubin occurs with hemolysis, both intravascular and extravascular, and following reabsorption of erythrocytes after massive intracorporeal hemorrhage. This form of hyperbilirubinemia, often called *hemolytic* or *prehepatic icterus,* occurs despite a normally functioning liver, as the rate of bilirubin production by the reticuloendothelial system temporarily exceeds the liver's ability to conjugate and excrete. Classically, this form of icterus is caused by the increased concentration of unconjugated bilirubin in the blood. However, on occasion, the concentration of conjugated bilirubin also is mildly increased in the blood as a result of hepatic "spillover" when the excessive bilirubin is processed by the liver or reabsorbed via the enterohepatic circulation. The presence and intensity of hemolytic icterus are determined by the rate and extent of erythrocyte destruction and the rate of uptake of bilirubin by the liver.

Impaired uptake and conjugation of bilirubin also result in increased blood levels of unconjugated bilirubin with subsequent icterus. This form of icterus is referred to as *retention* or *hepatic icterus* and is the most common form in horses with liver disease, usually the result of acute hepatocellular disease.[15, 20, 21] In horses, the presence of icterus is highly inconsistent with chronic hepatocellular disease.[14] In addition to hepatocellular disease, certain drugs, anorexia, or prematurity can impede bilirubin uptake and conjugation by hepatocytes, despite an otherwise normally functioning liver.[4, 14, 15, 20] Steroids can inhibit bilirubin uptake in all species. Heparin administration to horses sometimes results in icterus and is believed to be due in part to impaired uptake of bilirubin by hepatocytes.[14] Anorexia in horses causes variable degrees of hyperbilirubinemia and may be related to the half-life of ligandin.[14, 21] Ligandin is the intrahepatic protein responsible for extracting unconjugated bilirubin from albumin in the sinusoidal blood. The half-life of ligandin is relatively short (days) and starvation in other species reduces the hepatocytes' store of ligandin, thus impeding bilirubin uptake.[4] Premature and neonatal foals are also more susceptible to retention icterus, in the absence of hepatic disease. The cause of icterus in equine neonates is presumably a result of lower hepatocellular ligandin concentrations, compared with the adult.[54] In humans, inherited or congenital deficiencies in heptocellular binding proteins or the enzymes responsible for conjugation (glucuronyltransferase) may result in icterus (Gilbert's syndrome or Crigler-Najjar syndrome type II) without clinical signs.[21] Similar physiologic defects in bilirubin uptake and conjugation have been reported in the horse.[55]

If the excretion of conjugated bilirubin into the biliary tract is impeded, *regurgitation icterus* occurs.[20] Blockage of bile flow with resultant regurgitation icterus can accompany cholangitis, hepatitis, obstructive cholelithiasis, neoplastic infiltration, fibrosis, or hyperplasia of the biliary tract. Because conjugated bilirubin is water-soluble, this form of icterus may be accompanied by bilirubinuria.

In hepatocellular disease, icterus most often is the result of a combined increase in both unconjugated and conjugated bilirubin.[20] Of the two fractions, the majority of the increase in the total bilirubin is due to increased unconjugated bilirubin. Increases in the conjugated fraction greater than 25% of the total are usually indicative of hepatocellular disease, and increases greater than 30% are usually indicative of cholestasis.[15]

Weight Loss

Weight loss and failure to thrive are most consistently present during chronic hepatic insufficiency. However, chronic liver disease may be present without apparent weight loss. Weight loss is due to anorexia and the loss of normal hepatocellular metabolic activities.

Hepatogenic Photosensitization

Photosensitization refers to abnormally heightened reactivity of the skin to ultraviolet sunlight owing to the increased blood concentration of a photodynamic agent. In the case of hepatogenic photosensitization, the photodynamic agent is *phylloerythrin.* Phylloerythrin is normally formed in the gastrointestinal tract as a result of bacterial degradation of chlorophyll, absorbed into the general circulation, conjugated, and excreted by the liver.[56] During hepatic insufficiency, the blood concentrations of this photodynamic agent are increased. Subsequent exposure of phylloerythrin to ultraviolet light causes activation of electrons within the molecule to an excited state, with resultant free radical formation. The local production of free radicals causes cell membrane damage and necrosis. Ultraviolet light is absorbed most efficiently by unpigmented areas, thus the lesions of photosensitization are restricted to white skin. The skin first appears erythematous and edematous. Pruritus, pain, vesiculation, ulceration, necrosis, and sloughing may ensue.

Colic, Diarrhea, Ascites, Steatorrhea

Abdominal pain associated with acute hepatocellular disease is a result of acute hepatic swelling, or biliary obstruction (cholelithiasis).[4, 57] Signs of anterior abdominal pain include anorexia, bruxism, dog-sitting, recumbency, and rolling up onto the dorsum. A pain response may also be elicited by palpation over the last few ribs (especially on the right) or immediately caudal to the rib.

Diarrhea may infrequently accompany chronic hepatic insufficiency in horses.[22] Alterations in the intestinal microflora, portal hypertension, and deficiency of bile acids may be involved in the pathogenesis.[4] Though uncommon in horses, portal hypertension can lead to increased hydrostatic and oncotic pressure in the intestinal mucosa, with resultant water and protein loss into the lumen of the bowel and the peritoneal cavity (ascites).

Decreased excretion of bile may result in lipid malabsorption and excessive amounts of fat in the feces, or steatorrhea.[4] Steatorrhea subsequently may cause osmotic diarrhea. Because the normal equine diet is very low in fat, steatorrhea is rare in horses. Chronic cholestasis may cause clay-colored feces due to lack of fecal urobilinogen and stercobilin. This is rarely observed in adult herbivores, since the normal fecal color is generated primarily by plant chlorophylls and not by bilirubin metabolites.[15]

Hemorrhagic Diathesis

Because the liver is responsible for the synthesis of numerous factors involved in coagulation and fibrinolysis, abnormal hemostasis may be a sequela to hepatic insufficiency. Clinical signs may vary from petechial or ecchymotic hemorrhages, to hemorrhage after trauma or venipuncture, to spontaneous hemorrhage (epistaxis, melena, hemoptysis, hematuria, or hematomas).[4, 15, 20, 58, 59] Especially sensitive to hepatic failure is the synthesis of fibrinogen and the vitamin K–dependent factors (II, VII, IX, X, and protein C), which have relatively short half-lives. Factor VII has a half-life of only 4 to 5 hours. Other vitamin K–dependent factors and fibrinogen have half-lives in the range of 4 to 5 days. Since vitamin K is fat-soluble and requires bile acids for proper absorption from the intestinal tract, vitamin K–dependent factors are particularly affected during hepatic insufficiency when bile excretion is decreased.

During hepatic insufficiency, the synthesis of protein C and antithrombin III may be altered. Decreased plasma con-

centrations of these two anticoagulants would result in uncontrolled clot formation and consumption of other coagulation factors. In chronic hepatic disease, the plasma concentration of protein C is normal or decreased; however, antithrombin III may be normal, increased, or decreased.[58] Pregnant women with fatty livers have decreased antithrombin III activity, but patients with biliary cirrhosis or biliary obstruction have increased antithrombin III activity.[58] Horses with liver disease have increased antithrombin III activity, and should theoretically tend to bleed.[60] Alterations in the factors controlling fibrinolysis are variable in chronic liver disease.[58] Conditions that promote fibrinolysis, such as increased plasminogen and plasminogen activator, or decreased plasminogen activator inhibitor, α_2-antiplasmin, and α_2-macroglobulin, result in bleeding tendencies. Conditions that aid thrombus formation, such as decreased plasminogen, further promote consumptive coagulopathy. The fibrinolytic factors have not been evaluated in horses with liver disease.

Finally, the liver plays an important role in balancing normal hemostasis by Kupffer cell removal of activated coagulation factors and fibrin degradation products from the general circulation.[58] Failure to remove activated coagulation factors further promotes coagulation and fibrin degradation products interfere with platelet function and fibrin clot formation.

Fever

Horses with hepatic abscesses, acute hepatitis, chronic active hepatitis, obstructive cholelithiasis, fatty liver failure, or neoplasia may have constant or intermittent fevers.[57, 61–66]

Hemolysis

Hemolysis is rarely seen with fulminant hepatic failure in horses.[22] The exact cause of hemolysis is not known, but is believed to be the result of increased erythrocyte fragility.

Pruritus

Retention of bile acids and accumulation in the skin may cause pruritus. This finding is rarely reported in horses.[22]

Edema

Hypoalbuminemia and water retention can occur with chronic liver failure and may result in dependent edema. Because the half-life of albumin is relatively long (19–20 days) in the horse, edema is a rare clinical sign.[67] Ponies with hyperlipemia may develop dependent abdominal edema secondary to vascular thrombosis.[65]

Endotoxemia

The Kupffer cell plays an important role in removing bacterial endotoxin that is normally absorbed from the lumen of the intestinal tract and carried to the liver via the portal circulation.[19] Failure of Kupffer cell phagocytosis of endotoxin may result in clinical and laboratory evidence of endotoxemia.

Polydipsia, Polyuria, and the Hepatorenal Syndrome

Alterations in renal function, including deranged sodium concentrations, impaired water excretion, and urine concentrating ability, may accompany severe liver disease.[4, 68] Sodium retention results from increased blood aldosterone concentrations due to failure of hepatic biotransformation, and a decrease in the effective circulating blood volume as a result of portal hypertension and hypoalbuminemia. Sodium retention raises the osmolality of the extracellular fluid, thereby stimulating the thirst center. Polydipsia has been reported in horses with chronic liver disease.[69, 70] Despite the potential increase in exchangeable sodium, the serum sodium concentration is usually normal or decreased, as a result of superimposed water retention. The mechanism for water retention is multifactorial, but increased antidiuretic hormone, reduced effective circulating volume, and altered renal prostaglandin synthesis are most likely involved.[68] The urine concentrating ability is sometimes impaired as a result of reduced medullary interstitial urea, the net effect being polyuria[67] or isothenuria, or both.

Hepatorenal syndrome is characterized by acute azotemia and anuria and may occur in ponies with hyperlipemia and hepatic lipidosis[69] (see Hyperlipemia and Hepatic Lipidosis). The pathogenesis is obscure, but speculative causes include reduced effective circulating volume, decreased hepatic inactivation of renin, and endotoxemia.[68]

Diagnosis and Laboratory Findings of Hepatic Insufficiency

Historical information, as discussed under Specific Hepatic Diseases, may be useful in the diagnosis of certain types of hepatic insufficiency. The definitive diagnosis of hepatic disease in horses is confounded by nonspecific clinical signs and variable laboratory findings. Paramount to the laboratory diagnosis of hepatic insufficiency in horses is knowledge of the sensitivity and specificity of the tests. Because massive hepatic disease must be present before alterations are seen with some laboratory tests, and because different liver functions are variably altered by disease, the specificity of the laboratory diagnosis of hepatic disease increases with the magnitude of abnormal findings. Laboratory findings also may be useful for therapeutic and prognostic considerations.

Evaluation of Bilirubin

The *total bilirubin* concentration in the blood, as determined by the van den Bergh test, is a combination of both unconjugated and conjugated bilirubin. Because the diagnostic value of the bilirubin concentration, when used for evaluation of hepatic disease, depends on which subfraction is increased, the concentrations of both unconjugated and conjugated bilirubin must be determined.

The serum bilirubin concentration is stable for several days, if protected against sunlight.[15] The total bilirubin concentration is first determined in a chromogenic assay by reaction for 30 minutes with a diazo reagent (sulfanilic acid and sodium nitrite) and methyl alcohol.[15] Conjugated or direct reacting bilirubin is similarly determined over 5 min-

utes, without the addition of methyl alcohol. The amount of unconjugated bilirubin is then determined by the difference between the total bilirubin concentration and the direct reacting bilirubin. Because the unconjugated fraction is determined arithmetically, it is appropriately called indirect reacting bilirubin. In normal horses, the total bilirubin concentration is in the range of 0.2 to 5.0 mg/dL (3.4–85.5 μmol/L) with conjugated bilirubin in the range of 0 to 0.4 mg/dL (0–6.8 μmol/L).[20] As discussed above, increases in the unconjugated bilirubin fraction may occur without hepatic disease. Hemolysis, anorexia, intestinal obstruction, cardiac insufficiency, and the administration of certain drugs (steroids, heparin, halothane) may cause an increase in the unconjugated bilirubin concentration.[14] If the unconjugated bilirubin concentration is increased, the erythron should be concurrently evaluated to rule out hemolysis as the causative factor. Hemolysis may cause the unconjugated bilirubin concentration to rise as high as 80 mg/dL (1,368 μmol/L).[15] Complete anorexia can cause an increase in the unconjugated bilirubin concentration within 12 hours; however, it is unlikely to rise greater than 6 to 8 mg/dL (102.6–136.8 μmol/L) in horses suffering purely from anorexia.[15, 155] Finally, the age of the horse and concurrent drug therapy must be considered. Neonates normally have more unconjugated bilirubin than adults. The higher bilirubin concentration in foals most likely is caused by the turnover of fetal hemoglobin to adult hemoglobin, and the relative deficiency of liver binding and conjugating enzymes compared with the adult.[54] The unconjugated bilirubin fraction in foals can be further increased by concurrent prematurity or illness, in the absence of liver disease.

Keeping the above limitations of interpretation in mind, increases in the unconjugated bilirubin fraction in horses with hepatic disease are most likely to occur with acute hepatocellular disease.[14, 15, 20] It is rare for the unconjugated bilirubin fraction in acute hepatic disease to exceed 25 mg/dL (427.5 μmol/L).[15] An increase in the bilirubin concentration may be indicative of hepatic disease, but not necessarily failure. Furthermore, a normal bilirubin value, as commonly occurs in chronic hepatic disease, does not necessarily preclude the diagnosis of hepatic insufficiency.

An increase in the conjugated bilirubin fraction in horses more reliably is indicative of hepatic disease.[14, 15, 20] If the conjugated bilirubin concentration is greater than 25% of the total bilirubin value, hepatocellular disease should be suspected. If the conjugated bilirubin concentration is greater than 30% of the total value, cholestasis should be suspected.[15] Conjugated bilirubin is water-soluble and detectable in the urine only if blood concentrations become sufficiently increased to surpass the renal threshold.[16] Urine dipstick analysis is less sensitive than analysis with a diazo tablet.[16] Urobilinogen may be detected by dipstick analysis in normal horse urine and its presence indicates a patent bile duct.[16] Because urobilinogen is highly unstable, it must be determined on a fresh urine sample. Dilute or acidic urine may interfere with accurate determination of urobilinogen. Reagent strips are not sensitive enough to detect the absence of urobilinogen: Ehrlich's reagent must be used. The absence of urobilinogen is not necessarily indicative of liver disease, but may be compatible with failure of excretion of bilirubin into the intestine, biliary obstruction, failure of intestinal bacterial reduction (diarrhea, overuse of oral antimicrobials), or failure to reabsorb it from the ileum.[4] Increased concentrations of urobilinogen in the urine may be caused by the increased production of urobilinogen by intestinal bacteria, failure of the liver to remove it from the enterohepatic circulation, portosystemic shunting, or spillover following severe hemolysis.[4]

Serum Bile Acid Concentration

Because greater than 90% of bile acids are removed by the normal liver from the enterohepatic circulation, the blood concentration of bile acids may be increased with liver disease.[14, 71, 72] Serum bile acids are stable for at least 1 month if stored at −20 °C and are measured by radioimmunoassay or by an enzymatic colorimetric method. The serum concentration of bile acids is not affected by short-term fasting (<14 hours), but may be increased by more prolonged fasting.[73] Reported normal values for horses and ponies as determined by radioimmunoassay are 8.2 ± 1.6 μmol/L (n = 9)[70] and 5.3 ± 6.5 μmol/L (n = 51) for the colorimetric method.[71] Increased serum bile acid concentrations are highly specific for the presence of liver disease (may increase within 24–48 hours after onset of hepatic disease), but are not specific for the type of liver disease.[14, 72] Because bile acids are 90% restricted to the enterohepatic circulation, increases in the blood may occur as a result of shunting or decreased blood flow to the liver (first-pass effect), failure of the liver to remove bile acids from the enterohepatic circulation, failure of the hepatocytes to conjugate the bile acids for excretion, or failure of excretion with subsequent regurgitation of the bile acids into the blood (biliary obstruction). Fasting for longer than 3 days in horses caused an increase in the serum bile acid concentration of three times over baseline values.[73] Ligation of the bile duct caused a sixfold increase in serum bile acid concentration compared with fasted horses.[73] Carbon tetrachloride toxicity resulted in a threefold increase compared with fasted horses.[73] Concentrations of serum bile acids greater than 50 μmol/L in horses with pyrrolizidine toxicosis were associated with a grave prognosis.[70] A value less than 20 μmol/L appears to be a good predictor in ruling out liver disease.[71] Serum bile acid concentrations greater than 20 μmol/L appear to be indicative of chronic liver disease, but are less effective in detecting acute hepatic disease.[71] Bile acid concentrations are highest in biliary obstructive diseases and portosystemic shunts.

Tests of Protein Synthesis

The blood concentrations of protein or amino acids relate not only to the rate of synthesis by the liver but also to their half-life in the circulation. The half-life of albumin in horses is relatively long (19–20 days), thus a decrease in the albumin concentration is rarely detectable until greater than 80% of the liver mass is lost for more than 3 weeks.[15, 20, 67] It is unusual for the total serum protein to decrease below 5 g/dL (50 g/L) in chronic liver disease.[19] Hypoalbuminemia is a nonspecific finding in chronic liver disease, as it may occur secondary to endoparasitism, nephrosis, malnutrition, malabsorption, circulatory failure, and many other chronic diseases.[21, 67]

The globulin fraction is often increased in chronic hepatic disease as a result of decreased Kupffer cell mass. Loss of Kupffer cell function may result in wider dissemination of enteric-derived foreign antigens, and thus polyclonal gammopathy.[4, 12, 15] Although the globulin fraction may be increased, it is a nonspecific finding with chronic hepatic disease, as polyclonal gammopathy can occur secondary to numerous chronic diseases. A decreased serum albumin concentration concurrent with an increased globulin concentration in chronic hepatic disease causes the total plasma protein or serum protein to appear normal. Thus, serum protein fractionation is paramount. Fractionation of the components making up the total serum protein is most accurately determined by serum protein electrophoresis.[12]

The blood concentration of amino acids may be increased following acute hepatocellular necrosis or during protein catabolic states such as illness or starvation, in response to insulin or glucagon.[4] Fractionation of the blood amino acids and determination of the branched-chain amino acid:aromatic amino acid ratio is more useful than evaluating either fraction separately (see Hepatic Encephalopathy). Decreases in this ratio are indicative of hepatic insufficiency.[39] The risk of clinical signs of hepatic encephalopathy may be projected from the branched chain amino acid:aromatic amino acid (phenylalanine, tyrosine) ratio. A normal ratio falls between 3.5 and 4.5. The risk of hepatic encephalopathy is low, medium, or high if the ratio is 3.0 to 3.5, 2.5 to 3.0, and less than 2.5, respectively.[39]

Because the liver is primarily responsible for removing *ammonia* from the circulation and converting it to urea for renal excretion, increases in the blood ammonia concentration or a decrease in the BUN concentration (<9 mg/dL [6.43 mmol/L]) may be indicative of chronic hepatocellular disease.[19, 20] There is no correlation between the blood ammonia concentration and the severity of liver disease,[34] especially in horses, because of the compounding effects of ammonia-generating and urea-utilizing bacteria in the gastrointestinal tract, as well as the effects of the ration. If blood ammonia is to be determined, blood should be collected into heparin as an anticoagulant, and the test run immediately.[20] The effect of the ration can be evaluated by concurrently determining the blood ammonia concentration of a stablemate receiving a similar ration. Oral ammonia challenge tests have not been fully evaluated in horses; however, the sensitivity of the oral challenge test may be decreased because of the effect of enteric bacteria. Normal values for ammonia vary among laboratories, but have been reported in the range of 13 to 108 μg/dL (7.63–63.42 μmol/L).[22]

Because the liver is also responsible for the synthesis of certain coagulation factors, evaluation of hemostatic function may be useful. Changes in hemostatic function values are not specific for liver disease and must be evaluated in light of the other laboratory findings. The vitamin K–dependent factor with the shortest half-life is factor VII, thus abnormalities are frequently first observed in the *prothrombin time (PT)*. However, adequate evaluation of hemostatic function necessitates determination of the *activated partial thromboplastin time (APTT)*, the *fibrinogen* and *fibrin degradation products (FDP)* concentrations, and a platelet count. Typically, a 50% to 70% decrease in the blood concentration of the coagulation factors is necessary before a change in these clotting time–based assays is detectable.[20] Daily variation in the normal values for clotting times also hinders accurate detection of the abnormal. The clotting times may be more appropriately standarized if a clotting assay is concurrently determined on a normal horse. If the ratio of clotting time (PT or APTT) of the patient with suspected hepatic disease to the normal horse's value is greater than 1.3, the test may be interpreted as abnormal.[74] The sensitivity of coagulation factor deficiency during hepatic insufficiency may be increased by diluting the plasma[75] or by determining the concentration of specific factors, by either clot-based, chromogenic, or radioimmunologic assays. These assays are not widely available.

Hypofibrinogenemia cannot be detected by the heat block precipitation method, the most common method for determination of the plasma fibrinogen concentration.[12] The fibrinogen concentration is more accurately determined by a clotting assay using thrombin. Fibrinogen concentrations less than 100 mg/dL (1 g/L) are indicative of either decreased production or increased consumption. The FDP concentration, as determined by latex agglutination, may be increased during hepatic insufficiency owing to decreased removal by Kupffer cells. Concentrations of FDP greater than 16 μg/dL are indicative of increased production or reduced removal. The plasma concentration of several factors acting as anticoagulants or involved in fibrinolysis also may be altered in chronic liver failure (see Hemorrhagic Diathesis). Tests for these factors are primarily limited to academic and research institutions.

Tests of Carbohydrate Metabolism

Changes in the blood glucose concentration are rarely seen in horses with liver insufficiency.[19] Hyperglycemia may be seen early in disease, but hypoglycemia (glucose <60 mg/dL [3.33 mmol/L]) is more likely in chronic liver disease as anorexia progresses, glycogen stores are depleted, and gluconeogenesis and glycolysis are impaired by increased glucagon concentrations. If glucose is administered, often blood glucose levels will remain abnormally increased, indicative of tissue insulin resistance.[76] Both insulin receptor number and binding affinity for insulin have been found to be diminished in humans with chronic liver disease. Changes in the blood glucose concentration are not specific for liver disease and must be evaluated in the light of the other laboratory findings.

Tests of Lipid Metabolism

The concentration of blood triglycerides may become increased during hepatic insufficiency as a result of increased mobilization from adipose tissue to support energy-requiring processes, coupled with decreased clearance by the liver.[4, 15] In contrast, the VLDL and esterified cholesterol blood concentrations may be decreased because of failure of liver synthesis. Compared with other species, Equidae are thought to possess a greater clearance capacity for triglycerides, as well as a greater hepatic exporting capacity for VLDL. Thus, changes in the blood VLDL, esterified cholesterol, or triglyceride concentrations are rarely seen in horses.[21] An exception to this is the marked increase in blood triglyceride levels that occurs with hyperlipidemia syndrome (see Hyper-

lipidemia and Hepatic Lipidosis). Because blood lipid concentrations may be altered by nonhepatic diseases, these tests are neither sensitive nor specific for liver disease in horses.[15] The blood cholesterol and triglyceride concentrations are normally higher in neonates, compared with adults.[54]

Increased mobilization of triglycerides and fatty acid oxidation by the liver may result in increased production of *ketone bodies,* acetoacetate, and β-hydroxybutyric acid.[13] Although ketone bodies may be utilized for energy by peripheral tissues, these compounds are weak acids and increased levels in the blood may result in ketoacidosis. The pathway for ketone formation is poorly developed in horses, thus ketoacidosis is not common.[21] Ketoacidosis should be suspected in horses that are acidemic and have an abnormally high anion gap. Ketones may be quantitated in the blood or urine. Because the renal threshold of ketone bodies is low, ketonuria usually precedes ketonemia. Routine urine dipsticks only detect acetoacetate.[15]

Liver Enzymes

Acute hepatocellular necrosis or changes in hepatocyte membrane permeability result in the release of soluble cytosolic enzymes into the sinusoidal blood. Thus increased blood concentrations of these cytosolic enzymes may be indicative of active hepatic disease. Caution must be exercised when evaluating increases in these enzymes, as not all are liver-specific. Furthermore, some of these hepatocellular enzymes may be increased owing to induction by drugs. Most of these enzymes are quantitated colorimetrically, thus hemolysis or lipemia may interfere with accurate evaluation. Furthermore, wide variation in values can exist because of age differences, stage of hepatic disease, and laboratory methodology. In horses, the following cytosolic enzymes are liver-specific and are not inducible: iditol dehydrogenase (formerly sorbitol dehydrogenase), arginase, ornithine carbamoyltransferase, and glutamate dehydrogenase.[15, 20] Although increases in these enzymes in the blood are highly specific for heptocellular disease, they are not specific for the type of disease. Marked increases occur following acute hepatic necrosis. Mild increases in these enzymes may be seen subsequent to hepatic hypoxemia or toxemia resulting from endotoxemia, septicemia, transient intestinal disease, hyperthermia, or certain drugs (benzimidazole anthelmintics).[15, 19, 20]

Iditol dehydrogenase (IDH) has been widely used in the evaluation of acute liver disease in horses.[19, 54, 77] The short half-life of this liver cytosolic enzyme makes it ideal for the evaluation of acute ongoing disease. Blood levels of IDH start to decline within 4 hours of transient hepatic necrosis or anoxia. Its short half-life necessitates analysis within 12 hours of collection, or 48 hours if the serum is separated from blood and refrigerated.[55] Although mild variations exist between laboratories, the normal blood concentration of IDH in horses is usually less than 5 to 6 units/L.[22] Foals 2 to 4 weeks of age may have IDH concentrations slightly greater than those of adult horses.[54, 77] *Arginase (ARG)* is used in the Krebs-Henseleit cycle for urea synthesis. It is found in highest concentration in hepatocytes, though minute amounts also exist in renal tissue, brain, skin, testicles, and erythrocytes.[21] Increases in ARG are most indicative of acute hepatic necrosis. Like IDH, ARG has a very short half-life. *Glutamate dehydrogenase (GLDH)* is found in hepatocytes, renal tissue, brain, muscle, and intestinal cells. Like IDH and ARG, GLDH has the highest tissue concentration in the liver and increases of this enzyme in the blood can be considered specific for acute liver disease. The half-life of GLDH is 14 hours.[21]

Other cytosolic enzymes include aspartate aminotransferase, alkaline phosphatase, lactate dehydrogenase, alanine aminotransferase, and isocitrate dehydrogenase. These enzymes are also found in high concentrations in other tissues, or are inducible. Thus, increases in these enzymes are *not specific* for liver disease in horses. Because some of these enzymes are frequently reported in equine biochemical profiles, they may serve as a crude indicator of liver disease; however, the limitations of their usefulness must be recognized.

Aspartate aminotransferase (AST), formerly glutamic oxaloacetic transaminase (GOT), is a cytosolic- and mitochondrial-bound enzyme that catalyzes the reaction responsible for aspartate biosynthesis from carbohydrate.[20] Basically, all cells contain AST, but liver and skeletal muscle cells contain the highest concentrations. Cardiac muscle, erythrocytes, intestinal cells, and the kidney also are sources of AST. Hemolysis and lipemia will falsely increase the value of AST.[20] Increases are most frequently associated with muscle damage, but may be seen following acute hepatic necrosis. Often the AST concentration is normal in chronic hepatic disease.[19] The half-life of AST is relatively long and thus it may take greater than 2 weeks for the blood concentration to decrease following acute hepatic disease. The AST value is most useful when analyzed with other tissue-specific enzymes. For instance, if a muscle-specific enzyme, such as creatine phosphokinase, also is increased, an increase in AST most likely has its origin in muscle. Serial AST and IDH values can be useful for the determination of ongoing hepatic disease. If the IDH and AST values were both initially increased, but subsequent evaluation reveals a normal or decreasing IDH and elevated AST, then a favorable prognosis is indicated, as hepatic necrosis is most likely subsiding. The normal serum concentration of AST is 98 to 278 units/L.[22] *Isocitrate dehydrogenase (ICD)* has a distribution similar to AST.

Alanine aminotransferase (ALT), formerly glutamic pyruvic transaminase (GPT), is responsible for alanine synthesis from carbohydrate.[20] Increases may be seen with acute hepatic disease, but myositis will also increase blood levels. Hemolysis will falsely increase the value of this enzyme and microsomal enzyme inducers (i.e., glucocorticoids) will increase its production and release in the absence of liver disease. This enzyme is not useful for predicting liver disease in horses.[20]

Alkaline phosphatase (ALP) catalyzes the hydrolysis of monophosphate esters. This enzyme is bound to the mitochondrial membrane, thus it does not leak into the blood with changes in cell membrane permeability or necrosis. Increases in the blood concentration of this enzyme are secondary to induction.[20] Cholestasis and certain drugs, including glucocorticoids, primidone, and phenobarbital, will induce production and release of ALP. The ALP value is most likely to be increased in chronic or cholestatic liver diseases, rather than acute or hepatocellular disease. Other tissues beside the liver contain ALP, including bone, intestine, kidney, placenta, and leukocytes, thus increases are not necessarily indicative of cholestasis. Because of increased osteoblastic activity, foals have ALP values two to three times those of adults.[21] Pregnancy, hemolysis, and gastrointestinal disease will also cause increases in ALP.

Lactate dehydrogenase (LDH) is the name for five major isoenzymes located in liver, muscle, erythrocytes, intestinal cells, and renal tissue. Increases in LDH are not liver-specific unless the liver isoenzyme concentration is determined. Isoenzyme 5 (LDH-5) is a useful indicator of acute hepatocellular disease in horses.[78] It is stable at room temperature for 36 hours.

γ-Glutamyl transpeptidase or -transferase (GGT) is involved in glutathione metabolism and transfer of glutamyl groups.[20] γ-Glutamyl transpeptidase is primarily associated with microsomal membranes in the biliary epithelium. Production and release of GGT is induced by cholestasis. Renal tubule cells contain GGT, but this source is released into urine. The only other potentially significant source of GGT in the blood is pancreatic in origin. Because pancreatic disease is relatively rare in horses, the blood concentration of GGT is considered specific for hepatic disease in horses.[22] The half-life of GGT is approximately 3 days and it is stable in serum for 2 days at room temperature, or 30 days if frozen.[21] Mild increases may be seen following acute hepatocellular necrosis,[22] but increases are more persistent in chronic disease, especially with cholestasis.[19] Foals 2 weeks to 1 month old may have greater GGT values than adults.[54, 77] The wider variation in younger horses reflects the degree and extent of hepatic maturation. Normal values for GGT in adult horses are less than 30 units/L.[22]

In summary, evaluation for liver disease in horses should include quantitation of at least IDH or arginase, and GGT. However, normal values for these liver enzymes should not necessarily be interpreted as absence of liver disease.

Clearance of Foreign Dyes

In addition to clearance of endogenous substances from the blood, liver function can be evaluated following injection of an exogenous substance. One such exogenous substance that is removed by the liver, conjugated, and excreted into bile is *Bromsulphalein (BSP).*[15] Following intravenous injection of BSP 2.2 mg/kg body weight, a clearance half-life is determined by periodically obtaining heparinized blood samples over 12 to 15 minutes. Caution should be exercised when injecting BSP, as it can be thrombogenic and irritating if administered perivascularly. Blood samples for BSP quantitation should be collected from a site other than the injection site. Suggested collection times are 3, 6, 9, 12, and 15 minutes post injection. Collection of plasma at the suggested times is not crucial; however, it is important to record the exact time at which the samples were obtained to assure accurate determination of the half-life. The half-life of BSP, thus the rate of extraction by the liver, is determined by plotting the plasma concentrations against the collection times on semilog paper. The normal half-life of BSP in horses is 2.8 ± 0.5 minutes.[15]

The BSP half-life is prolonged when greater than 50% of the hepatic function is lost.[15, 20] It is a very useful test in horses, especially to distinguish hepatoencephalopathy from other causes of abnormal behavior or cerebral signs, and to test liver function in chronic liver disease when bilirubin, IDH, and GGT blood levels are normal. Proper interpretation of the BSP half-life must take into account the state of hepatic blood and bile flow, and the bilirubin and albumin concentrations.[20] If the hepatic blood flow is significantly decreased, as may occur with hepatic congestion or portosystemic shunts, the rate of delivery of BSP to the liver will be decreased, thus the half-life of BSP in the plasma will be prolonged. Because BSP is bound to albumin for delivery to the liver, if the blood concentration of albumin is markedly decreased, a higher proportion of unbound BSP will be delivered to the hepatocytes, will be bound to BSP, and thus the half-life of BSP will be shortened.[20] If the blood concentration of bilirubin is markedly increased, the bilirubin will compete with the BSP for binding sites and conjugating enzymes in the liver, thus prolonging the apparent half-life of BSP. If significant cholestasis is present, the BSP excreted into the biliary tract will be reabsorbed into the circulation, causing an apparent prolongation of its clearance. Thus, although a BSP clearance test is very useful as a test of hepatic function, the results must be interpreted in light of these limitations. Furthermore, because pharmaceutical-grade BSP is no longer commercially available, this test is basically limited to academic and research institutions.

It has been suggested that determination of the BSP clearance time is more useful in the detection of liver disease than the BSP half-life.[79] It has also been suggested that the porportionality transfer constants of clearance may be more useful in predicting hepatic disease than the BSP half-life alone.[80] The clearance time is the amount of dye irreversibly removed from the plasma per unit time. A dose of 5 mg/kg of BSP is given intravenously and heparinized blood samples are obtained 2, 5, 10, 15, 25, and 30 minutes post injection. The BSP clearance time in fed normal horses is 10 mL/min/kg and 6 mL/min/kg for horses fasted 3 days.[79]

The *indocyanine green* (*ICG:* Beckmann & Dickinson, Baltimore) clearance test has replaced the BSP clearance test in humans.[4] Basically, the procedure and the limitations are the same as the BSP clearance test. The ICG clearance time in fed horses is 3.5 ± 0.67 mL/min/kg, and 1.6 ± 0.57 mL/min/kg for fasted horses.[79] Although the clearance of ICG is an excellent predictor of hepatic blood flow and extraction rates, its current expense precludes its routine use in horses. Another disadvantage is that quantitation requires a spectrophotometer that reads infrared wavelengths. These limitations have hindered evaluation of ICG clearance times as a diagnostic test of liver insufficiency in horses.

Other Nonspecific Laboratory Findings

Increased formation and release of acidic metabolic products, including ketone bodies, lactate, pyruvate, and amino acids, contribute to acidemia. Other factors that may contribute to acidemia include diarrhea and loss of renal acidification due to impaired urea synthesis. Acidosis and anorexia both predispose to hypokalemia.

Although infrequently reported in horses, aldosterone and water retention may cause deranged concentrations of sodium and isosthenuria. (see Polydipsia, Polyuria, and the Hepatorenal Syndrome). Azotemia may occur with hyperlipemia.[69]

Cholangiohepatitis, chronic acitive hepatitis, or a focal hepatic abscess may cause an inflammatory leukogram, anemia of chronic disease, and hyperfibrinogenemia.[66] Primary polycythemia has been reported in horses with hepatocellular carcinoma.[81, 82] Because fibrinogen is synthesized by the liver, widespread chronic hepatitis may mask an increase in this acute phase reactant protein.

Diagnostic Imaging of the Liver

Ultrasonography is a safe, noninvasive imaging technique that uses the reflection of high-frequency sound waves from tissue interfaces to produce a visual image. Liver ultrasonography in horses is limited by the ribs, the depth and size of the liver, and its anatomical location deep to the diaphragm and lungs.[2] Mechanical sector or linear array scanners with 3.0-MHz crystals are most effective.[2] Ultrasonography should be used to assess the right and left sides of the liver, and the liver shape, size, position, and texture. Hepatic veins are more anechoic than portal veins and the biliary system is not normally visible. Liver ultrasonography is most useful for determining the general size of the liver; changes in the hepatic parenchyma, including abscesses, cysts, and neoplastic masses; and detecting dilated bile ducts or obstructions with choleliths. Abnormal intra- or extrahepatic blood flow or vasculature may be detectable. Ultrasonography is also useful for guiding biopsy instruments into the liver (see Liver Biopsy).[83]

Radionucleotide imaging also may be used to detect alterations in the hepatic parenchyma or blood flow.[84] Radionucleotide scanning noninvasively evaluates function, as well as yields structural information. Two radionucleotide scanning techniques are available to evaluate the liver: liver scan and biliary scan. In the liver scan, a technetium 99m (^{99m}Tc)–labeled sulfur colloid is injected intravenously. Technetium-99m is a gamma-emitting radioactive compound that is detected in the body by a gamma camera. After injection, the ^{99m}Tc sulfur colloid is phagocytosed by Kupffer cells. Subsequent scanning with the gamma camera detects the radioactive emissions from the ^{99m}Tc and resolves them into a two-dimensional image. Thus, alterations in blood flow (portosystemic shunt) or hepatic masses such as abscesses, cysts, and neoplasia may be detectable. In the biliary scan, ^{99m}Tc-labeled iminodiacetic acid is injected intravenously. The iminodiacetic acid is extracted by the hepatocytes, conjugated, and excreted in the bile.[85] Subsequent scanning images the biliary system and may be useful for the detection of biliary obstruction, including atresia, cholangitis, and cholelithiasis. Because radionucleotide imaging is somewhat expensive and requires a large gamma camera, this procedure is limited to research and academic institutions.

Operative mesenteric portography may be performed when a portosystemic shunt is suspected. In this procedure, a celiotomy is performed, radiopaque material is injected into a mesenteric vein, and rapid, sequential survey radiographs are obtained. Simultaneous opacification of the portal vein, azygous vein, and caudal vena cava or lack of filling of the intrahepatic portal system is indicative of portosystemic shunting.[84]

Liver Biopsy

A liver biopsy can yield important diagnostic, prognostic, and therapeutic information. The procedure is performed at the right 12th to 14th intercostal space, at the intersection of a line drawn from the tuber coxae to a point midway between the elbow and the point of the shoulder. The procedure must be performed in a sterile manner. The area should be clipped, aseptically prepared, and a local-acting anesthetic injected subcutaneously. A stab incision is then made with a no. 15 scapel blade. A Tru-Cut (Baxter-Travenol, St. Louis) or Franklin modified Vim-Silverman (Mueller & Co., Chicago) biopsy instrument is inserted and directed craniad and ventrad through the diaphragm into the liver. Samples should immediately be placed in formalin for histopathologic evaluation and, if necessary, in transport media for culture of microorganisms. Precautions to consider prior to performing the procedure include the risk of hemorrhage, pneumothorax, and peritonitis from bile leakage and colon or abscess puncture, and spread from infectious hepatitis. These complications may be reduced by performing a hemostasis profile to assess the risk of hemorrhage and by using ultrasonography to guide needle placement.[83]

Summary of Diagnostic Procedures

The most useful diagnostic tests for evaluation of hepatic disease in horses are quantitation of IDH, GGT, total and direct reacting bilirubin, bile acids, and the BSP half-life or clearance time. Although less useful in horses, additional tests of liver function may include quantitation of ALP, AST, albumin, fibrinogen, globulins, glucose, esterified triglycerides, ammonia, BUN, and amino acids. Serial testing of these indices may increase their diagnostic and prognostic value. Abnormal laboratory findings should be further investigated with ultrasonography and biopsy, following evaluation of a hemostasis profile.

Treatment of Hepatic Insufficiency

Management techniques for hepatic insufficiency are largely supportive. Specific therapies for specific liver diseases are discussed in more detail under Specific Hepatic Diseases. The basic goal of treatment is to maintain the animal until enough liver regeneration occurs to provide adequate function. Patients with severe hepatic fibrosis respond poorly since adequate regeneration often is not possible. Horses with signs of hepatic encephalopathy that are agitated, restless, or uncontrollable must be sedated to enable therapy; however, any medication should be used judiciously since most tranquilizers are metabolized by the liver or potentiate the abnormal neural function of hepatic encephalopathy. Xylazine or detomidine in small doses is safest and most effective in these instances. Fluid deficit and acid-base or electrolyte imbalances should be corrected by intravenous fluids. Since most horses with hepatic encephalopathy are anorectic and blood glucose may be decreased, continuous intravenous infusion of 5% dextrose at a rate of 2 mL/kg/hr can be beneficial.[86] If continued more than 24 to 48 hours, 2.5% to 5.0% dextrose in half-strength saline or Ringer's solution should be substituted.

Therapy should also be directed at reducing the production of toxic protein metabolites by enteric bacteria or by interfering with their absorption. The administration of mineral oil per nasogastric tube is safe and aids in reducing toxin absorption. Methods to reduce the production of ammonia and other enteric toxins include the oral administration of poorly absorbable antibiotics or lactulose. Neomycin has been recommended at a rate of 10 to 100 mg/kg PO every 6 hours.[62, 87] This treatment significantly alters the gastrointestinal flora, thus may cause diarrhea in some horses, and predisposes to salmonellosis because most *Salmonella* species are not sensitive to neomycin. Lactulose, a syrup containing lactose and other disaccharides, passes through the upper small intestine, then is metabolized by ileal and colonic bacteria to organic acids, thereby reducing luminal pH. Proposed beneficial mechanisms of action of lactulose include increased bacterial assimilation of ammonia, decreased ammonia production, ammonia trapping in the bowel lumen, enteric microflora changes, and osmotic catharsis.[24, 26] A dose of 0.3 mL/kg of lactulose syrup every 6 hours per nasogastric tube has been recommended for horses[87]; however, this therapy is expensive, usually causes diarrhea, and has not been adequately evaluated in horses. Many clinicians prefer not to use oral antimicrobials or lactulose, but to rely on institution of a low protein diet. Although oral concentrates of BCAAs can be formulated for horses[39] and intravenous preparations of BCAAs (Baxter Healthcare Corp., Deerfield, Ill.) are available, controlled clinical trials in humans have not shown this form of therapy to consistently ameliorate the signs of hepatic encephalopathy.[40]

Once the appetite returns, a horse with hepatic encephalopathy or chronic liver disease is best managed by dietary manipulation. The ration should be high in carbohydrates and low in protein, with the protein source optimally rich in BCAAs. A mixture of two parts beet pulp and one part cracked corn in molasses can be fed at a rate of 2.5 kg/100 kg body weight per day divided into six or more feedings.[87] Sorghum or milo can be substituted for the beet pulp. Multiple small feedings are optimal in horses with liver disease because of impaired gluconeogenesis. Oat hay is the best roughage, followed by other grass hay.[86] Grazing grass pastures should be encouraged provided horses can be protected from the sun. Alfalfa and legumes should be avoided because of their high protein content. Vitamins B_1, K_1, and folic acid should be administered parenterally on a weekly basis. Vitamin K therapy is most useful when cholestasis is present.[4]

A number of experimental drugs have been studied in humans and may have a future role in management of hepatic encephalopathy in horses. Regimens to stimulate hepatic regeneration include insulin and glucagon[88] and cytosolic extracts from regenerating liver.[89] None have been shown to be definitively effective in humans. As discussed above, benzodiazepine receptor antagonists have been suggested to induce clinical and electrophysiologic remissions of hepatic encephalopathy in humans with both acute and chronic liver failure.[24, 90] This neuropharmacologic approach to treatment of hepatic encephalopathy holds great promise, although it may not be economically feasible in horses.

If any drugs are to be administered to a horse with hepatic insufficiency, it may be necessary to alter dosage. Alterations in hepatic blood flow, albumin, and biotransformation during hepatic insufficiency may prolong the half-life, as well as the dosage interval. Drugs that rely heavily on the liver for metabolism and excretion, such as chloramphenicol, erythromycin, and corticosteroids, should be avoided.[18]

Prognosis

The prognosis for hepatic insufficiency in horses depends upon the severity and type of the underlying disease. Horses with acute hepatic failure have the best chance for hepatic regeneration, thus they have a guarded-to-fair prognosis if adequate and appropriate supportive care is given. Patients with severe hepatic fibrosis and chronic liver disease have a poor prognosis because of their inability to compensate for lost hepatic function. Pyrrolizidine alkaloid toxicosis, the most common cause of hepatic fibrosis in horses, results in mitotic arrest of hepatocytes and prevents regeneration. As the cells die they are replaced by fibrous tissue. The presence of severe encephalopathy, intravascular hemolysis, profound acidosis, or diarrhea markedly increase serum bile acid concentration. BSP half-life greater than 10 minutes, or decreased albumin, strongly suggests a poor prognosis. If the horse survives more than 5 days, the prognosis for this bout of encephalopathy is fair. Therapy is not warranted in horses with severe hepatic fibrosis.

SPECIFIC HEPATIC DISEASES

Acute Hepatic Diseases

Theiler's Disease

Sir Arnold Theiler first described this disease in South Africa in 1918 following vaccination of horses against African horse sickness with both live virus and equine-origin antiserum.[91] In 1934 and 1937, a similar disease was described in the United States following vaccination of horses against western equine encephalomyelitis, using both live virus and equine-origin antiserum.[63, 92, 93] Despite numerous accounts of this syndrome, the exact cause of Theiler's disease remains unclear. Today, this disease is one of the most commonly described causes of acute hepatic failure in horses.[22, 63] Theiler's disease is also referred to as *acute hepatic necrosis, serum-associated hepatitis,* and *serum sickness.*

Clinical Signs. Theiler's disease is limited to adult horses. The onset of clinical signs of hepatic failure in Theiler's disease is acute to subacute, and rapidly progresses over 2 to 7 days. Most horses are anorectic and icteric; hepatic encephalopathy is reported in 80% of the cases.[63] Photodermatitis, hemorrhagic diathesis, and bilirubinuria may be present. Although uncommon, some horses with Theiler's disease have an insidious history of chronic weight loss.[63]

Epidemiology and Pathogenesis. The disease typically occurs sporadically, but outbreaks involving multiple horses on a single farm over several months have been reported.[63] In the northeastern part of the United States, a pattern of seasonality may occur, with a larger percentage of cases presenting in summer and fall.[22, 63] Approximately 20% of horses with Theiler's disease have received an equine-origin biological 4 to 10 weeks prior to the onset of hepatic failure,

hence the name "serum-associated hepatitis." Equine-origin biologicals that have been associated with Theiler's disease include vaccines or antisera for African horse sickness, eastern and western encephalomyelitis, *Bacillus anthracis,* tetanus antitoxin, *Clostridium perfringens, Clostridium botulinum, Streptococcus equi,* influenza, equine herpesvirus type 1, and pregnant mare's serum.[19, 63]

Reports of outbreaks in association with parenteral injection of homologous live virus vaccine or antiserum suggest an infectious bloodborne viral cause.[63] The history, onset, clinical signs, and histopathologic findings of Theiler's disease appear most similar to hepatitis B virus in humans. Hepatitis B virus is present in all body fluids and excreta, and is transmitted primarily by parenteral injection.[94] Viral surface antigen or antibody to viral core protein is detectable in 75% to 90% of human patients with hepatitis B.[94] Newer techniques that detect viral DNA or DNA polymerase are even more sensitive and specific tests of infection. To date, these assays have been negative in horses with Theiler's disease. Furthermore, viral isolation on horses with Theiler's disease has been unsuccessful, the disease has not been transmitted experimentally by blood or tissue inoculation, and a large percentage of horses with Theiler's disease do not have a recent history of receiving an equine-origin biological.[95, 96] The sum of these negative findings does not necessarily exclude the possibility of a viral cause. However, if such exists, there must be other modes of transmission, infection, and establishment of disease.

Other suggested causes of Theiler's disease include exposure to hepatotoxic substances, such as mycotoxins (aflatoxin and rubratoxin), plant toxins (pyrrolizidine alkaloids, alsike clover), drugs, or chemicals.[19] However, these causes have not been uniformly demonstrable and usually are considered separate disease entities.

Aside from widespread tissue icterus, the pathologic findings are limited to the liver. The liver appears smaller than normal, but may be large in peracute cases. Although not pathognomonic, the histopathologic findings in Theiler's disease consistently include widespread centrolobular-to-midzonal hepatocellular necrosis.[95] A mild inflammatory infiltrate, primarily monocytes and lymphocytes, is present in the portal triads. The occasional finding of mild-to-moderate biliary hyperplasia and fibroblastic infiltration is evidence of a more chronic disease course than the clinical signs alone would suggest.[95]

Diagnosis. Recent inoculation with an equine-origin biological, coupled with an abrupt onset of clinical signs and laboratory evidence of hepatic insufficiency, is strongly suggestive of Theiler's disease. Bilirubinemia and bilirubinuria are usually present. Liver enzymes, including IDH, ARG, and AST, are increased. The BSP half-life, PT, and APTT are often prolonged. Hemolysis may occur terminally. The histopathologic findings on a liver biopsy offer the strongest diagnostic evidence of Theiler's disease.

Treatment. There is no specific treatment for Theiler's disease aside from general supportive care for hepatic insufficiency (see Treatment of Hepatic Insufficiency).

Prognosis and Client Education. The prognosis is poor to grave in horses with severe hepatic encephalopathy, hemorrhage, or hemolysis. Horses that survive longer than a week usually recover completely. A favorable prognosis is warranted if serial IDH concentrations are decreasing or clinical signs are waning. There is no preventive, aside from the judicious use of equine-origin antiserum.

Bacterial Hepatitis

Tyzzer's Disease. *Bacillus piliformis* is a motile, gramnegative, spore-forming, obligate intracytoplasmic bacterium that causes acute necrotizing hepatitis. The disease was first described by E.E. Tyzzer in 1917 in a colony of waltzing mice.[97] The first documented outbreak in foals occurred in Kentucky on a single farm between 1964 and 1973, fatally infecting 23 foals.[98]

Clinical Signs. In horses, the disease is limited to foals between the ages of 7 and 42 days.[99] The clinical signs are usually nonspecific and include loss of a suckle reflex, depression progressing to recumbency, fever, tachypnea, tachycardia, icterus, petechiation, diarrhea, dehydration, shock, seizures, and coma.[98-101] Often the foals are found dead without premonitory signs.

Epidemiology and Pathogenesis. Outbreaks of Tyzzer's disease are sporadic, thus it is not believed to be a contagious disease.[99] Seasonality has not been demonstrated. The disease has been reported in the United States, Canada, South Africa, England, New England, and Australia.[99, 100] Mice with Tyzzer's disease are infected by an oral route perinatally, with clinical signs and death occurring between 6 and 44 days of age.[100] Adult mice can be latent carriers, shedding the organism in the feces. In rodents and rabbits, administration of corticosteroids or sulfonamides may induce active disease.[100] The natural mode of transmission in horses is not definitely known, but, the distribution of lesions strongly suggests an oral route of infection. Because bacterial spores can survive in the soil for at least 1 year and can be recovered experimentally from the feces of adult horses, it has been suggested that foals are infected by ingesting spores in the feces of their dams, or in the soil.[99, 100]

Bacillus piliformis causes acute multifocal hepatitis and enteritis. Grossly, the liver is swollen with 1- to 5-mm white foci scattered throughout the parenchyma. Tissues are icteric and petechial hemorrhages are present in many tissues. Microscopically, the foci are areas of coagulative necrosis with an associated inflammatory infiltrate consisting of neutrophils, macrophages, and lymphocytes. The organisms, best demonstrated at the periphery of the lesions by Warthin-Starry or Dietrerle's silver stains, appear as long bacilli organized in bundles. In addition to hepatitis, enterocolitis, myositis, pleural effusion, pulmonary congestion and edema, and lymphoid necrosis or depletion may be present.[99, 100]

Diagnosis. The peracute onset and nonspecific signs confound antemortem diagnosis of Tyzzer's disease. Hematologic study may reveal hemoconcentration, leukopenia or leukocytosis, a left shift, and toxic neutrophils.[99] Other nonspecific laboratory findings include hyperfibrinogenemia, acidosis, hyperkalemia, and profound hypoglycemia.[99-101] Liver enzymes are increased, including IDH, GGT, AST, ALP, and LDH-5.[99-101]

The definitive diagnosis is determined at necropsy by demonstration of the organism intracytoplasmically. *Bacillus piliformis* is extremely fastidious and can only be grown in living tissue, such as embryonated chick eggs.[101] Differential diagnosis for hepatic failure in foals includes iron hepatotoxicity, perinatal equine herpesvirus type 1, bacteremia, atresia of the bile duct, and portosystemic shunt.

Treatment. In foals, there are no reports of successfully treated Tyzzer's disease. In rodents and rabbits, *B. piliformis* is sensitive to penicillin, tetracycline, erythromycin, and streptomycin.

Prognosis and Client Education. Tyzzer's disease in foals is considered invariably fatal. All reported cases have died within 48 hours of onset. There is no preventative.

Infectious Necrotic Hepatitis

Clostridium novyi type B is the cause of infectious necrotic hepatitis, or *black disease*. The disease is most common in sheep and cattle, but at least four cases have been documented in horses.[61, 102-104]

Clinical Signs. The onset of disease may be peracute with sudden death. Acute signs are progressive over 24 to 72 hours and include depression, reluctance to move, fever, icterus, petechiae, periods of recumbency, tachycardia, and tachypnea.[61, 102-104] Some affected horses remain standing until a short time before death.

Epidemiology and Pathogenesis. Reported cases of infectious necrotic hepatitis in horses have occurred in or adjacent to areas with a large population of sheep.[61, 102-104] In sheep and cattle, infectious necrotic hepatitis is the result of multiplication of *C. novyi* in areas of liver compromised by the migration of *Fasciola hepatica*.[102] This fluke normally does not infest horses, but migration of any parasite through the liver may predispose to infectious necrotic hepatitis. Horses with infectious necrotic hepatitis had parasitic infestations, though there was no direct evidence of migrating parasites in the liver at the time of necropsy. The onset of disease in one case occurred 48 hours after administration of mebendazole.[61]

The carcass blackens rapidly after death owing to engorgement of subcutaneous blood vessels; hence the name black disease. Often, necropsy findings include serosanguineous effusion in the pericardial sac, and the thoracic and abdominal cavities, widespread hemorrhages and icterus, and multifocal areas (1–2 mm) of coagulative hepatic necrosis. Smears or histologic sections of the hepatic lesions reveal large numbers of gram-positive rods.

Diagnosis. The acute and nonspecific nature of this disease makes antemortem diagnosis improbable. In reported cases, liver-specific enzymes and bilrubin were only mildly increased.[61, 102] An abdominocentesis was performed on one horse and revealed serosangineous peritonitis.[61] Definitive diagnosis is based on positive staining with fluorescein conjugated antiserum specific for *C. novyi,* or isolation of the organism at necropsy.[102] The organism is difficult to isolate and requires rapid tissue sampling and anaerobic conditions.

Treatment. Treatment with high doses of penicillin or ampicillin are indicated, in addition to general supportive care for hepatic insufficiency.

Prognosis and Client Education. All four reported cases of infectious necrotic hepatitis in horses were fatal.

Miscellaneous Causes of Bacterial Hepatitis

Primary bacterial hepatitis is rare in adult horses. Bacterial septicemia in neonates may result in multifocal hepatitis, though rarely accompanied by clinical signs of hepatic failure. Bacterial endotoxin, released during acute fulminant gram-negative infection, or absorbed from the gastrointestinal tract following mural damage, may cause hepatic hypoxemia. Because Kupffer cells normally phagocytose endotoxin, bombardment of the liver with endotoxin may temporarily impede the function of Kupffer cells.

Primary bacterial cholangiohepatitis has been reported in horses, though more commonly, it is secondary.[105, 106] *Secondary cholangiohepatitis* in horses is a sequela to biliary stasis, cholethiasis, chronic active hepatitis, hepatic neoplasia, pancreatitis, enterocolitis, intestinal parasitism, and intestinal obstruction. Clinical signs include anorexia, fever, and icterus. Hepatic encephalopathy may be present. Laboratory abnormalities may include leukocytosis and increased concentrations of IDH, ARG, GGT, and direct reacting bilirubin.[105] Definitive diagnosis is based on histopathologic findings on liver biopsy and bacterial isolation. Isolates are most commonly enteric organisms such as *Salmonella* species, *Escherichia coli,* and *Citrobacter, Aeromonas,* and *Acinetobacter* species.[56, 105, 106] Treatment includes general supportive care for hepatic failure (see Treatment of Hepatic Insufficiency) and 4 to 6 weeks of antimicrobial therapy. The antimicrobial therapy should be based on culture and sensitivity results. Recommended antimicrobials for bacterial cholangiohepatitis in horses include trimethoprim-sulfonamide, penicillin and gentamicin, ampicillin, and chloramphenicol.[57]

Viral Hepatitis

Equine Herpesvirus Infection in Foals

Pregnant mares infected with equine herpesvirus type 1 (EHV-1) may abort in the third trimester or deliver stillborn or weak foals. Some foals may appear normal at birth, but develop clinical signs of respiratory distress, icterus, fever, and severe depression.[107] Secondary bacterial septicemia is common. Pathologic lesions of aborted fetuses or neonatal foals are similar and include severe pulmonary congestion, pneumonitis, bronchiolitis, hyaline membrane disease, and intralobular coagulative hepatocellular necrosis.[107] Intranuclear, acidophilic inclusions are present in hepatocytes and biliary epithelium. There is no specific treatment. General supportive care and prophylactic administration of broad-

spectrum antimicrobials are indicated. The prognosis is poor to grave. Most affected foals die within a few days of birth. Vaccination of pregnant mares is only partially efficacious for prevention.

Equine Infectious Anemia

The causative organism of equine infectious anemia is a retrovirus which has a tropism for mononuclear phagocytes.[108] Although cyclic fever, anemia, icterus, edema, and weight loss are the systemic manifestations of the disease, the Kupffer cells in the liver are a major site of infection. Icterus is due to increased erythrocyte destruction, as well as acute hepatic necrosis.

Equine Viral Arteritis

This disease is caused by a togavirus and typically is manifest clinically by depression, fever, acute upper respiratory tract infection, abortion, petechiation, and edema. Following ingestion or inhalation, viral septicemia leads to vascular damage. Overt clinical signs of hepatic disease are rare, but vascular damage in the liver may cause icterus.[109]

Giant Cell Hepatopathy

A disease similar to human neonatal hepatitis has been reported in aborted midterm fetuses.[110] Histologically, there is disorganization of hepatic cords, multifocal necrosis, a mild mononuclear cell infiltrate, and a large hepatocyte syncytium with 8 to 10 nuclei. The cause in horses and humans is unknown, but is presumably viral. Viral and bacterial isolation, viral immunofluorescence, and serologic testing have been unsuccessful in horses. Giant-cell hepatopathy was reported in one foal with prolonged neonatal isoerythrolysis.[110]

Parasitic Hepatitis

Parasitic infestation may cause focal hepatic disease, but rarely overt hepatic insufficiency. Following their ingestion, as embryonated eggs, larvae of *Parascaris equorum* hatch in the small intestine, then migrate through the liver and lungs. Focal or diffuse hepatic fibrosis may result.[111] Migration of *Strongylus edentatus* or *Strongylus equinus* through the hepatic portal veins may cause focal hepatitis, subcapsular hemorrhage, and edema, followed by focal parenchymal fibrosis and capsular fibrin deposits.[111] Focal hepatic infarcts may occur secondary to thrombotic emboli due to migrating *Strongylus vulgaris* in mesenteric arteries. The canine cestode, *Echinococcus granulosa,* may form hydatid (larval) cysts in the liver, which are usually an incidental finding.[22]

Toxic Hepatopathy

There are numerous chemicals, drugs, mycotoxins, and plant toxins that are hepatotoxic, but these rarely cause acute hepatic failure in horses. Some substances cause fatty change, cloudy swelling, necrosis, mild inflammatory infiltration, and fibrosis, primarily in the centrolobular location, where the oxygen tension is lowest. Other substances cause the same lesions periportally, in the area of initial exposure. Some substances are directly hepatotoxic, others require biotransformation by the liver to toxic metabolites.

Chemical Hepatotoxins

Horses are rarely exposed to hepatotoxic chemicals in sufficient amounts to induce hepatic failure. Potential hepatotoxic chemicals include arsenic (pesticide), carbon tetrachloride (fumigant), chlorinated hydrocarbons (insecticide), monesin (ionophore), pentachlorophenols (wood preservative, herbicide, fungicide), phenol (disinfectant, wood preservative), phosphorus (fertilizer), and paraquat (herbicide).[112] All of these cause centrolobular necrosis, except phosphorus, which causes primarily periportal changes.

Drugs

There is a wide range of effects that pharmaceutical agents can have on the liver, depending on the drug type, dose, frequency, duration, and route of administration, age of the animal, diet, and concurrent treatment.[113] The hepatic damage may be acute or chronic, cholestatic, zonal, vascular, or hypersensitivity-mediated. Certain drugs alter hepatocellular permeability, without visible injury or loss of function.

Drugs that are intrinsically hepatotoxic reproducibly cause hepatocellular necrosis.[112, 114] Examples of intrinsic hepatotoxic drugs that cause zonal centrolobular necrosis include carbon disulfide and carbon tetrachloride.[112] These drugs cause hepatocellular damage in a dose-related manner and toxicity often results in hepatic failure. Anabolic steroids cause cholestasis with little or no evidence of hepatic damage or inflammation, resulting in mild icterus, which is completely and rapidly reversible once the drug is discontinued.[113, 114] Phenothiazines and macrolide antibiotics (erythromycin) cause cholestatic injury, which is accompanied by significant hepatocellular necrosis and periportal inflammation.[114] Recovery is usually expected after discontinuation of the drug. Some drugs, such as tetracycline, cause fatty infiltration of the liver, but rarely cause liver dysfunction.

Idiosyncratic hepatotoxicity has been reported following administration of erythromycin, rifampin, isoniazid, halothane, diazepam, sulfonamides, phenobarbital, phenytoin, and aspirin.[112, 114] Injury varies from mild focal hepatitis to massive necrosis. Idiosyncratic hepatopathy has a low incidence, is not dose-related, and often resolves upon discontinuation of the drug. Rarely, progressive liver failure ensues. Some idiosyncratic drug hepatopathies may have a pathogenesis similar to drug allergy. Others may be related to the liver's biotransformation properties. For example, if an individual has enhanced biotransformation of a certain drug, and the metabolite of the drug is more cytotoxic than the original unaltered drug, hepatic damage may ensue.

Finally, some drugs induce increased hepatic enzyme activities, or alter hepatocellular permeability, but do not cause significant hepatic damage or clinical signs. Examples include benzimidazole anthelmintics, phenobarbital, phenylbutazone, and corticosteroids.

Iron Toxicity in Foals

Acute, fatal toxic hepatopathy was reported in numerous newborn foals given an oral microbial inoculum.[115] The syndrome is reproducible if *ferrous fumarate* is given orally.[116] The incidence of hepatic failure was highest when the foals were given the inoculum prior to nursing. Colostrum contains abundant vitamin E, an essential cofactor for glutathione. Glutathione protects against free radical damage, a proposed mechanism for iron toxicity. Thus, presumably, foals that are given iron supplements prior to ingesting colostrum are most susceptible to iron toxicity.[116]

Clinical signs include hepatic encephalopathy, icterus, and peracute death. Laboratory abnormalities include increased blood concentrations of bilirubin, IDH, GGT, and ammonia, and reduced BCAA/AA ratio, decreased glucose, and prolonged PT. At necropsy, the liver was abnormally small and histologic study revealed massive hepatic necrosis with blood-filled reticulum. Some livers had mild biliary hyperplasia and periportal fibrosis.

Supportive therapy may prolong life, but most foals with iron hepatotoxicosis die. Those foals that survived recovered fully.

Mycotoxins

Mycotoxicosis is more common in ruminants than in horses. The two most common mycotoxins affecting horses are *aflatoxin,* produced by the molds *Aspergillus flavus* and *Aspergillus parasiticus,* and *rubratoxin,* produced by the mold *Penicillium rubrum. Aspergillus* species grow on a wide variety of feedstuffs if the temperature, moisture, and carbohydrate content are sufficient.[112] Aflatoxins impair protein synthesis and carbohydrate metabolism.

The degree of hepatic damage and extent of clinical signs depend on the duration and extent of exposure to the mycotoxin. Most horses refuse to eat moldy feed, thus hepatic failure is uncommon. Pathologic findings include hepatocellular necrosis, fatty change, biliary hyperplasia, periportal fibrosis, and megalocytosis.

There is no specific treatment for aflatoxicosis. Administration of activated charcoal or a cathartic shortly after ingestion may impede absorption. Mycotoxicosis is best prevented by avoiding moldy feed.

Acute Biliary Obstruction

Acute obstruction of the common bile duct causes icterus and signs of abdominal pain. Acute biliary occlusion may occur secondary to cholelithiasis (see below) or colon displacement. Intense icterus, colic, and increased concentrations of direct bilirubin (>85.5 μmol/L), GGT (>400 units/L) and bile acids (>150 units/L) were reported in two horses with acute colon displacements. These abnormalities quickly abated after surgical correction of the displaced colon.

Chronic Hepatic Diseases
Chronic Megalocytic Hepatopathy

Megalocytic hepatopathy occurs worldwide and is the most common cause of chronic liver failure in horses in certain parts of the United States.[22] It is caused by the ingestion of *pyrrolizidine alkaloid*–containing plants. The intoxication typically results in the delayed onset of chronic, progressive liver failure.

Clinical Signs. The development of clinical signs of liver disease is usually delayed 4 weeks to 6 months following the consumption of pyrrolizidine alkaloid–containing plants. However, there are individual differences in susceptibility, as not all horses consuming the plants develop clinical signs.[117] The onset of obvious hepatic failure, characterized by hepatic encephalopathy and photosensitization, is usually abrupt and occurs late in the disease despite the time interval since ingestion. Premonitory signs of insidious onset may include anorexia, weight loss, exercise intolerance, and mild-to-moderate icterus. Diarrhea, edema, polydipsia, pruritus, laryngeal hemiparalysis, and hemolysis also have been reported to occur late in the disease.[70, 117, 118] Sometimes oral ulcers and halitosis develop.[119] Although uncommon, if sufficient consumption occurs during a single exposure, abortion or clinical signs of liver failure may develop acutely.

Epidemiology and Pathogenesis. There are numerous species of pyrrolizidine alkaloid–containing plants (Table 13–2). In the United States, *Senecio jacobea,* and *Senecio vulgaris* are found primarily along the Pacific Coast and in the western states, *Amsinckia intermedia* in the West, and *Crotolaria sagittalis, Crotolaria spectabilis,* and *Heliotropium europaeum* primarily in the Southeast.

Pyrrolizidine alkaloid–containing plants are not palatable and horses will not typically consume them unless pastures are heavily contaminated or there is no alternative feed source. Some herbicides may increase palatability.[118] Pyrrolizidine alkaloids are quite stable and many intoxications occur following ingestion of contaminated hay, pellets, or grain. *Senecio vulgaris* is a common contaminant in alfalfa hay, especially at the first cutting. Not all parts of the plant contain pyrrolizidine alkaloids, and the concentration may vary with the season.[120] *Amsinckia* and *Crotolaria* species concentrate pyrrolizidine alkaloids in their seeds; thus intoxication may occur following ingestion of contaminated oat hay or grain screenings.[118]

Horses and cattle are relatively sensitive to pyrrolizidine alkaloid intoxication compared to goats and sheep. Consumption of the plants at a dose of 2% to 5% of a horse's body weight, fed at one time or over a few days, can result in acute toxicity.[118] The effects of pyrrolizidine alkaloids are cumulative, thus it is more common for toxicity to occur following chronic low-level exposure. There are over 100 different pyrrolizidine alkaloids, but only a few have proved to be toxic (see Table 13–2). The toxic pyrrolizidine alkaloids vary among plants, but they all cause the same basic lesion. Ingested pyrrolizidine alkaloids are carried to the liver via the portal circulation and are metabolized by the microsomal enzymes to toxic pyrrole derivatives.[119] Drugs that induce microsomal enzymes, such as mixed function oxidases, will increase the toxicity of pyrrolizidine alkaloids. The pyrroles are chemically highly reactive and capable of alkylating nucleic acids and protein. Consequently, cellular replication and protein synthesis are inhibited. Because the cells cannot divide, hepatocytes enlarge, forming megalocytes. When the megalocytes die, fibrosis ensues. When fibrosis becomes extensive, the liver shrinks, develops a firm texture, and failure is inevitable.

Hepatocytes surrounding the portal triads are usually affected first. When there is acute massive consumption, extensive centrolobular hepatocellular necrosis occurs. Fibrosis around the portal vessels can cause portal hypertension, ascites, and diarrhea. Endothelial cell swelling in the portal vein is especially common with *Crotalaria* species, further promoting veno-occlusion. Despite periportal fibrosis and veno-occlusion, portal hypertension rarely develops in horses, though it is a common manifestation of pyrrolizidine alkaloid toxicity in cattle.[118] Additional pathologic findings include myocardial necrosis, colitis, widespread hemorrhages, and adrenal cortical hypertrophy.[70] The toxic pyrrolizidine alkaloid in *Crotalaria* species, monocrotaline, also is pneumonotoxic and may cause hydrothorax, pulmonary edema, epithelialization, and pulmonary arteritis.[119]

Pyrrolizidine alkaloids are rapidly excreted in body fluids such as milk and urine.[119] The alkaloids can pass the placenta in pregnant animals, thus are potentially toxic to the fetus.[119]

Diagnosis. A presumptive diagnosis of megalocytic hepatopathy can be made from history of exposure to pyrrolizidine alkaloids, clinical signs, and laboratory evidence of hepatic

---

Table 13–2. Pyrrolizidine Alkaloid–Containing Plants

Species Name	Common Name	Alkaloids
Senecio jacobea	Tansy or common ragwort, stinking Willie	Jacobine, jacodine, senecionine
Senecio ridelli	Ridell's groundsel	Ridelline
Senecio longilobus	Threadleaf groundsel	Longilobine
Senecio vulgaris	Common groundsel	Senecionine, seneciphylline, retrosine
Senecio spartioides	Broom groundsel	Senciphylline
Senecio intergerrimus	Lamb's tongue groundsel	Intergerrimine
Amsinckia intermedia	Fiddleneck, fireweed, or tarweed	
Crotalaria species	Rattlebox	Monocrotaline, fulvine, crispatine
Echium plantagineum	Viper's bugloss	
Heliotropium europaeum	Common heliotrope or potato weed	Heliotrine, lassiocarpine

disease. Early in the disease, IDH and AST may be increased, but by the time clinical signs develop, these enzymes are often normal or only mildly increased. Because fibrosis occurs periportally, GGT and ALP are persistently increased. Bilirubin may be increased and the BCAA/AAA ratio may be decreased.[121] The BSP half-life is prolonged and serum bile acids are usually increased late in the disease.[70]

A definitive diagnosis of pyrrolizidine alkaloid intoxication requires a liver biopsy. The histopathologic findings of megalocytosis, biliary hyperplasia, and fibrosis are essentially pathognomonic. Pyrrolizidine alkaloids can be detected in feed by high-performance liquid chromatography.[70] Some pyrrolizidine alkaloids can be identified in liver tissue. Unfortunately, because of the prolonged delay in development of clinical signs, often the original source of contamination remains unidentified.

Treatment and Prognosis. There is no specific antidote for pyrrolizidine alkaloid intoxication. Despite general supportive care, death usually occurs within 10 days of the onset of obvious clinical signs of hepatic failure. A serum bile acid concentration greater than 50 μmol/L is suggestive of a grave prognosis.[70] Because regeneration is not possible, if extensive megalocytosis and fibrosis are present, treatment is not warranted. Treatment with branched-chain amino acids may decrease the severity of neurologic signs, but does not prevent death.[70] If clinical signs or histologic changes are mild, a low protein (grass or oat hay), high-energy (molasses concentrate grain) ration may be beneficial.

Attention should be directed toward asymptomatic horses that also may have consumed the plants. The source of contamination should be identified, either by identification of the plant in hayfields or pasture, or by analysis of feed, and the feed discontinued. Progress can be monitored by serial liver enzyme quantitation and biopsies.

Chronic Active Hepatitis

Chronic active hepatitis (CAH) in horses is an idiopathic, chronic, progressive hepatopathy characterized histopathologically by biliary hyperplasia, with concomitant periportal or biliary inflammation or both, and associated hepatocellular damage.

Clinical Signs. The onset of clinical signs of CAH is insidious. Signs are compatible with progressive liver failure and include depression, exercise intolerance, weight loss, anorexia, colic, icterus, and fever.[66] The signs may be intermittent. Although uncommon, some horses with CAH have moist exfoliative coronary dermatitis.[66]

Etiology and Pathogenesis. The exact cause of CAH in horses is not known. A similar syndrome occurs in humans and has been linked to autoimmune disease, chronic hepatitis B virus infection, non-A, non-B (viral) hepatitis, Wilson's disease, α₁-antitrypsin deficiency, and drug allergy.[94] Humans with autoimmune-associated CAH often have marked polyclonal gammopathy and hepatic actin and antinuclear antibodies. Histologic study of the liver reveals mononuclear and plasma cell infiltrates, large areas of necrosis, and fibrosis. Extrahepatic signs of autoimmune disease, including dermatitis, arthritis, and glomerulonephritis, may be present. Some horses with CAH have polyclonal gammopathy, but this is a nonspecific finding in many types of chronic hepatic disease and is not necessarily indicative of autoimmunity. Occasionally, horses with CAH have predominantly plasma and mononuclear cell infiltrates in the liver, suggestive of heightened humoral activity. The presence of coronary dermatitis in horses with CAH may be a manifestation of autoimmune disease, though this has not been confirmed by immunohistologic staining. There have been no reports of antinuclear antibodies in horses with CAH, and viral hepatitis, Wilson's disease, and α₁-antitrypsin deficiency have not been documented. Idiosyncratic drug hypersensitivity has been reported in horses, though not as a consistent feature of CAH.

In addition to the possibility of an autoimmune or hypersensitivity reaction, CAH in horses may be a manifestation of chronic cholangitis. Many horses with CAH have a suppurative inflammatory response involving the biliary system, in addition to periportal inflammation and hepatocellular necrosis.[66] Often the cholangiohepatitis is accompanied by biliary hyperplasia, fibrosis, and cholestasis. In some cases, coliform organisms have been isolated from the liver, suggestive of ascending infection from the gastrointestinal tract.

In a large number of horses, there is histopathologic evidence of fibrosis, acute inflammation, and hepatocellular necrosis, but no specific cause can be determined.

Diagnosis. The diagnostic criteria for CAH in humans include abnormally increased serum transaminase concentrations for greater than 6 months, abnormal immunologic findings, and characteristic histopathologic findings.[94] In horses, serum IDH and AST concentrations may be mildly increased, but GGT and ALP are often markedly increased in CAH. The serum bile acid, total protein, and bilirubin (especially the direct reacting fraction) concentrations may be increased. Bilirubinuria may be present and the BSP half-life is usually prolonged. Hematology may reveal an inflammatory leukogram, with or without a left shift.[66] Immunodiagnostics, including determination of the antinuclear antibody titer and anti-immunoglobulin immunofluorescent staining of skin lesions, may help confirm an autoimmune phenomenon.

In the face of clinical signs and the demonstration of significant laboratory findings indicative of liver disease, a liver biopsy should be obtained (see Liver Biopsy). A sample should be submitted for histopathologic examination, as well as bacterial isolation and antimicrobial sensitivity testing. The definitive diagnosis of CAH depends on the presence of characteristic histopathologic findings. Progressive periportal hepatocellular necrosis obscures and distorts the limiting plate, the cord of hepatocytes that surrounds the portal triad. As this destructive process continues, bands of necrotic hepatocytes and inflammatory cells connect one liver lobule to another or extend from the portal tract to the central vein. This feature is called *bridging necrosis*. As bridging necrosis progresses, fibrosis and cirrhosis prevail.

Treatment. General supportive care for hepatic failure (see Treatment of Hepatic Insufficiency) is indicated whenever clinical signs are apparent. Specific therapy for CAH depends on the histopathologic findings. If the liver biopsy reveals abundant plasma cells, or other diagnostic tests suggest autoimmune or hypersensitivity disease, corticosteroid therapy may be beneficial. In humans with autoimmune-associated CAH, corticosteroids improve appetite and attitude, reduce inflammation and serum transaminase concentrations, and hinder fibrosis. Despite short-term improvement, corticosteroids do not alter survival time and the long-term prognosis remains poor. In horses, initial treatment with dexamethasone at the dose rate of 0.05 to 0.1 mg/kg/day for 4 to 7 days, followed by a gradual reduction in dose rate over 2 to 3 weeks, has been suggested.[122] Additional treatment with prednisolone (1 mg/kg/day) may be necessary for several additional weeks.

If the liver biopsy reveals cholangitis, long-term (4–6 weeks) antimicrobial therapy is indicated. The choice of antimicrobial is best determined by culture and sensitivity results. Antimicrobials that are excreted in bile, such as chloramphenicol and ampicillin, or broad-spectrum antimicrobials such as penicillin and gentamicin or trimethoprim-sulfonamide, are recommended.[57] The decision for corticosteroid therapy should be carefully scrutinized in these cases of CAH.

Prognosis. The prognosis for CAH is variable, depending on the cause and duration of disease. The presence of cirrhosis warrants a grave prognosis.

Cholelithiasis

Cholelithiasis, or the formation of biliary calculi, occasionally results in hepatocellular disease in horses. Hepatic failure and clinical signs occur when multiple stones are present or the common bile duct is occluded.

Clinical Signs. Cholelithiasis occurs most commonly in adult, middle-aged horses (6–15 years old), though horses as young as 5 years old have been affected.[57] The most frequently reported clinical signs include icterus, abdominal pain, fever, depression, and weight loss.[57, 123–125] Signs of hepatic failure, such as photosensitization, petechial hemorrhages, and hepatic encephalopathy, have been uncommonly reported.[126] Clinical signs are often intermittent unless the common bile duct is occluded, whereupon persistent abdominal pain prevails.

Pathogenesis. The initial step in the formation of a cholelith is precipitation or aggregation of normally soluble constituents of bile: bilirubin, cholesterol, or bile acids. In humans 75% of bile stones are composed principally of cholesterol and 25% are composed principally of calcium bilirubinate. The majority of calcium bilirubinate choleliths in humans are associated with bacterial cholangitis.[126, 127] The majority of choleliths in horses consist principally of calcium bilirubinate, and are associated with cholangitis.[57]

The exact sequence of events leading to precipitation of bilirubin in bile is not entirely known; however, soluble, conjugated bilirubin becomes unconjugated by the enzyme β-glucuronidase, then combines with calcium, a normal constituent of bile, to form calcium bilirubinate. Excessive formation of unconjugated bilirubin causes the formation of columnar complexes of calcium bilirubinate that subse-

quently precipitate. β-Glucuronidase is synthesized by the bile duct epithelium, hepatocytes, and certain bacteria. The concentration of β-glucuronidase is normally very low in bile, plus an inhibitor, glucaro-1,4-lactone, is usually present.

Whether bacterial, biliary, or hepatic in origin, increased bile concentration of β-glucuronidase has been demonstrated in humans with bacterial infection cholangitis.[127] Because the majority of choleliths in horses are composed of calcium bilirubinate and many affected horses with cholelithiasis have documented bacterial cholangitis, it seems logical that cholelith formation in horses most likely occurs subsequent to bacterial infection. Furthermore, because enteric organisms are most commonly isolated from horses with cholelithiasis, infection presumably ascends from the intestinal tract. Horses may be more prone to ascending infection because they lack an exit port sphincter to prevent backflow of intestinal contents into the biliary tree. If bile flow is decreased for any reason, retrograde flow and infection are likely. However, the correlation of infection with cholelithiasis in horses does not necessarily prove causation. It is also plausible that the sequence of events is the initial presence of a stone, precipitating cholestasis and subsequent infection. Despite its origin, cholangitis is the likely cause of fever. Chronic cholestasis due to the presence of choleliths results in increased biliary pressure, a likely cause of abdominal discomfort. If biliary pressure is not resolved, pressure-induced periportal hepatocellular necrosis with subsequent fibrosis ensues.

At necropsy, tissues are icteric and the liver is mottled in appearance. The liver appears enlarged following acute biliary obstruction, and shrunken and firm with chronic cholestasis. Choleliths range in size, are single or multiple in number, usually green-brown in color (bilirubinate), and smooth-textured. Histopathologic study reveals periportal hepatocellular necrosis, fibrosis, biliary stasis, and biliary hyperplasia. Suppurative cholangitis is often present. Organisms isolated from the liver or bile consist of mixed populations of gram-negative coliforms.[57] Nonobstructive choleliths are subclinical and only recognized at necropsy.

Diagnosis. Cholelithiasis should be considered in the differential diagnosis in any horse with a history of fever, icterus, and abdominal pain, especially if accompanied by signs of hepatic failure. Hematology sometimes reveals leukocytosis due to mature neutrophilia, especially if cholangitis is present.[57, 123] Other nonspecific findings may include hyperproteinemia and hyperfibrinogenemia.[57, 123] The most common abnormal laboratory findings suggest cholestatic liver disease and include markedly increased GGT (>15 times normal); hyperbilirubinemia, with the direct reacting fraction greater than 25% of the total value; and bilirubinuria.[57, 123, 126, 128] Although not liver-specific, SAP is often markedly increased. Less commonly, IDH, ARG, AST, and LDH-5 are mildly increased and clotting times and the BSP half-life are prolonged.[57, 123, 124, 128] Serum bile acids have not been fully evaluated in horses with cholelithiasis, but in those horses whose bile acid concentrations were determined, the values were significantly increased.

Hepatic ultrasonography is quite helpful in the diagnosis of cholethiasis.[57] In one retrospective study of cholelithiasis, all horses (N = 8) with cholelithiasis had visibly dilated bile ducts, which appeared as thin-walled, anechoic structures.[57] The liver appeared enlarged with increased echogenicity. This contrasts with normal horses, in which the bile ducts are not detectable. In six out of eight horses evaluated, choleliths were observed as hyperechoic areas within the bile ducts. Choleliths were most commonly seen at the level of the right sixth to seventh intercostal space.

Obtaining a liver biopsy is useful for diagnostic, therapeutic, and prognostic purposes. The histopathologic findings of periportal fibrosis, biliary stasis and hyperplasia, and cholangitis are not pathognomonic for cholelithiasis; however, a liver biopsy may help rule out other causes of biliary stasis such as chronic active hepatitis or megalocytic hepatopathy.

Treatment. If clinical signs of liver failure are present, general supportive care is indicated (see Treatment of Hepatic Insufficiency). If the common bile duct is occluded, surgical intervention is necessary. Although cholelithotripsy may be accomplished in humans percutaneously, via endoscopy or laparotomy, exploratory laparotomy currently is the only available means for reduction of a common bile duct obstruction in horses.[57] Both choledocholithotripsy (the crushing of choleliths in the bile ducts) and choledochotomy (surgical formation of an opening into the bile duct) have been successfully performed in the horse.[125, 126, 129] If multiple choleliths are distributed throughout the biliary tree, these cannot be removed by surgery.

If cholangitis is present, long-term (4–6 weeks) treatment with antimicrobials may be beneficial. Antimicrobial selection should be guided by bacterial isolation and sensitivity results, obtained either via a liver biopsy or culture of the bile or cholelith obtained at surgery. Trimethoprim-sulfonamide has been used successfully; chloramphenicol, ampicillin, and penicillin-gentamicin also have been recommended.[57, 126] Dissolution of cholesterol choleliths in humans has been successful with long-term administration of bile acids.[130] Because choleliths in horses are composed primarily of biliary pigments, treatment with bile acids would most likely be unavailing.

Prognosis. The prognosis of cholelithiasis depends on the extent of hepatic fibrosis, severity of clinical signs, and number and location of choleliths. Extensive fibrosis, multiple choleliths accompanied by clinical signs of hepatic failure, and severe hepatic encephalopathy warrant a poor prognosis. If obstruction of the bile duct by a single cholelith requires a choledochotomy, the prognosis is guarded because of limited access to the bile duct in a horse, and the risk of choleperitoneum.

Chronic Cholangiohepatitis and Biliary Fibrosis

These changes are most commonly associated with chronic active hepatitis, chronic cholangiohepatitis, cholelithiasis, and pancreatitis (see above). Liver failure rarely results from primary idiopathic cholangitis or biliary fibrosis.[63] Therapy is supportive. Treatment of bacterial cholangiohepatitis is discussed elsewhere (see Bacterial Hepatitis; Chronic Active Hepatitis; Cholelithiasis). The prognosis depends on the degree of fibrosis. Extensive fibrosis warrants a grave prognosis.

Neonatal Acquired Biliary Obstruction

Healing duodenal ulcers located adjacent to the hepatopancreatic ampulla in neonatal foals may result in extrahepatic biliary stenosis.[22, 131] Clinical signs are compatible with gastroduodenal obstruction and include reduced suckling reflex, depression, prolonged recumbency, colic, bruxism, and firm feces. Nasogastric intubation often produces voluminous reflux. Duodenal stenosis may be confirmed radiographically by delayed gastric emptying of barium sulfate. Biliary stenosis should be suspected if the serum concentrations of conjugated bilirubin and GGT are increased. Cholangiohepatitis may develop due to chronic cholestasis and may be confirmed by histopathologic examination of a liver biopsy. Acquired biliary stenosis must be differentiated from congenital biliary atresia (see p. 735). Successful surgical correction of acquired biliary stenosis secondary to duodenal stricture has been described.[131]

Chronic cholangiohepatitis without biliary stenosis, another potential sequela to duodenitis or duodenal ulceration, should be considered in icteric foals with increased serum concentrations of conjugated bilirubin and GGT.[22] The diagnosis is confirmed by histopathologic examination. Treatment should consist of long-term antimicrobial therapy, directed by bacterial isolation and sensitivity results (see Bacterial Hepatitis).

Hyperlipemia and Hepatic Lipidosis

Hyperlipemia occurs primarily in ponies and minature horses, and may lead to fatty infiltration of the liver, often accompanied by clinical signs of liver failure and a poor prognosis. In ponies and miniature horses, obesity, stress, inability to satisfy metabolic energy demands, and hormonal imbalance are the major precipitating factors for hyperlipemia.[132–135]

Epidemiology and Clinical Signs. Female ponies, especially Shetland ponies, and miniature horses are most susceptible to hyperlipemia. The ponies are usually obese and have a recent history of stress or weight loss. Hyperlipemia is more common in late gestation or early lactation, and occurs more frequently during the winter months.[65] The onset of clinical signs of hyperlipemia is often acute and includes icterus, anorexia, weakness, severe depression, ataxia, muscular weakness, diarrhea, mild colic, fever, and dependent edema.[65, 132, 134] In severe cases, clinical signs of hepatic failure may prevail (see Clinical Signs of Hepatic Insufficiency). Sudden death due to hepatic rupture may occur.[133]

Pathogenesis. The liver serves a unique role in energy homeostasis (see Physiology), especially in large animals in which volatile fatty acids, and not glucose, are a major energy source. Glucose is primarily manufactured in the liver from fatty acids and amino acids and is stored as glycogen for future use. If intake is decreased or energy demands are increased, glycogen stores become depleted, and the major source of energy is provided by fatty acid oxidation. Obesity sets the stage for hyperlipemia by providing excessive adipose tissue stores of fatty acids, available for immediate and rapid mobilization. Fatty acid mobilization is usually first triggered by a stress or inability to maintain energy homeostasis. Concurrent diseases, such as chronic infection, parasitism, or neoplasia, or any stressful event, like transport or weaning, may precipitate fatty acid mobilization. Stress increases the release of catecholamines and glucocorticoids, both of which stimulate fatty acid release from the adipose tissue. A negative energy balance, as may occur during late gestation, early lactation, starvation, or secondary to anorexia induced by some other primary disease, exacerbates hyperlipemia by further promoting fatty acid mobilization.

After lipolysis of adipose tissue triglyceride occurs, free fatty acids, nonesterified fatty acids, and glycerol are released into the blood. The glyceride, fatty acids bound to albumin, and nonesterified fatty acids are carried to the liver, where the glyceride is converted to glucose (see Fig. 13–3). In the liver, fatty acids may be oxidized to acetyl coenzyme A and used in the tricarboxylic acid cycle; used in gluconeogenesis; resynthesized to triglycerides and stored in the liver; or used to make triglycerides that are released into the sinusoidal blood as VLDL (see Fig. 13–3). If the oxaloacetate supply is limited, acetyl coenzyme A is shuttled away from the tricarboxylic acid cycle and used to make ketone bodies. Because the equine liver is quite efficient in synthesizing triglycerides and exporting VLDL, hepatic lipidosis and ketosis are less common than in other species.[135] However, when fatty acid mobilization and synthesis of triglycerides exceed oxidation and VLDL formation, hepatic lipidosis ensues. Fat infiltration disrupts hepatic function and excessive amounts of fat in the liver can result in hepatic failure and even hepatic rupture.[133]

Hormonal factors may contribute to the development of hyperlipemia and hepatic lipidosis. Insulin normally impedes the development of hyperlipemia by inhibiting tissue hormone-sensitive lipase, the enzyme responsible for lipolysis of adipose tissue. Insulin also curtails the development of hyperlipemia by stimulating gluconeogenesis in the liver and by activating lipoprotein lipase, the endothelial enzyme responsible for adipose tissue uptake of fatty acid from VLDL in the blood. Despite often normal insulin levels, ponies appear to have a relative tissue insulin insensitivity compared with horses.[133] Considering the effects of insulin on fat metabolism, it is not surprising that ponies are more susceptible than horses to the development of hyperlipemia. Glucocorticoids, catecholamines, and progesterone may contribute to the development of hyperlipemia by opposing the biological actions of insulin (see Fig. 13–3). This may account for the high incidence of hyperlipemia during periods of increased cortisol levels (stress, pituitary adenoma, late pregnancy) and increased progesterone (pregnancy).

Necropsy findings include widespread fatty change in the liver, skeletal muscle, kidney, adrenal cortex, and myocardium.[65, 133] The liver and kidney are enlarged, yellow, friable, and greasy. One of every five ponies with hepatic lipidosis has a ruptured liver.[133] Microscopically, hepatocytes are engorged with lipid. The nucleus is often displaced and hepatocellular necrosis may ensue.

Vascular thrombosis can occur secondary to hyperlipemia and fat embolism, and may be seen in the lung, kidney, brain, and subcutaneous vessels. Subcutaneous thrombosis causes dependent edema. Renal nephrosis and necrotizing pancreatitis are sometimes present.[65, 133] Renal disease most likely is a sequela of occlusive thrombosis. The exact cause of pancreatitis is not known; however, hyperlipemia precedes pancreatitis. It is speculated that excessive lipid is deposited in and around the pancreas, which is subsequently hydrolyzed by pancreatic lipase, and released as free fatty acids. Free (unbound to albumin) fatty acids are cytotoxic and when the albumin binding capacity is exceeded, pancreatic vascular injury occurs.[136]

Compared with ponies and miniature horses, hyperlipemia rarely develops in horses, though *hyperlipidemia* (trigylcerides <500 mg/dL) may develop during azotemia.[134, 137] Azotemia prevents lipid removal from the blood by inhibiting lipoprotein lipase. The degree of hyperlipidemia is directly correlated with the degree of azotemia.[137] Mild hepatic lipidosis may ensue, but hyperlipidemia rarely results in clinically recognizable disease.

Diagnosis. Hyperlipemia should be considered in the differential diagnosis for any obese pony or miniature horse with clinical signs of severe depression, anorexia, ataxia, and icterus. The blood grossly appears opalescent. The blood concentrations of all lipids are increased, especially triglycerides (>500 mg/dl), nonesterified fatty acids, and VLDLs. Laboratory evidence of hepatic failure may include increased serum concentrations of IDH, GGT, bilirubin, and ammonia, and decreased glucose, BUN, and albumin.[132] The BSP half-life is prolonged. Oral and intravenous glucose challenge tests may reveal glucose intolerance due to insulin insensitivity. Metabolic ketoacidosis should be suspected if the anion gap is increased. A definitive diagnosis of hepatic lipidosis is confirmed by the concurrent demonstration of increased blood concentrations of lipid, laboratory evidence of hepatic dysfunction, and histopathologic findings of fatty infiltration in the liver. The serum concentrations of creatinine and electrolytes should be determined as an adjunct to therapy.

Treatment. The major therapeutic objectives for hyperlipemia and hepatic lipidosis include (1) treatment of hepatic failure, (2) improvement of energy intake and balance, (3) elimination of stress or treatment of concurrent disease, (4) inhibition of fat mobilization from adipose tissue, and (5) increased triglyceride uptake by peripheral tissues. Treatment of hepatic failure is addressed elsewhere (see Treatment of Hepatic Insufficiency). Intake of concentrated carbohydrate feed, such as molasses-coated grain and high-quality pasture or hay, should be encouraged. Anorectic ponies should receive 5% dextrose as a continuous infusion at a rate of 2 mL/kg/hour and gavage with gruel should be attempted. Blood glucose concentrations should be closely monitored since some ponies have glucose intolerance and excessive glucose will worsen acidosis and induce hypokalemia. Weaning suckling foals may help reduce stress and the energy demand imposed on lactating mares. Concurrent diseases amenable to therapy, such as parasitism, chronic infection, and musculoskeletal disease, should be appropriately treated with anthelmintics, antimicrobials, or analgesics, respectively.

In addition to supplying immediate energy, glucose therapy stimulates the release of insulin. Concurrent carbohydrate and insulin administration have been used successfully to manage hyperlipemia in ponies.[132, 138] The following regimen has been suggested for a 200-kg pony.[138] Day 1: Administer 30 IU of protamine zinc insulin IM and 100 g of glucose PO, both twice-daily; day 2: administer 15 IU of insulin IM twice-daily, and 100 g of galactose once. Galactose is slowly converted to glucose, thus lactic acid production is minimized. This regimen may be continued for 3 days. Blood glucose and insulin concentrations should be closely monitored. Nicotinic acid, thought to act by inhibiting of hormone-sensitive lipase, has been used in cattle with fatty liver; however, nicotinic acid has not been evaluated in ponies with hepatic lipidosis.

Heparin potentiates the activity of lipoprotein lipase and may increase triglyceride removal from the blood. Recommended dosages range from 100 to 250 IU/kg twice-daily,[138] but dosages as low as 40 IU/kg are temporarily beneficial.[132] Because of the potential for hemorrhage, heparin therapy should be used with discretion and monitored by daily hemostatic testing. If present, azotemia, acidosis, and electrolyte abnormalities should be addressed with appropriate fluid therapy.

It is unlikely that lipotropic agents, such as choline and methionine, are useful in horses with hyperlipemia, as triglyceride synthesis in the liver is usually sufficient.

Prognosis and Client Education. The prognosis of hyperlipemia is poor. Mortality has been estimated to occur in 60% to 100% of the cases.[132, 133] Prevention is best achieved by providing appropriate nutrition without inducing obesity, avoiding stress, and practicing good routine health care.

Hepatic Abscessation

Liver abscessation is uncommon in horses. Clinical signs of hepatic abscessation depend on the extent and location of the abscess(es); however, abscesses are unlikely to result in hepatic failure. Small solitary abscesses or multifocal microabscesses usually remain subclinical. Larger abscesses may be accompanied by weight loss, intermittent fever, and anorexia.

Hepatic abscessation in foals may be hematogenous in origin as a sequela to bacteremia, or ascending through the umbilical vein as a sequela to omphalophlebitis.[139] In the adult, bacteremia is uncommon and hepatic infection or abscessation more likely originates in the intestinal lumen and ascends the bile duct, or originates in the intestinal wall or mesenteric lymph nodes and carried to the liver via the portal blood. The latter is a likely sequela to primary abdominal or mesenteric abscessation due to *Streptococcus equi.* In one retrospective study of abdominal abscesses in horses, only 2 of 25 horses had solely hepatic abcesses, though some horses had abscesses involving several abdominal structures.[140]

Laboratory diagnosis of hepatic abscessation is difficult. Smaller abscesses may not result in sufficient hepatocellular damage to impede liver function. Laboratory abnormalities characteristic of chronic inflammation and infection, including anemia of chronic disease, hyperfibrinogenemia, hypergammaglobulinemia, and mature neutrophilia, may be seen with larger abscesses. Increased concentrations of liver-specific cytosolic enzymes or bile acids, or both, rarely occur.

Ultrasonography of the liver may reveal a focal hyperechoic area. A liver biopsy should be guided by ultrasound to avoid penetration of the abscess. Long-term antimicrobial therapy should be directed by culture and sensitivity results. Common isolates from abdominal abscesses in horses include *S. equi, Streptococcus zooepidemicus,* and *Corynebacterium pseudotuberculosis.*[140]

Hepatic Neoplasia

Primary hepatic neoplasia is quite rare in horses. A retrospective survey in 1952 indicated that hepatic tumors accounted for only 0.74% of all equine neoplasms.[141] Of the documented primary hepatic neoplasms in horses (cholangiocarcinoma, hepatocellular carcinoma, hepatoblastoma, and mixed hamartoma), cholangiocarcinoma is the most common.[64, 81, 82, 141–145] Hepatic neoplasia in horses is more likely to occur secondary to metastasis of some other primary tumor, especially lymphosarcoma.[2] Because clinical signs of hepatic failure usually are not apparent and laboratory findings are nonspecifically indicative of chronic inflammatory disease, antemortem diagnosis of hepatic neoplasia is difficult.

In one report, *cholangiocarcinoma* accounted for 9 of 10 primary liver neoplasms in horses.[141] Cholangiocarcinoma originates from the bile duct epithelium and is distinguished from hepatocellular carcinoma by its tendency to form multiple foci, its firm texture, and a whitish color produced by abundant fibrous stroma. The primary mass is typically solitary, with multiple intrahepatic secondaries. Extrahepatic metastasis is common with transperitoneal lymphatic spread to the peritoneum and diaphragm, and hematogenous spread to the lungs.[143] In humans, dogs, and cats, there is an etiologic relationship with liver fluke infestation.[143] Microscopically, cholangiocarcinoma is adenocarcinomatous, producing cuboidal or columnar-lined ductules and acini. The neoplastic bile ducts do not contain bile, but may contain mucus.

The clinical presentation and progression of cholangiocarcinoma in horses is not well documented, but it appears to be more common in older horses.[141] One case report describes a 10-year-old mixed-breed horse in which the presenting signs included anorexia, weight loss, pyrexia, mild icterus, tachypnea, severe dependent edema, and abdominal distention.[145] Abnormal clinicopathologic findings included mature neutrophilia; hyperfibrinogenemia; anemia; moderately increased serum bilirubin, GGT, and IDH concentrations; and nonseptic peritonitis and pleuritis. Neoplastic cells were not detected in the body cavity effusions. Definitive antemortem diagnosis of cholangiocarcinoma was made by histopathologic examination of a liver biopsy. Necropsy revealed multiple extrahepatic metastases, including the serosal surfaces of the intestine and spleen, diaphragm, omentum, pleural surfaces, and lung.

Hepatocellular carcinoma, or hepatoma, has been reported in three horses, all less than 3 years of age.[81, 82, 144] Hepatocellular carcinomas are usually solitary and multilobulated. Extrahepatic metastasis occurs transperitoneally and hematogenously to lungs. Microscopically, the neoplastic cells resemble hepatocytes and retain cord arrangement. However, the normal liver architecture is lost and sometimes the cells are difficult to differentiate. Mitotic figures are uncommon.

Possible etiologic factors in other species include heredity, parasitism, chemical and plant carcinogens, and viral hepatitis.[143]

Reported clinical signs of hepatocellular carcinoma in horses include depression, anorexia, weight loss, intermittent diarrhea, and abdominal distention.[81, 82, 144] Abnormal laboratory findings included absolute erythrocytosis, persistent hypoglycemia, sanguineous peritoneal effusion, and increased serum concentrations of IDH, GGT, SAP, and indirect reacting bilirubin. In one case, absolute erythrocytosis was attributed to erythropoietin secretion by the carcinoma (inappropriate secondary erythrocytosis).[82] The same horse had a high serum concentration of alpha-fetoprotein, a globulin normally synthesized only by embryonic fetal liver cells that is commonly detectable in human patients with hepatocellular carcinoma.

There is one case report of a three-year-old appaloosa gelding with malignant *hepatoblastoma*.[64] Clinical signs included emaciation, pyrexia, and pleural effusion. Laboratory abnormalities included mature neutrophilia, hypergammaglobulinemia, hyperfibrinogenemia, and increased serum concentrations of GGT and ASP. Necropsy revealed a large solitary hepatoblastoma, with several satellite nodules throughout the liver. Metastasis occurred to the omentum, mesentery, and lung. Histologically, the neoplastic cells consisted of mixed mesenchymal and epithelial cell types.

A *mixed hamartoma* was described in the liver of a late-term aborted equine fetus.[142] Histologically, the lesion appeared to be a proliferation of large hepatocyte-like cells with eccentric nuclei and voluminous cytoplasm; abnormal bile ducts; and fibroblastic fibrocystic interstitial tissue, with complete lack of structural organization.

Hepatic Amyloidosis

Amyloidosis refers to a group of diseases that are characterized by the extracellular deposition of a proteinaceous fibril substance, *amyloid,* in the tissues. Amyloid deposits are composed of nonbranching fibrils in β-pleated sheet conformation formed by the proteolytic cleavage of precursor proteins by the mononuclear phagocyte system. Depending on the organ of deposition, amyloid distorts normal tissue architecture and may lead to functional impairment. In horses, the liver and spleen are the most common organs involved in systemic amyloidosis.[55] Two forms of systemic amyloidosis exist and are distinguished by the type of precursor protein and subsequent protein fibril. The precursor in *reactive* or *secondary* systemic amyloidosis is serum amyloid protein AA, an acute phase protein produced by hepatocytes in response to chronic infection or inflammation. The AA fibrils are identified in tissues by green birefringence in polarized light, after staining with Congo red, which is lost after treatment with potassium permanganate. Most often in horses, hepatic amyloid deposits are AA fibrils and have been associated with severe parasitism or chronic infection and inflammation.[55, 146] One horse in which the liver was the principal organ of amyloid deposition presented for evaluation of chronic weight loss.[146] An antemortem diagnosis of hepatic amyloidosis was not made; however, laboratory abnormalities included severe hypoalbuminemia, polyclonal gammopathy, and large numbers of ascarid and strongylid eggs in the feces. Histopathologically, the liver revealed extracellular deposits of AA amyloid periportally and adjacent to the sinusoids in the space of Disse. The amyloid deposits were accompanied by hepatocytic atrophy and a mild mononuclear cell infiltrate.

Systemic primary, immunocytic, or *idiopathic amyloidosis* is due to the deposition of AL (amyloid light chain) fibrils. The precursor proteins in primary amyloidosis are the variable region of immunoglobulin light chains. The AL fibrils also stain with Congo red, but staining is retained after potassium permanganate treatment. *Local immunocytic amyloidosis,* with deposition in the upper respiratory mucosa or skin, is more common in horses than systemic primary amyloidosis. However, there is at least one reported case of systemic primary amyloidosis in a 14-year-old Thoroughbred mare, which presented for chronic weight loss and cutaneous nodules.[147] Amyloid (AL) deposits were identified in the liver, myocardium, spleen, gastrointestinal mucosa, pulmonary interstitium, pancreas, and arterial walls.

Hypoxemia

Right-sided heart failure causes the pressure in the caudal vena cava to rise. Retrograde pressure increases in the hepatic central veins cause hypoxemia and pressure necrosis of the adjacent hepatocytes. Chronic passive congestion may cause fatty change, atrophy, and fibrosis.

Congenital Abnormalities
Portosystemic Shunt

Portosystemic shunts may be intrahepatic or extrahepatic, congenital or acquired. There have been few reports of documented congenital extrahepatic portosystemic shunts in foals.[84, 148] The vascular shunts allow blood within the portal system to bypass the liver and drain into the systemic circulation, directly or indirectly, via the caudal vena cava or the azygous vein. In the reported cases, age at presentation varied between 2 and 6 months. Vague intermittent neurologic signs of blindness, ataxia, and severe depression were consistent with hepatic encephalopathy. Growth appeared to be stunted. These clinical signs are due to the altered hepatic blood flow and hepatic insufficiency secondary to hepatocellular atrophy.

Laboratory abnormalities in the reported cases varied, but the most consistent findings included a decreased BUN, prolonged BSP half-life, and increased blood ammonia concentration. Liver biopsies revealed hepatocellular atrophy and necrosis, fibrosis, and biliary hyperplasia.[84] Antemortem diagnosis was confirmed by operative mesenteric portography (see Diagnostic Imaging of the Liver). Surgical correction was unsuccessfully attempted in one case.[149] Necropsy examination revealed small firm livers. The location of the shunt(s) in reported cases was variable, but all were extrahepatic, involving a direct connection between the mesenteric veins and the caudal vena cava. Alzheimer type II astrocytes were seen in the brain in one case and were consistent with hepatic encephalopathy.[148]

Acquired portosystemic shunts are rare in horses. There is one report of an 11-year-old Thoroughbred presented with hepatic encephalopathy that subsequently was determined to have a functional portosystemic shunt secondary to vascular thrombosis of the portal vein.[149]

Biliary Atresia

There have been at least two documented cases of extrahepatic biliary atresia in foals.[150, 151] An antemortem diagnosis was not possible in either case; however, veterinary attention was sought at 4 weeks of age in both foals for anorexia, depression, lethargy, poor weight gain, colic, polydipsia, polyuria, pyrexia, and icterus. Laboratory evaluation of one of the foals was consistent with biliary obstruction, as indicated by a mildly increased serum concentration of IDH, and markedly increased concentrations of GGT and conjugated bilirubin.[151] Necropsy of both foals revealed a large, firm liver. Although not specifically documented in one case, both the entrance to the bile duct and the main bile duct were absent in the other foal.[151] Histologically, both livers appeared similar and consistent with extrahepatic biliary atresia. Bile canaliculi were present and distended, with associated degenerative hepatocytes. Biliary proliferation was extensive and surrounded by fibrous tissue with interdispersed islands of hepatocytes. There was no bile in the proliferative bile ducts and the portal triad ducts were absent.

In horses, it is speculated that extrahepatic biliary atresia is congenital. In humans, other causes suggested include neonatal sclerosing cholangiohepatitis, excretion of a biliary toxin, deficit of bile flow in utero, or lumen destruction due to ductal vascular insufficiency.[152] Despite the cause, extrahepatic biliary atresia induces intrahepatic biliary hypertrophy, an abortive attempt to establish continuity. The biliary hypertrophy displaces hepatocytes, causing periportal and perilobular hepatocellular degeneration, fibrous replacement, and ultimately, loss of normal hepatic architecture. Although an antemortem diagnosis was not possible in either equine case, hepatobiliary scintigraphy (see Diagnostic Imaging of the Liver) successfully detected total biliary obstruction in a neonatal lamb with biliary atresia.[85]

Serous Cysts

Serous hepatic cysts have been reported and usually are an incidental finding at necropsy.[17]

REFERENCES

1. Sisson S: Equine digestive tract. In Getty R, ed: *Sisson and Grossman's The Anatomy of Domestic Animals.* Philadelphia, WB Saunders, 1975, p 454.
2. Rantanen NW: *Diagnostic Ultrasound.* Philadelphia, WB Saunders, 1986, p 105.
3. Ham AW: *Histology.* Philadelphia, WB Saunders, 1974, p 686.
4. Iber FL: Normal and pathologic physiology of the liver. In Sodeman WA, Sodeman TM, eds: *Sodeman's Pathologic Physiology: Mechanisms of Disease.* Philadelphia, WB Saunders, 1985, p 875.
5. Lehninger AL: *Biochemistry.* New York, Worth, 1975, p 829.
6. Guyton AC: *Guyton Textbook of Medical Physiology.* Philadelphia, WB Saunders, 1986, p 937.
7. Guyton AC: *Guyton Textbook of Medical Physiology.* Philadelphia, WB Saunders, 1986, p 923.
8. Guyton AC: *Guyton Textbook of Medical Physiology.* Philadelphia, WB Saunders, 1986, p 909.
9. Guyton AC: *Guyton Textbook of Medical Physiology.* Philadelphia, WB Saunders, 1986, p 897.
10. McDermott WV: Metabolism and toxicity of ammonia. *N Engl J Med* 257:1076, 1957.
11. Lehninger AL: *Biochemistry.* New York, Worth, 1975, p 559.
12. Duncan JR, Prasse KW: *Veterinary Laboratory Medicine.* Ames, Iowa University Press, 1986, p 105.
13. Lehninger AL: *Biochemistry.* New York, Worth, 1975, p 543.
14. Engelking LR: Evaluation of equine bilirubin and bile acid metabolism. *Compend Contin Educ Pract Vet* 11:328, 1989.
15. Coles EH: *Veterinary Clinical Pathology.* Philadelphia, WB Saunders, 1988, p 129.
16. Coles EH: *Veterinary Clinical Pathology.* Philadelphia, WB Saunders, 1988, p 171.
17. MacLachlan NJ, Cullen JM: Liver, biliary system, and exocrine pancreas. In Thompson RG, ed: *Special Veterinary Pathology.* Philadelphia, BC Decker, 1988, p 229.
18. Papich MG, Davis LE: *Liver Disease.* Philadelphia, WB Saunders, 1985, p 77.
19. Reed S, Andrews FM. The biochemical evaluation of liver function in the horse. *Proc 32nd Ann Conv Am Assoc Equine Pract,* 1986, p 81.
20. Duncan JR, Prasse KW: *Veterinary Laboratory Medicine.* Ames, Iowa State University Press, 1986, pp 121–132.
21. Engelking LR, Paradis MR: Evaluation of hepatobiliary disease in the horse. In Doxey DL, ed: *Clinical Pathology and Diagnostic Procedures.* Philadelphia, WB Saunders, 1987, p 563.
22. Divers TJ: Liver disease and liver failure in horses. *Proc 29th Ann Conv Am Assoc Equine Pract,* 1983, p 213.
23. Fraser CL, Arieff AI: Hepatic encephalopathy. *N Engl J Med* 313:865, 1985.
24. Gammal SH, Jones EA: Hepatic encephalopathy. *Med Clin North Am* 73:793, 1989.
25. Scharschmidt BF: Acute and chronic hepatic failure and hepatic transplantation. In Wyngaarden JB, Smith LN, eds: *Cecil Textbook of Medicine.* Philadelphia, WB Saunders, 1988, p 852.
26. Zieve L: Hepatic encephalopathy. In Schiff L, Schiff ER, eds: *Diseases of the Liver.* Philadelphia, JB Lippincott, 1987, p 925.
27. Zieve L: Hepatic encephalopathy. In Schiff L, Schiff ER, eds: *Diseases of the Liver.* Philadelphia, JB Lippincott, 1982, p 433.
28. Lockwood AH, MacDonald JM, Reiman RE, et al: The dynamics of ammonia metabolism in man. Effects of liver disease and hyperammonemia. *J Clin Invest* 63:449, 1979.
29. Flannery DB, Hsia YE, Wolf B: Current status of hyperammonemia syndromes. *Hepatology* 2:495, 1982.
30. Bode J, Schafer K: Pathophysiology of chronic hepatic encephalopathy. *Hepatopathy* 32:259, 1985.
31. Lockwood AH: Ammonia-induced encephalopathy. In McCandless DW, ed: *Cerebral Energy Metabolism and Metabolic Energy.* New York, Plenum Press, 1985, p 203.
32. Bessman SP, Bessman AN: The cerebral and peripheral uptake of ammonia in liver disease with a hypothesis for the mechanism of hepatic coma. *J Clin Invest* 34:622, 1975.
33. Crossley IR, Wardle EN, Willams R: Biochemical mechanisms of hepatic encephalopathy. *Clin Sci* 64:247, 1983.
34. Pappas SC, Ferenci P, Scafer DF, et. al.: Visual evoked potentials in rabbit model of hepatic encephalopathy. II. Comparison of hyperammonemic encephalopathy, postictal coma and coma induced by synergic neurotoxins. *Gastroenterology* 86:546, 1984.

35. Cohn R, Castell DO: The effect of acute hyperammonemia on the encephalogram. *J Lab Clin Med* 68:195, 1966.

36. Jones EA, Schafer DF, Ferenci P, et al: The neurobiology of hepatic encephalopathy. *Hepatology* 4:1235, 1984.

37. Record CO, Mardini H, Bartlett K: Blood and brain mercaptan concentrations in hepatic encephalopathy. *Hepatology* 2:144, 1982.

38. Fischer JE, Baldessarine RJ: False neurotransmitters in hepatic failure. *Lancet* 2:75, 1971.

39. Gulick BA, Rogers QR, Knight HD: Plasma amino acid patterns in horses with hepatic disease. *Proc 21st Ann Conv Am Assoc Equine Pract*, 1978, p 517.

40. Alexander WF, Spinder E, Harty RF, et al: The usefulness of branched chain fatty acids with acute or chronic hepatic encephalopathy. *Am J Gastroenterol* 84:91, 1989.

41. Zieve L, Olsen RL: Can hepatic coma be caused by a reduction of brain noradrenalin or dopamine? *Gut* 18:688, 1977.

42. Morgan MY, Milson PJ, Sherlock S: Plasma ratio of valine, leucine, and isoleucine to phenylalanine, tyrosine in liver disease. *Gut* 19:1068, 1978.

43. Uribe M, Garcia-Ramos G, et al: Standard and higher doses of bromocriptine for severe chronic portal-systemic encephalopathy. *Am J Gastroenterol* 78:517, 1983.

44. Ferenci P, Jones EA, Hanbauer I: Lack of evidence for impaired dopamine receptor function in experimental hepatic coma in the rabbit. *Neuroscience* 65:60, 1986.

45. Tallman JF, Gallager DW: The GABA-ergic system: A locus of benzodiazepine action. *Annu Rev Neurosci* 8:21, 1985.

46. Levy LJ, Leek J, Losowsky MS: Evidence of gamma-aminobutyric acid as the inhibitor of gamma-aminobutyric binding in the plasma of humans with liver disease and hepatic encephalopathy. *Hepatogastroenterology* 32:171, 1987.

47. Bassett ML, Mullen KD, Schoolz B, et al: Increased brain GABA uptake in pre-coma encephalopathy in rabbit model of fulminant hepatic failure. *J Lab Clin Med* 102:870, 1985.

48. Schafer DF, Fowler JM, Jone EA: Colonic bacteria: A source of gamma-aminobutyric acid in blood. *Proc Soc Exp Biol Med* 167:301, 1981.

49. Madison JE, Dodd PR, Johnston GA, et al: Brain GABA receptor binding is normal in rats with thioacetamide induced hepatic encephalopathy despite elevated plasma GABA-like activity. *Gastroenterology* 93:1062, 1987.

50. Olsen SW, Wong EH, Staufer GB, et al: Biochemial pharmacology of the GABA receptor/ionophore protein. *FASEB J* 43:2773, 1984.

51. Study R, Barker J: Diazepam and (−) pentobarbital: Fluctuation analysis reveals different mechanisms for potentiation of gamma-aminobutyric acid responses in cultured central neurons. *Proc Natl Acad Sci U S A* 77:7486, 1981.

52. Basile AS, Gammal SH, Mullen KD: Differential responsiveness of cerebellar Purkinje neurons to GABA and benzodiazepine ligands in an animal model of hepatic encephalopathy in man. *J Neurosci* 8:2414, 1988.

53. Bassett ML, Mullen K, Skolnick P, et al: Amelioration of hepatic encephalopathy by pharmacologic antagonism of the GABA-A-benzodiazepine receptor complex in a rabbit model of fulminant heptic failure. *Gastroenterology* 93:1069, 1987.

54. Bauer JE, Asquith RL, Kivipelto J: Serum biochemical indicators of liver function in neonatal foals. *Am J Vet Res* 50:2037, 1989.

55. Andel AC, Gruys E, Kroneman J: Amyloid in the horse: A report of nine cases. *Equine Vet J* 20:277, 1988.

56. Scott DW: *Large Animal Dermatology.* Philadelphia, WB Saunders, 1988, p 65.

57. Johnston JK, Divers TJ, Reef VB, et al: Cholelithiasis in horses: Ten cases (1982–1986). *J Am Vet Med Assoc* 194:405, 1989.

58. Ratnoff OD: Disordered hemostasis in hepatic disease. In Schiff L, Schiff ER, eds: *Diseases of the Liver.* Philadelphia, JB Lippincott, 1987, p 187.

59. Valli VE: The hematopoietic system. In Jubb KVF, Kennedy PJ, Palmer N, eds: *Pathology of Domestic Animals.* Orlando, Fla, Academic Press, 1985, p 83.

60. Johnstone IB: Antithrombin III activity in normal and diseased horses. *Vet Clin Pathol* 17:20, 1988.

61. Gay CC, Lording PM, McNeil P, et al: Infectious necrotic hepatitis (black disease) in a horse. *Equine Vet J* 12:27, 1980.

62. Tennant BC, Hornbuckle WE: Diseases of the liver. In Anderson NV, ed: *Veterinary Gastroenterology.* Philadelphia, Lea & Febiger, 1980, p 593.

63. Tennant B: Acute hepatitis in horses: Problems of differentiating toxic and infectious causes in the adult. *Proc 21st Ann Conv Am Assoc Equine Pract*, 1978, p 465.

64. Prater PE, Patton CS, Held JP: Pleural effusion resulting from malignant hepatoblastoma in a horse. *J Am Vet Med Assoc* 194:383, 1989.

65. Gay CC, Sullivan ND, Wilkinson JS, et al: Hyperlipaemia in ponies. *Aust Vet J* 54:459, 1978.

66. Carlson GP. Chronic active hepatitis in horses. In *7th American College of Veterinary Internal Medicine Proceedings*, San Diego, May, 1989, p 595.

67. Pearson EG: Hypoalbuminemia in horses. *Compend Contin Educ Pract Vet* 12:555, 1990.

68. Epstein M: Renal complications in liver disease. In Schiff L, Schiff ER, eds: *Diseases of the Liver.* Philadelphia, JB Lippincott, 1987, p 903.

69. Byars TD: Chronic liver failure. In Robinson NE, ed: *Current Therapy in Equine Medicine.* Philadelphia, WB Saunders, 1987, p 112.

70. Mendle VE: Pyrrolizidine alkaloid-induced liver disease in horses: An early diagnosis. *Am J Vet Res* 49:572, 1988.

71. Pearson EW, Craig AM: Serum bile acids for diagnosis of chronic liver disease in horses. In *4th American College of Veterinary Internal Medicine Proceedings,* Washington, DC, 1986, May, p 10.

72. West HJ: Evaluation of total plasma bile acid concentration for the diagnosis of hepatobiliary disease in horses. *Res Vet Sci* 46:264, 1989.

73. Hoffman WE, Baker G, Rieser S, et al: Alterations in selected serum biochemical constituents in equids after induced hepatic disease. *Am J Vet Res* 48:1343, 1987.

74. Feldman BF: Acquired disorders of hemostasis. In *7th American College of Veterinary Internal Medicine Proceedings,* San Diego, May, 1989, p 33.

75. Badylak SF: *Hemostasis.* Philadelphia, WB Saunders, 1988, p 87.

76. Ockner RK: Hepatic metabolism in liver disease. In Wyngaarden JB, Smith LH, eds: *Cecil Textbook of Internal Medicine.* Philadelphia, WB Saunders, 1985, p 804.

77. Gossett KA, French DD: Effect of age on liver enzyme activities in serum of healthy quarter horses. *Am J Vet Res* 45:354, 1984.

78. Bernard W, Divers TJ, Ziemer E: Isoenzyme 5 of lactate dehydrogenase as an indicator of equine hepatocellular disease. *Vet Clin Pathol* 17:19, 1988.

79. Engelking LR, Answer MS, Lofstedt J: Hepatobiliary transport of indocyanine green and bromosulphthalein in fedland fasted horses. *Am J Vet Res* 46:2278, 1985.

80. West HJ: Clearance of bromosulphthalein from plasma as a measure of hepatic function on normal horses and in horses with liver disease. *Res Vet Sci* 44:343, 1988.

81. Jeffcott LB: Primary liver-cell carcinoma in a young thoroughbred horse. *J Pathol* 97:394, 1968.

82. Roby AA, Beech J, Bloom JC, Black M: Hepatocellular carcinoma associated with erythrocytosis and hypoglycemia in a yearling. *J Am Vet Med Assoc* 196:465, 1990.

83. Modransky PD: *Diagnostic Ultrasound.* Philadelphia, WB Saunders, 1986, p 115.
84. Buonanno AM, Carlson GP, Kantrowitz B: Clinical and diagnostic features of portosystemic shunt in a foal. *J Am Vet Med Assoc* 192:387, 1988.
85. Lofstedt J, Koblik PD, Jakowski RM, et al.: Use of hepatobiliary scintigraphy to diagnose bile duct atresia in a lamb. *J Am Vet Med Assoc* 193:95, 1988.
86. Carlson GP: The liver. In Mansmann RA, McAllister ES, Pratt PW, eds: *Equine Medicine and Surgery.* Santa Barbara, Calif, American Veterinary Publications, 1982, p 633.
87. Divers TJ: Therapy of liver failure. In Smith BP, ed: *Large Animal Internal Medicine.* St Louis, Mosby–Year Book, 1990, p 869.
88. Farivar M, Wands JR, Isselbacher KJ, et al: Beneficial effects of insulin and glucagon in fulminant murine viral hepatitis. *Lancet* 1:696, 1979.
89. Ohkawa M, Hayashi H, Chaudry IH, et al: Effects of regenerating liver cytosol on drug-induced hepatic failure. *Surgery* 97:455, 1985.
90. Ferenci P, Grimm G, Meryn S, et al: Successful long-term treatment of portal-systemic encephalopathy by the benzodiazepam antagonist flumazenil. *Gastroenterology* 96:240, 1989.
91. Theiler A: Acute liver atrophy and parenchymatous hepatitis in horses. In *Fifth and Sixth Research Directory of Veterinary Research, Department of Agriculture, Union of South Africa,* 1917 p 9.
92. Madsen DE: Equine encephalomyelitis. *Utah Acad Sci Arts Lett* 11:95, 1934.
93. Marsh H: Supplementary note to article on equine encephalomyelitis. *J Am Vet Med Assoc* 91:330, 1937.
94. Ockner RK: Acute viral hepatitis. In Wyngaarden JB, Smith LH, eds: *Cecil Textbook of Internal Medicine.* Philadelphia, WB Saunders, 1985, p 831.
95. Robinson M, Gopinth C, Hughes DL: Histopathology of acute hepatitis in the horse. *J Comp Pathol* 85:111, 1975.
96. Thomsett LR: Acute hepatic failure in a horse. *Equine Vet J* 3:15, 1971.
97. Tyzzer EE: A fatal disease of Japanese Waltzing mice caused by a spore-bearing bacillus. *J Med Res* 37:307, 1917.
98. Swerczek TW, Crowe MW, Prickett ME, et al: Focal bacterial hepatitis in foals. *Mod Vet Pract* 54:66, 1973.
99. Humber KA, Sweeney RW, Saik JE, et al: Clinical and clinicopathologic findings in two foals infected with *Bacillus piliformis. J Am Vet Med Assoc* 193:1425, 1988.
100. Turk MA, Gallina AM, Perryman LE: *Bacillus piliformis* infection (Tyzzer's disease) in foals in northwest United States: A retrospective study of 21 cases. *J Am Vet Med Assoc* 178:279, 1981.
101. Carrigan MJ, Pedrana RG, McKibbin AW: Tyzzer's disease in foals. *Aust Vet J* 61:199, 1984.
102. Sweeney HJ, Greg A: Infectious necrotic hepatitis in a horse. *Equine Vet J* 18:150, 1986.
103. Hollingsworth TC, Green VJ: Focal necrotizing hepatitis caused by *Clostridium novyi* in a horse. *Aust Vet J* 54:48, 1978.
104. Dumaresq JA: A case of black disease in the horse. *Aust Vet J* 15:53, 1939.
105. Schulz KS, Simmons TR, Johnson R: Primary cholangiohepatitis in a horse. *Cornell Vet* 80:35, 1990.
106. Thornberg LP, Kintner LD: Cholangiohepatitis in a horse. *Vet Med Small Anim Clin* 75:1895, 1980.
107. Hartley WJ, Dixon RJ: An outbreak of foal perinatal mortality due to equid herpesvirus type 1: Pathologic observations. *Equine Vet J* 11:214, 1979.
108. Claybough D: Equine infectious anemia: The clinical signs, transmission, and diagnostic procedures. *Vet Med* 85:1007, 1990.
109. Blood DC, Radostits OM: *Veterinary Medicine: A Textbook of the Diseases of Cattle, Sheep, Pigs, Goats, and Horses.* Philadelphia, Bailliere Tindall, 1989, p 884.
110. Car BD, Anderson WI: Giant cell hepatopathy in 3 aborted midterm equine fetuses. *Vet Pathol* 25:389, 1988.
111. Uhlinger CA, Brumbaugh GW: Parasite control programs. In Smith BP, ed: *Large Animal Internal Medicine.* St Louis, Mosby–Year Book, 1990, p 1513.
112. Pearson EG: Other hepatotoxins. In Smith BP, ed: *Large Animal Internal Medicine.* St Louis, Mosby–Year Book, 1990, p 853.
113. Adam SE: A review of drug hepatopathy in animals. *Vet Bull* 42:683, 1972.
114. Ockner RK: Toxic and drug-induced liver disease. In Wyngaarden JB, Smith LH, ed: *Cecil Textbook of Internal Medicine.* Philadelphia, WB Saunders, 1985, p 820.
115. Divers TJ, Warner A, Vaala WE, et al: Toxic hepatic failure in newborn foals. *J Am Vet Med Assoc* 183:1407, 1983.
116. Mullaney TP: Iron toxicity in neonatal foals. *Equine Vet J* 20:119, 1988.
117. Giles CJ: Outbreak of ragwort (*S. jacobaea*) poisoning in horses. *Equine Vet J* 15:248, 1983.
118. Pearson EG: Pyrrolizidine alkaloid toxicity. In Smith BP, ed: *Large Animal Internal Medicine.* St Louis, Mosby–Year Book, 1990, p 850.
119. McLean EK: The toxic actions of pyrrolizidine (*Senecio*) alkaloids. *Pharmacol Rev* 22:429, 1970.
120. Blood DC, Radostits OM: *Veterinary Medicine: A Textbook of the Diseases of Cattle, Sheep, Pigs, Goats, and Horses.* Philadelphia, Bailliere Tindall, 1989, p 1339.
121. Lessard P, Wilson WD, Alander HJ, et al: Clinicopathologic study of horses surviving pyrrolizidine alkaloid toxicosis. *Am J Vet Res* 47:1776, 1986.
122. Pearson EG: Chronic active hepatitis. In Smith BP, ed: *Large Animal Internal Medicine.* St Louis, Mosby–Year Book, 1990, p 849.
123. Scarratt WK, Fessler RL: Cholelithiasis and biliary obstruction in a horse. *Compend Contin Educ Pract Vet* 7:s428, 1985.
124. McDole MC: Cholelithiasis in a horse. *Equine Pract* 2:37, 1980.
125. Green DS, Davies JV: Successful choledocholithotomy in a horse. *Equine Vet J* 21:464, 1989.
126. Roussel AJ, Becht JL, Adams SB: Choledocholithiasis in a horse. *Cornell Vet* 74:166, 1984.
127. Bolt RJ: Pathophysiology of gallbladder disease. In Sodeman WA, Sodeman TM, eds: *Sodeman's Pathologic Physiology: Mechanisms of Disease.* Philadelphia, WB Saunders, 1985, p 910.
128. Leur RJ, Kroneman J: Three cases of cholelithiasis and biliary fibrosis in the horse. *Equine Vet J* 14:251, 1982.
129. Tulleners ER, Becht JL, Richardson DW, et al: Choledocholithotripsy in a mare. *J Am Vet Med Assoc* 186:1317, 1985.
130. Solovay RD: Choledocholithiasis and cholangitis. In Wyngaarden JB, Smith LH, eds: *Cecil Textbook of Internal Medicine.* Philadelphia, WB Saunders, 1985, p 859.
131. Orsini JA, Donawick WJ: Hepaticojejunostomy for treatment of common hepatic duct obstructions associated with duodenal stenosis in two foals. *Vet Surg* 18:34, 1989.
132. Naylor NJ: Treatment and diagnosis of hyperlipemia and hyperlipidemia. In *Proceedings of the American College of Veterinary Internal Medicine,* Salt Lake City, July 19, 1982, p 47.
133. Jeffcott LB, Field JR: Current concepts of hyperlipaemia in horses and ponies. *Vet Rec* 116:461, 1985.
134. Field JR: Hyperlipemia in a quarter horse. *Compend Contin Educ Pract Vet* 10:218, 1988.

135. Bauer JE: Plasma lipids and lipoproteins of fasted ponies. *Am J Vet Res* 44:379, 1983.
136. Zerbe CA: Canine hyperlipemias. In Kirk RW, ed: *Current Therapy. IX. Small Animal Practice.* Philadelphia, WB Saunders, 1986, p 1050.
137. Naylor JM, Kronfeld DS, Acland H: Hyperlipemia in horses: Effects of undernutrition and disease. *Am J Vet Res* 41:899, 1980.
138. Wensing TH, Schotman AJ, Kroneman J: Effect of treatment with glucose, galactose, and insulin in hyperlipemia in ponies. *Tijdschr Diergeneesk* 99:919, 1974.
139. Reef VB, Collatos C, Spencer PA, et al: Clinical, ultrasonographic, and surgical findings in foals with umbilical remnant infections. *J Am Vet Med Assoc* 195:69, 1989.
140. Rumbaugh GE, Smith BP, Carlson GP: Internal abdominal abscesses in horses: A study of 25 cases. *J Am Vet Med Assoc* 172:304, 1978.
141. Tamaschke C: Beiträge zur vergleichenden Onkologie der Haussäugetiere. *Wiss Z Humboldt Univ Math Naturwissenschaften Reihe* 1:37, 1952.
142. Roperto F, Galati P: Mixed hamartoma of the liver in an equine fetus. *Equine Vet J* 16:218, 1984.
143. Moulton JE: *Tumors in Domestic Animals.* Los Angeles, University of California Press, 1978.
144. Kanemaru T, Oikaura MI, Yoshihara T: Post-mortem findings of hepatocellular carcinoma in a racehorse. *Exp Rep Equine Health Lab* 15:8, 1978.
145. Mueller PO, Morris DD, Carmichael KP, et al: Cholangiocarcinoma in a horse. *J Am Vet Med Assoc* 201:899, 1992.
146. Vanhooser SL, Reinemeyer CR, Held JP: Hepatic AA amyloidosis associated with severe strongylosis in a horse. *Equine Vet J* 20:274, 1988.
147. Hawthorne TB, Bolon B, Meyer DJ: Systemic amyloidosis in a mare. *J Am Vet Med Assoc* 196:323, 1990.
148. Lindsay WA, Ryder JK, Beck KA, et al: Hepatic encephalopathy caused by a portacaval shunt in a foal. *Vet Med* 83:798, 1988.
149. Beech J: Portal vein anomaly and hepatic encephalopathy in a horse. *J Am Vet Med Assoc* 170:164, 1977.
150. Bastianello SS, Nesbit JW: The pathology of a case of biliary atresia in a foal. *J S Afr Vet Assoc* 58:89, 1986.
151. Leur RJ: Biliary atresia in a foal. *Equine Vet J* 14:91, 1982.
152. Witzleben CL, Buck BE, Schnaufer BE, et al: Studies on the pathogenesis of biliary atresia. *Lab Invest* 38:525, 1978.

Chapter 14

Equine Ophthalmology

David A. Wilkie, DVM, MS

EXAMINATION

The equine eye presents particular challenges in both its diagnostic and therapeutic approaches. However, the basic principles of a complete ophthalmic examination hold true. A list of the equipment required to perform a routine ophthalmic examination is provided in Table 14–1. The initial ophthalmic examination should take place in a well-lighted environment and should be performed prior to tranquilization. The examiner assesses facial, orbital, and eyelid symmetry, evaluates for the presence of ocular discharge (serous, mucoid, mucopurulent) or blepharospasm, and performs a cranial nerve evaluation, specifically cranial nerves II through VII. A complete ophthalmic examination includes assessment of pupillary light and menace response, maze testing, globe position and mobility, sensation of ocular and adnexal structures, and eyelid position and function. To accurately evaluate direct and consensual pupillary light re-sponses, a bright focal light source (3.5 V halogen) and a darkened examination area are often required.

Further examination or therapy may require some form of tranquilization, regional nerve blocks, and topical anesthesia. Xylazine (Rompun, Haver-Lockhart, Shawnee, KS) 0.5 to 1.0 mg/kg IV, in combination with butorphenol tartrate (Torbugesic, Bristol Laboratories, Inc., Evansville, Ind.) 0.01 mg/kg IV provide a synergistic analgesic effect and facilitate examination, sample collection, nasolacrimal irrigation, lavage tube placement, and minor surgical procedures. If determination of intraocular pressure (IOP) is to be performed, it should be noted that intravenous administration of xylazine will significantly lower the IOP.[1a]

Sensory innervation of the globe and adnexa is provided by the trigeminal nerve (cranial nerve V) and motor innervation is from the facial nerve (VII). The ophthalmic nerves blocked most frequently are the auriculopalpebral branch of cranial nerve VII and the supraorbital (frontal) branch of cranial nerve V. When blocked, these provide akinesia and anesthesia of the superior eyelid, respectively. The auriculopalpebral nerve can be palpated as it courses over the zygomatic arch in the area of the temporofrontal suture. Using a 25-gauge ⅝-in. needle, the nerve is blocked by injection of 3 to 5 mL of mepivacaine HCl (Carbocaine, Winthrop Laboratories, New York) over the zygomatic arch in this area. The supraorbital nerve is blocked as it emerges from the supraorbital foramen of the frontal bone. This foramen is palpated, a 25-gauge ⅝-in. needle is inserted into the foramen, and 2 mL of mepivacaine HCl is injected; another 2 to 3 mL is infiltrated subcutaneously as the needle is removed. Additional sensory nerves that are occasionally blocked include the infratrochlear, lacrimal, and zygomatic branches of cranial nerve V.[1a] Alternatively, local infiltration of anesthetic can be used to provide anesthesia of a specific area.

A complete ophthalmic examination can now be performed (see Table 14–1). If samples are required for bacterial or fungal culture or evaluation of tear production, these are obtained prior to instilling any topical solution or ointment on the eye. Measurement of the aqueous production of tears is done using commercially available Schirmer tear test strips, with normal wetting being 20 mm or greater in 30 seconds. Using a bright focal light source, examination of the conjunctiva, nictitans, cornea, anterior chamber, iris, pupil, and lens is now performed. The ocular media (cornea, aqueous humor, lens, and vitreous) are evaluated for clarity and transparency. The position and size of the lens, shape

---

Table 14–1. Basic Equipment for Equine Ophthalmic Examination*

Bright focal light source—3.5-V halogen light with Finoff illuminator
Direct ophthalmoscope
Indirect 20-di × 5 lens
Magnifying loupe
Dressing forceps
Open-ended urinary catheter (3.5F) for nasolacrimal catheterization
Catheter (5F) for cannulation of nasolacrimal duct at nares
Sterile fluorescein strips
Schirmer tear test strips
Sterile culture swabs
Kimura spatula for obtaining cytology
Glass slides
Sterile eyewash
Proparacaine 0.5% (Alcain)—topical anesthetic
Tropicamide 1% (Mydriacyl)—short-acting dilating agent
Sedation
   Xylazine (Rompun)
   Butorphenol tartrate (Torbugesic)
Mepivacaine HCl (Carbocaine)—local nerve blocks

*From Wilkie DA: Ophthalmic procedures and surgery in the standing horse. *Vet Clin North Am Equine Pract* 7:535–547, 1991.

and mobility of the pupil, and appearance of the corpora nigra are assessed. The cornea is examined for irregularities, vascularization, and pigmentation. Fluorescein staining of the cornea will detect the presence of corneal ulceration, and the appearance of fluorescein at the nares indicates a patent nasolacrimal system. Following instillation of topical anesthesia (proparacaine 0.5%, Alcaine, Alcon Laboratories, Fort Worth, Tex.), the nasalacrimal puncta can be cannulated using a 3.5F urinary catheter, and the nasolacrimal system irrigated. Alternatively, the nasolacrimal system can be irrigated in retrograde fashion, cannulating the duct using a 5F catheter at the nasal opening. Using thumb forceps the nictitans can be grasped and the palpebral and bulbar surfaces examined for foreign bodies, mass lesions, or other abnormalities. Conjunctival and corneal cells are collected for cytologic study using a Kimura spatula following topical anesthesia. If available, intraocular pressure can be determined using an applanation tonometer such as the Tonopen (Mentor O&O, Norwell, MA).

To examine the posterior segments of the eye (optic nerve, retinal blood vessels, and tapetal and nontapetal fundus), both direct and indirect ophthalmoscopy should be performed. The size and color of the optic nerve, number and size of retinal blood vessels, pigmentation of the nontapetal fundus, and the presence or absence of hypo- or hyperreflective changes of the tapetal fundus are evaluated.

OCULAR ULTRASONOGRAPHY

Technique

Ocular ultrasonography can be performed directly through the cornea, the eyelids, or by using an offset device. The optimal transducer for ocular ultrasonography is the 10-MHz probe, but a 7.5-MHz probe can be used. Sedation, auriculopalpebral nerve block, and topical anesthesia are generally required. Sterile K-Y jelly works well as a contact material provided the cornea is irrigated following its use.

Normal Anatomy

Unless an offset device is used, the cornea and a portion of the anterior chamber are lost in the near artifact. The anterior and posterior lens capsules are visible as an echodense line at the 12 and 6 o'clock positions, while the remainder of the lens is anechoic. The iris and the ciliary body are often visible. The vitreous body is normally anechoic. The posterior eye wall is visible as a concave echodensity with the optic nerve head seen as a very echodense area at the posterior pole with an anechoic optic nerve posteriorly. The orbital contents are best visualized using a 7.5-MHz transducer evaluating the extraocular muscle cone, optic nerve, and associated structures.

Indications

Ocular ultrasound is indicated for evaluation of intraocular contents when one or more of the ocular transmitting media are opaque. This includes opacification of the cornea, aqueous and vitreous humors, and the lens. The most common indications for ocular ultrasound are in eyes with a cataract to evaluate for the presence of a retinal detachment, following traumatic hyphema to assess posterior segment damage,

or in eyes with severe corneal opacification. In addition, orbital evaluation can be performed in instances of exophthalmos or orbital trauma.

EYELIDS

Congenital

Diseases of the equine eyelid are common. Congenital lesions include coloboma, agenesis, dermoid, and entropion.[2, 2a] Of these, entropion is the only disease seen frequently. Entropion, an inward rolling of the eyelid margin, results in facial hairs contacting the cornea leading to irritation, conjunctivitis, and possibly secondary corneal ulceration. Causes include premature or dehydrated foals with enophthalmos, ocular pain resulting in spastic entropion, and primary conformational problems. Manual reduction and frequent topical ocular lubrication with artificial tear ointment is the initial treatment of choice and may be the only treatment required in some foals, especially if the entropion is secondary to dehydration. If the entropion is severe, or does not respond to manipulation, two or three vertical temporary everting mattress sutures are placed to correctly position the eyelid.[2] Care is taken to avoid overcorrection and inability to close the eyelids during blinking. Suture placement is at and perpendicular to the eyelid margin, tacking this to the periocular skin over the orbital rim. Monofilament, 3–0 to 5–0 nylon suture is preferred; the sutures are removed after 10 to 14 days. Associated corneal disease must be treated to prevent secondary infection and subsequent scar formation. Entropion requiring more aggressive surgical intervention in the form of skin excision is rare. Severe or recurrent entropion is corrected by excising an elliptical portion of eyelid skin in the affected area and reapposing the skin edges (Hotz-Celsus procedure).

Acquired

Common acquired conditions involving the equine eyelid include trauma and neoplasia.

Trauma

Eyelid trauma includes both contusions and lacerations.[3] Commonly associated with eyelid trauma are corneal abrasions or lacerations, anterior uveitis, and if the trauma involves the medial canthus, nasolacrimal system damage. Eyelid contusions often result in blepharoedema and hemorrhage. Although this does not require therapy, recovery can be hastened by using systemic flunixin meglumine (Banamine, Schering Corp., Kenilworth, N.J.), cold compresses in the acute phase, and warm compresses beginning the day following the injury.

Eyelid lacerations are more serious and usually require immediate therapy. The vascular supply to the eyelid is extensive and many apparent avascular segments of eyelid will recover following repair. If possible, primary wound closure is preferred. All debris must be removed from the wound prior to closure. The eyelid surface and adjacent tissues are disinfected with a 1:25 to 1:50 dilution of povidone-iodine solution. Excessive tissue debridement should be avoided and under no circumstances should a pedicle of eyelid be amputated. Loss of eyelid margin, whether through trauma or iatrogenic, will result in severe, chronic corneal irritation, vascularization, ulceration, and fibrosis. In addition, it is difficult to reconstruct an eyelid margin from the adjacent skin following amputation of the normal eyelid margin.

Lacerated eyelids should be sutured using a two-layer closure, ensuring accurate anatomical apposition of the wound edges and eyelid margin. Surgical repair can be performed with sedation and local nerve blocks for minor repairs, but may require general anesthesia if the injury is severe. The deeper, conjunctival, layer is sutured first using 4-0 to 6-0 absorbable suture in a horizontal mattress pattern beginning away from and working toward the eyelid margin. Care is taken to avoid penetrating the conjunctiva so that the suture does not contact the cornea. The skin is closed with 4-0 to 6-0 nonabsorbable suture. The eyelid margin is the most important part of wound closure and is closed first to ensure accurate apposition. I prefer to use a cruciate suture pattern at the eyelid margin and a simple interrupted pattern for the remainder of the skin closure. Failure to perform a two-layer closure or achieve precise apposition of the eyelid margin may result in ulcerative keratitis or other secondary complication.[3a] Postoperative therapy includes systemic antibiotics for 5 to 7 days, tetanus toxoid, warm compresses, and flunixin meglumine if inflammation and swelling are a problem. Topical medication is not required for eyelid injuries unless there is associated corneal or anterior segment damage. Eyelid function must be evaluated and the eyelid must provide adequate protection to the cornea. If the blink response is impaired, the cornea should be protected with topical lubricants as often as possible. Advanced blepharoplastic techniques for repair of severe eyelid trauma with resulting loss of tissue are beyond the scope of this chapter, but are discussed in detail elsewhere.[2]

Neoplasia

The most common neoplasms of the equine eyelid are sarcoid and squamous cell carcinoma. In addition, melanoma, mast cell tumor, lymphosarcoma, basal cell carcinoma, and papilloma can affect the eyelid. The differential diagnosis for eyelid neoplasms includes parasitic diseases such as ocular habronemiasis and other causes of granulomatous skin disease. Treatment of eyelid neoplasia is dependent on location, size, tumor type, age and purpose of the horse, cost, surgical skill, and equipment available. Treatment modalities include surgical excision, radiation therapy, chemotherapy, hyperthermia, immunotherapy, cryosurgery, or a combination of these. The aim of therapy is to eliminate or halt progression of the tumor while maintaining eyelid function and preserving the eye and vision. Complete excision with primary closure is the optimal treatment, but often cannot be achieved owing to limitations on availability of tissue for reconstruction and the extensive and aggressive nature of many eyelid neoplasms. If eyelid margins cannot be apposed following tumor excision, more involved blepharoplastic techniques, such as advancement skin flaps, may be indicated (Fig. 14–1).

Squamous Cell Carcinoma

Squamous cell carcinoma involving the eyelid is usually erosive and ulcerative.[4] The medial canthus is the most

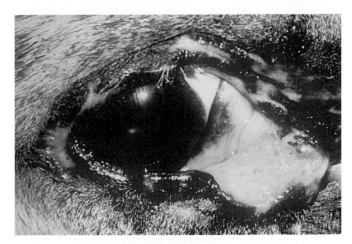

Figure 14–1. Squamous cell carcinoma involving the medial canthus and inferior eyelid of a 19-year-old appaloosa.

common site of origin (see Fig. 14–1). Invasion of adjacent soft and bony orbital tissue is possible, if untreated. Treatment of ocular squamous cell carcinoma is discussed in detail under Conjunctiva and Third Eyelid.

Sarcoid

Periocular sarcoid is the second most common eyelid neoplasm of the horse. The average age of an affected horse is 4 years and both smooth and warty-type sarcoids are seen. Orbital invasion and bony involvement are possible. Surgical excision is associated with frequent recurrence and is often combined with cryosurgery, hyperthermia, chemotherapy, or irradiation to ensure complete tumor destruction.

Intralesional immunotherapy, using cell wall extracts of bacillus Calmette-Guérin (BCG) in oil, has been used effectively in repeated injections 3 weeks apart. A total of four doses is usually required for complete tumor regression. Injection of cell wall extracts of BCG is associated with local inflammation and tumor necrosis. During this period of inflammation the globe must be protected to prevent corneal desiccation or ulceration. The use of live BCG organisms or whole killed organisms has been associated with anaphylactic reaction and death and is discouraged. Adverse systemic reactions to cell wall extracts of BCG are rare, but premedication with systemic corticosteroids is advised.

Intralesional chemotherapy with cisplatin in an oil-water emulsion has been reported to result in regression of equine sarcoid.[5] A series of four injections, spaced 2 weeks apart, with a mean dose of cisplatin of 0.97 mg/cm[3] of tumor mass resulted in tumor regression in all treated horses. In addition, 87% of sarcoid-treated horses were relapse-free at 1-year follow-up.

CONJUNCTIVA AND THIRD EYELID

The conjunctiva is divided into bulbar and palpebral surfaces. The conjunctiva merges with the cornea at the limbus, with the eyelid at the eyelid margin, and the bulbar and palpebral conjunctiva join to form the fornix. The conjunctiva has a normal resident flora of bacteria and fungi. The most common isolates from the equine conjunctiva vary according to geography, season of the year, and investigator.[6–8] In general, isolates of gram-positive organisms, *Corynebacterium, Bacillus, Staphylococcus,* and *Streptomyces,* are more common than gram-negative organisms from the normal equine conjunctiva.[7] Fungi are more commonly isolated in the summer and autumn and have been reported to be present in 95% of normal horse conjunctiva samples.[8] In addition, fungi are isolated more frequently from stabled horses, which likely relates to the immediate environmental and husbandry conditions.[7]

Congenital diseases of the equine conjunctiva are uncommon, conjunctival dermoid being the most common congenital abnormality. A dermoid is a congenital tumor of skin and associated glands, hair, and hair follicles that can affect the cornea and adjacent conjunctiva. If a dermoid is irritating the globe or adnexa, it should be surgically removed by performing a superficial keratectomy.

Unlike the small animal patient, infectious conjunctivitis is rare in the horse. Organisms reported to result in infectious conjunctivitis in the horse include equine herpesvirus type 2,[8a] *Mycoplasma* species, *Chlamydia, Moraxella equi,* and mycotic and viral agents.[2]

Foreign bodies and trauma are a common cause of conjunctival irritation and damage and are often associated with concurrent eyelid and corneal injuries. Treatment is directed toward eliminating the cause, treating any conjunctival or associated eyelid or corneal damage, and preventing secondary infection. A complete ophthalmic examination must be performed in all animals with evidence of ocular trauma. Conjunctival foreign bodies should be considered in any horse with a recurrent corneal erosion, ocular pain, or conjunctivitis. Examination of the superior and inferior fornices and the bulbar and palpebral surface of the nictitans should be performed following administration of topical 0.5% proparacaine. Magnification is essential to detect foreign bodies. In addition, irrigation of the nasolacrimal system may yield foreign material associated with chronic conjunctivitis or dacryocystitis.

Parasites

Common parasites of the equine conjunctiva include *Thelazia lacrymalis, Habronema* species, and *Onchocerca cervicalis.* In a necropsy sample, the prevalence of *Thelazia* in the conjunctival sac of horses is highest in young animals, with 43% of 1- to 4-year-old horses affected.[9] In most instances infection is not associated with clinical signs, but a chronic conjunctivitis, seromucoid discharge, and conjunctival nodules can occur.[2] The adult parasite may be visible on ophthalmic examination of the cornea and conjunctival fornix and larvae can be seen on examination of centrifuged samples of nasolacrimal washes. Treatment includes removal of the adult worms, irrigation of the nasolacrimal system, topical corticosteroids to control inflammation, and fly control. Topical organophosphates, echothiophate 0.03% to 0.06% b.i.d. or isoflurophate 0.025% s.i.d. for 7 days, have been reported to kill the parasite.[10] Systemic treatment with fenbendazole 10 mg/kg PO s.i.d. for 5 days is also reported to be effective in killing *Thelazia.*[11]

Ocular manifestations of equine cutaneous habronemiasis (ECH) result when the larvae of the *Habronema* sp. are deposited on or around the eye by the house or stable fly.[2, 12, 13] The resulting granuloma is associated with inflammation, intense pruritus, and epiphora. Yellow, caseous granules

are noted throughout the granulation tissue. Histologically, eosinophils and mast cells predominate.[2, 13] Diagnosis is made based on clinical signs, location, season of the year, and histologic findings. Clinical appearance can simulate squamous cell carcinoma. Histologically, the differential diagnosis is equine cutaneous mastocytosis.[2, 13] Ocular lesions are most common at the medial canthus and may involve the skin, nasolacrimal duct, third eyelid, or conjunctiva. Treatment of ECH is variable and no single treatment is routinely successful.[12] Surgical excision, cryosurgery, local and systemic corticosteroid therapy, systemic ivermectin (single dose, 0.2 mg/kg IM), various larvicidal treatments in the form of topical and systemic organophosphates, and various topical formulations containing ronnel or metrifonate with a dimethyl sulfoxide (DMSO) vehicle are used[2, 12, 13] (Table 14–2). DMSO serves as both a vehicle and has anti-inflammatory effects, possibly related to its ability to detoxify hydroxyl radicals generated by neutrophils. The aim of therapy is to kill the larvae while controlling the resulting inflammation. In addition, fly control is an essential part of an overall management program.

The *O. cervicalis* microfilaria is transmitted by the blood-sucking midge, *Culicoides nebeculosus.* Once transmitted, the immature microfilariae migrate through lymphatics and can travel to ocular and adnexal tissues. The prevalence of equine onchocerciasis increases with age, with an overall prevalence of 50% to 60%.[15–17] The prevalence of onchocerciasis on histologic examination of the lateral bulbar conjunctiva is 10.8%.[17] The presence of conjunctival microfilaria does not correlate with clinical abnormalities.[17] Ocular onchocerciasis has been proposed as a cause of keratitis, conjunctivitis, equine recurrent uveitis, and depigmentation of the temporal bulbar conjunctiva.[17] The pathogenesis is thought to involve the death of the microfilaria, release of antigens, and development of hypersensitivity in susceptible horses. Treatment is indicated in those horses with active conjunctivitis, keratitis, or uveitis attributable to onchocerciasis. Treatment includes anti-inflammatory agents such as topical corticosteroids and systemic flunixin meglumine, topical echothiophate iodide 0.025%, and systemic diethylcarbamazine, levamisole, or ivermectin[2] (Table 14–3).

Table 14–2. Topical Preparations Used in the Treatment of Equine Cutaneous Habronemiasis

Ingredients	Amount	Reference
Ronnel solution (33%)	60 mL	Vasey[12]
Thiabendazole (33%)	120 g	
9-Fluoroprednisolone acetate	60 mg	
Dimethyl phthalate (24%)	30 mL	
Dimethyl sulfoxide (DMSO)	500 mL	
Nitrofurantoin ointment	225 g	Rebhun et al.[13]
Ronnel solution	20 mL	
DMSO	20 mL	
Dexamethasone solution	20 mL	
Nitrofurazone ointment (0.2%)	135 g	Moore et al.[14]
Metrifonate (12.3%)	30 mL	
Dexamethasone (2 mg/mL)	30 mL	
DMSO	30 mL	

Table 14–3. Systemic Treatment of Ocular Onchocerciasis

Drug	Dose
Diethylcarbamazine	4.4–6.6 mg/kg/day PO for 21 days
Levamisole	1.1 mg/kg/day PO for 7 days
Ivermectin	0.2–0.5 mg/kg IM

Neoplasia

Neoplasms affecting the conjunctiva and third eyelid include squamous cell carcinoma (SCC), lymphosarcoma, melanocytoma, mastocytoma, hemangioma, and angiosarcoma.[2] Diagnosis and characterization of adnexal neoplasms is based on history, signalment, location, appearance, and histopathology. Surgical biopsy can be routinely performed with sedation, local nerve blocks, and topical anesthesia. Most adnexal neoplasms are either benign or locally invasive, the exception being ocular angiosarcoma, which is reported to have a high incidence of metastasis.[18] Treatment of adnexal neoplasms varies according to tumor type, location, and size; use of the animal; treatment modalities available; and cost. The aim of treatment is to eliminate the tumor, restore normal anatomy, and maintain function of the eye and associated structures.

Squamous Cell Carcinoma

Squamous cell carcinoma is the most common tumor of the equine eye and adnexa (Fig. 14–2). Involvement can be unilateral or bilateral with the third eyelid and medial canthus affected most frequently.[10, 19] Involvement of the corneal limbus, sclera, conjunctiva, and other adnexal structures has also been reported.[10, 19, 20]

The mean age of onset for SCC is 9.8 years for all horses compared with 3.8 years for ocular sarcoidosis.[20] The incidence of ocular SCC is higher in draft-breed horses and appaloosas than in light horses,[21, 22] and sexually intact males

and females have a decreased incidence.[21] It is hypothesized that adnexal hypopigmentation[20, 21] and increased exposure to actinic radiation[20, 21] may predispose to ocular SCC development.

Ocular SCC is malignant and locally invasive with the potential to metastasize.[22, 23] Metastases to local and cranial mediastinal lymph nodes, parotid salivary glands, and the thoracic cavity occur in 10% to 15% of patients.[22]

Treatment of ocular SCC is varied and must be designed for the individual patient. Surgical excision,[20] radiofrequency hyperthermia (RFH),[24] cryotherapy,[25] immunotherapy,[25] radiation therapy,[20, 23–25] intralesional chemotherapy,[5, 25a] laser surgery,[4] or a combination of these,[24, 25] all have been used with success. Location, size, and depth of the tumor, visual status, financial commitment, purpose of the animal, and the presence or absence of metastatic disease influence the choice of therapy.

If possible, complete surgical excision is curative and is the preferred therapy. Difficulty arises with surgical excision when preservation of the globe and ocular and adnexal anatomy and function are required. Complete excision of the third eyelid is possible. This can often be performed using sedation and local nerve blocks. The bulbar and palpebral margins of the third eyelid conjunctiva should be apposed following excision using 5-0 to 6-0 absorbable suture in a simple continuous pattern.

Most SCCs are radiosensitive and can be successfully treated with sources of beta or gamma radiation. The major disadvantage of less expensive modes of radiation therapy, such as strontium 90, a source of beta radiation, is the size limit of tumor amenable to treatment. With ^{90}Sr for example, half the beta radiation produced is lost after passage through 1 mm of soft tissue.[26] Thus treatment should be limited to lesions less than 2 mm deep,[26] such as corneal, scleral, or conjunctival SCC. It is most appropriate as an adjunct therapy following surgical removal of a corneal or conjunctival SCC. When used appropriately ^{90}Sr can achieve a nonrecurrence rate for SCC of 87.5% after 2 years.[26]

The use of interstitial radiotherapy for periocular SCC has been reported.[24, 26] Radioactive gold seeds (^{198}Au) were used to impart a medium-energy gamma ray (0.41 MeV) with a half-life of 93.3 hours[24] for a total recommended dose of 5,000 rads.[24] Success rates of 80% at 1 year and 70% at 2 years are reported.[26] Disadvantages of radioactive implants are substantial cost, limited availability, risks associated with human exposure, and the licensing restrictions on their handling.[24] Secondary complications of interstitial radiation therapy include temporary corneal opacity, local necrosis, hair loss, damage to normal structures, and local depigmentation.[24, 26] Although no retinal or lens changes have been reported following interstitial radiation treatment, the possibility of photoreceptor damage and cataractogenesis secondary to radiation therapy should be considered.

RFH involves the passage of a radiofrequency (2 MHz) electric current between two electrodes.[24] Tissue between these probes offers resistance resulting in thermal energy being transferred to the tissue.[24] Tissue temperature rises to 50 °C in a 1-cm^2 area[24] with the malignant cells exhibiting a greater sensitivity to thermal energy than normal cells. It is recommended that topical RFH not be used as the only mode of treatment in tumors extending deeper than 3 mm or greater than 4 to 5 cm in diameter.[27] Superficial eyelid SCCs or corneal and conjunctival SCCs are therefore most appropriate for treatment using RFH. Overlapping the fields

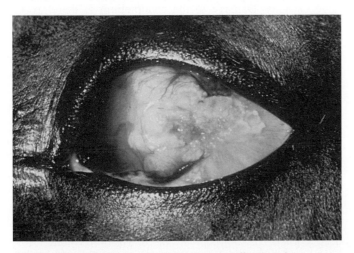

Figure 14–2. Squamous cell carcinoma affecting the temporal conjunctiva, limbus, and cornea.

of exposure should be avoided, especially in corneal tumors, as this creates a risk of excessive necrosis of normal tissue.[27]

Cryosurgery using nitrous oxide (-80 °C) or liquid nitrogen (-185 °C) in a single freeze– or double freeze–thaw cycle will result in tissue destruction. Cryodestruction is most indicated for treatment of eyelid SCC. Associated local depigmentation of skin and hair may be seen in the treated area. Thermocouples should be used and tissue temperatures of -25 °C are optimal.

Intralesional chemotherapy with cisplatin or bleomycin in an oil-water emulsion has been reported to result in regression of equine SCC.[5, 25a] Treatment is the same as previously described for eyelid sarcoidosis. Of those horses with adnexal SCC treated with intralesional cisplatin, 65–93% were relapse-free at 1 year.[5, 25a]

Regardless of the treatment used, frequent and continued follow-up examinations result in the greatest long-term success in the management of ocular and periocular SCC. Recurrence may occur at the initial site of involvement and must be distinguished from granulation tissue associated with the previous treatment. In addition, other sites and the opposite eye must be monitored for the development of new SCC lesions.

NASOLACRIMAL SYSTEM

The nasolacrimal system consists of the superior and inferior puncta and canaliculi, nasolacrimal sac, nasolacrimal duct, and nasal punctum located on the floor of the nasal vestibule.[28] The nasolacrimal system serves to carry tears from the medial canthus of the eye to the nasal vestibule. Abnormalities of the nasolacrimal system result in epiphora, an overflow of tears, secondary to an impairment in drainage of tears. Epiphora can be serous, mucoid, or mucopurulent. This must be differentiated from reflex lacrimation resulting from ocular irritation or inflammation. Examination of the nasolacrimal system includes placement of fluorescein stain in the conjunctival cul-de-sac and observing its appearance at the nasal opening. Irrigation of the nasolacrimal system can be performed antegrade from the eyelid punctum or retrograde from the nasal punctum. Topical anesthetic (0.5% proparacaine) is applied to the eye and a 3.5F open-ended feline urinary catheter is placed in the superior punctum. Sterile eyewash or saline (10–20 mL) is used to irrigate the system, first observing fluid passing out of the inferior punctum and subsequently, the nasal punctum. If irrigation is performed retrograde from the nasal punctum, a 5F or 6F urinary catheter is used and the volume of irrigating solution is increased. Radiographic imaging of the nasolacrimal duct, dacryocystorhinography, can be performed using contrast material injected into the duct from the superior eyelid punctum.[2, 28] Lateral and oblique radiographic views are best, and useful contrast materials include 60% barium sulfate (Novapaque, Picker Corp., Cleveland, OH) and 31% diatrizoate meglumine and diatrizoate sodium (Renovist II, Squibb Diagnostics). Indications for dacryocystorhinography include chronic epiphora, inability to irrigate the nasolacrimal duct, suspicion of a nasolacrimal foreign body, or evaluation of the nasolacrimal duct for congenital or acquired abnormalities.

Abnormalities of the nasolacrimal system can be congenital or acquired. In the horse, the most common congenital abnormality is atresia of the distal portion of the nasolacrimal duct and the nasal punctum, which results in mucoid epiphora at 3 to 4 months of age.[2, 29] Additional abnormalities include atresia of an eyelid punctum, abnormal placement of an eyelid punctum, and multiple nasal openings.[2] It is not known if these conditions are inherited. To correct an atretic nasal opening a catheter is passed from the inferior eyelid punctum to the level of the atresia. The end of the catheter is palpated in the nasal vestibule and an incision is made through the nasal mucosa overlying the catheter, exposing the catheter. The tubing is brought out the nasal opening and, along with the portion of tubing from the inferior punctum, is sutured to the skin of the face. The tubing is left in place for 3 to 4 weeks and topical broad-spectrum ophthalmic antibiotic solution is administered during this time.

Acquired conditions of the nasolacrimal system include dacryocystitis, foreign body obstruction, trauma, and involvement secondarily in neoplastic or inflammatory conditions of the medial canthus. Dacryocystitis appears as a mucopurulent ocular discharge without associated ocular inflammation. Dacryocystitis and foreign body obstructions are treated by nasolacrimal irrigation, as previously described, and bacterial and fungal culture with or without the aid of radiographic evaluation. Topical broad-spectrum ophthalmic antibiotic solution is administered following irrigation. Topical corticosteroids or systemic nonsteroidal anti-inflammatory drugs (NSAIDs) can also be used to help control swelling and inflammation. Traumatic or other damage to the nasolacrimal duct is best repaired at the time of injury and placement of a tube in the nasolacrimal duct for 3 to 4 weeks to maintain patency while healing occurs is recommended. Repair of the nasolacrimal duct is a referral procedure and requires general anesthesia. If the nasolacrimal duct cannot be made patent, treatment is either symptomatic therapy for the epiphora, or surgical trephination, conjunctivorhinotomy, to create a new outflow pathway for the tears.

CORNEA
Anatomy and Physiology

The cornea consists of the epithelium, stroma, Descemet's membrane, and endothelium. The epithelium is 7 to 15 cells in thickness and is replaced every 7 to 10 days. The corneal endothelium is a monolayer of cells with little to no regenerative capacity. Damage to the endothelium is therefore of great significance as complete repair is often not possible and results in permanent corneal edema. The cornea is transparent, avascular, and is supplied with sensory nerves from the ophthalmic branch of the trigeminal nerve. The epithelium and anterior stroma are richly innervated with sensory nerves, whereas the middle and inner cornea is less well supplied. Nutrition and waste removal are carried out by the tear film, aqueous humor, and diffusion to and from the scleral and conjunctival blood vessels. The cornea is maintained in a relative state of deturgescence by the mechanical barrier and pump mechanisms of the epithelium and endothelium. Interference with these barriers results in corneal edema, with endothelial damage being the more significant. Chronic irritation of the cornea results in superficial vascularization, while inflammation of the anterior uvea results in deep corneal vascularization. Vascularization is often followed by corneal pigmentation. Cellular infiltration of the cornea occurs in neoplastic, infectious, and inflammatory disease. All of these processes can occur alone or in combination, resulting in an alteration of corneal transparency. In addition, scar formation and noncellular infiltrates such as mineral and phospholipid deposits (corneal degeneration) will alter corneal transparency. It is essential to establish the cause of these changes and, if possible, eliminate it.

Ulcerative Diseases

Corneal ulceration is perhaps the most frustrating and potentially devastating disease of the equine eye. Of all species commonly treated in veterinary ophthalmology, the cornea of the horse is the slowest to heal, the most likely to become infected, and yields the poorest results. In addition, the size and temperament of the animal makes frequent treatment difficult for both owner and veterinarian. In most instances corneal ulceration is the result of an initial trauma, but secondary infection is common, especially in those eyes treated with topical corticosteroids following ulceration.

Clinical Signs and Diagnosis

A corneal ulcer is present when there is a break in the corneal epithelium. Clinically, this results in lacrimation, blepharospasm, photophobia, conjunctival hyperemia, corneal edema, and possibly miosis and aqueous flare. The diagnosis of a corneal ulcer is made based on these clinical signs and fluorescein staining of the cornea. Fluorescein stain will be retained by the underlying stroma and appear green in color. A bacterial and fungal culture should be submitted from all corneal ulcers in the horse. Cultures should be obtained from the margin of the ulcer itself, prior to instilling any therapeutic or diagnostic agents in the eye. Once a culture is obtained and the cornea has been fluorescein-stained, topical anesthetic is applied and a scraping is obtained from the ulcer for cytologic examination. The cells are placed on a glass slide and stained to examine for bacteria, fungal hyphae, and cell type. Gram's and Giemsa stains work well for examination. The presence of gram-negative rods indicates the possibility of an infection with a *Pseudomonas* sp. The presence of fungal hyphae is pathognomonic for mycotic keratitis, with *Aspergillus* spp.

being the most frequent corneal pathogens. Mixed bacterial and fungal infections are not uncommon.

A corneal ulcer should be characterized with regard to size, depth, and the presence or absence of cellular infiltration. In addition, the anterior chamber is examined for anterior uveitis. It is essential with all corneal ulcers to attempt to establish the cause of the ulceration and eliminate it (Fig. 14–3). The palpebral conjunctiva and bulbar surface of the nictitans are examined for the presence of a foreign body, the blink response and tear film are evaluated, and a complete history is obtained with regard to trauma and previous medication. Topical corticosteroids must not be administered in the presence of a corneal ulcer and a history of previous topical corticosteroid therapy increases the likelihood of infectious, especially fungal, keratitis.

Some specific types of corneal ulcers seen in the horse include indolent ulcers,[30] ulcers with eosinophilic cellular infiltrate,[30a] collagenase and mycotic ulcers, and possibly viral ulcerative keratitis.[2]

Routine Treatment

Treatment of an uncomplicated corneal ulcer involves controlling pain and inflammation, eliminating or preventing infection, and preventing secondary complications (see Table 14–7). Healing occurs by migration and mitosis of the adjacent epithelial cells and depending on the size of the ulcer should be complete in 2 to 6 days for an uncomplicated corneal ulcer. Complicated corneal ulcers are those that fail to heal in an appropriate time, are secondarily infected, have an ongoing source of irritation or reulceration, have a collagenase component, are associated with corneal vascularization, or are worsening despite appropriate treatment.

If miosis is observed, topical atropine 1% is administered to dilate the pupil, decrease the pain of anterior uveitis, and prevent posterior synechiae formation. Topical atropine is used as needed to dilate the pupil, but treatment frequency should not exceed four times daily. All topical ophthalmic medications are absorbed systemically and topical atropine can result in an ileus-type colic. While using topical atropine the intestinal motility should be evaluated by auscultation and the owner should observe for fresh fecal material in the stall each day. Systemic flunixin meglumine is indicated to

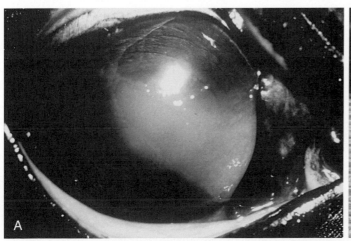
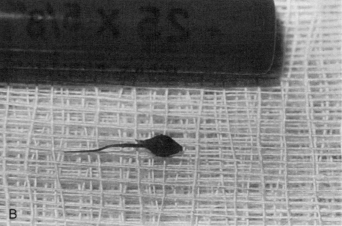

Figure 14–3. A, Chronic, superficial corneal ulcer. Note the shape and orientation of the corneal ulcer suggestive of a foreign body on the bulbar surface of the nictitans. **B,** Foreign body removed after examination of the bulbar surface of the nictitans.

suppress inflammation and control pain associated with a corneal ulcer. This, in combination with topical atropine, will help dilate the pupil.

Topical broad-spectrum antibiotics such as gentamicin (Gentafair, Pharmaderm, Melville, NY) or neomycin-bacitracin-polymyxin B (Neosporin, Burroughs Wellcome Co., Triangle Park, NC; AK-Spore, Akorn, Metairie, LA) are the initial antibiotics of choice. Ointments are preferred for their ease of administration and prolonged corneal contact time. Frequency of administration varies according to severity of the disease. When topical antibiotics are used prophylactically for an uncomplicated corneal ulcer treatment, three or four times daily is sufficient, but in severe infectious keratitis, therapy might be hourly. If infection with *Pseudomonas* sp. is suspected, then topical gentamicin, polymyxin B, ciprofloxacin, or preferably tobramycin 0.3% (Tobrex, Alcon Laboratories, Fort Worth, TX) is indicated every 2 to 4 hours. While gram-positive organisms predominate initially in equine infectious keratitis, intensive topical antimicrobial therapy results in a significant shift to gram-negative organisms and a change in susceptibility patterns.[30b] Additional treatment will vary according to the type and severity of the ulcer (see Complicated Ulcerative Diseases).

Do not administer topical corticosteroids to a horse with a corneal ulcer!

Complicated Ulcerative Diseases

Complicated corneal ulcers are those that require additional treatment over and above routine ulcer management, are infected, exhibit chronicity or recurrence, are in imminent danger of perforation, or have a collagenase component (Fig. 14–4). Secondary infection of a corneal ulcer is suggested by increasing corneal edema, interstitial keratitis associated with an increase in stromal inflammatory cells, corneal vascularization, purulent discharge, severe anterior uveitis, and stromal necrosis and liquefaction.

In many instances, complicated corneal ulcers require frequent and prolonged therapy, and some form of medication delivery system is indicated to ensure adequate treatment. Use of subpalpebral and nasolacrimal medication delivery systems has been described previously.[31] I prefer a

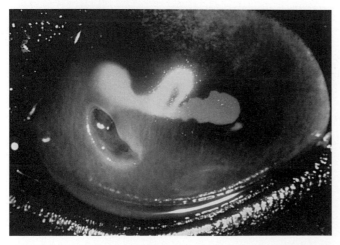

Figure 14–4. Deep corneal ulcer and descemetocele with associated focal corneal edema and miosis.

through-and-through subpalpebral lavage system, placement of which is described below.

Many complicated corneal ulcers require a combination of surgical and medical therapy to improve the likelihood of a successful outcome.

Indolent Corneal Ulceration

Indolent corneal ulcers are, by definition, chronic and superficial.[30, 32] Indolent ulcers often have a rim of loose or detached epithelium at the margin, focal corneal edema, moderate discomfort, and elicit minimal corneal vascularization. As with all chronic corneal ulceration, the eyelids, conjunctiva, and third eyelid must be examined thoroughly for the presence of foreign bodies, ectopic cilia, or other abnormality that might result in persistent ulceration.

The cause of indolent ulcers is suspected to be a failure in the attachment of the corneal epithelium to the underlying basement membrane. This attachment normally develops following epithelial migration and mitosis in the repair of a corneal ulcer. A basement membrane abnormality is suspected to be the underlying problem.

Treatment of indolent corneal ulcers includes removal of abnormal, loose epithelium and facilitation of epithelial attachment. Following sedation, auriculopalpebral nerve block, and topical anesthesia, the loose epithelial margins of the indolent ulcer are debrided to the point of normal attachment, using a cotton swab or cilia forceps. A superficial linear keratotomy is then performed using a 25-gauge needle. Using the beveled edge of the needle, a series of superficial, parallel horizontal and vertical grooves are placed in the cornea 0.5 to 1.0 mm apart. These extend through the basement membrane, and need only be deep enough to be visualized.

These areas serve as attachment sites for the migrating epithelium, shortening the healing time. Topical, broad-spectrum antibiotics are used every 6 hours and if miosis is present atropine 1% is used as needed to dilate the pupil. Use of a soft contact lens, 24–36 mm in diameter (OpTECH, Inc., Englewood, CO), may help protect the corneal epithelium from the shearing forces of the eyelid and third eyelid during healing, but is not essential. Topical hyperosmotics have been advocated for indolent corneal ulceration, but are of no benefit in my opinion and topical corticosteroids are contraindicated. Superficial keratectomy or a conjunctival pedicle graft, or both, can be used for indolent ulcers that fail to respond to debridement and superficial linear keratotomy.

Superficial Punctate Keratitis

Superficial punctate keratitis is characterized by multifocal, lacelike epithelial-to-subepithelial corneal opacities, some of which may be flourescein-positive, with mild corneal edema. Blepharospasm may be noted, but many horses are asymptomatic. The cause is unknown, but viral agents, specifically equine herpesvirus type 1, onchocerciasis, and immune-mediated causes have been proposed.[8a, 33, 34]

Treatment recommendations vary and include topical antibiotic-corticosteroid three to four times daily, topical cyclosporin A,[34a] or topical antiviral therapy, or a combination of these. Although the condition responds well to topical corticosteroids, recurrence is common and caution must be excercised when using topical corticosteroids in eyes with flourescein retention. Topical ophthalmic antiviral agents (idoxuridine and trifluridine) are administered every 2 to 4 hours until the lesions resolve. Therapy is then reduced to four times a day for 7 days.

Eosinophilic Keratoconjunctivitis

Eosinophilic keratitis may present with blepharospasm, chemosis, and conjunctivitis, but the hallmark feature is a yellow-white caseous plaque adherent to the limbal cornea with perilesional edema and corneal ulceration.[30a, 34b] Similar caseous material may also be found adherent to areas of ulcerated conjunctiva. Cytologically, the caseous material is predominantly eosinophils with a few mast cells.[30a] The lesion may be unilateral or bilateral and more than one lesion may be present within an eye. The condition appears seasonal, presenting in the spring and summer. The diagnosis is made based on clinical signs, season of the year, and cytology.

Untreated, eosinophilic keratoconjunctivitis is a chronic disease with healing by vascularization and scarring over several months. During this time secondary infection and acute exacerbation is possible. Treatment with topical corticosteroids has been described to reduced clinical signs, but mean time to resolution was 64 days, which is not significantly greater than without treatment.[30a] In addition, there is a risk of secondary bacterial or fungal infectious keratitis with the use of topical corticosteroids. Topical Iodoxamide 0.1% (Alomide, Alcon Laboratories, Forth Worth, TX) every 6–8 hours, fly control using fly masks, and superficial keratectomy may also be of benefit in resolving eosinophilic keratoconjunctivitis.

Mycotic Keratitis

All chronic corneal ulcers and ulcers that have been treated with topical corticosteroids must be considered as mycotic ulcers until proved otherwise. Mycotic keratitis is more common in the summer months and in warm climates.[35] Mycotic ulcers often have multifocal areas of cellular infiltrate and colonies of fungal organisms (Fig. 14–5). These appear as white lesions deep in the corneal stroma adjacent

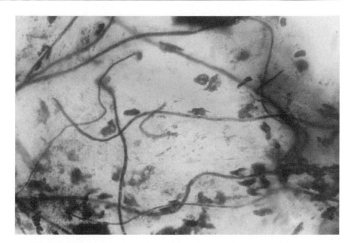

Figure 14–6. Corneal cytology from a horse with a combined infection with *Aspergillus* sp. and *Streptococcus* sp. Both filamentous hyphae and bacteria are present on cytologic examination.

to the ulcer and often appear 7 to 10 days following initial ulceration. These infiltrates are often fluorescein-negative. Diagnosis of mycotic keratitis is made based on history, clinical signs, cytology, culture, and, if possible, histopathologic examination of a biopsy sample (Fig. 14–6). Failure to see fungal elements on cytology or culture does not rule out mycotic keratitis. The most common isolate for eyes with keratomycosis is an *Aspergillus* sp.[35] *Fusarium* spp., *Penicillium* spp., and *Candida albicans* are also associated with keratomycosis. If in doubt, it is appropriate to treat for fungal infection.

In eyes where mycotic keratitis is suspected or documented, topical antifungals are indicated in addition to routine ulcer management. The only approved ophthalmic antifungal is natamycin 5% suspension (Natacyn, Alcon Laboratories, Forth Worth, TX), but it is often cost-prohibitive. Although not approved for ophthalmic use, the imidazole antibiotics (miconazole, ketoconazole) may have the best efficacy for the treatment of keratomycosis.[35] Miconazole 1% (Monistat IV, Janssen Pharmaceutica, Piscataway, N.J.) intravenous solution administered every 2 to 4 hours can be used topically for mycotic keratitis. An itraconazole-dimethyl sulfoxide ointment has also been used topically to treat keratomycosis.[35a] In addition, dilute povidone-iodine solution is fungicidal and can be applied to the cornea with a cotton swab once every 1 to 2 days. Iodine is irritating to corneal and conjunctival tissues and should be irrigated from the conjunctival cul-de-sac following application. All topical antifungal medications have limited ability to penetrate intact corneal epithelium, although miconazole is better than most. If the lesion is fluorescein-negative it may be necessary to debride the epithelium prior to medicating (see Corneal Stromal Abscess). Topical antifungal medication must be continued for a minimum of 3 to 4 weeks along with concurrent routine topical and systemic corneal ulcer management. Dermal antifungal preparations are not appropriate for topical use in the eye, but human vaginal antifungal preparations can be administered.

Many mycotic corneal ulcers are best managed using a combination of both surgical and medical management. Surgical debridement in the form of a partial-thickness keratectomy may help to remove much of the infected corneal

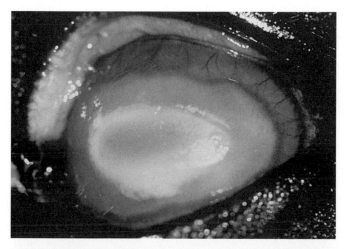

Figure 14–5. Mycotic keratitis. Deep corneal vascularization, stromal edema, and cellular infiltration are seen secondary to infection with *Aspergillus* sp.

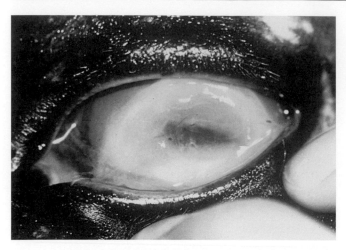

Figure 14–7. Severe melting caused by collagenase ulcer secondary to infection with *Pseudomonas aeruginosa*. Corneal malacia surrounds a large descemetocele.

stroma. This is performed under general anesthesia. The resulting ulcer can be managed medically or, more appropriately, a conjunctival pedicle graft[2, 36, 37] may be sutured to the ulcer to aid in healing or a penetrating keratoplasty performed for deeper lesions[37a] (see Corneal Surgery). The corneal vascularization provided by a conjunctival graft will facilitate healing. Most mycotic corneal ulcers will ultimately vascularize and scar to some degree. Topical corticosteroids have little if any effect on corneal scar formation and are not indicated, even following resolution of mycotic keratitis.

Collagenase Ulcers

Keratomalacia, or corneal melting, occurs as the result of host-derived collagenase (from neutrophils and keratocytes) and bacterial enzymes such as those produced by *Pseudomonas aeruginosa*.[37b] Collagenase ulcers progress rapidly and can result in corneal perforation within 24 hours (Fig. 14–7). Samples for bacterial and fungal culture and cytology should be obtained. Cytologic examination must include Gram's staining to examine for the presence of gram-negative rods suggestive of *Pseudomonas* spp. The topical antibiotic of choice for *Pseudomonas* is tobramycin 0.3% or ciprofloxacin (Ciloxan, Alcon Laboratories, Fort Worth, TX)[30b, 37b] every 1 to 2 hours. A topical anticollagenase such as acetylcysteine (Mucomyst, Mead Johnson Pharmaceutical, Evansville, Ind.) diluted to a 5% to 8% solution with artificial tears is administered every 2 to 4 hours to minimize collagenase activity. In addition, debridement and a conjunctival pedicle graft or penetrating keratoplasty are often indicated to repair the defect, aid in healing, and prevent corneal perforation.

Descemetocele

Descemet's membrane is the basement membrane of the endothelium and the last barrier to corneal perforation. Descemet's membrane does not stain with fluorescein and appears as a clearing in the center of an otherwise edematous corneal ulcer (see Fig. 14–4). As with all corneal ulcers in the horse, routine diagnostic procedures for a descemetocele

include culture and cytology. A descemetocele is a surgical emergency and likely requires referral to a veterinary ophthalmologist. Surgical management is designed to provide support to the weakened cornea and blood vessels and fibroblasts to repair the damage. This is achieved with a conjunctival graft or a lamellar or penetrating keratoplasty (see Corneal Surgery). Routine treatment for a corneal ulcer is used following surgery and is best delivered through a subpalpebral lavage system to avoid manipulation of the eyelids and corneal graft. The conjunctival graft can be debrided 2 to 4 weeks after surgery in an attempt to minimize scar formation by severing the blood supply to the graft tissue.

Corneal Perforation and Laceration

Causes of corneal perforation include rupture of a deep corneal ulcer or descemetocele, and trauma, both sharp and blunt. Depending on the cause of the perforation and severity of the damage, treatment involves primary repair, an intraocular prosthesis, or enucleation. If the horse is to be referred for consultation and treatment, self-trauma during transportation can be prevented through the use of cradles or other protective devices and sedation as required. The prognosis following a penetrating injury varies depending on the cause, size of the wound, location, depth of penetration, intraocular damage, and the presence or absence of infection or retained foreign objects. In general, perforating corneal wounds in the horse have a grave prognosis for vision and a guarded prognosis for cosmesis. They are always associated with secondary anterior uveitis and an iris prolapse is usually present (Fig. 14–8). Sequelae to a corneal perforation include corneal scar, anterior and posterior synechiae, cataracts, glaucoma, phthsis bulbi, blindness, and loss of the eye.

Primary repair of a corneal perforation is a referral procedure. Treatment includes repairing the rent, reestablishing the anterior chamber, preventing infection, and decreasing inflammation and pain. Removal of a penetrating object is best done at the time of repair. Tetanus toxoid is administered prior to repair. The aqueous humor, along with any retained foreign objects, should be cultured for aerobic bacteria and fungi. If iris tissue is protruding but appears viable and minimally contaminated, it is replaced. Contaminated,

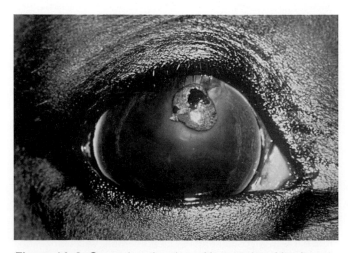

Figure 14–8. Corneal perforation with associated hyphema and iris prolapse.

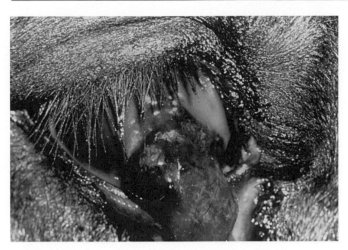

Figure 14–9. Corneal perforation secondary to blunt trauma. The lesion is explosive and expulsive with loss of intraocular contents. Enucleation is the treatment of choice.

nonviable iris is amputated using electrocautery to minimize hemorrhage. If electrocautery is not available, sharp excision can be performed and the bleeding controlled. If the lens capsule has ruptured secondary to trauma, the lens should be removed; lens protein is antigenic and may stimulate severe anterior uveitis. If wound margins can be apposed, the cornea is repaired with partial-thickness, simple interrupted 7-0 absorbable sutures. The anterior chamber is reformed with a balanced salt solution or, if unavailable, lactated Ringer's solution. Conjunctival grafts can be used to promote rapid corneal healing and vascularization and provide support. If a portion of cornea is missing, or the wound edges cannot be apposed, a corneal-scleral transposition or other type of graft procedure is required. Following surgery, topical broad-spectrum antibiotics are administered every 2 to 4 hours, topical atropine is used as needed, and systemic antibiotics and flunixin meglumine are also administered. Use of a subpalpebral lavage delivery system is indicated.

Blunt trauma, whether contusive, penetrating, or perforating, generally results in more severe ocular damage than injury from a sharp object[3] (Fig. 14–9). In contrast to sharp perforating injuries, blunt trauma results in a rapid increase in intraocular pressure, an explosive rupture from the inside outward, and the expulsion of the intraocular contents. The resulting rent in the fibrous tunic is often large and irregular, and portions of the cornea or sclera may be lost. The typical wound is one that originates at the limbus, extending forward into the cornea and posterior into the sclera. If the posterior portion of the eye ruptures, the horse may present with hyphema and decreased intraocular pressure and may require ocular ultrasound for accurate diagnosis.

Repair of these explosive ruptures is difficult and the treatment of choice may be enucleation. If cosmetic repair is important, an intraocular silicone prosthesis can be used in some patients provided there is sufficient tissue left to close the fibrous tunic.[2] This procedure should be performed as soon as possible following injury. If the injury is chronic and atrophy of the globe has occurred, placement of an intraocular prosthesis is not possible. The only cosmetic alternative in these horses is an orbital prosthesis, which is expensive, time-consuming, and requires frequent maintenance on the part of the owner.[2]

Technique for Placement of a Subpalpebral Lavage Delivery System

To facilitate topical medication in a horse with ocular pain or a fractious temperament, a subpalpebral lavage delivery system works well. This can be placed with sedation, auriculopalpebral and supraorbital nerve blocks, topical anesthesia, and appropriate equipment (Table 14–4). The through-and-through subpalpebral lavage technique described here is preferred over other subpalpebral lavage or nasolacrimal delivery systems.[31] This technique results in less irritation, fewer complications, and is less likely to become displaced.

Once the horse is sedated and nerve blocks have been performed, the superior eyelid is elevated and a 12-gauge hubless needle is directed superotemporally from the conjunctival surface. Care is taken to avoid traumatizing the cornea. The needle is always directed from conjunctiva out to skin to minimize the possibility of ocular trauma. The needle is placed as far temporal and into the conjunctival fornix as possible, while remaining anterior to the bony orbital rim. The needle is passed through the superior eyelid and out the skin. Silastic lavage tubing is passed through the needle and the needle is removed. Silastic tubing is preferred because of its low tissue reaction and pliable nature. The procedure is then repeated in the superonasal portion of the eyelid, again directing the needle outward from the conjunctiva and as far from the temporal hole as possible. This must be performed with a hubless needle to allow both needle passes to be directed away from the eye. The tubing is then passed through the needle and the needle is removed. A knot is tied in the medial portion of the tubing as it emerges from the skin of the superior eyelid. Enough throws are placed so that the tube will not migrate back through the eyelid, and they are made tight enough to occlude the lumen.

The amount of tubing on the inside of the eyelid adjacent to the palpebral conjunctiva is approximated. The tubing is pulled nasally and two or three small holes are made in that portion of the tubing midway between the two eyelid puncture wounds. Care is taken to avoid severing the tube. The tube is then pulled back into place.

The tubing is sutured to the skin of the lateral canthus

Table 14–4. Equipment Required for Placement of a Subpalpebral Lavage Delivery System*

Sedation
    Xylazine 100 mg/mL
    Butorphenol 10 mg/mL
Nerve blocks
    Mepivacaine 2%
    25-gauge needle
Topical anesthetic
    Proparacaine 1%
Hubless 12-gauge needle
Silastic tubing (0.065-mm outer diameter)
Tape, 1-in.
2-0 Vetafil suture
Feline urinary catheter, open-ended
Sterile injection cap
Tongue depressor

*From Wilkie DA: Ophthalmic procedures and surgery in the standing horse. *Vet Clin North Am Equine Pract* 7:535–547, 1991.

and to the forehead to prevent migration of the tubing. The tube can be attached to the halter or, in those animals that are extremely difficult to medicate, to the mane on the affected side. An open-ended feline urinary catheter is inserted in the end of the Silastic tubing and an injection cap is attached. This is then taped to a tongue depressor to provide support and the entire apparatus is attached to the halter, taking care to avoid kinking the tubing. The system should then be tested using sterile eyewash. The irrigating solution dripping over the cornea and running down the face is observed to be certain tube placement is correct. Also, note is taken of the volume of solution required to reach the eye. This indicates the volume of air that will be required to deliver the medication to the eye.

Medication used with a subpalpebral lavage system must be in solution, not ointment, form. The volume of medication used at each treatment time should be 0.1 mL and air must then be used to deliver this medication to the eye. The use of irrigating solution to deliver the medication will dilute the medication. Do not exceed 0.1 mL as this medication will be absorbed systemically and excessive volume will simply overflow onto the face. A 25-gauge needle works well for the injection of medication and will preserve the injection cap. Once daily the system should be irrigated with sterile eyewash to ensure its patency and to rinse away mucous buildup.

Complications from a subpalpebral lavage system include trauma during tube placement, improper placement of the delivery holes, irritation to the cornea from the tubing, and migration of the tubing. It is essential to always observe that the medication is reaching the cornea. Improper placement or migration of the tube can result in delivery of medication to the subcutaneous tissues and severe irritation. If corneal trauma occurs the tube must be removed and either replaced or an alternative means of medication found.

Corneal Surgery

Surgery, in the form of a superficial keratectomy, conjunctival graft, or corneal graft, may be indicated in addition to aggressive medical therapy for many complicated corneal ulcers. Corneal surgery must be performed using general anesthesia to optimize the outcome.

A superficial keratectomy provides a biopsy for histopathologic examination, debrides and debulks damaged and infected corneal stroma, and provides a bed for transplanting and suturing a conjunctival or corneal graft. A no. 64 Beaver blade or Martinez corneal dissector is used, first outlining the area to be excised, then undermining and removing the affected area of cornea. In general, 50% to 70% of the corneal thickness can be removed, but excision of 50% or more is an indication to reinforce the remaining cornea with a conjunctival or corneal lamellar graft. The thickness of the normal equine cornea is 1.0 to 1.5 mm, being thinnest centrally. The cornea will increase in thickness with disease as a result of edema, cellular infiltration, vascularization, and scar formation.

Conjunctival grafts include advancement, hood, bridge, pedicle, and complete conjunctival grafts.[36, 37] My preference is to perform a conjunctival pedicle graft for most focal corneal ulcers using the other types for more extensive lesions.[37] Prior to placement of a conjunctival graft, debridement of the affected cornea by superficial keratectomy is indicated. Bulbar conjunctiva is mobilized leaving an intact

blood supply. An attempt should be made to appose conjunctival and corneal epithelium at the edge of the graft and to place 6-0 to 7-0 Vicryl (polyglactin 910) sutures two-thirds depth into healthy cornea. Conjunctival grafts adhere to the underlying exposed corneal stroma providing the blood supply and cells required to repair and rebuild the damaged cornea. Opacification of the graft site will occur, but is generally less than would have occurred without surgery. Opacification can be minimized by trimming the graft, severing its blood supply, 2 to 3 weeks following the initial surgery.

Autologous and homologous lamellar corneal grafts, corneal-scleral transposition, and penetrating keratoplasty are more involved techniques reserved for the most severe corneal ulcers or for perforating corneal lesions.

Nictitating membrane or third eyelid flaps are of little or no benefit in the management of complicated and infected equine corneal disease and are, in many instances, contraindicated.

Nonulcerative Diseases

Nonulcerative corneal diseases include corneal scar, corneal edema, stromal abscessation, cellular and noncellular infiltrates, and a recently described nonulcerative keratouveitis.[38]

Corneal scars are not painful, have a history of prior corneal disease, and are associated with corneal vascularization. Topical corticosteroid therapy will not significantly decrease corneal scarring, but will predispose to infection and decrease healing in the event of a corneal ulcer. Tattooing of a corneal scar for ocular cosmesis is described,[2, 33] but not advised.

Cellular infiltration in the corneal stroma includes neoplastic and inflammatory cells. The most common corneal neoplasia is SCC (see Conjunctiva and Third Eyelid; Fig. 14–2). Corneal lymphosarcoma is also seen. Inflammatory cellular infiltration (neutrophils, lymphocytes, plasma cells, eosinophils) is seen in infectious keratitis (bacterial, mycotic) and is usually associated with corneal ulceration. However, a small, focal corneal ulcer can become infected and reepithelialize, resulting in a corneal stromal abscess. In addition, inflammatory corneal infiltration is seen with equine ocular onchocerciasis and nonulcerative keratouveitis.

Noncellular corneal infiltration or corneal degeneration is a sequela of previous corneal or limbal inflammation. Accumulations of mineral and phospholipids may remain within the corneal stroma following inflammation and appear as crystalline infiltration. These are rare, generally not painful, and do not require treatment. In some instances they predispose to corneal ulceration and can be removed with a superficial keratectomy.[2]

Corneal Edema

Corneal edema, if not associated with a corneal ulcer (fluorescein-negative), is the result of corneal endothelial damage. Blunt trauma to the globe can result in displacement of the corneal endothelium from the posterior surface of the cornea. This results in full-thickness, diffuse corneal edema, which may gravitate to the ventral cornea with time. In addition, diseases of the anterior uvea and aqueous humor, anterior uveitis and glaucoma, and anterior lens luxation can interfere with endothelial cell function, resulting in diffuse corneal edema. Although there is no specific treatment for corneal edema of endothelial origin, topical hyperosmotic agents such as sodium chloride 5% (Muro-128, Bausch & Lomb, Rochester, N.Y.) applied topically every 4 to 6 hours may decrease the severity of the edema and help prevent rupture of corneal bullae. In my opinion, this has only minimal efficacy. With time, the corneal endothelium may reattach or adjacent endothelial cells may hypertrophy, resulting in a decrease in corneal edema. During the period that the edema is present the cornea is compromised and at risk of ulceration. Topical corticosteroids are therefore to be avoided.

Nonulcerative Keratouveitis

A condition consisting of interstitial keratitis with peripheral corneal vascularization, edema, and cellular infiltrate and anterior uveitis (miosis, aqueous flare, iritis) has been described in five horses.[38] The pathogenesis of nonulcerative keratouveitis is unknown, but it is suggested that the anterior uveitis is secondary to interstitial keratitis and that an immune-mediated mechanism is involved. No infectious or neoplastic process is apparent. Histologically, nonulcerative keratouveitis is characterized by vascularization, fibroblasts, and inflammatory cells, predominantly lymphocytes. No infectious agents are seen on light or transmission electron microscopy.

Treatment is similar to that for equine recurrent uveitis and involves suppression of inflammation and control of ocular pain. Topical and subconjunctival corticosteroids, topical NSAIDs, topical cyclosporin A,[44a] topical mydriaticcycloplegics, and systemic NSAIDs are effective in controlling the symptoms, but some level of long-term maintenance therapy is usually required.

The differential diagnosis of nonulcerative keratouveitis comprises corneal stromal abscess, equine ocular onchocerciasis, and neoplasia.

Corneal Stromal Abscess

The usual cause of corneal stromal abscess formation is a focal, superficial corneal ulcer that allows opportunistic infection of the corneal stroma and then heals, trapping the microorganism. Topical antibiotic-corticosteroid therapy in eyes with corneal epithelial cell loss may predispose to stromal abscess formation.[2, 39, 39a] The lesion results in discomfort seen as photophobia, blepharospasm, and excessive lacrimation. A chronic, yellow-white, corneal stromal infiltrate with associated corneal edema and deep corneal vascularization is present.[39, 39a] Anterior uveitis may be present. Fluorescein staining of the cornea is often negative. Diagnosis is based on clinical signs. A corneal scraping should be obtained from the lesion, following removal of the overlying corneal epithelium, and submitted for cytology, bacterial culture and sensitivity, and fungal culture. Gram-positive cocci (Streptococcus and Staphylococcus spp.) have been reported to be the predominant organisms recovered,[39] but fungal stromal abscesses are also seen. Differential diagnosis is nonulcerative keratouveitis.

If the overlying epithelium is intact it should be removed prior to initiation of treatment to facilitate penetration of antibiotics. Topical antibiotics such as neomycin-bacitracin-polymyxin B or gentamicin are used every 4 hours pending culture and sensitivity results. In addition, some authors recommend subconjunctival injections of antibiotics.[2, 39] If anterior uveitis is present, topical atropine 1% is administered as needed to dilate the pupil, up to a maximum of four times a day. Systemic flunixin meglumine will help reduce ocular pain and secondary complications associated with inflammation. Topical corticosteroids are contraindicated. Resolution of the abscess may require 2 to 4 weeks and result in corneal scar formation.

A superficial keratectomy and conjunctival pedicle graft[39a] or penetrating keratoplasty[37a] are also appropriate and may result in a more rapid resolution and reduced corneal opacification than medical management alone.[39a] If a keratectomy is performed, the excised corneal stroma should be submitted for culture, cytology and/or histopathology as this will be more diagnostic than preoperative samples.[39a]

Equine Ocular Onchocerciasis

Onchcocerca cervicalis is a common equine parasite and has been implicated in conjunctivitis, peripheral keratitis, anterior uveitis, and peripapillary chorioretinitis. Corneal lesions result from Onchcocerca microfilariae that migrate to and die in the corneal stroma and that may incite an inflammatory response. The lesion begins peripherally at the temporal limbus, but can extend axially. Interstitial keratitis, manifested as corneal edema, vascularization, and subepithelial focal corneal opacities, occurs and may be associated with temporal bulbar conjunctival vitiligo, conjunctivitis, and anterior uveitis.[40] Diagnosis is made on the basis of history, clinical signs, and the presence of eosinophils on cytologic examination and microfilaria seen on conjunctival biopsy.[40] Microfilaria can be demonstrated cytologically by taking a biopsy of temporal bulbar conjunctiva, placing it on a slide with warm saline, and examining for the presence of motile microfilaria. The presence of microfilaria must be interpreted in combination with the clinical signs as microfilaria can be found in many horses without associated ocular disease.

Treatment includes suppression of ocular inflammation and microfilaricidal therapy (see Table 14–3). Inflammation is controlled with topical corticosteroids and systemic phenylbutazone or flunixin meglumine (see Table 14–7). If anterior uveitis is present, topical atropine 1% is used as needed to dilate the pupil. Pretreatment with anti-inflammatories for 2 to 3 days prior to administration of microfilaricides is indicated to minimize the ocular response to the dying microfilaria.

UVEA

Anatomy

The uvea is the middle, vascular tunic of the eye. It comprises the anterior portion, the iris and ciliary body, and the posterior choroid. Histologically, the uvea contains blood vessels, pigment cells, smooth muscle, and in the horse, a noncellular, fibrous tapetum in the choroid. The uvea is the primary site of the blood-ocular barrier, which has importance in the formation of the aqueous humor, serves as a barrier to bloodborne materials, and is an immunologic barrier to the internal components of the eye. This barrier is disrupted by inflammation (uveitis). Smooth muscles in the iris and ciliary body, under autonomic control, regulate pupil size and accommodation for near and far vision, respectively. In uveitis, spasm of these muscles results in constriction of the pupil and pain, seen clinically as miosis and photophobia. The ciliary body is the source of aqueous humor, which supplies nutrition to the cornea and lens. Aqueous humor is produced by both active and passive processes; its production is decreased by inflammation and by pharmacologic agents used in glaucoma therapy. The choroid supplies nutrition to the retina and also serves as a heat sink to protect the photoreceptors from the heat generated by light striking the retina. The tapetum, contained within the superior choroid, reflects light back across the retina, thereby maximizing the use of available light.

Abnormalities of the Pupil

The pupil of the horse is horizontally elliptical with the dorsal and ventral margins having pigmented prominences termed *corpora nigra*. The pupillary light reflex (PLR) in the horse is similar to that of other species with both a direct and consensual response. The afferent fibers of the PLR are carried in cranial nerve II and the efferent parasympathetic fibers are carried in cranial nerve III. Abnormalities in pupil response to a light stimulus result from afferent lesions involving the retina or optic nerve. Afferent abnormalities are associated with loss of vision in the affected eye. Efferent lesions are rare, but include damage to cranial nerve III with an associated ventrolateral strabismus, abnormalities of the iris itself as seen with synechiae, and glaucoma. Excited horses with sympathetic override, weak light source, and improper examination technique are also to be differentiated from an abnormal pupillary light response.

Sympathetic nerve fibers supply the dilator muscles of the iris. These fibers travel in the spinal cord, emerge in the ventral nerve roots at T1–2, course through the thorax, run in association with the internal carotid artery, synapse at the cranial cervical sympathetic ganglion, and travel to the eye with the ocular arteries. Damage to the sympathetic fibers results in Horner's syndrome. Clinical signs include ptosis, miosis, enophthalmos, protrusion of the third eyelid, and sweating on the affected side of the face and neck. Treatment is directed toward the primary disease, if possible. In some horses the clinical signs of Horner's syndrome will resolve without treatment.

Uveal Cysts

Cysts of the anterior uvea (iris, corpora nigra, and ciliary body) have been reported in the horse.[40a, 40b] They are usually heavily pigmented and may not transilluminate, making a uveal melanoma the most likely differential. Ocular ultrasonography will reveal these as cystic structures and confirm the diagnosis.

Treatment is not required unless the cysts are numerous or visually impairing. The cyst can be collapsed and/or aspirated by paracentesis or, if available, disrupted using laser energy delivered transcorneally.[40b]

Uveitis

Uveitis is an inflammation of the iris and ciliary body (anterior) and choroid (posterior). Uveitis is a common manifestation of many infectious and noninfectious diseases, both ocular and systemic, and as such it is essential to attempt to ascertain the cause. It is also essential to be able to differenti-

Table 14–5. Signs of Acute and Chronic Uveitis

Acute	Chronic
Miosis	Posterior synechiae
Photophobia	Cataract
Blepharospasm	Pigmentation of anterior lens capsule
Eyelid swelling	Atrophy of corpora nigra
Aqueous flare	Glaucoma
Corneal edema	Peripapillary depigmentation
Chorioretinitis	Phthisis bulbi
Keratitic precipitates	Blindness
Hypopyon	Lens luxation
Hypotony	

ate uveitis from other ophthalmic diseases resulting in a red and painful eye such as glaucoma, corneal ulceration, and conjunctivitis. Uveitis is reported as the leading cause of blindness in horses throughout the world.[33, 41]

Clinical Signs

Acute inflammation of the anterior uvea results in spasm of the iris and ciliary muscles, seen clinically as miosis and photophobia, and a breakdown in the blood-ocular barrier (Table 14–5). The primary mediators of intraocular inflammation are prostaglandins. Eyelids and conjunctiva may be swollen and hyperemic in the acute phase of anterior uveitis. Protein and cells leak into the anterior chamber, resulting in aqueous flare, hypopyon, and keratitic precipitates. Chronic inflammatory changes in the aqueous humor can result in secondary corneal endothelial and lens changes (e.g., corneal edema, cataract) and adhesions between the iris and adjacent lens or cornea, termed *synechiae* (Fig. 14–10). Inflammation of the choroid, because of its close association with the retina, usually also involves the retina and is termed *chorioretinitis*. Chorioretinitis, diagnosed by direct or indirect oph-

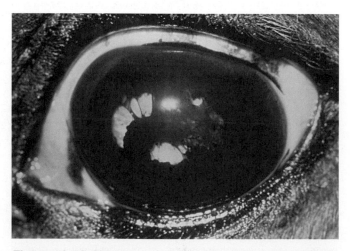

Figure 14–10. Numerous posterior synechiae and a cataract are seen secondary to chronic anterior uveitis. The corpora nigra are adhered to the anterior lens and result in distortion of the pupil margin.

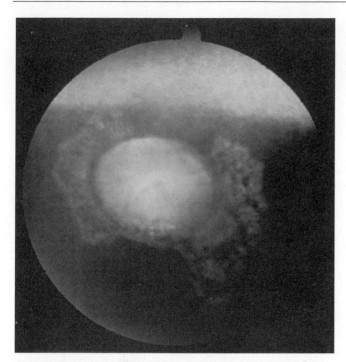

Figure 14–11. Peripapillary depigmentation, a so-called butterfly lesion, associated with the chorioretinitis of equine recurrent uveitis.

thalmoscopy, results in retinal and subretinal transudate and exudate, retinal vascular changes, hemorrhage, retinal detachment, and retinal degeneration. Choroidal depigmentation and areas of repigmentation or pigment clumping may be present (Fig. 14–11). Other chronic changes resulting from intraocular inflammation include secondary glaucoma, blindness, and phthisis bulbi. The development of intraocular changes secondary to uveitis is directly related to the duration and severity of the acute episode and is exacerbated by recurrent episodes of inflammation.

Etiology

The causes of anterior and posterior uveitis include primary ophthalmic as well as systemic diseases. Blunt or penetrating ocular trauma, intraocular neoplasia (primary or secondary), corneal ulceration, parasitic infiltration, and numerous systemic infectious diseases with associated septicemia, toxemia, immune-complex disease, and viremia are all associated with uveitis. Of the systemic infectious diseases implicated in equine uveitis, *Streptococcus equi* (strangles), *Leptospira interrogans* serogroup *pomona*,[43, 43a] and gram-negative sepsis are the most commonly seen. In addition to a complete ophthalmic examination, it is therefore essential to evaluate the entire animal through a complete physical examination and often laboratory testing. A complete ophthalmic evaluation must include fluorescein staining of the cornea; penlight examination to evaluate pupil size, aqueous humor content, lens position and transparency; and direct and consensual pupillary light responses. Direct (with or without indirect) ophthalmoscopic examination of the fundus is also essential. Failure to perform these routine diagnostic tests will result in misdiagnosis and incorrect therapy. It may also result in a failure to consider and examine for systemic disease, thereby placing the animal's health in jeopardy.

Primary ophthalmic diseases that result in anterior uveitis include corneal ulceration, lens-induced uveitis, and direct ocular trauma. Corneal ulceration results in secondary anterior uveitis through a reflex pathway involving the ophthalmic branch of cranial nerve V. Fluorescein staining of the cornea is therefore indicated in eyes with anterior uveitis. The lens is considered to be an immune-privileged site and as such is capable of stimulating an inflammatory reaction. Lens protein is exposed following traumatic rupture of the lens capsule or during the degenerative process of a hypermature cataract undergoing liquefaction and leakage. Either of these processes can result in anterior uveitis with rupture of the lens resulting in the more severe inflammation and, frequently, secondary glaucoma. Uveitis resulting from direct ocular trauma may be associated with rupture of the fibrous tunic of the eye, hyphema, lens luxation, corneal endothelial damage, retinal detachment, or proptosis. A complete ophthalmic examination is essential. If the anterior and posterior segments of the eye are not completely visible, then an ocular ultrasound examination is indicated, specifically to evaluate the position of the lens and retina and to look for changes in the echogenicity of the vitreous humor. In addition to a complete ophthalmic evaluation, the entire animal must be examined for signs of trauma to other body systems. Fractures and soft tissue damage of the head and neck, thoracic and abdominal trauma, fractures of the limbs, and neurologic changes involving the central nervous system are all potential complications seen in association with ocular trauma.

Systemic diseases resulting in anterior and posterior uveitis are numerous and include bacteremia, septicemia, disseminated mycoses, and the syndrome of equine recurrent uveitis. Infection with *Borrelia burgdorferi* has been reported to result in arthritis and panuveitis in a pony.[42] Foals with neonatal septicemia are especially prone to anterior and posterior uveitis. The uveitis in these foals is usually sterile. Systemic antimicrobial, topical and systemic anti-inflammatory, and topical atropine 1% therapy are the treatments of choice.

Equine Recurrent Uveitis

Equine recurrent uveitis (ERU, moon blindness, periodic ophthalmia) is the most common cause of blindness in horses, with Appaloosas at increased risk as compared with non-Appaloosas.[43a] It is believed to be an immune-mediated disease with numerous initiating or exacerbating factors[2, 43, 44] (Table 14–6). The clinical signs of ERU are similar to those

Table 14–6. Causative Agents Implicated in Equine Recurrent Uveitis

Leptospira interrogans serogroup *pomona*[43, 43a]
Onchocerca
Toxoplasma
Virus infection—adenovirus, influenza virus
Brucella
Streptococcus
Borrelia burgdorferi
Trauma
Other

of other causes of uveitis, the distinguishing feature being its recurrent nature. The frequency and severity of each recurrence are extremely variable. It is believed that even in times of clinical quiescence inflammation continues at a subclinical level resulting in further intraocular damage. Diagnosis is based on history and clinical examination. Although serologic evaluation for *Leptospira* species, *Brucella* species, or *Toxoplasma,* and conjunctival biopsies to evaluate for the presence of *Onchocerca cervicalis* have been advocated,[2] it is rare that the results of these tests alter individual therapy. This is in part due to the chronic nature of the disease and because the inciting cause may have begun years prior to development of uveitis, the clinical presentation may make definitive diagnosis difficult.

Treatment of the individual horse is directed toward suppression of inflammation, control of pain, and prevention of sequelae. In situations where the prevalence of ERU in a barn exceeds that normally expected, serologic testing and examination to attempt to determine the cause is indicated. Routine vaccination for *Leptospira* species is controversial and may be contraindicated in horses with active inflammation.

The prognosis for ERU varies according to the severity of uveitis, duration of episodes, response to treatment, and frequency of recurrence. Each episode results in some degree of intraocular damage and damage to the corneal endothelium, lens, and retina is cumulative, as repair of these tissues is difficult. In addition, damage often occurs at a subclinical level during the so-called inactive periods. Horses with evidence of previous uveitis, corneal edema, cataract, synechiae, pigment on the anterior lens capsule, atrophy of the corpora nigra, and degeneration of retina and optic nerve, should be considered ophthalmologically unsound. All animals that have had an episode of acute uveitis must be considered at risk for the development of chronic recurrent uveitis. All animals with chronic recurrent uveitis have a guarded prognosis for long-term maintenance of normal vision, with blindness often the end result.

Treatment

The treatment of any uveitis, acute or chronic, involves specific therapy determined by the cause of the uveitis and nonspecific therapy designed to decrease inflammation, pain, and prevent further intraocular damage. The initiation of specific therapy is dependent on correctly identifying the cause, whether a primary ophthalmic disease or a systemic problem. Failure to control intraocular inflammation may lead to severe secondary ophthalmic complications such as glaucoma, synechiae, cataract, retinal detachment, phthisis bulbi, and blindness.

Nonspecific therapy includes topical and systemic corticosteroids and NSAIDs to decrease inflammation, and atropine to dilate the pupil and decrease the pain of ciliary muscle spasm. Which medication to select, the frequency of treatment, and route of administration are dependent on the cause and severity of the uveitis and whether the uveitis is anterior, posterior, or both.

Topical medications for the treatment of anterior uveitis include atropine, corticosteroids, cyclosporin A, and NSAIDs. Topical atropine 1% is administered as needed to dilate the pupil, generally not more than four times a day. Intestinal motility should be monitored, as topical atropine can result in ileus and colic. Topical corticosteroids are used,

provided corneal ulceration is not present as determined by fluorescein stain. Prednisolone acetate 1% ophthalmic is the corticosteroid of choice, as it achieves the highest intraocular levels. Alternatively, dexamethasone 0.1% ophthalmic solution can be used. Frequency of administration varies according to severity, with initial frequency being every 4 to 6 hours and subsequently decreased as a response is seen. Topical corticosteroid therapy should be continued for several weeks after resolution of clinical signs. In addition, subconjunctival corticosteroids have been advocated in severe cases of anterior uveitis[2, 33] (Table 14–7). Topical NSAIDs are available (see Table 14–7), but little information exists regarding their efficacy in the treatment of ERU. My experience suggests some efficacy, but significantly less clinical response than seen with topical corticosteroids. Topical NSAIDs can be used in horses with anterior uveitis and associated corneal ulceration with less risk than corticosteroids. Topical corticosteroids and NSAIDs have a synergistic effect and can be used in combination. Topical antibiotics are not required unless a corneal ulcer is present; corticosteroids are then contraindicated. Topical cyclosporin A 0.2% ointment (Optimmune, Schering-Plough, Kenilworth, NJ) may be efficacious for the treatment of both active uveitis and as a long-term treatment to decrease the frequency and severity of subsequent recurrences.[34a] Topical medications can be delivered through a subpalpebral lavage system if required.

Systemic NSAIDs are used in conjunction with topical therapy. Flunixin meglumine is the systemic NSAID of choice for acute ocular inflammation. It can be used safely in the presence of corneal ulcer. Alternatively, phenylbutazone or aspirin can be used. Chronic administration of oral aspirin 25 mg/kg s.i.d. has been advocated to decrease the frequency and severity of recurrent episodes of uveitis.[2] Horses with active uveitis should be placed in a darkened stall to decrease discomfort, and exercise should be limited.

Glaucoma

Glaucoma, an elevation of intraocular pressure (IOP) to a level incompatible with the health of the eye, is rare in the horse. The reported normal intraocular pressure in the horse varies according to the technique used and whether sedation is employed, with sedation resulting in a decrease in IOP. An auriculopalpebral nerve block should be performed prior to determination of IOP in the horse. Normal values are reported to range from 20 to 30 mm Hg.[2] Measurement of IOP in the horse presents a challenge in that indentation tonometers, such as the Schiötz, are not well suited for use in the horse. Applanation tonometers, especially portable devices such as the Tonopen (Mentor O&O, Norwell, MA), are best suited for determination of equine IOP. As the use of such devices increases, the true incidence of equine glaucoma will become apparent. In our practice, determination of IOP is routinely performed as part of a complete ophthalmic examination. If determination of IOP is to be performed, it should be noted that intravenous administration of xylazine will significantly lower the IOP.[1a]

Although congenital and primary glaucoma have been reported in the horse, secondary glaucoma resulting from anterior uveitis, especially ERU, is the most common cause of equine glaucoma. The clinical signs of glaucoma in the horse are often more subtle than in other species. Acute glaucoma may result in pain (photophobia, blepharospasm,

Table 14–7. Commonly Used Ophthalmic Medications

Route	Category	Drug	Indication	Dose
Topical				
	Antibiotics	Gentamicin	Corneal ulceration	q2–6h
		Neomycin-bacitracin-polymyxin B	Corneal ulceration	q2–6h
		Tobramycin 0.3% (Tobrex)	Corneal ulceration	q2–6h
	Antifungals	Natamycin (Natacyn)	Corneal ulceration with suspected fungal keratitis	q2–4h
		Miconazole 1% IV, topical	Corneal ulceration with suspected fungal keratitis	q2–4h
	Anti-inflammatories			
	Corticosteroids	1.0% Prednisolone acetate (Econopred Plus)		1–6/day
		0.1% Dexamethasone solution (Decadron)		1–6/day
		0.05% Dexamethasone ointment (Decadron)		1–6/day
	Nonsteroidal	0.03% Flurbiprofen (Ocufen)		4/day
		1.0% Suprofen (Profenal)		4/day
	Parsympatholytics	Tropicamide 1%	Diagnostic agent to dilate the pupil	Single dose
		Atropine 1%	Therapeutic agent to dilate the pupil long-term	1–4/day
Subconjunctival	(do not exceed a volume of 1.0 mL)			
	Anti-inflammatories			
	Corticosteroids	Dexamethasone acetate		10–15 mg
		Betamethasone		5–15 mg
Systemic				
	Anti-inflammatories	Flunixin meglumine	Extra- or intraocular inflammation	1.1 mg/kg PO, IM, IV b.i.d.
		Phenylbutazone	Extra- or intraocular inflammation	2–4 mg/kg PO b.i.d.
		Aspirin	Extra- or intraocular inflammation	25 mg/kg PO, IV s.i.d./b.i.d.

lacrimation), corneal edema, linear corneal opacities, mydriasis (provided uveitis or posterior synechiae are not present), and decreased menace response. The linear opacities seen in equine glaucoma often extend from limbus to limbus and are areas of thinning of Descemet's membrane.[45] Similar linear opacities are also seen in normal horses, have been termed *band keratopathy,* and are not significant. In chronic glaucoma, corneal edema and corneal striae may be seen. Enlargement of the globe (buphthalmos), retinal degeneration, and blindness also occur.

Unfortunately, most glaucomatous horse eyes are presented late in the disease, resulting in a poor response to therapy. Medical treatment in acute glaucoma involves topical autonomic agents such as pilocarpine 2% (Isopto Carpine, Alcon Laboratories), timolol maleate 0.5% (Timoptic, Merck & Co., Inc., West Point, Pa.), dorzolamide 2% (Trusopt, Merck & Co.), and dipivefrin hydrochloride 0.1% (Propine, Allergan Pharmaceuticals, Irvine, Calif.). These are administered alone or in combination twice to four times daily in an effort to reduce IOP by increasing the outflow and decreasing production of aqueous humor. Of these agents, timolol maleate and dorzolamide are most effective and pilocarpine least effective. In the horse, because of the large percentage of uveoscleral outflow, careful use of topical atropine may actually reduce IOP in some eyes. Its use is controversial, however. Topical corticosteroids or systemic flunixin meglumine, or combined therapy, is indicated to control any concomitant inflammation or pain. Failure of topical therapy to control acute glaucoma indicates the need for surgical intervention. Surgery for the acute

patient includes cyclocryosurgery, and possibly cyclocoagulation using a neodymium:yttrium-aluminum-garnet (Nd:YAG) or diode laser.[46] Both of these procedures are designed to reduce the production of aqueous humor and decrease IOP. Cyclocoagulation is reported to have fewer intraocular side effects than cyclocryosurgery, but is not readily available. Surgical filtering procedures, designed to provide an alternative outflow pathway for aqueous humor, are generally unsuccessful in the horse.[2]

Treatment of chronic glaucoma is surgical and is designed to reduce discomfort. Enucleation or evisceration with insertion of an intraocular silicone prosthesis is the procedure of choice.[47]

Hyphema

Hyphema is blood in the anterior chamber of the eye (see Fig. 14–8). As is true of bleeding into other body cavities, blood in the anterior chamber of the eye does not usually clot. It is essential to remember that not all hyphema is the result of ocular trauma. Consideration must be given to systemic diseases that result in clotting disorders or intraocular inflammation.

If the hyphema is complete and precludes the evaluation of intraocular structures, ocular ultrasound is indicated to assess the lens position, retina, and posterior eye wall. The greatest resolution in ocular ultrasound is achieved with a 10-MHz or, if unavailable, 7.5-MHz probe. The probe can be placed directly on the cornea or imaging can be performed through the eyelid or an offset device. Provided no other intraocular damage is seen, hyphema will resolve, often without significant sequelae. If there is associated intraocular damage, potential sequelae include cataract, posterior synechiae, glaucoma, retinal detachment, and blindness (Fig. 14–12).

When hyphema results from a traumatic event, concurrent anterior uveitis is usually present. Although hyphema does not usually require therapy, the associated anterior uveitis does. As previously discussed, anterior uveitis is treated with topical atropine and systemic flunixin meglumine. If there is no corneal ulcer associated with the hyphema, topical corticosteroids may also be administered. Resolution of hyphema may require 7 to 21 days, and to decrease the incidence of rebleeding the horse should not be exercised during this time. Surgical intervention to remove the hyphema is rarely, if ever, indicated. In instances where lysis of a clot is beneficial, intracameral injection of tissue plasminogen activator (25 μg) (Activase, Genentech, Inc., South San Francisco, Calif.) may be indicated.[48]

LENS

The lens originates from surface ectoderm and is a clear, avascular, biconvex structure suspended posterior to the iris by lenticular zonules arising from the ciliary body. The lens depends on the aqueous and vitreous humors to supply nutrition and remove waste products. Examination of the lens should be performed in a darkened environment following dilatation of the pupil with tropicamide 1.0% (Mydriacyl, Alcon Laboratories). Using a bright focal light source the lens is evaluated for size, shape, location, and transparency. Abnormalities of the lens include congenital malformations, cataract, and luxation.

Congenital

Congenital disorders of the lens, other than cataract, are rare. Abnormalities of size (aphakia, microphakia), shape (coloboma, spherophakia), and location (luxation) are gener-

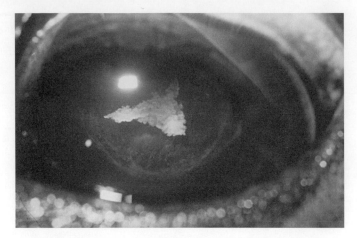

Figure 14–13. An incipient posterior cortical cataract.

ally seen in association with other ocular abnormalities such as microphthalmos, retinal dysplasia, or retinal detachment. These abnormalities can be uni- or bilateral and may or may not be inherited. Treatment is usually not required except for cataract and luxation. Breeding of affected animals should be discouraged.

Cataracts

A cataract is any opacity, of any size, involving the lens or its capsule (Figs. 14–13 and 14–14). Cataracts can be uni- or bilateral. Once diagnosed, cataracts are classified according to location and degree of lens affected (Table 14–8). This is done to help determine the cause, likelihood of progression, and to follow progression. These terms are only descriptive and are not mutually exclusive. For example, one such description might be an "anterior, cortical, axial, incipient cataract." In general, anterior, cortical, and equatorial cataracts are more likely to progress than nuclear and posterior cataracts. In addition, cataracts are classified on the basis of age of onset and, if possible, cause. Classification by age of onset includes congenital, juvenile, adult, and senile cataracts. Congenital cataracts are the most common congenital ocular anomaly in the horse, can be unilateral or

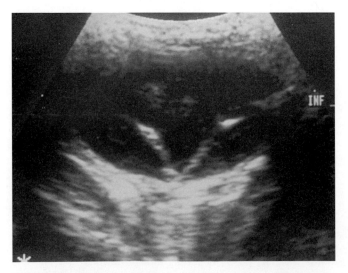

Figure 14–12. Ocular ultrasonography using a 7.5-MHz probe. A retinal detachment is observed with the retina remaining attached at the optic nerve and ciliary body.

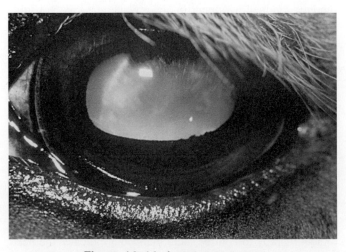

Figure 14–14. A mature cataract.

Table 14–8. Characterization of Cataracts

Location	Severity
Capsular	Incipient—earliest form, small vacuoles
Subcapsular	Immature—affecting most of lens, fundus visible
Cortical	Mature—entire lens affected, fundus not
Equatorial	visible
Axial	Hypermature—liquefying lens fibers, leaking
Nuclear	through lens capsule
Anterior/posterior	Morgagnian—entire cortex liquefied, nucleus settles ventrally

bilateral, and may only affect the nuclear portion of the lens.[49] Juvenile and adult cataracts, although acquired, can still be inherited.

Although many causes of cataracts exist in other species, most have not been documented in the horse. Potential causes of cataract formation include inherited, inflammatory, traumatic, metabolic, toxic, and nutritional abnormalities. Suspected inherited cataracts have been reported in several breeds of horses (Belgian, Morgan) and are thought to occur in other breeds, but are difficult to prove owing to the small number of offspring produced. It is important to remember that inherited cataracts are not necessarily congenital, nor are all congenital cataracts inherited. In general, if a cause of a cataract cannot be determined, and there is no evidence of intraocular inflammation, breeding of this animal should be discouraged. The most common cause of cataract formation in the horse is ERU.

Treatment of cataracts, if required, is surgical. The decision on whether to treat depends on the severity and cause of the cataract and the presence or absence of concomitant ocular disease. Cataracts that are unilateral or not severe enough to significantly interfere with vision generally do not require treatment. Cataracts resulting from intraocular inflammation, such as those seen in association with ERU, are not amenable to surgery. Treatment of cataracts seen in association with abnormalities of the retina, such as retinal detachment or degeneration, is not indicated. If the cataracts are bilateral, interfering with vision, and not the result of ERU or other intraocular inflammation, then surgical removal of the lens and its anterior capsule can be performed. Prior to cataract surgery, evaluation of retinal anatomy and function should be performed using ocular ultrasound and electroretinography. Foals with congenital cataracts should be operated on early (<6 months) to avoid possible deprivation amblyopia. Surgery is best performed using the technique of phacoemulsification.[50, 51] Controversy exists regarding unilateral cataract extraction in horses with a contralateral normal eye. Because artificial lens implants are unavailable for horses, cataract extraction results in some degree of postoperative hyperopia.[33] Although significant disparity in postoperative vision between eyes must result, one study suggests that such horses perform better following cataract surgery than as unilaterally blind horses prior to cataract extraction.[50] Cataract surgery is a referral procedure.

Luxation

Lens luxation and subluxation can be congenital or acquired. Acquired lens luxation occurs as the result of glaucoma and buphthalmos, trauma, or most frequently, uveitis, especially ERU. Once luxated, the lens can be displaced anteriorly or posteriorly. A posteriorly luxated lens results in liquefaction of the vitreous from lens movement. The lens will settle inferiorly, may or may not attach to the retina, and generally does not result in significant problems or require therapy. Anterior lens luxation results in anterior uveitis, trauma to the corneal endothelium resulting in diffuse corneal edema, and obstruction of the circulation of aqueous humor resulting in secondary glaucoma. Treatment of anterior lens luxation is surgical removal using an intracapsular extraction technique, provided the eye is visual. This is a referral procedure. In a blind eye, enucleation or intrascleral prosthesis is the treatment of choice.

FUNDUS

Examination of the equine fundus is best performed in a darkened environment following mydriasis. Both direct and indirect ophthalmoscopy can be used for examination of the equine fundus, although direct ophthalmoscopy is preferred for examination of the optic nerve and retinal blood vessels. Examination should include evaluation of the tapetal and nontapetal fundus, retina, retinal blood vessels, and optic nerve. Variations in the normal equine fundus are common and familiarity with these variations is essential.[10, 33, 49, 52] The horse has a paurangiotic retina (partially vascularized) with 30 to 60 small retinal vessels radiating from the margin of the optic disk. These vessels are visible for a distance of one to two disk diameters. The remainder of the equine retina is avascular, being supplied from the underlying choroidal blood vessels. The optic disk is situated in the nontapetal fundus, is oval, and salmon-pink in color. The fundus is divided into tapetal and nontapetal regions. The tapetum is situated in the dorsal fundus and is responsible for the characteristic yellow-green color of this portion of the fundus. Variations in tapetal color are related to coat color and include yellow, orange, and blue-green.[10, 49] The tapetum of the horse is fibrous and is penetrated by small choroidal vessels that appear as dark dots in the tapetum, termed the *stars of Winslow*. The ventral, nontapetal fundus is generally dark brown or black in color, but can appear lighter or nonpigmented depending on coat color.[10, 49]

Abnormalities on fundic examination include changes in size, shape, and color of the optic nerve and retinal vessels, elevation or depression of the optic nerve, hemorrhage, changes in tapetal reflectivity (hyper- and hyporeflective), and changes in pigmentation. Abnormalities that are hyperreflective often indicate thinning or loss of retinal tissue. Hyporeflective changes can indicate an increase in tissue thickness resulting from cellular infiltrates, edema, or folding of the retina, as seen in retinal dysplasia. Inflammation can result in depigmentation and pigment clumping in the nontapetal fundus and hyperpigmentation in the tapetal fundus. Equine motor neuron disease has been described to result in a mosaic pattern of yellow-brown pigmentation in the tapetal fundus accompanied by a horizontal band of pigment at the tapetal non-tapetal junction.[52a]

RETINA

Congenital Stationary Night Blindness

Equine night blindness (ENB) is a bilateral, congenital, nonprogressive retinal disease seen in appaloosa horses.[53] The degree of visual disturbance varies among horses with mildly affected horses exhibiting signs only in dark conditions, whereas severely affected horses are totally blind in the dark, exhibit apprehension in daylight, and may have a bilateral dorsomedial strabismus and nystagmus.[53] The diagnosis is suspected on history, breed of horse, clinical signs, and maze testing in an illuminated and darkened environment, but must be confirmed by electroretinogram, as the fundic examination in affected horses is normal. Electroretinography demonstrates an almost purely negative waveform in the scotopic (dark-adapted) response, characteristic of ENB.[53, 54] The results of the electroretinogram indicate an abnormality in signal transmission from the photoreceptor cells to the inner retina.[53] Although the inheritance of ENB in the appaloosa is not completely defined, it is suspected to be inherited as an autosomal recessive disease. There is no treatment.

Chorioretinitis

Inflammation of the retina and choroid in the horse is most often the result of ERU and may be associated with concomitant optic neuritis. In addition, the vascular nature of the choroid results in susceptibility to bloodborne disease, as is seen with bacteremia, septicemia, and viremia. This is most often seen in foals with pneumonia, strangles (*Streptococcus equi*), and other severe infectious diseases. Inflammation of the anterior portions of the eye, anterior uveitis, is often seen in association with chorioretinitis. Treatment of chorioretinitis includes systemic therapy for the primary infectious disease, if present, and flunixin meglumine to decrease inflammation. Topical treatment is only indicated if there is anterior uveal involvement. The sequelae of chorioretinitis include retinal degeneration, retinal detachment, and optic nerve atrophy.

Retinal Detachment

Retinal detachment can be congenital or acquired, partial or complete (Fig. 14–15). Since as the equine retina is almost totally dependant on the underlying choroid for its blood supply, detachment results in rapid and severe retinal degeneration. Common causes of retinal detachment in the horse include an inherited abnormality (associated with retinal dysplasia), ERU, and trauma. Congenital retinal detachment is often associated with other ocular abnormalities. Hyphema may be present in association with traumatic detachment, requiring ocular ultrasonography for definitive diagnosis. Treatment is limited to controlling the inciting disease and use of systemic anti-inflammatories.

Photic Headshaking

A condition of headshaking induced by exposure to light and eliminated by blindfolding, darkened environment, and contact lenses has been reported in the horse.[54a, 54b] The problem is usually seen in the spring and summer, is exacerbated by exercise, and may be accompanied by sneezing, snorting, and nasal rubbing.[54a] Differentials for photic headshaking include middle ear disorders, ear mites, guttural pouch mycosis, other ocular disorders, and nasal and dental disease.[54a] Ophthalmic examination in these animals is normal. It is hypothesized that an optic-trigeminal response is

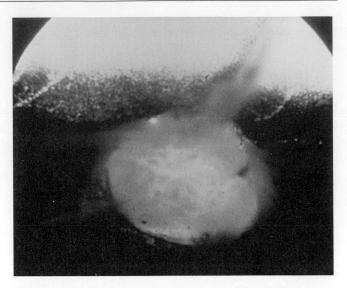

Figure 14–15. Gray folds of retina are observed overlying and adjacent to the optic nerve, indicating retinal detachment.

occurring with optic stimulation resulting in referred stimulation in areas innervated by the trigeminal nerve.[54a]

Treatment using cyproheptadine 0.3 mg/kg (Sidmark Laboratories Inc., East Hanover, NJ) every 12 hours has been effective in several horses.[54a, 54b] Cyproheptadine is an antihistamine (H_1 blocker) and a serotonin antagonist and is hypothesized to work in photic headshaking by moderating the trigeminal nerve sensation, having a central effect on melatonin or through anticholinergic activity.[54a]

OPTIC NERVE

The equine optic nerve is oval, salmon-pink in color, and located in the nontapetal region of the fundus. Arterioles and venules (30–60) extend a short distance from the optic nerve into the surrounding peripapillary retina. On direct ophthalmoscopic examination, the margin of the optic nerve is sharp and well-defined, as are the retinal blood vessels. Often the nerve fiber layer of the retina is visible as linear white streaks radiating outward from the optic nerve. Abnormalities of the optic nerve may appear as indistinct margins, pallor, vascular attenuation, peripapillary depigmentation, edema, hemorrhage, or proliferative changes.

Optic Atrophy

Trauma to the head of the horse has been associated with acute uni- or bilateral blindness as a result of optic nerve damage. The pupil in the affected eye will be dilated, but the remainder of the ophthalmic examination may be normal initially. Occasionally, retinal hemorrhage and papilledema are present. Fundic examination 3 to 4 weeks after the traumatic episode reveals optic nerve pallor and absence of retinal blood vessels, indicating atrophy[55] (Fig. 14–16). The cause of this lesion is hypothesized to be stretching of the optic nerve with subsequent rupture of the optic nerve axons[55] or trauma from bony fractures adjacent to the optic nerve. A small number of these horses may benefit from systemic anti-inflammatory therapy in the acute phase. The

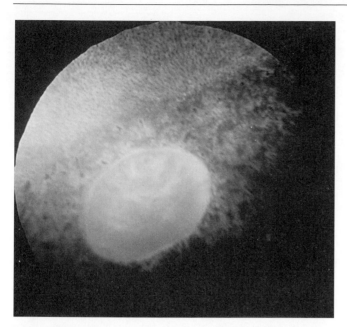

Figure 14–16. Severe optic nerve atrophy associated with head trauma. The optic nerve is pale and there is loss of peripapillary retinal blood vessels. The eye is not visual.

prognosis, however, is guarded and treatment is usually unrewarding. Optic nerve atrophy is also seen in association with ERU and as a result of chronic glaucoma.

Ischemic Optic Neuropathy

Ischemic optic neuropathy and resulting blindness is described following treatment of guttural pouch mycosis by arterial occlusion.[56] These horses are acutely blind with a fixed and dilated pupil on the affected side immediately following surgery. Blindness is thought to result from ischemia and infarction of the optic nerve and its associated fibers. The initial fundic examination is normal with abnormalities first seen 3 days following surgery. Indistinct optic disk margins suggesting papilledema or papillitis and raised, white lesions involving the optic nerve are the initial changes seen.[56]

Optic Nerve Hypoplasia

Horses affected with optic nerve hypoplasia have visual impairment or blindness and slow-to-absent pupillary light reflexes.[10, 49] This is a congenital abnormality and can be uni- or bilateral. Optic nerve hypoplasia may be seen in association with other ocular abnormalities, including cataracts, retinal detachment, and microphthalmos.[49] The optic disk appears small and pale with fewer retinal vessels than normal. Clinically, optic nerve hypoplasia can appear similar to acquired optic nerve atrophy. Definitive diagnosis can be made on histologic examination. No treatment is indicated and although the definitive cause is not known, the affected horse and possibly the sire and dam should not be used for breeding.

Other abnormalities of the optic nerve include bilateral optic neuropathy and blindness following severe hemorrhage[57] proliferative optic neuropathy seen in aged horses,[58] neoplasia of the optic nerve,[59] and optic neuritis, which may be seen in association with ERU.

ORBIT

The horse has a complete bony orbital rim, composed of the frontal, lacrimal, zygomatic, and temporal bones. The caudolateral and ventral walls of the equine orbit are fasciae. Abnormalities of the equine orbit are most often the result of trauma. The zygomatic arch and supraorbital process of the frontal bone and the medial orbital wall are most susceptible to injury. Damage to these areas can involve the supraorbital foramen and its associated nerve or the osseous portion of the nasolacrimal system, respectively.

The diagnosis of an orbital fracture is based on history, clinical signs, and radiographs. Radiographic evaluation of the equine orbit is technically difficult and often unrewarding. Oblique views, highlighting the area of greatest concern, are usually required. Care must be taken to evaluate the paranasal sinuses—the frontal, maxillary, and sphenopalatine—especially when subcutaneous emphysema is present.

Traumatic fractures of the orbit are often associated with concomitant injury of the globe and adnexa. Complete ophthalmic examination is essential. This must include assessment of facial symmetry, vision (menace response, maze testing), pupillary light reflex, fluorescein staining for the presence of a corneal ulcer, examination of the anterior chamber for hyphema and anterior uveitis, fundic examination evaluating the retina and optic nerve, assessment of globe and eyelid mobility, and nasolacrimal irrigation. Head trauma in the horse has been reported to result in acute blindness with fixed, dilated pupils as the result of optic nerve compression, stretching, or avulsion. In those eyes where ocular damage precludes examination of the posterior segment, ocular ultrasound is advised.

Blunt trauma to the orbit can result in a breakdown of the fibrous orbital septum and subsequent herniation of orbital fat. Clinically, this is a nonpainful swelling that appears at the time of or following orbital trauma. It is best treated surgically, removing or replacing the herniated portion of the orbital fat pad and attempting to surgically repair the rent in the septum.

Traumatic proptosis is rare in the horse because of the complete bony orbital rim. If the globe protrudes, it indicates severe head trauma, and thorough physical and neurologic examinations are required. Provided the optic nerve and extraocular muscles are intact, an exophthalmic globe should be replaced. This requires general anesthesia. Once the globe is replaced, a temporary tarsorrhaphy is performed to protect the eye until the swelling subsides. Systemic antibiotics and anti-inflammatory drugs are indicated to control postoperative complications.

Treatment of orbital trauma in the acute phase includes systemic anti-inflammatory therapy, systemic antibiotics, especially if a paranasal sinus is involved, and cold compresses. The anti-inflammatory of choice is systemic flunixin meglumine. Local therapy is required for the management of corneal exposure, ulceration, and anterior uveitis. If eyelid movement is impaired, either as the result of neurologic dysfunction or swelling of the eyelids, the cornea must be protected from exposure and desiccation using a topical, sterile ophthalmic lubricant applied as frequently as possible, or in the more severe cases, through the use of a temporary tarsorrhaphy. Topical broad-spectrum antibiotics are indicated in horses with corneal ulceration, and atropine is used to relieve the discomfort associated with anterior uveitis.

Although facial and orbital fractures in horses will often heal without surgery, they may do so in a manner that results in deformity and interferes with the normal function of the eye and adnexa. Therefore, surgical correction may be indicated, especially in those fractures that are displaced. Fractures that extend into a paranasal sinus must be considered as open fractures, as these sinuses contain resident bacterial and fungal flora. Early repair is associated with a more favorable cosmetic result, as skull fractures consolidate rapidly and the resulting fibrous callus may interfere with surgical reduction. Generous skin flaps in the surgical approach are advised because fractures are often more extensive than initially thought. Excessive periosteal dissection should be avoided, as periosteum provides both stability and blood supply to the damaged area.

Orbital neoplasia is rare and may result in exophthalmos, strabismus, and vision and pupil abnormalities. Skull radiographs, orbital ultrasound, cytologic examination of a fine needle aspirate, and histopathology are useful in confirming the diagnosis. Squamous cell carcinoma, lymphosarcoma, adenocarcinoma, medulloepithelioma, melanoma, and tumors of neuroendocrine origin have been described.[59a] Differentials would include trauma and orbital abscess/cellulitis. As most horses are presented late in the course of disease, orbital exenteration is often the treatment of choice.

REFERENCES

1. van der Woerdt A, Gilger BC, Wilkie DA, et al: Effect of auriculopalpebral nerve block and intravenous administration of xylazine on intraocular pressure and corneal thickness in horses. *Am J Vet Res* 56:155, 1995.
1a. Manning JP, St Clair LE: Palpebral, frontal, and zygomatic nerve blocks for examination of the equine eye. *Vet Med* 71:187, 1976.
2. Lavach JD: *Large Animal Ophthalmology.* St Louis, Mosby–Year Book, 1989.
2a. Barnett KC, Crispin SM, Lavach JD, et al: *Color Atlas and Text of Equine Ophthalmology.* St. Louis, Mosby-Wolfe, 1995.
3. Wilkie DA: Ocular injuries. In Robinson NE, ed: *Current Therapy in Equine Medicine,* ed 3. Philadelphia, WB Saunders, 1992, pp 587–591.
3a. van der Woerdt A, Wilkie DA, Gilger BC: Ulcerative keratitis secondary to single layer repair of a traumatic eyelid laceration in a horse. *Equine Pract* 18:33, 1996.
4. Lavach JD: Ocular neoplasia. In Robinson NE, ed: *Current Therapy in Equine Medicine,* ed 3. Philadelphia, WB Saunders, 1992, p 604.
5. Theon AP, Pascoe JR, Carlson GP, et al: Intratumoral chemotherapy with cisplatin in oily emulsion in horses. *J Am Vet Med Assoc* 202:261, 1993.
6. Whitley RD, Moore CP: Microbiology of the equine eye in health and disease. *Vet Clin North Am Large Anim Pract* 6:451, 1984.
7. Moore CP, Heller N, Majors LJ, et al: Prevalence of ocular microorganisms in hospitalized and stabled horses. *Am J Vet Res* 49:773, 1988.
8. Samuelson DA, Andresen TL, Gwin RM: Conjunctival flora in horses, cattle, dogs, and cats. *J Am Vet Med Assoc* 184:1240, 1984.
8a. Collinson PN, O'Reilly JL, Ficorilli N, et al: Isolation of equine herpesvirus type 2 (equine gammaherpesvirus 2) from foals with keratoconjunctivitis. *J Am Vet Med Assoc* 205:329, 1994.
9. Lyons ET, Tolliver BS, Drudge JH, et al: Eyeworms *(Thelazia lacrymalis)* in one- to four-year-old Thoroughbreds at necropsy in Kentucky (1984–1985). *Am J Vet Res* 47:315, 1986.
10. Riis RC: Equine ophthalmology. In Gelatt KN, ed: *Veterinary Ophthalmology.* Philadelphia, Lea & Febiger, 1981, p 586.
11. Lyons ET, Drudge JH, Tolliver SC: Controlled tests with fenbendazole in equids: Special interest on activity of multiple doses against natural infections of migratory stages of strongyles. *Am J Vet Res* 44:1058, 1983.
12. Vasey JR: Equine cutaneous habronemiasis. *Compend Contin Educ Pract Vet* 3:290, 1981.
13. Rebhun WC, Mirro EJ, Georgi ME, et al: Habronemic blepharoconjunctivitis in horses. *J Am Vet Med Assoc* 179:469, 1981.
14. Moore CP, Sarazan RD, Whitley RD, et al: Equine ocular parasites: A review. *Equine Vet J* 2:(suppl):76, 1983.
15. Cummings E, James ER: Prevalence of equine onchocerciasis in southeastern and midwestern United States. *J Am Vet Med Assoc* 186:1202, 1985.
16. Lyons ET, Tolliver SC, Drudge JH, et al: *Onchocerca* spp: Frequency in Thoroughbreds at necropsy in Kentucky. *Am J Vet Res* 47:880, 1986.
17. Schmidt GM, Krehbiel JD, Coley SC, et al: Equine ocular onchocerciasis: Histopathologic study. *Am J Vet Res* 43:1371, 1982.
18. Hacker DV, Moore PF, Buyukmichi NC: Ocular angiosarcoma in four horses. *J Am Vet Med Assoc* 189:200, 1986.
19. Dugan SJ, Roberts SM, Curtis CR, et al: Prognostic factors and survival of horses with ocular/adnexal squamous cell carcinoma: 147 cases (1978–1988). *J Am Vet Med Assoc* 198:298, 1991.
20. Gelatt KN, Myers VS, Perman V, et al: Conjunctival squamous cell carcinoma in the horse. *J Am Vet Med Assoc* 168:617, 1974.
21. Dugan SJ, Curtis CR, Roberts SM, et al: Epidemiologic study of ocular/adnexal squamous cell carcinoma in horses. *J Am Vet Med Assoc* 198:251, 1991.
22. Schwink K: Factors influencing morbidity and outcome of equine ocular squamous cell carcinoma. In *Proceedings of the American College of Veterinary Ophthalmology,* 1985, p 180.
23. Owen LN, Barnett KC: Treatment of equine squamous cell carcinoma of the conjunctiva using a strontium[90] applicator. *Equine Vet J* 2(suppl):105, 1983.
24. Wilkie DA, Burt JK: Combined treatment of ocular squamous cell carcinoma in a horse, using radiofrequency hyperthermia and interstitial [198]Au implants. *J Am Vet Med Assoc* 196:1831, 1990.
25. Rebhun WC: Treatment of advanced squamous cell carcinomas involving the equine cornea. *Vet Surg* 19:297, 1990.
25a. Theon AP, Pascoe JR, Madigan JE, et al: Comparison of intratumoral administration of cisplatin versus bleomycin for treatment of periocular squamous cell carcinomas in horses. *Am J Vet Res* 58:431, 1997.
26. Walker MA, Goble D, Geiser D: Two-year non-recurrence rates for equine ocular and periorbital squamous cell carcinoma following radiotherapy. *Vet Radiol* 27:146, 1986.
27. Grier RL, Brewer WG, Paul SR, et al: Treatment of bovine and equine ocular squamous cell carcinoma by radiofrequency hyperthermia. *J Am Vet Med Assoc* 177:5, 1980.
28. Latimer CA, Wyman M, Diesem CD, et al: Radiographic and gross anatomy of the nasolacrimal duct of the horse. *Am J Vet Res* 45:451, 1984.
29. Latimer CA, Wyman M: Atresia of the nasolacrimal duct in three horses. *J Am Vet Med Assoc* 184:989, 1984.
30. Cooley PL, Wyman M: Indolent-like corneal ulcers in 3 horses. *J Am Vet Med Assoc* 188:295, 1986.
30a. Yamagata M, Wilkie, DA, Gilger BC: Eosinophilic keratoconjunctivitis in seven horses. *J Am Vet Med Assoc* 209:1283, 1996.

30b. Moore CP, Collins BK, Fales WH: Antibacterial susceptibility patterns for microbial isolates associated with infectious keratitis in horses: 63 cases (1986–1994). *J Am Vet Med Assoc* 207:928, 1995.

31. Schoster JV: The assembly and placement of ocular lavage sysetms in horses. *Vet Med* May:60, 1992.

32. Rebhun WC: Chronic corneal epithelial erosions in horses. *Vet Med Small Anim Clin* 1635, 1983.

33. Davidson MG: Equine ophthalmology. In Gelatt KN, ed: *Veterinary Ophthalmology,* ed 2. Philadelphia, Lea & Febiger, 1991, p 576.

34. Miller TR: Punctate keratitis. In Robinson NE, ed: *Current Therapy in Equine Medicine,* ed 3. Philadelphia, WB Saunders, 1992, p 599.

34a. Gratzek AT, Kaswan RL, Martin CL, et al: Ophthalmic cyclosporine in equine keratitis and keratouveitis: 11 cases. *Eq Vet J* 27:327, 1995.

34b. Ramsey DT, Whitley HE, Gerding PA, et al: Eosinophilic keratoconjunctivitis in a horse. *J Am Vet Med Assoc* 205:1308, 1994.

35. Coad CT, Robinson NM, Wilhelmus KR: Antifungal sensitivity testing for equine keratomycosis. *Am J Vet Res* 46:676, 1985.

35a. Ball MA, Rebhun WC, Gaarder JE, et al: Evaluation of itraconazole-dimethyl sulfoxide ointment for treatment of keratomycosis in nine horses. *J Am Vet Med Assoc* 221:199, 1997.

36. Holmberg DL: Conjunctival pedicle grafts used to repair corneal perforations in the horse. *Can Vet J* 22:86, 1981.

37. Hakanson N, Lorimer D, Merideth RE: Further comments on conjunctival pedicle grafting in the treatment of corneal ulcers in the dog and cat. *J Am Anim Hosp Assoc* 24:602, 1988.

37a. Whittaker CJG, Smith PJ, Brooks DE, et al: Therapeutic penetrating keratoplasty for deep corneal stromal abscesses in eight horses. *Vet Comparative Ophthalmol* 7:19, 1997.

37b. Sweeney CR, Irby NL: Topical treatment of *Pseudomonas* sp. infected corneal ulcers in horses: 70 cases (1977–1994). *J Am Vet Med Assoc* 209:954, 1996.

38. Brooks DE, Millichamp NJ, Peterson MG, et al: Nonulcerative keratouveitis in five horses. *J Am Vet Med Assoc* 196:1985, 1990.

39. Rebhun WC: Corneal stromal abscesses in the horse. *J Am Vet Med Assoc* 181:677, 1982.

39a. Hendrix DVH, Brooks DE, Smith PJ, et al: Corneal stromal abscesses in the horse: a review of 24 cases. *Eq Vet J* 27:440, 1995.

40. Munger RJ: Equine onchocercal keratoconjunctivitis. *Equine Vet J* 2(suppl):65, 1983.

40a. Dziezyc J, Samuelson DA, Merideth R: Ciliary cysts in three ponies. *Eq Vet J* 22:22, 1990.

40b. Gilger BC, Davidson MG, Nadelstein B, et al: Neodymium:yttrium-aluminum-garnet laser treatment of cystic granula iridica in horses: 8 cases (1988–1996). *J Am Vet Med Assoc* 211:341, 1997.

41. Davidson MG: Anterior uveitis. In Robinson NE, ed: *Current Therapy in Equine Medicine,* ed 3. Philadelphia, WB Saunders, 1992, p 592.

42. Burgess EC, Gillette D, Pickett JP: Arthritis and panuveitis as manifestations of *Borrelia burgdorferi* infection in a Wisconsin pony. *J Am Vet Med Assoc* 189:1340, 1986.

43. Sillerud CL, Bey RF, Ball M, Bistner SI: Serologic correlation of suspected *Leptospira interrogans* serovar *pomona*–induced uveitis in a group of horses. *J Am Vet Med Assoc* 191:1576, 1987.

43a. Dwyer AE, Crockett RS, Kaslow CM: Association of leptospiral seroreactivity and breed with uveitis and blindness in horses: 372 cases (1986–1993). *J Am Vet Med Assoc* 207:1327, 1995.

44. Hines MT: Immunologically mediated ocular disease in the horse. *Vet Clin North Am* Large *Anim Pract* 6:501, 1984.

45. Brooks DE: Glaucoma. In Robinson NE, ed: *Current Therapy in Equine Medicine,* ed 3. Philadelphia, WB Saunders, 1992, p 602.

46. Nasisse MP, Davidson MG, MacLachlan NJ, et al: Neodymium:yttrium, alluminum, and garnet laser energy delivered transsclerally to the ciliary body of dogs. *Am J Vet Res* 49:1972, 1988.

47. Provost PJ, Ortenburger AI, Caron JP: Silicone ocular prosthesis in horses: 11 cases (1983–1987). *J Am Vet Med Assoc* 194:1764, 1989.

48. Martin C, Kaswan R, Gratzek A, et al: Ocular use of tissue plasminogen activator in companion animals. *Prog Vet Comp Ophthalmol* 3:29, 1993.

49. Munroe GA, Barnett KC: Congenital ocular disease in the foal. *Vet Clin North Am Large Anim Pract* 6:519, 1984.

50. Dziezyc J, Millichamp NJ, Keller C: Use of phacofragmentation for cataract removal in horses: 12 cases (1985–1989). *J Am Vet Med Assoc* 198:1774, 1991.

51. Dziezyc J, Millichamp NJ: Cataracts. In Robinson NE, ed: *Current Therapy in Equine Medicine,* ed 3. Philadelphia, WB Saunders, 1992, p 601.

52. Gelatt KN: Ophthalmoscopic studies in the normal and diseased ocular fundi of horses. *J Am Anim Hosp Assoc* 7:158, 1971.

52a. Jackson CA, Riis RC, Rebhun WC, et al: Ocular manifestations of equine motor neuron disease. *Proc Am Assoc Equine Pract* 41:225, 1995.

53. Rebhun WC, Loew ER, Riis RC, et al: Clinical manifestations of night blindness in the Appaloosa horse. *Compend Contin Educ Pract Vet* 6:S103, 1984.

54. Witzel DA, Joyce JR, Smith EL: Electroretinography of congenital night blindness in an Appaloosa filly. *J Equine Med Surg* 1:226, 1977.

54a. Madigan JE, Kortz G, Murphy C, et al: Photic headshaking in the horse: 7 cases. *Eq Vet J* 27:306, 1995.

54b. Wilkins PA: Cyproheptadine: Medical treatment for photic headshakers. *Comp Cont Ed* 19:98, 1997.

55. Martin L, Kaswan R, Chapman W: Four cases of traumatic optic nerve blindness in the horse. *Equine Vet J* 18:133, 1986.

56. Hardy J, Robertson JT, Wilkie DA: Ischemic optic neuropathy and blindness after arterial occlusion for treatment of guttural pouch mycosis in two horses. *J Am Vet Med Assoc* 196:1631, 1990.

57. Gelatt KN: Neuroretinopathy in horses. *J Equine Med Surg* 3:91, 1979.

58. Vestre WA, Turner TA, Carlton WW: Proliferative optic neuropathy in a horse. *J Am Vet Med Assoc* 181:490, 1982.

59. Bistner SI, Cambell RJ, Shaw D, et al: Neuroepithelial tumor of the optic nerve in a horse. *Cornell Vet* 73:30, 1983.

59a. Basher AWP, Severin GA, Chavkin MJ, et al: Orbital neuroendocrine tumors in three horses. *J Am Vet Med Assoc* 210:668, 1997.

Chapter 15

Diseases of the Reproductive Tract

15.1

Physiology of Gestation

Heidi M. Immegart, DVM, MS, PhD, Dip ACT
Walter R. Threlfall, DVM, MS, PhD, Dip ACT

EARLY GESTATION

Following ovulation, the formation of the corpus luteum (CL) begins and, with its development, the production of progesterone. The ovulated ovum is fertilized in the ampulla of the oviduct and is transported into the uterine lumen by days 5 and 6. Once in the uterus, the embryo migrates extensively through the horns and the body.[1, 2] This movement promotes widespread recognition of secreted embryonic factors that are responsible for maternal recognition of pregnancy and CL maintenance.[3, 4] Restriction of the mobility of this conceptus can result in failure to maintain the pregnancy.[5]

Fetal trophoblastic cells invade the maternal endometrium at approximately day 35 and are responsible for endometrial cup formation. The primary CL is the source of progesterone during early pregnancy and is responsible for maintenance of the pregnancy until the endometrial cups are functional and begin to produce equine chorionic gonadotropin (eCG). Although follicular development begins before endometrial cup formation and is considered to be due to follicle stimulating hormone (FSH) from the pituitary, eCG is most likely to be responsible for maturation and luteinization of these follicles into secondary CLs.[6] Ovulation of secondary follicles may or may not occur. The primary CL produces an increased amount of progesterone soon after endometrial cup formation, and then secondary CL formation results in a larger increase in progesterone.[7, 8] During the endometrial cup stage, the placenta also begins to produce progestogens. By day 100, ovarian sources of progestagens are no longer essential to maintain a pregnancy.[9] Endometrial cups are present until approximately day 120, when the maternal immune system reacts to the foreign trophoblastic cup cells.

Increases in conjugated estrogens can be detected starting at approximately day 35. This initial elevation in concentration has been associated with CL production of estrogens.[10–13] The continued increase in estrone sulfate concentrations after day 70 has been associated with the production of fetal steroids.[11, 12, 14] Thus, measurements of estrone sulfate between days 35 and 70 are not indicative of fetal viability, however, measurement is more accurate after day 70.[11] Urinary estrone sulfate concentrations reportedly were at nonpregnant levels 5 days after induced abortion at gestational day 44 or greater.[15]

The concentrations of eCG are significantly detectable by day 40 of gestation and peak between days 50 and 60.[13] Decreases in eCG can be detected starting at day 80 and continuing past day 150.[14] Determining pregnancy by the presence of eCG, however, may be misleading if fetal loss occurs after endometrial cup formation, since eCG production can be maintained until the time when maternal immunologic destruction would normally occur.[6]

MID TO LATE GESTATION

As pregnancy progresses, progesterone concentration decreases and is virtually undetectable in mid to late gestation.[15] Conventional techniques utilizing progesterone antiserum to detect progesterone appear to cross-react with other progestagens, whereas gas chromatography and mass spectometry reveal the undetectable levels of this specific hormone. The concentrations of progesterone metabolites such as 5α-dihydroprogesterone, pregnanes, pregnenes, and pregnenolone, however, remain high.[15, 16]

During mid to late gestation, high concentrations of estrogens are present in both the urine and the blood.[17] These estrogens are the common phenolic type (estrone and estradiol 17β) as well as the ring B unsaturated types (equilin and equilenin). The fetal gonads as well as a functional placental unit are required for the production of these steroids. Experimental fetal gonadectomy resulted in a rapid decline in estrogen concentration; however, pregnancy was maintained until approximately full term.[17]

Changes in the hemostatic profile have been reported to occur during the last 4 months of gestation. Increased plasma fibrinogen was noted during this time period as well as increased plasma factor VIIIC and circulating fibrinogen degradation products (FDP) during the last 2 weeks prepartum.[18] There were reportedly no significant changes in activated partial thromboplastin time (APTT) and prothrombin time assays determined in the same study.

At the end of gestation, progestogen concentrations increase, with a precipitous drop after parturition.[17] Estrogen concentrations decrease toward term, but estradiol-17β increases about 1 day pre-partum.[17, 19] Estrogen has been associated with normal production of prostaglandin which is important during labor. It has been detected that mares with low estrogen, following fetal gonadectomy, had weakened labor.[17] Prostaglandin metabolite concentrations steadily increase in late gestation, and there is a slight rise in the first stage of labor and a marked elevation during delivery.[17, 19, 20] Oxytocin concentrations also increase during the second stage of labor.[17] Since oxytocin is known to increase prostaglandin F_2 metabolite concentrations, it is thought that the combination of oxytocin and prostaglandin $F_{2\alpha}$ coordinate the contractions associated with productive labor.[17, 21]

Initial placentation in the equine pregnancy begins at approximately 10 days of gestation and is choriovitelline.[22] This structure is slowly replaced by a chorioallantoic placenta by days 30 to 40.[22–24] The placenta develops as the allantois expands from the hindgut over the dorsum of the amnion to surround it and eventually contact virtually the entire chorionic membrane as well. The endometrial cups form in the region called the chorionic girdle.[24] This region is on the chorion between the junction of the developing allantois and the yolk sac. Trophoblastic cells invade the maternal epithelium around day 35 and then secrete eCG.[26] The chorioallantoic membrane begins the formation of villous projections into the endometrium around day 40 gestation. Secondary branches of these villi develop by day 100, and by day 150, the microcotyledons, with tertiary branching, are fully developed.[22] Microcotyledons are thought to be the site of gas and small molecule exchange, because they have extensive fetal and maternal vasculature. These structures are present over the entire surface of the placenta, thus the classification of "diffuse microcotyledonary." The maternal endometrial cells, which are epithelial, are in contact with fetal chorionic cells and form layers of separation between maternal and fetal vascular endothelium and blood cells. The equine placenta is therefore also classified as "epitheliochorial." The intercotyledonary areas are located over the openings of the uterine glands. The uterine glands are secretory throughout pregnancy, and the chorioallantois demonstrates the capacity to uptake these secretions as well.[22, 25] It is thought that large water-soluble molecules are transferred in this area.

REFERENCES

1. Leith GS, Ginther OJ: Mobility of the conceptus and uterine contractions in the mare. *Therio* 244:701, 1985.
2. Ginther OJ: Dynamic physical interactions between the equine embryo and uterus. *Equine Vet J* Suppl 3:41, 1985.
3. Heap RB, Hamon M, Allen WR: Studies on oestrogen synthesis by the preimplantation equine conceptus. *J Reprod Fertil Suppl* 32:343, 1982.
4. Sharp DC, McDowell KJ, Weithenauer J, et al: The continuum of events leading to maternal recognition of pregnancy in mares. *J Reprod Fertil Suppl* 37:101, 1989.
5. Mcdowell KJ, Sharp DC, Grubaugh W, et al: Restricted conceptus motility results in failure of pregnancy maintenance in mares. *Biol Reprod* 39:340, 1988.
6. Allen WR: Hormonal control of early pregnancy in the mare. *Anim Reprod Sci* 7:283, 1984.
7. Squires EL, Wentworth BC, Ginther OJ: Progesterone concentration in blood of mares during the estrous cycle, pregnancy and after hysterectomy. *J Anim Sci* 39:759, 1974.
8. Holtan DW, Bett TM, Estergreen VL: Plasma progestins in pregnancy, post partum and cycling mares. *J Anim Sci* 40:359, 1975.
9. Sertich PL, Hinrichs K, Schiereck DE, et al: Periparturient events in ovariectomized embryo transfer recipient mares. *Int Cong Anim Reprod Artif Insem* 32:123, 1988.
10. Daels PF, DeMoraes JJ, Stabenfeldt GH, et al: The corpus luteum: Source of oestrogen during early pregnancy in the mare. *J Reprod Fertil Suppl* 44:501, 1991.
11. Stabenfeldt GH, Daels PF, Munro CJ, et al: An oestrogen conjugate enzyme immunoassay for monitoring pregnancy in the mare: limitations of the assay between days 40 and 70 of gestation. *J Reprod Fertil Suppl* 44:37, 1991.
12. Terqui M, Palmer E: Oestrogen pattern during early pregnancy in the mare. *J Reprod Fertil Suppl* 27:441, 1979.
13. Daels PF, Shideler S, Lasley BL, et al: Source of oestrogen in early pregnancy in the mare. *J Reprod Fertil* 90:55, 1990.
14. Kindahl H, Knudsen O, Madej A, et al: Progesterone, prostaglandin F-2 alpha, PMSG and oestrone sulphate during early pregnancy in the mare. *J Reprod Fertil Suppl* 32:353, 1982.
15. Kasman LH, Hughes JP, Stabenfeldt GH, et al: Estrone sulfate concentrations as an indicator of fetal demise in horses. *Am J Vet Res* 49:184, 1988.
16. Holtan DW, Goughton E, Silver M, et al: Plasma progestagens in the mare, fetus and newborn foal. *J Reprod Fertil Suppl* 44:517, 1991.
17. Hamon M, Clarke SW, Houghton E, et al: Production of 5 alpha-dihydroprogesterone during late pregnancy in the mare. *J Reprod Fertil Suppl* 44:529, 1991.
18. Pashen RL: Maternal and foetal endocrinology during late pregnancy and parturition in the mare. *Equine Vet J* 16:233, 1984.
19. Gentry PA, Feldman BF, O'Neill SL, et al: Evaluation of the haemostatic profile in the pre- and post parturient mare, with particular focus on the perinatal period. *Equine Vet J* 24:33, 1992.
20. Allen WR: Clinical and endocrinological aspects of parturition in the mare. Proc Ninth Bain-Fallon Memorial Lectures, The Mare and Foal 85, 1987.
21. Silver M, Barnes RJ, Comline RS, et al: Prostaglandins in maternal and fetal plasma and in allantoic fluid during the second half of gestation in the mare. *J Reprod Fertil Suppl* 27:531, 1979.
22. Barnes RJ, Comline RS, Jeffcott LB, et al: Foetal and maternal plasma concentrations of 13,14-dihydro-15-oxo-prostaglandin F in the mare during late pregnancy and at parturition. *J Endocrinol* 78:201, 1978.
23. Stemen DH: Placentatin in the mare. *J Reprod Fertil Suppl* 31:41, 1982.
24. Douglas RH, Ginther OJ: Development of the equine fetus and placenta. *J Reprod Fertil Suppl* 23:503, 1975.
25. Van Niekerk CH, Allen WR: Early embryonic development in the horse. *J Reprod Fertil Suppl* 23:495, 1975.
26. Samuel CA, Allen WR, Steven DH: Studies on the equine placenta. III: Ultrastructure of the uterine glands and the overlying trophoblast. *J Reprod Fertil* 51:433, 1977.

15.2

Accidents of Gestation

Heidi M. Immegart, DVM, MS, PhD, Dip ACT
Walter R. Threlfall, DVM, MS, PhD, Dip ACT

Gestational diseases such as hydropic conditions, uterine torsions, and ventral ruptures can result in loss of pregnancy and the death of mares. Infectious or toxic causes of fetal loss that have the potential to affect many mares in a herd can cause severe economic losses. Non-infectious causes of fetal loss may decrease the future ability of a mare to bear offspring. Early recognition of potential abnormalities of pregnancy can help to resolve the problem with minimal fetal, dam, and economic wastage.

Causes of abortion in mares include non-infectious problems as well as those due to infectious agents. The predominant cause of non-infectious abortion is twinning. Mares that become pregnant with twins will typically reabsorb one twin or terminate the pregnancy, usually during the embryonic stage of gestation.[1] Loss of a twin or both twins occurs due to a lack of sufficient uterine contact with one or both fetal membranes to support continued development and is most typically observed in unilateral twin pregnancies. In some cases, however, both embryos are established and develop into the fetal stage before they encounter a lack of nutrient supply and gaseous exchange through the placenta; this usually occurs in mares that have bilaterally located twins. One fetal membrane will typically cover a larger portion of the uterine surface than does the other, thus compromising the development of the smaller twin. When the placental exchange of oxygen, nutrients, and waste products is no longer supporting the smaller fetus, death occurs. The resultant prostaglandin $F_{2\alpha}$ release from the uterus due to fetal tissue autolysis frequently causes the abortion of both fetuses.[2] Abortion may be preceded by signs of impending delivery, such as mammary development and secretory activity plus relaxation of the pelvic ligaments.[3] When prepartum signs are observed, attempts to confirm the presence of a live fetus via transrectal palpation of fetal movement or transabdominal or transrectal ultrasonographic examination should be made. If a live fetus is present, Regumate (Hoescht Roussel, Agri-Vet Co., Somerville, NJ) can be administered in an attempt to maintain the pregnancy.[2, 4] Several mares carried the live twin fetus to term when treated. It was not known whether these mares would have maintained the pregnancy without supplementation of progestogen. The administration of exogenous progestogens does not guarantee that the pregnancy will be maintained, because many mares abort during treatment.[3]

Diagnosis of a twin pregnancy can be made utilizing transrectal ultrasonography. The presence of a twin pregnancy should be determined before endometrial cup formation at day 35 and ideally by day 20. Elimination of one twin is more likely to result in a single viable pregnancy when the procedure is performed earlier in the gestation and the twins are located bilaterally. Methods for eliminating one embryo or fetus include manually crushing one embryonic vesicle, transvaginal injection of hypertonic saline or potassium solution, or surgical removal.[5–11]

Infectious causes of abortion can be viral, bacterial, or fungal. The most commonly diagnosed cause of infectious abortion during late gestation is from equine herpes virus-1 (EHV-1) infection.[21] Subtype 1 is most frequently associated with abortions and neurologic disease; however, subtype 1 can also cause respiratory infections.[22] Abortion can occur 14 to 120 days after EHV-1 infection but occurs after the seventh month of gestation.[21] If near term, the fetus may die in utero from suffocation or may be born alive but weak. Typical lesions in aborted fetuses include 1-mm necrotic white foci in the liver with possible intranuclear eosinophilic inclusion bodies that are observed microscopically.[21, 22] When

the aborting mare belongs to a herd, it is imperative to isolate any pregnant mares as rapidly as possible from the area where the abortion occurred. The organism can be inhaled or ingested from material in the abortion area. A vaccination program utilizing a killed vaccine in the third, fifth, seventh, and ninth months of pregnancy can help to decrease the likelihood of this type of viral abortion.

Equine viral arteritis (EVA) has also been reported to cause abortion in horses. Clinical disease can usually be detected prior to abortion and can include fever, nasal and lacrimal discharge, and edema due to vasculitis.[21, 22] Abortion occurs approximately 23 to 57 days after exposure. Lesions in the fetus are usually minimal; however, the presence of arteritis is possible and may be particularly severe in the placenta.[21, 23] The EVA virus can be transmitted during breeding, because it is present in the semen of infected stallions. It can also be transmitted during contact with infected horses. Vaccines can be used to increase protection if administered prior to breeding susceptible mares that are to be bred to an infected stallion. Certain governmental regulations restrict the movement of EVA-positive horses to countries outside the United States. Due to positive titers following vaccination, these restrictions may limit vaccination of animals.

Although bacterial and fungal abortion are typically caused by an ascending placentitis that originates at the cervical pole, hematogenous spread of organisms is possible.[21, 24, 25] Organisms are typically in the anterior vagina and pass through the softened cervix during breeding or during gestational cervical relaxation. The most frequently reported bacteria are hemolytic streptococcal species; however, *Escherichia coli*, *Pseudomonas* species, *Klebsiella* species, *Staphylococcus* species, and *Taylorella equigenitalis* have been recovered from aborted fetuses and fetal membranes.[21, 24, 26] The most common fungal agents are *Aspergillus* spp., but *Mucor* spp., *Histoplasma capsulatum* spp., and *Candida* spp. have also been reported.[21, 25]

Bacterial placentitis can cause the fetus to die in utero due to placental insufficiency or due to septicemia.[21, 24] Alternatively, the fetus can be expelled alive but weak and small for its gestational age. The fetal condition is caused by the lack of a sufficient functional placental area for nutrient exchange. Fungal abortion is typified by the expulsion of an emaciated small fetus that may or may not have a characteristic dermatitis.[21, 25] With both bacterial and fungal abortions from cervical origin, the placenta has variably sized lesions associated with the cervical pole. Fungal hyphae can be readily detected microscopically.[21, 25] Bacteria may or may not be isolated from various tissues of the fetus, including fetal liver, eye, brain, lung or stomach contents, or the fetal membranes.

Systemic diseases can also cause abortion. Mares with colic have the potential for experiencing endotoxemia. Endotoxemia results in prostaglandin $F_{2\alpha}$ production and, if this release is sustained, can cause luteal regression in mares during the first trimester.[12–14] Flunixin meglumine and exogenous progestogens such as Regumate can be used to help prevent luteolysis and subsequent loss of pregnancy, although the success of treatment cannot be guaranteed.[15–18] When the mare is beyond 100 days of gestation, the placenta is the source of progestogens. Decreases in progestogens are detected in mares that exhibit colic in late gestation, and treatment with Regumate is warranted until endogenous progestogen concentrations return to normal. Pregnancy losses in mares with later gestation episodes of colic have been associated with increased severity of gastrointestinal compromise, corticosteroid concentrations at presentation, and hypoxia during surgical intervention.[19] Other diseases such as colitis can also result in abortion.[20] These types of abortions are not usually associated with future fertility problems because there is no long-term effect on the reproductive system.

Hydropic conditions in mares are uncommon; however, the consequences of their occurrence can be severe. Hydrops allantois is the abnormal accumulation of fluid in the allantoic cavity. Hydrops allantois has reportedly occurred from 6 to $10\frac{1}{2}$ months of gestation.[27–31] It can be presented as an abnormally large abdomen for the stage of gestation and typically has a relatively rapid onset from a few days to weeks' duration.[27, 28] The mares frequently have an amount of ventral edema owing to a pronounced compression of the epigastric vessels.[31] Transrectal palpation of the uterus reveals an abnormal amount of fluid that typically obscures palpation of the fetus.[31–33] Ventral abdominal rupture frequently results from the presence of an excessive weight of fetal fluid.[28, 32] Since mares affected with hydrops allantois typically abort, induction of parturition is the treatment of choice (see Chapter 15.8). Gradual release of allantoic fluid through an incision in the chorioallantois or through a uterine drain tube placed in the allantoic cavity has been suggested in order to reduce the speed of fluid loss and prevent splanchnic pooling of blood that may result in shock.[27, 31] Intravenous fluids can be administered during fluid release, and corticosteroids may be used to help prevent potential shock episodes.[32] For these cases, corticosteroids should be considered as the method for parturition induction. The mare should be monitored and assisted during delivery, because the overdistended uterus may be atonic (primary uterine inertia) and may not contract adequately to expel the fetus.[27] The cause of hydrops allantois is currently unknown; however, some reports suggest a potential hereditary component.[29] Although a cause and effect association is not clear, hydrops allantois has also frequently been accompanied by other abnormalities of pregnancy such as fetal anomalies, placentitis, multiple pregnancy, and placental insufficiency.[27–29, 31, 33, 34] Some mares have successfully produced normal offspring after hydrops allantois; however, many mares do not despite repeated attempts.

Hydrops amnion is the abnormal accumulation of fluid in the amnion and is rare in mares. One reported case involved a triplet pregnancy, and another case involved a torsion of the amnion and umbilical cord associated with a ruptured uterus.[33, 35] The cause of hydramnios has not been determined due to the infrequency of its occurrence; however, in other species it has been speculated to include fetal anomalies that decrease the capacity for normal fluid absorption and leakage of urine from the urachus into the amnion. As it is for hydrops allantois, the treatment of choice is induced parturition owing to the potential sequelae of uterine and ventral abdominal wall ruptures.

Uterine torsion can occur in mares during the last trimester of pregnancy and at parturition. Uterine torsion should be suspected in late pregnant mares that exhibit signs of colic that recur when analgesia subsides.[36–40] Transrectal palpation will reveal the tight band of the broad ligament coursing over the top of the uterus in the direction of the torsion.

Bowel may or may not be entrapped within the torsion. As the degree of torsion increases, vascular compromise to the uterus increases and the uterine wall will become edematous and friable.[41]

Several treatment options are available, and the choice will depend on the severity of the torsion, the condition of the uterus, the disposition of the mare, and the stage of gestation. The least invasive method of correction is to utilize a detorsion rod and obstetric chains placed on the fetal limbs. This method is only possible if the mare is at term and the cervix is relaxed. The next method of correction to consider is rolling the mare. The anesthetized mare is positioned laterally and is rolled in the same direction as the torsion.[40, 42, 43] Transrectal palpation should be used to monitor the effects of each roll. Do not, however, attempt to maintain an arm in the birth canal during rolling attempts. Several assistants are usually necessary to accomplish this procedure. Uterine rupture may occur before or at the time of anesthesia or during this treatment. Another approach is the standing flank incision, which can be used on a sedated mare to manually replace the uterus.[39, 41, 44] It is best to make the approach from the side toward which the uterus is rotated. This approach facilitates rocking the uterus up and pushing it away from the surgical site with a flat hand rather than pulling the uterus toward the incision with fingers. Although uncommon, rupture of the uterus or uterine artery can occur during this procedure as well as manual penetration of the uterine wall. A ventral midline approach can be used when concurrent gastrointestinal disturbances are present or the uterine torsion is present at stage I of labor and cannot be corrected by other methods.[39, 41, 45] The ventral midline laparotomy is ideal to allow proper realignment or repositioning of the uterus as well as to allow adequate exposure for observation and correction of gastrointestinal abnormalities and to perform a hysterotomy.

Fetal death can occur when torsion is present or after correction. Although many mares proceed to a normal delivery at term following correction, some uterine torsion corrections are followed by delivery of the fetus, whether or not it is at term.[39–41] Future reproductive capability depends on the extent of the damage to the uterus and decreases if uterine rupture occurs.

Ventral abdominal wall rupture can involve the prepubic tendon as well as the rectus abdominus, the obliques, and the transversus muscles. Ventral abdominal wall rupture has been associated more frequently with draft and unconditioned mares as well as twin and hydropic pregnancies.[46–50] Presentation can be similar for all types of ruptures; however, there is a typical stance associated with prepubic tendon rupture and transverse ruptures of the rectus abdominus.[46] Mares will accumulate ventral edema prior to the tear unless it is caused by trauma to the abdomen, in which case edema will develop afterward. When rupture of the prepubic tendon or transverse rupture of the abdominus has occurred, the mare will be reluctant to lie down and will stand with the tuber ischia elevated due to a lack of abdominal support of the pelvis.[46] The abdomen will appear to have dropped, and the mammary gland will be pulled cranially. Palpation of the ventral abdomen elicits a pain response, and edema may prevent specific identification of the ruptured site. The treatment of choice for pregnant mares with a ventral rupture is induced parturition.[46, 48] Assistance should be provided to the mare during delivery due to the reduction of the abdominal muscular contractions and will delay parturition. The prognosis for the recovery of a mare after ruptures of the prepubic tendon and after large ruptures of the abdominal muscles is poor since repair is virtually impossible and bowel herniation is problematic. Euthanasia may be the only treatment for these mares. For cases involving relatively small disruptions of the obliques or rectus muscles, induced parturition can be followed by repair of the rent.[48] Prognosis for a subsequent normal pregnancy, however, is poor due to a weakened abdominal wall.

Uterine ruptures can occur pre-partum in mares. Ruptures of this nature have been associated with abnormalities of pregnancy such as hydropic conditions, multiple pregnancies, and uterine torsion. In the case of hydrops and multiple pregnancies, an abnormal volume of uterine contents may contribute to the disruption of the uterine wall. With uterine torsion, the vascular compromise can result in edema and friability.[41] When this occurs, rupture of the uterus prior to treatment or during uterine manipulation is more likely to occur. Mares may appear uncomfortable prior to and immediately after rupture, and then the mares have a more normal attitude.[51, 52] Uterine rupture can be, but rarely has been, associated with significant hemorrhage.[53] Transrectal palpation of the uterus in many cases may not identify the fetus, but the uterus may be in a state of involution.[48, 52] Identification of the fetus in the cranial abdomen can be accomplished with a transabdominal ultrasonographic examination. Prompt surgical removal of the fetus is essential to prevent excessive peritonitis.[53] The prognosis for future reproduction will depend on the cause of the rupture and on the amount of associated uterine damage, peritonitis, and adhesion formation.

REFERENCES

1. Ginther OJ: Twin embryos in mares. II: Post fixation embryo reduction. *Equine Vet J* 21:171, 1989.
2. Roberts SJ, Myhre G: A review of twinning in horses and the possible therapeutic value of supplemental progesterone to prevent abortion of equine twin fetuses the latter half of the gestation period. *Cornell Vet* 73:257, 1983.
3. Le Blanc MM, Wolf GA: Twin abortions after repeated ultrasonographic diagnoses of a single fetus. *Compend Contin Educ Pract Vet* 6:641, 1984.
4. Neely DP: Progesterone/progestin therapy in the broodmare. *Proc Am Assoc Equine Pract* 34:203, 1988.
5. Hyland JH, Maclean AA, Robertson-Smith GR, et al: Attempted conversion of twin to singleton pregnancy in two mares with associated changes in plasma oestrone sulphate concentrations. *Aust Vet J* 62:406, 1985.
6. Stover SM, Pascoe DR: Surgical removal of one conceptus from the mare with a twin pregnancy. *Vet Surg* 16:103, 1987.
7. Chevalier-Clement F: Pregnancy loss in the mare. *Anim Reprod Sci* 20:231, 1989.
8. Pascoe DR, Stover SM: Surgical removal of one conceptus from fifteen mares with twin concepti. *Vet Surg* 18:141, 1989.
9. Macpherson ML, Homco LD, Blanchard TL, et al: Transvaginal ultrasound-guided allantocentesis for pregnancy reduction in the mare. *Therio* 168, 1993.
10. Roberts CJ: Termination of twin gestation by blastocyst crush in the broodmare. *J Reprod Fertil Suppl* 32:447, 1982.
11. Ginther OJ, Douglas RH: The outcome of twin pregnancies in mares. *Therio* 18:237, 1982.
12. Daels PF, Stabenfeldt GH, Kindahl H, et al: Prostaglandin release and luteolysis associated with physiological and pathological conditions of the reproductive cycle of the mare: A review. *Equine Vet J* 8(Suppl):29, 1989.
13. Kooistra LH, Ginther OJ: Termination of pseudopregnancy by administration of prostaglandin F2-alpha and termination of early pregnancy by administration of prostaglandin F2-alpha or colchicine or by removal of embryos in mares. *Am J Vet Res* 37:35, 1976.
14. Daels PF, Starr M Kindahl H, et al: Effect of *Salmonella typhimurium* endotoxin on PGF-2alpha release and fetal death in the mare. *J Reprod Fertil Suppl* 35:485, 1987.
15. Daels PF, Stabenfeldt GH, Hughes JP, et al: Effects of flunixin meglumine on endotoxin-induced prostaglandin F2-alpha secretion during early pregnancy in mares. *Am J Vet Res* 52:276, 1991.
16. Kendahl H, Daels P, Odensvik K, et al: Experimental models of endotoxaemia related to abortion in the mare. *J Reprod Fertil Suppl* 44:509, 1991.
17. Daels PF, Stabenfeldt GH, Hughes JP, et al: The role of PGF-2 alpha in embryonic loss following systemic infusion of *Salmonella typhimurium* endotoxin in the mare and the protective action of altrenogest and flunixin meglumine. *Proc Annu Meet Am Assoc Equine Pract* 34:169, 1988.
18. Daels PF, Stabenfeldt GH, Hughes JP, et al: Evaluation of progesterone deficiency as a cause of fetal death in mares with experimentally induced endotoxemia. *Am J Vet Res* 52:282, 1991.
19. Santschi EM, Slone DE, Gronwall R, et al: Types of colic and frequency of postcolic abortion in pregnancy mares: 105 cases (1984–1988). *J Am Vet Med Assoc* 199:374, 1991.
20. Santschi EM, Slone DE: Maternal conditions that cause high-risk pregnancy in mares. *Compend Contin Educ Pract Vet* 16:1481, 1994.
21. Acland HM: Abortion in mares: diagnosis and prevention. *Compend Contin Educ Pract Vet* 9:318, 1987.
22. Swerczek TW, Roberts AW: Equine rhinopneumonitis (equine herpesvirus) virus abortion. In Kirkbride CA, ed. *Laboratory Diagnosis of Livestock Abortion*. Ames, Iowa State University Press, 1990, p 217.
23. Johnson B, Baldwin C, Timoney P, et al: Arteritis in equine fetuses aborted due to equine viral arteritis. *Vet Pathol* 28:248, 1991.
24. Swerczek TW, Donahue JM: Equine bacterial abortions. In Kirkbride CA, ed. *Laboratory Diagnosis of Livestock Abortion*. Ames, Iowa State University Press, 1990, p 229.
25. Swerczek TW, Donahue JM: Equine mycotic placentitis. In Kirkbride CA, ed. *Laboratory Diagnosis of Livestock Abortion*. Ames, Iowa State University Press, 1990, p 224.
26. Hong CB, Donahue JM, Giles RC, et al: Etiology and pathology of equine placentitis. *J Vet Diagn Invest* 5:56, 1993.
27. Vandeplassche M, Bouters J, Spincemaille J, et al: Dropsy of the fetal sacs in mares: Induced and spontaneous abortion. *Vet Rec* Jul, 67, 1976.
28. Henry MM, Morris DD, et al: Hydrops allantois associated with twin pregnancy in a mare. *Equine Pract* 13:20, 1991.
29. Waelchli RO, Ehrensperger F: Two related cases of cerebellar abnormality in equine fetuses associated with hydrops of fetal membranes. *Vet Rec* Nov, 513, 1988.
30. Koterba AM, Haibel GK, Grimmet JB: Respiratory distress in a premature foal secondary to hydrops allantois and placentitis. *Compend Contin Educ Pract Vet* 5:121, 1983.
31. Blanchard TL, Varner DD, Buonanno AM, et al: Hydrops allantois in two mares. *Equine Vet Sci* 7:222, 1987.
32. Blanchard TL: Managing the mare with hydrallantois. *Vet Med* Aug, 790, 1989.
33. Allen WE: Two cases of abnormal equine pregnancy associated with excess foetal fluid. *Equine Vet J* 18:220, 1986.

34. Vandeplassche M: Obstetrician's view of the physiology of equine parturition and dystocia. *Equine Vet J* 12:45, 1980.

35. Honnas CM, Spensley MS, Laverty S, et al: Hydramnios causing uterine rupture in a mare. *J Am Vet Med Assoc* 193:334, 1988.

36. Barber SM: Torsion of the uterus—a cause of colic in the mare. *Can Vet J* 20:165, 1979.

37. Jones RD: Diagnosis of uterine torsion in a mare and correction by standing flank laparotomy. *Can Vet J* 17:111, 1976.

38. Wheat JD, Meagher DM: Uterine torsion and rupture in mares. *J Am Vet Med Assoc* 160:881, 1972.

39. Pascoe JR, Meagher DM, Wheat JD: Surgical management of uterine torsion in the mare: A review of 26 cases. *J Am Vet Med Assoc* 179:351, 1981.

40. Wichtel JJ, Reinertson EL, Clark TL: Nonsurgical treatment or uterine torsion in semen mares. *J Am Vet Med Assoc* 193:337, 1988.

41. Vasey JR: Uterine torsion. In McKinnon AO, Voss JL, eds. *Equine Reproduction.* Philadelphia, Lea & Febiger, 1993, p 457.

42. Guthrie RG: Rolling for correction of uterine torsion in a mare. *J Am Vet Med Assoc* 181:66, 1982.

43. Bowen JM, Gaboury C, Bousquet D: Non-surgical correction of a uterine torsion in the mare. *Vet Rec* Dec, 495, 1976.

44. Skjerven O: Correction of uterine torsion in the mare by laparotomy. *Nord Vet Med* 17:377, 1965.

45. Maxwell JAL: The correction of uterine torsion in a mare by caesarean section. *Aust Vet J* 55:33, 1979.

46. Roberts SJ: Diseases and accidents of the gestation period. In Roberts SJ, ed. *Veterinary Obstetrics and Genital Diseases (Theriogenology).* Woodstock, SJ Roberts, 1986, p 123.

47. Roberts SJ: Abortion and other gestational diseases in mares. In Morrow DA, ed. *Current Therapy in Theriogenology 2.* Philadelphia, WB Saunders, 1986, p 705.

48. Lofstedt RM: Miscellaneous diseases of pregnancy and parturition. In McKinnon AO, Voss JL, eds. *Equine Reproduction.* Philadelphia, Lea & Febiger, 1993, p 596.

49. Hanson RR, Todhunter RJ: Herniation of the abdominal wall in pregnant mares. *J Am Vet Med Assoc* 189:790, 1986.

50. Adams SB: Rupture of the prepubic tendon in a horse. *Equine Pract* 1:17, 1979.

51. Wheat JD, Meagher DM: Uterine torsion and rupture in mares. *J Am Vet Med Assoc* 160:881, 1972.

52. Honnas CM, Spensley MS, Laverty S, et al: Hydramnios causing uterine rupture in a mare. *J Am Vet Med Assoc* 193:334, 1988.

53. Hooper RN, Schumacher J, Taylor TS, et al: Diagnosing and treating uterine ruptures in mares. *Vet Med* Mar, 263, 1993.

15.3

Parturition Injuries

Walter R. Threlfall, DVM, MS, PhD, Dip ACT
Heidi M. Immegart, DVM, MS, PhD, Dip ACT

Injuries to the mare occur frequently at the time of parturition mainly because of the forceful and rapid delivery of the fetus. Some of these injuries are immediately life threatening, whereas others may not be noticed at the time of parturition and may only be observed and create problems with fertility later on. The following injuries are not a com-

plete listing of possible injuries but they serve to summarize the more commonly occurring problems.

DYSTOCIA

Dystocia is defined as an abnormal or difficult delivery that may or may not require assistance. Dystocia may result in injury or death to the mare or foal, and occurrences of dystocia in the mare are less than 1%. Certain breeds or the cross-breeding of animals of extreme size variation, where the mare is smaller, may increase this percentage. Although mares have fewer problems involving deliveries compared with the other domestic species; when present, these problems present as true emergencies. The reason for this is the rapid and very strenuous nature of the delivery process in this species.

Fetal causes of dystocia account for the majority of difficult deliveries. The main reason believed to be responsible for this is the postural abnormalities of the long fetal extremities. Abnormalities involving position and presentation can also occur but to a lesser degree. The fetus should be expelled from the uterus within 30 minutes and in the maximum time of 70 minutes after the rupture of the chorioallantoic membrane. Care should be taken when assisting in the extraction of a fetus to be certain that the uterus, cervix, vagina, vestibule, or vulvar lips are not lacerated by applying forced extraction too rapidly. The extraction of a fetus in an abnormal posture or position should not be attempted until the abnormality is corrected owing to the increased probability of injury to the fetus or dam. The round shape of the mare's pelvis compared with that of the cow reduces dystocias caused by large fetuses. Other less frequently encountered fetal causes of dystocia include fetal anasarca, ascites, fetal tumor, hydrocephalic fetus, fetal monster, and mummified fetus. Maternal causes of dystocia include uterine torsion, abnormally small pelvis, uterine inertia, immaturity, constriction of the cervix or vagina, and other causes unrelated to the fetus.

The approach to dystocia should not be hasty or heroic. A well-planned approach will be more successful than one that overlooks major points of information that are critical to a successful delivery. Important aspects of this approach consist of a complete history and a rapid complete physical examination. An obstetrician is often under the real or perceived pressure of the owner upon arrival at the dystocia and may be tempted to rush the approach. The procedure will be more successful if a reasonable time is taken to gather preliminary information and to do the physical examination.

The mare's behavior, posture, character of breathing, ability to rise and remain standing, response to stimulation, degree and frequency of straining, condition of the allantoischorion, presence of amnion, presence of visceral organs or fetal extremities protruding from the vulva, vulvar discharges, and the appearance of the vulva should all be noted. If possible prior to examination, the mare should be placed in a relatively dust-free quiet area. The mare's tail should be wrapped and secured to her neck with a cord.

The next procedure is to examine the reproductive tract and the fetus. The authors prefer to perform this procedure initially via transrectal palpation. This approach permits evaluation of the uterine body more anteriorly than may be possible via the vaginal canal, thus allowing assessment of the existence of uterine torsion, rupture of the uterine arteries, or uterine rupture on the dorsal surface. Fetal viability can also be assessed using the transrectal approach. Following the transrectal findings, the perineal area is washed. Using a sleeve and sterile lubricant, the vaginal, cervical, and uterine walls are examined for possible lacerations. This procedure should always be performed before examination of the fetus to eliminate the possibility of missing a significant lesion until after the delivery of the fetus.

The fetus should be palpated through the vaginal canal to determine its presentation, position, posture, and viability, only after the determination of the absence of lacerations. Several reflexes can be used to determine the viability of a fetus. Depression of the eyes should initiate either movement of the fetal head or, in a depressed fetus, only movement of the eye itself. A finger inserted deeply into the mouth should stimulate the sucking reflex. With a posterior presentation, a finger can be inserted into the fetal anus to detect movement of the entire fetus or simply contraction of the anal sphincter. The skin of the fetus can be pinched, or a limb can be flexed or extended maximally to stimulate a response and thus indicate fetal viability. A stethoscope on ultrasonographic examination can also be performed to determine the fetal heart beat or blood flow. The relative size of the fetus and that of the pelvis and birth canal should be approximated during this examination and determination of any fetal abnormalities that could compromise the delivery.

Fetal presentation refers to the relationship of the spinal axis of the fetus to the spinal axis of the dam. Anterior longitudinal presentation is when the fetal head is presented first at the vulva. Posterior presentation occurs when the rear limbs are presented first. Transverse presentation occurs when the mid-portion of the fetus is the first portion of the fetus to make contact with the cervix. Position, with the exceptions of transverse and vertical, is defined as the relationship of the dorsum of the fetus to the quadrant of the maternal pelvis. The possibilities that exist in longitudinal presentation are dorsosacral, right dorsoileal, dorsopubic, and left dorsoileal. Posture refers to the relationship of the fetal extremities to the fetal trunk and is not related to the dam. A normal delivery would be defined as an anterior longitudinal presentation, dorsosacral position, with the fetal head, neck, and forelimbs extended. Following the preceding examinations, the owner should be informed with regard to the prognosis of the mare and fetus and the cost of the recommended procedure before initiating therapy.

All genital examinations and obstetric procedures should be performed as sanitarily as feasible. Obstetric procedures are easiest in the standing position with an epidural anesthetic, unless the mare has been anesthetized and is in a dorsal recumbency position. Lateral recumbency is the most difficult position. Stocks are desirable to reduce side-to-side movement of the mare because mares may suddenly go from the standing position to the sternal or lateral recumbent position, thus making removal from stocks difficult. An anesthetized mare can be positioned with the rear quarters higher than the head on an incline, or the mare can be placed in a dorsal recumbent position with the rear feet elevated using a chain hoist (caution following epidural). This elevation permits the mare's abdominal viscera to move away from the pelvic area. The uterus and fetus will also move anteriorly, permitting more space around the fetus since it will be anterior to the pelvis.

Tranquilization of the mare may be accomplished with a combination of xylazine (0.5 to 1 mg/kg) and acepromazine (0.04 mg/kg) administered intravenously to obtain 30 to 40 minutes during which strong contractions will be absent or will diminish. This dosage may be repeated if necessary. Other agents such as butorphanol or dormosodan may also be used. The mare's condition must be known prior to the administration of any medication. The primary consideration to be made before administering any agent is what effect the agent may have on existing conditions, a decision later to anesthetize the mare, or the need to administer additional quantities or different agents to control straining.

General anesthesia for short-term usage can be induced with xylazine (1.1 mg/kg) intravenously and ketamine (2.2 mg/kg) intravenously and maintained with ketamine (2 mg/mL), xylazine (0.5 mg/mL), and guaifenesin (50 mg/mL) in 1 liter of 5% dextrose for up to 3 hours.[1] When procedures are to exceed 1 hour, it has been suggested that 1 mg/mL of ketamine and 0.25 mg/mL of xylazine be used with the 50 mg/mL of guaifenesin added. Recommended infusion rates of the 1-hour mixture were 2.21 to 2.67 mL/kg/hr. Recovery times ranged from 55 minutes to 3 hours. Reversal agents, such as yohimbine or tolazoline, have been suggested to reduce recovery times. If available, gas anesthesia may be indicated for a prolonged dystocia correction.

One of the challenging aspects of treating animals in dystocia is that only a limited number of methods are available for the correction. The most difficult aspect is to select the method that will achieve the obstetric objective of delivering a fetus that is alive with minimal trauma to the mare or to the fetus. The second most important aspect of successful management of dystocia is to have access to the mare early in the delivery process. The possibilities for correction of dystocia include mutation, forced extraction, fetotomy, laparotomy, and laparohysterotomy. Although euthanasia of the mare may be selected due to economics or to the physical condition of the mare at the time of arrival, it is not included as a treatment for dystocia because it does not fulfill the definition of mare and foal survivability.

The amount of assistance necessary will depend on the technique to be used for correction of dystocia. The minimal amount of assistance recommended for an obstetric procedure is two persons. One person will be at the head of the mare for the entire procedure, and one person will assist the obstetrician with equipment and with traction or fetotomy cuts when required. Generally, three or four assistants will help the procedure to go more rapidly and in some instances (e.g., a cesarean) may be required. In order to reduce the possibility of injury during mutation, forced extraction, or fetotomy, the obstetrician should always have an arm within the birth canal between the fetus and the mare.

The obstetric equipment recommended by the authors includes three obstetrical chains (60-inch), three obstetrical chain handles, a fetatome (Utrecht or flat tube model), a Krey hook, a wire introducer, two wire handles, a detorsion rod, a fetotomy finger knife, a rope snare, obstetric wire, a Kuhn crutch, rubber sleeves, buckets, stomach pump, uterine tube, and lubricant. The lubricant of choice is polyethylene polymer (J-Lube by Jorgensen Laboratories, Loveland, CO

80538), which comes in powder form and is water soluble. This lubricant can be mixed at the site of the dystocia and delivered into the uterus with a stomach pump and uterine tube. Although this equipment is not essential for every case of dystocia, its availability will improve the quality of the obstetric manipulation and will reduce the work required to obtain desirable results.

The most frequently used method of correction is mutation. Mutation is the procedure used to correct the malposture, position, and presentation followed by delivery of the fetus. This method should be the least traumatic and should be employed prior to the use of forced extraction. Mutation may not always be possible or indicated, depending on how long the mare has been in labor and the cause of dystocia.

Mutation involves returning the fetus to a normal presentation, position, and posture by repulsion, rotation, version, and adjustment or extension of the fetal extremities. It is primarily indicated when the fetus is alive, and the procedure can be performed in a relatively short time with a high probability of success. The authors have found that in cases of a dead fetus, fetotomy procedures to eliminate a postural abnormality are faster and less stressful on the mare and the obstetrician than attempts to mutate unless the dystocia has been of minimal duration and a sufficient area exists within the uterus to permit manipulation. The repulsion of the fetus into the abdominal cavity away from the pelvis helps to create more space in which to perform obstetric procedures. Lubrication is very important with all obstetric procedures including mutation and may make the difference between success or failure of the technique. The extension of the flexed limb is accomplished by repelling the proximal portion while the mid portion of the limb (carpus or tarsus) is rotated laterally. After this procedure the foot is brought medially and extended into the pelvis. If correction of the mutation is not possible in 15 to 20 minutes, another method of correction should be selected. Aftercare consists of uterine stimulants and intrauterine antibiotics or antiseptics.

Forced extraction is generally combined with mutation or fetotomy. Forced extraction is not intended to replace other techniques that could be utilized but is used to aid in the delivery process. Forced extraction, if used unwisely, will result in injury to the fetus and the mare's reproductive tract. Forced extraction involves the application of extractive force on the fetus within the uterus. Extractive force is used with uterine inertia, following corrective mutation, with inadequate cervical dilatation, in posterior presentations and in combination with a fetotomy. Extreme traction should never be applied in place of corrective mutation, a fetotomy, or a cesarean because of the possibility of trauma to the mare and fetus. The position and posture of the foal should be as near to the physiologic one as possible before forced extraction is applied. The traction placed on the fetus should be slightly dorsal and posterior until the forelimbs, head, and neck are at the vulvar lips. The direction of the traction is then directed more ventrally as more of the fetus is visible. The traction should mainly be directed ventrally by the time that the shoulders have passed through the vulvar lips.

When the operator is experienced and uses good judgment, forced extraction is relatively safe. It can cause various injuries, however, including damage to the head, limbs, and spinal cord of the fetus; damage to all areas of the birth canal and adjacent structures; eversion of the uterus;

and lacerations of the vagina, vulva, perineal body, and rectal floor. Aftercare following forced extraction may include uterine stimulants placed into the uterus or administered systemically. The use of antibiotics may be indicated to reduce the number of organisms introduced during the procedure. Broad-spectrum antibiotics are generally recommended for this purpose.

As soon as it becomes apparent that mutation is not going to be successful, another technique for correction should be attempted. Often a mistake made by the obstetrician is to continue using a technique beyond a reasonable time in anticipation that eventually it will be successful. Determination of the time to abandon one technique in favor of another is gained through experience and is always a challenge.

Fetotomy is indicated in many cases when the manipulative time and trauma to the mare can be reduced over that of mutation and when the fetus is dead. Fetotomy is the reduction in fetal size by removal of the extremities or by dissection of the body. Specific indications include the presence of a dead fetus in the absence of uterine contracture; a fetus that is not overly emphysematous; abnormalities in fetal presentation, position, or posture; the presence of an oversized fetus in relation to the maternal birth canal; the presence of fetal abnormalities such as ankylosis of the joints; and incomplete cervical dilatation. The decision to perform a fetotomy also depends on the veterinarian's opinion that there is or is not sufficient space in the dam's genital tract to perform the procedure and also on the experience of the obstetrician. The advantages of the fetotomy procedure include a reduction of fetal size; elimination of the need for a cesarean; minimal assistance necessary; decreased trauma to the mare; less infertility, recovery time, or after case than following a cesarean; more practical as a "field" technique than a cesarean; and monetarily advantageous to both the owner and the veterinarian.[2] A cesarean is the preferred approach by many veterinarians over that of a fetotomy in cases of a dead fetus. Reasons given vary from stretching the cervix; more physical exertion for the veterinarian; lacerations of the uterus, cervix, vagina, and operator; and the procedure being "too hard on the mare." A cesarean is generally not performed under farm situations with no technical assistance available; however, a fetotomy can be performed under these conditions. It has been recommended not to perform a fetotomy that requires more than one or two cuts in order to avoid severe injury to the genital tract.[3, 4] However, the duration of the fetotomy, the damage to the reproductive tract prior to the initiation of the fetotomy, and the correctness of the cuts have a major influence on the success of the procedure. The other consideration on the farm is what other options are available that will save the life of the mare. Furthermore, since most equine dystocias are due to single postural anomalies, only one or two cuts are generally necessary to permit delivery of the remainder of the fetus. Fetotomy procedures are usually less costly to the owner, because aftercare is considerably less and future reproductive capability is better.

A laparotomy is indicated primarily in cases involving uterine torsion when other methods of correction via the vagina were unsuccessful. Uterine torsion does occur in the equine and can be a cause of dystocia in the mare. The torsion may be evident months prior to the onset of labor and can be determined by prolonged colicky-like signs that fail to be allieved by therapy for gastrointestinal colic. The diagnosis can be made easily by transrectal palpation of the uterus and broad ligaments. The finding of one broad ligament traversing the midline to the opposite side dorsal to the uterus with the other broad ligament nonpalpable is sufficient information to make the diagnosis. The correction of the uterine torsion can be accomplished after a laparotomy and uterine manipulation.

Laparohysterotomy is another method to correct dystocia. A cesarean section refers to the delivery of a fetus through incisions in the abdominal wall and uterus of the dam. Such surgery is indicated when the fetus is alive and when it cannot be delivered otherwise. A cesarean is most advantageous when it is pre-planned or when the time and facilities are immediately available to permit delivery of the fetus while still alive.

Indications for cesarean include a previously fractured pelvis or another obstruction that caused a reduction in the pelvic diameter, a naturally occurring small pelvis, an absolutely large fetus, abdominal wall or prepubic tendon ruptures, uterine torsion that is not correctable by a vaginal approach or by rolling the mare, malpresentations that are not correctable by other methods, when a fetotomy cannot be performed, and fetal anomalies and live fetuses that cannot be delivered any other way.[5, 6]

One complication of a cesarean is rupture of the uterine artery during manipulation. The biggest problems encountered in regard to a cesarean are survival of the mare and foal and mare reproducibility. An elective cesarean gives the best prognosis. The additional preparation and possibly hoisting time required, once the decision has been made to do a cesarean, may reduce the success of the procedure.

The considerations involved in selecting a site for a cesarean section include the operative conditions and disposition of the animal. The surgeon's previous experience with operative sites is another important consideration. The possible operative sites include the right or left flank with the animal standing and use of sedation and local anesthesia. This approach, however, is seldom recommended owing to reduced exposure of the uterus, visible abdominal wall scarring, and possible movement of the mare. The flank approaches under general anesthesia are also options, but the reduced uterine exposure and visible scar following surgery are disadvantages. The primary advantage of using the left flank over the right flank is that the cecum is less of a problem and thus does not obstruct access to the uterus. However, the intestines may obstruct access and make the left flank approach difficult. With either standing flank approach, it is imperative that the animal remain standing and be quiet throughout the surgical procedure. Exposure of the uterus is not as good through a flank incision as it is through a ventral abdominal approach.

Possible operative sites in a recumbent animal include low approaches through either flank, paramedian, and midline. Low flank incisions are made medial to the fold of skin from the leg to the abdomen and lateral to the udder. The incision extends from the stifle region to the umbilicus and is somewhat parallel to the ribs; it should be long enough to enable delivery of the fetus. This approach provides good exposure of the uterus.

The paramedian incision is usually approximately 6 inches lateral to the midline and extends from a point just anterior to the udder cranially for a sufficient length to enable the delivery of a fetus. Excellent exposure of the uterus is obtained through a paramedian approach. There is less hemorrhage due to fewer muscles in this area than in the low flank area. For this same reason, there is less tissue to suture, and prolapse of the intestine through the incision during surgery is less likely. A longer incision is necessary for a paramedian approach than for a low flank approach, because the stretchable muscle mass at the incision site is less than in the flank.

The ventral midline incision is most commonly used and has the advantage of providing excellent exposure of the uterus. There is very little hemorrhage when this site is used. There may be one or two large veins that form an anastomosis from the right to the left subcutaneous abdominal veins in this area. These veins should be ligated before the ventral midline incision is made in the subcutaneous area. With this approach minimal suturing is required, primarily at the linea alba, subcutaneous area, and skin. The surgical site can become infected with any approach. Drainage from an infected incision on the ventral midline is excellent, whereas fistulous tracts may form when a high flank incision becomes infected.

Disadvantages of a ventral midline incision include the need for a longer surgical incision than with any other approach. This is primarily due to the inability of the linea alba to stretch, and thus any increase in the size of area for delivery must be achieved by making an incision. Subsequent herniation is a greater possibility with this approach than with a high flank approach but is not a major concern with proper suture patterns and material.

The aftercare of mares following a cesarean section should be provided on an individual basis; it is not feasible to treat all animals the same way and achieve good results. When delivery of a fetus is assisted, an antibiotic should be used to prevent subsequent metritis. The management of a retained placenta, which is another possible sequela, and metritis are described in Chapter 15.6. Administration of oxytocin is advisable in most cases to enhance uterine involution.

Following the correction of dystocia, the uterus should be examined to ensure that another fetus is not present. The tone of the uterine musculature should also be assessed. The birth canal should be palpated for evidence of lacerations. Recovery is much more rapid if lacerations are repaired immediately.

RUPTURED ARTERY NEAR THE TIME OF PARTURITION

The middle uterine or uterine, utero-ovarian and external iliac arteries supply the majority of blood to the uterus. If an arterial rupture is to occur, one of these bilaterally paired arteries usually ruptures during gestation, especially near parturition.[7, 8] The uterine artery is the artery that is most often affected, and the condition is, therefore, often described as a "ruptured uterine artery." The uterine artery is supported by the broad ligament as it travels from the origin near the aorta to the uterus. Near term the uterine artery can become approximately 2.5 cm in diameter, which is seven times its normal size. This increase in size is necessary to accommodate the increase in blood required to maintain fetal life and development. Although rupture of these arteries occurs most frequently in older mares,[7, 9–12] it can occur at any age. Age ranges listed in the literature are from 9 to 22 years with an average age of 16 years, but it has occurred in mares as young as 5 years of age. Although the rupture can occur on either side, the right side is affected more frequently than the left side.[8, 13] Rupture may be due to the displacement of the uterus to the left, which is caused by the location of the cecum.[13, 14] This displacement could increase the tension on the right uterine artery.[13, 14] It is believed that repeated increases and decreases in size, which occur during pregnancy and following parturition, create weakened areas within the arterial wall. The arterial wall of the older mare exhibits indications of a change in the collagen content and elastic fibers, which probably predisposes it to rupture.[9] The increased weight or pull on the arteries due to a distended uterus also adds to the insult on the arteries and could account for the arterial ruptures that occur before or at the time of parturition.[7] As the pressure increases in the vessel during labor or with stretching of the artery at the time of parturition or with assisted delivery, these weakened areas permit leakage of blood.[7] Although the mare may exhibit difficulty foaling,[7] this is not an essential part of the history that accompanies the rupture. If the hemorrhage occurs pre-partum, the first priority should be to deliver the foal as rapidly as possible and with the least trauma to the mare. Since these mares may be very anxious following delivery and may be unable to maintain a standing position, the foal should be close to, but not in the same area as, the mare.[7] It is important that the mare have contact with the foal so that she does not become more excited, but the mare should not be so close as to lie on the foal. It is critical that the mare remain calm.

If the tear is small and remains within the broad ligament, the blood may form a large hematoma and provide pressure on the bleeding area, thus controlling hemorrhage.[7, 9, 15] The mare may lose several gallons of blood and become weak with pale mucous membranes, but the mare may survive if the clot and vessel are not manipulated and the mare is quietly maintained in a stall. The mares that have a larger rupture in the vessel, and bleeding that is not confined to the broad ligament, lose larger amounts of blood into the abdominal cavity; these animals usually bleed to death internally before any assistance can be rendered.[7, 11] One of the important considerations of this condition is that no blood is observed externally[16]; all the bleeding flows into the peritoneal cavity. With the loss of blood the animal may show no signs other than white mucous membranes[11, 16, 17] and an increase in respiration and heart rate with a thready pulse.[7, 18] Animals may remain standing until they literally drop to the ground dead. If the blood loss is severe but slower, the mare will demonstrate signs of shock.[7, 11] She may exhibit increased respiration,[7] increased weakened pulse,[10, 17, 18] colicky signs,[7, 10, 11, 16–18] and cool moist skin[16–18] and appear depressed. In addition, the mare may stagger when attempting to walk or may have her head resting on the ground if one is lying down. She will "talk" to her foal but may not exhibit any other signs of maternal instinct, such as licking or nuzzling. Death can reportedly occur between minutes and 25 days postpartum. The normal range expected is less than 20 hours, unless the initially formed hematoma ruptures later and permits further hemorrhage.

This condition is most commonly fatal when severe hemorrhage occurs immediately. The mares that lose less blood and show signs early enough to seek assistance may be saved with fluids and the administration of corticosteroids for the shock.[7] Once the diagnosis has been made and depending on the extent of the hematoma, these animals should remain in the stall for 3 to 4 weeks and should not be examined rectally or vaginally during this time unless a deterioration in the mare's condition warrants an examination. Medications can be administered to the mare in an attempt to keep her quiet, but medications must be given carefully since further lowering of the blood pressure may cause additional medical problems. Medications to reduce some of the pain of the swelling of the hematoma within the broad ligament are also a consideration, depending on her condition. The process of palpating the hematoma or manipulating the uterus may cause the hemorrhaging to recommence. Surgery is generally not possible or advisable. The hemorrhage occurs so rapidly in animals with tears completely through the artery and into the peritoneal cavity that there is too little time to prepare and perform surgery. If there is time to do surgery, there is probably little need.

The care of mares that survive the initial hemorrhage is extremely important in that they must be maintained in a quiet environment.[7] It is contraindicated in the opinion of the authors to transport these animals to a veterinary hospital, because the ride may cause additional stress and increased blood pressure. This will cause unnecessary movement of the mare, which will in turn cause further hemorrhaging. The mare, although demonstrating colicky-like signs, should not be managed as a colicky mare might normally be in that she should not be forced to remain standing or to walk. This will hasten the deterioration of her condition and may cause a broad ligament containing hemorrhage to rupture into the abdominal cavity. It is also not recommended to transfuse these animals, because a transfusion will also increase blood pressure. It may be advisable in a severe case to wean the foal until the mare's condition is known to be non-critical, because during the nursing process oxytocin is released and causes uterine contractility; this stress may increase the likelihood of continued hemorrhage.

Mares that have had a rupture of the uterine artery and have survived may have an increased risk of rupture at subsequent pregnancies, and considerable thought should be given to the decision of whether or not to re-breed.[13, 18] It is thought that future ruptures may occur close to but not at the exact location of the initial tear. Therefore, the emotional and economic value of the mare should be weighed before re-breeding. Embryo transfer may be an option to eliminate further stretching and damage to the arteries, which could occur during a pregnancy.[10] Mares that have a rupture of the uterine artery may have fertility problems until the hematoma is resolved or possibly for a longer time.

Rupture of the uterine artery, or one of the other closely related arteries, is a major reason for death in older mares at or near the time or parturition.[9] Therefore, older mares should be observed for this condition more so than younger ones. The pale to white mucous membranes in combination with some discomfort are indications of arterial rupture. The first consideration should be the foal, whether the mare has started delivery or not. In some mares, a ruptured artery will occur prior to parturition, and the delivery of the foal should be accomplished in a speedy but non-damaging manner. Also, recall that observable blood externally is a rarity rather than a common occurrence. The presence of blood externally is more frequently associated with a laceration of the uterus, cervix, vagina, or vestibule. If a mare is of greater emotional value than potential economic value, do not breed her or consider an embryo transfer.[10]

INVAGINATION OF THE UTERINE HORN

Invagination of the uterine horn occurs during or immediately after stage two of parturition. As the placenta detaches from the endometrium, the apical end, which is the last portion to separate, pulls the ends of the uterine horns into the lumen of the uterus.[18] If this process continues, it results in uterine eversion.[18] If the process does not continue, the consequence is that a portion of the uterine horn is trapped within the lumen as the uterus contracts post-partum. This can result in colicky signs post-partum and may lead to ischemic necrosis of the horn if not corrected.[18, 19] The condition is diagnosed by transrectal palpation of the apical ends of the uterine horns. The condition may self-correct or may continue to cause slight to mild colicky pain for 1 to 3 days post-partum. Any time when colicky signs of a mild nature are present, this condition should be considered.[19] Successful treatment involves distention of the uterine lumen with large volumes of fluid until the horn is in its proper position and then to remove the fluid and administer 10 to 20 units of oxytocin once or twice.[9] Once ischemic necrosis has occurred, no treatment may be indicated other than to breed the mare only when she has breedable follicles on the opposite side. The authors have not observed this condition to occur bilaterally.

UTERINE EVERSION

Eversion of the uterus can occur in the mare and is considered to be more of a problem than in the cow,[18] owing to the potential rupture of the uterine arteries and damage to the endometrium.[19] Predisposing factors include the strong expulsive efforts developed by the mare, failure of the uterus to involute rapidly following delivery of the fetus, continued straining after delivery due to attempts to pass the placenta,[15] administration of large doses of oxytocin, and possibly hypocalcemia. Eversion is also more prevalent in mares that remain recumbent after parturition.

Eversion of the uterus has been associated with difficult deliveries in which excessive straining has occurred to expel the fetus and in mares that have uterine inertia after delivery.[16] Eversion can also occur immediately after a delivery in which excessive force has been used to extract the fetus. If excessive force is applied when the uterus is contracted around the fetus, the uterus can be everted or lacerated. Eversion may also occur following partial expulsion of a placenta, and its weight on the apical end of the uterine horns starts the process of invagination and possibly eversion.[18] Eversion can also occur when attempts are made to manually remove a retained placenta. One of the frequent occurrences after uterine eversion is rupture of the uterine artery.

In the authors' experience, uterine eversion is treated most satisfactorily by first administering an epidural anesthetic and then by cleansing the uterus and perineal area. Application of a sulfa-urea powder may help to remove fluid in the everted tissues and thus simplify replacement of the uterus. The mare's position is important in the success or failure of replacing an everted uterus. If the animal is standing, a cradle can be used to elevate the uterus so that a small portion of the everted uterine horn can be replaced each time that the hand is inserted into the birth canal. If the mare is recumbent or one administers a general anesthetic to place her in a recumbent position, the replacement procedure will be easier due to positioning and the elimination of all straining by the mare. It is generally easier to place the mare in dorsal recumbency and elevate the rear quarters by attaching ropes to the rear legs and lifting with a hoist. Before starting to reposition the uterus, the mare's general condition should be assessed; otherwise, she may die of other causes while the uterus is being replaced.

The prognosis for the animal's survival and her future reproductivity depends on the length of time that the uterus has been everted, the amount of uterus everted, the elasticity of the uterine arteries, and the amount of trauma to the endometrium. The uterus should be replaced as rapidly as is feasible and with as little trauma as possible even though relatively considerable pressure may be necessary.[19] This is best accomplished by exerting pressure on the uterus with the palm of the hand only[18] or with a closed fist[15] rather than with fingers that may penetrate the uterine wall.[18] The uterus is cleansed in such a manner that additional trauma to the endometrial surface is minimal. Replacement of the uterine horn should start with the area adjacent to the internal os of the cervix. If the uterus can be elevated, this assists replacement.[18] As a portion of uterine horn is replaced, another portion is selected for replacement. After most of the uterine horn has been returned into the abdominal cavity, its weight will help to pull the remaining portion into normal position.

Following replacement of the everted horn, the lumen of the uterus should be palpated to be certain that the apical end of the uterine horn is in a normal position. If any doubt exists regarding its repositioning, the uterus can be filled with a warm antiseptic solution to distend the horns.[19] The fluid can then be siphoned from the uterus.[15, 18, 19] Drugs that enhance myometrial contractions are indicated to stimulate uterine involution.[19] These agents include low doses of oxytocin. If the animal is suffering from hypocalcemia, supplementation of calcium will enhance uterine contractions and will help to prevent another eversion. After replacement of the uterus into the abdominal cavity, a solution of broad-spectrum antibiotics should be infused into it to reduce the probability of infection.[18] A hysterectomy is seldom indicated, but it may be advisable for mares with an everted uterus that is not replaceable and the animal has emotional value.[18]

UTERINE, CERVICAL, AND VAGINAL LACERATIONS

Lacerations or tears in the cervix and anterior vaginal wall may expose the peritoneal cavity to infection and may occasionally result in prolapse of intestines or the bladder.[18, 20]

Small lacerations in the dorsal wall of the uterus may contract and heal without suturing,[18] but larger wounds in the uterus, especially in the ventral areas, must be repaired. Whether or not to suture tears in the retroperitoneal portion of the vagina and vestibule involves making an estimate about the extent of damage and the feasibility of surgical closure of the laceration without abscess formation. When a tear in the vaginal wall is thought to be infected, it is best to debride the wound and leave it open to drain; local or systemic antibiotics should be administered as the lesion dictates for 3 to 5 days.[18] When bleeding occurs from the vaginal or vestibular wall, the involved vessel(s) should be isolated and ligated.

Lacerations, contusions, abrasions, and hematomas of the cervix, vagina, vestibule, and vulva are often preventable through professional management of dystocia. This involves obtaining veterinary services promptly in cases of difficult deliveries and using good judgment in the selection of the obstetric procedure to correct the dystocia.

VAGINAL PROLAPSE

Vaginal prolapse in the mare is uncommon, and most cases occur at the time of parturition unless caused by vaginal tumors or a persistent hymen.[21] The prolapse appears to be due to excessive straining and may be combined with a vaginal or vestibular laceration that causes additional irritation. With advancing age and multiple pregnancies, the supporting tissues of the vagina become stretched and are more relaxed, which accounts for more prolapses occurring in older mares.[22] In addition to the effect of hormones present in late gestation, which increase relaxation of the birth canal, the fetus and fetal fluids add to the pressure exerted on the vaginal wall during the immediate pre-partum period, especially when the animal is recumbent. Slight prolapse of the vaginal wall through the vulvar lips can become more exaggerated as this tissue becomes irritated; the animal will strain and cause additional prolapse of vaginal tissue.

The treatment of a prolapsed vagina is relatively easy once parturition has occurred. Treatment is focused on eliminating vaginal inflammation and infection if present. A thorough examination of the vagina should be performed to determine if any other abnormalities are present.

PROLAPSE OF THE RECTUM

Prolapse of the rectum is usually evident during the forceful stage II of parturition. The extreme abdominal pressure forces the rectum of some mares to be slightly prolapsed at parturition.[18] If prolapse is occurring and appears to be more than a few centimeters, it should be controlled by attempting to maintain pressure on the anus to reduce the amount of rectum that is being prolapsed.[18] The primary concerns are trauma to the rectum while prolapsed and tearing of the supporting mesentery and blood vessels if the prolapse is of considerable length.

URINARY BLADDER EVERSION

Although eversion of the urinary bladder is uncommon in the mare, it is not rare. An actual prolapse of the bladder may also occur through a laceration of the vaginal floor.[18] These terms are often used interchangeably when two distinct conditions are referred to. A prolapsed bladder can be differentiated from eversion of the bladder through the urethra by observing the serosal surface and by locating the ureters that lead to the bladder.[18, 23, 24] Any accumulation of urine within the bladder can be drained through a needle. The bladder can be replaced, and, in the case of a prolapsed bladder, the tear in the vaginal floor can be sutured.[18]

PERINEAL LACERATIONS

Perineal lacerations can result in infertility if they are not diagnosed and treated correctly. Although the laceration can occur in any mare, it is more frequent in mares experiencing their first foaling[25] and in mares that have had previous perineal surgeries.[18] The strenuous and rapid delivery accounts for the increased problem with this condition over the occurrence reported in other species.[26] Lacerations of the perineal area have been divided into four categories based on the extent of the laceration in relation to the tissue involved.[25, 27]

First-degree lacerations are of least concern because they only involve the vulvar labia.[25] However, it is not implied that since these lacerations are of lesser severity that they should be ignored. Because defects in the closure of the vulvar lips can result in vestibular, vaginal, and uterine contamination, these defects should be surgically repaired following the elimination of edematous swelling and the establishment of sufficient regeneration of tissue in the area for surgical correction to be successful.[27] The first-degree lacerations involve only the skin, the subcutaneous tissue in the perineal area, and the mucosa of the vestibule. Correction of these defects consists primarily of a modified Caslick surgery or a vulvoplasty.[28] The scar tissue edges of the laceration are removed and reposed, and a Caslick procedure is performed to the extent indicated to prevent pneumovagina.

The second-degree perineal laceration consists of a first-degree perineal laceration plus a laceration that involves the perineal body,[25, 27, 28] vestibular and vaginal mucosa,[28] and the tissue in the area of the vestibular sphincter.[25, 28] The second-degree perineal laceration is potentially more severe because there is a greater probability of uterine contamination due to the abnormal conformation of the tissue in this area. The mare may also be predisposed to urine pooling, depending on the exact location and extent of the laceration.[17] The surgical correction of these lacerations will be necessary for a mare to achieve optimal reproductive efficiency. This is generally accomplished after the edema has subsided and the surface has been covered with granulation tissue in the absence of infection.[28]

A third-degree perineal laceration involves the mucosa of the vestibule and the vagina,[25, 27, 28] the perineal body,[25, 27–30] the vulvar lips,[29, 30] the rectal mucosa,[25, 27–29] and the anal sphincter.[25, 28–30] These lacerations must obviously be repaired due to the potential fecal contamination of the uterus. The repair should also be postponed until the swelling has regressed[28, 29] and the surface has re-epithelialized, which is approximately 30 days or more.[28] Repair of these lacerations immediately may be tempting but is usually unsuccessful and appears not to be worth the expense.

The preparation of the mare is concerned primarily with the softening of the feces in order that following surgical correction firm feces passing through the area do not cause failure of the suture line.[25, 31] The best method to accomplish soft feces is to place the mare on grass pasture early in the spring. This is usually adequate to loosen the stool for surgery. Other methods of stool softeners such as mashes, mineral oil,[32, 33] and magnesium sulfate may be successful, but the authors have found none to be superior to green grass with a high moisture content.

The mare is placed in stocks, the tail is wrapped; the epidural area is clipped and scrubbed; and epidural anesthesia is administered.[25, 27, 29, 32] The tail is then secured to the stocks above the mare with a 2.5-cm rope in order to assist in maintaining the balance and weight of the mare during surgery.[29] Mares can be sedated or tranquilized with the agent of choice. The authors will generally utilize one of the following depending on the disposition of the mare: acepromazine maleate combined with xylazine, torbugesic, or morphine. The feces are removed from the rectum and vagina, then the internal and external areas are scrubbed thoroughly with an iodine scrub.[25, 29] For the surgical repair of the third-degree laceration, the authors recommend an equine surgical text.

The rectovaginal fistula is defined as a hole through the perineal body involving the vaginal or vestibular mucosa and the rectal mucosa. The vulvar lips and the anal sphincter are not involved.[29, 34, 35] Much of the same concerns expressed for a third-degree perineal laceration apply to the rectovaginal fistula in regard to contamination, time to surgery, and surgical repair. The repair of the fistula can be attempted with or without incising the perineal body; however, depending on the size and the location of the fistula, the degree of reported success is better if the fistula is converted to a third-degree laceration.[28]

VULVAR HEMATOMAS

Hematomas occurring lateral and ventral to the vulva occur in the mare at parturition, primarily due to trauma of blood vessels supplying this area by the fetus during expulsion or due to assistance given at the time of parturition.[15, 18] The hemorrhage may be minimal with an area 5 to 15 cm in diameter affected, or the area may be as large as 25 to 30 cm in diameter. Treatment varies depending on the size and interference with urination and vaginal access. Smaller hematomas are not treated locally; if any treatment is administered, it should be systemic antibiotics. The larger hematomas may require surgical intervention. The area is surgically prepared and anesthetized. An incision is made to remove the clot; local antibiotics are placed in the area; and the incision is sutured. Care must be taken if the hematoma is to be incised prior to the time of organization (7 to 10 days), because the hemorrhage may begin again. Waiting, if possible, until there is little probability of re-initiation of hemorrhage would be recommended. The area should be closed for primary intention healing if no contamination of the clot has occurred. If there is doubt or concern, a drain

tube may be placed in the area with second intention healing expected to occur.

NERVE PARALYSIS

Damage to the gluteal nerve may occur as the fetus passes through the pelvis of the mare and over the nerve.[18] The injury is usually unilateral, although bilateral damage is possible.[18] The characteristic signs of the condition include difficulty when rising or a lameness involving the affected limb.[18] As the lameness disappears or normal function returns, the gluteal muscles exhibit atrophy, causing a physical blemish that is easily identified.[18] The prognosis for return to function as a broodmare is usually excellent assuming that no other complications are present.[18] However, the atrophic area may remain visible due to failure of nerve and muscle regeneration.

Damage to the obturator nerve may result in more severe signs, including a failure to stand even with repeated efforts.[16] The mare may exhibit failure to control the rear quarters when attempting to stand, and the fetus should be removed from the stall if this is suspected.[16] The muscles involved with obturator paralysis are the obturator externus, pectineus, adductor, and gracilis. The primary problem is the failure of the mare to adduct her limbs and, therefore, a mechanism to maintain the limbs in a near-normal position is indicated so that further damage does not occur due to extreme abduction. This can be accomplished with leg straps to hold the affected limb in proximity to the opposite rear limb or with the aid of a sling.[18] If the damage to the obturator nerve is severe, the prognosis for future usefulness of the limb should be guarded.[18] This problem is not as common in the mare as it is in the cow.[18]

REFERENCES

1. Lin HC, Wallace SS, Robins RL, et al: A case report on the use of guaifenesin-ketamine-xylazine anaesthesia for equine dystocia. *Cornell Vet* 84:61, 1994.
2. Bierschwal CJ, deBois CHW: *The technique of fetotomy in large animals.* Bonner Spring, VM Publishing, 1983, p 11.
3. Vandeplassche M, Spincemaille J, Bouters R, et al: Some aspects of equine obstetrics. *Equine Vet J* 4:105, 1983.
4. Blanchard TL, Bierschwal CJ, Youngquist RS, et al: Sequelae to percutaneous fetotomy in the mare. *J Am Vet Med Assoc* 182:1127, 1983.
5. Roberts SJ: Parturition. In Roberts SJ, ed. *Veterinary Obstetrics and Genital Diseases*, ed 3. Woodstock, Davis & Charles, 1986, p 251.
6. Vaughn JT: Surgical management of abdominal crisis in the horse. *J Am Vet Med Assoc* 161:1199, 1972.
7. McCarthy PF, Hooper RN, Carter GK, et al: Postparturient hemorrhage in the mare: Managing ruptured arteries of the broad ligament. *Vet Med* 89:147, 1994.
8. Rooney JR: Internal hemorrhage related to gestation in the mare. *Cornell Vet* 54:11, 1964.
9. Rooney JR: Ruptured aneurysm of the uterine artery. *Mod Vet Pract* 60:316, 1979.
10. Kline RC: Mare and foal management. In Kline RC, ed. *Equine Reproduction and Genetics*. Toledo, The Ohio State University, 1989, p 23.

11. Rossdale PD: Difficult foaling. In Rossdale PD, ed. *Horse Breeding*. Woodstock, David & Charles, 1992, p 293.

12. Lofstedt RM: Miscellaneous diseases of pregnancy to parturition. In McKinnon AO, Voss JL, eds. *Equine Reproduction*. Philadelphia, Lea & Febiger, 1993, p 601.

13. Pascoe RR: Rupture of the utero-ovarian or middle uterine artery in the mare at or near parturition. *Vet Rec* 104:77, 1979.

14. Rooney JR: Internal hemorrhage related to gestation. *Cornell Vet* 54:11, 1964.

15. Allen WE: Other postpartum problems. In Chandler EA, ed. *Fertility and Obstetrics in the Horse*. Oxford, Blackwell Scientific, 1988, p 111.

16. Rose J, Pilliner S: Foaling problems and foal diseases. In Rose J, Pilliner S, eds. *Breeding the Competition Horse*. Oxford, Blackwell Scientific, 1993, p 85.

17. Walker DF, Vaughan JT: Surgery of the perineum, vagina and rectum. In Walker DF, Vaughan JT, eds. *Bovine and Equine Urogenital Surgery*. Philadelphia, Lea & Febiger, 1980, p 196.

18. Roberts SJ: Injuries and diseases of the puerperal period. In Roberts SJ, ed. *Veterinary Obstetrics and Genital Diseases*, ed 3. Woodstock, David & Charles, 1986, p 353.

19. Hooper RN, Blanchard TL, Taylor TS, et al: Identifying and treating uterine prolapse and invagination of the uterine horn. *Vet Med* 88:60, 1993.

20. Tulleners EP, Richardson DW, Reid BV: Vaginal evisceration of the small intestine in three mares. *J Am Vet Med Assoc* 186:385, 1985.

21. Allen WE: Non-infectious fertility in mares. In Chandler EA, ed. *Fertility and Obstetrics in the Horse*. Oxford, Blackwell Scientific, 1988, p 55.

22. Morel MCGD: Physical process of parturition. In Morel MCGD, ed. *Equine Reproductive Physiology, Breeding and Stud Management*. Ipswich, United Kingdom, Farming Press, 1993, p 96.

23. Vaughan JT: The genital system. In Oehme FW, Prier JE, eds. *Textbook of Large Animal Surgery*. Baltimore, Williams & Wilkins, 1974, p 507.

24. Haynes PF, MClure JR: Eversion of the urinary bladder: A sequel of third-degree perineal laceration in the mare. *Vet Surg* 9:66, 1980.

25. Colbern G, Asnes W, et al: Surgical management of perineal lacerations and rectovestibular fistulae in the mare: A retrospective study of 47 cases. *J Am Vet Med Assoc* 186:265, 1985.

26. Straub OC, Fowler ME: Repair of perineal lacerations in the mare and cow. *J Am Vet Med Assoc* 138:659, 1961.

27. Ansari M: Surgical repair of rectovestibular lacerations in mares. *Compend Contin Educ Pract Vet* 5:S139, 1983.

28. Trotter GW: Surgery of the perineum in the mare. In McKinnon AO, Voss JL, eds. *Equine Reproduction*. Philadelphia, Lea & Febiger, 1993, p 417.

29. Heinze CD, Allen AR: Repair of third-degree perineal lacerations in the mare. *Vet Scope* 11:12, 1966.

30. Hilbert B: Surgical repair of recto-vaginal fistulae in mares. *Aust Vet J* 57:85, 1981.

31. Bemis HE: A new operation for rectovaginal fistula. *North Am Vet* 30:37, 1930.

32. Vaughan JT: Surgery of the equine reproductive system. In Morrow DA, ed. *Current Therapy in Theriogenology*. Philadelphia, WB Saunders, 1980, p 806.

33. Teeter SM, Stillions MC: Dietary management of rectovaginal surgery. *Proc Am Assoc Equine Pract* 12:119, 1966.

34. Rossdale PD, Ricketts SW: Birth. In Rossdale PD, Ricketts SW, eds. *Equine Stud Farm Medicine*, ed 2. Philadelphia, Lea & Febiger, 1980, p 270.

35. Aanes WA: Surgical repair of third-degree perineal laceration and rectovaginal fistula in the mare. *J Am Vet Med Assoc* 144:485, 1964.

15.4

Uterine Disease and Therapy

Walter R. Threlfall, DVM, MS, PhD, Dip ACT
Heidi M. Immegart, DVM, MS, PhD, Dip ACT

For appropriate therapy of uterine disease, the diagnosis must be definitive. Examples of uterine disease include inflammatory and infectious endometritis, endometriosis, metritis, toxic metritis, pyometra, perimetritis, parametritis, endometrial scar tissue, endometrial glandular reduction, endometrial cysts, and uterine cysts.

Endometritis is an infection or inflammation of the endometrium. Infectious endometritis must be confirmed with signs of inflammation plus confirmation of the presence of organisms.[1] The most common causes for endometritis are insemination at the wrong stage of the estrous cycle, breeding too often, and not utilizing proper breeding hygiene. Infertility can also be a common sequela to abnormal parturition or after metritis and lacerations of the uterus. Uterine contamination and inflammation are normal occurrences at the time of parturition and should be distinguished from clinically significant endometritis. The inflammation or contamination that occurs at parturition can progress to a clinically significant condition, but generally the normal involutionary process of the uterus is responsible for eliminating contaminating organisms and reducing inflammation.

Endometriosis is a term that has been developed to describe the condition of the endometrium when degenerative changes have occurred in the absence of active inflammation. The lesions include endometrial fibrosis, lymphatic stasis, transluminal adhesions, and endometrial and uterine cysts. Lymphocytes, macrophages, and plasmacytes are the major cells observed in endometrial biopsies from these mares. This condition can occur at any age but is most frequently observed at age 14 or older. These animals are susceptible to recurrent endometrial inflammation or to infection after breeding or contamination and, therefore, should be managed accordingly.

Endometrial fibrosis is not a specific uterine disease; however, because of its importance as an abnormality, it is listed separately. The importance is primarily in the understanding that much of the fibrosis that occurs is preventable if action is taken early. Mares should be reproductively efficient at an early age to help avoid the pressure for production at an older age. Endometrial cysts are due to dilated endometrial glands and rarely exceed 2 to 3 mm. Uterine cysts are due to accumulations of lymph following blockage of lymph ducts. These cysts may exceed 15 cm in diameter. Both types increase in occurrence with the age of the mare.

Metritis is an extension of endometritis into the myometrial layers of the uterus. The uterus will have a tendency to increase in size and decrease in tone. There may be an accumulation of fluid in the lumen of the uterus. The endometrial folds may become less defined on palpation or endoscopic examination. Acute toxic metritis is seen less frequently in the mare than in the cow and is characterized by signs of metritis plus systemic involvement that can include signs of increased temperature, depression, loss of appetite, laminitis, and other signs representative of a toxemia or septicemia. Toxic metritis may lead to perimetritis or parametritis. This condition is observed primarily within 5 days of parturition. Perimetritis indicates that the infection or inflammation has progressed to the serosal surface of the uterus. Parametritis denotes further peritoneal spread of the infection or inflammation to the broad ligaments and other tissue surrounding the uterus.

Pyometra is characterized by an accumulation of pus within the lumen of the uterus in addition to the persistence of a corpus luteum beyond its normal life span during the seasonally polyestrous period. Pyometra in the mare results in the expected increased and sustained level of progesterone. The failure of estrus may be due to an altered capability of the endometrium to produce or release prostaglandin $F_{2\alpha}$. These mares may, during winter, have no functional corpus luteum present. Mares with pyometra generally do not exhibit systemic clinical signs, and the volume of fluid retained in the uterus varies greatly. A uterus distended with purulent material, which is incapable of drainage due to cervical adhesions, has also been referred to as pyometra. However, if the corpus luteum is not maintained during the seasonally polyestrous time of year, this mare may be able to self-correct or to respond to treatment if the cervix is opened and maintained open. This mare would be expected to continue to cycle during the polyestrous season and, therefore, the condition would be correctly defined as a metritis that has cervical adhesions. The presence of a retained corpus luteum is an important distinction between pyometra and metritis with fluid. Mares with pyometra generally develop cervical adhesions and closure of the cervix, if the condition has been present for prolonged periods. A mare with metritis may eventually develop pyometra; however, as long as she continues to cycle, she stands a much better probability of recovery than would a mare with pyometra. Due to the absence of systemic involvement, this condition may not be detected for years in non-brood mares, and owners only seek veterinary assistance when they note a copious intermittent vulvar discharge.

DIAGNOSIS

Diagnosis of uterine disease depends on an examination for breeding soundness. The first portion of the breeding soundness examination is a complete and accurate history. The history should include all known reproductive activity. Omissions of information may lead to omissions of indicated tests or the inclusion of diagnostic aids that are not necessary. The examination includes transrectal palpation and ultrasonographic examination of the reproductive tract; uterine culture; endometrial biopsy; endometrial cytology, if indicated; digital examination of the cervix; examination of the vagina, vestibule, and vestibular sphincter; and assessment of vulvar conformation. Endoscopic examination of the reproductive tract may be indicated following the results of the preceding diagnostic tests.

The importance of the complete battery of diagnostic tests becomes evident when one realizes their significance with regard to the various uterine abnormalities. The confirmation of the diagnosis of endometritis, endometrial fibrosis, or endometriosis must include an endometrial culture and endometrial biopsy or endometrial cytology. It has been suggested that the diagnosis can be based solely on the observation of purulent exudate from the cervix with "substantial proof" that cervicitis is not present. However, the authors do not believe that cervicitis can be eliminated using this technique. Transrectal palpation of the uterus cannot, by definition, diagnose endometritis, because only the endometrium is involved.

Bacterial infection of the uterus is a significant cause of reduced fertility in mares.[2] Since bacteria gain access to the uterus during breeding, parturition, and intravaginal cervical manipulations and from poor vulvar conformation, attention must be given to these areas to reduce the possibility of contamination. The prevention of infection is far superior to the treatment. Cultures of the uterus must be just that—a culture of the lumen of the uterus and not of the vagina or the cervix. There is no correlation between cultures of the lumen of the uterus and cultures of the vagina or cervix. Uterine cultures can be taken during any stage of the estrous cycle or during winter anestrus with excellent correlation to ones obtained during estrus. The cervix is easily dilated during any reproductive stage, even pregnancy, and this is not a recommended time to culture! Cultures must be obtained utilizing proper technique including proper perineal preparation, sterile or bacteria-free sleeves, sterile lubricant, suitable environment, and use of a guarded culture rod. The authors prefer the Accu-CulShure rod (ACCU-MED Corporation, 270 Marble Avenue, Pleasantville, NY 10570-2982). The obtainment of cultures using an unguarded culture rod is possibly worse than no culture. An unguarded culture rod may come in contact with organisms within the vagina or cervix that do not reflect the uterine environment. Therefore, treatment of the uterus for vaginal contaminants may occur.

Many clinicians at present disregard the significance of uterine cultures in the absence of other clinical signs of infection. Although some studies demonstrate major differences in conception rates between "clinically normal" uninfected mares and "clinically normal" streptococcal infected mares, there is some question as to the accuracy of this report. The conception rates for these two groups were 80% and 52% respectively, based on a total of 225 Thoroughbred mares. The classification of a "clinically normal" infected mare utilized cultures and "thorough vaginal and cervical examinations," but this study did not involve endometrial biopsies—thus one is not sure as to the "normal."

Many organisms can create a problem in the uterus, but *Streptococcus zooepidemicus* accounts for two thirds of all uterine infections. Uterine cultures that reveal mixed organisms are usually indicators of contamination rather than uterine infection. Susceptibility tests of organisms cultured should be performed in order to determine the best antibiotic for therapy. It should be recognized that the lumen of the normal non-pregnant uterus is bacteriologically sterile. The majority of younger mares are resistant to uterine infection and prolonged inflammation as evidenced by a return to normal within 96 hours of an exposure to an irritant or potentially pathogenic organism.[3]

Endometrial biopsy has added greatly to our diagnostic

and prognostic capability. The use of this diagnostic aid should be mandatory for any mare that has been bred and failed to deliver a viable fetus. This diagnostic test is probably more important than a culture. However, a biopsy without a culture does not give the veterinarian all the information needed to manage the reproductive events including treatment. Mares may have inflammatory endometritis or endometriosis without infection, and this condition would not be known without the endometrial biopsy. Mares with infection and only biopsy results available would not provide information on which antibiotics to use.

Endometrial cysts and uterine cysts are diagnosed by transrectal palpation of the uterus or by ultrasonographic examination. Endometrial cysts are caused by an accumulation of fluid in the endometrial glands, and these cysts do not exceed 2 to 3 mm. Uterine cysts are due to a blockage of lymph ducts and can exceed 12.5 cm. The diagnosis of metritis is made possible by the use of rectal examination for size, tone, and presence of fluid. Ultrasonographic examination may also be used for conformation. A speculum examination, uterine culture, endometrial cytology, and endometrial biopsy should provide information regarding the cause of enlargement. By definition, the uterine tone or size will be abnormal with metritis and, therefore, diagnostic aids to indicate this are very meaningful. Systemic signs are apparent with toxic metritis, but the uterine size will be larger than normal and the tone will be decreased.

Perimetritis and parametritis are more severe than the nontoxic metritis because they are no longer within the uterus. The inflammation or infection has progressed through the uterine wall following metritis, perimetritis, or parametritis and can be diagnosed by the palpation of adhesions on the uterine surface or surrounding tissue, by pain elicited from palpation of this area, or by a peritoneal tap indicating the presence of inflammation or infection with no other site as a possibility.

Pyometra is diagnosed by the presence of large quantities of fluid present within the uterus and the presence of a retained functional corpus luteum during the seasonally polyestrous time of the year. The fluid may exceed 15 gallons. The cervix may become involved as the development of transluminal adhesions form. These adhesions will prevent drainage of the fluid. The success of treatment is extremely poor with pyometra and, therefore, must be distinguished from metritis, which may also involve an accumulation of fluid within the uterus.

PRETREATMENT CONSIDERATIONS

Many mares may not warrant treatment for uterine disease if their endometrial biopsy results indicate an extremely poor reproductive prognosis. Furthermore, it should be stated that prevention of uterine infection with proper foaling and breeding practices should supersede any consideration regarding therapy. Once uterine disease is established, early detection and immediate treatment of the cause is recommended. Uterine infections and inflammation account for a significant proportion of infertility in mares. Therefore, uterine disease and treatment have received considerable attention and effort in an attempt to reduce infertility. Most veterinarians agree that elimination of pathogenic organisms,

reduction in uterine size, improvement of uterine tone, elimination of uterine fluid, and elimination of inflammation are all desirable in a treatment program. However, opinions differ with regard to the methods used to obtain these objectives.

It is reported that a normal mare's uterine lumen that is artificially exposed to large numbers of pathogenic organisms can return to a non-contaminated, non-infected, and non-inflamed status within a few days. However, the mare that no longer has a normal uterine defense mechanism may require longer to eliminate the bacterial organisms or may not be able to do so without assistance. Therapy, therefore, is valuable for reducing lost reproductive time and for assisting the abnormal mare. Some authors have recommended sexual rest as a treatment for metritis.[4] This aids in elimination of additional bacterial contamination that occurs at breeding and permits the mare to cycle. The bacterial resistance of the reproductive tract is highest during estrus and, therefore, mares that cycle normally have repeated periods of high resistance.

Extreme caution should be taken when using local uterine therapy. The treatment selected should not pose a greater danger to reproductive health than does the disease itself. Extra-label use of numerous products as intrauterine medications in mares is common, despite the lack of information as to their potentially damaging properties.

Mares that appear more susceptible to endometritis must be handled with greater care than normal mares. Recommendations for these problem mares include intrauterine infusions of semen extender containing an antibiotic before natural service and possibly the day after breeding.[4] Opinions as to treatment objectives and anticipated responses are varied and stimulate much controversy. One basic principle should always be remembered: only treat the abnormal. The treatment of reproductively "normal" mares reduces fertility.

THERAPY

Surgical correction of problems such as pneumovagina should always precede any other form of therapy, because often the abnormal conformation is responsible for the uterine infection. The Caslick surgical procedure, named after its describer, is recommended whenever mares have a faulty vulvar conformation that leads to pneumovagina.[5] This routinely used procedure has greatly improved fertility by elimination of chronic contamination, especially in Thoroughbreds. Many infected mares become free of infection after this procedure without any other therapy. Any abnormality, such as third-degree perineal lacerations, rectovaginal fistula, cervical lacerations, and urine pooling, which can be eliminated by surgery, should be corrected to improve the likelihood of breeding success.

Hormonal preparations for the treatment of uterine disease have included estrogens, oxytocin, and prostaglandin $F_{2\alpha}$. Estrogen has been recommended as a means of enhancing uterine involution.[6] It has been described that estrogen, when administered to the mare systemically followed by oxytocin, would exogenously produce a situation similar to estrus. However, the clinical significance of these effects currently are questioned by the authors and, therefore, we no longer utilize this hormone for treatment of uterine abnormalities.

Oxytocin can definitely increase contractility of the uterus, thus increasing tone, decreasing size, and aiding in the mechanical clearance of the uterine lumen. Although oxytocin can enhance contractility at any stage of the estrous cycle, maximal effects occur when the uterus is under the influence of endogenous estrogenic stimulation. Prostaglandin $F_{2\alpha}$ is commonly used in cows with pyometra to evacuate the uterus and to re-establish cycling activity.[7] It is also gaining acceptance as a treatment for metritis and endometritis in the mare. Prostaglandin $F_{2\alpha}$ will short cycle a mare with a corpus luteum. The subsequent estrus will increase her resistance to infection. Prostaglandin $F_{2\alpha}$ may also have a direct beneficial effect on the myometrium by increasing uterine contractility. It appears that this hormone and oxytocin are the two that currently may have the most potential in treatment of uterine abnormalities.

The major indications for the use of antiseptics are to reduce the size and increase the tone of the uterus by virtue of direct irritation. They have also been used to decrease the viscosity of uterine fluid to aid in its expulsion. Furthermore, in conditions of chronic inflammation without infection, they are capable of changing the inflammatory status to that of an acute one. Antibiotics have no value in this situation unless they are irritating. Antiseptic preparations are also generally, as the name implies, antibacterial and possibly antifungal. A partial list of antiseptic agents used in the past includes acriflavine, bismuth subnitrite, boric acid, charcoal, chlorine, iodine and iodine solutions, iodoform, perborate, vinegar, and silver oxide. Although Lugol's infusion (10% solution) used in three mares resulted in an endometrium that was "virtually altered" and contained blood, serosanguinous fluid, and fibrin strands and furthermore required over 21 days for the endometrium to return to normal, iodine in the form of Lugol's solution is the authors' preference.[8] This previous report, however, is in contrast to other research[9] and to the authors' clinical case reports (unpublished) evaluated with ultrasonographic, endoscopic, and endometrial biopsy evaluations on a daily to every other day basis. In the cow, the infusion of dilute Lugol's solution (2%) is capable of chemical irritation to the uterus sufficient to cause regression of the corpus luteum, depending on the stage of the estrous cycle, and regeneration of the endometrium 5 days later.[10] Whenever one is using chemical curettage as an intrauterine treatment, one must remember not to inflict further damage by too harsh or too concentrated a treatment solution.[11]

Chlorhexidine suspension has been available for intrauterine infusion of the cow's uterus. Chlorhexidine solution, however, should never be placed into the uterus of the mare. The most serious abnormalities observed in reproductive tracts of mares presented to The Ohio State University have had, in the history, treatment with chlorhexidine solution. These results have also been reported by Voss and associates.[4] Other less detrimental substances are equally effective, and chlorhexidine solution is not warranted. Before utilizing any irritant, be certain that it will not do more damage than good.

Mechanical curettage has been utilized as a possible treatment for uterine abnormalities and has been very successful in humans. One report of uterine curettage involved 17 infertile mares. Following curettage, 16 mares conceived and eight of these mares produced live foals.[12] The authors have never used mechanical curettage but have been able to visualize endoscopically the appearance of the endometrium after this procedure. The appearance of multiple strands of endometrium detached from the uterine lumen has been the reason why the authors have never used it.

Assuming the cause of the uterine abnormality is an infectious organism and the organism has been identified and the antibiotic sensitivity of the organism determined, treatment can be initiated. If one is uncertain as to whether the condition is caused by an infection or if the organism is not sensitive to the antibiotic instilled, additional money will be wasted and additional reproductive time will be lost. Uterine therapy can be accomplished by the local instillation of antibiotics directly into the uterus. The other approach involves systemic antibiotic treatment.

The first consideration regarding intrauterine infusion is the choice of the most effective antibiotic. With regard to the use of antibiotics to eliminate bacterial infections, one should remember that bacterial cultures and antibiotic susceptibilities are the best way to approach the problem of an efficacious antibacterial selection. Combinations of antibiotics should be avoided with uterine therapy, because they often have little value due to drug incompatibility.[13] The same can be said for antibiotic and antiseptic combinations[14] or of these combinations plus hormonal or other "preparations" to be used on an intrauterine basis. The antibiotics most commonly utilized for intrauterine infusion are penicillin, tetracycline, amikacin,[15] gentamicin,[16] ampicillin, streptomycin, ticarcillin, chloramphenicol,[17] nitrofurazone, polymyxin B, neomycin, and the sulfonamides.[13] The antibiotics that are effective against most pathogenic organisms generally are penicillin, ampicillin, chloramphenicol, ticarcillin, gentamicin, and amikacin.

The majority of reports of equine uterine infections have dealt with how and when infections occur as well as the organisms responsible for the infection. The success of the intrauterine medications has been based on the production of a foal the following year,[17] conception rates,[16] the elimination of the organism from the uterus, or by an improvement in uterine size and tone. The following have been suggested as more common risks associated with local antibiotic therapy in the uterus: changes in the "normal" flora of the horse and development of resistant strains of microorganisms owing to "*indiscriminate*" use of antibiotics.[4] One observation reported in the literature[18] and made by these authors is that some mares treated successfully for streptococcal infection or for bacterial contaminants with various local antibiotics will re-culture a pure growth of *Pseudomonas* sp.

It has been reported for penicillin that plasma concentrations can be increased by decreasing the volume infused, by expelling air from the vagina after infusion, and by infusing 10% Lugol's solution into the uterus before the penicillin.[19] Penicillin is thought to be one of the most effective antibiotics available,[20] and this can be understood when examining the organisms responsible for equine uterine infection. In this article it was recommended that intrauterine treatments be administered "at 24 hour intervals in order to maintain a therapeutic level." It requires approximately 60 mL of fluid to cover the endometrial surface of a normal mare's uterus.[21] Most veterinarians, however, report using quantities from 100 to 500 mL for the abnormal uterus. The primary objective is to infuse sufficient volume to obtain complete endometrial contact by the substance in use. Up until the mid to late 1960s, uterine treatment as well as cultures were performed only while the mare was in heat. A slow transition away from that practice has occurred with no attributable damage to the mare.[7] The frequency of antibiotic infusion into the uterus has probably been determined in the past on a "convenience" basis rather than being based on sound medical judgment. The most popular clinical treatments have included daily infusions with recommended or larger than systemic doses for 3 to 5 days,[9, 20] or infusions every other day for two to five treatments. It is generally not practical to infuse mares more frequently than once a day. Frequency of treatment, however, should probably be based on the length of time that the antibiotic is active in the uterus. Davis and Abbitt[13] suggested that "correct usage" of antibiotics was essential if treatment was to be successful and resistance avoided. Placement of an Indwelling Uterine Infusor (Fort Dodge Loratones, Fort Dodge, IA 50501) in mares to facilitate more frequent treatments has been described.[22]

Some investigators have presented the argument that local antibiotic therapy is a technique held over from the days of local antiseptic therapy and compare the uterus to the udder with regard to higher tissue levels being present in the udder after systemic therapy than local treatment.[22] It was also noted in favor of systemic therapy that intrauterine infused antibiotics are rapidly absorbed in normal animals. However, in cows with endometritis, absorption other than to the endometrium is reduced. In cattle, one supporting argument for systemic versus local therapy has been a report in which the intramuscular route of oxytetracycline administration resulted in substantial concentrations in the oviduct, ovaries, and so forth. With intrauterine therapy, high concentrations occur in the endometrium and myometrium with no detectable quantities in other reproductive tract tissues at 24 hours after treatment.[23] The intrauterine route, however, had very high luminal and endometrial concentrations for 72 hours following treatment. This has also been found to be true for ticarcillin.[24]

The basic question to be addressed is what tissues are involved in the uterine infection being treated? If the infection involves deeper layers of the uterus and other genital tissues, systemic therapy would be necessary. If, however, the infection is limited to the endometrium, then local therapy is probably warranted due to very high sustained levels of antibiotic in the lumen and endometrium. It has been suggested that in the case of severe endometritis, antibiotics may be retained and degraded in the uterine lumen.[23] The fact that antibiotics are not absorbed into the circulation does not indicate that they are degraded nor that they are not as beneficial locally as systematically administered antibacterial agents. It is questionable that local therapy for endometritis would be less successful than systemic therapy.[4] More severe conditions such as toxic or septic metritis, pyometra, or perimetritis may, however, deserve systemic therapy if antibiotics alone are to be used in treatment. Antibiotics are only effective if infection is the cause or if the antibiotic is irritating and noninfectious endometritis is the cause.

The organisms most commonly present within the infected uterus are *Streptococcus* spp, hemolytic *Escherichia coli*, *Klebsiella* sp., *Staphylococcus* sp., *Proteus* sp., *Pseudomonas* sp., and *Corynebacterium* sp.[25] β-Hemolytic streptococcal organisms account for an estimated 65% of all equine uterine

infections. Hemolytic *E. coli*, *Proteus* sp., *Pseudomonas* sp., and *Klebsiella* sp. account for an additional 30%.[26–29]

Most treatments have consisted of eliminating the initial cause and then allowing the mare to self-correct or infusing iodine solutions (e.g., Nystatin Oral Suspension [USP Morton Grove Pharmaceuticals, Inc., Morton Grove, IL 60053] or amphotericin B). The *Candida* sp. appear to be the most common organism associated with fungal uterine infection.[30] The success of treatment with Lugol's solution and mycostatin is represented by a report in which 6 of 13 infected mares receiving either or both conceived when bred on the heat following treatment.[31] Of the non-treated controls, one of three conceived after 3 months of repeated breedings. Nystatin was reportedly used on one mare for the treatment of a *Candida rugosa* infection that had followed successful treatment of a *Pseudomonas aeruginosa* infection with carbenicillin.[22] However, the discharge continued and the organism was still present. The organism was then treated with 0.3% iodine solution, but the discharge continued for an additional 6 weeks. Four months later the mare was cultured and no bacterial or fungal organisms were present. She was bred and conceived. Amphotericin B has been used to treat successfully *Monosporium apiospermum*[32] and has been used clinically for *Candida* sp. Another report suggested using 200 mg of amphotericin B or 2.4 million units of intrauterine nystatin (mycostatin) daily for 4 days.[34] Gentian violet has also been used successfully on two mares that had a mold infection.[4]

Uterine flushes have proved useful in the past by rinsing fluid out of the uterus, stimulating blood flow to the uterus, improving tone, and decreasing size.[12] Hot saline (40 to 45 °C), used to enhance the myometrial tone, provided a rapid but transient effect in cases of myometrial atony and endometrial atrophy to enhance the myometrial tone.[35] Also saline flushes at day 6 of the cycle[36] have been shown to induce luteal regression, whereas this did not occur at day 1 or day 11 of the cycle. Uterine flushes on alternate days for 9 days with warm and cold salt solutions have been successful as a uterine therapy for infection.[37] There appears to be an advantage of this technique in older mares with enlarged uteri.[1, 38–40]

Probably one of the most important and promising aspects in the prevention and treatment of uterine infection concerns the local immune responses and natural local defense mechanisms of the uterus. The loss of the local immune response could be and probably is the reason why some mares become infected following bacterial contamination of the uterus and others do not. These natural uterine mechanisms have been separated into cellular and non-cellular. The cellular mechanism involves the phagocytes. The non-cellular factors include opsonins, thermal stabile factors, and the leukocytic tide.

Immunoglobulins within the uterine luminal fluid of normal and abnormal mares have been reported to include IgA, IgG, IgG(T), and IgM.[33, 40, 41] A comparison has indicated that mares with reduced fertility (lowered resistance) had increased amounts of IgA, IgG, and IgG(T). Insufficient data were obtained to determine a difference for IgM. Earlier work had failed to demonstrate the presence of IgG(T) and IgM but did report the presence IgGa, IgGb, and IgGc.[42] A more recent report indicated that although IgA was increased, IgG and IgG(T) were not elevated in infected mares.

The differences may be due in part to the differences in abnormal animals selected in each study.

It has been reported that the infected uterus of a mare has lost its ability to eliminate contaminating organisms and overcome infections.[41] The mechanisms involved are not understood. This loss of ability is possibly related to failures in the immune system. The uterus of a normal maiden mare responds rapidly to experimental inoculation of *Streptococcus zooepidemicus* organisms.[43] In contrast, the older chronically infected mare may show little or no response.

It has been suggested that a practical method to overcome inadequate immune defense mechanisms of the uterus is to place substances, such as colostrum or plasma that already contains these antibodies, into the uterine lumen. In a group of 20 infertile mares, colostrum was infused into the uterus in an attempt to improve uterine resistance to infection.[11] During the mating estrus, 120 mL of colostrum and 380 mL of normal saline were infused into each mare. Of these 20 mares, 15 were diagnosed pregnant at 40 days after the last breeding date. Four of six mares diagnosed pregnant and followed to term had normal foals. There is one report of a mare that developed serum sickness after an intrauterine plasma infusion.[44]

Enzyme preparations used locally to enhance recovery from pyometra have also been reported.[4] Products such as pepsin, papain, urea, and yeast have been utilized in the uterus because of their possible effect on tissue debris. However, the ability of these products to enhance recovery is doubtful. Intrauterine dimethyl sulfoxide (DMSO) has been used for several different purposes.[4] Studies as to its effect on the uterus indicate that it is a severe irritant causing ulceration and inflammation after an infusion.[45] DMSO also did not have any beneficial effect in reducing scar tissue. When 120 mL of DMSO was applied cutaneously twice daily for 10 days, the systemic changes noted included hemoglobin depression, reduction in platelets, and decreased sedimentation rate but no change in prothrombin clotting time.[46] Marked "alterations" occurred in sorbitol dehydrogenase and serum glutamic oxaloacetic transaminase levels. There were no local changes. DMSO has been shown to be "mildly" antifungal and antibacterial.[21] This same report noted that skin exposed to once daily treatments with DMSO "rapidly became tolerant" to the irritating properties of this product.

RE-EVALUATION

Re-examination of infected mares following therapy is as important as the original diagnosis of a problem. Therapy of any type is rarely 100% effective, and therefore re-evaluation is necessary to ascertain success. The length of time between uterine therapy and subsequent culture has been recommended to be 30 days. The authors have used a figure of 14 days after the last treatment, and the results have been excellent.

PREVENTION

Mares that are susceptible to uterine infection at breeding should be bred as few times as necessary to obtain conception. Palpation of these mares and breeding one time close to, but before ovulation, is recommended.[36] Daily intrauterine infusions following breeding until the cervix closes has been recommended for mares that become infected following natural service. However, the routine use of post-breeding infusions on all mares (normal and abnormal) may decrease foaling rates in the normal mares.[17] Mares with chronic or recurrent uterine infections should only be bred utilizing antibiotic-treated semen extender or by the minimum contamination technique.[42]

SUMMARY

The reduction of uterine size, elimination of fluid, and improved tone should be accomplished before antibiotic therapy commences. This can be accomplished with flushes, hormones, or antiseptics. Antibiotic treatment guidelines should be based on culture and sensitivity of all mares treated. General or routine treatment of all problem mares with the same antibiotic will not ensure the best treatment results. In order to obtain maximal treatment efficacy, mares must be handled as individuals. Guidelines recommended by these authors include using antibiotics indicated by sensitivity tests. These antibiotics are administered by intrauterine instillation according to systemic dose recommendations of the pharmaceutical company. Daily infusions are administered with the volume sufficient to obtain complete endometrial contact with the infused material. This generally ranges from 250 to 1,000 mL. The infusion is performed after the mare's tail is wrapped and held or tied to one side and the perineal area has been thoroughly cleansed. A sterile sleeve, treatment rod, and lubricant are used for the infusion. Medication is placed in the uterus per gravity flow by connecting the free end of the rod to the inverted bottle via a sterile simplex. Uterine therapy, as is the case with uterine biopsy and culture, can be performed at any time during the estrous cycle or during anestrus. Two weeks after therapy, the uterus is re-cultured to determine the effectiveness of the treatment. Most, if not all, of the preceding techniques have had application to the treatment of infertility. The only summary that one can make from the available information is that at present there is no single treatment for all uterine diseases. One of the most important challenges that must be met is not to simply treat the infection successfully but to subsequently manage mares so that they will not become re-infected.

REFERENCES

1. Asbury AC: Infectious and immunologic considerations in mare infertility. *Compend Contin Educ Pract Vet* 9:585, 1987.
2. Vandeplassche M, Spincemaille J, Bouters R: Aetiology, pathogenesis and treatment of retained placenta in the mare. *Equine Vet J* 3:144, 1971.
3. LeBlanc MM: Breakdown in uterine defense mechanisms in the mare: Is a delay in physical clearance the culprit? *Therio* 121, 1994.
4. Jackson RS, Skewes AR, Voss JL, et al: Equine infertility—Doctor to doctor seminar. Kenilworth, Schering, 1972, p 4.
5. Caslick EA: The vulva and the vulvo-vaginal orifice and its relation to genital health of the Thoroughbred mares. *Cornell Vet* 27:172, 1937.

6. Varachin M: Endometritis: A common cause of infertility in mare. *J Reprod Fertil Suppl* 23:353, 1975.

7. Gustafsson B, Backstrom G, Edquist LE: Treatment of bovine pyometra with prostaglandin F₂: An evaluation of a field study. *Therio* 6:45, 1976.

8. Mather EC, Refsal KR, Gustafsson BK, et al: The use of fiberoptic techniques in clinical diagnosis and visual assessment of experimental intrauterine therapy in mares. *J Reprod Fertil Suppl* 27:293, 1979.

9. Woolcock JB: Equine bacterial endometritis—diagnosis, interpretation and treatment. Symposium on Equine Reproduction. *Vet Clin North Am Large Animal Pract* 2:241, 1980.

10. Seguin BE, Morrow DA, Louis TM: Luteolysis, luteostasis, and the effect of prostaglandin F₂ in cows after endometrial irritation. *Am J Vet Res* 35:57, 1974.

11. Dewes HF: Preliminary observations on the use of colostrum as a uterine infusion in Thoroughbred mares. *N Z Vet J* 28:7, 1980.

12. Ellsworth KS: A practical approach to the treatment of endometritis. *Proc Am Equine Pract* 18:490, 1972.

13. Davis LE, Abbitt B: Clinical pharmacology of antibacterial drugs in the uterus of the mare. *J Am Vet Med Assoc* 170:204, 1977.

14. Threlfall WR: Treatment of uterine infection in the mare. Proceedings of the Symposium on Mare Infertility, Western States Veterinary Conference, February, 1984, p 15.

15. Caudle AB, Purswell BJ, Williams DJ, et al: Endometrial levels of amikacin in the mare after intrauterine infusion of amikacin sulfate. *Therio* 19:433, 1983.

16. Houdeshell JW, Hennessey PW: Gentamicin in the treatment of equine metritis. *Vet Med Small Animal Clin* 67:1348, 1972.

17. Wearly WK, Murdick PW, Hensel JD: A five year study of the use of post-breeding treatment in mares in a Standardbred stud. *Proc Am Assoc Equine Pract* 1971, p 89.

18. Hughes JP, Loy RG: The relation of infection to infertility in the mare and the stallion. *Equine Vet J* 7:155, 1975.

19. Allen WE, Clark AR: Absorption of sodium benzylpenicillin from the equine uterus after local Lugol's iodine treatment, compared with absorption after intramuscular injection. *Equine Vet J* 10:174, 1978.

20. Blanchard TL, Woods GL: Reproductive management of the barren mare. *Compend Contin Educ Pract Vet* II:5141, 1980.

21. Northway RB: A treatment regimen for equine cervicitis and metritis. *Vet Med Small Animal Clin* 68:269, 1973.

22. Roberts SJ: *Veterinary Obstetrics and Genital Diseases*, ed 2. Ithaca, Roberts, 1971, p 538.

23. Gustafsson BK, Ott RS: Current trends in the treatment of genital infections in large animals. *Compend Contin Educ Pract Vet* 3:147, 1981.

24. Lock TF, DiPiertro JA, Ott RS, et al: Distribution of ticarcillin in the reproductive tract of pony mares following parenteral and intrauterine administration. Proceedings of the 61st Annual Meeting on Research Work and Disease, Conference of Research Workers in Animal Disease. Chicago, IL, Dec., 1980, p 16.

25. Bain AM: The role of infection in infertility in the Thoroughbred mare. *Vet Rec* 78:168, 1966.

26. Shin SJ, Lein DH, Aronson AL, et al: The bacteriological culture of equine uterine contents, in-vitro sensitivity of organisms isolated and interpretation. *J Reprod Fertil Suppl* 27:307, 1979.

27. Asbury AC: Endometritis in the mare. In Morrow DA, ed. *Current Therapy in Theriogenology 2*. Philadelphia, WB Saunders, 1986, p 718.

28. Ricketts SW, Mackintosh ME: Role of anaerobic bacteria in equine endometritis. *J Reprod Fertil Suppl* 35:343, 1987.

29. Hinrichs K, Cummings MR, Sertich PL, et al: Clinical significance of aerobic bacterial flora of the uterus, vagina, vestibule, and clitoral fossa of clinically normal mares. *J Am Vet Med Assoc* 193:72, 1988.

30. Zafracas AM: *Candida* infection of the genital tract in Thoroughbred mares. *J Reprod Fertil Suppl* 23:349, 1975.

31. Abou-Gabal M, Hogle RM, West JK: Pyometra in a mare caused by *Candida rugosa*. *J Am Vet Med Assoc* 170:177, 1977.

32. Reid MM, Frock IW, Jeffrey DR, et al: Successful treatment of a maduromycotic fungal infection of the equine with amphotericin B. *Vet Med Small Animal Clin* 72:1194, 1977.

33. Asbury AC, Halliwell REW, Foster GW, et al: Immunoglobulins in uterine secretions of mares with differing resistance to endometritis. *Therio* 14:299, 1980.

34. Doyle AW, O'Brien HV: Genital tract infection with *Candida albicans* (monilia) in a Thoroughbred mare. *Irish Vet J* 23:90, 1969.

35. Kenney RM, Ganjam VK: Selected pathological changes of the mare's uterus and ovary. *J Reprod Fertil Suppl* 23:335, 1975.

36. Arthur GH: *Veterinary Reproduction and Obstetrics*, ed 4. London, Bailliere-Tindall, 1975, p 467.

37. Ginther OJ, Meckley PE: Effect of intrauterine infusion on length of diestrus in cows and mares. *Vet Med Small Animal Clin* 67:751, 1972.

38. Ricketts SW: Uterine abnormalities. In Robinson NE, ed. *Current Therapy in Equine Medicine II*. Philadelphia, WB Saunders, 1987, p 503.

39. Asbury AC: Large-volume uterine lavage in the management of endometritis and acute metritis in mares. *Compend Contin Educ Pract Vet* 12:1477, 1990.

40. Asbury AC: Failure of uterine defense mechanisms. In Robinson NE, ed. *Current Therapy in Equine Medicine 2*. Philadelphia, WB Saunders, 1987, p 508.

41. Williamson P, Dunning A, O'Connor J, et al: Immunoglobulin levels, protein concentrations and alkaline phosphatase activity in uterine flushings from mares with endometritis. *Therio* 19:441, 1983.

42. Kenney RM, Khaleel SA: Bacteriostatic activity of the mare's uterus: A progress report on immunoglobulins. *J Reprod Fertil Suppl* 23:357, 1975.

43. Evans MJ, Hamer JM, Gason LM, et al: Factors affecting uterine clearance of inoculated materials in mares. *J Reprod Fertil Suppl* 35:327, 1987.

44. Tully RC: Use of exogenous equine plasma. *J Am Vet Med Assoc* 188:1140, 1986.

45. Frazer GS, Rosol JR, Threlfall WR, et al: Histopathologic effects of dimethyl sulfoxide on the horse endometrium. *J Am Vet Med Assoc* 49:1774, 1988.

46. Edds GT, Kirkham WW: Dimethyl-sulfoxide: Tests for safety in horses. *J Am Vet Med Assoc* 150:1305, 1967.

15.5

Postpartum Period

Walter R. Threlfall, DVM, MS, PhD, Dip ACT
Heidi M. Immegart, DVM, MS, PhD, Dip ACT

The post-partum period is of extreme importance to the mare since the events of this period will determine the general and reproductive health of the mare. The normal uterine involution free of any abnormalities is essential since most mares will be considered for foal heat breeding, which will occur between 3 and 18 days post-partum. Although any injury that occurs at parturition will affect the post-partum period, this chapter specifically addresses the post-partum period exclusive of the conditions under parturition injuries.

RETAINED FETAL MEMBRANES

Retained fetal membranes is reported to be the most common post-partum problem in the mare.[1] Although the passage of the fetal membranes is actually considered to be part of the events of stage III parturition, when delayed it is no longer a portion of the normal parturition process and is considered to occur within the post-partum period. Retained fetal membranes, also referred to as retained after birth or retained placenta, have multiple definitions in the literature. All authors consider retained fetal membranes to be a failure of passage of part or all of the allantochorionic membrane with or without the amniotic membrane within a specific period of time. It is the length of time post-partum, however, that creates the disagreement. The reported times vary to include 30 minutes,[2] 1 hour,[3] 1.5 hours,[2] 2 hours,[4] 3 hours,[5] and 6 to 12 hours.[6]

The occurrence of this condition is difficult to assess due to the lack of a specific post-partum time interval in the definition. It is, however, reported to occur after parturition in mares between 2% and 10.5%.[7] Draft mares[8, 9] and mares experiencing dystocia,[7] prolonged gestation,[10] hydrops,[11] and a cesarean[7] have a higher incidence. Retained fetal membranes have been reported to occur at a higher incidence in association with abortion, stillbirth, and twinning in light-weight horses; however, one report indicated no increase with these conditions if they occurred in the absence of dystocia.[12] This same report stated that the occurrence of retained fetal membranes did not differ between the birth of a weak or diseased foal and that of a healthy foal. There was no influence on retained membranes due to the sex of the foal. There may be an influence of the mare's age on retained fetal membranes on some farms; the reason for this effect is not known. Mares older than 15 years of age may have a significantly higher incidence of retained fetal membranes than do younger mares. The time of year appeared to influence the incidence of retained fetal membranes only on certain farms, and there was a higher incidence after March 31 in the Northern hemisphere. Barren or maiden mares from the previous year had no difference involving the incidence of retained placenta after foaling than did mares that had foaled the previous year. Artificial insemination during foal heat did not influence the retained fetal membrane occurrence compared with mares that were artificially bred at heats following the foal heat. It has been reported that mares bred naturally have an increased occurrence of retained fetal membranes compared with mares that were naturally bred at later heats after parturition.[13]

The specific causes for retained fetal membranes are unknown. The microcotyledons are tightly adhered by the seventh month of gestation.[7] This attachment prevents complete separation of the fetal membranes unless the microvilli are released. It is reported that either the gravid horn[14, 15] or the nongravid horn allantochorion of a retained fetal membrane is attached to the endometrium, thus preventing expul-

sion. A third report stated that it is neither horn but actually the body of the uterus that remains attached.[16] The generalized opinion today is that areas of the fetal membrane near the tip of the non-pregnant horn have failed to separate. Mechanical interference or hormonal imbalance may be possible causes for this condition. Allantochorion thickness, length of villi, and degree of attachment of the placenta increase from the gravid horn to the nongravid horn. An explanation for these characteristics includes the presence of more developing microvilli in uterine horns than in the body; furthermore, the microvilli are more branched and larger in the non-pregnant horn.[17] Folding of the fetal membrane and endometrium within the nongravid horn is also more pronounced.[18] Lastly, uterine involution occurs at a slower rate in the non-gravid horn than in the gravid horn. These events, working in combination or alone, may help to explain the slower release of the fetal membranes from the non-gravid horn. Edema is also reported to be partially responsible for retention.[19]

Infection, bloodborne or ascending after cervical relaxation, and inflammatory endometritis during pregnancy could induce choriouterine adherences and delay separation of the placenta.[2] Mares that have uterine infections before breeding, become infected at breeding, or are bred to an infected stallion may have retarded fetal membrane separation at the next parturition.[2]

Many authors believe that retained fetal membranes are primarily due to uterine inertia and hormonal imbalance, because mares affected with retained fetal membranes do not exhibit the signs of colic associated with post-partum uterine contractions.[20] This hormonal imbalance could result in abnormal myometrial activity. Excellent results obtained with treatment of retained fetal membranes with oxytocin suggest a possible deficiency or a lack of this hormone in the circulation.[7, 21]

The signs of a mare with a retained placenta may include the visualization of the fetal membranes protruding from the vulva, no membrane visible due to only a portion of the fetal membrane remaining attached to the endometrium, and the failure of post-partum mild to slight colic.[2] The treatment for retained fetal membranes includes tying the membranes up away from the hocks.[22] This procedure will reduce the probability of injury to the foal.[2] It also reduces the probability that the mare will step on the placenta, causing it to tear or causing the tip of the uterine horn to invaginate within itself or to evert through the vulva.

Treatments for retained fetal membranes vary with advantages and disadvantages of each. The most conservative and superior treatment in the authors' opinion is the use of oxytocin. Oxytocin can be administered by intravenous drip[19] or intramuscularly.[3, 23] Dosages range from 20 to 12 units and can be repeated at 1.5- to 2-hour intervals until passage of the placenta. The reported disadvantage of the bolus form of administration includes intense and only spasmodic contractions when "large" doses were administered and were believed to be of no value.[7] Colic was reported to be more of a problem with bolus administration than with intravenous administration, although cramping may have been dose related.[21] These authors have not encountered excessive colic with 20 units of oxytocin administered intramuscularly every 1 to 2 hours. Colicky signs, if they occur, can be eliminated with sedation or analgesics.[24]

Antibiotics have been frequently used in the therapy of retained fetal membranes. One author has recommended oxytetracycline hydrochloride in capsule form as the antibiotic of choice.[25] In the authors' experience, use of powdered antibiotics (or antibiotics in capsule or tablet form) is considered undesirable because the antibiotic is unable to make contact with much of the endometrial surface for prolonged periods, if ever. Many antibiotics have been utilized in the treatment of retained fetal membranes such as sulfanilamide,[24] penicillin,[24] polymyxin, amikacin, ticarcillin, and others.[19] It has been recommended that the administration of intrauterine antibiotics should commence at approximately 8 hours after delivery. An important reason given for the use of antibiotics in the uterus of a mare with retained fetal membranes is to aid in controlling the numbers of contaminating bacteria. However, the information available indicates that treated mares have a significantly higher pregnancy rate than do mares untreated[12]; however, due to a higher pregnancy loss, both groups had the same foaling percentage the following year. In a study of intrauterine therapy combined with systemic antibiotic therapy versus only oxytocin therapy, 5 hours after treatment, 55% of the intrauterine-treated mares had not passed the placenta in comparison with 19% for those treated with oxytocin alone.[12]

Although numerous methods are described for the manual removal of the retained fetal membranes,[7, 12, 22, 24] the authors do not recommend this technique. Although reported by many as the treatment of choice, manual removal of a placenta is not without undesirable side effects and has many potential undesirable complications. Hemorrhage is one of the more frequent complications following manual removal of the retained fetal membranes.[7] This hemorrhage can be life threatening when large quantities of blood are lost. Blood in the uterus serves as an excellent medium for bacteria to grow and multiply. Also, venous emboli from the uterine veins have been reported as a possible disadvantage of manual removal.[7] Invagination or intussusception of the uterine horn can occur at the site of attachment of the membranes to the endometrium. Manual removal of the fetal membranes has also been listed as a cause of delayed uterine involution.[7] In addition, it has been noted that accumulation of fluid within the uterus is greater following manual removal than with more conservative therapy.[24] The separation of the microvilli from the remainder of the membranes was attributed to the increased occurrence of tissue debris, endometritis, laminitis, uterine spasm, and delayed involution.[24] At least one previous report acknowledged that manual removal should be discouraged due to the induced trauma, hemorrhage, and infection.[25] However, it was then recommended as an acceptable treatment after other methods had failed.

It has been suggested in the literature and by the authors that manual removal of the placenta can result in permanent damage to the endometrium.[19] The authors have observed an increase in damage in several mares that had normal fertility until manual removal of retained fetal membranes occurred. These animals often had a decrease in endometrial biopsy classification to a IIB or III based on the presence of scar tissue. The cervix has been reported to remain open longer when the membranes were manually removed.[7] It has been suggested that manual removal of the placenta has been continued from a time when draft horses predominated and retained placentas were more of a problem,[24] but no reason was given for the continued use of this technique when it has been shown to be detrimental. Other methods of treatment that have been suggested with variable degrees of success include the infusion of antiseptics, infusion of iodine and warm water into the uterus and inside the placenta,[3] placement of 10 to 12 liters of povidone iodine into the allantochorionic space followed by closure of the hole in this membrane,[26] flushing and siphoning of fluid from the uterus,[22, 24] infusing the uterus with 42 °C water,[27] and flushing the uterus with large volumes of saline containing antibiotics. There is much controversy regarding therapy for retained fetal membranes, but the literature has provided more information on which to base our therapeutic judgement. Tetanus protection in the form of antitoxin or, as preferred by the authors, toxoid is recommended.[24]

Although the complications of a retained placenta in the mare have been of major concern to veterinarians, early and proper treatment of the retained membranes considerably reduces or eliminates that concern. The complicating factors associated with retention of the membranes include metritis, laminitis, septicemia, or death.[26] The occurrence of acute metritis and laminitis, as described in heavy breeds, are not as commonly seen in Thoroughbreds and other light breeds. A study of 356 retained placentas in Standardbreds treated without manual removal reported no cases of laminitis, toxemia, septicemia, or acute metritis.[12] Postparturient laminitis is associated more with a systemic acute metritis with or without a retained placenta.[28, 29]

Some recommend treating any animal with retained fetal membranes in order to prevent laminitis. Recommended treatments have included cold water or ice to hooves, suitable supportive footing, uterine and systemic antibiotic therapy in order to prevent septic metritis, antihistamines,[24] phenylbutazone,[19] nonsteroidal anti-inflammatory drugs, and tranquilizers.[19] Although some have recommended flushing a septic or toxic uterus or manually removing the placenta, these authors are opposed to both practices. The disadvantages of both techniques are that the treatment itself will increase absorption of septic or toxic material during removal and flushing, and the mare's condition will deteriorate before she can improve. This action can result in more damage to the feet or in death. Excellent results have been obtained with conservative therapy involving systemic therapy and supportive care plus antibiotic therapy of the uterus on the first day or possibly the first 2 days. The conservative approach is based on helping the mare to establish the uterine barrier, which develops by approximately day 3 postpartum in the normal mare. This assistance is accomplished primarily by systemic antibiotics, anti-inflammatory agents such as phenylbutazone (Butazolidin) or flunixin meglumine, and systemic fluids if necessary. This approach will result in an improvement of the mare's condition within 24 to 48 hours. Once this improvement has occurred, uterine therapy can be initiated. Frequent temperature and complete blood count monitoring in mares treated in this manner will demonstrate slight subclinical relapses in progress after every uterine manipulation for 2 to 3 days. However, this result is more desirable than the less conservative therapies.

No differences in pregnancy rates have been reported after the first breeding or after the breeding season, pregnancy loss rates, and foaling rates between normal foaling mares without retained fetal membranes and mares with retained fetal membranes.[12] This lack of a difference was evident regardless of the duration of time that the placenta was retained. No manual removal was used in this study.

All fetal membranes should be thoroughly examined after delivery. The placenta is usually passed in an everted position. The allantoic membrane is examined for roughened areas, thickened areas, missing segments, or any other unusual appearance. Once the amnion has been examined for abnormalities, the placenta is returned to its natural position with the chorionic membrane outermost. The chorion is examined very closely since this is a mirror image of the endometrium. The first and possibly most important point of examination is to determine if it is complete or if holes are present. It should be adequately determined that there are no portions missing or that this would be an indication for uterine therapy. The next examination of the chorion is to determine the presence of thickened areas, segments devoid of villinous attachments, the presence of plaques, ante-mortem discolorations, or similar abnormalities.

The examination of the mare's udder may be indicated especially if the foal demonstrates continued nursing or the history indicates a lactational problem with the mare. The administration of oxytocin for treatment of a retained placenta may also create a leakage of colostrum or milk from the udder. An external examination of the mare's genitalia is indicated within the first day or two post-partum to determine if lacerations have occurred. If not performed at that time, examinations must be performed at the time of the foal heat examination. Repairs of such lacerations are generally performed 25 to 30 days after parturition.[30]

Since the mare was likely vaccinated during the end of her ninth month of gestation for rhinopneumonitis, influenza, and tetanus,[31–33] the only vaccination recommended for the mare following parturition is for rhinopneumonitis. This is to reduce the probability of the mare becoming infected with the herpes virus. The foal is vaccinated for influenza, rhinopneumonitis, and tetanus as soon as possible after delivery.[32, 33] The authors have found that this is particularly easy and less stressful to the neonate if achieved before the foal stands. The use of active immunization for tetanus has the advantage over passive protection of antitoxin in that antibody concentrations are increasing at the time when incubation of the organism and toxin production is occurring. The administration of antitoxin creates maximal antitoxin availability immediately and is minimal at the time when needed most. If antitoxin is to be administered to the neonate, it would appear most advisable to do so at 7 to 10 days after birth.

DELAY OF UTERINE INVOLUTION POST-PARTUM

Delay of uterine involution post-partum will significantly influence the fertility until the uterus has achieved an environment suitable for sperm survival and transport and for survival of the embryo. A normal uterus post-partum should have excellent tone for the first 1 to 3 days. The tone of the uterus will decrease to good and usually maintains this tone until pregnant or until the second post-partum estrus when the tone may lessen. The size of the uterus will be in excess

of 15 cm immediately after parturition and reduces in size thereafter. The size at 9 to 10 days will be approximately 10 to 15 cm in diameter, dependent on the age of the mare and the number of previous foals. The vulvar discharge should be most noticeable during the first 24 hours post-partum and reduces during the next 5 to 8 days until no discharge is present.[34] The color of the discharge will be hemorrhagic initially and will become more yellow and serous with time.[35] An ultrasonographic examination of the uterus will also reveal a reduction of fluid within the uterus until only estrual edema is present at 8 to 10 days post-partum.[36] Any alteration in this normal involution suggests a potential problem and may account for a reduction in fertility.

HYPOCALCEMIA

Lowered blood calcium can occur in the lactating broodmare but is much less common than in the dairy cow. It is observed primarily in the excellent lactating mare that is receiving grass or grass hay as her source of nutrients.[2] The signs of hypocalcemia in the mare are similar to those seen in other species, including nervousness,[2] atypical respirations,[2] muscle spasms,[2, 30] and failure of the pupils to constrict when exposed to bright light. The condition may be confused to some extent with tetanus, because the post-partum mare can also have a clostridial infection of the uterus as the source of tetanus toxins. The treatment of the condition is the careful administration of calcium.[2, 30, 37]

REFERENCES

1. Asbury AC: Management of the foaling mare. *Proc Am Assoc Equine Pract* 18:487, 1972.
2. Roberts SJ: Injuries and diseases of the puerperal period. In Roberts SJ, ed: *Veterinary Obstetrics and Genital Diseases*, ed 3. Woodstock, David & Charles, 1986, p 353.
3. White TE: Retained placenta. *Mod Vet Pract* 61:87, 1980.
4. Shipley WD, Bergen WC: Care of the foaling mare and foal. *Vet Med* 64:63, 1969.
5. Sager FC: Examination and care of the genital tract of the broodmare. *J Am Vet Med Assoc* 115:450, 1949.
6. Wright JG: Parturition in the mare. *J Comp Pathol* 53:212, 1943.
7. Vandeplassche M, Spincemaille J, Bouters R: Aetiology, pathogenesis and treatment of retained placenta in the mare. *Equine Vet J* 3:144, 1971.
8. Jennings WE: Some common problems in horse breeding. *Cornell Vet* 31:197, 1941.
9. Williams WL: *The Diseases of the Genital Organs of Domestic Animals*, ed 3. Ithaca, Williams, 1943, p 552.
10. Blanchard TL, Bierschwal CJ, Youngquist RS, et al: Sequelae to percutaneous fetotomy in the mare. *J Am Vet Med Assoc* 182:1127, 1983.
11. Vandeplassche M, Bouters R, Spincemaille J, et al: Dropsy of the fetal sacs in mares: Induced and spontaneous abortion. *Vet Rec* 99:67, 1976.
12. Provencher R, Threlfall WR, Murdick PW, et al: Retained fetal membranes in the mare: A retrospective study. *Can Vet J* 29:903, 1988.
13. Jennings WE: Twelve years of horse breeding in the army. *J Am Vet Med Assoc* 116:11, 1950.
14. Van der Kaay FC: Cursus Nota's. Faculteit Diergeneeskunde, Utrecht, deel II, 1945, p 37.

15. Alhnelt E: *Tiergeburtshilte,* ed 2. Berlin, P. Pary, 1960, p 638.
16. Derivauz J: *Obstetrique Veterinaire.* Paris, Vigot Frères, 1957, p 333.
17. Vandeplassche M, Spincemaille J, Bouters R, et al: Some aspects of equine obstetrics. *Equine Vet J* 4:105, 1972.
18. Arthur GH: *Wright's Veterinary Obstetrics,* ed 3. Baltimore, Williams & Wilkins, 1964, p 341.
19. Held JP: Retained placenta. In Robinson NE, ed. *Current Therapy in Equine Medicine,* ed 2. Philadelphia, WB Saunders, 1987, p 547.
20. Berthelon M, Tournut J: Retention of the placenta in domestic animals. *Rev Med Vet* 104:529, 1953.
21. Cox JE: Excessive retainment of the placenta in a mare. *Vet Rec* 89:252, 1971.
22. Allen WE: *Fertility and Obstetrics in the Horse.* Boston, Blackwell Scientific, 1988, p 104.
23. Hafez ESE: *Reproduction in Farm Animals,* ed 5. Philadelphia, Lea & Febiger, 1987, p 418.
24. Arthur GH, Noakes DE, Pearson H: *Veterinary Reproduction and Obstetrics,* ed 5. London, Bailliere Tindal, 1982, p 250.
25. Neely DP, Liu IKM, Hillman RB: *Equine Reproduction.* Nutley, Veterinary Learning Systems, 1983, p 87.
26. Burns SJ, Judge NG, Martin JE, et al: Management of retained placenta in mares. *Proc Am Assoc Equine Pract* 23:381, 1977.
27. Sager FC: Management and medical treatment of uterine disease. *J Am Vet Med Assoc* 153:1567, 1968.
28. Adams OR: *Lameness in Horses,* ed 3. Philadelphia, Lea & Febiger, 1974, p 248.
29. Threlfall WR, Carleton CL: Treatment of uterine infections in the mare. In Morrow DA, ed. *Current Therapy in Theriogenology,* ed 2. Philadelphia, WB Saunders, 1986, p 730.
30. Allen WE: Other post-partum problems. In Chandler EA, ed. *Fertility and Obstetrics in the Horse.* Boston, Blackwell Scientific, 1988, p 110.
31. Morel MCGD: Management of the pregnant mare. In Morel MCGD, ed. *Equine Reproductive Physiology, Breeding and Stud Management.* Ipswich, United Kingdom, Farming Press, 1993, p 241.
32. Evans JW, Borton A, Hintz H, et al: Horse-breeding problems and procedures. In Evans JW, Borton A, Hintz H, et al, eds. *The Horse,* ed 2. New York, WH Freeman, 1990, p 390.
33. Rossdale PD: Abnormalities and disease. In Rossdale PD, ed. *Horse Breeding.* Woodstock, David & Charles, 1992, p 237.
34. Koskinen E, Katila T: Uterine involution, ovarian activity and fertility in the postpartum mare. *J Reprod Fertil Suppl* 35:733, 1987.
35. Roberts SJ: Parturition. In Roberts SJ, ed. *Veterinary Obstetrics and Genital Diseases,* ed 3. Woodstock, David & Charles, 1986, p 245.
36. McKinnon AO, Squires EL, Harrison LA, et al: Ultrasonographic studies on the reproductive tract mares after parturition: Effect of involution and uterine fluid on pregnancy rates in mares with normal and delayed first postpartum ovulatory cycles. *J Am Vet Med Assoc* 192:350, 1988.
37. Morel MCGD: Physical process of parturition. In Morel MCGD, ed. *Equine Reproductive Physiology, Breeding and Stud Management.* Ipswich, United Kingdom, Farming Press, 1993, p 96.

15.6

Normal Parturition

Walter R. Threlfall, DVM, MS, PhD, Dip ACT
Heidi M. Immegart, DVM, MS, PhD, Dip ACT

The average length of gestation for the mare is approximately 340 days.[1] This average varies considerably and may range from 315 to 400 days. The average gestation is influenced by the season with winter term deliveries usually being longer than summer term dates.[2, 3] The effect of light on the length of gestation has been reported by the utilization of artificial lighting programs, which provide 16 hours of light and are capable of reducing the gestation by 10 days.[4] Male fetuses have been reported to have a slightly longer gestation than do females.[5] When a large variation from the average occurs, there should always be some concern and possible indication for examination. The definition of eutocia is a "normal delivery"[6] or a safe easy delivery without significant injury to either the fetus or the mare. Since foaling is the climax of much waiting and hoping and may have been preceded by long periods of concentrated effort and considerable expense, the importance of this event cannot be underestimated or diminished.

Mare Pre-partum Changes

During the first two thirds of gestation, maintenance rations that adequately maintain the mare in a healthy (not fat and not thin) condition are adequate. Proper nutrition and exercise are extremely important during the third trimester of gestation in order to ensure that the mare is prepared for the delivery process. The abdominal cavity gradually increases in size in most mares. The front portion may appear to enlarge first; however, as the mare approaches parturition, the ventral abdominal wall or the fetus is said to "drop." This indicates that the enlargement is more toward the mare's pelvis and generally occurs during the last month of pregnancy. "Dropping" actually occurs as part of the relaxation process of the abdominal muscles and may be important for the correct positioning and expulsion of the fetus. It is more pronounced in older mares that have had several foals. Progesterone concentrations in the peripheral plasma are less than 1 ng/mL during the last half of gestation and as a result make the measurement of this hormone useless for determining deficiencies or for predicting the time of parturition.[7] Other progestogens, such as 20α-hydroxy-5α-pregnen-3-1 and 5α-pregnane-3β,20α-diol, decrease during the last 24 hours prior to parturition.[7, 8]

Pre-partum changes in the mare include enlargement of the udder 4 to 6 weeks prior to delivery.[5, 9] This time varies with the individual animal and depends somewhat on the number of previous pregnancies, if any. The udder becomes more rounded as it enlarges. Enlargement and edema of the udder and the abdominal wall immediately anterior to the udder are apparent 2 to 3 weeks prior to foaling.[5] Waxing or the appearance of a sebaceous-like secretion on the teat ends surrounding the sphincter should appear as the mare approaches parturition. However, waxing has been observed to occur as early as 4 weeks before delivery and may not occur in some mares.[5, 10, 11] Waxing generally occurs with regularity in the same animal at approximately the same time prior to parturition. The teats will fill and distend usually 2 to 14 days prior to parturition but may not be observed.[1] Some mares will drip or stream colostrum prior to parturition.[5] This is undesirable, because once the colostrum is lost from the udder it is not replaced, and a substitute colostrum should be made available for the foal following delivery.

Relaxation of the tail head and pelvic ligaments occur gradually over several weeks pre-partum.[5, 9] During this same period the vulva is relaxing and the opening elongates.[5] One to 3 weeks prior to foaling, the relaxation becomes apparent in the flank area, and the mare appears somewhat "gaunt" in this area. Approximately 7 to 10 days later, the gluteal muscles and the muscles adjacent to the tail head relax and appear less evident and the bones in that area become more pronounced. The ultrasonographic character of the fluids within the uterus also change during the last 10 days of gestation, and echogenic particles appear.[12] The vagina and vulva are relaxing, and the amount of mucus increases. The vaginal wall may appear reddened; this generally occurs within 24 hours of parturition. The cervix becomes completely relaxed, and the uterus increases in the frequency and strength of contraction. The shape of the pelvic canal is elongated, and the opening nearest the cervix is larger than the opening nearest the vulva. In addition, the diameter of the canal is not round but is somewhat oval, and the greatest diameter is in a dorsolateral to dorsoventral direction. Since some mares foal with only a few of these normal signs, the clinical prediction as to the exact time of foaling is difficult to estimate without further diagnostic testing (as described under induced parturition). Body temperature has been suggested as a possible method to determine the time of parturition before the onset of stage I of labor.[11, 13] However it has been further delineated that although changes in body temperature, as observed at 6-hour intervals with the use of an electronic rectal thermometer, were not adequate to predict parturition,[14] the use of telemetry with a computerized system recording core body temperatures at 15-minute intervals could be useful in the prediction of parturition.[15]

Sweating initiated in the shoulder area combined with frequent observations of the flank area by the mare are indicators that stage I of labor is occurring. Kicking, biting of the flank, or other signs of mild colic frequently occur during this period. During this stage the final positioning and posturing occur. The front feet and the nose make an excellent wedge to aid in cervical dilatation. This is also assisted by the fetal fluid putting pressure on the cervical opening as the pressure increases. The increase in pressure is first due to the increased uterine activity. As the pressure increases and the cervix starts to dilate, this stimulation of the cervix causes the release of oxytocin. Oxytocin increases the uterine contractions and indirectly stimulates the abdominal muscles to contract and further increase the uterine pressure. Restlessness increases as the mare approaches parturition. Before this increase mares may demonstrate de-creased activity, which could last for several weeks. Personality changes are obvious as the time of parturition approaches. This is especially true during the 24 hours pre-partum. Distractions of any kind should be minimized during this period. Myometrial activity changes pre-partum have been reported,[15–17] and pre-partum changes are associated with the prediction of parturition.

FETAL CHANGES

The fetus is in a variety of presentations until approximately the sixth month of gestation, when the fetus aligns itself in an anterior presentation. The presentation may change after this stage and, therefore, cannot be used reliably to determine the presentation of the fetus until parturition actually begins. The fetus assumes various positions, including a dorsosacral position for longer durations as it approaches term.[17] As parturition approaches, the head and forelimbs can be palpated in the pelvic canal of the mare and may sometimes be alongside the cervix with pressure on the vaginal wall. The fetal heart rate prior to the onset of parturition is approximately 76 beats/min and increases occur with increased activity.[12] The increases may be 40 beats/min, and the accelerations may average one per minute. The activity of the fetus is most pronounced during the period of 5 to 72 hours pre-partum. The fetal cardiac rate per minute during the 24 hours prior to delivery is approximately 62, and during stage I and stage II the cardiac rate is between 54 and 60 beats/min.[18] The heart rate of the neonate averages over 100 beats/min.

PARTURITION

There is no need to wrap the mare's tail, wash the perineal area, or wash the udder. These procedures, although recommended by some, mainly serve only to disrupt the mare and have no medical basis. However, cleaning the stall and maintaining reasonable cleanliness are especially important immediately pre-partum and post-partum. This cleaning could include disinfecting stalls between mares but is not practical with most farm facilities. In order for disinfectants to be effective, all organic material must be removed. This is usually only feasible with a high-pressure sprayer and requires that relatively nonporous material be used in the construction of stalls, including the floor. The size of the stalls should be at least 12 × 12 feet or larger, and the stalls should be bedded preferably with relatively large quantities of straw. Other types of bedding material may promote bacterial growth or may be too dusty for use with neonates or with mares immediately post-partum. If a Caslick procedure has been performed to improve the vulvar conformation, this area should be opened in preparation for foaling approximately 14 days prior to the due date or as determined by visual assessment of the mare's impending parturition.

The beginning of stage I of parturition is difficult to determine because its onset is not marked by any single event or by a change in the mare.[19] The beginning of stage I is rather vague and variable. As the normal mare approaches foaling, she may have a decrease in activity during the day before the night of foaling. It has been reported that approximately 85% of mares foal between 7:00 PM and 9:00 AM, and most mares foal between 11:00 PM and 4:00 AM.[11, 20, 21] Two hours prior to foaling, the mare may become restless and show signs of colic. She may paw the ground and stop eating for short periods of time, which is an indication of pain. Increased switching or movement of the tail is also usually observed as the mare approaches parturition. Sweating may begin in the area of the front shoulder, and then sweating becomes evident over the entire side and the neck. Milk may be seen squirting from the teats. This activity is associated with release of oxytocin and apparent uterine pain and is not constant, but intermittent corresponding with the contractions. The periods may last from 1 or 2 minutes up to 20 minutes. These events may not be observed in older mares, even though the entire period may take several hours. This explains how the mare is able to foal during the 30 minutes when an observer may be absent. The mare should be observed but left undisturbed unless problems arise. The average range for this period is 1 to 4 hours. Any disturbances may delay the foaling and result in complications.

Internally, during this period, the mare's uterus begins more active with contractions beginning at the end of the uterus near the ovary and progressing posteriorly toward the cervix. These contractions force the fetus and fetal fluids surrounding the fetus against the cervix; the pressure causes the cervix to further dilate. The outermost portion of the placenta (chorioallantoic membrane) ruptures, and the allantoic fluid escapes. This fluid is the fetal urine and is water-like in consistency. This marks the end of stage I.

Stage II signs are more apparent. The mare lies down during most of this period; she may be up and down several times and is generally sweating. When in the recumbent position, all legs may be extended with the head stretched outward away from the body. The mare may bite her flank or chew on hay or straw. During stage II of labor the mare will frequently urinate and defecate to permit more area in the pelvis and due to the pressure applied by the contracting uterus and the abdominal wall. Some mares may roll, apparently in an attempt to lessen the pain or position the fetus. The average time for this period is 20 minutes, calculated from the time of chorioallantoic membrane rupture until the delivery of the fetus. It is abnormal for mares to continue this stage of labor for longer than 70 minutes, and such a delay would indicate that problems are likely to be present and that fetal death is likely to occur.[1, 19] It is generally recommended that mares be given 20 minutes before one becomes alarmed. Some normal progression in the delivery process should be occurring during this period. Hopefully, assistance can be obtained within the remaining time.

During stage II, the innermost portion of the placenta, called the amniotic membrane, which contains amniotic fluid, is seen protruding from the vulva. This is sometimes referred to as a "water-bag." The amniotic membrane should be visible at the vulvar lips within 5 to 10 minutes following the rupture of the chorioallantoic membrane if she has not been disturbed during the delivery process. Once this structure is seen, the fetus has entered the birth canal sufficiently to stimulate strong abdominal contractions. As the foal is pushed posteriorly by the abdominal and uterine contractions, the feet of the fetus are observed through the amniotic membrane. Rupture of the membrane does not usually occur

until the fetus is at least mid-way or completely out of the birth canal. Although most mares foal in the recumbent position, it is acceptable for parturition to occur in the standing position. If the foal is delivered and the amniotic membrane remains intact as the foal struggles following delivery, the membrane should be incised and removed from the area of the fetal nose and mouth. The normal delivery posture of the fetus is one forelimb extending approximately 4 inches in front of the other and the soles of both feet directed ventrally. This off-setting of the feet results in a slight angling of the shoulders and, thus, reduces the width of this area as it passes through the mare's pelvis. While the foal is passing through the vulvar lips and is surrounded by the amnion, the observer can determine the offset position of the hooves and can note that the soles are ventral. If the soles are not directed ventrally, immediate attention is indicated. The head is resting on the forelimbs in the area of the carpal joints. The head and the neck are extended. If the nose of the fetus has not appeared by the time that the carpal joints are observable, immediate intervention is indicated. The vertebra of the fetus are located near to the vertebra of the mare; the position is close to a dorsosacral position but slightly off toward the ilium. This position permits the fetus to take advantage of the greater pelvic diameter. As the fetus is expelled further, the rear limbs are extended so that the rear hooves are the last part of the fetus that is delivered. Any variation from this normal position, such as failure to observe one of the feet or the head and neck, indicates a postural abnormality and a difficult delivery. The anterior half of the fetus should be expelled within an average of 20 to 30 minutes with a maximum of 70 minutes following the rupture of the chorioallantoic membrane. Because the mare's delivery is so forceful, she may severely injure herself by pushing the fetus out and tearing her tissue in the process. Also, anything that slows down the delivery process is detrimental, because the placenta separates rapidly and thus eliminates the fetal supply of oxygen. This probably accounts for the poor survival rate of foals when the mare was in need of assistance and none was immediately available.

The red blood cell count of the normal neonate should average approximately $11.9 \times 10^{12}/L$.[22] The packed cell volume should approximate 0.42 L/L. The hemoglobin should average 14.2 ± 0.2 g/dL. The mean cell volume should be 35.0 ± 1 fL. The normal white blood cell count should be $7.8 \pm 0.3 \times 10^9/L$. The ratio of neutrophils to lymphocytes at birth is greater than 2.5, and this ratio continues to increase for 24 hours. If this ratio is extremely low (less than 1.0), it indicates fetal immaturity and a poor prognosis.

The mare should be permitted to lie quietly in the stall for up to 1 hour if she so desires following parturition. However, if she jumps up rapidly following delivery, it is not necessarily a reason to panic. It has not been demonstrated that abdominal wall damage occurs to the fetus when this occurs. The determination of hemorrhage from the umbilicus, although not common, should be made. Although once advised that large volumes of fetal blood could be lost from the placenta and care must be taken to ensure that the cord remained attached to the placenta,[23] a more recent scientific study revealed that blood flow through the umbilical vessels ceases by the time that the umbilical cord is visible at the vulvar area of the mare.[24] After delivery of the fetus and after the mare has accepted the foal and is resting, the cleaning of the stall and observation of the mare and foal are the two most important managerial tasks that one can do. Stage III of parturition begins with the expulsion of the foal and ends weeks later when uterine involution is complete. The fetal membranes should be expelled within 3 hours after delivery. Administration of antibiotics to the foal or mare are not recommended nor indicated. The instillation of antibiotics, irritants, or other substances into the uterus is also not recommended unless there is an abnormality that indicates their use. The time-honored practices of routinely administering an enema or treating the umbilical area of the fetus with iodine do not appear to be necessary. The quantity of fluid utilized in most enemas to foals is inadequate to be of value. The occurrence of failure to pass meconium is relatively low. Therefore, the routine use of enemas is not cost effective, and the observation of foals for signs of failure to pass meconium and treatment with larger quantities of warm soapy water using an enema tube are much more effective. The placement of iodine or other substances on the umbilicus has not been demonstrated to be effective clinically. A report on the reduction of bacteria in the umbilical area following treatment with iodine did not suggest any differences in the clinical occurrence of umbilical infections.[25] The authors of this chapter have managed more than 1,500 foalings in which nothing was placed on the umbilicus and no cases of infections have occurred in the umbilical area. Stall cleanliness was managed to eliminate the major causes of environmental contamination. Because of uterine inflammation and infection and laminitis associated with retained fetal membranes, it is generally recommended to treat the mare if the placenta has not been passed within 3 hours.

REFERENCES

1. Rossdale PD, Ricketts SW: *Equine Stud Farm Management*, ed 2. Philadelphia, Lea & Febiger, 1980, p 213.
2. Hintz HF, Hintz RL, Van Vleck LD: Length of gestation periods in Thoroughbred mares. *J Equine Med Surg* 3:289, 1979.
3. Howell C, Rollins WC: Environmental sources of variation in the gestational length of the horse. *J Anim Sci* 10:789, 1951.
4. Hodge SL, Kreider JL, Potter GD, et al: Influence of photoperiod on the pregnant and postpartum mare. *Am J Vet Res* 43:1752, 1982.
5. Evans JW, Torbeck RL: *Breeding Management and Foal Development*. Tyler, Equine Res, 1982, p 392.
6. *Dorland's Illustrated Medical Dictionary*, ed 23. Philadelphia, WB Saunders, 1957, p 481.
7. Holtan DW, Houghton E, Silver M, et al: Plasma progesterone in the mare, fetus and newborn foal. *J Reprod Fertil Suppl* 44:517, 1991.
8. Haluska GJ, Currie WB: Variation in plasma concentrations of estradiol-17beta and their relationship to those of progesterone, 13, 14-dihydro-15-ketoprostaglandin F2 alpha and oxytocin across pregnancy and at parturition in pony mares. *J Reprod Fertil* 84:635, 1988.
9. Arthur GH: *Veterinary Reproduction and Obstetrics*, ed 4. London, Bailliere Tindall, 1975, p 131.
10. Peaker M, Rossdale PD, Forsyth IA, et al: Changes in mammary development and the composition of secretion during late pregnancy in the mare. *J Reprod Fertil Suppl* 27:555, 1979.
11. Haluska GJ, Wilkins K: Predictive utility of prepartum temperature change in the mare. *Equine Vet J* 21:116, 1989.
12. Adams-Brendenmuehl C, Pipers FS: Antepartum evaluation of the equine fetus. *J Reprod Fertil Suppl* 35:565, 1987.
13. Shaw EB, Houpt KA, Holmes DF: Body temperature and behaviour of mares during the last weeks of pregnancy. *Equine Vet J* 20:199, 1988.
14. Ammons SF, Threlfall WR, Kline RC: Equine body temperature and progesterone fluctuations during estrus and near parturition. *Theriogenology* 31:1007, 1989.
15. Cross DT, Threlfall WR, Kline RC: Telemetric monitoring of body temperature in the horse mare. *Theriogenology* 36:855, 1991.
16. Haluska GJ, Lowe JE, Currie WB: Electromyographic properties of the myometrium of the pony mare. *J Reprod Fertil* 81:471, 1987.
17. Haluska GJ, Lowe JE, Currie WB: Electromyographic properties of the myometrium correlated with the endocrinology of the pre-partum and the post-partum periods and parturition in pony mares. *J Reprod Fertil Suppl* 35:553, 1987.
18. Too K, Kanagawa H, Kawata K: Fetal and maternal electrocardiograms during parturition in the mare. *J Vet Res* 15:5, 1967.
19. Roberts SJ: *Veterinary Obstetrics and Genital Diseases (Theriogenology)*, ed 3. Woodstock, David Charles, 1986, p 251.
20. Rossdale PD, Short RV: The time of foaling in Thoroughbred mares. *J Reprod Fertil* 13:341, 1969.
21. Bain AM, Howey WP: Observations on the time of foaling in Thoroughbred mares in Australia. *J Reprod Fertil Suppl* 23:545, 1975.
22. Jeffcott LB, Rossdale PD, Leadon DP: Haematological changes in the neonatal period of normal and induced premature foals. *J Reprod Fertil Suppl* 32:537, 1982.
23. Rossdale PD: Clinical studies on the newborn Thoroughbred foal. 1: Perinatal behavior. *Br Vet J* 123:470, 1967.
24. Doarn RT, Threlfall WR, Kline R: Umbilical blood flow and the effects of premature severance in the neonatal horse. *Theriogenology* 28:789, 1987.
25. Lavin RT, Madigan JE, Walker R, et al: Effects of disinfectant treatments on the bacterial flora of the umbilicus of neonatal foals. 6th International Proceedings of the Symposium on Equine Reproduction, Caxambu-Minas Gerais, Brazil, 1994, p 19.

15.7

Monitoring Gestation

Heidi M. Immegart, DVM, MS, PhD, Dip ACT
Walter R. Threlfall, DVM, MS, PhD, Dip ACT

It is frequently of concern to the veterinarian to be able to assess the maturity and fetal well-being of horses. These occasions may arise due to diseases or injuries sustained by the mare, suspected abnormal pregnancies, or the desire to induce parturition. Although some techniques have been applied to the horse, the limitations of each should be recognized as well as their potential.

The simplest method for determining the presence and viability of a fetus is by transrectal palpation of the mare's uterus. During the last trimester of gestation, the fetal head and forelimbs, if in anterior presentation, can be readily detected and fetal movement can usually be elicited following gentle transrectal ballotment or fetal manipulation. Lack of fetal movement, however, should not be the only determinant of fetal viability, because "sleep" periods of the fetus are not accompanied by activity.[1] Re-evaluation at a different time or by another method is warranted before fetal death can be diagnosed. Transrectal palpation can also be used to detect the presence of abnormally large volumes or decreased quantities of allantoic fluid (hydrallantois) associated with fetal death. This subject is further discussed in Chapter 15.6.

An assessment of fetal cardiac function has been determined by utilizing a transcutaneous electrocardiogram (ECG) and transabdominal ultrasonographic examination.[2-5] ECGs have been useful for detecting the presence of one or multiple viable fetuses as well as fetal heart rate and the presence of fetal arrhythmias.[2, 5] A bipolar lead is placed with the positive electrode on the mare's dorsal midline and the negative probe ideally on the ventral midline 6 inches cranial to the mammary gland.[2, 3] The ventral probe has been placed laterally in the flank cranial to the left stifle with little loss of trace clarity for mares that resent the midline probe.[2] Some limitations of fetal ECG include the small amplitude of the fetal tracing, variability in the lead configuration producing the best tracing, and variability of the normal heart rate between the fetus and the mare as well as difficulties with mare restraints.[6, 7] Real-time and Doppler ultrasonography have also been used to determine fetal heart rate.[1, 4] The location of the fetal heart may be altered as fetal activity results in changes of the chest location within the mare's abdomen. Fetal heart rates have been reported to range from 60 to 120 beats/min, with a consistent decrease in the rate as term approaches.[2, 3, 5] This coincides with an increase in maternal heart rate towards term. Increased fetal activity has been associated with an increased heart rate of 10 to 25 beats/min for 30 to 60 seconds' duration; however, some bouts of activity were not associated with an increased heart rate.[4] Larger increases and longer durations of increase were detected in some fetuses, but the normalcy of this was unknown. Three fetuses in which this exaggerated heart rate response was detected were delivered within 48 hours.[4] The maternal heart rate was not associated with the fetal heart rate and would increase independently.[3, 5] Persistent fetal tachycardia or bradycardia are indications of fetal abnormalities. An initial tachycardia followed by bradycardia were reported in a fetus immediately prior to death and abortion. Fetal arrhythmias may also indicate cardiac abnormalities or impending fetal death.[2, 4, 5]

Ultrasonography can also be used to assess the echogenicity of the fetal fluid and the size of the fetal aorta. Echogenic particles have been detected in normal late gestation pregnancies and have tended to increase in size as the pregnancy progresses.[4] Measurements of fetal aortic diameter have been correlated, with significant relationships, to body weight, girth, and hip height.[4] The clinical significance of this measurement currently remains unknown.

Maturation of the pulmonary system is considered crucial for the well-being of the fetus as a neonate following parturition. Therefore, assessment of fetal maturity by an evaluation of amniotic fluid for surfactant phospholipids has been attempted.[8-11] It has been reported that fetal lung maturity and surfactant film formation are not present at 300 days of gestation and, in some cases, are also not present at what is considered term (335 days) in the horse.[12] Another report indicates that pulmonary phospholipids increase between days 100 and 150 of gestation, after which these phospholipids remain constant.[13] This report suggested that lung maturation begins when the phospholipids increase at the end of the first trimester. The technique of ultrasound-guided amniocentesis was utilized to obtain samples for evaluation of percent phosphotidyl glycerol, the lecithin to sphingomyelin ratio, and cortisol concentration.[9] In this study, the factors studied were not reliable predictors of fetal maturity. Complications of the procedure included inadvertent allantoic fluid sampling and premature delivery after the procedure.[8, 11] Because of the variability of the results and the lack of predictive value as well as the possible complications of sampling, pre-term amniotic fluid sampling is currently not useful.

Methods for monitoring the preterm mare to predict when foaling will occur include an evaluation of mammary gland development and its secretions and perineal/pelvic structure relaxation. These methods are discussed in Chapter 15.6. Body temperature changes, which are measured by rectal probes, have not been as useful in mares as in dogs, since the significant temperature decrease apparent by radiotelemetric body core readings are not routinely detected.[14, 15]

Aids are available to allow rapid detection of parturition once it has started. The Foalert (Foalert, Inc., Route 5, Box 295 A, East Cherokee Drive, Canton, GA 30114) and the Birth-Alert units (Profitable Breeding Corp., 9877 Simonds Road, Corfu, NY 14036) provide a source of transmitted signals to indicate when parturition has commenced. These systems provide a means for detecting delivery with fewer distractions to the mare. Video systems with remote monitoring also allow the mare more privacy during the peri-parturient period. This may be beneficial for mares that are easily distracted and will temporarily delay parturition until the environment is undisturbed.

REFERENCES

1. Adams-Brendemuehl C: Fetal assessment. In Koterba AM, Drummond WH, Kosch PC, eds. *Equine Clinical Neonatology*. Philadelphia, Lea & Febiger, 1990, p 16.
2. Parkes KD: Fetal electrocardiography in the mare as a practical aid to diagnosing singleton and twin pregnancy. *Vet Rec* Jan:25, 1977.
3. Holmes JR, Darke PGG: Foetal electrocardiography in the mare. *Vet Rec* Jun:651, 1968.
4. Adams-Grendemuehl C, Pipers FS: Antepartum evaluation of the equine fetus. *J Reprod Fertil Suppl* 35:565, 1987.
5. Colles CM, Parkes RD, May CJ: Foetal electrocardiography in the mare. *Equine Vet J* 10:32, 1978.
6. Buss DD, Asbury AC, Chevalier L: Limitations in equine fetal electrocardiography. *J Am Vet Med Assoc* 177:174, 1980.
7. Larks SD, Holm LW, Parker HR: A new technique for the demonstration of the fetal electrocardiogram in the large domestic animal (cattle, sheep, horse). *Cornell Vet* 50:459, 1960.
8. Schmidt AR, Williams MA, Carleton CL, et al: Evaluation

of transabdominal ultrasound-guided amniocentesis in the late gestational mare. *Equine Vet J* 23:261, 1991.

9. Williams MA, Schmidt AR, Carleton CL, et al: Amniotic fluid analysis for ante-partum foetal assessment in the horse. *Equine Vet J* 24:236, 1992.

10. Tulley RT, Paccamonti DL: Concentrations in equine amniotic fluid during the 1st third of gestation. *J Vet Intern Med* 6:137, 1992.

11. Williams MA, Goyert NA, Goyert GL, et al: Preliminary report of transabdominal amniocentesis for the determination of pulmonary maturity in an equine population. *Equine Vet J* 20:457, 1988.

12. Pattle RE, Rossdale PD, Schock C, et al: The development of the lung and its surfactant in the foal and in other species. *J Reprod Fertil Suppl* 23:651, 1975.

13. Aridson G, Astedt B, Ekelund L, et al: Surfactant studies in the fetal and neonatal foal. *J Reprod Fertil Suppl* 23:663, 1975.

14. Ammons SF, Threlfall WR, Kline RC: Equine body temperature and progesterone fluctuations during estrus and near parturition. *Therio* 31:1007, 1989.

15. Cross DT, Threlfall WR, Kline RC: Body temperature fluctuations in the periparturient horse mare. *Therio* 37:1041, 1992.

15.8

Induced Parturition

Walter R. Threlfall, DVM, MS, PhD, Dip ACT
Heidi M. Immegart, DVM, MS, PhD, Dip ACT

REASONS FOR PARTURITION INDUCTION

Parturition induction permits observation and professional assistance, if necessary, at the time of foaling. There are primarily two reasons to induce parturition. The first reason is for medical indications. It is of most value when used for mares that have a history of difficult deliveries or that have had injuries, or illnesses occur that could possibly endanger the life of the mare or the foal if not assisted immediately at the time of parturition. Among the clinical indications for induced parturition are rupture of the prepubic tendon, rupture or weakening of the abdominal wall, after surgical correction of third-degree perineal lacerations or rectovaginal fistulas, previous fracture of the pelvis with narrowing of the birth canal, history of premature placental separation, prolonged gestation, near-term colic, or uterine inertia.[1-5] Induction of parturition also permits opening of a Caslick procedure immediately before delivery and replacement immediately post-partum, thus reducing contamination of the reproductive tract. Furthermore, if an episiotomy is indicated to prevent vulvar lacerations, it can be performed when indicated. Induced parturition in mares that have produced previous foals with neonatal isoerythrolysis can be easily managed by removal of the foal immediately following delivery.

The second reason for the induction of parturition is for convenience.[6, 7] Most mares reportedly foal at night.[8] The induction of parturition is becoming an accepted method for permitting the owner, manager, or veterinarian to be present at the time of delivery in non-problem mares. The value of induced parturition in labor savings is brought about by the elimination of "foal watchers," people hired to observe mares near-term, or by the elimination of frequent observations throughout the night with the possibility of missing the onset of foaling.[9] The expenses incurred in the induction of parturition are easily offset by the labor savings plus the guarantee that a veterinarian in addition to the owner, manager, or some other farm employee will be present at the time of parturition. The convenience factor also applies to certain research projects involving parturition and neonatal physiology and for the educational value of being able to provide a demonstration of parturition. Induction of parturition has also been utilized when the primary intention was to provide a nurse mare for a valuable foal.[10] There has been no association of parturition induction with impaired future reproductive efficiency.[11] Owners must be aware of the problems with dysmature or premature foals if the delivery occurs prior to the time when the foal is mature.[12] (Additional information is found in Chapter 18.)

GENERAL CONSIDERATIONS

Some general criteria to consider before induction of parturition include knowledge of the gestation length that should exceed 320 days. The mare's previous gestation lengths can be utilized to some extent to determine term, but the effect of the time of year should be considered. Mares that foal in January, February, and March have longer gestation periods than do mares that foal in April, May, and June. Pre-partum changes such as perineal and cervical relaxation have been used to predict parturition[4, 13] but may not be accurate enough for predicting the time to induce parturition.[10] Although relaxation of the pelvic ligaments can also be used as an indicator of approaching parturition, it is less noticeable than udder changes, and more experience is necessary to detect the subtle changes.[14] Mares should be introduced into the foaling environment at least 3 to 4 weeks prior to induction if possible. This permits the mare to be exposed to the organisms in the new environment as well as become accustomed to her new surroundings. The mare should be placed in a clean stall bedded with straw in a quiet area of the barn. A recto-genital examination of the mare at this time will usually permit an evaluation of the fetal presentation, position, and posture as well as the viability status of the fetus. Since this is an elective procedure and the time of delivery is predetermined, a tail wrap is applied to the mare and the perineal area is washed prior to the administration of the inducing agent.

The determination of the fetal presentation, position, and posture plus a physical examination of the mare must be performed again immediately prior to the induction. The fetus should be presented in an anterior longitudinal presentation and slight dorsoileal position with the head and neck extended. Although the final delivery position and posture will occur as the mare enters stage I of parturition,[11] the presentation will have already been determined. A posterior presentation would indicate the importance of assistance much earlier in the delivery process than would an anterior presentation. If the head and feet are not in the proper posture, it is very probable that correction of this posture will occur before delivery without assistance. The authors do not advise intervention once the delivery has been induced, unless it is apparent that the progress is slower than normal or is abnormal. Assistance that is premature or too aggressive may result in delay of the parturition process or cervical lacerations.

Many significant changes occur in the udder generally during the last 2 weeks of gestation.[4, 13] The increased size of the udder is influenced by the age of the mare and by the number of previous foals. The udder should be evaluated daily for a change, and the secretion present within the udder should be evaluated once the mare appears to be close to delivery. The evaluation process can be initiated 2 weeks or more before parturition without harmful affects to the mare or foal. Mares, especially young ones, carrying their first foal, may have to be acclimated to the examination procedure and removal of secretion from the udder. The secretion characteristics will change from a cloudy or straw-colored fluid to a smokey-gray color, and finally, a few hours to a few days before parturition, the color becomes opaque-white.[7, 9] The consistency changes from a viscous nature a few weeks prior to delivery to a more fluid consistency as parturition approaches. Although waxing usually occurs, the time at which it is observed varies considerably and may not be seen until the mare is in the first stage of labor.

Sodium and chloride concentrations decrease during late gestation, and lactose, potassium, citrate, phosphate, calcium, magnesium, and protein increase in lactational secretion. A scoring system for the use of a combination of calcium, potassium, and sodium in pre-term lactational secretions has been described for use to determine when the fetus is mature and thus when parturition could be induced.[15] It was suggested that the determination of calcium alone in lactational secretions pre-partum could be used to predict the time of parturition.[16] Changes in electrolytes in mammary secretions pre-partum have been reported to be effective in determining the time of parturition in mares or the times when the mare is not going to foal.[15, 17–21] Mammary secretions during gestation have been reported to be an indicator of fetal maturity and can reportedly be used as an indicator of impending parturition.[19, 22]

Sofchek test strips (Environmental Test Systems, Elkhart, IN 46514), Predict-a-Foal Mare Foaling Predictor Kit (Animal Healthcare Products, Vemon, CA 90058),[17] and Titrets Calcium Hardness Test Kit (CHEMetrics, Inc., Calverton, VA 22016)[23] have been compared to determine their capability to predict parturition.[24] Mares were able to be induced with no detrimental effect on the fetus when the results of the tests were as follows: Sofchek—$\geq$ 250 ppm; Titrets—$\geq$ 250 ppm, and Predict-a-Foal—$\geq$ 4-color change. The probability of mares foaling within 24 hours without intervention or induction once the previous concentrations or findings were observed were 79%, 53%, and 59%, respectively. Sofchek was reportedly fairly subjective with the color changes that were not consistent with the manufacturer's standard. The Predict-a-Foal was easier to interpret but had a large variation in results between samples. The Titrets were found to have the least variation. Mares in this study were sampled once daily until the Sofchek indicated the

hardness to be equal to 120 ppm, and then sampling with all tests occurred twice daily.

Although as the mare approaches parturition the cervix is expected to be relaxing, parturition can be induced in a mare with a closed cervix. However, some veterinarians hesitate to induce parturition unless the cervix is dilated 3 to 4 cm because of the concern regarding possible lacerations.[7] All vaginal examinations, pre-partum, partum, or post-partum must be performed properly to avoid contamination of the reproductive tract. This should include tail wrap, tail tie, perineal washing and drying, and the use of a sterile sleeve and sterile lubricant. Although some prefer to do a speculum examination for the determination of the degree of cervical relaxation, the authors prefer to digitally palpate the external os and the lumen of the cervix.

CONTRAINDICATIONS

Contraindications to parturition induction include conditions that indicate that expulsion of the fetus is not possible through a pelvic lumen greatly reduced in size and where a cesarean would be a better approach for delivery. Induction of parturition should never be performed if there is doubt as to the delivery of a viable fetus, which due to the induction procedure may not survive. Any abnormal condition affecting the mare prior to the anticipated induction of parturition should be brought to the attention of the owner, and a decision should be made as to whether to proceed with the induction. Conditions such as increased body temperature, abnormal vulvar discharges, and abnormal presentation of the fetus (e.g., transverse) should influence the decision to induce and may affect the outcome.

METHOD OF INDUCTION

The most commonly utilized agent to induce parturition has been oxytocin by intravenous or intramuscular administration.[3, 5, 7, 10, 25, 26] If the cervix is closed, the administration of estradiol cypionate (4 to 6 mg) or diethylstilbestrol has been used 12 to 24 hours in advance of oxytocin administration to aid in relaxation.[5, 10] Oxytocin also has the capability of inducing cervical relaxation in a mare with a closed or nearly closed cervix. When utilizing oxytocin for cervical relaxation, the best results are obtained when it is administered as a 10-unit dose intravenously every 15 to 30 minutes. Four to six repetitions of administration may be required. If dilatation occurs without delivery, the dosage of oxytocin can be increased to 20 units.

The dosage of oxytocin administered varies with the degree of cervical relaxation. If the cervix is relaxed at least 2 cm internal diameter, it has been recommended by several authors to administer 40 to 60 units of oxytocin as an intravenous bolus. Delivery of the fetus should occur within 90 minutes. In a pluriparous mare the sequence may be more rapid, and stage II is completed within 30 minutes from the time of oxytocin administration. In many practices oxytocin has been traditionally administered intramuscularly[4, 5, 7, 10, 25] or intravenously (by a drip and/or a bolus). Much of the recent literature has reiterated the observation that the mare's response (both in speed and violence) is proportional to the dose of oxytocin given. The higher the dose of oxytocin, the faster will be the delivery of the fetus.[5] Oxytocin was used to induce parturition in six mares within approximately 34 minutes, and all foals were delivered normal and healthy.[25] None of the mares had a retained placenta, and all lactated normally. The dose of oxytocin was 40 or 60 IU.

In mares with at least 2 cm of cervical dilatation and other signs of impending delivery, the administration of 20 IU of oxytocin[22] is followed in approximately 5 to 10 minutes with restlessness and slight colicky pains, which include tail movements and looking at her flank. Within 20 minutes, the mare will exhibit more frequent walking, frequent defecation will be occurring, the tail will be held partially up for long periods of time, frequent urinations will occur, repeated movement from the standing position to the recumbent position will occur, and sweat will appear in the area of the shoulders. These actions will become more pronounced, and the sweating will extend to other areas of the body. The chorioallantoic membrane will rupture approximately 30 minutes following administration of oxytocin. Delivery of the fetus will begin approximately 30 to 60 minutes following administration and will take approximately 30 to 40 minutes. The placenta should be passed within 3 hours or the animal should receive additional oxytocin as a treatment for the retained fetal membranes. Therefore, the authors prefer to administer 20 IU of oxytocin intramuscularly to induce parturition in mares with a minimum of 2 cm dilatation and have not had any of the following reported problems.

Reportedly oxytocin is dangerous for the induction of parturition because it has the capability to induce parturition whether the fetus is mature or not. The response of the mare is to release larger quantities of prostaglandin than occurs during a natural parturition and thus is a pharmacologic not a physiologic induction.[27] Fetal heart rate increases higher with oxytocin induction than with normal delivery,[28] but no association has been made to this observation and a detrimental influence on the fetus. Fetal membrane retention has occurred as an undesirable effect in two of three mares when oxytocin was given by slow intravenous drip for longer than 3 hours.[29] Four of five mares induced with oxytocin produced foals that were weaker than normal, and one had to be "destroyed."[1] Cases of malposition have been reported after induction with oxytocin.[30] It, therefore, has been recommended by some authors to examine the fetus 20 minutes after the administration of oxytocin to determine the fetal position and to correct any malposture or malposition.[7] The authors believe that some of these problems could and do occur in natural deliveries as well as following induction. Some of the side effects associated with induction may be related to dose or intravenous administration of an overdosage.

Initially, prostaglandin $F_{2\alpha}$ reportedly failed to induce parturition in the mare.[31] Prostaglandin $F_{2\alpha}$ can also cause very strong myometrial contractions and may jeopardize foal survival due to early placental separation and fetal weakness.[4, 31–33] Fluprostenol, a prostaglandin $F_{2\alpha}$ analogue, was reportedly capable of inducing parturition in mares.[3, 34] Fluprostenol causes less myometrial stimulation than prostaglandin $F_{2\alpha}$ and, therefore, has been successfully used for induction. Mares with a closed cervix can be induced with fluprostenol at a dose of 1 μg/lb. The time to delivery should be approximately 4 hours.[34, 35] Fluprostenol was administered to 17 ponies, horses, and donkeys to induce parturition in order to determine the correlation of prostaglandin F metabolites to parturition. These metabolites increased and peaked during the maximal expulsive efforts of parturition after injection in mares that delivered within 90 minutes following the injection. If parturition required longer than 90 minutes, the prostaglandin FM increased at various times following the injection and peaked before the maximal expulsive efforts.[36]

Thirty-three mares were induced to foal with prostalene or fenprostalene following prefoaling mammary secretion determination. Tests were performed to determine the content of calcium carbonate or the total hardness of the secretion. Mares were monitored beginning 10 days prior to the expected foaling date, and the secretion was checked daily for 3 days and then twice daily until parturition.[37] Twenty-three mares served as controls and were monitored but not induced. All mares given fenprostalene delivered within 3.9 hours following injection without complications. Seventy-five percent of mares receiving prostalene delivered without difficulty within 3.7 hours, and the remainder delivered within 30 to 56 hours after the injection.

Combinations of fenprostalene (Bovilene TM Syntex Agribusiness, West Capital, Des Moines, IA) followed by oxytocin in 5 i.u. doses at 20-minute intervals has been recommended as a means to reduce the approximate 4-hour time interval following the prostaglandin analogue administration until delivery. The oxytocin is administered 1 hour after the initial injection, and the delivery time is more predictable.[22, 27]

Glucocorticoids have reportedly failed to induce parturition in the mare.[29] Combinations of $PGF_{2\alpha}$ and flumethasone, a synthetic glucocorticoid, has been reported to successfully induce parturition.[38] Dexamethasone, 100 mg at 24-hour intervals until parturition occurs, has been utilized but with less reliability than oxytocin. The average induction time of 4 ± 1.6 days was considered to be undesirable since qualified assistance probably would not be present when required.[39] Since suppression of the immune response is a disadvantage of corticosteroid therapy, it is thought that the use of this substance to induce parturition may be undesirable.[3, 31, 39]

SUMMARY

The mare should have a current tetanus vaccination or should have a booster immediately after induction of parturition if not possible prior to it. It is imperative that following the delivery of the fetus the mare's reproductive tract be examined for the presence of a second fetus or lacerations and to determine the uterine tone.

The assessment of the foal's survival rests with the veterinarian, and even though the history may be inaccurate, one must be certain that the induction will not result in a premature foal being delivered and that sufficient colostrum is available. As described previously, all mares approaching term should be monitored for pelvic and perineal relaxation as well as udder development and milk secretion once or twice a day. Parturition in the mare is very rapid, whether natural or induced. It is, therefore, essential that if a mare is to be induced the veterinarian performing the procedure remain with the mare until parturition is complete and the foal, mare, and placenta, if possible, have been examined. If a fetus is presented with malposture or malposition or has any other problem, the veterinarian should be present to assist. Although foaling problems can and do occur without induction of parturition, induced deliveries may be evaluated more critically and induction be held accountable for unrelated problems. When used only in mares near term at a 20 i.u. dosage administered intravenously, oxytocin has remained the authors' preferred method of induction because of its safety and rapid action.

REFERENCES

1. Jeffcott LB, Rossdale PD: A critical review of current methods for induction of parturition in the mare. *Equine Vet J* 4:308, 1977.
2. Hillman RB, Laser SA: Induction of parturition. *Vet Clin North Am Large Animal Pract* 2:333, 1980.
3. Jeffcott LB, Rossdale PD: A critical review of current methods for induction of parturition in the mare. *Equine Vet J* 9:208, 1977.
4. Hillman RB: Induction of parturition in the mare. In Morrow DA, ed. *Current Therapy in Theriogenology*. Philadelphia, WB Saunders, 1980, p 753.
5. Hillman RB: Induction of parturition in mares. *J Reprod Fertil Suppl* 23:641, 1975.
6. Purvis AD: Oxytocin used to induce a mare to deliver: Elective induction of labor and parturition in the mare. Proceedings of the 18th Annual Convention of American Association Equine Practice, San Francisco, 1972, p 113.
7. Purvis AD: The induction of labor in mares as a routine breeding farm practice. Proceedings of the 23rd Annual Convention of the American Association of Equine Practice Vancouver, 1977, p 145.
8. Bain AM, Howey WP: Observations on the time of foaling in Thoroughbred mares in Australia. *J Reprod Fertil Suppl* 23:545, 1975.
9. Jeffcott LB, Rossdale PD: A critical review of current methods for induction of parturition in the mare. *Equine Vet J* 9:208, 1977.
10. Purvis AD: Elective induction of labor and parturition in the mare. *Proceedings of the American Association of Equine Practice,* San Francisco, 1972, p 113.
11. Roberts SJ: *Veterinary Obstetrics and Genital Diseases*, Vol 46. Ann Arbor, Edwards Brothers, 1971, p 204.
12. Silver M, Fowden AL: Induction of labour in domestic animals: Endocrine changes and neonatal survivability. In Kunzel W, Jensen A, eds. *The Endocrine Control of the Fetus*. Berlin, Springer-Verlag, 1988, p 403.
13. Hillman RB, Laser SA: Induction of parturition. *Vet Clin North Am Large Animal Pract* 2:333, 1988.
14. Neely DP, Liu IKM, Hillman RB: *Equine Reproduction*. Belvidere, Hoffman-LaRoche, 1983, p 80.
15. Ousey JC, Dudan FE, Rossdale PD: Preliminary studies of mammary secretions in the mare to assess fetal readiness for birth. *Equine Vet J* 16:259, 1984.
16. Peaker M, Rossdale PD, Forsyth IA, et al: Changes in mammary development and the composition of secretion during late pregnancy in the mare. *J Reprod Fertil Suppl* 27:555, 1979.
17. Brook D: Evaluation of a new test kit for estimating the foaling time in the mare. *Equine Pract* 9:34, 1987.
18. Cash RSG, Ousey JC, Rossdale PD: Rapid strip test method to assist management of foaling mares. *Equine Vet J* 17:61, 1985.
19. Leadon DP, Jeffcott LB, Rossdale PD: Mammary secretions in normal spontaneous and induced premature parturition in the mare. *Equine Vet J* 16:256, 1984.
20. Ousey JC, Dudan FE, Rossdale PD, et al: Effects of fluprostenol administration in mares during late pregnancy. *Equine Vet J* 16:264, 1984.
21. Ousey JC, Delclaux M, Rossdale PD: Evaluation of three strip tests for measuring electrolytes in mares' prepartum mammary secretions and for predicting parturition. *Equine Vet J* 21:196, 1989.
22. Leadon DP, Jeffcott LB, Rossdale PD, et al: A comparison of agents for inducing parturition in mares in the previable and premature periods of gestation. *J Reprod Fertil Suppl* 32:597, 1982.
23. Ley WB, Hoffman JL, Meacham TN, et al: Daytime management of the mare. 1: Prefoaling mammary secretion testing. *J Equine Vet Sci* 9:88, 1989.
24. Ley WB, Hoffman MS, Crisman MV, et al: Daytime foaling management of the mare. 2: Induction of parturition. *J Equine Vet Sci* 9:95, 1989.
25. Hillman RB, Ganjam VK: Hormonal changes in the mare and foal associated with oxytocin induction of parturition. *J Reprod Fertil Suppl* 27:541, 1979.
26. Pashen RL: Oxytocin—the induction agent of choice in the mare? *J Reprod Fertil Suppl* 32:645, 1982.
27. Pashen RL: Low doses of oxytocin can induce foaling at term. *Equine Vet J* 12:85, 1980.
28. Adams-Brendenmuehl C, Pipers FS: Antipartum evaluation of the equine fetus. *J Reprod Fertil Suppl* 35:565, 1987.
29. Rossdale PD, Jeffcott LB: Problems encountered during induced foaling in pony mares. *Vet Rec* 97:371, 1975.
30. Klug E, von Lepel JD: Uber die Moglichkeit der Gebuntseinleitung beim pferd mit oxytocin. *DTW Dtsch Tierarztl Wochenschn* 81:349, 1974.
31. Alm CC, Sullivan JJ, First NL: The effect of corticosteroid (dexamethasone), progesterone, estrogen, and prostaglandin F2 alpha on gestation length in normal and ovarietomized mares. *J Reprod Fertil Suppl* 23:637, 1975.
32. Bristol F: Induction of parturition in near-term mares by prostaglandin F2 alpha. *J Reprod Fertil Suppl* 32:644, 1982.
33. Townsend HGG, Tabel H, Bristol FM: Induction of parturition in mares: Effect on passive transfer of immunity to foals. *J Am Vet Med Assoc* 182:255, 1983.
34. Rossdale PD, Jeffcott LB, Allen WR: Foaling induced by a synthetic prostaglandin analogue (fluprostenol). *Vet Rec* 99:26, 1976.
35. Allen WR, Pashen RL: The role of prostaglandins during parturition in the mare. *Acta Vet Scan Suppl* 77:279, 1981.
36. Rossdale PD, Pashen RL, Jeffcott LB: The use of synthetic prostaglandin analogue (fluprostenol) to induce foaling. *J Reprod Fertil Suppl* 27:521, 1979.
37. Ley WB, Hoffman MS, Crisman MV, et al: Daytime foaling management of the mare. 2: Induction of parturition. *Equine Vet Sci* 9:95, 1989.
38. van Niekerk CH, Morgenthal JC: Plasma progesterone and estrogen concentrations during induction of parturition with flumethasone and prostaglandin. Proceedings of the 8th International Congress on Animal Reproduction, Vol 3, 1976, p 386.
39. Alm CC, Sullivan JJ, First NL: Induction of premature parturition by parenteral administration of dexamethasone in the mare. *J Am Vet Med Assoc* 165:721, 1974.

15.9

Stallion Functional Disorders

Heidi M. Immegart, DVM, MS, PhD, Dip ACT
Walter R. Threfall, DVM, MS, PhD, Dip ACT

In order for stallions to produce offspring, they must have the capacity to produce fertile ejaculates and the ability to deliver the semen to the mare. If either portion of this system fails, poor conception rates will result. Even when a horse can produce an ejaculate with good fertilizing capability, a number of functional disorders may occur which reduce the potential of the ejaculate being appropriately delivered or collected. Examples such as poor libido, overly aggressive sexual behaviors, and failure to mount, achieve erection, intromission, and ejaculation will be considered in relation to breeding potential.

Libido is defined by *Stedman's Medical Dictionary* as "sexual desire" and is measured in stallions by the behaviors of sexual interest in and desire to copulate with mares in estrus.[1] These behaviors include initial courtship activity with sniffing, Flehman response, and vocalizations as well as mounting and copulatory activity. Erection should occur with the appropriate olfactory, visual, and auditory stimuli followed by intromission and ejaculation. Failure at any point in the progression from sexual arousal to ejaculation may indicate a behavioral or functional problem with the stallion that should be evaluated in order to attempt to correct the situation.

LIBIDO

The intensity of libido in individual stallions can be influenced by genetics, environment, management, sensory input, and previous experience.[2] Low levels of libido have been associated with "novice" breeders, performance animals, horses expected to breed in a new or distracting environment or without appropriate sensory stimulation as well as stallions having experienced a breeding accident or those being "overused" or abused.[3, 4] To evaluate a horse's libido, it is important to provide a clean, comfortable environment with good footing and no distractions. In addition, a source of adequate stimulation is necessary. A cooperative mare in strong behavioral estrus or ovariectomized mares that are administered estradiol cypionate 24 hours prior to exposure can supply the olfactory and visual stimuli for the stallion.[5] Phantoms or mares that are not in heat may not supply adequate stimulation, and uncooperative females may even intimidate certain stallions.

For stallions with low libido, a detailed history is helpful to provide information about training, previous breeding experiences, changes in routine, handling, and onset of the problem.[6] From the history, it is often possible to determine what events contributed to the inappropriate behavior. Inexperienced stallions often express lower libido during their first few breeding encounters.[3, 4] This can be due to the previous administration of severe disciplinary actions for displays of sexual behavior during training and performance.[2] Positive reinforcement from good experiences and appropriate handling are usually adequate to intensify libido expression at future breedings.[4] Hand mating outdoors may aid some shy animals. Pen mating can be used initially to overcome inhibition that may arise from human intervention. Visual cues such as watching other stallions breed or being watched by other stallions can aid the hesitant breeder.[6] Patience with these animals is extremely important in order to overcome the behavioral problems. Stallions that have not had adequate socialization with other horses may also initially have a lack of appropriate libido.[2] Some horses reared in the absence of other horses will inappropriately display sexual interest in humans.[3] This situation is representative of abnormal behavioral patterns and can be dangerous to the person or people involved.

When a stallion has a history of normal breeding behavior followed by a decrease in libido, events surrounding the change in behavior should be elicited. Changes in the handling or handler, the environment, or the breeding routine can inhibit the horse's expression of sexual interest. Similarly, bad breeding experiences involving punishment or trauma can decrease a stallion's interest in breeding.[2-4] In these situations, providing the stallion with positive experiences, proper environment with good handling techniques, and a cooperative teaser mare can help to re-establish confidence. A change in environment may help a stallion with an unpleasant association in the usual breeding place; however, some stallions are inhibited when out of the routine breeding area.

Some stallions display a deficiency of libido when breeding opportunities are presented too frequently.[2] The maximal number of breedings will be different for each stallion; however, overuse depression of libido should be considered when a rigorous breeding schedule is enforced. Overuse decreases in libido can be eliminated by increasing the amount of time between breedings.[2] Overuse of the young stallion may have a more permanent effect than on an older experienced stallion.

Stallions with a libido problem should be examined to determine whether there are deficits in sensory organs (eyes, ear, or nose), abnormalities of the reproductive tract, or points of pain.[3, 4] Problems with these organs could decrease the horse's desire or ability to breed comfortably and thus result in depressed libido. Treatment of physical ailments will frequently be accompanied by a return of libido with positive reinforcement during breeding.[3, 4] An endocrine evaluation could involve the determination of luteinizing hormone, FSH, testosterone, and estradiol concentrations; however, the role of these hormones in the regulation of sexual behavior has not been adequately determined.[7, 8] Injected testosterone as well as estradiol restored libido in treated geldings.[9] The treatment of low libido with androgens or anabolic steroids is not recommended in stallions because these hormones feed back on the hypothalamic-pituitary-gonadal axis and cause suppression of endogenous testosterone production and spermatogenesis. The use of human chorionic gonadotropin will increase testosterone; however, the potential for reducing endogenous FSH release due to androgen feedback may decrease spermatogenesis because of decreased stimulation of Sertoli cell function.[10] The use of GnRH is controversial for improvement of libido. Some reports have indicated that testosterone production or libido are increased whereas others have demonstrated no change.[11–13]

For selected stallions, psychotropic drugs, such as diazepam, have been administered prior to semen collection. Diazepam, 0.05 mg/kg with a maximum dose of 20 mg, can be infused slowly intravenously approximately 10 minutes before breeding in order to help eliminate inhibitions that the horse may experience.[11] These inhibitions may be associated with the novice stallion, with stallions having negative experiences, or with horses being collected with an artificial vagina after extensive natural service. The tricyclic antidepressants, imipramine and clomipramine, may be useful because an increase in sexual motivation has been demonstrated by treated stallions.[11, 14]

Some stallions exhibit excessive aggressive behavior during breeding. This savagery can be directed at the mare or the handler. The behavior is sometimes expressed at each breeding, but it may be intermittent depending on what stimulus triggers the activity. Horses with these tendencies require strict discipline and adequate restraint to ensure the safety of the mare and the handlers. Safety devices such as breeding shields on the mare and a muzzle on the stallion can prevent wounds inflicted through biting. Chain shanks applied over the nose, under the lip, or through the mouth or bridles can be used to direct the stallion's attention away from destructive behavior and toward breeding. Stallions that cannot be adequately restrained and controlled should be gelded or euthanized to prevent injury to humans and other horses. Stallions must be disciplined when unruly contrary to some suggestions that this control may result in the previously described lack of libido in an abused animal.

Aggression can also result from sexual frustration due to the inability to attain full erection or ejaculation with repeated sexual stimulation. In these circumstances, treatment of the underlying problem can eliminate the expression of the undesired behavior.

FAILURE TO ACHIEVE ERECTION

In order for the penis to become erect, psychogenic stimulation as well as neurovascular responses must occur. The process of erection involves increases in arterial blood flow to the penis, relaxation of the cavernous spaces to permit filling with blood, and restricted venous outflow.[15, 16] This is at least partially achieved by contraction of the ischiocavernosus and bulbospongiosus muscles.[17, 18] The exact mechanism that produces this result has not been completely elicited for the horse. Suppressed libido may result in failure to achieve erection; however, some horses with a normal libido do not have complete penile tumescence. Nocturnal observation of the horse at rest for signs of erection and masturbation can help to differentiate whether the horse has the ability to achieve an erection but is inhibited by the surroundings or by the presence of people.[19] Depressed libido was discussed in the previous section. When a good libido is present in the absence of an erection, neurologic or vascular disturbances should be considered for evaluation.

Polyneuritis equi has been reported to cause impotence in a stallion due to damage to the ventral roots of the second and third sacral nerves that contain preganglionic parasympathetic fibers.[20] These nerves are thought to be partially responsible for production of an erection. Damage to the vasculature, including the corpus cavernosum penis from previous trauma or scarring, can prevent normal penile engorgement.[21, 22] Diagnostic aids used to determine the cause of erection failure in men have not been tested in the equine. Similarly, the usual treatment modalities in humans have not been tested for safety or efficacy in horses. Some stallions that cannot achieve full erections can be stimulated to ejaculate into an artificial vagina or a mare with assisted intromission.[6, 21]

FAILURE TO MOUNT/ACHIEVE INTROMISSION

Some stallions that display normal libido and erection have difficulty mounting the mare or achieving intromission. Difficulty or inability to mount or instability while mounted can often be attributed to hind limb or pelvic lameness or ataxia. These stallions may be hesitant to mount or may dismount prematurely. Anti-inflammatory agents, such as phenylbutazone, have been used to decrease pain.[3, 4] When appropriate, the underlying source of pain or instability should be treated. For breeds that allow artificial insemination, collection of semen into an artificial vagina from either the horse mounting a phantom of reduced height or with the stallion standing on all feet can facilitate continued use of the animal as a breeder.[23, 24] For breeds not permitting artificial insemination, selection of shorter cooperative mares or providing elevated footing for the stallion in relation to the mare can alleviate some of the stress and discomfort for the horse.

Penile deviations due to previous trauma such as lacerations, contusions, or scarring can interfere with normal intromission.[22] Massage and directing the penis into the mare or an artificial vagina can be used to achieve the natural service or semen collection, respectively.

FAILURE TO EJACULATE

Ejaculation involves emission of the semen components into the pelvic urethra and expulsion of the ejaculate to the exterior. The process of discharging semen into the urethra is controlled by the sympathetic nervous system. Specifically, it is the stimulation of the α-adrenergic receptors with simultaneous suppression of the β-adrenergic receptors, which leads to normal ejaculation. α-Adrenergic stimulation not only stimulates the smooth muscle of the epididymis and accessory glands to contract and expel their contents but also controls closure of the smooth muscle of the neck of the bladder, preventing urine outflow and retrograde ejaculation.[22, 25, 26] The movement of semen through the urethra is due to contraction of the muscles surrounding the urethra.[26] The paired pudendal nerves of the somatic nervous system are responsible for stimulation of these muscles, which include the ischiocavernosus, bulbospongiosus, urethralis, and other striated muscles of the pelvis. Stimulation for ejaculation is dependent on afferent sensory input primarily from the dorsal nerve of the penis. This nerve carries impulses from the genital region during copulation.

Copulatory activity without subsequent ejaculation is a relatively common problem in stallions. The presence of the disorder may be undetected in some horses under natural service conditions, because tail flagging and urethral pulsations can be present in some affected animals.[6, 22] This condition is often associated with normal or increased intensity of libido. The lack of ejaculation can be intermittent or delayed with several mounting and thrusting episodes preceding ejaculation, or it can be continuous with a complete lack of ejaculation. These stallions can become fatigued or frustrated following repeated attempts at copulation without ejaculation.[27] Frustration may be evidenced by behavioral changes such as aggression or loss of sexual interest.

Ejaculatory failure can be caused by any dysfunction in the normal control of semen emission and expulsion. Psychogenic inhibition can occur when stallions have been abused or have had previous breeding accidents at or near the time of ejaculation.[25] Stallions that are taken to a new environment or that have been overused may also exhibit ejaculatory failure. These horses should be treated similarly to horses with low libido; that is, expose the horses to positive experiences or, in the case of overuse, by a decrease in breeding activity.

Organic causes of ejaculatory failure include a lack of stimulation of the glans penis during coitus, damage to the innervation of the penis, pneumovagina of the mare, or lack of adequate erection or thrusting by the stallion.[28] Decreased sensation to the glans may be overcome by an increased temperature and pressure of water in the artificial vagina and increased pressure on the base of the penis during semen collection.[21, 29] Ejaculatory failure was also reported for two stallions with aortic-iliac thrombosis.[30, 31] Both stallions benefitted from an exercise program to increase hind limb strength.

Other problems can involve the lack of sympathetic nervous stimulation or antagonistic parasympathetic stimulation of emission or expulsion. Pharmacologic manipulation of stallions affected in this fashion can be of value.[27] Treatment consists of using α-adrenergic agonists with β-adrenergic antagonists or anticholinergics. L-norepinephrine (a potent alpha stimulator), 0.01 mg/kg intramuscularly, 15 minutes prior to and carazolol (a β-blocker), 0.015 mg/kg, 10 minutes before breeding have been used to correct ejaculatory dysfunction in several stallions.[32] Carazolol has been reported to be of value but is not available in the United States. These treatments should not be used in horses with chronic obstructive pulmonary disease because of the potential to cause bronchoconstriction. The tricyclic antidepressants imipramine and clomipramine have been used in horses with ejaculatory dysfunction to produce erection, masturbation, and even ejaculation.[6, 25] The activity of these drugs is thought to be due to alpha and possibly anticholinergic activity.

Some horses exhibit sexual satiety following apparent lack of ejaculation or ejaculation of fluid without spermatozoa. This can potentially occur when there is an obstruction to emission of spermatozoa into the pelvic urethra, when semen is ejaculated retrograde into the bladder, or when no spermatozoa are being produced by the testes. Although retrograde ejaculation has not been documented in horses, it is recognized in other species and can be detected by the presence of sperm in the contents of the bladder post-breeding.[26]

Spermatozoal obstruction can occur when there is an abnormal accumulation of sperm in the ductus deferens, ampulla, or epididymis.[33] Frequent ejaculation with massage of the ampulla via transrectal palpation can help to dissolve the occlusion. Regularly scheduled ejaculation should occur following return to normal ejaculated semen quality and to prevent re-obstruction.[34] Prostaglandins and oxytocin have not been successful at alleviating blockage of the ejaculatory ducts, and one study concluded that $PGF_{2\alpha}$ made stallions unsafe due to muscle weakness after injection.[4, 25, 34] When no blockage is present and there is continued azoospermia, the lack of spermatozoal production by the testes can be detected by examining a biopsy of the testes.[35, 36] When testicular causes for azoospermia are present, it is necessary to treat the underlying cause of decreased spermatogenesis, if possible.

Masturbation has been considered by some to be a behavioral problem that is dysfunctional in breeding stallions. This behavior in stallions has been studied, and it was not accompanied by ejaculation. Thus, it does not decrease available sperm stores for actual breeding. Masturbation is also a normal behavior of stallions at rest and can be used to distinguish between organic and psychogenic causes of erection failure.[19, 37]

REFERENCES

1. Basmajian JV, Burke MD, Burnett GW, et al: *Stedman's Medical Dictionary*, ed 24. Baltimore, Waverly Press, 1982, p 783.
2. Roberts SJ: Infertility in male animals (andrology). *In* Roberts SJ, ed. *Veterinary Obstetrics and Genital Diseases (Theriogenology)*, ed 3. Ann Arbor, Edwards Brothers, 1986, p 752.
3. McDonnell SM: Normal and abnormal sexual behavior. *Vet Clin North Am Equine Pract* 8:71, 1992.
4. McDonnell S: Reproductive behavior of the stallion. *Vet Clin North Am Equine Pract* 2:535, 1986.
5. Voss JL, Wotowey JL: Hemospermia. Proceedings of the Annual Meeting of the American Association of Equine Practice, Vol 18, 1972, p 103.
6. Pickett BW, Voss JL, Squires IL: Impotence and abnormal sexual behavior in the stallion. *Therio* 8:329, 1977.
7. Irvine CHG, Alexander SL, Hughes JP: Sexual behavior and serum concentrations of reproductive hormones in normal stallions. *Therio* 23:607, 1985.
8. Burns PJ, Douglas RH: Reproductive hormone concentrations in stallions with breeding problems: Case studies. *Equine Vet Sci* 5:40, 1985.
9. Thompson DL, Pickett BW, Squiers EL, et al: Sexual behavior, seminal pH and accessory sex gland weights in geldings administered testosterone and(or) estradiol-17 beta. *J Anim Sci* 51:1358, 1980.
10. Amman RP: Effects of drugs or toxins on spermatogenesis. In McKinnon AO, Voss JL, eds. *Equine Reproduction*. Philadelphia, Lea & Febiger, 1993, p 831.
11. McDonnell SM, Garcia MC, Kenney RM: Pharmacological manipulation of sexual behaviour in stallions. *J Reprod Fertil Suppl* 35:45, 1987.
12. Montovan SM, Daels PP, Rivier J, et al: The effect of a potent GnRH agonist on gonadal and sexual activity in the horse. *Therio* 33:1305, 1990.
13. Pozor MA, McDonnell SM, Kenney RM, et al: GnRH facilitates copulatory behaviour in geldings treated with testosterone. *J Reprod Fertil Suppl* 44:666, 1991.
14. McDonnell SM, Garcia MC, Kenney RM: Imipramine-induced

15. Bartels JE, Beckett SD, Brown BG: Angiography of the corpus cavernosum penis in the pony stallion during erection and quiescence. *Am J Vet Res* 45:1464, 1984.
16. Lue TF, Tanagho EA: Physiology of erection and pharmacological management of impotence. *J Urol* 137:829, 1987.
17. Beckett SD, Hudson RS, Walker DF, et al: Blood pressures and penile muscle activity in the stallion during coitus. *Am J Physiol* 225:1072, 1973.
18. Beckett SD, Walder DF, Hudson RS, et al: Corpus spongiosum penis pressure and penile muscle activity in the stallion during coitus. *Am J Vet Res* 36:431, 1975.
19. Wilcox S, Dusza K, Houpt K: The relationship between recumbent rest and masturbation in stallions. *Equine Vet Sci* 11:23, 1991.
20. Held JP, Vanhooser S, Prater P, et al: Impotence in a stallion with neuritis cauda equina: A case report. *Equine Vet Sci* 9:67, 1989.
21. Love CC, McDonnell SM, Kenney RM: Manually assisted ejaculation in a stallion with erectile dysfunction subsequent to paraphimosis. *J Am Vet Med Assoc* 200:1357, 1992.
22. Varner DD, Schumacher J, Blanchard TL, et al: Sexual behavior dysfunction. In Varner DD, Schumacher J, Blanchard TL, et al, eds: *Diseases and Management of Breeding Stallions*, Goleta, American Veterinary Punblications, 1991, p 159.
23. McDonnell SM, Love CC: Manual stimulation collection of semen from stallions: Training time, sexual behavior and semen. *Therio* 33:1201, 1990.
24. Crump J, Crump J: Stallions ejaculation induced by manual stimulation of the penis. *Therio* 31:341, 1989.
25. McDonnell SM: Ejaculation physiology and dysfunction. *Vet Clin North Am* 8:57, 1992.
26. Thomas AJ: Ejaculatory dysfunction. *Fertil Steril* 39:445, 1983.
27. Klug E, Deegen E, Lazarz B, et al: Effect of adrenergic neurotransmitters upon the ejaculatory process in the stallion. *J Reprod Fertil Suppl* 32:31, 1982.
28. Rasbech NO: Ejaculatory disorders of the stallion. *J Reprod Fertil Suppl* 23:123, 1975.
29. Tischner M, Kosiniak K, Bielanski W: Analysis of the pattern of ejaculation in stallions. *J Reprod Fertil* 41:329, 1974.
30. McDonnell SM, Love CC, Martin BB, et al: Ejaculatory failure associated with aortic-iliac thrombosis in two stallions. *J Am Vet Med Assoc* 200:954, 1992.
31. McDonnell SM, Love CC: Xylazine-induced ejaculation in stallions. *Therio* 36:73, 1991.
32. Klug E. Ejaculatory failure. In Robinson NE, ed. *Current Therapy in Equine Medicine 2*. Philadelphia, WB Saunders, 1987, p 562.
33. Varner DD, Schumacher J, Blanchard TL, et al: Diseases of the epididymis. In Varner DD, Schumcher J, Blanchard TL, et al, eds. *Diseases and Management of Breeding Stallions*. Goleta, Calif, American Veterinary Publications, 1991, p 233.
34. McDonnell SM: Pharmacologic manipulation of sexual behavior. In McKinnon AO, Voss JL, eds. *Equine Reproduction*, Philadelphia, Lea & Febiger, 1993, p 825.
35. Threlfall WR, Lopate C: Testicular biopsy. In McKinnon AO, Voss JL, eds. *Equine Reproduction*. Philadelphia, Lea & Febiger, 1993, p 943.
36. Threlfall WR, Lopate C: Testicular biopsy. *Therio* 65, 1987.
37. Tischner M: Patterns of stallions sexual behaviour in the absence of mares. *J Reprod Fertil Suppl* 32:65, 1982.

15.10

Semen Abnormalities

Heidi M. Immegart, DVM, MS, PhD, Dip ACT
Walter R. Threlfall, DVM, MS, PhD, Dip ACT

Normal ejaculation occurs in fractions that can be associated with the products of specific reproductive organs.[1] The pre-ejaculatory fraction consists mainly of the secretory products of the bulbourethral gland. The sperm-rich fraction consists of the products of the epididymis, ductus deferens, ampulla, and prostate as well as the spermatozoa. The third fraction, or gel, is mainly the product of the vesicular glands. During normal ejaculation, smooth muscle contractions synchronously cause emission of these seminal components into the pelvic urethra for expulsion, and they maintain bladder sphincter closure. Abnormalities of the different ductular and glandular portion of the urogenital tract as well as the testes can have adverse effects on the semen and its fertilizing capacity.

HEMOSPERMIA

Hemospermia is the presence of blood in the ejaculate. This is usually apparent grossly as a pink to red discoloration of the semen or as red blood cells present in the ejaculate at the time of semen evaluation.[2, 3] Blood draining from the mares vulva following natural service can also be an indication of this problem.[4] Blood in the ejaculate decreases the fertilizing capacity of the spermatozoa. Stallions that have blood in every ejaculate tend to be infertile[5]; however, when bleeding is intermittent, the unaffected ejaculates may have normal fertility.[4] Some stallions will have an associated pain reaction when ejaculating a hemospermic sample.[5] It has been determined that the presence of red blood cells and not blood serum is responsible for hindering fertility.[4, 5]

There are many causes of hemospermia, and it can occur at any point in a horse's breeding career. Causes for hemospermia are urethritis, lacerations, or lesions of the urethra or external penis, glans, and urethral process, and cutaneous habronemiasis around the glans and urethral process.[4] Hemospermia has also been associated with inflammation or infection of the seminal vesicles and ampulla as well as the epididymitis or epididymal sperm granulomas. Protrusion of blood vessels into the urethra due to increased compression from stallion rings can result in contamination of the semen with blood.[2] Trauma to the penis during intromission can cause hemospermia.[2, 6] This could be caused by a rupture of tissue surrounding the corpus spongiosum penis, which is responsible for the creation of pressures in excess of 600 mm Hg during coitus.[7]

Diagnosis of the cause of hemospermia first involves an examination of the external portions of the penis and glans for lacerations or other lesions. Lacerations of the penis or prepuce can be caused by the tail hairs of the mare or breeding stitches as well as improper artificial vagina placement and self-injury from kicking. Other lesions, such as habronemiasis and other proliferative processes, can be traumatized and bleed during breeding or semen collection.[4] Examination of the urethra for evidence of urethral lesions can be performed with a flexible fiberoptic endoscope through which direct visualization of the entire urethra is possible.[4] Lesions may appear as plaques, rents, lacerations, inflammatory sites, ulcerations or growths, and also as strictures, prolapsed subepithelial vessels, and varicosities.[2, 8] Most lesions appear as inflammatory processes or varicosities and are located in the pelvic urethra. In some cases multiple lesions occur in both the penile and pelvic urethra.[2, 8] Urethral cultures may reveal the presence of potentially pathogenic organisms. In some cases, *Pseudomonas aeruginosa*, *Streptococcus* sp., and *E. coli* have been cultured from the urethra. Urethral cytologic examination can be used to detect viral inclusion bodies; however, this technique has not been highly successful. Strictures can be viewed on endoscopic examination, but contrast urethrograms have also been useful to detect the presence and location of one or more strictures in the urethra.[2]

Treatment for hemospermia has inconsistent results in returning the stallion to normal (prehemospermic) fertility. Sexual rest has resulted in some horses recovering and having no blood in the ejaculate.[8] Many of these apparently recovered horses will start to ejaculate blood when used again in a breeding program. Treatment of stallions with positive cultures has been controversial due to the low probability of the antibiotic penetrating adequately into the site of infection. Urinary acidifiers, in conjunction with oral methenamine (10 g/day), have also been administered to some stallions without a recurrence of hemospermia during treatment.[2] One stallion was treated in this manner for 2 years. Both formalin and furosemide have been used and have resulted in a decrease in blood in the ejaculate.[2, 6] When treatment was discontinued, however, the blood was apparent again in the semen. Surgical intervention to release strictures or to open the urethra for local treatment have been successful in some horses. Unfortunately, many horses fail to respond to any treatment. Unilateral castration may be appropriate for cases of chronic unilateral epididymitis or sperm granuloma. See Chapter 15.12 for descriptions of these disease processes and their diagnosis.

UROSPERMIA

Urospermia is the presence of urine in the ejaculate. Usually this is grossly apparent as a distinct yellowish color or urine-like odor to the ejaculate. This condition, however, may frequently be unrecognized since urine contamination cannot always be detected visibly.[9] The presence of urine in the ejaculate has detrimental effects on spermatozoal motility and conception rates from such ejaculates.[9] This is thought to be caused by an adverse pH and osmolarity as well as by some undetermined factors.[10]

The causes of urospermia are not completely understood. One cause of urospermia may be due to stimulation of bladder contraction simultaneously with stimulation of ejaculation via the hypogastric nerve. The hypogastric nerve is thought to be responsible for ejaculation; however, under some circumstances, stimulation of this nerve also causes bladder contraction.[9] Thus, urination occurs simultaneously with ejaculation. Another possible cause is a lack of adequate smooth muscle contraction of the neck of the bladder.[10, 11] This is a function of α-adrenergic stimulation and has been associated with retrograde ejaculation in other species. Although retrograde ejaculation has not been documented in horses, it is possible that some urine could be voided into the ejaculate through an open bladder sphincter.

In general, most horses do not have urine in each ejaculate; however, it can be a random occurrence.[9] This may be attributable to the degree of bladder distention at the time of ejaculation, when less or no urine might be voided soon after micturition.

For situations in which urospermia is suspected but not supported by gross changes in the ejaculate color, odor, or volume, azostix and multistyx have been found to be accurate for the detection of urine contamination.[12] Modifications for appropriate use of each test were found to prevent most false-positive results and negative results. The azostix pad should be examined only after 10 seconds have elapsed, then rinsed with distilled water and read. A green color to the pad indicates urine as measured by urea nitrogen. The multistix test strip should be placed horizontally for 3.5 minutes before reading. An orange color to the nitrogen pad is indicative of the presence of urine. It has been recommended that a laboratory test for creatinine or urea nitrogen in the ejaculate should be performed when the test strips indicate the presence of urine.[12]

Treatment for urospermia has mainly involved the practice of inducing urination prior to semen collection or breeding or waiting until the horse urinates spontaneously.[13] This may not be a convenient measure on some breeding farms. The use of pharmacologic agents such as an α-adrenergic stimulator have been used to prevent retrograde ejaculation in humans; however, the use of these agents needs to be tested for efficacy in the stallion.[14]

IMMUNE INFERTILITY

Spermatozoa develop in an immunologically privileged and protected space within the seminiferous tubules. Under normal conditions, the blood testis barrier prevents interaction between immune cells and developing germ cells. The leukocytes present in the testicular interstitium consist of macrophages and around the tubules of the rete consist mainly of suppressor T cells.[15, 16] Thus, haploid cells that are "foreign" to the body do not trigger a large immune response to their presence. It is possible, however, for the blood-testis barrier to be breached in some situations of trauma or granuloma formation and spermatozoa to be extravasated into tissues and exposed to immune cells. When this occurs, there is the potential for antibody formation against the antigens present on the haploid germ cells. If these antibodies are present in the ejaculate, they can bind to spermatozoa and alter the fertilizing capacity of these cells by inhibiting normal motility or normal membrane changes that occur during capacitation and the acrosome reaction. Not all antibodies, however, alter fertility because they may bind to sites on the sperm that do not inhibit normal function.[17–19]

Most of the knowledge in the area of immune-mediated

infertility applies to humans; however, two reports of possible immune-mediated infertility have been reported in stallions.[20, 21] Both horses had experienced testicular trauma after which spermatozoal motility was virtually absent. Sperm-immobilizing assays were performed to detect the presence of antibodies in the seminal plasma. Both horses responded to corticosteroid treatment with increases in spermatozoal motility and decreases in spermatozoal immobilization.

Relatively little is known about infertility due to an immune response to spermatozoa in horses. This should be considered in cases in which the potential for extravasation of germ cells is present and other more common causes of reduced fertility are not apparent.

INFECTIOUS AGENTS AND INFLAMMATORY PRODUCTS

It has long been recognized that venereal transmission of disease occurs at breeding and can affect fertility. This is not only due to the presence of the organisms on the contacting surfaces of the genitalia of the mare and stallion but also to the presence of pathogenic organisms in the semen. Because no physical contact is necessary for the transmission of these organisms from the stallion to the mare, breeders using artificial insemination programs as well as those using natural service need to be aware of this possibility.

Both bacteria and viral agents have been transmitted via the semen from apparently normal stallions that do not display outward signs of disease. Bacterial agents include *Pseudomonas* sp., *Klebsiella* sp., and *Streptococcus* sp.[6, 22] The presence of these organisms in the ejaculate can cause either conception failure or early embryonic death with or without concomitant endometritis in mares.[23–25] It has also been demonstrated that addition of bacterial products to equine semen samples significantly reduces spermatozoal motility.[25] *Pseudomonas* sp. are ubiquitous and can establish an inappropriate colonization of the reproductive organs when commensal organisms are reduced or during debility.[26] It is unknown how many locations these bacteria can be harbored in the internal reproductive tract; however, they have been cultured from the seminal vesicles and the urethra of stallions.[27] Contamination of an ejaculated sample can occur, also, due to poor management of the artificial vagina, inadequate penile washing, and careless handling of ejaculate. For cases in which the stallion is shedding bacteria, treatment of the horse has previously resulted in a low probability of success.[23, 24, 27] It is best to treat the semen by dilution with an extender containing an antibiotic to which the bacteria are sensitive.[24] For natural service, it is best to infuse the mare's uterus with the same extender immediately prior to breeding. Cultures of the extended ejaculate, 20 to 30 minutes following extension, can indicate if the antibiotic is working appropriately.[24]

Viral pathogens can also be excreted in the ejaculate and cause infertility or disease in mares. The best known example is equine arteritis virus (EVA). Upon the initial infection, edema may be present around the eyes, genitalia, and limbs; however, stallions that appear to have recovered will shed the organism in the ejaculate.[28] Shedding of the virus into the ejaculate can last up to several years following exposure.[28–31] Serum titers for EVA can be used to detect exposure; how-

ever, semen viral isolation is necessary to determine the status of ejaculatory contamination.[32] Ejaculates containing EVA have the potential to infect and cause disease symptoms in mares that do not have immunity to this virus through previous exposure or vaccination.[31, 33] The virus can survive during cooling and freezing processes and thus can still be a problem with shipped or cryopreserved semen samples.[30, 32] The occurrence of clinical signs compatible with EVA in mares bred to a stallion indicates that an evaluation of EVA titers and semen viral isolation are necessary. A modified live vaccine has been tested in stallions with no detectable passage of virus in the ejaculate and no titer formation in the mares that were subsequently bred.[34] Due to the restrictions on the transport of horses with titers to EVA into some countries, vaccination may not be the best option for some breeding animals.

REFERENCES

1. Varner DD, Schumacher J, Blanchard TL, et al: Reproductive anatomy and physiology. In Varner DD, Schumacher J, Blanchard TL, et al, eds: *Diseases and Management of Breeding Stallions*. Goleta, American Vet, 1991, p 1.
2. Voss JL, Pickett BW: Diagnosis and treatment of hemospermia in the stallion. *J Reprod Fertil Suppl* 23:151, 1975.
3. Voss JL, Wotowey JL: Hemospermia. Proceedings of the Annual Meeting of the American Association of Equine Practice, 1972, Vol 18, p 103.
4. McKinnon AO, Voss JL, Trotter GW, et al: Hemospermia of the stallion. *Equine Pract* 10:17, 1988.
5. Voss JL, Pickett BW, Shideler RK: The effect of hemospermia on fertility in horses. *Proc Int Cong Anim Reprod Artif Insem* 8:1093, 1976.
6. Scoggins RD: Hemaspermia: A case report. *Equine Vet Sci* 9:176, 1989.
7. Beckett D, Walder DF, Hudson RS, et al: Corpus spongiosum penis pressure and penile muscle activity in the stallion during coitus. *Am J Vet Res* 36:431, 1975.
8. Sullins KE, Berone JJ, Voss JL, et al: Treatment of hemospermia in stallions: A discussion of 18 cases. *Compend Contin Educ Pract Vet* 10:1396, 1988.
9. Nash JG, Voss JL, Squires EL: Urination during ejaculation in a stallion. *J Am Vet Med Assoc* 176:224, 1980.
10. Makler A, David R, Blumenfeld Z, et al: Factors affecting sperm motility. VII: Sperm viability as affected by change of pH and osmolarity of semen and urine specimens. *Fertil Steril* 36:507, 1981.
11. Beckett SD, Walder DR, Hudson RS, et al: Corpus spongiosum penis pressure and penile muscle activity in the stallion during coitus. *Am J Vet Res* 36:431, 1975.
12. Althouse GC, Seager SWJ, Varner DD, et al: Diagnostic aids for the detection of urine in the equine ejaculate. *Therio* 31:1141, 1989.
13. Varner DD, Schumacher J, Blanchard TL, et al: Diseases affecting semen. In Varner DD, Schumacher J, Blanchard TL, et al, eds. *Diseases and Management of Breeding Stallions*. Goleta, American Vet, 1991, p 335.
14. Kaufman DG, Nagler AM: Specific nonsurgical therapy in male infertility. *Urol Clin North Am* 14:489, 1987.
15. Barratt CLR, Bolton AE, Cooke ID: Functional significance of white blood cells in the male and female reproductive tract. *Hum Reprod* 5:639, 1990.
16. Russell LD, Ettlin RA, Sinha Hikim AP, et al: Mammalian spermatogenesis. In Russell LD, Ettlin RA, Sinha Hikim AP,

et al, eds. *Histological and Gistopathological Evaluation of the Testis.* Clearwater, Cache River Press, 1990, p 1.

17. Zouari R, De Almeida M, Feneux D: Effect of sperm-associated antibodies on the dynamics of sperm movement and on the acrosome reaction of human spermatozoa. *J Reprod Immunol* 22:59, 1992.

18. Cross NL, Moore S: Regional binding of human anti-sperm antibodies assessed by indirect immunofluorescence. *Hum Reprod* 5:47, 1990.

19. De Almeida M, Zouari R, Jouannet P, et al: In-vitro effects of anti-sperm antibodies on human sperm movement. *Hum Reprod* 6:405, 1991.

20. Zhang J, Ricketts SW, Tanner SJ: Antisperm antibodies in the semen of a stallion following testicular trauma. *Equine Vet J* 22:138, 1990.

21. Papa FO, Alvarenga MA, Lopes MD, et al: Infertility of autoimmune origin in a stallion. *Equine Vet J* 22:145, 1990.

22. Cooper WL: Methods of determining the site of bacterial infections in the stallion reproductive tract. *Therio* 1, 1979.

23. Hughes JP, Asbury AC, Loy RG, et al: The occurrence of *Pseudomonas* in the genital tract of stallions and its effects on fertility. *Cornell Vet* 57:53, 1967.

24. Blanchard TL, Varner DD, Love CC, et al: Use of a semen extender containing antibiotic to improve the fertility of a stallion with seminal vesiculitis due to *Pseudomonas aeruginosa. Therio* 28:541, 1987.

25. Rideout MI, Burns SJ, Simpson RB: Influence of bacterial products on the motility of stallion spermatozoa. *J Reprod Fertil Suppl* 32:35, 1982.

26. Bowen JM, Tobin N, Simpson RB, et al: Effects of washing on the bacterial flora of the stallion's penis. *J Reprod Fertil Suppl* 32:41, 1982.

27. Balnchard TL, Varner DD, Hurtgen JP, et al: Bilateral seminal vesiculitis and ampullitis in a stallion. *J Am Vet Med Assoc* 192:525, 1988.

28. Timoney PJ, McCollum WH: Equine viral arteritis. *Can Vet J* 28:693, 1987.

29. Timoney PJ, McCollum WH, Murphy TW, et al: The carrier state in equine arteritis virus infection in the stallion with specific emphasis on the venereal mode of virus transmission. *J Reprod Fertil Suppl* 35:95, 1987.

30. Neu SM, Timoney PJ, McCollum WH: Persistent infection of the reproductive tract in stallions experimentally infected with equine arteritis virus. *Proc Int Conf Equine Infect Dis* 5:149, 1988.

31. Timoney PJ, McCollum WH, Robers AW: Detection of the carrier state in stallions persistently infected with equine arteritis virus. Proceedings of the Annual Meeting of the American Association of Equine Practice, 1986, Vol 32, p 57.

32. Little TV, McCollum WH, Timoney PJ: Persistent equine arteritis virus infection in the stallion. *Therio* 151, 1991.

33. McCollum WH, Timoney PJ, Roberts AW, et al: Response of vaccinated and non-vaccinated mares to artificial insemination with semen from stallions persistently infected with equine arteritis virus. *Proc Int Conf Equine Infect Dis* 5:13, 1988.

34. Timoney PJ, Umphenour NW, McCollum WH: Safety evaluation of a commercial modified live equine arteritis virus vaccine for use in stallions. *Proc Int Conf Equine Infect Dis* 5:19, 1988.

15.11

Accidents of Breeding

Heidi M. Immegart, DVM, MS, PhD, Dip ACT
Walter R. Threlfall, DVM, MS, PhD, Dip ACT

Natural service involves the physical contact of the mare and the stallion in which either animal may incur injuries. Adequate restraint of both horses and the use of protective devices can help to minimize some of the potential risk involved.

Some of the injuries inflicted on the mare include lacerations and contusions of the trunk and neck from the stallion during mounting. Stallions that are shod should have protective boots placed on their feet to decrease the likelihood of lacerations. Breeding capes should be used to protect the mare from stallions that tend to bite excessively while mounted. These capes can also be useful as a better grip for stallions to stabilize themselves than by grasping the mare's neck with their teeth. Lacerations or contusions of the head of the mare should be prevented by adequate training of the stallion in mounting technique and controlled handling.

Injuries inflicted during intromission can include vaginal, cervical, and rectal lacerations.[1] Vaginal and cervical lacerations occur when the penile length of the stallion exceeds the expandable space of the vagina and thrusting by the stallion tears the cranial vaginal wall or cervix. Blood on the stallion's penis or blood coming from the mare's vulva following breeding are indications that this may have occurred. A vaginal examination will confirm the diagnosis. Peritonitis will occur if the laceration perforates the peritoneum due to the presence of the ejaculate and bacteria in the peritoneal cavity. Treatment should be geared toward minimizing this outcome by use of appropriate antibiotics and anti-inflammatory agents. The vaginal wall will heal without suture; however, the mare should be kept quiet with minimal abdominal exertions for 3 to 5 days.

These lacerations can be avoided by utilizing a breeding roll to prevent complete penetration of the penis of the stallion. This device should be used when a small mare is being bred to a large stallion or to a stallion with a large penis.

Inappropriate intromission into the rectum can result in tears of the rectal wall. Rectal intromission has been reportedly associated with the use of novice stallions as well as pre-breeding transrectal palpations. Following the palpation procedure, the anal sphincter may be more relaxed and more readily penetrated by the stallion's penis. Rectal tearing should be suspected if the stallion has blood on his penis and the mare has blood coming from the rectum following service. These injuries constitute life-threatening emergencies and should be treated immediately as should any case of rectal laceration. This situation can be avoided by assisting entry of the stallion's penis into the vestibule and not permitting natural service for approximately 3 hours after a transrectal examination.

Injuries to the mare may also result from the use of certain breeding restraint techniques. Breeding hobbles are frequently used to protect the stallion from kicks; however, situations where stallions become entangled in the straps can result in disaster. Appropriate timing for breeding can eliminate the potential for kicking by some mares. The authors prefer to use a twitch and moderate tranquilization with xylazine and acepromazine for restraining the less than cooperative mare that cannot be artificially inseminated. The use of breeding stocks or gates in front of the mare should never be recommended because this can also result in injuries. Mares that cannot move forward when mounted are more likely to have vaginal tearing during forceful intromission.

Vulvar lacerations can occur during breeding when a Caslick suture does not allow adequate space for penile penetration. The use of breeding stitches can help prevent this, or the Caslick surgical repair can be opened prior to breeding.

Rupture of the remnant of the hymen may occur in maiden mares during breeding. Blood may be seen on the stallion's penis and coming from the mare's vulva following service. A vaginal examination should be used to differentiate this injury from a vaginal laceration. On occasion, young mares will associate the pain of the first breeding, when hymen remnant tissue was torn, to future situations and may be less than cooperative. Manual breakdown of the hymen 2 weeks prior to (but not immediately before) a natural service can prevent this problem.

Injuries to the stallion can include kicks to the penis, prepuce, scrotum, inguinal area, legs, or body by an inadequately restrained mare. Such injuries to the reproductive organs are covered in Chapter 15.9 on reproductive tract abnormalities in stallions. Rupture of the tunica albuginea of the penis may also occur if the mare makes a sudden lateral movement during copulation. Poor footing in the breeding or semen collection area can result in instability during mounting. The stallion is more likely to slip or fall during mounting, which can result in injury. Stallions that have negative experiences like this may be reluctant to breed after that experience. Breeding hobbles used on the mare may cause injury to the stallion if his legs become entangled. The mare's tail should be diverted to the side to prevent the hair from lacerating the stallion's penis or prepuce. If a tail-rope is tied around the mare's neck, it should be tied with a quick-release knot. This allows rapid release and prevents a situation in which the stallion's leg is caught during breeding or dismounting.

REFERENCE

1. Williams WL: *Diseases of the Genital Organs of Animals.* Ithaca, Press of Andrus and Church, 1921, p 210.

15.12

Stallion Reproductive Tract Neoplasms

Walter R. Threlfall, DVM, MS, PhD, Dip ACT
Heidi M. Immegart, DVM, MS, PhD, Dip ACT

PENIS AND PREPUCIAL TUMORS

Penal and prepucial neoplasms occur infrequently in the stallion and can be observed as variable appearing lesions. The size and the location of the lesion will vary due to cause and duration. Since the origin of the covering tissue of the penis and prepuce is common to the remainder of the skin, it is possible to have neoplasms with a variety of cell origins affecting the prepuce. The most frequently encountered neoplasm of the penis and prepuce is squamous cell carcinoma.[1–7] Another tumor that has been reported to affect this area is the fibrosarcoma.[8] Other tumors include angiomas, hemangioma, mastocytoma, sarcoids, melanomas, and papillomas. Sarcoids involving the skin of horses are common, but they involve the penis and prepuce less frequently. The most common differential considerations from tumors are the granulomatous reactions that accompany Habromena megastoma larva migrating through this area (cutaneous habronemiasis—summer sores) or the granulomatous reaction after trauma to the area. The diagnosis of habronemiasis is best made after histologic encysted larvae or a large number of eosinophils infiltrating the area.

Although early in the developmental process of the squamous cell carcinoma the only indication may be a loss of pigment,[9] squamous cell carcinoma lesions usually become ulcerated and may be malodorous. However, these lesions occur at a later stage of development and are not present initially. The squamous cell carcinoma is a slow-growing tumor that may eventually metastasize to the regional lymph nodes and the lungs. The lymph nodes may ulcerate, and the presence of cellulitis and edema will be present in the area of the penis and prepuce. The definitive diagnosis of squamous cell carcinoma should be based on histopathologic conformation of a tissue sample taken when the tumor was removed. Lesions of the glans penis may be multiple and can involve the majority of the glans and surrounding tissue.[10, 11] Stallions have a lower incidence of neoplasia than do geldings, and a lack of pigment on the penis and prepuce has been associated with increases in the occurrence of tumors.[4, 11]

Treatment

The method utilized to treat the condition is based primarily on the size of the lesion and on the use of the animal. The treatment may include local removal of the lesion, amputation of the penis, or euthanasia in cases that have progressed to severe regional lymph node involvement, ulceration, and edema. Successful use of 5-fluorouracil on small lesions has been reported.[12] The lesion may be removed with a scalpel being certain to incorporate a normal-appearing border around the lesion to help ensure that the lesion does not reappear at the site. If possible, it is recommended to have the tissue edges of the excised tissue examined for the absence of abnormal cells. Small lesions can easily be removed with sedation and local anesthesia with the horse in the standing position.[13] Cryosurgery has also been recommended for the removal of squamous cell carcinomas from the penis and prepuce. Cryosurgery has certain advantages, such as absence of bleeding and suturing, but has the disadvantages of delayed healing, loss of large areas of covering tissue due to sloughing following the freezing of the lesion, and potential damage to the urethra if the freezing of tissue penetrates too deeply.[14-16] As the lesion increases in size, it may be necessary to perform a reefing operation on the penis or prepuce; a circumscribed area encircling the penis is completely removed and the remaining normal tissue is reapposed and sutured. When severe lesions exist only on the glans penis, it has been recommended that the glans be removed utilizing a surgical procedure called Vinsot's. This procedure is apparently not advisable in breeding stallions owing to stricture formation and possible loss of the sensation contributing to the stimulation of the ejaculatory response. Furthermore, phallectomy and en bloc resection, although suitable for geldings, are not acceptable for breeding stallions due to the loss of ejaculation capability.[17] Phallectomy is the procedure in which a large portion of the penis is amputated. En bloc resection is the removal of the entire prepuce and all of the penis that is not firmly attached to the pelvis.[5] Modifications in this technique have included the removal of a shorter portion of the penis with the remainder being rotated 180 degrees and sutured ventral to the ischium. This procedure has reportedly eliminated some of the difficulties involved with the urethrostomy, which is required with en bloc resection.[18] It also includes the removal of lymph nodes and surrounding tissue. An opening is established in the perineal area for urination. Recurrence of the squamous cell carcinoma is frequent regardless of treatment.[1, 7]

Sarcoids occasionally occur on the penis and prepuce of the male horse and represent the location of approximately 8% of sarcoids.[19] It has been suggested that there is a familial correlation to sarcoids.[20] This has been further defined to demonstrate a correlation between increased risk and the presence of the major histocompatibility complex encoded class II allele ELA W13.[19] These benign tumors[21] are highly associated with wounds or trauma to the area and have been linked to an infectious cause.[22-30] Treatment of the sarcoid may not be necessary but is usually indicated owing to the size or the contamination of the ejaculate at the time of ejaculation. Treatments that have been successful at least to some degree include surgical removal,[31] cryotherapy,[32] brachytherapy,[33, 34] hyperthermia,[35] hyperthermia combined with radiotherapy,[34] local immunostimulation,[36, 37] and chemical agents such as podophyllum[38, 39] and 5-fluorouracil.[38, 40, 41] Melanomas of the penis and prepuce appear similar to the characteristic neoplasms observed in the perineal area of the horse. The lesions are generally small and smooth on the surface. Although normally expected in the gray horse, they may appear in any colored animal. However, when the tumor does occur in other than the gray animal, its rate of growth and spread is more rapid.[29, 42-44] Melanomas on the prepuce and penis are generally not removed owing to the slow growth and absence of lesions that would interfere with copulation.[45] However, the age of the stallion at the time of appearance and the value of the animal should enter into the appropriate method of handling the case. Chemotherapy as a treatment of melanomas may be possible but cannot be recommended at this time owing to the absence of information regarding the effect on spermatogenesis.[46]

Papillomas of this area are considered to be benign cauliflower-shaped lesions.[29] This neoplasm can be treated successfully with surgical removal, freezing, or waiting until immunity develops and the lesions regress. The treatment depends greatly on the available equipment and the time of year in relationship to the stallion being used as a breeder. This neoplasm has been reported to have the capability to become malignant.[29]

TESTICULAR TUMORS

Testicular tumors are rare in the stallion.[7] Testicular tumors are subdivided into those of primary or secondary origin. The primary tumors that are more commonly reported include those of germinal and non-germinal origin.[47] Germinal neoplasms include the seminoma, teratoma, teratocarcinoma, and embryonic carcinoma. The seminoma is the most frequently reported testicular tumor of the stallion.[7, 47] The seminoma is generally considered to be benign, but metastasis and invasiveness are more prevalent in the equine than in other domestic species.[7, 48] The seminoma has been reported to be bilateral.[49]

The teratoma has been considered to be the most "important" testicular tumor in the stallion.[5] These tumors may also be bilateral.[1, 7] The teratoma can occur during the first 5 years of life, and the tissue within consists of bone, cartilage, skin, hair, epithelial ducts, dentigerous cysts, mammary tissue, and nerves.[1, 7] The teratocarcinoma[50] and the embryonic carcinoma[51] are both rare in the equine.

Non-germinal testicular tumors including the Leydig cell tumor and the Sertoli cell tumor are rare in the stallion.[7, 47, 52, 53] During the examination of testes at any time careful palpation for size, symmetry, and consistency must be emphasized. In addition, if any abnormalities are suspected, an ultrasonographic examination should be performed. An ultrasonographic evaluation of any testicular enlargement is indicated to further delineate the nature and the extent of the lesion.[54] If further information regarding the lesion is necessary, a split needle biopsy can be performed.[55] If confirmation of the lesion as neoplastic is made, the involved testis should be removed. As is the case involving the removal of all tumors, the adjacent tissue and the removed cord should be examined histologically for the presence of metastasis of the tumor. Although metastasis of the tumor to the regional lymph nodes is possible, it probably will not change the course of therapy. The removal of the affected testis may provide additional time during which the stallion can be used for breeding or for semen to be collected and frozen for future use.[56] Chemotherapy is generally not practical or economically feasible and has a detrimental effect on fertility.

REFERENCES

1. Cotchin E: A general survey of tumors in the horse. *Equine Vet J* 9:16, 1977.
2. Sundberg JP, Burnstein T, Page EH, et al: Neoplasms of Equidae. *J Am Vet Med Assoc* 170:150, 1977.
3. Jubb KVF, Kennedy PC: *Pathology of Domestic Animals*, Vol 2. New York, Academic Press, 1970, p 443.
4. Vaughn JT: Surgery of the testes. In Walker DF, Vaughn JT, eds. *Bovine and Equine Urogenital Surgery*. Philadelphia, Lea & Febiger, 1980, p 52.
5. Vaughn JT: Surgery of the male equine reproductive system. In Morrow DA, ed. *Current Therapy in Theriogenology*, Vol 2. Philadelphia, WB Saunders, 1986, p 740.
6. Baker JR, Leyland A: Histological survey of tumors of the horse with particular reference to those of the skin. *Am J Vet Res* 96:419, 1975.
7. Moulton JE: Tumors of the male genital system. In Moulton JE, ed. *Tumors in Domestic Animals*, ed 2. Berkeley, University of California Press, 1978, p 309.
8. Hall WC, Nielson SW, McEntee K: Tumors of the prostate and penis. *Bull WHO* 53:247, 1976.
9. Bowen JM: Management of the breeding stallion. In Morrow DA, ed. *Current Therapy in Theriogenology 2*. Philadelphia, WB Saunders, 1986, p 644.
10. Ladds PW: The male genital system. In Jubb DVF, Kennedy PC, Palmer N, eds. *Pathology of Domestic Animals*, Vol 3, ed 2. Orlando, Academic Press, 1985, p 409.
11. Stannard AA, Pulley LT: Tumors of the skin and soft tissues. In Moulton J, ed. *Tumors in Domestic Animals*, ed 2. Berkeley, University of California Press, 1978, p 16.
12. Fortier LA, Mac Harg MA: Topical use of 5-fluorouracil for treatment of squamous cell carcinoma of the external genitalia of horses: 11 cases. *J Am Vet Med Assoc* 205:1183, 1994.
13. Threlfall WR: Squamous cell carcinoma of the penis. In White NA, Moore JN, eds. *Current Practice of Equine Surgery*. Philadelphia, JB Lippincott, 1990, p 730.
14. Stick JA, Hoffer RE: Results of cryosurgical treatment of equine penile neoplasms. *J Equine Med Surg* 2:505, 1978.
15. Joyce JR: Cryosurgical treatment of tumors of horses and cattle. *J Am Vet Med Assoc* 168:226, 1976.
16. Threlfall WR: Squamous cell carcinoma of the penis. In White NA, Moore JN, eds. *Current Practice of Equine Surgery*. Philadelphia, J B Lippincott, 1990, p 730.
17. Danks AG: *Williams Surgical Operations*. Ithaca, 1943, p 86.
18. Markel MD, Wheat JD, Jones K: Genital neoplasms treated by en bloc resection and penile retroversion in horses: 10 cases (1977–1986). *J Am Vet Med Assoc* 192:396, 1988.
19. Marti E, Lazary S, Antczak DF, et al: Report on the first international workshop on equine sarcoid. *Equine Vet J* 25:397, 1993.
20. James US: A family tendency to equine sarcoids. *Southwest Vet* 21:235, 1968.
21. Strafuss AC, Smith JE, Dennis SM, et al: Sarcoid in horses. *Vet Med Small Animal Clin* 68:1246, 1973.
22. Olson C. Equine sarcoid: A cutaneous neoplasm. *Am J Vet Res* 9:333, 1948.
23. Olson C Jr, Cook RH: Cutaneous sarcoma-like lesions of the horse caused by the agent of bovine papilloma. *Proc Soc Exp Biol Med* 77:281, 1951.
24. Ragland WL, Keown GH, Gorham JR: An epizootic of equine sarcoid. *Nature* 210:1399, 1966.
25. Ragland WL, Spencer GR: Attempts to relate bovine papilloma virus to the cause of equine sarcoid: Immunity to bovine papilloma virus. *Am J Vet Rec* 29:1363, 1968.
26. Ragland WL, Spencer GR: Attempts to relate bovine papilloma virus to the cause of equine sarcoid: Equidae innoculated

27. intradermally with bovine papilloma virus. *Am J Vet Res* 30:743, 1969.
28. Ragland WL, Keown GH, Spencer GR: Equine sarcoid. *Equine Vet J* 2:2, 1970.
29. Voss JL: Transmission of equine sarcoid. *Am J Vet Res* 30:183, 1969.
30. Montes LF, Vaughn JT: Tumors. In *Atlas of Skin Diseases of the Horse*. Philadelphia, WB Saunders, 1983, p 119.
31. McFadyean J: Equine melanomatosis. *J Comp Pathol* 46:186, 1933.
32. Brown MP: Surgical treatment of the equine sarcoid. In Robinson NE, ed. *Current Therapy in Equine Medicine*. Philadelphia, WB Saunders, 1983, p 537.
33. Joyce JR: Cryosurgery for removal of equine sarcoids. *Vet Med Small Animal Clin* 70:200, 1975.
34. Wyn-Jones G: Treatment of equine cutaneous neoplasia by radiotherapy using iridium 192 liner sources. *Equine Vet J* 15:361, 1983.
35. Turrel JM, Stover SM, Gyorgyfalvy J: Iridium-192 interstitial brachytherapy of equine sarcoid. *Vet Radiol* 26:20, 1985.
36. Hoffman KD, Kainer RA, Shideler RK: Radiofrequency current-induced hyperthermia for treatment of equine sarcoid. *Equine Pract* 5:24, 1983.
37. Wyman M, Rings MD, Tarr J, et al: Immunotherapy in equine sarcoid: A report of 2 cases. *J Am Vet Med Assoc* 171:449, 1977.
38. Rebhun WC: Immunotherapy for sarcoids. In Robinson NE, ed. *Current Therapy in Equine Medicine*, ed 2. Philadelphia, WB Saunders, 1987, p 637.
39. Roberts D: Experimental treatment of equine sarcoid. *Vet Med Small Animal Clin* 65:67, 1970.
40. Metcalf JW: Improved technique in sarcoid removal. *Am Assoc Equine Pract Proc* 17:45, 1971.
41. Turrel JM, Kitchell B, Luck EE, et al: Preliminary results of therapeutic drug-matrix implants for equine sarcoid and canine mast cell tumor. *Proc Vet Cancer Soc Meet*, May 1985, p 22.
42. Bertone AL, McClure JJ: Therapy for sarcoids. *Compend Contin Educ Pract Vet* 12:262, 1990.
43. McFadyean J: Equine melanomatosis. *J Comp Pathol* 46:186, 1933.
44. Lerner AB, Cage GW: Melanomas in horses. *Yale J Biol Med* 46:646, 1974.
45. Runnells RA, Benbrook EA: Malignant melanomas of horses and mules. *Am J Vet Res* 2:340, 1941.
46. Neely DP: Physical examination and genital diseases of the stallion. In Morrow DA, ed. *Current Therapy in Theriogenology*. Philadelphia, WB Saunders. 1980, p 694.
47. McClure RD: Endocrine investigation and therapy. *Urol Clin North Am* 14:471, 1987.
48. Morse MJ, Whitmore WF: Neoplasms of the testis. In Walsh PC, Gittes RF, Perlmutter AD, et al, eds. *Campbell's Urology*, Vol 2, ed 5. Philadelphia, WB Saunders, 1986, p 1535.
49. Pandolfi F, Roperto F: Seminoma with multiple metastases in a zebra (Equus zebra) x mare (Equus caballus). *Equine Vet J* 15:70, 1983.
50. Gibson GW: Malignant seminoma in a Welsh pony stallion. *Compend Contin Educ Pract Vet* 6:296, 1984.
51. Shaw DP, Roth JE: Testicular teratocarcinoma in a horse. *Vet Pathol* 23:327, 1986.
52. Valentine BA, Weinstock D: Metastatic testicular embryonal carcinoma in a young horse. *Vet Pathol* 23:92, 1986.
53. Rahaley RS, Gordon BJ, Leiopold HW, et al: Sertoli cell tumor in a horse. *Equine Vet J* 15:68, 1983.
54. Smith HA: Interstitial cell tumor of the equine testis. *J Am Vet Med Assoc* 124:356, 1954.
55. Nachtsheim DA, Scheible FW, Gosink B: Ultrasonography of testis tumors. *J Urol* 129:978, 1983.
56. Threlfall WR, Lopate C: Testicular biopsy. *Therio* 65, 1987.

56. Hoagland TA, Ott KM, Dinger JE, et al: Effects of unilateral castration on morphological characteristics of the testis in one-, two-, and three-year-old stallions. *Therio* 26:397, 1986.

15.13

Mastitis

Nigel Perkins, BVSc, MS, Dip ACT
Walter R. Threlfall, DVM, MS, PhD, Dip ACT

Mastitis is defined as inflammation of the mammary gland.[1] Although injury of any type will produce an inflammatory response, for practical purposes mastitis is usually defined as being caused by the presence of microbes within the mammary gland.[1] It has been reported that a nematode, cephalobus, was responsible for mastitis in a mare.[2]

The incidence of mastitis in the mare is considered to be much lower than in the cow.[3] This may partially be explained by the relatively smaller size and concealed position of the gland and the presence of smaller teats with less exposure to trauma and infection.[3] In addition, the equine gland has a relatively small milk capacity, and because foals often nurse several times per hour, the gland is frequently emptied in the lactating mare. Large amounts of milk are thus prevented from accumulating in the glands at any one time.[3] The possibility of greater resistance to infection in the equine mammary gland because of differences in endocrine environment or local immunity has been suggested, although this remains to be demonstrated. Possible routes of invasion of the mammary gland by bacteria include hematogenous, percutaneous, or most commonly directly via the teat canal.[1]

Equine mastitis has been reported in lactating mares,[4–7] non-lactating mares,[5, 8] and in foals.[5, 9] The condition is considered by some authors to be most prevalent in the period immediately after weaning, when continued milk production results in the accumulation of secretion within the mammary gland.[3, 8] However, in a review of 28 cases of equine mastitis, 44% occurred in lactating mares, 28% in mares within 8 weeks of weaning a foal, and 28% in mares that had not lactated within the previous 12 months.[4] A similar study of 17 cases of equine mastitis reported 29% of cases in lactating mares, 24% in immature fillies (2 months to 2 years of age), and 47% in non-lactating mares.[5] Cases have also been reported within days of foaling,[4, 5] after injury to the teat or mammary gland,[4, 5, 8] and after an incision into the mammary gland during abdominal surgery.[4] Eleven of 17 cases in a series were presented for investigation with mastitis as the primary complaints.[5] The primary complaint in the remaining six cases were sick foal (two cases), weight loss (two cases), abortion (one case), and chronic diarrhea (one case).[5]

Most cases of equine mastitis have been clinical cases. The incidence of subclinical mastitis in mares is unknown as is the possibility of long-term adverse effects on subse-quent milk production due to mastitis. It is possible that mastitis could adversely affect subsequent mammary gland function and result in reduced foal growth during future lactational periods compared with mares without any history of mastitis.[9, 11]

SIGNS

Disorders of the mammary gland are usually evidenced by abnormalities in size or secretion of one or both glands. The most common sign of equine mastitis is increased size of the affected gland(s).[4, 5] Other signs observed in mares affected with mastitis include firmness; heat; pain on palpation; purulent, serous or bloody discharge from affected gland(s); edema between hindlimbs and occasionally extending forward under the abdomen; unilateral hindlimb lameness on the limb adjacent to the affected gland; circumduction of the hindlimb adjacent to the affected gland; and reluctance to allow the foal to nurse in lactating mares with a foal.[4–9] Affected mares often show normal temperature, pulse, and respiratory rate and continue to eat normally[5, 8] although some mares may show systemic signs of disease as evidenced by fever, anorexia, depression, and elevations in pulse and respiratory rate.[4, 7, 9] The secretion from affected glands is usually changed in appearance and may appear as copious clear or serous fluid early in the stages of the disease or as a thick, non-flocculent, purulent discharge with or without the presence of blood.[5–9]

DIAGNOSIS

The diagnosis of clinical mastitis depends on the results of the physical examination and laboratory tests. Tranquilization, sedation, physical restraint, and in some cases even general anesthesia may be necessary for a complete examination of the mammary gland and for initiation of treatment.[8]

A sample of secretion from the affected lobe(s) or gland(s) should be obtained in an aseptic manner after careful preparation of the teat's surface. Each mammary gland in the mare is divided by a fibrous septum into two lobes with separate teat cisterns and openings at the teat's orifice.[4, 10] As a result, mastitis may involve one or both lobes of one or both glands. For this reason it is recommended that an attempt be made to obtain separate samples of secretion from each lobe in order to further define the lobe(s) and gland(s) affected. Milk samples collected in this manner should be subjected to aerobic culture and sensitivity and cytologic examination in an attempt to confirm the diagnosis of mastitis and identify the organisms involved. Anaerobes are not currently considered to be a significant cause of equine mastitis and therefore anaerobic culture is not routinely recommended.[4, 5] The combination of culture and cytology is considered to be necessary to diagnose mastitis, because up to 30% of samples of mammary gland secretions from cases of mastitis may fail to produce bacterial growth when cultured.[4]

Cytologic examination of smears of whole milk may aid in the diagnosis of subclinical and clinical mastitis.[6] Slides for cytologic examination may be fixed in alcohol and stained with a commercial cell stain such as Dif-Quik. Lactating mares have a secretion that is almost non-cellular, although a few neutrophils may be seen.[11] After weaning, smears may contain large macrophages with marked cytoplasmic vacuolation (foam cells), small dark cells resembling small lymphocytes, macrophages, and low numbers of neutrophils.[11] Smears from mares with mastitis contain large numbers of degenerated and non-generated neutrophils, necrotic debris, and unrecognizable degenerated cells. Subclinical mastitis may be diagnosed based on cytologic evidence of inflammation without clinical signs. The incidence of subclinical mastitis in the mare is unknown but is likely to be more common than clinical mastitis, as is reported for the cow.[11]

The identification of causative bacteria in cases of mastitis is considered to be important because both gram-negative and gram-positive bacteria have been cultured from animals with mastitis.[4, 5] In cultures of milk samples from 37 cases of equine mastitis, 30 cases cultured aerobic bacteria and 26 of the 30 positive cultures were of a single isolate.[4, 5] More gram-positive bacteria (23 or 68%) were recovered than gram-negative (11 or 32%).[4, 5] Bacteria may be seen on cytologic examination of milk smears, and a direct Gram stain of mammary secretions may provide a rapid method of identifying gram-positive or gram-negative bacteria and permit earlier selection of antibiotics than would be possible with a culture and sensitivity test. However, gram staining of 18 milk samples from cases of mastitis resulted in identification of bacteria in only six cases (33%).[4]

A hematologic examination of peripheral blood samples may provide additional information regarding the severity and the course of the disease, and two of 12 (17%) cases of mastitis indicated leukocytosis and neutrophilia and six (50%) with elevated fibrinogen.[4] Hematologic changes in uncomplicated cases of mastitis are likely to be mild or non-detectable, and the presence of changes may suggest concurrent disease.[5]

Streptococcus zooepidemicus is the most common bacterial isolate from equine mastitis cases, accounting for 11 of 34 isolates (32%). Other bacteria isolated include *Staphylococcus* spp. (14.7%), *Actinobacillus* spp. (5.9%), *Pseudomonas aeruginosa* (2.9%), *Enterobacter aerogenes* (2.9%), *Pasteurella ureae* (2.9%), *Streptococcus viridans* (2.9%), *Streptococcus agalactiae* (2.9%), *Corynebacterium* spp. (2.9%), and *Bacillus* spp. (2.9%).[4, 5]

It is important to consider neoplasia as a differential diagnosis for enlargement of the mammary gland. Neoplasia of the equine mammary gland is considered to be rare, and tumors are likely to be benign.[1] In cases in which the mammary gland is enlarged, aerobic culture is negative and the gland does not respond to an initial course of broad-spectrum antibiotics, anti-inflammatory drugs, and hydrotherapy, one should suspect mammary gland neoplasia or hyperplasia.[12] A definitive diagnosis of mammary gland neoplasia depends on a histologic examination of biopsy samples. The most common equine mammary gland tumor is the adenocarcinoma[13] with other reported tumors including lymphosarcoma[14] and carcinoma.[12] Some cases may present with severe systemic signs that are attributable to multiple neoplastic metastases involving abdominal and thoracic organs with the primary neoplasia involving the mammary gland.[12, 13]

TREATMENT

All treatments for mastitis should be combined with stripping of the affected lobes in an attempt to physically remove bacteria and necrotic debris. Stripping may be combined with hot packing and hydrotherapy.[9] Subclinical and mild clinical cases of equine mastitis with minimal gland swelling may be treated by local therapies alone, instilled into each affected lobe. Teats should be cleaned and disinfected prior to treatment. Lactating cow intramammary preparations represent convenient and relatively inexpensive methods of treating cases of equine mastitis. The choice of product should depend on the results of culture and sensitivity tests. A commercial dry cow product with residual antibiotic activity may be used after cessation of lactating cow therapy.[4] Intramammary infusions of injectable antibiotics such as gentamicin (100 to 150 mg) or polymyxin-B, diluted in 100 to 200 mL of sterile saline, have also been used to treat cases of equine mastitis.[4, 8] Local treatments may be infused into the teat orifice via a bovine teat cannula. Some authors recommend caution in inserting syringe tips into teat orifices in the mare owing to the small size of the teat orifices compared with those of the cow and the subsequent risk of trauma to the teat orifice and streak canal.[4]

The decision to utilize systemic antibiotics as a treatment for mastitis may depend on the severity of the mastitis and the disposition of the mare. The choice of antibiotic should again depend on the culture and sensitivity results. In the absence of culture results, a broad-spectrum antibiotic should be chosen. The wide range of organisms isolated from mastitis secretions and the unpredictable sensitivity patterns of gram-negative organisms suggest that penicillin alone may not be the optimal choice of antibiotic.[4, 5] The use of combinations such as oral trimethoprim-sulphonamide products and penicillin-gentamicin combinations should provide a broad spectrum of activity and are considered to be the treatments of choice. Nonsteroidal anti-inflammatory drugs such as phenylbutazone may be combined with other treatments in an attempt to minimize inflammation and reduce pain and swelling. Furosemide has been administered to mares with mastitis in an attempt to reduce associated edema.[4]

The response to effective therapy is usually rapid. A significant improvement in the nature of mammary gland secretions is seen within 3 days of the initiation of therapy and the mammary gland is almost normal with 1 week.[4, 5, 8, 9] It is recommended that treatments be continued for 5 to 7 days or until 24 hours after clinical resolution of the disease. There is little available information regarding the long-term follow-up on mares with mastitis. Recurrence of mastitis in the same gland does not appear to be a significant problem. One mare in a series of 28 cases was reported to have had mastitis in the same gland twice in 2 years.[4] The incidence of chronic mastitis persisting in a non-lactating gland and becoming clinically apparent with the resumption of lactation is not known. Mares have been reported with clinical mastitis within days of foaling, and this information would support the presence of subclinical mastitis in these mares prior to foaling.[4, 5] Chronic mastitis may have an adverse effect on milk production and on normal fetal and neonatal development. One mare is reported to have aborted at 10 months of gestation, 5 days after diagnosis of acute mastitis due to *S. zooepidemicus*.[4] No evidence of bacterial infection of the placenta or fetus was reported at necropsy and, therefore, any direct association between the mastitis and subsequent abortion in this case remains questionable. However, the possibility of bacteremia or septicemia originating in the mammary gland and resulting in placentitis or septic metritis of pregnancy and abortion remains a possibility.

CONTROL

Few recommendations can be made regarding the control and prevention of equine mastitis. It is recommended that mares be observed carefully for signs of mastitis after weaning, when the foal appears unthrifty or when there is an untimely death of a suckling foal. Inspection and palpation of the mammary glands should comprise part of the routine physical examination of the mare since mastitis occurs in barren and non-lactating mares.

REFERENCES

1. Jubb K, Kennedy P, Palmer N: *Pathology of Domestic Animals*, ed 3. San Diego, CA, Academic Press, 1985, P 527.
2. Greiner E, Mays M, Smart Jr. G, et al: Verminous mastitis in a mare caused by a free-living nematode. *J Parasitol* 77:320, 1991.
3. Jackson P: Equine mastitis: Comparative lessons. *Equine Vet J* 18:88, 1986.
4. McCue P, Wilson W: Equine mastitis—a review of 28 cases. *Equine Vet J* 21:351, 1989.
5. Perkins NR, Threlfall WR: Mastitis in the mare. *Equine Vet Educ* 5:192, 1993.
6. Freeman K: Cytological evaluation of the equine mammary gland. *Equine Vet Educ* 5:212, 1993.
7. Reese G, Lock T: Streptococcal mastitis in a mare. *J Am Vet Med Assoc* 173:83, 1978.
8. Roberts M: *Pseudomonas aeruginosa* mastitis in a dry- nonpregnant pony mare. *Equine Vet J* 18:146, 1986.
9. Pugh D, Magnusson R, Modransky P, et al: A case of mastitis in a young filly. *Equine Vet Sci* 5:132, 1985.
10. Noden D, De Lahunta A: *The Embryology of Domestic Animals: Developmental Mechanisms and Malformations*. Baltimore, MD, Williams & Williams, 1985.
11. Freeman K, Roszel J, Slusher S, et al: Cytologic features of equine mammary fluids: Normal and abnormal. *Compend Contin Educ* 10:1090, 1988.
12. Munson L: Carcinoma of the mammary gland in a mare. *J Am Vet Med Assoc* 191:71, 1987.
13. Foreman J, Weidner J, Perry B, et al: Pleural effusion secondary to thoracic metastatic mammary adenocarcinoma in a mare. *J Am Vet Med Assoc* 197:1193, 1990.
14. Anonymous: Mammary gland lymphosarcoma in a mare. *Vet Med* 1:21, 1991.

Chapter 16

The Urinary System

16.1

Anatomy and Development

Harold C. Schott II, DVM, PhD

ANATOMY

The urinary system of the horse, like that of most mammals, consists of paired kidneys and ureters, the bladder, and the urethra. With the exception of the abdominal portion of the urinary bladder, the entire urinary tract is located in the retroperitoneal space. In a newborn foal, each kidney weighs about 175 g. In an adult horse, the left kidney weighs 600 to 700 g and the right kidney is usually 25 to 50 g heavier, although this is not a consistent finding and the reverse relation may be observed.[1, 2] Thus, the kidneys account for approximately 0.65% to 0.75% and 0.27% to 0.37% of the total body weight of the foal and adult horse, respectively.[1, 3] The right kidney is located immediately below the dorsal extent of the last two or three ribs and the first lumbar transverse process. It is shaped like a horseshoe and measures about 15 cm in length, 15 cm in width, and 5 to 6 cm in height (dorsal to ventral). Craniolaterally, it is embedded into the liver, and its more craniad position in comparison to the left kidney prevents it from being accessible on rectal palpation. The left kidney is bean shaped, with the cranial pole at the level of the hilus of the right kidney. It is about 18 cm long, 10 to 12 cm wide, and 5 to 6 cm in height. Owing to its more caudal location, the caudoventral aspect of the left kidney can routinely be palpated during rectal examination. The blood supply to the kidneys comes from one or more renal arteries branching from the aorta. Accessory renal arteries (which generally enter caudally) may arise from the caudal mesenteric, testicular or ovarian, or deep circumflex iliac arteries.[1, 2]

The ureters are 6 to 8 mm in diameter and travel about 70 cm to their insertions in the dorsal bladder neck or trigone, close to the urethra. The distal 5 to 7 cm of each ureter courses within the bladder wall. This intramural segment of the ureter functions as a one-way valve to prevent vesicoureteral reflux with progressive bladder distension. The urinary bladder lies on the pelvic floor when empty but can increase in size and drop forward over the pelvic brim when distended. The bladder can accommodate up to 3 to 4 L of urine before micturition is stimulated. In the foal, the bladder is attached to the ventral abdominal wall by the urachus and remnants of the umbilical arteries. Consequently, when empty, the bladder is commonly a band-shaped structure in a neonatal foal. During the first few months of life this ventral attachment loosens as the urachal remnant becomes the middle ligament and the umbilical arterial remnants become the round ligaments of the free border of the paired lateral ligaments of the bladder.[1]

The urethra is about 2 to 3 cm long in a mare and 75 to 90 cm in a male. In the intact male, the pelvic urethra, which is 10 to 12 cm long, widens in an elliptical pattern to a diameter of 5 cm across and 2 to 3 cm from dorsal to ventral. A rounded dorsal prominence, the colliculus seminalis, is located immediately caudal to the urethral orifice and is the site of the common openings of the ductus deferens and ducts of the seminal vesicles. The openings of the prostatic ducts are on two groups of small papillae lateral to the colliculus seminalis. Between 2 and 3 cm farther caudad, the ducts of the bulbourethral glands open in paired dorsal lines. The smaller openings of the ducts of the lateral urethral glands open at the same level on the lateral aspect of the urethra.[1]

The surface of each kidney is covered by a fibrous capsule that is easily peeled from the normal kidney. The equine kidney consists of an outer cortex slightly wider than the inner medulla. The cortex is dotted with dark spots—renal corpuscles or glomeruli within Bowman's capsules. In horses, the corticomedullary junction is less distinct than in other species and is typically a deep red color that is well-contrasted against the paler medulla and red-brown cortex. This region undulates along renal pyramids (cortex) and renal columns (medulla). The pyramids are subdivisions of the renal parenchyma, which are separated by arcuate arteries at the level of the corticomedullary junction. The equine kidney contains a total of 40 to 60 pyramids arranged in four parallel rows. The renal pelvis is the dilated proximal portion of the ureter. Microscopic examination reveals numerous small openings of the collecting ducts (ducts of Bellini). Additionally, the renal pelvis and proximal ureter are lined with both compound tubular mucus glands and goblet cells that secrete thick, viscid mucus that is usually found in the renal pelvis and urine of normal horses.[1, 4]

The functional unit of the kidney is the nephron. Each nephron is composed of a renal corpuscle (glomerulus within Bowman's capsule), a proximal tubule (convoluted and straight components), an intermediate tubule (loop of Henle), a distal convoluted tubule, a connecting tubule, and cortical, outer medullary, and inner medullary collecting ducts (Fig. 16–1). There are two populations of nephrons: (1) superficial (or cortical) nephrons possessing a short loop of Henle and

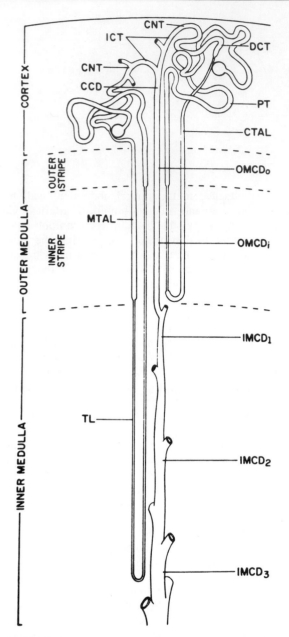

Figure 16–1. Diagram of a superficial and juxtamedullary nephron. Key: PT, proximal tubule; TL, thin limb of Henle's loop; MTAL, medullary thick ascending limb of Henle's loop; CTAL, cortical thick ascending limb of Henle's loop; DCT, distal convoluted tubule; CNT, connecting segment; ICT, initial collecting tubule; CCD, cortical collecting duct; $OMCD_0$, collecting duct in outer stripe of outer medulla; $OMCD_1$, collecting duct in inner stripe of outer medulla; $IMCD_1$, outer third of inner medullary collecting duct; $IMCD_2$, middle third of inner medullary collecting duct; and $IMCD_3$, inner third of inner medullary collecting duct. (From Tisher CC, Madsen KM: Anatomy of the kidney. *In* Brenner BM, Rector FC, eds. The Kidney, ed 4, vol. 1. Philadelphia, WB Saunders, 1991, p. 9.)

(2) juxtamedullary nephrons with a long loop of Henle. There are gradations between these two general categories of nephrons as well as species variation in the ratio of short looped nephrons to long ones. For example, in humans there

are seven times more short than long looped nephrons, whereas essentially 100% of nephrons in dogs and cats have long loops.[5] From information collected over a range of other species, each kidney of the horse can be estimated to contain approximately 4 million nephrons,[6] but there is little information on the ratio of short to long looped nephrons in horses. Histologically, the equine nephrons are similar in most respects to those of other mammalian species; however, the diameter and epithelial height of the tubule and collecting duct segments are comparatively larger. In addition, the equine macula densa (segment of the ascending loop of Henle that lies in close association with the juxtaglomerular apparatus of the afferent arteriole) appears more prominent than that of other mammals.[7] Whether these subtle histologic differences are accompanied by functional differences has not been investigated.

Relative to its size, the mammalian kidney has a richer innervation than almost any other organ.[8] Although the neuroanatomy of the equine kidney has not been well studied, autonomic nerves course from the aorticorenal and renal ganglia along the major renal vessels into the kidneys.[1] These nerves are predominantly sympathetic, as the kidneys appear to be poorly supplied by cholinergic nerves. Although the best-recognized effect of renal nerves is control of renal vascular resistance (for regulation of renal blood flow over a wide range of perfusion pressures), they also act directly on renal tubules and juxtaglomerular cells. For example, low-frequency stimulation of renal nerves (below the threshold for vasoconstriction) increases proximal tubular sodium reabsorption and renin release by activation of α_1 adrenoceptors.[9] In addition to α- and β-adrenoceptors, the renal cortex is rich in dopaminergic adrenoceptors, and activation of the latter leads to dilatation of renal arterioles. Presence of these receptors is the basis for use of dopamine in an attempt to improve renal blood flow in acute renal failure.[10, 11] Renal adrenoceptors can also be activated unintentionally by administration of drugs. A common clinical example is the diuresis induced by administration of the α_2-agonists xylazine and detomidine. Although the diuresis has been attributed to a transient hyperglycemia and glucosuria, the latter is often absent.[12, 13] An alternative explanation may be drug binding to α_2-adrenoceptors located on collecting duct epithelium. Activation of these receptors can lead to antagonization of the effects of antidiuretic hormone on cortical collecting ducts, which results in diuresis.[14] More recently, renal afferent nerves have been identified, and these nerves appear to play a role in the pathogenesis of hypertension in species affected by this disorder.[8]

Autonomic innervation of the ureters, bladder, and urethra is important to ureteral peristalsis and micturition. The equine ureteral smooth muscle contains both α_1- and β_2-adrenoceptors, which induce contraction and relaxation, respectively, when activated by norepinephrine.[15] Recent studies of the innervation of the equine ureter demonstrated greater densities of adrenergic neurons in the proximal (renal pelvis) and intravesicular (bladder wall) portions of the ureter.[16] Increased densities in these regions are consistent with the suspected pacemaker activity of the renal pelvis, which initiates ureteral peristalsis and the sphincterlike function of the distal segment of the ureter. The sympathetic nerve supply to the urinary bladder is provided via the hypogastric nerve, with preganglionic fibers arriving from spinal seg-

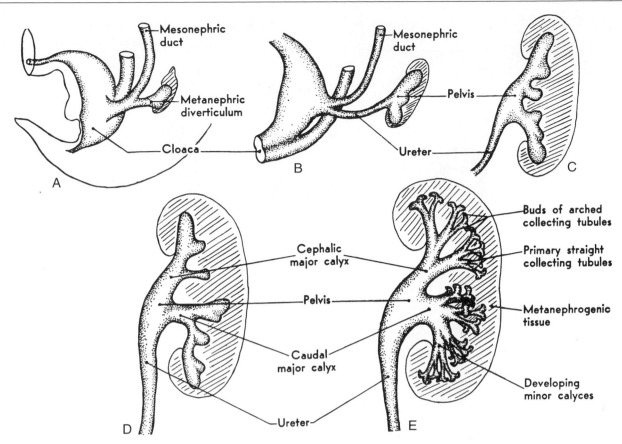

Figure 16–2. Progression of the differentiation and development of the metanephric diverticulum into the collecting system of the mature kidney. **A,** Metanephric diverticulum originates from the caudal end of the mesonephric duct. **B,** It develops craniad, and intermediate mesoderm (metanephrogenic tissue, hatched lines) collects about its cranial end. **C–E,** The metanephric diverticulum becomes the ureter and renal pelvis and the metanephrogenic tissue becomes the collecting system and parenchyma of the mature kidney. (From Patten BM, Carlson BM: Foundations of Embryology, ed 3. New York, McGraw-Hill, 1974, p. 509.)

ments L1–4 to synapse in the caudal mesenteric ganglion. Postganglionic fibers supply the bladder (β_2-adrenergic receptors) and proximal urethra (primarily α_1- and some α_2-adrenergic receptors).[17, 18] In addition to adrenergic innervation, the equine bladder is also innervated by cholinergic and peptidergic nerve fibers.[19] Parasympathetic innervation originates in the sacral segments of the spinal cord with neurons joining to form the pelvic nerve.[17, 18] There are many complex interneuronal connections between sympathetic and parasympathetic nerves in the wall of the bladder, as well as small adrenergic cells that facilitate interaction between sympathetic and parasympathetic pathways.[20] As a result, complete denervation of the bladder is virtually impossible. Somatic innervation of the lower urinary tract is primarily to the striated muscle of the external urethral sphincter via a branch of the pudendal nerve, which originates from the sacral cord segments (S1–2).[1]

DEVELOPMENT

The embryonic upper urinary tract arises from bilateral primordial mesonephric ducts and intermediate mesoderm.[21] The metanephric diverticulum originates from the caudal end of each mesonephric duct and develops craniad to become the ureter and renal pelvis. The advancing metanephric diverticuli collect about their ends intermediate mesoderm (metanephrogenic tissue), which becomes the collecting system and parenchyma of the mature kidney (Fig. 16–2). The vascular supply is derived from a branch of the aorta (renal artery) that invades the metanephrogenic tissue. The urinary bladder develops as a dilated proximal portion of the allantois. The bladder is separated from the hindgut by the craniocaudad growth of the urorectal fold, which divides the rectum from the urogenital sinus. The latter structure gives rise to the urethra (Fig. 16–3). The mesonephric and metanephric ducts initially open into the urogenital sinus, but as development continues the distal segments of the mesonephric ducts are absorbed into the bladder wall and the openings of the metanephric ducts are pulled craniad to their final site in the dorsal bladder neck.[21]

The fate of the mesonephric tubules (mesonephros) and mesonephric ducts varies with gender. Paired paramesonephric ducts (müllerian ducts) arise parallel to the mesonephric ducts in both sexes. In the female, they fuse distally to become the vagina and uterine body, whereas proximally they remain separate to give rise to uterine horns and oviducts. The mesonephric ducts regress into vestigial remnants

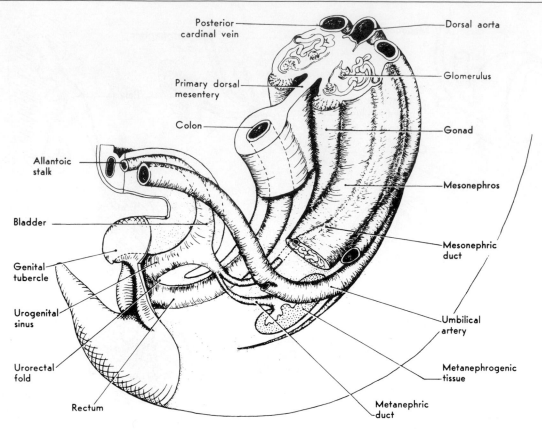

Figure 16–3. Developing urogenital tract of the young mammalian embryo. (From Patten PM, Carlson BM: Foundations of Embryology, ed 3. New York, McGraw-Hill, 1974, p. 513.)

termed the *epoöphoron* proximally (near the ovaries) and *Gartner's canals* distally (near the vagina and uterus) (Fig. 16–4). In the male, sexual differentiation of the gonads and production of androgenic steroid hormones lead to regression of the müllerian ducts. The duct system of the male reproductive tract is appropriated from the mesonephros and mesonephric ducts (also termed *wolffian ducts*). Androgenic steroid hormones also stimulate these structures to develop into the seminiferous tubules, epididymis, and ductus deferens. The distal portion of the mesonephric duct becomes the ejaculatory duct, the terminal portion of the ductus deferens.[21]

DEVELOPMENTAL MALFORMATIONS OF THE URINARY TRACT

Anomalies of the urinary tract are uncommon in horses. A survey by Höfliger revealed a similar frequency of unilateral renal agenesis (0.07%) in horses[22] and humans (0.10%).[5] In contrast, horseshoe kidneys (attached at the cranial or caudal poles) are the most common anomaly in humans (0.25%) but have rarely been described in horses.[5, 23]

Renal Agenesis, Hypoplasia, and Dysplasia

Renal agenesis, which may be unilateral or bilateral, results from failure of the metanephric duct to fuse with the meta-

nephrogenic mesodermal tissue. Although unilateral anomalies have been described more frequently, this may simply reflect the incompatibility of bilateral agenesis with postnatal life.[22, 24–26] Brown described a foal with bilateral renal agenesis in which severe azotemia was detected shortly after birth. Bilateral ureteral dysgenesis and cryptorchidism, agenesis of the right adrenal gland, and atresia ani accompanied the renal agenesis in this foal.[26] Unilateral defects may be incidental findings in otherwise healthy horses[27] or may be detected during examination of the reproductive tract, since many have associated anomalies of that system. Occasionally, unilateral agenesis may result in clinical renal disease if a problem arises in the contralateral kidney. Johnson described a 4-year-old quarter horse with unilateral renal agenesis and a ureterolith causing contralateral hydronephrosis. The gelding was presented for weight loss, pollakiuria, and stranguria. In addition to the renal anomaly, unilateral agenesis of the ipsilateral testicle was also found on necropsy.[25] Renal agenesis may be a familial disorder in several species.[23, 28] Although there is no information to suggest a hereditary basis in horses, repeat matings should probably be discouraged if such an anomaly is detected.

Renal hypoplasia is diagnosed when one kidney is at least 50% smaller than normal or when the total renal mass is decreased by more than one third.[23] Renal hypoplasia is a quantitative defect caused by a reduced mass of metanephrogenic tissue or by incomplete induction of nephron formation by the metanephric duct. The condition may be confused with renal dysplasia. Unilateral renal hypoplasia is usually

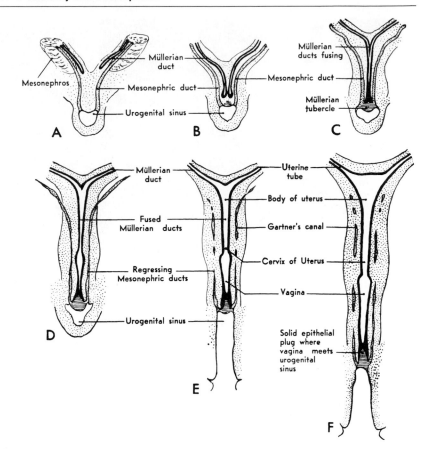

Figure 16–4. Development of the mesonephric tubules (mesonephros) and mesonephric ducts into the female reproductive tract. **A, B,** Paired paramesonephric ducts (müllerian ducts) arise parallel to the mesonephric ducts in both sexes. **C–E,** In females, they fuse distally to become the vagina and uterine body but remain separate proximally to give rise to uterine horns. **D, E,** The mesonephric ducts regress into vestigial remnants termed *Gartner's canals.* (From Patten BM, Carlson BM: Foundations of Embryology, ed 3. New York, McGraw-Hill, 1974, p. 497.)

associated with contralateral hypertrophy and normal renal function whereas bilateral hypoplasia generally leads to chronic renal failure.[23, 28] Andrews described bilateral renal hypoplasia in a foal presented after death and in three young horses with chronic renal failure that had poor growth from birth. Anomalies in these four horses were limited to the upper urinary tract.[29]

Renal dysplasia is disorganized development of renal tissue due to anomalous differentiation, intrauterine ureteral obstruction, fetal viral infection, or teratogens.[23, 30] Bilateral dysplasia usually leads to renal failure. In general, dysplastic kidneys are normal in size unless concurrent hypoplasia exists or the animal lives for months to years before developing renal failure. Roberts reported a case of bilateral renal dysplasia in a 19-month-old pony gelding.[31] The pony was presented for weight loss over a 3-month period, and clinicopathologic assessment revealed chronic renal failure. A small, firm, and nodular left kidney was palpated per rectum. At necropsy, the kidneys weighed 280 g each (33% smaller than normal for body weight) and were nodular. Renal dysplasia was suspected since glomeruli in the collapsed areas of the kidneys were small, tubules were immature, and inflammatory cells were scant. Three similar cases of bilateral renal dysplasia resulted in chronic renal failure in horses from 14 months to 7 years of age.[32, 33] At necropsy, the kidneys were small and irregular, the cortex and medulla were not well-delineated, and immature glomeruli and primitive tubules were found on histologic examination (Fig. 16–5). Zicker described renal dysplasia in a 2-day-old foal presented for diarrhea and depression.[34] Clinicopathologic

assessment revealed azotemia, hyponatremia, hypochloremia, and urinary sodium wastage. At necropsy, the kidneys were normal in size (380 g), but histologic examination revealed immature glomeruli, hypoplastic tubules and vasa recta, and extensive myxomatous connective tissue occupying 90% of the total medullary volume. Renal dysplasia may also be a unilateral problem that does not result in renal failure. Recently, Jones found ureteropelvic polyps to be the cause of unilateral hydronephrosis and renal dysplasia in a Trakehner colt.[35] Poor growth and hematuria of several weeks' duration were the presenting complaints. Ureteral obstruction by the polyps was the suggested cause of renal dysplasia, as urinary tract obstruction has been found in a large percentage of cases of human renal dysplasia.[30]

Renal Cysts

One or more renal cysts are occasionally discovered as incidental findings on necropsy examination. The cysts may arise from any portion of the nephron but are more often observed in the cortex than in the medulla. The pathogenesis is not known, but a defect in the basement membrane that allows tubular dilatation is suspected. Renal cysts vary in size from microscopic to as large as the organ itself and routinely have a clear to slightly opaque wall and contain a thin, clear fluid. Congenital cysts are easily differentiated from acquired cysts (secondary to obstruction) by the extensive scarring that accompanies the latter. Renal cysts may also develop as a consequence of drug therapy (i.e., long-acting corticosteroids) or exposure to certain chemicals.[23, 28]

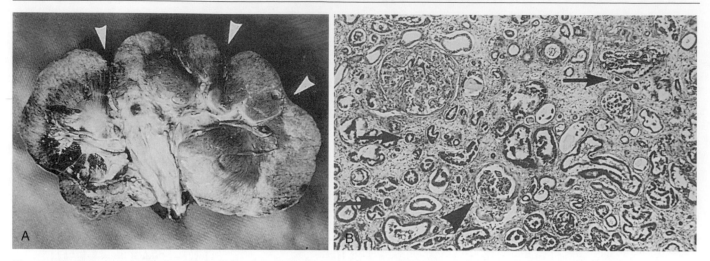

Figure 16–5. A, Longitudinal section of the right kidney from a 7-year-old Arabian gelding with renal dysplasia shows focal, irregular thinning of the cortex *(arrows),* resulting in a nodular surface and poor delineation of the corticomedullary junction. **B,** Histologic section of same kidney (Masson's trichrome stain, original magnification ×35) reveals an immature glomerulus *(large arrowhead)* and primitive tubules *(arrows)* surrounded by persistent mesenchyme. (From Ronen N, van Amstel SR, Nesbit JW, van Rensburg IBJ: Renal dysplasia in two adult horses: Clinical and pathological aspects. Vet Rec 132:269, 1993.)

Polycystic Kidney Disease and Glomerulocystic Disease

Polycystic kidney disease is a disorder in which numerous, variably sized cysts are found throughout the cortex and medulla. With glomerulocystic disease, cysts are microscopic and limited to Bowman's spaces. Cysts of the bile duct and pancreas may also be observed with polycystic kidney disease, and both conditions have been described in stillbirths in many species, including foals.[23] There are two major types of human polycystic kidney disease: (1) a rare congenital or infantile form inherited as an autosomal-recessive trait (which may be found in stillbirths), and (2) a more common adult form inherited as an autosomal-dominant trait which leads to renal insufficiency in later life in association with dramatically enlarged, cystic kidneys.[36, 37] A genetic cause has been proposed in some domestic animal species, but patterns of inheritance have not been established. Ramsay described polycystic kidneys in a 9-year-old Thoroughbred mare that presented for anorexia and weight loss. Clinicopathologic assessment revealed chronic renal failure, and euthanasia was performed. At necropsy, the kidneys were grossly enlarged and each weighed 12 kg (Fig. 16–6).[38] A similar case of bilateral polycystic kidney disease was described in a 15-year-old pony that presented with a 4-week history of hematuria and moderate weight loss. Evaluation revealed azotemia and presence of large masses in the area of both kidneys on rectal examination and dramatically enlarged polycystic kidneys weighing 11.4 and 9.1 kg, respectively, were found at necropsy.[39] Bertone reported a third case of adult polycystic kidney disease in a 10-year-old paint gelding that presented for weight loss.[40] The horse was mildly azotemic, and several 2- to 15-cm diameter cysts were imaged in both kidneys during ultrasonographic examination. In humans, polycystic kidneys are believed to result in renal failure as cysts expand (sometimes under pressure) and compress adjacent normal renal tissue. Altered compliance of tubular basement membranes and proliferation of

renal tubular epithelium result in outflow obstruction and proximal ballooning, leading to renal cyst formation.[37] In some human cases, pressure within cysts may be five to 10 times higher than surrounding interstitial tissue pressures. Bertone found no increase in pressure in several cysts catheterized percutaneously in a gelding with polycystic kidney disease but differences in sodium concentrations suggested that the sampled cysts had arisen from different segments of the renal tubule.[40] Euthanasia was performed after a prolonged hospital course (235 days), and the kidneys were not grossly enlarged except where distorted by large cysts.

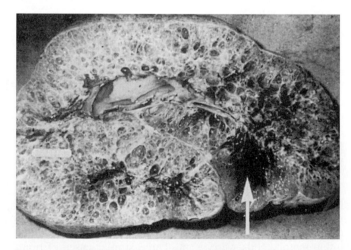

Figure 16–6. Longitudinal section of the left kidney (35 cm long, 25 cm wide, 20 cm deep, and weighing 12 kg; white bar is scale of 3 cm) from a 9-year-old Thoroughbred mare with polycystic kidneys. A calculus is located in the renal pelvis, and the arrow demonstrates the only grossly normal-looking renal parenchyma. (From Ramsey G, Rothwell TLW, Gibson KT, et al. Polycystic kidneys in an adult horse. Equine Vet J 19:243, 1987.)

Vascular Anomalies

Anomalies of the vascular supply to the equine urinary tract are rare but may result in hematuria, hemoglobinuria, partial ureteral obstruction, or hydronephrosis.[28, 41] Latimer described a distal aortic aneurysm and associated extrarenal arterioureteral fistula in a 5-month-old colt presented for intermittent hematuria, colic, and lameness.[42] Partial ureteral obstruction and hydronephrosis were observed on the affected side. Intrarenal vascular anomalies, termed *renal arteriovenous malformations,* are similarly rare (reported frequency of 0.04% in humans).[43] Interestingly, these vascular malformations may be silent until later in life, when varying degrees of hematuria and flank pain may ensue. The anomalous vessels are often tortuous and may be focally enlarged and devoid of elastic tissue. Hematuria and hemoglobinuria are thought to arise from areas where the anomalous vessels lie close to the collecting system.[43, 44] With vascular anomalies, an attempt should be made to determine the extent of the defect (unilateral or bilateral) via ultrasonographic examination, contrast radiographic studies, or cystoscopy (visualization that hematuria is coming from only one ureteral orifice). When a unilateral defect is documented in the absence of azotemia, unilateral nephrectomy or selective renal embolization has been recommended to prevent possible fatal exsanguination through the urinary tract[41, 42]; however, conservative treatment may be considered if the urinary tract bleeding is minor and has not resulted in anemia.

A large vascular anomaly resulting in transient hemoglobinuria was recently reported in a quarter horse colt.[45] Over several weeks, the large anomalous vascular structure (Fig. 16–7) spontaneously filled with a thrombus so that specific treatment (a nephrectomy) was not pursued. Severe adult-onset, idiopathic renal hemorrhage was also recently described in two horses.[46] Whether or not this latter syndrome was the consequence of congenital renal vascular malformations was not determined (see Hematuria).

Pendulant Kidney

A pendulant kidney is a rare anomaly in the horse.[47] Rectal examination reveals an extremely mobile kidney that is attached to the dorsal body wall by a thin band of tissue. Although a pendulous kidney could result from extreme weight loss, hydronephrosis, or perirenal trauma, the condition is usually thought to be congenital. The abnormality is an incidental finding unless displacement or rotation leads to partial or complete ureteral obstruction.

Ectopic Ureter

Although ureteral ectopia occurs rarely in the horse,[48] it is the most commonly reported developmental anomaly of the equine urinary tract.[49–62] Ectopic ureters may develop when (1) the ureteric bud (metanephric duct) either fails to be incorporated into the urogenital sinus or fails to migrate craniad, to the bladder neck, or (2) the mesonephric duct fails to regress. In the former case, the ectopic ureter opens near the urethral papilla in females or into the pelvic urethra near the colliculus seminalis in males, whereas in the latter, the ureter may open anywhere along the vagina, cervix, or uterus (but only in females since this portion of the mesonephric duct becomes the wolffian duct system in males). In 14 reported cases of ectopic ureter in horses, 12 (86%) were females[49–52, 56–61]; however, this sex distribution may reflect easier recognition in females of the presenting complaint of urinary incontinence rather than a true sex predilection. Incontinence is more often recognized in females because in males urine entering the pelvic urethra may pass retrograde into the bladder. Although no breed predilection has been established, quarter horses may be at greater risk; the condition has been reported in five quarter horses, two standardbreds, two Thoroughbreds, two Appaloosas, an Arabian, a Clydesdale, and a shire.

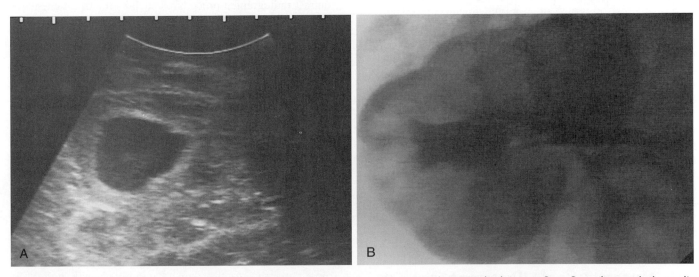

Figure 16–7. Ultrasonographic image of the right kidney of a 9-day-old quarter horse colt shows a 2 × 3 cm hypoechoic cavity on a dorsal oblique view. **A,** A swirling pattern, similar in appearance to blood in the ventricles of the heart, was consistent with an arteriovenous malformation. **B,** In a selective nephrogram of the right kidney of the same colt at 20 days of age, immediately after injection of contrast a dilated vascular space was demonstrated (contrast appears dark owing to reverse gray scale), and the renal cortical tissue abaxial to this structure appeared to have reduced capillary phase contrast. (From Schott HC, Barbee DD, Hines MT, et al. Renal arteriovenous malformation in a Quarter Horse foal. J Vet Intern Med 10:204, 1996.)

In horses with ureteral ectopia, urinary incontinence is generally apparent from birth and affected animals are presented for extensive scalding of the hindlimbs. With unilateral ectopia horses also void normally, as the other ureter enters the bladder in the appropriate location. Renal function is usually normal, but the affected ureter may be markedly dilated. Urine pooling in the vagina and uterus was a complicating factor in one case.[57] To determine the site of the ectopic ureteral orifice(s), visual examination of the vestibule and vagina (using a blade speculum) is initially performed to look for intermittent urine flow from the area of the urethral papilla. Ectopic ureteral openings usually are not apparent unless urine flow is seen. Endoscopy may be helpful in females (while inflating the vestibule and vagina with air and using a hand to form a seal at the vulva) and is required in males to visualize the ectopic ureteral opening. Intravesical placement of methylene blue dye was performed in one filly to provide evidence for ureteral ectopia. Continued dribbling of clear urine (from the ectopic ureter) followed by passage of blue, discolored urine indicated that only one ureter emptied into the bladder but provided no information on the location of the opening of the ectopic ureter.[50] Intravenous administration of dyes—including sodium fluorescein (10 mg/kg IV; yellow-green color), indigotindisulfonate (indigo carmine, 0.25 mg/kg IV; blue-purple color), azosulfamide (2.0 mg/kg IV; red color), or phenolsulfonphthalein (1.0 mg/kg IV; red color)—to discolor the urine may help locate ectopic ureteral openings.[63] Contrast radiography (excretory urography or retrograde contrast studies) has been used to detail renal architecture and the course of the ureters in affected animals.[51]

Treatment has included surgical reimplantation of the ectopic ureter into the bladder or unilateral nephrectomy. Before surgery it is imperative to determine whether the condition is unilateral or bilateral, which side is affected if unilateral, and whether urinary tract infection is present. Further, attempts should be made to rule out other anomalies, especially of the reproductive tract. If the problem is bilateral (5 of 14 cases), presence of a normal micturition response should be established by measuring the intravesicular pressure response to progressive distension until the fluid infused is voided spontaneously. This provides an estimate of bladder volume and ensures competency of the urethral sphincter before reimplantation. Among 10 cases in which surgical correction has been described, reimplantation of ectopic ureters (unilateral and bilateral) was successful in establishing a functional urinary system in seven,[51, 52, 59, 60] but three died of postoperative complications.[52, 59] In contrast, all three cases treated by unilateral nephrectomy had a favorable outcome.[56, 57] Since affected ureters are often dilated and tortuous, surgical reimplantation is difficult and may not result in a functional ureteral orifice. Consequently, when the problem is unilateral nephrectomy of the affected side may be the preferred treatment option.[64, 65]

Ureteral Defects (Ureterorrhexis)

Retroperitoneal accumulation of urine and uroperitoneum have been described in four foals with unilateral or bilateral ureteral defects.[54, 55, 66–69] A single defect was found in one foal and bilateral defects in the others; multiple defects were apparent in one ureter. In affected foals, ultrasonographic examination may reveal fluid accumulation around the kidneys or farther caudad within the retroperitoneal space, and excretory urography may identify the site of the defects.[68–70] The latter examination has not routinely been pursued since exploratory celiotomy was generally performed shortly after a diagnosis of uroperitoneum was established. Catheterization of the ureters via a cystotomy and retrograde injection of methylene blue allowed localization of the defect(s), and surgical correction was successfully performed in two cases by suturing the defect around an indwelling catheter. In all cases the defects have been limited to the proximal third of the ureter.

The cause of these ureteral defects is not known. Traumatic disruption was suggested in one case in which histologic examination of the margins of the defect revealed hemorrhage and proliferation of immature connective tissue.[65] Since the retroperitoneal location of the ureters provides good protection against trauma and because the ureters are normally under low pressure, the defects are more likely developmental malformations. A sex predilection is not apparent: two foals of each sex have been affected.

Rectourethral and Rectovaginal Fistulas

If the urorectal fold fails to completely separate the primitive hindgut from the urogenital sinus, a rectourethral fistula may be found in a colt or a rectovaginal fistula or a persistent cloaca in a filly. These anomalies are rare in horses and, when present, are usually associated with atresia ani and other anomalies, including agenesis of the coccygeal vertebrae and tail, scoliosis, adherence of the tail to the anal sphincter area, angular limb deformities, and microphthalmia.[54, 55, 71–75] Evidence for a fistula is passage of fecal material from the vagina or urethra. In fillies rectovaginal fistulas may be detected by digital palpation of the dorsal vagina, but in colts a definitive diagnosis usually requires contrast radiographic procedures such as a barium enema or a retrograde urethrogram. Surgical correction of atresia ani and fistulas have been performed successfully in several foals, but multiple surgical procedures have generally been required. In humans there is evidence that these anomalies are hereditary, and in one report several foals born with atresia ani were sired by the same stallion.[76] Consequently, affected horses should not be used for breeding after surgical correction of the anomalies.

Bladder Defects

Uroperitoneum may result from bladder rupture during parturition in foals (most commonly males)[77] or as a consequence of urachal leakage secondary to infection of the umbilical structures.[78] In addition, Wellington described uroperitoneum in two foals that were full brothers.[79] Urine entered the abdomen from a dorsal defect in both colts, and smooth margins to the defects combined with a lack of appreciable inflammation provided evidence in favor of anomalous development rather than trauma. Other authors have suggested that some cases of uroperitoneum are likely associated with anomalous bladder defects owing to the size, location, or lack of apparent inflammation of the margins of the defects.[54, 75, 80–82] For example, Bain described uroperitoneum in a foal in which the ventral portion of the bladder was absent between the lateral ligaments (umbilical artery remnants) from the umbilicus to the urethra.[80]

Anomalous fusion of the bladder to the inner umbilical ring (absence of the urachus) has been described in one foal.[83] The malformation precluded normal contraction and evacuation of the bladder, and a megavesica—a markedly enlarged bladder—developed. The clinical appearance was similar to that of uroperitoneum, and surgical separation of the bladder from the umbilical ring restored normal anatomic and functional integrity of the bladder. A similar case with a markedly distended bladder was reported in a foal evaluated for abdominal distension[54] that was attributed to an adhesion of the bladder to the urachus or umbilical remnant. An enlarged, flaccid bladder was also described in a foal undergoing exploratory celiotomy for suspected urinary tract disruption.[78] Adhesions to the abdominal wall were not reported, and the foal survived following the surgery during which 50% of the distended bladder was resected. In addition to bladder distension, persistent attachment of the bladder to the area of the umbilicus via a urachal remnant was reported to cause pollakiuria and dysuria in a 15-month-old Thoroughbred filly.[84] We have also seen post-partum bladder rupture in a mare in which a persistent urachal attachment was suspected to be a contributing factor.

Excessive bladder distension or megavesica has been further described in four stillborn foals[85] and one neonatal foal.[86] In the latter foal and in another recent report,[87] chronic bladder distension appeared to lead to loss of smooth muscle in the dorsal bladder wall and replacement with collagen. The result was bladder rupture during parturition. Although these reports are similar to an early report by Rooney describing the dorsal bladder wall as the anatomic weak link and likely area for rupture,[77] they differ in that chronic distension of the bladder in utero with smooth muscle loss is not recognized in more typical bladder ruptures in neonatal foals. It is not clear why bladder distension should occur in utero without obstruction of the lower tract (not found in these cases). Although an excessively long umbilical cord (longer than 85 cm) may lead to urachal obstruction,[85, 88] urine produced in utero could, alternatively, drain into the amniotic cavity via the urethra. Thus, this latter form of megavesica remains poorly characterized and poorly understood.

Patent Urachus

The urachus is the conduit through which fetal urine passes from the bladder into the allantoic cavity. Normally, the urachus closes at the time of parturition, but incomplete closure is the most common malformation of the equine urinary tract. Patent urachus occurs more commonly in foals than in other domestic species.[28] Greater than average length or partial torsion of the umbilical cord has been suggested to cause tension on the attachment of the umbilical cord to the body wall. The result is dilatation of the urachus and subsequent failure to close at birth.[54, 55, 85, 88, 89] Patent urachus results in a persistently moist umbilicus after birth, from which urine may leak, as drips or as a stream, during micturition. It is important to distinguish this malformation

from septic omphalitis, which can also result in urine leakage from the umbilicus within a few hours to days after birth. Patent urachus has been referred to as a congenital problem and the latter as an acquired one, but both may result in urine leakage from the urachus from birth. Neither is life threatening, but local sepsis is often accompanied by more severe illness, including septicemia or localized infection, particularly in joints.

The congenital patent urachus traditionally has been treated with frequent (two to four times daily) chemical cauterization of the urachus with swabs dipped in a concentrated phenol or 7% iodine solution or with silver nitrate applicators.[90] Since the urachus may close spontaneously in a number of cases, and because these agents desiccate and irritate tissue (and may predispose to infection) the rationale for this approach has been questioned.[89] In a recent study comparing the effects of disinfectant solutions on the bacterial flora of the umbilicus of normal foals, use of a 7% iodine solution was observed to cause rapid desiccation of the umbilical tissue and subsequent development of a patent urachus when the stump fell off a few days later.[91] Consequently, in the absence of apparent infection, no local treatment may be specifically indicated, but affected foals are frequently given prophylactic antibiotics. For acquired patency (which may be associated with local infection or septicemia), broad-spectrum antibiotic therapy is indicated and resolution of the systemic disease may be accompanied by elimination of the umbilical infection and closure of the urachus. Chemical cauterization is contraindicated with local sepsis, as it may increase the risk of urachal rupture and development of uroperitoneum.[92] If no decrease in urine leakage is observed after 5 to 7 days of medical therapy or if ultrasonography reveals abnormalities of multiple structures in the umbilicus,[93, 94] surgical exploration and resection of the urachus and umbilical vessels may be indicated. In a retrospective study of 16 foals treated for sepsis of umbilical cord remnants, six of nine (67%) survived after surgical resection and antibiotic treatment whereas only three of seven (43%) survived after antibiotic treatment alone.[95] Although this series of 16 foals is often cited in support of surgical intervention, it should be emphasized that it studied a small number of foals and that the cases were evaluated over 10 years (1975 to 1985), during which many aspects of neonatal care improved. In a more recent retrospective report of 33 foals with umbilical remnant infections, no difference in survival was observed between foals treated with antibiotics in combination with surgical resection or with antibiotic therapy alone.[94] Further, emphasis was placed on the insensitivity of palpation of the umbilicus in detection of umbilical remnant infection (in comparison with ultrasonographic examination) and the poor outcome of cases in which the umbilical vein was involved. Finally, in addition to the possibility of omphalitis leading to urachal rupture and development of uroperitoneum, urachal leakage may also occur into the abdominal musculature and subcutaneous tissues and lead to swelling and cellulitis of the ventral abdominal wall.[96, 97] In both instances surgical intervention is usually required.

REFERENCES

1. Sisson S: Equine urogenital system. In Getty R, ed. *Sisson and Grossman's The Anatomy of Domestic Animals,* ed 5. Philadelphia, WB Saunders, 1975, p 524.

2. Schummer A, Nickel F, Sack WO: *The Viscera of the Domestic Animals,* ed 2. New York, Springer-Verlag, 1979, p 298.

3. Webb AI, Weaver BQM: Body composition of the horse. *Equine Vet J* 11:39–47, 1979.

4. Calhoun ML: Comparative histology of the ureters of domestic animals. *Anat Rec* 133:365, 1959.

5. Tisher CC, Madsen KM: Anatomy of the kidney. In Brenner BM, Rector FC, eds. *The Kidney,* ed 4, Vol 1. Philadelphia, WB Saunders, 1991, p 3.

6. Rytand DA: The number and size of mammalian glomeruli as related to kidney and to body weight, with methods for their enumeration and measurement. *Am J Anat* 62:507, 1938.

7. Yadava RP, Calhoun ML: Comparative histology of the kidney of domestic animals. *Am J Vet Res* 19:958, 1958.

8. DiBona GF: The function of renal nerves. *Rev Physiol Biochem Pharmacol* 94:75, 1982.

9. DiBona GF: Neural regulation of renal tubular sodium reabsorption and renin secretion. *Fed Proc* 44:2816, 1985.

10. Trim CM, Moore JN, Clark ES: Renal effects of dopamine infusion in conscious horses. *Equine Vet J* Suppl 7:124, 1989.

11. Denton MD, Chertow GM, Brady HR: "Renal-dose" dopamine for the treatment of acute renal failure: Scientific rationale, experimental studies and clinical trials. *Kidney Int* 49:4, 1996.

12. Thurmon JC, Steffey EP, Zinkl JG, et al: Xylazine causes transient dose-related hyperglycemia and increased urine volume in mares. *Am J Vet Res* 45:224, 1984.

13. Trim CM, Hanson RR: Effects of xylazine on renal function and plasma glucose in ponies. *Vet Rec* 118:65, 1986.

14. Gellai M: Modulation of vasopressin antidiuretic action by renal α_2-adrenoceptors. *Am J Physiol* 259:F1, 1990.

15. Prieto D, Hernandez M, Rivera L, et al: Catecholaminergic innervation of the equine ureter. *Res Vet Sci* 54:312, 1994.

16. Labadía A, Rivera L, Costa G, García-Sacristán A: Alpha and beta adrenergic receptors in the horse ureter. *Rev Española Fisiol* 43:421, 1987.

17. Labadía A, Rivera L, Prieto D, et al: Influence of the autonomic nervous system in the horse urinary bladder. *Res Vet Sci* 44:282, 1988.

18. Prieto D, Benedito S, Rivera L, et al: Autonomic innervation of the equine urinary bladder. *Anat Histol Embryol* 19:276, 1990.

19. Prieto D, Benedito S, Rodrigo R, et al: Distribution and density of neuropeptide Y-immunoreactive nerve fibers and cells in the horse urinary bladder. *J Auto Nerv Sys* 27:173, 1989.

20. de Groat WC, Booth AM: Physiology of the urinary bladder and urethra. *Ann Intern Med* 92:312, 1980.

21. Patten BM, Carlson BM: *Foundations of Embryology,* ed 3. New York, McGraw-Hill, 1974, p 497.

22. Höflinger VH: Zur Kenntnis der kongenitalen unilateralen Nierenagenesie bei Haustieren II. Ihr Vorkommen bei den einzelnen Tierarten. *Schweizer Arch Tierheilkunde* 13:330, 1971.

23. Maxie MG: The urinary system. In Jubb KVF, Kennedy PC, Palmer N, eds. *Pathology of Domestic Animals,* ed 3, Vol 2. San Diego, Academic Press, 1985, p 343.

24. Huston R, Saperstein G, Leipold HW: Congenital defects in foals. *J Equine Med Surg* 1:146, 1977.

25. Johnson BD, Klingborg DJ, Heitman JM, et al: A horse with one kidney, partially obstructed ureter, and contralateral urogenital anomalies. *J Am Vet Med Assoc* 169:217, 1976.

26. Brown CM, Parks AH, Mullaney TP, et al: Bilateral renal dysplasia and hypoplasia in a foal with an imperforate anus. *Vet Rec* 122:91, 1988.

27. Schott HC, Papageorges M, Hodgson DR: Diagnosis of renal disease in the nonazotemic horse. Abstract #15. *J Vet Intern Med* 3:116, 1989.

28. Jones TC, Hunt RD: *Veterinary Pathology.* Philadelphia, Lea & Febiger, 1983, p 1443.

29. Andrews FM, Rosol TJ, Kohn CW, et al: Bilateral renal hypoplasia in four young horses. *J Am Vet Med Assoc* 189:209, 1986.

30. Taxy JB: Renal dysplasia: A review. *Pathol Annu* 20:139, 1985.

31. Roberts MC, Kelly WR: Chronic renal failure in a young pony. *Aust Vet J* 56:599, 1980.

32. Anderson WI, Picut CA, King JM, Perdrizet JA: Renal dysplasia in a Standardbred colt. *Vet Pathol* 25:179, 1988.

33. Ronen N, van Amstel SR, Nesbit JW, et al: Renal dysplasia in two adult horses: Clinical and pathological aspects. *Vet Rec* 132:269, 1993.

34. Zicker SC, Marty GD, Carlson GP, et al: Bilateral renal dysplasia with nephron hypoplasia in a foal. *J Am Vet Med Assoc* 196:2001, 1990.

35. Jones SL, Langer DL, Sterner-Kock A, et al: Renal dysplasia and benign ureteropelvic polyps associated with hydronephrosis in a foal. *J Am Vet Med Assoc* 204:1230, 1994.

36. Grantham JJ: Polycystic kidney disease: A predominance of giant nephrons. *Am J Physiol* 244:F3, 1983.

37. Gardner KD: Pathogenesis of human cystic renal disease. *Annu Rev Med* 39:185, 1988.

38. Ramsey G, Rothwell TLW, Gibson KT, et al: Polycystic kidneys in an adult horse. *Equine Vet J* 19:243, 1987.

39. Scott PC, Vasey J: Progressive polycystic renal disease in an aged horse. *Aust Vet J* 63:92, 1986.

40. Bertone JJ, Traub-Dargatz JL, Fettman MJ, et al: Monitoring the progression of renal failure in a horse with polycystic kidney disease: Use of the reciprocal of serum creatinine concentration and sodium sulfanilate clearance half-time. *J Am Vet Med Assoc* 191:565, 1987.

41. Divers TJ: Diseases of the urinary system. In Colahan PT, Mayhew IG, Merritt AM, Moore JN, eds. *Equine Medicine and Surgery,* ed 4, Vol 2. Goleta, CA, American Veterinary Publications, 1991, p 1539.

42. Latimer FG, Magnus R, Duncan RB: Arterioureteral fistula in a colt. *Equine Vet J* 23:483, 1991.

43. Crotty KL, Orihuela E, Warren MM: Recent advances in the diagnosis and treatment of renal arteriovenous malformations and fistulas. *J Urol* 150:1355, 1993.

44. Takaha M, Matsumoto A, Ochi K, et al: Intrarenal arteriovenous malformation. *J Urol* 124:315, 1980.

45. Schott HC, Barbee DD, Hines MT, et al: Renal arteriovenous malformation in a Quarter Horse foal. *J Vet Intern Med* 10:204, 1996.

46. Schott HC, Hines MT: Severe urinary tract hemorrhage in two horses (Letter). *J Am Vet Med Assoc* 204:1320, 1994.

47. Keller H: Diseases of the urinary system. In Wintzer HJ, ed. *Equine Diseases: A Textbook for Students and Practitioners.* New York, Springer-Verlag, 1986, p 148.

48. Baker JR, Ellis CE: A survey of post mortem findings in 480 horses 1958 to 1980: (1) Causes of death. *Equine Vet J* 13:43, 1981.

49. Ordidge RM: Urinary incontinence due to unilateral ureteral ectopia in a foal. *Vet Rec* 98:384, 1976.

50. Rossdale PD, Ricketts SW: *Equine Stud Farm Medicine,* ed 2. London, Baillière Tindall, 1980, p 409.

51. Christie B, Haywood N, Hilbert B, et al: Surgical correction of bilateral ureteral ectopia in a male Appaloosa foal. *Aust Vet J* 57:336, 1981.

52. Modransky PD, Wagner PC, Robinette JD, et al: Surgical correction of bilateral ectopic ureters in two foals. *Vet Surg* 12:141, 1983.

53. Modransky PD: Neoplastic and anomalous conditions of the urinary tract. In Robinson NE, ed. *Current Therapy in Equine Medicine 2.* Philadelphia, WB Saunders, 1987, p 720.

54. Richardson DW: Urogenital problems in the neonatal foal. *Vet Clin North Am: Equine Pract* 1:179, 1985.

55. Robertson JT, Embertson RM: Surgical management of congenital and perinatal abnormalities of the urogenital tract. *Vet Clin North Am: Equine Pract* 4:359, 1988.

56. Houlton JEF, Wright IM, Matic S, Herrtage ME: Urinary incontinence in a Shire foal due to ureteral ectopia. *Equine Vet J* 19:244, 1987.

57. Sullins KE, McIlwraith CW, Yovich JV, et al: Ectopic ureter managed by unilateral nephrectomy in two female horses. *Equine Vet J* 20:463, 1988.

58. MacAllister CG, Perdue BD: Endoscopic diagnosis of unilateral ectopic ureter in a yearling filly. *J Am Vet Med Assoc* 197:617, 1990.

59. Pringle JK, Ducharme NG, Baird JD: Ectopic ureter in the horse: Three cases and a review of the literature. *Can Vet J* 31:26, 1990.

60. Squire KRE, Adams SB: Bilateral ureterocystostomy in a 450-kg horse with ectopic ureters. *J Am Vet Med Assoc* 201:1213, 1992.

61. Blikslager AT, Green EM, MacFadden KE, et al: Excretory urography and ultrasonography in the diagnosis of bilateral ectopic ureters in a foal. *Vet Radiol Ultrasound* 33:41, 1992.

62. Blikslager AT, Green EM: Ectopic ureter in horses. *Compend Contin Educ Pract Vet* 14:802, 1992.

63. Rossoff IS: *Handbook of Veterinary Drugs and Chemicals*, ed 2. Taylorville, IL, Pharmatox Publishing, 1994.

64. Walker DF, Vaughan JT: *Bovine and Equine Urogenital Surgery*. Philadelphia, Lea & Febiger, 1980, p 170.

65. DeBowes RM: Kidneys and ureters. In Auer JA, ed. *Equine Surgery*. Philadelphia, WB Saunders, 1992, p 768.

66. Stickle RL, Wilcock BP, Huseman JL: Multiple ureteral defects in a Belgian foal. *Vet Med Small Anim Clin* 70:819, 1975.

67. Richardson DW, Kohn CW: Uroperitoneum in the foal. *J Am Vet Med Assoc* 182:267, 1983.

68. Robertson JT, Spurlock GH, Bramlage LR, Landry SL: Repair of ureteral defect in a foal. *J Am Vet Med Assoc* 183:799, 1983.

69. Divers TJ, Byars TD, Spirito M: Correction of bilateral ureteral defects in a foal. *J Am Vet Med Assoc* 192:384, 1988.

70. Divers TJ: Diseases of the renal system. In Smith BP, ed. *Large Animal Internal Medicine*. St. Louis, CV Mosby, 1990, p 872.

71. Gideon L: Anal agenesis with rectourethral fistula in a colt. *Vet Med* 72:238, 1977.

72. Chaudhry NI, Cheema NI: Atresia ani and rectovaginal fistula in an acaudate filly. *Vet Rec* 107:95, 1980.

73. Kingston RS, Park RD: Atresia ani with an associated urogenital tract anomaly in foals. *Equine Pract* 4(1):32, 1982.

74. Furie WS: Persistent cloaca and atresia ani in a foal. *Equine Pract* 5(1):30, 1983.

75. Crowe MW, Swerczek TW: Equine congenital defects. *Am J Vet Res* 46:353, 1985.

76. Fuchsloser RK, Rusch K: Atresia recti bei einem Vollblutfohlen. *Deutsch Tierärztl Wchnschr* 78:519, 1971.

77. Rooney J: Rupture of the urinary bladder in the foal. *Vet Pathol* 8:445, 1971.

78. Adams RA, Koterba AM, Cudd TC, et al: Exploratory celiotomy for suspected urinary tract disruption in neonatal foals: A review of 18 cases. *Equine Vet J* 20:13, 1988.

79. Wellington JKM: Bladder defects in newborn foals. *Aust Vet J* 48:426, 1972.

80. Bain AM: Diseases of foals. *Aust Vet J* 30:9, 1954

81. Pascoe RR. Repair of a defect in the bladder of a foal. *Aust Vet J* 47:343, 1971.

82. Blood DC, Radostits OM: *Veterinary Medicine: A Textbook of the Diseases of Cattle, Sheep, Pigs, Goats, and Horses*, ed 7. Philadelphia, Baillière Tindall, 1989, p 396.

83. Dubs VB: Megavesica zufolge Urachusmangel bei einem neugeborenen Fohlen. *Schweiz Arch Tierheilk* 118:395, 1976.

84. Dean PW, Robertson JT: Urachal remnant as a cause of pollakiuria and dysuria in a filly. *J Am Vet Med Assoc* 192:375, 1988.

85. Whitwell KE, Jeffcott LB: Morphological studies on the fetal membranes of the normal singleton foal at term. *Res Vet Sci* 19:44, 1975.

86. Rossdale PD, Greet TRC: Mega vesica in a newborn foal. *Int Soc Vet Perinatol Newsletter* 2(2):10, 1989.

87. Oikawa M, Yoshihara T, Katayama Y, et al: Ruptured bladder associated with smooth muscle atrophy of the bladder in a neonatal foal. *Equine Pract* 15(7):38, 1993.

88. Whitwell KE: Morphology and pathology of the equine umbilical cord. *J Reprod Fertil* Suppl 23:599, 1975.

89. Turner TA, Fessler JF, Ewert KM: Patent urachus in foals. *Equine Pract* 4(1):24, 1982.

90. Brown CM, Collier MA: Bladder diseases. In Robinson NE, ed. *Current Therapy in Equine Medicine*. Philadelphia, WB Saunders, 1983, p 567.

91. Lavan RP, Madigan J, Walker R, et al: Effect of disinfectant treatments on the bacterial flora of the umbilicus of neonatal foals. Proceedings of the 40th Annual Meeting of the American Association of Equine Practitioners, 1994, p 37.

92. Ford J, Lokai MD: Ruptured urachus in a foal. *Vet Med Small Anim Clin* 77:94, 1982.

93. Reef VB, Collatos C: Ultrasonographic examination of normal umbilical structures in the foal. *Am J Vet Res* 49:2143, 1988.

94. Reef VB, Collatos C, Spencer PA, et al: Clinical, ultrasonographic, and surgical findings in foals with umbilical remnant infections. *J Am Vet Med Assoc* 195:69, 1989.

95. Adams SB, Fessler JF: Umbilical cord remnant infections in foals: 16 cases (1975–1985). *J Am Vet Med Assoc* 190:316, 1987.

96. Madigan JE: *Manual of Equine Neonatal Care*. Woodland, CA: Live Oak, 1987, p 170.

97. Lees MJ, Easley KJ, Sutherland JV, et al: Subcutaneous rupture of the urachus, its diagnosis and surgical management in three foals. *Equine Vet J* 21:462, 1989.

16.2

Renal Physiology

Harold C. Schott II, DVM, PhD

The kidneys of all species, including those of horses, perform two essential functions in the maintenance of homeostasis: elimination of nitrogenous and organic waste products and control of body water content and ion composition. In addition, the kidneys are important endocrine organs, which produce renin, erythropoietin, and the active form of vitamin D. They also play an important role in the degradation and excretion of a number of other hormones, including gastrin and parathormone. To gain an understanding of the pathophysiologic alterations associated with renal disorders in horses, it is important first to review some aspects of normal renal physiology in this species.

PRODUCTION AND ELIMINATION OF NITROGENOUS AND ORGANIC WASTES

The two most commonly recognized waste products excreted in urine are urea and creatinine, but many other nitrogenous

Table 16–1. Compounds Excreted by the Kidneys

Urea	Creatinine
Phenols	Pyridine derivatives
Indoles	Guanidino compounds
Skatoles	β_2-Microglobulin
Hormones	Hippurate esters
Polyamines	Aliphatic amines
Trace elements	Aromatic amines
Serum proteases	Middle molecules

or organic wastes are produced each day and subsequently eliminated by the kidneys (Table 16–1).[1]

Urea Metabolism

A molecule of urea is produced in the liver from two ammonium ions which are liberated during catabolism of amino acids. For each urea molecule the carbon atom is derived from bicarbonate. One ammonium ion is cleaved from an amino acid via an α-ketoglutarate–dependent trans-amination coupled to oxidative deamination of glutamate. The second ammonium ion is derived from aspartate in the urea cycle.[2] Urea synthesized in the liver is released into the blood, and clearance by the kidneys represents the major pathway (75% to 100%) of excretion.[3] Extrarenal urea excretion include losses in sweat and through the gastrointestinal tract. With normal intestinal function, enteric excretion is minimal owing to enterohepatic recirculation (reabsorption of ammonia from the degradation of urea by bacterial ureases and subsequent reformation of urea in the liver).[3]

In humans, inborn errors of metabolism due to deficiency of a specific transaminase or of one of the five enzymes of the urea cycle can result in accumulation of ammonia and other intermediates of amino acid catabolism. These disorders are typically inherited as autosomal-recessive traits, and the consequence is moderate to severe mental retardation since the accumulated intermediates can be toxic to the central nervous system (ammonia) or can act as false neurotransmitters (aromatic amines).[1] Since in these disorders urea production is limited, blood urea nitrogen concentration (BUN) is often low.[2] Such defects in metabolism are rare in domestic animals[4] and have not been reported for horses.

BUN depends on age, diet, rate of urea production, and renal function. For example, a low BUN is typically found in neonatal foals secondary to an anabolic demand for amino acids.[5] Next, investigations of nitrogen utilization in ponies have demonstrated that urea production is proportional to dietary protein content. Similarly, urinary urea excretion increases in parallel with urea production.[6, 7] As a result, with increased levels of dietary protein or when urea is supplemented in the diet, BUN may increase twofold or greater.[8–10]

In humans and small animals, BUN is routinely higher in samples collected postprandially since diets are typically high in protein.[3] Postprandial elevation of BUN has not been described in horses or other herbivores. Fasting, on the other hand, leads to enhanced protein catabolism to meet energy demands and increased BUN in horses.[11] In ponies, however, BUN decreases with fasting.[12] This opposite response suggests differences in the metabolic responses of horses and ponies to anorexia, consistent with a greater capacity of ponies to mobilize and utilize fat during starvation. Other causes of protein catabolism, including fever, infection, trauma, myositis, burns, and corticosteroid therapy, can also produce an increase in BUN.[3] Finally, a decrease in renal blood flow (RBF) or renal function produces an increase in BUN. The former may occur with dehydration or during periods of anesthesia or exercise; the latter is a reflection of renal disease.[3] With short bouts of moderate to intensive exercise, BUN often does not change,[10, 13] but during prolonged exercise, it can increase by 50% or more, owing to the combined effects of decreased RBF and protein catabolism.[14, 15]

The majority of renal nitrogen excretion occurs in the form of urea in urine. It is important to recognize that urea excretion is completely passive and that the high concentrations achieved in urine are merely a consequence of medullary tonicity produced by the countercurrent-multiplier function of the loop of Henle. Thus, although variations in dietary protein intake lead to parallel changes in urea excretion, the idea that low-protein diets decrease the work load on the kidney is a fallacy.[3] Urinary urea nitrogen concentrations can vary from as low as 50 mg/dL in neonatal foals or horses with primary polydipsia to greater than 2500 mg/dL in normal horses on high-protein diets. Total daily urea excretion usually ranges between 100 and 300 g per day in horses with normal renal function.[5]

Creatinine Metabolism

Creatinine is produced by the nonenzymatic, irreversible cyclization and dehydration of creatine. Creatine is produced indirectly from three amino acids in the kidney, liver, and pancreas and subsequently is transported to other organs such as muscle and brain, where it is phosphorylated to store energy in the form of phosphocreatine.[3, 16] In humans, 1.5% to 2% of the creatine pool is converted to creatinine daily and results in fairly constant excretion of creatinine within a given individual.[3] With normal renal function, there is a direct relationship between daily creatinine production, serum creatinine concentration (Cr), and creatinine excretion, all three being proportional to total muscle mass. This is supported by the fact that Cr is 30% higher in human males than in females and by the finding that urinary creatinine excretion is correlated to body size across a wide range of animal species.[3, 17] Creatinine is excreted principally in urine, but sweat and the gastrointestinal tract are secondary routes of excretion.[3] In contrast to urea, enterohepatic recycling of creatinine does not occur, and the gastrointestinal tract may represent a major route of excretion when renal function is compromised. For example, in a group of azotemic human patients, between 15% and 65% of radiolabeled creatinine was found to be excreted through the intestine.[18] Creatinine excreted by this route is rapidly degraded by bacteria so that little is found in feces.

Like BUN, Cr can vary with age, activity level, and renal function. In contrast, dietary protein intake has little influence on Cr in horses.[8] Newborn foals routinely have Cr values 30% to 50% higher than those measured in the mare, and values as high as 20 to 30 mg/dL have been measured in some premature or asphyxiated foals.[5] These high values may be the result of limited diffusion of creatinine across the placenta. For example, the Cr in equine amniotic fluid collected at term is proportionately much greater than urea nitrogen concentration (Cr, 10.1 mg/dL; UN, 38.8 mg/dL).[19] If the foal appears healthy and all other laboratory values are within reference ranges, a serum Cr value in the range of 5 to 15 mg/dL should not cause alarm. In most healthy foals with normal renal function, Cr decreases to values below 3.0 mg/dL within the first 3 to 5 days of life.[18] After the first week of life, Cr is actually lower in foals than in adults.[9] This is due to the combined effect of rapid growth and the fact that skeletal muscle comprises a smaller percentage of body weight in foals than in adult horses. Other nonrenal factors that may influence Cr include fasting, rhabdomyolysis or muscle wasting consequent to disease, and exercise. Although fasting can increase the measured value for Cr, a substantial portion of this increase is actually due to other compounds (possibly ketones) that increase during fasting and are measured as noncreatinine chromagens in the commonly used Jaffé colorimetric assay for Cr determination (see Examination of the Urinary System).[9, 11, 20] In contrast, the increase in Cr (up to 80% in some reports) associated with various types of exercise is likely the combined result of increased release of creatine from muscle and decreased urinary creatinine excretion during the exercise bout.[9, 11, 13–15]

Creatinine is freely filtered at the glomerulus and is concentrated to values of 100 to 300 mg/dL in equine urine. This results in a total daily urine excretion of 15 to 25 g of creatinine.[21, 22] In comparison to urea, creatinine excretion is responsible for only one tenth as much urinary nitrogen excretion. Minor species and sex differences have been reported for renal tubular handling of creatinine with a weak proximal tubular secretory mechanism in humans and male dogs (accounting for 7% to 10% of total urinary creatinine excretion).[3, 16] To determine whether tubular secretion of creatinine occurs in equine kidneys, Finco instrumented anesthetized ponies with ureteral catheters and performed simultaneous inulin and exogenous creatinine clearance studies.[23] Since inulin is freely filtered at the glomerulus and neither secreted nor reabsorbed by renal tubules, inulin clearance (Cl_{In}) provides a standard of comparison for creatinine clearance (Cl_{Cr}). Tubular secretion of creatinine should result in a greater value for Cl_{Cr} than for Cl_{In}, whereas the opposite should occur with tubular reabsorption of creatinine. To magnify any minor tubule secretion of creatinine, stop-flow studies were performed by temporarily occluding the ureteral catheters. During obstruction, tubular lumen pressure increased and tubuler flow decreased. As a consequence, fluid remained in contact with tubule epithelium for a prolonged period, enhancing local tubule secretory or resorptive processes. Analysis of a series of urine samples collected after release of ureteral occlusion revealed no differences in tubular handling of inulin or creatinine, leading to the conclusion that creatinine was neither reabsorbed nor secreted by equine kidneys. In contrast, simultaneous measurement of endogenous Cl_{Cr} and Cl_{In} in several horses with chronic renal failure (authors' unpublished observations) has revealed higher values for Cl_{Cr}, indicating that tubule secretion of creatinine may develop in horses as renal function declines (see

Chronic Renal Failure). Whether or not significant excretion of creatinine occurs in sweat or through the gastrointestinal tract has not been investigated in horses.

Metabolism of Other Nitrogenous and Organic Compounds

Although the kidneys excrete a number of nitrogenous and organic wastes in addition to urea and creatinine (see Table 16–1), these compounds are quantitatively unimportant in terms of nitrogen balance.[1] Two of the more commonly recognized molecules are ammonia and uric acid. In proximal tubule epithelial cells, ammonium ions and α-ketoglutarate are produced from glutamine. Subsequent metabolism of α-ketoglutarate results in generation of two bicarbonate molecules that are returned to the systemic circulation. Ammonium ions are secreted in exchange for sodium into the tubule lumen, where they remain trapped, since tubules are relatively impermeable to ammonium ions. Further, since the pK_a for ammonia is greater than 9.0, the vast majority of tubule ammonia remains in the form of ammonium ions, even in relatively alkaline equine urine. Although ammonium ion excretion is of little significance in overall nitrogen excretion, it plays an important role in acid (hydrogen ion) excretion. In fact, glutamine metabolism and ammonium ion excretion can increase severalfold in response to metabolic acidosis.[24] Although urinary ammonium concentration is not routinely measured, it can be estimated because it is directly related to the urinary anion gap ($[Na^+ + K^+] - Cl^-$) in human patients with normal anion gap metabolic acidosis.[25] More important, impairment of this proximal tubule acid secretion pathway contributes to development of metabolic acidosis in patients with renal insufficiency.

Uric acid is a product of purine nucleotide degradation and is the major nitrogenous waste product formed in amphibians and reptiles. In mammals, however, uric acid excretion (most in the ionic form of urate) is comparatively unimportant in terms of overall nitrogen excretion.[26] Uric acid metabolism has received little attention in veterinary species with the exception of Dalmation dogs. This breed exhibits high urate excretion rates and is predisposed to uric acid stone formation; however, this problem is a consequence of decreased hepatic uricase activity rather than any abnormality in renal urate handling.[27] Finally, hyperuricemia (leading to gout in humans) can also be attributed to a lack of uricase activity in human tissues and greater renal reabsorption of urate as compared with other mammalian species. Thus, crystallization of urate in tissues appears to be limited to humans.[26] Urate metabolism has been little studied in horses, although Keenan observed that plasma concentrations increased dramatically in response to exercise (from less than 1 μmol/L at rest to 150 to 200 μmol/L 1 hour after racing) and that these increases were accompanied by a transient increase in urinary urate excretion (from less than 40 μmol/L at rest to 250 to 1270 μmol/L after racing).[13]

The proximal tubule is also the major site of excretion (by tubular secretion) of a number of endogenous organic anions and cations.[26] The anions share the common pathway measured by p-aminohippurate clearance, the substance traditionally used to measure effective renal plasma flow (since more than 90% is excreted via this pathway). A number of exogenous compounds are also excreted via these pathways—acetazolamide, furosemide, probenecid, penicillin G, sulfadiazine, salicylate, atropine, cimetidine, and neostigmine. Thus, administration of these compounds can interfere with tubular secretion of endogenous organic wastes or other exogenous products by healthy kidneys.[28] More important, pharmacokinetics of these products vary widely in patients with renal insufficiency. Combined with the fact that anion binding to plasma proteins is decreased with azotemia, dosing protocols of many medications must be readjusted for patients with renal failure.

BODY WATER AND ELECTROLYTE BALANCE

Body Fluids: Volume and Composition

Water accounts for 60% of total body weight, equivalent to 300 L in a 500-kg horse.[29-31] About 200 L of total body water is intracellular fluid, and the remaining 100 L is extracellular fluid. Extracellular fluid is divided between plasma (4% to 6% of body weight, ≈ 25 L), interstitial fluid and lymph (10% to 12% of body weight, ≈ 45 L), and transcellular fluid (6% to 10% of body weight, ≈ 30 L, the majority in the lumen of the gastrointestinal tract). Despite marked differences in ion composition (Table 16–2), the extracellular fluid and intracellular fluid exchange water freely to maintain osmotic equilibrium.[32]

From the values in Table 16–2, the total amount of exchangeable sodium, potassium, and chloride in the body fluids of a 500-kg horse can be estimated: ≈ 16,000 mEq, ≈ 28,800 mEq, and ≈ 10,800 mEq, respectively (including gastrointestinal fluid ion contents). These values are accurate except for that of sodium which may be twice as great;

Table 16–3. Water Balance in Hay Fed Horses in a Cool Climate

Water Intake (L)		Water Loss (L)	
Consumption	23.6	Feces	14.0
Hay	1.1	Urine	4.9
Metabolic	2.7	Insensible	8.5
Total	27.4	Total	27.4

Data from Tasker JB: Fluid and electrolyte studies in the horse. III. Intake and output of water, sodium, and potassium in normal horses. *Cornell Vet* 57:649, 1967.

however, 40% to 50% is sequestered in bone and is not readily available to buffer sodium alterations in body fluids.[29-31] Thus, the 16,000-mEq estimate is accurate for the exchangeable sodium content in body fluids. Similarly, body fluid contents of calcium, magnesium, and phosphorus can be estimated at ≈ 1000 mEq (20 g), ≈ 6875 mEq (84 g), and ≈ 8150 mEq (140 g), respectively (excluding gastrointestinal fluid ion contents, since these vary with the amount and solubility of the dietary source). As for sodium, the values underestimate the total body content of calcium, magnesium, and phosphorus, since more than 99%, 70%, and 85%, respectively, are contained in the skeleton.[33]

Water Balance

Appropriate water balance maintains plasma osmolality in a relatively narrow range (270 to 300 mOsm/kg) and is achieved by matching daily water intake with water loss.[34-36] Water is provided from three sources: (1) free water intake (drinking); (2) water in feed; and (3) metabolic water (Table 16–3). Most water is consumed by drinking (about 85%), but feed and metabolic water provide about 5% and 10% of daily water, respectively. Water is lost by three routes: (1) in urine; (2) in feces; and (3) as insensible losses (evaporation) across the skin and respiratory tract (Table 16–3). Investigations of water balance have revealed a maintenance water requirement of 60 to 65 mL/kg per day or 27 to 30 L/day for a 500-kg horse.[34, 37] These values are consistent with traditional recommendations that 5 to 10 gallons/day of fresh water be provided to a stabled horse under mild environmental conditions.[38] Urinary and fecal water losses range from 20% to 55% and 30% to 55%, respectively, of the total daily water loss.[34, 37, 39, 40] The remaining (insensible) loss accounted for up to 15% to 40% of daily water loss, despite mild ambient conditions and the lack of observed sweating in most studies of water balance.

Water drinking and urine production are the mechanisms by which water balance is finely tuned; however, they can vary widely between individual horses and are also affected by age, environmental conditions, level of exercise, and diet. Often, for example, neonatal foals daily consume milk in excess of 20% of their body weight.[41] This equates to fluid intake approaching 250 mL/kg per day. Next, water intake by horses increased 15% to 20% when ambient temperature increased from 13 °C to 25 °C.[42] Under conditions of high ambient temperature and humidity, urine concentration may

Table 16–2. Approximate Ionic Compositions (mEq/L) of Plasma, Interstitial Fluid, and Intracellular Fluid (Skeletal Muscle)

Electrolyte	Plasma	Interstitial Fluid	Skeletal Muscle Cell
Cations			
Na^+	140	143	10
K^+	4.0	4.1	142
Ca^{++}	5.5	2.4	4.0
Mg^{++}	1.1	1.1	34
Total	147.6	150.6	190
Anions			
Cl^-	100	113	4
HCO_3^-	25	28.2	12
$H_2PO_4^-$, HPO_4^{-2}	2.0	2.3	40
Protein	14	0.0	50
Other	6.6	7.1	84*
Total	147.6	150.6	190

*This largely represents organic phosphates such as ATP.

Adapted from Rose BD: Physiology of body fluids. In Clinical Physiology of Acid-Base and Electrolyte Disorders, ed 3. New York, McGraw-Hill, 1989, p 20.

also increase to conserve water whereas fecal water content tends to remain fairly stable, at $\approx$ 75% of fecal weight. Exercising horses, especially endurance horses and racing horses treated with furosemide, can increase water consumption by 100% to 200% to replace body water lost in sweat (and urine). Horses and ponies on all-roughage diets also drink more and have greater daily fecal water loss (owing to greater daily fecal volume) than animals fed a large amount of concentrate or complete pelleted diets.[39, 40] Diets high in nitrogen (protein) and calcium, such as legume hays, typically increase urine volume by 50% or more and are associated with a similar increase in urinary nitrogen excretion. These diets are relatively more digestible, so that fecal water excretion generally decreases, consequent to a decrease in total fecal material.[6, 11, 39, 40] Although high dietary levels of salt have been suggested to increase drinking and promote diuresis, no increase in water consumption or urine volume was observed in ponies fed five to ten times the daily salt requirement (equivalent to about 350 g of sodium chloride for a 500-kg horse).[43] The effects of water access, continuous versus intermittent, have received less attention, although a recent study showed no difference in water balance in horses provided water three times daily as compared with horses that had continuous access to water.[44] Further, most water is drunk within the hour after feeding,[45] and feral horses and ponies often drink only once or twice daily.[46] Thus, it is unlikely that horses require continuous access to water. An obvious exception is a patient with renal insufficiency, which should have access to fresh water at all times.

There are two main stimuli for thirst: increased plasma osmolality and hypovolemia or hypotension.[47] The former is mediated through osmoreceptors in the hypothalamus that have a rather high threshold for activation (about 295 mOsm/kg) in humans. Hemodynamic stimuli are mediated by both low- and high-pressure baroreceptors. Both osmotic and hemodynamic stimuli can produce their dipsogenic effect, in part, by activating a local renin-angiotensin-aldosterone system in the central nervous system.[48]

Renal water reabsorption is controlled principally by the action of arginine vasopressin (antidiuretic hormone) on the collecting ducts.[49] Vasopressin is produced in the neurosecretory neurons of the supraoptic nuclei, packaged in granules, and transported down axons for storage in the neurohypophysis (pars nervosa or posterior pituitary). As for thirst, an increase in plasma osmolality and hypovolemia or hypotension are the stimuli for vasopressin release. Osmoreceptors for vasopressin release are also located in the hypothalamus, adjacent to the osmoreceptors mediating thirst. Activation of these receptors is the signal for vasopressin release from the neurohypophysis. Further, these osmoreceptors are not equally sensitive to all plasma solutes. For example, increases in plasma sodium concentration and infusion of mannitol are potent stimuli, whereas increases in plasma glucose and urea concentrations are weak stimuli. These differences have led to the suggestion that osmoreceptor activation is caused by an osmotic water shift that produces cell shrinkage (which would be greater for sodium and mannitol than for glucose or urea). There also appears to be a threshold value for activation of osmoreceptors signaling vasopressin release; however, this threshold appears to be highly variable between individuals. In addition, the threshold for vasopressin release in humans is significantly lower

(270 to 285 mOsm/kg) than that for thirst. Thus, vasopressin release can be thought of as the initial line of defense against a mild increase in plasma osmolality, whereas thirst and drinking are secondary responses to even greater increases.

Studies in horses, ponies, and donkeys have demonstrated that both increased plasma osmolality (induced by water deprivation or infusion of hypertonic saline) and hypovolemia (induced by furosemide administration) are stimuli for thirst.[44, 49-53] Further, after a period of water deprivation, dehydrated ponies, horses, and donkeys appear to be able to replace water deficits within 15 to 30 minutes of gaining access to water. The increases in plasma osmolality and vasopressin concentration associated with water deprivation are also corrected in this same period of time, indicating that imbibed water is rapidly absorbed from the gastrointestinal tract.[50] Although increases in plasma vasopressin concentration have been measured in horses and ponies during water deprivation,[50, 54] vasopressin also appears to be a "stress hormone" in equidae, since substantially greater concentrations (10-fold greater than those induced by water deprivation) have been measured after application of a nose twitch, nasogastric intubation, or exercise.[55, 56] Thus, increases in plasma vasopressin concentration subsequent to water deprivation would be expected to vary in horses, and it may sometimes be difficult to separate osmotic effects from "stress" effects.

Once released, vasopressin acts on V_2 receptors on the basolateral membrane of collecting duct epithelial cells, leading to insertion of water channels (transmembrane proteins) in the apical membrane.[47] These channels increase the water permeability of the apical membranes and lead to increased water reabsorption. Action of V_2 receptors is mediated by activation of adenyl cyclase and a stimulatory transmembrane G protein. Of interest, V_2-receptor activation can be antagonized by activation of adjacent α_2-adrenoceptors and by a prostaglandin E_2–mediated effect on an inhibitory G protein.[57, 58] Although effects of these antagonists vary with species and have not yet been studied in horses, it is likely that the diuresis associated with administration of α_2-agonists to horses[59, 60] may be attributed to vasopressin antagonism at the collecting duct.

As mentioned above, most water drinking in equidae occurs periprandially; thus, feeding practices affect timing of water intake.[45] As the horse eats a large meal once or twice daily, both increased plasma sodium concentration and decreased plasma volume (owing to a shift of fluid into the bowel) stimulate thirst and vasopressin release. The result is a simultaneous increase in water intake and a decrease in urine output.[61] In addition, hypovolemia further stimulates activation of the renin-angiotensin-aldosterone system, which leads to enhanced renal sodium conservation as an additional means of restoring plasma volume. Although the increase in plasma sodium concentration with meal feeding is rather small (1% to 3%), the decrease in plasma volume is much greater (5% to 25%). The magnitude of this fluid shift (and the degree of activation of the renin-angiotensin-aldosterone system) can be largely attenuated by feeding multiple small meals four to six times throughout the day.[62, 63] Thus, more frequent feeding causes less perturbation of body fluids and likely has a protective effect against development of some forms of colic.

Although balance of daily water intake and output is

Table 16–4. Water and Electrolyte Balance in Horses Receiving a Low-Sodium Diet (Alfalfa-Timothy Hay)

	Intake	Urinary Loss	Fecal Loss	Unmeasured*
Tasker (1967)†				
Water (L)	27.4	4.9	14	8.5 (31%)
Sodium (mEq)	329	7	116	206 (63%)
Potassium (mEq)	3930	2196	993	741 (19%)
Groenendyk et al (1988)§				
Water (L)	27.6‡	9.9	7.2	10.5 (38%)
Sodium (mEq)	986	527	253	206 (21%)
Potassium (mEq)	3320	2661	504	155 (5%)
Chloride (mEq)	3008	2347	174	487 (16%)

*Unmeasured losses include insensible water losses as well as electrolyte losses thought to occur in sweat; value in parenthesis is the percentage represented by these unmeasured losses.
†Tasker JB: Fluid and electrolyte studies in the horse. III. Intake and output of water, sodium, and potassium in normal horses. *Cornell Vet* 57:649, 1967.
‡Water intake includes imbibed water (23.6 L), water in feed (1.1 L), and metabolic water (2.9 L).
§Groenendyk S, English PB, Abetz I: External balance of water and electrolytes in the horse. *Equine Vet J* 20:189, 1988.

critical for maintenance of homeostasis, it warrants mention that equidae tolerate water deprivation quite well.[64–70] For example, after horses were deprived of water for 72 hours (which resulted in body weight loss in excess of 10%), the majority of the weight lost (90% of which was assumed to be water) was recovered within the first hour of their being provided access to water.[67] Similarly, even greater body weight losses (approaching 20%) induced by water deprivation and desert walking in donkeys and burros were largely replaced within the first few minutes after water was provided.[65, 66] Thus, in terms of water balance, equidae (especially donkeys and burros) can truly be considered desert-adapted animals.[70, 71] An important reason for their ability to tolerate water deprivation appears to be a substantial intestinal reserve of water and electrolytes that can be called upon during periods of dehydration for the maintenance of plasma volume.[72, 73] Despite rapid fluid replacement by equidae that have been dehydrated by water deprivation, horses that become dehydrated as a consequence of prolonged exercise or diarrheal disease (colitis) often do not drink. This can be attributed to the fact that these conditions produce loss of both body water and osmoles in the form of sweat or diarrhea. As a result, plasma osmolality does not increase and osmotic thirst stimulus is not produced. In human endurance athletes this state of mild to moderate dehydration that does not induce thirst has been called "voluntary dehydration,"[74] and, although it is not well-documented, a similar response appears to occur in endurance horses. Another form of voluntary dehydration, which may be accompanied by increases in plasma osmolality and protein concentration, has also been described anecdotally in postfoaling mares.

Electrolyte Balance

Intake and loss of electrolytes must also be appropriately matched to maintain body content of electrolytes within relatively narrow ranges. This balance is most important for the exchangeable ions (Na^+, K^+, and Cl^-), as these have minimal tissue (skeletal) reserves that can be called on during times of need. An exception is the fluid and electro-

lyte reserve in the lumen of the gastrointestinal tract, which may be able to provide replacement of 10% or more of the body content of these electrolytes.[73] Electrolytes are provided from three sources: in feed; in water (usually minimal amounts); and in the form of a number of dietary supplements. Electrolytes are also lost by three routes: in urine; in feces; and in sweat (insensible losses; Table 16–4). Investigations of electrolyte balance have revealed that most horses that eat predominantly hay or pasture grass ingest excess potassium and chloride. In contrast, sodium intake is variable and with some diets may be marginal.[34, 36, 37] A maintenance requirement for sodium of 0.4 to 0.8 mEq/kg per day or 200 to 400 mEq per day (6 to 12 g per day) for a 500-kg horse has been suggested[37, 52]; however, exercising horses, which lose 500 to 1000 mEq of sodium per hour in sweat or are treated with furosemide have greater dietary requirements to replace such losses.[36] Thus, addition of 50 to 75 g of common salt (which provides 850 to 1275 mEq, since 1 g NaCl provides ≈ 17 mEq Na^+) is both a safe and economic method of providing daily supplemental sodium and chloride to athletic horses.

The data from the water and electrolyte balance studies performed by Tasker and by Groenendyk (see Table 16–4) provide a good illustration of the equine kidneys' capacity to conserve sodium when dietary intake is low (Tasker's data at top) in comparison to when intake is unlimited (Groenendyk's data at bottom).[34, 37] Further, these studies demonstrate that urinary excretion is the major route for loss of both potassium and chloride. Although dietary intake of potassium is usually excessive, equine kidneys do not appear to have a great capacity to conserve potassium during periods of food and water deprivation or with anorexia associated with disease.[34, 36, 75] Thus, urinary potassium concentration and total excretion can remain substantial in the face of decreased intake. Consequently, with decreased feed intake horses can develop significant total body potassium depletion and often benefit from supplemental dietary potassium (25 to 50 g per day of KCl provides 375 to 750 mEq, since 1 g KCl provides ≈ 15 mEq K^+).

In horses, the stimuli for electrolyte intake ("salt appetite") have received much less attention than has water balance. Houpt found that horses whose sodium intake was marginal (250 mEq per day) and that were treated with furosemide ate more salt in the hours after treatment than did placebo-treated horses on the same diet[52]; however, salt intake (which was comparable for eating salt from a block and drinking a 0.9% sodium chloride solution) was excessive in both treatment groups (in excess of 100 g). Thus, salt appetite, unlike water intake, is not closely regulated to balance intake with losses. In fact, when salt is available ad libitum, it appears that horses consume more than their maintenance needs. The excess is eliminated by increasing urinary sodium excretion. Although this apparently excessive salt appetite may seem inappropriate, it could also be considered advantageous for exercising horses, which have a much greater daily salt requirement.

RENAL REGULATION OF BODY WATER CONTENT AND ION COMPOSITION

The kidneys are the organs responsible for fine tuning body water content and ion composition within relatively narrow ranges. The important components of renal regulation of water and ion content include renal blood flow, glomerular filtration, and tubular modification of glomerular filtrate to produce the final urine.

Renal Blood Flow

At rest, the kidneys receive about 15% to 20% of the cardiac output, or about 7.5 to 10 L per minute for an average-sized horse.[76, 77] This relatively high tissue perfusion, 500 to 600 mL/min per 100 g of kidney, in comparison to 50 to 100 mL/min per 100 g of brain tissue, is necessary for the kidney to function both as an effective filter and as a regulator of extracellular fluid composition. Further, tubule resorption of glomerular filtrate requires energy. Since more than 99% of the filtrate is reabsorbed, the kidneys' metabolic rate is high (second only to the heart's), and despite the fact that the kidneys account for less than 1% of body weight they are responsible for about 10% of whole body oxygen utilization.[78] Next, renal blood flow (RBF) is preferentially distributed to the renal cortex. In fact, renal medullary blood flow, which is derived entirely via the vasa recta which arise from the efferent arterioles of juxtamedullary glomeruli, accounts for less than 20% of total RBF.[77] As a consequence, the inner medullary tissue normally functions in a relatively hypoxic environment.

RBF of horses has been measured by a variety of techniques including p-aminohippurate clearance (Cl_{PAH}, by classic clearance techniques involving timed urine collections and by plasma disappearance curves), clearance of radionuclides, microsphere injection, and use of ultrasonic Doppler flow probes placed around the renal artery (Table 16–5).[76, 77, 79–92] The latter technique does not provide absolute blood flow values but rather measures changes in RBF from a baseline value.[92] Recently, plasma disappearance curves for ^{131}I-orthoiodohippuric acid (^{131}I-OIH) were documented in normal horses in an attempt to establish a radionuclide technique for rapid and noninvasive measurement of RBF in

hospitalized horses.[90] Although this study demonstrated that the radionuclide technique compared well with Cl_{PAH} (the gold standard), its future use in a clinical setting will likely remain limited owing to expense (about $100 per measurement).[93]

Both intrinsic and extrinsic factors play a role in the control of RBF. The former include autoregulation and action of renal nerves; the latter, vasoconstrictors (catecholamines, renin-angiotensin system, arginine vasopressin) and vasodilators (prostaglandins, atrial peptides, dopamine, bradykinin, adenosine).[94] Although not unique to the kidney, autoregulation of blood flow is a physiologic response that maintains RBF in the normal range through a rather wide range of perfusion pressures (75 to 180 mm Hg in humans). This response is independent of neural or hormonal mechanisms and is attributed to a myogenic response to changes in arterial wall tension. The local action of renal nerves or release of vasoconstrictor substances leads to an increase in renal vascular resistance. This may occur in response to disease states (hypovolemic or endotoxic shock), drugs (anesthesia), or physical stress (exercise). RBF may or may not decrease, depending on the degree of vasoconstriction. For example, during low-intensity exercise renal vascular resistance increases to divert a greater portion of the cardiac output to the working muscles. Thus, the fraction of cardiac output delivered to the kidneys decreases; however, since cardiac output also increases in response to exercise, total RBF remains unchanged.[87] In contrast, during halothane anesthesia in ponies, redistribution of cardiac output occurs without an increase in cardiac output. Under these circumstances, renal vasoconstriction is accompanied by a decrease in renal blood flow to about 60% of the awake value at 1.0 to 1.5 minimal alveolar concentration of halothane. As the plane of anesthesia deepens (to 2.0 minimal alveolar concentration), a greater increase in renal vascular resistance (or degree of vasoconstriction) further decreases RBF to about 25% of the awake value, likely owing to further vasodilatation of other vascular beds and a mild decrease in cardiac output.[83]

When RBF decreases, counteracting vasodilatory mediators are usually released in an attempt to ameliorate the decrease in RBF. The best-studied of these vasodilatory mediators include renal prostaglandins (PGI_2 and PGE_2) and dopamine. While the role of renal prostaglandins in the control of basal or resting renal blood flow is thought to be insignificant, renal prostaglandins are important mediators of vasodilatation in response to a number of vasoconstrictive stimuli.[95] Further, the production of renal prostaglandins is several times greater in medullary tissue, so that action of these mediators leads to a greater increase in inner cortical (region of juxtamedullary glomeruli) and medullary blood flow. In light of this fact, it is not surprising that the lesion associated with nonsteroidal antiinflammatory drug toxicity is renal medullary crest necrosis (secondary to ischemia).[96, 97]

With or without renal vasoconstriction, activation of dopamine receptors (DA_1 type) leads to renal vasodilatation. Since the receptors are located on most renal arterioles, blood flow increases in both the renal cortex and the medulla. For this reason dopamine infusions may be of benefit in the treatment of acute renal failure, as this catecholamine has been shown to increase RBF and urine output by 30% to 190% in normal horses.[92] Finally, peptides recently iso-

Table 16–5. Reported Values for Effective Renal Plasma Flow and Renal Blood Flow in Horses and Ponies

Investigator	Animals (No.)	Method[a]	Effective Renal Plasma Flow (mL/min/kg [range])	Renal Blood Flow (mL/min/kg[b])
Knudsen (1959)[79]	1 ♀ horse	$Cl_{Diodrast}$	6.91 ± 0.81	13.2 ± 1.6
Paul (1973)[80 c]	1 ♀ pony	$Cl_{131I-o-HA}$	Bolus injection: 12.85 ± 1.81	21.7 ± 3.1
			Constant infusion: 11.45 ± 1.25	19.4 ± 2.1
	3 ♀ horses	$Cl_{131I-o-HA}$	Bolus injection: 11.97 ± 2.63	20.2 ± 4.4
			Constant infusion: 9.56 ± 1.84	16.2 ± 3.1
Zatzman et al (1982)[81]	6 ♀ ponies	Cl_{PAH}	12.09 ± 0.34 (7.86–21.62)	20.4 ± 0.6
	2 ♀ horses		9.59 ± 0.86 (4.75–19.78)	16.2 ± 1.4
Hood et al (1982)[82]	5 ♀ and ♂g[d] horses	$Cl_{131I-o-HA}$	8.24 ± 2.88 (5.66–12.89)	13.9 ± 4.9
Brewer et al (1990)[85]	8 ♀ horses	Cl_{PAH}	Bolus injection: 12.0 ± 1.7	20.3 ± 2.9
	4-day-old foals		Bolus injection: 15.2 ± 1.5	25.7 ± 2.7
	5 horse foals (3 ♂, 2 ♀)		Infusion (Cl-plasma): 18.2 ± 2.0	30.8 ± 3.4
	3 pony foals (1 ♂, 2 ♀)		Infusion (Cl-urine): 11.9 ± 1.9	20.1 ± 3.2
Hinchcliff et al (1990)[86]	6 ♀ horses	Cl_{PAH}	8.5–10.8[e]	14.4–18.3
Schott et al (1991)[87]	6 ♀ horses	Cl_{PAH}	11.9 ± 1.0	20.0 ± 1.7
Held and Daniel (1991)[88]	6 horses[f]	$Cl_{131I-o-HA}$	6.26 (4.33–6.80)	10.58 (7.32–11.50)
Matthews et al (1992)[90]	8 ♀ horses	Cl_{PAH}	9.65 ± 0.84 (5.60–12.54)	16.31 ± 1.42
		$Cl_{131I-o-HA}$	11.32 ± 1.03 (7.82–15.71)	19.14 ± 1.74
Staddon et al (1979)[77]	4 ponies[f]	Microspheres	—	208 ± 58[g,h]
Parks and Manohar (1983)[76]	11 ponies[f]	Microspheres	—	548 ± 87[g]
Manohar and Goetz (1985)[83]	8 ponies[f]	Microspheres	—	483 ± 79[g]
Manohar (1987)[84]	11 ponies[f]	Microspheres	—	670 ± 50[e,g]
Armstrong et al (1992)[89]	3 horses (♀, ♂, and ♂g)	Microspheres	—	535 ± 93[g]
Manohar et al (1995)[91]	9 horses[f]	Microspheres	—	589.5 ± 50[g]

[a]$Cl_{Diodrast}$, clearance of 3,5-diiodo-4-pyridine-N-acetic acid; $Cl_{131I-o-HA}$, clearance of ^{131}I-o-iodohippurate; Cl_{PAH}, clearance of p-aminohippurate.

[b]RBF values presented have been calculated from effective renal plasma flow (ERPF) data using extraction ratios (ER) of 0.80 for Diodrast and 0.91 for ^{131}I-o-iodohippurate and p-aminohippurate: RBF = (ERPF/ER)/(1-hematocrit); hematocrit was assumed to be 0.35.

[c]Other horses and ponies were also studied following bolus injection of ^{131}I-o-iodohippurate and yielded ERPF values of 16.93 ± 6.05 and 10.65 ± 2.73 mL/min/kg for ponies and horses, respectively; these values corresponded to a RBF of 28.6 ± 10.2 mL/min/kg in ponies and 18.0 ± 4.6 mL/min/kg in horses.

[d]♂g = gelding.

[e]Values estimated from figure.

[f]Sex not reported.

[g]RBF values for microsphere studies are expressed in units of mL/min/100 g of kidney tissue; a value of 500 mL/min/100 g would correlate to a RBF value of 18 mL/min/kg (or 3.6 and 9 L/min for a 200-kg pony or a 500-kg horse, respectively).

[h]Values reported are for ponies under general anesthesia (halothane in oxygen); these authors also reported that renal medullary blood flow was 2.6–18.8% of total RBF in two ponies.

lated from the atrial myocardium have been demonstrated to have vasodilatory, diuretic, and natriuretic (increasing sodium excretion) effects on the kidneys. Owing to their effects on sodium excretion, the peptides have been termed "atrial natriuretic factor(s)." Similar atrial peptides have been found in equine plasma and their concentrations increase in response to increases in atrial pressure (distension).[98]

Glomerular Filtration

Approximately 20% of the blood entering the glomeruli passes through small pores in the filtration barrier into Bowman's capsule. The primary force driving filtration is glomerular capillary transmural hydraulic pressure. A relatively constant pressure across the glomerular capillary wall is maintained by greater resistance in the arteriole leaving the glomerulus (efferent arteriole) than in the arteriole entering the glomerulus (afferent arteriole). This difference in vascular resistance generates the hydraulic pressure that forces plasma water out of the glomerular capillaries.[99] The filtration barrier is made up of three layers: endothelium of the glomerular capillaries, basement membrane, and foot processes of the epithelial cells (podocytes) lining Bowman's capsule. The pore size of the filtration barrier, about 8 to 10 nm in diameter, prevents filtration of cells and larger proteins. As a result, the fluid that enters Bowman's capsule is an ultrafiltrate that is essentially identical to plasma except that it has less than 0.05% of the protein content of plasma. Interestingly, the diameter of albumin is about 6 nm, so its size should not prevent filtration. Glycosaminoglycans containing heparan sulfate and sialic acid residues impart a significant negative charge to the filtration barrier. Thus, charge repulsion of albumin (which is similarly negatively charged) may be more important than molecular size in preventing significant loss of albumin into the filtrate; however, with metabolic disturbances (metabolic acidosis) the glomerular charge barrier can be neutralized and transient proteinuria can be observed in the absence of structural damage to the glomerular barrier.[100]

Glomerular filtration rate (GFR), by definition, is the volume of plasma filtered per unit of time and is commonly described in milliliters per minute per kilogram of body weight. The GFR of horses and ponies is in the range of 1.6 to 2.0 mL/kg per minute, some authors reporting slightly higher values for ponies. This range is similar to those of other animals and humans. For a 500-kg horse this value equals 800 to 1000 mL per minute or about 1200 to 1400 L per day. This value represents filtration of the total plasma volume 60 to 70 times per day. Since urine production is about 10 L per day, more than 99% of the glomerular filtrate is reabsorbed.

Like RBF, GFR has been measured in horses by a variety of techniques, including inulin clearance (Cl_{IN}, by classic clearance techniques), clearance of endogenous or exogenous creatinine, and clearance or plasma disappearance of radionuclides (Table 16–6).[21–23, 79–82, 85, 87, 90, 101–109] Plasma disappearance curves for ^{99m}Tc-diethylenetriaminopentaacetic acid (^{99m}Tc-DTPA) have also been documented to compare well in normal horses with Cl_{IN} (the gold standard).[90] Although this technique is less expensive ($\approx$ \$35 per measurement) than ^{131}I-OIH,[93] clinical use is limited by availability of nuclear medicine capabilities and expense (since multiple measurements must be performed to assess disease progression or response to treatment).

The mechanisms responsible for control of RBF (autoregulation, neural input, hormonal factors) also play a role in control of GFR. In addition, GFR is further affected by factors such as plasma protein concentration (oncotic pressure) and alterations in the filtration barrier. As discussed above, there is a balance between action of vasoconstrictor and vasodilator substances during periods of decreased RBF. Interestingly, GFR decreases less than RBF with moderate to severe renal vasoconstriction. This sparing effect on GFR has long been attributed to greater vasoconstrictive effects of angiotensin II on efferent arterioles in comparison to afferent arterioles.[110] Such a response could increase the glomerular capillary transmural hydraulic pressure driving filtration and would be manifested by an increase in filtration fraction. In fact, the latter response has been documented in exercising horses.[87] More recently, however, other vasoconstrictors (endothelins) and vasodilators (endothelium-derived relaxing factors/nitric oxide) have been shown to play a role in the control of glomerular capillary hemodynamics and filtration, so that a singular role for angiotensin II is likely an oversimplified explanation for the sparing effect on GFR.[111]

Renal Tubular Function

Once the glomerular filtrate enters the renal tubule, it is modified extensively in the process of becoming the final product excreted into the renal pelvis. A complete review of renal tubule function is beyond the scope of this text; however, a few general concepts warrant mention, and a number of specific aspects are addressed elsewhere in this chapter. First, the majority of glucose, amino acid, electrolyte, and water reabsorption occurs across epithelial cells lining the proximal tubule; however, these substances are not all reabsorbed to the same extent. For example, this tubule segment is responsible for reabsorption of essentially all filtered glucose and amino acids, about 90% of filtered bicarbonate, about 70% of filtered sodium, and about 60% of filtered chloride.[112] Furthermore, at the end of the proximal tubule fluid is no more concentrated than it was in Bowman's space. Tubular sodium concentration is relatively unchanged, whereas tubular chloride concentration has actually increased (owing to preferential bicarbonate reabsorption). Despite limited modification of these tubule fluid components, net reabsorption of between 60% and 80% of the total filtered load of sodium, chloride, and water occurs within the proximal tubule. Proximal tubular epithelial cells are also responsible for secretion of ammonium ions and a number of organic anions and cations, as described above.

Tubule fluid passing into the loop of Henle becomes progressively more concentrated (hypertonic) as it travels to the inner medulla, since the descending limb is permeable to water, urea, and electrolytes (the latter to a lesser degree).[113] In contrast, the ascending limb is relatively impermeable to water but actively reabsorbs sodium, chloride, and potassium via the apical $Na^+/K^+/2Cl^-$ cotransporter (blocked by furosemide), which is coupled to Na^+/K^+ ATPase on the basolateral membrane. As a result, fluid leaving this nephron segment is actually less concentrated (hypotonic) than the original filtrate. The loop of Henle is responsible for reabsorption of an additional 15% to 20% of filtered sodium and chloride, along with addition of urea to the tubular fluid. More important, Henle's loop is responsible for generation of the medullary osmotic gradient via countercurrent multiplication. This function is a consequence of the combined effects of different permeability characteristics of the descending and ascending limbs of the loop of Henle and active removal of sodium and chloride in the ascending limb.

The distal tubule is quantitatively less important in reabsorption of electrolytes and water; however, it is the nephron segment where the final qualitative changes in urine occur.[114] For example, the distal tubule is an important site of calcium, potassium, and acid excretion. The latter two are typically exchanged for sodium under the influence of aldosterone. Tubule fluid passes from the distal tubule into the outer or cortical collecting ducts, which are impermeable to urea. In addition to further modification of fluid in the cortical collecting ducts, tubular urea concentration increases steadily as water is removed (under the influence of vasopressin) as fluid travels to the inner medulla. In contrast, in the absence of vasopressin (as with diabetes insipidus), the collecting ducts are impermeable to water and hypotonic urine is produced. The collecting ducts remain impermeable to urea (which accounts for up to 50% of the osmoles in urine) except for the innermost medullary segments, which allow urea to be recycled into the interstitium for maintenance of the medullary osmotic gradient.

Reabsorption of glomerular filtrate by renal tubules requires a close association with the vascular system which will carry reabsorbed solute and water to the circulation. Proximal tubules are adjacent to peritubular capillaries, which have a tremendous capacity to accommodate the massive flux of solute and water across proximal tubule epithelial cells. Equally important in maintenance of the medullary osmotic gradient are the vasa recta, hairpin capillaries that travel deep into the renal medulla in association with the loops of Henle derived from the population of juxtamedullary nephrons. Blood flow through these capillaries is typically slow, allowing for countercurrent exchange of sol-

Table 16–6. Reported Values for Glomerular Filtration Rate in Horses and Ponies

Investigator	Animals (No.)	Method[a]	GFR (mL/min/kg [range])	Cl_{CRend}/Cl_{IN} Ratio
Ketz et al (1956)[b]	Not reported[b]	Cl_{IN}	0.83 ± 0.13[c,d]	1.02
		Cl_{CRend}	0.85 ± 0.22[c,d]	
Poulson (1957)[b]	1 horse[e]	Cl_{IN}	1.4	——
Knudsen (1959)[79]	12 ♀ horses	Cl_{IN}	1.66 ± 0.33[c] (1.17–2.28)	0.88 ± 0.11
		Cl_{CRend}	1.46 ± 0.24[c] (1.10–1.65)	
Paul (1973)[80f]	1 ♀ pony	$Cl_{125I-iothalamate}$	Bolus injection: 5.43 (1 study)	——
			Constant infusion: 6.10 ± 1.27	
	3 ♀ horses	$Cl_{125I-iothalamate}$	Bolus injection: 4.20 ± 1.13	
			Constant infusion: 3.14 ± 0.53	
Rawlings and Bisgard (1975)[101]	13 ponies[e]	Cl_{CRend}	1.93 ± 0.37[c] (1.36–2.70)	——
	9 − no NaCl suppl		2.06 ± 0.34[c] (1.64–2.70)	
	4 − + NaCl suppl		1.63 + 0.27[c] (1.36–1.99)	
Traver et al (1977)[102]	7 ♀ horses	Cl_{CRend}	3.68 ± 1.18[c] (2.07–4.99)	——
Gelsa (1979)[103]	4 ♀ horses	Cl_{IN}	1.65 ± 0.07[c] (1.34–2.04)	0.96 ± 0.02
		Cl_{CRend}	1.62 ± 0.03[c] (1.29–2.15)	
Zatzman et al (1982)[80g]	6 ♀ ponies	Cl_{IN}	1.92 ± 0.06[c] (0.64–3.37)	0.86[c]
		Cl_{CRend}	2.24 ± 0.06[c] (1.04–4.15)	
	2 ♀ horses	Cl_{IN}	1.86 ± 0.14[c] (0.71–3.68)	1.11[c]
		Cl_{CRend}	1.67 ± 0.13[c] (0.68–3.09)	
Hood et al (1982)[82]	12 ♀ and ♂ g horses	$Cl_{99mTc-DTPA}$	1.93 ± 0.27 (1.39–2.53)	——
Snow et al (1982)[104]	4 ♂ g[h] horses	Cl_{CRend}	1.34 ± 0.51[c] (1.01–2.10)	——
Lane and Merritt (1983)[105]	1 ♀ pony	Cl_{CRend}	1.15 ± 0.08	——
	4 horses (1 ♂ g, 3 ♀)	Cl_{CRend}	1.45 ± 0.21[c]	
Morris et al (1984)[21]	10 ♂ g horses	Cl_{CRend}	1.88 ± 0.46	——
Gronwall (1985)[106i]	12 ♀ horses	Cl_{CRend}	1.48 ± 0.04	——
Finco and Groves (1985)[23j]	1 ♂ pony	Cl_{14C-IN}	1.74 ± 0.15	0.61 ± 0.11
		Cl_{CRend}	1.06 ± 0.10	
	4 ponies (2♂, 2♀)	Cl_{14C-IN}	1.66 ± 0.38[c] (1.34–2.22)	1.02 ± 0.07[c]
		Cl_{CRex}	1.70 ± 0.39[c] (1.43–2.27)	
Kohn and Stasser (1986)[22]	6 ♀ horses	Cl_{CRend}	1.92 ± 0.51 (1.49–2.74)	——
Smith et al (1988)[107k]	2 ♀ horses	Cl_{CRend}	Awake horses: 2.65[c]	——
			During anesthesia: 1.32[c]	
			Following anesthesia: 2.50[c]	
Brewer et al (1990)[85]	8 ♀ horses	Cl_{IN}	Bolus injection: 1.63 ± 0.33	
	4-day-old foals	Cl_{CRend}	2.81 ± 0.55	1.00[c,l]
	5 horse foals (3♂, 2♀)	Cl_{IN}	Bolus injection: 2.30 ± 0.34	
	3 pony foals (1♀, 2♀)		Infusion (Cl-plasma): 2.56 ± 0.30	
			Infusion (Cl-urine): 2.82 ± 0.32	
McKeever et al (1991)[108]	6 ♀ horses	Cl_{CRrex}	2.56 ± 0.60[c]	——
Schott et al (1991)[87]	6 ♀ horses	Cl_{IN}	1.88 ± 0.67	——
Matthews et al (1992)[90]	8 ♀ horses	Cl_{IN}	1.83 ± 0.21 (0.89–2.95)	——
		$Cl_{99mTc-DTPA}$	1.79 ± 0.18 (1.08–2.51)	
Walsh and Royal (1992)[109]	12 ♀ horses	Cl_{IN}	1.55 ± 0.04[c] (0.98–2.22)	——
		$Cl_{99mTc-DTPA}$	1.47 ± 0.27[c] (0.91–1.82)	
		$Cl_{99mTc-DTPA(cam)}$	1.55 ± 0.22[c,m]	

[a]Cl_{IN}, inulin clearance; Cl_{CRend}, endogenous creatinine clearance; $Cl_{125I-iothalamate}$, clearance of ^{125}I-iothalamate; Cl_{CRex}, exogenous creatinine clearance; Cl_{14C-IN}, clearance of ^{14}C-inulin; $Cl_{99mTc-DTPA}$, clearance of ^{99m}Tc-diethylenepentaacetic acid; $Cl_{99mTc-DTPA(cam)}$, clearance of ^{99m}Tc-diethylenetriaminopentaacetic acid determined by serial imaging at the body surface with a gamma camera.

[b]Data from Knudsen.[79]

[c]Values have been calculated from original data.

[d]Low GFR values were attributed to rapidly declining plasma inulin concentrations (non–steady-state conditions) during the urine collection periods.

[e]Gender not reported.

[f]Other horses and ponies were also studied following bolus injection of ^{125}I-iothalamate and yielded GFR values of 5.39 ± 1.79 and 3.44 ± 1.11 mL/min/kg for ponies and horses, respectively.

[g]Attempts at measuring GFR by plasma disappearance after bolus injection of inulin were unsuccessful.

[h]♂ g, gelding.

[i]Value is for control group; GFR was not different after phenylbutazone administration (1.36 ± 0.04 mL/min/kg) or phenylbutazone and furosemide administration (1.44 ± 0.12 mL/min/kg) but was reported to increase to 1.75 ± 0.16 mL/min/kg after water loading (25 L) and to 1.77 ± 0.18 mL/min/kg after water loading and phenylbutazone administration.

[j]Ponies were anesthetized during the studies.

[k]Mares studied before, during, and after 1.2 MAC halothane anesthesia.

[l]Value calculated from urinary clearance values for inulin and creatinine.

[m]Despite correction for differences in depth (right kidney closer to lateral body surface than left kidney) the clearance of ^{99m}Tc-diethylenepentaacetic acid determined by serial imaging at the body surface with a gamma camera showed a greater (≈60% total) GFR by the right kidney in comparison to the left kidney (≈40% of total); since similar differences have not been demonstrated in microsphere studies of renal blood flow (in which both kidneys receive equal blood flow), this technique requires further refinement before it can be used to provide accurate measures of GFR in horses.

ute in the medullary interstitium, which is necessary for generation and maintenance of medullary hypertonicity. Urea leaving the descending limb of Henle and being recycled across the innermost portion of the medullary collecting duct is responsible for about half of this medullary hypertonicity.

These basic aspects of tubular function have a number of important clinical implications. First, most renal tissue functions in a state of relative hypoxia. For proximal tubule epithelial cells, which are in a well-perfused portion of the kidney, relative hypoxia can be attributed to their extremely high metabolic rate. The inner medulla receives only a small fraction of total RBF which results in a normally hypoxic local environment. Thus, any degree of renal hypoperfusion is also accompanied by a decrease in proximal tubular metabolic rate and exacerbation of medullary hypoxia. Next, although the distal tubule and collecting ducts are responsible for reabsorption of less than 5% of the total glomerular filtrate, a decrease in reabsorption of only 1% to 2% can be quantitatively significant and lead to dramatic polyuria (see Polyuria and Polydispsia). Finally, generation of a maximal medullary concentration gradient requires both slow flow of tubular fluid for countercurrent multiplication and slow flow of blood through the vasa recta to maximize countercurrent exchange. Thus, conditions that increase tubule flow rates (high-volume intravenous fluids) or increase vasa recta blood flow (endogenous PGI_2 and PGE_2 production consequent to renal hypoperfusion) compromise the medullary concentration gradient (partial medullary washout) and lead to increased urinary sodium excretion.

Excretion of Solute and Water

Renal function is traditionally thought of in terms of glomerular filtration, tubular modification of the filtered fluid, and excretion of the final urine. This concept accommodates excretion of nitrogenous and organic wastes and the major aspects of regulation of body water content and ionic balance. Urine concentration and volume are also affected by solute excretion, and another way to think about renal function is in terms of total solute and water excretion. For example, a horse could produce 6 L of urine daily with an osmolality of 900 mOsm/kg to excrete 5400 mOsm of solute or, if the solute load were doubled to 10,800 mOsm, 12 L of urine with an osmolality of 900 mOsm/kg could be produced to eliminate the additional solute. Thus, urine osmolality reflects the kidney's ability to dilute or concentrate the final urine but does not necessarily provide an accurate estimate of the "quantitative ability" to excrete solute or retain water. These functions are assessed by calculating the osmolal (C_{osm}) and free water clearances (C_{H_2O}).[115] Like other clearances, these calculations require measurement of urine flow (via timed urine collection) and measurement of both plasma and urine osmolality.

These measures of renal solute and water handling are conceptualized by considering urine to have two components: (1) that which contains all the urinary solute in a solution that is isosmotic to plasma (C_{osm}, usually expressed in milliliters per minute or liters per day); and (2) that which contains free water without any solute (C_{H_2O}, also expressed in milliliters per minute or liters per day). The sum of these two components is the actual urine flow rate in milliliters per minute or liters per day. Since urine is typically more concentrated than plasma, C_{H_2O} typically has a negative value, indicative of water conservation. In fact, the inverse of free water clearance is termed "renal water reabsorption." Returning to the above example, excretion of the 5400 osmoles would require production of 18 L of urine that is isosmotic with plasma (using a value of 300 mOsm/kg for plasma). However, since 6 L of concentrated urine was actually produced during the period measured, the kidneys have quantitatively reabsorbed 12 L of free water per day. In contrast, despite production of urine with an identical urine osmolality (900 mOsm/kg), excretion of 10,800 mOsm would require production of 36 L of urine isosmotic with plasma. Free water clearance would be −30 L per day (i.e., 30 L per day of free water would be reabsorbed by the kidneys). Thus, although concentrated urine will always have a negative C_{H_2O} value indicative of renal water reabsorption, and dilute urine will always have a positive value for C_{H_2O}, indicative of renal water excretion; quantitative assessment of renal solute and water handling requires measurement of both osmolal and free water clearances.

Excretion of free water by the kidney occurs by generation of hypotonic tubule fluid in the ascending limb of Henle's loop, and the amount or volume of free water produced depends on the amount of tubule fluid presented to that segment. Free water is consequently excreted by keeping the collecting ducts relatively impermeable to water (lack of vasopressin). Assessment of C_{H_2O} is most helpful in patients with hyponatremia and hypoosmolality that cannot be attributed to another primary disease process (diarrhea or bladder rupture). For hyponatremia to develop, water excretion must be defective. For example, hyponatremia can develop with prerenal failure (hypovolemia) or with oliguric renal failure secondary to decreased GFR and amount of filtrate presented to the loop of Henle. Hyponatremia and hypoosmolality may also develop with use of loop diuretics because less free water is generated in the ascending limb of Henle's loop owing to blockade of the apical $Na^+/K^+/2 Cl^-$ cotransporter (smaller amounts of solute are removed). A final cause of true hyponatremia may be the syndrome of inappropriate vasopressin secretion (SIADH, syndrome of inappropriate antidiuretic hormone secretion). Although the latter condition has not been documented in horses, it may play a role in the development of hyponatremia in an occasional foal.[116]

REFERENCES

1. May RC, Kelly RA, Mitch WE: Pathophysiology of uremia. In Brenner BM, Rector FC, eds: *The Kidney*, ed 4, Vol 2. Philadelphia, WB Saunders, 1991, p 1997.
2. Dimski DS: Ammonia metabolism and the urea cycle: Function and clinical implications. *J Vet Intern Med* 8:73, 1994.
3. Finco DR: Kidney function. In Kaneko JJ, ed: *Clinical Biochemistry of Domestic Animals*, ed 3. New York, Academic Press, 1980, p 337.
4. Strombeck DR, Meyer DJ, Freedland RA: Hyperammonemia due to a urea cycle enzyme deficiency in two dogs. *J Am Vet Med Assoc* 166:1109, 1975.
5. Brewer BD: The urogenital system. Section two: Renal disease. In Koterba AM, Drummond WH, Kosch PC, eds: *Equine Clinical Neonatology*. Philadelphia, Lea & Febiger, 1990, p 446.

6. Prior RL, Hintz HF, Lowe JE, Visek WJ: Urea recycling and metabolism of ponies. *J Anim Sci* 38:565, 1974.

7. Hintz HF, Schryver HF: Nitrogen utilization in ponies. *J Anim Sci* 34:592, 1972.

8. Reitnour CM, Treece JM: Relationship of nitrogen source to certain blood components and nitrogen balance in the equine. *J Anim Sci* 32:487, 1971.

9. Landwehr K: Untersuchungen über die Beeinflussung von Kreatinin und Harnstoff im Blutplasma des Pferdes durch extrarenale Faktoren. Inaugural-Dissertation Tierärztliche Hochschule Hannover, 1986.

10. Miller PA, Lawrence LM: The effect of dietary protein level on exercising horses. *J Anim Sci* 66:2185, 1988.

11. Patterson PH, Coon CN, Hughes IM: Protein requirements of mature working horses. *J Anim Sci* 61:187, 1985.

12. Baetz AL, Pearson JE: Blood constituent changes in fasted ponies. *Am J Vet Res* 33:1941, 1972.

13. Keenan DM: Changes of blood metabolites in horses after racing, with particular reference to uric acid. *Aust Vet J* 55:54, 1979.

14. Snow DH, Kerr MG, Nimmo MA, Abbott EM: Alterations in blood, sweat, urine and muscle composition during prolonged exercise in the horse. *Vet Rec* 110:377, 1982.

15. Rose RJ, Ilkiw JE, Arnold KS, et al: Plasma biochemistry in the horse during 3-day event competition. *Equine Vet J* 12:132, 1980.

16. Narayanan S, Appleton HD: Creatinine: A review. *Clin Chem* 26:1119, 1980.

17. Gärtner VK, Reulecke W, Hackbarth H, Wollnik F: Zur Abhängigkeit von Muskelmasse und Körpergröße im Verleich von Maus, Ratte, Kaninchen, Hund, Mensch und Pferd. *Dtsch Tierärztl Wschr* 94:52, 1987.

18. Jones JD, Burnett PC: Creatinine metabolism in humans with decreased renal function: Creatinine deficit. *Clin Chem* 20:1204, 1974.

19. Schott HC, Mansmann RA: Biochemical profiles of normal equine amniotic fluid at parturition. *Equine Vet J* Suppl 5:52, 1988.

20. Mascioli SR, Bantle JP, Freier EF, Hoogwerf BJ: Artifactual elevation of serum creatinine level due to fasting. *Arch Intern Med* 144:1575, 1984.

21. Morris DD, Divers TJ, Whitlock RH: Renal clearance and fractional excretion of electrolytes over a 24-hour period in horses. *Am J Vet Res* 45:2431, 1984.

22. Kohn CW, Strasser SL: 24-Hour renal clearance and excretion of endogenous substances in the mare. *Am J Vet Res* 47:1332, 1986.

23. Finco DR, Groves C: Mechanism of renal excretion of creatinine by the pony. *Am J Vet Res* 46:1625, 1985.

24. Rose BD: Regulation of acid-base balance. In Rose BD, ed: *Clinical Physiology of Acid-Base and Electrolyte Disorders,* ed 3. New York, McGraw-Hill, 1989, p 286.

25. Goldstein MB, Bear R, Richardson RMA, et al: The urine anion gap: A clinically useful index of ammonium excretion. *Am J Med Sci* 292:198, 1986.

26. Grantham JJ, Chonko AM: Renal handling of organic anions and cations; excretion of uric acid. In Brenner BM, Rector FC, eds: *The Kidney,* ed 4, Vol 2. Philadelphia, WB Saunders, 1991, p 483.

27. Gronwall R, Brown MP: Probenicid infusion in mares: Effect on para-aminohippuric acid clearance. *Am J Vet Res* 49:250, 1988.

28. Foreman JW: Renal handling of urate and organic acids. In Bovée KC, ed: *Canine Nephrology.* Media, PA, Harwal, 1984, p 135.

29. Carlson GP: Thermoregulation and fluid balance in the exercising horse. In Snow DH, Persson SGB, Rose RJ, eds: *Equine Exercise Physiology.* Cambridge, Granta Editions, 1983, p 291.

30. Carlson GP: Hematology and body fluids in the equine athlete: A review. In Gillespie JR, Robinson NE, eds: *Equine Exercise Physiology 2.* Davis, CA, ICEEP Publications, 1987, p 393.

31. Schott HC, Hinchcliff KW: Fluids, electrolytes, and bicarbonate. *Vet Clin North Am: Equine Pract* 9:577, 1993.

32. Rose BD: Physiology of body fluids. In Rose BD, ed: *Clinical Physiology of Acid-Base and Electrolyte Disorders,* ed 3. New York: McGraw-Hill, 1989, p 3.

33. Simensen MC: Calcium, phosphorous, and magnesium metabolism. In Kaneko JJ, ed: *Clinical Biochemistry of Domestic Animals,* ed 3. New York: Academic Press, 1980, p 575.

34. Tasker JB: Fluid and electrolyte studies in the horse. III. Intake and output of water, sodium, and potassium in normal horses. *Cornell Vet* 57:649, 1967.

35. Carlson GP: Fluid and electrolyte dynamics in the horse. *Proc Annu Vet Med Forum Am Coll Vet Intern Med* 4:7–29, 1986.

36. Rose RJ: Electrolytes: Clinical applications. *Vet Clin North Am: Equine Pract* 6:281, 1990.

37. Groenendyk S, English PB, Abetz I: External balance of water and electrolytes in the horse. *Equine Vet J* 20:189, 1988.

38. Hinton M: On the watering of horses: A review. *Equine Vet J* 10:27, 1978.

39. Fonnesbeck PV: Consumption and excretion of water by horses receiving all hay and hay-grain diets. *J Anim Sci* 27:1350, 1968.

40. Cymbaluk NF: Water balance of horses fed various diets. *Equine Pract* 11(1):19, 1989.

41. Martin RG, McMeniman NP, Dowsett KF: Milk and water intakes of foals sucking grazing mares. *Equine Vet J* 24:295, 1992.

42. Caljuk EA: Water metabolism and water requirements of horses. *Nutr Abst Rev* 32:574, 1962.

43. Schryver HF, Parker MT, Daniluk PD, et al: Salt consumption and the effect of salt on mineral metabolism in horses. *Cornell Vet* 77:122, 1987.

44. Cymbaluk NF, Freeman DA, Schott HC, et al: Intermittent versus continuous watering: Effects on water balance and hydration status. Proceedings of the 42nd Annual Meeting of the American Association of Equine Practice, 1996, p 330.

45. Sufit E, Houpt KA, Sweeting M: Physiological stimuli of thirst and drinking patterns in ponies. *Equine Vet J* 17:12, 1985.

46. Keiper RR, Keenan MA: Nocturnal activity patterns of feral ponies. *J Mammol* 61:116, 1980.

47. Robertson GL, Berl T: Pathophysiology of water metabolism. In Brenner BM, Rector FC, eds: *The Kidney,* ed 4, Vol 1. Philadelphia, WB Saunders, 1991, p 667.

48. Andersson B, Augustinsson O, Bademo E, et al: Systemic and centrally mediated angiotensin II effects in the horse. *Acta Physiol Scand* 129:143, 1987.

49. Houpt KA: Drinking: The behavioral sequelae of diuretic treatment. *Equine Pract* 9(9):15, 1987.

50. Houpt KA, Thorton SN, Allen WR: Vasopressin in dehydrated and rehydrated ponies. *Physiol Behav* 45:659, 1989.

51. Jones NL, Houpt KA, Houpt TR: Stimuli of thirst in donkeys *(Equus asinus). Physiol Behav* 46:661, 1989.

52. Houpt KA, Northrup A, Wheatley T, Houpt TR: Thirst and salt appetite in horses treated with furosemide. *J Appl Physiol* 71:2380, 1991.

53. Irvine CHG, Alexander SL, Donald RA: Effect of an osmotic stimulus on the secretion of arginine vasopressin and adrenocorticotropin in the horse. *Endocrinology* 124:3102, 1989.

54. Sneddon JC, van der Walt J, Mitchell G, et al: Effects of dehydration and rehydration on plasma vasopressin and aldosterone in horses. *Physiol Behav* 54:223, 1993.

55. McKeever KH, Hinchcliff KW, Schmall LM, et al: Plasma renin activity and aldosterone and vasopressin concentrations during incremental treadmill exercise in horses. *Am J Vet Res* 53:1290, 1992.

56. Nyman S, Hydbring E, Dahlborn K: Is vasopressin a "stress hormone" in the horse? *Pferdeheilkunde* 12:419, 1996.

57. Gellai M: Modulation of vasopressin antidiuretic action by renal α_2-adrenoceptors. *Am J Physiol* 259:F1, 1990.

58. Kinter LB, Huffman WF, Stassen FL: Antagonists of the antidiuretic activity of vasopressin. *Am J Physiol* 254:F165, 1988.

59. Thurmon JC, Steffey EP, Zinkl JG, et al: Xylazine causes transient dose-related hyperglycemia and increased urine volume in mares. *Am J Vet Res* 45:224, 1984.

60. Trim CM, Hanson RR: Effects of xylazine on renal function and plasma glucose in ponies. *Vet Rec* 118:65, 1986.

61. Clarke LL, Argenzio RA, Roberts MC: Effect of meal feeding on plasma volume and urinary electrolyte clearance in ponies. *Am J Vet Res* 51:571, 1990.

62. Youket RJ, Carnevale JM, Houpt KA, Houpt TR: Humoral, hormonal and behavioral correlates of feeding in ponies: The effects of meal frequency. *J Anim Sci* 61:1103, 1985.

63. Clarke LL, Ganjam VK, Fichtenbaum B, et al: Effect of feeding on renin-angiotensin-aldosterone system of the horse. *Am J Physiol* 254:R524, 1988.

64. Tasker JB: Fluid and electrolyte studies in the horse. IV. The effects of fasting and thirsting. *Cornell Vet* 57:658, 1967.

65. Yousef MK, Dill DB, Mayes MG: Shifts in body fluids during dehydration in the burro, *Equus asinus. J Appl Physiol* 29:345, 1970.

66. Maloiy GMO: Water economy of the Somali donkey. *Am J Physiol* 219:1522, 1970.

67. Carlson GP, Rumbaugh GE, Harrold D: Physiological alterations in the horse produced by food and water deprivation during periods of high environmental temperatures. *Am J Vet Res* 40:982, 1979.

68. Brobst DF, Bayly WM: Responses of horses to a water deprivation test. *Equine Vet Sci* 2:51, 1982.

69. Genetzky RM, Lopanco FV, Ledet AE: Clinical pathologic alterations in horses during a water deprivation test. *Am J Vet Res* 48:1007, 1987.

70. Sneddon JC, van der Walt JG, Mitchell G: Water homeostasis in desert-dwelling horses. *J Appl Physiol* 71:112, 1991.

71. Sneddon JC: Pysiological effects of hypertonic dehydration on body fluid pools in arid-adapted mammals. How do Arab-based mammals compare? *Comp Biochem Physiol* 104A:201, 1993.

72. Webb AI, Weaver BMQ: Body composition of the horse. *Equine Vet J* 11:39, 1979.

73. Meyer H, Coenen M: Influence of exercise on the water and electrolyte content of the alimentary tract. *Proc Equine Nutr Physiol Symp* 11:3, 1989.

74. Sawka MN, Pandolf KB: Effects of body water loss on physiologic function and exercise performance. In Gisolfi CV, Lamb DR, eds: *Perspectives in Exercise Science and Sports Medicine, Volume 3: Fluid Homeostasis During Exercise.* Carmel, IN, Benchmark Press, 1990, p 1.

75. Rumbaugh GE, Carlson GP, Harrold D: Urinary production in the healthy horse and in horses deprived of feed and water. *Am J Vet Res* 43:735, 1982.

76. Parks CM, Manohar M: Distribution of blood flow during moderate and strenuous exercise in horses. *Am J Vet Res* 44:1861, 1983.

77. Staddon GE, Weaver BMQ, Webb AI: Distribution of cardiac output in anaesthetised horses. *Res Vet Sci* 27:38, 1979.

78. Gullans SR, Hebert SC: Metabolic basis of ion transport. In Brenner BM, Rector FC, eds: *The Kidney,* ed 4, Vol 2. Philadelphia, WB Saunders, 1991, p 76.

79. Knudsen E: Renal clearance studies on the horse I: Inulin, endogenous creatinine and urea. *Acta Vet Scand* 1:52, 1959.

80. Paul JW: A comparative study of renal function in horses and ponies and a study of the pharmacokinetics of oxytetracycline in the horse. MS Thesis, The Ohio State University, 1973.

81. Zatzman ML, Clarke L, Ray WJ, et al: Renal function of the pony and horse. *Am J Vet Res* 43:608, 1982.

82. Hood DM, Amoss MS, Gremmel SM, Hightower D: Renovascular nuclear medicine in the equine: A feasability study. *Southwest Vet* 35:19, 1982.

83. Manohar M, Goetz TE: Cerebral, renal, adrenal, intestinal, and pancreatic circulation in conscious ponies and during 1.0, 1.5, and 2.0 minimal alveolar concentrations of halothane-O_2 anesthesia. *Am J Vet Res* 46:2492, 1985.

84. Manohar M: Furosemide and systemic circulation during severe exercise. In Gillespie JR, Robinson NE, eds: *Equine Exercise Physiology 2.* Davis, CA, ICEEP Publications, 1987, p 132.

85. Brewer BD, Clement SF, Lotz WS, Gronwall R: A comparison of inulin, para-aminohippuric acid, and endogenous creatinine clearances as measures of renal function in neonatal foals. *J Vet Intern Med* 4:301, 1990.

86. Hinchcliff KW, McKeever KH, Schmall LM, et al: Renal and systemic hemodynamic responses to sustained submaximal exertion in horses. *Am J Physiol* 258:R1177, 1990.

87. Schott HC, Hodgson DR, Bayly WM, Gollnick PD: Renal responses to high intensity exercise. In Persson SGB, Lindholm A, Jeffcott LB, eds: *Equine Exercise Physiology 3.* Davis, CA, ICEEP Publications, 1991, p 361.

88. Held JP, Daniel GB: Use of nonimaging nuclear medicine techniques to assess the effect of flunixin meglumine on effective renal plasma flow and effective renal blood flow in healthy horses. *Am J Vet Res* 52:1619, 1991.

89. Armstrong RB, Essén-Gustavsson B, Hoppeler H, et al: O_2 delivery at $\dot{V}O_{2max}$ and oxidative capacity in muscles of Standardbred horses. *J Appl Physiol* 73:2274, 1992.

90. Matthews HK, Andrews FM, Daniel GB, et al: Comparison of standard and radionuclide methods for measurement of glomerular filtration rate and effective renal blood flow in female horses. *Am J Vet Res* 53:1612, 1992.

91. Manohar M, Goetz TE, Saupe B, et al: Thyroid, renal, and splanchnic circulation in horses at rest and during short-term exercise. *Am J Vet Res* 56:1356, 1995.

92. Trim CM, Moore JN, Clark ES: Renal effects of dopamine infusion in conscious horses. *Equine Vet J Suppl* 7:124, 1989.

93. Matthews HK, Andrews FM, Daniel GB, Jacobs WR: Measuring renal function in horses. *Vet Med* 88:349, 1993.

94. Dworkin LD, Brenner BM: The renal circulations. In Brenner BM, Rector FC, eds: *The Kidney,* ed 4, Vol 2. Philadelphia, WB Saunders, 1991, p 164.

95. Dunn MJ, Zambraski EJ: Renal effects of drugs that inhibit prostaglandin synthesis. *Kidney Int* 18:609, 1980.

96. Gunson DE: Renal papillary necrosis in horses. *J Am Vet Med Assoc* 182:263, 1983.

97. Gunson DE, Soma LR: Renal papillary necrosis in horses after phenylbutazone and water deprivation. *Vet Pathol* 20:603, 1983.

98. McKeever KH, Hinchcliff KW, Schmall LM, et al: Atrial natriuretic peptide during exercise in horses. In Persson SGB, Lindholm A, Jeffcott LB, eds: *Equine Exercise Physiology 3.* Davis, CA, ICEEP Publications, 1991, p 368.

99. Maddox DA, Brenner BM: Glomerular ultrafiltration. In Brenner BM, Rector FC, eds: *The Kidney,* ed 4 Vol 2. Philadelphia: W.B. Saunders, 1991, p 205.

100. Kanwar YS: Biology of disease: Biophysiology of glomerular filtration and proteinuria. *Lab Invest* 51:7, 1984.

101. Rawlings CA, Bisgard GE: Renal clearance and excretion of endogenous substances in the small pony. *Am J Vet Res* 36:45–48, 1975.

102. Traver DS, Salem C, Coffman JR, et al: Renal metabolism of

endogenous substances in the horse: Volumetric vs. clearance ratio methods. *J Equine Med Surg* 1:378, 1977.

103. Gelsa H: The renal clearance of inulin, creatinine, trimethoprim and sulphadoxine in horses. *J Vet Pharmacol Therap* 2:257, 1979.

104. Snow DH, Munro CD, Nimmo MA: Effects of nandrolene phenylpropionate in the horse: (1) Resting animal. *Equine Vet J* 14:219, 1982.

105. Lane VM, Merritt AM: Reliability of single-sample phosphorous fractional excretion determination as a measure of daily phosphorous renal clearance in equids. *Am J Vet Res* 44:500, 1983.

106. Gronwall R: Effect of diuresis on urinary excretion and creatinine clearance in the horse. *Am J Vet Res* 46:1616, 1985.

107. Smith CM, Steffey EP, Baggott JD, et al: Effects of halothane anesthesia on the clearance of gentamicin sulfate in horses. *Am J Vet Res* 49:19, 1988.

108. McKeever KH, Hinchcliff KW, Schmall LM, Muir WW: Renal tubular function in horses during sustained submaximal exercise. *Am J Physiol* 261:R553, 1991.

109. Walsh DM, Royal HD: Evaluation of ^{99m}Tc-labeled diethylenetriaminopentaacetic acid for measuring glomerular filtration rate in horses. *Am J Vet Res* 53:776, 1992.

110. Steinhausen M, Endlich K, Wiegman DL: Glomerular blood flow. *Kidney Int* 38:769, 1990.

111. Lüscher TF, Bock HA, Yang Z, Dierderich D: Endothelium-derived relaxing and contracting factors: Perspectives in nephrology. *Kidney Int* 39:575, 1991.

112. Rose BD: Proximal tubule. In Rose BD, ed: *Clinical Physiology of Acid-Base and Electrolyte Disorders*, ed 3. New York, McGraw-Hill, 1989, p 86.

113. Rose BD: Loop of Henle and the countercurrent mechanism. In Rose BD, ed: *Clinical Physiology of Acid-Base and Electrolyte Disorders*, ed 3. New York: McGraw-Hill, 1989, p 116.

114. Rose BD: Functions of the distal nephron. In Rose BD, ed: *Clinical Physiology of Acid-Base and Electrolyte Disorders*, ed 3. New York, McGraw-Hill, 1989, p 139.

115. Rose BD: Regulation of plasma osmolality. *In* Rose BD, ed: *Clinical Physiology of Acid-Base and Electrolyte Disorders*, ed 3. New York, McGraw-Hill, 1989, p 248.

116. Lakritz J, Madigan J, Carlson GP: Hypovolemic hyponatremia and signs of neurologic disease associated with diarrhea in a foal. *J Am Vet Med Assoc* 200:1114, 1992.

16.3

Examination of the Urinary System

Harold C. Schott II, DVM, PhD

HISTORY AND PHYSICAL EXAMINATION

To begin the evaluation of a horse with urinary tract disease, a complete history should be collected and a thorough physical examination performed. Important historical information includes duration and type of clinical signs, number of horses affected, diet, medications administered, and response to treatment. Water intake and urine output should also be assessed. For example, owners may mistake pollakiuria (fre-

quent urination) for polyuria (increased urine production) and distinguishing between the two is helpful for forming a diagnostic plan. Pollakiuria is frequently seen in females during estrus or with cystic calculi or cystitis in either sex. In contrast, polyuria more often accompanies renal disease, pituitary adenoma, behavior problems (primary polydipsia), diabetes insipidus, or diabetes mellitus. Astute owners may note increased thirst after exercise or a change in the urine, such as a clearer stream, to support polydipsia and polyuria.

Water intake can be determined over 24 hours by turning off any automatic watering devices and providing a known volume of water to the horse.[1] Water intake can vary widely with environmental conditions, level of activity, and diet (see Renal Physiology), so that repeated measurements over several 24-hour periods may be more rewarding in documenting average daily water consumption. Urine output, which should range between 5 and 15 L in a horse with normal renal function, is more difficult to determine. Urine collection harnesses can be applied for 24-hour urine collections[2–5]; alternatively, indwelling Foley catheters attached to a collection apparatus can be used to quantify urine output in mares. Although horses used for research tolerate these devices fairly well, they have limited application to clinical patients. A fairly practical collection device for geldings and stallions can be constructed by cutting off the bottom of a large plastic bottle, which is then padded and fitted over the prepuce. The opening of the bottle is covered with a rubber tube and clip, and urine can be removed every few hours.[6] During the collection period, horses are usually tied or restrained in stocks to minimize interference with the collection device.

The most common presenting complaints for horses with urinary tract disease are weight loss and abnormal urination. Other clinical signs vary with the cause and site of the problem and may include fever, anorexia, depression, ventral edema, oral ulceration, excessive dental tartar, colic, or scalding or blood staining of the perineum or hindlegs. Although lumbar pain and hindlimb lameness have been attributed to urinary tract disease, a musculoskeletal problem is the usual cause of these clinical signs. Decreased performance may be an early presenting complaint for renal disease, but poor performance is likely a result of changes associated with uremia (mild anemia and lethargy) rather than a consequence of renal pain. An occasional horse with urolithiasis or renal neoplasia may have a history of recurrent colic. Prolonged or repeated posturing to urinate and dysuria or hematuria would be important findings to implicate the urinary tract as the probable source of abdominal pain in such patients.

In addition to a thorough physical examination, rectal palpation should be included in the evaluation of all horses with suspected urinary tract disease. The bladder should be palpated to determine size, wall thickness, and presence of cystic calculi or mural masses. If the bladder is full, palpation should be performed again after bladder catheterization or voiding. The caudal pole of the left kidney can be palpated for size and texture. The ureters generally are not palpable unless enlarged or obstructed by disease, but the dorsal abdomen (retroperitoneal course of ureters) and trigone should be palpated to determine if they can be detected. Dilatation of a ureter may occur with pyelonephritis or ureterolithiasis, and in mares palpation of the distal ureters through the vaginal wall may be more rewarding. The reproductive tract should also be palpated to assess whether a reproductive problem could be causing the clinical signs.

HEMATOLOGY AND SERUM BIOCHEMISTRY

A complete blood count that reveals an elevated white blood cell count and total protein or fibrinogen concentration would support an inflammatory or infectious disease process. Mild anemia (packed cell volume 20% to 30%) consequent to decreased erythropoietin production and a shortened red blood cell life span may be observed in horses with chronic renal failure.

Blood urea nitrogen (BUN) and serum creatinine (Cr) concentrations are the most commonly utilized indices of renal function, specifically glomerular filtration rate (GFR).[7-9] It is important to remember that BUN and Cr do not increase until the majority of nephrons (generally considered about 75%) become nonfunctional.[10] Although this commonly used percentage is based on studies of partially nephrectomized laboratory animals, several clinical reports in which unilateral nephrectomy was successfully used to manage disorders of the upper urinary tract support a similar renal reserve capacity in horses.[11-15] In addition, renal function remained within normal ranges and body weight was maintained after experimental unilateral nephrectomy in ponies[16] and in horses (R. DeBowes, personal communication, 1991). Thus, measurement of BUN and Cr is of little use in evaluating early or minor changes in GFR. Once elevated, however, small increases in BUN and Cr are more sensitive indicators of further deterioration in GFR, as doubling of BUN or Cr can be interpreted as a 50% decline in remaining renal function (Fig. 16–8).

Urea can be measured by a variety of methods that are broadly categorized as direct or indirect analyses.[7, 8] The direct method is the diacetyl monoxime reaction, in which urea reacts with diacetyl after hydrolysis of diacetyl monoxime to diacetyl and hydroxylamine. Urea concentration is determined spectrophotometrically by measuring the yield of the yellow diazine reaction product. Indirect analysis is based on enzymatic conversion of urea to ammonia and carbonic acid by urease. There are several methods for subsequently determining ammonia concentration, and the one utilized most often is the enzyme-coupled reaction with glutamate dehydrogenase. Although the term "*blood* urea nitrogen" is widely accepted, it is important to remember that the actual measurement reported is the urea concentration in serum or plasma.

Cr can also be assayed by several methods, but the one employed most often is Jaffé's reaction, which is a colorimetric assay based on the formation of a complex between creatinine and alkaline picrate.[7-9] Unfortunately, a number of other substances in plasma or serum contribute to the yellow color, which leads to a 20% overestimate of actual Cr in humans and in horses.[17] These noncreatinine chromagens include glucose, pyruvate, acetoacetate, fructose, uric acid, and ascorbic acid. Interference by noncreatinine chromagens is greatest when Cr is in the normal range, which leads to a high coefficient of variation in repeated measurements of the same sample. With azotemia, Cr measurement by Jaffé's

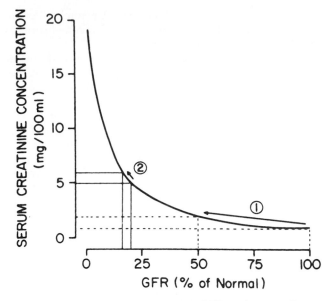

Figure 16–8. Relationship between GFR and serum Cr. When renal function is normal, a large decrease in GFR (as with acute renal failure) results in a relatively minor increase in serum Cr *(arrow 1)*. In contrast, when renal function is decreased (as with chronic renal failure) a much smaller decrease in GFR results in a similar increase in serum Cr *(arrow 2)*. (From Brezis M, Rosen S, Epstein FH: Acute renal failure. In Brenner BM, Rector FC, eds: *The Kidney,* ed 4, Vol 1. Philadelphia, WB Saunders, 1991, p 994.)

reaction becomes more accurate, as the contribution from noncreatinine chromagens does not increase significantly (noncreatinine chromagens are responsible for less than 5% of the color development when Cr is greater than 5.0 mg/dL). Noncreatinine chromagens do not interfere significantly with urine Cr measurement.

In addition to the factors discussed in the preceding section that influence urea and creatinine metabolism (see Renal Physiology), spurious increases in Cr may be reported in various metabolic disorders or after administration of certain cephalosporin antibiotics.[8] When such increases in Cr are thought to be factitious, "true" Cr can be measured by several methods. These include use of an automated analyzer that distinguishes creatinine and noncreatinine chromagens by their different rates of color development or performance of the creatinine imidohydrolase enzyme assay. The latter yields ammonia, which can be quantified by colorimetric methods. As an example, Cr measured by the Jaffé reaction increased 16% after horses were fasted for 3 days; however, when serum was analyzed by the enzymatic method, no increase in Cr was detected.[17] In addition to spurious increases in Cr, other substances can cause spurious decreases in serum Cr. The most common one is bilirubin, which, when elevated above 5.0 mg/dL, may decrease measured Cr by 0.1 to 0.5 mg/dL.[8]

The reporting of serum or plasma urea and creatinine concentrations also varies between different countries. In the United States, BUN and Cr are reported in milligrams per deciliter whereas in other parts of the world they are reported in standard international units of millimoles and micromoles per liter, respectively. Conversion of BUN from milligrams per deciliter to millimoles per liter and of Cr from milligrams per deciliter to micromoles per liter is accomplished by multiplying by 0.357 and 88, respectively.[8]

Azotemia can be prerenal in origin, owing to decreased renal perfusion; may be attributable to primary renal disease; or may accompany obstructive diseases or disruption of the urinary tract (postrenal azotemia).[10, 18] Thus, BUN and Cr should be interpreted in light of hydration status of the patient, presenting complaint, and physical findings. In general, animals with prerenal azotemia tend to have smaller increases in BUN and Cr than animals with intrinsic renal failure, whereas animals with postrenal failure may have the greatest degree of azotemia.[19] Unfortunately, BUN and Cr can cover a wide range of values for all three categories of azotemia so, specific ranges do not identify types of azotemia.[19-22] In an attempt better to characterize azotemia, use of the BUN-Cr ratio has also been examined. In theory, it should be higher for prerenal azotemia (owing to increased reabsorption of urea with low tubule flow rates) and postrenal azotemia (owing to preferential diffusion of urea across peritoneal membranes in cases of uroperitoneum) than for azotemia associated with intrinsic renal failure. As for categorical values for BUN and Cr, BUN-Cr ratios measured in azotemic dogs with naturally occurring diseases were distributed over wide, nondiscriminatory ranges for all three types of azotemia.[19, 20] In horses, the BUN-Cr ratio has more often been used to separate acute renal failure from chronic renal failure. In the acute form, Cr tends to increase proportionately more than BUN, leading to a BUN-Cr ratio less than 10:1.[23] In contrast, with chronic renal failure, the BUN-Cr ratio often exceeds 10:1.[24] Although a clear explanation for this difference has not been established, it may be related to different volumes of distribution for urea and creatinine. Urea, a nonpolar molecule, diffuses freely into all body fluids, whereas creatinine, a charged molecule, likely requires longer to diffuse out of the extracellular fluid space. Thus, a sudden decrease in renal perfusion leads to a greater increase in Cr than in BUN. Muscle breakdown or damage, as with rhabdomyolysis, may be an additional factor contributing to the rapid increase in serum Cr. Further, the BUN-Cr ratio value provides only a suggestion of the duration of azotemia in horses, as exceptions can be found for both acute and chronic renal failure. Finally, the BUN-Cr ratio may also be useful in assessing adequacy of dietary protein intake in cases of chronic renal failure (see Chronic Renal Failure).[24]

The terms "prerenal azotemia" and "prerenal failure" are used to describe the reversible increase in BUN and Cr associated with renal hypoperfusion.[10, 18, 22, 25] Although these terms are firmly entrenched in both human and veterinary medical literature, they likely contribute to the failure to recognize the renal damage that accompanies a number of medical and surgical conditions. This can be attributed to the large renal functional reserve. In fact, in many cases of prerenal failure, altered glomerular and tubule function can be demonstrated by proteinuria and cast formation, impaired concentrating ability, and changes in electrolyte excretion.[26, 27] Although such functional alterations are usually reversible, a degree of permanent nephron loss can occur and it could explain the finding of microscopic evidence of renal disease in as many as one third of equine kidneys examined.[28] Thus, it may be more appropriate to consider "prerenal failure" as

a transient and reversible period of compromised renal function that can lead to permanent, but clinically silent, decreased renal functional mass. Further, periods of decreased renal blood flow or prerenal failure are accompanied by a number of compensatory renal responses that are mobilized to preserve renal blood flow (autoregulatory response of the afferent arterioles) and GFR (increase in filtration fraction due to angiotensin II–mediated efferent arteriolar constriction). In addition, increased intrarenal production of vasodilatory prostaglandins (PGI_2 and PGE_2) is an important response to renal ischemia that maintains or even increases medullary blood flow (see Renal Physiology). Thus, prerenal failure can also be considered as a period of decompensation from the numerous renal compensatory responses to hypoperfusion.[29]

Prerenal azotemia is traditionally differentiated from intrinsic renal failure by assessing urinary concentrating ability. With prerenal azotemia, maintenance of urinary concentrating ability is demonstrated by a urine specific gravity above 1.020 and urine osmolality exceeding 500 mOsm/kg. In contrast, urinary concentrating ability is typically lost with intrinsic renal failure, and urine specific gravity and osmolality are less than 1.020 and 500 mOsm/kg, respectively, in the face of dehydration.[30] Such assessment is challenging, however, because it is valid only when performed on urine collected before initiation of fluid therapy or administration of any of a number of medications (α_2-receptor agonists, furosemide) that can affect urine flow and concentration.[31-34] In addition to these measures of urinary concentrating ability, urine-serum ratios of osmolality, urea nitrogen, and creatinine concentrations, and fractional sodium clearance may provide useful information to differentiate prerenal azotemia from intrinsic renal failure (Table 16–7).[30, 31] For example, urine–serum Cr ratios in excess of 50:1 (reflecting concentrated urine) and fractional sodium clearance values below 1% (indicating adequate tubule function) would be expected in horses with prerenal azotemia, whereas ratios less than 37:1 and clearance values greater than 0.8% were reported in a group of horses determined to have primary renal disease.[30] Although these values can be helpful, the data in Table 16–7 illustrate that renal hypoper-

Table 16–7. Diagnostic Indices That May Be Useful for Separating Prerenal from Renal Azotemia in Horses

Diagnostic Index	Normal Horses	Prerenal Azotemia	Renal Azotemia
Urine osmolality (mOsm/kg)	727–1456	458–961	226–495
Uosm/Posm	2.5–5.2	1.7–3.4	0.8–1.7
Uun/Pun	34.2–100.8	15.2–43.7	2.1–14.3
UCr/PCr	2.0–344.4	51.2–241.5	2.6–37.0
FCl$_{Na}$	0.01–0.70	0.02–0.50	0.80–10.10

Key: Uosm, urine osmolality; Posm, plasma osmolality; Uun, urine urea nitrogen; Pun, plasma urea nitrogen; UCr, urine creatinine; PCr, plasma creatinine; FCl$_{Na}$, fractional sodium clearance.

(Adapted from Grossman BS, Brobst DF, Kramer JW, et al: Urinary indices for differentiation of prerenal azotemia and renal azotemia in horses. *J Am Vet Med Assoc* 180:284, 1982.)

fusion is accompanied by a progressive loss of concentrating ability, since the ranges of these ratios tends to be lower for horses with prerenal azotemia than for clinically normal horses. Thus, these data also support the concept that the progression from prerenal failure to intrinsic renal failure is associated with decompensation of the intrarenal responses to hypoperfusion.[29] Clinically, this decompensation is recognized as persistence of azotemia, whereas prerenal azotemia rapidly resolves (by 30% to 50% within 24 hours and completely by 72 hours) in response to fluid therapy and other supportive treatments.

In patients at risk for developing acute renal failure, including horses with serious gastrointestinal disorders, rhabdomyolysis, and those receiving nephrotoxic medications, serial assessment of urine specific gravity or osmolality, sodium concentration, and fractional sodium clearance may be useful in identifying significant changes in renal function before the onset of azotemia. Similarly, if urine flow rate is determined during a timed urine collection period, assessment of renal water reabsorption (free water clearance, see Renal Physiology) can be a sensitive predictor of impending renal failure.[35–37] Unfortunately, monitoring these parameters is often complicated by use of intravenous fluid support in such patients. Although intravenous fluids can complicate interpretation of many of these indices of renal function, Roussel found that the urine-plasma osmolality ratio remained greater than 1.7:1 in healthy horses receiving 20 L of an intravenous polyionic solution over a 4-hour period.[31] Thus, serial measurement of urine specific gravity or osmolality may provide useful information for patients at high risk for acute renal failure.

Postrenal azotemia resulting from obstruction or disruption of the urinary tract is usually suspected on the basis of clinical signs, including dysuria and renal colic. With bladder rupture, however, some affected foals and adult horses continue to void urine although progressive abdominal distension usually accompanies development of uroperitoneum. Urinary tract disruption is most often confirmed by measuring a twofold or greater value for peritoneal creatinine concentration in comparison to serum creatinine concentration. In an occasional foal with a urachal problem or a gelding with a disrupted urethra, postrenal azotemia may be accompanied by considerable swelling in the abdominal wall or in the prepuce, respectively.

In addition to screening for azotemia and concentrating ability, the laboratory data base should include serum electrolyte, protein (albumin and globulin), and glucose concentrations and muscle enzyme activity.[8, 18, 21–25] Hyponatremia and hypochloremia are fairly common in horses with renal disease. Serum potassium concentration may be normal or may be elevated in cases of acute or chronic renal failure. Hyperkalemia is often most extreme and most serious with urinary tract disruption and uroperitoneum. Calcium and phosphorus concentrations vary in horses with renal disease. Hypercalcemia and hypophosphatemia are often found in horses with chronic renal failure, especially those fed alfalfa hay (see Chronic Renal Failure), whereas hypocalcemia and hyperphosphatemia are more common with acute renal failure. With protein-losing glomerulopathies, albumin tends to be lost to a larger extent than the higher-molecular weight globulin. Low total protein and albumin concentrations can be found in severe cases of chronic renal disease, whereas

other horses may have an increased globulin concentration consistent with a chronic inflammatory response. Hyperglycemia (values above 150 to 175 mg/dL) secondary to stress, exercise, sepsis, pituitary adenoma, or diabetes mellitus can result in glucosuria.[38, 39] Finally, when pigmenturia is a complaint, muscle enzyme activity measurements are helpful in differentiating myoglobinuria from hematuria or hemoglobinuria.

URINALYSIS

Urinalysis should be performed whenever urinary tract disease is suspected. Urine can be collected as a midstream catch during voiding, via urethral catheterization, or via cystocentesis in foals. Unlike cows, horses cannot easily be stimulated to urinate, but they often urinate within a few minutes after being placed in a freshly bedded stall. Manual compression of the bladder during rectal palpation may stimulate urination after the rectal examination is completed. Color, clarity, odor, viscosity, and specific gravity should be evaluated at the time of collection.[40, 41] Normal equine urine is pale yellow to deep tan and is often turbid owing to large amounts of calcium carbonate crystals and mucus. It is not uncommon for urine appearance to change during urination, especially toward the end of micturition, when more crystals tend to be voided. If pigmenturia or hematuria is present, noting the timing and duration of passage of discolored urine may help localize the source. Pigmenturia throughout urination is most consistent with myonecrosis or a bladder or kidney lesion, whereas passage of discolored urine at the start or end of urination is more often seen with lesions of the urethra or accessory sex glands (see Hematuria).

Assessment of Urine Concentration

Urine specific gravity (sp gr) is a measure of the number of particles in urine and is a useful estimate of urine concentration. Although determination of specific gravity with a refractometer is quick and easy (reagent strips should not be used to measure it in horses),[40] it is important to recognize that urine concentration is most accurately determined by measurement of urine osmolality. This is because the presence of larger molecules in urine, such as glucose or proteins, leads to overestimation of urine concentration by assessment of specific gravity. Clinically, this is a problem in patients with diabetes or heavy proteinuria.[42] Urine specific gravity is used to separate urine concentration into three categories: (1) urine that is more dilute than serum (hyposthenuria or specific gravity less than 1.008 and osmolality less than 260 mOsm/kg); (2) urine and serum of similar osmolality (isosthenuria or specific gravity of 1.008 to 1.014 and osmolality of 260 to 300 mOsm/kg); and (3) urine that is more concentrated than serum (specific gravity above 1.014 and osmolality above 300 mOsm/kg). Although urine of most normal horses is relatively concentrated (three to four times more concentrated than serum with specific gravity of 1.025 to 1.050 and an osmolality of 900 to 1200 mOsm/kg), occasionally a normal horse produces dilute or highly concentrated urine. For example, in response to water deprivation of 24 to 72 hours' duration, horses with normal renal function often produce urine with a specific gravity greater than 1.045 and an osmolality greater than 1500 mOsm/kg.[43–45] In contrast, foals typically have hyposthenuric urine consequent to their mostly milk diet.[46] Although the constant polyuria decreases the neonate's ability to generate a large osmotic gradient in the medullary interstitium, dehydrated foals can still produce urine with a specific gravity more than 1.030. With chronic renal insufficiency the ability to produce either concentrated (specific gravity greater than 1.025) or dilute (specific gravity less than 1.008) urine is lost. Thus, horses with chronic renal failure typically manifest isosthenuria. As discussed above, urine specific gravity is helpful in differentiating prerenal from renal azotemia in horses that present with dehydration or shock secondary to a number of disorders.

Reagent Strip Analysis

The pH of equine urine is usually alkaline (7.0 to 9.0).[40, 41, 47] Vigorous exercise or bacteriuria can result in acidic pH. Bacteriuria can impart an ammonia odor to the urine secondary to breakdown of urea by bacteria with urease activity. Concentrate feeding generally decreases urine pH toward the neutral value.[47] Similarly, the more dilute the urine sample is, the closer the pH is to 7.0. The dilute urine produced by foals typically has a neutral pH and is relatively free of crystalline material. Occasionally, aciduria is detected in a dehydrated or anorectic horse. Although aciduria has typically been attributed to metabolic acidosis, many patients may actually have hypochloremic metabolic alkalosis accompanied by paradoxical aciduria. The mechanism for paradoxic aciduria is likely similar to that described in ruminants with abomasal outflow obstruction.[48] Briefly, after all chloride has been reabsorbed from the glomerular filtrate, further sodium reabsorption occurs by exchange with (excretion of) potassium or hydrogen ions. Thus, paradoxical aciduria is most likely to occur with concomitant hypokalemia or whole-body potassium depletion.

Commercially available urine reagent strips can yield false-positive results for protein when alkaline samples are tested. Thus, proteinuria is better assessed by performing the semiquantitative sulfosalicylic acid precipitation test or by specific quantification with a colorimetric assay (such as the Coomassie Brilliant Blue dye method[49] or other assays that are routinely used on cerebrospinal fluid). In normal mares, a mean value of 3.2 mg/kg (1.6 g) per day and a range of 3.6 to 22.3 mg/kg (1.8 to 11.2 g) per day for urinary protein excretion have been reported by the authors[50] and by Kohn and Strasser,[51] respectively. These values translate into urinary protein concentrations of less than 100 mg/dL in the majority of normal horses. Comparison of the quantitative protein result (mg/dL) to urine creatinine concentration (mg/dL) in the form of a urine protein–creatinine ratio (UP:UCr) is also recommended. This technique is more practical since it obviates timed urine collection. Although a normal range has not yet been reported for horses, values in excess of 1.0:1 and 3.5:1, respectively, are considered above normal for dogs[52] and indicative of nephrotic range proteinuria in humans.[8] Thus, a UP-UCr ratio above 2:1 likely supports significant proteinuria in an equine patient. Proteinuria may occur with glomerular disease, bacteriuria, or pyuria, or may transiently follow exercise.[50]

Normal equine urine should not contain glucose. Although the renal threshold for glucose has not been thoroughly evaluated in horses, an early study by Link suggested that it may be lower (about 150 mg/dL) than that of small animals and humans.[53] Thus, glucosuria can accompany hyperglycemia associated with the causes described above or with administration of dextrose-containing fluids or parenteral nutrition products.[38, 39] In addition, glucosuria may accompany sedation with α_2 agonists or exogenous corticosteroid administration.[32, 33] When glucosuria is detected in the absence of hyperglycemia, primary tubule dysfunction should be suspected. Glucosuria has more often been detected in horses with acute renal failure (mostly in experimental models of nephrotoxicity) than in those with chronic renal disease. Unlike ruminants, ketones are rarely detected in equine urine, even in advanced catabolic states or with diabetes mellitus. A positive result for blood on a urine reagent strip can reflect the presence of hemoglobin, myoglobin, or intact red blood cells (RBCs) in the urine sample. Evaluation of serum for hemolysis and of urine sediment for RBCs, combined with an ammonium sulfate precipitation test to detect myoglobin,[54] can be rewarding in differentiating between these pigments (see Hematuria). Finally, bilirubinuria is occasionally detected on reagent strip analysis of equine urine. Bilirubinuria is associated with intravascular hemolysis, hepatic necrosis, and obstructive hepatopathies. In most instances, hemolysis and hepatic disease are detected by abnormal biochemical data such as elevated serum bilirubin concentration and increased hepatic enzyme activity.

Sediment Examination

Sediment examination is probably the most underutilized diagnostic technique available for evaluation of urinary tract disorders in horses. Unfortunately, a major limitation is that sediment should be examined within 30 to 60 minutes after collection. To perform sediment examination, 10 mL of fresh urine should be centrifuged (usually in a conical plastic tube) at 1000 rpm for 3 to 5 minutes. The supernatant urine is discarded (or can be used for quantitative protein determination), and the pellet is resuspended in the few drops of urine remaining in the tube. A drop of sediment is transferred to a glass slide, and a coverslip is applied. The sediment is first examined at low power to evaluate for casts, and subsequently high-power examination is used to quantify erythrocytes, leukocytes, and epithelial cells and to determine whether or not bacteria are present. Casts are molds of Tamm-Horsfall glycoprotein and cells that form in tubule lumens and subsequently pass into the bladder. They are rare in normal equine urine but may be associated with inflammatory or infectious processes. Casts are relatively unstable in alkaline urine; thus, evaluation of urine sediment should be performed as soon as possible after collection, to ensure accurate assessment. Fewer than five RBCs should be seen per high-power field (hpf) in an atraumatically collected urine sample. Increased numbers of urinary RBCs can result from inflammation, infection, toxemia, neoplasia, or exercise (see Hematuria). Pyuria (more than 10 white blood cells per high-power field is most often associated with infectious or inflammatory disorders and normal equine urine should have few bacteria, if any. The absence of

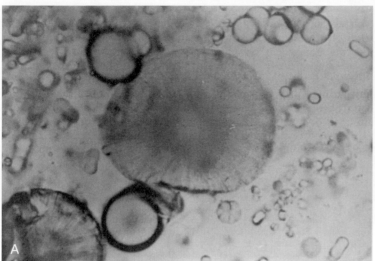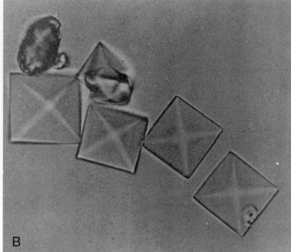

Figure 16–9. Crystals commonly observed in equine urine sediment (original magnification × 160). **A,** Large, round calcium carbonate crystals (*center* and *lower left*) and smaller calcium phosphate crystals *(oblong).* **B,** Calcium oxalate dihydrate crystals. (Reproduced from Osborne CA, O'Brien TD, Ghobrial HK, et al: Crystalluria: Observations, interpretations, and misinterpretations. *Vet Clin North Am: Small Anim Pract* 16:45, 1986.)

bacteria on sediment examination does not rule out their presence, however, and bacterial culture of urine collected by catheterization or cystocentesis (foals) should be performed when cystitis or pyelonephritis is suspected. Finally, equine urine is rich in crystals. The majority of these are calcium carbonate crystals of variable size, but calcium phosphate crystals and occasional calcium oxalate crystals can also be seen in normal equine urine (Fig. 16–9).[40, 41, 55] Addition of a few drops of a 10% acetic acid solution may be necessary to dissolve crystals for accurate assessment of urine sediment.[40]

Enzymuria

More than 40 enzymes have been detected in urine of various species. Measuring urinary concentrations of some have been found to be diagnostically relevant in some situations. Factors to consider when endeavoring to quantitate and interpret urine enzyme levels are discussed in detail in a separate segment at the end of this section on diagnostic evaluation.

Fractional Clearance of Electrolytes

Urinary electrolyte losses, which reflect tubule function, can be expressed as excretion rates (total amount of electrolyte excreted during a given time period, expressed as milliequivalents per minute) or as clearance rates. Determination of clearance rates utilizes the same clearance concept used for measurement of GFR. In brief, a clearance rate (Cl_A) is a measure of the volume of plasma that is completely cleared of the substance in question (A) during a given time period. It is calculated by performing timed urine collection (to determine urine flow in milliliters per minute) and measuring the concentration of the desired substance in plasma and urine (creatinine or inulin for determination of GFR)[8]:

$$Cl_A = \frac{Urine\,[A]}{Plasma\,[A]} \times Urine\,flow$$

As with protein, urinary clearance of many substances, including electrolytes, is often compared to that of creatinine.[8] Basically, a substance that is largely filtered across the glomerulus but neither reabsorbed nor secreted by renal tubules (inulin) will have a clearance rate similar to that of creatinine. In contrast, a substance that is either poorly filtered (larger molecule) or reabsorbed to a great extent by renal tubules (sodium or chloride) will have a lower clearance value than that of creatinine. Similarly, clearance values for substances that are eliminated by both filtration and tubular secretion (potassium) may exceed that measured for creatinine. An advantage of comparing the clearance of a substance (A) to creatinine clearance (expressed as a fraction of creatinine clearance) is that it obviates timed urine collection, as the urine flow factor is cancelled out in the calculation:

$$\frac{Cl_A}{Cl_{Cr}} = \frac{\frac{Urine\,[A]}{Plasma\,[A]} \times Urine\,flow}{\frac{Urine\,[Cr]}{Plasma\,[Cr]} \times Urine\,flow}$$

which, by rearrangement and expression as a percentage becomes

$$\frac{Cl_A}{Cl_{Cr}} = \left(\frac{Plasma\,[Cr]}{Urine\,[Cr]} \times \frac{Urine\,[A]}{Plama\,[A]}\right) \times 100$$

This calculation is called the "fractional creatinine clearance value."[8, 56] More often, however, the term "fractional excretion" has been used to describe this value. Although most sources recommend that blood and urine samples be collected at the same time for determination of fractional

Table 16–8. Fractional Electrolyte Clearance Values for Horses and Ponies

Sodium	Potassium	Chloride	Phosphorus	Calcium	Investigators
Adults					
0.16 ± 0.24	27.0 ± 14.6	0.17 ± 0.11	NR	NR	Rawlings and Bisgard (1975)[57] *
0.02–1.00	15–65	0.04–1.60	0.00–0.50	NR	Traver et al (1976)[58]
0.11–0.87	10.8–28.5	NR	0.07–0.74	NR	Traver et al (1977)[60]
0.01–0.70	NR	NR	NR	NR	Grossman et al (1982)[30]
0.27 ± 0.02	38.52 ± 7.26	1.01 ± 0.24	NR	1.49 ± 1.58	Morris et al (1984)[61]
0.0–0.46	23.9–75.1	0.48–1.64	0.04–0.16	NR	Kohn and Strasser (1986)[51]
0.032–0.52	23.3–48.1†	0.59–1.86	0–20†	0.0–6.72†	Brobst and Parry (1987)[62]
0.034 ± 0.095	42.4 ± 9.8	0.352 ± 0.190	0.710 ± 0.250	NR	Genetzky et al (1988)[45]
0.04–0.52	35–80	0.70–2.10	0.00–0.20	NR	Harris et al (1988)[76]
0.0002–2.43	1.0–42.7‡	0.012–3.47	0.023–2.77	NR	Edwards et al (1989)[41]
NR	NR	NR	0.115–0.302	NR	Lane and Merritt (1983)[70]
NR	NR	NR	0.08–5.53†	2.10–4.60†	Caple et al (1982)[71]
NR	NR	NR	0.61–0.75	11–33	Cuddeford et al (1990)[72] §
Foals					
0.31 ± 0.18	13.26 ± 4.49	0.42 ± 0.32	3.11 ± 3.81	2.85 ± 3.26	Brewer et al (1991)[63]
After furosemide *administration*					
12.0	207	9.5			Traver et al (1976)[58]

*Values calculated from data provided.

†Fractional clearance of potassium may exceed upper limit on high potassium diets; a fractional clearance of phosphorus exceeding 4% suggests excessive dietary intake; and a fractional clearance for calcium should exceed 2.5% with adequate intake.

‡Low range attributed to low urine potassium concentrations determined by ion specific electrodes.

§Fractional clearance value for magnesium reported at 7–30.

clearance values, serum electrolyte and creatinine concentrations are usually fairly stable (except in patients with prerenal azotemia or acute renal failure), so blood values measured within a few days of the urine sample can be used in the clearance calculations. As a consequence, it is acceptable to leave a specimen cup for the client to use to collect a voided sample, obviating bladder catheterization in many cases.

As previously discussed (see Renal Physiology), the equine kidneys function to conserve more than 99% of filtered sodium and chloride ions. In contrast, potassium ions are poorly conserved except during periods of whole-body potassium depletion (anorexia, prolonged exercise). Thus, normal fractional clearance values are less than 1% for sodium but are considerably higher for potassium (Table 16–8).[30, 41, 45, 51, 57–64] Increases in fractional sodium and chloride clearance values may reflect an appropriate renal regulatory response to dietary excess, as with psychogenic salt consumption.[65] Alternatively, increases in fractional clearance values, specifically for sodium and phosphorous, can also be early indicators of renal tubule damage[30, 66–68]; however, results of these calculations must be interpreted in light of fluid therapy since fractional clearance values can be artifactually increased in horses receiving intravenous polyionic solutions.[31] Similarly, medication (furosemide) or light exercise can also result in increased urine flow and fractional sodium and chloride clearance values.[69]

The kidneys play an important role in equine calcium and phosphorus homeostasis, and renal loss of these ions varies with dietary intake. Thus, fractional clearances of calcium and phosphorous have been used to assess adequacy of dietary intake.[58–60, 62, 64, 70–75] Although diet is more appropri-

ately evaluated on a herd basis by feed analyses of hay and concentrates, fractional clearances may be useful in individual animals or when feed analysis is impractical (forage consists of pasture). Determination of fractional calcium and phosphorus clearances has received limited study with a focus on young racing horses.[70–75] For example, excessive dietary phosphorus intake (which can lead to nutritional secondary hyperparathyroidism) leads to increased fractional clearance of phosphorus. Evaluation of fractional calcium clearance is hampered by the fact that the majority of calcium in equine urine is in the form of calcium carbonate crystals. To determine a reliable measure of urinary calcium concentration, the entire contents of the bladder must be collected during voiding or via catheterization to ensure that both the initial crystal-poor and final crystal-rich fractions are collected. Subsequently, a well-mixed aliquot of urine is treated with acetic acid or nitric acid to solubilize the crystals.[64] In one report, fractional calcium and phosphorus clearance values above 2.5% and less than 4% were considered consistent with adequate dietary intake (adequate calcium intake with phosphorus intake that was not excessive).[71] Unfortunately, since the ranges for fractional calcium and phosphorus clearances can be quite wide in normal horses (see Table 16–8), measurement of these clearances may not be sensitive enough to detect minor dietary imbalances.

Determination of fractional electrolyte clearance values has also been advocated in the evaluation of horses with recurrent rhabdomyolysis.[76–78] Low sodium and potassium clearances have been reported in some affected horses. Whether these low fractional clearance values reflected total body electrolyte depletion (as a consequence of repeated bouts of exercise in hot weather or repeated furosemide

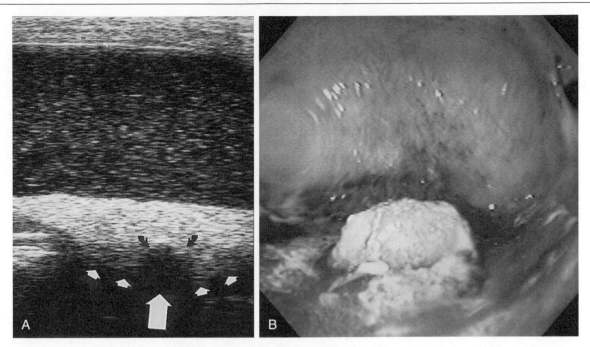

Figure 16–10. Transrectal ultrasonographic and cystoscopic images of the bladder of a miniature horse mare with recurrent cystitis and urolithiasis. **A,** The ultrasonographic image shows a layer of echogenic crystalline material in the ventral aspect of the bladder (*small, white arrows* outline ventral bladder wall) and presence of a small cystolith (outlined by *small black arrows* and *large white arrow*). **B,** After lavage of the urine sediment, cystoscopy confirmed presence of a small urolith, which was amenable to removal by digital manipulation.

administration) or a true physiologic predisposition to rhabdomyolysis was not determined. Nevertheless, low fractional clearance values document the need for electrolyte supplementation in equine athletes. Harris also described another population of horses that exhibited recurrent rhabdomyolysis that had increased fractional phosphorus clearance and reportedly responded to dietary supplementation with ground limestone.[77] Thus, although determination of fractional electrolyte clearances may be helpful in the evaluation of horses with recurrent rhabdomyolysis, only a small portion of affected horses are likely to show significant clinical improvement in response to dietary electrolyte supplementation alone. Finally, a note of caution is warranted when ion-specific electrodes (instead of a flame photometer) are used to measure urinary potassium concentration, as components of animal urine can interfere with the ion-specific electrode and lead to spurious low values. This problem can usually be avoided by performing the analysis on urine diluted with water.[79]

IMAGING TECHNIQUES

Ultrasonography

Ultrasonographic examination of the urinary tract can be performed transrectally or transabdominally.[80–85] Bladder imaging is best performed transrectally using a 5-mHz probe. It is important to remember the character of equine urine while imaging the bladder, as it will be an inhomogeneous, echogenic fluid owing to the presence of mucus and crystals. The latter can appear as echogenic material in the ventral aspect of the bladder. Presence of a cystic calculus can also

be confirmed, since calculi have a highly echogenic surface and produce an acoustic shadow (Fig. 16–10). Similarly, masses in the bladder wall may be both imaged and palpated during the examination.

The right kidney is triangular or horseshoe shaped and is best imaged transabdominally via the dorsolateral extent of the last two or three intercostal spaces (Fig. 16–11). The left kidney is bean shaped and lies deep to the spleen. It can be imaged via the last two intercostal spaces or via the para-

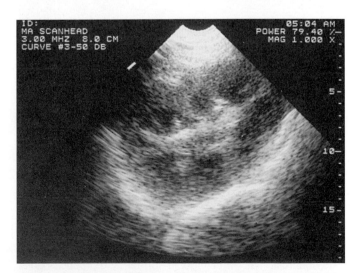

Figure 16–11. Transabdominal ultrasonographic image of a normal right kidney: the renal medulla is more echolucent than the renal cortex, except for the renal pelvis, which varies in echogenicity.

lumbar fossa. Because the left kidney is deeper than the right kidney, it can be difficult to image completely and is best examined with a 2.5- or 3-mHz probe. The size and shape of both kidneys, architecture, and echogenicity of the parenchyma should be assessed systematically. This includes imaging the kidneys in dorsal, sagittal, transverse, and transverse oblique anatomic planes.[85] In acute renal failure the kidneys may be normal or enlarged, and abnormalities of parenchymal detail are not often detected. When present, abnormal findings may include perirenal edema, widening of the renal cortex, and loss of a distinct corticomedullary junction.[81, 82, 84, 86] Chronic renal failure can result in kidneys that are smaller and more echogenic than normal. Cystic or mineralized areas in renal parenchyma can be associated with chronic renal disease or congenital anomalies. Calculi in the renal pelvis generally cast an acoustic shadow and can result in hydronephrosis of the affected kidney (Fig. 16–12).[81, 82, 84] Occasionally, one or both kidneys cannot be imaged owing to presence of gas-filled bowel between kidney and abdominal wall. Reexamination at a later time is generally required for successful imaging in such cases.

Radiography

Radiography is rarely used to evaluate urinary tract disease in adult horses. Diagnostic radiographs of the urinary tract usually can be obtained only in foals or miniature horses. Excretory urography is useful to identify a nonfunctional kidney or hypoplastic kidneys or ectopic ureters.[87–91] The procedure is used infrequently and requires general anesthesia. Retrograde contrast studies can also be utilized to evaluate the ureters in mares[92]; however, they have most often been used in foals suspected of having an ectopic ureter or a ruptured bladder. Contrast radiographic studies can also help to identify strictures or masses in the urethra or bladder,

but endoscopy is generally more useful for these problems. In small animals, abdominal survey radiographs are most useful for assessing kidney size and shape, whereas ultrasonography provides more information about parenchymal changes associated with renal disease.[93] Thus, use of a standardized protocol for ultrasonographic evaluation of the equine kidneys should provide essentially the same amount of information as the combined use of survey radiography and ultrasonography in small animal patients.[85] Unfortunately, the additional information gained from intravenous pyelography is not available for full-sized horses.

Nuclear Scintigraphy

Nuclear scintigraphy is an additional imaging modality often used to assess renal anatomy and function in humans and small animals. Various radionuclides and pharmaceuticals can be used, depending on the type of scintigraphic examination being pursued.[94–96] In fact, scintigraphy is routinely used for quantitative measurement of GFR in these species. Walsh and Royal compared use of renal scintigraphy (using 99-metastable technetium [^{99m}Tc] tagged to diethylenetriaminopentaacetic acid [DTPA]—similar to inulin in that it is neither secreted nor reabsorbed after filtration) for measurement of GFR in horses but found greater variability in comparison to GFR values measured by plasma disappearance of inulin or the same radionuclide (^{99m}Tc-DTPA).[97] Nevertheless, renal scintigraphy utilizing ^{99m}Tc-DTPA can provide qualitative information about renal function and is the only method currently available for assessing split renal function (assessing individual kidney function) in horses. Renal scintigraphy has also been performed with ^{99m}Tc tagged to glucoheptanate (GH, taken up by the proximal tubule epithelial cells to provide anatomic detail) to provide qualitative information about renal anatomy and function (Fig. 16–13).[98] Thus, renal scintigraphy may be used to document the presence of a functional kidney in horses when multiple ultrasonographic examinations have been complicated by interfering bowel or when information about individual kidney function is desired.

Endoscopy

Endoscopy of the urinary tract is an extremely useful diagnostic aid when the complaint is abnormal urination.[40, 99–101] A flexible endoscope with an outside diameter of 12 mm or less and a minimum length of 1 m is adequate for examination of the urethra and bladder of an adult horse of either sex. Cold sterilization of the endoscope should be performed before endoscopy of the lower urinary tract. Tranquilization of the patient is recommended, and the distal end of the penis or the vulva should be cleansed thoroughly. The endoscope is passed just as a catheter is, using the air control intermittently to inflate the urethra or bladder. Normal urethral mucosa is pale pink with longitudinal folds. When dilated with air the mucosa flattens and may appear redder than normal, and a prominent vascular pattern may be apparent. Passage of a catheter before endoscopy (for sample collection or to empty the bladder) can produce mild irritation and erythema of the urethral mucosa. These should not be mistaken for abnormal findings. The regions of the ischial arch

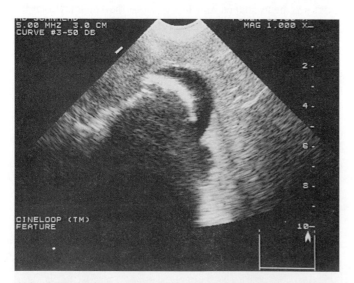

Figure 16–12. Transrectal ultrasonographic image of the left kidney of a mare with nephrolithiasis and hydronephrosis. The nephrolith has an echogenic surface and produces an acoustic shadow. The echolucent crescent moon–shaped structure is a fluid-filled remnant of the renal parenchyma, consistent with hydronephrosis.

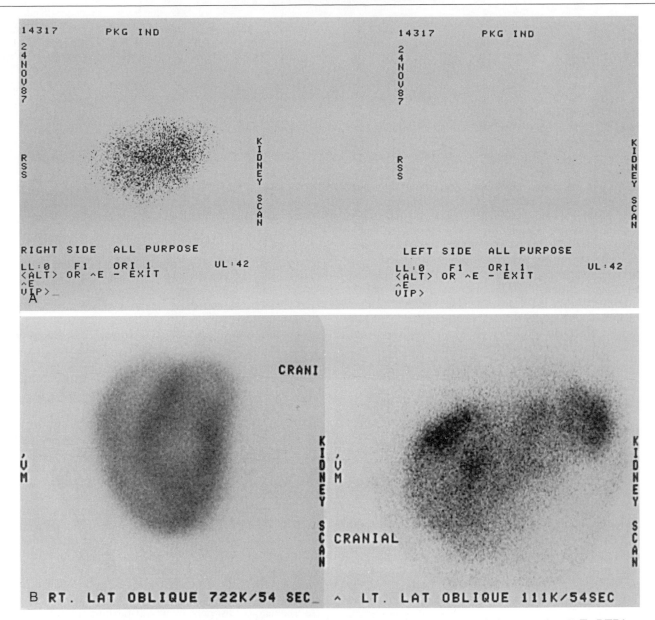

Figure 16–13. Renal scintigraphic images of horses with renal disease. **A,** Renal scintigraphic image using ^{99m}Tc-DTPA revealed absence of functional left renal tissue, in comparison to an image of the right kidney, in a stallion with chronic renal failure. A nonfunctional hypoplastic left kidney was found on necropsy examination. **B,** Renal scintigraphic image using ^{99m}Tc-GH in a gelding with unilateral left-sided pyelonephritis revealed inhomogeneous uptake of the radionuclide and lesser count emission over the same time in comparison to the normal right kidney. The scintigraphic study, which provided both anatomic and functional information, supported pursuit of unilateral nephrectomy, rather than prolonged antibiotic administration, as the treatment of choice for this horse.

(where the urethra begins to widen into the ampullar portion) and of the colliculus seminalis (in the roof of the pelvic urethra just distal to the urethral sphincter) should be examined closely, as these are common sites of posturination or postbreeding hemorrhage in geldings or stallions (see Hematuria). Subsequent passage of the endoscope through the urethral sphincter and air distension allows evaluation of the bladder for calculi, inflammation, and masses (see Fig. 16–10). Viewing the ureteral openings in the dorsal aspect of the trigone can help determine the source of hematuria or pyuria (see Hematuria). A small volume of urine should pass from each ureteral opening approximately once each minute.

Ureteral catheterization to obtain urine samples from each kidney can be performed by passing sterile polyethylene tubing via the biopsy channel of the endoscope. Additionally, biopsy of masses in the bladder or urethra can be performed.

SPECIALIZED DIAGNOSTIC TECHNIQUES

Ureteral Catheterization

With development of high-resolution videoendoscopic equipment, retrograde instrumentation of the bladder, ureter, and renal pelvis is rapidly replacing surgical exploration for diagnostic evaluation and therapeutic management of urinary tract disorders in humans and dogs.[102–105] Similarly, retrograde ureteral catheterization and instrumentation can be a valuable technique for evaluation and treatment of horses with unilateral disorders of the upper urinary tract.[106–108] In addition to localization of unilateral renal hemorrhage, pyelonephritis, and neoplasia; ureteral catheterization further enables retrograde pyelography.[92] As mentioned above, this technique may be successfully accomplished in both male and female horses during cystoscopic examination.[40, 99–101]

In mares the ureters can also be catheterized manually without endoscopic guidance.[109] After preparation of the vulva, the bladder is catheterized and urine is drained. The bladder catheter is removed and the urethra is dilated manually until two fingers can be passed into the bladder. The ureteral orifices can be palpated dorsally as small, soft projections. This done, a catheter is placed between the fingertips, passed through the urethra, and directed into the ureter (Fig. 16–14). A relatively rigid catheter with a rounded end (No. 8 to 10 French polypropylene catheter) facilitates passage into the ureter. After the catheter is advanced 5 to 10 cm into the ureter, a syringe is attached to the other end of the catheter and a urine sample collected. During sampling, the catheter is held in place and the fingertips occlude the ureteral opening to minimize loss of urine around the catheter.

Water Deprivation and the Antidiuretic Hormone Challenge Test

Water deprivation is a simple test to determine whether hyposthenuric polyuria is due to a behavior problem such as primary (psychogenic) polydipsia or is the result of central or nephrogenic diabetes insipidus (DI).[6] A water deprivation test should not be performed in an animal that is clinically dehydrated or azotemic. Baseline urinalysis (sample collected by catheterization to empty the bladder at the start of the test) and measurement of BUN, Cr, and body weight should be performed before removal of water (food does not

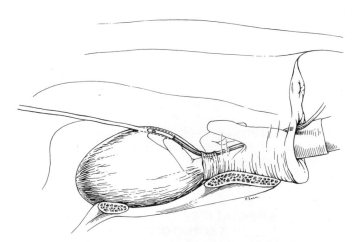

Figure 16–14. Manual placement of a polypropylene catheter into the ureter of a mare. (From Schott HC, Hodgson DR, Bayly WM: Ureteral catheterisation in the horse. *Equine Vet Educ* 2:140, 1990.)

necessarily need to be removed, but this may help prevent gastrointestinal complications of water deprivation). Urine specific gravity and weight loss are measured after 12 (usually overnight) and 24 hours. Horses with normal renal function typically produce urine with a specific gravity above 1.045 and an osmolality above 1500 mOsm/kg in response to water deprivation of 24 to 72 hours' duration.[43–45] Practically, the test can be stopped when urine specific gravity reaches 1.025 or greater. Further, the test should be stopped if more than 5% of body weight is lost or clinical evidence of dehydration becomes apparent. With long-standing primary polydipsia, affected horses may not be able to fully concentrate urine (to a specific gravity above 1.025), owing to partial washout of the medullary interstitial osmotic gradient. It is of little benefit to extend the test period beyond 24 hours for such patients; however, affected horses should respond more favorably to water deprivation (producing urine with a higher specific gravity) after a period of partial water deprivation (termed a "modified water deprivation test") during which daily water intake is restricted to 40 mL/kg for several days, which should allow time for restoration of the medullary interstitial osmotic gradient.[6] Horses with central or nephrogenic diabetes insipidus cannot concentrate urine in response to a water deprivation test.[6, 110–112] When these problems are suspected, patients should be monitored every few hours, as significant dehydration may ensue within 6 hours of water deprivation.

In the absence of azotemia or clinical signs of early renal failure, inability to concentrate urine in response to water deprivation supports a diagnosis of diabetes insipidus; however, the test does not distinguish between the neurogenic and nephrogenic forms of the disorder. These can be differentiated by exogenous administration of vasopressin (antidiuretic hormone).[110–112] Typically, intramuscular administration of 0.2 IU/kg of exogenous vasopressin (Pitressin Synthetic, Parke-Davis) should produce an increase in urine specific gravity to more than 1.025 for 12 hours or more in horses with central diabetes insipidus while little to no response is observed with nephrogenic diabetes insipidus. Another protocol that may maximize the ability to detect a response to exogenous vasopressin would be intramuscular administration of 60 IU every 6 hours over a 24-hour period (see Polyuria and Polydipsia). Use of the synthetic vasopressin analog desmopressin (DDAVP), which is more potent than endogenous vasopressin, has essentially replaced the use of exogenous vasopressin in the diagnostic evaluation and treatment of diabetes insipidus in humans and dogs. However, DDAVP is expensive, and its use has not yet been described in horses.

A final test for evaluating polyuria and polydipsia is an intravenous challenge with hypertonic saline (Hickey-Hare test).[113] The goal is to produce an increase in plasma osmolality, which should trigger release of endogenous vasopressin. One protocol for the test would be to measure plasma osmolality and endogenous vasopressin concentrations before and within 30 minutes after administration of 1 to 2 mL/kg of a 7.5% sodium chloride solution. A normal response, expected in horses with primary polydipsia, would be concurrent increases in plasma vasopressin concentration and urine specific gravity. Horses with nephrogenic diabetes insipidus would also respond with an increased plasma vasopressin concentration; those with neurogenic diabetes insipidus would not. Urine specific gravity would not be expected to increase in response to hypertonic saline administration with either form of diabetes insipidus. Plasma vasopressin concentrations could similarly be evaluated before and at the end of a water deprivation test.[114, 115] Unfortunately, however, assays for plasma vasopressin concentration are not currently available at commercial laboratories. Thus, pursuit of this diagnostic test requires cooperation of a research laboratory.

Quantitative Measures of Renal Function

As mentioned above, azotemia does not develop until more than 75% of nephrons cease to function; therefore, measurement of BUN and Cr, although readily available, provides a poor reflection of smaller declines in renal function. A number of methods are available to quantitate renal function in horses.[40, 116] Basically, these tests can be separated into plasma disappearance curves or clearance studies involving use of timed urine collections. Generation of plasma disappearance curves requires collection of an initial blood sample, intravenous administration of one of a number of compounds (inulin, creatinine, sodium sulfanilate, phenolsulfonphthalein [phenol red], or radionuclides), and collection of a series of further blood samples over the subsequent 60 to 90 minutes.[97, 116–121] Results can be expressed in terms of an elimination half-life in minutes or as clearance values in milliliters per kilogram per minute. Mean elimination half-lives of 39.5 ± 4.4 and 16.4 ± 2.3 minutes have been reported for sodium sulfanilate and phenolsulfonphthalein, respectively, in healthy horses.[117, 118] The difference in these values can be explained by the fact that phenolsulfonphthalein is eliminated by tubular secretion, in addition to glomerular filtration, and is consequently cleared more rapidly from plasma.[118] Plasma elimination half-times are most useful when measured sequentially throughout the course of renal disease; for example, Bertone reported a progressive increase in the sodium sulfanilate elimination half-time from 90 to 150 minutes during a 240-day course of chronic renal failure in a horse with polycystic kidney disease.[122]

When plasma disappearance curves are used to estimate GFR as a clearance value, the compound being used must meet all the requirements of a filtration agent[119–121]: (1) no significant binding to plasma proteins; (2) ability to be freely filtered across the glomerulus; and (3) absence of tubular reabsorption or secretion. The gold standard compound is inulin.[8, 116] More traditionally, GFR has been measured by timed urine collection periods (to measure urine flow rate) and measurement of plasma and urine concentrations of a test compound that meets the requirements listed above.[8, 116] There are several protocols for performing urine clearance studies. Ideally, the urine collection period should span 24 hours, although for practicality, shorter collection periods may be used.[6, 116] For all protocols, the bladder is documented to be empty at the start of the collection period by catheterization or observation of voiding. All urine produced during the study period is collected and pooled into one sample. The bladder should again be emptied via catheterization at the end of the collection period, and the total volume of urine produced is recorded and an aliquot of the pooled urine sample assayed for the test substance. Similarly, the concentration of the test substance is measured in a blood sample collected near the midpoint of the urine collection

period. For urine collections of 12 to 24 hours, endogenous creatinine is the test substance used because it is the only one that does not have to be given by steady intravenous infusion during the collection period. GFR is calculated as the clearance of creatinine,

$$GFR = \frac{Urine\ [Cr]}{Plasma\ [Cr]} \times urine\ flow$$

with the modification that the result is usually divided by body weight (in kilograms) to express GFR in term of milliliters per minute per kilogram. Although endogenous creatinine is a convenient test substance, its use typically underestimates GFR because noncreatinine chromagens in serum artifactually increase the value in the denominator.[116] Similarly, significant tubular secretion of creatinine can be one of the compensatory responses to renal failure. This can lead to overestimation of GFR calculated using endogenous creatinine clearance. Despite these limitations, the endogenous creatinine clearance technique for measurement of GFR can provide useful information, especially when it is performed on several occasions during the course of renal failure (see Chronic Renal Failure).

To avoid the limitations of endogenous creatinine clearance as a measure of GFR, a number of filtration markers (inulin, creatinine, radionuclides) can be administered as an intravenous infusion throughout the urine collection period.[120, 121, 123–128] The infusion is started as a bolus, to increase the plasma concentration of the test substance to the desired level (for example, the desired plasma concentration for exogenous creatinine is 5 to 10 mg/dL, to minimize the influence of noncreatinine chromagens), and subsequently is continued as a steady infusion throughout the remainder of the collection period. This type of study is usually performed for a shorter period with the horse restrained in stocks. The bladder should be emptied at the start of the study, and urine is collected after two or three 30-minute intervals. A catheter should be passed, and the bladder should be emptied completely at the end of each 30-minute period. Alternatively, an indwelling bladder catheter can be used for the entire collection. After urine volumes are measured, an aliquot of each urine sample and a blood sample collected at the midpoint of each urine collection period are assayed for the test substance and GFR is calculated as the mean value for the two or three collection periods. For all practical purposes, these types of GFR measurements (with the exception of exogenous creatinine clearance) are usually limited to research studies, since commercial laboratories do not offer inulin assays. This shorter protocol can also be used for GFR determination using endogenous creatinine as the test substance, without the need for an intravenous infusion. The results of a number of studies measuring GFR in normal horses were presented in the previous section of this chapter (see Renal Physiology).

Renal Biopsy

Renal biopsy is a useful diagnostic technique for identifying the affected region of the nephron, the type of lesion, and the chronicity and severity of disease.[8, 129–131] Although a relatively safe procedure when performed with ultrasonographic guidance, it has risks, including perirenal hemorrhage or hematuria and, less commonly, penetration of bowel. In humans, perinephric hematomas are common and have been detected in 57% to 85% of patients on the day after biopsy. Microscopic hematuria occurs in virtually all patients for the first couple of days after biopsy, and gross hematuria is observed in 5% to 10% of patients. Most of these complications are inconsequential, but in 1% to 3% of patients they have resulted in the need for postbiopsy transfusions.[8] Similar complications have been reported anecdotally in horses. Thus, renal biopsies remain controversial in both human and equine renal failure patients.[132–134] They should be approached with caution and are indicated only when the results would alter the therapeutic plan or prognosis. There is limited information about the impact of renal biopsy results on therapy and outcome of renal disease in humans; however, in one prospective study biopsy results were found to influence physicians' decisions on about half of cases when the technique was performed.[135] In general, renal biopsy is pursued more aggressively in humans with acute renal insufficiency than in those with chronic renal insufficiency, especially when it is difficult to determine the type of renal disease based on results of urinalysis and sediment examination.[8] In the equine patient, a renal biopsy is performed with the horse sedated and restrained in a stocks. Penetration of the needle (a Tru-cut biopsy needle or, preferably, a triggered biopsy device) into the renal parenchyma is imaged sonographically by triangulating the ultrasound beam with the biopsy instrument and the kidney. The tissue collected should be placed in formalin for histopathologic and electron microscopic evaluation. Additional samples can be collected for bacterial culture and for immunofluorescence testing (placed in Michel's medium or quick-frozen after coating with a preservative such as Tissue-Tek). Appropriate sample processing should be determined beforehand by contacting the pathologist who will examine the biopsy samples.

Although renal biopsy results could provide useful diagnostic and prognostic information about the type of renal disease in horses with acute renal failure (glomerulonephritis, tubular necrosis, interstitial nephritis), they have more often been used to document the presence of chronic disease in horses with chronic renal failure. In most cases of chronic renal failure, the inciting cause cannot be detected unless it can be associated with a historical event or immunofluorescence testing is pursued. This limitation can be attributed to the fact that significant renal disease develops before onset of azotemia. Pathologic lesions are widespread at this point, and involvement of all nephron segments and the interstitium often leads to the interpretation of end-stage kidney disease. In occasional cases the results may help separate infectious (pyelonephritis) or congenital (renal dysplasia) from nonspecific causes of renal failure. Although such results could be useful in the therapeutic approach to these patients, the limitations and risks of renal biopsy should be considered before performing this technique in horses with chronic renal failure.

Urodynamic Procedures

Cystometrography and urethral pressure profiles are used to evaluate detrusor and urethral muscle function, respectively. Both techniques involve measurement of intraluminal pressure during inflation of the bladder or urethra. These techniques have been useful for diagnosis of myogenic and neurogenic disorders of the bladder and urethra in dogs and humans.[136] The procedures have been performed experimentally in normal horses and ponies,[137–139] but little information is available about use of these techniques in clinical cases (see Urinary Incontinence and Bladder Dysfunction).

REFERENCES

1. Sneddon JC, Colyn P: A practical system for measuring water intake in stabled horses. *J Equine Vet Sci* 11:141, 1991.
2. Vander Noot GW, Fonnesbeck PV, Lydman RK: Equine metabolism stall and collection harness. *J Anim Sci* 24:691, 1965.
3. Warwick IS: Urine collection apparatus for male horses. *J Sci Technol* 12:181, 1966.
4. Tasker JB: Fluid and electrolyte studies in the horse. II. An apparatus for the collection of total daily urine and feces from horses. *Cornell Vet* 56:77, 1966.
5. Harris P: Collection of urine. *Equine Vet J* 20:86, 1988.
6. Roussel AJ, Carter GK: Polydipsia and polyuria. In Brown CM, ed: *Problems in Equine Medicine.* Philadelphia, Lea & Febiger, 1989, p 150.
7. Finco DR: Kidney function. In Kaneko JJ, ed: *Clinical Biochemistry of Domestic Animals,* ed 3. New York: Academic Press, 1980, p 337.
8. Levey AS, Madaio MP, Perrone RD: Laboratory assessment of renal disease: Clearance, urinalysis, and renal biopsy. In Brenner BM, Rector FC, eds: *The Kidney,* ed 4, Vol 2. Philadelphia, WB Saunders, 1991, p 919.
9. Perrone RD, Madias NE, Levey AS: Serum creatinine as an index of renal function: New insights into old concepts. *Clin Chem* 38:1933, 1992.
10. Osborne CA, Polzin DJ: Azotemia: A review of what's old and what's new. Part I. Definition of terms and concepts. *Compend Contin Educ Pract Vet* 5:497, 1983.
11. Irwin DHG, Howell DW: Equine pyelonephritis and unilateral nephrectomy. *J So Afr Vet Assoc* 51:235, 1980.
12. Trotter GW, Brown CM, Ainsworth DM: Unilateral nephrectomy for treatment of a renal abscess in a foal. *J Am Vet Med Assoc* 184:1392, 1984.
13. Juzwiak JS, Bain FT, Slone DE, et al: Unilateral nephrectomy for treatment of chronic hematuria due to nephrolithiasis in a colt. *Can Vet J* 29:931, 1988.
14. Sullins KE, McIlwraith CW, Yovich JV, et al: Ectopic ureter managed by unilateral nephrectomy in two female horses. *Equine Vet J* 20:463, 1988.
15. Jones SL, Langer DL, Sterner-Kock A, et al: Renal dysplasia and benign ureteropelvic polyps associated with hydronephrosis in a foal. *J Am Vet Med Assoc* 204:1230, 1994.
16. Tennant B, Lowe JE, Tasker JB: Hypercalcemia and hypophosphatemia in ponies following bilateral nephrectomy. *Proc Soc Exp Biol Med* 167:365, 1981.
17. Landwehr K: Untersuchungen über die Beeinflussung von Kreatinin und Harnstoff im Blutplasma des Pferdes durch extrarenale Faktoren. Inaugural-Dissertation Tierärztliche Hochschule Hannover, 1986.
18. Koterba AM, Coffman JR: Acute and chronic renal disease in the horse. *Compend Contin Educ Pract Vet* 3:S461, 1981.
19. Finco DR, Duncan JR: Evaluation of blood urea nitrogen and serum creatinine concentrations as indicators of renal dysfunction: A study of 111 cases and a review of related literature. *J Am Vet Med Assoc* 168:593, 1976.
20. Osborne CA, Polzin DJ: Azotemia: A review of what's old

and what's new. Part II. Localization. *Compend Contin Educ Pract Vet* 5:561, 1983.

21. Brobst DF, Grant BD, Hilbert BJ, et al: Blood biochemical changes in horses with prerenal and renal disease. *J Equine Med Surg* 1:171, 1977.
22. Bayly WM: A practitioner's approach to the diagnosis and treatment of renal failure in horses. *Vet Med* 86:632, 1991.
23. Divers TJ, Whitlock RH, Byars TD, et al: Acute renal failure in six horses resulting from haemodynamic causes. *Equine Vet J* 19:178, 1987.
24. Divers TJ: Chronic renal failure in horses. *Compend Contin Educ Pract Vet* 5:S310, 1983.
25. Tennant B, Dill SG, Rebhun WC, King JM: Pathophysiology of renal failure in the horse. *Proc Annu Conv Am Assoc Equine Pract* 31:627, 1985.
26. Grauer GF: Clinicopathologic evaluation of early renal disease in dogs. *Compend Contin Educ Pract Vet* 7:32, 1985.
27. Allen TA, Fettman MJ: Comparative aspects of nonoliguric renal failure. *Compend Contin Educ Pract Vet* 9:293, 1987.
28. Banks KL, Henson JB: Immunologically mediated glomerulitis of horses. II. Antiglomerular basement membrane antibody and other mechanisms of spontaneous disease. *Lab Invest* 26:708, 1972.
29. Badr KF, Ichikawa I: Prerenal failure: A deleterious shift from renal compensation to decompensation. *N Engl J Med* 319:623, 1988.
30. Grossman BS, Brobst DF, Kramer JW, et al: Urinary indices for differentiation of prerenal azotemia and renal azotemia in horses. *J Am Vet Med Assoc* 180:284, 1982.
31. Roussel AJ, Cohen ND, Ruoff WW, et al: Urinary indices of horses after intravenous administration of crystalloid solutions. *J Vet Intern Med* 7:241, 1993.
32. Thurmon JC, Steffey EP, Zinkl JG, et al: Xylazine causes transient dose-related hyperglycemia and increased urine volume in mares. *Am J Vet Res* 45:224, 1984.
33. Trim CM, Hanson RR: Effects of xylazine on renal function and plasma glucose in ponies. *Vet Rec* 118:65, 1986.
34. Gellai M: Modulation of vasopressin antidiuretic action by renal α_2-adrenoceptors. *Am J Physiol* 259:F1, 1990.
35. Baek SM, Brown RS, Shoemaker WC: Early prediction of acute renal failure and recovery: I. Sequential measurements of free water clearance. *Ann Surg* 177:253, 1973.
36. Baek SM, Makabali GG, Brown RS, Shoemaker WC: Freewater clearance patterns as predictors and therapeutic guides in acute renal failure. *Surgery* 77:632, 1975.
37. Kosinski JP, Lucas CE, Ledgerwood AM: Meaning and value of free water clearance in injured patients. *J Surg Res* 33:184, 1982.
38. Taylor FGR, Hillyer MH: The differential diagnosis of hyperglycemia in horses. *Equine Vet Educ* 4:135, 1992.
39. Chapman DI, Haywood PE, Lloyd P: Occurrence of glycosuria in horses after strenuous exercise. *Equine Vet J* 13:259, 1981.
40. Kohn CW, Chew DJ: Laboratory diagnosis and characterization of renal disease in horses. *Vet Clin North Am: Equine Pract* 3:585, 1987.
41. Edwards DJ, Brownlow MA, Hutchins DR: Indices of renal function: Reference values in normal horses. *Aust Vet J* 66:60, 1989.
42. Rose BD: Physiology of body fluids. In Rose BD, ed: *Clinical Physiology of Acid-Base and Electrolyte Disorders*, ed 3. New York, McGraw-Hill, 1989, p 3.
43. Rumbaugh GE, Carlson GP, Harrold D: Urinary production in the healthy horse and in horses deprived of feed and water. *Am J Vet Res* 43:735, 1982.
44. Brobst DF, Bayly WM: Responses of horses to a water deprivation test. *Equine Vet Sci* 2:51, 1982.
45. Genetzky RM, Lopanco FV, Ledet AE: Clinical pathologic

46. Martin RG, McMeniman NP, Dowsett KF: Milk and water intakes of foals sucking grazing mares. *Equine Vet J* 24:295, 1992.
47. Wood T, Weckman TJ, Henry PA, et al: Equine urine pH: Normal population distributions and methods of acidification. *Equine Vet J* 22:118, 1990.
48. Gingerich DA, Murdick PW: Paradoxic aciduria in bovine metabolic alkalosis. *J Am Vet Med Assoc* 166:227, 1975.
49. Bradford MM: A rapid and sensitive method for the quantification of microgram quantities of protein utilizing the principle of protein-dye binding. *Anal Biochem* 72:248, 1976.
50. Schott HC, Hodgson DR, Bayly WM: Haematuria, pigmenturia and proteinuria in exercising horses. *Equine Vet J* 27:67, 1995.
51. Kohn CW, Strasser SL: 24-hour renal clearance and excretion of endogenous substances in the mare. *Am J Vet Res* 47:1332, 1986.
52. Grauer GF, Thomas CB, Eicker SW: Estimation of quantitative proteinuria in the dog, using the urine protein-to-creatinine ratio from a random, voided sample. *Am J Vet Res* 46:2116, 1985.
53. Link RP: Glucose tolerance in horses. *J Am Vet Med Assoc* 97:261, 1940.
54. Blondheim SH, Margoliash E, Shafrir E: A simple test for myohemoglobinuria (myoglobinuria). *JAMA* 167:453, 1958.
55. Mair TS, Osborn RS: The crystalline composition of normal equine urine deposits. *Equine Vet J* 22:364, 1990.
56. Constable PD: Letter to the editor. *J Vet Intern Med* 5:357, 1991.
57. Rawlings CA, Bisgard GE: Renal clearance and excretion of endogenous substances in the small pony. *Am J Vet Res* 36:45–48, 1975.
58. Traver DS, Coffman JR, Moore JN, et al: Urine clearance ratios as a diagnostic aid in equine metabolic disease. *Proc Annu Conv Amer Assoc Equine Pract* 22:177, 1976.
59. Coffman J: Percent creatinine clearance ratios. *Vet Med/Small Anim Clin* 75:671, 1980.
60. Traver DS, Salem C, Coffman JR, et al: Renal metabolism of endogenous substances in the horse: Volumetric vs. clearance ratio methods. *J Equine Med Surg* 1:378, 1977.
61. Morris DD, Divers TJ, Whitlock RH: Renal clearance and fractional excretion of electrolytes over a 24-hour period in horses. *Am J Vet Res* 45:2431, 1984.
62. Brobst DF, Parry BE: Normal clinical pathology data. In Robinson NE, ed: *Current Therapy in Equine Medicine 2*. Philadelphia, WB Saunders, 1987, p 725.
63. Brewer BD, Clement SF, Lotz WS, Gronwall R: Renal clearance, urinary excretion of endogenous substances, and urinary indices in healthy neonatal foals. *J Vet Intern Med* 5:28, 1991.
64. King C: Practical use of urinary fractional excretion. *J Equine Vet Sci* 14:464, 1994.
65. Divers TJ, Whitlock RH, Byars TD, et al: Acute renal failure in six horses resulting from haemodynamic causes. *Equine Vet J* 19:178, 1987.
66. Bayly WM, Brobst DF, Elfers RS, et al: Serum and urine biochemistry and enzyme changes in ponies with acute renal failure. *Cornell Vet* 76:306, 1986.
67. Hinchcliff KW, McGuirk SM, MacWilliams PS: Gentamicin nephrotoxicity. *Proc Annu Conv Amer Assoc Equine Pract* 33:67, 1987.
68. Buntain BJ, Coffman JR: Polyuria and polydipsia in a horse induced by psychogenic salt consumption. *Equine Vet J* 13:266, 1981.
69. Schott HC, Bayly WM, Hodgson DR: Urinary excretory responses in exercising horses: Effects on fractional excretion

values. *Proc Annu Meet Assoc Equine Sports Med* 11:23, 1992.

70. Lane VM, Merritt AM: Reliability of single-sample phosphorous fractional excretion determination as a measure of daily phosphorous renal clearance in equids. *Am J Vet Res* 44:500, 1983.

71. Caple IW, Doake PA, Ellis PG: Assessment of the calcium and phosphorous nutrition in horses by analysis of urine. *Aust Vet J* 58:125, 1982.

72. Cuddeford D, Woodhead A, Muirhead R: Potential of alfalfa as a source of calcium for calcium deficient horses. *Vet Rec* 126:425, 1990.

73. Caple IW, Bourke JM, Ellis PG: An examination of the calcium and phosphorous nutrition of Thoroughbred racehorses. *Aust Vet J* 58:132, 1982.

74. Mason DK, Watkins KL, McNie JT: Diagnosis, treatment and prevention of nutritional secondary hyperparathyroidism in Thoroughbred race horses in Hong Kong. *Equine Pract* 10(3):10, 1988.

75. Ronen N van Heerden J, van Amstel SR: Clinical and biochemistry findings, and parathyroid hormone concentrations in three horses with secondary hyperparathyroidism. *J South Afr Vet Assoc* 63:134, 1992.

76. Harris P, Colles C: The use of creatinine clearance ratios in the prevention of equine rhabdomyolysis: A report of four cases. *Equine Vet J* 20:459, 1988.

77. Harris PA, Snow DH: Role of electrolyte imbalances in the pathophysiology of the equine rhabdomyolysis syndrome. In Persson SGB, Lindholm A, Jeffcott LB, eds: *Equine Exercise Physiology 3*. Davis, CA, ICEEP Publications, 1991, p 435.

78. Beech J, Lindborg S: Potassium concentrations in muscle, plasma, and erythrocytes and urinary fractional excretion in normal horses and those with chronic intermittent exercise-associated rhabdomyolysis. *Res Vet Sci* 55:43, 1993.

79. Brooks CL, Garry F, Swartout MS: Effect of an interfering substance on determination of potassium by ion-specific potentiometry in animal urine. *Am J Vet Res* 49:710, 1988.

80. Traub-Dargatz JL, McKinnon AO: Adjunctive methods of examination of the urogenital tract. *Vet Clin North Am: Equine Pract* 4:339, 1988.

81. Rantanen NW: Diseases of the kidneys. *Vet Clin North Am: Equine Pract* 2:89, 1986.

82. Reef VB: Ultrasonic evaluation of large animal renal diseases. *Proc Annu Vet Med Forum Am Coll Vet Intern Med* 4:2–45, 1986.

83. Penninck DG, Eisenberg HM, Teuscher EE, Vrins A: Equine renal ultrasonography: Normal and abnormal. *Vet Radiol* 27:81, 1986.

84. Kiper ML, Traub-Dargatz JL, Wrigley RH: Renal ultrasonography in horses. *Compend Contin Educ Pract Vet* 12:993, 1990.

85. Hoffman KL, Wood AKW, McCarthy PH: Sonographic-anatomic correlation and imaging protocol for the kidneys of horses. *Am J Vet Res* 56:1403, 1995.

86. Bayly WM, Elfers RS, Liggitt HD, et al: A reproducible means of studying acute renal failure in the horse. *Cornell Vet* 76:287, 1986.

87. Christie B, Haywood N, Hilbert B, et al: Surgical correction of bilateral ureteral ectopia in a male Appaloosa foal. *Aust Vet J* 57:336, 1981.

88. Modransky PD, Wagner PC, Robinette JD, et al: Surgical correction of bilateral ectopic ureters in two foals. *Vet Surg* 12:141, 1983.

89. Houlton JEF, Wright IM, Matic S, Herrtage ME: Urinary incontinence in a Shire foal due to ureteral ectopia. *Equine Vet J* 19:244, 1987.

90. Sullins KE, McIlwraith CW, Yovich JV, et al: Ectopic ureter

91. managed by unilateral nephrectomy in two female horses. *Equine Vet J* 20:463, 1988.

91. Blikslager AT, Green EM, MacFadden KE, et al: Excretory urography and ultrasonography in the diagnosis of bilateral ectopic ureters in a foal. *Vet Radiol Ultrasound* 33:41, 1992.

92. Rapp HJ, Tellhelm B, Spurlock SL: Die röntgenologische Darstellung der Harnableitenden wege der Stute mit Hilfe retrograder Kontrastmittelgabe. *Pferdeheilkunde* 3:309, 1987.

93. Konde LJ, Park RD, Wrigley RH, Lebel JL: Comparison of radiography and ultrasonography in the evaluation of renal lesions in the dog. *J Am Vet Med Assoc* 188:1420, 1986.

94. Kogan BA, Hattner RS: Radionuclide imaging. In Tanagho EA, McAninch JW, eds: *Smith's General Urology*, ed 12. Norwalk, Appleton & Lange, 1988, p 142.

95. Blaufox MD: Procedures of choice in renal nuclear medicine. *J Nucl Med* 32:1301, 1991.

96. Twardock AR, Krawiec DR, Lamb CR: Kidney scintigraphy. *Semin Vet Med Surg (Small Anim)* 6:164, 1991.

97. Walsh DM, Royal HD: Evaluation of ^{99m}Tc-labeled diethylenetriaminopentaacetic acid for measuring glomerular filtration rate in horses. *Am J Vet Res* 53:776, 1992.

98. Schott HC, Roberts GD, Hines MT, Byrne BA: Nuclear scintigraphy as a diagnostic aid in the evaluation of renal disease in horses. *Proc Annu Conv Amer Assoc Equine Pract* 39:251, 1993.

99. Sullins KE, Traub-Dargatz JL: Endoscopic anatomy of the equine urinary tract. *Compend Contin Educ Pract Vet* 11:S663, 1984.

100. Rapp HJ, Sernetz M: Urethroskopie und Ureterenkatheterisierung bei der Stute. *Pferdeheilkunde* 1:197, 1985.

101. Schott HC, Varner DD: Urinary tract. In Traub-Dargatz JL, Brown CM, eds: *Equine Endoscopy*, ed 2. St. Louis, CV Mosby, 1997, p 187.

102. Huffman JL, Bagley DH, Lyon ES: Extending cystoscopic techniques into the ureter and renal pelvis. *JAMA* 250:2002, 1983.

103. Thuroff JW: Retrograde instrumentation of the urinary tract. In Tanagho EA, McAninch JW, eds: *Smith's General Urology*, ed 12. Norwalk, Appleton & Lange, 1988, p 154.

104. Ensor RD, Boyarksy S, Glenn JF: Cystoscopy and ureteral catheterization in the dog. *J Am Vet Med Assoc* 149:1067, 1966.

105. Senior DF, Newman RC: Retrograde ureteral catheterization in female dogs. *J Am Anim Hosp Assoc* 22:831, 1986.

106. Schott HC, Papageorges M, Hodgson DR: Diagnosis of renal disease in the nonazotemic horse. Abstract #15. *J Vet Intern Med* 3:116, 1989.

107. MacHarg MA, Foerner JJ, Phillips TN, Barclay WP: Two methods for the treatment of ureterolithiasis in a mare. *Vet Surg* 13:95, 1984.

108. Rodger LD, Carlson GP, Moran ME, et al: Resolution of a left ureteral stone using electrohydraulic lithotripsy in a Thoroughbred colt. *J Vet Intern Med* 9:280, 1995.

109. Schott HC, Hodgson DR, Bayly WM: Ureteral catherisation in the horse. *Equine Vet Educ* 2:140, 1990.

110. Filar J, Ziolo T, Szalecki J: Diabetes insipidus in the course of encephalitis in the horse. *Medycyna Weterynaryjna* 27:205, 1971.

111. Breukink HJ, Van Wegen P, Schotman AJH: Idiopathic diabetes insipidus in a Welsh pony. *Equine Vet J* 15:284, 1983.

112. Schott HC, Bayly WM, Reed SM, Brobst DF: Nephrogenic diabetes insipidus in sibling colts. *J Vet Intern Med* 7:68, 1993.

113. Irvine CHG, Alexander SL, Donald RA: Effect of an osmotic stimulus on the secretion of arginine vasopressin and adrenocorticotropin in the horse. *Endocrinology* 124:3102, 1989.

114. Houpt KA, Thorton SN, Allen WR: Vasopressin in dehydrated and rehydrated ponies. *Physiol Behav* 45:659, 1989.

115. Sneddon JC, van der Walt J, Mitchell G, et al: Effects of dehydration and rehydration on plasma vasopressin and aldosterone in horses. *Physiol Behav* 54:223, 1993.

116. Matthews HK, Andrews FM, Daniel GB, Jacobs WR: Measuring renal function in horses. *Vet Med* 88:349, 1993.

117. Brobst DF, Bramwell K, Kramer JW: Sodium sulfanilate clearance as a method of determining renal function in the horse. *J Equine Med Surg* 2:500, 1978.

118. Hinchcliff KW, McGuirk SM, MacWilliams PS: Pharmacokinetics of phenolsulfonphthalein in horse and pony mares. *Am J Vet Res* 48:1256, 1987.

119. Hood DM, Amoss MS, Gremmel SM, Hightower D: Renovascular nuclear medicine in the equine: A feasibility study. *Southwest Vet* 35:19, 1982.

120. Matthews HK, Andrews FM, Danile GB, et al: Comparison of standard and radionuclide methods for measurement of glomerular filtration rate and effective renal blood flow in female horses. *Am J Vet Res* 53:1612, 1992.

121. Brewer BD, Clement SF, Lotz WS, Gronwall R: A comparison of inulin, para-aminohippuric acid, and endogenous creatinine clearances as measures of renal function in neonatal foals. *J Vet Intern Med* 4:301, 1990.

122. Bertone JJ, Traub-Dargatz JL, Fettman MJ, et al: Monitoring the progression of renal failure in a horse with polycystic kidney disease: Use of the reciprocal of serum creatinine concentration and sodium sulfanilate clearance half-time. *J Am Vet Med Assoc* 191:565, 1987.

123. Knudsen E: Renal clearance studies on the horse I: Inulin, endogenous creatinine and urea. *Acta Vet Scand* 1:52, 1959.

124. Gelsa H: The renal clearance of inulin, creatinine, trimethoprim and sulphadoxine in horses. *J Vet Pharmacol Ther* 2:257, 1979.

125. Zatzman ML, Clarke L, Ray WJ, et al: Renal function of the pony and the horse. *Am J Vet Res* 43:608, 1981.

126. Schott HC, Hodgson DR, Bayly WM, Gollnick PD: Renal responses to high intensity exercise. In Persson SGB, Lindholm A, Jeffcott LB, eds: *Equine Exercise Physiology 3.* Davis, CA, ICEEP Publications, 1991, p 361.

127. Finco DR, Groves C: Mechanism of renal excretion of creatinine by the pony. *Am J Vet Res* 46:1625, 1985.

128. McKeever KH, Hinchcliff KW, Schmall LM, Muir WW: Renal tubular function in horses during sustained submaximal exercise. *Am J Physiol* 261:R553, 1991.

129. Osborne CA, Fahning ML, Schultz RH, Perman V: Percutaneous renal biopsy in the cow and the horse. *J Am Vet Med Assoc* 153:563, 1968.

130. Bayly WM, Paradis MR, Reed SM: Equine renal biopsy: Indications, technique, interpretation, and complications. *Mod Vet Pract* 61:763, 1980.

131. Modransky PD: Comparative evaluation of ultrasound-directed biopsy techniques in the horse. M.S. Thesis, Washington State University, 1983.

132. Striker GE: Controversy: The role of renal biopsy in modern medicine. *Am J Kidney Dis* 1:241, 1982.

133. Morel-Maroger L: The value of renal biopsy. *Am J Kidney Dis* 1:244, 1982.

134. Donadio JV: The limitations of renal biopsy. *Am J Kidney Dis* 1:249, 1982.

135. Turner MW, Hutchinson TA, Barre PE, et al: A prospective study on the impact of renal biopsy in clinical management. *Clin Nephrol* 26:217, 1986.

136. Gleason DM, Bottaccini MR, Drach GW: Urodynamics. *J Urol* 115:356, 1976.

137. Clark SE, Semrad SD, Bichsel P, Oliver JE: Cystometrography and urethral pressure profiles in healthy horse and pony mares. *Am J Vet Res* 48:552, 1987.

138. Kay AK, Lavoie JP: Urethral pressure profilometry in mares. *J Am Vet Med Assoc* 191:212, 1987.

139. Ronen N: Measurements of urethral pressure profiles in the male horse. *Equine Vet J* 26:55, 1994.

16.4

Urinary Enzymes

Warwick M. Bayly, BVSc, MS

The diagnosis of renal disease in horses traditionally has been based on clinical history and examination and the results of a number of laboratory tests such as (1) measurement of serum urea nitrogen (UN) and creatinine (Cr) concentrations; (2) routine urinalysis, including urine specific gravity and examination of urine sediment; and (3) fractional excretion of urine electrolytes. Because these tests are relatively insensitive, it is estimated that approximately 65% to 70% of nephrons are dysfunctional before clinically significant changes in these variables are detectable. As a result, many cases of renal disease are not diagnosed until severe—possibly irreversible—renal damage has occurred. This is especially so since routine urinalysis has regressed from close microscopic examination of the fluid to the use of reagent sticks for a semiquantitative measure of protein, hemoglobin, pH, glucose, bilirubin, and ketone bodies.

The tubules of the kidneys are metabolically very active, being responsible for the absorption or excretion of a wide range of substances. The transport of these compounds is facilitated by a variety of enzymes, which generally can be found in large amounts in the brush borders of tubule cells or in lysosomes. Regular turnover of these cells and release of endocytotic vesicles of lysosomotrophic agents and lysosomes into the tubule lumen result in the presence of enzymes in urine (enzymuria).[1] Known lysosomotrophic agents include aminoglycosides, bile acids, mannitol, dextran, some radiographic contrast media, heavy metals, and cephalosporins. Following filtration, these substances are taken up via endocytosis into the tubule cells (primarily proximal cells) and combine with lysosomes. Agents that are not broken down by the acid hydrolases in the lysosomes are subsequently extruded into the tubule lumen as "residual bodies." Inflammatory swelling of tubule epithelial cells or their accelerated destruction results in elevated urinary activity of lysosomal and brush border enzymes. Because of their high metabolic rate, tubular epithelial cells are particularly susceptible to perfusion injury and toxin-induced change, with the result that determination of the concentrations of certain urinary enzymes can provide biochemical evidence of renal cell dysfunction a number of days before changes are likely to develop in the traditionally utilized parameters.[2–5]

Other potential sources of enzymuria are (1) serum, as low–molecular weight proteins like amylase and β-microglobulins may be filtered by the glomeruli (and are normally reabsorbed in the proximal tubules), and renal parenchymal damage resulting in effusion of protein into tubule lumina; (2) postrenal genitourinary tract epithelium, which generally makes a negligible contribution to the overall urine enzyme concentration (unless they become neoplastic) because of their low enzyme content; and (3) secretions from the sex glands, which is why intact males tend to have higher activities of lactate dehydrogenase (LDH) and *N*-acetyl-β-D-glucosaminidase (NAG).

Although more than 40 enzymes have been detected in the urine of different species, only a few appear to be diagnostically relevant. To be useful clinically, a urinary enzyme must have measurable activity in the kidneys, must appear to have measurable activity within fairly narrow limits in the urine of healthy horses, must be a large enough protein (molecular weight over 60 Kd) so that it is not filtered by the glomerulus, and must increase in activity early enough in the course of progressive renal injury to permit corrective action but not so early that there is a significant risk of prematurely discontinuing or altering essential therapy. Its activity should also remain fairly stable in urine for at least several days under easily achievable conditions. In humans and dogs, a number of enzymes, including NAG, LDH, β-glucuronidase, alanine aminopeptidase (AAP), alkaline phosphatase (AP), leucine aminopeptidase (LAP), γ-glutamyl transferase (GGT), and kallikrein have been demonstrated to be sensitive indicators of early renal damage.[2–4, 6, 7] Investigations of horses have been fewer, and consequently, less is specifically known about the clinical value of urinary enzyme activity measurements. Normal values have been established for activity of GGT, AP, NAG, LDH, and kallikrein in the equine species.[8–12] Attempts to assay aspartate aminotransferase and alanine aminotransferase activity were unsuccessful, activities of these enzymes apparently being below detectable limits in normal horses.[9]

Alkaline phosphatase and GGT are membrane-associated enzymes found principally in the brush border of the proximal tubular epithelium.[3–7, 13] Distally, their activity is negligible.[13] They are active in other tissues, but because they are not filtered by the glomerulus (in the absence of significant proteinuria) elevated activity in urine is assumed to originate from the kidneys. Their measurable baseline activity in urine is believed to be due to normal cell turnover.[3] Lactate dehydrogenase is a "more ubiquitous" tubular epithelial enzyme, being as active in the distal tubules and medullary papillae as it is proximally.[6–13] Consequently, LDH activity has been studied extensively in conjunction with nonsteroidal antiinflammatory drug nephrotoxicity. *N*-acetyl-β-D-glucosaminidase is a proximal tubular epithelial cell lysosome.[3–13] Only GGT, AP, LDH, and NAG have been assayed in the urine of horses known or believed to have some form of renal dysfunction. Determination of NAG concentrations can be difficult in normal equine urine owing to its alkalinity, and normal values may be below detectable assay limits, especially if a spectrophotometric, rather than a fluorometric method is used.[14–17] Published normal activity values for these enzymes are as follows: GGT, 0 to 25 IU/g Cr; AP, 0 to 28 IU/g Cr; LDH, 0 to 12 IU/g Cr; and NAG, <1 IU/g Cr (<2 IU/L urine).

The principal reason for the slow development of the use of urinary enzyme assays in clinical veterinary medicine has been the difficulty involved in assaying enzymes in a fluid that varies in volume and composition and that represents a hostile environment for many enzymes. For example, periods of diuresis or antidiuresis can cause variations in the degree of enzymuria. Determination of enzymes excreted over a 24-hour period would have greater value, but for clinically diagnostic purposes 24-hour urine collections from horses are not practical. This potential problem can be overcome by expressing the activity of a specific enzyme in a single urine specimen in terms of the urinary Cr concentration in the same sample, owing to the constancy of Cr excretion.[8, 18, 19] Care must be taken to express both variables in the same units. This minimizes volume-related variations in results, and greatly enhances the clinical value of analysis from a randomly collected specimen.

Other factors that must be considered when measuring urine enzyme activity include the conditions under which the urine sample has been stored, diurnal variation, gender- and age-linked variations, influences of pH, and other potential naturally occurring inhibitors or promoters of enzyme activity in urine (e.g., albumin, mucoproteins, proteolytic agents, amino acids, ammonia). Effects on equine urine of these various compounds has been incompletely studied. However, it is well-established that freezing can have deleterious effects on the activity of all enzymes, particularly GGT, and that, the colder the temperature, the more rapid the degeneration of the enzyme activity.[8] Consequently, to obtain the most accurate results, assays should be performed as soon as possible after collection, and certainly within 72 hours. If storage is necessary, refrigeration (~4 °C) is the best condition under which to maintain the sample.

Mild diurnal variations in activity have been demonstrated for GGT and AP. Although activity appears to be greatest in the early morning, variations are relatively mild; so values fall within the normal range, regardless of the time of sample collection, especially when expressed in terms of Cr excretion.[9]

Urinary pH definitely appears to affect urinary NAG activity. In species that tend to have a slightly acidic or neutral urinary pH, assay of NAG is considered one of the most clinically valuable tests available. However, its activity appears to be very susceptible to pH changes. In humans who had been administered nephrotoxic medications, NAG activity became indetectable when pH was greater than 8.[20] Tests that we conducted on the urine of normal horses (pH 7.5 to 8.5) produced values that were below the lower limit of sensitivity for the assay (i.e., below 2 IU/L).[21] Another study on the effect of monensin toxicosis in horses demonstrated that NAG activity increased as pH decreased, values of 7 IU/L coinciding with pH values of about 7.[10]

Certain amino acids and ammonia have been identified as natural inhibitors of lysosomal enzymes such as AAP and NAG in the urine of humans, dogs, and rats,[22, 23] and techniques have been developed to remove these agents from the urine by gel filtration before enzyme activity is assayed.[24] In human urine, these substances account for about 50% of the removable inhibitory potential. Gel-filtered samples can also be kept much longer without the inhibition-induced changes. While such filtration procedures are not routinely conducted with equine urine, given the large concentration of mucoproteins and other potentially bioactive agents normally found in the urine of this species, future refinements in assay techniques may incorporate such a step and lead to the development of normal ranges of activity quite different from those listed above. At the present time, however, relating specific urinary enzyme activity to Cr gives results that consistently fall into the broad range of values shown. It is also noteworthy that a commercially available serum assay for GGT yields accurate results when applied to unfiltered horse urine.[8] Similar validation has not been undertaken for AP.

Urinary enzyme activity may also be enhanced by the manner in which it is handled or by the urinary concentration of other substances such as urea and electrolytes. Enzyme activity enhancement is most likely to occur during the first 24 hours of storage. When equal quantities of GGT were added to horse urine, horse serum, and physiologic saline, GGT activity was significantly greater in urine than in other solutions.[8] Loss of the inhibitory action of urea, loss of certain protective molecules during storage, digestion or hydrolysis of particulate matter in urine, and changes in urinary electrolyte concentrations could all contribute to this apparent enhancement phenomenon. With respect to GGT, it has also been demonstrated in rats that the form of GGT in urine shifts from a membrane-bound form to a more soluble form in the face of cellular alkalosis and alkalinization of the urine.[25] Given the alkaline nature of horse urine, this may be responsible for part of the reported increase in GGT activity following short-term storage of urine from this species. Increases in urinary GGT and AP activity have been demonstrated clinically and experimentally in horses known to have received gentamicin and neomycin for 5 to 10 days[26, 27] and in horses with diarrhea, acute abdominal crises, and endotoxic shock. In the latter instances, it has been assumed that increased enzymuria has been indicative of some degree of renal ischemia. Five consecutive days of furosemide administration has also been demonstrated to produce moderate increases in GGT and AP activity,[21] with AP increasing more rapidly. Water deprivation for 48 hours failed to induce any changes in GGT, AP, or LDH activity.[12] It may be that the apparent effect of the furosemide on the degree of enzymuria was related to changes in urine electrolyte concentrations induced by the diuretic.

Theoretically, assessment of changes in the urinary activity of selected enzymes could help the clinician identify what segment of the kidney exhibits the greatest dysfunction or damage. Although NAG, GGT, and AP are associated principally with proximal tubule function, LDH is usually associated with distal tubular epithelial cells, and increases in LDH activity are believed to indicate distal tubule damage and renal papillary necrosis. Thus far, relatively little has been done to investigate LDH activity in equine urine, although one study designed to evaluate the effects of administration of 8.8 mg/kg phenylbutazone by mouth for 6 consecutive days indicated no change in urinary LDH activity.[12]

Increased enzymuria is most likely to occur in the acute stages of renal disease, when tubular epithelial enzymes are being lost at increased rates in association with hydropic change or exfoliation. Thus, elevations in urinary enzyme activity are principally indicative of acute tubule damage; however, apparent increases in urine enzyme–Cr ratios must be evaluated carefully. There is no well-established threshold for determining when an elevation in urinary enzyme activity is clinically significant, although it has been suggested that activity of GGT over 25 IU/g of Cr suggests tubular nephrosis.[8] Given the wide range of estimates for mean urinary

GGT activity in the literature and the small sample sizes on which those estimates have been based, it is questionable whether 99% of normal horses have urinary GGT activity within 3 standard deviations of the small population mean, as has been suggested.[8] Hinchcliff and coworkers make the distinction between an elevated level of urinary GGT activity (over 25 IU/g Cr) and a clinically significant increase, and urge caution when interpreting urinary GGT–Cr ratios between 25 and 100 IU/g Cr.[26]

Horses with chronic renal disease may have normal or reduced enzyme activity, which reflects the cellular changes that occur in nephrons in response to chronic active inflammation. Just as traditional parameters such as serum UN and Cr concentrations may be normal during the early stages of acute disease, urinary enzyme activities may not reflect renal dysfunction later in the disease course, when results of serologic tests and urinalysis are likely to be abnormal. Possible reasons for this phenomenon are that so much destruction of tubular epithelium has occurred that there is no longer a source of elevated enzyme activity or that regenerating tubular epithelial cells are refractory to the effects of the toxin. The former explanation seems more likely.

In summary, determination of urinary enzyme activity may be of considerable use in the clinical setting. Assessment of enzymuria can be a useful adjunct to the more traditional tests of renal function. It is recommended that practitioners consider assay of urinary enzyme activity when they have reason to suspect reduced renal function secondary to nephrosis (as after exposure to nephrotoxins) or when monitoring a horse's status in conjunction with treatment of conditions such as diarrhea and endotoxic shock, which may lead to ischemia and prerenal failure. To provide the best service, regular monitoring is advised until the resolution of the case becomes clear. Reasonable access to a laboratory is needed to ensure prompt analysis of samples for accuracy of results and to maximize the benefit that measuring urinary enzyme activity provides over more traditional tests of kidney function.

REFERENCES

1. Burchardt U, Peters JE, Neef L, et al: Der diagnostiche Wert von Enzymbestimmugen im Harn. *Z Med Labor Diag* 18:190, 1977.
2. Raab WP: Diagnostic value of urinary enzyme determinations. *Clin Chem* 18:5, 1972.
3. Price RG: Urinary enzymes, nephrotoxicity and renal disease. *Toxicology* 23:99, 1982.
4. Stroo WE, Hook JB: Enzymes of renal origin in urine as indicators of nephrotoxicity. *Toxicol Appl Pharm* 39:423, 1977.
5. Bayly WM, Brobst DF, Elfers RS, et al: Serum and urine biochemistry and enzyme changes in ponies with acute renal failure. *Cornell Vet* 76:306, 1986.
6. Prescott LF: Assessment of nephrotoxicity. *Br J Clin Pharmacol* 13:303, 1982.
7. Mahrun D, Paar D, Bock KD: Lysosomal and brush-border enzymes in urine of patients with renal artery stenosis and with essential hypertension. *Clin Biochem* 12:228, 1978.
8. Adams R, McClure JJ, Gossett KA, et al: Evaluation of a technique for measurement of γ-glutamyltransferase in equine urine. *Am J Vet Res* 46:147, 1986.
9. Brobst DF, Carroll RJ, Bayly WM: Urinary enzyme concentrations in healthy horses. *Cornell Vet* 76:229, 1986.

10. Amend J, Nicholson R, King R, et al: Equine monensin toxicosis: Useful ante-mortem and post-mortem clinicopathologic tests. *Proc Ann Conv Am Assoc Equine Pract* 31:361, 1985.

11. Giusti EP, Sampaio AM, Michelacci YM, et al: Horse urinary kallikrein I: Complete purification and characterization. *Biol Chem* 369:387, 1988.

12. Schmitz DG, Green RA: Effects of water deprivation and phenylbutazone administration on urinary enzyme concentrations in healthy horses. *Proc Ann Conv Am Assoc Equine Pract* 33:103, 1987.

13. Guder W, Ross B: Enzyme distribution along the nephron. *Kidney Int* 26:101, 1984.

14. Jung K, Pergande M, Schreiber G, et al: Stability of enzymes in urine at 37°C. *Clin Chim Acta* 131:185, 1983.

15. Goren M, Wright R, Osborne S, et al: Two automated procedures for N-acetyl-β-D-glucosaminidase determination evaluated for detection of drug-induced tubular nephrotoxicity. *Clin Chem* 32:2052, 1986.

16. Leaback D, Walker P: Studies on glucosaminidase 4. The fluorometric assay of N-acetyl-β-D-glucosaminidase. *Biochem J* 78:151, 1961.

17. Irie A, Tabuchi A, Ura T: Influence of pH and temperature on the activities of the urinary enzymes. *Jpn J Clin Pathol* 13:441, 1985.

18. Vestergaard P, Leverett R: Constancy of urinary creatinine excretion. *J Lab Clin Med* 51:211, 1958.

19. Werner M, Heilbron DC, Mahrun D, et al: Patterns of urinary enzyme excretion in healthy subjects. *Clin Chim Acta* 29:437, 1970.

20. Mahrun D, Fuchs I, Mues G, et al: Normal limits of urinary excretion of eleven enzymes. *Clin Chem* 22:1567, 1976.

21. Akins JA: Evaluation of Equine Urinary N-Acetyl-β-D-Glucosaminidase, Gamma-Glutamyltransferase, and Alkaline Phosphatase as Markers for Early Renal Tubular Damage. MS thesis, Washington State University, 1989.

22. Mattenheimer H, Frolke W, Grotsch H, et al.: Identification of inhibitors of urinary alanine aminopeptidase. *Clin Chim Acta* 160:125, 1986.

23. Reusch C, Vochezer R, Weschta E: Enzyme activities of alanine aminopeptidase (AAP) and N-acetyl-β-D-glucosaminidase (NAG) in healthy dogs. *J Vet Med A* 38:90, 1991.

24. Werner A, Mahrun D, Atoba A: Use of gel filtration in the assay of urinary enzymes. *J Chromatog* 40:234, 1969.

25. Welbourne TC, Phifer T, Thomas M, et al.: Gamma-glutamyltransferase release by the post ischemic kidney: Multiple forms and cellular Ph. *Life Sci* 33:1141, 1983.

26. Hinchcliff KW, McGuirk SM, MacWilliams PS: Gentamicin nephrotoxicity. *Proc Ann Conv Am Assoc Equine Pract* 33:67, 1987.

27. Edwards DJ, Love DN, Rause J, et al.: The nephrotoxic potential on neomycin in the horse. *Equine Vet J* 21:206, 1989.

16.5.

Acute Renal Failure

Warwick M. Bayly, BVSc, MS

Acute renal failure (ARF) is a clinical syndrome associated with abrupt reduction in glomerular filtration rate (GFR). Sustained reduction in GFR is associated with failure of the kidneys to excrete nitrogenous wastes causing azotemia, and with disturbances in fluid, electrolyte, and acid-base homeostasis. The human medical literature is full of various terms and definitions for different forms of ARF. Veterinary medical definitions are somewhat simpler. Basically, ARF can result from decreased renal perfusion without associated cell injury (prerenal failure), obstruction or disruption of the urinary outflow tract (postrenal failure), or ischemic or toxic damage to the tubules, tubular obstruction, acute glomerulonephritis leading to a primary reduction in the filtering capacity of the glomeruli, or tubulointerstitial inflammation and edema. Any of these intrarenal causes can be associated with intrinsic renal failure. Prerenal azotemia and ischemic tubular insults or necrosis represent a continuum, the former resulting in the latter when perfusion is sufficiently compromised to result in death of tubule cells.[1] Classically, ARF has been associated with oliguria, and occasionally anuria, and these are certainly the most commonly noted clinical signs associated with this disease in horses; however, nonoliguric forms of ARF, particularly intrinsic renal failure, exist. These are characterized by slower development of azotemia, lower peaks in serum creatinine concentrations, more subtle increases in urinary sodium clearance, and a more rapid recovery of renal function in response to treatment. Nonoliguric renal failure seems to be diagnosed rarely in horses, although it is not uncommon to recognize mildly azotemic horses that have apparently normal urine output. In some cases, localized proximal tubule damage and reduced solute reabsorption may actually lead to enhanced distal delivery of filtrate, which may result in polyuric ARF.

In horses, ARF is usually prerenal or renal in origin and most often is due to hemodynamic or nephrotoxic insults.[2] With the exception of bladder rupture in the neonate, postrenal failure is uncommon in horses. Identification and correction of the cause of ARF is important, as in the early stages of failure renal dysfunction is frequently reversible, whereas, established ARF often requires extensive supportive care and carries a guarded prognosis. By identifying patients at increased risk and attempting to interrupt the cycle of events leading to ARF, it may be possible to reduce the incidence of this condition.

ETIOLOGY

Prerenal failure is associated with conditions that result in decreased cardiac output or increased renal vascular resistance, or both, and is the most common cause of reversible azotemia. In horses, the most common causes of reduced cardiac output (and therefore, reduced renal perfusion) are associated with diarrhea, endotoxemia, acute blood loss, septic shock, and prolonged exercise. The resultant reductions in renal blood flow (RBF), GFR, and urine output usually result in azotemia and retention of water and electrolytes. Anesthesia may also decrease cardiac output enough to result in a degree of prerenal azotemia. Nonsteroidal antiinflammatory drugs (NSAIDs) can also precipitate prerenal azotemia in patients with decreased RBF.[3] Although prostaglandins play only a minor role in maintenance of RBF in the normal state, PGE_2 and PGI_2 are important vasodilatory mediators of RBF under conditions of reduced renal perfusion. Thus, administration of NSAIDs to dehydrated or toxemic patients may contribute further to renal hypoperfusion by exacerbating a decrease in RBF. In some cases, this may be sufficient to produce ischemic renal parenchymal damage also, thus causing intrinsic renal failure. Generally, the parenchymal lesion associated with NSAID toxicity is medullary crest or papillary necrosis. Such lesions develop because the renal medulla normally receives much less blood flow than the renal cortex, with the result that it is much more susceptible to NSAID-induced changes in RBF.

In humans, intrinsic renal diseases that lead to ARF are generally categorized according to the primary site of injury—tubules, interstitium, glomeruli, or vessels.[1] Acute tubular necrosis (ATN) is the form of intrinsic renal failure recognized most often in horses, interstitial and primary glomerular disease being recognized occasionally, and vascular disease almost never. Ischemia, especially when associated with microvascular coagulation (which often leads to irreversible cortical necrosis[4]) and nephrotoxins, probably are the most common causes of equine ATN. Important nephrotoxins include aminoglycoside antibiotics and NSAIDs. Less commonly, ATN develops consequent to exposure to endogenous pigments (myoglobin or hemoglobin), heavy metals such as mercury (contained in some counterirritants) or vitamin D or K_3.[5-8] Use of aminoglycosides, particularly gentamicin, is a relatively common cause of equine ATN.[9] Toxicity is a result of damage to proximal tubular epithelial cells that is mediated by impaired cell organelle function. Administration of potentially nephrotoxic agents such as NSAIDs or furosemide (which can exacerbate hypovolemia) can increase the risk of aminoglycoside nephrotoxicity.

Myoglobinuria and hemoglobinuria have both been associated with development of ARF in horses (pigment nephropathy).[10] Myoglobinuric nephrosis can be secondary to exertional rhabdomyolysis, heat stroke, or extensive crush injuries. Causes of intravascular hemolysis and hemoglobinuria include incompatible blood transfusions, immune-mediated hemolytic anemia, fulminant hepatic failure, and toxicosis from ingesting onions (*Allium* species) or withered red maple leaves (*Acer rubrum*). Although the mechanism of pigment-induced renal injury is still ill-understood, increased hydroxyl radical formation associated with reduction of ferrous iron compounds, and tubular obstruction by casts of heme proteins are likely contributing factors. That pigment nephropathy is uncommon in well-hydrated horses suggests a possible link to renal perfusion. It has been suggested that both myoglobin and hemoglobin can induce renal vasoconstriction.

Acute interstitial nephritis is not often recognized, but is believed usually to result from an allergic reaction to drugs such as the β-lactam and sulfa antibiotics. Autoimmune and embolic or ascending bacterial infections may also be associated with the condition, which is characterized by edema and inflammatory cell infiltration of the interstitium. Tubules frequently contain white and red blood cells, which pass into the lumen through the disrupted tubular basement membrane.

Glomerulonephritis is quite often identified post mortem in aged horses[11, 12] and apparently is most often immune mediated. It often results in subacute or nonoliguric renal failure. While theoretically reversible with immunosuppressive agents, in horses such undertakings are usually impractical and are rarely tried for long.

Postrenal obstructive failure can develop subsequent to disease of the renal pelves, ureters, bladder, or urethra. The severity of the failure depends on the extent of the obstruction. Frequently, problems are not recognized in horses until urine output is obviously reduced or renal function impaired to the point where systemic problems are manifested. Although a neurogenic bladder can cause a functional obstruction, postrenal failure in horses is most often a consequence of intraluminal blockage by uroliths. These can cause obstruction anywhere in the urinary outflow tract.[13, 14] Other possible intraluminal causes include neoplasia or stricture formation. Extraluminal obstructive lesions such as retroperitoneal tumors or adhesions or bladder displacements are also occasionally associated with development of postrenal failure.

PATHOPHYSIOLOGY

The pathophysiology of equine ARF has received little study, and it is assumed that the mechanisms at work are essentially the same as those identified in experimental studies of other animal species. Several mechanisms have been demonstrated to be involved in the development of ARF, the actual pathogenesis being complex and somewhat dependent on the cause of the disease. Multiple factors probably operate in different combinations at different times and in different nephrons. These different mechanisms are discussed below in relation to the type of failure with which they are associated (i.e., prerenal, intrinsic, and postrenal failure).

The pathophysiology of prerenal failure and ischemic ARF tend to involve the same processes. Toxins that cause ATN also share many pathophysiologic features with ischemic ARF.[15] The heterogeneity of intrarenal blood flow is an important factor in the development of this condition. The kidneys are particularly susceptible to ischemic and toxic injury because of their unique anatomic and physiologic features. Although they receive approximately 20% of the cardiac output, only about 10% to 20% of total RBF reaches the medulla via the vasa recta. This low medullary blood flow is necessary to ensure a functional countercurrent mechanism in this region of the kidney; however, it also creates a large corticomedullary oxygen gradient and renders the renal medulla relatively hypoxic and highly susceptible to ischemic injury. Conversely, the renal cortex receives 80% to 90% of total RBF and is particularly susceptible to toxins.

Hypovolemia triggers compensatory systemic and renal responses. The systemic responses include activation of the autonomic nervous system and renin-angiotensin system and release of antidiuretic hormone (ADH). Peripheral vasoconstriction is one of the effects of these responses. Renal responses to decreases in circulating blood volume have several phases. Initially, there is increased tubular reabsorption of sodium and water, which is mediated by both nerves and hormones. This is usually associated with reduced clearance of urea and an associated increase in serum urea nitrogen concentration in the face of preservation of GFR, which in turn maintains the plasma creatinine concentration in the normal range. More severe hypovolemia overcomes renal autoregulation, RBF being redistributed from the cortex to the medulla and GFR declining. The renal circulatory changes further enhance tubule solute reabsorption in the face of the decreased GFR. The net effect is production of relatively small amounts of concentrated urine, a high urine-plasma creatinine ratio, and low fractional sodium clearance.[16]

A further reduction in RBF results in a syndrome considered intermediate between the prerenal and intrinsic ischemic forms of ARF. Urine concentrating ability is apparently disrupted earlier than is sodium reabsorptive capability, with the result that urine osmolality decreases and output increases, but fractional sodium clearance stays quite low. Patients may appear to be mildly polyuric.[17] With more severe or prolonged renal hypoperfusion and ischemic insult, urinary sodium and fractional sodium clearance start to increase and the animal develops nonoliguric—and then oliguric—ARF. These changes are associated with progressively more severe tubule necrosis, as the ARF progresses from prerenal to renal. The more severe the insult is, the poorer the prognosis.

Intrarenal vasoconstriction is caused by an imbalance between vasoconstrictive and vasodilating factors (systemic or local) that act on small renal vessels in particular. These mediators include the vasodilator nitric oxide and the constrictor endothelin. Hypercalcemia is associated with increases in free calcium in the vascular smooth muscle and leads to enhanced vascular tone. Vasopressin and angiotensin II have also been shown to induce marked vasoconstriction under certain experimental conditions, as have endotoxins and myoglobin. Some nephrotoxins—gentamicin, heavy metals, radiographic contrast agents—can cause renal vasoconstriction in addition to having direct toxic effects on the proximal tubules.[18–20]

The prostaglandins PGE_2 and PGI_2 are potent mediators that are responsible for a critical vasodilating response in the face of reduced RBF when activation of the renin-angiotensin system alone would result in further vasoconstriction. Synthesis of these renal prostaglandins is stimulated by increases in circulatory concentrations of angiotensin II. Consequently, the vasoconstrictive effects of stimulating the renin-angiotensin system are usually blunted somewhat by concomitant increases in PGE_2 and PGI_2; however, in the face of increased angiotensin II and simultaneous inhibition of prostaglandin synthesis (e.g., due to an NSAID), a marked increase in renal vascular resistance results.[21]

The reduction in GFR associated with reduced renal perfusion is associated with a number of mechanisms involving the glomeruli, vasculature, and tubules. In the initial phases, a reduction in glomerular capillary hydrostatic pressure is associated with a net drop in RBF and a rise in renal vascular resistance. The latter phenomenon is usually associated with afferent arteriolar vasoconstriction and efferent arteriolar vasodilatation. Initially, this is reversible with volume expansion. Later (2 days or more), restoration of RBF does not necessarily improve GFR, and a drop in RBF is associated with a disproportionately greater drop in GFR.[22] Even when vasoconstriction is reversed, GFR may not improve; this reflects loss of RBF autoregulation. This disproportionate reduction in GFR suggests a fall in the ultrafiltration coefficient of the glomeruli secondary to a reduction in total filtering area. The mechanism for this is unclear, but it may be associated with increases in angiotensin II concentration,

as this agent is known to induce mesangial contraction and a drop in the ultrafiltration coefficient.[23]

In addition to the aforementioned vascular changes that can affect GFR, the possible effects on GFR in the juxtamedullary region of even mild changes in RBF warrant specific mention. The glomeruli and adjacent straight portion of the proximal tubule and thick ascending limbs of Henle's loops in this region are apparently particularly susceptible to hypoxia (i.e., ischemia), owing to their high oxygen requirements. Swelling of endothelial and tubule cells secondary to prolonged ischemia in this region results in increased vascular resistance and continued compromise of the medullary circulation, even when cortical RBF has been restored.[15, 24]

GFR can also be compromised to a significant extent by obstruction of tubular lumina by casts of cellular debris and inflammatory cells. Increased intratubular pressure decreases the net driving pressure for glomerular filtration in the same way that obstruction of the urinary outflow tract can ultimately lead to a lower GFR. One of the reasons that agents that accelerate the solute excretion rate (e.g., furosemide and mannitol) may be therapeutic adjuncts has been that they are believed to help disperse these luminal blockages.

Tubuloglomerular feedback is a regulatory mechanism that lowers GFR whenever solute (most notably sodium chloride) concentrations at the macula densa are increased. In ARF, impaired transport in the thick ascending limb of the loop of Henle in the context of preserved glomerular response to signals from the macula densa, results in a decrease in GFR. This feedback is a normal protective mechanism that is mediated principally by the renin-angiotensin system, although prostaglandin, intracellular calcium, and adenosine may play a role in signal transmission or regulation. In essence, the mechanism serves to prevent massive fluid losses associated with a reduction of tubular reabsorptive capacity; however, in cases of renal hypoperfusion and ischemia, the effect is the opposite, as basically, the feedback mechanism exacerbates the effects of already reduced RBF.

Proximal tubule cells undergo morphologic changes relatively early in cases of ischemia. They lose their brush borders and polarity, and the integrity of their tight junctions is disrupted, probably secondary to alterations in the actin and microtubular cytoskeletons.[25, 26] Under these conditions the glomerular filtrate is able to leap back to the peritubular circulation, thus reducing the net (or effective) GFR. This mechanism is thought to be an important source of GFR reduction only in more severe cases of ischemia or nephrotoxin exposure.

Tubule cells involved in solute reabsorption have a very high metabolic rate and a high demand for oxygen. The existence of the corticomedullary oxygen gradient makes these cells very vulnerable to the effects of hypoxia and ischemia, the thick ascending limb of the loop of Henle in the outer medulla being most susceptible.[27] Early in ischemic and toxic ARF there are decreases in adenosine triphosphate (ATP) and adenosine diphosphate (ADP) tissue levels with associated elevations in adenosine monophosphate (AMP) and inorganic phosphate concentrations. Much of the AMP is broken down further to adenosine and then to xanthine. Adenosine is a potent constrictor of cortical blood flow and probably enhances the effect of the tubuloglomerular feedback system. ATP depletion in tubular cells inhibits cell volume regulation, and the resultant swelling probably contributes to luminal obstruction and increased vascular resistance. Na^+-K^+-ATPase is redistributed from the basolateral to the apical membrane of the tubule cells, thus reducing the ability of the cells to extrude sodium into the peritubular fluid and circulation.[28] Redistribution of integrins to the apical surface contributes to the breakdown of tight junctions.[29] Depletion of ATP in tubule cells also leads to an increase in cytosolic calcium concentration. In addition to being a vasoconstrictor, calcium activates proteases and phospholipases, interferes with mitochondrial energy metabolism, and can break down the cytoskeleton.[1, 30] Administration of calcium channel blockers has helped ameliorate ARF in some experimental situations.[31]

Reperfusion of renal tissue after a period of ischemia is associated with rapid production of oxygen free radicals and with marked tissue damage. Xanthines, neutrophils, phospholipase A_2, mixed-function oxidases, and mitochondrial electron transport are all associated with the production of these oxidants.[32] Phospholipase A_2 hydrolyzes phospholipids in cell and mitochondrial membranes to free fatty acids and lysophospholipids as well as producing arachidonic acid. Arachidonate is in turn converted to eicosanoids that are both vasoconstricting and chemotactic for neutrophils.[33] Cell membranes are particularly susceptible to phospholipase activity following reperfusion. Reperfusion injury is a major consideration in transplant surgery; however, the role it plays in the pathogenesis of prerenal and ischemic ARF is not clear.

Many of the cellular biochemical and structural changes seen in conjunction with the ischemic form of ARF are also important parts of the pathogenesis of ATN associated with exposure to nephrotoxins. Toxin-associated dysfunction and necrosis of cells result in increased tubular pressure and a decreased glomerular capillary hydrostatic pressure gradient. Loss of reabsorptive capability triggers tubuloglomerular feedback and further reduces GFR by lowering RBF secondary to vasoconstriction and a decrease in the glomerular ultrafiltration coefficient. Transepithelial back-leak of solutes into the circulation further interferes with the excretory function of the kidneys.

Acute Tubular Necrosis. Many agents are recognized to have potential nephrotoxic effects.

Aminoglycoside-induced renal toxicity results from accumulation of these agents within the renal cortex. Streptomycin is the least nephrotoxic of the aminoglycosides, whereas gentamicin and kanamycin are intermediate nephrotoxins. Neomycin is the most nephrotoxic. Most cases of aminoglycoside toxicity are associated with conditions that cause reduced renal perfusion, as the healthy kidney can usually tolerate some degree of aminoglycoside overdosing. After filtration at the glomerulus, aminoglycosides bind to phospholipase on the brush border of proximal tubules and are subsequently reabsorbed by pinocytosis. Accumulation of these antibiotics interferes with lysosomal, mitochondrial, and Na^+/K^+-ATPase function by inhibiting phospholipase A activity. Binding to the brush border is saturable with the result that sustained exposure of the proximal cells to the drug (as with multiple daily dosing regimens) results in greater accumulation of the drug and increased nephrotoxicity. As a result, once daily dosing may attenuate the risk of nephrotoxicosis while maintaining or improving therapeutic efficacy

(because it results in higher peak concentrations).[34, 35] Many mild cases of aminoglycoside toxicity are notably associated with nonoliguric ARF and, therefore, may go unrecognized in horses.

Some cephalosporins, like cephaloridine, have considerable nephrotoxic potential. These agents cause necrosis due to mitochondrial toxicity secondary to accumulation of the antibiotic in the cell.[36]

Not all cases of ATN are due to direct toxic changes in tubule cells. For instance, whether myoglobin and hemoglobin are truly nephrotoxic is still debatable. The principal characteristics of pigment nephropathy caused by these agents are tubule obstruction and reduced RBF (due to the direct vasoconstrictor effects of the pigment). Whether obstruction is of a physical nature, due to pigment accumulation, or reflects aggregation of sloughed cells is not clear. Myoglobin tends to be associated with nephropathy more frequently than hemoglobin. Patients often quickly become oliguric, presumably because of the widespread tubule obstruction.

Acute Interstitial Nephritis. It can be difficult to distinguish between drug-induced ATN and acute interstitial nephritis, and the latter is rarely diagnosed in horses. This may be a particular problem when continued use of antibiotics is indicated. With ATN, the dosing regimen may be altered, whereas with interstitial nephritis, short-term corticosteroid therapy is often of benefit in humans. Interstitial nephritis is often marked by eosinophiluria and eosinophilia, and is more likely associated with the presence of red cells than is ATN. The exact immune mechanism by which interstitial nephritis develops is unclear, although it is thought most likely to be due to delayed cell-mediated hypersensitivity or the presence of anti–tubule basement membrane antibodies.[37] The prognosis is usually grave in horses with acute interstitial nephritis.

Acute Glomerulonephritis. Acute glomerular nephropathy is relatively rare in horses, but when it occurs, it is usually manifested by the nephrotic syndrome, although hematuria and oliguria are sometimes observed. Deposits of gamma globulin and complement are found along the basement membrane (global form) or in the mesangial area (mesangioproliferative form).[38] Group C streptococcal antigens have been identified in conjunction with equine glomerulonephritis, and equine infectious anemia viral antigen-antibody complexes have been recognized in the glomeruli of horses that were not in renal failure.[12, 39] Deposition of immune complexes activates the complement cascade. Formation of C_3b and C_5a causes platelet aggregation and attracts neutrophils. Tissue damage results from deposition of complement per se, and inflammation associated with neutrophil activation and release of reactive oxygen radicals, proteases, elastases, and other lysozymes. These enzymes, plus platelet-activator factor and leukotriene B_4, increase vascular permeability and up-regulate expression of adhesion molecules, thus promoting further inflammation.[33] Severe reduction in GFR results from large drops in the glomerular permeability coefficient, which is associated with the widening of Bowman's spaces secondary to inflammation and deposition of immune complexes.

The pathophysiology of postrenal ARF was referred to

above. Basically, increases in ureteral pressure—for any reason—result in GFR reduction owing to a drop in the glomerular capillary hydrostatic pressure gradient, some tubular back-leak, a decrease in the glomerular permeability coefficient, and ultimately, reduction in RBF.

CLINICAL SIGNS

In the majority of horses with hemodynamically mediated (i.e., prerenal or ischemic) ARF, clinical signs are usually referable to the primary problem, such as acute colic or enterocolitis, sepsis, coagulopathies, rhabdomyolysis, or heavy metal poisoning, rather than to renal dysfunction. Therefore, the predominant clinical signs are often dehydration (with or without diarrhea), depression, and anorexia. Other signs can include tachycardia, hyperemic mucous membranes, pyrexia, mild abdominal pain, and laminitis. Because clinical signs usually relate to the inciting problem, ARF may not be suspected or detected unless the veterinarian specifically evaluates renal function as part of the workup for a more obvious disease. In general, the clinical manifestations of ARF reflect the systemic effects of toxic substances usually excreted in the urine (i.e., uremia is generally reflected by anorexia and depression), urinary tract dysfunction, and derangements of fluid, electrolyte, and acid-base balance. Signs of encephalopathy may be observed in horses with severe azotemia.

Although oliguria is considered the hallmark of ARF, in horses urine production is variable. Oliguria frequently occurs in the early stages of hemodynamically mediated ARF and is the most frequently reported clinical sign that is directly related to urinary tract dysfunction. As outlined in the section on Pathophysiology, however, nonoliguric and polyuric stages of prerenal and intrinsic ARF can also be associated with renal hypoperfusion. Anuria is rare. Nonoliguric or polyuric ARF can also be associated with exposure to nephrotoxins (ATN), and polyuria is common during the recovery phase of ARF, regardless of its cause. The magnitude of azotemia tends to be lower in nonoliguric than in oliguric ARF, possibly indicating less severe damage in the former condition. Similarly, nonoliguric ARF is associated with a more favorable prognosis.

Patients with ARF are often initially treated with large volumes of intravenous or oral fluids for the primary disease. In these cases, oliguria may progress to polyuria. When significant renal damage has been sustained, persistence of oliguria in the face of fluid administration is usually manifested as failure to produce a significant volume of urine in response to fluid therapy. There is also minimal change in the degree of azotemia in the initial 24 to 36 hours of treatment. If these patients are not carefully monitored, fluid retention may lead to development of subcutaneous and pulmonary edema. Soft feces, due to fluid retention, may also be observed in patients with oliguric ARF.

Postrenal or obstructive uropathy is usually characterized by mild to severe abdominal pain and pollakiuria and stranguria (see section on Urolithiasis).

DIAGNOSIS

Increases in plasma urea nitrogen and creatinine concentrations (i.e., azotemia) are frequently the initial findings that suggest compromised renal function. Azotemia simply reflects a reduction in GFR; it has almost no differential diagnostic value. Once recent development of azotemia is established, the equine internist must proceed systematically to differentiate between six possible syndromes associated with ARF: prerenal ARF, ischemic ARF, ATN, acute interstitial nephritis, acute glomerulonephritis, and obstructive (postrenal) ARF. A useful way to go about this is first to try to rule out pre- and postrenal ARF. If this is possible, the patient must have a type of intrinsic ARF and further diagnostic efforts are directed at identifying the disease subtypes.

As described in greater detail later (see Urolithiasis), the diagnosis of postrenal obstructive disease is usually based on a combination of clinical signs, history, and the results of rectal palpation, ultrasonography, and urinary tract endoscopy. The frequency and volume of urination can vary with these cases, and total obstruction causes anuria. Salt and water reabsorption are often impaired as the problem persists. This results in hyponatremia (i.e., plasma sodium concentrations in the low normal range). While the mechanisms for this sodium wasting are not completely clear, it is apparently related to impaired function of the ascending limb of Henle's loop, and an increased medullary blood flow secondary to prostaglandin release. Both of these events greatly diminish the magnitude and effect of the medullary countercurrent–concentrating mechanisms. Prostaglandin also directly inhibits the effect of ADH.[40]

Measurement of specific gravity in the azotemic horse is a commonly practiced means of detecting prerenal ARF. In these cases, the value is usually above 1.025 and often as high as 1.055. In humans a number of reliable indices can be used to differentiate renal azotemia from prerenal azotemia.[41–43] These are based on urine osmolality and the ratio of urine to plasma osmolality (U/P_{osm}), urine sodium concentration and fractional sodium clearance, and ratios of urine to plasma urea concentration (U/P_{UN}) and urine to plasma creatinine concentrations (U/P_{Cr}). Fractional sodium clearance, in particular, is a good indicator of solute reabsorption and proximal tubule function, whereas U/P_{Cr}, and to a lesser extent U/P_{UN}, are useful indices of the ability of the tubules to reabsorb water. The utility of these indices in horses has also been investigated and has been shown to have considerable differential diagnostic value.[16] While these tests are relatively discriminatory, there is some degree of overlap between them with respect to prerenal and parenchymal or intrinsic problems. It must also be borne in mind that they do not allow differentiation between intrinsic and postrenal disease. A number of horses with prerenal (nonoliguric) ARF have urine osmolality below 360 mOsm. A small percentage of horses in prerenal ARF have U/P_{Cr} below 30 (usually above 50) and fractional sodium clearance above 0.80% (usually below 0.50%), most likely owing to the unrecognized existence of tubule damage before volume depletion or because of a natriuretic effect of some treatments such as diuretics or intravenous fluids. Natriuresis is particularly likely to be induced in conjunction with bicarbonate administration, as sodium cations are lost with unreabsorbed bicarbonate anions. In these cases, the determination of the fractional chloride clearance may be a better indicator of the response of the kidney to hypoperfusion.

No parameter reliably differentiates between prerenal and ischemic ARF, owing to the pathophysiologic continuum between these diseases. At one end is reduced GFR with preserved tubule function and concentrating mechanisms. This form of disease is readily reversible with appropriate therapy. Additional or more prolonged decreases in GFR lead to disturbances in tubule function and slower reversal of damage, until the other end of the spectrum is reached, where there is complete and irreversible loss of renal function. Assessment of urine specific gravity before initiation of fluid therapy is helpful in differentiating prerenal from renal failure. As normally functioning kidneys would maximally preserve salt and water in response to a transient decrease in RBF with prerenal failure, urine specific gravity and osmolality are greater than the values associated with serum, whereas, the urine produced by horses with intrinsic ARF is often isosthenuric (specific gravity below 1.020). In a clinical situation, assessment of the response to fluid therapy is the most practical way to differentiate prerenal failure from intrinsic forms of ARF. Azotemia caused by prerenal problems should resolve quickly with replacement of fluid deficits and restoration of renal perfusion. Also, in prerenal failure volume repletion should restore renal function, with the result that the magnitude of azotemia should decrease by 50% or more during the first day of therapy. In contrast, fluid therapy usually does not lead to prompt resolution of azotemia associated with intrinsic problems. Application of the measurement of U/P_{Cr} and U/P_{UN} ratios is limited to use on urine samples collected before initiation of fluid therapy or the first urine sample voided after fluid therapy has been started.

In prerenal ARF, electrolyte and acid-base abnormalities generally reflect problems caused by a primary disease (e.g., enterocolitis, colic, blood loss). Most frequently, horses are mildly acidotic, hyponatremic, and hypochloremic. Plasma concentrations of potassium and calcium vary according to what disease is causing renal hypoperfusion. Potassium concentration is also affected to some extent by urine output, hyperkalemia being most common in association with oliguria and anuria.

The technique for biopsy of the left kidney has been well-described.[44] Its main indication is to help differentiate between types of intrinsic renal disease when it is felt that this distinction will have therapeutic and prognostic relevance. Often, ischemic failure and ATN can be diagnosed without biopsy. The primary complication associated with the biopsy procedure is renal hemorrhage, which can be quite severe. Ultrasonographic guidance and use of a spring-loaded biopsy instrument may reduce the risk of complications. Ultrasonography also allows biopsy of the right kidney. As the knowledge of equine renal physiology and pathology improves and advances in molecular genetics lead to techniques that supplant or supplement standard histopathologic methods, the diagnostic usefulness of renal biopsy may increase. For example, the use of immunosuppressive agents in the treatment of some forms of renal parenchymal disease (e.g., interstitial nephritis) may be dictated by biopsy results.

Identification of subtypes of intrinsic ARF often depend on analysis of urine and urine sediment. The availability of a history of exposure to ischemic insults or potential nephrotoxins like aminoglycosides certainly helps in this regard, but determination of the severity of the condition and its prognosis still generally relies on the analysis of urine. Ischemic tubule disease is quite similar to ATN. In both cases there is slight to moderate proteinuria with specific gravities usually below 1.020 and urine osmolality below 350 mOsm. Fractional sodium clearance is nearly always greater than 1.0, regardless of urine output. Granular casts are frequently seen, particularly with ATN. Enzymuria and phosphaturia are frequently prominent early in the course of ATN.[45, 46] Plasma sodium and chloride concentrations are usually low. Plasma concentrations of calcium and inorganic phosphate are highly variable: increases, decreases, and normal values are all possible, depending on the horse's diet, the nephrotoxin, and the location and severity of damage to the nephron.[39, 45]

It is important to remember that GFR is reduced in cases of ATN. This is most likely due to the increase in presentation of sodium and chloride at the macula densa secondary to dysfunction of proximal sodium reabsorption. Stimulation of the macula densa results in release of renin and local production of angiotensin II, thus increasing renal vascular resistance and lowering RBF. The low GFR may mask the absolute magnitude of the damage in tubule function; however, if renal sodium reabsorption is studied carefully over time in cases of ATN, it appears that this defect improves more rapidly than that of GFR.[47]

Acute interstitial nephritis is not often recognized in horses; however, in a study conducted about 20 years ago, it was diagnosed in approximately one eighth of all human patients who needed renal biopsy for diagnosis of unexplained ARF.[48]

The disease is characterized by edema and diffuse or focal patches of interstitial inflammation. In human medicine, the number of drugs, toxins, and infectious agents known to induce this disease is growing. There is no reason to believe that similar agents are not capable of causing the same disease in equidae. Inflammatory cells surround the tubules and can move between epithelial cells into tubule lumina. As a result, white blood cell casts are quite common. The leukocytes are also capable of disrupting the tubule basement membrane, making cell repair much less likely. This is an important distinguishing feature between ATN and interstitial nephritis. With the former disease, the basement membrane usually stays intact. Reduction of GFR and azotemia probably result from the interstitial edema, intratubular obstruction, and release of vasoactive agents.

Acute interstitial nephritis and ATN have similar fractional sodium clearance, U/P_{Cr}, and U/P_{osm} values; however, the urine sediment may be quite different for each disease. Sterile pyuria and microscopic hematuria are commonly seen with interstitial nephritis, although red blood cell casts are rare. Mild proteinuria and eosinophiluria are also common. Eosinophiluria generally seems to be limited to renal interstitial disease—mainly drug-induced interstitial nephritis, but also chronic pyelonephritis and systemic lupus erythematosus.[49, 50] It may or may not be accompanied by eosinophilia. Eosinophils in equine urine should be relatively easy to observe using Wright's stain, given the alkaline nature of the fluid. Occasionally, fevers are believed to be associated with the development of interstitial nephritis. This is a relatively nonspecific clinical sign that might be quite misleading if the animal is being treated with antibiotics for an infection. What might be seen if the patient is closely monitored is an initial reduction or resolution of the fever after the onset of antimicrobial therapy followed by recurrence of the fever and development of azotemia. If this happens, acute interstitial nephritis should be on the rule-out list.

Acute glomerulonephritis is usually characterized by the nephrotic syndrome. Proteinuria is moderate to severe, and the urine is usually concentrated. Urine osmolality and U/P_{osm} are comparable to those seen with prerenal ARF and are higher than those values normally seen in ATN. Urinary sodium concentration and fractional sodium clearance tend to be much lower than with other intrinsic renal and postrenal causes of ARF. U/P_{UN} and U/P_{Cr} values are often similar to those associated with prerenal failure and higher than those in ischemic, tubular, interstitial, or postrenal disease. Renal tubular secretion of creatinine is increased in glomerulonephritis, with the result that serum creatinine concentrations may not rise very quickly and urea nitrogen-to-creatinine ratios stay high, as they frequently do with prerenal problems. Therefore, while urinary indices should make possible differentiation of acute glomerulonephritis from other parenchymal and postrenal diseases, they overlap much with those associated with prerenal ARF. ARF due to acute glomerulonephritis is going to be differentiated from that caused by hypoperfusion on the basis of the marked proteinuria and red cell numbers usually associated with the former disease. Red cell casts are more common with glomerulonephritis than with other intrinsic causes of ARF. Some causes of postrenal ARF may also manifest red cell casts, but the proteinuria is not normally as great in those situations.

TREATMENT

Initially, treatment of horses with ARF should focus on reversing the inciting or underlying cause and correcting fluid and electrolyte imbalances. Early identification of patients at risk and prevention of problems by rapid restoration and accurate maintenance of intravascular fluid volume, glomerular filtration, and urine production, with fluids, and possibly diuretics, is obviously preferable to treatment. The importance of prevention cannot be overstated. Initial fluid deficits should be corrected over the first 6 to 12 hours of treatment. Physiologic saline or a balanced electrolyte solution is the fluid of choice unless the patient is hypernatremic, as may be the case in prerenal ARF or acute glomerulonephritis. In the event of hypernatremia, a 0.45% sodium chloride–2.5% dextrose solution is recommended. The addition of 50 to 100 g of dextrose per liter of fluid to saline or polyionic fluids helps address the calorie needs of anorectic horses. If fluid administration is begun early in the course of the disease or if the problem is not severe, diuresis should result. When this occurs, intravenous fluid therapy is maintained at 40 to 80 mL/kg per day until serum creatinine concentration decreases dramatically. The rate of fluid administration is then reduced to 10 to 20 mL/kg per day until the creatinine concentration is normal or the horse is eating and drinking adequately.

In the event that the horse remains oliguric 10 to 12 hours after starting fluid therapy, administration of dopamine in 5% dextrose slowly (3 to 5 µg/kg per minute may improve RBF and urine output. Blood pressure should be monitored during dopamine infusion, as the drug can induce marked hypertension. Administration should be discontinued if blood pressure starts to rise. Restarting the infusion at a lower rate

can be attempted when pressure has returned to normal. Blood pressure may also increase owing to overhydration of oliguric patients who are receiving isotonic fluids. Regular monitoring of body weight, hematocrit, and serum total protein concentration, central venous pressure, and lung sounds is important if problems due to overhydration are to be avoided.

The use of diuretic agents such as mannitol and loop diuretics for treatment of ARF is somewhat controversial. Furosemide and ethacrynic acid are the loop diuretics most commonly used. Furosemide is a particularly potent short-acting agent that acts by blocking the $Na^+/K^+/2Cl^-$ cotransporter in the ascending limb of the loop of Henle. In addition to promoting diuresis, cotransporter inhibition may also protect these tubule cells by reducing their metabolic rate—and thus oxygen demand in the face of limited oxygen availability secondary to hypoperfusion. To be effective, loop diuretics must gain access to the tubule lumina. Therefore, they may be of limited value in prerenal or ischemic problems, although the potential protective effect of furosemide on the especially vulnerable cells of the thick ascending limb may warrant its administration. Also, loop diuretic administration may exacerbate or induce volume depletion in cases of ARF that are characterized by isosthenuria or polyuria (such as early ATN), thus making the condition worse and rendering the patient more susceptible to the effects of nephrotoxins like gentamicin. Loop diuretics appear to be most beneficial when used in cases characterized by tubule obstruction (e.g., pigmenturia), as the diuretic-induced increase in solute retention apparently helps flush these blockages and casts from the tubules.

While loop diuretics have no direct effect on GFR, 20% mannitol (0.25 to 1.0 g/kg) given over 15 to 20 minutes may help combat oliguria by increasing RBF and GFR. This occurs secondary to reductions in plasma protein concentration and oncotic pressure. These changes in turn result from the systemic effects of the increase in intravascular osmolality induced by the mannitol. Mannitol may also induce synthesis of the vasodilator PGE_2 and release of atrial natriuretic peptide, which would also increase RBF and GFR. Once filtered, the agent also acts as an osmotic diuretic, thus decreasing urine solute concentration and boosting urine volume. Consequently, it can also be very effective in the treatment of conditions characterized by tubular obstruction and swelling of tubule cells.

Hyperkalemia is relatively uncommon in equine ARF, except in some postrenal cases. When present, it is usually mild and responds to administration of potassium-free intravenous fluids. When hyperkalemia (above 6.5 mEq/L) persists, correction of any associated acidosis with sodium bicarbonate and/or administration of glucose (up to 10% solution) usually helps. In the worst—or most refractory—cases, insulin may be necessary. Potassium supplementation (potassium chloride 20 to 40 mEq/L) may be necessary during the polyuric phase of recovery from ARF.

Calcium metabolism is often disrupted in cases of equine ARF, with hypocalcemia and hyperphosphatemia or hypercalcemia and hypophosphatemia having been variously reported. Hypercalcemia usually resolves with a switch to a grass or grass hay diet—and time. Hypocalcemia probably results for a number of reasons, including skeletal resistance to parathyroid hormone during the early stages of ARF and deficiency of 1,25-dihydroxycholecalciferol, which results either from down-regulation of renal 1,25-hydroxylase by the hyperphosphatemia, or dysfunction of this enzyme secondary to renal parenchymal damage, or both.[46, 51] Hypoalbuminemia and enhanced deposition of calcium in injured tissues, as can occur in cases of rhabdomyolysis, are other factors to consider. Administration of a calcium salt as part of the intravenous fluid therapy protocol is usually sufficient to correct this.

Severe uremia often decreases red blood cell life span and induces platelet dysfunction. Consequently, anemia (possibly due also to decreased production of erythropoietin) and bleeding tendencies may be associated with ARF. These may require treatment with transfusions, synthetic erythropoietin, or conjugated estrogens.

As aminoglycoside toxicity is one of the more commonly recognized causes of equine ARF,[4, 9, 52] continued aminoglycoside use in horses with ARF warrants specific attention. Gentamicin and amikacin are the aminoglycoside antibiotics most often used in equine practice, and their pharmacokinetics have been well-studied in healthy animals. There are large interindividual and age variations in the volume of distribution and clearance of these drugs in normal horses, and this variability is even greater in diseased ones. Therefore, when aminoglycoside antibiotics are needed by patients with ARF, monitoring serum trough concentrations of the drug to adjust the dosing interval is strongly indicated, as it provides the best protection against exacerbating renal damage. Renal dysfunction associated with aminoglycoside toxicity is usually indicated by an increase of at least 0.3 mg/dL in serum creatinine concentration. When this occurs, discontinuing therapy or increasing the dosing interval should be considered. It is important to remember that changes in urine sediment and development of enzymuria, mild proteinuria, glucosuria, and decreased urine-concentrating ability develop a number of days before serum creatinine concentration increases and are good indicators of the development of aminoglycoside nephrotoxicity. The problem can usually be addressed successfully by maintaining or increasing intravenous fluid therapy to guard against renal hypoperfusion and by appropriately adjusting the dosing interval with the antibiotic.

PROGNOSIS

The prognosis for equine ARF depends on the underlying cause, the duration of renal failure, the response to initial treatment, and the development of secondary complications such as diarrhea, thrombophlebitis, and laminitis. Generally speaking, the duration of ARF before beginning therapy is the most important determinant of prognosis. Of the primary causes of ARF, severe ischemic failure and acute interstitial nephritis probably carry the worst prognosis in horses. ARF of any cause, however, should be associated with a reduced or poor prognosis in the event that early interruption of the pathophysiologic events leading to the ARF is not achieved or that the animal displays prolonged oliguria or anuria (longer than 12 hours) after institution of vigorous therapy. Most cases of postrenal ARF carry a favorable prognosis, provided the initiating disease is treated successfully. When discussing prognosis with horse owners practitioners must always bear in mind that a successful outcome is not always associated with complete return of normal function. Many horses live long after a bout of ARF but never fully regain the ability to concentrate urine as well as they did before the disease; or else they remain constantly polyuric. ATN, secondary to nephrotoxicity in particular, carries a favorable prognosis when tubule basement membranes remain intact.

REFERENCES

1. Thadhani R, Pascual M, Bonventre JV: Acute renal failure. *N Engl J Med* 334:1448, 1996.
2. Divers TJ: Acute renal failure. In Robinson NE, ed. *Current Therapy in Equine Medicine 2*. Philadelphia, WB Saunders, 1987, p 693.
3. Shankel SW, Johnson DC, Clark PS, et al: Acute renal failure and glomerulopathy caused by nonsteroidal anti-inflammatory drugs. *Arch Intern Med* 152:986, 1992.
4. Divers TJ, Whitlock RH, Byars TD, et al: Acute renal failure in six horses resulting from haemodynamic causes. *Equine Vet J* 19:178, 1987.
5. Schmitz DG: Toxic nephropathy in horses. *Compend Contin Educ Pract Vet* 10:104, 1988.
6. Markel MD, Dyer RM, Hattel AL: Acute renal failure associated with application of a mercuric blister in a horse. *J Am Vet Med Assoc* 185:92, 1984.
7. Harrington DD, Page EH: Acute vitamin D_3 toxicosis in horses: Case reports and experimental studies of the comparative toxicity of vitamins D_2 and D_3. *J Am Vet Med Assoc* 182:1358, 1983.
8. Rebhun WC, Tennant BC, Dill SG, et al: Vitamin K_3–induced renal toxicosis in the horse. *J Am Vet Med Assoc* 184:1237, 1984.
9. Riviere JE, Traver DS, Coppoc GL: Gentamicin toxic nephropathy in horses with disseminated bacterial infection. *J Am Vet Med Assoc* 180:648, 1982.
10. Brown C: Equine nephrology. *Vet Annu* 26:1, 1986.
11. Morris DD: Glomerulonephritis. In Robinson NE, ed. *Current Therapy in Equine Medicine 2*. Philadelphia, WB Saunders, 1987, p 702.
12. Banks KL, Henson JB: Immunologically mediated glomerulitis of horses II: Antiglomerular basement membrane antibody and other mechanisms in spontaneous disease. *Lab Invest* 26:708, 1972.
13. Ehnen SJ, Divers TJ, Gillette D, et al: Obstructive nephrolithiasis and ureterolithiasis associated with chronic renal failure in horses. *J Am Vet Med Assoc* 197:249, 1990.
14. Laverty S, Pascoe JR, Ling GV, et al: Urolithiasis in 68 horses. *Vet Surg* 21:56, 1992.
15. Brezis M, Rosen F: Hypoxia of the renal medulla—its implications for disease. *N Engl J Med* 332:647, 1995.
16. Grossman BS, Brobst DF, Kramer JW, et al: Urinary indices for differentiation of prerenal azotemia and renal azotemia in horses. *J Am Vet Med Assoc* 180:284, 1982.
17. Miller PD, Krebs RA, Neal BJ, et al: Polyuric prerenal failure. *Arch Intern Med* 140:907, 1980.
18. Baylis C: The mechanism of the decline in glomerular filtration in gentamicin induced acute renal failure in the rat. *J Antimicrob Chem* 6:381, 1980.
19. Flamenbaum W, McNeil JS, Kotchen TA, et al: Experimental acute renal failure induced by uranyl nitrate in the dog. *Circulation Res* 31:682, 1972.
20. Katzberg RW, Morris TW, Schulman G, et al: Reactions to intravenous contrast media, Part II: Acute renal response in euvolemic and dehydrated dogs. *Radiology* 147:331, 1983.
21. Levenson DJ, Simmons CD Jr., Brenner BM: Arachidonic

acid metabolism, prostaglandins, and the kidney. *Am J Med* 72:354, 1982.

22. Reineck HJ, O'Connor GJ, Lifschitz MD, et al: Sequential studies on the pathophysiology and glycerol-induced acute renal failure. *J Lab Clin Med* 96:356, 1980.

23. Dworkin LD, Ichikawa I, Brenner VN: Hormonal modulation of glomerular function. *Am J Physiol* 244:F95, 1983.

24. Frega NS, DiBona DR, Guertter B, et al: Ischemic renal injury. *Kidney Int* 10:517, 1976.

25. Molitoris BA: Ischemia-induced loss of epithelial polarity: Potential role of the actin cytoskeleton. *Am J Physiol* 260:F769, 1991.

26. Abbate M, Bonventre JV, Brown D: The microtubule network of renal epithelial cells is disrupted by ischemia and reperfusion. *Am J Physiol* 267:F971, 1994.

27. Venkatachalam MA, Bernard DB, Donohoe DF, et al: Ischemic damage and repair in the rat proximal tubule: Differences among the S1, S2, and S3 segments. *Kidney Int* 14:31, 1978.

28. Molitoris BA, Dahl R, Geerde SA: Cytoskeleton disruption and apical redistribution of proximal tubule Na$^+$/K$^+$ATPase during ischemia. *Am J Physiol* 263:F483, 1992.

29. Goligorsky MS, DiBona GF: Pathogenetic role of Arg-Gly-Asp-recognizing integrins in acute renal failure. *Proc Natl Acad Sci USA* 90:5700, 1993.

30. Kribben A, Widder ED, Wetzels JFM, et al: Evidence for role of cytosolic free calcium in hypoxia-induced proximal tubule injury. *J Clin Invest* 93:1922, 1994.

31. Bonventre JV: Mechanisms of ischemic acute renal failure. *Kidney Int* 43:1160, 1993.

32. Johnson KJ, Weinberg JM: Postischemic renal injury due to oxygen radicals. *Curr Opin Nephrol Hypertension* 2:625, 1993.

33. Klausner JM, Paterson IS, Goldman G, et al: Postischemic renal injury is mediated by neutrophils and leukotrienes. *Am J Physiol* 256:F794, 1989.

34. Hinchcliff KW, McGuirk SM, MacWilliams TS: Gentamicin nephrotoxicity. *Proc Am Assoc Equine Pract* 33:67, 1988.

35. Hostetler K, Hall L: Aminoglycoside antibiotics inhibit lysosomal phospholipase A and C from rat liver in vitro. *Biochim Biophys Acta* 710:506, 1982.

36. Blantz RC: Intrinsic renal failure: Acute. In Seldin DW, Giebsich G, eds. *The Kidney: Physiology and Pathophysiology.* New York, Raven Press, 1985, p 1875.

37. Galpin J, Shinaberger J, Stanley T, et al: Acute interstitial nephritis due to methicillin. *Am J Med* 17:756, 1978.

38. McCausland IP, Milestone BA: Diffuse mesangioproliferative glomerulonephritis in a horse. *NZ Vet J* 24:239, 1976.

39. Divers TJ, Timoney JF, Lewis RM, et al: Equine glomerulonephritis and renal failure associated with complexes of Group-C streptococcal antigen and IgG antibody. *Vet Immunol Immunopathol* 32:93, 1992.

40. Shimizu K, Kurosawa T, Maeda T, et al: Free water excretion and washout of renal medullary urea by prostaglandin E$_1$. *Jpn Heart J* 10:437, 1969.

41. Eliahou HD, Bata A: The diagnosis of acute renal failure. *Nephron* 2:287, 1965.

42. Miller TR, Anderson RG, Linas SL, et al: Urinary diagnostic indices in acute renal failure. *Ann Intern Med* 89:47, 1978.

43. Espinel CH, Gregory AW: Differential diagnosis of acute renal failure. *Clin Nephrol* 13:73, 1980.

44. Bayly WM, Paradis MR, Reed SM: Equine renal biopsy: Indications, technique, interpretations and complications. *Mod Vet Pract* 61:763, 1980.

45. Bayly WM, Brobst DF, Elfers RS, et al: Serum and urinary biochemistry and enzyme changes in ponies with acute renal failure. *Cornell Vet* 76:306, 1986.

46. Elfers RS, Bayly WM, Brobst DF, et al: Alterations in calcium, phosphorus, and C-terminal parathyroid hormone levels in equine acute renal disease. *Cornell Vet* 76:317, 1986.

47. Meroney WH, Rubini MD: Kidney function during acute tubular necrosis: Clinical studies and a theory. *Metabolism* 8:1, 1959.

48. Wilson DM, Turner DR, Cameron JS, et al: Value of renal biopsy in acute intrinsic renal failure. *Br Med J* 2:459, 1976.

49. Simenhoff NL, Guild WR, Gammin GJ: Acute diffuse interstitial nephritis. *Am J Med* 44:618, 1968.

50. Ruffing KA, Hoope SP, Blend D, et al: Eosinophils in urine revisited. *Clin Nephrol* 41:163, 1994.

51. Llach F, Felsenfeld AJ, Haussler MR: Pathophysiology of altered calcium metabolism in rhabdomyolysis-induced acute renal failure. Interactions of parathyroid hormone, 25-hydroxycholecalciferol and 1,25-dihydroxycholecalciferol. *N Engl J Med* 305:117, 1981.

52. Sweeney RW, MacDonald M, Hall J, et al: Kinetics of gentamicin elimination in two horses with acute renal failure. *Equine Vet J* 20:182, 1988.

16.6

Chronic Renal Failure

Harold C. Schott II, DVM, PhD

PREDISPOSING CONDITIONS

Chronic renal failure (CRF) is recognized infrequently in horses. For dogs and cats the prevalence of CRF has been reported to be 0.9% and 1.6%, respectively,[1] whereas the Veterinary Medical Data Base at Purdue University reported that only 515 of 442,535 horses admitted to participating veterinary teaching hospitals during the years 1964 through 1996 had CRF (prevalence of 0.12%). In actuality, this may be an underestimate, since when a diagnosis of CRF is established for a horse, it may likely be destroyed without presentation to a veterinary teaching hospital. As in dogs and cats, CRF appears to be a greater problem in older horses: the prevalence increased to 0.23% in horses older than 15 years. The 0.51% prevalence for intact males over 15 years of age also suggests that stallions may be at greater risk.

Although the clinical syndrome of CRF is uncommon, one widely cited abattoir study revealed that 16% of 45 horses examined had glomerular lesions on light microscopy and 42% (22 of 53 horses examined) exhibited deposits of immunoglobulin or complement on immunofluorescence staining.[2] Although these findings suggest that as many as one third of horses may show microscopic evidence of renal disease, only one of the horses in this survey exhibited signs of CRF. This disparity can be attributed to a large renal reserve capacity, as clinical signs of renal failure do not become apparent until two thirds to three fourths of functional nephrons have been lost.[3] Although this "rule of thumb" is based on studies of partially nephrectomized laboratory animals, support for similar renal reserve capacity in horses is found in several clinical reports of unilateral nephrectomy used successfully to manage disorders of the upper urinary tract.[4–8] In addition, after experimental unilateral nephrectomy in ponies[9] and horses (R. DeBowes, personal communication, 1991), renal function remained within normal ranges and body weight was maintained.

Disorders of the kidneys leading to CRF may be congenital or acquired. In horses younger than 5 years whose history includes no event that might have been complicated by acute renal failure (ARF), a congenital renal disorder should be suspected—renal agenesis, hypoplasia, dysplasia, polycystic kidney disease.[10–19] While each of these congenital abnormalities is occasionally recognized, acquired disease consequent to glomerular or tubular injury is more often the cause of CRF in horses.[20–26] Acquired disease is usually insidious in onset, and renal injury may have been initiated years earlier. Thus, identifying the cause of CRF is challenging because many horses have evidence of advanced glomerular and tubular disease, termed "end-stage kidney disease," by the time clinical signs of CRF develop. Nevertheless, knowing the various causes of CRF affords a better overall understanding of CRF in horses.

Glomerulonephritis

Glomerular injury is a common precipitant of renal insufficiency and CRF in horses. Although immune-mediated glomerular injury is most often implicated in glomerulonephritis (GN), glomerular integrity can be disrupted by a number of unrelated disease processes, including ischemia, toxic insults, and infection.[27] These mechanisms usually lead to significant vascular and tubulointerstitial changes in addition to glomerular injury. Thus, the designation "GN" is typically reserved to denote renal disease of which immune-mediated glomerular damage is suspected to be the initiating factor in development of renal failure. Until the last decade, GN was considered a rare cause of CRF in domestic animals; interstitial nephritis was more often implicated.[28–30] Refinement of histologic examination with immunofluorescence staining techniques and electron microscopic examination of renal tissues has led to increased recognition of both subclinical and clinically significant glomerulonephritis.[30]

A brief review of the "subgross" anatomy of the glomerulus will shed light on the pathophysiology of GN. The renal corpuscle, or glomerulus, is comprised of a tuft of glomerular capillaries surrounded by epithelial cells that line Bowman's capsule. The root that supports the pedicle of the glomerular capillary network is similar to the mesenteric root that supports the intestinal tract, and Bowman's capsule is analogous to the peritoneum (Fig. 16–15A). On a microscopic level, components of the glomerulus include capillary endothelial cells, mesangium (cells and matrix), glomerular basement membrane (GBM), and visceral epithelial cells. At the vascular pedicle, the latter become contiguous with parietal epithelial cells which line Bowman's space, much as mesothelial cells covering bowel serosa and mesentery become contiguous with the peritoneum at the mesenteric root.[27] Glomerular capillary endothelial cells are somewhat unique in that they are fenestrated with pores that represent the initial barrier for passage of blood components into the urinary space (Fig. 16–15B). The mesangium, which lies between endothelial and epithelial cells, is the support structure of the glomerular capillaries, analogous to the mesen-

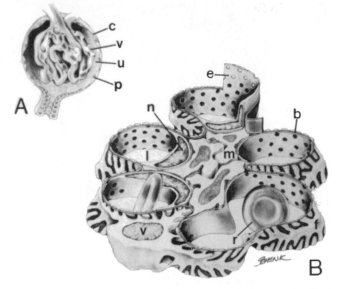

Figure 16–15. Subgross anatomy of a renal corpuscle. **A,** A renal corpuscle with a tuft of glomerular capillaries surrounded by Bowman's capsule *(c)* shows visceral *(v)* and parietal *(p)* epithelial cells separated by the urinary space *(u)*. **B,** Cross-section of a portion of a glomerulus shows the nucleus *(n)* and fenestrations *(e)* of capillary endothelial cells, the glomerular basement membrane *(b)*, mesangial cells *(m)* separated by mesangial matrix, and the nucleus *(v)* and foot processes *(f)* of a visceral epithelial cell. A red blood cell *(r)* is in the lumen *(l)* of one of the glomerular capillaries. (From Osborne CA, Hammer RF, Stevens JB, et al.: The glomerulus in health and disease: A comparative review of domestic animals and man. Adv Vet Sci Comp Med 21:207, 1977.)

teric tissue supporting bowel. Mesangial cells are a component of the reticuloendothelial system and phagocytize macromolecular substances, among them are fragments of "old GBM" or larger molecules that pass through endothelial cell pores but cannot subsequently pass through the GBM. In addition, mesangial cells have contractile elements that allow them to participate in regulation of glomerular hemodynamics. Furthermore, these cells proliferate in response to glomerular injury and can release a number of cytokines that modulate the glomerular inflammatory response.[31] The GBM lies between endothelial and epithelial cells and surrounds glomerular capillaries, except where mesangium is present (Fig. 16–16A). Returning to the abdominal cavity analogy, the GBM would lie beneath bowel serosa except in the area of mesenteric attachment, which would contain mesangial cells and matrix. The GBM consists of a central electron-dense layer, the lamina densa, and two thinner, more electron-lucent layers, the lamina rara externa and the lamina rara interna (Fig. 16–16B).[27, 32] The main components of the GBM are collagen-like molecules and matrix glycoproteins. These are produced principally by visceral epithelial cells, and normal GBM undergoes steady turnover and removal of debris by mesangial cells. The visceral epithelial cells, also called "podocytes" cover the "uriniferous duct" side of the GBM. They have many cytoplasmic extensions called "foot processes," which form extensive interdigitations with foot

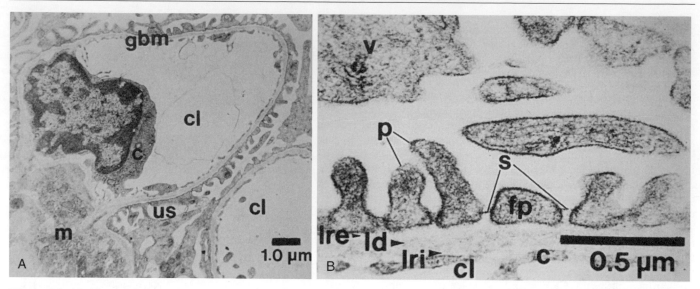

Figure 16–16. Electron micrograph of a normal glomerulus. **A,** Low-power magnification illustrates patent capillary lumens *(cl)* separated from the urinary space *(us)* by fenestrated endothelial cell cytoplasm *(c)*, the glomerular basement membrane *(gbm)*, and foot processes of visceral epithelial cells. Mesangial cells and matrix *(m)* are also apparent (bar = 1.0 μm). **B,** Higher power magnification reveals the ultrastructural features of the filtration barrier including, from bottom to top, the capillary lumen *(cl)* and endothelial cell cytoplasm *(c)*; the lamina rara interna *(lri)*, lamina densa *(ld)*, and lamina rara externa *(lre)* of the glomerular basement membrane; and cytoplasm *(v)*, foot processes *(fp)*, and slit diaphragms *(s)* of the visceral epithelial cells. Deposits of glomerular polyanion or glycosaminoglycans *(p)* can be seen on the foot processes (bar = 0.5 μm). (From Osborne CA, Hammer RF, Stevens JB, et al.: The glomerulus in health and disease: A comparative review of domestic animals and man. Adv Vet Sci Comp Med 21:207, 1997.)

processes of adjacent epithelial cells. The narrow gap between foot processes—the filtration slit or slit pore—is bridged by a thin membrane—the slit pore diaphragm.[27, 32]

The filtration barrier of the glomerulus consists of fenestrated endothelial cells, GBM, and slit pores between epithelial cell foot processes. These structures constitute a size-selective and charge-selective filtration barrier. Although all components of this barrier are anionic (i.e., they repel anionic macromolecules), the GBM is thought to be the principal agent of the permeability characteristics of the filtration barrier. The GBM is rich in glycosaminoglycans, containing heparan sulfate and sialic acid residues. These strongly anionic molecules are responsible for its negative "charge barrier," which limits filtration of anionic macromolecules, predominantly albumin.[32, 33]

GN is initiated by deposition of circulating immune complexes along the GBM and in the mesangium, leading to complement activation and leukocyte infiltration and adherence. Release of oxidants and proteinases by neutrophils and macrophages; production of eicosanoids, cytokines, and growth factors by macrophages and mesangial cells; and platelet aggregation and activation of coagulation factors lead to endothelial and epithelial cell swelling (with fusion of foot processes), formation of microthrombi in glomerular capillaries, and mesangial cell proliferation.[27, 33] Immune complexes can be deposited in a subendothelial, intra-GBM, or subepithelial site, depending on their size and charge properties. On electron microscopic examination these immune complexes appear as electron-dense granular deposits (Fig. 16–17A), and staining with anti–immunoglobulin G (IgG) and anticomplement (C3) antibodies reveals an irregular (granular or "lumpy bumpy") immunofluorescence stain-

ing pattern (Fig. 16–17B).[2, 27, 33] The GBM proliferates to surround the immune deposits, leading to irregular thickening of the filtration barrier. Despite widening of the filtration barrier, both the size-selective and charge-selective filtration properties are compromised, and microscopic hematuria and proteinuria result. In rare instances, GN may be attributed to a true autoimmune disorder in which autoantibodies directed against GBM components are produced. Electron microscopic examination in these cases also reveals GBM thickening with predominantly subepithelial electron-dense deposits (Fig. 16–18A) and immunofluorescence staining shows a more regular or smooth, linear pattern of immunofluorescence (Fig. 16–18B).[27, 34, 35] Autoimmune GN, accompanied by proteinuria, has also been described as one of the manifestations of systemic lupus erythematosus in horses.[36] Another immune mechanism of GN in horses is production of mixed or monoclonal cryoglobulins and deposition of antibody-antibody immune complexes along the glomerular GBM.[37, 38] Cryoglobulinemia is associated with a number of diseases in humans[37, 39] but has been described in only a few horses.[38, 40] Deposition of antibody-antibody immune complexes along the GBM may be a more important precipitant of GN than was previously recognized, since electron microscopic examination is required to demonstrate characteristic fibrillar or crystalline intracapillary and subendothelial deposits associated with the condition.[37] Regardless of what immune mechanism leads to glomerular injury, the end result is thickening of the filtration barrier, retarded glomerular filtration rate, and development of CRF in severe cases.

Although a number of terms are used to describe the specific morphologic changes associated with glomerular injury, GN is most broadly categorized histologically as

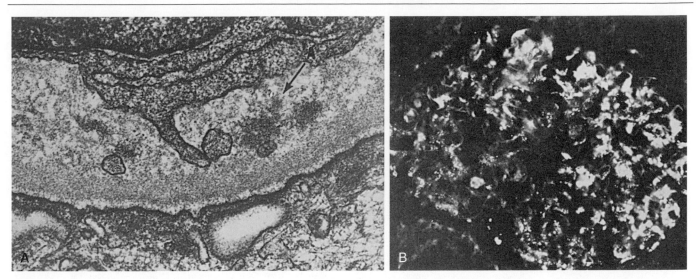

Figure 16–17. Immune-mediated glomerulonephritis in a horse 165 days after experimental infection with equine infectious anemia virus. **A,** An electron micrograph ($\times$32,500) shows endothelial cell swelling *(top),* thickening of the glomerular basement membrane with electron-dense immune deposits in a predominantly subendothelial location *(arrow),* and fusion of foot processes of the visceral epithelial cells. **B,** Immunofluorescent staining with fluorescein-tagged antiequine IgG antibody ($\times$100) demonstrates granular or "lumpy-bumpy" deposits of IgG along the glomerular basement membrane and in the mesangium. (From Banks KL, Henson JB, McGuire TC: Immunologically mediated glomerulitis of horses. I. Pathogenesis in persistent infection by equine infectious anemia virus. Lab Invest 26:701, 1972.)

proliferative or membranous.[27, 30, 33] Proliferative (or mesangioproliferative) GN describes glomerular injury associated with influx of inflammatory cells and proliferation of mesangial cells. The predominant histologic finding is increased cellularity in glomeruli (Fig. 16–19A, B). This lesion tends to be associated with the more acute stages of GN during which immune complexes are being deposited in a predomi-

nantly subendothelial site. "Membranous GN" describes glomerular injury accompanied by marked thickening of the capillary wall and GBM, and the predominant histologic finding is increased periodic acid–Schiff (PAS) stained material in the mesangial area and on the GBM (Fig. 16–19C). Thickening of the GBM can further be seen with a methenamine silver stain.[27, 30] Membranous GN tends to be associ-

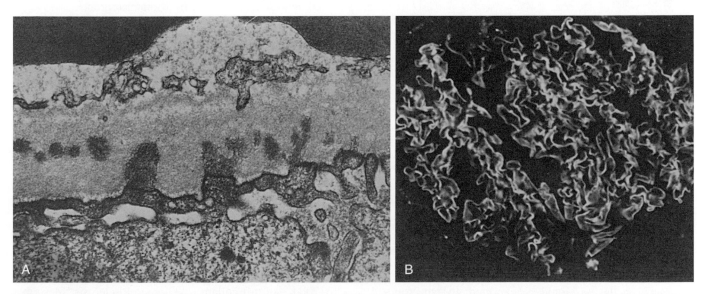

Figure 16–18. Spontaneous immune-mediated glomerulonephritis in a horse. **A,** An electron micrograph ($\times$22,750) shows a red blood cell in the capillary lumen *(top),* relatively normal fenestrated endothelial cytoplasm, thickening of the glomerular basement membrane with electron-dense immune deposits in a predominantly subepithelial location, and fusion of foot processes of the visceral epithelial cells. **B,** Immunofluorescent staining with fluorescein-tagged antiequine IgG antibody ($\times$160) demonstrates smooth, linear deposits of IgG. (From Banks KL, Henson JB, McGuire TC: Immunologically mediated glomerulitis of horses. II. Antiglomerular basement membrane antibody and other mechanisms of spontaneous disease. Lab Invest 26:708, 1972.)

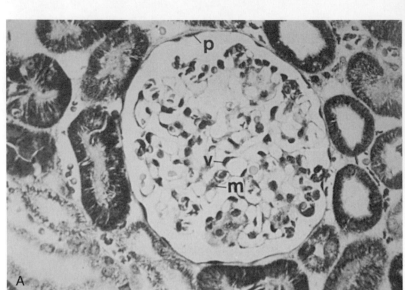

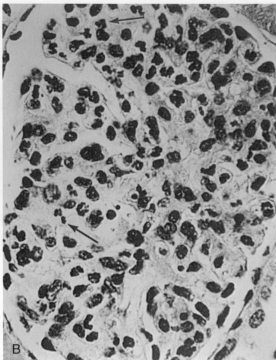

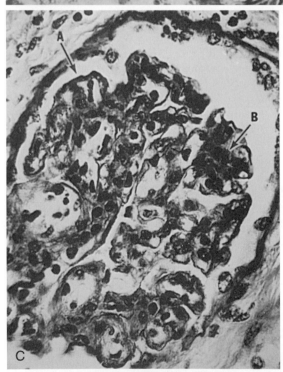

Figure 16–19. Histologic changes in equine glomerulonephritis. **A,** Photomicrograph of a normal glomerulus. Bowman's capsule is lined by flattened parietal epithelial cells *(p)*. Visceral epithelial cells *(v)* are adjacent to the glomerular basement membrane, which is of uniform thickness. Mesangial cells *(m)* are entirely surrounded by glomerular capillaries (×100 periodic acid–Schiff). **B,** Photomicrograph demonstrates proliferative glomerulonephritis in a horse after experimental infection with equine infectious anemia virus. There is a combination of neutrophil infiltration *(arrows)* and mesangial cell proliferation (×160 hematoxylin-eosin). **C,** Photomicrograph demonstrates membranous glomerulonephritis in a horse after experimental infection with equine infectious anemia virus. The glomerular basement membranes are thickened, **A,** and mesangial areas contain periodic acid–Schiff–positive material, **B,** (×160 periodic acid–Schiff). (**A,** from Osborne CA, Hammer RF, Stevens JB, et al.: The glomerulus in health and disease: A comparative review of domestic animals and man. Adv Vet Sci Comp Med 21:207, 1977. **B** and **C,** from Banks KL, Henson JB, McGuire TC: Immunologically mediated glomerulitis of horses. I. Pathogenesis in persistent infection by equine infectious anemia virus. Lab Invest 26:701, 1972.)

ated with more soluble immune complexes or autoantibodies that can pass through the GBM and localize in a predominantly subepithelial site, resulting in less infiltration of inflammatory cells. As would be expected, the spectrum of lesions can be seen in naturally occurring GN leading to varying histologic descriptions of the disease (membranoproliferative GN). As glomerular injury progresses, proliferation of the parietal epithelium also occurs, likely in response to filtration of macromolecules and cellular debris. Lesions associated with parietal cell proliferation can include lay-

ering of epithelial cells (termed "crescents") on the inner aspect of Bowman's capsule (Fig. 16–20A), adhesion formation between the glomerular tuft and Bowman's capsule (Fig. 16–20B), and tuft collapse. "Glomerulosclerosis" describes the end stage of progressive, irreversible glomerular injury in which replacement of glomerular components with hyaline material is visible on histologic examination (Fig. 16–20C).[27]

Specific histologic categorization of GN provides etiologic and prognostic information for humans with renal failure attributable to glomerular disease.[31, 39] Subcategorization of

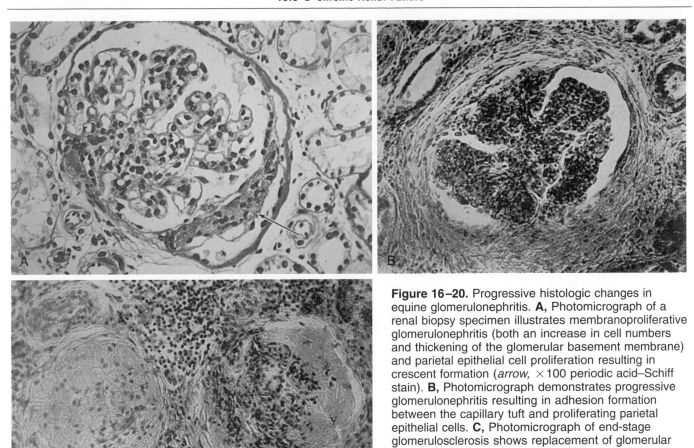

Figure 16–20. Progressive histologic changes in equine glomerulonephritis. **A,** Photomicrograph of a renal biopsy specimen illustrates membranoproliferative glomerulonephritis (both an increase in cell numbers and thickening of the glomerular basement membrane) and parietal epithelial cell proliferation resulting in crescent formation (*arrow,* ×100 periodic acid–Schiff stain). **B,** Photomicrograph demonstrates progressive glomerulonephritis resulting in adhesion formation between the capillary tuft and proliferating parietal epithelial cells. **C,** Photomicrograph of end-stage glomerulosclerosis shows replacement of glomerular components with hyaline material (more complete in glomerulus on the left). (**A,** from Osborne CA, Hammer RF, Stevens JB, et al.: The glomerulus in health and disease: A comparative review of domestic animals and man. Adv Vet Sci Comp Med 21:207, 1977. **B** and **C,** from Fincher MG, Olafson P: Chronic diffuse glomerulonephritis in a horse. Cornell Vet 24:356, 1934.)

glomerulopathies has also been performed in a prospective study of naturally occurring canine chronic renal disease. Although classifications—including focal GN, mesangioproliferative GN, endocapillary proliferative GN, crescentic GN, and sclerosing GN—could be made; histologic findings were not prognostically useful.[41] This study also revealed that glomerular disease was responsible for 52% of canine CRF; however, an inciting disease (vegetative endocarditis) could be identified in only 1 of 31 dogs with GN.

GN also appears to be an important cause of CRF in horses.[42] Of 59 reported cases of CRF attributable to acquired disease, GN was identified as the inciting cause of CRF in 31 (53%) (Table 16–9).[20–22, 37, 38, 43–55] It may also be the initiating disease process in cases of end-stage kidney disease (ESKD) when gross and histopathologic changes are so extensive that a primary mechanism of renal injury cannot be identified. A number of systemic inflammatory and infectious disease processes are thought to be accompanied by GN in horses, but progression to CRF appears to be a rare sequela. For example, experimental *Leptospira pomona* infection produced subacute GN characterized by hypercellularity and edema of capillary tufts,[56] but leptospirosis is a rare cause of clinical renal disease in horses.[57] Similarly, experimental infection with equine infectious anemia (EIA)

virus produced histologic and immunofluorescent evidence of GN in 75% and 87% of infected horses, respectively.[34] Immunoglobulins with anti-EIA activity were eluted from glomeruli collected from experimentally infected horses, but none of the horses showed clinical signs of renal disease. Poststreptococcal GN is a well-recognized cause of GN in humans,[31] and Roberts speculated that GN in a horse with chronic pleuritis and purpura hemorrhagica was likely a consequence of circulating immune complexes involving streptococcal antigens.[58] Recently, Divers provided support for this hypothesis by eluting group-C streptococcal antigens from immune complex deposits in glomeruli collected from a horse with CRF.[55] Finally, an occasional case of equine GN may be a consequence of true autoimmune disease and, in one instance, anti-GBM antibody was eluted from glomeruli with linear GBM immunofluorescent staining pattern isolated from a horse.[2] Little information is available about histopathologic subcategories of GN in horses, although several reports have attempted to make comparisons to glomerular lesions that have been better characterized in other species.[37, 53, 59] No reports have attempted to correlate histologic changes with the degree of renal failure in horses. Thus, assessment of the severity of renal disease associated with GN in horses is currently based more on clinical find-

Table 16–9. Causes of Chronic Renal Failure in 70 Horses (Excluding Reports of Congenital Renal Failure and Experimental Induction of Chronic Renal Failure)

Congenital Disorders (11/70 = 16%)	Cases (no.)	References [no. cases]
Renal agenesis/contralateral obstruction and hydronephrosis	1	Johnson et al (1976) [1][10]
Renal hypoplasia	3	Andrews et al (1986) [3][12]
Renal dysplasia	4	Roberts and Kelly (1980) [1], Anderson et al (1988) [1], Ronen et al (1993) [2][13–15]
Polycystic kidney disease	3	Scott and Vasey (1986) [1], Ramsay et al (1987) [1], Bertone et al (1987) [1][17–19]
Acquired Disorders (59/70 = 84%)*		
GN	31	Fincher and Olafson (1934) [1], Frank and Dunlop (1935) [1], Kadás and Százados (1974) [1], McCausland and Milestone (1976) [1], Brobst et al (1977) [1], Tennant et al (1978) [1], Brobst et al (1978) [1], Roberts and Seiler (1979) [1], Dobos-Kovács (1981) [1], Koterba and Coffman (1981) [2], Tennant et al (1982) [5], Morris and Lee (1982) [2], Waldvogel et al (1983) [1], Divers (1983) [1], Scarratt and Sponenberg (1984) [2], Sabnis et al (1984) [7], Maede et al (1991) [1], Divers et al (1992) [1][20–22, 37, 38, 43–55]
CIN	2	Webb and Knight (1977) [1], Brobst et al (1982) [1][74, 75]
With obstructive nephrolithiasis and/or ureterolithiasis	11	Byars et al (1989) [1], Hope et al (1989) [1], Ehnen et al (1990) [7], Hillyer et al (1990) [1], Laing et al (1992) [1][68–72]
With pyelonephritis	8	Tennant et al (1978) [1], Tennant et al (1982) [1], Divers (1983) [1], Held et al (1986) [1], Carrick and Pollitt (1986) [1], Sloet van Oldruitenborgh (1988) [1], Mair et al (1989) [1], Hamlen (1993) [1][20, 22, 51, 63–67]
With papillary necrosis	2	Divers (1983) [1], Gunson (1983) [1][22, 78]
ESKD	5	Andrews (1971) [1], Buntain et al (1979) [1], Brobst et al (1982) [1], Alders and Hutchins (1987) [1], Snyder and Batista da Cruz (1984) [1][75, 81–84]

*In many reports of acquired renal disease leading to CRF, histopathologic changes involve both glomeruli and interstitium. Categorization in this table is based on authors' conclusions in these reports. When severe lesions involved both glomeruli and interstitium, a categorization of ESKD was made.

ings (e.g., body condition, degree of azotemia) than on histologic changes in a renal biopsy sample.

Chronic Interstitial Nephritis

Tubulointerstitial disease is usually a consequence of acute tubular necrosis secondary to ischemia, sepsis, or exposure to nephrotoxic compounds. Hypovolemia associated with acute blood loss, colic, diarrhea, or sepsis can lead to renal hypoperfusion and ischemic damage.[60] Severe localized infection (e.g., pleuritis, peritonitis) or septicemia may also be accompanied by tubule damage. Aminoglycoside antibiotics, nonsteroidal antiinflammatory drugs (NSAIDs), vitamin D, vitamin K_3, acorns, and heavy metals such as mercury are all potentially nephrotoxic.[61] Intravascular hemolysis or rhabdomyolysis can also lead to acute tubular damage secondary to the nephrotoxic effects of hemoglobin or myoglobin (see Acute Renal Failure). In horses tubulointerstitial disease culminating in CRF can be caused by ascending urinary tract infection resulting in pyelonephritis[20, 22, 51, 62–67] or bilateral obstructive disease due to ureteroliths or nephroliths.[22, 68–73] In other cases a cause of the tubule disease may not be identified.[74, 75] Finally, although this has not yet

been described in horses, immune mechanisms, including anti–tubular basement membrane disease, can lead to chronic interstitial nephritis (CIN) in humans.[76]

CIN is most strictly defined by clinical signs of renal disease associated with histologic changes of tubular damage and an interstitial inflammatory cell infiltrate (Fig. 16–21). Inflammatory cells include lymphocytes, monocytes, and occasional plasma cells. Neutrophils are uncommon; however, eosinophilic infiltrates suggest drug reactions in human patients.[76] Major glomerular and vascular lesions are not apparent. The hallmark that distinguishes CIN from acute tubular and interstitial disease is interstitial fibrosis.

Although CIN has a fairly strict histologic definition, a number of disease processes can lead to tubular damage. For all practical purposes, CIN is used as a catch-all term for extraglomerular causes of CRF in horses. As a consequence, gross findings in horses with CIN can vary dramatically. For example, analgesic nephropathy (NSAID toxicity, of which phenylbutazone has the greatest nephrotoxic potential[77]) can produce papillary necrosis[78, 79] manifested by hematuria[80] in the early stages of disease, whereas chronic disease may be associated with nephrolithiasis and hydronephrosis. The area of papillary necrosis serves as a nidus for stone formation,

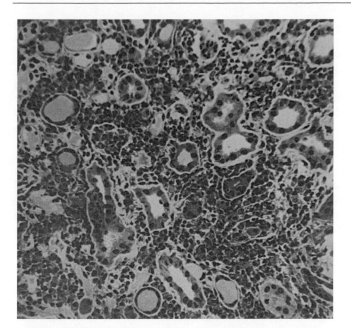

Figure 16–21. Histologic changes in interstitial nephritis. The interstitium contains dense infiltrates of lymphocytes and plasma cells superimposed on moderate interstitial fibrosis and tubular atrophy (×275 hematoxylin-eosin). (From Bennett WM, Elzinga LW, Porter GA: Tubulointerstitial disease and toxic nephropathy. In Brenner BM, Rector FC, eds. The Kidney, ed 4, Vol. 2. Philadelphia, WB Saunders, 1991, p. 1434.)

and subsequent obstructive disease leads to hydronephrosis.[70, 73] Similarly, upper urinary tract infection can lead to minor or major changes in the architecture of the kidneys and to variable histologic changes.

Using CIN as a broad category for "non-GN causes" of CRF in horses, this group of tubulointerstitial diseases was responsible for 39% (23 of 59) of the previously reported cases of CRF in horses (see Table 6–9). Although, in theory, CIN would be expected to be accompanied by greater evidence of tubular dysfunction (e.g., enzymuria, glucosuria, increased fractional clearance of sodium), abnormal measures of tubule function have not regularly been detected. Similarly, microscopic hematuria and proteinuria, the hallmarks of glomerular disease, would not be expected.

End-Stage Kidney Disease

ESKD describes the severe gross and histologic changes in kidneys collected from animals in the final stages of CRF. Grossly, the kidneys typically are pale, shrunken, and firm, and they may have an irregular surface and an adherent capsule. Histologically, severe glomerulosclerosis is observed, and hyalinization accompanied by extensive interstitial fibrosis. The end-stage lesions make it virtually impossible to determine the initiating cause of renal disease. In several cases with a pathologic description consistent with ESKD the underlying cause of renal injury could not be established.[75, 81–84]

Chronic Renal Failure of Other Causes

Several early cases of CRF in horses were attributed to oxalate poisoning because oxalate crystals were observed in

renal tubules.[74, 81] Horses appear to be more resistant than other domestic species to oxalate-induced renal damage,[85] however, and experimental administration of various forms of oxalate (in large doses) produce hypocalcemia and gastrointestinal signs rather than renal failure.[86] In fact, the early reports of "oxalate nephropathy" in horses failed to demonstrate that the affected horses had been exposed to oxalates.[74, 81] Furthermore, long-term ingestion of plants containing oxalate produces fibrous osteodystrophy (oxalates bind calcium in the intestinal tract, decreasing intestinal calcium absorption), but renal damage in affected horses has been minimal.[87] It is now recognized that formation of oxalate crystals in diseased equine kidneys is a secondary change likely related to stasis of urine in damaged renal tubules.[49]

Amyloidosis is an unusual cause of CRF in horses.[85, 88] Amyloid deposits associated with systemic disease are typically comprised of aggregates of the amino-terminal fragment of serum amyloid A protein, an acute-phase protein.[89–92] Concentrations of serum amyloid A increase nonspecifically in a variety of inflammatory disease processes, and chronic elevations can result in amyloid deposition (AA type) in a variety of tissues, a condition termed "systemic reactive amyloidosis."[93, 94] Incidence and tissue localization of amyloid exhibit considerable species variation. Dogs appears to be affected most often, but the fact that it is a familial disease in Abyssinian cats implies a genetic basis for the disease.[94] Amyloid deposits accumulate as stacks of protein in a β-pleated sheet conformation and are identified in tissue samples by their extracellular location and homogeneous, eosinophilic appearance when stained with hematoxylin and eosin. They are birefringent when viewed under polarized light, and staining with alkaline Congo red solution imparts a characteristic green color.[93, 94] Amyloid deposition in the kidney is most common in dogs and cattle, and renal amyloidosis is a significant cause of CRF in dogs.[94] In horses, localized amyloidosis of the upper airway or skin is more common than systemic amyloidosis.[93] In the localized form, amyloid deposits are composed of immunoglobulin light chains (AL-type). Although there have been reports of systemic reactive amyloidosis consequent to heavy parasite infestation in horses, renal involvement was minimal or not apparent.[95, 96] Systemic amyloidosis has most often been recognized in horses hyperimmunized for antiserum production, and hepatic and splenic involvement may be more common than renal involvement in these horses.[85, 88, 90]

A final acquired cause of CRF, renal neoplasia, is discussed in greater detail elsewhere in this chapter. Although horses with renal neoplasia may present with weight loss, the tumors are usually unilateral and development of CRF is uncommon.

UREMIC TOXINS AND THE UREMIC SYNDROME

Regardless of the underlying cause of nephron loss, the ensuing renal insufficiency leads to development of azotemia and its clinical manifestation, the uremic syndrome.[97–99] The uremic syndrome is a multisystem disorder that develops as a result of the effects of uremic toxins on cell metabolism and function. Although the uremic syndrome was originally attributed to the effects of increased blood urea nitrogen concentration (BUN), it is now known that there are a number of nitrogenous compounds that accumulate in CRF and contribute to alterations of cell metabolism and function. In fact, there is poor correlation between the severity of the uremic syndrome and the magnitude of azotemia. For example, urea administered to humans with normal renal function results simply in fluid shifts, osmotic diuresis, and increased thirst.[98] Urea toxicity has also been studied in nephrectomized dogs and in human CRF patients sustained by dialysis. Increasing the dialysate's urea concentrations to maintain BUN at artificially higher values has produced variable results. For example, BUN values up to about 150 mg/dL were associated with few clinical signs, whereas lethargy, weakness, anorexia, vomiting, and a bleeding diathesis (due to platelet dysfunction) were produced when BUN was increased to values exceeding 175 to 200 mg/dL.[99] Excess circulating urea can also spontaneously degrade to ammonia, carbonate, or cyanate. Cyanate can react with the N-terminal amino groups on a number of proteins and, by altering tertiary structure, interfere with enzyme activity and structural integrity of cell membranes.[99] Thus, accumulation of urea is likely responsible for some, but not all, of the signs of uremic syndrome.

Creatinine and other guanidino compounds also accumulate in renal failure. These compounds are strong organic bases that contain an amidino group ($N—C≡NH$).[99] With CRF, urinary excretion of creatinine and other guanidino compounds may actually increase (owing to tubular secretion) but not enough to prevent increases in blood concentrations. For example, we have found that in naturally occurring cases of equine CRF (authors unpublished data) endogenous creatinine clearance, when measured simultaneously with inulin clearance, overestimates glomerular filtration rate (GFR) by 50% to 100%. These data indicate that tubular secretion of creatinine, which Finco was unable to document in healthy ponies,[100] either is initiated by or is quantitatively much greater with CRF. Although metabolic pathways have not been fully elucidated, guanidino compounds appear to be produced predominantly in the liver and their concentration in blood and tissues increases with either decreased renal function or increased dietary protein intake.[98] The relationship between guanidino compounds and the syndrome of uremia is also unclear. For example, administration of methylguanidine to healthy dogs results in weight loss, neurologic signs, and anemia, but only when blood concentrations are an order of magnitude greater than those in spontaneous cases of CRF.[99] In contrast, administration of another guanidino compound, guanidinopropionic acid, leads to hemolysis by depleting erythrocyte glutathione concentrations (supporting a role for this uremic toxin in the anemia of CRF).

Products of intestinal bacterial metabolism, including secondary methylamines (from metabolism of choline and lecithin), aromatic amines (from metabolism of tyrosine and phenylalanine), polyamines (from metabolism of lysine and ornithine), and tryptophan breakdown products (indole, skatole, indoleacetic acid, and others), can all contribute to the clinical signs associated with the uremic syndrome. Some of these compounds have been studied thoroughly (e.g., the inhibitory effect of the polyamine spermine on erythropoiesis), whereas others are ill-understood but likely contribute to altered neuromuscular and neurologic function.[97–99]

Another group of larger "uremic toxins" have been termed "middle molecules."[98, 99] These compounds are higher–molecular weight compounds (500 to 3000 daltons) that are more readily removed from uremic patients by peritoneal dialysis than by hemodialysis. These compounds are not well-characterized, and their existence is supported more by the difference in clinical response to peritoneal dialysis and hemodialysis in uremic human patients awaiting renal transplantation.

In addition to nitrogenous compounds, abnormal metabolism of hormones and trace minerals also accompanies the decline in renal function associated with both acute and chronic renal failure. Secondary hyperparathyroidism (leading to osteodystrophy) and insulin insensitivity are well-recognized endocrine contributions to the uremic syndrome in human and small animal patients.[98, 99, 101, 102] Endocrine dysfunction can be attributed to several factors: (1) decreased production of renal hormones (erythropoietin, vitamin D_3); (2) decreased hormone clearance prolonging plasma half-life (parathormone, gastrin); (3) decreased hormone production (testosterone); (4) tissue insensitivity (insulin, parathormone); and (5) hypersecretion to reestablish homeostasis (parathormone).[99] With regard to trace minerals, uremia may be accompanied by aluminum toxicity and zinc deficiency. Aluminum may contribute to some of the neurologic signs associated with azotemia (especially with acute renal failure), whereas zinc has been implicated in testicular atrophy and abnormal taste in uremic human patients.[98, 99]

Clearly, as so many potential uremic toxins exert their effects as renal function declines, it is unlikely that a single compound, or even a few, will ever be identified as the primary cause of the uremic syndrome in patients with CRF. Furthermore, it is more likely that these compounds together impair basic cell function in a number of tissues and that the signs of uremia are more reflective of multisystem organ dysfunction. Methylation of a number of membrane proteins has recently received considerable attention as one of the common mechanisms of cell dysfunction.[103] What is truly remarkable, however, is the tremendous adaptive capacity of the failing kidneys to maintain sodium and water balance within relatively narrow ranges until GFR declines to 20% of the normal value or less.[104]

CLINICAL SIGNS OF CHRONIC RENAL FAILURE

Horses with CRF present relatively late in the disease course, when their owners note lethargy, anorexia, and weight loss. A history of months to years of polydipsia (PD) in some cases supports renal disease of long duration. In other animals preexisting disease (colic, colitis, pleuropneumonia) or prolonged medication (aminoglycoside antibiotics or NSAIDs) may provide important information about the initiation and duration of renal failure. In the majority of cases, however, the onset is insidious and it is not possible to identify a precipitating event or guage the duration of renal disease.

Chronic weight loss is the most common presenting complaint of horses with CRF.[20–26] Partial anorexia, ventral edema, polyuria/polydipsia (PU/PD), rough hair coat, lethargy, poor athletic performance are other owner concerns. In addition, horses with advanced CRF may have a characteristic odor that likely reflects the combined effects of uremic halitosis and increased urea in sweat. For the 70 horses presented in Table 16–9, weight loss, ventral and peripheral edema, and PU/PD, respectively, were reported in 53 of 63 (84%), 24 of 56 (43%), and 21 of 48 (44%) of the cases. Lethargy and weight loss can be attributable to several factors. An increase in the concentration of nitrogenous wastes in blood can have a direct central appetite-suppressant effect that can lead to partial or complete anorexia.[98, 99] Next, as azotemia develops, excess urea diffuses across gastrointestinal epithelium where it is metabolized to ammonia and carbon dioxide by bacterial urease. In the oral cavity, excess ammonia can lead to excessive dental tartar formation (Fig. 16–22), gingivitis, and oral ulcers. In the gastrointestinal tract, excess urea and ammonia can lead to ulceration and mild to moderate protein-losing enteropathy, and severely uremic animals may produce soft feces.[1, 98, 99] The prolonged half-life of gastrin (eliminated through the kidneys) may contribute further to ulcer formation owing to increased gastric acid secretion.[99] Finally, as the combined effects of uremic toxins render the affected patient "catabolic," body mass declines as body reserves are tapped to meet basal energy requirements.[98, 99]

Mild ventral edema with CRF may be attributable to three factors: decreased oncotic pressure, increased vascular permeability, and increased hydrostatic pressure. Since albumin accounts for approximately 75% of plasma colloid oncotic pressure, decreases in albumin concentration (below about 2.0 g/dL) can decrease plasma oncotic pressure despite a normal total plasma protein concentration.[105, 106] The effects of uremic toxins on endothelial cell membranes can alter vascular permeability, which contributes to edema.[98, 99] Chronic renal insufficiency can lead to renal hypoxia and hypoperfusion, which stimulate renal juxtaglomerular cells to release renin. Activation of the renin-angiotensin system tends to elevate blood (and capillary hydrostatic) pressure and contribute to edema. Activation of the renin-angiotensin system also leads to increased sodium reabsorption in both the proximal (direct effect of angiotensin II) and distal (effect of aldosterone) tubules.[106] Sodium retention leads to expansion of circulating volume—another factor in edema formation. Alterations in blood pressure in horses with CRF have not been routinely evaluated as they have in small animal[1] and human patients, nor have increased circulating concentrations of angiotensin II or aldosterone been documented. As a result, the nephrotic syndrome (characterized by edema, hypoalbuminemia, and heavy proteinuria) is not as well-documented in horses as in small animals and humans with CRF. However, horses with CRF appear less at risk for the significant pleural effusion or ascites that can accompany the nephrotic syndrome in small animals.[1]

PU/PD are variable findings in horses with CRF. The degree of PU/PD is theoretically related to the degree of tubulointerstitial damage; however, the degree of PU does not appear to be correlated with the magnitude of azotemia in clinical cases. Typically, PU is not as severe with CRF as with diabetes insipidus or psychogenic water drinking and may not be noticed by an owner (see Polyuria and Polydipsia). The wide variation in water intake in normal horses and common use of automatic waterers and large stock tanks also make it more difficult to observe PD. The mechanisms of PU with CRF can include (1) increased tubule flow rate in surviving nephrons; (2) decreased medullary hypertonicity; and (3) impaired response of collecting ducts to vasopressin (acquired nephrogenic diabetes insipidus). Although all these mechanisms may contribute to the PU of CRF, which may be most important is not known.[1, 107]

An early complaint for horses with CRF is sometimes poor performance. Poor performance may be related to mild anemia (packed cell volume 25% to 30%) and lethargy. Although the anemia of CRF has been attributed to several factors, including blood loss, decreased erythrocyte survival time, nutritional deficiencies, and decreased erythropoeitin activity, the latter has clearly emerged as the principal cause of anemia in humans and small animals with CRF.[1, 108, 109] In fact, administration of recombinant human erythropoietin (rhEPO) to patients awaiting kidney transplant has been one of the most significant advances in management of human CRF, as it has eliminated the need for blood transfusions, improved exercise capacity, and decreased morbidity associated with the uremic syndrome.[108, 109] Administration of rhEPO has also benefitted anemic dogs and cats with CRF; although both species may need iron supplementation to support erythropoiesis.[1, 108] The response has often been only temporary, as many small animal patients develop refractory anemia consequent to production of anti-rhEPO antibodies within a few weeks to months after initiation of treatment.[1] Plasma concentrations of erythropoietin have been determined in normal horses[110] and rhEPO administration (15 IU/kg, IV, three doses per week for 3 weeks) has been reported to increase the hematocrit in splenectomized horses[111]; however, there are no reports of rhEPO administration to horses with CRF. Further, moderate to severe anemia has been anecdotally reported to develop after repeated rhEPO administration to racehorses,[112] suggesting that anti-rhEPO antibodies would also limit its effectiveness in the treatment of CRF in horses.

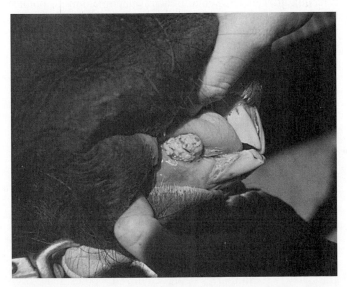

Figure 16–22. Excessive dental tartar on the canine tooth and lower corner incisor of a horse with chronic renal failure.

Table 16–10. Abnormal Laboratory Values Reported for Horses with Chronic Renal Failure

Parameter	Number*	Percent
BUN:Cr > 10	29/34	85
BUN:Cr > 15	17/34	50
Anemia (PCV < 30%)	12/30	40
Hypoalbuminemia (alb < 2.5 g/dL)	12/14	86
Hypoalbuminemia (alb < 2.0 g/dL)	7/14	50
Hyponatremia (Na$^+$ < 135 mEq/L)	26/40	65
Hyperkalemia (K$^+$ > 5.0 mEq/L)	23/41	56
Hypochloremia (Cl$^-$ < 95 mEq/L)	19/41	46
Hypercalcemia (Ca^{++} > 13.5 mg/dL)	26/39	67
Hypophosphatemia (P < 1.5 mg/dL)	17/36	47
Acidosis (pH < 7.35)	3/5	60

*Number, number of reports with this laboratory finding/total number of reports in which this laboratory parameter was reported.

DIAGNOSIS AND LABORATORY EVALUATION

A diagnosis of CRF is established when persistent isosthenuria (specific gravity of 1.008 to 1.014) accompanies azotemia and typical clinical signs.[21–26, 113] Rectal palpation of the left kidney may be normal or may reveal a kidney that is small or firm with an irregular surface. Less often, the kidneys and/or ureters may be enlarged if obstructed by uroliths or if infection or neoplasia is present. The ratio of BUN to creatinine (BUN-Cr ratio) in horses with CRF is typically greater than 10:1 (Table 16–10); that for horses with prerenal azotemia or ARF is often less than 10:1.[22] This difference can be attributed, in part, to different volumes of distribution for urea (all body fluids) and creatinine (primarily the extracellular fluid space). As a consequence, with acute reductions in renal blood flow the increase in serum creatinine concentration is usually greater, on a relative or percentage basis, than the increase in BUN concentration. It should be emphasized, however, that BUN is influenced by dietary protein intake so that BUN-Cr values do not always distinguish acute renal failure from CRF. In fact, BUN-Cr ratio can also be used to assess adequacy of dietary protein intake in the management of horses with CRF as a value greater than 15:1 can reflect excessive protein intake.[24]

In addition to azotemia, further abnormal laboratory data accompanying CRF can indicate mild anemia, hypoalbuminemia, hyponatremia, hyperkalemia, hypochloremia, hypercalcemia, hypophosphatemia, and metabolic acidosis (see Table 16–10). A nonregenerative anemia is related in large part to a deficient supply of the renally secreted glycoprotein, erythropoietin; however, reduced erythrocyte life span may be another significant contributor to anemia. Normally, equine erythrocytes have a life span of 140 to 155 days.[112] With uremia, erythrocyte life span is shortened because excessive nitrogenous waste products alter the integrity of erythrocyte membranes and the function of ion channels, which regulate erythrocyte volume.[99] These less resilient erythrocytes are more likely to be removed from the circulation by the reticuloendothelial system.

The electrolyte alterations associated with CRF reflect loss of tubule function. Since sodium, chloride, bicarbonate, and phosphate are conserved by renal tubules; CRF is accompanied by excessive urine loss of these electrolytes. Although fractional electrolyte clearance values (see Examination of the Urinary System) may remain within normal ranges or increase only slightly in horses with CRF, significant daily urinary loss of electrolytes may still occur. As an example, consider a horse with CRF and serum creatinine and sodium concentrations of 5.0 mg/dL and 130 mEq/L, respectively. If the horse is producing 20 L of urine daily with respective creatinine and sodium concentrations of 50 mg/dL and 12.5 mEq/L, the fractional clearance of sodium is 1.0% and daily urinary sodium loss 250 mEq. An increase in urinary sodium concentration to 25 mEq/L secondary to a further decrease in tubular reabsorption would result in an increase in fractional sodium clearance to 2% but would represent an additional 250 mEq of daily sodium loss in the urine. The latter value would approach 1% to 2% of the exchangeable sodium in the body and would require an additional 15 g of salt intake daily to accommodate this loss. This example illustrates the importance of providing adequate access to salt, in addition to water, to horses with CRF.

Hypercalcemia and hypophosphatemia (Williams-Smith syndrome) are fairly common findings in horses with CRF (see Table 16–10) and the degree of hypercalcemia appears to vary with the amount of calcium in the diet.[20, 48, 51, 114] In humans with ESKD, hypercalcemia is an occasional finding attributed to hyperparathyroidism, vitamin D supplementation, or use of calcium-containing dialysate solutions. Further, the osteodystrophy of CRF is associated with aluminum deposition in bone, which has been speculated to reduce skeletal buffering capacity for increases in serum calcium concentration and, thereby, contribute to hypercalcemia.[115] Since the equine kidney is an important route of calcium excretion (via calcium carbonate crystals), impaired tubule function in the face of continued intestinal absorption is the most common explanation for calcium accumulation in blood. This is supported by the rapid development of hypercalcemia after experimental bilateral nephrectomy in ponies fed alfalfa hay (Fig. 16–23).[9] In addition, Brobst reported that parathormone concentrations were below the lower limit of detection in horses with CRF and concluded that hyperparathyroidism did not play a role in development of hypercalcemia[75]; however, parathormone clearance by the kidney is reduced with CRF and may be associated with a change in the regulatory set point for calcium in uremic humans.[115] With the exception of Brobst's measurement of parathormone in horses with CRF,[75] little information is available about calcium metabolism or osteodystrophy in horses with CRF. Further, it is not known whether hypercalcemia in horses with CRF is associated with exacerbation of renal disease or tissue mineralization. Nevertheless, the effect of dietary calcium can be demonstrated by changing the type of hay fed to horses with CRF. Horses whose serum calcium concentrations exceed 20 mg/dL on a diet of mostly alfalfa can have their serum calcium concentrations return to the normal range within a few of days after changing the diet to grass hay.[19, 22] Similarly, nephrectomized ponies fed grass hay did not become hypercalcemic.[22] The cause of hypophosphatemia in horses with CRF also remains undocumented, although it has been explained by the law of mass

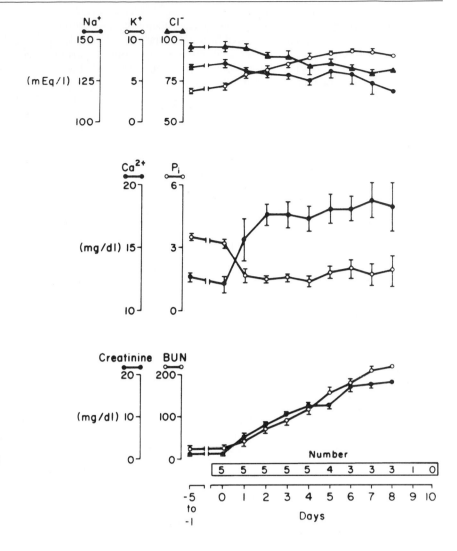

Figure 16–23. Changes in serum electrolyte concentrations, BUN, and serum Cr following bilateral nephrectomy in Shetland ponies. (From Tennant B, Lowe JE, Tasker JB: Hypercalcemia and hypophosphatemia in ponies following bilateral nephrectomy. Proc Soc Exp Biol Med 167:365, 1981.)

action, which leads to a decrease in serum phosphate concentration in association with hypercalcemia.[114, 115] A similar response is not observed in horses that eat *Cestrum diurnum* (leading to a syndrome of hypervitaminosis D): they develop hypercalcemia without hypophosphatemia.[116] Another possibility that has been suggested is that hypophosphatemia may be a consequence of long-standing anorexia associated with CRF.[75] Regardless of the cause, clinical problems associated with hypophosphatemia have not yet been recognized in horses with CRF.

A degree of metabolic acidosis accompanies CRF in humans and small animals and is attributed to decreased ability of failing kidneys to excrete hydrogen ions and regenerate bicarbonate.[1, 99] Normally, acid-base balance is maintained by reabsorption of filtered bicarbonate and excretion of hydrogen ions in combination with ammonia and phosphate. As renal function declines in the early stages of renal failure, hydrogen ion excretion via renal ammoniagenesis and ammonium excretion increases. As renal failure progresses both compromised renal ammoniagenesis and decreased medullary recycling of ammonia due to structural renal damage likely contribute to impaired ammonium excretion. Since hepatic glutamine synthesis is required for renal ammoniagenesis, the earlier increase in ammonium excretion may contribute to protein malnutrition in patients with CRF.[1] Metabolic acidosis also contributes to a number of the clinical signs of the uremic syndrome and may exacerbate some of the electrolyte alterations (e.g., hyperkalemia) of CRF. Metabolic acidosis has been reported in a limited number of horses with CRF (see Table 16–10); however, in the authors' experience and that of others,[21, 75] most horses with CRF have normal acid-base status or are alkalotic until the terminal stages of the disease, when metabolic acidosis typically develops. Metabolic alkalosis has been attributed to enhanced bicarbonate reabsorption and production, in association with hypochloremia and increased renal ammoniagenesis, respectively. In some instances, hypochloremic metabolic alkalosis may be accompanied by paradoxical aciduria.[75] The mechanism of paradoxic aciduria is likely similar to that of hypochloremic metabolic alkalosis in ruminants with abomasal outflow obstruction.[117] Briefly, after all chloride has been reabsorbed from the glomerular filtrate, further sodium reabsorption occurs by exchange with (excretion of) potassium or hydrogen ions. Thus, paradoxical aciduria is most likely to occur with concomitant hypokalemia or whole-body potassium depletion.

Horses with CRF can also develop hypercholesterolemia and hyperlipidemia (hypertriglyceridemia), and an occasional animal has grossly lipemic plasma (hyperlipemia).[22, 24, 113] In fact, Naylor reported a positive correlation between serum triglyceride and creatinine concentrations in a group of azotemic horses.[118] With azotemia, hyperlipidemia can develop as a result of increased synthesis, decreased degradation, or increased mobilization of triglycerides from fat stores.[119] Decreased lipoprotein lipase activity has received the most attention in horses, likely since heparin treatment (40 IU/kg, SC, every 8 hours) has been recommended to stimulate lipoprotein lipase in an attempt to clear the serum.[24, 120] Hypercholesterolemia and hyperlipidemia increase the risk of atherosclerotic cardiovascular disease in humans with CRF.[119] Further, they stimulate mesangial cell proliferation and matrix production in diseased glomeruli and thus accelerate progression to glomerulosclerosis.[121]

The failing kidneys have a tremendous adaptive capacity to maintain tubule function until GFR is quite low.[104] In the authors' experience, tubular dysfunction resulting in significant sodium or phosphorous wasting (manifested by increased fractional clearance values), glucosuria, or enzymuria is more common with acute renal failure than with CRF. When present, however, abnormal tubule function rarely leads to values for fractional sodium clearance in excess of 5%.[71, 84, 122] In contrast, loss of concentrating ability resulting in isosthenuria is a consistent feature of CRF that usually develops before azotemia. The associated polyuria may or may not be observed by the client, but water balance is usually well maintained through PD. PU typically results in urine that is clear and essentially devoid of crystals and mucus. Sediment examination is generally unremarkable, but increased numbers of red or white blood cells may occur with nephro- or ureterolithiasis or pyelonephritis, respectively. Gross hematuria further supports lithiasis or neoplasia. A quantitative urine culture should be included in the minimum data base of all horses with CRF, as bacteriuria may not always be accompanied by pyuria.

Alterations in the integrity of the highly anionic glomerular filtration barrier can also lead to loss of protein, predominantly albumin, in the urine. Few quantitative data are available on urinary protein loss in horses with CRF since in most previous reports proteinuria was assessed using urine reagent strips. Reagent strip results of + + + or + + + + correlate with protein concentrations of 100 to 300 to 1000 to 2000 mg/dL, depending on which reagent strip is used. In a proteinuric horse that is producing 20 L of urine daily, these values would yield a wide range of urinary protein loss—20 to 400 g daily. The latter value would approach 25% of the total protein content of plasma and, so, is not realistic. In humans with CRF, urinary protein loss exceeding 3.5 g per day (50 mg/kg per day for a 70-kg person) is classified as nephrotic-range proteinuria, and some patients with heavy proteinuria may lose in excess of 15 g per day (more than 200 mg/kg per day).[123] The upper limit of acceptable urinary protein excretion in dogs is 20 mg/kg per day.[124] Using these values, estimates for the upper acceptable limits for urinary protein loss and nephrotic-range proteinuria in a 500-kg horse would be 10 and in excess of 25 g per day, respectively. These values agree well with a mean value of 3.2 mg/kg (1.6 g per day) and a range of 3.6 to 22.3 mg/kg (1.8 to 11.2 g) per day in normal mares reported by the authors[125] and by Kohn and Strasser,[126] respectively. Another way to document proteinuria is by determining the urinary

protein–urinary creatinine ratio (in milligrams per deciliter). This technique is more practical, since it avoids a timed urine collection period. Although a normal range has not yet been reported for horses, values in excess of 1.0:1 and 3.5:1 are considered above normal and indicate nephrotic-range proteinuria in dogs[124] and humans,[123] respectively. Thus, a urine protein-creatinine ratio greater than 2.0:1 likely supports significant proteinuria in a horse with CRF. Finally, a horse with CRF and heavy proteinuria (more than 200 mg/ kg per day) could excrete as much as 100 g of protein daily (5% to 7% of total plasma protein). Proteinuria of this magnitude can increase urine specific gravity to 1.020 or greater. It would certainly be great enough to lead to a decline in serum albumin (and total protein) concentration, despite increased hepatic albumin production. In some horses with CRF and a normal total plasma protein concentration, increased globulin concentration offsets mild hypoalbuminemia, whereas in other cases hyperglobulinemia can actually result in an increase in total plasma protein concentration.

Another diagnostic test used on horses with CRF is renal ultrasonography that allows evaluation of kidney size and the presence of cysts or nephroliths. Horses with ESKD typically have small kidneys that are more echogenic than normal (owing to sclerosis and possible tissue mineralization).[127–129] Cystoscopy can be a useful diagnostic adjunct to qualitatively assess urine production by each kidney and is particularly useful when ultrasonographic imaging fails to identify a kidney.[129] Renal scintigraphy is another imaging option to detect functional renal tissue that may not be apparent by ultrasonography.[130] Renal biopsy using ultrasonographic guidance can be performed to document renal disease. Unfortunately, since most horses are presented for evaluation in the later stages of disease, biopsy results typically reveal glomerular, tubular, and interstitial lesions consistent with ESKD. Rarely do the lesions provide information about the inciting cause of the renal disease unless immunofluorescence testing is pursued. This requires placing a sample in Michel's fixative, in addition to the sample placed in formalin for routine histopathologic examination. In some cases, renal biopsy results supporting pyelonephritis or a congenital anomaly (dysplasia) as the cause of CRF are useful in developing a therapeutic plan.

The severity of CRF in affected horses can be assessed at many levels of sophistication. The magnitude of azotemia is the most readily available and practical parameter but a relatively insensitive one.[123] Azotemia becomes apparent only after 75% or more of renal function is lost. Further, the degree of azotemia can vary with nonrenal factors such as diet, body mass, and hydration. In general, creatinine concentration is a more reliable measure than BUN, and doubling of creatinine roughly correlates to a 50% decline in GFR (see Fig. 16–8). Serum creatinine concentrations in the range of 5 to 10 mg/dL indicate a marked decline in renal function, and values exceeding 15 mg/dL are consistent with a grave prognosis. In contrast, horses with a creatinine concentration below 5 mg/dL may exhibit few clinical signs and can be managed for months or years (Fig. 16–24). Plotting the inverse of serum creatinine concentration (1/Cr) over time has also been used to monitor progression of CRF in humans[131, 132] and in one horse,[19] in an attempt to predict the end point of the disease process (Fig. 16–25). Unfortunately, these plots are subject to considerable variation (ow-

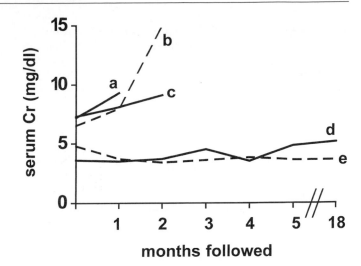

Figure 16–24. Serum Cr in five horses with chronic renal failure. The three horses with an initial Cr above 5 mg/dL (a-c) had rapid progression of renal disease over a 1- to 2-month period, necessitating euthanasia, whereas the two horses with an initial Cr below 5 mg/dL (d-e) were maintained with supportive care for longer than 18 months.

ing to changes in tubular secretion of creatinine) and have not proven to be of any more value than monitoring creatinine over time.[131, 132]

Measurement of GFR provides the most accurate quantitative assessment of renal function, but it is rarely pursued since it is more time consuming and technically demanding than measurement of serum creatinine concentration. Al-

though a number of methods are available to measure GFR,[133] measurement of endogenous creatinine clearance (Cl_{Cr}) or the plasma disappearance of exogenous creatinine, sulfanilate,[19, 134] or 99-metastable technetium tagged to diethylenetriaminepentaacetic acid (^{99m}Tc-DTPA)[135] are the most practical methods in a clinical setting. The former requires timed urine collections, whereas the latter may require spe-

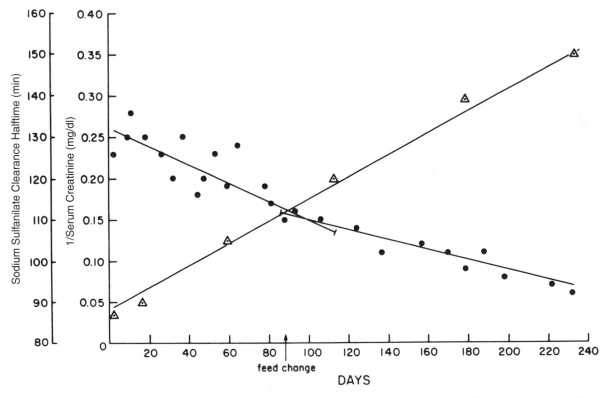

Figure 16–25. The inverse of the serum creatinine concentration *(filled circles)* and the whole-blood sodium sulfanilate clearance half-time in a horse with chronic renal failure associated with polycystic kidney disease. The slope of the line describing the reciprocals of serum creatinine concentration from day 1 to day 98 was significantly different ($P < 0.05$) from that from day 99 to 235 and the slope change was associated with a change from alfalfa to grass hay. (From Bertone JJ, Traub-Dargatz JL, Fettman MJ, et al: Monitoring the progression of renal failure in a horse with polycystic kidney disease: Use of the reciprocal of serum creatinine concentration and sodium sulfanilate clearance half-time. J Am Vet Med Assoc 191:565, 1987.)

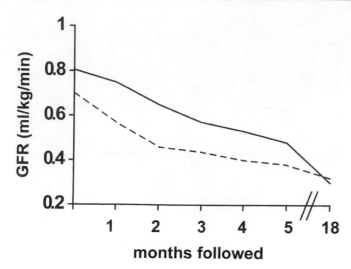

Figure 16–26. GFR as measured by endogenous creatinine clearance (Cl$_{Cr}$, *solid line*) and inulin clearance (Cl$_{In}$, *dashed line*) in a mare (horse e in Fig. 16–24) with chronic renal failure. GFR declined steadily over the 18-month period despite minimal change in serum creatinine concentration. In comparison to Cl$_{In}$, Cl$_{Cr}$ overestimated GFR until the terminal stage of the disease process. This difference likely reflects tubule secretion of creatinine in the earlier stages of chronic renal failure, which subsequently diminished during the final weeks of the disease course.

cial assays or nuclear medicine capabilities (see *Examination of the Urinary System*). Horses in the earlier stages of CRF can develop tubular creatinine secretion, which could lead to overestimation of GFR measured by the Cl$_{Cr}$ technique. As renal disease progresses, however, Cr excretion can decrease faster than GFR declines, owing to loss of compensatory secretion. Despite these limitations, repeated measurement of Cl$_{Cr}$ in a single animal can be useful for monitoring progression of CRF over time (Fig. 16–26).

PROGRESSION OF CHRONIC RENAL FAILURE

One of the hallmarks of CRF is the progressive nature of the disease,[136] and progression appears to be largely independent of the inciting cause, owing to final common pathways of renal injury. The response to a decrease in renal functional mass is a compensatory increase in filtration (termed "single nephron GFR") and tubule function (e.g., Cr secretion, ammoniagenesis) by remaining nephrons.[104, 136, 137] The increase in single-nephron GFR is the result of increased glomerular capillary blood flow and hydrostatic pressure leading to glomerular hyperfiltration. Hyperfiltration is associated with increased permeability of the GBM and proteinuria. Further, increased filtration of macromolecules leads to activation and proliferation of mesangial and epithelial cells and, eventually progression to glomerulosclerosis.[104, 136, 137]

A number of studies investigating the mechanisms of "glomerular hypertension" have demonstrated that activation of the renin-angiotensin system (RAS) and angiotensin

II (AII) production are of considerable importance, as AII is a potent constrictor of glomerular efferent arterioles.[136–138] Activation of the intrarenal RAS can produce significant glomerular hypertension without producing increases in systemic AII concentration or blood pressure. In fact, administration of specific AII receptor antagonists or angiotensin-converting enzyme (ACE) inhibitors have been demonstrated to decrease glomerular capillary hydrostatic pressure and the magnitude of proteinuria in experimental studies of renal disease.[138–140] ACE inhibitors have helped to control hypertension and proteinuria in small animals,[1, 141] but there are no reports of use of ACE inhibitors in horses with CRF.

The role of dietary protein in the progression of CRF has been the subject of a number of investigations in humans and small animals with a variety of renal diseases.[136, 137, 142–147] It has been well-established that clinical signs of uremia can be ameliorated by decreasing dietary protein content; however, it remains controversial whether decreasing dietary protein slows progression of renal disease. Increased dietary protein has been demonstrated to increase activation of the RAS; therefore, decreasing dietary protein could be protective, for the reasons discussed in the preceding paragraph. Next, a decrease in protein intake leads to production of smaller amounts of urea and other nitrogenous wastes. In theory, the work load on the kidneys is similarly decreased. Since all work (aerobic adenosine triphosphate production and utilization) is associated with a degree of free radical production, greater protein intake would generate more free radicals. Free radicals appear to be especially injurious to diseased kidneys, since their scavenging mechanisms are compromised. Increased dietary protein also requires increased ammoniagenesis by renal tubules to excrete the associated proton load; however, ammoniagenesis can lead to noninflammatory, nonimmune complement activation in proximal tubule epithelial cells. This proinflammatory consequence of ammoniagenesis can be ameliorated by supplementation with sodium bicarbonate. In summary, excessive dietary protein leads to a greater degree of uremia and has the potential to exacerbate renal damage in CRF by several mechanisms.

In contrast, protein-calorie malnutrition is strongly associated with increased morbidity and mortality in human CRF patients.[148] This can be attributed to increased protein catabolism when dietary protein intake is marginal to low. In humans, a number of serum components, including prealbumin, cholesterol, and insulin-like growth factor; plasma and muscle amino acid profiles; and body composition measurements have been studied as potential indices of nutritional status; however, serum albumin concentration is the most practical and most extensively studied nutritional index. In addition to heavy proteinuria, hypoalbuminemia can also be attributed to protein-calorie malnutrition. Further, a BUN-Cr ratio less than 10:1 may be another indication of inadequate protein intake. Thus, current dietary recommendations call for dietary protein and calories at levels that meet or slightly exceed predicted requirements, which should render nitrogen balance neutral.[148] Finally, a critically important but often overlooked aspect of nutritional management of CRF patients is provision of a very palatable diet.[1, 148] Feeding smaller meals more frequently and varying the diet help to increase food intake in CRF patients of all species.

Experimental studies of CRF in horses are limited to the

reports by Roberts and coworkers that describe the effects of prolonged daily dosing of horses with mercury compounds.[149-152] In these four reports, each involving a single horse, the subjects were destroyed between 85 and 191 days after mercury administration began. Anorexia, weight loss, and nonpruritic urticaria were the major clinical signs. The renal lesion was CIN, which was accompanied by a decrease in concentrating ability and an increase in water consumption. Additional tubule dysfunction included glucosuria in all four horses and a variable degree of proteinuria. Of interest, the clinical signs and tubular dysfunction preceded the development of azotemia in all horses and there was no increase in excretion of sodium or chloride. The final report focused principally on the effects on renal function, and azotemia did not develop until the final week of life, and GFR (assessed by endogenous Cl_{Cr}) decreased to 35% of the highest measured value on the day before euthanasia.[152] Aciduria and increased phosphate excretion, in addition to glucosuria and proteinuria, were also detected during the final week of life.

TREATMENT OF CHRONIC RENAL FAILURE

At the time of presentation most horses with CRF exhibit obvious weight loss and other clinical signs. Owing to the progressive and irreversible nature of the renal disease, the long-term prognosis is grave. Specific corrective treatment for CRF (renal transplantation) is not available for horses, and maintenance by peritoneal dialysis or hemodialysis is practical only for valuable breeding animals. Pyelonephritis could be considered an exception, since antibiotic treatment could, in theory, lead to resolution of infection and improved renal function. Unfortunately, significant renal damage has usually occurred by the time the diagnosis is established in most cases of bilateral pyelonephritis, so that the prognosis for a return to normal renal function is guarded to poor. In contrast, the short-term prognosis may be more favorable. Some horses with CRF may maintain serum creatinine concentration below 5 mg/dL for months with minimal deterioration. It is difficult to predict which patients will deteriorate more rapidly, but the recent history and initial ability to counteract weight loss with improved management are useful indicators. Laboratory analysis of blood samples at 2- to 4-week intervals to follow the degree of azotemia and serum electrolyte alterations may be useful in monitoring disease progression. In general, animals that are eating well and maintain reasonable body condition carry the best short-term prognosis and may still be able to perform some limited work. Their utility as breeding animals may be reduced because azotemia and eventual weight loss would reduce the chance for normal conception and gestation. The goal in each case is provide appropriate supportive care and to monitor the horse closely so as to provide humane euthanasia before the patient develops uremic decompensation.

As previously discussed, once significant renal disease is established, irreversible decline in GFR and progression of renal failure generally ensue.[136, 137] Thus, management of the equine patient afflicted with CRF involves palliative efforts to minimize further loss of renal function. The goals are to prevent complicating conditions (e.g., by providing plenty of water and salt), to discontinue administration of nephrotoxic agents, and to provide a palatable diet to encourage appetite and minimize further weight loss.[22-26, 153] Intravenous fluid therapy to promote diuresis, usually with 0.9% sodium chloride solution, is of much greater benefit in cases of acute, reversible renal failure but may also benefit patients that suffer a sudden exacerbation of CRF. Intravenous fluid therapy must be administered cautiously, as horses with CRF can develop significant peripheral or pulmonary edema.

Supportive care can include supplementation of sodium chloride (50 to 75 g per day) or sodium bicarbonate (50 to 150 g per day).[153] Bicarbonate is preferred when serum bicarbonate concentration is consistently below 20 mEq/L. Supplemental electrolytes may need to be added to bran mash, as horses may not get enough salt from licking a block. If electrolyte supplementation aggravates ventral edema, supplementation should be limited or discontinued. Edema is not usually a significant problem, and mild edema should be tolerated (rather than treated with diuretics, which could be ineffective or lead to further electrolyte wastage) unless it interferes with ambulation. Substituting high-calcium and high-protein feed sources such as alfalfa hay with good-quality grass hay and carbohydrates (corn and oats) may help control hypercalcemia and the level of azotemia. Ideally, the hay and grain should contain an adequate, but not excessive, amount of protein (less than 10% crude protein), which should maintain the BUN-Cr ratio in a target range between 10:1 and 15:1.[22] It is important to provide unlimited access to fresh water and to encourage adequate energy intake by feeding a variety of palatable feeds. In fact, if appetite for grass hay deteriorates, it is preferable to offer less ideal feeds such as alfalfa hay or increased amounts of concentrate to meet energy requirements and reduce the rate of weight loss. Often horses will continue to graze at pasture when their appetite for hay is diminished. Administration of B vitamins or anabolic steroids for their touted appetite-stimulating effects may benefit some animals. Although dietary fat is calorie dense, supplementation must be approached judiciously in patients with hyperlipidemia and hypercholesterolemia.

Administration of corticosteroids or NSAIDs can limit the intrarenal inflammatory response associated with renal failure and may also attenuate renal injury. For example, administration of meclofenamate limited proteinuria in a group of human patients with severe manifestations of the nephrotic syndrome[154]; however, nonspecific blockade of prostaglandin production by corticosteroids and most available NSAIDs has the adverse effect of decreasing production of important renal vasodilating agents (prostaglandin E_2 and prostacyclin). Production of these prostanoids increases during periods of renal vasoconstriction or ischemia, to maintain intrarenal blood flow, particularly to the renal medulla. With excessive or long-term NSAID administration, renal papillary necrosis develops secondary to medullary ischemia.[78, 79] Thus, the negative effects of corticosteroids and NSAIDs on renal blood flow outweigh possible benefits, and they are not recommended for the management of CRF in horses.

The progressive renal injury that occurs in CRF is associated with continued damage to glomerular and tubular membranes mediated by ongoing activation of the inflammatory cascade. In theory, treatment with antioxidant medications and free radical scavengers could be of benefit, but experimental data in horses do not bear this out. Similarly, there has been considerable interest in the role of dietary fatty acids as precursors of eicosanoids. Specifically, dietary supplementation with sources rich in omega-3 fatty acids (linolenic acid), as compared with omega-6 fatty acids (linoleic acid), appear to decrease generation of more damaging fatty acid metabolites during activation of the inflammatory cascade. In horses, dietary supplementation with omega-3 fatty acids (in the form of linseed oil) has been effective at ameliorating the effects of endotoxin in studies in vitro[155–157] and supplementation with fish oil (another rich source of omega-3 fatty acids) slowed the progression of renal failure in laboratory animals.[158, 159] Unfortunately, the effects of endotoxin in vivo were not ameliorated by feeding linseed oil in preliminary equine studies[160] and the possible benefits of feeding omega-3 fatty acids to horses with CRF are not known at this time.

Recently, attention has been directed to use of more specific antiinflammatory or immunosuppressant medications to limit renal injury in immune-mediated glomerulonephritis. For example, inhibition of thromboxane synthetase activity (thromboxane A_2 activity is a potent vasoconstricting agent and platelet activator) was demonstrated to limit renal histologic and functional changes in a canine model of immune-mediated glomerulonephritis.[161] Similarly, cyclosporine was used as an adjunctive treatment in a prospective study of naturally occurring canine glomerulonephritis. Unfortunately, renal function declined in cyclosporine-treated dogs, as it did in control dogs. The lack of any beneficial effect, in combination with adverse reactions to cyclosporine, led to the conclusion that cyclosporine was of no use for treating CRF.[162] As these studies demonstrate, specific manipulation of the inflammatory or immune response can limit renal injury when medications can be administered before or early in the course of renal disease; however, with long-standing, naturally occurring disease, such treatments are much less likely to significantly retard progression of renal failure. Finally, other investigators are currently focusing on developing therapeutic strategies that may modulate or limit renal fibrosis. Their studies of the effects of cytokines, lymphokines, and proteoglycans on matrix synthesis and degradation by mesangial cells and on fibroblast activation in damaged glomeruli may lead to novel treatment options in the future.[163, 164]

REFERENCES

1. Polzin DJ, Osborne CA, Bartges JW, et al: Chronic renal failure. In Ettinger SJ, Feldman EC, eds. *Textbook of Veterinary Internal Medicine,* ed 4, vol 2. Philadelphia, WB Saunders, 1995, p 1734.
2. Banks KL, Henson JB: Immunologically mediated glomerulitis of horses. II. Antiglomerular basement membrane antibody and other mechanisms of spontaneous disease. *Lab Invest* 26:708, 1972.
3. Osborne CA, Polzin DJ: Azotemia: A review of what's old and what's new. Part I. Definition of terms and concepts. *Compend Contin Educ Pract Vet* 5:497, 1983.
4. Irwin DHG, Howell DW: Equine pyelonephritis and unilateral nephrectomy. *J So Afr Vet Assoc* 51:235, 1980.
5. Trotter GW, Brown CM, Ainsworth DM: Unilateral nephrec-

tomy for treatment of a renal abscess in a foal. *J Am Vet Med Assoc* 184:1392, 1984.
6. Juzwiak JS, Bain FT, Slone DE, et al: Unilateral nephrectomy for treatment of chronic hematuria due to nephrolithiasis in a colt. *Can Vet J* 29:931, 1988.
7. Sullins KE, McIlwraith CW, Yovich JV, et al: Ectopic ureter managed by unilateral nephrectomy in two female horses. *Equine Vet J* 20:463, 1988.
8. Jones SL, Langer DL, Sterner-Kock A, et al: Renal dysplasia and benign ureteropelvic polyps associated with hydronephrosis in a foal. *J Am Vet Med Assoc* 204:1230, 1994.
9. Tennant B, Lowe JE, Tasker JB: Hypercalcemia and hypophosphatemia in ponies following bilateral nephrectomy. *Proc Soc Exp Biol Med* 167:365, 1981.
10. Johnson BD, Klingborg DJ, Heitman JM, et al: A horse with one kidney, partially obstructed ureter, and contralateral urogenital anomalies. *J Am Vet Med Assoc* 169:217, 1976.
11. Brown CM, Parks AH, Mullaney TP, et al: Bilateral renal dysplasia and hypoplasia in a foal with an imperforate anus. *Vet Rec* 122:91, 1988.
12. Andrews FM, Rosol TJ, Kohn CW, et al: Bilateral renal hypoplasia in four young horses. *J Am Vet Med Assoc* 189:209, 1986.
13. Roberts MC, Kelly WR: Chronic renal failure in a young pony. *Aust Vet J* 56:599, 1980.
14. Anderson WI, Picut CA, King JM, Perdrizet JA: Renal dysplasia in a Standardbred colt. *Vet Pathol* 25:179, 1988.
15. Ronen N, van Amstel SR, Nesbit JW, van Rensburg IBJ: Renal dysplasia in two adult horses: Clinical and pathological aspects. *Vet Rec* 132:269, 1988.
16. Zicker SC, Marty GD, Carlson GP, et al: Bilateral renal dysplasia with nephron hypoplasia in a foal. *J Am Vet Med Assoc* 196:2001, 1990.
17. Ramsey G, Rothwell TLW, Gibson KT, et al: Polycystic kidneys in an adult horse. *Equine Vet J* 19:243, 1987.
18. Scott PC, Vasey J: Progressive polycystic renal disease in an aged horse. *Aust Vet J* 63:92, 1986.
19. Bertone JJ, Traub-Dargatz JL, Fettman MJ, et al: Monitoring the progression of renal failure in a horse with polycystic kidney disease: Use of the reciprocal of serum creatinine concentration and sodium sulfanilate clearance half-time. *J Am Vet Med Assoc* 191:565, 1987.
20. Tennant B, Kaneko JJ, Lowe JE, Tasker JB: Chronic renal failure in the horse. *Proc Annu Conv Am Assoc Equine Pract* 23:293, 1978.
21. Koterba AM, Coffman JR: Acute and chronic renal disease in the horse. *Compend Contin Educ Pract Vet* 3:S461, 1981.
22. Divers TJ: Chronic renal failure in horses. *Compend Contin Educ Pract Vet* 5:S310, 1983.
23. Divers TJ: Chronic renal failure. In Robinson NE, ed: *Current Therapy in Equine Medicine 2*. Philadelphia, WB Saunders, 1987, p 698.
24. Divers TJ: Diseases of the renal system. In Smith BP, ed: *Large Animal Internal Medicine*. St. Louis, CV Mosby, 1990, p 872.
25. Whitlock RH: Chronic renal failure. In Robinson NE, ed: *Current Therapy in Equine Medicine 3*. Philadelphia, WB Saunders, 1992, p 628.
26. Pringle J, Ortenburger A: Diseases of the kidneys and ureters. *In* Kobluk CN, Ames TR, Geor RJ, eds: *The Horse, Diseases and Clinical Management*. Philadelphia, WB Saunders, 1995, p 583.
27. Osborne CA, Hammer RF, Stevens JB, et al: The glomerulus in health and disease: A comparative review of domestic animals and man. *Adv Vet Sci Comp Med* 21:207, 1977.
28. Langham RF, Hallman ET: The incidence of glomerulonephritis in domesticated animals. *J Am Vet Med Assoc* 49:471, 1949.

29. Slauson DO, Lewis RM: Comparative pathology of glomerulonephritis in animals. *Vet Pathol* 16:135, 1979.

30. Winter H, Majid NH: Glomerulonephritis—an emerging disease? *Vet Bull* 54:327, 1984.

31. Glassock RJ, Adler SG, Ward HJ, Cohen AH: Primary glomerular diseases. In Brenner BM, Rector FC, eds: *The Kidney,* ed 4, Vol 1. Philadelphia, WB Saunders, 1991, p 1182.

32. Tisher CC, Madsen KM: Anatomy of the kidney. In Brenner BM, Rector FC, eds: *The Kidney,* ed 4, Vol 1. Philadelphia: WB Saunders, 1991, p 3.

33. Grauer GF, DiBartola SP: Glomerular disease. In Ettinger SJ, Feldman EC, eds: *Textbook of Veterinary Internal Medicine,* ed 4, Vol 2. Philadelphia, WB Saunders, 1995, p 1760.

34. Banks KL, Henson JB, McGuire TC: Immunologically mediated glomerulitis of horses. I. Pathogenesis in persistent infection by equine infectious anemia virus. *Lab Invest* 26:701, 1972.

35. Banks KL: Animal model of human disease. Antiglomerular basement antibody in horses. *Am J Pathol* 94:443, 1979.

36. Geor RJ, Clark EG, Haines DM, Napier PG: Systemic lupus erythematosus in a filly. *J Am Vet Med Assoc* 197:1489, 1990.

37. Sabnis SG, Gunson DE, Antonovych TT: Some unusual features of mesangioproliferative glomerulonephritis in horses. *Vet Pathol* 21:574, 1984.

38. Maede Y, Inaba M, Amano Y, et al: Cryoglobulinemia in a horse. *J Vet Med Sci* 53:379, 1991.

39. Glassock RJ, Cohen AH, Adler SG, Ward HJ: Secondary glomerular diseases. In Brenner BM, Rector FC, eds: *The Kidney,* ed 4, Vol 1. Philadelphia, WB Saunders, 1991, p 1280.

40. Traub-Dargatz J, Bertone A, Bennett D, et al: Monoclonal aggregating immunoglobulin cryoglobulinaemia in a horse with malignant lymphoma. *Equine Vet J* 17:470, 1985.

41. MacDougall DF, Cook T, Steward AP, Cattell V: Canine chronic renal disease: Prevalence and types of glomerulonephritis in the dog. *Kidney Int* 29:1144, 1986.

42. Morris DD: Glomerulonephritis. In Robinson NE, ed: *Current Therapy in Equine Medicine 2.* Philadelphia, WB Saunders, 1987, p 702.

43. Fincher MG, Olafson P: Chronic diffuse glomerulonephritis in a horse. *Cornell Vet* 24:356, 1934.

44. Frank ER, Dunlap GL: Chronic diffuse glomerulo-tubular nephritis in a horse. *North Am Vet* 16:20, 1935.

45. Kadás I, Százados I: Membrano-proliferative diffuse glomerulonephritis in a horse. *Dtsch Tierarztl Wschr* 81:618, 1974.

46. McCausland IP, Milestone BA: Diffuse mesangioproliferative glomerulonephritis in a horse. *NZ Vet J* 24:239, 1976.

47. Brobst DF, Grant BD, Hilbert BJ, et al: Blood biochemical changes in horses with prerenal and renal disease. J Equine Med Surg 1:171, 1977.

48. Brobst DF, Lee HA, Spencer GR: Hypercalcemia and hypophosphotemia in a mare with renal insufficiency. *J Am Vet Med Assoc* 173:1370, 1978.

49. Roberts MC, Seiler RJ: Renal failure in a horse with chronic glomerulonephritis and renal oxalosis. *J Equine Med Surg* 3:278, 1979.

50. Dobos-Kovács M: Chronic, diffuse, membrane-proliferative glomerulonephritis and its complications in a horse. *Magyar Állatorvosok Lapja* 36:533, 1981.

51. Tennant B, Bettleheim P, Kaneko JJ: Paradoxic hypercalcemia and hypophosphotemia associated with chronic renal failure in horses. *J Am Vet Med Assoc* 180:630, 1982.

52. Morris DD, Lee JW: Renal insufficiency due to chronic glomerulonephritis in two horses. *Equine Pract* 4(8):21, 1982.

53. Waldvogel A, Wild P, Wegmann C: Membranoproliferative glomerulonephritis in a horse. *Vet Pathol* 20:500, 1983.

54. Scarratt WK, Sponenberg DP: Chronic glomerulonephritis in two horses. *J Equine Vet Sci* 4:252, 1984.

55. Divers TJ, Timoney JF, Lewis RM, Smith CA: Equine glomerulonephritis and renal failure associated with complexes of group-C streptococcal antigen and IgG antibody. *Vet Immunol Immunopathol* 32:93, 1992.

56. Morter RL, Williams RD, Bolte H, Freeman MJ: Equine leptospirosis. *J Am Vet Med Assoc* 155:436, 1969.

57. Hogan PM, Bernard WV, Kazakevicius PA, Fitzgerald MR: Acute renal disease due to *Leptospira interrogansa* in a weaning. *Equine Vet J* 28:331, 1996.

58. Roberts MC, Kelly WR: Renal dysfunction in a case of purpura haemorrhagica in a horse. *Vet Rec* 110:144, 1982.

59. Wimberly HC, Antonovych TT, Lewis RM: Focal glomerulosclerosis-like disease with nephrotic syndrome in a horse. *Vet Pathol* 18:692, 1981.

60. Divers TJ, Whitlock RH, Byars TD, et al: Acute renal failure in six horses resulting from haemodynamic causes. *Equine Vet J* 19:178, 1987.

61. Schmitz DG: Toxic nephropathy in horses. *Compend Contin Educ Pract Vet* 10:104, 1988.

62. Boyd WL, Bishop LM: Pyelonephritis of horses and cattle. *J Am Vet Med Assoc* 90:154, 1937.

63. Held JP, Wright B, Henton JE: Pyelonephritis associated with renal failure in a horse. *J Am Vet Med Assoc* 189:688, 1986.

64. Carrick JB, Pollitt CC: Chronic pyelonephritis in a brood mare. *Aust Vet J* 64:252, 1987.

65. Sloet van Oldruitenborgh-Oosterbaan MM, Klabec HC: Ureteropyelonephritis in a Fresian mare. *Vet Rec* 122:609, 1988.

66. Mair TS, Taylor FGR, Pinsent PJN: Fever of unknown origin in the horse: A review of 63 cases. *Equine Vet J* 21:260, 1989.

67. Hamlen H: Pyelonephritis in a mature gelding with an unusual urinary bladder foreign body: A case report. *J Equine Vet Sci* 13:159, 1993.

68. Byars TD, Simpson JS, Divers TJ, et al: Percutaneous nephrostomy in short-term management of ureterolithiasis and renal dysfunction in a filly. *J Am Vet Med Assoc* 195:499, 1989.

69. Hope WD, Wilson JH, Hager DA, et al: Chronic renal failure associated with bilateral nephroliths and ureteroliths in a two-year-old Thoroughbred colt. *Equine Vet J* 21:228, 1989.

70. Ehnen SJ, Divers TJ, Gillette D, et al: Obstructive nephrolithiasis and ureterolithiasis associated with chronic renal failure in horses: Eight cases (1981–1987). *J Am Vet Med Assoc* 197:249, 1990.

71. Hillyer MH, Mair TS, Lucke VM: Bilateral renal calculi in an adult horse. *Equine Vet Educ* 2:117, 1990.

72. Laing JA, Raisis AL, Rawlinson RJ, Small AC: Chronic renal failure and urolithiasis in a 2-year-old colt. *Aust Vet J* 69:199, 1992.

73. Divers TJ: Nephrolithiasis and ureterolithiasis in horses and their association with renal disease and failure. (Editorial) *Equine Vet J* 21:161, 1989.

74. Webb RF, Knight PR: Oxalate nephropathy in a horse. *Aust Vet J* 53:554, 1977.

75. Brobst DF, Bayly WM, Reed SM, et al: Parathyroid hormone evaluation in normal horses and horses with renal failure. *Equine Vet Sci* 2:150, 1982.

76. Bennett WM, Elzinga LW, Porter GA: Tubulointerstitial disease and toxic nephropathy. In Brenner BM, Rector FC, eds: *The Kidney,* ed 4, Vol 2. Philadelphia: WB Saunders, 1991, p 1430.

77. MacAllister CG, Morgan SJ, Borne AT, Pollet RA: Comparison of adverse effects of phenylbutazone, flunixin meglumine, and ketoprofen in horses. *J Am Vet Med Assoc* 202:71, 1993.

78. Gunson DE: Renal papillary necrosis in horses. *J Am Vet Med Assoc* 182:263, 1983.

79. Gunson DE, Soma LR: Renal papillary necrosis in horses

after phenylbutazone and water deprivation. *Vet Pathol* 20:603, 1983.

80. Behm RJ, Berg IE: Hematuria caused by medullary crest necrosis in a horse. *Comp Contin Educ Pract Vet* 9:698, 1987.

81. Andrews EJ: Oxalate nephropathy in a horse. *J Am Vet Med Assoc* 159:49, 1971.

82. Buntain B, Greig WA, Thompson H: Chronic nephritis in a pony. *Vet Rec* 104:307, 1979.

83. Alders RG, Hutchins DR: Chronic nephritis in a horse. *Aust Vet J* 64:151, 1987.

84. Snyder JR, Batista de Cruz J: Chronic renal failure in a stallion. *Comp Contin Educ Pract Vet* 6:S134, 1984.

85. Maxie MG: The urinary system. In Jubb KVF, Kennedy PC, Palmer N, eds: *Pathology of Domestic Animals,* ed 3, Vol 2. San Diego: Academic Press, 1985, p 343.

86. Stewart J, McCallum JW: The anhydraemia of oxalate poisoning in horses. *Vet Rec* 56:77, 1944.

87. Walthall JC, McKenzie RA: Osteodystrophia fibrosa in horses at pasture in Queensland: Field and laboratory investigations. *Aust Vet J* 52:11, 1976.

88. Jakob W: Spontaneous amyloidosis of animals. *Vet Pathol* 8:292, 1971.

89. Nunokawa Y, Fujinaga T, Taira T, et al: Evaluation of serum amyloid A protein as an acute-phase reactive protein in horses. *J Vet Med Sci* 55:1011, 1993.

90. Husebekk A, Husby G, Sletten K, et al: Characterization of amyloid protein AA and its serum precursor SAA in the horse. *Scand J Immunol* 23:703, 1986.

91. Sletten K, Husebekk A, Husby G: The amino acid sequence of an amyloid fibril protein AA isolated from the horse. *Scand J Immunol* 26:79, 1987.

92. Sletten K, Husebekk A, Husby G: The primary structure of equine serum amyloid A (SAA) protein. *Scand J Immunol* 30:117, 1989.

93. van Andel ACJ, Gruys E, Kroneman J, Veerkamp J: Amyloid in the horse: A report of nine cases. *Equine Vet J* 20:277, 1988.

94. DiBartola SP, Benson MD: The pathogenesis of reactive systemic amyloidosis. *J Vet Intern Med* 3:31, 1989.

95. Hayden DW, Johnson KH, Wolf CB, Westermark P: AA amyloid–associated gastroenteropathy in a horse. *J Comp Pathol* 98:195, 1988.

96. Vanhooser SL, Reinemeyer CR, Held JP: Hepatic AA amyloidosis associated with severe strongylosis in a horse. *Equine Vet J* 20:274, 1988.

97. Bovée KC: The uremic syndrome. *J Am Anim Hosp Assoc* 12:189, 1976.

98. Wills MR: Uremic toxins, and their effect on intermediary metabolism. *Clin Chem* 31:5, 1985.

99. May RC, Kelly RA, Mitch WE: Pathophysiology of uremia. In Brenner BM, Rector FC, eds: *The Kidney,* ed 4, Vol 1. Philadelphia, WB Saunders, 1991, p 1997.

100. Finco DR, Groves C: Mechanism of renal excretion of creatinine by the pony. *Am J Vet Res* 46:1625, 1985.

101. Malluche H, Faugere MC: Renal bone disease 1990: An unmet challenge for the nephrologist. *Kidney Int* 38:193, 1990.

102. Nagode LA, Chew DJ: Nephrocalcinosis caused by hyperparathyroidism in progression of renal failure. *Semin Vet Med Surg (Small Anim)* 7:202, 1992.

103. Perna AF, Ingrosso D, Galletti P, et al: Membrane protein damage and methylation reactions in chronic renal failure. *Kidney Int* 50:358, 1996.

104. Hayslett JP: Functional adaptation to reduction in renal mass. *Physiol Rev* 59:137, 1979.

105. Pearson EG: Hypoalbuminemia in horses. *Compend Contin Educ Pract Vet* 12:555, 1990.

106. Rose BD: Edematous states. In Rose BD, ed: *Clinical Physiology of Acid-Base and Electrolyte Disorders,* ed 3. New York, McGraw-Hill, 1989, p 416.

107. Bovée KC: Functional responses to nephron loss. In Bovée KC, ed: *Canine Nephrology.* Media, PA, Harwal, 1984, p 531.

108. Eschbach JW, Adamson JW: Hematologic consequences of renal failure. In Brenner BM, Rector FC, eds: *The Kidney,* ed 4, Vol 2. Philadelphia, WB Saunders, 1991, p 2019.

109. Ersley AJ: Erythropoeitin. *N Engl J Med* 324:1339, 1991.

110. Jaussand P, Audran M, Gareau RL: Kinetics and haematological effects of erythropoietin in horses. *Vet Res* 25:568, 1994.

111. McKeever KH, McNally BA, Kirby KM, et al: Effects of erythropoeitin on plasma and red cell volume, $\dot{V}_{O_{2max}}$, and hemodynamics in exercising horses. *Med Sci Sports Exer* 25:S25, 1993.

112. Geor RJ, Weiss DJ: Drugs affecting the hematologic system of the performance horse. *Vet Clin North Am: Equine Pract* 9:649, 1993

113. Bayly WM: A practitioner's approach to the diagnosis and treatment of renal failure in horses. *Vet Med* 86:632, 1991.

114. Matthews HK, Kohn CW: Calcium and phosphorous homeostasis in horses with renal disease. *Proc Annu Vet Med Forum Am Coll Vet Intern Med* 11:623, 1993.

115. Coburn JW, Slatopolsky E: Vitamin D, parathyroid hormone, and the renal osteodystrophies. In Brenner BM, Rector FC, eds: *The Kidney,* ed 4, Vol 2. Philadelphia: WB Saunders, 1991, p 2036.

116. Krook L, Wasserman RH, Shively JN, et al: Hypercalcemia and calcinosis in Florida horses: Implication for the shrub *Cestrum diurnum* as the causative agent. Cornell Vet 65:26, 1975.

117. Gingerich DA, Murdick PW: Paradoxic aciduria in bovine metabolic alkalosis. *J Am Vet Med Assoc* 166:227, 1975.

118. Naylor JM, Kronfeld DS, Acland H: Hyperlipemia in horses: Effects of undernutrition and disease. *Am J Vet Res* 41:899, 1980.

119. Anderson S, Garcia DL, Brenner BM: Renal and systemic manifestations of glomerular disease. In Brenner BM, Rector FC, eds: *The Kidney,* ed 4, Vol 2. Philadelphia, WB Saunders, 1991, p 1831.

120. Naylor JM: Hyperlipemia. In Robinson NE, ed: *Current Therapy in Equine Medicine 2.* Philadelphia, WB Saunders, 1987, p. 114.

121. Gröne HJ, Hohbach J, Gröne EF: Modulation of glomerular sclerosis and interstitial fibrosis by native and modified lipoproteins. *Kidney Int* 49(Suppl 54):S18, 1996.

122. Grossman BS, Brobst DF, Kramer JW, et al: Urinary indices for differentiation of prerenal azotemia and renal azotemia in horses. *J Am Vet Med Assoc* 180:284, 1982.

123. Levey AS, Madaio MP, Perrone RD: Laboratory assessment of renal disease: Clearance, urinalysis, and renal biopsy. In Brenner BM, Rector FC, eds: *The Kidney,* ed 4, Vol 2. Philadelphia, WB Saunders, 1991, p 919.

124. Grauer GF, Thomas CB, Eicker SW: Estimation of quantitative proteinuria in the dog, using the urine protein-to-creatinine ratio from a random, voided sample. *Am J Vet Res* 46:2116, 1985.

125. Schott HC, Hodgson DR, Bayly WM: Haematuria, pigmenturia and proteinuria in exercising horses. *Equine Vet J* 27:67, 1995.

126. Kohn CW, Strasser SL: 24-hour renal clearance and excretion of endogenous substances in the mare. *Am J Vet Res* 47:1332, 1986.

127. Rantanen NW: Diseases of the kidneys. *Vet Clin North Am: Equine Pract* 2:89, 1986.

128. Kiper ML, Traub-Dargatz JL, Wrigley RH: Renal ultrasonography in horses. *Compend Contin Educ Pract Vet* 12:993, 1990.

129. Traub-Dargatz JL, McKinnon AO: Adjunctive methods of

examination of the urogenital tract. *Vet Clin North Am: Equine Pract* 4:339, 1988.

130. Schott HC, Roberts GD, Hines MT, Byrne BA: Nuclear scintigraphy as a diagnostic aid in the evaluation of renal disease in horses. *Proc Annu Conv Amer Assoc Equine Pract* 39:251, 1993.

131. Levey AS: Measurement of renal function in chronic renal disease. *Kidney Int* 38:167, 1990.

132. Walser M: Progression of chronic renal failure in man. *Kidney Int* 37:1195, 1990.

133. Matthews HK, Andrews FM, Daniel GB, Jacobs WR: Measuring renal function in horses. *Vet Med* 88:349, 1993.

134. Brobst DF, Bramwell K, Kramer JW: Sodium sulfanilate clearance as a method of determining renal function in the horse. *J Equine Med Surg* 2:500, 1978.

135. Matthews HK, Andrews FM, Danile GB, et al: Comparison of standard and radionuclide methods for measurement of glomerular filtration rate and effective renal blood flow in female horses. *Am J Vet Res* 53:1612, 1992.

136. Klahr S, Schreiner G, Ichikawa I: The progression of renal disease. *N Engl J Med* 318:1657, 1988.

137. Meyer TW, Scholey JW, Brenner BM: Nephron adaptation to renal injury. In Brenner BM, Rector FC, eds: *The Kidney*, ed 4, Vol 2. Philadelphia, WB Saunders, 1991, p 1871.

138. Yoshioka T, Mitarai T, Kon V, et al: Role for angiotensin II in an overt functional proteinuria. *Kidney Int* 30:538, 1986.

139. Heeg JE, de Jong PE, van der Hem GK, de Zeeuw D: Reduction of proteinuria by angiotensin converting enzyme inhibition. *Kidney Int* 32:78, 1987.

140. Keane WF, Anderson S, Aurell M, et al: Angiotensin converting enzyme inhibitors and progressive renal insufficiency: Current experience and future directions. *Ann Intern Med* 111:503, 1989.

141. Brown SA, Walton C, Crawford P, Bakris G: Long-term effects of antihypertensive regimens on renal hemodynamics and proteinuria in diabetic dogs. *Kidney Int* 43:1210, 1993.

142. Ihle BU, Becker GJ, Whitworth JA, et al: The effect of protein restriction on the progression of renal insufficiency. *N Engl J Med* 321:1773, 1989.

143. Mitch WE: Dietary protein restriction in patients with chronic renal failure. *Kidney Int* 40:326, 1991.

144. Fouque D, Laville M, Boissel JP, et al: Controlled low protein diets in chronic renal insufficiency: Meta-analysis. *B Med J* 304:216, 1992.

145. Klahr S, Level AS, Beck GJ, et al: The effects of dietary protein restriction and blood-pressure control on the progression of chronic renal disease. *N Engl J Med* 330:877, 1994.

146. Polzin DJ, Osborne CA, Hayden DW, Stevens JB: Influence of reduced protein diets on morbidity, mortality, and renal function in dogs with induced chronic renal failure. *Am J Vet Res* 45:506, 1984.

147. Brown SA, Finco DR, Crowell WA, Navar LG: Dietary protein intake and the glomerular adaptations to partial nephrectomy in dogs. *J Nutr* 121:S125, 191.

148. Ikizler TA, Hakim RM: Nutrition in end-stage renal disease. *Kidney Int* 50:343, 1996.

149. Seawright AA, Roberts MC, Costigan P: Chronic methylmercurialism in a horse. *Vet Hum Toxicol* 20:6, 1978.

150. Roberts MC, Ng JC, Seawright AA: The effects of prolonged daily low level mercuric chloride dosing in a horse. *Vet Hum Toxicol* 20:410, 1978.

151. Roberts MC, Seawright AA, Ng JC: Chronic phenylmercuric acetate toxicity in a horse. *Vet Hum Toxicol* 21:321, 1979.

152. Roberts MC, Seawright AA, Ng JC, Norman PD: Some effects of chronic mercuric chloride intoxication on renal function in a horse. *Vet Hum Toxicol* 24:415, 1982.

153. Divers TJ: Management of chronic renal failure in the horse. *Proc Annu Conv Am Assoc Equine Pract* 31:1, 1985.

154. Velosa JA, Torres VE, Donadio JV: Treatment of severe nephrotic syndrome with meclofenamate: An uncontrolled pilot study. *Mayo Clin Proc* 60:586, 1985.

155. Morris DD, Henry MM, Moore JN, Fischer JK: Effect of dietary linolenic acid on endotoxin-induced thromboxane and prostacyclin production by equine peritoneal macrophages. *Circ Shock* 29:311, 1989.

156. Henry MM, Moore JN, Feldman EB: The effect of dietary alpha linolenic acid on equine monocyte procoagulant activity and eicosanoid synthesis. *Circ Shock* 32:173, 1990.

157. Morris DD, Henry MM, Moore JN, Fischer JK: Dietary alpha linolenic acid reduces endotoxin-induced production of tumor necrosis factor activity by peritoneal macrophages. *Am J Vet Res* 52:528, 1991.

158. Barcelli UO, Weiss M, Pollack VE: Effects of dietary prostaglandin precursor on the progression of experimentally induced chronic renal failure. *J Lab Clin Med* 100:786, 1982.

159. Scharschmidt LA, Gibbons NB, McGarry L, et al: Effects of dietary fish oil on renal insufficiency in rats with subtotal nephrectomy. *Kidney Int* 32:700, 1987.

160. Henry MM, Moore JN, Fischer JK: Influence of an omega-3 fatty acid–enriched ration on *in vivo* responses of horses to endotoxin. *Am J Vet Res* 52:523, 1991.

161. Longhofer SL, Frisbie DD, Johnson HC, et al: Effects of thromboxane synthetase inhibition on immune complex glomerulonephritis. *Am J Vet Res* 52:480, 1991.

162. Vaden SL, Breitschwerdt EB, Armstrong PJ, et al: The effects of cyclosporine versus standard care in dogs with naturally occurring glomerulonephritis. *J Vet Intern Med* 9:259, 1995.

163. Müller GA, Schettler V, Müller CA, Strutz F: Prevention of progression of renal fibrosis: How far are we? *Kidney Int* 49(Suppl 5):S75, 1996.

164. Davies M, Kastner S, Thomas GJ: Protcoglycans: Their possible role in renal fibrosis. *Kidney Int* 49(Suppl 54):S55, 1996.

16.7

Urinary Tract Infections

Harold C. Schott II, DVM, PhD

In humans, bacterial urinary tract infections (UTIs) are among the most common infections.[1] In contrast, bacterial UTIs appear to be uncommon in horses.[2–7] As in other species, ascending UTIs are more common, although septic nephritis may be an occasional consequence of septicemia, especially in neonatal foals.[8] Mares are at higher risk for UTIs than geldings or stallions, owing to their shorter urethra.

Development of a UTI requires initial urethral colonization with pathogenic bacteria, entry of pathogens into the bladder, and subsequent multiplication in the bladder.[1, 9] Urethral colonization involves adherence to uroepithelial cells, typically by fecal bacteria which possess fimbrial adhesins (pili) that bind to specific glycolipid receptors on uroepithelial cells. Not surprisingly, pathogenic *Escherichia coli* are rich in these specific surface adhesins whereas nonpathogenic *E. coli* have few specific surface adhesins. Further characterization of human pathogenic *E. coli* strains by their somatic (O), flagellar (H), and capsular (K) antigens has revealed that a small number of *E. coli* strains are responsible for a large percentage of UTIs.[1, 10, 11] Normal vulvar and preputial flora protect against urethral colonization by pathogenic bacteria, but any anatomic defect leading to turbulent urine flow compromises maintenance of normal flora and may increase the likelihood of colonization by pathogens.[12, 13] Although broodmares have not been proven to be at greater risk, intercourse is a well-established risk factor for development of UTIs in women. In addition, human prostatic secretions contain a heat-stable, cationic protein that has potent antibacterial activity.[1] Thus, stallions may be at lower risk than geldings for UTIs.

Once a pathogen has colonized the distal urethra, rapid proliferation between micturitions allows invasion of the proximal urethra and bladder, which do not have a protective flora. Host defenses in the bladder include immunoglobulins in urine and a mucopolysaccharide layer rich in glycosaminoglycans covering the uroepithelial surface.[10, 11] Production of protective glycosaminoglycans is under hormonal control by estrogen and progesterone in rabbits.[14] Thus, lack of these hormonal effects has been suggested as an explanation for the increased risk for UTIs in prepubertal and postmenopausal women and in spayed dogs.[9] Further, women with recurrent UTIs have been speculated to have decreased concentrations of secretory immunoglobulin A (IgA) in their urine.[15] Although continued urine production dilutes proliferating bacteria, once pathogens have gained access to the bladder the rate of replication far outweighs any dilution effect allowing the UTI to become established.[1] Although antibiotic therapy is highly effective in eliminating most UTIs, recurrent UTIs can be a challenge to manage. In addition to thorough evaluation to eliminate predisposing factors in these patients, additional approaches to prevention may be considered. For example, fimbrial vaccines have been shown to be effective against experimental UTIs in monkeys.[10]

URETHRITIS

Bacterial urethritis has been described as a cause of hemospermia in stallions[16, 17]; however, with the exception of traumatic, parasitic (habronemiasis), or neoplastic conditions of the penis or urethra that interfere with urine flow, we are unaware of documented cases of primary bacterial urethritis resulting in dysuria.[18, 19] Further, it is likely that hemospermia attributable to urethritis in a number of previous cases was probably a consequence of proximal urethral defects, which have become easier to identify with high-resolution videoendoscopy (see Hematuria).[20] Bacterial infections of accessory sex glands or the prepuce may also cause dysuria. Accessory sex gland infections are generally limited to intact males and are more likely to cause infertility or hemospermia than dysuria.[21, 22] Preputial infections can occur secondary to trauma, presence of a foreign body, habronemiasis, or neoplasia, and affected horses typically present with a malodorous, swollen sheath. Examination of the sheath and penis, in combination with biopsy of abnormal tissue, allows diagnosis of the primary problem. An occasional older gelding may develop recurrent sheath swelling or infection that cannot be attributed to a primary disease process. The pathogenesis of this problem is not known, although fat accumulation, poor hygiene, and inactivity may be contributing factors. Treatment involves repeated sheath cleaning, application of topical anti-inflammatory and antibacterial ointments, and, when involvement is more severe, systemic antibiotic administration.

CYSTITIS

Bacterial cystitis is usually a secondary problem that may accompany alterations in urine flow due to urolithiasis, bladder neoplasia, bladder paralysis, an anatomic defect of the bladder or urethra, or instrumentation of the urinary tract (e.g., catheterization, endoscopy).[2–7, 12, 13, 23–27] Dysuria may be manifested by pollakiuria, stranguria, hematuria, or pyuria. Scalding and accumulation of urine crystals may be observed on the perineum of affected mares or on the front of the hindlimbs of affected male horses. These findings should not be confused with normal estrus activity in an occasional mare. Although nosocomial UTIs are a well-documented problem in hospitalized human[1] and small animal patients,[28] this complication has not been well-recognized in equine patients except for ill neonatal foals. Diagnostic evaluation includes physical and rectal examinations and collection of a urine sample for urinalysis and quantitative bacterial culture. In the absence of uroliths or other bladder masses, transrectal palpation of the bladder is usually within normal limits; however, endoscopic and/or ultrasonographic examination of the bladder may be helpful in assessing mucosal damage and wall thickening in horses with cystitis.[29, 30] Since normal equine urine is rich in mucus and crystals, gross examination may be unrewarding, but sediment examination may reveal increased numbers of white blood cells (more than 10 leukocytes per high-power field [hpf]) and presence of bacteria in some, but not all, cases of cystitis. Normal sediment examination results do not rule out UTI. A definitive diagnosis requires quantitative culture results exceeding 10,000 colony-forming units (cfu)/mL in a urine sample collected by midstream catch or urethral catheterization.[5, 7, 31] For best results, urine sediment should be evaluated within 30 to 60 minutes of collection and samples for culture should be cooled during transport, since bacterial numbers may increase in samples left at room temperature. Organisms that may be recovered on culture include *E. coli*, *Proteus*, *Klebsiella*, *Enterobacter*, *Streptococcus*, or *Staphylococcus* species, *Pseudomonas aeruginosa*, and rarely *Corynebacterium renale*.[2–7, 25] Isolation of more than one organism is not uncommon. *Salmonella* spp. have occasionally been isolated from the urine of apparently healthy horses, and *Candida* infections of the lower urinary tract have also been documented in sick neonatal foals receiving broad-spectrum antibiotics.[4, 5]

Successful treatment of bacterial cystitis requires correction of predisposing problems such as urolithiasis and administration of systemic antibiotics. Ideally, selection of an antibiotic is based on the results of susceptibility testing of isolated organisms and the initial recommended course of treatment has traditionally been at least one week.[2–7] A trimethoprim-sulfonamide combination, ampicillin, penicillin, and an aminoglycoside, or ceftiofur can be initial choices. In humans with uncomplicated cystitis, single-dose antimicrobial therapy, which is less costly and is associated with fewer adverse effects, has a success rate comparable to that of longer-term conventional therapy (75% or greater). Further, relapse following single-dose therapy is not accompanied by more severe clinical signs or more extensive urinary tract involvement[1]; however, if clinical signs recur after treatment is discontinued, repeat urine culture should be performed along with additional diagnostic evaluation to determine a cause for altered urine flow or bacterial persistence.

Treatment of recurrent UTI usually requires long-term medication (4 to 6 weeks) and ease of administration and cost become additional considerations in antibiotic selection. Trimethoprim-sulfonamide combinations and the penicillins are excreted via the kidneys and concentrated in urine. Although results of in vitro susceptibility testing of isolated pathogens may reveal resistance, these drugs may have effective antimicrobial activity against the causative organisms owing to the high concentrations achieved in urine.[7] Metabolism of the antibiotic should be another consideration. For example, sulfamethoxazole is largely metabolized to inactive products before urinary excretion whereas sulfadiazine is excreted largely unchanged in urine.[32]

Additional treatments for recurrent UTI can include supplementation with 50 to 75 g of loose salt to the diet[7] or provision of warm water during cold weather in an attempt to increase water intake and urine production. Administration of the urine-acidifying agent ammonium chloride (20 to 40 mg/kg per day by mouth) has also been recommended in cases of both cystitis and urolithiasis.[23] Use of ammonium chloride at this dose, however, has not produced a consistent decrease in urine pH. Recently, use of larger oral doses of ammonium chloride (60 to 520 mg/kg per day),[33–35] methionine (1 g/kg, every 24 hours), vitamin C (1 to 2 g/kg per day),[36] or ammonium sulfate (175 mg/kg per day)[37] were more successful in reducing urine pH below 6.0 in a limited number of horses; however, at these doses medications were usually unpalatable and had to be administered by dose syringe or stomach tube. Adding grain to the diet is another simple way to decrease urine pH, although the decline is modest and urine pH typically remains greater than 7.0.[36] A final treatment aid is bladder lavage. This procedure most benefits horses with accumulations of large amounts of crystalloid material in the bladder, a condition that has been termed "sabulous urolithiasis."[37] Although a number of antiseptics can be added to the sterile polyionic lavage fluid, the most important consideration is adequate volume to completely flush the crystalline debris from the bladder. Concurrent cystoscopy is a useful tool to assess the efficacy of bladder lavage.

There is one report of experimental induction of cystitis in equids.[38] After chemical irritation of the bladder mucosa, 2.5×10^{13} cfu of *Proteus mirabilis* were instilled into the bladders of nine female ponies. Three days later, all ponies demonstrated stranguria and culture results yielded 20,000 to 100,000 cfu/mL of *P. mirabilis*. Sediment examination revealed increased numbers of white blood cells (more than 10/hpf) in seven of nine ponies, and bacteria were observed in all samples (although in low numbers of 1 to 3/hpf). In two untreated ponies, the cystitis resolved spontaneously between 2 and 4 weeks after inoculation; however, resolution

was complete within 3 to 6 days in ponies treated with a trimethoprim/sulfadiazine combination.

Epizootics of cystitis have also been reported in the southwestern United States[25, 39] and in Australia.[40] In the former reports, a syndrome of ataxia and urinary incontinence was associated with ingestion of Sudan grass and Johnson grass (hybrids of *Sorghum* species). Both problems were attributed to sublethal intoxication with hydrocyanic acid in the plants, which resulted in demyelination of the lower spinal cord and bladder paralysis. Pyelonephritis was often the cause of death in affected horses.[39] Another outbreak of cystitis, manifested by hematuria more than incontinence, occurred in the Northern Territories and Western Australia in 1963.[40] The kidneys and ureters were not affected and ataxia was not observed in these horses. The problem, which resulted in loss of more than 200 horses, began shortly after the end of the wet season. Affected horses were on range pasture and, although this was not proven, a fungal toxin was suspected since sporidesmin (a toxin produced by *Pithomyces chartarum*) was known to cause bladder lesions in sheep and cattle. An environmental cause was further substantiated when no additional cases developed in 1964, after a "dry" wet season.

PYELONEPHRITIS

Upper UTIs involving the kidneys and/or ureters are rare in horses.[3–5, 7] The course of the distal segment of the ureters in the dorsal bladder wall creates a physical barrier or valve to prevent vesicoureteral reflux (VUR), a prerequisite for ascending pyelonephritis.[1] VUR is more common in children since the intramural portion of the distal ureter lengthens with growth. Further, congenital VUR is often recognized in families. This suggests a genetic tendency for the problem, which has been associated with developmental anomalies of the intramural insertion of one or both ureters.[1] More obvious problems that interfere with this barrier and increase the risk for VUR and associated upper UTIs include ectopic ureter or bladder distension, which may occur with bladder paralysis or urethral obstruction. Over time, VUR leads to progressive ureteral dilatation and renal scarring (Fig. 16–27). This explains the common finding of ureteral dilatation in young horses with ectopic ureters and provides further support for unilateral nephrectomy, rather than reimplantation of the ureter, as the treatment of choice for ectopic ureter.[41, 42] In addition to VUR, intrarenal reflux is also required to initiate renal damage predisposing the parenchyma to ascending infection. The renal papillae contain collections of papillary duct openings. These are typically conical structures that protrude into the renal pelvis. Similar to the protective nature of the intramural ureteral segment against VUR, this morphology protects against intrarenal reflux; however, in human infants and young pigs a second type of large, concave, "refluxing" papillae have also been described in the areas of the renal pelvis most often affected with renal scarring.[1] Thus, both VUR and intrarenal reflux are important in development of pyelonephritis.

The role of recurrent lower UTI in the development of pyelonephritis is less clear. For example, pyelonephritic scarring (without infection) can develop following high-pressure urinary tract obstruction (urethrolithiasis) and predispose to

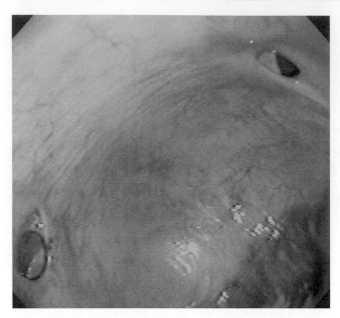

Figure 16–27. Endoscopic image of the bladder of a pony mare with recurrent cystitis and pyelonephritis. The ureteral openings were easily distended by insufflation of the bladder with air. Ureteral dilatation was the result of long-term vesiculoureteral reflux.

future upper UTI. In contrast, many cases of recurrent cystitis never proceed to involve the upper urinary tract.[1] Since the kidneys are densely vascular organs, septic nephritis may develop in association with septicemia in neonatal or adult horses.[8] Unless renal involvement is extensive, the upper UTI may go undetected but could lead to development of nephrolithiasis or chronic renal failure months to years later. As in the bladder, defense mechanisms within the normal kidney act to minimize bacterial colonization and proliferation. Efficacy of renal clearance varies with the species of bacteria entering the kidney. In addition, obstruction to urine flow (unilateral ureterolithiasis or nephrolithiasis) increases, rather than decreases, the risk of bacterial proliferation in the obstructed kidney.

Pyelonephritis in horses has been described in association with urolithiasis, recurrent cystitis, and bladder paralysis.[3–5, 7, 24, 39] Other causes have included accidental amputation of the penis during castration,[43] foreign bodies in the bladder,[44] and lower urinary tract neoplasia.[26, 45] With pyelonephritis, dysuria is manifested by hematuria or pyuria rather than stranguria and pollakiuria (as for cystitis). In addition, horses with upper UTIs generally have other clinical signs, including fever, weight loss, anorexia, or depression.[3–5, 7, 44–52] Upper UTIs can also be accompanied by nephrolithiasis and/or ureterolithiasis.[52] In such cases it is unclear whether lithiasis or infection develops first or whether both are consequences of VUR, intrarenal reflux, and renal parenchymal damage. In an occasional case, small uroliths may travel down the ureter and lead to recurrent urethral obstruction with renal colic as the presenting complaint.

As for cystitis, diagnostic evaluation includes physical and rectal examinations, urinalysis, and a quantitative urine culture. Careful palpation may allow detection of an enlarged ureter and/or kidney, although the kidney may also become shrunken in long-standing cases. In addition to the organisms causing cystitis, *Actinobacillus equuli, Streptococcus equi, Rhodococcus equi,* or *Salmonella* spp. can also be isolated from horses with hematogenous septic nephritis.[5, 8] In horses with upper UTIs, a complete blood count and serum biochemistry profile should be performed to assess the systemic inflammatory response and renal function. Finally, cystoscopy (including watching for urine flow from each ureteral opening) and/or ultrasonographic imaging of the bladder, ureters, and kidneys are helpful adjunctive diagnostic procedures.[29, 30] Ureteral catheterization (by passing polyethylene tubing via the biopsy channel of the endoscope or by using a No. 8–10 French polypropylene catheter, which can be passed blind in mares) may allow collection of urine samples from each ureter to distinguish unilateral from bilateral disease.[53]

Treatment for upper UTIs includes a prolonged course of appropriate systemic antibiotics (selected on the basis of susceptibility testing results on isolated pathogens). In select cases with unilateral disease, surgical removal of the affected kidney and ureter may be considered.[47, 54, 55] Prerequisites for a nephrectomy include documentation of unilateral disease by normal laboratory results for renal function (absence of azotemia), recovery of insignificant numbers of bacteria (fewer than 10,000 cfu/mL) from urine collected from the ureter leading to the nonaffected kidney, and ultrasonographic evidence of abnormal structure (e.g., fluid-filled structures, nephrolithiasis) in the affected kidney. Alternatively, poor response to several weeks of appropriate antimicrobial therapy or recurrence of clinical signs of pyelonephritis are additional indications for nephrectomy. Unfortunately, successful treatment of bilateral pyelonephritis is rare, but the poor prognosis is likely related to failure to establish the diagnosis until relatively late in the disease course.

PARASITIC INFECTIONS OF THE URINARY TRACT

Parasitic lesions associated with the nematodes *Strongylus vulgaris, Halicephalobus* (previously *Micronema*) *deletrix,* and *Dioctophyma renale* are occasionally found in equine kidneys.[56] Although larval migration of *S. vulgaris* in the renal artery and parenchyma is considered aberrant,[57] it was found in more than 20% of horses in one abattoir survey.[58] Passage through renal tissue may result in infarction or subcapsular or pelvic hemorrhage when parasites localize in these sites.[58] Although rare, *H. deletrix* infection is often life threatening owing to central nervous system involvement leading to a variety of neurologic deficits that generally require euthanasia.[59–63] It has been suggested that *H. deletrix* may be the most important cause of verminous meningoencephalomyelitis in horses.[64] Only the female parasite has been identified in equine tissues, typically in highly vascular organs. Large, granulomatous lesions that are full of the rhabditiform nematodes are usually found in the kidneys. The life cycle of *H. deletrix* is unknown, but the apparent saprophyte appears to have worldwide distribution. The finding of gingival lesions and oral granulomas in some horses suggests that ingestion is the likely route of infection. Attempts to find either nematode larvae or eggs in urine have been unsuccessful, and it is unclear whether the horse is an accidental host or is important for the parasite's life cycle.[59] The free-living form is found in decaying organic debris (e.g., tree stumps) and has also been described to affect humans.[63] Ante-mortem diagnosis has not been made, and cerebrospinal fluid cytologic changes in affected horses cannot differentiate between nematodiasis and protozoal encephalomyelitis.[62] Renal involvement is typically inapparent, although one affected horse demonstrated a 2-week course of stranguria and polyuria before onset of neurologic deficits.[60] *Dioctophyma renale* is a large, bright red nematode, and the female may reach 100 cm in length. The typical hosts are carnivorous species, but the parasite occasionally affects horses that ingest the intermediate host (annelid worm) while grazing or drinking from natural water sources.[65] Once localized in the kidney, the parasite may live 1 to 3 years, and eggs are shed in the urine. It completely destroys the renal parenchyma, and death of the parasite leads to shrinking of the host kidney into a fibrous mass. Occasionally, hydronephrosis and/or renal hemorrhage may be a serious complication of parasitic infection.[66, 67]

In contrast to the nematodes, infection with *Klossiella equi*, a coccidian parasite, appears common, yet there are no reports of clinical disease associated with this coccidial infection.[68–73] Although disorders accompanied by immunosuppression have been suggested to increase its likelihood, *K. equi* infection is still considered an incidental finding in affected horses. The life cycle has not been fully elucidated, but it has been proposed that ingested sporocysts (or sporozoites) enter the bloodstream and undergo schizogony in endothelial cells of the glomeruli. Merozoites are released into the urinary space and undergo one or more additional rounds of schizogony in tubular epithelial cells. Eventually, a population of merozoites develop into microgametes and macrogametes. There is little evidence of an inflammatory response to parasite replication in renal tissues. Sporogony follows with the subsequent release of sporocysts into the urine.[69, 73] Although *K. equi* has not been associated with clinical disease, it warrants mention that it has been found worldwide in horses, ponies, donkeys, burros, and zebras and a recent post-mortem survey of 47 horses in Australia revealed six (12.8%) to be infected.[73]

REFERENCES

1. Rubin RH, Tolkoff-Rubin NE, Cotran RS: Urinary tract infection. Pyelonephritis, and reflux nephropathy. In Brenner BM, Rector FC, eds. *The Kidney*, ed 4, Vol 2. Philadelphia, WB Saunders, 1991, p 1369.
2. R Brown CM, Collier MA: Bladder diseases. In Robinson NE, ed. *Current Therapy in Equine Medicine*. Philadelphia, WB Saunders, 1983, p 567.
3. Hodgson DR: Cystitis and pyelonephritis. In Robinson NE, ed. *Current Therapy in Equine Medicine 2*. Philadelphia, WB Saunders, 1987, p 708.
4. Boy MG: Cystitis and pyelonephritis. In Robinson NE, ed. *Current Therapy in Equine Medicine 3*. Philadelphia, WB Saunders, 1992, p 616.
5. Divers TJ: Diseases of the renal system. In Smith BP ed. *Large Animal Internal Medicine*. St. Louis, CV Mosby, 1990, p 872.
6. Ortenburger A, Pringle J: Diseases of the bladder and urethra. In Kobluk CN, Ames TR, Geor RJ, eds. *The Horse, Diseases and Clinical Management*. Philadelphia, WB Saunders, 1995, p 597.
7. Divers TJ. Diagnosis and management of urinary tract infections in the horse. *Proceedings of a Symposium on Trimethoprim/Sulfadiazine, Clinical Application in Equine Medicine*. Princeton Junction: Veterinary Learning Systems, 1984, p 31.
8. Robinson JA, Allen GK, Green EM, et al: A prospective study of septicaemia in colostrum-deprived foals. *Equine Vet J* 25:214–219.
9. Senior DF: Bacterial urinary tract infections: Invasion, host defenses, and new approaches to prevention. *Compend Contin Educ Pract Vet* 7:334, 1985.
10. Roberts JA: Bacterial adherence and urinary tract infection. *South Med J* 80:347, 1987.
11. Reid G, Sobel JD: Bacterial adherence in the pathogenesis of urinary tract infection: A review. *Rev Infect Dis* 9:470, 1987.
12. Johnson PJ, Goetz TE, Baker GJ, et al: Treatment of two mares with obstructive (vaginal) urinary outflow incontinence. *J Am Vet Med Assoc* 191:973, 1987.
13. Sertich PL, Hamir AN, Orsini P, et al: Paraurethral lipoma in a mare associated with frequent urination. *Equine Vet Educ* 2:121, 1990.
14. Mulholland SG, Qureshi SM, Fritz RW, et al: Effect of hormonal deprivation on the bladder defense mechanism. *J Urol* 127:1010, 1982.
15. Reidasch G, Heck P, Rauterberg E, et al: Does low urinary sIgA predispose to urinary tract infection? *Kidney Int* 23:759, 1983.
16. Voss JL, Pickett BW: Diagnosis and treatment of haemospermia in the stallion. *J Reprod Fertil* Suppl 23:151, 1975.
17. Sullins KE, Bertone JJ, Voss JL, et al: Treatment of hemospermia in stallions: A discussion of 18 cases. *Compend Contin Educ Pract Vet* 10:1396, 1988.
18. Schumacher J: Surgery of the prepuce and penis. In Auer JA, ed. *Equine Surgery*. Philadelphia, WB Saunders, 1992, p 703.
19. Schumacher J, Varner DD: Neoplasia of the stallion's reproductive tract. *In* McKinnon AO, Voss JL, eds. *Equine Reproduction*. Philadelphia, Lea & Febiger, 1993, p 871.
20. Schumacher J, Varner DD, Schmitz DG, et al: Urethral defects in geldings with hematuria and stallions with hemospermia. *Vet Surg* 24:250, 1995.
21. Blanchard TL, Varner DD, Hurtgen JP, et al: Bilateral seminal vesiculitis and ampullitis in a stallion. *J Am Vet Med Assoc* 192:525, 1988.
22. Taylor TS, Varner DD: Diseases of the accessory sex glands of the stallion. In Auer JA, ed. *Equine Surgery*. Philadelphia, WB Saunders, 1992, p 723.
23. DeBowes RM, Nyrop KA, Boulton CH: Cystic calculi in the horse. *Compend Contin Educ Pract Vet* 6:S268, 1984.
24. Laverty S, Pascoe JR, Ling GV, et al: Urolithiasis in 68 horses. *Vet Surg* 21:56, 1992.
25. Adams LG, Dollahite JW, Romane WM, et al: Cystitis and ataxia associated with sorghum ingestion. *J Am Vet Med Assoc* 155:518, 1969.
26. Fischer AT, Spier S, Carlson GP, et al: Neoplasia of the urinary bladder as a cause of hematuria. *J Am Vet Med Assoc* 186:1294–1296, 1985.
27. Holt PE, Mair TS: Ten cases of bladder paralysis associated with sabulous urolithiasis in horses. *Vet Rec* 127:108, 1990.
28. Wise LA, Jones RL, Reif JS: Nosocomial canine urinary tract infections in a veterinary teaching hospital (1983–1988). *J Am Anim Hosp Assoc* 26:148, 1990.
29. Sullins KE, Traub-Dargatz JL: Endoscopic anatomy of the equine urinary tract. *Compend Contin Educ Pract Vet* 6:S663, 1984.
30. Traub-Dargatz JL, McKinnon AO: Adjunctive methods of examination of the urogenital tract. *Vet Clin North Am Equine Pract* 4:339, 1988.

31. Kohn CW, Chew DJ: Laboratory diagnosis and characterization of renal disease in horses. *Vet Clin North Am Equine Pract* 3:585, 1987.

32. Nouws JFM, Firth EC, Vree TB, et al: Pharmacokinetics and renal clearance of sulfamethazine, sulfamerazine, and sulfadiazine and their N_4-acetyl and hydroxy metabolites in horses. *Am J Vet Res* 48:392, 1987.

33. Johnson PJ, Crenshaw KL: The treatment of cystic and urethral calculi in a gelding. *Vet Med* 85:891, 1990.

34. Robertson JT, Buffington CA: Surgical removal of uroliths. In White NA, Moore JN, eds. *Current Practice of Equine Surgery.* Philadelphia, JB Lippincott, 1990, p 734.

35. Mair TS, Holt PE: The aetiology and treatment of equine urolithiasis. *Equine Vet Educ* 6:189, 1994.

36. Wood T, Weckman TJ, Henry PA, et al: Equine urine pH: Normal population distributions and methods of acidification. *Equine Vet J* 22:118, 1990.

37. Remillard RL, Modransky PD, Welker FH, et al: Dietary management of cystic calculi in a horse. *J Equine Vet Sci* 12:359, 1992.

38. Divers TJ, Byars TD, Murch O, et al: Experimental induction of *Proteus mirabilis* cystitis in the pony and evaluation of therapy with trimethoprim-sulfadiazine. *Am J Vet Res* 42:1203, 1981.

39. Van Kempen KR: Sudan grass and sorghum poisoning of horses: A possible lathyrogenic disease. *J Am Vet Med Assoc* 156:629, 1970.

40. Hooper PT: Epizootic cystitis in horses. *Aust Vet J* 44:11, 1968.

41. Modransky PD, Wagner PC, Robinette JD, et al: Surgical correction of bilateral ectopic ureters in two foals. *Vet Surg* 12:141, 1983.

42. Pringle JK, Ducharme NG, Baird JD: Ectopic ureter in the horse: Three cases and a review of the literature. *Can Vet J* 31:26, 1990.

43. Roberts MC: Ascending urinary tract infection in ponies. *Aust Vet J* 55:191, 1979.

44. Hamlen H: Pyelonephritis in a mature gelding with an unusual urinary bladder foreign body. *J Equine Vet Sci* 13:159, 1993.

45. Sloet van Oldruitenborgh-Oosterbaan MM, Klabec HC: Ureteropyelonephritis in a Fresian mare. *Vet Rec* 122:609, 1988.

46. Boyd WL, Bishop LM: Pyelonephritis of cattle and horses. *J Am Vet Med Assoc* 90:154, 1937.

47. Irwin DHG, Howell DW: Equine pyelonephritis and unilateral nephrectomy. *J South Afr Vet Assoc* 51:235, 1980.

48. Tennant B, Bettleheim P, Kaneko JJ: Paradoxic hypercalcemia and hypophosphotemia associated with chronic renal failure in horses. *J Am Vet Med Assoc* 180:630, 1982.

49. Held JP, Wright B, Henton JE: Pyelonephritis associated with renal failure in a horse. *J Am Vet Med Assoc* 189:688, 1986.

50. Carrick JB, Pollitt CC: Chronic pyelonephritis in a brood mare. *Aust Vet J* 64:252, 1987.

51. Mair TS, Taylor FGR, Pinsent PJN: Fever of unknown origin in the horse: A review of 63 cases. *Equine Vet J* 21:260, 1989.

52. Divers TJ: Chronic renal failure in horses. *Compend Contin Educ Pract Vet* 5:S310, 1983.

53. Schott HC, Hodgson DR, Bayly WM: Ureteral catheterisation in the horse. *Equine Vet Educ* 2:140, 1990.

54. DeBowes RM: Kidneys and ureters. In Auer JA, ed. *Equine Surgery.* Philadelphia, WB Saunders, 1992, p 768.

55. Trotter GW, Brown CM, Ainsworth DM: Unilateral nephrectomy for treatment of a renal abscess in a foal. *J Am Vet Med Assoc* 184:1392, 1984.

56. Keller H: Diseases of the urinary system. In Wintzer HJ, ed. *Equine Diseases: A Textbook for Students and Practitioners.* New York, Springer-Verlag, 1986, p 148.

57. Cranley JJ, McCullagh KG: Ischaemic myocardial fibrosis and aortic strongylosis in the horse. *Equine Vet J* 13:35, 1981.

58. Poynter D: The arterial lesions produced by *Strongylus vulgaris* and their relationship to the migratory route of the parasite in its host. *Res Vet Sci* 1:205, 1960.

59. Rubin HL, Woodard JC: Equine infection with *Micronema deletrix. J Am Vet Med Assoc* 165:256, 1974.

60. Alstad AD, Berg JE, Samuel C: Disseminated *Micronema deletrix* infection in the horse. *J Am Vet Med Assoc* 174:264, 1979.

61. Blunden AS, Khalil LF, Webbon PM: *Halicephalobus deletrix* infection in a horse. *Equine Vet J* 19:255, 1987.

62. Darien BJ, Belknap J, Nietfeld J: Cerebrospinal fluid changes in two horses with central nervous system nematodiasis *(Micronema deletrix). J Vet Intern Med* 2:201, 1988.

63. Angus KW, Roberts L, Archibald DRN, et al: *Halicephalobus deletrix* infection in a horse in Scotland (Letter). *Vet Rec* 131:495, 1992.

64. Lester G: Parasitic encephalomyelitis in horses. *Compend Contin Educ Pract Vet* 14:1624, 1992.

65. Cheng TC: *General Parasitology.* New York, Academic Press, 1973, p 616.

66. Smits GM, Misdorf W: *Dioctophyma renale* beim Hund in den Neiderlanden. *Zbl Vet Med B* 12:327, 1965.

67. Szwejkowski H: Sektionsbild der Dioctophymease der Hunde. *Arch Exp Vet Med* 14:1184, 1960.

68. Newberne JW, Robinson VB, Bowen NE: Histological aspects of *Klossiella equi* in the kidney of a zebra. *Am J Vet Res* 19:304, 1958.

69. Vetterling JM, Thompson DE: *Klossiella equi* Baumann, 1946 (Sporozoa: Eucoccidia: Adeleina) from equids. *J Parasitol* 58:589, 1972.

70. Todd KS, Gosser HS, Hamilton DP: *Klossiella equi* Baumann, 1946 (Sporozoa: Eucoccidiorida) from an Illinois horse. *Vet Med Small Animal Clin* 72:443, 1977.

71. Lee CG, Ross AD: Renal coccidiosis of the horse associated with *Klossiella equi. Aust Vet J* 53:287, 1977.

72. Austin RJ, Dies KH: *Klossiella equi* in the kidneys of a horse. *Can Vet J* 22:159, 1981.

73. Reppas GP, Collins GH: *Klossiella equi* infection in horses; sporocyst stage identified in urine. *Aust Vet J* 72:316, 1995.

16.8

Obstructive Disease of the Urinary Tract

Harold C. Schott II, DVM, PhD

The majority of cases of obstructive urinary tract disease in horses are due to urolithiasis. Urinary tract displacement, trauma, and neoplasia are other causes.[1-4] Urinary tract obstruction can result in a variety of clinical signs, depending on the site and degree of obstruction. Incomplete obstruction can result in dysuria, incontinence, and mild abdominal pain, whereas complete obstruction usually results in moderate to severe pain, termed "renal colic." A further complication of complete obstruction is rupture of the bladder or urethra. Signs of pain subside after rupture but are replaced by depression and inappetence, which accompany postrenal acute renal failure. In some cases of disruption of the urinary tract, progressive abdominal distension and/or enlargement of the penis and prepuce may also be observed.

EPIDEMIOLOGY OF UROLITHIASIS

The epidemiology of urolithiasis varies with species.[5–8] Lower urinary tract stones predominate in veterinary species whereas upper urinary tract stones are more common in people. Historically, lower urinary tract stones were a more substantial problem in humans as well, and they remain the more common form of urolithiasis in underdeveloped countries. The shift in prevalence from lower to upper urinary tract stones appears to have accompanied industrialization but the reasons for the shift are not entirely clear.[8]

From 1970 to 1989, urolithiasis was responsible for 0.11% of equine admissions to 22 veterinary teaching hospitals and accounted for 7.8% of the diagnoses of urinary tract disease.[5] Male horses, especially geldings, are predisposed to urolithiasis (75% of all cases), but a breed predisposition has not been described. This sex predilection has been attributed to the shorter, distensible urethra of the mare, which likely permits voiding of small calculi.[6] Urolithiasis is typically an adult disease and the mean age of affected horses is about 10 years.[5] Nevertheless, young horses can be affected, and the authors have seen bilateral nephrolithiasis in a weaning foal (likely a consequence of neonatal septicemia) and dysuria in a 3-month-old colt due to multiple cystoliths which formed on sutures used for repair of a ruptured bladder as a neonate. Uroliths are most common in the urinary bladder (60%), although they may also develop in the kidneys (12%), ureters (4%), and urethra (24%).[5] Of interest, as many as 10% of affected horses have had uroliths in multiple locations.[5] Uroliths can vary quite dramatically in size. In one mare, a cystolith weighing more than 6 kg was detected as an apparently incidental finding in a horse destroyed for a limb fracture.[9]

PATHOPHYSIOLOGY OF UROLITHIASIS

In general, two steps are required for calculus formation: (1) nucleation and (2) crystal growth.[10–13] Factors that contribute to precipitation of urinary crystals and nucleation include supersaturation of urine; prolonged urine retention; genetic tendencies to excrete larger amounts of calcium (hypercalciuria), uric acid (hyperuricosuria), or oxalates (hyperoxaluria); and inhibitors and promoters of crystal growth. For two or more ions in a solution to precipitate into a crystal, the product of their individual ion activities must exceed the equilibrium solubility product (K_{sp}). A supersaturated solution is one in which the ion activity product exceeds the K_{sp}. A mildly supersaturated solution is termed "metastable," as crystals tend to precipitate and dissolve at similar rates, so that crystal growth does not occur and the solution remains clear. Once the ion activity product exceeds a critical value (formation product ratio), however, precipitation outpaces dissolution and rapid crystal growth can be seen as the solution becomes cloudy.[10–13] Normal human urine is typically supersaturated with respect to one or more ion activity products; however, the formation product ratios are considerably higher in urine (10 times greater than K_{sp}) than they are

in an aqueous solution, owing to the presence of inhibitors of crystal growth.[10] This explains why observation of crystals in urine sediment examination is common yet calculus formation is uncommon. Further, although K_{sp} values are constant for each type of crystal, they vary with temperature and pH. Typically, cooling promotes crystal formation (as when samples are refrigerated), whereas effects of pH vary with the type of calculus (acidification leads to dissolution of calcium crystals but promotes crystallization of urate crystals).[11] Next, any problem resulting in urine retention or incomplete bladder emptying increases the chance of crystal growth. Although not described for horses, genetic variations in ion excretion rates are well-documented risk factors for human and canine urolithiasis. For example, hypercalciuria is inherited as an autosomal dominant trait in humans and is responsible for 30% to 40% of nephroliths.[10] Similarly, dogs with cystine urolithiasis have an inherited defect in renal tubular transport of cystine while Dalmatians are afflicted with urate stones because of a defect in uric acid metabolism in the breed.[7]

Normal urine is rich in a number of inhibitors of crystal growth including pyrophosphate, citrate, magnesium ions, glycosaminoglycans, and several glycoproteins including nephrocalcin.[10, 11, 13] The degree of inhibitory activity varies with crystal type; for example, pyrophosphate is responsible for 50% of the inhibitory activity against calcium phosphate stone formation in human urine but has a much less inhibiting effect on calcium oxalate stone formation.[10] Although poorly documented, inhibitors of crystal growth in equine urine, including its high mucus content, likely play an important protective role against calculus formation. This would seem especially true in light of the substantial urinary excretion of calcium carbonate crystals by normal horses. Similar to the risk associated with increased ion excretion, it should not be surprising that defects in inhibitor activity have also been documented in syndromes of human urolithiasis.[10, 11] Other urine components may act as promoters of crystal growth. These principally include organic matrix components of calculi: matrix substance A, uromucoid, and a number of serum proteins.[11, 12] Finally, some urine components may have both inhibitor and promoter activity. For example, Tamm-Horsfall glycoprotein, a protein secreted in the ascending limb of the loop of Henle that forms the backbone of urine casts, has been shown to be a promoter of struvite crystal formation in feline urine.[14] In contrast, it also inhibits calcium oxalate crystal aggregation, and a group of human patients with calcium oxalate urolithiasis were recently demonstrated to have an abnormality in Tamm-Horsfall mucoprotein.[15]

Since normal urine of most species is typically supersaturated and is in balance between crystal precipitation and dissolution, spontaneous nucleation rarely initiates calculus growth. Rather, nucleation generally requires stasis of urine flow, increasing the chance of contact between crystalloid material and uroepithelium (as occurs in areas of the renal pelvis) or a damaged uroepithelial surface.[11–14] The latter results in local activation of inflammatory and clotting pathways, producing a nidus for local crystal adherence.[16] In addition, desquamated epithelial cells, leukocytes, or necrotic debris may provide a nidus for crystal growth at more distal sites in the urinary tract. Tissue damage from a variety of causes is likely the most important factor for the develop-

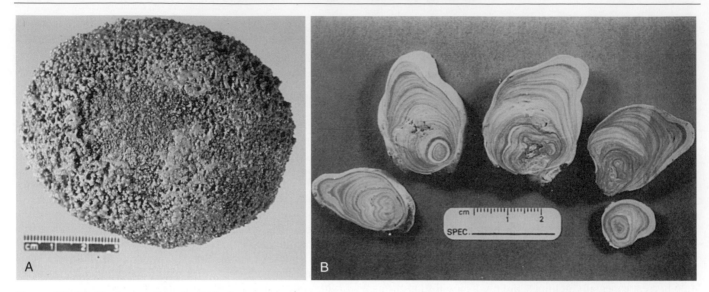

Figure 16–28. Equine cystic calculi: **A,** the more common flattened, sphere-shape type of bladder calculus, which is usually spiculated; **B,** the less common form of gray, smooth-surfaced calculus, which may be more irregular in shape. (B from DeBowes RM: Surgical management of urolithiasis. Vet Clin North Am Equine Pract 4:461, 1988.)

ment of uroliths in horses. For example, after urinary tract instrumentation (e.g., catheterization, endoscopy), areas of traumatized uroepithelium are rapidly covered with a fine layer of crystalline material. This material usually resolves spontaneously unless infection develops. Similarly, nephroliths may form in the renal medulla or pelvis consequent to papillary necrosis accompanying phenylbutazone toxicity. Once crystal growth has been initiated around a nidus, equine urine has the disadvantage of being highly alkaline, favoring crystallization of most urolith components, especially calcium carbonate.

In horses there are two basic forms of uroliths, and both are primarily composed of calcium carbonate.[6, 17] More than 90% are yellow-green, spiculated stones that can easily be fragmented (Fig. 16–28A). Less commonly, uroliths are gray-white, smooth stones that are more resistant to fragmentation (Fig. 16–28B). The latter stones often contain phosphate in addition to calcium carbonate. The crystalline composition of normal equine urine sediment (calcium carbonate crystals predominate, although calcium oxalate and phosphate crystals can also be found) and uroliths is similar: calcium carbonate ($CaCO_3$) in the form of calcite (a hexagonal crystal form of $CaCO_3$) is most common, followed by vaterite (a metastable, hexagonal crystal form in which $CaCO_3$ is partially replaced by magnesium or to a lesser extent by manganese, strontium, and sulfur). Other less common components include aragonite (an orthorhombic crystal form of $CaCO_3$), weddellite (calcium oxalate dihydrate), struvite (magnesium ammonium phosphate hexahydrate), hydroxyapatite, and uric acid (Table 16–11).[17–22] Neumann recently examined the cut surface of a number of equine uroliths by scanning electron microscopy and described a pattern of irregular, concentric bands around the core (Fig. 16–29A) that were separated by small spherules of crystalline material (Fig. 16–29B).[17] This

Table 16–11. Published Results of X-Ray Crystallographic Analysis of Equine Urinary Calculi

Reference	Sutor and Wooley (1970)	Grünberg (1971)	Mair and Osborn (1986)	Neumann et al. (1994)
Total number of calculi	4	157	18	17
Calcite	2	58	2	11
Calcite/vaterite	1	11	9	5
Calcite/aragonite	1	—	—	1
Calcite/weddellite	—	63	4	—
Calcite/whewellite	—	2	—	—
Calcite/hydroxyapatite	—	8	—	—
Calcite/octacalcium phosphate	—	5	—	—
Calcite/struvite	—	3	—	—
Calcite/gypsum	—	2	—	—
Calcite/vaterite/weddellite	—	2	2	—
Calcite/whewellite/weddellite	—	3	—	—
Calcite/vaterite/sodium acid urate	—	—	1	—

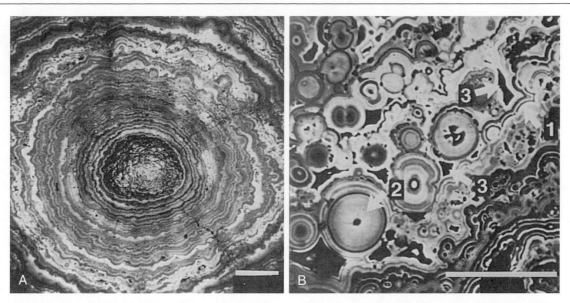

Figure 16–29. Scanning electron microscopic appearance of the cut surface of equine cystic calculi. **A,** Lower-power micrograph reveals the intricate pattern of concentric banding around the core (bar = 500 μm). **B,** Higher-power micrograph reveals the ultrastructural features, including bands *(1)*, spherules *(2)*, and primary porosity in black *(3)* (bar = 50 μm). (From Neumann RD, Ruby AL, Ling GV, et al.: Ultrastructure and mineral composition of urinary calculi from horses. Am J Vet Res 55:1357, 1994.)

pattern suggested that calculus growth occurs by accretion of preexisting microscopic spherules (the crystals already present in normal equine urine) on the surface of the growing urolith rather than by de novo crystal formation at the urolith's surface. Further, banding was speculated to represent growth through incorporation of organic matrix on the urolith's surface at times when fewer spherules were present in urine. The gaps between adjacent spherules result in "porosity" to the urolith. Since precipitation and dissolution occur simultaneously during growth of urinary calculi, porosity allows exposure of inner aspects of the urolith to urine, which can lead to dissolution as urine composition changes. Neumann described two types of porosity observed by electron microscopy: primary porosity, consisting of the original pores or gaps between spherules, and secondary porosity, which developed consequent to dissolution of inner areas of the uroliths. Greater dissolution or secondary porosity developed preferentially in areas of the urolith with higher magnesium content (vaterite). More extensive development of secondary porosity theoretically leads to increased urolith fragility, which has the therapeutic benefit of increasing the chance that the urolith can be crushed or fragmented before removal.

The role of urinary tract infection (UTI) in the development of urolithiasis appears to vary with species.[7, 10, 12] Struvite urolithiasis in humans and dogs appears to be almost exclusively a consequence of UTI, whereas the majority of struvite uroliths in cats and sheep are not associated with infection.[12] In addition to contributing to uroepithelial injury and nidus formation, UTI with urease-positive bacteria (*Proteus* species and coagulase-positive staphylococci are most common) allows splitting of urea into two ammonia molecules, which are rapidly hydrolyzed to ammonium ions (a component of struvite crystals).[10, 12, 13] In a review of 68 horses with urolithiasis, Laverty reported positive urine cul-

ture results in only two of 19 horses in which urine culture was performed[5]; however, culture of material from the centers of 30 calculi yielded positive results from 19 (63%), and a variety of different bacterial species were isolated. Only one of 28 calculi examined in this study contained struvite. The significance of finding bacteria in the center of equine calcium carbonate uroliths is not known, especially for isolates other than coagulase-positive staphylococci and *Proteus* species, and culture of an appropriately collected sample of urine is always preferred over culture of a calculus.[5, 23] Nephroliths and/or ureteroliths are also found in some, but not all, cases of pyelonephritis.[24-27] Laing described a 2-year-old colt with bilateral nephrolithiasis and chronic renal failure. A *Proteus* species was recovered from urine, and the nephroliths were composed principally of calcium carbonate but also contained lesser amounts of struvite.[27] In contrast, Ehnen found evidence of infection in only one of eight horses with nephro- and/or ureterolithiasis and chronic renal failure.[28] In the authors' experience, the presence of stones in the upper urinary tract or presence of multiple uroliths warrants concurrent evaluation for UTI, as we have seen two horses with recurrent urinary tract obstruction with urethroliths that were ultimately determined to be sequelae of unilateral pyelonephritis. A similar case was described by Holt in which a renal calculus and abscess were found 5 months after removal of a cystic calculus.[29]

NEPHROLITHIASIS AND URETEROLITHIASIS

Renal or ureteral calculi were rarely described as a cause of equine urolithiasis before the last decade[30]; however, there have been a number of recent reports[5, 26-28, 31-35] describing nephrolithiasis and ureterolithiasis in horses. In Laverty's review of 68 horses with urolithiasis, 16% had uroliths in the kidneys and ureters and a few horses with cystic calculi also had calculi in the upper urinary tract.[5] Of interest, nine of 15 horses with nephroliths in this review were stallions; three were geldings and three, mares. It is not clear whether there is a true increase in prevalence of nephrolithiasis and ureterolithiasis or whether these conditions have become easier to document with the simultaneous development of ultrasonographic imaging as a diagnostic tool for equine medicine. It has been speculated, but not documented, that young racehorses may be at greater risk of developing renal calculi owing to the common use of nonsteroidal antiinflammatory drugs (and risk for development of papillary necrosis) in these athletes.[28] The important point is that upper urinary tract lithiasis should not be overlooked in horses.

Nephroliths may develop around a nidus associated with a variety of renal diseases, including polycystic kidney disease (Fig. 16–6), pyelonephritis (Figure 16–30A), papillary necrosis (Figure 16–30B), or neoplasia. At present, data on upper urinary tract stones in horses are insufficient to know whether they develop spontaneously (in the absence of tissue damage) as in humans or whether they differ significantly in mineral composition from cystic calculi. Although nephrolithiasis and/or ureterolithiasis are quite painful conditions in humans, horses with nephroliths or ureteroliths often remain asymptomatic until bilateral obstructive disease leads to development of acute or chronic renal failure. Upper urinary tract stones may also be an incidental finding at necropsy.[30] When clinical signs are present, nonspecific presenting complaints consistent with uremia (poor performance, lethargy, inappetance, and weight loss) are more common than signs of obstructive disease (colic, stranguria, hematuria). In an occasional horse, a stone or nidus may pass down the ureter and lead to urethral obstruction and signs of acute obstructive disease. Rectal palpation may reveal an enlarged kidney or ureter (or bladder with urethral obstruction), and ureteral calculi may be palpable in an enlarged ureter. Since normal ureters are not palpable on rectal examination, the entire course of the ureters (retroperitoneally along the dorsal abdominal wall to the dorsolateral aspects of the pelvic canal to their insertion at the dorsal bladder neck) should be carefully palpated, since it can be easy to overlook an enlarged ureter.

Diagnosis of renal and ureteral calculi is usually made during rectal or ultrasonographic examination (Fig. 16–31). Although ultrasonographic imaging may provide information on the presence, number, and location of calculi, stones smaller than 1 cm diameter can be missed despite complete examination. Other ultrasonographic findings to support upper tract lithiasis include dilatation of the renal pelvis or proximal ureter and, in longstanding cases, hydronephrosis.[36, 37] Although azotemia generally accompanies bilateral disease, horses with unilateral disease often maintain normal renal function. For reasons detailed above, a quantitative urine culture should be performed in all horses with nephrolithiasis or ureterolithiasis to assess possible intercurrent UTI.

Since most horses with nephrolithiasis and/or ureterolithiasis are in chronic renal failure by the time the diagnosis is established,[28, 38, 39] few cases are amenable to treatment. Thus, there are few reports of successful management of horses with renal and ureteral calculi. Removal of the calculus, limited to horses with unilateral disease or mild azotemia, has been the only effective means of treatment.[31, 33, 35] In the absence of azotemia, nephrectomy is the preferred technique for management of unilateral renal calculi.[33] Further, removal of the affected kidney and ureter should eliminate any associated upper urinary tract infection or chance of recurrence. The approach involves a dorsal flank incision, rib resection, and blunt retroperitoneal dissection to expose the kidney.[40–42] In one horse with mild azotemia, nephrotomy (via a similar approach as a nephrectomy) was successfully performed to remove obstructing calculi in the renal pelvis and proximal ureter.[28] Unfortunately, there was little improvement in azotemia, and the horse was destroyed a few weeks later.[28] Ureteral calculi have also been removed by ureterolithectomy via both ventral celiotomy and paralumbar approaches.[31, 34]

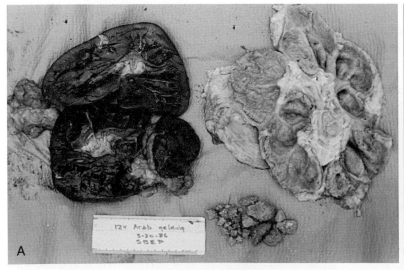
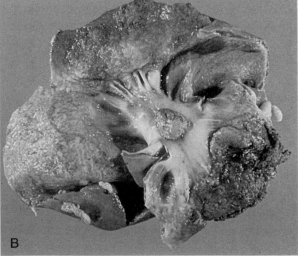

Figure 16–30. A, Multiple nephroliths developed in association with unilateral pyelonephritis in a gelding that presented for repeated urethral obstruction. **B,** A small nephrolith lodged in the renal pelvis resulted in ureteral obstruction and development of hydronephrosis in a standardbred gelding that had a history of phenylbutazone therapy for 4 years.

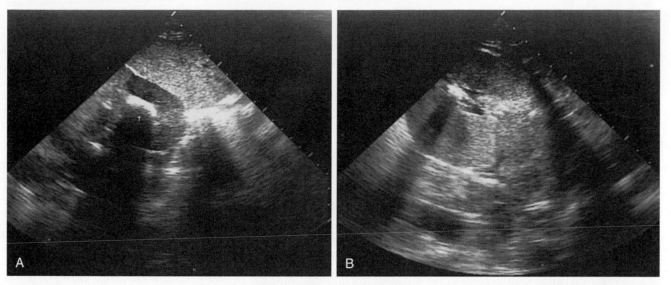

Figure 16–31. Ultrasonographic images of the left, **A,** and right, **B,** kidneys of a 10-month-old Arabian filly that developed bilateral nephrolithiasis and chronic renal failure as sequelae of neonatal septicemia. The nephroliths are highly echogenic and cast acoustic shadows in both kidneys.

A basket stone dislodger (Dormia Stone Dislodger, V Mueller Co, Division of American Hospital Supply Co, McGow Park, IL) introduced through a vestibulourethral approach and guided by rectal palpation has also been used for removal of distal ureteral calculi in the mare.[31] Medical management (antibiotics, grass hay, and salt to promote diuresis) of bilateral ureterolithiasis was attempted in a 3-year-old Thoroughbred filly with incomplete ureteral obstruction and mild azotemia.[34] After 4 weeks, deterioration of clinical signs and more severe azotemia prompted ureterolithectomy to remove stones from the left ureter. Percutaneous nephrostomy was successfully used for placement of a catheter in the right renal pelvis (to establish percutaneous urine flow) for short-term management of azotemia in the postoperative period. Unfortunately, the filly was destroyed after developing cecal impaction 6 days later, and necropsy examination revealed a shrunken, nonfunctional left kidney and a previously undetected nephrolith in the right kidney. This case demonstrated the feasibility and potential benefits of accessing the renal pelvis of the horse via percutaneous nephrostomy.[43, 44]

Rodger recently described the use of electrohydraulic lithotripsy through a ureteroscope to successfully disintegrate a single, unilateral ureterolith in a horse with evidence of bilateral renal disease.[35] Electrohydraulic lithotripsy is a means of converting electrical energy into mechanical energy, which can be directed to fragment the urolith.[35, 45, 46] Basically, the device produces an electrical discharge arc (a spark) between two electrodes at the tip of the instrument. The heat associated with the discharge causes a small amount of the liquid medium (urine) to burst into gas bubbles, and the associated shock wave fractures the urolith. The end of the instrument must be kept adjacent to the urolith yet away from the mucosa, which could be disrupted by the same shock waves that destroy the calculus. Although the technique has not been highly successful for treatment of canine uroliths,[47] equine uroliths may be more amenable

to its use since they are commonly quite porous (and fragile). Although electrohydraulic lithotripsy has been effective in the treatment of selected equine cystoliths[45, 46] and one ureterolith,[35] the expense of the equipment and availability of other surgical options will likely limit its use to selected cases that are not amenable to routine surgical treatments. A more recent development in upper tract stone removal for humans and dogs is extracorporeal shock wave lithotripsy (ESWL).[44] This noninvasive technology uses a reflector to focus the energy from a shock wave generated outside the body on a nephrolith in situ and has proven quite efficacious in the treatment of human nephrolithiasis. Although ESWL and laser technology have not yet been attempted in horses, they provide future treatment options for equine nephrolithiasis and ureterolithiasis.

CYSTIC CALCULI

Cystic calculi are the most commonly recognized form of equine uroliths.[1–6, 29] Cystoliths are typically flattened, sphere-shaped stones with a spiculated or smooth surface. Dysuria consequent to the presence of cystoliths may include hematuria, stranguria, pollakiuria, pyuria, or incontinence. Hematuria may be more apparent after exercise. An affected male horse may demonstrate stranguria by repeatedly dropping its penis and posturing to urinate but voiding little or no urine. An affected mare may also repeatedly posture to urinate and demonstrate winking, and these signs could be confused with estrus activity. Less common signs include an irritable attitude, recurrent colic, and loss of condition; one burro presented for recurrent rectal prolapse.[48]

The diagnosis of cystic calculi is usually made by palpation of the bladder per rectum. Bladder uroliths are usually large enough to be detected easily; however, if the bladder is distended, it may be necessary to empty it by passing a catheter to facilitate palpation of the stone. Bladder catheter-

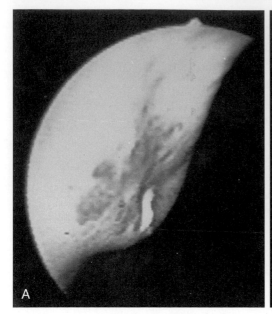
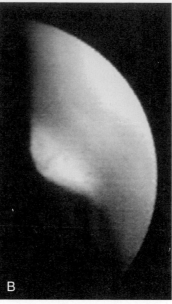

Figure 16–32. View of the abnormal left, **A**, and normal right, **B**, ureteral openings of a horse with unilateral pyelonephritis and recurrent cystic calculi. The diagnosis was confirmed by culture of urine samples collected from each ureter.

ization also allows assessment of urethral patency and collection of samples for urinalysis and quantitative culture. A complete blood count and serum biochemical profile should be performed to document whether anemia, inflammation, or azotemia has developed. Cystoscopic examination is helpful in assessing the severity of damage to the bladder mucosa and any asymmetry in appearance or function of the ureteral openings (Fig. 16–32).[49, 50] Since it is not uncommon for calculi to be in multiple sites in the urinary tract, thorough evaluation of the upper urinary tract is warranted for all cases of cystic urolithiasis.

In contrast to upper urinary tract lithiasis, many reports[45, 46, 48, 51–66] and several reviews[5, 6, 29, 40, 67, 68] detail the clinical signs and surgical options for management of cystic calculi. The size of the calculus, gender of the horse, and surgeon's preference play a role in treatment selection. The preferred technique in males, especially for larger stones, is laparocystotomy through a ventral midline or paramedian incision with the horse in dorsal recumbency under general anesthesia. For removal of smaller cystoliths, a perineal urethrotomy can be performed in the standing male horse with the use of local or epidural anesthesia. The urethra is catheterized to facilitate identification of the urethra and an incision is made at the level of the ischial arch. After the urethra has been incised, forceps are used to grasp and remove the calculus and the bladder is lavaged free of remaining debris. Removal of larger calculi may be attempted via this approach by using a lithotrite to crush the urolith into smaller fragments. The urethral incision can be closed but is usually allowed to heal by second intention. Although this approach can be performed at less expense and avoids the risks of general anesthesia, the risk of complications is greater. Complications include urethral trauma and stricture formation,[29, 69, 70] uretherolith formation at the surgical site,[5, 71] development of a urethral diverticulum,[71] and persistent urine passage through a fistula at the surgical site.[70, 72] The distensible urethra of the mare allows retrieval of cystic calculi via this route in many cases. Using sedation and epidural anesthesia, the stone can be removed intact with forceps or by direct grasping if the surgeon has small hands. A spiculated urolith may be crushed with a lithotrite to ease removal. Spiculated stones or urolith fragments can further be manipulated into a sterile plastic bag or palpation sleeve to minimize trauma to the urethral mucosa during removal. If necessary, the urethral lumen can also be enlarged by performing sphincterotomy in the dorsal aspect of the urethra.[73] A pararectal (Gökels) approach for a dorsal cystotomy[40, 66] and electrohydraulic lithotripsy,[45, 46] as described for ureterolithiasis, have also been used in male and female horses to treat cystic calculi.

Following surgical removal of cystoliths, systemic antibiotics and an antiinflammatory agent are administered for a minimum of 1 week. As for cystitis, antibiotic selection should be based on susceptibility testing of recovered isolates. If culture results are negative, a sulfonamide-trimethoprim combination would be an appropriate selection. An early report by Lowe described excellent long-term results—and no recurrence—after cystic calculi were removed by laparocystotomy in four horses.[71] Similar low rates of recurrence have been echoed in several reviews of equine urolithiasis.[6, 29, 40, 67] In contrast to these favorable reports (most which do not provide supporting data), Laverty reported that clinical signs of urolithiasis recurred in 12 of 29 horses (41%) for which follow-up data were available. The interval between episodes of recurrence was 1 to 32 months (mean 13 months). As initially described in 1965 by Lowe,[71] Laverty also found greater recurrence of cystic calculi after treatment by perineal urethrotomy (seven of 15 horses), in comparison to laparocystotomy. Other complications of cystic calculi, unrelated to the surgical approach, have included vesicoureteral reflux and renal failure[74] and concurrent urolithiasis at other sites.[5] Although a more common complication of urethral obstruction,[69] bladder rupture may also occur consequent to cystic urolithiasis. We have also seen a case of squamous cell carcinoma of the bladder which was associated with a large cystic calculus and development of uroperitoneum consequent to bladder rupture (Fig. 16–33).

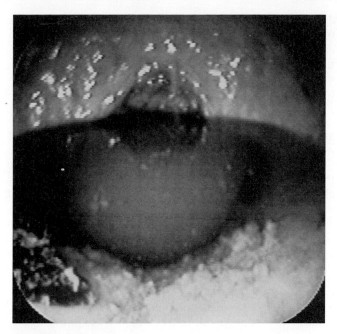

Figure 16–33. A large urolith is present in the bladder below the surface of the pool of urine. The cystolith was accompanied by bacterial cystitis and squamous cell carcinoma of the bladder.

Postoperative recommendations that may help prevent recurrence include control of UTI and use of urinary acidifiers, although the benefits of the latter are not well-documented (detailed under Cystitis).[6, 64, 67, 68, 75] Other considerations for decreasing recurrence include dietary modifications to decrease calcium excretion and to promote diuresis. Changing the diet from a high-calcium hay such as alfalfa to grass or oat hay would decrease dietary calcium and, thus, should decrease urinary calcium excretion, since fecal calcium excretion is relatively constant in horses.[76] This dietary change should decrease total calcium excretion, and it may decrease urinary nitrogen excretion and daily urine volume.[77] The latter changes could enhance supersaturation of urine. In theory, diuresis should be promoted by addition of 50 to 75 g of loose salt daily to the concentrate portion of the diet; however, in a study of ponies fed sodium chloride as 1%, 3%, or 5% of the total dry matter of the diet (1% approximates 75 g of sodium chloride for a 500-kg horse), no differences in water intake, urine production, or calcium excretion were observed.[78] Another factor that affects urine pH and urine calcium excretion is dietary cation–anion balance ($DCAB = [Na + K] - [Cl + S]$). A lower DCAB has been associated with both a decrease in urine pH and an increase in urinary calcium excretion.[79–81] DCAB is usually lowered by increasing the amount of grain in the diet, changing to lower-quality hay, or adding one or more minerals to the diet (e.g., ammonium chloride, calcium chloride, ammonium sulphate). It should not be surprising that supplements that decrease DCAB are familiar as urinary acidifying agents. Since a diet low in both calcium and DCAB could result in a negative calcium balance, a possible long-term effect could be decreased skeletal calcium content.

Despite the success of dietary management (low-protein,

phosphorous, and magnesium) for medical dissolution of canine[82] and feline[83] uroliths, dietary management is unlikely to replace surgical treatment of cystic urolithiasis in horses. This can be attributed to the fact that dietary management for small animals has been directed at struvite urolithiasis and that such stones are not common in horses. Dietary management should not, nevertheless, be overlooked as one of the postoperative recommendations for urolithiasis, as it could decrease the risk of recurrence. At the least, legume hays and dietary supplements containing calcium should be avoided, and the diet could be supplemented with 50 to 75 g loose salt daily. These dietary manipulations, in conjunction with administration of ammonium sulfate as a urine-acidifying agent, were effectively used by Remillard to manage one recurrent case of equine urolithiasis.[84]

URETHRAL CALCULI

Urethral calculi are primarily a problem of male horses,[1–6, 69, 71, 85, 86] although they have been detected in a few mares.[5] In the absence of predisposing urethral damage or stricture formation, urethroliths are usually small cystoliths passed into the urethra. Thus, most urethroliths initially lodge where the urethra narrows as it passes over the ischial arch. They may slowly pass farther down the urethra, until complete obstruction produces signs of renal colic. An obstructing urethral calculus should be considered when male horses show colic signs and frequently posture to urinate. Occasionally, blood may be seen on the end of the urethra. Palpation of the penis may reveal repeated urethral contractions or a firm mass in the urethra. Rectal palpation reveals a distended bladder that is turgid—unlike the flaccid bladder distension of bladder paralysis. If the bladder ruptures, colic signs are supplanted by progressive depression and anorexia consequent to the development of postrenal acute renal failure.[5, 69, 85, 86] The diagnosis is confirmed by passage of a urinary catheter that is obstructed by the urolith or by endoscopic examination of the urethra. Suspected bladder rupture can be confirmed by measuring a twofold or greater increase in peritoneal fluid creatinine concentration, in comparison to serum creatinine concentration.

Calculi lodged at the ischial arch can be removed through a perineal urethrotomy. Passage of a catheter into the bladder, if that is not achieved before surgery, is necessary to ensure a patent urinary tract after stone removal. The urethrotomy is allowed to heal by second intention, and temporary use of an indwelling bladder catheter usually is not necessary. Calculi lodged in the distal urethra can often be removed from a sedated horse by gentle transurethral crushing of the urolith with a hand or forceps. When the calculus is lodged distal to the ischial arch and cannot be palpated in the distal portion of the penis, general anesthesia and positioning the horse in dorsal recumbency are generally necessary for surgical removal of the stone. The urethra may be closed or allowed to heal by second intention. Follow-up endoscopic examination of the urethra allows assessment of urethral healing and possible stricture formation (Fig. 16–34). Further treatment includes administration of antibiotics and antiinflammatory agents until dysuria resolves. Although initial treatment of urinary tract obstruction due to a urethrolith is relatively straightforward, the prognosis for affected

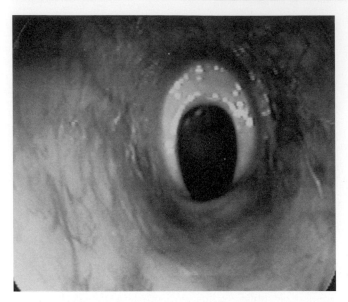

Figure 16–34. Stricture formation in the urethra at the level of the ischial arch formed as a complication of a perineal urethrotomy.

horses should remain guarded since there are a number of potential complications of perineal urethrotomy (described above). Further, a substantial number of horses have had poor outcomes owing to associated bladder rupture and peritonitis[5, 69, 85] or upper urinary tract lithiasis or pyelonephritis.[5, 29]

SABULOUS UROLITHIASIS

Another form of equine urolithiasis termed "sabulous urolithiasis" has also been described in a limited number of horses.[29, 87] Sabulous (Greek for *sand*) urolithiasis refers to the accumulation of large amounts of crystalloid urine sediment in the ventral aspect of the bladder. This condition is a secondary problem, consequent to bladder paralysis or other physical or neurologic disorders interfering with complete bladder emptying.[88–90] Affected horses usually present for evaluation of urinary incontinence or hindlimb weakness and ataxia, and accumulation of urine sediment in a distended bladder may be detected during rectal palpation. Symptomatic treatment includes repeated bladder lavage, medications that promote bladder emptying, and broad-spectrum antibiotics, but the condition carries a poor prognosis unless the primary problem resulting in bladder paralysis can be resolved (see Urinary Incontinence).

BLADDER DISPLACEMENT

Displacement of the urinary bladder is a rare cause of obstruction and dysuria.[91–95] In mares, two types of bladder displacement can occur: (1) extrusion through a tear in the floor of the vagina; or (2) true prolapse with eversion of the bladder.[96] Urethral obstruction may also occur with vaginal or uterine prolapse. In male horses, scrotal herniation of the bladder has been described, but this type of bladder displacement is extremely rare.[97] Bladder displacements are typically a consequence of repeated abdominal contractions or straining. Thus, they are most often associated with parturition and, to a lesser extent, with colic. Perineal lacerations, consequent to trauma or foaling, may lead to extrusion while excessive straining without laceration leads to prolapse/eversion. Since the bladder turns inside out with the latter problem, the diagnosis is established by recognizing the appearance of the bladder mucosa and ureteral openings. Eversion does not always result in obstruction.

With urethral obstruction, a catheter should be passed into the bladder prior to correction of the displacement. In the absence of obstruction, extrusions are corrected during repair of the perineal or vaginal laceration. A course of broad-spectrum antibiotics and an antiinflammatory agent should be instituted since pelvic abscess and peritonitis are potential complications. Manual reduction of bladder eversions may be successful in some cases, but, more often than not, urethral sphincterotomy may be needed to replace the bladder.[95] In some cases, reduction via laparotomy may be necessary as the everted bladder may be filled with the pelvic flexure, complicating manual reduction.[94] A purse-string suture placed in the area of the external urethral sphincter may be of benefit to prevent recurrence of the prolapse, and medical treatment should include broad-spectrum antibiotics and an antiinflammatory agent, since UTI is a potential complication.

PENILE TRAUMA

Urinary tract obstruction is an occasional complication of penile trauma and/or paraphimosis, and patency of the urethra should be considered in all cases of penile injury. Causes may include blunt trauma, breeding injuries, use of stallion rings, sedation with phenothiazine tranquilizers, or laceration during castration.[98–101] In addition to preputial swelling, injury may result in a penile hematoma or possible paraphimosis.[102, 103] In one report, hematoma formation in the corpus spongiosum penis of a quarter horse stallion resulted in complete obstruction and bladder rupture.[104] In addition to ensuring patency of the urinary tract, treatment includes administration of antibiotics and antiinflammatory agents until the majority of swelling resolves. Lacerations of the urethra may be closed primarily or left to heal by second intention, depending on location and condition of the wound. Since stricture formation is a possible complication, some wounds may be better treated by phallectomy than by urethral repair.[100]

REFERENCES

1. DeBowes RM: Obstructive urinary tract disease. In Robinson NE, ed. *Current Therapy in Equine Medicine 2.* Philadelphia, WB Saunders, 1987, p 713.
2. Divers TJ: Diseases of the renal system. In Smith BP, ed. *Large Animal Internal Medicine.* St. Louis, CV Mosby, 1990, p 872.
3. Ford TS: Obstruction and rupture of the urinary tract. In Robinson NE, ed. *Current Therapy in Equine Medicine 3.* Philadelphia, WB Saunders, 1992, p 613.

4. Ortenburger A, Pringle J: Diseases of the bladder and urethra. *In* Kobluk CN, Ames TR, Geor RJ, eds. *The Horse, Diseases and Clinical Management.* Philadelphia, WB Saunders, 1995, p 597.
5. Laverty S, Pascoe JR, Ling GV, et al: Urolithiasis in 68 horses. *Vet Surg* 21:56, 1992.
6. DeBowes RM, Nyrop KA, Boulton CH: Cystic calculi in the horse. *Compend Contin Educ Pract Vet* 6:S268, 1984.
7. DiBartola, Chew DJ: Canine urolithiasis. *Compend Contin Educ Pract Vet* 3:226, 1981.
8. Sutor DJ, Wooley SE, Illingsworth JJ: A geographical and historical survey of the composition of urinary stones. *Br J Urol* 46:393, 1974.
9. Wharrier J: Cystic calculus in the horse (Letter). *Vet Rec* 76:187, 1964.
10. Coe FL, Favus MJ: Nephrolithiasis. In Brenner BM, Rector FC, eds. *The Kidney,* ed 4, Vol 2. Philadelphia, WB Saunders, 1991, p 1728.
11. Smith LH: The medical aspects of urolithiasis: An overview. *J Urol* 141:707, 1989.
12. Osborne CA, Polzin DJ, Abdullahi SU, et al: Struvite urolithiasis in animals and man: Formation, detection, and dissolution. *Adv Vet Sci Comp Med* 29:1, 1985.
13. Senior DF, Finlayson B: Initiation and growth of uroliths. *Vet Clin North Am: Small Animal Pract* 16:19, 1986.
14. Buffington CA, Blaisdell JL, Sako T: Effects of Tamm-Horsfall glycoprotein and albumin on struvite crystal growth in urine of cats. *Am J Vet Res* 55:965, 1994.
15. Hess B, Nakagawa Y, Parks JH, et al: Molecular abnormality of Tamm-Horsfall glycoprotein in calcium oxalate nephrolithiasis. *Am J Physiol* 260:F569, 1991.
16. See WA, Williams RD: Urothelial injury and clotting cascade activation: Common denominators in particulate adherence to urothelial surfaces. *J Urol* 147:541, 1992.
17. Neumann RD, Ruby AL, Ling GV, et al: Ultrastructure and mineral composition of urinary calculi from horses. *Am J Vet Res* 55:1357, 1994.
18. Sutor DJ, Wooley SE: Animal calculi: An x-ray diffraction study of their crystalline composition. *Res Vet Sci* 11:299, 1970.
19. Grünberg W: Carbonate urinary calculi in herbivorous domestic animals. *Zbl Vet Med A* 18:767, 1971.
20. Mair TS, Osborn RS: The crystalline composition of normal equine urine deposits. *Equine Vet J* 22:364, 1990.
21. Mair TS: Crystalline composition of equine urinary calculi. *Res Vet Sci* 40:288, 1986.
22. Osborne CA, Sanna JJ, Unger LK, et al: Analyzing the mineral composition of uroliths from dogs, cats, horses, cattle, sheep, goats, and pigs. *Vet Med* 84:750, 1989.
23. Ruby AL, Ling GV: Bacterial culture of uroliths: Techniques and interpretation of results. *Vet Clin North Am Small Animal Pract* 16:325, 1986.
24. Boyd WL, Bishop LM: Pyelonephritis of cattle and horses. *J Am Vet Med Assoc* 90:154, 1937.
25. Held JP, Wright B, Henton JE: Pyelonephritis associated with renal failure in a horse. *J Am Vet Med Assoc* 189:688, 1986.
26. Hillyer MH, Mair TS, Lucke VM: Bilateral renal calculi in an adult horse. *Equine Vet Educ* 2:117, 1990.
27. Laing JA, Raisis AL, Rawlinson RJ, et al: Chronic renal failure and urolithiasis in a 2-year-old colt. *Aust Vet J* 69:199, 1992.
28. Ehnen SJ, Divers TJ, Gillette D, et al: Obstructive nephrolithiasis and ureterolithiasis associated with chronic renal failure in horses: Eight cases (1981–1987). *J Am Vet Med Assoc* 197:249, 1990.
29. Holt PE, Pearson H: Urolithiasis in the horse—a review of 13 cases. *Equine Vet J* 16:31, 1984.
30. Jackson OE: Renal calculi in a horse. *Vet Rec* 91:7, 1972.
31. MacHarg MA, Foerner JJ, Phillips TN, et al: Two methods for the treatment of ureterolithiasis in a mare. *Vet Surg* 13:95, 1984.
32. Hope WD, Wilson JH, Hager DA, et al: Chronic renal failure associated with bilateral nephroliths and ureteroliths in a two-year-old Thoroughbred colt. *Equine Vet J* 21:228, 1989.
33. Juzwiak JS, Bain FT, Slone DE, et al: Unilateral nephrectomy for treatment of chronic hematuria due to nephrolithiasis in a colt. *Can Vet J* 29:931, 1988.
34. Byars TD, Simpson JS, Divers TJ, et al: Percutaneous nephrostomy in short-term management of ureterolithiasis and renal dysfunction in a filly. *J Am Vet Med Assoc* 195:499, 1989.
35. Rodger LD, Carlson GP, Moran ME, et al: Resolution of a left ureteral stone using electrohydraulic lithotripsy in a Thoroughbred colt. *J Vet Intern Med* 9:280, 1995.
36. Rantanen NW: Diseases of the kidney. *Vet Clin North Am Equine Pract* 2:89, 1986.
37. Kiper ML, Traub-Dargatz JL, Wrigley RH: Renal ultrasonography in horses. *Compend Contin Educ Pract Vet* 12:993, 1990.
38. Divers TJ: Chronic renal failure in horses. *Compend Contin Educ Pract Vet* 5:S310, 1983.
39. Divers TJ: Nephrolithiasis and ureterolithiasis in horses and their association with renal disease and failure (Editorial). *Equine Vet J* 21:161, 1989.
40. DeBowes RM: Surgical management of urolithiasis. *Vet Clin North Am Equine Pract* 4:461, 1988.
41. DeBowes RM: Kidneys and ureters. In Auer JA, ed. *Equine Surgery.* Philadelphia, WB Saunders, 1992, p 768.
42. Pringle J, Ortenburger A: Diseases of the kidneys and ureters. *In* Kobluk CN, Ames TR, Geor RJ, eds. *The Horse, Diseases and Clinical Management.* Philadelphia, WB Saunders, 1995, p 583.
43. Donner GS, Ellison GW, Ackerman N, et al: Percutaneous nephrolithotomy in the dog: An experimental study. *Vet Surg* 16:411, 1987.
44. Mulley AG: Management of nephrolithiasis: New approaches to "surgical" kidney stones. *Annu Rev Med* 39:347, 1988.
45. MacHarg MA, Foerner JJ, Phillips TN, et al: Electrohydraulic lithotripsy for treatment of a cystic calculus in a mare. *Vet Surg* 14:325, 1985.
46. Eustace RA, Hunt JM: Electrohydraulic lithotripsy for treatment of cystic calculus in two geldings. *Equine Vet J* 20:221, 1988.
47. Senior DF: Electrohydraulic shock-wave lithotripsy in experimental canine struvite bladder stone disease. *Vet Surg* 13:143, 1984.
48. Snyder JR, Pascoe JR, Williams JW: Rectal prolapse and cystic calculus in a burro. *J Am Vet Med Assoc* 187:421, 1985.
49. Sullins KE, Traub-Dargatz JL: Endoscopic anatomy of the equine urinary tract. *Compend Contin Educ Pract Vet* 6:S663, 1984.
50. Traub-Dargatz JL, McKinnon AO: Adjunctive methods of examination of the urogenital tract. *Vet Clin North Am Equine Pract* 4:339, 1988.
51. Kendrick JW: Cystic calculi in a horse. *Cornell Vet* 40:187, 1950.
52. Usenik EA, Larson LL, Sauer F: Cystotomy and removal of a urolith in a Shetland mare. *J Am Vet Med Assoc* 128:453, 1956.
53. Menon MN, Lingam UM: Laparo-cystotomy in a horse. *Indian Vet J* 35:482, 1958.
54. Lowe JE: Suprapubic cystotomy in a gelding. *Cornell Vet* 50:510, 1960.
55. Furness TR: Cystic calculus in a three-year-old gelding. *Can Vet J* 1:221, 1960.

56. Wright JG, Neal PA: Laparo-cystotomy for urinary calculus in a gelding. *Vet Rec* 72:301, 1960.

57. Lowe JE: Surgical removal of equine uroliths via the laparo-cystotomy approach. *J Am Vet Med Assoc* 139:345, 1961.

58. Reed DG: Suprapubic cystotomy in a stallion. *Can J Comp Med Vet Sci* 28:95, 1964.

59. Williams KR: Laparo-cystotomy in a gelding. *Vet Rec* 76:83, 1964.

60. Williams PFB: Removal of an urinary calculus from a gelding. *NZ Vet J* 27:223, 1979.

61. Mair TS, McCaig J: Cystic calculus in a horse. *Equine Vet J* 15:173, 1983.

62. Belling TH: Equine laparocystotomy. *Equine Pract* 5(1):16, 1983.

63. Kaneps AJ, Shires GMH, Watrous BJ: Cystic calculi in two horses. *J Am Vet Med Assoc* 187:737, 1985.

64. Johnson PJ, Crenshaw KL: The treatment of cystic and urethral calculi in a gelding. *Vet Med* 85:891, 1990.

65. Crabbe BG, Bohn AA, Grant BD: Equine urocystoliths. *Equine Pract* 13(1):12, 1991.

66. van Dongen PL, Plenderleith RW: Equine urolithiasis: Surgical treatment by Gökels pararectal cystotomy. *Equine Vet Educ* 6:186, 1994.

67. Mair TS, Holt PE: The aetiology and treatment of equine urolithiasis. *Equine Vet Educ* 6:189, 1994.

68. Robertson JT, Buffington CA: Surgical removal of uroliths. *In* White NA, Moore JN, eds. *Current Practice of Equine Surgery,* Philadelphia: J.B. Lippincott, 1990, p 734.

69. Sullins KE, Bertone JJ, Voss JL, et al: Treatment of hemospermia in stallions: A discussion of 18 cases. *Compend Contin Educ Pract Vet* 10:1396, 1988.

70. Dyke TM, Maclean AA. Urethral obstruction in a stallion with possible synchronous diaphragmatic flutter. *Vet Rec* 121:425, 1987.

71. Lowe JE: Long-term results of cystotomy for removal of uroliths from horses. *J Am Vet Med Assoc* 147:147, 1965.

72. Trotter GW, Bennett DG, Behm RJ: Urethral calculi in five horses. *Vet Surg* 10:159, 1981.

73. Firth EC: Urethral sphincterotomy for delivery of vesical calculus in the mare: A case report. *Equine Vet J* 8:99, 1976.

74. Crabbe BG, Grant BD: Complications secondary to a chronic urocystolith. *Equine Pract* 13(3):8, 1991.

75. Wood T, Weckman TJ, Henry PA, et al: Equine urine pH: Normal population distributions and methods of acidification. *Equine Vet J* 22:118, 1990.

76. Schryver HF, Hintz HF, Lowe JE: Calcium and phosphorous in the nutrition of the horse. *Cornell Vet* 64:493, 1974.

77. Cymbaluk NF: Water balance of horses fed various diets. *Equine Pract* 11(1):19, 1989.

78. Schryver HF, Parker MT, Daniluk PD, et al: Salt consumption and the effect of salt on mineral metabolism in horses. *Cornell Vet* 77:122, 1987.

79. Hintz HF: Dietary cation-anion balance. *Equine Pract* 13(10):6, 1991.

80. Wall DL, Topliff DR, Freeman DW, et al: Effects of dietary cation-anion balance on urinary mineral excretion in exercised horses. *J Equine Vet Sci* 12:168, 1992.

81. Cooper SR, Kline KH, Foreman JH, et al: Effects of dietary cation-anion balance on blood pH, acid-base parameters, serum and urine mineral levels, and parathyroid hormone (PTH) in weanling horses. *J Equine Vet Sci* 15:417, 1995.

82. Osborne CA, Polzin DJ, Kruger JM, et al: Medical dissolution of canine struvite urocystoliths. *Vet Clin North Am Small Animal Pract* 16:349, 1986.

83. Osborne CA, Lulich JP, Kruger JM, et al: Medical dissolution of feline struvite urocystoliths. *J Am Vet Med Assoc* 196:1053, 1990.

84. Remillard RL, Modransky PD, Welker FH, et al: Dietary management of cystic calculi in a horse. *J Eq Vet Sci* 12:359, 1992.

85. McCue PM, Brooks PA, Wilson WD: Urinary bladder rupture as a sequela to obstructive urethral calculi. *Vet Med* 84:912, 1989.

86. Gibson KT, Trotter GW, Gustafson SB: Conservative management of uroperitoneum in a gelding. *J Am Vet Med Assoc* 200:1692, 1992.

87. Holt PE, Mair TS: Ten cases of bladder paralysis associated with sabulous urolithiasis in horses. *Vet Rec* 127:108, 1990.

88. Hooper PT: Epizootic cystitis in horses. *Aust Vet J* 44:11, 1968.

89. Adams LG, Dollahite JW, Romane WM, et al: Cystitis and ataxia associated with sorghum ingestion. *J Am Vet Med Assoc* 155:518, 1969.

90. VanKempen KR: Sudan grass and sorghum poisoning of horses: A possible lathyrogenic disease. *J Am Vet Med Assoc* 156:629, 1970.

91. Boulton CH: Urinary tract displacement. In Robinson NE, ed. *Current Therapy in Equine Medicine 2.* Philadelphia, WB Saunders, 1987, p 715.

92. Pascoe JR, Pascoe RRR: Displacements, malpositions, and miscellaneous injuries of the mare's urogenital tract. *Vet Clin North Am Equine Pract* 4:439, 1988.

93. Donaldson RS: Eversion of the bladder in a mare. *Vet Rec* 92:409, 1973.

94. Haynes PF, McClure JR: Eversion of the urinary bladder: A sequel to third-degree perineal laceration in the mare. *Vet Surg* 9:66, 1980.

95. Alvarenga J, Oliveira CM, Correia da Silva LCL: Prolapse with eversion of the urinary bladder in a mare. *Equine Pract* 17(8):8, 1995.

96. Vaughan JT: Equine urogenital surgery. In Jennings PB, ed. *The Practice of Large Animal Surgery.* Vol 2. Philadelphia, WB Saunders, 1984, p 1136.

97. Noone JP: Scrotal herniation of the urinary bladder in the horse. *Irish Vet J* 20:11, 1966.

98. Robertson JT: Conditions of the urethra. In Robinson NE, ed. *Current Therapy in Equine Medicine 2.* Philadelphia, WB Saunders, 1987, p 719.

99. Wheat JD: Penile paralysis in stallions given propiopromazine. *J Am Vet Med Assoc* 148:405, 1966.

100. Yovich JV, Turner AS: Treatment of a postcastration urethral stricture by phallectomy in a gelding. *Compend Contin Educ Pract Vet* 8:S393, 1986.

101. Todhunter RJ, Parker JE: Surgical repair of urethral transection in a horse. *J Am Vet Med Assoc* 193:1085, 1988.

102. Gibbons WJ: Hematoma of penis. *Mod Vet Pract* 45:76, 1964.

103. Memon MA, McClure JJ, Usenik EA: Preputial hematoma in a stallion. *J Am Vet Med Assoc* 191:563, 1987.

104. Firth EC: Dissecting hematoma of corpus spongiosum and urinary bladder rupture in a stallion. *J Am Vet Med Assoc* 169:800, 1976.

16.9.

Hematuria

Harold C. Schott II, DVM, PhD

Hematuria can be a presenting complaint for a variety of disorders of the urinary tract, including vascular malformation, urinary tract infection, urolithiasis, and neoplasia. In addition to these problems, which are discussed elsewhere in this chapter, there are several other specific causes of hematuria. These range from microscopic hematuria accompanying exercise to more severe conditions that can result in life-threatening urinary tract hemorrhage.

Although values have not been determined in horses, normal human urine contains about 5000 (range 2000 to 10,000) red blood cells (RBCs) per milliliter.[1] This range of RBC excretion should yield negative results on reagent strip analysis and a report of not more than 5 RBCs per high-power field (hpf) on sediment examination.[2] Increases in RBC excretion may lead to microscopic or macroscopic hematuria. Microscopic hematuria, which implies an increase in RBC excretion that cannot be seen grossly, is usually associated with increases in the range of 10,000 to 2,500,000 RBC per milliliter urine. On sediment examination at least 10 RBC/hpf should be apparent. Reagent strip analysis results can range from trace to $+++$. It is important to realize that reagent strip results, which utilize the peroxidase-like activity of hemoglobin and myoglobin to oxidize a chromogen in the test pad, do not differentiate between hemoglobin and myoglobin.[2] Thus, positive results are not specific for hematuria and may be more appropriately termed "pigmenturia." Despite this limitation, reagent strips can be used to differentiate hematuria from hemoglobinuria or myoglobinuria when the color change is limited to scattered spots on the test pad. This pattern implies that intact RBCs were adsorbed onto the pad, underwent lysis, and produced a localized color change due to hemoglobin activity on the chromogenic substrates. Ability to differentiate hematuria from excretion of the heme pigments is limited to a threshold of 250,000 to 300,000 RBCs per milliliters urine, unless urine samples are diluted with normal saline. Other limitations of reagent strip analysis include false-positive reactions when urine samples are contaminated with oxidizing agents (e.g., disinfectants) or false-negative reactions when urine samples contain vitamin C or have been preserved with formalin.[2]

Macroscopic or gross hematuria indicates RBC excretion in excess of 2,500,000 to 5,000,000 RBC per milliliters urine (or about 0.5 mL blood per liter of urine).[1-4] Macroscopic hematuria can be differentiated from other causes of pigmenturia by centrifuging a sample of urine to produce a red cell pellet and yellow supernatant urine. Quantification of erythrocyte numbers in macroscopic hematuria is of little clinical value. In contrast, urinary RBC numbers may provide diagnostic and prognostic information in cases of microscopic hematuria in humans.[1] However, accurate counts are complicated by variations in urine concentration. In concentrated urine (specific gravity over 1.020), RBCs tend to become crenated, owing to osmotic shift of water out of the cells. In urine with a specific gravity below 1.010, osmotic swelling and dilution of hemoglobin lead to "ghost cell" formation.[1, 5] Further, many RBCs will lyse in dilute urine (especially alkaline urine) so that RBC excretion is vastly underestimated. Reagent strip analysis can be useful in dilute urine samples to detect hemoglobin released from lysed erythrocytes.[4]

Microscopic examination of urine sediment in cases of hematuria is helpful in distinguishing glomerular from nonglomerular bleeding. The hallmark of glomerular bleeding is a substantial variation in RBC size, shape, and hemoglobin content (termed "dysmorphism"), while bleeding from other sites produces a more uniform population of urinary erythrocytes.[1, 4, 6] Dysmorphism is attributed to membrane deformation, which occurs as erythrocytes traverse the glomerular filtration barrier.[7] Urinary RBCs in normal persons are typically dysmorphic, indicating glomerular origin, but the excretion rate is low.[1] Thus, urinary RBC morphologic characteristics must be interpreted in combination with urinary RBC numbers to determine significance.[6] The volume of dysmorphic cells tends to be lower than that of erythrocytes of nonglomerular origin, so that measurement of mean corpuscular volume has also been used to separate glomerular from nonglomerular bleeding.[8] The presence of RBC or hemoglobin casts is also pathognomonic for glomerular bleeding.[1, 4, 5] These casts are formed as urinary RBCs and hemoglobin from the proximal portion of the nephron (glomerulus) combine with Tamm-Horsfall mucoprotein secreted in the ascending limb of the loop of Henle. Since both urinary RBCs and casts deteriorate rather rapidly in urine samples, other methods of detecting glomerular hematuria such as immunocytochemical staining for Tamm-Horsfall glycoprotein have been developed but have not gained widespread use.[9]

Noting the timing of hematuria is usually a more practical means of initially localizing the site of urinary tract hemorrhage.[5] Hematuria throughout urination is consistent with hemorrhage from the kidneys, ureters, or bladder, whereas hematuria at the beginning of urination is often associated with lesions in the distal urethra. Hematuria at the end of urination is usually the result of hemorrhage from the proximal urethra or bladder neck. A thorough diagnostic evaluation, including physical examination, rectal palpation, analyses of blood and urine, endoscopy of the lower tract, and ultrasonography, is usually rewarding in establishing the source and cause of urinary tract hemorrhage.

UTI, although relatively uncommon in horses, may result in hematuria. With infection of the upper urinary tract, partial anorexia, weight loss, and fever may be additional presenting complaints, whereas horses with cystitis generally manifest stranguria and/or pollakiuria; however, hematuria has been the presenting complaint in several reports of cystitis and pyelonephritis.[10-13] The presence of uroliths at any level of the urinary tract may cause mucosal irritation and hemorrhage, resulting in hematuria.[14-16] Typically, affected horses also show signs of renal colic or painful urination (stranguria or pollakiuria), especially with uroliths in the bladder or urethra. Finally, neoplasia of the kidneys, ureters, bladder, or urethra may also result in hematuria as the presenting complaint.[17-19] These conditions are discussed in detail in other sections in this chapter.

DRUG TOXICITY

Nephrotoxicity, particularly that secondary to administration of nonsteroidal anti-inflammatory drugs (especially phenylbutazone), may result in microscopic or gross hematuria.[20-24] The historical or current use of nephrotoxic medications supports this diagnosis, and discontinuation of the nephrotoxic agent and supportive care are the appropriate treatments.

URETHRAL DEFECTS

Although a recognized cause of hemospermia in stallions, defects or tears of the proximal urethra at the level of the

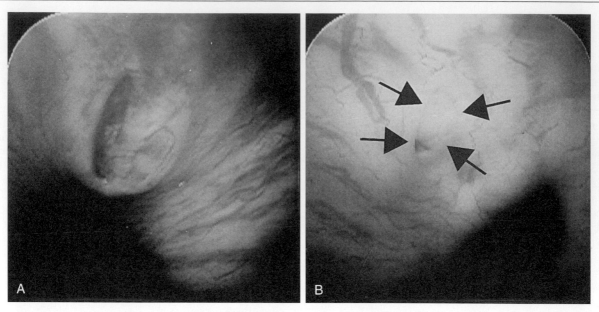

Figure 16–35. Endoscopic images of urethral defects or tears at the level of the ischial arch. **A,** A more acute lesion (hematuria of 2 weeks' duration) is surrounded by a raised rim of tissue. **B,** A chronic lesion (hematuria of 6 months' duration) is flat to recessed *(between arrows)*. There is minimal evidence of inflammation around both lesions.

ischial arch are a more recently described cause of hematuria in geldings.[25, 26] Since the defects are difficult to detect without high-resolution videoendoscopic equipment, it is likely that lesions may have been missed in previous reports of urethral bleeding.[27, 28] Consequently, hematuria has been attributed to urethritis or hemorrhage from "varicosities" of the urethral vasculature.[25, 28] Since the vasculature underlying the urethral mucosa becomes quite prominent when the urethra is distended with air during endoscopic examination, especially in the proximal urethra (to the point that blood can be seen flowing in the submucosal vasculature), it would be easy to suspect that hemorrhage could arise from apparent urethritis or urethral varicosity.

Urethral defects or tears typically result in hematuria at the end of urination, in association with urethral contraction.[25, 26] Affected horses generally void a normal volume of urine that is not discolored. At the end of urination, a series of urethral contractions results in squirts of bright red blood. Occasionally, a smaller amount of darker blood may be passed at the start of urination. In most instances, the condition does not appear painful or result in pollakiuria. Interestingly, the majority of affected stallions with hemospermia and geldings with hematuria have been quarter horses or quarter horse crosses that have been free of other complaints.[26, 28] Treatment with antibiotics for suspected cystitis or urethritis has routinely been unsuccessful, although hematuria has resolved spontaneously in approximately half of the cases seen by the authors.

Examination of affected horses is often unremarkable. In comparison, horses with hematuria due to neoplasms involving the distal urethra or penis are usually presented with additional complaints such as pollakiuria, a foul odor to the sheath, or presence of a mass in the sheath or on the penis. With urethral defects, laboratory analysis of blood reveals normal renal function, although mild anemia can be an occasional finding. Urine samples collected midstream or by

bladder catheterization appear grossly normal. Urinalysis may have normal results, or there may be an increased number of red blood cells on sediment examination, a finding that would also result in a positive reagent strip result for blood. Bacterial culture of urine yields negative results.

The diagnosis is made via endoscopic examination of the urethra, during which a lesion is typically seen along the dorsocaudal aspect of the urethra at the level of the ischial arch (Fig. 16–35A). With hematuria of several weeks' duration, the lesion appears as a fistula communicating with the vasculature of the corpus spongiosum penis (Fig. 16–35B). External palpation of the urethra in this area is usually unremarkable but can help localize the lesion because external digital palpation can be seen via the endoscope as movements of the urethra.

Although the pathophysiology of this condition remains unclear, it has been speculated that the defect is the result of a "blowout" of the corpus spongiosum penis (cavernous vascular tissue surrounding the urethra) into the urethral lumen (Fig. 16–36).[26] Contraction of the bulbospongiosus muscle during ejaculation causes a dramatic increase in pressure in the corpus spongiosum penis, which is essentially a closed vascular space during ejaculation. The bulbospongiosus muscle also undergoes a series of contractions to empty the urethra of urine at the end of urination; thus the defect into the urethra may develop by a similar mechanism in geldings. Once the lesion has been created, it is maintained by bleeding at the end of each urination, and the surrounding mucosa heals by formation of a fistula into the overlying vascular tissue. An explanation for the consistent location along the dorsocaudal aspect of the urethra at the level of the ischial arch has not been documented but may be related to the anatomy of the musculature supporting the base of the penis and an enlargement of the corpus spongiosum penis in this area. Further, there is narrowing of the lumen of the urethra at the distal extent of the ampullar portion of

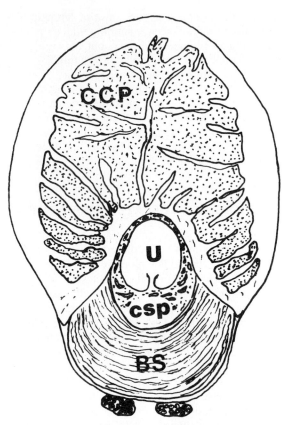

Figure 16–36. Cross-sectional diagram of the equine penis at the level of the ischial arch shows a defect between the corpus spongiosum penis *(csp)* and the urethral lumen *(U)*. The corpus spongiosum penis is a cavernous tissue surrounding the urethra, which is distinct from the corpus cavernosum penis *(CCP)*; it is also adjacent to the bulbospongiosus muscle *(BS)* caudally. (From Schumacher J, Varner DD, Schmitz DG, Blanchard TL: Urethral defects in geldings with hematuria and stallions with hemospermia. Vet Surg 24:250, 1995.)

the urethra, which may also contribute to the location of the defects. An anatomic predisposition in quarter horses has not been documented but could be speculated based on an apparently increased risk in this breed. In addition, some of the affected horses have asymmetry to the musculature under the tail in this area, supporting a possible developmental defect (Fig. 16–37).

Since hematuria may resolve spontaneously, no treatment may be required initially. If hematuria persists longer than a month or if significant anemia develops, a temporary sub-ischial urethrotomy has been successful in a number of affected geldings. With sedation and epidural or local anesthesia, a vertical incision is made down to a catheter placed in the urethra. The surgical wound requires several weeks to heal, and moderate hemorrhage from the corpus spongiosum penis is apparent for the first few days after surgery. Additional treatment consists of local wound care and prophylactic antibiotic treatment (typically a trimethoprim-sulfonamide combination) for 7 to 10 days. Hematuria should resolve within a week following this procedure. Recently, incising into the corpus spongiosum penis but not into the

urethral lumen has been a successful treatment.[26] This treatment option provides support for the "blowout" cause and lessens the risk of urethral stricture formation. Further, it decreases the chance of a permanent fistula forming at the site, a surgical complication that has occurred in a couple of geldings.

IDIOPATHIC RENAL HEMATURIA

Macroscopic hematuria, often accompanied by passage of blood clots and development of life-threatening anemia, has been reported in a limited number of adult horses.[29] Similar conditions of recurrent renal hemorrhage, unassociated with trauma or other obvious causes of hematuria, have been described as idiopathic renal hematuria or benign essential hematuria in humans and dogs.[30–36] In these species hematuria is more commonly a unilateral than a bilateral problem, similar to what has been observed in the few affected horses. The pathophysiology remains ill-understood, but in humans macroscopic hematuria has been associated with immune-mediated glomerular damage (acute post-infectious glomerulonephritis, membranoproliferative glomerulonephritis, and immunoglobulin A [IgA] nephropathy or Berger's disease), thin basement membrane nephropathy, and the loin pain–hematuria syndrome.[30] The cause of the latter syndrome is suspected to be a nonglomerular, microvascular disease that may be associated with abnormal platelet function.[30, 33] Al-

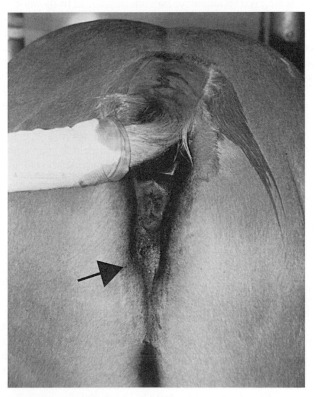

Figure 16–37. Perineum of paint gelding with hematuria associated with a proximal urethral defect; note the asymmetry of the perineal musculature at the level of the ischial arch. (Arrow shows where asymmetry is more prominent on left side.)

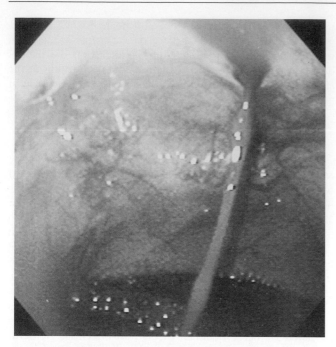

Figure 16–38. Endoscopic image of a large blood clot exiting the right ureteral opening of a gelding with idiopathic renal hematuria.

though hematuria has been recognized with systemic disease in horses,[37] patients affected with idiopathic renal hematuria appear to have spontaneous, severe hematuria in the absence of other signs of disease. Neither UTI nor lithiasis has been detected, and the magnitude of hematuria has resulted in the need for repeated blood transfusions in three of five horses examined by the authors. Cystoscopic examination revealed unilateral hematuria (Fig. 16–38) in all five horses, but the problem subsequently developed in the contralateral kidney in one mare subjected to nephrectomy. Four horses either suffered a fatal hemorrhage or were destroyed within 3 months of the initial observed bout of hematuria. The fifth horse developed chronic renal failure after a 2-year course of intermittent hematuria, prompting a decision for euthanasia. Two mares had dilated renal pelves containing blood clots at necropsy examination, and histologic changes included evidence of prior infarcts (not apparently associated with the hemorrhage). Minimal light microscopic evidence of glomerular disease was detected. In one case the inner medullary collecting ducts were filled with blood, suggesting leakage from the vasculature at this level.

The diagnosis of idiopathic renal hematuria is made by exclusion of systemic disease, alterations in hemostasis, and other causes of hematuria. Physical examination may reveal tachycardia, tachypnea, and pale membranes consistent with acute blood loss. Rectal palpation may reveal an enlarged, irregular bladder, owing to the presence of blood clots. Azotemia is uncommon. Endoscopic examination is important to document that hematuria is originating from the upper urinary tract and to determine whether hemorrhage is unilateral or bilateral. Repeated examinations may be required to answer the latter question. Ultrasonographic imaging is necessary to rule out nephrolithiasis or ureterolithiasis and may occasionally reveal a distended vascular space

or renal vascular anomaly as the cause of hematuria. Renal biopsy and immunofluorescence staining may help document immune-mediated glomerular injury, but the significance of such results is not well-understood at this time.

Treatment for idiopathic hematuria consists of supportive care for acute blood loss, including blood transfusions. The condition may be self-limiting in some patients so that supportive treatment is warranted. With severe and recurrent hematuria of unilateral renal origin, nephrectomy may be indicated, but owners should be warned that there is a risk of hematuria developing in the contralateral kidney.

EXERCISE-ASSOCIATED HEMATURIA

Exercise is accompanied by increased filtration of red blood cells and protein across the glomerular barrier in a large percentage of human and equine athletes.[3, 38] Typically, the hematuria is microscopic, but occasionally gross discoloration of urine may be observed. Gross hematuria may more often be a consequence of bladder erosions, which may be traumatically induced by the abdominal contents pounding the bladder against the pelvis during exercise. Detection of focal bladder erosions or ulcers with a contrecoup distribution and a history of emptying the bladder immediately before the exercise bout would be characteristic for this problem. A diagnosis of exercise-associated hematuria should be one of exclusion after diagnostic evaluation has ruled out other causes of hematuria such as presence of a cystolith.

PIGMENTURIA ASSOCIATED WITH SYSTEMIC DISEASE

With any systemic disease that may lead to alterations in hemostasis or vascular permeability, hematuria or hemoglobinuria may develop. Discolored urine has the potential to be accompanied by a degree of nephrotoxicity, owing to interaction of iron ions of the heme molecules with proximal tubular epithelial cells. With transient pigmenturia (as with exercise-associated hematuria), changes in renal function may not be apparent, but with more severe disease processes and hemolysis, acute renal failure may develop. In humans, development of acute renal failure in association with diseases complicated by coagulopathies or disseminated intravascular coagulation has been termed the "hemolytic-uremic syndrome." The syndrome is recognized more commonly in infants and children than in adults. A similar syndrome has been described in a limited number of horses.[37] Similarly, hemolysis and hemoglobinuria may be recognized with liver disease or immune-mediated hemolytic anemias consequent to infection (*Streptococcus equi*) or drug treatments. Finally, conditions accompanied by extensive rhabdomyolyis may also result in pigmenturia. Assessment of muscle enzyme activity in these cases is usually rewarding in establishing myoglobin as the most likely cause of pigmenturia. In addition, the Blondheim test (ammonium sulfate precipitation) can be used to differentiate myoglobinuria from hemoglobinuria.[39]

REFERENCES

1. Levey AS, Madaio MP, Perrone RD: Laboratory assessment of renal disease: clearance, urinalysis, and renal biopsy. In Brenner BM, Rector FC, eds. *The Kidney,* ed 4, Vol 1. Philadelphia, WB Saunders, 1991, p 919.
2. Osborne CA, Stevens JB: *Handbook of Canine and Feline Urinalysis.* St. Louis, Ralston Purina Company, 1981, p 91.
3. Schott HC, Hodgson DR, Bayly WM: Haematuria, pigmenturia and proteinuria in exercising horses. *Equine Vet J* 27:67, 1995.
4. Fairley KF, Birch DF: Microscopic urinalysis in glomerulonephritis. *Kidney Int* 44, Suppl 42:S9, 1993.
5. Hitt ME: Hematuria of renal origin. *Compend Contin Educ Pract Vet* 8:14, 1986.
6. Pollock C, Pei-Ling L, Györy AZ, et al: Dysmorphisms of urinary red blood cells—value in diagnosis. *Kidney Int* 36:1045, 1989.
7. Jai-Trung L, Hiroyoshi W, Hiroshi M, et al: Mechanism of hematuria in glomerular disease: An electron microscopic study in a case of diffuse membranous glomerulonephritis. *Nephron* 35:68, 1983.
8. Gibbs DD, Lynn KL: Red cell volume distribution curves in the diagnosis of glomerular and non-glomerular hematuria. *Clin Nephrol* 33:143, 1990.
9. Janssens PMW: New markers for analyzing the cause of hematuria. *Kidney Int* 46(Suppl 47):S115, 1994.
10. Boyd WL, Bishop LM: Pyelonephritis of cattle and horses. *J Am Vet Med Assoc* 90:154, 1937.
11. Hooper PT: Epizootic cystitis in horses. *Aust Vet J* 44:11, 1968.
12. Johnson JK, Neely DP, Latterman SA: Hematuria caused by abdominal abscessation in a foal. *J Am Vet Med Assoc* 191:971, 1987.
13. Bernard WV, Williams D, Tuttle PA, Pierce S: Hematuria and leptospiruria in a foal. *J Am Vet Med Assoc* 203:276, 1993.
14. DeBowes RM, Nyrop KA, Boulton CH: Cystic calculi in the horse. *Compend Contin Educ Pract Vet* 6:S268, 1984.
15. Laverty S, Pascoe JR, Ling GV, et al: Urolithiasis in 68 horses. *Vet Surg* 21:56, 1992.
16. Juzwiak JS, Bain FT, Slone DE, et al: Unilateral nephrectomy for treatment of chronic hematuria due to nephrolithiasis in a colt. *Can Vet J* 29:931, 1988.
17. Fischer AT, Spier S, Carlson GP, et al: Neoplasia of the urinary bladder as a cause of hematuria. *J Am Vet Med Assoc* 186:1294, 1985.
18. Owen RR, Haywood S, Kelly DF: Clinical course of renal adenocarcinoma associated with hypercupraemia in a horse. *Vet Rec* 119:291, 1986.
19. West HJ, Kelly DF, Ritchie HE: Renal carcinomatosis in a horse. *Equine Vet J* 19:548, 1987.
20. Abraham PA, Matzke GR: Drug-induced renal disease. In DiPiro JT, Talbert RL, Hayes PE, Yee GC, Posey LM, eds. *Pharmacotherapy: A Pathophysiologic Approach.* New York, Elsevier, 1989, p 543.
21. Gunson DE: Renal papillary necrosis in horses. *J Am Vet Med Assoc* 182:263, 1983.
22. Gunson DE, Soma LR: Renal papillary necrosis in horses after phenylbutazone and water deprivation. *Vet Pathol* 20:603, 1983.
23. Behm RJ, Berg IE: Hematuria caused by renal medullary crest necrosis in a horse. *Compend Contin Educ Pract Vet* 9:698, 1987.
24. Edwards JF, Carter GK: Severe renal pelvic necrosis and hematuria of Arabian horses associated with possible analgesic nephrosis. *Proc 42nd Ann Mtg Am Coll Vet Pathol* 1991, p 45.
25. Lloyd KCK, Wheat JD, Ryan AM, et al: Ulceration in the proximal portion of the urethra as a cause of hematuria in horses: four cases (1978–1985). *J Am Vet Med Assoc* 194:1324, 1989.
26. Schumacher J, Varner DD, Schmitz DG, et al: Urethral defects in geldings with hematuria and stallions with hemospermia. *Vet Surg* 24:250, 1995.
27. Voss JL, Pickett BW: Diagnosis and treatment of haemospermia in the stallion. *J Reprod Fertil* Suppl 23:151, 1975.
28. Sullins KE, Bertone JJ, Voss JL, et al: Treatment of hemospermia in stallions: A discussion of 18 cases. *Compend Contin Educ Pract Vet* 10:1396, 1988.
29. Schott HC, Hines MT: Severe urinary tract hemorrhage in two horses (Letter). *J Am Vet Med Assoc* 204:1320, 1994.
30. Glassock RJ, Adler SG, Ward HJ, et al: Primary glomerular diseases. *In* Brenner BM, Rector FC, eds. *The Kidney,* ed 4, Vol 1. Philadelphia, WB Saunders, 1991, p 1182.
31. Pardo V, Berian MG, Levi DF, et al: Benign primary hematuria: Clinicopathologic study of 65 patients. *Am J Med* 67:817, 1979.
32. Lano MD, Wagoner RD, Leary FJ: Unilateral essential hematuria. *Mayo Clin Proc* 54:88, 1979.
33. Aber GM, Higgins PM: The natural history and management of the loin pain/hematuria syndrome. *Br J Urol* 54:613, 1982.
34. Stone EA, DeNovo RC, Rawlings CA: Massive hematuria of nontraumatic renal origin in dogs. *J Am Vet Med Assoc* 183:868, 1983.
35. Holt PE, Lucke VM, Pearson H: Idiopathic renal hemorrhage in the dog. *J Small Animal Pract* 28:253, 1987.
36. Kaufman AC, Barsanti JA, Selcer BA: Benign essential hematuria in dogs. *Compend Contin Educ Pract Vet* 16:1317, 1994.
37. Morris CF, Robertson JL, Mann PC, et al: Hemolytic uremic-like syndrome in two horses. *J Am Vet Med Assoc* 191:1453, 1987.
38. Abarbanel J, Benet AE, Lask D, Kimche D: Sports hematuria. *J Urol* 143:887, 1990.
39. Blondheim SH, Margoliash E, Shafrir E: A simple test for myohemoglobinuria (myoglobinuria). *JAMA* 167:453, 1958.

16.10.

Polyuria and Polydipsia

Harold C. Schott II, DVM, PhD

For small animals, polyuria and polydipsia (PU/PD) have been defined as urine output in excess of 50 mL/kg per day and fluid intake of more than of 100 mL/kg per day.[1, 2] These values would equate to 25 L of urine production and 50 L of water consumption for a 500-kg horse. In comparison to normal values for daily urine production and water consumption of 5 to 15 L and 20 to 30 L, respectively,[3–10] these definitions of PU/PD appear applicable to horses as well. It is important to remember that urine production and water consumption vary with age, diet, work load, environmental temperature, and gastrointestinal water absorption. For example, urine production increases by 50% to 100% when the diet is changed from a grass to a legume hay.[11] Although this increase in urine production has been associated with higher dietary protein intake and urinary nitrogen excretion,[12] increases in calcium intake and urinary calcium excretion may be another contributing factor. Similarly, horses exercised heavily, stabled in hot climates, or with chronic diarrhea may have a water intake in excess of 100 L per day yet produce normal volumes of urine.[13]

A brief review of water turnover by the equine kidneys provides insight into how a small change in renal water reabsorption can lead to a dramatic increase in urine production (polyuria). In normal horses, glomerular filtration rate exceeds 1000 L per day, a volume that is 10 times greater than the total extracellular fluid volume; however, approximately 99% of this water is reabsorbed in the renal tubules and collecting ducts, resulting in production of between 5 and 15 L of urine daily. The result is urine that is three to four times more concentrated than plasma (urine osmolality 900 to 1200 mOsm/kg urine and specific gravity 1.025 to 1.050). Further, urea (in urine) has replaced sodium (in plasma) as the most important solute. If only 98% of water is reabsorbed, urine volume would double and the additional water would result in more dilute urine (urine osmolality 450 to 600 mOsm/kg urine and specific gravity 1.015 to 1.025). If water reabsorption decreased to 96% of filtered water, approximately 40 L of urine would be produced with a urine osmolality of 225 to 300 mOsm/kg and a specific gravity of 1.005 to 1.010 (Table 16–12). In the latter case, urine is more dilute than plasma (hyposthenuria) and the kidneys are actively excreting or losing water. Under certain conditions, active water excretion by the kidneys is important for maintenance of plasma osmolality in the normal range. The best example is a neonatal foal that may ingest a volume of milk in excess of 20% of its body weight daily.[14] This equates to a fluid intake approaching 250 mL/kg per day, and failure to produce a large volume of hyposthenuric urine could result in water retention, decreased plasma osmolality, and clinical hyponatremia (manifested by neurologic signs).

Determining that a horse is producing more urine than normal is often difficult, especially in horses kept at pasture. Owners may report that a horse is polyuric when in fact it is the frequency of urination which has increased (pollakiuria) rather than the volume. Pollakiuria occurs with conditions such as cystitis and urolithiasis or during estrus in the mare. Horses housed in stalls bedded with straw are difficult to evaluate, as excessive urine may not be obvious to the casual observer. For those bedded on shavings or sawdust, excessively wet bedding may be easier to recognize, but this is a subjective impression. In an occasional horse, polyuria may be so severe that urine may flow from the stall into the barn aisle. When there is doubt as to whether or not a horse has PU/PD, it may be necessary to document water consumption over one or more 24-hour periods.[6] Further, urine production can be quantified by collecting urine over a 12- or 24-hour period. For geldings and stallions, a collection device can be constructed by cutting off the bottom of a large plastic bottle which is then padded and fitted over the prepuce. The opening of the bottle is covered with a rubber tube and clip and urine can be removed every few hours. In mares, an indwelling Foley catheter can be placed in the bladder or a urine collection harness can be applied.[15–19] During the collection period, horses are usually tied to minimize interference with the collection device.

The major causes of polyuria in horses include renal failure, pituitary adenoma (Cushing's disease), and primary or "psychogenic" polydipsia.[15, 20] Less common causes include excessive salt consumption, central and nephrogenic diabetes insipidus, diabetes mellitus, sepsis and/or endotoxemia, and iatrogenic causes (sedation with α_2-agonists, corticosteroid therapy, or diuretic use).

RENAL FAILURE

In horses with acute renal failure, there is usually a transient period of anuria or oliguria. If horses survive the acute phase of renal disease, tubule damage results in a subsequent period during which impaired concentrating ability results in polyuria.[15, 21] Urine is frequently hyposthenuric during this period of tubular repair. Horses recovering from acute renal failure should be provided adequate water, salt, and a low-nitrogen (protein) and calcium diet. Such a diet can be achieved by feeding good-quality grass hay or nonlegume pasture. Repair of tubules and return of concentrating ability may take several weeks. Although these animals appear to have normal renal function after this recovery period, a permanent reduction in total renal function likely persists as most animals can maintain apparently normal health with only about 30% to 50% of functioning nephrons.

Chronic renal failure may develop consequent to damage from nephrotoxins. In addition, immune-mediated mecha-

---

Table 16–12. Relationship of the Percentage of Water Filtered That Is Reabsorbed to Daily Urine Output and Renal Water Absorption

Glomerular Filtration Rate (L/day)	Filtered Water Reabsorbed (%)	Urine Production (L/day)	Urinary Osmole Excretion	Urine Osmolality (mOsm/kg)	Renal Water Reabsorption* (L/day)
1000	99	10	10,000 mosmoles	1000	23.3
1000	98	20	10,000 mosmoles	500	13.3
1000	96	40	10,000 mosmoles	250	−6.7

*Renal water reabsorption (the inverse of free water clearance) is a calculated volume of water that is retained or lost by the kidney. It is calculated from actual urine volume, and the calculated volume of urine required to excrete all osmoles in urine that is isosmotic with plasma. In this table a urine osmolality value of 300 mOsm/kg is assumed to be isosmotic to plasma, 1 kg of water is assumed to equal 1 L of water, and a total of 10,000 osmoles is assumed to be excreted daily. Thus, when 98% of filtered water is reabsorbed, the 20 L of urine produced (if isosmotic) would contain 6000 mosmoles. Since an additional 13.3 L of water would be needed to excrete the remaining 4000 mosmoles (as isosmotic urine), the kidneys are considered to be actively reabsorbing 13.3 L of water.

nisms, chronic infection, and nephrolithiasis may also give rise to chronic renal failure.[21–23] Also, horses that do not recover from the ischemic renal damage occurring with hypovolemic or endotoxic shock may also progress to chronic renal failure. Signs are variable and include polyuria and polydipsia in some, but not all, cases. When present, PU/PD is usually moderate in comparison to the dramatic increases in urine production observed with primary polydipsia or diabetes insipidus. Most horses with chronic renal failure also exhibit other signs, including poor performance, weight loss, and ventral edema. A variable degree of azotemia is present and urinalysis reveals isosthenuria (urine is isosmotic with plasma [260 to 300 mOsm/kg] with a specific gravity of 1.008 to 1.014).

The mechanisms of polyuria consequent to acute and chronic renal failure are not entirely clear.[24] Increased tubular flow rate in surviving nephrons is one possible mechanism that would result in less time for water removal from tubular fluid. Next, medullary hypertonicity may decrease, owing to diminished transport of sodium and chloride out of tubular fluid passing through the ascending limb of Henle's loop (diluting segment of the nephron) along with increased blood flow through the remaining medullary tissue. A third possibility is impaired response of collecting ducts to vasopressin (acquired nephrogenic diabetes insipidus). Although all these mechanisms may contribute to the polyuria of renal failure, it is not known which may be most important. Further, since hyposthenuric urine can be produced during the recovery phase of acute renal failure, the mechanism(s) of polyuria are somewhat different for acute and chronic renal failure.

PITUITARY ADENOMA

Pituitary adenomas are common in older horses and result in a syndrome of hyperadrenocorticism (Cushing's disease).[25–33] Although the most consistent clinical sign is hirsutism, hyperadrenocorticism is often accompanied by polydipsia and polyuria. In addition, affected horses may show weight loss, lethargy, laminitis, and recurrent infections. An occasional horse may have neurologic signs, including blindness and/or seizures. Diagnosis is based on presence of excessive hair growth, one or more of the other clinical signs, and supportive laboratory data. In addition to hyperglycemia, there is often neutrophilia, lymphopenia, and mild anemia. Serum activity of hepatic enzymes may also be elevated. The diagnosis may be confirmed by several endocrinologic tests, including measurement of elevated plasma adrenocorticotropin (ACTH) concentration,[34] a failure of plasma cortisol concentration to decrease (suppress) after dexamethasone administration,[25, 26, 35] or an exaggerated cortisol response to administration of thyrotropin-releasing hormone.[36] Treatment with serotonin antagonists (cyproheptadine) or dopamine agonists (bromocriptine or pergolide) may modify the clinical signs but does not achieve a cure, as the pituitary lesion will continue to grow slowly.[25, 26, 37]

In one review of 17 horses with Cushing's disease due to pituitary adenoma, PU/PD was found in 13 (76%)[33]; however, in another series of 21 cases of pituitary adenoma, PU/PD was not a historical complaint in any of the affected horses.[32] Thus, the PU/PD associated with Cushing's disease is generally less severe than that observed with primary polydipsia or diabetes insipidus. Pituitary adenomas may lead to polyuria by several mechanisms. First, polyuria may be a consequence of actions of hormones derived from proopiomelanocortin, most specifically ACTH. Hyperadrenocorticism resulting from excessive ACTH activity on the adrenal cortex can lead to hyperglycemia, which may exceed the renal tubular threshold for reabsorption. The renal threshold for glucose in horses appears to be lower than in small animals (about 150 mg/dL).[38] When plasma glucose concentrations exceed this threshold value, the resultant glucosuria can lead to an osmotic diuresis. Although commonly implicated as the cause of polyuria in horses with pituitary adenomas, glucosuria was found in only one of five affected horses in a recent clinical report.[32] Further, horses with hyperglycemia and glucosuria may still be able to concentrate their urine in response to water deprivation.[29] A second mechanism implicated in the development of polyuria is antagonism of the action of vasopressin on the collecting ducts by cortisol. Although frequently cited as the mechanism of polyuria in canine hyperadrenocorticism, experimental evidence to support this mechanism is lacking in both dogs and horses. Further, there is considerable species heterogeneity in the effects of corticoids on vasopressin activity and in some species a primary dipsogenic effect may be more important. Next, growth of the adenoma may lead to impingement on the posterior pituitary and hypothalamic nuclei (located immediately dorsal to the pituitary gland), the sites of vasopressin storage and production, respectively. Decreased vasopressin production and release would result in a partial central diabetes insipidus as a third mechanism for polyuria.[26] Central diabetes insipidus, however, is not the cause of polyuria in all cases as some affected horses can concentrate their urine when deprived of water.[29] Consequently, PU/PD seen in many, but not all, horses with pituitary adenomas is likely the combined result of several mechanisms.

PRIMARY POLYDIPSIA

Although rare, primary or "psychogenic" polydipsia is probably the most common cause of PU/PD in adult horses for which clients will have a primary complaint of excessive water consumption and urination.[15, 20] This can be attributed to the fact that horses that exhibit this problem are generally in good body condition and are not azotemic. Further, the magnitude of polyuria typically is much greater than that observed with either renal failure or a pituitary adenoma. Owners may report that horses with primary polydipsia drink two to three times more water than their stablemates and their stalls are often flooded with urine. In some instances, primary polydipsia appears to be a stable vice that reflects boredom in affected horses, while in other cases it may develop following a change in environmental conditions, stabling, diet, or medication administration. Anecdotally, it is reported to be more common in southern states during periods of high temperature and humidity. In humans, primary polydipsia can be a compulsive behavior associated with mental illness or it may be caused by a primary abnormality in the osmoregulation of thirst, in which case it is referred to as "dipsogenic diabetes insipidus."[39] The latter may be idiopathic, or it may be secondary to neurologic disease involving the hypothalamic osmoreceptors regulating thirst. Excessive water consumption causes expansion and dilution of body fluids, leading to a decrease in plasma osmolality and suppression of vasopressin release. With low plasma vasopressin concentrations, collecting ducts become impermeable to water and hyposthenuria is induced to allow rate of water excretion to balance intake. In humans, the magnitude of polydipsia and resultant polyuria vary considerably between affected persons, and similar variation, although undocumented, likely occurs in affected horses as well.

The diagnosis of primary polydipsia is made by exclusion of renal failure and hyperadrenocorticism. In addition, other factors such as salt supplementation and medication administration must be excluded. Diabetes insipidus is excluded, and the diagnosis is confirmed by demonstrating urine-concentrating ability after water deprivation.[7, 9] Specific gravity should exceed 1.025 after water deprivation of sufficient duration (12 to 24 hours) to produce a 5% loss in body weight. In cases of long-standing polyuria, the osmotic gradient between the lumen of the collecting tubule and the medullary interstitium may be diminished (medullary washout). In these cases vasopressin activity may not lead to an increase in urine specific gravity to values greater than 1.020. Consequently, in horses with primary polydipsia of several weeks' duration that fail to concentrate their urine after 24 hours' water deprivation, a modified water deprivation test may be tried. This is performed by restricting water intake to approximately 40 mL/kg per day for 3 to 4 days. By the end of this time, urine specific gravity should exceed 1.025 in a horse that has had medullary washout. If the urine specific gravity remains in the isosthenuric range (1.008 to 1.014), the polyuric horse should be further evaluated for early chronic renal failure, in which urine-concentrating ability may be compromised before the onset of significant azotemia. In theory, this could occur when between two thirds and three fourths of functional nephrons have been lost. Subtle signs of decreased performance and mild weight loss would also support early renal failure. Finally, horses with primary polydipsia typically produce hyposthenuric urine. Although such dilute urine would be an unlikely finding in the early stages of chronic renal failure, it could be found in the polyuric recovery phase following acute renal failure. In the latter instance, a thorough history should reveal whether any event that may have been complicated by acute renal failure may have recently affected the horse.

Management of horses with primary polydipsia is empirical. As it is a diagnosis of exclusion, once it has been established that the horse is not suffering from a significant renal disease, it is safe to consider restricting water intake to meet maintenance, work, and environmental requirements of the horse. In addition, steps should be taken to improve the attitude of the horse by reducing boredom. Increasing the amount of exercise or turning the horse out to pasture are possible options, as is providing a companion or toys in the stall. Also, increasing the frequency of feedings or the amount of roughage in the diet may increase the time spent eating and thus reduce the habitual drinking.

EXCESSIVE SALT CONSUMPTION

In an occasional case of apparent primary polydipsia, PU/PD may be attributed to excessive salt consumption and is manifested by increased fractional sodium clearance. Such "psychogenic salt eaters" appear to be less common than "psychogenic water drinkers," as the former would have to consume a substantial amount of salt to develop polyuria. In fact, the authors are aware of only one well-documented report of psychogenic salt eating in which a yearling paint filly drank in excess of 500 mL/kg per day and had excessive urination when provided free access to salt.[40] The fractional clearances of sodium (3.4%) and chloride (2.6%) were increased, supportive of excessive intake. Although salt intake was not quantified for this filly, it may have exceeded 10% of the dry matter intake and appeared to be causally associated with muscle fasciculations and a stilted gait. Such a high intake is suggested, since no increases in water consumption or urine volume were detected in one study in which ponies were fed diets containing 1%, 3%, and 5% of sodium chloride.[41] The 5% sodium chloride diet contained five to ten times the daily requirement of sodium chloride and was similar to feeding about 350 g sodium chloride daily to a 500-kg horse. Similar to cases of primary polydipsia, the filly described in this report was able to concentrate urine in response to water deprivation, and successful management was achieved by limiting water intake to 50 mL/kg per day and preventing access to salt.

DIABETES INSIPIDUS

Diabetes insipidus (DI) results in PU/PD as a consequence of vasopressin deficiency or insensitivity of the renal collecting duct epithelial cells to vasopressin. In humans, vasopressin deficiency, or neurogenic DI, is the more common form of DI, both hereditary and acquired forms being described.[39, 42, 43] The hereditary form appears to result from decreased numbers of neurosecretory neurons in the supraoptic nuclei of the hypothalamus and is inherited in an autosomal-dominant fashion. However, PU/PD does not develop until after the first few years of life in affected persons, suggesting progressive loss of neurosecretory tissue. The acquired form of neurogenic DI results from degeneration of neurons in the supraoptic nuclei secondary to trauma, vascular abnormalities, infection, or a variety of tumors.[39, 42, 43] As with the hereditary form, PU/PD is not usually manifested until 80% to 90% of the neurosecretory neurons are destroyed.

In equidae, two well-documented cases of neurogenic DI have been described.[44, 45] Neither animal could concentrate urine in response to water deprivation, but administration of exogenous vasopressin resulted in an increase in urine concentration and a decrease in urine volume. In a Welsh pony in which the condition was considered idiopathic, the absence of an increase in plasma vasopressin concentration after water deprivation (in comparison to control ponies) further supported a diagnosis of neurogenic DI.[44] Acquired neurogenic DI secondary to encephalitis was confirmed histologically in the other horse.[45] Two other reports of DI in horses more likely described cases of primary polydipsia, since both animals demonstrated an ability to concentrate urine during water deprivation or had random urine specific gravities above 1.020.[46, 47]

Nephrogenic DI is the result of resistance of the cortical and medullary collecting ducts to the antidiuretic action of vasopressin.[39, 42, 43] In the absence of systemic disease, it is most commonly a familial disorder in humans with an X-linked semirecessive mode of inheritance. As such, the disorder is carried by females and expressed in male offspring.[48] We previously described nephrogenic DI in sibling Thoroughbred colts, suggesting that an inherited form of nephrogenic DI may also occur in horses.[49] These colts could not increase urine concentration in response to water deprivation, although they did show appropriate increases in plasma vasopressin concentration. Further, minimal response to exogenous vasopressin administration confirmed resistance of the cortical and medullary collecting ducts to the antidiuretic action of vasopressin. Nephrogenic DI may also be acquired consequent to drug therapy or a variety of metabolic, infectious, or mechanical (postobstruction) disorders. Anomalous or neoplastic disorders resulting in structural deformation of the kidneys are another potential cause of nephrogenic diabetes insipidus.[39, 42, 43]

With respect to pathophysiology, the neurogenic and nephrogenic forms of DI are similar to each other. Polyuria due to a lack of vasopressin activity results in net water loss and an increase in plasma osmolality. As plasma osmolality increases, stimulation of thirst results in a compensatory increase in water consumption. In normal individuals and those with nephrogenic DI, the increase in plasma osmolality is sensed by osmoreceptors in the hypothalamus, which subsequently provide the signal for vasopressin release. As little as a 1% increase in plasma osmolality (about 3 mOsm/kg) results in a 1 pg/mL increase in plasma vasopressin concentration. In normal individuals, this small change is substantial enough to increase urine osmolality and decrease urine flow. With greater increases in plasma osmolality, more vasopressin is secreted. In humans, urine osmolality approaches a maximum after an increase in vasopressin concentration to about 5 pg/mL (from a resting value of about 1.0 pg/mL).[39, 43]

Limited studies in ponies and horses suggest that a similar degree of vasopressin release occurs in response to minor increases in plasma osmolality[50–52]; however, vasopressin also appears to be a "stress hormone" in horses since substantially greater concentrations (10-fold higher than those induced by water deprivation) have been measured after application of a nose twitch, nasogastric intubation, or exercise.[53] Thus, increases in plasma vasopressin concentration consequent to water deprivation would be expected to be variable in horses, and it may be difficult to separate osmotic effects from stress effects in an individual horse. A word of caution is also warranted about subjecting horses with suspected DI to water deprivation. Since urine-concentrating ability may show minimal improvement with either form of DI, affected horses may continue to excrete excess water in the face of water deprivation. As a result, they may become substantially dehydrated (10% to 15%) within the first 12 hours of water deprivation. Thus, horses with suspected DI should be carefully monitored during the period of water deprivation to decrease the risk of inducing serious hypertonic dehydration. In addition to assessing the effects of water deprivation on urine-concentrating ability and plasma vasopressin concentrations, the final diagnostic manipulation is often administration of exogenous vasopressin. A suggested regimen for an adult horse is administration of 60 IU of exogenous vasopressin (pitressin synthetic, Parke-Davis) in oil every 6 hours in combination with monitoring urine specific gravity.

The medullary interstitial osmotic gradient develops as a consequence of countercurrent exchange, and the magnitude of the gradient is inversely related to tubular flow. Medullary washout may occur with the high tubular flow rates that can accompany renal disease. Although partial medullary washout may contribute to the concentrating defect in DI, the rapid response to exogenous vasopressin administration in cases of neurogenic DI (increase in urine osmolality to 900 mOsm/kg or greater) indicates that the medullary concentration gradient is not severely compromised.[39, 54] This further explains why in some cases of DI urine osmolality can be greater than plasma osmolality after water deprivation. The mechanism for this response is thought to be a decrease in tubule flow rate which allows more time for passive water extraction from the hypoosmotic tubular fluid. With nephrogenic DI, mild improvement in urine-concentrating ability (an increase in urine osmolality up to 500 mOsm/kg) may also be observed in response to exogenous vasopressin administration. This response has been attributed to partial sensitivity of the collecting ducts to vasopressin as well as vasopressin activity at other portions of the renal tubule.[39, 42]

Treatment of DI is directed at managing polydipsia and polyuria. With neurogenic DI, recovery of vasopressin secretion is rare once the secretory neurons have degenerated to the degree that PU/PD becomes apparent. Consequently, treatment consists of hormone replacement. In the past, intramuscular injection of pitressin tannate in oil every 2 to 3 days was successful in limiting polyuria; however, development of resistance or allergic reactions was an occasional problem. With the development of potent vasopressin analogs (desmopressin), effective treatment by nasal insufflation is now available.[39] The use of desmopressin for diagnosis and treatment of neurogenic DI in small animals has been described.[54, 55] Largely by chance, other oral medications, including chlorpropamide and clofibrate, have been found efficacious in treating neurogenic DI. The mechanism of action of these drugs is uncertain, but they are thought to potentiate the effect of vasopressin on the collecting ducts.[39, 54]

With nephrogenic DI, replacement hormone therapy is ineffective, and the only practical form of treatment for many years has been to restrict sodium and water intake or to administer thiazide diuretics. The latter treatment may reduce polyuria by 50% in many cases.[39] Thiazide diuretics inhibit sodium reabsorption in the distal tubule (diluting segment of the nephron) and increase solute delivery to the collecting duct. The mechanism by which such therapy paradoxically benefits patients with nephrogenic DI is ill-understood. Explanations include enhanced proximal tubular fluid reabsorption (via glomerulotubular balance) and decreased glomerular filtration and tubular flow (via a greater osmotic stimulus to the macula densa and subsequent tubuloglomerular feedback).[39, 43] Recently, treatment with prostaglandin inhibitors or amiloride has decreased polyuria in patients with nephrogenic DI. The former agents probably work by decreasing renal blood flow and glomerular filtration while the latter drug, a sodium channel blocker, is thought to act in a manner similar to the thiazide diuretic's.[39]

DIABETES MELLITUS

Diabetes mellitus (DM) is a state of chronic hyperglycemia usually accompanied by glucosuria.[56, 57] The resultant osmotic diuresis is an occasional cause of PU/PD in horses that has been described to result in a water intake in excess of 80 L per day.[58] Type I (insulin-dependent) diabetes mellitus results from a lack of insulin that in humans is usually attributable to viral or autoimmune disease. Persons with type II (non–insulin-dependent) diabetes mellitus have normal to high insulin concentrations but their tissues are insulin insensitive. Thus, the response to an oral carbohydrate load or an intravenous glucose challenge is impaired, resulting in prolonged hyperglycemia.[56] The mechanism of insulin resistance is not well-documented for horses but may be the result of decreased numbers of insulin receptors or lack of insulin receptor activation in response to insulin binding. The most common cause of equine non–insulin-dependent DM is pituitary adenoma.[27–31] With Cushing's disease, elevated plasma cortisol concentrations appear to antagonize the effect of insulin, leading to hyperglycemia and glucosuria.

Although uncommon, there are a few reports of both insulin-dependent and non–insulin-dependent DM that were not caused by a pituitary adenoma and that resulted in polyuria and polydipsia as one of the presenting complaints.[58–62] Diagnostic evaluation reveals consistent hyperglycemia but negative dexamethasone suppression test results (a normal decrease of plasma cortisol to low concentrations). Treatment in most instances is supportive, although replacement insulin therapy may be helpful in cases in which measured serum insulin concentrations are low (insulin-dependent DM). Insulin therapy may even be of some benefit in cases with elevated serum insulin concentrations, as pharmacologic doses may overcome, in part, the insulin insensitivity. In such cases, synthetic insulin products may be preferred over protamine zinc insulin, as one horse with a pituitary adenoma and secondary DM developed antiinsulin antibodies and had a relapse in clinical signs after 7 weeks of insulin therapy.[31]

SEPSIS AND/OR ENDOTOXEMIA

PU/PD has also been reported as clinical signs in horses with sepsis or endotoxemia, although other clinical signs such as fever, abdominal pain, and weight loss predominate.[63] The mechanism is unclear but may be a consequence of endotoxin-induced prostaglandin production. Prostaglandin E_2 is a potent renal vasodilating agent in laboratory animals and it antagonizes the effects of antidiuretic hormone on the collecting ducts.[64] Some horses with chronic gram-negative bacterial infections (such as peritonitis or pleuritis) may have low-grade or intermittent endotoxemia as a mechanism for polyuria, similar to the polyuria observed with canine pyometra.[65]

IATROGENIC POLYURIA

Finally, polyuria can be iatrogenic, secondary to a number of management practices or medical treatments. The most obvious iatrogenic cause is fluid therapy, for which polyuria is a desired response. Polyuria has also been observed with exogenous corticoid administration, although as for pituitary adenomas the mechanism remains unclear. People and dogs appear to experience a potent thirst response to exogenous corticoids; thus, polydipsia may be an important cause of the polyuria observed. In horses receiving long-term dexamethasone treatment for immune-mediated disorders, profound glucosuria (2 to 3 g/dL) may be observed and lead to osmotic diuresis in these patients. Finally, transient diuresis or polyuria accompanies sedation with the α_2-agonists xylazine and detomidine.[66, 67] Although these agents cause hyperglycemia, and occasionally glucosuria, a more likely mechanism for the transient polyuria is the existence of α_2-adrenoreceptors on collecting duct epithelial cells. Activation of these receptors is another mechanism by which actions of vasopressin can be antagonized.[68]

REFERENCES

1. Grauer GF: The differential diagnosis of polyuric-polydipsic diseases. *Compend Contin Educ Pract Vet* 3:1079, 1981.
2. Hughes D: Polyuria and polydipsia. *Compend Contin Educ Pract Vet* 14:1161, 1992.
3. Tasker JB: Fluid and electrolyte studies in the horse. III. Intake and output of water, sodium, and potassium in normal horses. *Cornell Vet* 56:649, 1967.
4. Fonnesbeck PV: Consumption and excretion of water by horses receiving all hay and hay-grain diets. *J Animal Sci* 27:1350, 1968.
5. Groenendyk S, English PB, Abetz I: External balance of water and electrolytes in the horse. *Equine Vet J* 20:189, 1988.
6. Sneddon JC, Colyn P: A practical system for measuring water intake in stabled horses. *J Equine Vet Sci* 11:141, 1991.
7. Rumbaugh GE, Carlson GP, Harrold D: Urinary production in the healthy horse and in horses deprived of feed and water. *Am J Vet Res* 43:735, 1982.
8. Morris DD, Divers TJ, Whitlock RH: Renal clearance and fractional excretion of electrolytes over a 24-hour period in horses. *Am J Vet Res* 45:2431, 1984.
9. Brobst DF, Bayly WM: Responses of horses to a water deprivation test. *Equine Vet Sci* 2:51, 1982.
10. Kohn CW, Strasser SL: 24 hour renal clearance and excretion of endogenous substances in the mare. *Am J Vet Res* 47:1332, 1986.
11. Cymbaluk NF: Water balance of horses fed various diets. *Equine Pract* 11(1):19, 1989.
12. Prior RL, Hintz HF, Lowe JE, et al: Urea recycling and metabolism of ponies. *J Animal Sci* 38:565, 1974.
13. Carlson GP: Fluid and electrolyte dynamics in the horse. *Proc Annu Vet Med Forum Am Coll Vet Intern Med* 5:7–29, 1987.
14. Martin RG, McMeniman NP, Dowsett KF: Milk and water intakes of foals sucking grazing mares. *Equine Vet J* 24:295, 1992.
15. Roussel AJ, Carter GK: Polydipsia and polyuria. In Brown CM, ed. *Problems in Equine Medicine.* Philadelphia, Lea & Febiger, 1989, p 150.
16. Vander Noot GW, Fonnesbeck PV, Lydman RK: Equine metabolism stall and collection harness. *J Anim Sci* 24:691, 1965.
17. Warwick IS: Urine collection apparatus for male horses. *J Sci Technol* 12:181, 1966.
18. Tasker JB: Fluid and electrolyte studies in the horse. II. An apparatus for the collection of total daily urine and faeces from horses. *Cornell Vet* 56:77, 1966.
19. Harris P: Collection of urine. *Equine Vet J* 20:86, 1988.
20. Whitlock RH: Polyuria. In Robinson NE, ed. *Current Therapy in Equine Medicine 3.* Philadelphia, WB Saunders, 1992, p 620.
21. Koterba AM, Coffman JR: Acute and chronic renal disease in the horse. *Compend Contin Educ Pract Vet* 3:S461, 1981.

22. Tennant B, Kaneko JJ, Lowe JE, et al: Chronic renal failure in the horse. *Proc Annu Conv Amer Assoc Equine Pract* 23:293, 1978.
23. Divers TJ: Chronic renal failure in horses. *Comp Contin Educ Pract Vet* 5:S310, 1983.
24. Bovée KC: Functional responses to nephron loss. In Bovée KC, ed. *Canine Nephrology.* Media, PA, Harwal, 1984, p 531.
25. Beech J: Tumors of the pituitary gland (pars intermedia). In Robinson NE, ed. *Current Therapy in Equine Medicine 2.* Philadelphia, WB Saunders, 1987, p 182.
26. Love S: Equine Cushing's disease. *Br Vet J* 149:139, 1993.
27. King JM, Kavanaugh JF, Bentinck-Smith J: Diabetes mellitus with pituitary neoplasms in a horse and a dog. *Cornell Vet* 52:133, 1962.
28. Loeb WF, Capen CC, Johnson LE: Adenomas of the pars intermedia associated with hyperglycemia and glycosuria in two horses. *Cornell Vet* 56:623, 1966.
29. Green EM, Hunt EL: Hypophyseal neoplasia in a pony. *Compend Contin Educ Pract Vet* 7:S249, 1985.
30. Horvath CJ, Ames TR, Metz AL, et al: Adrenocorticotropin-containing neoplastic cells in a pars intermedia adenoma in a horse. *J Am Vet Med Assoc* 192:367, 1988.
31. Staempfli HR, Eigenmann EJ, Clarke LM: Insulin treatment and development of anti-insulin antibodies in a horse with diabetes mellitus associated with a functional pituitary adenoma. *Can Vet J* 29:934, 1988.
32. van der Kolk JH, Kalsbeek HC, van Garderen E, et al: Equine pituitary neoplasia: a clinical report of 21 cases (1990–1992). *Vet Rec* 133:594, 1993.
33. Hillyer MH, Taylor FGR, Mair TS: Diagnosis of hyperadrenocorticism in the horse. *Equine Vet Educ* 4:131, 1992.
34. Couëtil L, Paradis MR, Knoll J: Plasma adrenocorticotropin concentration in healthy horses and in horses with clinical signs of hyperadrenocorticism. *J Vet Intern Med* 10:1, 1996.
35. Dybdal NO, Hargreaves KM, Madigan JE, et al: Diagnostic testing for pituitary pars intermedia dysfunction in horses. *J Am Vet Med Assoc* 204:627, 1994.
36. Beech J, Garcia M: Hormonal response to thyrotropin-releasing hormone in healthy horses and in horses with pituitary adenoma. *Am J Vet Res* 46:1941, 1985.
37. Beech J: Treatment of hypophysial adenomas. *Compend Contin Educ Pract Vet* 16:921, 1994.
38. Link RP: Glucose tolerance in horses. *J Am Vet Med Assoc* 97:261, 1940.
39. Robertson GL, Berl T: Pathophysiology of water metabolism. In Brenner BM, Rector FC, eds. *The Kidney,* ed 4, Vol 1. Philadelphia, WB Saunders, 1991, p 667.
40. Buntain BJ, Coffman JR: Polyuria and polydipsia in a horse induced by psychogenic salt consumption. *Equine Vet J* 13:266, 1981.
41. Schryver HF, Parker MT, Daniluk PD, et al: Salt consumption and the effect of salt on mineral metabolism in horses. *Cornell Vet* 77:122, 1987.
42. Coggins CH, Leaf A: Diabetes insipidus. *Am J Med* 42:806, 1967.
43. Robertson GL: Differential diagnosis of polyuria. *Annu Rev Med* 39:425, 1988.
44. Breukink HJ, Van Wegen P, Schotman AJH: Idiopathic diabetes insipidus in a Welsh pony. *Equine Vet J* 15:284, 1983.
45. Filar J, Ziolo T, Szalecki J: Diabetes insipidus in the course of encephalitis in the horse. *Medycyna Weterynaryjna* 27:205, 1971.
46. Chenault L: Diabetes insipidus in the equine. *Southwest Vet* 22:321, 1969.
47. Satish C, Sastry KNV: Equine diabetes insipidus—a case report. *Indian Vet J* 55:584, 1978.
48. Forssman H: Two different mutations of the X-chromosome causing diabetes insipidus. *Am J Human Genet* 7:21, 1955.
49. Schott HC, Bayly WM, Reed SM, et al: Nephrogenic diabetes insipidus in sibling colts. *J Vet Intern Med* 7:68, 1993.
50. Houpt KA, Thorton SN, Allen WR: Vasopressin in dehydrated and rehydrated ponies. *Physiol Behav* 45:659, 1989.
51. Irvine CHG, Alexander SL, Donald RA: Effect of an osmotic stimulus on the secretion of arginine vasopressin and adrenocorticotropin in the horse. *Endocrinology* 124:3102, 1989.
52. Sneddon JC, van der Walt J, Mitchell G, et al: Effects of dehydration and rehydration on plasma vasopressin and aldosterone in horses. *Physiol Behav* 54:223, 1993.
53. Nyman S, Hydbring E, Dahlborn K: Is vasopressin a "stress hormone" in the horse? *Pferdeheilkunde* 12:419, 1996.
54. Greene CE, Wong P, Finco DR: Diagnosis and treatment of diabetes insipidus in two dogs using two synthetic analogs of antidiuretic hormone. *J Am Anim Hosp Assoc* 15:371, 1979.
55. Kraus KH: The use of desmopressin in diagnosis and treatment of diabetes insipidus in cats. *Compend Contin Educ Pract Vet* 9:752, 1987.
56. Corke MJ: Diabetes mellitus: The tip of the iceberg (Editorial). *Equine Vet J* 18:87, 1986.
57. Taylor FGR, Hillyer MH: The differential diagnosis of hyperglycemia in horses. *Equine Vet Educ* 4:135, 1992.
58. Muylle E, van den Hende C, DePrez P, et al: Non-insulin dependent diabetes mellitus in a horse. *Equine Vet J* 18:143, 1986.
59. Siegel ET: Diabetes mellitus in a horse. *J Am Vet Med Assoc* 149:1016, 1966.
60. Jeffrey JR: Diabetes mellitus secondary to chronic pancreatitis in a pony. *J Am Vet Med Assoc* 153:1168, 1968.
61. Baker JR, Richie HE: Diabetes mellitus in the horse: a case report and review of the literature. *Equine Vet J* 6:7, 1974.
62. Ruoff WW, Baker DC, Morgan SJ, et al: Type II diabetes mellitus in a horse. *Equine Vet J* 18:143, 1986.
63. Traver DS, Moore JN, Coffman JR, et al: Peritonitis in a horse: A cause of acute abdominal distress and polyuria-polydipsia. *J Equine Med Surg* 1:36, 1977.
64. Kinter LB, Huffman WF, Stassen FL: Antagonists of the antidiuretic activity of vasopressin. *Am J Physiol* 254:F165, 1988.
65. Hardy RM, Osborne CA: Canine pyometra: Pathophysiology, diagnosis and treatment of uterine and extra-uterine lesions. *J Am Anim Hosp Assoc* 10:245, 1974.
66. Thurmon JC, Steffey EP, Zinkl JG, et al: Xylazine causes transient dose-related hyperglycemia and increased urine volume in mares. *Am J Vet Res* 45:224, 1984.
67. Trim CM, Hanson RR: Effects of xylazine on renal function and plasma glucose in ponies. *Vet Rec* 118:65, 1986.
68. Gellai M: Modulation of vasopressin antidiuretic action by renal α_2-adrenoceptors. *Am J Physiol* 259:F1, 1990.

16.11

Renal Tubular Acidosis

Warwick M. Bayly, BVSc, MS

It is well-recognized that horses with acute or chronic renal failure are frequently acidotic. These animals are almost invariably azotemic, hypochloremic, and normo- or hyperkalemic and frequently have marked abnormalities on urinalysis. A less frequent renal disease associated with acidosis is renal tubular acidosis (RTA). RTA is a clinical syndrome of impaired renal acidification characterized by a hypokalemic, hyperchloremic acidosis without azotemia. Affected horses frequently have normal urinalysis. The condition has been well-described in humans,[1-3] and several case reports documenting its existence in horses have appeared since the mid-1980s.[4-7]

The causes and pathogenic mechanisms responsible for the development of RTA are ill-understood. In humans it may be primary (genetic or idiopathic) or secondary to a variety of conditions, including hyperglobulinemia, various autoimmune disorders, kidney disease such as polynephritis and obstructive uropathy, cirrhosis, drug- or toxin-induced nephropathies (including amphotericin B toxicity), metabolic disorders involving nephrocalcinosis, and a number of genetically transmitted diseases. All reported equine cases have apparently been idiopathic as no signs of primary renal, hepatic, or autoimmune disease, or disturbance of calcium metabolism have been evident, and there has been no history of access to toxins. In some cases, however, low-grade renal tubular disease has been suspected because of mild proteinuria.

It is generally agreed that there are three types of RTA.[8] Type I, which is also known as "distal or classic" RTA, arises from the inability of the cells of the distal tubule to establish a steep hydrogen ion gradient between the blood and the urine. This results from failure of normal hydrogen ion (H^+) excretion from the distal tubules. In many cases, this gradient may be less than 10:1. It is not clear whether this is because of an insufficient number of proton-secreting pumps in the distal nephron, or because H^+ diffuses back across the lumenal membrane after it has been secreted. Accelerated potassium (K^+) secretion occurs owing to the existing electrochemical driving forces in the distal nephron and the lack of protons to offset them. As well as having high urinary K^+ clearances, patients may be hypercalciuric and hyperphosphaturic, although in horses this may be difficult to assess. Equine urinary concentrations of K^+ and calcium in particular, are quite high. In humans, about 70% of adults with distal RTA develop some form of urolithiasis.[9] This has not been recognized in the few reported equine cases, and may not be, given the marked differences between the two species.

Type II, or proximal, RTA is caused by a failure of bicarbonate ion (HCO_3^-) resorption in the proximal tubule. This part of the nephron usually reabsorbs the bulk of the filtered HCO_3^- via sodium (NA^+)-H^+ exchange and the subsequent breakdown of carbonic acid to carbon dioxide (CO_2) and water under the influence of carbonic anhydrase. Disruption of normal Na^+-H^+ exchange or carbonic anhydrase activity therefore results in excess flow of HCO_3^- to the distal tubule where the ability to resorb the anion is relatively poor. This bicarbonaturia also results in accelerated K^+ secretion and hypokalemia. In people with this form of the disease it has been suggested that there is a reduction in the threshold concentration at which HCO_3^- is reabsorbed from the proximal nephron. As a result, reabsorption is resumed once serum HCO_3^- concentration drops below this threshold and a new steady state is said to develop. More likely, because of the urinary HCO_3^- loss, plasma HCO_3^- concentration decreases, as does glomerular filtration of

HCO_3^-. Eventually a point is reached where the distal tubule can handle the amount of HCO_3^- presented. Urine pH may start to decrease because of the lower amount of HCO_3^- being excreted. A new steady plasma HCO_3^- concentration is established, albeit considerably below the normal range, and acid-base homeostasis may gradually return. Consequently, the type II condition often appears to be self-limiting in humans.[10] This form of the disease occurs rarely by itself in humans and is almost always associated with other signs of proximal tubule dysfunction such as defective resorption of glucose, amino acids, and phosphate (Fanconi's syndrome). Type II RTA has been reported in two horses.[4]

Type IV RTA is characterized by hyperkalemic, hyperchloremic acidosis and is quite common in humans, but it has not been reported in horses. It is apparently associated with hypoaldosteronism or resistance of the distal nephron cells to the effects of aldosterone. As a result, there is a reduction in the renal clearance of both K^+ and H^+. The associated natriuresis may ultimately lead to a reduced ability to concentrate urine due to "washout" of the medullary concentrating gradient, if the condition becomes chronic. Another form of RTA (type III) which had formerly been described as having characteristics of both type I and type II RTA is now considered to be a variation of type I.[8]

Differentiating between the distal (H^+ retention) and proximal (HCO_3^--wasting) forms of RTA is theoretically important if the approach to the human form of the disease is any guide. This is because, in humans, the two types differ with respect to clinical severity, treatment, and prognosis.[11] In horses, the ability to differentiate between the forms of the disease appears to be less critical, as treatment does not seem to differ much according to the suspected type of RTA. Some differential characteristics of the two types of the disease are summarized in Table 16–13. In people with type II RTA, plasma HCO_3^- concentrations tend to be higher than those associated with the distal form of the disease. This does not appear to be the case in horses, as all the cases we have seen, plus those that have been described in the literature, have been severely acidotic (HCO_3^- concentrations of 10 mmol/L or less). In horses, differentiation between the distal and proximal types of the condition has been based on measurement of the urine pH. Evaluation of urine ammonium excretion, urine net charge or anion gap, and urinary P_{CO_2} have not been reported in horses, although they are regarded as critical to the specific differentiation of RTA in people.[12-14] Owing to the alkalinity of normal equine urine, measurement of urine P_{CO_2} is probably of little benefit. With type I RTA, urine pH tends to stay high (i.e., in the normal to alkaline range). In type II it is generally neutral or slightly acidic. A suggested way of making this differentiation is to assess the urinary response to the administration of the urine-acidifying agent ammonium chloride (0.1 g/kg). Typically, this solution is given orally and should lower the urine pH below 7.0, which it supposedly does in normal horses and those with type II RTA. In cases of distal (type I) RTA, the urine pH remains high in the face of the increased acid load. Because the administration of such acidifying agents could potentially worsen the degree of acidosis in cases of type II RTA because of reduced buffering capacity, it is not recommended that this test be performed until at least partial replacement of the HCO_3^- deficit has been attempted. In our hands, the ammonium chloride challenge

Table 16–13. Features Used to Differentiate Type I and Type II Renal Tubular Acidosis

Variable	Type I	Type II
Acidosis	Severe	Less severe, self-limiting
Hypokalemia	Severe	Mild to moderate
Glycosuria, proteinuria	Absent	Often present
Urine pH during		
Mild/mod acidosis	Inappropriately high	Inappropriately high
Severe acidosis	Inappropriately high	Normal
Effect of alkali administration	Decreases or worsens hypokalemia, depending on stage of disease	Worsens hypokalemia
Amount of HCO_3^- needed to correct acidosis	Low	High
Ammonium chloride challenge	Failure to excrete acid (urine does not acidify)	Urine pH decreases
Bicarbonate loading	Filtered bicarbonate is reabsorbed	Bicarbonate is lost in the urine

test has proven unreliable, having failed to acidify the urine of normal healthy horses even when given intravenously in a 4-L solution. The dose and rate of administration may need to be increased before it can be considered a worthwhile test. A more suitable alternative may be to infuse sodium sulfate as is sometimes done in humans.[1] We could find no reports of this test's use in horses.

Another diagnostic option that may be worthy of investigation in horses is calculation of the urine net charge. As in any body fluid, the sum of urinary cations must equal the sum of its anions. Therefore, in urine,

$$Na^+ + K^+ + Ca^{++} + Mg^{++} + NH_4^+ = Cl^- + HPO^{--} + SO^{--} + \text{other urine buffers} + \text{organic anions}.$$

In humans, Ca^{++} and Mg^{++} tend to be present in urine in small, quite constant quantities. Excretion of phosphate, sulfate, titratable buffers, and organic anions is also relatively constant and exceeds the Ca^{++} and Mg^{++} by an amount that is referred to as the "urine anion gap" (AG_u). Thus,

$$Na^+ + K^+ - Cl^- = AG_u - NH_4^+$$

($Na^+ + K^+ - Cl^-$) is referred to as the "urine net charge" and reflects the excretion of ammonium (NH_4^+).[13] Given the aforementioned plasma electrolyte and acid-base abnormalities, it has been shown that type II RTA likely exists when the urine net charge is negative (i.e., $Cl^- > [Na^+ + K^+]$) because $NH_4^+ > AG_u$. In other words, H^+ continues to be secreted normally from the distal tubule, and plenty of NH_4^+ is being produced. When ($Na^+ + K^+$) > Cl^-, the net charge is positive, indicating that NH_4^+ excretion is low, owing to failure to excrete H^+ (i.e., type I or distal RTA exists).

Horses with RTA usually present with a history of severe, progressive weakness, depression, and anorexia. Various other signs such as chronic weight loss, ataxia, dysphagia, and periodic collapse have also been noted. The latter three signs may all be manifestations of severe weakness, which is probably due to the severe hypokalemia. The reduced K^+ concentration may also be associated with bradycardia.

On clinical examination, affected horses are usually afebrile. Mild icterus is quite common, presumably because of the anorexia, although marked indirect hyperbilirubinemia and increases in serum concentrations of γ-glutamyltransferase and alkaline phosphatase have been observed. Although cirrhosis of the liver has been associated with the development of RTA in humans, the equine cases of which we are aware have demonstrated no clinicopathologic changes that are compatible with severe liver disease. Sulfobromophthalein clearance half-time was normal in the one case in which it was measured.[5]

RTA should be suspected whenever a horse has a severe hyperchloremic metabolic acidosis in the absence of any obvious cause of extrarenal hypovolemia such as diarrhea or small intestinal ileus. In such cases the plasma anion gap is usually widened, while it remains normal with RTA. (However, hypoalbuminemia may mask widening of the anion gap because albumin is normally responsible for much of the normal anion gap.[15] Therefore, its value should be smaller in hypoalbuminemic horses.) Azotemia has not been recognized in cases of equine RTA, although signs of tubular dysfunction such as mild proteinuria and increases in fractional K^+ clearance and urine γ-glutamyltransfcrase activity have been observed. The results from renal biopsy and ultrasonic examination of the kidneys are normal.

Definitive diagnosis of RTA is based on the demonstration of severe hypokalemia (2.3 mmol/L or less) and a urine pH that is generally either neutral or alkaline in the face of a severe acidosis (venous blood pH below 7.15), although slight aciduria could theoretically be observed with type II RTA. Hypokalemia in the face of severe acidosis is extremely uncommon. Classically, the reverse is expected, owing to intracellular buffering of H^+ and the reciprocal role of H^+ and K^+ in maintaining the electrical neutrality of the extracellular fluid. Occasionally, serum chloride concentrations are in the high normal range rather than being increased. Blood gas measurement usually reveals some degree of compensatory respiratory alkalosis (P_{CO_2} = 25–35 torr).

The differential diagnosis of RTA includes those of any animal that presents with sudden weakness, depression, and possible collapse: cardiovascular failure, neurologic disease (including rabies), hypoglycemia, and peracute toxemia or endotoxemia. All of these can usually be ruled out on the basis of a thorough physical examination that finds nothing to support their possible existence. These findings, plus demonstration of the aforementioned electrolyte and acid-base abnormalities, are very suggestive of RTA. Conditions such as hypokalemic periodic paralysis, Addison's disease, adenoma of the pars intermedia of the pituitary, and chronic corticosteroid or diuretic abuse could cause some of these clinicopathologic disturbances, but not the combination of hyperchloremia, acidosis, hypokalemia, and a normal plasma anion gap.

It is important that the disease be promptly recognized and therapy instituted quickly, as the untreated condition is potentially fatal. All reported equine cases of RTA have responded satisfactorily to treatment, as have the cases we have seen. While the ability to differentiate between type I and type II RTA may be important in humans from a therapeutic perspective, it has not seemed to be essential in horses. Regardless of the suspected type of the disease, treatment of the condition in horses is associated with HCO_3^- and K^+ replacement therapy. Although the administration of $KHCO_3$ would seem to be ideal, the lack of ready availability of this substance and the need for prompt therapy means that treatment usually involves a combination of oral potassium chloride and intravenous sodium bicarbonate and potassium chloride. It must be emphasized that sodium bicarbonate should not be given without some form of potassium supplementation, to ensure that the hypokalemia does not get worse. Generally, a steady improvement in the patient's condition is seen following 12 to 24 hours of treatment. All fluids are usually given four to six times per day for the first 48 hours while intravenous fluids are frequently given at a slow but steady rate. Inclusion of glucose or dextrose in the latter helps to promote uptake of potassium by the cells. The serum chloride concentration usually decreases as HCO_3^- concentration increases. In our experience, a steady improvement is seen in HCO_3 values, and these tend to improve more rapidly than the potassium concentrations. Serum concentrations of the latter appear to be slower to return to normal, possibly because intracellular stores are replaced first. It is impossible to estimate the total potassium deficit before the onset of treatment because of the huge intracellular deficit these animals suffer. In our experience, total deficits of this cation frequently exceed 4000 mmol.

With the correction of the acid-base and electrolyte disturbances, muscle strength and appetite generally return within 48 hours of the onset of treatment. At this point, potassium supplementation can usually be reduced and subsequently discontinued once the horse's forage intake has returned to normal. It is obviously very important that the horse be given a diet that includes ample amounts of good-quality hay, owing to the high potassium content of this feedstuff. Bicarbonate therapy generally continues longer, although intravenous assistance is usually discontinued with return of the animal's appetite. Periodic rechecking of the animal is advised until it becomes clear that its condition is stable. Long-term follow-up of cases we have seen and those that have been reported in the literature suggest that the prognosis is favorable.

REFERENCES

1. Gennari FJ, Cohen JJ: Renal tubular acidosis. *Annu Rev Med* 29:521, 1978.
2. Coe FL, Brenner BM: Renal tubular acidosis. In Isselbacher KJ, et al, eds. *Harrison's Principles of Internal Medicine,* ed 9. New York, McGraw-Hill, 1980.
3. Morris RC, Sebastian A: Disorders of the renal tubule that cause disorders of fluid, acid-base and electrolyte metabolism. In Maxwell MH, Kleeman DR, eds. *Clinical Disorders of Fluid and Electrolyte Metabolism,* ed 3. New York, McGraw-Hill, 1980, pp 883–946.
4. Trotter GW, Miller D, Parks A, et al: Type II renal tubular acidosis in a mare. *J Am Vet Med Assoc* 188:1050, 1986.
5. Hansen TO: Renal tubular acidosis in a mare. *Compend Contin Educ Pract Vet* 8:864, 1986.
6. Ziemer EL, Parker HR, Carlson GP, et al: Renal tubular acidosis in two horses: diagnostic studies. *J Am Vet Med Assoc* 190:289, 1987.
7. van der Kolk JH, Kalsbeek HC: Renal tubular acidosis in a mare. *Vet Rec* 133:44, 1993.
8. Rose BD: Clinical Physiology of Acid-Base and Electrolyte Disorders, ed 3. New York, McGraw-Hill, 1989, p 527.
9. Van den Berg CJ, Harrington TM, Bunch TW, et al: Treatment of renal lithiasis associated with renal tubular acidosis. *Proc Eur Dial Transplant Assoc* 20:473, 1983.
10. Battle D: Renal tubular acidosis. Symposium on acid-base disorders. *Med Clin North Am* 67:859, 1983.
11. Kauffman CE, Selsenfelv HA, Vanatta JV, et al: Potassium. In Frolich ED, ed. *Pathophysiology: Altered Regulatory Mechanisms in Disease.* Philadelphia, JB Lippincott, 1984, pp 249–255.
12. Halperin ML, Richardson RMA, Bear R, et al: Urine ammonium: The key to the diagnosis of distal renal tubular acidosis. *Nephron* 50:1, 1988.
13. Goldstein MB, Bear R, Richardson RMA, et al: The urine anion gap: A clinically useful index of ammonium excretion. *Am J Med Sci* 292:198, 1986.
14. Rodriguez-Soriano J, Vallo A: Renal tubular acidosis. *Pediatr Nephrol* 4:268, 1990.
15. van Leeuwen AM: Net cation equivalency (base-binding power) of the plasma proteins. *Acta Med Scand* 176(Suppl 422):36, 1964.

16.12.

Neoplasia of the Urinary Tract

Harold C. Schott II, DVM, PhD

Although neoplasia of the urinary tract is uncommon in horses,[1-6] there are reports of tumors involving both the upper and lower urinary tract in this species. Renal neoplasms, which represent fewer than 1% of all equine tumors, include adenomas, renal cell carcinomas, and nephroblastomas.[7] Renal adenomas are small, well-circumscribed lesions in the renal cortex, which are usually incidental necropsy findings.[8] The best-described renal tumor in the horse is renal cell carcinoma or adenocarcinoma.[9-16] These lesions arise from epithelium of the proximal convoluted tubules in most cases. In humans, renal cell carcinomas are known as the "internist's tumor" because of their diverse and often obscure presenting signs. Although a classic triad of symptoms including flank pain, gross hematuria, and palpable renal mass has been described, it is seen in fewer than 10% of affected humans at presentation.[17] Similarly, affected horses usually have nonspecific presenting complaints, including poor performance, depression, weight loss, and/or recurrent colic (Table 16–14). Signs that increase suspicion of a primary urinary tract problem include hematuria (7 of 12 cases in Table 16–14) and detection of a palpable mass on rectal examination (8 of 12 cases in Table 16–14). Renal cell carcinomas are typically unilateral, and normal renal function is maintained by the contralateral kidney. Although

Table 16–14. Clinical Features of 12 Horses with Renal Cell Carcinoma

Breed	Age (yr)	Sex	Unilateral or Bilateral	Presenting Complaint	Weight Loss	Pain/ Colic	Hematuria	Palpable Mass on Rectal Examination?	Azotemia	Post-Mortem Findings	Reference
American saddlebred	15	G	Bilateral	Recurrent colic	Yes	Yes	No	Yes	No	25-cm diameter mass, renal calculus, metastases to liver and other kidney	Berggren (1980)
Albino	10	F	Unilateral, left	Abortion and ascites	No	No	No	Yes	Mild	75-cm diameter, 31-kg mass, metastases to peritoneum	Haschek et al. (1981)
Standardbred	16	F	Unilateral, right	Weight loss, hematuria	Yes	No	Yes	Yes	No	30-cm diameter, 8-kg mass, adhesions to liver and bowel, no metastases	Haschek et al. (1981)
Thorough-bred	6	F	Unilateral, left	Weight loss	Yes	No	Yes	Yes	Mild	35-cm diameter, 20-kg mass, hemoperi-toneum, no metastases	Pomroy (1981)
Thorough-bred	16	F	Unilateral, right	Weight loss, soft feces	Yes	No	No	No	Mild	Metastases to liver and lungs	van Amstel et al. (1984)
Pony	15	G	Unilateral, left	Weight loss, hematuria	Yes	No	Yes	Yes	No	6.6-kg mass, metastases to liver and lungs	Brown and Holt (1986)
Pony	10	G	Unilateral, right	Weight loss, back pain, colic, PU/PD	Yes	Yes	Yes	No	No	6-cm diameter mass, hemoperi-toneum, no metastases	Brown and Holt (1986)
Thorough-bred	4	G	Unilateral, left	Respiratory noise	No	No	NR	NR	No	30-cm diameter mass, local invasion of sublumbar muscles	Brown and Holt (1986)
Grade	7	G	Unilateral, right	Hematuria, followed by weight loss and colic	Yes	Yes	Yes	No	Mild	40-cm diameter, 23-kg mass, hemothorax and hemoperi-toneum, metastases to liver and lungs	Brown and Holt (1986)
Thorough-bred	9	F	Unilateral, right	Recurrent colic, weight loss	Yes	Yes	No	Yes	No	30-cm diameter mass, metastases to omentum and muscle	Van Mol and Fransen (1986)
Shire	4	F	Unilateral, right	Hematuria, followed by weight loss	Yes	Yes	Yes	Yes	No	65-cm diameter, 47.7-kg mass, adhesion to liver and bowel, no metastases	Owen et al. (1986)
Grade	14	F	Unilateral, left	Pyrexia, hematuria, diarrhea	Yes	No	Yes	Yes	No	5-kg mass; metastases to liver, pancreas, and lungs	West et al. (1987)

G, gelding; F, mare; PU/PD, polyuria and polydipsia; NR, not reported.

nephrectomy is the treatment of choice in humans, tumors are typically quite large and adherent to surrounding organs by the time they are detected in horses. Thus, surgical removal usually is not possible. Further, frequent metastases (8 of 12 cases in Table 16–14) are another indication that renal adenocarcinoma is usually not a treatable disease. This can be attributed to the fact that clinical signs of intraabdominal neoplasia in horses often are not apparent until the disease is quite advanced.[18] In one report of renal carcinoma, clinical signs of the tumor were absent until the horse was anesthetized for laryngeal surgery. After an uncomplicated surgery, the horse was repositioned for recovery but died shortly thereafter. Compression of the caudal vena cava by a large renal carcinoma was suspected to lead to a decrease in venous return as the cause of sudden death.[19] Other neoplastic diseases that may affect the kidneys include nephroblastoma,[20–22] transitional cell carcinoma,[18, 23] and squamous cell carcinoma.[24] Nephroblastoma (Wilms' tumor) is an embryonal tumor that arises in primitive nephrogenic tissue or in foci of dysplastic renal tissue, whereas the latter tumor types arise from the uroepithelium of the renal pelvis or ureter.[8] Neoplastic involvement of the upper urinary tract may also occur with dissemination of lymphosarcoma, hemangiosarcoma, melanoma, or adenocarcinoma arising from other tissues in the abdomen.[2, 7, 8, 18, 25] Finally, although they are not truly cancerous disease processes, mucinous hyperplasia of the renal pelvic and proximal ureteral uroepithelium or ureteropelvic polyp formation can also lead to development of a tissue mass in the area of either kidney, ureteral obstruction, and hydronephrosis.[26, 27]

In addition to rectal palpation for a mass in the area of either kidney and examination of urine for red blood cells (hematuria), ultrasonographic evidence of a tissue mass destroying the normal architecture of the kidney would support renal neoplasia. Unfortunately, attempts to establish a definitive antemortem diagnosis were successful in only two previous reports. In the first case, neoplastic cells were detected on analysis of a sample of peritoneal fluid,[12] while percutaneous biopsy of the tissue mass in a second horse demonstrated neoplastic tissue. Thus, these procedures are warranted in all horses with a mass consistent with a renal neoplasm. In addition to analyzing urine for hematuria, cytologic examination of urine for neoplastic cells is also warranted.[28]

The most common presenting complaint for bladder neoplasia is hematuria.[28–30] Unlike dogs, in which transitional cell carcinoma is the most commonly described bladder neoplasm, squamous cell carcinoma has been reported most frequently in horses.[28, 29] Other types of bladder neoplasms affecting horses include transitional cell carcinoma, lymphosarcoma, leiomyosarcoma, and fibromatous polyps. In contrast to cattle, which develop bladder neoplasia in association with chronic ingestion of bracken fern and other plants (enzootic hematuria), dietary factors have not been incriminated in development of bladder cancer in horses.[8] Diagnosis of bladder neoplasms can be established by palpation or ultrasonographic imaging of a bladder mass, endoscopic examination and biopsy (Fig. 16–39), and urine cytology. Treatment has included partial bladder resection or intravesicular instillation of 5-fluorouracil, but successful outcomes have not been reported.[28] Again, a poor prognosis is likely related to the extensive bladder involvement by the time clinical signs are noted.

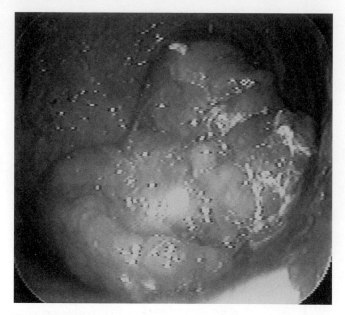

Figure 16–39. Leiomyosarcoma of the urinary bladder resulted in hematuria. (Courtesy of Dr. R. MacKay, University of Florida.)

Tumors of the urethra and external genitalia are the most common urinary tract neoplasms of horses. Although there are reports of a paraurethral lipoma[31] and fibrosarcomas[32] resulting in frequent urination or dribbling and urinary tract infection, respectively, tumors of the external genitalia are more common than urethral tumors.[33–35] Tumors affecting the external genitalia include squamous cell carcinoma, sarcoid, melanoma, mastocytoma, hemangioma, and papillomas or warts. Habronemiasis used to be a significant cause of genital lesions before the use of ivermectin, and it should remain on the differential list since it can be distinguished from squamous cell carcinoma or sarcoid only by examination of a biopsy sample. Breeds with nonpigmented genitalia (Appaloosas and paints) appear to be predisposed to squamous cell carcinoma. Similarly, a predilection for geldings and stallions has been associated with a carcinogenic potential of smegma.[36] Affected horses may have a malodorous sheath or hematuria if the distal urethra is involved. Urinary tract obstruction is uncommon unless the tumors are quite large. Diagnosis is by visual examination and collection of a biopsy sample. Collection of the latter is often performed by complete excision of the lesion. In addition to surgical excision, a rather high rate of recurrence has led to use of a number of adjunctive therapies, including immunotherapy, cryotherapy, hyperthermia, and radiation therapy. Since all treatment combinations have had variable success, some authors recommend aggressive surgical treatment early in the course of the disease.[37] Most recently, local injection of cisplatin, a cytotoxic antineoplastic agent, has been used with a high success rate to treat equine sarcoid and squamous cell carcinoma.[38, 39]

REFERENCES

1. Modransky PD: Neoplastic and anomalous conditions of the urinary tract. In Robinson NE, ed. *Current Therapy in Equine Medicine 2.* Philadelphia, WB Saunders, 1987, p 720.

2. Divers TJ: Diseases of the renal system. In Smith BP, ed. *Large Animal Internal Medicine.* St. Louis, CV Mosby, 1990, p 872.
3. Keller H: Diseases of the urinary system. In Wintzer HJ, ed. *Equine Diseases: A Textbook for Students and Practitioners.* New York, Springer-Verlag, 1986, p 148.
4. Brown CM: Equine nephrology. *Vet Annu* 26:1, 1986.
5. Sundberg JP, Burnstein T, Page EH, et al: Neoplasms of equidae. *J Am Vet Med Assoc* 170:150, 1977.
6. Cotchin E: A general survey of tumors in the horse. *Equine Vet J* 9:16, 1977.
7. Madewell BR, Theilen GH: Tumors of the urogenital tract: Part 1. Tumors of the urinary tract. In Theilen GH, Madewell BR, eds. *Veterinary Cancer Medicine,* ed 2. Philadelphia, Lea & Febiger, 1987, p 567.
8. Maxie MG: The urinary system. In Jubb KVF, Kennedy PC, Palmer N, eds. *Pathology of Domestic Animals,* ed 3, Vol 2. San Diego, Academic Press, 1985, p 343.
9. Berggren PC: Renal adenocarcinoma in a horse. *J Am Vet Med Assoc* 176:1252, 1980.
10. Haschek WM, King JM, Tennant BC: Primary renal cell carcinoma in two horses. *J Am Vet Med Assoc* 179:992, 1981.
11. Pomroy W: Renal adenocarcinoma in a horse. *Equine Vet J* 13:198, 1981.
12. Van Amstel SR, Huchzermeyer, Reyers F: Primary renal cell carcinoma in a horse. *J South Afr Vet Assoc* 55:35, 1984.
13. Brown PJ, Holt PE: Primary renal cell carcinoma in four horses. *Equine Vet J* 17:473, 1985.
14. Van Mol KAC, Fransen JLA: Renal carcinoma in a horse. *Vet Rec* 119:238, 1986.
15. Owen RR, Haywood S, Kelly DF: Clinical course of renal adenocarcinoma associated with hypercupraemia in a horse. *Vet Rec* 119:291, 1986.
16. West HJ, Kelly DF, Ritchie HE: Renal carcinomatosis in a horse. *Equine Vet J* 19:548, 1987.
17. Garnick MB, Richie JP: Renal neoplasia. In Brenner BM, Rector FC, eds. *The Kidney,* ed 4, Vol 2. Philadelphia, WB Saunders, 1991, p 1809.
18. Traub JL, Bayly WM, Reed SM, et al: Intraabdominal neoplasia as a cause of chronic weight loss in the horse. *Compend Contin Educ Pract Vet* 5:S526, 1983.
19. Robertson SA, Waterman AE, Lane JG, Brown PJ: An unusual cause of anaesthetic death in a horse. *Equine Vet J* 17:403, 1985.
20. Nyka W: Sur une tumeur renal du cheval issue du blastème métanéphrique. *Bull Cancer* 17:241, 1928.
21. Köhler H: Nephroblastom in der Niere eines Pferds. *Dtsch Tierärztl Wschr* 84:400, 1977.
22. Jardine JE, Nesbit JW: Triphasic nephroblastoma in a horse. *J Comp Pathol* 114:193, 1996.
23. Servantie J, Magnol JP, Regnier A, et al: Carcinoma of the renal pelvis with bony metaplasia in a horse. *Equine Vet J* 18:236, 1986.
24. Vivotec J: Carcinomas of the renal pelvis in slaughter animals. *J Comp Pathol* 87:129, 1977.
25. Carrick JB, Morris DD, Harmon BG, Faezi M: Hematuria and weight loss in a mare with pancreatic adenocarcinoma. *Cornell Vet* 82:91, 1992.
26. Kim DY, Cho DY, Snider III TG: Mucinous hyperplasia in the kidney and ureter of horse. *J Comp Pathol* 110:309, 1994.
27. Jones SL, Langer DL, Sterner-Kock A, et al: Renal dysplasia and benign ureteropelvic polyps associated with hydronephrosis in a foal. *J Am Vet Med Assoc* 204:1230, 1994.
28. Fischer AT, Spier S, Carlson GP, Hackett RP: Neoplasia of the urinary bladder as a cause of hematuria. *J Am Vet Med Assoc* 186:1294, 1985.
29. Lloyd KCK, Wheat JD, Ryan AM, Matthews M: Ulceration in the proximal portion of the urethra as a cause of hematuria in horses: Four cases (1978–1985). *J Am Vet Med Assoc* 194:1324, 1989.
30. Sweeney RW, Hamir AN, Fisher RR: Lymphosarcoma with urinary bladder infiltration in a horse. *J Am Vet Med Assoc* 199:1177, 1991.
31. Sertich PL, Hamir AN, Orsini P, et al: Paraurethral lipoma in a mare associated with frequent urination. *Equine Vet Educ* 2:121, 1990.
32. Sloet van Oldruitenborgh-Oosterbaan MM, Klabec HC: Ureteropyelonephritis in a Fresian mare. *Vet Rec* 122:609, 1988.
33. Walker DF, Vaughan JT: *Bovine and Equine Urogenital Surgery.* Philadelphia, Lea & Febiger, 1980, p 125.
34. Schumacher J: Surgery of the prepuce and penis. In Auer JA, ed. *Equine Surgery.* Philadelphia, WB Saunders, 1992, p 703.
35. Schumacher J, Varner DD: Neoplasia of the stallion's reproductive tract. In McKinnon AO, Voss JL, eds. *Equine Reproduction.* Philadelphia, Lea & Febiger, 1993, p 871.
36. Plaut A, Kohn-Speyer AC: The carcinogenic action of smegma. *Science* 105:656, 1947.
37. Markel MD, Wheat JD, Jones K: Genital neoplasms treated by en bloc resection and penile retroversion in horses: 10 cases (1977–1986). *J Am Vet Med Assoc* 192:396, 1988.
38. Théon AP, Pascoe JR, Carlson GP, et al: Intratumoral chemotherapy with cisplatin in oily emulsion in horses. *J Am Vet Med Assoc* 202:261, 1993.
39. Théon AP, Pascoe JR, Meagher DM: Perioperative intratumoral administration of cisplatin for treatment of cutaneous tumors in Equidae. *J Am Vet Med Assoc* 205:1170, 1994.

16.13

Urinary Incontinence and Bladder Dysfunction

Warwick M. Bayly, BVSc, MS

Loss of control of bladder function is a relatively infrequent problem in horses. When it is recognized, it is usually because a degree of incontinence develops, which, by definition, means that intravesicular pressure exceeds resting urethral pressure. Although there are a number of recognized abnormalities of bladder emptying that can afflict people, dysfunctions of equine bladder control and micturition tend to fall into one of three categories, with the extent to which they are recognized, depending upon clinical signs. Basically, the three types of problems are (1) the reflex or upper motor neuron (UMN) bladder (also known as "spastic or autonomic"); (2) paralytic or lower motor neuron (LMN) bladder; and (3) the myogenic or nonneurogenic bladder. Either of the last two conditions can be associated with the atonic bladder syndrome, which is probably appropriate given the similarity of clinical signs and subsequent treatment once either of the two types of conditions is recognized. In fact, although signs of UMN bladder problems are initially different from those of the other two groups, this condition in horses is also not usually recognized until a degree of incontinence develops. A final form of bladder neuropathy that has been described in humans and dogs, but not in horses, is reflex dyssynergia. In this condition, there is loss of coordination of detrusor contraction and urethral relaxation, with the result that the animal may make efforts to urinate but fail to do so. Such cases frequently appear very similar to those of urethral obstruction and must be distinguished from them.

While treatment options are limited and tend to be the same, regardless of what type of condition is responsible for the incontinence, determining the origin of the problem is prognostically important. To accomplish this, the internist needs to have a good working knowledge of how micturition is normally controlled.

CONTROL OF MICTURITION

From a neurologic perspective, the bladder can be regarded as having a body and an outlet, which can be further divided into the neck (or trigone) and the proximal urethra. Functionally, it alternates between filling and storage and emptying and elimination phases.[1] Dysfunction in any of these areas or phases may result in clinical problems. Somatic innervation is primarily to the striated muscle of the urethra via a branch of the pudendal nerve, which originates from the sacral cord (S1–2). Other branches of this nerve go to the anal sphincter and perineum. The sympathetic nerve supply is provided via the hypogastric nerve, with the preganglionic fibers arriving from L1–4 and synapsing in the caudal mesenteric ganglion. From there, postganglionic fibers supply the bladder (β_2-receptors) and proximal urethra (primarily α_1- and some α_2-adrenergic receptors).[2] Parasympathetic innervation originates in the sacral cord also, with neurons combining to form the pelvic nerve. There are many complex interneuronal connections between sympathetic and parasympathetic nerves in the wall of the bladder, as well as small adrenergic cells that facilitate contact between sympathetic and parasympathetic pathways.[3] As a result, complete denervation of the bladder is virtually impossible. During the filling phase there is an increase in tone of the smooth and striated muscles that together comprise the external and internal urethral sphincters. These muscles are innervated by the pudendal nerve and the sympathetic nerves, respectively. Continence is maintained by contraction of these muscles during filling. While the striated muscle forms a definite sphincter around the pelvic urethra, the anatomic existence of a bona fide internal sphincter is debatable.[4] However, the restriction to urine outflow that follows stimulation of the α-adrenergic receptors at the neck of the bladder has a sphincterlike effect. The smooth muscle of the bladder, referred to as the "detrusor muscle," is innervated by both the parasympathetic pelvic nerve and β_2-adrenergic postganglionic fibers.

The storage or filling phase is dominated by sympathetic nerve activity and provides an excellent example of the effects of reciprocal innervation.[5] During filling, the detrusor muscle relaxes owing to α-receptor–mediated inhibition of pelvic nerve afferents and stimulation of sympathetic β_2 receptors in the smooth muscle of the bladder body. The latter is a reflex response that involves sensory input from bladder stretch and pressure receptors via the afferent pelvic

nerve fibers to the sacral cord, interneurons in the cord, and pre- and postganglionic sympathetic axons in the hypogastric nerve. Relaxation of this muscle allows accumulation of large volumes of urine with little or no increase in intravesicular pressure.

Intravesicular pressure starts to rise once detrusor muscle fibers are fully stretched. Receptors in the bladder wall detect these increases, and impulses are transmitted via the pelvic nerve and ascending spinoreticular cord tracks to the pons, cerebrum, and cerebellum, where they are interpreted as the sensation of bladder fullness. Signals responsible for voluntary micturition originate in the cerebrum and exert their influence via the brainstem, from which upper motor neurons descend in reticulospinal tracts to the sacral parasympathetic nuclei. This triggers the emptying phase. From these sacral segments, pelvic nerve impulses stimulate detrusor muscle contraction, action potentials traveling via parasympathetic ganglia in the pelvic plexus or bladder wall to postganglionic fibers that stimulate the smooth muscle. Depolarization waves spread throughout the bladder via tight junctions, resulting in a strong, coordinated, contractile process. Simultaneous inhibition of the pudendal nerve and hypogastric α- and β_2-sympathetic activity further facilities detrusor muscle activity and relaxation of the external and internal urethral sphincters, respectively. Part of this inhibitory activity represents reflex neuronal activity linking pelvic and pudendal nerve axons in the sacral cord and inhibiting internuncial connections between sacral segments and the sympathetic neurons in the lumbar cord. Urethral sphincter relaxation is also coordinated centrally in a number of areas, including the cerebellum. Detrusor muscle contraction pulls the bladder neck open, and micturition occurs. The emptying phase ends when the bladder stretch receptors sense that the bladder is empty and afferent parasympathetic (pelvic nerve) impulses cease. Pelvic nerve efferent activity also stops, and pudendal motor and sympathetic nerve activity resumes (as it is no longer inhibited), with the result that the detrusor muscle relaxes and external and internal urethral sphincter tone is restored.

CLINICAL SIGNS OF BLADDER DYSFUNCTION

It can be seen that control of bladder function is complex and that there are many sites from which disruption of normal micturition could originate. In reality, problems are usually detected in horses only when a degree of incontinence develops. This is usually manifested as constant or periodic dribbling of urine from the vulva or penis. In chronic cases there is frequently evidence of scalding and associated depilation of the perineum in mares and of the ventral abdomen in males, as well as the insides of the rear limbs in all animals. Any activity that results in increased intraabdominal pressure, such as coughing or exercise, may exacerbate signs or else be associated with their initial observation. Adult horses develop these problems much more frequently than do foals.

Academically, it may seem important to be able to differentiate between the different neurogenic forms of bladder dysfunction and those of myogenic origin. In reality, the clinical signs and treatments tend to be the same, regardless of cause. UMN disease is characterized by increased urethral resistance, despite the presence of a full bladder. This may make catheterization or manual emptying of the bladder via rectal compression very difficult. The condition usually occurs in association with broad, deep spinal cord lesions. In horses, these problems are rarely recognized in such cases because of the severe nature of associated clinical problems such as recumbency and myopathies. Frequently, such situations are deemed incompatible with life. (It is possible that a focal lesion due to a disease like equine protozoal myeloencephalopathy or an aberrant parasite migration could result in the development of spastic bladder without associated neurologic signs.)

In the event that horses suffering from this type of problem are able to stand, or are kept in a sling, or have an isolated problem, in time they may develop the ability to urinate reflexively. This reflex develops owing to the stimulation of pressure receptors connected to pelvic nerve afferents, which reflexively activate pelvic (parasympathetic) nerve efferents and the pudendal nerve. This activation results in detrusor muscle contraction and relaxation of the striated urethral muscle (external sphincter) leading to relatively frequent urination, especially if there are regular increases in abdominal pressure, as may occur with any movement. These patients usually have some residual volume in the bladder after these voiding episodes. In such cases, urine dribbling is usually reported to occur intermittently, which is an important part of differentiating this type of dysfunction from paralytic (i.e., LMN) causes of incontinence.

With respect to the LMN bladder, lumbosacral trauma, equine herpes virus-1 myeloencephalitis, and cauda equina neuritis are probably the most common causes of this type of dysfunction, although in some parts of the world Sudan grass toxicity[6] and sorghum cystitis-ataxia (enzootic ataxia cystitis)[6, 7] are major problems. Tumors of the lumbosacral spinal cord, such as lymphosarcoma and melanomas, are also capable of inducing paralytic bladder. Finally, iatrogenic paralysis secondary to epidural administration of alcohol has occasionally been reported in show horses. As this practice is taboo, it is impossible to know how frequently the procedure leads to this problem.

With a paralytic (LMN) bladder, it is usual to see other signs of LMN and lumbosacral dysfunction, including all or some of the following: loss of anal sphincter tone, tail paralysis, analgesia or hypalgesia over the perineum, atrophy of the muscles of the hip and hind leg, and hindlimb weakness. Damage to the pudendal nerve and loss of external urethral sphincter integrity are, therefore, particularly important in the development of this problem. The bladder is quite atonic and distended with the urethral muscles relaxed, which results in urine dribbling due to overflow from the bladder. This incontinence may appear continuous, which helps to differentiate it from spastic (UMN) dysfunction. Sometimes the penis or vulva may appear paralyzed also. The prognosis is usually very poor owing to the development of secondary cystitis and general damage to the bladder wall and the detrusor muscle.

Myogenic problems are seen mainly in geldings. While they can occur secondary to obstructive effects of cystic calculi and cystitis, the problem generally lacks a specific identifiable cause. It generally develops slowly, in association with the accumulation of large amounts of sabulous or mucoid urinary sediment or sludge in the bladder. This is mainly comprised of calcium carbonate crystals. In time, the weight and volume of this material, when coupled with those of normal urine accumulation, progressively stretch the detrusor muscle. Incontinence is not normally noted until the cranial aspect of the bladder begins to protrude over the edge of the pubis. This results in craniad and ventrad displacement of the sediment, with the result that the bladder muscle is stretched beyond its normal modulus of elasticity and normal contraction and micturition is no longer possible. Severe distension and stretching also leads to a breakdown in tight junctions that prevents depolarizing waves from passing from muscle fiber to muscle fiber. Eventually, overdistension becomes so marked that the ability to maintain sphincter function is lost and incontinence develops. These cases usually occur without any other signs of neurologic disease; however, owing to the lack of any identifiable cause or specific pathophysiologic mechanism, it could in fact be that specific focal lesions of a peripheral nerve, such as the hypogastric nerve, may lead to a similar syndrome. Certainly, retention of urine in the bladder for any period results in the deposition of large quantities of sediment which, in turn, exacerbate the problem. It is important to recognize that part of the problem in cases of myogenic atony may stem from secondary cystitis, which develops secondary to retention of urine for any period. The urea in retained urine breaks down to ammonia, which is very irritating to the mucosal wall. Subsequent inflammation helps to damage the bladder musculature further.

Cystitis and chronic urethritis, per se, can be nonneurogenic, nonmyogenic causes of apparent incontinence. Irritation of stretch receptors in the bladder wall apparently causes regular stimulation of stretch receptors in parasympathetic afferents and stimulates detrusor contractions that cannot be voluntarily inhibited. This results in an apparent marked increase in the frequency of urination (pollakiuria) and an inability to control when it occurs. It is frequently referred to as "urge incontinence." Urge incontinence may also be seen in association with a unilateral ectopic ureter in which the bladder is much smaller than usual (owing to disuse) and incapable of storing a normal volume of urine. The frequency of micturition is again increased.

Hypoestrogenism has also been reported as a cause of nonneurogenic incontinence in an 18-year-old female Shetland pony.[8] A similar condition has been noted in older spayed bitches. The pathophysiologic mechanism of the condition is not known, although it is probably linked to a modulating effect of estrogen on the affects norepinephrine exerts on α-adrenergic receptor activity in the internal urethral sphincter.[9] In the documented case, the patient responded well to small doses (2 mg) of estradiol cypionate given intramuscularly every other day.

A transient postoperative condition that results in urine retention following abdominal or perineal operations has been noted in humans.[10] The cause has not been explained, although it has been hypothesized that there may be reflex depression of parasympathetic nerves that are responsible for detrusor muscle stimulation. This condition is distinct from that which may be associated with pain and reluctance to contract abdominal muscles following surgery. Whether such a condition exists in horses is unknown.

DIAGNOSIS

Careful general physical and neurologic examinations are the basis for characterization of the type of bladder dysfunction that exists in the equine patient, as well as serving as the basis for any efforts aimed at identifying a cause. While never good, the prognosis appears to be most positive in cases in which marked increases in intravesicular pressure can still be generated. Therefore, performance of tests aimed at evaluating bladder and urethral pressure-generating capacities may be diagnostically useful. Cystometry, which involves the inflation of the bladder with volumes of sterile water, isotonic saline, or carbon dioxide, has been described in horses and pony mares.[11, 12] Briefly, a large-gauge (No. 30 French) catheter is introduced into the bladder and connected via a three-way stopcock to an infusion pump and pressure transducer. The pressure transducer is connected to a chart recorder. The bladder is filled until micturition occurs. Intravesicular pressure is recorded continuously. There is usually a gradual increase in pressure related to the infusion of fluid until the pressure suddenly rises, reflecting the onset of detrusor muscle contraction. The pressure at the point of this sharp increase is regarded as the contraction threshold. In normal horses, this threshold is about 90 ± 20 cm H_2O.[11] The urethral pressure profile is determined in the same test by using a catheter with multiple side openings and positioning the tip at the urethral sphincter. The catheter is then filled with fluid and withdrawn at a constant rate while recording the intraurethral pressure. Normal values are usually greater than 50 cm H_2O. Pressures were significantly lower in recordings of three incontinent mares.[12] While these tests have not been widely utilized, they have considerable prognostic potential. Put simply, it seems that the higher the pressures, the better is the prognosis. The distance over which "high" pressure is present in the urethra can also be determined from these tests. This may also be important, as it gives some further information on the integrity of the urethral sphincters.

TREATMENT

Some cases of UMN disease recover gradually, especially if a specific cause can be determined and treated. A major complication with paralytic and myogenic forms of bladder dysfunction is that cases often are not recognized until the atonia is irreversible. By that time, the prognosis tends to be poor and identification of an initiating cause is difficult—and likely irrelevant. In such cases, the treatment is often futile; however, this can often only be definitively determined by assessing the response to attempted treatment. Regardless of whether dealing with UMN, LMN, or myogenic disorders, treatment tends to be the same with respect to the bladder.

If a definitive cause such as equine herpes virus-1 myeloencephalitis or equine protozoal myeloencephalopathy is identified, then that disease's specific treatment should be instituted. With respect to bladder dysfunction, the basic aim is to provide support while hoping for spontaneous recovery. This may take a long time (e.g., months in cases of pelvic nerve damage). A basic aim of therapy is to avoid retention of urine because of secondary problems that this entails. Therefore, promotion of bladder emptying is an important

goal. This may be attempted by regular catheterization or the use of an indwelling catheter. (In males, such catheters are normally inserted via a perineal urethrostomy.) While facilitating drainage, intermittent or indwelling catheterization appears to predispose to secondary bacterial cystitis and therefore should not be used without some forethought. Some horses that are chronically incontinent seem to survive comfortably without any catheterization procedures.[7] Antimicrobial therapy is important for treating any incontinence cases but is especially critical when indwelling or regular catheterization is involved.

The α-adrenergic blocker phenoxybenzamine may be given (0.7 mg/kg per os every 6 hours) to eliminate any urethral resistance, thus facilitating emptying in either the reflex UMN problem or in situations of marked atonic overdistension. Bethanechol chloride is a parasympathomimetic agent that is resistant to the action of acetylcholinesterase and apparently has a selective effect on the smooth muscle of the gastrointestinal tract and bladder. It is used principally to stimulate detrusor muscle activity. It acts by stimulating postganglionic parasympathetic effector cells rather than motor end plates. The recommended dose ranges from 0.25 to 0.75 mg/kg subcutaneously three times a day. It is recommended that clinicians start with the smallest dose. This drug reportedly has varying results.[13] It has no effect when the bladder is completely atonic or areflexic. If the muscle is capable of generating weak contractions, then bethanechol may be useful. Whether or not contractions are possible could be determined with cystometry. While it can increase intravesicular pressure, whether or not bethanecol helps evacuate the bladder also depends on the status of the urethral sphincter and striated muscle. It must be remembered that drugs such as phenoxybenzamine and bethanechol can have undesired side effects in other body systems. The use of general muscle relaxants as well as an α-adrenergic blocker may be useful for achieving urethral muscle relaxation. Diazepam (0.2 to 0.5 mg/kg IV) and dantrolene are the most commonly used relaxants. Diazepam is quite effective in large doses, which also usually result in sedation. Dantrolene (10 mg/kg per os loading dose; 2.5 mg/kg per os maintenance every 6 hours) slows release of calcium from the sarcoplasmic reticulum, and has been tried in dogs, with varying effects.

Surgical removal of the sabulous sludge found in a number of these cases has been tried via perineal urethrostomy or cystotomy, with poor results.[14] Removal via cystotomy is not recommended because of difficulties in evacuating the material without contaminating the peritoneal cavity. Perineal urethrotomy, combined with irrigation with large volumes of fluid while the horse is anesthetized, seems to be the most effective way of removing this material. However, the prognosis is still poor, owing to chronic irreversible changes in the bladder wall, which seem to prohibit any possible return of normal detrusor muscle function.

REFERENCES

1. Khanna OMP: Disorders of micturition. *Urology* 8:316, 1976.
2. Labadia A, Rivera L, Costa G, et al: Influence of the autonomic nervous system in the horse urinary bladder. *Res Vet Sci* 44:282, 1988.

3. de Groat WC, Booth AM: Physiology of the urinary bladder and urethra. *Ann Intern Med* 92:312, 1980.

4. Brorasmussen F, Sorensen AH, Bredahl E, et al: The structure and function of the urinary bladder. *Urol Internat,* 19:280, 1965.

5. Learmonth JR: Contribution to neurophysiology of urinary bladder in man. *Brain* 54:147, 1930.

6. VanKampen KR: Sudan grass and sorghum poisoning of horses: A possible lathyrogenic disease. *J Am Vet Med Assoc* 156:629, 1970.

7. Adams LG, Dollahite JW, Romaine WM, et al: Cystitis and ataxia associated with sorghum ingestion by horses. *J Am Vet Med Assoc* 155:518, 1969.

8. Madison JB: Estrogen-responsive urinary incontinence in an aged pony mare. *Compend Contin Educ Pract Vet* 6:S390, 1984.

9. Hodgson DJ, Dumas S, Bolling DR, et al: Effect of estrogen on sensitivity of the rabbit bladder and urethra to phenylephrine. *Invest Urol* 16:67, 1978.

10. Starr I, Ferguson LK: Beta-methylcholine-urethane. Its action in various normal and abnormal conditions, especially postoperative urinary retention. *Am J Med Sci* 200:372, 1940.

11. Clark ES, Semrad SD, Bichsel T, et al: Cystometrography and urethral pressure profiles in healthy horse and pony mares. *Am J Vet Res* 48:552, 1987.

12. Kay AD, Lavoie JP: Urethral pressure profilometry in mares. *J Am Vet Med Assoc* 191:212, 1987.

13. Finkbeiner AE: Is bethanechol chloride clinically effective in promoting bladder emptying? A literature review. *J Urol* 134:443, 1985.

14. Holt PE, Mair TS: 10 cases of bladder paralysis associated with sabulous urolithiasis in horses. *Vet Rec* 127:108, 1990.

Chapter 17

Endocrine Disease

17.1

The Hypothalamus

Stephen M. Reed, DVM, Dip ACVIM

The hypothalamus serves an important regulatory function for other portions of the brain. In horses there appear to be no significant primary lesions of the hypothalamus, although it has been suggested that at least part of the cause of the clinical signs of pituitary adenoma in horses is pressure on the hypothalamus. The hypothalamus is the primary source for many releasing hormones that influence the action of other glands in the body. For example, the median eminence of the hypothalamus is the source of corticotropin-releasing hormone, thyrotropin-releasing hormone, luteinizing-releasing hormone, and melanocyte-stimulating hormone-releasing factor, as well as several release-inhibiting hormones.

The hypothalamus, as an endocrine organ, contains approximately 20 pairs of nuclei, which are located very close to the pituitary gland. Anatomically, the hypothalamus lies within the sella turcica of the sphenoid bone, separated by a reflection of the dura mater known as the *diaphragma sellae*. It is also closely associated with the optic chiasm. This very close association has important anatomic as well as functional significance and may play a role in several clinically important problems of horses.

The hypothalamus is located above the pituitary gland and acts somewhat like an avenue of communication between the pituitary and the central nervous system. It is the site of the thirst center in animals, where osmoreceptors detect changes in osmolality and sodium concentration in the extracellular fluid. When osmolality is increased, the animal is stimulated to drink. Similarly, these receptors act through the hormone vasopressin to stimulate active water reabsorption in the kidney and to concentrate urine.

The hypothalamus also contains cells that act to release neurotransmitters in response to local heating or cooling. These areas are important in the maintenance of normal body temperature. Damage to the hypothalamus might therefore result in loss of thermoregulatory capacity. The mechanisms for control of this are partially regulated by prostaglandin-mediated actions on the hypothalamus, as injection of prostaglandins into the hypothalamus induces fever.

17.2

Pituitary Adenomas: Equine Cushing's Disease

Stephen M. Reed, DVM, Dip ACVIM

Abnormalities of the endocrine system have been reported to be quite rare in horses; however, observation of clinical signs such as obesity, laminitis, poor hair coat or hirsutism, and appetite changes is not uncommon. Many of these clinical signs are suspected to be the result of endocrine abnormalities. The conditions that have received the most attention include hyper- and hypoadrenocorticism, hypothyroidism, pancreatic disorders, and pheochromocytoma.

Cushing's disease in horses is similar to the syndrome in humans because both are characterized by excessive production and secretion of adrenocorticotropin (ACTH), but, unlike the human lesions, the tumors involve the intermediate lobe of the pituitary and only rarely arise from the anterior lobe. Clinical signs associated with adenomas of the pars intermedia may be somewhat variable because of excess production of other pro-opiolipomelanocortin (POMC) peptides.[1, 2] Cushing's disease is a common clinical syndrome in horses, although, many times a tumor is identified at post-mortem examination in elderly horses that did not previously demonstrate clinical signs. The underlying cause of Cushing's syndrome is associated with pituitary adenomas of the pars intermedia. This condition is reported in all breeds and in both sexes, although in several studies it appeared to be more common in females.[3-6] Two recent reports demonstrated approximately equal occurrence in males and females.[7, 8] The tumor is often associated with increasing age and can be an incidental finding in older horses at necropsy. Affected horses often lose condition despite a ravenous appetite. The clinical signs can often be quite obvious, yet accurate diagnosis is sometimes very difficult.

Cushing's disease is defined as pituitary-dependent hyperadrenocorticism.[2] The tumor has been described as a *pituitary adenoma, diffuse adenomatous hyperplasia*, and *chromophobe adenoma* (i.e., the tumor itself has not been well-defined). The cells of pituitary adenomas are sometimes difficult to distinguish but are reported most closely to resemble hyperplastic melanotrophs.[7-9] The clinical signs of pituitary adenoma in horses include polyuria and polydipsia, along with a long, poor-quality hair coat and hirsutism. The long hair coat is often associated with very dry and scaly skin and does not shed out, regardless of the time of year. In one case report involving 21 cases of pituitary neoplasia, 6 horses were presented for the primary complaint of colic.[7] Affected horses frequently have a weak and pendulous abdomen and lose muscle mass along the dorsum of the back. The pot-bellied appearance is due to a lack of tone in the abdominal musculature. The muscle wasting along the dorsal midline and elsewhere results in prominence of the croup, tuber coxae, and tuber sacrale regions.

Many affected horses are prone to repeated infections of the skin and other body systems associated with increased susceptibility to pathogens, along with severe, chronic laminitis. The cause of these problems may be related to the elevated resting blood glucose concentration in affected horses. Recently, there has been discussion of this on the equine clinicians' network among veterinarians, in an attempt to explain the bulging supraorbital fat pads often observed in horses with pituitary adenoma. One possible explanation might be redistribution of fat to this site, although the exact mechanism is not known.

Horses that are stalled are the ones most likely to have obvious polyuria and polydipsia. In some early work it was suggested that the tumor might be nonfunctional and that most or all of the clinical signs were the result of compression by the mass on the hypothalamus and anterior pituitary.[10] However, although the exact mechanism is not yet fully understood, one possible phenomenon that may lead to the development of the tumor is a loss of dopaminergic innervation to the intermediate lobe of the pituitary.[7, 9] The underlying cause of the clinical signs is thought to be the lesion in the pituitary, as in humans and other mammalian species, rather than pressure on the hypothalamus or loss of an intrinsic control mechanism.[11]

In 70% of horses with a neoplasm of the pituitary gland there is gross enlargement combined with histologic evidence of the tumor, which consists of trabecular to sinusoidal cell arrangement with a small amount of fibrous tissue and blood vessels.[6] In many cases the tumor does not maintain a distinct boundary between the pars intermedia, which sometimes results in compression of the pars distalis and the pars nervosa.[6]

DIAGNOSIS

When a horse is examined that appears to have many of these clinical signs it is reasonable to assume that the horse has a pituitary adenoma; however, it is important to attempt to confirm this diagnosis with appropriate clinicopathologic data and/or special diagnostic testing. The clinical signs and age of the horse can be useful in arriving at a diagnosis of pituitary adenoma. The average age is reported to be 19 to 21 years, although, affected horses as old as 40 years have been described.[5, 7, 8, 12] By comparison, the average age of horses with severe weight loss and poor hair coat of other causes, such as lymphosarcoma or squamous cell carcinoma, has been reported to be 10 years.[13, 14] This observation notwithstanding, it is critical that the veterinarian carefully examine the horse for other possible causes of weight loss, poor hair coat, and poor performance, to rule out conditions such as pleuropneumonia, renal failure, granulomatous enter-

itis, or neoplasia of other body systems. Owners who are unaware or do not care about the well-being of their animal may have a horse in very poor physical condition. Poor dental care, parasites, and underlying systemic illness may lead to such an animal. Horses that drink excessively and urinate frequently may have underlying renal or bladder disease, or these signs could be a result of psychogenic polydipsia, which is a nonpathologic cause of increased water consumption and excessive urination.

Some clinical signs, such as hirsutism, are reported in 85% of horses with pituitary adenoma. Many affected horses have a shaggy hair coat that fails to shed at the appropriate time. Horses with adrenal exhaustion or insufficiency may also have an abnormal hair coat.[15] In addition, horses with pituitary adenoma are sometimes plagued by repeated infections of the skin and other organs, likely as a result of the hypercortisolism and hyperglycemia.[8] Horses with equine Cushing's disease have frequent bouts of laminitis, which are not always responsive to treatment.

To confirm the diagnosis, endocrine function tests such as ACTH stimulation and dexamethasone suppression and others may be helpful. Before the performance of any function tests the veterinarian can examine the resting cortisol level. There appears to be wide variation in the normal resting values of cortisol, which may be affected by time of day, level of stress, and recent exercise the horse has received.[16, 17] The diurnal variation for resting plasma cortisol is marked by higher morning values.[18] Loss of the normal diurnal variation has been suspected in horses with pituitary adenoma, although there appears to be enough variation among normal horses that this is not a very useful tool to assist in the diagnosis of pituitary adenoma. Still, a suspicion of a pituitary adenoma may be achieved through the detection of elevated resting cortisol levels, loss of the normal diurnal rhythm of cortisol, exaggerated response to ACTH, or poor response to dexamethasone suppression testing.

Less frequently performed tests include measurement of resting insulin levels, intravenous glucose tolerance testing, and insulin tolerance tests Regulation of blood glucose levels in horses with pituitary adenoma is often abnormal, resulting in insulin-resistant hyperglycemia.[16, 17]

Sojka and Levy noted that measurement of plasma ACTH concentration was valuable in the diagnosis of pituitary-dependent hyperadrenocorticism.[19] The values of ACTH in affected horses were reported to be approximately six times greater than those of normal controls.[19] The authors reported that the samples had to be handled in a very special fashion, which began by collection in cold ethylenediamine tetraacetate (EDTA) tubes, which were quickly separated and then rapidly frozen at −70 °C.

The ACTH stimulation test is performed by examining the level of plasma cortisol before and 8 hours after intramuscular administration of 1 IU/kg of ACTH gel. Synthetic ACTH gel may be administered intravenously at a dose of 100 IU/kg. Samples should be collected before and 2 hours after the intravenous injection.[17, 20, 21] Results in a normal horse reveal a two- to threefold increase in the cortisol levels by 8 hours after injection. If a horse has an active pituitary adenoma the response is very exaggerated and may result in a four- to sixfold increase in cortisol.[17, 19–21] Sojka indicated that, when results of this test are observed in a horse with an elevated resting ACTH level, the results led to a more accurate diagnosis of horses with pituitary-dependent hyperadrenocorticism.[19]

The dexamethasone suppression test may be helpful in the evaluation of pituitary adrenocortical function. Performance of this test involves administration of 40 μg/kg of dexamethasone intramuscularly followed by sampling of the cortisol concentration in plasma. A normal horse demonstrates 80% depression 1 hour after injection[17, 19, 22] This depression of cortisol persists for approximately 24 hours in normal horses. In horses with pituitary adenoma the response is much more modest, indicating lack of response of the pars intermedia to glucocorticoid feedback.[22, 23]

Dybdal has described an overnight dexamethasone suppression test that has excellent sensitivity and specificity.[22] In the performance of this test a resting cortisol value is taken at 5:00 PM, followed by intramuscular injection of 40 μg/kg. The "postdexamethasone" collection should be at noon the following day.

There is also a combined dexamethasone suppression and ACTH stimulation test, which can be a more practical and efficient means for evaluating the pituitary adrenal axis; however, the test does not discriminate between a normal horse and a horse with pituitary adenoma. The procedure involves collecting a resting sample of plasma cortisol followed by administration of 10 mg of dexamethasone. Three hours after the dexamethasone, the plasma cortisol level is measured again and the horse is given 100 IU of synthetic ACTH intravenously. The third plasma cortisol level is collected 2 hours later. Normal horses exhibit a 70% reduction in plasma cortisol followed by an increase to about twice baseline values.[19, 22]

In 1985, Beech and Garcia demonstrated a unique response to thyroid-releasing hormone injection in horses with equine Cushing's disease. Injection of thyroid-releasing hormone resulted in release of ACTH and a subsequent rise in the plasma cortisol level. Performance of this test involves intravenous administration of 1 mg of thyroid-releasing hormone followed by recognition of increased levels of plasma cortisol, which begins within 15 minutes and lasts approximately 90 minutes.[16, 19] The increase in plasma cortisol is likely a result of release of ACTH or corticotropin-like intermediate lobe peptide (CLIP) from the pituitary, with subsequent action on the adrenal gland.

Pathophysiology of Equine Cushing's Disease

The pituitary gland of the horse is the source of several hormones, and some of them have a common precursor known as POMC, which is contained in both the pars intermedia and the pars distalis and is the important common source of many substances secreted by the pars intermedia and pars distalis. The pars intermedia of the pituitary gland of horses is the source of ACTH, melanocyte-stimulating hormone (MSH), beta endorphins (β-END) and CLIP. The pars intermedia is responsible for only 2% of the ACTH, however, while in the pars distalis pro-opiolipomelanocortin is processed into ACTH, β-END, β-lipotropin (β-LPH), and α-lipotropin (α-LPH).[7, 9, 11]

Many of the clinical signs, as well as the abnormal laboratory values, that are found in horses with pituitary adenoma may be a result of oversecretion of the POMC peptides. For example, Millington has suggested that the docile or lethargic behavior of many affected horses may be a result of the increased levels of β-endorphin and increased levels of insulin could result from hypersecretion of CLIP.[7, 11, 24] Hypersecretion of ACTH in some but not all horses with pituitary adenoma leads to adrenocortical hyperplasia and oversecretion of cortisol in some horses, which partially explains the variations in clinical signs among affected horses.[8, 25]

The production of these hormones in the pars distalis is at least partially under the control of corticotropin-releasing factor and arginine vasopressin from the hypothalamus;[19, 26] however, in the pars intermedia, hormone production is under more direct influence of dopamine and other neurotransmitters from the hypothalamus.[27] The two important neurotransmitters responsible for the production and release of these hormones are dopamine and serotonin.[7, 11, 19]

In horses with adenoma of the pituitary gland, the pars intermedia is the source for hypersecretion of this precursor substance, which leads to many of their clinical signs. The resultant effect of tumors of the pars intermedia is to produce excessive ACTH, production of which is unaffected by the negative feedback usually exerted by glucocorticoids released by the adrenal glands.[7, 9, 11, 28] In most older horses this gland is hypertrophic, and following the development of an adenoma the gland is insensitive to negative feedback by glucocorticoid.

Clinical Laboratory Testing

Diagnosing a pituitary adenoma in a horse is sometimes a significant challenge, although a presumptive diagnosis can often be based on the clinical signs and preliminary laboratory data. Initial testing should include a complete blood count, a serum chemistry profile, and urinalysis. Many horses with pituitary adenoma show evidence of either absolute or relative neutrophilia with lymphopenia.[1, 3, 4] Less commonly, such horses may show eosinopenia, although this is sometimes difficult to detect since, in our laboratory, evidence of eosinophils in normal horse blood is uncommon. Some horses may show evidence of mild anemia, whereas others show leukocytosis associated with chronic antigen stimulation, infection, or increased glucocorticoid concentration.

The chemistry profile shows evidence of hyperglycemia, which is persistent and should be detected on repeated samples. In most horses the serum glucose level is high enough so that glucosuria may be observed. Although insulin-resistant hyperglycemia can be observed in horses with Cushing's disease, it is also possible for similar levels of blood glucose in horses to be associated with stress. Some horses demonstrate hyperlipidemia.[29]

The underlying problem in horses with a pituitary adenoma is pituitary-dependent hyperadrenocorticism. Adrenal steroid secretion is under corticotrope control. As a result of excess secretion of ACTH by corticotropes in the pars distalis of the pituitary gland, horses with pituitary adenoma overproduce and oversecrete POMC in the pars intermedia. This results in increased levels of MSH, β-END, and ACTH and leads to loss of normal control and regulation of cortisol.[3, 7, 29]

The diagnosis of pituitary adenoma in the horse or recognition of pituitary-dependent hyperadrenocorticism can be suggested by the clinical signs. Additional testing to help confirm the diagnosis might include all or some of the following. Resting plasma cortisol is one, although there is significant variability in this value—as in response to stress, exercise, or low blood sugar. The range is wide enough that the cortisol value of many horses with pituitary adenoma may be within the normal range. Other tests to consider are serum glucose concentration and urine specific gravity and glucose concentration and plasma endogenous ACTH concentration, as well as results from diagnostic tests described above.

TREATMENT

Horses with pituitary tumors are difficult not only to diagnose but also to treat. The clinical signs vary and, because the condition is observed primarily in older horses, it is important to treat the tumor and many of the intercurrent conditions. Attention needs to be given to selection of excellent-quality feed, to deworming, to dental care, and especially to the hooves (since many affected horses have laminitis). It is also important to pay particular attention to the skin and hair coat, realizing that many horses cannot properly shed their winter coat and thus are prone to skin infections. The most difficult complication to manage is the laminitis, a problem complicated by overfeeding of energy-dense hay or grain, which can exacerbate the condition, or by the high levels of cortisol and of blood glucose in affected horses.

Medical management of equine Cushing's disease involves the use of one of two types of drugs: either dopamine agonists or serotonin antagonists. Bromocriptine and pergolide are the two most commonly used dopamine agonists.[31–35] The goal of therapy is to help reestablish a balance between the neurotransmitters dopamine and serotonin, which are responsible for the secretion of many of the POMC peptides and cortisol. Bromocriptine can be given either orally (although oral absorption is poor) or by subcutaneous injection.[11, 30] Oral pergolide has been shown to have similar beneficial effects in the treatment of horses and ponies with pituitary tumors.[3, 4] In a study by Beech that involved horses and ponies between 250 and 500 kg, a clinical response was noted with a total dose of 1 to 5 mg/animal. The response was usually observed with 3 to 4 weeks.

At Ohio State we have utilized cyproheptadine with good success in more than 25 horses. Cyproheptadine acts to inhibit secretion of ACTH by the par intermedia through anti-serotonin pathways. This drug should initially be administered at 0.25 mg/kg daily for 2 to 3 weeks. If there is no change in the clinical signs and no reduction in plasma ACTH levels the dosage frequency should be increased to twice a day for 1 month, at which time the ACTH measurement is repeated. In most horses the polyuria and polydipsia begin to decrease in frequency within 1 to 2 weeks after the initiation of treatment. It has been our experience that some horses require dosages as high as 0.36 mg/kg twice a day before a change in the clinical signs is observed. In horses that require high doses to achieve clinical improvement it is a good idea to reduce the dose after approximately 30 days, so long as the clinical response remains favorable. In horses that fail to respond to very high doses of cyproheptadine switching to bromocriptine or pergolide is recommended. For a few horses it may be necessary to use both drugs

simultaneously. The longest period I have had a horse in remission and on treatment is 6 years. Some personal complications I have observed include a fracture of the radius following strenuous exercise in one horse. This horse had such severe laminitis that it had not walked out of its stall for nearly a year. Following treatment with cyproheptadine the horse improved so much that it began to play in the paddock each day and fractured the radius. Post-mortem examination revealed evidence of severe osteoporosis in all long bones, possibly the result of prolonged inactivity.

In horses that respond to treatment, the first signs of improvement are a reduction in the frequency of urination and a decrease in water drinking. These are often followed by improvement of the laminitis. Failure to shed the winter hair coat often requires clipping the coat, but thereafter the hair remains normal.

REFERENCES

1. Couetil LL: New development in equine Cushing's disease. *Equine Pract* 18(9):28–32, 0000.
2. Love S: Equine Cushing's disease. *Br Vet J* 149:139–153, 1993.
3. Beech J: Tumors of the pituitary gland (pars intermedia). In Robinson NE, ed. *Current Therapy in Equine Medicine 2*. Philadelphia, WB Saunders, 1987, pp 182–185.
4. Beech J: Tumors of the pituitary gland. In Robinson NE, ed. *Current Therapy in Equine Medicine 1*. Philadelphia, WB Saunders, 1983, pp 164–169.
5. Henrichs M, Baumgartner W, Capen CC: Immunocytochemical demonstration of pro-opiomelanocortin-derived peptides in pituitary adenomas of the pars intermedia in horses. *Vet Pathol* 27:419–425, 1990.
6. Boujon CE, Bestetti GE, Meier HP, et al. Equine pituitary adenoma: A functional and morphological study. *J Comp Path* 109:163–178, 1993.
7. van der Kolk JH, Kalsbeek HC, van Garderen E, et al: Equine pituitary neoplasia: A clinical report of 21 cases (1990–1992). *Vet Rec* 133:594–597, 1993.
8. Hillyer MH, Taylor FGR, Mair TS, et al: Equine pituitary tumors. *Equine Vet Educ* 4:131–135, 1992.
9. Millington WR, Dybdal NO, Dawson R Jr, et al: Equine Cushing's disease: Differential regulation of β-endorphin processing in tumors of the intermediate pituitary. *Endocrinology* 123:1598–1604, 1988.
10. Loeb WF, Capen CC, Johnson LE: Adenomas of the pars intermedia associated with hyperglycemia and glycosuria in two horses. *Cornell Vet* 15:623–639, 1966.
11. Orth DN, Holscher MA, Wilson MG, et al: Equine Cushing's disease: Plasma immunoreactive pro-opiolipomelanocortin peptide and cortisol levels basally and in response to diagnostic tests. *Endocrinology* 110:1430–1441, 1982.
12. Dybdal NO, Hargreaves KM, Gribble DH: Equine Cushing's disease: Diagnosis using the single dose dexamethasone suppression test. *Proceedings of the 4th Annual Forum American College Veterinary Internal Medicine*, 1986, p 14.
13. van der Hoven R, Franken P: Clinical aspects of lymphosarcoma in the horse: A clinical report of 16 cases. *Equine Vet J* 15:49–53, 1983.
14. Rebhun WC, Bertone A: Equine lymphosarcoma. *J Am Vet Med Assoc* 184:720–722, 1984.
15. Dowling PM: Adrenal exhaustion and skin disease in horses. *J Am Vet Med Assoc* 203:1166–1170, 1993.
16. Beech J, Garcia MC: Hormonal response to thyrotropin-releasing hormone in healthy horses and in horses with pituitary adenoma. *Am J Vet Res* 46:1941–1943, 1985.

17. Beech J: Evaluation of thyroid, adrenal and pituitary function. *Vet Clin North Am Equine Pract* 3:649–661, 1987.
18. Bottoms GD, Roesel OF, Rausch FD, et al: Circadian variation in plasma cortisol and corticosterone in pigs and mares. *Am J Vet Res* 33:785–790, 1972.
19. Sojka JE, Levy M: Evaluation of endocrine function. *Vet Clin North Am Equine Pract* 11:415–435, 1995.
20. Eiler H, Goble D, Oliver J: Adrenal gland function in the horse: Effect of cosyntropin (synthetic) and corticotropin (natural) stimulation. *Am J Vet Res* 40:724–726, 1979.
21. Eiler H, Oliver J, Goble D: Combined dexamethasone suppression cosyntropin (synthetic ACTH-) stimulation test in the horse: A new approach to testing of adrenal gland function. *Am J Vet Res* 41:430–434, 1980.
22. Dybdal NO, Hargreaves KM, Madigan JE, et al: Diagnostic testing for pituitary pars intermedia dysfunction in horses. *J Am Vet Med Assoc* 204:627–632, 1994.
23. Sojka JE, Johnson MA, Bottoms GD: The effect of starting time on dexamethasone suppression test results in horse. *Dom An Endo* 10:1–5, 1993.
24. Wilson MG, Nicholson WE, Holscher MA, et al: Pro-opiolipomeloanocortin peptides in normal pituitary, pituitary tumor, and plasma of normal and Cushing's horses. *Endocrinology* 110:941–954, 1982.
25. Beech J, Garcia MC: In Colahan PT, Mayhew IG, Merritt AM, et al, eds. *Equine Medicine and Surgery.* Goleta, Calif, American Veterinary Publications, 1991, pp 1737–1751.
26. Taylor AL, Fishman LM: Corticotropin-releasing hormone. *N Engl J Med* 319:213–221, 1998.
27. Fischer JL, Moriarty CM: Control of bioactive corticotropin release from the neurointermediate lobe of the rat pituitary *in vitro. Endocrinology* 100:1047–1054, 1977.
28. Moore JN, Steiss J, Nicholson WE, et al: A case of pituitary adrenocorticotropin-dependent Cushing's syndrome in the horse. *Endocrinology* 104:576–582, 1979.
29. van der Kolk JH, Wensing HC, Kalsbeek HC, et al: Lipid metabolism in horses with hyperadrenocorticism. *J Am Vet Med Assoc* 206:1010–1012, 1995.
30. Dybdal NO: Endocrine disorders. In Smith B, ed. *Large Animal Internal Medicine.* St. Louis, CV Mosby, 1990, pp 1296–1302.
31. Beck DJ: Effective long term treatment of a suspected pituitary adenoma with bromocriptine mesylate in a pony. *Am J Vet Res* 46:1941–1943, 1985.
32. Beech J: Treatment of hypophyseal adenomas. *Compend Contin Educ Pract Vet* 4:119–121, 1994.
33. Krieger DT, Amorosa L, Linick F: Cyproheptadine-induced remission of Cushing's disease. *N Engl J Med* 293:893–896, 1975.
34. Munoz MC, Doreste F, Ferrer O, et al: Pergolide treatment for Cushing's syndrome in a horse. *Vet Rec* 139:41–43, 1996.
35. Peters D: Low dose pergolide mesylate treatment for equine hypophyseal adenomas (Cushing's syndrome). *Proc Am Assoc Equine Pract* 41:154–155, 1995.

17.3

Thyroid Gland

Wendy M. Duckett, DVM, MS

THYROID FUNCTION

An understanding of the function of the thyroid gland and of the physiologic effects of thyroid hormones is important in recognizing, diagnosing, and managing thyroid dysfunction. The relative importance of the thyroid glands is reflected in the large volume of blood flow—4 to 6 mL per minute per gram of tissue, which is greater than the blood flow to the kidneys.[1]

Iodine and Hormone Metabolism

One major function of the thyroid is to actively trap and conserve iodine against a large concentration gradient.[1–3] Iodine can be absorbed in its soluble form, iodide (I^-), via the intestinal mucosa or any moist body surface such as other mucosa or broken skin.[3] Once in the thyroid follicle, the iodide is oxidized and reacts with tyrosyl residues on the storage protein thyroglobulin, to form inactive precursors, monoiodotyrosine (MIT), and diiodotyrosine (DIT). Coupling of these precursors results in synthesis of the active iodothyronines, thyroxine (T_4) and triiodothyronine (T_3). When needed, T_4 and T_3 are cleaved from the thyroglobulin, picked up by the follicular cells by a process of endocytosis, and transported into the circulation.[1, 3] Hormone synthesis and release are controlled by iodine availability and the anterior pituitary hormone thyroid-stimulating hormone (TSH). TSH release is in turn mediated by the hypothalamic thyrotropin-releasing factor (TRF). In addition to an intrinsic autoregulatory mechanism controlling rate of hormone production and iodine levels, the thyroid, pituitary, and hypothalamus participate in a classic negative feedback mechanism of control. The feedback regulation of TSH secretion is closely related to the circulating concentrations of unbound (free) thyroid hormones (fT_4 and fT_3).[1, 3]

The circulating thyroid hormones are T_4, T_3, and reverse T_3 (rT_3). T_4 and T_3 are the biologically active hormones. Reverse T_3 and T_3 are both deiodination products of T_4. All of the circulating T_4 is derived directly from the thyroid gland. Only 10% to 20% of the circulating T_3 is secreted directly from the gland. The majority is derived from 5'-monodeiodoninase degradation of T_4 peripherally. This is referred to as "T_3 neogenesis." In adults, most rT_3 is derived by peripheral 5'-monodeiodinase degradation of T_4.[1] In the fetus, 5'-monodeiodoninase activity is retarded, so that T_3 neogenesis is low, but 5'-monodeiodinase activity is accelerated, resulting in high levels of rT_3. A switch in enzyme activity occurs at birth, owing partly to the influence of glucocorticoids.[1] The hormones circulate in the blood bound to transport proteins. Thyroid-binding globulin (TBG) is the major protein; T_4-binding prealbumin (TBPA) and albumin bind to a lesser degree. In horses, the percentages of circulating T_4 bound to TBG, TBPA, and albumin were found to be 61%, 22%, and 17%, respectively.[4] T_3 is bound to TBG and albumin but not to TBPA. The hormones are reversibly bound to the transport proteins. It is the hormones in their unbound or free state that can readily traverse capillary endothelium[5] and are available to exert their biologic effects at the peripheral tissues. The protein-binding properties thus in part determine the biologic activity of each hormone. T_3 is much more potent than T_4, and it has a shorter half-life. T_4 has much greater protein-binding affinity; T_3 is therefore more readily available to interact with receptors at peripheral tissues. T_4 is sometimes thought of in terms of a prohormone. The half-life of T_4 in horses is approximately 50 hours.[6]

Metabolic degradation of the thyronine ring after deiodination includes deamination, decarboxylation, and conjugation.

The enzymes responsible for the production of T_3 and rT_3 are also responsible for their destruction. Five-monodeiodinase is responsible for the production of rT_3 from T_4 and the degradation of T_3, whereas, 5'-monodeiodininase activity results in the production of T_3 from T_4 and the degradation of rT_3. There are two classes of 5'-monodeiodoninase. Type I is located in the liver and kidney and is inhibited noncompetitively by propylthiouracil (PTU). Type II is located in the central nervous system and is not affected by PTU.[1] Type II 5'-monodeiodinase is also found in the brown fat of neonates and is responsive to rT_3.[7] Metabolites are excreted via the urine, and some are conjugated and enter the enterohepatic circulation. Most iodide is returned to the thyroid gland.

The thyroid is also the site of production of calcitonin, secreted by the C cells, which are interspersed among the thyroid follicles. Calcitonin is involved in calcium homeostasis.[1, 3, 8]

Hormone Activity

T_3, whether directly transported into the cell or derived intercellularly from T_4, is considered to be the effector in target cells. The mitochondria and nucleus are the intracellular sites of action that result in the thermogenesis, increased oxygen consumption, increased protein synthesis, increased metabolic rate, increased carbohydrate absorption and glucose metabolism, stimulation of growth and maturation and erythropoiesis, increased lipid metabolism and conversion of cholesterol into bile salts, activation of lipoprotein lipase, increased sensitivity of adipose tissue to lipolysis, stimulation of heart rate, cardiac output and blood flow, increased neural transmission, and cerebral and neuronal development in young animals.[2, 3]

EXTRATHYROID FACTORS THAT AFFECT THYROID FUNCTION AND TESTING

Many endogenous and exogenous factors can affect thyroid function and sometimes test results. Awareness of these factors and interactions can help with test interpretation and the establishment of an accurate diagnosis.

Age

There are certain age-related differences in thyroid hormone levels in horses. Foals have very high levels as compared with adults, which decrease further with advanced age.[9–14]

Gender

The correlation of gender and thyroid hormone levels appears to be variable. In one study, T_4 levels were not significantly influenced by sex: males had slightly higher T_3 values than females.[14] Serum thyroid hormone concentrations may be lower for stallions and geldings than for females,[10, 15] but others report no gender differences.[16–19] Lower thyroid hormone concentrations have been reported in mares than in stallions.[20] The level of free T_4 was found to be higher in stallions than in other horses.[21] Mares tested at all stages of the estrous cycle were found to show no statistically significant differences according to stage of the cycle.[17] T_4 levels, however, were decreased following ovulation, which is the converse of the hormone pattern seen in other species following ovulation. Individual variations were found to be greater than variations within the estrous cycle.[17] Higher than normal serum hormone concentrations were reported during pregnancy in mares,[22] which finding is consistent with those in other species.[1] This may be due in part to increased TBG levels during pregnancy.[1] Furthermore, it was found that the levels vary with stage of gestation. T_4 levels were statistically significantly higher in the mares between days 49 to 55 of gestation as compared with those in advanced stages. T_3 did not vary statistically significantly with gestational stage in mares.[23] One investigator found that hormone levels in mares at midgestation were no different from normal.[15] The high hormone levels were believed to be due more to the effect of the cold.[24] No significant differences in stages of gestation or in pregnant versus nonpregnant mares was found in one study.[6]

Other Hormones

Glucocorticoids inhibit endogenous TRH secretion and decrease the response of TSH to TRH. Glucocorticoids also inhibit peripheral deiodination in adults. In neonates, glucocorticoids enhance conversion of T_4 to T_3. Glucocorticoids decrease serum TBG and increase TBPA.[1] Catecholamines enhance the rate of deiodination of T_4 to T_3 and have a potentiating effect.[25] Estrogen enhances TBG production, and androgens tend to suppress it.[1]

Breed

There has been no evidence of thyroid hormone level differences among breeds.[14, 16]

Daily Rhythm

A daily rhythm in equine thyroid hormone levels has been identified.[26, 27] In adult geldings, T_4 was found to peak around 4:00 PM (mean, 2.43 ± 0.81 µg/dL) at levels significantly higher than the lowest T_4 values around 4:00 AM (mean, 1.79 ± 0.63 µg/dL). T_3 was shown to peak between 8:00 AM and 4:00 PM ($\sim 54 \pm 13$ ng/dL) at levels significantly different than the lowest T_3 around midnight (mean, 38.71 ± 10.81 ng/dL).[27] Higher levels of T_4 between 5:00 and 8:00 PM than at 8:00 AM have also been reported.[26]

Extrathyroidal Illness

Aberrations in thyroid hormone levels are associated with illness and must be distinguished from thyroid dysfunction. Extrathyroid illness, also referred to as "low T_3 syndrome" or "euthyroid sick syndrome" is characterized by decreased T_3 levels, usually in association with normal or increased T_4 levels. In cases of calorie deprivation, systemic illness, fever, chronic liver disease, renal failure, trauma, surgery, and anesthesia, decreased 5'-monodeiodinase activity results in decreased T_3 neogenesis.[1, 28, 29] Extrathyroid illness can result in a low T_4 state in addition to low T_3.[28] This state is associated with increased mortality in people. One mechanism may be inhibition of hormone secretion by tumor necrosis factor (TNF). In these cases of low hormone levels associated with nonthyroid illness, stimulation tests should elicit a normal response. In low T_3 syndrome there is a reciprocal increase in rT_3 because the suppressed enzyme, 5'-monodeiodinase, which is responsible for T_3 neogenesis, is also the enzyme that degrades rT_3.[1]

Season

Thyroid activity increases while horses are becoming acclimatized to colder temperatures.[6, 30, 31]

Weaning

In a study to evaluate the effect of weaning on thyroid function, no difference in hormone levels was found between abrupt and gradual weaning methods.[19]

Activity

Interest in the relationship of thyroid function and muscle metabolism has prompted investigation in race horses. Irvine[9, 32] found the T_4 secretion rate (TSR) to be increased in horses in full training, whereas protein-bound iodine (PBI) was decreased. This decrease in PBI was not consistent with the finding of increased PBI in human athletes.[15] T_4 levels were found to be markedly increased in the latter stages of training, and the proposal was made that T_4 measurement might be used to monitor the training reserves in racehorses.[33] Another investigator found very low T_4 concentrations in healthy thoroughbreds and concluded that serum T_4 values were an unreliable indicator of thyroid function and that T_3 was a more accurate one.[34] He found no correlation between T_4 and T_3 concentrations and racing performance. Another investigator documented substantial increases in T_4 within 30 minutes after exercise but no differences in T_3.[18, 22] Significant increases in T_3 and T_4 levels were found 1 hour after swimming.[35]

Feeding

Feeding a high-energy and high-protein diet to weanlings 6 to 8 months of age was found to stimulate thyroid gland secretion initially, and then peripheral conversion of T_4 to T_3 resulted in a relative T_4 decrease 3 hours after a meal.[36] It was found to be the soluble carbohydrate (glucose) rather than protein portion of the diet that increased thyroid hormone response in weanlings.[37] It was found that the accelerated T_4 to T_3 conversion following the high-carbohydrate meal correlated with the increased insulin secretion that followed the glucose rise.[38] Insulin also accelerates deiodination of T_3 thus shortening its duration of effectiveness.[39] Further, this response was found to be age related. By the time the animals were 12 to 14 months of age, feeding the high-carbohydrate and high-protein diet no longer affected thyroid hormone concentrations.[38] One study on the effects of meal frequency and T_3 levels observed a hormone rise after meals, the rise being greater when animals were given one feeding a day than after six feedings a day.[40]

Exogenous Compounds

Substances that exert their goitrogenic effect by blocking or competing with iodide uptake are thiocyanate and perchlorate. Iodide oxidation and coupling of iodotyrosines are inhibited by drugs such as sulfonamides, phenylbutazone, phenothiazines, thiouracils, thiopental, and methimazole. Soybean meal, linseed meal and plants of the Brassica family contain goitrogenic substances.[2, 3] Phenylbutazone administration decreasing thyroid hormone levels in horses is documented.[26] In those cases, stimulation-response tests were normal. Exogenous and endogenous glucocorticoids have the same effects—suppressing pituitary TSH secretion, decreasing the response of TSH to TRH, inhibiting monodeionination (except in the perinatal period), inhibiting TBG, and decreasing release of hormone from the gland.[1, 41] Propylthiouracil, in addition to affecting iodine metabolism, inhibits peripheral conversion of T_4 to T_3. In humans, aspirin in therapeutic doses lowers TSH response to TRH.[41] Phenobarbital increases the metabolic clearance of thyroid hormones.[7] Reserpine, a catecholamine-depleting agent, inhibits secretion of TSH and inhibits deiodination.[25] Antipyrine has antithyroid activity.[1] Anabolic steroids can have an inhibitory effect on TBG levels;[1] however, in one study it was found that short-term anabolic steroid use did not significantly affect horses' thyroid function tests.[42] Exogenous compounds containing iodine or iodides are of particular interest. Iodine excess—as well as deficiency—can cause thyroid dysfunction and interfere with thyroid tests. Horses are exposed to iodine or iodide compounds in the form of feedstuffs, expectorants, leg paints, shampoos, injectable counterirritants, radiographic contrast media, and the antiprotozoal drug iodochlorhydroxyquin. Individuals can respond to excessive amounts of iodine by either suppressing or accelerating hormone production. Iatrogenic hypothyroidism subsequent to cleansing of an open wound with povidone iodine is documented in humans.[43] When large amounts of iodide inhibit proteolysis and hormone release from the gland, resulting in decreased thyroid function, it is known as the "Wolf-Chaikoff effect." The second way an individual can respond to large amounts of iodide is by accelerated production—which produces elevated levels—of thyroid hormone. This is referred to as "jodbasedow thyrotoxicosis."[1, 44]

FUNCTION TESTS AND DIAGNOSTICS
Direct Tests

Irvine[30] was one of the first investigators to develop and use quantitative thyroid function tests for horses. TSR was calculated after injecting iodine[131] and plotting the fall of PBI. The volume of distribution was calculated by extrapolation from the disappearance curve to zero time. The product of volume of distribution and the PBI was used to calculate the T_4 pool. From the half-life of protein-bound ^{131}I, the fractional turnover of the pool, and thus the daily loss of T_4, was obtained. Assuming loss and replacement to be equal, the amount was designated the TSR. This method of measurement was not clinically practical.[9]

PBI was for years the standard determination for estimating serum hormone concentrations.[3, 15] All iodine, hormonal or not, is measured. This measurement is influenced greatly by substances containing iodine and by iodine in the diet.

Hormone Levels

Competitive protein-binding assays are the basis for the determination of total T_4 and, indirectly, TBG and fT_4 levels.[3] Another readily available method for determining total hormone levels is radioimmunoassay. Species-specific test kits must be used if results are to be accurate.[45] This technique has been used to measure horses' thyroid hormones since 1978[16] and is validated for horses.[46] Immunoassay of TBG and TSH levels is done routinely in human medicine but is not readily available for horses at this time. Radioimmunoassay quantification of T_4 and T_3 is not affected by the presence of hemolysis of the blood sample.[47] Enzyme-linked immunosorbent assay (ELISA) techniques are available to measure hormone levels.[3] The big advantage of this method is that no radioactive agents are required. The most precise way to quantify the actual amount of hormone available to target tissues is to determine the unbound or free fractions.[24] Because amounts are minute, accurate measurement techniques are tedious and not universally available in practice.[21] Normal thyroid hormone levels generally have a wide range of values and vary among laboratories and measurement techniques (Table 17–1). For most consistent results the practitioner should always use the same laboratory and become familiar with its values. Ratios of circulating hormones may be indicative of dysfunction. In general, among species, the ratio of circulating total T_4 to T_3 is 20:1. In horses, it was found to be 23:1.[21] The ratio of fT^4 to fT_3 was found to be 1.83:1 in horses.[21] An increased ratio T_3 to T_4 has been associated with hypothyroidism in dogs[48] and in humans.[1] With iodine deficiency, the thyroid produces and secretes more T_3 as a way of conserving iodine, thus increasing the T_3–T_4 ratio.[1] If the rT_3 value is available in addition to T_4 and T_3 values, certain patterns may be suggestive and supportive of dysfunction. For instance, rT_3 may be increased in hyperthyroidism and euthyroid sick syndrome.[1] Because rT_3 is a breakdown product of T_4, its levels depend on the T_4 levels. Thus, rT_3 may be increased along with T_4 in hyperthyroidism. In euthyroid sick syndrome the activity of 5'-monodeiodinase is decreased. This is the enzyme responsible for T_3 neogenesis and rT_3 breakdown; therefore, in that syndrome, T_3 is decreased and rT_3 is increased. Likewise, in hypothyroidism, where T_4 is decreased, rT_3 may also be decreased.[1]

There are no direct tests to evaluate the impact of thyroid hormones on the target tissues. The most direct measure of metabolic activity is basal metabolic rate (BMR). Routine determination of BMR is not clinically practical.[3]

Indirect Tests

Serum cholesterol is elevated in humans and dogs with hypothyroidism.[3] This is not a specific response to thyroid dysfunction. Increased cholesterol levels have been found in some hypothyroid horses but not others, so this is not a reliable indicator in horses.[30, 49] A normochromic, nonresponsive anemia of chronic disease, once again, is not specific but may be seen with hypothyroidism.[3] This finding of anemia responsive to thyroid supplementation has been documented in horses.[49–51] Low body temperature and bradycardia may indicate hypothyroidism.

Trophic Response Tests
Thyroid-Stimulating Hormone

Trophic hormone response tests are useful to help differentiate primary from secondary thyroid dysfunction, and they remove the variability of endogenous and exogenous factors that influence other tests. The TSH stimulation test protocol is to inject 5 IU of TSH intravenously and compare pre- and postinjection hormone levels. In normal horses, T_4 peaks 3 to 4 hours after injection.[52] T_4 peaks at 4 hours, at a level 2.4 times the preinjection value. T_3 doubles within 30 minutes and peaks at 2 hours at a level five times baseline.[48]

Table 17–1. Thyroid Hormone Levels in Adult Horses*

Investigators	Total T_4 (μg/dL)	Total T_3 (ng/dL)	fT_4 (pg/mL)	fT_3 (pg/mL)
Chen & Riley, 1981	1.76	98.69		
Reap et al., 1978	1.63 ± 0.51 (0.95 − 2.38)	77.1 ± 45.75 (31 − 158)		
Kallfelz & Lowe, 1970	(1.46 − 3.38)			
McBride et al., 1985	1.79 ± 0.17	62 ± 4.3		
Thomas & Adams, 1978	1.57 ± 0.62 (0.30 − 3.70)			
Anderson et al., 1988	1.56 ± 0.081	67.7 ± 10.2	5.9 ± 0.39	3.22 ± 0.18
Duckett et al., 1989	2.13 ± 0.76 (0.93 − 4.31)	47.38 ± 13.66 (13.30 − 97.40)		

*Mean ± SD; ranges in parentheses.

Normal responses are characterized by a rise in T_3 that antedates the T_4 rise and is also greater. When 5 IU TSH was given intramuscularly, T_4 peaked at 2 times baseline value 6 to 12 hours after injection, and T_3 peaked in 1 to 3 hours.[26] The suggested protocol for intravenous TSH response test is to measure hormone levels at baseline and 4 hours after injection.[48] The suggested protocol if the TSH is given intramuscularly is to measure hormone levels at baseline and 3 and 6 hours after injection.[26] The protocol for 1-day-old foals is to measure T_3 levels at baseline and 1 and 3 hours after intravenous injection of 5 IU of TSH. A normal response is a 50% increase by 3 hours. T_4 values were too variable.[53] An insufficient increase in hormone indicates a primary thyroid problem. The ability to perform a TSH challenge test may be limited by the cost or availability of the TSH.

Thyroid-Releasing Hormone

TRH challenge tests have been done in horses.[54-56] TRH is administered intravenously, 1 mg to horses and 0.5 mg to ponies. An inadequate hormone response to TRH would occur in primary or secondary hypothyroidism. In normal animals, T_4 peaks at 4 hours and T_3 at 2 hours after TRH injection.[55] In a second study, T_3 had increased significantly at 1 to 2 hours after TRH injection and peaked at 2 to 4 hours. T_4 increased by 2 hours and peaked at 4 to 10 hours. Both hormones should increase two- to threefold in a normal response. The suggested protocol is an intravenous dose of 1 to 3 mg TRH with hormone measurements at baseline and 4 to 5 hours later. At higher levels of TRH side effects such as salivation, urination, defecation, vomiting, pupillary constriction, tachycardia, and tachypnea can be seen.[56] The TRH challenge test has also been used as a diagnostic aid in the evaluation of pituitary adenomas in horses.[54]

Imaging

Pertechnetate (technetium 99m) is a diagnostically useful compound that is taken up by the iodine-trapping mechanism.[3] Scintigraphic imaging has been used clinically to evaluate the thyroid glands of horses.[57] Abnormal uptake patterns have been seen with thyroid carcinoma in horses.[58-60] Ultrasonographic evaluation of the glands can differentiate solid structures from cystic ones.[1]

Biopsy

Aspirate or biopsy sampling can help differentiate cysts, neoplasia, hyperplastic goiter, colloidal goiter, and inflammation.

Physical Features of the Gland

Physically, horses' thyroid glands are two discrete, firm lobes located at the caudal aspect of the larynx. The remnant of an isthmus that connects the caudal poles at the level of the third to sixth tracheal ring, if it is present at all, is a fibrous band in the horse.[3, 61] The weight of the glands as a ratio of grams of thyroid tissue per kilogram of body weight is largest for fetuses and foals (mean, 0.28 g/kg; range, 0.12 to 0.67) and diminishes progressively with age. The weight ratio for adults is, an average, 0.08 g/kg (range, 0.01 to 0.15).[62] The normal total gland weight for foals is around 15.[63] The glands are very vascular, being supplied by two major arteries arising from the external carotid and subclavian arteries, supplying, respectively, the cranial and caudal poles. On palpation, a bruit may be felt when blood flow is accelerated, for instance during pregnancy.[1] Gland size does not parallel function, and other tests must be used to establish an accurate diagnosis.

HYPOTHYROIDISM

Hypothyroidism occurs in two entities because of the actions of thyroid hormone on cell differentiation and metabolic rate regulation.[5] Liver, muscle, kidney, heart, salivary glands, and pancreatic tissue are sensitive targets of thyroid hormone action.[1] Hypothyroidism can manifest in many ways, and diagnosis may be a challenge. Hypothyroidism, or thyroprivia, results when thyroid tissue is removed or function suppressed. Hypothyroidism can be classed as primary, secondary or tertiary. Primary gland dysfunction can be caused by iodine deficiency (endemic goiter) or excess (Wolff-Chaikoff effect), thyroiditis, neoplasia, biochemical defects, thyroid agenesis, or ingestion of goitrogenic compounds, which can block hormone synthesis. Of these, iodine excess, iodine deficiency, and neoplasia have been reported as causes of hypothyroidism in horses. Secondary hypothyroidism occurs as a consequence of pituitary (trophoprivic) or hypothalamic dysfunction. There are reports of hypothyroid activity in horses with pituitary adenoma,[50, 64] but all horses with pituitary adenoma do not have concomitant hypothyroidism.[54] "Tertiary hypothyroidism" denotes a defect in hormone utilization at the peripheral tissues. It has not been identified or reported in horses. In one report a defect in T_4 to T_3 deiodination was suspected, and a hair coat started to grow when T_3 supplementation was implemented.[65] In many of the reported cases of hypothyroidism in horses, a specific cause has not been identified.

Hypothyroidism in Foals

The consequences of inadequate circulating thyroid hormone is potentially devastating and life threatening to fetus and foal. The poor prognosis is associated with the essential role of thyroxine in normal growth and development. Chances of recovery are unlikely once critical developmental stages are passed. Function test results may be within normal limits at the time of examination, making it difficult to confirm a previous transient or in utero deficit.[5]

Signs

The majority of clinical signs thus far reported in hypothyroid foals are attributable to the crucial role of T_4 in the development and maturation of the nervous and musculoskeletal systems. Physeal dysgenesis[66]; weakness, death, or incoordination in newborns[11]; defects in ossification with tarsal bone collapse[67, 68]; hypoplastic carpal bones, common digital extensor tendon rupture, forelimb contracture, and mandibular prognathism[69, 70]; stillbirths, weakness, and long haircoat[71]; weak suckle reflex[72]; and premature, weak foals that die shortly after birth[63] have been reported. Thyroid hormones are required for the biochemical maturation, hypertrophy, and capillary penetration of growing cartilage. T_3 may act indirectly to promote chondrogenesis by stimulating anterior pituitary synthesis and secretion of growth hormone. An age-related, "carbohydrate diet–responsive" insulin–T_4–T_3 interaction has been identified that may play a role in cartilage maturation defects in weanlings.[73] Thyroxine also plays a role in maturation of the lungs and in surfactant production.[1] There is one report in the literature of a foal with respiratory distress syndrome and hypothyroidism.[74] Doige and McLaughlin[75] described two foals that died in respiratory distress. Neonatal thermogenesis is also T_4 dependent[5]; thus, cold intolerance could be a problem. In one study, when young growing animals were thyroidectomized, physeal plate closure and incisor eruption were delayed. Very young foals suffered severe growth retardation and died.[76] In a second study in which day-old foals were thyroidectomized, lethargy, depression, and rough, dry hair coats were seen.[77]

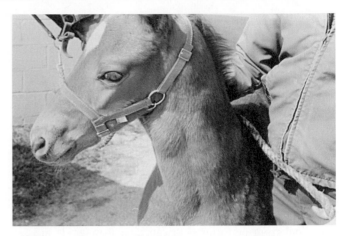

Figure 17–1. Goiter in a foal. The dam was inadvertently given a ration that contained too much iodide. (Courtesy of Debra Ann Knight, PhD.)

Cause

The major cause of hypothyroidism in foals is believed to be nutritional. Congenital thyroid enlargement (goiter) (Fig. 17–1) with decreased function is associated with both inadequate iodine intake and excessive iodine intake by the mare. T_4 is transported transplacentally and via the milk.[78] No cases of hypothyroidism due to an inborn error of metabolism have been described in foals. There are several reports in the literature of goiter and hypothyroidism in foals associated with ingestion of excessive amounts of iodine in kelp-supplemented rations.[63, 71, 72, 78, 79] The dams of these foals may or may not be affected. Feeding 40 mg or more of iodine daily can produce this syndrome.[79]

Diagnosis

Foals that exhibit any of the signs mentioned above, with or without enlarged glands, are suspect. The mare and her nutrition should be examined. Because enlargement of the thyroid gland alone does not automatically imply hypo- or hyperthyroidism, function tests should be done to confirm a diagnosis. One crucial point to remember is that very high thyroid hormone levels are normal in foals (Table 17–2). Not only is there is a powerful central drive to stimulate the thyroid axis late in gestation,[5] but TBG levels are increased in neonates[1] and hormone protein binding is more pronounced in neonates than in adults.[5] Thyroid hormone levels measured in umbilical cord blood of newborn foals were found to be 14, 5, 7, and 3 times adult levels, respectively for total T_4, fT_4, total T_3, and fT_3.[5] For most of fetal life, T_4 is deiodinated to rT_3, and levels of T_3 are negligible and those of T_4 and rT_3 high. At birth, rT_3 production is decreased and the deiodination pathway leads to T_3. Foals' plasma rT_3 levels fall rapidly as T_3 rises for 24 to 48 hours after birth, plateaus for 2 to 3 days, then declines to parallel the T_4 value.[5] There is a decline in T_4 levels during the first 16 days of life. Free T_4 levels declined over the first 3 months of life.[11] In term foals, serum T_3 levels are elevated far above adult levels for the first 6 to 12 hours; by 24 hours they have declined significantly. Premature foals' rT_3 levels

Table 17–2. Thyroid Hormone Levels in Foals*

Investigators	Age	Total T_4 (µg/dL)	Total T_3 (ng/dL)	fT_4 (pg/mL)	fT_3 (pg/mL)
Chen & Riley, 1981	1.5 – 4 mo	4.02 ± 0.19 (2.9 – 5.25)	192.86 ± 8.54 (135 – 270)		
Dudan et al., 1987	5 min	29.3			
	48 hr	20.5			
Irvine & Evans, 1975	1 – 10 hr	28.86	991	12.12	2.99
Shaftoe et al., 1988	1 day	13.63 ± 5.12 (4.4 – 25.1)	366 ± 22.54 (26 – 732)		

*Mean ± SD; ranges in parentheses.

are lower than those of term foals, but a further decline is not observed up to 48 hours. This observation is consistent with a surge of 5'-deiodination resulting in T_3 production and rT_3 degradation about 6 to 12 hours after birth for term foals. Deiodination is impaired in preterm foals.[80] McCall and coworkers[19] found T_3 levels in foals 4 months of age comparable to adult levels; however, mean T_4 levels were higher at 2.9 μg/dL.

Hypothyroidism in Adult Horses

Hypothyroidism in adults, unlike that in foals, is not life threatening. The following conditions that have been attributed to thyroid dysfunction certainly serve to prevent an individual from performing to capacity. Low-grade anemia responsive to thyroid supplementation has been described in thyroidectomized horses[49, 50] and in racehorses with myopathy.[51] Hypothermia (low normal body temperature) was reported in thyroidectomized animals.[49] Reproductive problems in mares are irregular and absent estrus cycles.[49, 63] Thyroidectomized mares could conceive and carry a foal to term.[81] Stallions exhibit decreased libido.[49, 65] Thyroidectomized stallions had decreased total sperm count but normal semen characteristics and testicular histology, and they could sire foals.[76, 81] Bradycardia, obesity, and lethargy were seen in mares whose thyroid function was suppression owing to ingestion of excess iodine.[63] Lethargy, rear limb edema, coarse haircoat, and decreased appetite were seen in thyroidectomized mares.[81] One case describes failure to grow a normal hair coat in a stallion.[65] Alopecia attributed to iodinism and low circulating thyroid hormone values were documented in a horse being treated with an expectorant containing iodide and topical povidone iodine.[82] The hair coat grew and thyroid function returned to normal when the medications were discontinued. One report described agalactia associated with decreased thyroid function.[83] TRH has been shown to stimulate pituitary secretion of prolactin in many species. Mares, however, do not show a prolactin response following TRH injection.[83, 84] Poor performance in racehorses during the season when ambient temperatures are increasing may be related to seasonal thyroid function changes. At this time hormone levels may drop too low to support optimal muscle performance.[32]

Hypothyroidism has been implicated as a cause of anhidrosis. In one study, mean T_3 and T_4 values were found to be lower in anhidrotic horses than in unaffected horses.[85] Another report found that thyroid function was not abnormal in some horses selected from a group affected with anhidrosis.[86] Whether or not hypothyroidism is a cause or a contributing factor in laminitis has yet to be proven.[87]

Treatment of Hypothyroidism

When the diagnosis is low circulating hormone levels or hyperplastic goiter, whether dietary intake of iodine is adequate *must be ascertained.* The National Research Council recommends a minimum daily intake of 0.1 mg/kg of feed. Total daily intake of 1 to 2 mg iodine per animal has also been reported.[63] The soils of some geographic areas are low or marginal in iodine, for instance, the Great Lakes Region. Iodinated casein or thyroprotein, 5 g orally per day, re-

versed the effects of thyroidectomy in adults.[76] Iodinated casein, 5 to 10 g orally per day, reversed the thyroid-associated anemia and myopathy in racehorses.[51] Desiccated thyroid extract, 2 mg/kg body weight orally per day, has been used successfully.[71] The responses to the iodinated casein and thyroid extract may not be consistent, as hormone levels in the products can vary.

Hormone supplementation with T_4 should be effective unless there is a deiodination defect. A starting dose of 20 μg T_4 orally per kilogram body weight daily is recommended.[18] If T_3 is to be supplemented, an oral dose of 1 mg/kg body weight once a day is recommended.[88]

The animal should be monitored for clinical response to therapy, which can take at least 2 weeks. Hormone levels should be monitored periodically and function and dosages reassessed, particularly if the desired response is not achieved.

HYPERTHYROIDISM

Very few reports of equine hyperthyroidism are documented. A syndrome of tremors, excitability, tachycardia, sweating, and weight loss in spite of a good appetite has been described in racehorses.[32, 89] Plasma hormone levels were elevated, and the horses improved markedly in response to antithyroid treatment of 1 g potassium iodide orally per day.[30, 32] The use of thyroidectomy as a means of behavior modification for high-strung, unmanageable horses has had variable success.[76] In these cases it was not stated whether a diagnosis of hyperthyroidism was confirmed by hormone levels or function tests. High levels of thyroid hormones can be seen in physiologic states not associated with abnormal clinical signs—such as pregnancy[23] and the well-documented high levels needed for normal fetal growth and development.[11, 14] There are no reports of hyperthyroidism associated with neoplasia or an autoimmune condition in horses. Horses are, however, at risk for accelerated thyroid hormone production owing to exposure to increased quantities of iodine, as in expectorants, counterirritants, and contrast media, drugs (e.g., iodochlorhydroxyquin), and leg paints and shampoos containing iodine. This is called the jodbasedow phenomenon.[1, 44] It is recognized in human medicine that certain persons (such as those with multinodular goiter) are predisposed to this effect. It would be typified in a horse by transiently elevated thyroid hormones that return to normal after the source of the excess iodine is discontinued. People who respond this way to excessive iodine would not be expected to respond to the supplemental potassium iodide that causes suppression of thyroid hormone production in others (Wolff-Chaikoff effect). In a racehorse that shows appropriate signs and elevated hormone levels, it is imperative to determine if an iodine compound has been used or if the horse may have received a TSH "jug." If severe distress of thyrotoxicosis is present, administration of glucocorticoids should alleviate the signs.[1]

THYROID TUMORS

Tumors of the thyroid in horses tend to occur more frequently in lightweight breeds than in draught horses and, in general, more often in aged horses than in young ones.[90] Based on immunohistochemical techniques, three cell types are distinguished in the thyroid glands of horses. The first are undifferentiated and do not react to antibodies; the second are parafollicular cells, which have calcitonin-positive secretory granules; and the third type are thyroglobulin-positive follicular epithelial cells. There are also three classifications of cell aggregations. One is ultimobranchial remnant (UBR) embedded in thyroid tissue without compression of adjacent cells. The second is nodular hyperplasia of the ultimobranchial remnant (UBH) that compresses adjacent follicular cells. The third cell aggregation classification is adenoma of the ultimobranchial segment (UBA) surrounded by fibrous capsule. It was found in horses that all cell aggregations had undifferentiated cells that retained embryonic characteristics such as those of UBR.[90]

Adenoma

Adenoma is the most common neoplasia of the equine thyroid.[91–97] It is an age-related phenomenon, occurring mainly in horses older than 16 years. It is benign, usually unilateral, and is not associated with thyroid dysfunction. Occasionally its size may warrant surgical excision. Prognosis is good. Horses with thyroid adenoma or hypophyseal adenoma were found to have exaggerated insulin responses following oral glucose tolerance testing and failed to maintain cortisol suppression 24 hours after a dexamethasone suppression test. These findings were observed also in preclinical cases that were diagnosed at necropsy.[96]

Adenocarcinoma

Malignant neoplasia of the thyroid occur less frequently. In three reported cases of thyroid adenocarcinoma, one horse was euthyroid and two hypothyroid on the basis of serum T_3 and T_4 concentrations.[58–60] One case of thyroid carcinoma with systemic metastasis and concurrent pituitary adenoma is reported.[98] There is one report of a horse with a diagnosis of carcinoma and adenoma in the same gland. The low T_3 level seen with this horse was felt to be due to euthyroid sick syndrome, as the TSH stimulation response was normal.[95]

Medullary Carcinoma

Medullary carcinoma (C-cell or parafollicular cell tumors) have been reported in horses.[61, 99] In these cases, the youngest horse was 8 years old and the tumors were unilateral. In two horses, a complaint of constant gulping was alleviated by surgical removal of the enlarged glands, and the horses returned to athletic function.[61] A third horse had no associated clinical signs.[99] Thyroid function tests were not done. In other species, familial multiple endocrine neoplasia, hypocalcemia, lameness, and amyloid can be associated with medullary carcinoma. C-cell hyperplasia has been described in horses as young as 3 years.[93] Electron microscopy or immunohistochemical techniques may be necessary to distinguish C-cell tumors from other thyroid neoplasias.

Treatment

In circumstances that warrant surgical excision, prognosis is best when the condition is unilateral and there is no concurrent systemic abnormality. Potential complications of the surgery include infection, hemorrhage, laryngeal hemiplegia on the side of the surgery, and scar tissue at the surgical site. The horse's parathyroid glands are not connected to the thyroids, and hypocalcemia is not a complication.[61] When hypo- or hypercalcemic states were induced in bilaterally thyroidectomized horses, normocalcemia was not achieved until T_4 was supplemented, suggesting that the absence of calcitonin alone was not responsible for the abnormal calcium homeostasis.[8]

REFERENCES

1. Ingbar SH: The thyroid gland. In Wilson JD, Foster DW, eds. *Williams' Textbook of Endocrinology,* 7th ed. Philadelphia, WB Saunders, 1985, p 682.
2. Capen CC, Martin SL: The thyroid gland. In McDonald LE, ed. *Veterinary Endocrinology and Reproduction.* Philadelphia, Lea and Febiger, 1989, p 58.
3. Kaneko JJ: Thyroid function. In Kaneko JJ, ed. *Clinical Biochemistry of Domestic Animals.* San Diego, Academic Press, 1989, p 630.
4. Larsson M, Pettersson T, Carlström A: Thyroid hormone binding in serum of 15 vertebrate species: Isolation of thyroxine-binding globulin and prealbumin analogs. *Gen Compar Endocrinol* 58:360, 1985.
5. Irvine CHG: Hypothyroidism in the foal. *Equine Vet J* 16:302, 1984.
6. Katovich M, Evans JW, Sanchez O: Effects of season, pregnancy and lactation on thyroxine turnover in the mare. *J Anim Sci* 38:811, 1974.
7. Ferguson DC: The effect of nonthyroidal factors on thyroid function tests in dogs. *Compend Contin Ed Practic Vet* 10:1365, 1988.
8. Argenzio RA, Lowe JE, Hintz HF, et al: Calcium and phosphorus homeostasis in horses. *J Nutrition* 204:18, 1974.
9. Irvine CHG: Thyroxine secretion rate in the horse in various physiological states. *J Endocrinol* 39:313, 1967a.
10. Motley JS: Use of radioactive triiodothyronine in the study of thyroid function in normal horses. *Vet Med Small Anim Clinician* 67:1225, 1972.
11. Irvine CHG, Evans MJ: Postnatal changes in total and free thyroxine and triiodothyronine in foal serum. *J Reprod Fertil Suppl* 23:709, 1975.
12. Irvine CHG, Evans MJ: Hypothyroidism in foals. NZ *Vet J* 25:354, 1977.
13. Khan VTS: Studies on thyroidal states in equines during normal and certain disturbed conditions of reproduction. *Mysore J Agr Sci* 14:1382, 1980.
14. Chen CL, Riley AM: Serum thyroxine and triiodothyronine concentrations in neonatal foals and mature horses. *Am J Vet Res* 42:1415, 1981.
15. Irvine CHG: Protein bound iodine in the horse. *Am J Vet Res* 28:1687, 1967.
16. Thomas CL, Adams JC: Radioimmunoassay of equine serum for thyroxine: Reference values. *Am J Vet Res* 39:1239, 1978.
17. Kelley ST, Oehme FW, Brandt GW: Measurement of thyroid gland function during the estrous cycle of nine mares. *Am J Vet Res* 35:657, 1974.
18. deMartin BW: Study on the thyroid function of thoroughbred

horses by means of "in vitro" ^{125}I-T$_3$ modified and ^{125}I-T$_4$ tests. *Rev Fac Med Vet Zootec Univ S Paulo* 12:107, 1975a.

19. McCall CA, Potter GD, Kreider JL, et al: Physiological responses in foals weaned by abrupt or gradual methods. *Equine Vet Sci* 7:368, 1987.

20. Reap M, Cass C, Hightower D: Thyroxine and triodothyronine levels in ten species of animals. *Southwest Vet* 31:31, 1978.

21. Anderson RR, Nixon DA, Akasha MA: Total and free thyroxine and triiodothyronine in blood serum of mammals. *Comp Biochem Physiol* 89A:401, 1988.

22. deMartin BW: Study on the thyroid function of male and female thoroughbred horses in different times after winning races at the Hippodrome Cidade Jardim, with the use of "in vitro" ^{125}I-T$_3$, and ^{125}I-T$_4$ tests. *Rev Fac Med Vet Zootec Univ S Paulo* 14:199, 1977.

23. deMartin BW: Study on the thyroid function of thoroughbred females in varying stages of pregnancy using "in vitro" tests ^{125}I-T$_3$ and ^{125}I-T$_4$. *Rev Fac Med Vet Zootec Univ S Paulo* 12:121, 1975.

24. Irvine CHG: Measurement of free and total T$_4$ and T$_3$ in domestic animals. In Stockigt JR, Nagatake S, eds. *Thyroid Research VIII.* New York, Pergamon, 1980, p 252.

25. Galton VA: Thyroid hormone–catecholamine interrelationships. *Endocrinology* 77:278, 1965.

26. Morris DD, Garcia M: Thyroid-stimulating hormone: Response test in healthy horses, and effect of phenylbutazone on equine thyroid hormones. *Am J Vet Res* 44:503, 1983.

27. Duckett WM, Manning JP, Weston PG: Thyroid hormone periodicity in healthy adult geldings. *Equine Vet J* 21:125, 1989.

28. Ferguson DC: Effect of nonthyroidal factors on thyroid function tests in the dog. In Proceedings 7th Annual American College of Veterinary Internal Medicine Forum. San Diego, 1989, p 930.

29. Beech J: Evaluation of thyroid, adrenal and pituitary function. *Vet Clin: Equine Pract* 3:649, 1987.

30. Irvine CHG: Thyroid function in the horse. In American Association of Equine Practitioners Proceedings, 1966, p 197.

31. McBride GE, Christopherson RJ, Sauer W: Metabolic rate and plasma thyroid hormone concentrations of mature horses in response to changes in ambient temperature. *Can J Anim Sci* 65:375, 1985.

32. Irvine CHG: The role of hormones in exercise physiology. In Snow DH, Persson SGB, Rose RJ, eds. Equine exercise physiology. Cambridge, Granta Editions, 1983, p 377.

33. Takagi S, Ito K, Shibata H: Effects of training on plasma fibrinogen concentration and thyroid hormone level in young race horses. *Exper Results Equine Health Lab* 11:94, 1974.

34. Blackmore DJ, Greenwood RES, Johnson C: Observations on thyroid hormones in the blood of thoroughbreds. *Res Vet Sci* 25:294, 1978.

35. Garcia MC, Beech J: Endocrinologic, hematologic, and heart rate changes in swimming horses. *Am J Vet Res* 47:2004, 1986.

36. Gupta S, Glade MJ: Hormonal responses to high and low planes of nutrition in weanling Thoroughbreds. *Equine Vet Data* 4:170, 1983.

37. Biesik LM, Glade MJ: Changes in serum hormone concentrations in weanling horses following gastric infusion of sucrose or casein. *Nutrition Rep Int* 33:651, 1986.

38. Glade MJ, Reimers TJ: Effects of dietary energy supply on serum thyroxine, tri-iodothyronine and insulin concentrations in young horses. *J Endocrinol* 104:93, 1985.

39. Glade MJ, Luba NK: Serum triiodothyronine and thyroxine concentrations in weanling horses fed carbohydrate by direct gastric infusion. *Am J Vet Res* 48:578, 1987.

40. Youket RJ, Carnevale JM, Houpt KA, et al: Humoral, hormonal and behavioral and correlates of feeding in ponies: The effects of meal frequency. *J Anim Sci* 61:1103, 1985.

41. Hershman JM: Use of thyrotropin-releasing hormone in clinical medicine. *Med Clin North Am* 62:313, 1978.

42. Morris DD, Garcia MC: Effects of phenylbutazone and anabolic steroids on adrenal and thyroid gland function tests in healthy horses. *Am J Vet Res* 46:359, 1985.

43. Prager EM, Gardner RE: Iatrogenic hypothyroidism from topical iodine-containing medications. *West J Med* 130:553, 1979.

44. Goldberger J, Goldberger S: Iatrogenic thyroid dysfunction. *Hosp Pract* 24(9):30, 1989.

45. Hanauer G, Schroth HJ: Serum effects on thyroxine and triiodothyronine levels. *J Am Vet Med Assoc* 34:790, 1987.

46. Reimers TJ, Cowan RG, Davidson HP, et al: Validation of radioimmunoassays for triiodothyronine, thyroxine, and hydrocortisone (cortisol) in canine, feline, and equine sera. *Am J Vet Res* 42:2016, 1981.

47. Reimers TJ, Lamb SV, Bartlett SA, et al: Effects of hemolysis and storage on quantification of hormones in blood samples from dogs, cattle, and horses. *Am J Vet Res* 52:1075, 1991.

48. Oliver JW, Held JP: Thyrotropin stimulation test—new perspective on value of monitoring triiodothyronine. *J Am Vet Med Assoc* 187:931, 1985.

49. Lowe JE, Baldwin BH, Foote RH, et al: Semen characteristics in thyroidectomized stallions. *J Reprod Fertil Suppl* 23:81, 1975.

50. Lowe JE, Kallfelz FA: Thyroidectomy and the T$_4$ test to assess thyroid dysfunction in the horse and pony. *Proc 16th Am Assoc Eq Pract Conv*, 135, 1970.

51. Waldron-Mease E: Hypothyroidism and myopathy in racing thoroughbreds and standardbreds. *J Equine Med Surg* 3:124, 1979.

52. Held JP, Oliver JW: A sampling protocol for the thyrotropin-stimulation test in the horse. *J Am Vet Med Assoc* 184:326, 1984.

53. Shaftoe S, Schick MP, Chen CL: Thyroid-stimulating hormone response tests in one-day-old foals. *J Equine Vet Sci* 8:310, 1988.

54. Beech J, Garcia M: Hormonal response to thyrotropin-releasing hormone in healthy horses and in horses with pituitary adenoma. *Am J Vet Res* 46, 1941, 1985.

55. Lothrop CD, Nolan HL: Equine thyroid function assessment with the thyrotropin-releasing hormone response test. *Am J Vet Res* 47:942, 1986.

56. Chen CL, Li WI: Effect of thyrotropin releasing hormone (TRH) on serum levels of thyroid hormones in thoroughbred mares. *J Equine Sci* 6:58, 1986.

57. Hillidge CJ, Theodorakis MC, Duckett WM: Scintigraphic evaluation of equine thyroid function. *Proc 27th Am Assoc Eq Pract Conv*, 1981, p 477.

58. Joyce JR, Thompson RB, Kyzar JR, et al: Thyroid carcinoma in a horse. *J Am Vet Med Assoc* 168:610, 1976.

59. Hillidge CJ, Sanecki RK, Theodorakis MC: Thyroid carcinoma in a horse. *J Am Vet Med Assoc* 181:711, 1982.

60. Held JP, Patton CS, Toal RL, et al: Work intolerance in a horse with thyroid carcinoma. *J Am Vet Med Assoc* 187:1044, 1985.

61. Lucke VM, Lane JG: C-cell tumours of the thyroid in the horse. *Equine Vet J* 16:28, 1984.

62. Dimock WW, Westerfield C, Doll ER: The equine thyroid in health and disease. *J Am Vet Med Assoc* 104:313, 1944.

63. Drew B, Barber WP, Williams DG: The effect of excess dietary iodine on pregnant mares and foals. *Vet Rec* 97:93, 1975.

64. Green EM, Hunt EL: Hypophyseal neoplasia in a pony. *Compend Contin Ed Pract Vet* 7:S249, 1985.

65. Stanley O, Hillidge CJ: Alopecia associated with hypothyroidism in a horse. *Equine Vet J* 14:165, 1982.

66. Vivrette SL, Reimers TJ, Krook L: Skeletal disease in a hypothyroid foal. *Cornell Vet* 74:373, 1984.

67. Rooney JR: Endocrine disease. In Huntington PJ, ed: *Equine Diagnostics and Therapeutics: Proceedings of the Tenth Bain-*

Fallon Memorial Lectures. May 1988, Adelaide, Australia, p 76.

68. Shaver JR, Fretz PB, Doige CE, et al: Skeletal manifestations of suspected hypothyroidism in two foals. *J Equine Med Surg* 3:269, 1979.

69. McLaughlin BG, Doige CE: Congenital musculoskeletal lesions and hyperplastic goitre in foals. *Can Vet J* 22:130, 1981.

70. McLaughlin BG, Doige CE, McLaughlin PS: Thyroid hormone levels in foals with congenital musculo-skeletal lesions. *Can Vet J* 27:264, 1986.

71. Conway DA, Cosgrove JS: Equine goitre. *Irish Vet J* 34:29, 1980.

72. Baker JR: Case of equine goitre. *Vet Rec* 112:407, 1983.

73. Glade MJ: The role of endocrine factors in equine developmental orthopedic disease. *Proc 23rd Am Assoc Eq Pract Conv,* p 170, 1987.

74. Murray MJ: Hypothyroidism and respiratory insufficiency in a neonatal foal. *J Am Vet Med Assoc* 197:1635, 1990.

75. Doige CE, McLaughlin BG: Hyperplastic goitre in newborn foals in Western Canada. *Can Vet J* 22:42, 1981.

76. Lowe JE, Baldwin BH, Foote RH, et al: Equine hypothyroidism: The long term effects of thyroidectomy on metabolism and growth in mares and stallions. *Cornell Vet* 64:276, 1974.

77. McLaughlin BG, Doige CE: A study of ossification of carpal and tarsal bones in normal and hypothyroid foals. *Can Vet J* 23:164, 1982.

78. Driscoll J, Hintz HF, Schryver HF: Goiter in foals caused by excessive iodine. *J Am Vet Med Assoc* 173:858, 1978.

79. Baker HJ, Lindsey JR: Equine goiter due to excess dietary iodine. *J Am Vet Med Assoc* 153:1618, 1968.

80. Dudan FE, Ferguson DC, Little TV, et al: Circulating serum thyroxine (T_4), triiodothyronine (T_3) and reverse T_3 (rT_3) in neonatal term and preterm foals (Abstract). In *Proceedings of the 5th Annual Veterinary Medical Forum,* San Diego, 1987, p 881.

81. Lowe JE, Foote RH, Baldwin BH, et al: Reproductive patterns in cyclic and pregnant thyroidectomized mares. *J Reprod Fertil Suppl* 35:281, 1987.

82. Fadok VA, Wild S: Suspected cutaneous iodinism in a horse. *J Am Vet Med Assoc* 183:1104, 1983.

83. Thompson FN, Caudle AB, Kemppainen RJ, et al: Thyroidal and prolactin secretion in agalactic mares. *Theriogenology* 25:575, 1986.

84. Thompson DL, Nett TM: Thyroid stimulating hormone and prolactin secretion after thyrotropin releasing hormone administration to mares: Dose response during anestrus in winter and during estrus in summer. *Domest Anim Endocrinol* 1:263, 1984.

85. Poomvises P, Gesmankit P, Tawatsin A, et al: Studies on serum triiodothyronine and thyroxine in anhidrotic horses. *Centaur* II(4):139, 1986.

86. Mayhew IG, Ferguson HO: Clinical, clinicopathologic, and epidemiologic features of anhidrosis in central Florida thoroughbred horses. *J Vet Intern Med* 1:136, 1987.

87. Hood DM, Hightower D, Amoss MS, et al: Thyroid function in horses affected with laminitis. *Southwest Vet* 38:85, 1987.

88. Chen CL, McNulty ME, McNulty BA, et al: Serum levels of thyroxine and triiodothyronine in mature horses following oral administration of synthetic thyroxine (Synthroid®). *J Equine Vet Sci* 4:5, 1984.

89. deMartin BW: Study on the thyroid function of Thoroughbred horses using ^{131}I-TBI: *Rev Fac Med Vet Zootec Univ S Paulo* 10:35, 1973.

90. Tateyama S, Tanimura N, Moritomo Y, et al: The ultimobranchial remnant and its hyperplasia or adenoma in equine thyroid gland. *Jpn J Vet Sci* 50:714, 1988.

91. Schlotthauer CF: The incidence and types of disease of the thyroid gland of adult horses. *J Am Vet Med Assoc* 78:211, 1931.

92. Cubillos V, Norambuena L, Espinoza E: Cell growth and thyroid neoplasia in horses. *Zbl Vet Med* 28:201, 1981.

93. Hopper LD, Kennedy GA, Taylor WA: Diagnosing and treating thyroid adenoma in a horse. *Vet Med* 82:1252, 1987.

94. Yoshikawa T, Yoshikawa H, Oyamada T, et al: A follicular adenoma with C-cell hyperplasia in the equine thyroid. *Jpn J Vet Sci* 46:615, 1984.

95. Hovda LR, Shaftoe S, Rose ML, et al: Mediastinal squamous cell carcinoma and thyroid carcinoma in an aged horse. *J Am Vet Med Assoc* 197:1187, 1990.

96. Ralston SL, Nockels CF, Squires EL: Differences in diagnostic test results and hematologic data between aged and young horses. *Am J Vet Res* 49:1387, 1988.

97. Damodaran S, Ramachandran PV: A survey of neoplasms in equidae. *Centaur* II(4):161, 1986.

98. Chiba S, Okada K, Numakunai S, et al: A case of equine thyroid follicular carcinoma accompanied with adenohypophyseal adenoma. *Jpn J Vet Sci* 49:551, 1987.

99. Van Der Velden MA, Meulenaar H: Medullary thyroid carcinoma in a horse. *Vet Pathol* 23:622, 1986.

17.4

Disorders of Calcium Metabolism

Clara K. Fenger, DVM, MS, Dip ACVIM

Calcium plays an important and diverse role in physiology. Its contributions range from structural support of the body in bone, to helping determine the membrane threshold potential of excitable cells, to acting as a cofactor in enzymatic reactions. Clinical signs associated with abnormal calcium homeostasis are attributable to the malfunctioning of one or more of the processes in which it is involved.

Calcium comprises about 1.5% of the body by weight. The majority is in the form of hydroxyapatite in bone, and the remainder is divided between the intra- and extracellular fluid compartments. The presence of this large quantity of calcium in bone represents a relatively limitless reservoir for the maintenance of plasma ionized calcium. Therefore, most diseases associated with abnormal ionized calcium concentration are the result of abnormal calcium regulation rather than an absolute deficiency or excess.

Ionized calcium in plasma is maintained at about 5.4 mEq/L (6 mg/dL), whereas that in interstitial fluid is about 2.5 mEq/L (2.8 mg/dL). The total plasma calcium concentration, which includes protein-bound, complexed, and ionized calcium, is usually 11 to 13 mg/dL but may vary, depending on protein concentration, pH, and other factors. The cytosolic calcium is maintained at about 10^{-4} mEq/L, in several intracellular reservoirs: (1) mitochondria, (2) endoplasmic (or sarcoplasmic) reticulum, and (3) calcium-binding proteins, such as calmodulin. This significant concentration gradient of calcium between the interstitial and intracellular compartments permits calcium to perform a number of important intracellular functions. Minuscule changes in calcium conductance across the cell membrane mediated by signals such as hormone binding or membrane voltage changes result in a cascade of intracellular events, which underscore calcium's role as a second messenger. Because of this important role, the body controls ionized (free) plasma calcium within narrow limits.

AN OVERVIEW OF CALCIUM IN PHYSIOLOGY

Structural and Storage Roles in Bone

Bone contains the majority of the calcium in the body. Calcium is stored in two general reservoirs: a small, accessible pool and a larger, stable and slowly exchangeable pool. The larger pool consists of insoluble hydroxyapatite within a structural matrix of protein. This forms the structural support of the body—the skeleton—and is constantly remodeled by a balance of osteogenesis and osteolysis. Remodeling occurs along lines of stress. This larger pool turns over more rapidly during phases of growth thus the greater requirement for calcium at that time.[1]

The smaller pool of calcium consists of soluble complexes of calcium and phosphorus present on the surfaces of bone. This pool is available to be mobilized for the maintenance of plasma ionized calcium or for conversion to the more stable hydroxyapatite. Any hormonal regulation of calcium concentration has an impact on this reservoir of calcium.

The maintenance of an adequate quantity of calcium in conjunction with bone formation is essential for osteogenesis. Since the bone has a high calcium, the diffusion gradient would encourage osteolysis. Bone circumvents this problem by maintaining a low calcium concentration in the canalicular fluid. The bone lining cells, which are formed from osteoblasts, cover the surfaces of the bone and actively transport calcium out of this canalicular fluid to the space directly surrounding the bone. Active alkaline phosphatase in these cells cleaves phosphate extracellularly, which increases the amount of phosphate in the same space. The result of this is precipitation of calcium and phosphorus on the surface of bone. This removes the calcium from the fluid to maintain the gradient and provides a calcium-phosphorus complex of intermediate solubility. This property allows this substance to be readily mobilized into plasma or further catalyzed into hydroxyapatite.[1]

Calcium Membrane Channels

The large calcium concentration differentials across most cell membranes create a strong driving pressure for inward flux of calcium. Therefore, small increments in calcium conductance permit entry of calcium ions into the cytosol, initiating a cascade of secondary effects. Calcium may enter through channels of three different types. A minimal quantity of calcium enters cells through cation channels, which are specific for other cations, such as fast sodium channels. The majority of calcium enters through calcium-specific channels, which are either voltage gated or ligand gated. Voltage-gated channels are opened when the membrane potential of an excitable cell reaches a certain degree of depolarization. Examples of this type are found in nerves, muscle, and some endocrine cells. Ligand-gated channels are often associated

with a G protein–receptor complex. The hormone receptor is complexed to a G protein, whose alpha subunit is bound to guanosine diphosphate (GDP). Upon hormone binding, the GDP is replaced by a guanidine triphosphate, resulting in the separation of the alpha-subunit from the beta-gamma subunit. The alpha-subunit activates phospholipase C, which hydrolyzes the membrane phospholipid phosphatidylinositol 4,5-diphosphate into inositol triphosphate (IP_3) and diacylglycerol. Both of these products act as second messengers. The IP_3 opens calcium channels, which can be on the cell membrane or the endoplasmic reticulum. Both types of channels are involved with the amplification of signals mediated by calcium and are discussed further below.

Calcium may also be transported across cell membranes by transport proteins. The active transport protein of calcium exchanges two hydrogen ions for one calcium at the cost of one adenosine triphosphate (ATP) molecule. Calcium is also transported out of cells by an antiport protein that trades two sodium ions for one calcium ion. This protein is indirectly driven by the Na^+-K^+-ATPase pump, because the sodium is moved along its concentration gradient, while calcium is moved against its concentration gradient.

Calcium as a Second Messenger

Calcium plays a role in many intracellular functions, particularly by amplifying hormonal or voltage-gated signals. Through a combination of voltage-gated and ligand-gated channels, a signal can result in a relatively large increase in intracellular calcium. Either alone or in association with calmodulin, this intracellular calcium can act as a cofactor for many enzymes and precipitate a cascade of events.

Calmodulin was once believed to be a storage protein for calcium but is now recognized to have a facilitatory function for a number of enzymes. Inactive until bound with calcium, calmodulin activates multiple protein kinases, including phosphorylase kinase, which is important for glycogen breakdown in muscle, myosin light chain kinase in smooth muscle cells, which is important for smooth muscle contraction, and the calcium-calmodulin kinases. Further discussion of these functions follows.

Membrane Potentials

Cell membrane resting potentials are determined by the distribution of diffusible ions on either side of the membrane, their respective permeabilities (conductances), and equilibrium potentials. The ions that are usually present in equilibrium across cell membranes, such as chloride, do not contribute to the resting membrane potential. Because sodium and potassium are subject to great electrochemical gradients they almost completely determine the magnitude of the resting membrane potential. These electrochemical gradients are maintained by the Na^+-K^+-ATPase pump, which exchanges three sodium ions for two potassium ions. The physiologic importance of the resting membrane potential is underscored by the fact that 33% of the resting metabolic rate is due to energy consumed by this ion pump.

The resting membrane is relatively impermeable to calcium; therefore, calcium contributes little to the resting membrane potential. This relative impermeability, in concert with the large differential concentration of free calcium across the membrane, permits calcium to perform important cell functions. A small increment in calcium conductance results in a rapid increase in intracellular calcium. This phenomenon allows calcium to play important roles in excitable cells, including determination of membrane threshold potential, amplification of signals as a second messenger, coupling of muscle excitation, and contraction and release of neurotransmitters.

Excitable cells are notable for their ability to propagate a signal in the form of an action potential. An action potential is a self-propagating change in sodium conductance that results from the summation of excitatory stimuli to a threshold potential. Membrane excitability is the difference between the resting membrane potential and the threshold potential. The threshold potential is determined by the extracellular free calcium concentration. Increased extracellular free calcium increases the threshold potential, which stabilizes the membrane by decreasing its excitability, whereas decreased extracellular calcium decreases the threshold potential, increasing excitability. The mechanism of calcium antagonism of hyperkalemia depends on this phenomenon: hyperkalemia increases resting membrane potential closer to threshold, thus increasing membrane excitability, whereas calcium administration raises the threshold potential, stabilizing membrane excitability.[2]

Neurons

In addition to its effects on membrane excitability, calcium is required for the release of neurotransmitters. When the neuronal action potential reaches the nerve terminal, voltage-dependent calcium channels in the presynaptic membrane open. This increase in calcium conductance increases the intracellular free calcium concentration. Both free calcium and the calcium-calmodulin complex act within the presynaptic terminal to mobilize the actin and myosin of the microtubular network. Vesicles containing the neurotransmitter are thus moved to the presynaptic membrane, where the contents are released. This effect requires the presence of only a small amount of calcium in the extracellular fluid and is therefore unlikely to contribute to clinical signs associated with abnormalities of extracellular free calcium.

Skeletal Muscle

In the myocyte, calcium plays several roles. First, extracellular free calcium determines the threshold potential, as in other excitable cells. Second, the small increase in intracellular calcium with excitation is amplified by intracellular events, resulting in excitation-contraction coupling. In addition, the intracellular calcium acts as a cofactor for enzymes important in energy release. Abnormalities of the functions of calcium in muscle are often the first clinical signs attendant on hypocalcemia. Both increased membrane excitability and muscle weakness may be observed, whereas impairment of cofactor function of calcium is less evident because less calcium is needed for this action.

In skeletal muscle, the muscle action potential extends down T tubules to continue within the sarcoplasmic reticulum. This opens voltage-dependent calcium channels, creating a net flux of calcium from both the extracellular compartment through the cell membrane and the intracellular calcium stores through the sarcoplasmic reticulum into the cytosol. About 90% to 95% of intracellular calcium required for contraction is released by intracellular stores. The free calcium in the cytosol combines with troponin C, which causes a conformational change in the molecule and frees myosin-binding sites on the actin molecule, resulting in contraction. Therefore, the higher the concentration of cytosolic calcium, the greater the number of free binding sites and the greater the force of contraction.[3] Muscle contraction is terminated by the active pumping of cytosolic calcium back into the sarcoplasmic reticulum, resulting in muscle relaxation.

The calcium cascade functions not only to initiate contraction but also to activate glycogenolysis, providing energy for ATP generation. Calcium activates phosphorylase kinase, which phosphorylates several muscle enzymes. Phosphorylation of the inactive phosphorylase b results in the active phosphorylase a, which is responsible for the breakdown of glycogen. Phosphorylation inactivates glycogen synthase, simultaneously arresting glycogen synthesis. Therefore, calcium acts in active skeletal muscle to both initiate contraction and provide the energy to sustain it.

Cardiac Muscle

In the cardiac myocyte, calcium also mediates excitation-contraction coupling; however, the mechanism is slightly different than in skeletal muscle. The action potential extends down T tubules, where voltage-gated calcium channels are opened. This influx of calcium diffuses to the sarcoplasmic reticulum, where it triggers ligand-gated channels to release additional calcium. As in skeletal muscle, intracellular stores of calcium are responsible for the majority of the increase with excitation.

Calcium also contributes to the spontaneous depolarization of cardiac muscle through a slow cation channel.[3, 4] Spontaneous depolarization is the result of a gradual increase in conductance of both sodium and calcium, the affinity for sodium being greater. Once threshold is achieved, fast sodium channels open, resulting in the fast upstroke (phase 0) of the cardiac action potential. As the membrane potential passes the -30 to -40 mV mark, voltage-gated calcium channels open, allowing calcium influx into the cell. These calcium channels remain open for a relatively long time, resulting in the plateau (phase 2) of the cardiac action potential. This calcium influx is then available for excitation-contraction coupling.

Clinical signs of hypocalcemia are manifested by cardiac muscle as a result of abnormal ionized calcium concentration. Hypocalcemia decreases the rate of the slow inward calcium current, prolonging the plateau phase of the cardiac action potential and the QT and ST segments of the electrocardiogram (ECG). With profound hypocalcemia, this results in slowing the heart rate, heart block, and arrhythmias, as well as decreasing the strength of contraction, or contractility, owing to lack of calcium to bind troponin C. Hypercalcemia, such as that induced by rapid administration of calcium for treatment of hyperkalemia, shortens the QT and ST segments, flattens the T wave, and may cause first-degree heart block. Severe hypercalcemia may cause asystole or ventricular arrhythmias, increasing heart rate and contractility. Therefore, it is always advisable to monitor heart rate whenever calcium is administered.

Smooth Muscle Cells

Smooth muscle cells, such as those found in the vasculature and the gastrointestinal tract, also require calcium for excitation-contraction coupling. Cell membranes of smooth muscle cells contain voltage-dependent calcium channels. These can be activated by electrical stimulation, hormonal influences, or a combination of the two. Once opened, the cytosolic calcium concentration increases in calcium-triggered calcium release similar to the phenomenon seen in skeletal and heart muscle. In the vascular smooth muscle, calcium enters and binds to calmodulin, which activates myosin light-chain kinase. This enzyme is responsible for the phosphorylation of myosin, which is required for the activation of smooth muscle myosin.[3]

Other Cells

Many cells utilize calcium as a second messenger, stimulated either by hormone binding or electrical impulses. An example of hormone-stimulated action can be found in the parietal cells in the stomach. Acetylcholine binding activates calcium channels to increase cytosolic free calcium. This increase in calcium causes an increase in acid secretion. An example of electrical stimulation can be found in the β cells of the islets of Langerhans. Glucose entry depolarizes the membrane, resulting in an increase in calcium conductance. This calcium influx activates the microtubule system to facilitate release of insulin from storage vesicles in the cytosol. The examples of both types of calcium channels are innumerable, but abnormalities in this role for calcium seldom result in clinical signs. The absolute amount of calcium required for these functions is so minute that these functions are unimpaired, even in the face of profound hypocalcemia.

Coagulation

In addition to its effects on intracellular events, calcium is clotting factor IV, an important cofactor in coagulation. Calcium is a required cofactor for the serine proteases, including factors II, VII, IX, X, XI, XII and XIII. These serine proteases are present as proenzymes that share the common feature of a serine residue at their active site. After the proenzymes of factors II, VII, IX and X are produced in the liver, they are enzymatically altered by the vitamin K–mediated carboxylation of glutamic acid residues. The result of this carboxylation is the creation of a calcium-binding site, to which calcium must be bound if enzyme function is to continue.

The amount of calcium required for coagulation is miniscule. Therefore, decreasing ionized calcium concentration would kill the animal from its other effects before dropping low enough to interfere with coagulation. Further discussion of hemostasis may be found in Chapter 11.

Lactation

An important role for calcium is in the nutrition of neonates. At the onset of lactation, the daily calcium requirement of mares more than doubles. Calcium is concentrated within the mammary gland of all species, but mares have one of the lowest calcium levels, at 17 mM, just over half that of cows. Despite the high total calcium content of milk, the ionized calcium content is similar to that of plasma. The majority of calcium present in milk is complexed to organic bases and casein.

Calcium is concentrated in the mammary gland by an active mechanism. Ionized calcium is actively transported into the Golgi apparatus of mammary secretory cells. In the Golgi system, the calcium is complexed to citrate and other multivalent anions, thus preventing formation of a large concentration gradient. Vesicles containing the complexed calcium are "exocytosed" into the lumen. Some of this complexed calcium remains in solution in the milk, and some is incorporated into the casein and fat micelles.[5]

Ionized Calcium Metabolism

Plasma free calcium depends on the balance of (1) calcium influx from the intestine and bone, (2) calcium efflux into the gastrointestinal tract, bone, and urine, and (3) the degree of protein binding in the plasma. In contrast to sodium, potassium, and chloride, which are almost completely absorbed from the intestine, intestinal absorption of calcium and phosphorus is incomplete. Regulation of the serum concentrations of these other electrolytes is determined principally by secretion and reabsorption at the renal tubule. Regulation of serum calcium and phosphorus occurs at several levels: intestinal absorption, flux between the skeletal stores and plasma, and excretion in the urine.

Calcium is absorbed in the small intestine. Absorption is most efficient in the duodenum, although it occurs throughout the length of the small intestines. The majority of absorption occurs in the jejunum, because of its length. Absorption occurs via two mechanisms: (1) active transport and (2) facilitated diffusion. Active transport is a saturable mechanism of calcium uptake but may be increased by the vitamin D–stimulated increase in protein synthesis in intestinal cells. Facilitated diffusion increases with calcium intake and is neither saturable nor energy dependent. The presence of lactose or fatty acids in intestinal chyme enhances absorption of calcium, whereas phosphate, oxalates, and phytates chelate calcium. These substances create obligatory intestinal calcium losses. There are also small obligatory losses through the bile.

Once absorbed, calcium is subject to regulation in the kidneys. Free calcium is freely filtered through the glomerulus, but reabsorption occurs throughout the entire renal tubule. The proximal convoluted tubule reabsorbs 65% of the filtered calcium and is not influenced by hormone regulation. Proximal tubule reabsorption depends on the anions present in the filtrate, and the $2 Na^+-1 Ca^{++}$ antiporter. Therefore, if a large concentration of anions is present, obligatory losses of calcium will be larger at this point. In addition, if sodium is being conserved, as during hypovolemia, calcium will be reabsorbed. In horses, which normally have alkaline urine, the bicarbonate in the urine tends to bind the calcium, resulting in high urine losses of calcium; however, diets are usually rich in calcium, which offsets this effect. The ascending loop of Henle reabsorbs about 25% of the free calcium. The distal convoluted tubule is responsible for the final 10% of absorption and is the only site that is hormonally regulated. Parathyroid hormone (PTH) increases the uptake of calcium at this site, probably by stimulating adenyl cyclase to increase intracellular cyclic adenosine monophosphate (cAMP). Vitamin D is also needed for this effect, although it appears to have a "permissive" effect rather than an active role.

Bone acts as a reservoir for calcium in the body. Two mechanisms achieve transfer of calcium from bone to plasma. The classic mechanism is the action of osteoclasts, large, multinucleate cells that stem from monocytic precursors. They function as part of the normal turnover process of bone, creating resorption bays in bone and absorbing the minerals and the protein matrix. The ruffled border of the osteoclast overlies the resorption bay, creating hydrogen ions and oxygen radicals to dissolve the hydroxyapatite and the protein matrix, respectively. This releases calcium, phosphorus, and amino acids into the extracellular fluid. The size of the ruffled border changes, depending on different hormonal signals. PTH and prostaglandin E increase the surface area of the ruffled border, whereas calcitonin decreases it.

The number of osteoclasts can also be modulated. PTH stimulates undifferentiated monocyte precursors to proliferate and develop into osteoclasts. PTH, interleukin 1, tumor necrosis factor, and other cytokines can increase the rate of development of committed precursors into osteoclasts.

Hormonal regulation of calcium homeostasis is mediated in these tissues by PTH, vitamin D, and calcitonin. In response to low plasma calcium, the net result of PTH and the active form of vitamin D, calcitriol, is to increase intestinal absorption, bone resorption, and renal reabsorption. Calcitonin acts to lower plasma calcium in response to elevated plasma concentrations. Abnormal plasma concentrations of ionized calcium occur as a result of either (1) failure or delayed correction of abnormal calcium balance or (2) resetting of the regulating mechanisms to a new set point.

Parathyroid Hormone

PTH is a single polypeptide chain produced in the chief cells of the parathyroid gland and released principally in response to decreased plasma ionized calcium concentration. Other stimulators of PTH release include adrenergic agonists, prostaglandin E, magnesium, and vitamin D metabolites. Low serum magnesium concentration and 1,25-dihydroxycholecalciferol (calcitriol or vitamin D) inhibit PTH secretion. PTH is metabolized in the liver into several fragments. The amino-terminal fragment retains some biologic activity, whereas the carboxyl-terminal fragment is inactive.[6, 7] In the circulation the half-life is less than 20 minutes.

PTH acts to increase plasma calcium concentration in three ways: (1) stimulates bone resorption in the presence of 1,25-dihydroxycholecalciferol, (2) stimulates renal conversion of 25-hydroxycholecalciferol to the active calcitriol, and (3) augments active renal reabsorption of ionized calcium in the distal convoluted tubule. PTH stimulates cAMP production in its effector cells, although this may not be the sole mechanism, since both PTH and calcitonin increase cAMP in renal tubule cells, with widely differing results. In bone, PTH stimulates activity and proliferation of osteoclasts while inhibiting osteoblasts, which results in an increase in both plasma calcium and phosphorus. PTH acts on the proximal tubule cells to stimulate the conversion of 25-hydroxycholecalciferol to calcitriol, although the renal conversion of vitamin D to calcitriol may not be as important for calcium homeostasis in horses as it is in other species. Even after total nephrectomy, horses continue to exhibit hypercalcemia.[7, 8] PTH also acts on the distal convoluted tubule to increase calcium uptake and inhibit phosphorus and bicarbonate reabsorption. The net result of PTH secretion is increase of both calcium and phosphorus in plasma from resorption of bone—and indirectly from increased intestinal absorption due to vitamin D effects—and increased fractional excretion of bicarbonate and phosphate.

Vitamin D

Vitamin D_3 (cholecalciferol) is produced in mammalian skin by ultraviolet irradiation of a cholesterol derivative, 7-dehydrocholesterol. Transport of this compound in the plasma is like that of other steroid hormones, bound to plasma proteins (principally albumin) but also lipoproteins, and a specific binding protein. It is converted to 25-hydroxycholecalciferol in the liver, under minimal regulation. The active form, calcitriol, is formed by the action of 1α-hydroxylase in mitochondria of renal proximal convoluted tubule cells. This enzyme is the step that is most closely regulated. In the proximal convoluted tubule cells, PTH serves as the primary stimulus of 1α-hydroxylase, whereas in the short, straight segment calcitonin is the primary regulator. In addition, low plasma phosphorus, low plasma calcium, calcitonin, growth hormone, estrogen, and prolactin increase 1α-hydroxylase activity. High plasma phosphorus, hypercalcemia, metabolic acidosis, excessive intake of strong anions,[9] high concentrations of calcitriol, and low plasma insulin inhibit 1α-hydroxylase activity.

In the face of low plasma calcium, calcitriol is produced to offset this problem. Calcitriol binds to nuclear receptors in effector cells, stimulating mRNA synthesis. The increased mRNA increases protein synthesis. The primary effector cells are the intestinal cells, which respond by increasing production of the active transport protein of calcium. This increases the maximal rate of calcium absorption. Other effector cells include the proximal renal tubule cells, which respond by facilitating calcium reabsorption, and osteoblasts, which respond by increasing active transport of calcium into the extracellular fluid. Calcitriol also acts on the parathyroid cells as a feedback inhibitor of PTH release.

In addition to its effects on calcium metabolism, calcitriol also plays an interesting role in circulating monocytes. This hormone stimulates monocyte conversion into macrophages and is released from activated macrophages under the influence of interferon-γ and interleukin 2. The adaptive significance of this release is not known, but calcitriol excess has been identified in chronic granulomatous processes in humans.

Calcitonin

Calcitonin is produced in the parafollicular cells (C cells), which are interspersed throughout the thyroid gland. The primary stimulant of calcitonin is high plasma calcium, but β-adrenergic agents, dopamine, estrogen, gastrin, cholecystokinin, glucagon, and secretin all stimulate calcitonin release. Calcitonin is broken down in the kidney, and the circulating half-life is about 5 to 10 minutes.

Receptors for calcitonin are found in bone and kidney. Calcitonin directly inhibits ionized calcium flux from osteoclasts, osteoblasts, and renal tubule cells via increased adenyl cyclase activity. The net result is a rapid drop of plasma calcium. The calcitonin response is rapid and short lived, suggesting that it provides protection against postprandial hypercalcemia.

Other Substances Affecting Calcium

Several cytokines and endotoxin have been shown to affect osteoclast activity, resulting in a change in bone resorption. Interleukin 1 (IL-1) and tumor necrosis factor (TNF), two cytokines that have been implicated in endotoxic shock, stimulate osteoclastic bone resorption. Interferon-γ, which is also released during endotoxic shock, antagonizes this effect of IL-1 and TNF. Prostaglandin E also increases bone resorption by osteoclast stimulation. Endotoxemia appears to cause hypocalcemia.

CLINICAL PATHOLOGY

Plasma calcium exists in diffusible and nondiffusible forms. About 10% of the plasma calcium is complexed to bicarbonate, citrate, and other organic bases, and 50% to 60% is in the active, extracellular form, ionized calcium; this 60% to 70% is the diffusible calcium pool. The other 30% to 40% of plasma calcium is nondiffusible, bound to plasma proteins, particularly albumin. The nondiffusible calcium is not filtered at the glomerulus. Neither complexed nor protein-bound calcium is available to influence membrane potentials, enter cells through calcium channels, or provide feedback on calcium homeostasis. Only the ionized calcium plays a role in these physiologic processes; therefore, if ionized calcium is normal, there will be no clinical signs of calcium deficiency, regardless of the total plasma calcium concentration.

The percentage of plasma calcium present as ionized calcium depends upon plasma albumin and hydrogen ion concentrations (pH). A low plasma albumin concentration results in a low total calcium concentration, despite a normal ionized calcium concentration (i.e., the fraction of ionized calcium rises). Low pH results in the displacement of calcium from albumin by hydrogen ions, thus increasing ionized calcium concentration. Conversely, alkalosis results in the dissociation of the weak acid residues on albumin, increasing its calcium binding and decreasing free and ionized calcium concentrations. The ionized calcium concentration cannot be estimated from the pH or albumin concentration and thus must be measured directly.[10]

Routine laboratory measurement of calcium in blood includes measurement of total calcium by spectrophotometric techniques or ionized calcium using an ion-specific elec-

trode. The advantage of monitoring total calcium is that no special sample handling is required; however, the actual concentration of biologically active calcium is not measured. The measurement of free calcium requires anaerobic sample collection and an ion-specific electrode.[11] The normal range should be about 50% of the normal range for total calcium, or 6 to 6.25 mg/dL.

Both PTH and calcitriol can be measured by radioimmunoassay and can be determined by several different specialty laboratories. The normal range for PTH differs between laboratories. Therefore, care should be taken to use a laboratory that has experience with equine samples.

DISORDERS OF CALCIUM

Hypocalcemia

The clinical signs associated with mild hypocalcemia are attributable to an increase in membrane excitability of excitable tissue, including the heart and skeletal muscle. With more severe hypocalcemia, the strength of contraction of skeletal muscle decreases resulting in flaccid paralysis. The specific signs observed may differ with the clinical syndrome.

Clinical Signs

Synchronous Diaphragmatic Flutter

Synchronous diaphragmatic flutter (SDF) has been recognized for 160 years and has been associated with colic,[12] lactation tetany,[13] shipping, thoracic hematoma,[14] blister beetle toxicosis,[15] urethral obstruction,[16] but most often with athletic stress, particularly endurance exercise.[17] Horses are among the few mammals that use sweating as a primary means of thermoregulation.[18] During exercise, equine sweat glands respond to both circulating and locally released catecholamines at beta₂-receptors.[19] After prolonged exercise, particularly in the heat, large quantities of sodium, chloride, potassium, and calcium are lost in hypertonic secretions.[20]

The resultant hypocalcemia lowers the threshold potential of the phrenic nerve, thus allowing depolarization of the right atrium to stimulate an action potential in the nerve as it crosses the heart. SDF "flutter" is evident as a rhythmic movement, or "tic," of the flank of the horse that is synchronous with the heartbeat.[14] Contraction of the diaphragm coincides with depolarization of the right atrium.

In addition to actual calcium losses with prolonged exercise, the associated alkalosis results in greater calcium binding, which further reduces the amount of ionized calcium. A disproportionate amount of chloride is lost in sweat, which causes hypochloremic metabolic alkalosis. Hydrogen ions compete with calcium for sites on albumin, and, therefore, in alkalosis a smaller proportion of the total calcium is present in ionized form. This association with alkalosis is not limited to metabolic alkalosis, since horses with respiratory alkalosis may also exhibit SDF.[14] This suggests that it is the alkalosis, rather than the hypochloremia, that contributes to SDF.

Hypocalcemic Tetany

The lower threshold potential increases membrane excitability by decreasing the amount of stimulation required to generate a self-propagating action potential. This is manifest in skeletal myocytes as tetany (excessive muscle contractions). Cardiac myocytes respond to hypocalcemia with tachycardia and arrhythmias, although slowing of the heart rate may be observed owing to the decrease in the slow inward calcium current. There are two recognized clinical syndromes associated with hypocalcemic tetany: lactation tetany and transit tetany. Mares about 10 days post partum eating a low-calcium ration are at risk, particularly draft horses that are worked during lactation. Horses transported for long distances also develop hypocalcemia.[13]

Hypocalcemic Seizures

Hypocalcemia in humans may precipitate grand mal–type seizures, particularly in children. This has also been recognized clinically in foals. The patient exhibits a normal interictal period and a characteristic electroencephalogram (EEG). In most human cases and in foals, an underlying cause for the hypocalcemia was not determined. Clinical signs usually improve with calcium treatment, although relapses that require repeated treatment may occur. In such cases euthanasia may be the ultimate outcome. Necropsy has failed to reveal any abnormalities. Others respond to a single calcium infusion and experience no recurrence.

Treatment

Treatment of hypocalcemia is similar whatever the cause. Ideally, the ionized calcium deficit can be determined from the measured ionized calcium value:

$$\frac{(6 - [Ca^{++}])(ECF)}{[Ca^{++}]/[Ca_{tot}]} =$$

The difference between the measured ionized calcium and normal ($\sim$ 6 to 7 mg/dL) is multiplied by the extracellular fluid (ECF) volume, then divided by the fraction of total calcium present in ionized form. For example, a 450-kg horse with an ionized calcium level of 4.5 mg/dL and a total calcium of 10 mg/dL would have an ECF calcium deficit of 4500 mg:

$$\frac{(6\ mg/dL - 4.5\ mg/dL)\ (0.3)\ (450\ L)}{0.45} = 4500\ mg$$

This amount should be given slowly, intravenously—no faster than 1 mg/kg per hour. The problem with this method of calcium supplementation is that the ionized calcium value must be known, and few practitioners have the capability of measuring it. An alternative is to calculate the deficit based on total measured calcium.

If neither measurement is available, calcium may be administered intravenously slowly to effect, but heart rate should be monitored carefully. Solutions of choice contain either calcium borogluconate or calcium chloride. While the latter agent is, theoretically, preferred, practical experience has shown there is little or no difference between clinical responses to each preparation. Solutions containing calcium should never be added to fluids containing bicarbonate as insoluble calcium carbonate complexes result. If a horse is suspected to be hypocalcemic and is anorectic, empiric addition of 200 mg/kg/day by mouth or in intravenous fluids may help prevent hypocalcemia.

Hypoalbuminemic, hypocalcemic horses might not need calcium supplementation unless they are clinically hypocalcemic, as ionized calcium concentrations may be normal. Particular care needs to be taken in such cases if the horse is acidemic as the percentage of ionized calcium increases in these situations and administration of calcium may be harmful.

Specific Causes of Hypocalcemia

Hypoparathyroidism

Hypoparathyroidism may be primary, the type that results from abnormal production, release, or binding of PTH. In humans, this is associated with hypocalcemia and hyperphosphatemia and normal renal function. This has not been recognized in horses. Secondary hypoparathyroidism is the result of hypomagnesemia.[21] Magnesium ions are required for PTH release from the chief cells of the parathyroid gland; therefore the hypocalcemia found in this situation is profound. Hypomagnesemia should always be included in the differential diagnosis of hypocalcemia.

Vitamin D Deficiency

Primary vitamin D deficiency is not a recognized disease syndrome in horses; however, since it could occur secondary to intestinal malabsorption or to chronic renal or hepatic failure, it is a theoretical possibility. The hepatic enzyme that is responsible for the conversion of vitamin D to 25-hydroxycholecalciferol is a member of the P_{450} microsomal enzyme system. Therefore, drugs or toxins that disable this enzyme system could result in vitamin D deficiency. Despite this possibility, horses that have been completely nephrectomized and therefore lack of 1-α-hydroxylase still remained hypercalcemic. This suggests that calcitriol contributes little to calcium homeostasis in horses.

Pancreatic Necrosis

The cause of hypocalcemia with this rare condition is unclear, but in humans it is considered to be associated with deposition of calcium in regions of saponification of peripancreatic fat (fat necrosis). Pancreatitis principally causes colic in horses but has been recognized to cause hypocalcemia.

Oxalate Toxicity

Oxalates chelate divalent cations, which process renders them inaccessible to the intestinal cells and, thus, they are lost in the feces. Oxalates are present in several tropical grasses, several species of toxic weeds, and alfalfa hay. The grasses include buffel (*Cenchrus cilaris*), pangola (*Digitaria decumbens*), setaria (*Setaria spachhelata*), and kikuyu (*Penisetum clandestinum*). Toxic weeds include rhubarb (*Rheum rhapneticum*), halogeton (*Halogeton glomeratus*), greasewood (*Sacrobatus vermiculatus*), and soursob (*Oxalis cernua*). The oxalates in alfalfa do not interfere with calcium absorption, because of the large quantity of calcium present[22]; however, other oxalate-containing plants do not have enough calcium, so hypocalcemia and secondary hyperparathyroidism have developed separately in horses grazing pastures affected with toxic plants.

Tetracycline Administration

Rapid intravenous administration of tetracycline and its related compounds can result in recumbency or even death in horses and other animals. Tetracycline is a calcium chelator that, if administered rapidly intravenously, may bind the free calcium required for normal conduction in the myocardium, resulting in severe arrhythmias. In these cases total calcium is normal, but the ionized calcium value is low. Treatment consists of intravenous calcium.

Furosemide Administration

Furosemide is commonly administered to horses, both to treat various diseases and to prevent exercise-induced pulmonary hemorrhage. Owing to its blocking action on the chloride cotransporter in the thick ascending loop of Henle, furosemide causes an increase in chloruresis. Cations that accompany the chloride loss include hydrogen and calcium ions. Both acidic urine and excessive excretion of strong anions result in increased urinary loss of calcium. Calcium, potassium, and chloride remain low for at least 8 hours after intramuscular administration of a single dose (1 mg/kg) of furosemide.[23]

Bicarbonate Overdose

Long-term administration of bicarbonate has been a relatively common practice in racehorses and horses that suffer repeated bouts of exertional rhabdomyolysis (ER). These uses have, however, recently fallen into disfavor owing to the introduction of regulations prohibiting prerace administration of bicarbonate and the realization that there are more effective ways of treating ER. This practice has gained favor despite the lack of experimental evidence to support a beneficial effect. It results in a chronic bicarbonate load presented to the renal tubule for removal. This load presents an obligatory cation excretion, which includes calcium. The most common presentation for hypocalcemia of this origin is synchronous diaphragmatic flutter.

Other Conditions Associated with Hypocalcemia

Cantharidin (blister beetle) toxicosis, acute renal failure, and severe exertional rhabdomyolysis may be associated with hypocalcemia and hypomagnesemia.[21, 24] The mechanism of the hypocalcemia in the first two diseases is likely to be excessive losses coupled with the effect of low magnesium on PTH release. Uremia also interferes with the intestinal absorption of calcium and magnesium. In exertional rhabdomyolysis, part of the calcium loss may be due to calcium influx into the damaged myocytes. Further discussion of these diseases can be found in Chapters 12, 16, and 19.

Severe colic and colitis can be associated with hypocalcemia. The mechanism for this association is probably continued renal excretion of calcium in the face of decreased intestinal absorption. These horses are usually anorectic owing to pain or have malabsorption secondary to severe diarrhea. Since horses are habitually in a state of calcium excess due to the high calcium content of most hay, sudden removal of all intake results in acute calcium deprivation. The animals, unable to readjust rapidly, develop hypocalcemia. Often, there are no overt clinical signs with this mild hypocal-

cemia, and within a few days the animal should be able to adjust; however, hypocalcemia may contribute to poor gastrointestinal motility, and supplementation may be helpful for these horses.

Hypercalcemia

In equine medicine, hypocalcemia is a more common problem than hypercalcemia. Clinical signs associated with hypercalcemia are generally attributable to the underlying disease process; however, hypercalcemia causes dystrophic mineralization of soft tissues, particularly the kidneys. Additional clinical signs related to organ failure can be observed if this mineralization is severe.

Treatment

Chronic hypercalcemia is rare, and clinical signs are usually referable to organ failure in mineralized tissues. Treatment should be directed at the underlying cause and should include supportive care of involved organs. Acute, severe hypercalcemia is potentially life threatening and should be addressed immediately. This should consist primarily of intravenous fluids for the purpose of volume expansion, to prevent obligatory absorption of calcium with sodium retention. Administration of an alkalinizing solution would increase the obligatory urinary losses of calcium.

If the hypercalcemia is considered to be immediately life threatening, magnesium can be used as a calcium blocker. Slow intravenous administration of magnesium sulfate is safe up to 30 mg/kg and causes sedation. This is a theoretical contingency, since this condition has not been reported.

Specific Disease Conditions

Hypervitaminosis D

Ingestion of certain toxic plants (*Cestrum* and *Solanum* spp.) or oversupplementation with feed additives may result in hypervitaminosis D. The toxic principles in these plants have homology with calcitriol, the active form of vitamin D. Therefore, they are able to circumvent the renal regulation by α_1-hydroxylase and act unchecked on intestinal absorption.

Clinical signs are insidious and include weight loss, depression, tachycardia, polyuria, and polydipsia. Clinical pathology findings may include a normal or a high free calcium concentration. Signs are attributable to extensive soft tissue mineralization, including renal calcinosis. Treatment is unrewarding in most cases but should include removal of sources of toxin and limitation of sources of calcium and phosphorus.

Hyperparathyroidism

Primary Hyperparathyroidism. Primary hyperparathyroidism occurs as the result of a hypersecretory parathyroid gland. In humans, this is most often caused by parathyroid adenomas but can also result from chief cell hyperplasia or carcinoma. This disease reflects upward resetting of the serum free calcium set point. Functional parathyroid adenomas have been identified in older horses. Primary hyperparathyroidism has been reported in a horse[25] with generalized medullary osteonecrosis; however, serum total calcium, ionized calcium, and renal fractional excretion of calcium were all within normal limits.

Secondary Hyperparathyroidism. Nutritional secondary hyperparathyroidism is a commonly recognized clinical syndrome in horses. It is seen in animals that either ingest excessive phosphorus or consume plants containing oxalate for a long time. The hyperphosphatemia results in excessive PTH activity and inhibition of renal 1α-hydroxylase and, therefore, excessive osteoclast activity with increased bone absorption. The weakened bone then remodels with fibrous tissue, a phenomenon known as "osteodystrophic fibrosa." The classic clinical sign is enlargement of the maxilla, sometimes accompanied by partial respiratory obstruction.[26] Horses walk with a stiff gait and may exhibit shifting leg lameness, loose teeth, and possibly pathologic fractures.[27] Chronic excessive sweat losses may contribute to nutritional secondary hyperparathyroidism with nutritional status is borderline.[27]

Diagnosis of nutritional secondary hyperparathyroidism is based predominantly on clinical signs and a history of inadequate calcium intake, such as high-grain rations with grass hay. Serum calcium tends to be low, and serum phosphorus high, although both values may remain within the normal range. More valuable is the measurement of urine fractional excretions of calcium and phosphorus. Calcium fractional excretion drops below 2.5% with inadequate calcium intake. Excessive phosphorus intake is reflected by fractional excretion over 4%.[28]

Prevention of nutritional secondary hyperparathyroidism depends on proper nutritional management. A calcium-phosphorus ratio of 1:1 to 2:1 is recommended for maintenance, but a ratio as high as 6:1 is required for treatment once a horse shows clinical signs. Animals suffering excessive stress, such as increased sweat losses, should be maintained on a higher Ca:P ratio.[27]

Paraneoplastic Syndrome. Malignant mesenchymoma, lymphosarcoma, and gastric squamous cell carcinoma may each be associated with hypercalcemia in horses.[29–31] The mechanism for this in horses has not been investigated, but in humans hypercalcemia of malignancy is associated with hypercalcemia, decreased PTH, increased bone resorption, and increased renal tubular reabsorption. A PTH-like factor has been identified from these tumors. In addition, both tumor necrosis factor and interleukin 1 are increased in some animals that have tumors, suggesting a possible role for these cytokines in hypercalcemia of malignancy.

Other Diseases Associated with Hypercalcemia. Both acute and chronic renal failure can be associated with hypercalcemia. Acute nephrosis is accompanied by an elevation in serum PTH and transient hypercalcemia. In the acute model, the increase is transient, whereas in the chronic renal failure model the hypercalcemia is persistent. This increase in plasma calcium is likely due to persistent absorption of calcium through the intestines with failure of calcium excretion. In acute nephrosis, the hypercalcemia coincides with oliguria.[7] These findings suggest that renal conversion of vitamin D is not as important in horses as in other species,

since other species usually respond to renal failure with hypocalcemia. Further discussion of renal failure is found in Chapter 16.

Thyroid hormone increases the rate of bone turnover, which can lead to elevated serum ionized calcium. Hyperthyroidism is not a recognized clinical syndrome in horses, but routine thyroid hormone supplementation has become common practice. Therefore, iatrogenic hyperthyroidism could develop, and excessive tissue deposition of calcium may become more prevalent.

REFERENCES

1. Parfitt AM, Simon LS, Villaneuva AR, et al: Procollagen type I carboxy-terminal extension peptide in serum as a marker of collagen biosynthesis in bone. Correlation with iliac bone formation and comparison with total alkaline phosphatase. *J Bone Mineral Res* 2:427, 1987.
2. Junge D: *Nerve and Muscle Excitation.* Sunderland, Sinaur Associates, 1981.
3. McCall D: Basic mechanisms of action of calcium blocking agents. *Curr Probl Cardiol* 10(8):6, 1985.
4. Antman EM, Stone PH, Muller JE, et al: Calcium channel blocking agents in the treatment of cardiovascular disorders. Part I: Basic and clinical electrophysiological effects. *Ann Intern Med* 93:875, 1980.
5. Davies DT, Holt C, Christie WW: The composition of milk. In *Biochemistry of Lactation.* New York, Elsevier, 1982, p 96.
6. Bayly WM, Brobst DF, Reed SM: A model for the study of acute nephrosis, with specific reference to calcium and phosphorus homeostasis. *Proc Am Assoc Equine Pract* 31:649, 1985.
7. Elfers RS, Bayly WM, Brobst DF, et al: Alterations in calcium, phosphorus and C-terminal parathyroid hormone levels in equine acute renal disease. *Cornell Vet* 76:317, 1986.
8. Tennant B, Lowe JE, Tasker JB: Hypercalcemia and hypophosphatemia in ponies following bilateral nephrectomy. *Proc Soc Exp Biol Med* 167:365, 1981.
9. Greger JL, Kaup SM, Behling AR: Calcium, magnesium and phosphorus utilization by rats fed sodium and potassium salts of various inorganic anions. *J Nutrition* 121:1382, 1991.
10. Kohn CW: Failure of pH to predict ionized calcium percentage in healthy horses. *Am J Vet Res* 51:1206, 1990.
11. Endres DB, Rude RK: Mineral and bone metabolism. In Burtis CA, Ashwood ER, eds. *Tietz Textbook of Clinical Chemistry,* 2nd ed. Philadelphia, WB Saunders, 1986, p 1897.
12. Kaneps AJ, Knight AP, Bennett DG: Synchronous diaphragmatic flutter associated with electrolyte imbalances in a mare with colic. *Equine Pract* 2(3):18, 1980.
13. Baird JD: Lactation tetany (eclampsia) in a Shetland pony mare. *Aust Vet J* 47:402, 1971.
14. Mansmann RA, Carlson GP, White NA, et al: Synchronous diaphragmatic flutter in horses. *J Am Vet Med Assoc* 165:265, 1974.
15. Schoeb TR, Panciera RJ: Blister beetle poisoning in horses. *J Am Vet Med Assoc* 173:75, 1978.
16. Dyke TM, Maclean AA: Urethral obstruction in a stallion with possible synchronous diaphragmatic flutter. *Vet Rec* 121:425, 1987.
17. Carlson GP, Mansmann RA: Serum electrolyte and plasma protein alterations in horses used in endurance rides. *J Am Vet Med Assoc* 165:262, 1974.
18. Jenkinson DM: Comparative physiology of sweating. *Br J Dermatol* 88:397, 1973.

19. Warner AE, Mayhew IG: Equine anhidrosis: A survey of affected horses in Florida. *J Am Vet Med Assoc* 180:627, 1982.

20. Kerr MG, Snow DH: Composition of sweat of the horse during prolonged epinephrine (adrenaline) infusion, heat exposure, and exercise. *Am J Vet Res* 44:1571, 1983.

21. Knochel JP: Neuromuscular manifestations of electrolyte disorders. *Am J Med* 72:521, 1982.

22. Hintz HF, Schryver HF, Doty J, et al: Oxalic acid content of alfalfa hays and its influence on the availability of calcium, phosphorus and magnesium to ponies. *J Anim Sci* 58:939, 1984.

23. Freestone JF, Carlson GP, Harrold DR, et al: Influence of furosemide treatment on fluid and electrolyte balance in horses. *Am J Vet Res* 49:1899, 1988.

24. Schmitz DG: Cantharidin toxicosis in horses. *J Vet Intern Med* 3:208, 1989.

25. Fenger CK, Bertone JJ, Biller D, et al: Generalized medullary infarction in the long bones of a horse. *J Am Vet Med Assoc* 202:621, 1993.

26. Robertson JT, Fenger CK: Diseases of the nasal passages. In Robinson NE, ed. *Current Veterinary Therapy in Equine Medicine III*. Philadelphia, WB Saunders, 1992, p 270.

27. Mason DK, Watkins KLL, McNie JT: Diagnosis, treatment and prevention of nutritional secondary hyperparathyroidism in thoroughbred race horses in Hong Kong. *Equine Pract* 10(3):10, 1988.

28. Denny JEFM: Equine blood serum calcium and phosphorus concentrations in progressive nutritional hyperparathyroidism. *J S Afr Vet Assoc* 56:123, 1985.

29. McCoy DJ, Beasley R: Hypercalcemia associated with malignancy in a horse. *J Am Vet Med Assoc* 189:87, 1986.

30. Mair TS, Yeo SP, Lucke VM: Hypercalcaemia and soft tissue mineralisation associated with lymphosarcoma in two horses. *Vet Rec* 126:99, 1990.

31. Karcher LF, Le Net JL, Turner BF, et al: Pseudohyperparathyroidism in a mare associated with squamous cell carcinoma of the vulva. *Cornell Vet* 80:153, 1990.

17.5

Diseases of the Adrenal Glands

Luis Rivas, DVM, MS, Dip ACVIM

FUNCTIONAL PHEOCHROMOCYTOMA

Pheochromocytomas are tumors of the chromaffin (dark-staining) cells of the adrenal medulla. These tumors, although rare, have been reported in most domestic animals, and they may or may not be functional (i.e., secrete catecholamines at a rate sufficient to cause clinical signs).[1] Most of the few articles reporting pheochromocytomas in horses include the description of functional tumors because of the dramatic clinical picture,[2] although it is suspected that most of the pheochromocytomas in horses, as in other species, are nonfunctional and therefore undiagnosed.[3] Both epinephrine and norepinephrine have been identified as the predominant catecholamines produced by equine pheochromocytomas.[4]

Functional pheochromocytomas in horses have no breed or gender predilection, and have been described only in horses older than 12 years.[2] Because clinical signs exhibit acute onset and rapid progression and are the result of intense adrenergic stimulation, the clinical picture resembles that of more common diseases such as colic, rhabdomyolysis, acute laminitis, impending colitis, and hyperkalemic periodic paralysis. The clinical signs most often observed are anxiety, tachycardia, tachypnea, profuse sweating, muscle fasciculations, and mydriasis (with intact pupillary light reflex). Occasionally, horses may also show abdominal pain from large hematomas or gastric and intestinal distension secondary to ileus (sometimes colonic gas distension is detectable on rectal palpation), hyperthermia, dry, pale mucous membranes, increased capillary refill time, bladder paralysis, and ataxia. Noninfectious abortion has also been reported in one mare at 271 days' gestation.

Hematologic abnormalities induced by a functional pheochromocytoma have been poorly documented. Increased hematocrit and a "stress leukogram" (mature neutrophilia with lymphopenia) or leukopenia with neutropenia and a leftward shift have been described. Epinephrine-mediated splenic contraction, rather than dehydration, seems responsible for the increased hematocrit.[1-3, 5] Epinephrine and epinephrine-induced steroid release are responsible for the stress leukogram; however, if there is a concurrent focus of inflammation and necrosis (especially after the rupture of the adrenal tumor), neutropenia with a leftward shift may be the laboratory hematologic finding.[2, 3]

The serum biochemical profile of horses with a functional pheochromocytoma is similar to that for other, more common diseases. Azotemia and metabolic acidosis with hyperkalemia are among the most consistently abnormal clinicopathologic findings. It is believed that intense renal and muscular vasoconstriction induced by catecholamines results in reduced renal blood flow (causing azotemia) and reduced muscle blood flow (causing lactic acidosis and exit of potassium from cells). A combination of hyponatremia, hyperkalemia, hypocalcemia, and hyperphosphatemia suggests acute renal failure and has been reported in horses with pheochromocytoma without evidence of renal lesions at necropsy.[2, 3] Hyperkalemia, hypocalcemia, and hyperphosphatemia could in part be the result of prolonged muscle fasciculations and ischemia, although serum concentrations of creatine kinase (CK) were normal or only mildly increased.[1-3, 5] Hyperglycemia and glycosuria were also found frequently, likely the results of the glycogenolytic action of epinephrine.

Because functional pheochromocytomas are rare and because the clinical and clinicopathologic abnormalities they induce are nonspecific, they are rarely sought ante mortem. A functional pheochromocytoma may, however, be suspected when an older horse has a paroxysmal attack of anxiety, sweating, and muscle tremors, along with azotemia, metabolic acidosis, hyperkalemia, and hyperglycemia. Once other common diseases have been ruled out (colic, impending colitis, acute laminitis, rhabdomyolysis, hypersegmented neutrophil), a more specific diagnosis may be pursued, with the understanding that the poor prognosis for this condition may not justify the expense. Documentation of a high serum concentration of catecholamines or their metabolites in urine is difficult because of the extremely labile nature of these substances and the need for sophisticated instruments.[1, 2, 5, 6]

Alternatively, ultrasonographic evaluation and measurement of blood pressure can support the diagnosis.

If diagnosis is achieved ante mortem, adrenalectomy may be attempted. Surgery may be extremely difficult because of the anatomic proximity of the adrenals and major vessels, the risk of induction of fatal arrhythmias (interaction between catecholamines and anesthetic agents),[3] and the complications of prolonged muscle ischemia and recumbency.[1, 5] It has been suggested that hypotensive agents be used before induction of anesthesia, to stabilize blood pressure.[2, 3]

Functional pheochromocytomas in horses do not appear to metastasize; most of them are unilateral (no predilection for right or left) and tend to bleed. Although the capsule initially may contain the hemorrhage and preclude aspiration of hemorrhagic fluid during abdominocentesis, at necropsy the tumor is frequently found to be ruptured.

HYPOADRENOCORTICISM

Also called "adrenal insufficiency" or "steroid letdown syndrome," hypoadrenocorticism is poorly documented in horses. Naturally occurring hypoadrenocorticism may be secondary to adrenal atrophy following conditions such as colic and endotoxemia, as the gland is a shock organ.[7] However, most cases of hypoadrenocorticism involve sudden discontinuation of prolonged administration of exogenous glucocorticoids[7] or anabolic steroids.[8] The steroids suppress production of pro-opiomelanocortin (POMC) peptides by pituitary corticotropins, and the (glucocorticoid and gonadocorticoid producing) zona fasciculata of the adrenal gland will atrophy for lack of stimulus by adrenocorticotropin (ACTH). The (mineralocorticoid producing) zona glomerulosa is usually preserved, since its main stimulant is angiotensin II, although biochemical abnormalities in some cases of adrenal insufficiency (see below) may be explained by its malfunction. The amount and duration of exogenous steroid treatment that induces adrenocortical atrophy is not known: as little as 4 mg of dexamethasone may suppress the pituitary-adrenal axis for 18 to 24 hours,[7] whereas 0.088 mg/kg of dexamethasone every 5 days for six treatments did not modify the response to ACTH stimulation, even though is reduced cortisol levels for up to 4 days.[9]

Clinical signs include depression, anorexia, weight loss, mild abdominal discomfort, poor hair coat, and lameness.[7, 8, 10] Serum biochemical analysis may be normal,[8] or hyponatremia, hypochloremia, hyperkalemia, and hypoglycemia may be observed.[7] Presumptive diagnosis is based on history of prolonged steroid administration and on clinical signs. Since cortisol has a short half life and its concentration may show great daily fluctuation, its measurement does not provide a reliable indicator of adrenal cortical function. Instead, an ACTH stimulation test is performed[10]: cortisol concentration (heparinized blood collection tube) is measured before and 8 hours after intramuscular administration of 1 IU/kg of ACTH gel, or is measured before and 2 hours after intravenous administration of 100 IU of aqueous ACTH. An increase in cortisol two to three times the baseline value is expected in normal horses.

Treatment of hypoadrenocorticism in horses involves rest (strict avoidance of any stress, including surgery) and steroid supplementation. A case of hypoadrenocorticism secondary to anabolic steroid administration was successfully treated with 300 mg of prednisone, orally, for 9 months.[8] This therapeutic regimen supplied the needed glococorticoids without further depressing adrenal cortical function.

HYPERADRENOCORTICISM

Hyperadrenocorticism resulting from pituitary dysfunction is discussed in detail elsewhere in this text. Iatrogenic[11] and adrenal hyperadrenocorticism,[12] although far less common than pituitary hyperadrenocorticism, have also been described in horses.

Iatrogenic hyperadrenocorticism was induced in a horse after first injecting 12 mg of triamcinolone acetonide, followed by two injections of 200 mg, all within 6 weeks.[11] Clinical signs (depression, polyuria/polydipsia, weight loss, laminitis) and blood and urinalysis abnormalities (stress leukogram, hyperglycemia, glycosuria) were the same as in pituitary-dependent hyperadrenocorticism; however, elevated concentrations of gamma-glutamyltransferase (GGT), alkaline phosphatase (ALP), and bile acids (suggesting hepatopathy) have been reported only in iatrogenic hyperadrenocorticism. Diagnosis is based on historical data and on subnormal cortisol concentrations—both baseline (0 µg/dL) and following ACTH administration (suggestive of adrenal suppression). Treatment for this condition (other than discontinuing administration of exogenous steroids) has not been tried. Steroid-induced hepatopathy was reversible in this case.

Adrenal-dependent hyperadrenocorticism is diagnosed by a negative dexamethasone suppression test and a delayed peak concentration of cortisol (at 12 hours instead of 8) following ACTH gel administration.[12] Treatment for this condition has not been tried.

REFERENCES

1. Yovich JV, Horney FD, Hardee GE: Pheochromocytoma in the horse and measurement of norepinephrine levels in horses. *Can Vet J* 25:21–25, 1984.
2. Duckett WM, Snyder JR, Harkema JR, et al: Functional pheochromocytoma in a horse. *Compend Contin Educ Pract Vet* 9:1118–1121, 1987.
3. Johnson PJ, Goetz TE, Foreman JH, et al: Pheochromocytoma in two horses. *J Am Vet Med Assoc* 206:837–841, 1995.
4. Gelberg H, Cockerell GL, Minor RR: A light and electron microscopic study of a normal adrenal medulla and a pheochromocytoma from a horse. *Vet Pathol* 16:395–404, 1979.
5. Yovich JV, Ducharme NG: Ruptured pheochromocytoma in a mare with colic. *J Am Vet Med Assoc* 183:462–464, 1983.
6. Hardee GE, Lau JW, Semrad SD, et al: Catecholamines in equine and bovine plasmas. *J Vet Pharmacol Ther* 5:279–284, 1982.
7. Dybdal NO: Endocrine disorders. In Smith BP, ed. *Large Animal Internal Medicine*. St Louis, CV Mosby, 1996, p 1449.
8. Dowling PM, Williams MA, Clark TP: Adrenal insufficiency associated with long-term anabolic steroid administration in a horse. *J Am Vet Med Assoc* 203:1166–1169, 1993.
9. MacHarg MA, Bottoms GD, Carter GK, et al: Effects of multiple intramuscular injections and doses of dexamethasone on plasma cortisol concentrations and adrenal responses to ACTH in horses. *Am J Vet Res* 46:2285–2287, 1985.

10. Sojka JE, Levy M: Evaluation of endocrine function. *Vet Clin North Am Equine Pract* 11:415–435, 1995.
11. Cohen ND, Carter GK: Steroid hepatopathy in a horse with glococorticoid-induced hyperadrenocorticism. *J Am Vet Med Assoc* 200:1682–1684, 1992.
12. Traver DS, Bottoms GD: Adrenal dysfunction. *Proc 24th Am Assoc Equine Pract* 499–514, 1981.

17.6

Endocrine Pancreas

Luis Rivas, DVM, MS, Dip ACVIM

DIABETES MELLITUS

Characterized by chronic hyperglycemia and glycosuria, diabetes mellitus results from either hypoinsulinemia or subnormal response of tissues to insulin (insulin resistance). Diabetes mellitus is rare in horses and most frequently is associated with insulin resistance induced by pituitary adenomas.[1–5] Pituitary dysfunction is discussed in detail elsewhere in this text.

Insulin resistance and resultant diabetes mellitus may be induced by other hormone imbalances, as suspected in a mare with bilateral granulosa cell tumors.[6] Although the exact cause of diabetes mellitus was not determined in this case, the lack of pituitary and pancreatic lesions, together with abnormal glucose and insulin tolerance tests, suggested that insulin resistance was present and possibly related to the release of hormones by the ovarian tumors.[6] Idiopathic insulin resistance has been demonstrated in another mare with diabetes mellitus, hyperinsulinemia, normal plasma concentration of growth hormone, and no lesions in pituitary or adrenal glands.[7]

Hypoinsulinemia, a less common cause of diabetes mellitus in horses, is the result of chronic pancreatitis induced by parasite migration, most commonly *Strongylus equinus* larvae.[8–11] Since invasion of the pancreas by *S. equinus* larvae occurs around 7 weeks after infection, insulin-dependent diabetes mellitus can be observed in younger animals.[10]

Diabetes mellitus should be considered when horses exhibit polyuria and polydipsia, progressive weight loss in spite of polyphagia, and rough haircoat. These clinical signs are typical of horses with functional pituitary adenoma but are also observed in other insulin resistance–related diseases and in cases of hypoinsulinemia.

Chronic hyperglycemia with glycosuria defines diabetes mellitus. Therefore, to reach a correct diagnosis, temporary hyperglycemia due to a high-carbohydrate diet, strenuous exercise, steroid treatment, sedation with xylazine or detomidine or anesthesia with halothane must not be present.[12] Ketone odor, ketonemia, and ketonuria have variously been reported in diabetic ponies (regardless of the cause) and in a horse with idiopathic insulin resistance.[3, 4, 7–9] Laboratory abnormalities suggestive of cholestasis may be present in insulin dependent diabetes mellitus when an inflamed pancreas compresses the common bile duct.[10]

The first goal after the diagnosis of diabetes mellitus (chronic hyperglycemia and glycosuria) is to rule out a functional pituitary adenoma by means of a dexamethasone suppression test or a TRH stimulation test. Only then is a glucose tolerance test indicated to characterize the pathogenesis of other types of diabetes mellitus. Intravenous administration of glucose is preferred over oral testing, to prevent the confounding effects of gastrointestinal motility.[13] A 50% solution of glucose, 0.5 g/kg, is administered intravenously, and serum concentrations of glucose and insulin are measured. In a normal horse, insulin is released immediately and glucose returns to baseline value within 3 hours. In the case of primary insulin-dependent diabetes mellitus, insulin concentration does not rise and glucose concentration remains elevated. In the case of insulin resistance, the concentration of insulin rises but the return of glucose concentration to normal is delayed more than 3 hours.

Alternatively, an insulin tolerance test can be performed.[3, 4, 6, 9, 14] Soluble (regular) insulin, 1 to 8 IU/kg, is administered intravenously, and plasma concentration of glucose is determined every 15 minutes for 3 hours. Failure of insulin to lower the concentration of glucose to normal values suggests insulin-resistant diabetes mellitus.

Serum insulin concentration, measured by radioimmunoassay, may aid in the diagnosis of diabetes mellitus.[5, 6] Elevated concentration suggests insulin resistance and reduced concentration insulin-dependent diabetes mellitus.

Treatment of diabetes mellitus secondary to a functional pituitary adenoma is discussed in detail elsewhere in this text. Treatment with insulin (lente) was attempted in a valuable stallion with pituitary adenoma.[5] Relief of symptoms was initially achieved for 6 weeks, but subsequent worsening of hyperglycemia, polyuria, and polydipsia, along with swelling at the injection sites and development of antibodies against porcine and bovine insulin, suggested refractoriness to treatment either by exacerbation of the hyperadrenocorticism or insulin interference by antibodies.[5] Treatment with insulin was also successful for 6 weeks in a case of insulin-dependent diabetes mellitus.[9] When treatment was discontinued, clinical signs of diabetes mellitus developed again.[9] During the treatment of insulin-dependent diabetes mellitus it is possible to observe hypoglycemic shock that quickly responds to intravenous administration of dextrose.[9] There are no reports on long-term insulin therapy in horses.

HYPERINSULINISM

Excessive insulin in blood may induce hypoglycemic shock. Hyperinsulinemia with accompanying hypoglycemia may be the result of therapeutic[9] or fraudulent[15, 16] injections of insulin, or secondary to increased release of endogenous insulin by a pancreatic tumor.[17]

Depending on the degree of hypoglycemia, the affected horse may show trembling, ataxia, tachycardia, tachypnea, mydriasis, nystagmus, profuse sweating, unawareness of surroundings followed by recumbency, violent seizures, coma and death. Injection of insulin may be suspected in insured horses that suddenly show these clinical signs.[15, 16] Hyperinsulinism secondary to pancreatic neoplasia has been documented only in a 12-year-old pony, and it appears that onset is insidious and that signs wax and wane, depending on several stimuli (especially feeding).[17] Differentiation between endogenous (pancreatic neoplasia) and exogenous (injected) insulin is done by high-pressure liquid chromatography.[16]

REFERENCES

1. King JM, Kavanaugh JF, Bentinck-Smith J: Diabetes mellitus with pituitary neoplasms in a horse and dog. *Cornell Vet* 52:133–145, 1962.
2. Loeb WF, Capen CC, Johnson LE: Adenomas of the pars intermedia associated with hyperglycemia and glycosuria in two horses. *Cornell Vet* 623–639, 1966.
3. Tasker JB, Whiteman CE, Martin BR: Diabetes mellitus in the horse. *J Am Vet Med Assoc* 149, 1966.
4. Baker JR, Ritchie HE: Diabetes mellitus in the horse: A case report and a review of the literature. *Equine Vet J* 6:7–10, 1974.
5. Staempfli HR, Eigenmann EJ, Clarke LM: Insulin treatment and development of anti-insulin antibodies in a horse with diabetes mellitus associated with a functional pituitary adenoma. *Can Vet J* 29:934–936, 1988.
6. McCoy DJ: Diabetes mellitus associated with bilateral granulosa cell tumors in a mare. *J Am Vet Med Assoc* 188:733–735, 1986.
7. Ruoff WW, Baker DC, Morgan SJ, et al: Type II diabetes mellitus in a horse. *Equine Vet J* 1:143–144, 1986.
8. Bulgin MS, Anderson BC: Verminous arteritis and pancreatic necrosis with diabetes mellitus in a pony. *Compend Contin Educ Pract Vet* 5:S482–S485, 1983.
9. Jeffrey J: Diabetes mellitus secondary to chronic pancreatitis in a pony. *J Am Vet Med Assoc* 153:1168–1175, 1968.
10. Collobert C, Gillet JP, Sorel P, et al: Chronic pancreatitis associated with diabetes mellitus in a standardbred race horse: A case report. *Equine Vet Sci* 10:58–61, 1990.
11. Riggs WL: Diabetes mellitus secondary to chronic necrotizing pancreatitis in a pony. *Southwest Vet* 25:149–152, 1972.
12. Stockham SL: Interpretation of equine serum biochemical profile results. *Vet Clin North Am Equine Pract* 11:391–414, 1995.
13. Sojka JE, Levy M: Evaluation of endocrine function. *Vet Clin North Am Equine Pract* 11:415–435, 1995.
14. Muylle E, van den Hende C, Deprez P, et al: Non–insulin-dependent diabetes mellitus in a horse. *Equine Vet J* 18:145–146, 1986.
15. Meirs DA, Taylor BC: Insulin induced shock. *Equine Pract* 2:47–49, 1980.
16. Given BD, Mostrom MS, Tully R, et al: Severe hypoglycemia attributable to surreptitious injection of insulin in a mare. *J Am Vet Med Assoc* 193:224–226, 1988.
17. Ross MW, Lowe JE, Cooper BJ, et al: Hypoglycemic seizures in a Shetland pony. *Cornell Vet* 73:151–169, 1983.

Chapter 18

Diseases of Foals

18.1

Neonatal and Perinatal Diseases

Clara K. Fenger, DVM, MS, Dip ACVIM

Causes of foal wastage, including neonatal septicemia, diarrhea, and neonatal maladjustment syndrome, have been identified for many years.[1-3] Despite this, veterinary intervention in these diseases was minimal before the early 1980s. During this same time period, significant advances in veterinary reproduction were occurring. The natural progression from the study of protecting and nurturing the conceptus was to the study of protecting and safeguarding the neonate. Clinicians began in the 1980s to devote more time and effort to adapting the lessons from human neonatology to the therapy of the equine neonate.[4] As more clinicians adopt this approach, and improve their ability to diagnose and treat early neonatal disease, the cost of treatment is declining, which should ultimately increase the availability of this service to horse breeders.[5] This new approach has ushered in the era of equine neonatal intensive care, and necessitates that all practitioners have an understanding of the basis for identification, diagnosis, and treatment of neonatal disease.

EVALUATION OF THE PREGNANT MARE AND FETUS PRIOR TO DELIVERY

Many of the problems that lead to diseased neonates or abortion begin in utero, and therefore adequate vigilance prior to parturition may prevent the potential loss of the foal. Identification of high-risk mares is an important management consideration. Conditions that place mares in this category include poor general state of health, advanced age, previous difficulty conceiving, previous abnormal foals, poor perineal conformation, premature lactation, prolonged transport during late gestation, and previous or concurrent disease.

The general health of the mare is important for the health of the fetus. The mare provides nutrients to the foal, and removes metabolites via the placenta. Epitheliochorial placentation prevents most macromolecules, including immunoglobulins, from crossing this barrier, but oxygen, carbon dioxide, energy substrates, and small molecules readily diffuse into the placental circulation. Therefore, the maintenance of these nutritional substances in the mare is essential

to the health of the fetus. Any disease process in the mare, and particularly those that result in abnormal hemodynamic parameters, hypoxia, or catabolism, compromises the fetus. Endotoxins, in particular, diffuse across the placenta, and frequently result in death of the fetus. Therefore, every precaution should be undertaken to identify and minimize systemic disease in the gravid mare.

Poor perineal conformation, in which the vulvar lips lie more than 25% above the pelvis, can result in aspiration of air and fecal material into the vaginal vault. The result is vaginitis, and, potentially, ascending placentitis. This condition may be accompanied by a vulval discharge, but may also be completely asymptomatic. This is often associated with fertility problems, because chronic infection also results in early embryonic loss, scarring of the uterus, placental insufficiency, and abortion. Therefore, the identification of poor perineal conformation prior to breeding is important so that a perineoplasty (Caslick's or Gadd's procedure) may be performed. Once a mare with poor perineal conformation is bred and found to be in foal, regular evaluation should continue until parturition. The mare should be regularly evaluated for evidence of vulval discharge, and for evidence of cervical relaxation.

Mares that are advanced in age have a significantly lower live foaling rate than younger mares.[6] Scarring of the uterus and chronic endometritis secondary to multiple pregnancies, and the progressively worsening perineal conformation associated with aging may contribute to this phenomenon. These factors also contribute to potential loss of the foal.

Premature lactation contributes to foal losses by contributing to failure of passive transfer, as discussed in detail in Chapter 1.

Prolonged transport contributes to high-risk neonates for several reasons. First, transport may result in immunosuppression in horses.[7] This predisposes to respiratory viruses, which also contribute to immunosuppression. Endogenous glucocorticoid release by the mare may contribute to premature parturition. While this hormonal change alone has not been implicated as a cause of premature parturition in mares, it may contribute in concert with other factors. Prolonged transport also predisposes horses to hypocalcemia, by an unknown mechanism. Transport for the purpose of foaling the mare on a farm where she will be rebred in the foal heat is a common practice. This may result in failure to protect a foal against the environmental pathogens of this new environment. Humoral immunity in the foal comes exclusively from the mare's colostrum. The immunoglobulins in the mare's colostrum will be against pathogens from the home farm environment if transported in late gestation.

Every pregnant mare should be evaluated for these risk

factors. Some of these factors, such as prolonged transport, can be actively avoided during late gestation. Others, such as poor perineal conformation, may be managed and carefully monitored, so that potential problems with the foal might be limited. If a pregnant mare does exhibit evidence of being in a high-risk category, evaluation of the viability of the fetus should be performed. In early pregnancy, evaluation includes primarily rectal examination, ultrasound, and measurement of progesterone concentrations. Further discussion of these procedures in early pregnancy may be found in Chapter 15. In late gestation, prepartum evaluation of the fetus includes rectal examination, ultrasonography, fetal electrocardiogram (ECG), and amniocentesis.

Prepartum Evaluation of the Fetus

Mares in which no risk factors have been identified do not routinely require prepartum evaluation of the fetus. However, in mares identified as high-risk individuals, the fetus should be evaluated for viability. Unfortunately, the ability to diagnose an impending premature parturition does not necessarily result in prevention.

The first step in the evaluation of the fetus should be rectal palpation. This examination should include evaluation of the cervix, uterus, and gastrointestinal tract, in addition to evaluation of the fetus. The cervix should remain tight throughout gestation, until the mare enters labor. The uterus in late gestation will be large and fluid-distended, and usually pulled far forward into the abdomen. The fetus should be gently stimulated by ballottement, and will often move in response to gentle stimulus. However, some normal fetuses may fail to respond. If a limb can be isolated, it may be gently pinched, because the withdrawal reflex is intact in utero in late term.[8]

The rectal examination requires minimal equipment, and provides a gross evaluation of fetal viability. Nonetheless, if a high-risk mare requires constant monitoring, multiple rectal palpations with manipulation of the fetus may be harmful. Alternatively, a biophysical profile of the late-gestation fetus may be determined ultrasonographically. Fetal heart rate, fetal aortic diameter, fetal fluid quantities, uteroplacental contact, uteroplacental thickness, and fetal activity are all associated with perinatal morbidity and mortality.[9, 10] The ultrasonogram is performed transabdominally, and requires a window from the udder caudally to the xiphoid cranially, and laterally to the skinfolds of the flank. A low-frequency probe (e.g., 3 MHz) provides depth of view for imaging the fetal heart, whereas detailed imaging of the endometrium and placenta requires a high-frequency probe (e.g., 7.5 MHz).

The ultrasound examination includes evaluation of the size of the fetus, the fetal heart rate, the amniotic and allantoic fluid, and placental thickness. Large amounts of allantoic fluid with echogenic particles are normally seen. The amniotic fluid may be difficult to image. It lies close to the fetus, primarily between the front legs, surrounding the head and neck, and may also contain echogenic particles.[9] The uteroplacental unit should be 8 to 16 mm in thickness.[10] Fluid should not be detectable between the placenta and uterine wall.

Specific abnormalities of the fetus are difficult to detect by ultrasound, but this method provides an unparalleled view of the placenta. Thickening of the placenta beyond the normal range results from edema and cellular infiltration secondary to placentitis. Fluid between the placenta and the uterus represents premature placental separation, and may result from placentitis or hemorrhage. Mares with this condition should be treated for placentitis, and confined to a stall to prevent further separation. The placenta should be repeatedly evaluated to determine whether the separation is continuing. If so, induction of labor may be considered. Calcification of the placenta secondary to chronic placentitis is visible as acoustic shadowing.[9]

Ultrasound is valuable for determining fetal viability, but is expensive and time-consuming. The fetal heart rate can also be determined by the fetal ECG. Electrodes are placed on the skin of the mare to maximize the size of the fetal QRS complex. The position of the fetus may change, and therefore optimal electrode placement may vary between subsequent evaluations. The left leg electrode is placed near the heart base of the mare. The right arm and left arm electrodes are placed on the torso in the transverse plane around the flank of the mare, usually starting in the right and left flank region. These electrodes are then moved until a maximal fetal QRS is seen. The amplitude of the maximized fetal QRS is about 0.05 to 0.1 mV, and is therefore seen as a small peak overlying the ECG of the mare.[11] The acquisition of a high-quality ECG is essential, because the fetal ECG is easily lost in artifact. This technique permits the repeated evaluation of fetal heart rate.

The fetal heart rate can be detected beginning at about 160 days of gestation.[12] The rate is highly variable at this stage, from 80 to 160 beats per minute (bpm), with an average of 120 bpm. Fetal heart rates become less variable, and gradually decrease over the course of gestation. Normal fetal heart rate in the last few months of gestation ranges from 65 to 115 bpm. While the range for normal fetal heart rates is wide, the range for any individual fetus is narrow. Therefore, regular monitoring of the fetal heart rate can be of great value clinically. Transient tachycardia may be observed to correspond with movement of the fetus, but persistent tachycardia is associated with fetal distress. Bradycardia, particularly progressive slowing of the heart rate, is suggestive of fetal hypoxia. Further discussion of diagnosis and treatment of impending abortion may be found in Chapter 15.

Prediction of Parturition

The detection of high-risk neonates would increase appreciably if parturition could be predicted within a limited time frame. This would significantly streamline broodmare management, and improve foal survival. In addition, the determination of readiness for birth would permit accurate timing of elective cesarean section or induced labor. Despite these advantages, few accurate methods of predicting parturition have been found.

Determination of the gestational age provides a gross prediction of parturition. However, gestational length varies considerably, from 315 to 365 days (mean, 340.7 days) for Thoroughbreds.[8] Miniature horses appear to have a longer gestational length, commonly exceeding 365 days. These large windows of time limit the utility of gestational age for prediction of parturition.

Fetal pulmonary maturity can be evaluated in humans by the determination of the lecithin:sphingomyelin ratio from amniotic fluid phospholipids, but this appears to be of limited value in horses. This ratio, as well as the percentages of amniotic sphingomyelin, cortisol, and creatinine concentrations have been shown to have no relationship to birth readiness in foals.[13, 14] Additionally, amniocentesis in horses, even with ultrasound guidance, is associated with a high rate of abortion, which limits the use of this technique in a clinical setting.[15]

Physical appearance of the mammae, including enlargement of the glands and presence of "wax" on the surface of the teats, are commonly used as predictors of parturition. Unfortunately, both of these factors may occur up to a week prior to parturition, and as many as 15% of mares may fail to exhibit these signs.[16] The precolostrum begins as a serum-colored fluid and gradually changes to the typical cloudy-white color of colostrum as parturition approaches. This color change has been used as a predictor of parturition. However, this color change may occur as soon as 4 days before parturition, and as many as 77% of mares fail to have this color change before parturition.[16]

Electrolyte concentration of the precolostrum has been used effectively to determine readiness for birth. Prior to parturition, the composition of the mammary secretion relatively closely reflects that of the mare's serum, but as parturition approaches, these constituents gradually change. The most consistent change immediately preceding parturition is a rapid rise in colostral calcium above 10 mmol/dL.[16] The evaluation of precolostrum may be performed by laboratory analysis of electrolytes, or, more simply, by the use of hard water test kits. These kits determine calcium concentration of precolostrum by the presence of a color change on the strip. This method appears to be most accurate, although the date of parturition can only be predicted within 1 day. Additionally, both false-negatives, where the precolostrum fails to increase in calcium content prior to parturition,[16] and false-positives, where precolostrum indicates readiness but the foal is actually dysmature,[17] are known to occur.

RISK FACTORS OF THE NEWBORN FOAL

Early recognition of an abnormality is often the most important factor determining the ultimate outcome of disease in the foal. Therefore, the most important examination that a foal receives occurs the first time it is seen in the field. This examination includes a careful examination of the mare, the placenta, and each body system of the foal to identify potential problems. Any abnormality, no matter how slight, should raise suspicion of serious disease. Neonates can deteriorate rapidly, even when they appear normal at birth.

The Mare

A thorough physical and gynecologic examination of the mare should be performed soon after parturition. In addition to determining the condition of the mare, this examination may lead to the identification of potential disease in the foal. A thorough history should include the mare's past breeding and foaling success, evidence of premature lactation, presence of disease during gestation, or dystocia. Any history that places the mare in a high-risk category, as described above, including repeated breedings to get a mare in foal, or previous abortions, increases the likelihood of disease of her current foal.

Physical examination should reveal the presence of current systemic disease. Respiratory disease, such as severe obstructive pulmonary disease, may result in profoundly low arterial oxygen tension (PaO_2) values, and placental insufficiency. Low blood pressure, as occurs during shock, may decrease circulation to the uterus, similarly resulting in placental insufficiency. Endotoxemia, enteritis, or gram-negative sepsis commonly results in premature parturition. Conditions that cause severe catabolism, such as chronic laminitis, infection, or neoplasia, may result in starvation of the fetus and a malnourished foal.

The gynecologic examination should be performed to determine the condition of the mare's reproductive tract, and to identify the possibility of infection. Post foaling, the uterus is a mixture of lochia and bacteria, which is rapidly cleared as the uterus involutes. The lochia is normally dark brown. Evidence of suppurative exudate may reflect an infection that was present before parturition, and may have caused a placentitis. In cases where the placenta is not available for evaluation, this may be the only evidence of an in utero infection of the foal.

Passive transfer of immunity by the ingestion of an adequate quantity of mare's colostrum with adequate IgG concentration is another significant risk factor. The epithelio-chorial placentation of the horse precludes the transfer of passive immunity in utero. Therefore, the entire humoral immunity of the immunologically naive foal is a consequence of the ingestion of colostrum. Colostrum is created in the mammary gland during the final few days of gestation under the influence of estrogen and progesterone. The mare concentrates immunoglobulins in the colostrum against a concentration gradient from the plasma. The colostrum contains primarily IgG and IgG(T), with some IgA and IgM.[18, 19]

High-quality colostrum contains at least 3,000 mg/dL of IgG, which has a specific gravity of 1.050.[20, 21] Unfortunately, the quality of an individual mare's colostrum is difficult to predict. Colostral IgG concentration varies considerably between individuals and between breeds, with Arabians having higher IgG concentrations (9,691 ± 1,639 mg/dL) than Standardbreds (8,329 ± 6,207 mg/dL) and Thoroughbreds (4,608 ± 2,138 mg/dL).[21, 22] Qualitative examination of the colostrum, mare parity, age, month of parturition, retention of the placenta, assisted delivery, and the mare's serum IgG concentration have no relationship to the quality of colostrum.[21, 23] Premature lactation, wherein the initial colostrum is lost, is associated with low-quality colostrum. However, some of these mares will still have colostrum of adequate quality, because the colostrum continues to be formed in the 24 hours preceding parturition. This condition often occurs as a premonitory sign of another problem, such as placental insufficiency. Repeated vaccination of the mare, with vaccination in the 10th month of gestation, increases the colostral IgG, but does not predict the final IgG concentration.[22] Since colostral quality cannot be predicted, the only method of determining colostral IgG concentration is by measurement of IgG, either directly by radial immunodiffusion (RID), or indirectly by specific gravity. The RID must be performed in the laboratory, and requires a minimum of 24 hours to complete. Therefore, the specific gravity measurement by Colostrometer (Lane Manufacturing Inc., Denver) is superior in determining colostral quality. Further discussion of the importance of colostrum is found below under Colostrum Intake.

A related risk factor is the dam's mothering ability. Normally, the dam will encourage the foal to rise and nurse, but if the mare rejects the foal, the foal will fail to ingest colostrum. Occasionally, the mare will accept the foal, but fail to allow it to nurse. This is most common in maiden mares. In these cases, it may be necessary to restrain the mare to allow the foal to nurse. Twitching or hobbling the mare may be effective. Some farms have stocks or stalls with kicking boards placed so that the mare cannot injure the foal during nursing. Most mares ultimately accept their foals, although this may take several days. Occasionally, a mare cannot be coerced to do so. In this case, the foal must be raised as an orphan (see Chapter 5).

The Placenta

Examination of the placenta may reveal evidence of abnormalities before birth that lead to a high-risk neonate. Abnormalities of the placenta can lead to hypoxia or starvation of the foal due to impaired diffusion of nutrients across the abnormal membrane (placental insufficiency). This may result in the death and abortion of the fetus, delayed intrauterine growth (dysmaturity), or damage to specific organs. Conditions that can be detected by gross examination of the placenta include placentitis, avillous regions, and edematous regions. Any of these abnormalities may result in placental insufficiency or premature placental separation. The normal amnion is thin and transparent. Infection may result in thickening of this membrane. However, abnormalities of the allantochorion are more easily detected. The villous surface should appear pink and velvety, with minimal avillous regions. The cervical star, where the chorion does not contact the endometrium, is avillous, and is normally disrupted during parturition by the foal.

Placentitis may result in placental insufficiency or overt infection of the fetus. Often, ascending placentitis may be diagnosed on the basis of thickening and suppurative infiltrate in the region surrounding the cervical star. Hematogenous infection of the placenta is more likely when the abnormal placenta is distributed in other regions. Avillous regions may result from either endometrial fibrosis or the presence of a second placenta, as in the case of twins. The ingestion of fescue late in gestation may result in edema of the placenta, and premature placental separation. Any questionable regions of the placenta should be sampled for culture and for histopathologic evaluation. Additional discussion of placental abnormalities may be found in Chapter 15.

Colostrum Intake

Failure of passive transfer (FPT) of immunoglobulins from the dam to the foal results from lack of quality or quantity of colostrum, or both. Equine placentation is epitheliochorial, which precludes the transfer of immunoglobulins from the mare to the fetus in utero. Therefore, the foal relies upon absorption of immunoglobulins from the colostrum for humoral immunity. The neonatal foal is immunocompetent at birth, but immunologically naive, meaning that the ability to respond to antigens exists, but has not yet been challenged. Minimal IgG and IgM are present in the presuckle serum, and result from preparturient immunologic stimulation.[19] The foal may begin producing immunoglobulin immediately, but this is not reflected in the circulation for 10 to 14 days. Therefore, equine neonates depend upon passive transfer of colostral antibodies for the majority of their immunologic protection against the pathogens they encounter in the first few days of life.

IgG is selectively absorbed by specialized epithelial cells in the small intestine of the foal.[19] These cells engulf the colostrum, which then enters the circulation through the lymphatic vessels. Over the course of 24 to 48 hours, these cells are replaced, resulting in the loss of the ability to absorb immunoglobulins. Maximal absorptive capacity occurs in the first 8 hours post parturition, while maximum blood levels occur at about 18 hours of age. The half-life of IgG in nondiseased foals is about 12 to 25 days,[18] but when challenged by infection, the foal's IgG concentration declines rapidly. The foal's serum IgG concentration is significantly correlated with the colostral IgG concentration.[23]

The diagnosis of FPT is based on the detection of IgG in the serum of the foal. The most accurate method is the single RID, which quantitates equine IgG by comparison of the radius of diffusion of serum IgG in agar with a known IgG concentration. This is accurate, but requires an overnight incubation, which makes it an impractical test for clinical use. Sodium sulfite, refractance, and serum electrophoresis have all been evaluated and determined to be of limited benefit in determining serum IgG concentration in horses.[24] The zinc sulfate turbidity test is based on the chemical property of IgG to precipitate in a 20% solution of zinc sulfate. The optical density of the resulting solution can be measured, and correlates well ($r = .875$) with IgG concentration. Hemolysis in the blood sample interferes with the test.[24, 25] A highly specific and sensitive test is the semiquantitative enzyme-linked immunosorbent assay (ELISA) (CITE-Foal IgG Test, AgriTech Systems, Inc., Portland, Me.). This test is easy to perform, specific for immunoglobulins, and the results are immediate.[26]

Partial failure of passive transfer has been reported to occur in 2.9% to 24% of foals.[20, 21, 23, 27, 28] Despite this high rate of occurrence, there is not a similar high rate of occurrence of septicemia in these foals. This discrepancy is due to the contribution of other factors to the development of disease in the neonate. Good management practices, including observed foalings in which the foal is born into a clean environment, result in a minimal pathogen challenge. Colostral-derived immunoglobulins probably play a smaller role in the development of disease in these foals. The less clean the environment of the foal, the more likely partial failure of passive transfer will result in disease.

Measurement of serum IgG concentration by semiquantitative methods is a reasonable component of routine postfoaling management on broodmare farms. However, since partial failure of passive transfer does not necessarily result in disease, the added expense may not always be warranted. In cases where the cleanliness of the environment is in question, or the foal falls into a high-risk category, the serum

IgG concentration should definitely be measured. Since peak serum IgG concentration occurs 18 hours after ingestion of colostrum, this test should be performed on serum taken at least 12 hours after first suckle. At this point, if the sample is below 800 mg/dL, the foal can be given additional colostrum or, alternatively, plasma intravenously.

Agalactia or death of the dam results in the need for colostrum from an alternative source. Ideally, up to 250 mL of colostrum can be harvested from every mare that foals, immediately after its own foal has nursed for the first time. This colostrum can be stored frozen at -4 °F (-20 °C) for at least 1 year, and serves as the basis for a colostrum bank. This provides the optimal source of colostrum, because these mares are exposed to the same environment in which the foal was born, and therefore provides the best protection. Ideally, this colostrum should be tested for alloantibodies to ensure that it will not precipitate neonatal isoerythrolysis (see Chapter 11). Bovine colostrum has been substituted for equine colostrum and provides short-term protection against environmental pathogens. However, these antibodies have a half-life of only 4 days, compared to the normal, approximately 20 days, of equine colostrum. This could lead to a large window of risk to the neonate before it has made sufficient immunoglobulins. If the foal is determined to be in a high-risk category, and also has partial or complete failure of passive transfer, plasma transfusion is warranted. This is discussed below with respect to treatment of septicemia in foals.

EVALUATION OF THE EQUINE NEONATE

Examination of the mare and placenta provides valuable information regarding possible risk factors for the foal. However, the most important examination is of the foal itself. Careful evaluation of each organ system may provide clues to the presence of infection, birth trauma, or congenital developmental anomalies. Any abnormality, no matter how slight, warrants aggressive therapy, because disease in the neonate progresses rapidly. In some foal diseases, such as congenital intestinal aganglionosis, normal physical findings do not guarantee a normal foal. Therefore, vigilance, early detection, and aggressive therapy are the best defenses against neonatal mortality. Normal physical findings are listed in Table 18–1.

Behavioral Adaptation

Normal foals become sternal within seconds, and stand within 2 hours of parturition. The suckle reflex is often present at birth, and should be exhibited within 20 minutes of birth.[8] Most normal foals nurse by 2 hours of age, but may take as long as 4 hours to nurse.[8] Defecation occurs soon after standing, and may immediately follow the first successful attempt to nurse.[29] External visual, auditory, and tactile stimuli result in exaggerated responses by the foal, and this persists for the first few weeks of life.[30]

Neurologic Adaptation

Foals are nonresponsive while in the birth canal, but respond to external stimuli immediately after parturition. The righting reflex is exhibited before the foal has been completely ex-

Table 18–1. Normal Physical Examination Findings in Neonatal Foals

Examination	Normal Findings
Mentation	Bright, alert, responsive
Rectal temperature	37.2°–38.5 °C
Rectum	Should be evidence of meconium on thermometer or perineum
Heart rate	65–135 beats/min
Heart sounds	Normal rhythm; may have patent ductus arteriosus (machinery murmur) or benign systolic murmur (auscultable left heart base)
Respiratory rate	20–40 breaths/min
Respiratory sounds	Bronchovesicular sounds may seem louder than in the adult
Respiratory effort	Biphasic respiratory effort should not be forced
Mucous membrane color	Pink
Capillary refill	1 sec

pelled from the birth canal. The withdrawal reflex is present in the fetus, but is absent while the foal is in the pelvic canal during delivery. However, this reflex returns immediately after the hips pass through the delivery canal.[8] The pupillary light reflex[8] and blink reflex in response to bright light[30] are present essentially at birth, although the menace response may require 2 weeks to develop.[30] The pupillary angle in foals is ventromedial to the palpebral fissure, and becomes gradually dorsomedial as the foal ages to 1 month. Abnormalities in this position may be related to neurologic disease. The remainder of the cranial nerve responses are fully developed.[30]

The stance and gait of foals also differ from the adult. Foals tend to have a wide-based stance, and a hypermetric, exaggerated gait.[30] The spinal reflexes, including those of the biceps, triceps, extensor carpi radialis tendon, patellar tendon, gastrocnemius, and cranial tibial reflexes tend to be exaggerated. The crossed extensor reflex, in which pinching of a limb elicits flexion (withdrawal) of that limb and extension of the contralateral limb, is present by 3 weeks of age.[30] Tail tone, and the anal and perineal reflexes are similar to those of the adult.

Thermoregulation is developed in foals within a wide range of temperatures. Neonatal foals are able to thermoregulate normally in ambient temperatures as low as 38 °F (3.3 °C).[31] Normal rectal temperature is maintained between 99 °F and 102 °F (37.2°–38.9 °C). Foals lack brown adipose tissue, and increase their temperature by shivering, although this requirement results in a marked increase in oxygen consumption.[31] Failure to maintain rectal temperature within these limits is a sign of neurologic or systemic disease. Some draft-breed foals are born with the inability to thermoregulate, despite being otherwise normal.

Cardiovascular Adaptation

Within the first 5 minutes following parturition, the foal's heart rate may be low, between 30 and 80 bpm. This rapidly increases to 65 to 135 bpm.[8, 32] A continuous murmur is normally auscultable over the base of the left side of the heart, which is attributable to the ductus arteriosus. This murmur is loudest within the first 12 hours of life, and usually becomes undetectable by the fourth day of life.

Fetal circulation includes multiple adaptations to minimize blood flow through nonfunctional vascular beds. Lung and liver functions at this stage are fulfilled by the placenta, rendering these organs relatively nonfunctional. A large proportion of the pulmonary circulation is shunted to the systemic circulation through the ductus arteriosus and foramen ovale. Following birth, these shunts gradually close and pulmonary vascular resistance and pulmonary arterial pressure decrease to normal adult values. By the end of the first day of life, pulmonary vascular resistance decreases by 75% (from 400 to 100 absolute resistance units), and pulmonary arterial pressure decreases from an average of 40.3 to 27.5 mm Hg.

Pulmonary Adaptation

The respiratory rate of the foal immediately after birth exceeds that of the adult, being as high as 75 breaths per minute.[33] This rate rapidly decreases by about 50% within the first hour but remains slightly higher than the adult rate. The respiratory effort also differs from the adult. The compliant nature of the foal's rib cage requires that both inspiration and expiration have active components.[34] The significance of this is that pressure on the chest or abdomen in foals during restraint may result in impairment of respiration. Minute ventilation in foals is more than double the resting adult value, which is probably required to ventilate a larger percentage of dead space[35] and maintain a higher metabolic rate.[34] Occasionally, normal foals will exhibit hyperpnea during the first few weeks of life, although hyperpnea is usually associated with pulmonary abnormalities.

Gastrointestinal and Nutritional Adaptation

Evaluation of the gastrointestinal tract in the normal foal is usually confined to auscultation of borborygmi, visual examination for evidence of milk reflux at the nostrils, and normal passage of the meconium. The suckle reflex is present almost immediately after birth, and normal foals will nurse within 2 hours of being born. Passage of meconium usually occurs shortly thereafter. Borborygmi in foals are similar to those in adults, and should be auscultable in all four quadrants.

The foal's digestive tract is capable of digesting milk without difficulty, and may even be more efficient at absorbing substances than the adult tract.[36] Foals usually nurse small amounts frequently, which naturally prevents excessive distention of the stomach. This pattern should be emulated when feeding very young, orphaned foals. The predominant source of carbohydrate in mare's milk is lactose, which is parallelled by the high quantity of lactase in the foal's small intestine.[37] The quantity of this enzyme decreases soon after weaning. Feeding of other disaccharides should be avoided in the young foal, because the absence of adequate enzymes for their digestion results in gas production and colic. Mares have low concentrations of fat in the milk compared with other species, and the carbohydrates and fat contribute almost equally to the energy content of the milk.[38] These factors should be considered when formulating feed supplementation programs for orphaned foals (see Chapter 5).

Defecation usually occurs within the first few hours of life, often within minutes of the first meal.[29] The first feces consist of meconium, which is the residual material left from swallowed amniotic fluid, sloughing of intestinal cells, and bile and intestinal secretion during gestation. This material has a dark-brown appearance and should be easily distinguished from the lighter-brown color of milk feces, which first appear about 10 hours after the first meal.[39] The consistency is usually soft, but formed, although it may be present as hard pellets or as diarrhea. Many normal foals have some difficulty passing meconium, and require enemas.

Hepatic microsomal enzymes in foals are less active than in the adult, which is similar to neonates of other species.[36] These enzyme systems mature rapidly, and approach adult levels by 6 to 12 weeks.

Musculoskeletal Adaptation

Horses are a species with neonatal precocity, which is likely to have evolved for the purpose of enabling escape from predation shortly after birth. This suggestion is supported by the finding that foals have a well-developed musculoskeletal system when born. Foals are able to stand within several hours of birth, and have legs about 75% of their adult length. The bones themselves should be well ossified, and incomplete ossification is a sign of dysmaturity.[40]

The uterus provides the fetus with a protected environment in which to grow and develop. However, the lack of weight-bearing of the fetus within the uterus fails to provide adequate stimuli for stress remodeling of the bones and associated soft tissue structures. Therefore, many foals are born with some degree of angular limb deformity due to tendon or ligamentous laxity, which corrects itself rapidly within the first week of life.[41] Severe deviation (>15 degrees) or deformity that persists beyond 1 week of age warrants intervention.

Normal Clinical Pathology

Just as neonates of many species differ from adults in their clinical chemistry profile, a separate set of normal values should exist for foals at each stage of development. Laboratories vary in the techniques used to measure blood constituents, and therefore each laboratory should ideally develop its own reference values. This is often unrealistic, particularly in private laboratories, where blood from only a few foals is evaluated annually.

Normal values have been established for many of the blood constituents and parameters that are commonly measured. These are listed in Tables 18–2, 18–3, and 18–4. These values should be used if reference values for foals are not available from the laboratory. Birth values in these tables correspond to presuckle values.

Concentrations of many blood constituents are not significantly different between foals and adult horses. These include the electrolytes sodium, potassium, and chloride; total

Table 18–2. Normal Hematologic Values*†

	Age			
	Birth	1–2 days	1 mo	2 mo
RBC × 10⁶/µL	7.9–12.3	8.7–13.3	7.6–10.9	7.4–14.2
PCV (vol %)	36–51	28–46	28–42	30–49
Hemoglobin (g/dL)	13–17.8	10.2–16.4	10.1–14.9	10.6–16.6
MCV (fl)	33–35	30–50	31–46	31–43
MCH (pg)	12–18	10–19	13–15	11–16
MCHC (g/dL)	29–38	31–38	34–38	34–39
Platelets × 10³/µL	60–500	100–500	100–500	100–500
WBC × 10³/µL	3.2–14	5.01–12.6	5.0–12.6	5.5–12.7
Band neutrophils × 10³/µL	0–800	0–600	0–500	0–400
Segmented neutrophils × 10³/µL	1.8–8.9	2.0–10.2	2.0–9.3	2.0–9.5
Lymphocytes × 10³/µL	0.6–5.0	0.6–5.0	1.6–6.2	2.3–7.2
Monocytes × 10³/µL	0.02–43	0.02–0.39	0.02–0.63	0.02–0.61
Eosinophils × 10³/µL	0	0–0.07	0–0.4	0–0.5
Fibrinogen (mg/dL)	70–360‡	66–426	144–652	130–682
Total iron-binding capacity (µg/dL)	470–555	205–513	435–695	429–669
Serum iron (µg/dL)	400–490	58–370	49–266	67–295
Serum ferritin (ng/dL)	70–110	120–250	50–90	40–100
Transferrin saturation (%)	69–100	20–100	10–50	10–55

*Data from references 43, 44, and 46.
†RBC, red blood cells; PCV, packed cell volume; MCV, mean corpuscular volume; MCCH, mean corpuscular volume of hemoglobin; WBC, white blood cells.
‡Presuckle value is not available, so this value is taken from foals less than 12 hours old, but after first colostral meal.

Table 18–3. Normal Serum Clinical Chemistry Values*

	Age			
	Birth	1–2 days	1 mo	2 mo
Protein (g/dL)	3.6–7.2	4.4–7.6	4.6–6.6	5.0–6.5
Albumin (g/dL)	1.7–3.6	2.3–3.4	2.0–3.5	2.2–4.0
Bilirubin total (mg/dL)	0.8–5.4	0.5–4.3	0.7–2.5	1.2–2.2
Bilirubin direct (mg/dL)	0.2–1.2	0.2–1.9	0.1–1.5	0.2–0.9
Blood urea nitrogen	0.5–22	0–29.4	4.9–12.1	4.3–14.7
Creatinine (mg/dL)	0.7–3.7	0.4–3.6	1.2–2.2	1.2–2.6
Glucose (mg/dL)	48.2–62.6	108–223	115–156	90–143
Cholesterol (mg/dL)	33–331	100–478	100–200	100–150
Calcium, total (mg/dL)	10.6–14.6	9.6–13.6	10.7–12.9	9.4–13.4
Phosphorus (mg/dL)	4.0–8.0	3.4–7.4	6.0–8.0	6.0–8.0
Alkaline phosphatase (IU/L)	655–2,803†	530–2,700	99–759	132–688
Aspartate aminotransferase (IU/L)	100–300†	85–460	200–450	250–500
Creatine phosphokinase (IU/L)	24–120	25–350	40–162	40–162
γ-Glutamyltransferase (IU/L)	8–36†	10–38	13–80	3–50
Lactate dehydrogenase (IU/L)	10–961†	596–1,134	498–1,066	484–804
Sorbitol dehydrogenase (IU/L)	0.2–4.7†	0.6–3.8	1.0–6.1	0.5–3.6

*Data from Sato et al.[44]
†Data from Bauer et al.[45]

Table 18–4. Normal Arterial Blood Gas Values for Foals*

	Age	
	Birth	1–2 days
pH (units)	7.348–7.412	7.366–7.420
O_2 tension (mm Hg)	68.3–83.6	75–89.4
CO_2 tension (mm Hg)	38.6–48.3	42.1–48
HCO_3 (mEq/L)	24.5–26.9	19–27.4
Total CO_2 (mEq/L)	21–33	21–33
Base excess (mEq/L)	− 0.4–3.2	− 7.3–3.9

*Data from references 49, 56.

magnesium; and albumin. The blood coagulation pathway in the equine neonate is fully developed at birth, with prothrombin and activated partial thromboplastin times equivalent to adult values. However, foal platelet aggregation differs from adults, with a delayed response to epinephrine within the first 12 hours, a delayed response to adenosine diphosphate (ADP) on the first day, and a delayed response to collagen in the first 3 days.[42]

A number of blood parameters are different in the presuckle newborn owing to changes that occur after ingestion of colostrum. Protein concentration before ingestion of colostrum is low in foals because of low globulin concentrations. Total protein remains below the adult reference range until after about 6 months of age, which is similar to the profile seen with growth in other species.[43] Both blood glucose and cholesterol are low in the presuckle newborn, and increase dramatically after the first meal, reflecting the intestinal absorption of this high caloric food.

Glucose concentration in foals exhibits much greater variability than in adults. Hepatic enzyme systems are not completely developed in foals, which may lead to inefficient regulation of plasma glucose. Foals also have minimal body reserves of glycogen, which is the normal source of readily available carbohydrate in adults. Therefore, blood glucose depends heavily upon the time between milk meals. The higher cholesterol content of blood in foals than in adults probably also results from the ingestion of milk, as milk has a higher fat content than the normal foods of adult horses.

The blood constituents that alter with age usually change as a result of specific events associated with maturity. Alkaline phosphatase (ALP) and serum phosphorus concentrations are higher in foals than in adult horses. Higher osteoblastic activity associated with bone growth is responsible for this difference.[44] A corresponding change in calcium is not evident, probably because ionized calcium is tightly regulated within narrow limits. Intestinal pinocytosis and liver activity may also contribute to serum ALP activity.[45]

Bilirubin is relatively high in young foals; values decrease to approach normal adult levels by the end of the first month. This same phenomenon is observed in some other species (humans, monkeys), and is known to be caused by immature hepatic function. While this may contribute to the higher

bilirubin values in horses as well, diminished hepatic uptake because of lack of enteral nutrition in utero may be contributory. This is the same mechanism that results in hyperbilirubinemia in anorectic adult horses.

Mean corpuscular volume (MCV) of foals is relatively high, although not significantly higher than for adults. Higher MCVs have been identified in premature and dysmature foals. Fetal hematopoiesis occurs in the fetal liver, spleen, and lymph nodes, and does not switch to the bone marrow until shortly before parturition. Cells made in these extramedullary centers are larger than those from bone marrow, which probably accounts for the larger cells in dysmature foals. During growth, erythrocytes gradually decrease in size, reaching a nadir at about 4 months, when the cells are microcytic, compared to adult cells. This gradual decrease in the size of erythrocytes has been attributed to a relative iron deficiency in foals. Serum ferritin is low before suckling, and increases markedly after ingestion of colostrum. Colostrum contains an average of 354 ng/mL ferritin, and this concentration drops off after the first day. Foal serum ferritin mirrors this change. After the initial peak of ferritin following colostrum ingestion, there is a gradual decrease to a minimal value at about 1 month.[46] A relatively low serum ferritin persists until 5 months, and is attributed to a demand for iron for growth (>85% increase in body weight).[46] This iron profile is unaffected by iron supplementation.[47]

Foals tend to have much higher blood neutrophil counts than adults, and these values gradually decrease over the first 4 months of life.[46] A concomitant rise in lymphocytes results in approximately no change in total white blood cell (WBC) numbers. These changes are thought to be the result of a decrease in the total blood pool of neutrophils, and a gradual maturation of the lymphoid system.[46] The neutrophil:lymphocyte ratio should be greater than 2.5:1 at birth, and gradually approaches 1:1 by the third to fourth month of life.[46, 48]

The relatively high packed cell volume (PCV) found in foals after birth is similar to that found in other species. The placenta is relatively hypoxic, because the fetus must compete with the dam's blood for oxygen. Therefore, erythropoietin concentrations are high. Additionally, the fetus normally shares its total blood volume with the placenta, and most of that blood volume shifts to the foal before the umbilicus is severed. Therefore, the newborn has relatively more red blood cells (RBCs) than immediately prior to parturition.[46] Stress associated with birth, and subsequent splenic contraction probably also add a minor contribution to this relatively high PCV. The rapid decline in erythrocytes after birth is probably related to colostrum ingestion, and the absorption of both fluids and osmotically active proteins. Additionally, erythrocytes gradually decrease in number over the course of the first 2 to 4 weeks, due to some physiologic destruction as well as an increase in plasma volume secondary to growth.[46]

Fibrinogen concentration increases in normal foals over the course of the first 5 months. The reason for this increase is not known. The finding is consistent among surveys, suggesting that the trend is not associated with subclinical disease.[46] One explanation is that the hepatic enzyme systems first mature, and then overreact to stimuli inducing acute phase reactants. These stimuli could include the normal bombardment of the immune system by environmental bacteria, parasites, and pathogens.

Both arterial[49] and mixed venous (i.e., pulmonary arterial)[50] oxygen tensions differ depending upon the body position of the foal (i.e., lateral, sternal, or standing), although these differences rapidly decrease as the foal ages. The mixed venous oxygen tension (Pvo_2) is usually consistent among body positions by day 5. The Pao_2 is lower in the recumbent foal than the standing foal, and lower still for foals in lateral vs. sternal recumbency. In normal foals, these differences diminish by the end of the first week, but in foals with disease, they may persist much longer.

NEONATAL INTENSIVE CARE
Background

In the early 1980s, as mentioned, the approach to treatment of foals with severe disease shifted. Veterinary clinicians began to adapt the intensive care techniques and methods used in human neonatal medicine to the treatment of equine neonates.[4] Since the implementation of intensive care in equine neonatal medicine, the survival of neonatal patients has increased,[4, 5, 51] while the average daily cost of treatment has decreased.[5]

Long-term performance of foals that survive treatment in the neonatal intensive care unit (NICU) does not appear to differ from that of the general population.[51] Qualitatively, some of these foals were still small as yearlings, compared with stablemates, but were able to overcome this discrepancy by their second year.[51] Of those animals that matured into adults, most were considered useful as athletes.[5, 51] These data suggest that neonatal intensive care medicine is valuable to the equine industry, and increasingly cost-effective.

Triage

Many disease conditions can be treated on the farm, depending upon the abilities and motivation of the field veterinarian and farm manager. However, intensive care is most effectively administered in a hospital setting. The decision to transfer an equine neonate to an intensive care facility should be made early in the course of treatment to provide the best possible prognosis.

It is the responsibility of the field veterinarian to stabilize the foal for transfer. If the foal is standing, and able to nurse, minimal therapy before shipping is necessary. If the foal is recumbent and depressed, an attempt should be made to stabilize the foal before shipping. First, a complete physical examination should be performed. The presence of any immediately life-threatening conditions should be identified, and treatment initiated, if possible. A critical problem in depressed foals is inability to nurse, either from a loss of the suckle reflex, or inability to reach the mammae. Foals, like other neonatal animals, have minimal body reserves for the maintenance of blood glucose, and therefore rapidly become hypoglycemic when food is withheld. Therefore, initial therapy for this type of foal involves the administration of colostrum if the foal is younger than 24 hours, and milk if the foal is older. This oftens require placement of a stomach tube. The foal's temperature should be monitored, and, if hypothermic, hot-water bottles should be used to warm the foal during shipping. Shock should be treated prior to and during shipping by the administration of intravenous fluids, ideally a 2.5% dextrose, 0.45% saline solution. This provides an isosmotic replacement fluid that permits fluid therapy without excessive sodium load. Other balanced salt solutions with glucose added are adequate alternatives if half-strength saline-dextrose is not available. The classic shock dose of fluids (30 mL/kg) cannot be rapidly administered to a foal because of the risk of causing pulmonary edema.

The NICU clinician must rapidly assess the foal's therapeutic requirements. Affected neonates are often presented as critical emergencies. Therefore, the initial physical examination may need to be brief, permitting rapid identification of immediately life-threatening conditions. This initial examination should assess overall appearance, mental state, temperature, pulse, respiration, and mucous membranes. The presence of any gross abnormalities, such as unconsciousness, severe respiratory distress, bloating, or colic warrants immediate intervention. These conditions are discussed in detail below. Once life-threatening conditions have been addressed, a thorough physical examination and history are performed.

Critical foals may be divided into several categories for supportive care. Hospital protocols differ widely and, these categories represent only one of many acceptable schemes for dividing hospitalized foals. First, foals that are able to nurse should be allowed to nurse the mare. Foals will more readily suckle a teat than a bottle. In addition, the risk of aspiration or aerophagia is greater with a bottle. This group includes foals that are able to stand and nurse and do not require continuous intravenous fluids. These foals may remain with the mare, as long as the dam is tolerant of intervention by hospital staff.

The second group includes foals able to stand and nurse intermittently. These foals are often recumbent for long periods and require intravenous fluids. Hospitalization may be in proximity to the mare so the mare can maintain some contact, but the foal is separated so that fluids and other treatment may be readily administered. This form of care may be provided by a number of different methods. A stall may be segregated using boards or straw bales. A mobile foal bed may be rolled in front of the mare's open stall door. An alternative method involves the confinement of the mare in stocks adjacent to the foal bed. Using any of these methods, the recumbent foal can be managed intensively, with ready access to the dam for milk.

The third group includes the most intensively managed cases. These foals are usually recumbent most of the time, and cannot nurse the mare. Therefore, intensive management is most easily provided separate from the mare. This improves the ability of the clinician to maintain cleanliness, monitor intake and output, and is safer for all foal handlers. However, this method of providing care is not without its disadvantages. If the mare and foal are separated long enough, the mare may not accept the foal. Nonetheless, for the severely affected foal, intensive care is most effectively administered with the foal physically separated from the mare.

Initial Evaluation of the Critical Foal

Effective NICUs must have a standard protocol for initial evaluation and treatment of critical neonates. This protocol

Table 18–5. Crash Cart Supplies

Fluid Administration	Sampling and Preparation Supplies
Catheter	Clippers with no. 40 blade
Suture and/or Superglue	Heparin and syringes for blood gases
IV solution administration set	Blood tubes
Extension set	Scrub
Fluids	Alcohol
0.45% NaCl with 2.5% dextrose	
50% dextrose	Blood culture bottles
Bicarbonate	Glucostix
Respiratory Support	**Emergency Drugs**
Nasotracheal tubes	Diazepam
Ambu bag	Prednisolone sodium succinate
Oxygen tank	Doxapram
Insufflation tube	Dopamine
Demand valve	Dobutamine
Humidifier	Xylazine
	Butorphanol
Nursing Care	
	Nutritional Support
Fleece pads	
Absorbent "diapers"	Flexible nasogastric tube
Heat lamp	Milk replacer
Hot-water bottles or pad	
Zinc oxide	

should be designed to facilitate rapid identification of any immediately life-threatening conditions, as well as the collection of a standard group of blood samples. The diversity of clinical presentations that may accompany septicemia dictates that all foals be considered septic upon initial evaluation and treated as medical emergencies. Implementation of the protocol is facilitated by advance preparation in the form of a foal crash cart. Supplies that should be readily available in this form are listed in Table 18–5. Standardization of evaluation optimizes patient care by preventing inadvertent omissions, and permits comparison of cases.

Every clinical protocol must begin with a physical examination. In the critical neonate, the initial physical examination may be brief, limited to the identification of level of consciousness, presence of shock, depth and rate of respiration, and rectal temperature. These parameters are important for the detection of conditions requiring immediate attention.

Unconsciousness may be due to inadequate blood pressure, hypoxemia, hypoglycemia, electrolyte imbalances, or sepsis. Regardless of the underlying cause of the foal's condition, immediate administration of dextrose is indicated. Foals that have been ill for any length of time are likely to be hypoglycemic, which may contribute to the loss of consciousness, or seizure activity. The presence of seizure activity requires immediate therapy with diazepam 0.01 mg/kg IV bolus dose, repeated to effect, up to 0.1 mg/kg total

dose, or phenobarbital 10 mg/kg IV bolus dose, followed by 2 mg/kg IV repeated to effect, up to 20 mg/kg total dose. Shock, regardless of the underlying cause, warrants immediate administration of fluids. Oxygen insufflation may need to be instituted immediately if the foal is in respiratory distress. Analgesia may be required if the foal is colicky. Hypothermia may contribute to low blood pressure due to bradycardia, as well as increasing the foal's glucose utilization by inducement of shivering. Therefore, heating pads, heat lamps, or hot-water bottles may be required.

Venous blood should be drawn for a standard set of laboratory tests, including a complete blood count, fibrinogen, serum electrolytes, ionized calcium, creatinine, bilirubin concentration, blood gas analysis, immunoglobulin quantitation, and immediate blood glucose estimate. Arterial blood may be taken from the greater metatarsal, facial, or carotid arteries for blood gas analysis. Completion of these tests may require some time, but an immediate estimate of the blood glucose concentration is essential. Hypoglycemia is common in foals that have not nursed for several hours, and contributes to dementia, unconsciousness, and seizures.

After these samples are collected, the neck should be clipped using no. 40 clipper blades for the placement of a jugular catheter. Clipping the region is preferable to shaving, because neonatal skin is sensitive and highly susceptible to razor burn. The site should be prepared as for surgery, and local anesthesia infiltrated subcutaneously to facilitate catheter placement. Blood should be withdrawn through this prepared site for inoculation of blood culture, either by needle, immediately before catheter placement, or through the catheter.

Catheter placement in the early stage of foal evaluation permits the immediate institution of therapy for severely life-threatening conditions. This includes the administration of high-volume isotonic fluids, or hypertonic saline for the reestablishment of adequate blood pressure, and the administration of glucose-containing fluids for the correction of hypoglycemia. Often fluid therapy must be instituted prior to receiving serum chemistry results. In this case, 2.5% dextrose, 0.45% saline is an adequate choice until the electrolyte concentrations are known and the fluids can be adjusted appropriately. Fluids may be administered as a shock dose (30 mL/kg rapid gravity drip IV) if significant respiratory distress is not evident. Rapid fluid administration may result in pulmonary edema if a respiratory problem is present. For further discussion of fluid therapy, see Chapter 4.

After any immediately life-threatening conditions have been addressed, a thorough physical examination should be completed. Special consideration is given to the respiratory system, umbilicus, joints, and eyes. Diseases of the respiratory system are responsible for 44% of the mortality of foals under 1 week of age.[52] Moisture of the end of the umbilicus may reveal a patent urachus. The presence of any enlarged joints should raise suspicion of infection, and arthrocentesis should be performed for cytologic evaluation and culture. Further discussion of respiratory distress, oxygen therapy, umbilical diseases, and enlarged joints may be found below. An ophthalmologic examination should be performed to determine the presence of hypopion or hyphema. Uveitis is a common sequela to septicemia, and may lead to glaucoma or phthisis bulbi. Once the physical examination is completed, and initial therapy instituted, a sepsis score should be calculated to determine the likelihood of sepsis.[53]

Pharmacologic therapy should be individualized to meet the specific needs of the animal. However, certain therapies are similar among most critical foals. Gastric ulceration is a serious complication of disease in foals and may lead to perforation and death. Therefore, all critical foals should be placed on antiulcer medication. If the gastrointestinal tract is determined to be normal, the foal may be medicated orally. The specific medication used is at the clinician's discretion, but may be ranitidine 4.4 mg/kg b.i.d. or t.i.d., sucralfate 1 to 4 g t.i.d. or q.i.d., or omeprazole 0.5 mg/kg q.i.d. (see below). If the foal has gastrointestinal disease, including colic or diarrhea, cimetidine 5 mg/kg IV q.i.d. may be used.[54]

The severe consequences of septicemia warrant the use of a broad-spectrum antibiotic in all suspect foals. The sepsis score provides a sound basis for initiation of antibiotic therapy, but even a low sepsis score may fail to identify sepsis. The antibiotic combination of choice may differ depending on regional clinical experience.

SUPPORTIVE CARE OF THE RECUMBENT FOAL

Supportive care of the recumbent foal is similar, regardless of the condition. In particular, recumbency may lead to compromise of multiple systems that require special consideration. Vigilance is essential to management.

One of the most important considerations in recumbent foals is body position. Normal foals are hypoxemic in the first week of life,[31, 49, 55, 56] and lateral recumbency further lowers the PaO_2, by approximately 14 mm Hg.[49] Recumbency increases pressure on the dependent lung, resulting in atelectasis and ventilation-perfusion mismatching. This decrease in PaO_2 with recumbency does not adversely affect normal foals, but may be a significant factor in compromised foals. Therefore, diseased foals, and particularly those with respiratory compromise, should be maintained in sternal recumbency. If sternal recumbency cannot be achieved, foals should be turned frequently.

Recumbent foals tolerate PaO_2 values of 50 mm Hg without requiring oxygen supplementation. In foals with PaO_2 values less than 50 mm Hg, but with normal arterial carbon dioxide tension ($PaCO_2$) values (<50 mm Hg), oxygen insufflation is indicated. Neurologically abnormal foals with borderline values of PaO_2 are likely to drop below critical levels during seizures, and therefore may benefit from oxygen insufflation. Oxygen insufflation should be humidified and may be administered by nasal, pharyngeal, or transtracheal routes at a rate of 10 L/min. Nasal or pharyngeal oxygen insufflation should be administered by small-bore flexible tubing, which can be sutured in place via a suture through the nares. Specialized transtracheal catheters may be placed through the midcervical trachea, and sutured in place. Transtracheal catheters deliver oxygen at the carina, reducing the oxygen flow rates necessary to achieve adequate oxygenation. This system should be considered in foals refractory to intranasal oxygen therapy.[57] Further discussion of oxygen supplementation is found below.

Hypoxemia in combination with hypercapnia ($PaCO_2$ >50 mm Hg) results from hypoventilation. In foals, this may be due to central nervous system (CNS) depression, excessive respiratory effort because of surfactant deficiency, or pneumonia. The decision to artificially ventilate the foal should be made very carefully. Artificial ventilation requires a moribund or heavily sedated patient. It is associated with multiple complications, including depression of cardiac output, oxygen toxicity, and bronchopulmonary dysplasia.[58] An alert foal with a borderline $PaCO_2$ should be monitored closely. If the $PaCO_2$ progressively increases, then artificial ventilation should be instituted.

Foals are born with the ability to thermoregulate,[59] but critical foals are often hypothermic because of sepsis or CNS depression. A temperature increase of 1 °F requires a 10% increase in oxygen consumption. This results in a significant energy drain on an already catabolic animal. The temperature of the foal should be monitored at least every hour, and hot-water bottles, heat lamps, or heating pads used to increase the core temperature. Electric heating pads should be avoided because of the risk of burning the foal.

Normal neonatal foals gain 1 to 2 lb/day[60] and ingest about 25% of their body weight in mare's milk divided among frequent small feedings per day. This provides about 100 Mcal/day of energy for maintenance and growth (see Chapter 5). Diseased foals require less energy for maintenance because they are not active, but they are often anorectic, catabolic, and losing weight. Therefore, these foals still require approximately 100 Mcal/day of energy. In addition, foals require frequent milk intake for the maintenance of blood glucose. Nutritional support should be instituted early in the course of therapy.

Ideally, nutritional support should be provided by the mare. Milking the mare every 4 hours is required to maintain milk production. Neonates should be fed at least every 2 hours. If the foal can stand with help, and an effective suckle reflex is present, the foal can be placed on the mare. More commonly, foals that are critically ill cannot nurse and must be fed by bottle or stomach tube. Small-bore flexible stomach tubes are available for use as indwelling foal feeding tubes. These may be passed by endoscopic guidance or blindly. The placement of the tube in the esophagus may then be confirmed by radiography or endoscopy.

The total daily energy requirement should be divided among at least 12 feedings. If this is tolerated, the feedings may be gradually increased in quantity and decreased in frequency. On the other hand, if the foal exhibits bloat or colic, the feeding should be decreased, and the foal fed gradually. Feeding by gradual continuous drip may prevent colic in some foals that are intolerant to bulk feedings.

Accurate recording of the milk and fluid input, fecal and urinary output, and weight are essential in the neonate. Moribund foals may not exhibit observable signs with colic, and the only sign of a serious gastrointestinal abnormality may be lack of fecal output. Bloat can be monitored by using a "bloat rope." The girth of the foal's abdomen at the level of the 16th or 17th rib can be measured using a measuring tape, or marked on a piece of baling twine. This girth is then measured every 2 hours. An increase of 2 in. is regarded as abnormal.

Total parenteral nutrition (TPN) should be considered in the foal that cannot tolerate enteral feeding. The decision to institute TPN should be made as soon as the enteral route of feeding is determined to be ineffective. The longer that a neonate is in a catabolic state, the less effective TPN becomes. TPN should be administered through a dedicated central venous catheter. Catheters designed for long-term maintenance, such as Silastic catheters, are less thrombogenic than conventional Teflon catheters. Further discussion on instituting TPN may be found in Chapter 5.

Ophthalmic lesions develop commonly in critically ill foals. Evaluation of the eyes should be performed at least twice-daily. Uveitis, manifested by hypopyon and hyphema, is a common sequela of septicemia. Cataracts, glaucoma, and phthisis bulbi may ensue. Corneal ulcers may develop secondary to entropion. Dehydration causes sinking of the globe and inward folding of the lids. Treatment can consist of procaine penicillin subcutaneously in the lid to engorge the lid, or suture or staples. Foals should be kept in sternal recumbency as much as possible. If they remain in lateral recumbency, they should be turned every few hours. Further discussion of the treatment of uveitis and corneal ulcers may be found in Chapter 14.

Nursing care of the recumbent foal includes management of bed sores and urine scalding. Bed sores are common in recumbent animals, but are particularly prevalent in premature foals. Prevention is difficult, but should consist of thick padding and frequent removal of soiled bedding. Bed sores and urine scalding should be treated topically with astringents to encourage callous formation. Classically, zinc oxide (Desitin) may be used, but aluminum simethicone (Maalox) is equally effective.

The musculoskeletal system of horses is designed for immediate use by the foal after birth. Prolonged recumbency leads to severe joint and tendon laxity. Once the foal begins standing, this may result in angular limb deformities and collapse of immature cuboidal bones. Premature and dysmature foals commonly have incomplete ossification of the cuboidal bones of the carpi and tarsi. Physical therapy during intensive care, in the form of passive flexion and extension of the limbs, may limit some of the joint and tendon laxity. Radiography of the carpi and tarsi should be performed soon after admission, and repeated when the foal begins to stand. As the time spent standing increases, splinting or sleeve casts may be indicated to prevent permanent angular limb deformities.

PHARMACOLOGY

The effect of a pharmacologic agent is achieved when therapeutic concentrations are achieved in the tissue of interest. The dosage required to accomplish this depends upon the pharmacokinetics of the drug. Special consideration must be made when prescribing drugs for neonates to account for possible differences in drug properties, and the metabolic response of the foal. Neonates and adults differ in their response to pharmacologic agents and dosages cannot simply be extrapolated. Premature and dysmature foals may differ even more and careful monitoring and adjustment of drug therapy is necessary in these patients. Drug efficacy may also differ between foals and adults. The organisms that infect foals are often different from those that infect adults, requiring a different spectrum of antibiotic activity. Toxicity of drugs may differ between foals and adults. For example,

foals appear to be more susceptible to the formation of gastric ulcers in response to nonsteroidal anti-inflammatory drugs (NSAIDs).[61] Foals may also be more susceptible to the toxic effects of overdosing. Dosages should be adjusted according to response to therapy, clinical chemistry indices, and serum drug levels, when possible.

Gastrointestinal absorption in foals is indiscriminately high immediately after birth, while specialized epithelial cells engulf colostrum. After these cells slough, the foal intestinal tract becomes similar to that of the adult.[36] The predominantly milk diet of young foals is probably responsible for the differential absorption observed for some drugs, as compared to the adult. The high calcium content may prevent the absorption of chelating compounds, such as tetracycline. In addition, foals may have less intestinal fermentation than adults, which results in differences in bacterial degradation of some pharmacologic agents. This may account for the higher absorption of some oral medications by foals.[62] Several oral antibiotics with inconsequential bioavailability in adults can be used effectively in foals. Cephradine, a first-generation cephalosporin effective against most gram-positive bacteria, *Listeria,* and *Pasteurella,* achieves therapeutic concentrations after oral administration in foals.[63] Penicillin V[62] and amoxicillin[64] 30 mg/kg PO q.8h. also may be effectively administered to foals.

Drug distribution is also different in foals and adults. Water makes up a higher percentage of the foal's weight (70%–75%) than in adults (50%–60%), and is primarily distributed to the extracellular fluid. This leads to a higher volume of distribution of drugs to the extracellular fluid, requiring a higher dose to achieve the same plasma levels.[36] An example is phenylbutazone, which has a higher volume of distribution in foals (0.190–0.401 L/kg) than in adults (0.152 L/kg).[65] Albumin, which is a common carrier of hydrophobic compounds, is present in lower concentrations in foals than in adults. Therefore, the dosage of drugs that are highly protein-bound must be lower in foals because an adequate unbound (active) concentration will be present despite a lower total (bound plus unbound) drug concentration. Foals also have higher permeability of the blood-brain barrier, which increases drug distribution to cerebrospinal fluid (CSF).[36] Therefore, lower doses are required to achieve the same drug levels in CSF, and drugs with a high risk for CNS toxicity should be avoided.

Foals are metabolically mature compared to neonates of other species. Renal function appears to mature within the first 2 days of life, and drugs that are metabolized and excreted by this route have kinetics similar to those of adults. Urinary pH of foals, in contrast to adult horses, is acidic, which favors the reabsorption of weak organic acids with pK_a values in the pH 5 to 7 range.[36] Weak organic bases may be excreted at a higher rate because of the same mechanism. The normally rapid maturation of renal function may not apply to premature or septic neonates. Renal function should be monitored in neonates, and drug dosages adjusted accordingly.

Liver biotransformation ability does not appear to be fully mature in the foal at birth.[66] Metabolism of substances by the liver occurs predominantly by microsomal oxidative reactions, and glucuronide conjugation, but also includes acetylation, hydroxylation, ester hydrolysis and sulfate conjugation. Glucuronide conjugation develops by the first week of age, as shown by maturation of the chloramphenicol oxidation pathway.[67] Microsomal pathways approach the adult metabolic capacity by 8 to 12 weeks after birth.[36] An example of this phenomenon can be seen with salicylates. Between the ages of 7 days and 28 days, the apparent volume of distribution of salicylate for a foal decreased from 0.283 L/kg to 0.210 L/kg. Kinetics are first-order, and the half-life decreased significantly by 28 days of age. This change in the half-life of salicylate was attributed to the increase in liver biotransformation with maturity.[66] The delay in maturation of hepatic metabolism may also be responsible for the prolonged half-life of phenylbutazone in foals, which ranged from 6.4 to 22.1 hours compared to 7.9 hours in adults.[65] Drugs, such as trimethoprim, which normally have a high "first-pass" effect, will therefore have higher bioavailability in foals compared to adults.[36] There may be additional differences in metabolic capacity between premature foals and normal foals.

Sedation and anesthesia present special problems in neonates. The refractory nature of foals necessitates the use of sedation for many procedures that would not require sedation in the adult. However, foals often respond unpredictably. In addition to metabolic concerns, the electroencephalographic pattern of foals differs from that of adults until about 3 to 6 months.[68] This may contribute to the response of foals to sedation and anesthesia. Therefore, special consideration must be taken when approaching sedation and anesthesia of the equine neonate.

The 2'-agonists are effective for sedation and anesthetic premedication in adults, and may be used in foals. These agents may be administered intravenously or intramuscularly. Both the dose and the route of administration affect both the type of side effects and the duration of effect. Xylazine 1.1 mg/kg IV produces safe and predictable sedation in normal foals,[69] but may be dangerous in neonates at less than half the dose (0.44–0.55 mg/kg IV).[70, 71] Detomidine 10 to 40 mg/kg IV also produces predictable sedation, but can be arrhythmogenic 5 to 10 minutes after administration.[72] The 2'-agonists should be used sparingly in diseased foals, because compromised foals may die when stressed under sedation.

Healthy foals may be safely anesthetized with either isoflurane or halothane,[73] but isoflurane is probably safer in compromised individuals. Anesthetic induction by anesthetic gas via nasotracheal intubation in foals eliminates the requirement for a separate induction agent.[74] These foals usually require xylazine sedation before the nasotracheal tube is passed. Ventilation under general anesthesia is depressed, and most foals will be hypercapnic. In addition, 42% of foals undergoing anesthesia for colic surgery require oxygen insufflation for more than 8 hours to maintain PaO_2 above 60 mm Hg.[75]

Specific pharmacokinetic studies have not been performed in foals for all therapeutic agents. Dosing regimens for some of the drugs that have been studied are included in Table 18–6. Despite the lack of a complete understanding of pharmacokinetics in foals, intelligent decisions can be made based on the principles outlined above. Probably the most important guiding premise for the use of drugs in foals is careful monitoring of the patient's condition, and flexibility in the clinician's plan to accommodate changes in the clinical picture.

THE WEAK OR DEPRESSED FOAL

Weakness and depression in the neonatal foal have many causes. The clinical presentation can range from mild depression of the suckle reflex to the extreme case of the recumbent, moribund foal. Many foal diseases share this clinical presentation, which may confound a diagnosis. Depression stems from different physiologic abnormalities that affect the CNS. Commonly, endotoxic or hypovolemic shock, hypoglycemia, low blood oxygen content, and electrolyte abnormalities are major contributors. Neonatal maladjustment syndrome results from birth asphyxia and may be accompanied by intracranial bleeding. Bilirubin in sufficient quantities in the CNS can cause seizures and depression. Some causes of depression are listed in Table 18–7. Prematurity and dysmaturity and septicemia are discussed below. Other causes of weakness or depression are discussed under Foal Seizure Disorders. Congenital equine herpesvirus type 1, influenza virus, and equine arteritis virus can cause weakness in foals, with high mortality. Primary muscular and neuromuscular disorders can cause profound weakness and are discussed below.

Prematurity and Dysmaturity

Horses are precocious animals, whose normal, mature, term offspring are able to stand, nurse, and escape predation within hours of birth. Immature foals are unable to adapt physiologically. Multiple body systems may be involved, but most commonly, clinical signs are due to immaturity of the respiratory and central nervous systems.

Foals that lack maturity are classified into three groups, although these groups cannot be readily differentiated on the basis of clinical presentation. (1) Premature foals are those born before 320 days of gestation; (2) dysmature foals are full term, but have characteristics of prematurity, resulting from some form of placental insufficiency; (3) immature foals are full-term foals that lack maturity, but exhibit no evidence of placental insufficiency.[76] Foals of any group may be considered small-for-gestational-age. The significance of the classification of these groups is that prematurity is more likely to be identified early by the owner if he or she knows the breeding date. Therefore, dysmature or immature foals may have a delayed prognosis.

Lack of maturity results in a spectrum of clinical and clinicopathologic abnormalities. Some of these are listed in Table 18–8. Classically, these foals are weak, with a soft, silky hair coat, and exhibit a depressed suckle reflex.

Septicemia

Septicemia is responsible for the majority of deaths of horses younger than 7 days of age.[51, 77–80] Septicemia is a systemic disease caused by hematogenous spread of microorganisms or their byproducts throughout the body. The clinical picture of septicemia in foals is widely variable due to the involvement of multiple body systems.

Pathogenesis

Systemic bacterial infection of the neonate may develop as a result of in utero infection, placentitis, or postparturient

Table 18–6. Drugs and Dosages for Neonatal Foals

Therapeutic Class, Agent	Dosage		
	Route	Foal	Frequency
Nonsteroidal Anti-Inflammatory Drugs			
Phenylbutazone	PO, IV	2.2 mg/kg	q24h
Flunixin meglumine	PO, IM	1.1 mg/kg	q24h
Steroids			
Prednisolone sodium succinate	IV	5–10 mg/kg	NA
Antibiotics			
Penicillin			
Penicillin G sodium	IV	15–30,000 IU/kg	q6h
Procaine penicillin G	IM	25,000 IU/kg	q24h
Ampicillin sodium	IV, IM	15–30 mg/kg	q6–8h
Pivampicillin	PO	30–50 mg/kg	q8h
Amoxicillin sodium	IV, IM	15–30 mg/kg	q6–8h
Amoxicillin trihydrate oral suspension	PO	25–40 mg/kg	q8h
Amoxicillin-clavulanate	IV	15–25 mg/kg	q6–8h
Amoxicillin-clavulanate oral suspension	PO	20–30 mg/kg	q8h
Ticarcillin sodium	IV, IM	40–60 mg/kg	q8h
Ticarcillin-clavulanate	IV	50 mg/kg	q6–8h
Cephalosporins			
Cephradine	PO	25 mg/kg	q6–8h
Cefotaxime sodium	IV, IM	15–25 mg/kg	q8–12h
Cefoperazone sodium	IV, IM	20–30 mg/kg	q8–12h
Ceftiofur sodium	IM	1 mg/kg	q12h
Aminoglycosides			
Gentamicin sulfate	IV, IM	2–4 mg/kg	q8–12h
Amikacin sulfate	IV, IM	4–8 mg/kg	q8–12h
Trimethoprim-sulfonamide, parenteral	IV	24 mg/kg	q12h
Trimethoprim-sulfonamide, tablets	PO	15–30 mg/kg	q12h
Metronidazole	PO	15–25 mg/kg	q12h
Chloramphenicol sodium succinate	IV	25 mg/kg	q6–8h
Chloramphenicol palmitate	PO	40–50 mg/kg	q8h
*Anticonvulsants**			
Diazepam	IV	0.1–0.4 mg/kg	p.r.n.
Phenobarbital	IV, PO	20 mg/kg loading, then 10 mg/kg	q8–12h
Phenytoin	IV, PO	1–5 mg/kg, then 1–5 mg/kg	q2–4h q12h
Primidone	PO	20–40 mg/kg	q12–24h
Sedatives			
Xylazine	IV, IM	1.1 mg/kg	NA
Diazepam	IV	0.05–0.1 mg/kg	NA

*Data from Beech J: Therapeutics in the neonate. *Proc Am Assoc Equine Pract* 28:359, 1982.

oral, respiratory, or umbilical inoculation. Septicemia results when the immunity of the foal is overcome by bacterial challenge. The lymphocytes of foals are able to respond to antigenic stimulation by day 80 of gestation,[81] but neutrophil function may not be fully developed until after the fourth month of life.[82] Therefore, the fetus or foal is not well prepared to combat infectious agents.

The route of infection may be difficult to identify. About half of neonates that become septic are infected in utero, and about half are infected after birth.[78] Regardless of the

Table 18–7. Factors Causing Central Nervous System Depression

Primary System Involved	Factor	Specific Disease
Cardiovascular	Shock	Sepsis
	Hypovolemia	Sepsis, dehydration
	Anemia	Neonatal isoerythrolysis, chronic disease
Respiratory	Hypoxia	Pneumonia, patent ductus arteriosus, foramen ovale, hypoventilation, prolonged recumbency
	Hypercapnea	Hypoventilation
Nervous	Primary defect	Hydrocephalus, congenital anomalies
Other	Hypoglycemia	Sepsis, lack of enteral nutrition
	Hyperbilirubinemia	Neonatal isoerythrolysis
	Edema	Neonatal maladjustment, inappropriate fluid therapy

Table 18–9. Organisms Causing Septicemia

Common Isolates	Factors Influencing Antibiotic Choice
Gram-negative	
Escherichia coli	Usually require sensitivity for antibiotic choice
Actinobacillus equuli	Commonly susceptible to amikacin
Salmonella spp.	Commonly resistant to gentamicin
Klebsiella	Commonly resistant to aminoglycosides
Gram-positive	
Streptococcus spp.	Usually susceptible to penicillin
Staphylococcus aureus	Usually resistant to penicillin
Clostridium spp. (anaerobe)	May be resistant to penicillin, susceptible to metronidazole

original route of infection, sepsis is commonly accompanied by serologically diagnosed FPT, which is defined as a serum IgG concentration of less than 400 mg/dL. The primary problem may be FPT in combination with an overwhelming bacterial challenge at birth, or a combination of these factors.[79] Some evidence indicates that partial FPT is relatively common, and not necessarily related to sepsis. However, most septic foals exhibit low serum IgG, and routine monitoring of IgG status in neonates results in decreased overall mortality from sepsis.[80] These disparate results indicate that management schemes that minimize the environmental accumulation of pathogens may be of greatest importance in preventing sepsis. An alternative explanation for the associa-

tion of low serum IgG with sepsis is that the overwhelming infection consumes the IgG that is present despite the ingestion of adequate quantity and quality of colostrum. Consumption of immunoglobulins at the site of infection may result in persistently low serum IgG concentrations despite repeated plasma transfusion.

The prevalence of each bacterial species has shifted over time.[83] Most commonly, however, the bacteria recovered from septic foals are gram-negative organisms (Table 18–9). Many of the clinical signs observed during sepsis are, therefore, secondary to the associated endotoxemia. Endotoxins are potent nonspecific stimulators of macrophages. Unfortunately, this commonly results in inappropriate immune responses with excessive production of immune mediators, including tumor necrosis factor (TNF), interleukin-1 (IL-1) and interleukin-6 (IL-6). High serum TNF activity has been

Table 18–8. Examinations to Assess Maturity

Examination	Dysmature,* Premature	Septicemic	Neonatal Maladjustment Syndrome (NAS)*
Mentation	Depressed, obtunded	Depressed, obtunded	Depressed, obtunded
Suckle reflex	Present or absent	Probably absent	Absent
Willingness to stand	Depressed	Depressed	Depressed
Temperature	Normal, low	High, normal, low	Normal
Heart rate	High, normal, low	High, normal, low	Normal
Head	Domed forehead	Normal	Normal
Hair coat	Short, silky	Normal	Normal
Ears	Lack of rigidity	Normal	Normal
Ossification of carpal and tarsal bones	Incomplete	Complete	Complete

*Dysmaturity or NMS may be accompanied by septicemia, which can complicate the clinical picture.

associated with high mortality in septic foals,[84] and both TNF and IL-6 are observed to rise in endotoxin-infused foals.[85, 86] At the high TNF activity observed in sepsis, TNF causes direct myocardial depression, hypotension, hypoglycemia, and disseminated intravascular coagulation (DIC). A comprehensive overview of the immunologic changes in endotoxemia is presented in Chapters 1 and 12.

Clinical Signs

Clinical signs associated with septicemia are nonspecific, and vary from mild depression to moribundity. Foals that develop septicemia are often normal at birth. Early in the course of the disease, the foal may be slightly depressed, and nurse less frequently. The first sign may be distention of the udder on the mare. Even the trained layperson may miss these signs. The foal usually becomes progressively depressed, and sleeps more often than a normal foal. If the foal survives the initial bacteremia, the bacteria commonly seed the foal's organs, and signs of multiple system involvement develop. Often, the initial septicemic episode is not witnessed, and the foal will be presented with multiple system involvement. The appearance of an acute lameness from a septic joint often results in the owner's assumption that the mare stepped on the foal. The time course of septicemia can be highly variable, progressing rapidly to death in some cases, progressing slowly in others.

A thorough physical examination should reveal the extent of the septicemia. In foals with immediately life-threatening conditions, the complete physical examination may need to be postponed until after a brief examination, sample collection, and the institution of lifesaving measures. The severely moribund or seizuring foal should be treated immediately. If possible, a baseline temperature, pulse rate, and respiratory rate should be taken, but only if this can be accomplished without delaying immediate treatment. Once the foal has been stabilized, the remainder of the examination can be completed.

General attitude and mentation are commonly depressed, but foals can be bright, alert, and responsive in the face of sepsis. Foals that are brighter in attitude are often those in which the original septic episode has been missed, but bacterial seeding of joints or other organs has already occurred. Septic foals are probably transiently febrile during the course of disease, but are often hypothermic when presented to the attending veterinarian. Even normal foals are not able to thermoregulate in temperature extremes. Mucous membranes may be pale, icteric, congested, or cyanotic, depending upon concurrent disease conditions. Capillary refill time will commonly be slow, indicating poor peripheral perfusion.

Tachycardia and tachypnea are commonly present secondary to hypovolemia and hypoperfusion from shock. Hemoconcentration, dehydration, and acidemia contribute in many cases. Despite tachypnea, many of these foals will be hypoxemic and hypercapnic from hypoventilation, ventilation-perfusion mismatch, and right-to-left shunting of blood. Hypoventilation occurs as a result of depression of the respiratory centers in the brainstem. Ventilation-perfusion mismatch occurs secondary to pulmonary infection, as well as atelectasis of dependent lung regions. Right-to-left shunting of blood occurs primarily through the ductus arteriosus (PDA), which is patent for the first few days in the normal foal, and may remain patent much longer in septic foals. PDA can be readily identified on auscultation as a continuous "machinery" murmur heard best over the left heart base.

Pulmonary auscultation may reveal conclusive evidence of pulmonary disease with crackles, wheezes, or pronounced bronchial sounds. However, foals may have completely normal lung sounds even in the face of advanced pulmonary parenchymal disease. Therefore, chest radiography is always recommended. Careful examination of the foal's nose, mouth, and palate should be performed to determine if aspiration of milk is contributing to any respiratory involvement. Meconium staining of the skin may indicate meconium aspiration.

Examination of the gastrointestinal tract includes investigation of the perineum for the presence of fecal or meconium staining. Digital rectal examination should be performed to ensure that feces are being moved through the intestinal tract. The abdomen may be evaluated by external palpation, ultrasonography, and radiography. Colic pain in neonatal foals may not be evident, particularly in foals with altered mentation. Therefore, the abdomen should be carefully examined for evidence of distention.

A complete ocular examination should be performed looking for uveitis, hyphema, and entropion. Uveitis and hyphema commonly result secondary to bloodborne infection of the globe. Foals, like adults, may develop permanent blindness and glaucoma secondary to uveitis. Dehydration of the pliable foal skin commonly results in entropion and secondary corneal ulceration from abrasion by the eyelashes. The menace response cannot be used as an indicator of vision in foals at this age, because this response does not develop for several weeks in normal foals.

The umbilicus should be carefully palpated for evidence of infection, which is characterized by enlargement, heat, or discharge. A clear discharge commonly results from a patent urachus, whereas a purulent discharge results from abscessation of the umbilical structures. Ultrasound examination of the umbilicus is warranted even in the absence of abnormal findings on physical examination. The umbilical arteries and vein may be abscessed in the absence of external evidence. In addition, many septic foals ultimately develop a patent urachus even when the urachus was closed during the first examination.

Potentially the greatest threat to the septic foal is the development of septic arthritis. Multiple joint or physeal involvement greatly worsens the prognosis for recovery to athletic soundness. Early detection of any and all infected joints is therefore one of the most important purposes of the physical examination. Many septic foals are presented to the attending veterinarian with a single-limb lameness and a clearly distended and infected joint. The extent of the infection, however, may not be obvious. Subtle joint capsule distention can be detected by careful and repeated joint palpation. If possible, radiographs of the most commonly affected physes, the distal physes of the radius and tibia, are performed early in the diagnostic evaluation. These can be used for comparison as the disease progresses.

The complete physical examination may not be completed until well after lifesaving treatment has been initiated. However, once it has been completed for the baseline evaluation, the entire examination should be repeated frequently. Septicemia, bacteria and toxins in the bloodstream, is constantly seeding new organs, joints, and regions of already infected organs. Therefore, the absence of a clinical sign at the initial examination does not preclude its existence in a subsequent examination. It is only when the foal no longer has a new problem every day that the light at the end of the tunnel is in sight.

Diagnosis and Clinical Pathology

Antemortem definitive diagnosis of septicemia depends upon the recovery of bacteria from the blood of the foal. A looser definition could include the recovery of bacteria from any body fluid, most commonly joint fluid. However, in many cases, bacteria cannot be recovered. The sepsis score, described by Brewer and Koterba,[53] is commonly used to determine the likelihood of sepsis. This scoring system has a sensitivity of 93% and specificity of 89%.[53] The use of this scoring system is extremely valuable, but the treatment of any suspect foal as a septicemic case is recommended because 7% of cases are falsely negative with this scoring system.

Blood cultures should be performed in all neonatal foals where sepsis is suspected or even possible. Blood cultures may not always be positive when generalized sepsis is present, but they are estimated to be positive in 60% to 81% of cases, and are invaluable in directing antibiotic therapy.[78, 87] Ideally, blood cultures should be taken prior to the initiation of antibiotic therapy. False-positive blood cultures may result from failure to properly prepare the skin site from which the sample is taken. Usually it is simplest to clip the hair from over the jugular vein using a no. 40 clipper blade, and then perform a 5- to 10-minute surgical scrub. A catheter should be placed using sterile technique, and the first 10 mL of blood removed from the catheter used for the blood cultures. Alternatively, the blood can be withdrawn directly from the preparation site. If this is done, the needle should be removed and replaced with a new sterile needle before the sample is introduced into the culture receptacle, or skin bacteria are likely to be introduced. Blood culture bottles or tubes should be used according to the manufacturer's instructions. Usually, the culture bottle has a rubber stopper punctured by a needle for the introduction of the blood sample. The rubber stopper should be covered with alcohol-soaked gauze until immediately before the blood is injected into the bottle.

Serum immunoglobulin (IgG) concentration should be measured early in the diagnostic workup in foals over 8 hours of age. Before this age, the history will be more valuable in determining the possibility of FPT. A foal may have nursed sufficiently to achieve a high serum concentration of IgG, but this will not yet be reflected by complete absorption. The IgG determination may be made using the zinc sulfate turbidity test, but ELISA is preferred. The availability of this test with high specificity and sensitivity for detecting IgG has rendered the less effective method of zinc sulfate turbidity virtually obsolete. Complete FPT is defined as less than 200 mg/dL IgG, whereas 200 to 400 mg/dL IgG is considered to be partial FPT. Sick foals with less than 800 mg/dL IgG should be supplemented with plasma.

Septicemia in foals may be associated with any number of disorders, which may change rapidly over the course of the disease. Potentially the most common abnormality, and certainly one of the most immediately life-threatening, is hypoglycemia. Foals have minimal glycogen stores, which are essentially exhausted during the anaerobic period in which they are in the birth canal. A foal that fails to nurse will therefore develop low blood glucose. A compounding factor in septic foals is endotoxemia, which depresses blood glucose by enhanced peripheral uptake of glucose and depressed hepatic gluconeogenesis. Hypoglycemia should be assumed to contribute to the clinical picture in a foal that is moribund or seizuring. Dextrose should be administered as part of the immediate lifesaving treatment in these cases. Ideally, an estimate of blood glucose should first be obtained, but only if the result can be read immediately.

Prerenal azotemia usually accompanies sepsis because of dehydration and hypovolemia. This can progress to primary renal damage from the sepsis itself, DIC, prolonged decreases in renal blood flow, or complications from treatment with aminoglycoside antibiotics and NSAIDs. Therefore, creatinine and serum urea nitrogen concentrations should be monitored frequently, and drug dosages of both aminoglycosides and NSAIDs adjusted if azotemia is persistent.

Electrolyte abnormalities vary widely depending upon the primary organ systems involved. Decreased renal blood flow and dehydration are almost invariably present. Sodium and chloride concentrations can be highly variable, depending upon the presence or absence of diarrhea, the degree of dehydration, renal compromise, and administration of fluids, milk replacer, or electrolyte solutions prior to admission. Potassium concentration may be high, normal, or low, because potassium concentration depends upon both renal excretion and enteral intake of milk, both of which are depressed in sepsis.

Blood gas abnormalities are common in septic foals. Arterial and mixed venous blood gas determinations are of value in the diagnostic workup. Arterial blood gas values are most valuable for determining pulmonary function. Most septic foals are hypoxemic, although some of these blood gas values may be artifactual due to the difference in blood gas values between standing, sternal, and lateral recumbency. Pao_2 values greater than 70 mm Hg are considered normal, but values greater than 50 mm Hg may be normal if the sample was taken with the foal in lateral recumbency.[50] Hypercapnia may result from hypoventilation, which occurs because of cerebral depression. Mixed venous blood gases are valuable for determining tissue oxygen consumption and assessing acidosis. Mild-to-severe metabolic acidosis occurs in sepsis from the production of lactate in underperfused peripheral tissues. Often, the acidosis is mixed, with respiratory acidosis occurring secondary to ventilation-perfusion mismatch because of pneumonia, right-to-left shunting through a PDA, or hypoventilation. Pvo_2 values (i.e., those obtained ideally from the pulmonary artery) less than 25 mm Hg indicate that peripheral oxygen consumption is limited by oxygen delivery. This may result from decreased oxygenation of blood in the lungs, or decreased peripheral perfusion. This information is valuable in directing therapy. If arterial blood gas values indicate hypoxemia and hypercapnia, but peripheral oxygenation is sufficient, ventilation of the foal may be unnecessary. This is a particularly valuable use of Pvo_2, because artificial ventilation decreases cardiac output, and often requires that the foal be heavily sedated.

Any blood chemistry value may be abnormal in sepsis, depending upon the specific body system involved. Bilirubin may be increased, although large increases in bilirubin are more likely to be associated with neonatal isoerythrolysis. Muscle enzymes (aspartate aminotransferase [AST] and creatine phosphokinase [CPK]) may be mildly elevated after prolonged recumbency; however, high muscle enzymes can be associated with nutritional muscular dystrophy (white muscle disease) (see Chapter 8). Liver enzyme concentrations (AST, sorbitol dehydrogenase, and γ-glutamyltransfer) will increase with bacterial hepatitis, and will also increase mildly with endotoxemia.

The WBC count may be normal, increased, or decreased. Normal or low total WBC counts with a neutropenia and left shift are common during bacteremia.[78] The WBC count and differential are valuable as a baseline. The differential is extremely important, because often the neutrophil:lymphocyte ratio will be inverted, which is misleading if only the total count is taken into consideration. In addition, toxic changes and Döhle's bodies in neutrophils may be the primary hematologic evidence of sepsis.

RBC counts are usually normal at presentation, although anemia often develops in chronic infections. If anemia is observed, other conditions, such as neonatal isoerythrolysis or blood loss, should be considered. Fibrinogen concentration increases in response to IL-1 and IL-6 stimulation of the liver. An increased fibrinogen concentration in the first 24 hours of life is indicative of a congenital infection.[78]

Treatment

Treatment of neonatal septicemia is supportive care and appropriate antimicrobial therapy. Depressed foals with altered mentation should be considered medical emergencies. A brief physical examination should identify any immediately life-threatening conditions. Blood cultures should be taken from a sterilely prepared region over the jugular vein. The neck is clipped with a no. 40 clipper blade. Shaving with a razor is not recommended, because foal skin is easily irritated, and the razor often causes skin irritation, which interferes with future catheter placement. Catheter choice is important, because septicemia often leads to a hypercoagulable state and venous thrombosis. It is preferred to use a less thrombogenic catheter (e.g., MILA polyethylene catheter) and maintain it for long periods of time. After catheter placement, 10 mL of jugular venous blood is withdrawn for culture, a complete blood count (CBC), serum chemistry, and determination of immunoglobulin and fibrinogen concentrations. One drop of blood can be placed on a Glucostix for blood glucose determination. Immediately after catheter placement, broad-spectrum antibiotic and fluid therapy should be instituted. The foal's body temperature should be determined, and measures instituted to gradually return the temperature to normal. Every 1 °C increase in temperature requires a 10% increase in oxygen consumption. Energy expended in bringing temperature from below normal to normal also increases oxygen consumption. Excessive heat applied to the skin surface will result in vasodilation, which may shunt blood away from vital internal structures to the skin. Therefore, heat should be applied gradually at first, and should include heating of intravenous fluids before administration.

Fluid therapy in neonatal sepsis is directed at restoring and maintaining tissue perfusion and supporting blood glucose levels. Replacement fluids with glucose added should be administered as soon as a catheter has been placed in order to combat shock and hypoglycemia. Usually, this precedes the results of the serum electrolyte analysis. Nonetheless, any polyionic fluid will improve renal blood flow, and will be appropriate as the initial fluid therapy before the electrolyte concentrations are known. The use of 0.45% saline with 2.5% to 5.0% dextrose is an excellent first-choice fluid to initiate fluid replacement for shock. This fluid combination permits the administration of glucose and electrolytes in an isotonic formulation. Alternatively, hypertonic saline 7% at 2 to 5 mL/kg administered over 10 minutes will improve both cardiac output and renal blood flow. Shock is accompanied by poor peripheral perfusion and endothelial swelling, which can be directly counteracted by hypertonic saline. However, this must be followed by appropriate isotonic fluid administration to prevent exacerbation of the dehydration. Fluid administration rates of 30 to 40 mL/kg/hr should be sufficient to combat shock.[88]

The foal should be carefully monitored during the rapid administration of intravenous fluids, because neonates are much more susceptible to developing pulmonary edema from excessive fluid administration than adults. Otherwise, fluids are administered on the basis of estimated deficit and maintenance requirements (see Chapter 4.3.).

The terminology of partial or complete FPT is used for convenience, because some foals infected in utero may have complete passive transfer of maternal immunoglobulins, but ultimately consume the immunoglobulins at the site of infection, resulting in a low plasma immunoglobulin concentration. Treatment of low immunoglobulin concentration consists of replacement therapy, regardless of the cause. Plasma or plasma products are usually used. Multiple commercial products are available. These products are free from anti-RBC antibodies, equine infectious agents, and often contain concentrated immunoglobulins. Some products are derived from horses that have been hyperimmunized against various agents, most notably endotoxin. This can be particularly valuable, as gram-negative organisms are usually suspected of causing the problem. If plasma is needed, and these products are not available, plasma can be separated from an adult donor. If neonatal isoerythrolysis can be ruled out, the dam is a reasonable donor. Alternatively, a gelding that has never been transfused can be used.

With neonatal sepsis, the clinician cannot wait for the results of culture and sensitivity testing before initiating antimicrobial therapy. The choice of antimicrobials in the treatment of sepsis or suspected sepsis depends upon the susceptibility patterns of bacterial isolates in the region. This may differ from region to region depending upon the antimicrobial usage in the area. The guidelines to use in choosing an antimicrobial are: (1) the spectrum should cover both gram-negative and gram-positive organisms; (2) the antimicrobial should be bactericidal, rather than bacteriostatic; (3) the agent should be able to penetrate the tissues of primary concern. Commonly, a penicillin and aminoglycoside combination is chosen, but the specific aminoglycoside used should be chosen with some knowledge of the regional microbial susceptibility. Amikacin generally provides a greater spectrum of activity and less nephrotoxicity than gentamicin. Widespread use of gentamicin has generated widespread resistance, which has limited its clinical efficacy.

Adequate nutrition is essential to the septic foal. If the intestines are functional, the foal should be fed enterally. If a suckle reflex is present, the foal can be fed on the mare or by bottle. Care must be taken if the foal is fed by bottle to prevent aspiration. If the suckle reflex is absent or inadequate, the foal should be fed by feeding tube. Several types of nasogastric feeding tubes are available for enteral feeding. Various types of material are used for nasogastric feeding, and all are sufficient for short-term or single-use feeding. When the tube is to be maintained chronically, flexible polyethylene feeding tubes are ideal. These cause minimal irritation at the pharynx, yet are stiff enough to remain in place. The tip should be positioned in the distal esophagus, because interference with the cardia of the stomach may result in abnormal motility patterns. The tube can be secured with suture at the nares. Milk or milk replacer should be fed at 2- to 4-hour intervals. Some neonates may not be able to tolerate the larger volumes associated with feedings of this frequency. In these cases, the foal can be fed more often. Occasionally, a constant slow drip may prevent colic in these foals. Further discussion of neonatal nutritional support may be found in Chapter 5.

Careful monitoring is as important as therapy in the care of septic foals. All input and output of the animal should be recorded. Often, these animals are too depressed to exhibit signs of colic if an impaction or volvulus occurs. Therefore, if the foal becomes bloated, or output does not keep pace with input, intestinal obstruction could be a problem. If the foal is on the mare, then the mare's udder should be monitored regularly for distention, which suggests that the foal has failed to nurse regularly.

Neonatal Isoerythrolysis

Neonatal isoerythrolysis results from the ingestion of alloantibodies in the colostrum from the dam, and subsequent loss of RBCs by both intra- and extravascular hemolysis. Weakness of the foal results from low blood oxygen content. Clinical examination reveals profoundly icteric mucous membranes and serum. A complete discussion of this disease is provided in Chapter 11.

Botulism

Botulism is a neuromuscular disease caused by the anaerobic organism *Clostridium botulinum*. In adults, the clinical disease is usually caused by the ingestion of the preformed toxin, but in foals up to 8 months of age, the organism can live in focal regions of the gastrointestinal tract, such as gastric ulcers and necrotic foci within the liver.[89] These live organisms elaborate toxin, leading to toxicoinfectious botulism, or the "shaker foal syndrome."

Clostridium botulinum elaborates an epsilon toxin which binds to the presynaptic membrane of motor neurons to interfere with the release of acetylcholine. The result is generalized muscular weakness. This may manifest itself in foals as tremors, which led to the name, "shaker foal syndrome." Alternatively, the foals may be found dead, or recumbent and unable to rise. Mortality is higher than 90%.

This clinical syndrome has been recognized since the 1940s, although the causative organism was not identified until 1980.[89]

Clinical signs resulting from the profound, progressive weakness include pupillary dilatation, dysphagia, tremors of the limbs, recumbency, and terminal respiratory distress. Death ensues from respiratory paralysis, usually within a few days, although some animals may linger longer. Rare cases may recover. These are usually treated foals greater than 4 weeks of age.[89]

Treatment includes antibiotics because the toxicoinfectious form of botulism is caused by live organisms in specific lesions in the foal. Penicillin or metronidazole is effective. Botulinum antitoxin is available and should be administered early in the course of disease. A detailed discussion of botulism is provided in Chapter 19.

Nutritional Muscular Dystrophy (White Muscle Disease)

Nutritional muscular dystrophy in foals is probably caused by a dietary deficiency of vitamin E or selenium, or both, in the dam. Large areas of the United States, including the Northwest, the Great Lakes region, New England, and the southeastern Atlantic Coast are selenium-deficient. There are two forms of the disease. The fulminant form results in rapid death from arrhythmias brought on by myocardial degeneration, or in circulatory collapse from exhaustion. The subacute form affects the respiratory musculature more severely. Mildly affected animals may appear ataxic and uncoordinated because of skeletal muscle weakness. Dysphagia may result from degeneration of the tongue and pharyngeal muscles and is often the first clinical sign. Aspiration pneumonia may be a significant problem because of inability to swallow.

The pathophysiology of this disease involves lack of selenium, which in glutathione peroxidase provides protection against oxygen free radical damage. Oxygen free radicals are normal byproducts of oxidative metabolism. Normally, scavengers protect the cells from membrane lipid peroxidation by the free radicals. Glutathione peroxidase reduces lipid hydroperoxides to alcohol, while vitamin E inactivates the free radicals. Insufficient vitamin E and selenium result in membrane damage, and ultimately cell death.

The clinicopathologic findings vary depending upon the course. During active muscle damage, high serum concentrations of muscle enzymes are present, including creatine kinase (CK), AST, and lactic dehydrogenase (LDH). These are elevated in about 75% of cases. Other clinical signs may be referable to concurrent disease, including dysphagia and pneumonia.[90] Nutritional muscular dystrophy is discussed in greater detail in Chapter 8.

FOAL SEIZURE DISORDERS

Disorders of foals that are accompanied by seizures overlap significantly with those that cause weakness and depression. Seizures have been associated with multiple clinical conditions, including sepsis, prematurity, hypoxia, and neonatal isoerythrolysis. Mechanisms for these seizures include hypoglycemia, hypoxia, and cerebral edema.[91] Prolonged seizures result in further hypoxic damage to the CNS, and effort should be directed at immediate control. Treatment must be aimed at the underlying condition, although palliative therapy can be achieved in most cases with diazepam 0.05 to 0.4 mg/kg IV every 30 minutes, or phenobarbital 20 mg/kg IV loading dose, then 10 mg/kg q.12 h. Other anticonvulsant agents are listed in Table 18–6. Hypoglycemia is a common problem, regardless of other mitigating factors, and therefore bolus treatment with dextrose should be used in emergency situations. Administration of water-soluble glucocorticoids will rapidly mobilize glucose and provide anti-inflammatory protection to the CNS.

Peripartum Asphyxia Syndrome or Neonatal Maladjustment Syndrome

The term *neonatal maladjustment syndrome (NMS)* was coined to describe a primary neurologic disorder of neonatal foals.[92] However, many foals that had sepsis, prematurity, or other conditions were indiscriminately diagnosed with NMS, which brought the use of the term into question. In 1994 the descriptive term *peripartum asphyxia syndrome (PAS)* was used to describe this condition.[93] NMS/PAS is commonly associated with sepsis, because of failure to nurse and other abnormal behaviors which predispose the foal to disease. Nonetheless, NMS/PAS results from a specific cause, fetal asphyxia.

Pathogenesis

All causes of equine fetal asphyxia have not been identified, and NMS/PAS may occur in apparently normal births. However, NMS/PAS does appear to be associated with several abnormal conditions, including disease in the mare, abnormalities of the placenta, meconium aspiration, heart defects, and difficult parturition.[93] All of these events result in insufficient oxygen delivery to the CNS during a defined time period, culminating in hemorrhage, edema, and necrosis. Dystocia may also result in subdural hemorrhage.[94] Chronic administration of trimethoprim-sulfamethoxazole and pyrimethamine to mares in late gestation has also been associated with NMS/PAS foals. The specific mechanism has not been elucidated, but it is likely to be related to abnormal development of the CNS secondary to inhibition of folic acid metabolism and synthesis.

Equine fetal asphyxia has not been studied, but research in human fetal asphyxia has been applied to foals.[93] Fetal asphyxia in humans results in hypoxic and ischemic damage to the CNS. This results in accumulation of toxic concentrations of the excitatory amino acids glutamate and aspartate. Glutamate stimulates the opening of sodium channels, which permits inward flux of sodium, chloride, and the passive flux of water, resulting in neuronal swelling. High levels of glutamate also activate calcium channels resulting in high intracellular calcium and the production of oxygen free radicals.[93] Reperfusion injury probably also plays a role in the pathogenesis.

Clinical Signs

The clinical picture associated with NMS/PAS is widely variable, and should reflect the structures affected. Depression is probably the most consistently observed sign, usually accompanied by partial or complete lack of a suckle reflex. Generally, NMS/PAS foals sleep excessively, exhibit generalized hypotonia, and have subtle seizure activity, manifest by randomly directed suckling behavior, paddling, Cheyne-Stokes and apneic breathing patterns, and abnormal eye movement.[93] Foals may also exhibit grand mal epileptic seizures, which can be life-threatening and warrant immediate pharmacologic intervention. These seizures are associated with focal cortical damage, which may be the result of ischemia, edema, or hemorrhage. Moderately severe NMS/PAS can be characterized by vestibular signs, including compulsive circling and head tilt. Severe NMS/PAS is associated with profound depression, hypotonia, seizures, and apneic breathing. This is associated with a grave prognosis.[93]

Treatment

The NMS/PAS foal often has complications with problems other than the neurologic signs. Hypoxic damage secondary to fetal asphyxia may affect any organ system. In addition, failure of passive transfer is common because of the foal's inability to stand and nurse. Therefore, a physical examination and collection of a minimal database should be completed. Support of any and all organ systems affected should be performed in addition to treatment of the neurologic condition.

Seizure activity, particularly of the grand mal type, requires immediate attention, because prolonged seizures perpetuate the CNS damage. Anticonvulsant drugs and dosages have been mentioned. Fluid therapy should be conservative, because excessive fluid administration may exacerbate cerebral edema. Dextrose in water, either 2.5% with 0.45% saline or as an isotonic 5% solution, is indicated in most cases because of the presence of hypoglycemia. Once enteral feeding is initiated and tolerated by the foal, the foal will usually be able to maintain blood glucose above 70 mg/dL, and intravenous dextrose can be discontinued. Dimethyl sulfoxide (DMSO) 1 g/kg IV in a 10% solution is a valuable adjunct in decreasing cerebral edema. The use of mannitol should be avoided because of the common presence of subdural hemorrhage.

Hypoventilation is a common problem in these foals. The presence of hypercapnia will exacerbate the cerebral edema, and therefore artificial ventilation may be indicated. Hyperventilation using positive pressure ventilation will decrease the carbon dioxide and relieve some of the cerebral edema. Artificial ventilation will also impede cardiac output and may be difficult to maintain in a thrashing foal. Therefore the total clinical picture must be considered before initiating this form of assistance.

Liver Disease and Hepatic Encephalopathy

Severe liver disease may result in neurologic signs, including seizures, ataxia, and depression. This is usually associated with increased serum liver enzyme, ammonia, and bile acid concentrations. In neonatal foals, liver damage is most commonly a sequela to septicemia. Primary liver disease is uncommon, but has resulted from ferrous sulfate administration and *Bacillus piliformis* infection (Tyzzer's disease). Oral administration of ferrous sulfate in a probiotic formula to foals before colostrum ingestion has resulted in massive hepatocellular necrosis and liver failure.[95] The probiotic formula that was implicated has been taken off the market.

Tyzzer's disease is usually fatal, and affects foals from 7 to 42 days of age.[96] Mares appear to be the carriers of the causative organism, and should not be used as nurse mares after their own foals die.[97] The first sign of Tyzzer's disease in foals is often sudden death. The incubation period is probably 3 to 7 days, but the clinical course of the disease is most commonly very short, usually 2 to 12 hours. Some depression may be apparent for up to 2 days. Affected foals may exhibit fever and icterus, although the clinical period is commonly missed. Histologic hepatic lesions include numerous hemorrhagic foci of necrosis bounded by filamentous bacterial rods.[96]

Hepatic encephalopathy in older foals is uncommon, but may be caused by ascending bacterial hepatitis or portosystemic shunt (see Chapter 13). Portosystemic shunt is rare, but has been reported in a 6-month-old foal.[98] Signs included poor weight gain, depression, lethargy, and ataxia. Serum chemistry was consistent with an hepatic lesion, as reflected by increased serum ammonia, bile acids, and liver enzyme concentrations. Further discussion of hepatic disease may be found in Chapter 13.

Other Neurologic Diseases

There are several neurologic diseases that are congenital in horses. A congenital encephalopathy associated with mild-to-moderate spongiform degeneration with axonal swelling confined to the white matter, and most prominent in the lateral funiculi, was identified in several offspring of a single dam, suggesting a heritable condition. Clinical signs included coarse tremors of the rearlimbs that disappeared when anesthetized or sleeping.[99] Cerebellar abiotrophy of Arabians has been positively identified as a heritable trait associated with severe gross tremors and lack of fine motor control. This condition is evident from birth (see Chapter 9.7).

Spinal ataxia has been identified in foals as well. Equine cervical vertebral myelopathy (CVM), degenerative myelopathy (EDM), and protozoal myeloencephalopathy (EPM) have all been identified in foals. Usually these conditions require at least several months to become evident. Therefore, ataxia in younger foals should be regarded as arising from a different cause, although EPM has been identified in foals as young as 2 months of age.

RESPIRATORY DISTRESS

Respiratory distress is characterized by labored respiratory efforts and hypoxemia or hypoxia. Hypoxemia is subnormal blood oxygen tension. Hypoxia (lack of oxygen at the tissue level) may occur in the presence or absence of hypoxemia. Hypoxia may result from hypoxemia, hypoperfusion, or subnormal oxygen-carrying capacity of the blood (either anemia or abnormal hemoglobin).

There are five mechanisms by which hypoxemia may develop in animals. These are (1) low inspired oxygen ten-

sion, (2) hypoventilation (or abnormal ventilation), (3) ventilation-perfusion mismatch, (4) diffusion impairment, and (5) right-to-left shunting of blood, either intrapulmonary or intracardiac. Diseased neonatal foals commonly suffer from arterial hypoxemia. Often this is due to hypoventilation, to CNS depression caused by sepsis, NMS, or other neurologic conditions. Ventilation-perfusion mismatch is also seen, and may be worsened with recumbency. The effect of mismatching is worse in foals with pneumonia or bronchopulmonary dysplasia.[58] Diffusion impairment is not commonly seen, but may be a contributor in premature foals with surfactant deficiency. Surfactant deficiency probably contributes its greatest effect by increasing the work of ventilation, thereby causing hypoventilation. Right-to-left shunting through the foramen ovale and ductus arteriosus may contribute to hypoxemia in very young foals, and may increase with recumbency.[50] This condition is exacerbated by pulmonary hypertension, which may occur as a result of reversion to fetal circulation in response to stress. Persistence of fetal circulation in the neonate has also been reported.[100] This condition may be mimicked by pulmonic valve stenosis, which should be considered if the condition worsens as the foal ages.[101]

Bacterial Pneumonia

Neonatal foals commonly develop pneumonia secondary to sepsis. Primary pneumonia of other cause also occurs, although usually in an older age group. Duration of protection from passive immunity depends upon the quantity and type of immunoglobulins received in the colostrum. Usually, serum immunoglobulins are lowest about the sixth week of life, which is the most critical period for the initial development of pneumonia. Pneumonia has been estimated to occur in 9% of all foals under 6 months of age, and results in the death of 1% of the total foal crop.[102]

Predisposing Conditions

Management factors probably contribute greatly to foal pneumonia. Lack of ventilation predisposes foals to chemical irritation from ammonia, and stagnant air prolongs contact of foals with opportunistic pathogens. Transportation of foals to foreign surroundings should be avoided if possible, so that the immunoglobulin protection of the foal matches the profile of the pathogens in the environment. Stress, particularly during the critical period of low immunoglobulin concentration (6–12 weeks), should be avoided.

Bacterial pneumonia is commonly secondary. Viral upper respiratory disease commonly results in secondary bacterial colonization of the lungs. Migrating ascarids also contribute to foal pneumonia, and can be prevented by routine deworming of the dam within 1 month of foaling. Ascarids most commonly infect foals by the transmammary route. Often, the pneumonia will fail to respond until the migrating ascarids have been addressed. Foals may be dewormed with ivermectin, which is larvicidal to ascarids.

The most frequently isolated bacterium in foal pneumonia is *Streptococcus zooepidemicus*. This gram-positive organism is present in the upper respiratory tract of normal horses, and commonly becomes an opportunistic pathogen. Additional organisms that can be isolated, either alone or in mixed infections, include *Actinobacillus equuli, Pasteurella, Klebsiella pneumoniae, Salmonella,* and *Bordetella bronchiseptica.* Sensitivity patterns of these gram-negative organisms are not predictable, and tracheal wash for culture and sensitivity is necessary.

Rhodococcus equi is a common cause of severe pneumonia in foals. Infection occurs during the first few weeks of life, but does not develop into the fulminant infection until about 2 to 4 months. The organism is a soil contaminant and is enzootic on some farms. Often, affected farms will lose a percentage of the foal crop to this disease every year.

The ability of the young animal to fight this infection is dependent upon the immunoglobulin opsonization of the organism. Foal phagocytes are able to ingest *R. equi,* but fail to kill the organism, permitting it to proliferate. The ability of the foal's immune cells to kill the bacteria depends upon the presence of the opsonizing antibodies.[103] Both adult and neonatal equine phagocytic cells are capable of ingesting and killing *R. equi,* although a small percentage of foals exhibit significantly lower killing ability.[104] Other phagocytic cell functions, including random migration, iodination, and ingestion, appear to be less efficient in foals than in adult horses.[82] The combination of these factors may contribute to the susceptibility of foals to this disease. Complete discussion of *R. equi* pneumonia is covered in the next section of this chapter.

Viral Pneumonia

Viral respiratory infections of horses are usually limited to relatively mild respiratory signs, which become significant when associated with secondary bacterial infection. However, a syndrome of fulminant viral pneumonia may occur in foals that is caused by several different viruses. While these cases are usually sporadic, they may occur in an epizootic form, and the definitive diagnosis of the causative agent is important for herd health.

Diagnosis is most commonly based on a fourfold rise in antibody titer against a specific virus. A definitive diagnosis may also be made from virus isolation, or demonstration of inclusions in tissues.[105] These latter techniques have limited availability, and are usually performed in specialized research laboratories, although the recent application of an antigen ELISA for influenza[106] may be the beginning of a new era in stallside diagnosis of respiratory viruses. A nasal swab can be tested for the presence of influenza nucleoprotein using the Directogen FLU-A kit (Becton-Dickinson, Franklin Lakes, NJ).

Equine herpesvirus type 1 (rhinopneumonitis; EHV-1) usually results in a mild respiratory disease in young adults, or abortion in late-term pregnant mares. Occasionally, foals may be born affected. They may either be weak at birth or become affected later. The early signs are weakness and loss of the suckle reflex. This progresses to respiratory distress and diarrhea, with secondary bacterial infection.[107] This form of EHV-1 is usually refractory to antimicrobial therapy, and is associated with thymic necrosis and lymphopenia. For further discussion, see Chapter 2.2.

Adenovirus may be isolated from both normal and diseased horses. It predominantly causes fatal respiratory dis-

ease in Arabian foals with combined immunodeficiency (CID) (see Chapter 1.4). Other foals may be affected, but do not succumb to the disease.[108] In CID foals, adenovirus causes fatal pneumonia, while non-CID foals exhibit less severe clinical signs. Signs are similar to those associated with pneumonia from other causes, including fever, tachypnea, and increased respiratory effort, with auscultable abnormalities distributed primarily cranioventrally. About 25% of the affected foals also have diarrhea. CID foals are lymphopenic, and do not respond to infection with a rise in antibody titer, whereas non-CID foals develop a rise in antibody titer by 10 days.[108] Intranuclear inclusions can be detected in conjunctival and nasal epithelial cells.[109] Adenovirus may predispose foals to secondary bacterial infection, and be a significant factor in the pathogenesis of foal pneumonia.[108]

Equine influenza virus most commonly causes a mild upper respiratory infection in young horses. However, it may cause a severe, rapidly progressive viral pneumonia in foals. Diagnosis may be made from a nasal swab by use of the aforementioned Directogen Kit.

Equine arteritis virus (EVA) is usually manifest in a group of previously naive mares as abortion storms, affecting 40% to 60% of mares[110] (see Chapter 15). Affected foals are born weak, but the disease is usually not fatal.[111, 112] Infection may occur horizontally, or vertically, which is usually associated with abortion. EVA has been implicated in viral pneumonia leading to death in neonatal foals.[110, 113] Clinical signs include acute onset of respiratory distress, with severely decreased lung compliance and pulmonary edema.

Other Conditions Associated with Respiratory Distress

Respiratory distress is not necessarily associated with primary pulmonary disease. Tachypnea, or apparent panting, can be associated with abnormal thermoregulatory mechanisms. Some draft foals born in hot weather exhibit pyrexia with apparent tachypnea. The pyrexia is not responsive to NSAIDs, and the foals are anhidrotic, as determined by a terbutaline skin test. The high body temperature and panting respond to body clipping, alcohol, or cold-water soaks, and the use of fans to lower temperature. Draft-breed foals appear to grow out of this condition. A similar condition is also seen in foals treated with erythromycin and rifampin for *R. equi,* although the primary pneumonia may contribute to the tachypnea in those cases.

Respiratory distress may result from primary cardiac anomalies, or severe anemia, as in neonatal isoerythrolysis. Severe cardiac anomalies that result in cardiac failure or severe right-to-left shunting is usually accompanied by dependent edema, jugular pulses, and cyanosis. Primary cardiac diseases are discussed in Chapter 7. Neonatal isoerythrolysis is discussed in Chapter 11.

COLIC

Colic in the young foal must be evaluated similarly to that in the adult. However, both the size and age of the animal require special consideration. Clinical examination reveals an animal that is in pain, tachycardic, and that may have a grossly distended abdomen. Cardiovascular status should be evaluated, including membrane color and capillary refill time. The abdomen should be percussed and ballottement performed for detection of gas or fluid. The presence of meconium in the rectum should be noted. Foals, unlike adult horses, may fail to show severe colic in the presence of a severe lesion, and conversely may exhibit refractory pain in the presence of a minimal lesion. Rectal palpation is an essential part of the colic examination of the adult, but cannot be performed on young foals. Alternative diagnostic methods for evaluation of the abdominal viscera are easily applied to foals, and include radiography and ultrasonography.

Abdominocentesis may be attempted with either an 18-gauge 2.5-cm needle[114] or with a teat cannula after local anesthesia and stab incision.[115] In foals with colic, excessive bowel distention may increase the chance of bowel puncture, which should be taken into consideration when deciding whether to perform an abdominocentesis.[75] Foals are about seven times more likely to develop complications secondary to abdominocentesis than adults.[115] Sufficient fluid may not be recovered in about 25% of normal foals.[114] Peritoneal fluid cytology in foals is similar to that in adults, except for a lower total WBC count. A WBC count up to 3,000/μL is normal.[114]

Ultrasonography of the foal abdomen is most easily performed with the foal in the standing position. Free fluid in the abdomen can be detected as anechoic fluid surrounding the viscera. In contrast to adults, foals usually have minimal gas in the chyme in the intestinal lumen, and therefore the abdominal viscera are readily evaluated ultrasonographically. Gas in the lumen of the bowel appears as bright echoes, which shadow deeper structures. Gas-filled bowel loops are associated with ileus or obstruction.[75] Intussusception may be diagnosed by abdominal ultrasonography. A characteristic target-shaped structure can be identified in the abdomen.[116] Volvulus may be suspected when the small intestine is visualized by ultrasound as large, chyme-filled loops of bowel with minimal peristaltic activity. The walls of compromised bowel will be edematous and hypoechoic.[117]

Radiography is also a valuable technique for determining the location of the lesion in the colicky foal, with a 96% sensitivity and 71% specificity.[118] Meconium impactions can nearly always be identified. Intestinal distention is easily detected, but it is difficult to differentiate the cause as functional or mechanical. Contrast studies may be of value in suspected diseases of the orad gastrointestinal tract, but of limited value in the aborad segment because often the decision to perform surgery must be made before the contrast material moves that far. Even in the case of orad lesions, such as gastric ulcers, the restriction of the veterinary clinician to a few radiographic views limits this technique.

Meconium Retention

The most common cause of colic in the neonatal foal is meconium impaction. Foals have abdominal distention with gas, which may be percussed. Affected foals will strain frequently to defecate, evidenced by a kyphotic posture (humped back), with the rearlimbs placed under the body, and the tail extended. This condition is often easily treated by warm, soapy-water enemas (50–100 mL with mild soap).

These are performed by passing a lubricated flexible rubber tube into the rectum. Fluid should not be forced in under pressure, but rather by gravity flow through a funnel. This minimizes the chance of rectal tears. Repeated enemas increase the risk of damage to the rectal mucosa. If two enemas do not resolve the impaction, mineral oil should be administered by nasogastric tube. If colic persists, surgery should be considered.

Specific anesthetic considerations are discussed above, and surgical technique may be found elsewhere.[119] There is a tendency for younger foals to develop more adhesions than older foals.[120]

Obstruction

Intussusception, volvulus, displacement, diaphragmatic hernia, and other intraluminal obstructions are all seen in foals. Large colon torsions in foals may be associated with enteritis and diarrhea instead of failure of fecal passage.[75]

Gastroduodenal Ulceration

Gastric ulceration is a significant problem in foals and is of particular concern in foals with diarrhea.[121, 122] About 50% of foals younger than 90 days of age have some gastric ulceration, regardless of disease history. Foals with a history of disease also develop ulceration on the glandular portion of the stomach.[123] About 25% of older foals (>90 days of age) develop gastric ulceration with clinical disease, whereas only 3% of normal foals develop ulcers.[123, 124] Ulceration on the margo plicatus is usually subclinical and may be observed in both affected and healthy foals. Foals exhibiting clinical signs of ulcers have greater involvement of the glandular region of the stomach.[125] The greater susceptibility of foals to ulcer disease may be related to a higher gastric acidity (pH may approach 1).[126]

Clinical Signs

Gastroduodenal ulceration of foals has four common clinical forms. Foals may ultimately exhibit all of these syndromes, although usually the signs at any given moment are in a single category. The first form is asymptomatic ulceration. About 3% of normal foals have ulceration of the margo plicatus which is associated with clinical signs.[123] Despite this, death from exsanguination secondary to this form of gastric ulceration has been reported.[127]

The second ulcer syndrome is of symptomatic, active ulcers, manifest by colic in the foal. This constitutes the classic clinical syndrome, accompanied by bruxism, ptyalism, and rolling, particularly with the tendency to remain in dorsal recumbency.[122] Occasionally, foals with ulcers will spontaneously reflux, although this is more commonly seen in animals with duodenal ulceration. Diarrhea often develops. Nursing will usually continue, but the foal will often fail to ingest a normal volume, and periods of nursing will be interrupted by periods of colic. Clinical signs are often referable to the primary disease process, but tachycardia may be present as a result of colic pain. Pressure applied over the paracostal and xiphoid regions may elicit a pain response.[121]

The third clinical syndrome results from perforating ulcers, which cause severe peritonitis, and usually result in death. Clinical signs are caused by endotoxemic shock, and rapidly progress to death. Rare foals may be saved by surgery if the perforating ulcers are small and contained in the omentum.[129] Further discussion of endotoxic shock may be found in Chapter 12.7.

Pyloric obstruction may occur during the active stage of symptomatic ulcers, or may become a problem after the active clinical signs have abated. Healing ulcers may result in fibrous tissue replacement of normal mucosa, submucosa, and muscularis. Strictures, segmental ulcerative duodenitis, and diffuse thickening of the duodenum may be sequelae to ulcer disease in foals, and ultimately result in abnormal gastric emptying.[123] In patients with active disease, clinical signs are similar to those described above, but these patients have copious nasogastric reflux, and may reflux spontaneously. These foals are often 3 to 5 months of age.[123] Occasionally, horses up to 18 months of age may show signs of pyloric outflow obstruction, which can be attributed to ulcer disease as foals. Further discussion of ulcers may be found in Chapter 12.3.

Diagnosis

The classic appearance of bruxism, ptyalism, and dorsal recumbency in foals is highly suggestive of gastric ulceration. However, some foals fail to show these classic signs. Therefore, gastric ulceration should be included in the differential diagnosis of any colicky foal. The high morbidity of diseased foals warrants consideration of prophylactic therapy, even in the absence of clinical signs.

Diagnostic tests which may aid in the diagnosis of ulcer disease include a hemogram, an occult blood test, and abdominocentesis. A hemogram is nonspecific, but may reflect blood loss anemia, or neutropenia associated with ulcer perforation into the abdomen. The presence of occult blood in feces or gastric reflux is highly suggestive of ulcer disease, although many foals with ulcers will be occult blood–negative. Abdominocentesis may reflect severe ulceration with leakage of bowel contents into the peritoneal cavity. A definitive diagnosis can be achieved by gastroendoscopy, although most commercially available endoscopes are unable to visualize the foal stomach because of length or diameter limitations.[123]

Treatment

The rationale for the treatment of ulcers in foals is based on decreasing the gastric acidity and improving mucosal protection. A detailed description of ulcer treatment can be found in Chapter 12.3. Hospitalized foals at risk for the development of ulcers may be treated with histamine $H_{\alpha 2}$ receptor antagonists or the mucosal protectant sucralfate. Some clinicians advocate the use of both in high-risk foals. Foals that exhibit clinical signs should be treated with both drugs. The H_2 blocker most commonly used is ranitidine, which may be administered at 2.2 mg/kg PO q.12h. Alternatively, cimetidine may be used, although the dose is higher, and it must be administered more frequently. However, cimetidine is available in a parenteral formulation which may be valuable in foals that are refluxing. Sucralfate 20 mg/kg,

PO q.6 h. forms an adherent gel, which, upon exposure to gastric acid, coats the surface of the ulcer. In addition, sucralfate stimulates the local mucosal release of prostaglandin E_2 (PGE$_2$), which has a cytoprotective effect.[129]

Additional pharmacologic treatment for ulcers includes bismuth subsalicylate, antacids, omeprazole, 16,16-dimethyl PGE$_2$, and omega-3 fatty acids. Anecdotally, bismuth subsalicylate diminishes colic pain after administration. This effect is attributed to a coating effect. Both antacids and omeprazole exert their action by decreasing gastric acidity. Antacids directly neutralize acid, although their duration of action is short, and their presence may interfere with the absorption of cimetidine.[125] Omeprazole directly inhibits the K$^+$, H$^+$-pump on the gastric acid–secreting parietal cells. Omeprazole is now available in the United States. Both 16,16-dimethyl PGE$_2$ and omega-3 fatty acids increase the local concentration of PGE$_2$. Omega-3 fatty acids are present in relatively high amounts in corn oil.

Treatment of perforating gastric ulcers is unrewarding. Diffuse peritonitis in foals carries a grave prognosis. When the ulcer is contained by the omentum, resection of the affected portion of the stomach may be successful,[128] but successful surgical intervention in these cases is rare.[75]

Delayed gastric emptying due to fibrosis of the pylorus is associated with a poor prognosis unless surgery is performed. A pyloric bypass is the recommended treatment.[130]

Congenital Defects

Atresia

Developmental anomalies of the gastrointestinal system account for 3.1% of deaths in late-term fetuses and newborn foals.[131] Acute colic develops within a few hours of birth (2–26 hours; mean, 8.2). There is an absence of meconium staining, and the condition may be diagnosed by barium enema or colonoscopy if the blind end is not too far proximal. If much of the small colon is present, barium enema may be normal. Abdominocentesis will be normal unless the involved intestine is compromised. Atresia may be associated with other congenital abnormalities. Surgical correction may be attempted, but success is elusive. There are three types of colonic atresia: (1) membrane atresia, (2) cord atresia, and (3) blind-end atresia, with a short bowel and a gap. The suspected cause is a loss of blood supply during development.[132, 133]

Lethal White Syndrome

All-white foals born of overo-overo matings of paint horses may suffer from congenital aganglionosis of the terminal ileum, cecum, and colon. Foals appear normal at birth, but develop fatal colic within a few days. The foals lack normal propulsive motility of the affected bowel, and therefore develop meconium impactions of the ileum. The mechanism may be due to abnormal migration of the neural crest cells during development. Both melanocytes and myenteric ganglion cells are of neural crest origin in the embryo.[134]

ENTERITIS

Enteritis is commonly associated with abdominal pain in foals. In addition, serious intestinal obstructions, such as colonic volvulus, may be associated with diarrhea. Diarrhea is predominantly a problem of foals between the age of 1 week and 2 months.[135] Mild diarrheas associated with foal heat or nutritional changes from overconsumption of milk or coprophagy probably occur in all foals. More serious diarrheal diseases may occur in as many as 50% of foals worldwide.[135] Viruses, bacteria, and parasites all contribute to this problem, and treatment for diarrhea is similar, regardless of the cause. Supportive care for foals was discussed earlier in this chapter. Specific pharmacologic treatment of diarrheal diseases is presented in Chapter 12.10 and 12.11.

Foal Heat Diarrhea

Foal heat diarrhea usually occurs between the age of 5 and 14 days. This diarrhea is usually mild and transient. Mentation and attitude are usually maintained as bright, alert, and responsive during these mild forms of diarrhea, and no specific therapy is indicated. Several mechanisms for foal heat diarrhea have been proposed, but none have been substantiated. The temporal relationship to the mare's first estrus has prompted investigation of changes in milk composition, but no changes have been found.[136] In addition, foals that have been taken off mare's milk will still exhibit foal heat diarrhea.

Strongyloides westeri infection, which occurs via transmammary infection, was once considered a possible cause, but is now known not to be involved. The prevalence of *S. westeri* infection in foals before the availability of thiabendazole, and later ivermectin, was about 90%, which made this nematode a leading suspect in foal heat diarrhea. However, the use of effective anthelmintics has lowered the prevalence of *S. westeri* infection in foals to 6%,[137] without a corresponding decrease in foal heat diarrhea.

Nutritional changes in the foal's diet have been suspected as the cause of foal heat diarrhea. Coprophagy, which commonly begins around the time of the mare's first heat, has also been suspected. Anecdotal experience suggests that foals experience diarrhea even when reared in isolation. The definitive cause of foal heat diarrhea remains elusive.

Rotaviruses

Rotaviruses infect neonates of many different species. An equine rotavirus appears to be a significant pathogen of foals, being found in 30% to 40% of diarrheal foals up to 3 months of age in every region of the world.[135, 138–143] The RNA genome of rotaviruses consists of 11 separate strands of double-stranded RNA. The rotaviruses are grouped into major serogroups according to complement fixation, ELISA, immune electron microscopy, and hemagglutination. Serogroups are further grouped into serotypes determined by differences in specific epitopes on the outer capsid proteins. The G serotype is determined by specific epitopes on the VP-7 capsid protein. Foal rotaviruses are all classified as serogroup A, and are predominantly of the G3 serotype, although additional serotypes have been identified. In addition, some rotavirus isolates remain untyped, suggesting the existence of additional serotypes. Foal rotavirus isolates are more similar to one another than to rotavirus isolates from

other species, suggesting that equine rotavirus has evolved as a specific pathogen of horses.[138]

Rotaviral diarrhea is typically observed in groups of foals where large numbers of foals and mares are housed temporarily, such as large nurseries where mares are shipped with their foals to the breeding shed. Serotyping of these viruses suggests that the stress of shipping on the foals permits infection with endemic rotaviruses, rather than the introduction of new rotaviruses with incoming stock.[138] Rotaviruses are commonly found in the diarrheal feces of foals affected with other pathogens, and can also be detected in foals with no clinical signs. Nonetheless, experimental inoculation of these viruses to foals consistently results in clinical disease, supporting circumstantial evidence that they are legitimate pathogens.

Clinical Signs

The clinical course of infection begins as anorexia and depression and rapidly progresses to profuse watery diarrhea. Foals are commonly febrile and dehydrated, and may experience electrolyte abnormalities. Younger foals tend to have more severe symptoms, and may require intensive care, whereas older foals may act primarily as carriers for dissemination of the virus. Severity and types of clinical symptoms may be related to the strain of rotavirus.[144] Signs may vary from severe, profuse watery diarrhea, to mild pasty feces, to constipation. Duration of clinical signs is from 1 to 12 days, and some cases may actually suffer from chronic diarrhea indefinitely, although the systemic disease is minimal.

Pathogenesis

There are several mechanisms of the diarrhea associated with rotavirus infection. Rotavirus replicates within intestinal epithelial cells, and results in denudation of the intestinal villi. Since the villi have a primary absorbing function, and the crypts have a primary secretory function, the result is that secretion exceeds absorption. In addition, rotavirus interferes with the production of disaccharidases, including lactase. In addition, the sodium-glucose cotransporter is impaired. This results in failure to absorb sugars, and ultimately, osmotic diarrhea.

Diagnosis

Rotavirus is not shed in large amounts in the feces of diarrheal foals. Therefore, the detection level of any single diagnostic test is only about 33% of known infected foals. Several ELISA-based test kits are available (e.g., Rotazyme II, Abbott Laboratories, North Chicago, Ill.). Direct detection is by polyacrylamide gel electrophoresis or electron microscopy. Detection methods for rotavirus must be applied to multiple affected foals for the purpose of detecting an outbreak, or several different methods of detection must be used to confirm disease in any given animal.[135] Additionally, rotavirus is commonly found in combination with other infections in foals with diarrhea.

Other Viral Diarrheas

Coronaviruses have been implicated in serious diarrheal diseases in most domestic species, but no specific equine coronaviruses have been identified. Nonetheless, coronavirus-like particles have been found in feces of three foals dying of diarrheal disease, suggesting a possible, as yet undefined, role for coronavirus in foal diarrhea.[145]

Equine adenovirus is usually considered a mild pathogen of the respiratory tract of foals, but has been found associated with diarrhea.[109] An antigenically distinct equine adenovirus has been identified in foals with diarrhea, although most of those foals had concurrent rotaviral infection.[146] A definitive role for adenovirus in foal diarrhea has not been established.

Parvovirus-like particles have been identified in the feces of a foal with severe diarrhea, although transmission studies were not done. The duration of the diarrhea was about 2.5 weeks. Culture for *Salmonella* species was negative, and electron microscopy revealed only parvovirus-like particles on several occasions.[147] No other reports have suggested a parvovirus as the cause of equine diarrhea, and treatment consisted of supportive care and TPN.

Bacterial Diarrhea

Necrotizing Enteritis

Necrotizing enteritis is caused by infection with *Clostridium perfringens* type C, or *Clostridium difficile*. This disease is characterized by acute onset of abdominal pain, dehydration, recumbency, and profuse, watery diarrhea. The presence of bloody feces presages a poor prognosis. Diagnosis is by anaerobic culture of intestinal contents, demonstrating the presence of large numbers of gram-positive rods. *Clostridium perfringens* type C has been identified in foals in North America and Australia, and the organism is subtyped by mouse inoculation. The presence of both α- and β-toxins indicates type C *Clostridium perfringens*.[148] *Clostridium difficile* has also been associated with necrotizing enteritis in foals.[149] This bacterium appears to be transmitted by a transmammary route to the foal, and certain mares may be carriers. Treatment consists of muzzling the foal and providing an alternative milk source for 48 to 72 hours. After this period, the foals appear to be less susceptible to the organism.

Salmonella

Salmonella species are a cause of neonatal septicemia in neonates, but may cause diarrhea in a slightly older age group.

Escherichia coli

There is no relationship between the presence of *E. coli* in the feces and diarrhea in foals.[135] This is probably due to the ubiquitous presence of *E. coli* subtypes in the feces of animals. *Escherichia coli* serogroups may contain both nonpathogenic and pathogenic organisms.[150] Simple diagnostic tests for detection of pathogenic strains are not commercially available. *Escherichia coli* may cause diarrhea by one of three different mechanisms: (1) the elaboration of enterotoxin; (2) mucosal invasion; (3) the destruction of the small-intestinal brush border with subsequent malabsorptive diarrhea. Enterotoxigenic *E. coli* causes the classic hypersecretory diarrhea by the action of specific binding of bacterial pili to small-intestinal cells, and the elaboration of enterotoxins, which stimulate intracellular cyclic adenosine monophosphate (cAMP) in the cells. This results in an imbalance between secretion and absorption, and ultimately, hypersecretion of electrolytes into the intestinal lumen. Hypersecretory *E. coli* diarrhea in foals has not been identified. Enteroinvasive *E. coli* binds and migrates through the mucosa, stimulating an inflammatory response. The third mechanism of diarrhea is caused by enteropathogenic *E. coli,* which results in the loss of intestinal microvilli without concurrent loss of enterocytes. This causes loss of function of the microvilli, and therefore malabsorption of luminal constituents and fluid.[151] Enteropathogenic *E. coli* is capable of causing brush border depletion of equine intestines under experimental conditions, but has not yet been implicated in clinical disease.

Other Bacterial Diarrheas

Bacteroides fragilis may be a cause of diarrhea in young foals, mainly those less than 7 days old.[152] The presence of enterotoxin is determined by the injection of isolated *B. fragilis* into intestinal loops of anesthetized rabbits, and subsequent observation for signs of enteritis.[153] Of 40 diarrheal foals 10 (25%) were infected with enterotoxigenic *B. fragilis,* although dual infections with rotavirus or *Salmonella* species occurred in some of the affected foals. One foal died.[152] This study could not conclude that *B. fragilis* was the definitive cause of the diarrhea, but this organism should be included as a potential cause of diarrhea in young foals.

Aeromonas hydrophila was found in 9% of foals with diarrhea in a survey in Britain. This organism was not found at all in normal foals, or in foals under 1 week of age. Highest prevalence was found in foals aged between 1 week and 1 month.[135] *Aeromonas hydrophila* elaborates an enterotoxin that can be a significant cause of chronic diarrhea in human infants.

Streptococcus durans is an enterococcus that has been identified in the small intestines of foals that died from both natural and experimental infections. This gram-positive coccus is found extensively throughout the small-intestinal mucosal surface. Colonization of the mucosal surface appears to permit proliferation of nonpathogenic *E. coli* in the lumen of the intestines, resulting in high bacterial counts of *E. coli* in the feces of these foals. The significance of this bacterium as a pathogen in foals is unknown.[154]

Parasitic Causes of Diarrhea

Nematodes

Strongyloides westeri is the most common parasitic infection of young foals, affecting as many as 90% of young foals. Transmission is transmammary, and therefore foals can acquire a patent infection as early as 8 to 12 days of age.[155, 156]

The source of the parasites in the mammary gland is thought to be larvae that were ingested when the dam was a foal.[156] *Strongyloides westeri* infections are self-limiting, and the adult worms will be cleared by the foal before 1 year of age. This organism has been anecdotally implicated in foal heat diarrhea, but there is no scientific basis for this observation. Diagnosis of a patent infection can be confirmed by the presence of embryonated eggs on fecal flotation. The number of eggs per gram does not correlate with severity of diarrhea, and therefore need not be performed.[155] Effective treatment of suspected *S. westeri* diarrhea can be achieved by benzimidazole anthelmintics or ivermectin. Ivermectin is also effective against the tissue stage in the mammary gland, and pretreatment of the mare can decrease transmission to the suckling foal.

Diarrhea in young foals caused by *Strongylus vulgaris* results primarily from the migration of the L4 larval stage through the arterioles of the submucosa of the ileum, cecum, and ventral colon. At about 2 weeks after ingestion of the infective larvae (L3), the migrating L4 larvae reach the cranial mesenteric artery. After this point, clinical signs reflect thromboembolic colic.[155] Diagnosis of *S. vulgaris* infection is based on farm deworming history, clinical signs, and clinicopathologic changes. Peripheral leukocytosis with neutrophilia and eosinophilia, hypoalbuminemia, and hyperglobulinemia are consistent with migrating larvae. The prepatent period of *S. vulgaris* is about 6 months. Therefore, fecal flotation is of little value in the diagnosis of this disease in foals.[155] Anthelmintics effective against migrating *S. vulgaris* include ivermectin at the label dose, oxfendazole administered as two doses on alternate days at the label dose, fenbendazole 10 mg/kg/day for 5 days, and thiabendazole 440 mg/kg/day for 2 days. The dosages for the last two are higher than the manufacturers' recommended dose.

Equine small strongyles comprised over 40 species, mostly cyathostomes, including multiple genera. These species are passed into the environment in the feces, where they develop into the infective L3 larval stage. These are ingested, and penetrate the intestinal mucosa and submucosa, where they develop into the encysted L4 stage. These encysted larvae can remain in a hypobiotic state for long periods of time. The sudden emergence of these encysted larvae can result in diarrhea.[155] Strongyles are probably an uncommon cause of diarrhea in young foals.

Protozoa

Cryptosporidium species are responsible for gastroenteritis and diarrhea in many animal species and, unlike other coccidia, are not host-specific. These organisms have been implicated in foal diarrhea,[157] but can be isolated from feces of diarrheal and normal foals at the same rate.[135, 158] Similar to other coccidia, the sporozoites emerge from ingested oocysts and undergo schizogony and gametogony within the intestinal epithelial cells. Unlike other coccidia, *Cryptosporidium* species may autoinfect the host. The oocysts that are released into the lumen of the small intestine may release sporozoites before being passed into the feces. The incubation period is 3 to 7 days, with a clinical course of 5 to 14 days.[159] This condition is usually self-limiting in the immunocompetent patient, but immunocompromised patients, such as septic and

premature foals, are at high risk for serious complications.[157, 160] However, normal foals may shed *Cryptosporidium* oocysts in the feces, and therefore the presence of oocysts does not prove that this is the cause of the diarrhea.[159] Treatment consists of supportive therapy to prevent dehydration and concomitant complications. Cryptosporidiosis is a zoonotic disease, and extreme care should be taken in handling these patients. In addition, care should be taken to prevent the spread to other compromised hospital patients.

Other protozoa may be found in horses, but are incidental, and experimental infection is not associated with diarrhea.[161] *Eimeria leukarti* is adapted to the small intestine of horses and causes a mild self-limiting infection of juvenile horses.[155] Oocysts are commonly found in the feces of normal foals.[162] With repeated sampling of feces, over 90% of foals eventually shed *E. leukarti*.[163]

Trichomonas equi is a common parasite of the equine large intestine. While this protozoan has been implicated in diarrhea, the clinical disease cannot be duplicated through transmission studies, which sheds doubt on its role as a pathogen.[159] This organism is often found in the feces of horses with chronic diarrhea, but this is probably because the chronic fluidity encourages the proliferation of the flagellate, rather than the other way around.[159]

Giardia species are likely to be host-specific, with *Giardia equi* infecting horses. The prevalence is unknown. It can be detected in the feces of clinically normal foals,[164] and has been associated with chronic diarrhea in an adult.[165] The diarrhea results from enteritis and malabsorption.[159] Diagnosis is based on the presence of cysts in feces as detected by flotation in a 33% zinc sulfate solution.[159] In cases where no other pathogen can be identified, treatment with metronidazole 5 mg/kg PO t.i.d. for 10 days may be effective.[165]

URINARY TRACT DISORDERS
Uroperitoneum

Uroperitoneum results from the leakage of urine from the urinary tract into the peritoneal space. The source of the urine may be anywhere in the urinary tract, but most commonly from a tear in the urinary bladder or urachus.[75] Ureteral anomalies or rupture may be the source of the urine leakage.[166, 167]

Usually, the defect is present at birth, although affected foals initially appear normal at birth. Some foals may develop the defect post parturition, secondary to trauma[167] or septicemia and cystitis.[75] Rarely, older foals may develop a uroperitoneum secondary to other disease processes.[168] Stranguria, demonstrated by an increase in the frequency and decrease in the volume of urination, is often the first clinical sign observed. The stimulus for micturition in these foals is usually abdominal distention, because the bladder is not distended. The presence of a stream of urine does not rule out the presence of uroperitoneum, because the foal may be able to accumulate some urine in the bladder, and partially evacuate it. Foals will strain to urinate in a lordotic posture, with the rearlimbs placed caudally. The appearance of foals straining to defecate includes cranially placed limbs and a kyphotic posture. Despite these differences, these two conditions are commonly mistaken for one another.

Additional clinical signs are referable to electrolyte abnormalities and azotemia. The accumulation of urine in the abdominal cavity results in failure to regulate the blood constituents. Often, abdominal distention is grossly evident, and the excess fluid may be palpated in the abdominal cavity. Serum chemistry reveals hyponatremia, hyperkalemia, hypochloremia, and azotemia, which result from the equilibration of plasma with urine in the peritoneal fluid.[169] Depression results from electrolyte abnormalities, and the direct effect of azotemia on the CNS. Cardiac arrhythmias, particularly bradycardia, may be seen as a result of the hyperkalemia. Both urea and creatinine accumulate in the blood, although an increased serum creatinine concentration may be more consistent in foals.[169] This combination of chemistry values is highly suggestive of uroperitoneum. However, prerenal causes, renal failure, and functional or structural blockage of the urethra may cause similar serum abnormalities, without the presence of uroperitoneum.[75] In addition, foals with concurrent disease may not conform to the classic clinical chemistry profile for this condition. A ratio of peritoneal fluid creatinine to serum creatinine greater than 2:1 will confirm the presence of urine in the abdomen,[75] and should be performed in every suspected case of uroperitoneum. Urea is a small molecule and rapidly equilibrates across the peritoneum, but the larger molecule, creatinine, equilibrates at a slower rate. Early in the course of disease, these serum and peritoneal abnormalities may not be present.[75]

Further diagnostic techniques are required to determine the site of the leakage. These include ultrasonography, contrast radiography, migration of dye from the bladder into the peritoneal cavity, and exploratory celiotomy. Ultrasonography of the abdomen is extremely valuable. The presence of an abnormality on a sonogram is diagnostic, although inability to detect one does not rule out any possibilities. The ultrasound examination is carried out with the foal in the standing position. A large volume of free fluid in the abdomen can be readily appreciated as anechoic fluid surrounding the viscera. This finding alone does not confirm the diagnosis of uroperitoneum, because ascitic fluid will have the same appearance.[75] If the bladder is filled with urine, it can be seen as a thin-walled structure filled with anechoic fluid. If the bladder is small, it appears as a thick-walled deflated structure in the pelvic inlet. A residual volume of urine may or may not be present. Often, a tear in the bladder wall can be directly visualized, although if the bladder is small, the tear may not be readily apparent.[117] When the urachus is the source of the rupture, the subcutaneous tissues may also be filled with urine. This is seen as anechoic fluid between tissue planes in the ventral abdomen. The tear in the urachus should be easily visualized. Ureteral tears may be more difficult to detect with ultrasound.

Bladder catheterization will often result in the collection of urine. The instillation and subsequent recovery of a known volume of sterile fluid has been advocated by some clinicians, but is not considered reliable.[169] The infusion of a sterile nontoxic dye, such as new methylene blue, into the bladder, and its subsequent presence in peritoneal fluid is diagnostic of a ruptured bladder or urachus. Other causes of uroperitoneum will not result in leakage of dye into the abdominal cavity.

Radiography of the abdomen may reveal free fluid in the abdomen, or thickening of the ventral abdominal wall.[75] Contrast radiography may identify the site of the abnormal-ity. Contrast cystography may demonstrate leakage into the abdomen from the bladder. The bladder should be catheterized and evacuated. Contrast material should be instilled into the empty bladder. Radiographs should be taken immediately. This technique may reveal leakage of contrast through either a bladder or urachal defect.[75] Excretory urography may identify a ureteral defect as the source of urine, but is nonspecific, and may not add significant information if surgery is an option.

Uroperitoneum, regardless of pathogenesis, requires surgery. Therefore, it is only necessary to perform as many diagnostic tests as needed to be confident that the animal has uroperitoneum. At surgery, the bladder, urachus, and ureters should be carefully evaluated.

Ruptured Bladder

The most common source of uroperitoneum in foals is a ruptured bladder. This condition is usually seen in male foals, although it also occurs in females. The mechanism proposed for development of uroperitoneum is high intraluminal pressure in males during parturition.[170] The smaller urethral diameter of the male produces greater resistance to passive urine flow than the larger urethra of the female.

In some animals, the tear in the dorsal bladder wall can be visualized by ultrasound. The differential diagnosis includes meconium impaction for the straining, but the electrolyte abnormalities will not be present. Uroperitoneum can also exist due to ureteral tears or ectopic ureters.[117] If the tear cannot be visualized by ultrasonography, contrast radiography can be performed. If contrast material is seen leaking into the peritoneal cavity from the bladder, the diagnosis is confirmed. An additional diagnostic technique is instillation of sterile new methylene blue dye through a sterile urinary catheter into the bladder. The presence of the dye in abdominal fluid is diagnostic of a ruptured bladder. A 3-month-old colt with a ruptured bladder secondary to a urethral calculus has been reported.[168]

Ureteral Abnormalities

Uroperitoneum may result from congenital defects or tears in the ureters. In these cases, the ureters terminate in the retroperitoneal space, which causes accumulation of urine. The urine may then leak into the peritoneal cavity, resulting in uroperitoneum. Surgical repair may be successful.[171]

Intravenous pyelography can rule out ureteral tears or ectopic ureters.

UMBILICAL DISORDERS

The umbilical cord provides the link between the fetus and the placenta. The umbilical vein carries nutrients and oxygen from the placenta to the fetus and the umbilical arteries carry carbon dioxide and waste products from the fetus to the placenta. Urine produced in the fetus is expelled into the allantois through the urachus. The umbilical cord breaks at parturition, at which point the muscular arteries constrict, and the urachus and umbilical vein also close. The defect in the body wall at this point fibroses, and the external structures scar, leaving the umbilicus. Several conditions may affect the umbilicus of the neonate.

Omphalitis and Omphalophlebitis

Generalized infection of the equine neonate may be introduced via the umbilicus. Foals infected by this route are usually normal at birth, although the infection probably occurs shortly after birth. External swelling, purulent discharge, ventral edema, and a patent urachus may be evident in some foals, but many will not exhibit these external signs. In these foals, omphalitis may be suspected based on evidence of bacterial seeding of other organs.

Careful palpation of the umbilicus should be a part of every physical examination of the neonate. Despite this, some cases of omphalitis may not be accompanied by external signs. Therefore, if this condition is suspected, further diagnostic tests are necessary.

Diagnosis of omphalitis and confirmation of the extent of involvement can be made by ultrasonographic evaluation. This is most easily performed with the foal in the standing position. The superficial nature of the umbilical structures necessitates the use of a high-frequency transducer with an offset (7.5 MHz). The umbilical vein and arteries can be readily identified in the normal foal during the first month of life, and may be identified in the foal up to 2 months of age. The umbilical vein is a thin-walled, blood-filled structure, which extends cranially along the ventral abdomen from the umbilical stump to the liver. The umbilical vein should appear hypoechoic and less than 10 mm in diameter. The umbilical arteries are paired structures with thick walls, which extend caudally from the umbilical stump to become the round ligaments of the bladder. In contrast to the umbilical vein, the arteries have no lumen owing to contraction of the muscular walls when the umbilical cord breaks. These are seen as relatively echodense paired structures, which should measure less than 13 mm in diameter. If infected, these structures may have a fluid-filled center, reflecting suppurative debris, but most commonly, infected structures appear larger than expected. The urachus is the most commonly infected structure.[172] This is not usually visualized in the normal foal, but, if infected, it appears as a structure located between the umbilical arteries. Viewed in longitudinal section, the apex of the bladder can be seen tapering to a point rather than a round border. Usually, more than one structure is affected.[172, 173]

Omphalophlebitis is most effectively treated surgically. The entire infected section must be removed, including that cranial to the liver and caudal to the bladder. The apex of the bladder should be resected, because the blood supply to the tip runs with the urachus, and the apex may slough if it is not removed. In cases where the structures are less than twice the normal size, and there is no evidence of bacteremia and seeding of joints or other organs, medical treatment can be attempted, and can be successful. It is not recommended in cases with septicemia, because additional organs remain at risk as long as the nidus of infection remains. If medical therapy is chosen, ultrasonography should be repeated at 3- to 5-day intervals to monitor efficacy. If this shows worsening of signs, then therapy should be reevaluated.[117]

Hernias

Umbilical hernias form because of the failure of the umbilical stump to completely heal after birth. This process can be influenced by genetics, umbilical infection, or excessive intraabdominal pressure during the first few days post parturition. Hernias must be differentiated from umbilical infections. The contents of the hernial sac should be reducible, and not hard and painful. Foals with omphalophlebitis will often show some signs of infection, including fever, purulent discharge, or evidence of sepsis.

Small umbilical hernias are likely to close by themselves as the animal matures. If these fail to close by 6 to 12 months, correction should be attempted. Large hernias are at risk of incarcerating bowel and should be closed early in the foal's life.

Hernia repair may be performed by open or closed reduction techniques. Closed reduction must be confined to smaller defects, and includes hernia clamps and local injection of an irritant material. Clamping the hernial sac crushes the tissue, disrupting the blood supply to the sac. This tissue subsequently necroses and sloughs, and the defect is closed by fibrous tissue. Disadvantages of this method include the potential for bowel entrapment, infection, adhesions, and cutaneous myiasis. The injection of an irritant material, such as iodine in oil, results in a local inflammatory response. This method has a high rate of failure. In addition, the inadvertent injection of the material into the abdominal cavity could result in adhesions and colic. Because of the risk associated with these methods of closed reduction, open reduction and herniorrhaphy are the recommended treatment of umbilical hernias.

REFERENCES

1. Mahaffey LW, Rossdale PD: Convulsive and allied syndromes in newborn foals. *Vet Rec* 69:1277, 1957.
2. Platt H: Septicemia in the foal. A review of 61 cases. *Br Vet J* 129:221, 1973.
3. Dimock WW, Edwards PR, Bruner DW: Infections observed in equine fetuses and foals. *Cornell Vet* 37:89, 1947.
4. Brewer BD: Equine neonatal intensive care: Success or failure? *Compend Contin Educ Pract Vet* 12:415–418, 1990.
5. Freeman L, Paradis MR. Evaluating the effectiveness of equine neonatal care. *Vet Med* 921, 1992.
6. McDowell KJ, Powell DG, Baker CB: Effect of book size and age of mare and stallion on foaling rates in Thoroughbred horses. *J Equine Vet Sci* 12:364, 1992.
7. Anderson NV, DeBowes RM, Nyrop KA, et al. Mononuclear phagocytes of transport stressed horses with viral respiratory disease. *Am J Vet Res* 46:2272, 1985.
8. Rossdale PD: Clinical studies on the newborn thoroughbred foal. I. Perinatal behavior. *Br Vet J* 123:470, 1967a.
9. Adams-Brendemuehl CS, Pipers FS: Antepartum evaluations of the equine fetus. *J Reprod Fertil Suppl* 35:565, 1987.
10. Reef VB, Worth LT, Vaala WE: Transabdominal fetal monitoring: The development of a biophysiologic profile for the equine fetus. *Proc Am Coll Vet Intern Med* 11:701, 1993.
11. Buss DD, Asbury AC, Chevalier L: Limitations in equine fetal electrocardiogrphy. *J Am Vet Med Assoc* 177:174, 1980.
12. Colles CM, Parkes RD, May CJ: Foetal electrocardiography in the mare. *Equine Vet J* 10:32, 1978.
13. Williams MA, Schmidt AR, Carleton CL, et al. Amniotic

fluid analysis for ante-partum foetal assessment in the horse. *Equine Vet J* 24:236, 1992.

14. Paradis MR: Lecithin/sphingomyelin ratios and phosphatidylglycerol in term and premature equine amniotic fluid (abstract). *Annu Vet Med Forum* 5:789, 1987.

15. Schmidt AR, Williams MA, Carleton CL, et al. Evaluation of transabdominal ultrasound guided amniocentesis in the late gestational mare. *Equine Vet J* 23:261, 1991.

16. Peaker M, Rossdale PD, Forsyth IA, et al. Changes in mammary development and the composition of secretions during late pregnancy in the mare. *J Reprod Fertil Suppl* 27:555, 1979.

17. Stewart JH, Rose RJ, Young IH, et al. The distribution of ventilation-perfusion ratios in the lungs of a dysmature foal. *Equine Vet J* 22:442, 1990.

18. MacDougall DF: Immunoglobulin metabolism in the neonatal foal. *J Reprod Fertil Suppl* 23:739, 1975.

19. McGuire TC, Crawford TB: Passive immunity in the foal: Measurement of immunoglobulin classes and specific antibody. *Am J Vet Res* 34:1299, 1973.

20. LeBlanc MM, McLaurin BI, Boswell R: Relationships among serum immunoglobulin concentration in foals, colostral specific gravity, and colostral immunoglobulin concentration. *J Am Vet Med Assoc* 189:57, 1986.

21. Kohn CW, Knight D, Hueston W, et al. Colostral and serum IgG, IgA, and IgM concentrations in Standardbred mares and their foals at parturition. *J Am Vet Med Res* 195:64, 1989.

22. Pearson RC, Hallowell AL, Bayly WM, et al. Times of appearance and disappearance of colostral IgG in the mare. *Am J Vet Res* 45:186, 1984.

23. Morris DD, Meirs DA, Merryman GS: Passive transfer failure in horses: Incidence and causative factors on a breeding farm. *J Am Vet Med Assoc* 46:2294, 1985.

24. Rumbaugh GE, Ardans AA, Ginno D, et al. Measurement of neonatal equine immunoglobulins for assessment of colostral immunoglobulin transfer: Comparison of single radial immunodiffusion with zinc sulfate turbidity test, serum electrophoresis, refractometry for total serum protein, and the sodium sulfite precipitation test. *J Am Vet Med Assoc* 172:321, 1978.

25. LeBlanc MM, Hurtgen JP, Lyle S: A modified zinc sulfate turbidity test for the detection of immune status in newly born foals. *J Equine Vet Sci* 10:36, 1990.

26. Bertone JJ, Jones RL, Curtis CR: Evaluation of a test kit for determination of serum immunoglobulin G concentration in foals. *J Vet Intern Med* 2:181, 1988.

27. Perryman LE, McGuire TC: Evaluation for immune system failures in horses and ponies. *J Am Vet Med Assoc* 176:1374, 1980.

28. Baldwin JL, Cooper WL, Vanderwall DK, et al. Prevalence (treatment days) and severity of illness in hypogammaglobulinemic and normogammaglobulinemic foals. *J Am Vet Med Assoc* 198:423, 1991.

29. Waring GH: Onset of normal behavioral patterns in the newborn foal. *Equine Pract* 4:587, 1982.

30. Adams R, Mayhew IG: Neurological examination of newborn foals. *Equine Vet J* 16:306, 1984.

31. Rossdale PD: Blood gas tension and pH values in the normal Thoroughbred foals at birth and in the following 42 hours. *Biol Neonate* 13:18, 1968.

32. Green SL: A problem-oriented approach to the physical examination of neonatal foals. *Vet Med* 66, 1992.

33. Rossdale PD: Measurements on pulmonary ventilation in normal newborn Thoroughbred foals in the first three days of life. *Br Vet J* 125:157, 1969.

34. Koterba AM, Kosch PC: Respiratory mechanics and breathing pattern in the neonatal foal. *J Reprod Fertil Suppl* 35:575, 1987.

35. Gillespie JR: Post-natal lung growth and function in the foal. *J Reprod Fertil Suppl* 23:667, 1975.

36. Baggot JD, Short CR: Drug disposition in the neonatal animal with particular reference to the foal. *Equine Vet J* 16:364, 1984.

37. Roberts MC, Hill FWG, Kidder DW: The development and distribution of small intestinal disaccharidases in the horse. *Res Vet Sci* 17:42, 1974.

38. Ullrey DE, Struthers RD, Hendricks DG: Composition of mare's milk. *J Anim Sci* 25:271, 1966.

39. Campbell ML, Ackerman N, Peyton LC: Radiographic gastrointestinal anatomy of the foal. *Vet Radiol* 25:194, 1984.

40. Adams R, Poulos P: A skeletal ossification index for neonatal foals. *Vet Radiol* 29:217, 1988.

41. Wagner PC, Watrous BJ. Equine pediatric orthopedis: Part 3—tendon laxity and rupture. *Equine Pract* 12:19, 1990.

42. Clemmons RM, Dorsey-Lee MR, Gorman NT, et al: Haemostatic mechanisms of the newborn foal: Reduced platelet responsiveness. *Equine Vet J* 16:353, 1984.

43. Ekman L, Persson SGB, Ullberg L: The levels of some blood constituents in Standardbred horses during their first year of life. In *Proceedings of the First International Symposium on Equine Hematology of the American* Association of Equine Practitioners, 1975, pp 289.

44. Sato T, Katsuichi O, Kubo M: Hematological and biochemical values of Thoroughbred foals in the first six months of life. *Cornell Vet* 69:3, 1979.

45. Bauer JE, Asquith RL, Kivipelto J: Serum biochemical indicators of liver function in neonatal foals. *Am J Vet Res* 50:2037, 1989.

46. Harvey JS, Asquith RL, Sussman WA, et al: Serum ferritin, serum iron and erythrocyte values in foals. *Am J Vet Res* 48:1348, 1987.

47. Altmann DH, Harvey JW, Asquith RL, et al: Hematologic development in foals receiving intra-venous iron supplementation. *J Equine Vet Sci* 11:103, 1991.

48. Jeffcott LB, Rossdale PD, Freestone J, et al: An assessment of wastage in Thoroughbred racing from conception to 4 years of age. *Equine Vet J* 14:185, 1982.

49. Stewart JH, Rose RJ, Barko AM: Respiratory studies in foals from birth to seven days old. *Equine Vet J* 16:323, 1984.

50. Madigan JE, Thomas WP, Backus KQ, et al: Mixed venous blood gases in recumbent and upright positions in foals from birth to 14 days of age. *Equine Vet J* 24:399, 1992.

51. Baker SM, Drummond WH, Lane TJ, et al: Follow-up evaluation of horses after neonatal intensive care unit. *J Am Vet Med Assoc* 189:1454, 1986.

52. Dwyer RM, Powell D, Lyons ET, et al: The aetiology of infectious diarrhea in Thoroughbred foals in central Kentucky. *Equine Vet J* 5(Suppl):59, 1988.

53. Brewer BD, Koterba AM: Development of a scoring system for the early diagnosis of equine neonatal sepsis. *Equine Vet J* 20:18, 1988.

54. Geor RJ, Papich MG: Medical therapy for gastrointestinal ulceration in foals. *Compendium Continuing Educ Pract Vet* 12:403, 1990.

55. Rossdale PD: Some parameters of respiratory function in normal and abnormal newborn foals with special reference to levels of PaO_2 during air and O_2 inhalation. *Res Vet Sci* 11:270, 1970.

56. Rose RJ, Rossdale PD, Leadon DP: Blood gas and acid base status in spontaneously delivered, term and induced, premature foals. *J Reprod Fertil Suppl* 32:521, 1982.

57. Hoffman AM, Viel L: A percutaneous transtracheal catheter system for improved oxygenation in foals with respiratory distress. *Equine Vet J* 24:239, 1992.

58. Freeman KP, Cline JM, Simmons R, et al: Recognition of

bronchopulmonary dysplasia in a newborn foal. *Equine Vet J* 21:292, 1989.

59. Rossdale PD: Clinical studies on the newborn thoroughbred foal. III. Thermal stability. *Br Vet J* 124:18, 1968b.

60. Hintz HF: Growth rate of horses. In *Proceedings of the 24th Annual Convention of the American Association of Equine Practitioners,* 1978, p 455.

61. Traub JL, Gallina AM, Grant BD, et al: Phenylbutazone toxicosis in a foal. *Am J Vet Res* 44:1410, 1983.

62. Baggot JD, Love DN, Love RJ, et al: Oral dosage of penicillin V in adult horses and foals. *Equine Vet J* 22:290, 1990.

63. Henry MM, Morris DD, Lakritz J, et al: Pharmacokinetics of cephradine in neonatal foals after single oral dosing. *Equine Vet J* 24:242, 1992.

64. Baggot JD, Love DN, Stewart J, et al: Bioavailability and disposition kinetics of amoxicillin in neonatal foals. *Equine Vet J* 20:125, 1988.

65. Wilcke JR, Crisman MV, Sams RA, et al: Pharmacokinetics of phenylbutazone in neonatal foals. *Am J Vet Res* 54:2064, 1993.

66. Davis LE, Westfall BA, Short CR: Biotransformation and pharmacokinetics of salicylate in newborn animals. *Am J Vet Res* 34:1105, 1973.

67. Adamson PJW, Wilson WD, Baggot JD, et al: Influence of age on disposition kinetics of chloramphenicol in equine neonates. *Am J Vet Res* 52:426, 1991.

68. Mysinger PW, Redding RW, Vaughan JT, et al: Electroencephalographic patterns of clnically normal sedated and tranquilized newborn foals and adult horses. *Am J Vet Res* 46:36, 1985.

69. Carter SW, Robertson SA, Steel CJ, et al: Cardiopulmonary effects of xylazine sedation in the foal. *Equine Vet J* 22:384, 1990.

70. Koterba AM, Drummond WH, Kosch PC: Intensive care of the newborn foal. *Vet Clin North Am Equine Pract* 3, 1985.

71. Beech J: Therapeutics in the neonate. *Proc Am Assoc Equine Pract* 28:359, 1982.

72. Oijala M, Katila T: Detomidine (Dormosedan) in foals: Sedative and analgesic effects. *Equine Vet J* 20:327, 1988.

73. Steffey EP, Willits N, Wong P, et al: Clinical investigation of halothane and isoflurane for induction and maintenance of foal anesthesia. *J Vet Pharmacol Ther* 14:300, 1991.

74. Webb AI: Nasal intubation in the foal. *J Am Vet Med Assoc* 185:48, 1984.

75. Adams R, Koterba AM, Brown MP, et al: Exploratory celiotomy for gastrointestinal disease in neonatal foals: A review of 20 cases. *Equine Vet J* 20:54, 1988.

76. Rossdale PD, Ousey JC, Silver M, et al: Studies on equine prematurity 6: Guidelines for asessment of foal maturity. *Equine Vet J* 16:300, 1984.

77. Morris DD: Bacterial infection of the newborn foal. Part I. Clinical presentation, laboratory findings and pathogenesis. *Compendium Continuing Educ Pract Vet* 6:S332, 1984.

78. Koterba AM, Brewer BD, Tarplee FA: Clinical and clinicopathological characteristics of the septicemia neonatal foal: A review of 38 cases. *Equine Vet J* 16:376, 1984.

79. Carter GK, Martens RJ: Septicemia in the neonatal foal. *Compendium Continuing Educ Pract Vet* 8:S256, 1986.

80. Cohen ND: Causes of and farm management factors associated with disease and death in foals. *J Am Vet Med Assoc* 195:1759, 1994.

81. Perryman LE, McGuire TC, Torbeck RL: Ontogeny of lymphocyte function in the equine fetus. *Am J Vet Res* 41:1197, 1980.

82. Coignoul FL, Bertram TA, Roth JS, et al: Functional and ultrastructural evaluation of neutrophils from foals and lactating and non-lactating mares. *Am J Vet Res* 45:898, 1984.

83. Brewer BD, Koterba AM: Bacterial isolates and susceptibility patterns in foals in a neonatal intensive care unit. *Compendium Continuing Educ Pract Vet* 12:1773, 1990.

84. Morris DD, Moore JN: Tumor necrosis factor activity in serum from neonatal foals with presumed septicemia. *J Am Vet Med Assoc* 199:1584, 1991.

85. Allen GK, Green EM, Robinson JA, et al: Serum necrosis factor alpha concentrations and clinical abnormalities in colostrum-fed and colostrum-deprived neonatal foals given endotoxin. *Am J Vet Res* 54:1404, 1993.

86. Robinson JA, Allen GK, Green EM, et al: Serum interleukin-6 concentrations in endotoxin-infused neonatal foals. *Am J Vet Res* 54:1411, 1993.

87. Wilson WD, Madigan JE: Comparison of bacteriologic culture of blood and necropsy specimens for determining the cause of foal septicemia. *J Am Vet Med Assoc* 195:1759, 1989.

88. Morris DD: Bacterial infection of the newborn foal. Part II. Diagnosis, treatment, and prevention. *Compendium Continuing Educ Pract Vet* 6:S436, 1984.

89. Swerczek TW: Toxicoinfectious botulism in foals and adult horses. *J Am Vet Med Assoc* 176:217, 1980.

90. Moore RM, Kohn CW: Nutritional muscular dystrophy in foals. *Compendium Continuing Educ Pract Vet* 13:476, 1991.

91. Kortz GD, Madigan JE, Lakritz J, et al: Cerebral oedema and cerebellar herniation in four equine neonates. *Equine Vet J* 24:63, 1992.

92. Rossdale PD: Modern concepts of neonatal disease in foals. *Equine Vet J* 4:117, 1972.

93. Vaala WE: Peripartum asphyxia. *Vet Clin North Am Equine Pract* 10:187, 1994.

94. Rossdale PD, Leadon D: Equine neonatal disease: A review. *J Reprod Fertil Suppl* 23:658, 1975.

95. Divers TJ, Watner A, Vaala WE, et al: Toxic hepatic failure in newborn foals. *J Am Vet Med Assoc* 183:1407, 1983.

96. Turk MAM, Gallina AM, Perryman LE: *Bacillus piliformis* infection (Tyzzer's disease) in foals in northwestern United States: A retrospective study of 21 cases. *J Am Vet Med Assoc* 178:279, 1981.

97. Swerczek TW, Crowe MW, Prickett ME, et al: Focal bacterial hepatitis in foals: Preliminary report. *Mod Vet Pract* 54:66, 1973.

98. Buananno AM, Carlson GP, Kantrowitz B: Clinical and diagnostic features of portosystemic shunt in a foal. *J Am Vet Med Assoc* 192:387, 1988.

99. Seahorn TL, Fuentealba IC, Illanes OG, et al: Congenital encephalomyelopathy in a Quarter Horse. *Equine Vet J* 23:394, 1991.

100. Cottril CM, Cudd TA: Foal neonatal intensive care: Experience during four years of private veterinary practice. *Clin Res* 36:70A, 1988.

101. Hinchcliff KW, Adams WM: Critical pulmonary stenosis in a newborn foal. *Equine Vet J* 23:318, 1991.

102. Report of foal pneumonia panel. *AAEP Newslett* 2:76, 1978.

103. Yager JA, Foster SF, Zink MC, et al: In vitro bactericidal efficacy of equine polymorphonuclear leukocytes against *Corynebacterium equi. Am J Vet Res* 47:438, 1986.

104. Martens JG, Martens RJ, Renshaw HW: *Rhodococcus (Corynebacterium) equi* bactericidal capacity of neutrophils from neonatal and adult horses. *Am J Vet Res* 49:295, 1988.

105. Coggins L, Kemen MJ: Viral respiratory infections of horses: Some viruses affecting the horse. *J Am Vet Med Assoc* 166:80, 1975.

106. Chambers TM, Shortridge KF, Li PH, et al: Rapid diagnosis of equine influenza by the Directigen FLU-A enzyme immunoassay. *Vet Rec* 135:275, 1994.

107. Bryans JT, Swerczek TW, Darlington RW, et al: Neonatal foal disease with perinatal infection by equine herpesvirus 1. *J Equine Med Surg* 1:20, 1977.

108. McChesney AE, England JJ: Adenoviral infection in foals. *J Am Vet Med Assoc* 166:83, 1975.

109. McChesney AE, England JJ, Adcock JL, et al: Adenovirus infection in suckling Arabian foals. *Pathol Vet* 7:547, 1970.

110. Vaala WE, Hamir AN, Dubov EJ, et al: Fatal, congenitally acquired infection with equine arteritis virus in a neonatal thoroughbred. *Equine Vet J* 24:155, 1992.

111. Golnik W, Michalak T: Choroby zahazna. I. Iniwzyjne. *Med Weter* 35:605, 1979.

112. Golnik W, Michalska Z, Michalak T: Natural equine viral arteritis in foals. *Schweiz Arch Tierheilkd* 123:523, 1981.

113. Doll ER, Knappenberger RE, Bryans JT: An outbreak of abortion caused by the equine arteritis virus. *Cornell Vet* 47:69, 1957b.

114. Behrens E, Parraga ME, Nassif A, et al: Reference values of peritoneal fluid from healthy foals. *J Equine Vet Sci* 10:348, 1990.

115. Tulleners EP: Complications of abdominocentesis in the horse. *J Am Vet Med Assoc* 182:232, 1983.

116. Bernard WV, Reef VB, Reimer JM, et al: Ultrasonographic diagnosis of small intestinal intussusception in three foals. *J Am Vet Med Assoc* 194:395, 1989.

117. Reef VB: The use of diagnostic ultrasound in the horse. *Ultrasound Q* 9:1, 1991.

118. Fischer AT, Kerr LV, O'Brien TR: Radiographic diagnosis of gastrointestinal disorders in the foal. *Vet Radiol* 28:42, 1987.

119. Ross MW, Hanson RR: Large intestine. In Auer JA, ed. *Equine Surgery*. Philadelphia, WB Saunders, 1992, p 402.

120. Lundin CL, Sullins KE, White NA, et al: Induction of peritoneal adhesions with small intestinal ischaemia and distention in the foal. *Equine Vet J* 21:451, 1989.

121. Rebhun WC, Dill SG, Power HT: Gastric ulcers in foals. *J Am Vet Med Assoc* 180:404, 1982.

122. Becht JL, Byars TD: Gastroduodenal ulcers in foals. *Equine Vet J* 18:307, 1986.

123. Murray MJ: Endoscopic appearance of gastric lesions in foals: 94 cases (1987–1988). *J Am Vet Med Assoc* 195:1135, 1989.

124. Wilson JH: Gastric and duodenal ulcers in foals. A retrospective study. In *Proceedings of the Second Symposium on Equine Colic Research*. 1986, p 149.

125. Murray MJ: Regional gastric pH measurement in horses and foals. *Equine Vet J* 7(Suppl):73, 1988.

126. Furr MO, Murray MJ, Ferguson DC: The effects of stress on gastric ulceration, T_3, T_4, reverse T_3 and cortisol in neonatal foals. *Equine Vet J* 24:37, 1992.

127. Traub-Dargatz J, Bayly W, Riggs M, et al: Exsanguination due to gastric ulceration in a foal. *J Am Vet Med Assoc* 186:280, 1985.

128. Probst CW, Schneider RK, Hubbell JA, et al: Surgical repair of a perforating gastric ulcer in a foal. *Vet Surg* 12:93, 1983.

129. Brooks WS: Sucralfate: Non-ulcer uses. *Am J Gastroenterol* 80:206, 1985.

130. Doran R, Allen D, Orsini JA: Small Intestine. In Auer JA, ed: *Equine Surgery*. Philadelphia, WB Saunders, 1992, p 365.

131. Crow MW, Swerczek TW: Equine congenital defects. *Am J Vet Res* 46:353, 1985.

132. Cho DY, Taylor HW: Blind-end atresia coli in two foals. *Cornell Vet* 76:11, 1986.

133. Estes R, Lyall W: Congenital atresia of the colon: A review and report of four cases in the horse. *J Equine Med Surg* 3:495, 1979.

134. Hultgren BD: Ileocolonic aganglionosis in white progeny of overo spotted horses. *J Am Vet Med Assoc* 180:289, 1982.

135. Browning GF, Chalmers RM, Snodgrass DR, et al: The prevalence of enteric pathogens in diarrhoeic Thoroughbred foals in Britain and Ireland. *Equine Vet J* 23:405, 1991.

136. Johnston RH, Kamstra LD, Kohler PH: Mares' milk composition as related to "foal heat" scours. *J An Sci* 31:549, 1970.

137. Lyons ET, Drudge JH, Tolliver SC, et al: Anthelmintic resistence in equids. In *Resistance of Parasites to Antiparasitic Drugs: Round Table Conference,* ICOPA VII, Paris, 1990, p 67.

138. Snodgrass DR, Browning GF: Characterization of equine rotavirus. In *Equine Infectious Diseases VI: Proceedings of the Sixth International Conference*. R & W, 1991, p 219.

139. Kanitz CL: Identification of an equine rotavirus as a cause of neonatal foal diarrhea. *Proc Am Assoc Equine Pract* 22:155, 1976.

140. Conner ME, Darlington RW: Rotavirus infection of foals. *Am J Vet Res* 41:1699, 1980.

141. Studdert MJ, Mason RW, Patten BE: Rotavirus diarrhea of foals. *Aust Vet J* 54:363, 1978.

142. Strickland KL, Lenihan P, O'Connor MG, et al: Diarrhea in foals associated with rotavirus. *Vet Rec* 111:421, 1982.

143. Imagawa H, Wada R, Hirasawa K, et al: Isolation of equine rotavirus in cell cultures from foals with diarrhea. *Jpn J Vet Sci* 46:1, 1984a.

144. Tzipori S: The relative importance of enteric pathogens affecting neonates of domestic animals. *Adv Vet Sci Comp Med* 29:103, 1985.

145. Bass EP, Sharpee RL: Coronavirus and gastroenteritis in foals. *Lancet* 2:822, 1975.

146. Studdert MJ, Blackney MH: Isolation of an adenovirus antigenically distinct from equine adenovirus type I from diarrheic foal feces. *Am J Vet Res* 43:543, 1982.

147. Baker JC, Ames TR: Total parenteral nutritional therapy of a foal with diarrhoea from which parvovirus-like particles were identified. *Equine Vet J* 19:342, 1987.

148. Dickie CW, Klinkerman DL, Petrie RJ: Enterotoxemia in two foals. *J Am Vet Med Assoc* 173:306, 1978.

149. Jones RL, Adney WS, Alexander AF, et al: Hemorrhagic necrotizing enterocolitis associated with *Clostridium difficile* infection in four foals. *J Am Vet Med Assoc* 193:76, 1988.

150. Davies ME: Some studies on equine strains of *Escherichia coli*. *Equine Vet J* 10:115, 1978.

151. Batt RM, Embaye H, Hunt J, et al: Ultrastructural damage to equine intestinal epithelium induced by enteropathogenic *Escherichia coli*. *Equine Vet J* 21:373, 1989.

152. Myers LL, Shoop DS, Byars TD: Diarrhea associated with enterotoxigenic *Bacteroides fragilis* in foals. *Am J Vet Res* 48:1565, 1987.

153. Myers LL, Firehammer BD, Shoop DS, et al: *Bacteroides fragilis*: A possible cause of acute diarrheal disease in newborn lambs. *Infect Immun* 44:241, 1984.

154. Tzipori S, Hayes J, Sims L, et al: *Streptococcus durans*: An unexpected enteropathogen of foals. *J Infect Dis* 150:589, 1984.

155. Lyons ET, Drudge JH, Tolliver SC, et al: The role of intestinal nematodes in foal diarrhea. *Vet Med* 86:320, 1991.

156. Lyons ET, Drudge JH, Tolliver SC: On the life cycle of *Strongyloides westeri* infections in the equine. *J Parasitol* 59:780, 1973.

157. Poonacha KB, Tuttle PA: Intestinal cryptosporidiosis in two Thoroughbred foals. *Equine Pract* 11:6, 1989.

158. Coleman SV, Klei TR, French DD, et al: Prevalence of *Cryptosporidium* sp in equids in Louisiana. *Am J Vet Res* 50:575, 1989.

159. Lyons ET, Granstrom DE, Drudge JH, et al: The role of intestinal protozoa in foal diarrhea. *Vet Med* 86:193, 1991a.

160. Snyder SP, England JJ, et al: Cryptosporidiosis in immunodeficient Arabian foals. *Vet Pathol* 15:12, 1978.

161. Barker IK, Remmler O: The endogenous development of *Eimeria leukarti* in ponies. *J Parasitol* 58:112, 1972.

162. McQueary CA, et al: Observations on the life cycle and prevalence of *Eimeria leukarti* in horses in Montana. *Am J Vet Res* 38:1673, 1977.

163. Lyons ET, Drudge JH, Tolliver SC: Natural infection with *Eimeria leukarti:* Prevalence of oocysts in feces of horse foals on several farms in Kentucky during 1986. *Am J Vet Res* 49:96, 1988.

164. Bemrick WJ: *Giardia* in North America. *Vet Med Small Anim Clin* 63:163, 1968.

165. Kirkpatrick CE, Skand DL: Giardiasis in a horse. *J Am Vet Med Assoc* 197:163, 1985.

166. Robertson JT, Spurlock GH, Bramlage LR, et al: Repair of a ureteral defect in a foal. *J Am Vet Med Assoc* 183:799, 1983.

167. Stickle RL, Wilcock BP, Huseman JL: Multiple ureteral defects in a Belgian foal. *Vet Med Small Anim Clin* 70:819, 1975.

168. Vacek JR, MacHarg MA, Phillips TN, et al: Struvite urethral calculus in a three-month old Thoroughbred colt. *Cornell Vet* 82:275, 1992.

169. Richardson DW: Urogenital problems in the neonatal foal. *Vet Clin North Am Equine Pract* 1:179, 1985.

170. Rooney JR: Rupture of the urinary bladder in the foal. *Vet Pathol* 8:445, 1971.

171. Divers TJ, Byars TD, Spirito M: Correction of bilateral ureteral defects in a foal. *J Am Vet Med Assoc* 192:384, 1988.

172. Reef VB, Collatos CA, Spencer PA, et al: Clinical, ultrasonographic and surgical findings in foals with umbilical remnant infections. *J Am Vet Med Assoc* 195:69, 1989.

173. Reef VB, Collatos CA: Ultrasonography of umbilical structures in clinically normal foals. *Am J Vet Res* 49:2143, 1988.

18.2

Pneumonia and Other Disorders Associated with *Rhodococcus equi*

Joseph J. Bertone, DVM, MS, Dip ACVIM

Rhodococcus equi–associated bronchopneumonia of young foals was originally identified in 1923.[1, 2] Relative to other causes, pneumonia associated with this organism has distinct clinical features, including its insidious nature. *Rhodococcus equi (R. equi)* pneumonia can progress to severe and extensive lung involvement prior to the development of clear clinical signs. Careful observation of foals coupled with management practices that reduce the risk of disease can reduce mortality.

TAXONOMIC CLASSIFICATION

Magnusson[1] and Miessner and Wetzel[2] were the first to report on disease associated with this organism. They proposed that it be placed in the genus *Corynebacterium* and given the species name *equi*. *Corynebacterium equi* was the recognized and accepted name for many years, although it was more structurally related to the mycobacteria than to other coryneform organisms.[3, 4] Evidence in support of *C. equi* reclassification into the genus *Rhodococcus,* a nocardioform actinomycete, was presented in the 1970s and included

structural, biochemical, and habitat similarities between *C. equi* and *Rhodococcus coprophilus*.[5, 6] The genus *Rhodococcus* is characterized by a rod-to-coccus morphologic change that occurs during the growth cycle. Other more detailed biochemical similarities exist as well.[7] In 1980, *R. equi* was established as a new species and added to the approved list of bacterial names, but the organism continued to be referenced as *C. equi*.[8] Studies in the early 1980s, using DNA reassociation and antigen analysis by rocket immunoelectrophoresis, also supported the reclassification of *C. equi* to *R. equi*.[9, 10]

MICROBIOLOGICAL CHARACTERISTICS

Staining Characteristics, Microscopic and Colony Morphology

On microscopy, *R. equi* is a gram-positive, pleomorphic bacillus, generally less than 1 μm in diameter and 2 μm in length. The organism is often clumped with formation of L and V shapes that resemble Chinese characters.[11] They have a polysaccharide capsule and a peptidoglycan cell wall composed of sugars and amino acids, similar to other gram-positive bacteria.[12, 13] The cell wall of *R. equi* bears substantial structural similarities, the presence of mycolic acid being of particular importance, to the cell walls of the genera *Mycobacterium* and *Nocardia*. These similarities give it acid-fast staining characteristics under some growth environments.[5] Mycolic acid contributes to the development of granulomas in infections with all three genera.

Rhodococcus equi commonly forms smooth, shiny, mucoid, irregular-to-round colonies.[12] The size and shape of *R. equi* colonies varies with the culture environment and age.[14] Colonies less than 48 hours old range from 1 to 3 mm in diameter and have a white or gray cast. Decreased synthesis of capsular material in old, compared with young, colonies is associated with a change in colony morphology from smooth to rough and from white to salmon-pink. Variations from this typical appearance include rough, dry colonies and the development of yellow, red, or brown pigment.[12, 15]

Rhodococcus equi is a nonmotile organism without flagella, but with surface pili evident on electron microscopy. The significance of these structures is unknown.[13] However, cell surface appendages in isolates of *R. equi* from human beings have been associated with virulence and bacterial and β-lactam resistance. Their exact role is unclear.[16]

Biochemical Tests and Metabolic Requirements

Rhodococcus equi is a relatively nonreactive organism in standard, microbiological, biochemical tests. It is gram-positive and catalase-positive, nonproteolytic, and does not oxidize or ferment any standard test carbohydrate or alcohol. These organisms tend to be negative for gelatin and coagulated serum liquefaction, negative for ammonia and indole production, negative for the oxidase reaction, and negative for oxidation or fermentation of sugars and alcohols. They are often positive to nitrate reduction, lipase, and phosphatase activity. *Rhodococcus equi* is CAMP-positive with *Staphylococcus aureus* and *Corynebacterium pseudotuberculosis*.[1, 12, 17]

Rhodococcus equi does not seem to have many metabolic requirements for survival and pathogenicity. The organism can be subcultured on simple agar media for at least 15 years and still retain its virulence.[14] *Rhodococcus equi* organisms can use a wide variety of carbon sources that include many short-chain fatty acids, pyruvate, and L- and D-lactate.[18, 19] *Rhodococcus equi* is classified as an obligate aerobe and grows well from 10° to 40 °C (50°–104 °F).[13, 18, 20]

Diffusible Substances

Rhodococcus equi elaborates a diffusible substance that enhances the hemolytic activity of several other bacterial species. This forms the basis of a serum hemolysin inhibition test and the aforementioned CAMP test. The substance is a phospholipase that hydrolyzes the phospholipids of mammalian erythrocyte membranes.[3, 20–22] Its significance in the pathogenesis of disease associated with this organism is unclear.

Serotypes

Rhodococcus equi has been classified into serotypes. It is doubtful that there is a correlation between serotype and pathogenicity.[23–25]

EPIZOOTIOLOGY

An understanding of the epizootiology of infection with *R. equi* is important in the effective control of the organism. Appropriate management based on manure removal, and resolution of dirt paddocks and other contributors to a dusty environment can prevent spread and subsequent infection.

Habitat and Source of Infection

Rhodococcus equi is widespread in herbivores and their environment. The organism has been isolated on every continent except Antarctica. The organism is frequently isolated from soil, where it is known to survive for considerable periods.[26–29] *Rhodococcus equi* is a saprophytic soil inhabitant whose optimal multiplication depends on environmental temperature, volatile fatty acids found in herbivore manure, and soil pH.[5, 12, 30–32] The highest numbers of *R. equi* are found in the surface soil on infected horse farms.[33] Growth temperature varies from a minimum of 10 °C (50 °F) to a maximum of 40 °C (104 °F). Optimal growth occurs between 30 °C (86 °F) and 37 °C (98.6 °F).[30, 31, 33]

Cultures of *R. equi* have been recovered from feces of horses, cattle, goats, deer, pigs, sheep, and other domestic animals.[21, 32, 34] Feces from wild birds are often positive on culture, but the organism is rarely found in the manure of chickens.[34] The organism rarely appears in feces from dogs, cats, and humans.[34, 35] The organism can easily be isolated from soil with and without a history of fecal contamination.[20, 36, 37] There can be a 10,000-fold increase in *R. equi* numbers in herbivore manure under dry warm conditions.[11, 30]

Rhodococcus equi is an obligate aerobe. Therefore, it is unlikely that it multiplies in the relatively anaerobic environment of the large bowel of horses and other herbivores.[11, 32, 38]

There is no evidence that there is intestinal multiplication of organisms in mature horses. It is most likely that their presence in adult horse feces results from passive accumulation from the environment. *Rhodococcus equi* can multiply in the intestinal tracts of foals up to 12 weeks of age.[39] Multiplication in foals is probably facilitated by coprophagy. This behavior seems to be one mechanism by which virulent organisms concentrate on farms where foals are raised.[20]

Exposure

The major route of exposure appears to be dust aerosols. Most horses are naturally challenged by *R. equi* and develop immunologic evidence of exposure, horses on endemically affected farms having the most widespread and highest antibody concentrations.[40] The widespread antibody titers found in horses would intuitively lead one to assume that the disease is widely and diffusely disseminated. However, *R. equi* infection varies from endemic to sporadic and in many cases does not manifest as bronchopneumonia. The annual variation in new cases of *R. equi* pneumonia can be explained, in large part, by differences in environmental factors. The organism is readily isolated from the air on infected farms on dry windy days.[31, 41] The infection is most common in climates with very hot seasons. Variation in *R. equi* strain pathogenicity may contribute to the sporadic-to-endemic nature of the disease.[25] The process is amplified with high-risk management practices such as concentrated facilities, dusty paddocks, incomplete manure removal, and the presence of larger numbers of virulent strains of *R. equi*, as seen on endemically affected farms.[42, 43]

Environmental Resistance

Rhodococcus equi is considerably resistant to environmental exposure even though it does not form spores. Pasture soil free of *R. equi* can be contaminated experimentally and subsequently yield isolates for 12 months.[29] The organism is resistant to desiccation, sunlight exposure, and hypochlorous acid, is relatively resistant to acids and bases in general, and is susceptible to phenol and merbromin.[5, 14, 20] Isolation of *R. equi* from contaminated sources is aided by the use of selective media containing nalidixic acid and novobiocin-actidione (cycloheximide)-potassium tellurite.[12, 36, 41, 44] These agents inhibit the growth of contaminating organisms in laboratory culture.

Infection in Other Species

There are numerous reports of isolation of *R. equi* from nonequine species, including pigs,[45, 46] buffalo,[47] goats,[48–51] sheep,[52] deer,[34] cats,[53] dogs,[54] koala bears,[55] seals,[56] marmosets,[57] guinea pigs,[58] alligators, and crocodiles.[59] A comprehensive table is presented in a recent review article.[7] The disease was a fairly common problem in pigs, but the number of reports have declined in association with decreased numbers of pasture-reared animals.

Zoonosis

The opportunistic nature of the organism is evident in human disease caused by *R. equi*. Most cases of *R. equi* infection in humans occur during or immediately after periods of immunosuppression induced by chemotherapy,[60] or are identified in patients with acquired immunodeficiency syndrome (AIDS).[60–65] The source of infection in these patients is unclear. Only a small fraction of infected human patients have had an association with herbivorous animals, or their manure.[7, 60] Under normal conditions the organism is not pathogenic for immunocompetent humans, but exceptions have been reported.[66–68]

PATHOGENESIS

Susceptibility of foals to *R. equi* relates to a combination of factors that includes extensive respiratory challenge, declining maternally derived antibody, and absence of fully competent cellular immune mechanisms. Experimental induction of disease in foals has been attempted with some reports of success by intratracheal and nasal inoculation.[12, 20, 27, 69, 70] Experimentally induced clinical disease is indistinguishable from the spontaneous condition.[12, 20, 69, 71–73] Massive exposure by oral inoculation of live *R. equi* organisms can induce intestinal and pulmonary lesions.[70] In one study, subcutaneous inoculation of *R. equi* induced local abscesses, but no pulmonary lesions.[69] Other postulated routes of infection have been discussed. It has been proposed that ingested contaminated helminth larvae migrate to the lung and infect the pulmonary parenchyma, or they migrate into the bowel wall and the organism spreads to the lung via the bloodstream.[26, 28] Other postulated routes include in utero infection,[28, 29] and hematogenous spread of the organism from an infected umbilicus soon after birth.[74]

Opportunism

Rhodococcus equi is an opportunistic organism with low pathogenicity evident in the fact that the organism is relatively ubiquitous in the environment, and yet *R. equi* pneumonia occurs sporadically in foals and is rare in adult horses.[7, 12, 20, 42, 72, 75–77] The opportunistic nature of the organism is evident in human disease where the organism is isolated from immunosuppressed persons, as mentioned above.[60–65] Immunosuppression has been proposed as a necessary condition in the development of natural infection with this organism.[32, 60, 72, 75, 76, 78, 79] The majority of equine cases involve young foals from 2 to 6 months of age. This is a time when maternal antibody concentration begins to wane.[80, 81] In addition, foals with combined immunodeficiency seem to be at high risk for *R. equi* pneumonia in conjunction with *Pneumocystis carinii*.[26, 82]

Intracellular Survival

The ability of *R. equi* to multiply in and destroy alveolar macrophages is basic to its pathogenicity. Histologically, lesions of *R. equi* pneumonia are characterized by numerous polymorphonuclear leukocytes and macrophages, many of which contain ingested bacteria.[72, 76] *Rhodococcus equi* survives within macrophages with associated granulomatous inflammation. These lesions become suppurative with subsequent macrophage destruction.[72] Organisms appear to evade

killing in macrophages by preventing phagosome-lysosome fusion and causing nonspecific degranulation of lysosomes.[29, 73, 76, 83–86] In vitro studies revealed that equine alveolar macrophages and neutrophils ingested *R. equi*, but the organism maintained viability hours later.[78, 86] This reaction seems to be related to a surface component of *R. equi* that decreases bactericidal activity by blockade of lysosomal degranulation.[78] Failure of lysosome-phagosome fusion has been associated with defective intracellular killing of a number of organisms.

Immune Responses

Sensitized lymphocytes enhance macrophage and neutrophil ingestion and killing of *R. equi* by producing specific opsonizing antibody for the organism.[84, 87, 88] These reactions demonstrate the importance of both cellular and humoral immune mechanisms in protection against infection. Some foals require the presence of antibody for phagocytic ingestion which may predispose these foals to *R. equi* infection when antibody is not present.[88]

Anti-*R. equi* antibody has been identified, with gel diffusion, passive hemagglutination, and enzyme-linked immunosorbent assay (ELISA) in serum from naturally infected and experimentally inoculated horses. The antibody appears to be directed primarily at surface and capsular antigens of the organism.[23, 81, 89] The intestinal tract is probably the major source of antigenic stimulation.[31, 90–92] The majority of equine cases occur in foals from 2 to 6 months of age. This is a time when maternal antibody concentration begins to wane, decreasing the antibody enhancement of uptake and killing of organisms by macrophages and neutrophils.[80, 81] Furthermore, the severity of *R. equi* pneumonia is related to the concentration of specific antibody in foals.[81] The success of immunoprophylaxis with specific immune plasma also demonstrates the importance of the humoral response.[93] However, concentrations of antibody detected by ELISA correlate poorly with opsonizing activity and chemiluminescence assays.[94] Part of the protective effect of immune plasma may result from nonspecific factors in plasma, including lymphokines and interferons.[93]

The importance of the cell-mediated immune response in resistance to *R. equi* appears evident.[23, 29, 73, 75, 76, 95] Lymphocyte blastogenesis studies detected *R. equi*–specific lymphocytes in horses.[27, 70, 96] Humoral responses to *R. equi* occur in conjunction with cell-mediated immunity as evidenced by mitotic responses of sensitized equine lymphocytes to specific *R. equi* capsular and cell wall antigens and delayed-type hypersensitivity skin reactions.[79, 89] On farms with epizootic *R. equi* pneumonia, cell-mediated immune responses are not uniformly aggressive. The results of lymphocyte blastogenesis assays do not correlate with clinical conditions. The majority of affected foals and adults are categorized as non-reactors. Data suggest that endogenous interferon-γ (IFN-γ) and tumor necrosis factor-alpha (TNF-α) are involved in the cell-mediated immunologic response to *R. equi*.[97] In a recent study, it was demonstrated that athymic nude mice are unable to clear *R. equi* and that CD4 + - and CD8 + -positive T cell subsets play a particularly important role in bacteria clearance.[98, 99]

Virulence Factors

Murine models have been developed to study the virulence of *R. equi*,[100] and have shown that clinical isolates from foals have a higher median lethal dose (LD$_{50}$) than most soil isolates.[41] Survival of mice intravenously infected is related to hepatic and splenic clearance of the organism and to phagocytosis and intracellular killing by macrophages.[101, 102] Based on data from experimental infections, clinical isolates are more pathogenic than environmental isolates and strains vary in virulence potential.[103–106] A 15- to 17-kDa protein, as defined by a monoclonal antibody and encoded by a large 80- to 90-kb plasmid, is found in virulent strains of organisms.[25, 103–107] Strains of *R. equi* with longer-chain mycolic acids are more lethal to mice and induce a more severe granulomatous reaction than strains with shorter-chain mycolic acids.[108] Other implicated virulence factors include capsular polysaccharide[109] and cholesterol oxidase and choline phosphohydrolase exoenzymes (*equi* factors).[110] Attachment of *R. equi* to both murine and equine macrophages is mediated by the surface receptor Mac-1 (complement receptor type 3).[111] A heat-stable surface component of *R. equi* inhibits the oxygen-dependent cytotoxic mechanisms of adult horse neutrophils against *Staphylococcus aureus*.[78] In addition, a water-soluble fraction obtained from *R. equi* blocks degranulation of mast cells.[112, 113] The importance of these substances in the manifestation of clinical disease has not been clearly defined.

Necropsy Findings

The characteristic gross necropsy lesion of foals infected with *R. equi* is a bilateral bronchopneumonia with severe coalescing abscess formation (Fig. 18–1). Generalized miliary abscesses are also common (Fig. 18–2), but irregular multifocal involvement of the ventral lung fields with abscesses ranging from a few millimeters to greater that 10 cm in diameter is more typical (see Fig. 18–1). Mucopurulent exudate often clogs the airways in affected regions. The pulmonary parenchyma around the abscesses usually is congested or consolidated. A bronchial and mediastinal lym-

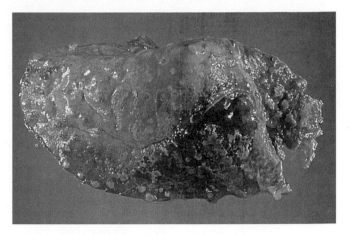

Figure 18–2. Miliary, pulmonary abscesses found at necropsy in the lung of a foal with *Rhodococcus equi* infection.

phadenopathy with abscesses also occurs. *Rhodococcus equi* can be cultured from the exudate and abscess fluid in pure or mixed culture. Pleural empyema can occur, but inflammation of the pleura is unusual even when there is extensive pulmonary involvement.[20, 42]

Pyogranulomatous reactions predominate on histologic evaluation of lungs infected with *R. equi*. Abscesses have a necrotic central core with a collar of degenerating neutrophils. The tissue surrounding the core is infiltrated with macrophages, occasional giant cells, and lymphocytes. Peripheral to the abscesses there is congestion, edema, alveolar infiltration by macrophages and neutrophils, acute suppurative bronchitis and peribronchitis, and bronchiolar fibrinopurulent material. Bacterial organisms within the affected structures may be gram-negative, but the predominant organisms will be gram-positive and pleomorphic. The organisms may have acid-fast staining qualities. *Rhodococcus equi* may be free within the alveolar lumen and in the cytoplasm of macrophages.[11, 12, 42, 114]

Gastrointestinal lesions are variable and may be located along the length of the intestinal tract (Fig. 18–3). Lesions include villous atrophy, mucosal necrosis, diphtheritic membranes, ulcerative enterocolitis, and mesenteric lymphadenitis and abscess formation. Histopathologic findings of gastrointestinal tract lesions are characterized by infiltration of phagocytic cells into the lamina propria, necrosis of the submucosa and villi, and mucosal ulceration. Peyer's patches seem to be especially at risk for lesion development. The lymph nodes that drain the affected areas of intestine contain numerous giant cells, large numbers of *R. equi*–laden macrophages, and necrotic debris. Of foals that are necropsied, almost half will show multifocal ulcerative colitis and typhlitis over the area of the Peyer's patches with granulomatous or suppurative inflammation of colonic or mesenteric lymph nodes, or both.[11, 12, 20, 42, 71, 114, 115] Peritonitis may occur and the organism can be isolated from peritoneal fluid in some cases. In unusual cases, only the intestine is involved.

An apparently immune-mediated synovitis or arthritis occurs. Septic physitis and other forms of osteomyelitis have been seen. Disease in mature horses is similar pathologically to that in foals, but occurs rarely. Lung abscesses in adults

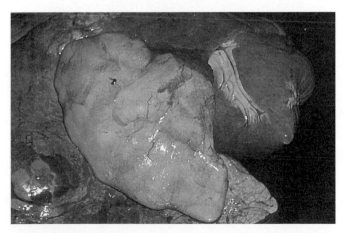

Figure 18–1. A large, loculated, singular, pulmonary abscess found at necropsy in the lung of a foal with *Rhodococcus equi* infection.

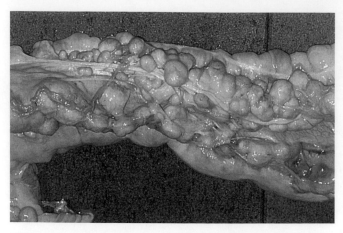

Figure 18–3. Extensive abscess formation in the colonic mesenteric lymph nodes found in a foal with *Rhodococcus equi* infection.

tend to be localized and rupture of these abscesses may result in pleuropneumonia in adult horses.[42]

CLINICAL SYNDROMES
Bronchopneumonia

Rhodococcus equi organisms most often induce a chronic bronchopneumonia in young foals. Foals are affected up to 6 months of age. The lesion development is often insidious with early signs that include depression, lethargy, and fever as high as 41 °C (106 °F). These signs can progress for weeks until the foal dies from asphyxiation or septicemia.[20, 42] The disease is sporadic in nature, except on farms where *R. equi* infection is endemic.[20, 75] Foals will continue to nurse, but often lose weight. If a cough is present, it may vary from a quiet, intermittent, deeply resonant, and moist cough (i.e., light cough into the feed and bedding), to a frequent, paroxysmal, unproductive hack (i.e., honk), accompanied by groaning and discomfort. On auscultation, moist, loud breath sounds with crackles and wheezes may be heard, but lungs may auscultate normally. A mucopurulent nasal discharge is common, but often does not occur.[42]

Foals may present in acute respiratory distress when the lung infection has been undetected and lung involvement is extensive. These foals can present with severe acute respiratory distress, tachypnea, nostril flaring, abdominal breathing, and cyanosis. The lungs are often severely affected.[20]

The development of lung disorders coupled with compensatory mechanisms is associated with a difficult early clinical diagnosis of *R. equi* bronchopneumonia. If respiratory disease is detected early, the degree of lung involvement can be minimal. During the subclinical period preceding signs of pneumonia, foals with *R. equi* may be detected by a combination of twice-daily temperature monitoring and weekly thoracic auscultation, with rebreathing, and evaluation of plasma fibrinogen concentration.[96] Despite this intensive monitoring program, some affected foals go undetected until fulminant pneumonia develops.

Intestinal Disease

The intestinal form of *R. equi* infection, which results in enteritis and abscess formation, is not as common as the pneumonic syndrome. Clinical signs associated with enteric disease due to *R. equi* are diarrhea, dehydration, and weight loss or poor growth, or all of these. The abdominal fluid may be increased in volume, and have increased protein and white blood cell concentration. Lesions in the intestine may occur alone, but are most often seen with pulmonary disease.[12, 20, 83, 114, 116] Foals with diarrhea associated with *R. equi* have a poor prognosis because of the massive granulomatous inflammation of the colonic mucosa and submucosa and mesenteric lymph nodes.[42]

Nonseptic Synovitis

Chronic, active, nonseptic synovitis in a foal should be a red flag for this condition. Foals are rarely lame and synovial fluids are often normal, or may have slightly elevated white blood cell or protein concentrations.[43]

Sporadic Abscesses

In rare instances, *R. equi* is associated with ulcerative lymphangitis, suppurative and nonsuppurative arthritis, nephritis, mastitis, abortion, osteomyelitis, hepatitis, nephritis, and retrobulbar abscess formation[12, 26, 29, 117-123] (Fig. 18–4). Disease in adult horses is rare, but is similar to disease in foals.[52, 115, 116, 124, 125]

DIAGNOSIS

Diagnosis of *R. equi* pneumonia in foals is usually based on positive culture, tracheal wash, Gram's stain, cytology, and

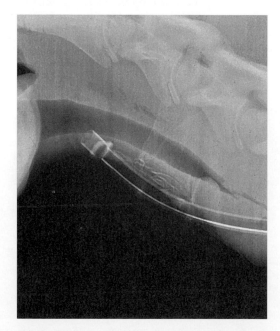

Figure 18–4. Radiograph of a foal with airway obstruction secondary to a cervical abscess associated with *Rhodococcus equi.*

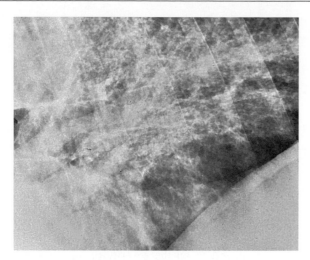

Figure 18–5. Typical thoracic radiograph of a foal with *Rhodococcus equi* infection.

the presence of clinical and radiographic findings consistent with this condition[20, 42, 126] (Fig. 18–5). Most other bacterial pneumonic conditions of foals require fairly similar therapy based on culture and cytology of transtracheal wash fluids (Fig. 18–6). Since *R. equi* infection often presents as a critical acute or chronic condition and treatment is fairly specific, rapid diagnosis and the initiation of treatment are essential. On farms with historical disease, this is simpler, especially when the odds of this bacterial association become higher. However, it represents a dilemma on farms with no history of *R. equi* infection where there is no reason to expect disease due to this organism. On endemic farms, the incidence of pneumonia due to *R. equi* is greater than that associated with other causes, and a presumptive diagnosis can be based on the results of clinical examination, tracheal wash cytology, and response to treatment with erythromycin and rifampin. Definitive diagnosis is still based on positive culture of the organism.

Clinical Signs

Many of the signs evident with *R. equi* pneumonia are seen with other pneumonic conditions in foals. Signs of depression, weight loss, abnormal thoracic percussion and auscultation, dyspnea, and fever can be seen. Increased neutrophil counts and fibrinogen levels can be evident, but these changes can be evident in foals with other causes of pneumonia and can be within normal limits in affected foals. Diarrhea may occur alone or with signs of respiratory disease.

Culture

Transtracheal wash cytology and culture are required for a positive diagnosis of this condition.[7, 20, 42, 126] Transtracheal wash fluid is the most desirable sample to evaluate, but care should be taken, since many of these foals are respiratory-compensated to their limit. Bronchoalveolar lavage is not recommended because of the stress to the foal and little data to suggest that this adds to diagnostic success in this condi-

tion. If a foal is severely distressed, other options are available. Percutaneous tracheal aspirate without lavage may be all that is necessary for culture and cytology. Large gram-positive pleomorphic (rod-to-coccus) organisms on tracheal wash cytology are highly suggestive of *R. equi* infection. The organism is often not seen in large numbers, so careful and complete examination of the sample slide is necessary. *Rhodococcus equi* can be isolated on aerobic culture. Nasal swabs may be positive for the bacterium, but, because of its widespread presence in the environment, recovery of the organism from this site should not be considered diagnostic.

Radiography and Ultrasonography

Lung radiographic changes progress from a prominent interstitial pattern, to dense patchy alveolar opacities (cotton balls), to lung consolidation and abscesses[20, 42, 126] (Fig. 18–3). Radiography may be used to assess the extent of lesions and response to treatment. Radiographically, the resolution of abscesses and consolidation can be followed.[127–129] Ultrasonography may be useful to detect abscesses adjacent to the thoracic wall.

Immunologic Tests

Immunologic tests that detect the cholesterol oxidase exoenzyme of *R. equi* include agar gel diffusion, synergistic hemolysis inhibition, and radial immunodiffusion. These tests seem to be useful in the later stages of disease.[40, 130–133] ELISA also seems to be useful, but antigens have not been defined.[24] Western blot analysis can be used to identify virulent isolates from horses and their environments.[25, 41, 134] Problems with serologic testing for this disease include (1) foals with exposure and no clinical disease may develop antibodies and be serologically positive, (2) passive transfer of antibody may result in false-positive seroreactivity, (3) foals with early infection are often not positive, and (4) standardized tests of proven sensitivity and specificity are not available commercially.[7, 42] Other immune disorders must be considered in this condition and a complete blood count and immunoglobulin testing may be warranted.

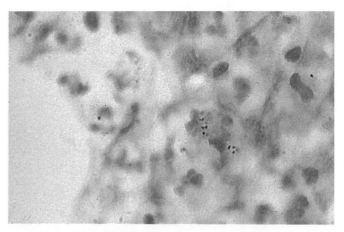

Figure 18–6. Transtracheal wash from a foal with *Rhodococcus equi* infection. The organisms are evident in the central portion of the photograph.

TREATMENT
Antibiotics

Early recognition of pneumonia with isolation and treatment of infected foals will reduce loss and prevent the spread of virulent organisms. In many cases, the insidious nature of *R. equi* pneumonia delays diagnosis and greatly complicates treatment.[7, 29, 42, 75, 126, 135] Standard therapy involves the use of a combination of erythromycin and rifampin. Rarely have other antibiotics been as useful in the therapy of this condition. This is most likely because in vitro sensitivity is often not a good indicator of in vivo success, especially with fibrous encapsulated abscess formation and when dealing with an intracellular organism. Antibiotics that the organism is sensitive to and that are lipophilic seem to be a necessary combination for positive clinical results. Erythromycin and rifampin fill those requirements. The combination has additive or synergistic activity,[136] excellent penetration of alveolar macrophages (unlike aminoglycosides and β-lactam drugs), and can be administered orally for prolonged periods. Use of the combination reduces the likelihood of development of resistance to either drug. Penicillin-gentamicin is synergistic against the organism in vitro,[137] but clinical use of these drugs was associated with high mortality of diseased foals.[126, 138] If disease is seen very early in the progression, trimethoprim-sulfamethoxazole may be used, but poor abscess penetration and resistance (in vitro) would make this a poor second choice.[137, 139] There is such a large range of sensitivity seen with chloramphenicol (minimal inhibitory concentration [MIC] from 1.6 to 50 μg/mL) that this too is a poor second choice.[7]

Dosages for the erythromycin-rifampin combination range from 5 to 10 mg/kg orally one to two times daily for rifampin,[43, 134, 140–144] and between 10 and 37.5 mg/kg orally two to four times daily for erythromycin.[43, 136, 141, 144–146] Questions have been raised regarding the salt or ester of erythromycin that may be used. In one study, the pharmacokinetics were no different for the ester (estolate, ethylsuccinate) and the salts (phosphate, stearate).[145] This does not coincide with data from humans. However, findings in horses may be explained by the more neutral pH of equine gastric contents.[145] It was also shown in this study that doses of estolate and phosphate at 37.5 mg/kg gave levels above the reported MIC_{90} for *R. equi* of 0.25 μg/mL[143, 147] for over 12 hours. In addition, the phosphate is often less expensive to use. Rifampin at 5 mg/kg two times per day and erythromycin 25 mg/kg three times per day, or 37.5 mg/kg two times per day is a useful starting dosage. The length of treatment will depend on the clinical response, the return of the complete blood count and fibrinogen concentrations to normal, and resolution of radiographic abnormalities. It can last 30 to 60 days.[20, 148]

In rare circumstances, foals receiving the oral combination of erythromycin and rifampin may develop severe diarrhea in the first days of treatment. In this case, the drug should be withdrawn, and foals treated to restore fluid losses. Partial anorexia, mild colic, and bruxism may also occur. One author identified an idiosyncratic reaction that occurs during times of high ambient temperatures (>30 °C, >86 °F) with the use of this drug combination. Signs of this response were reported to include severe tachypnea and hyperthermia (40°–41 °C, 104°–105.8 °F).[42] Studies in mice indicate that erythromycin alone is not useful in treatment.[16, 149] Strains of *R. equi* have been identified that are resistant to rifampin.[150, 151]

Supportive and Other Therapy

Additional supportive therapy includes intravenous polyionic fluids for dehydrated foals. Foals with respiratory distress will benefit from nasal insufflation of oxygen. Hyperimmune serum may also aid in the treatment of afflicted foals. Because of the chronicity of disease, nebulization will have little effect under most circumstances. Antiulcer and anti-inflammatory medication should be considered.

Long-Term Prognosis

Prognosis is dependent on the severity of lung lesions and response to initial therapy. If the foal survives, and therapy is administered until thoracic radiographic changes and other complications resolve, foals will grow to be normal. In one study, adult horses that had *R. equi* pneumonia as foals were evaluated and appeared to have no residual effect of the disease.[152]

PREVENTION
Hyperimmune Serum

Intravenous administration of hyperimmune plasma may be beneficial on farms with endemic disease. Foals may be tested for low concentrations of antibody to *R. equi* and then treated with plasma as an antibody source.[81, 153] Foals should be given plasma in the first month of life. This practice may significantly reduce the incidence of *R. equi* pneumonia.[42, 93, 154, 155]

Immunization

Field studies by Magnusson in 1923 and 1924 failed to show the value of vaccination with broth cultures of *R. equi*.[1] Vaccination of foals with a formalin-killed *R. equi* bacterin do not protect them against heavy intratracheal challenge.[27] However, oral immunization of young foals with a nonattenuated clinical isolate of *R. equi* did protect against aerosol challenge.[156] This finding supports the notion that intestinal exposure of foals to *R. equi* results in a form of natural vaccination. This hypothesis was supported by the fact that *R. equi*–specific IgG levels rise in foals after oral administration of *R. equi*.[24, 31] As yet, a practical method for immunization has not been developed.

Management

Foals are at risk for disease when exposed to large numbers of organisms concomitant with the absence of protective antibody or with immunosuppression.[20, 81] Conditions that cause stress should be avoided and include overcrowding, excessive handling, and poorly ventilated and dusty environments. Frequent collection and disposal of manure is simple and may do a lot to reduce environmental contamination and the prevalence of the disease. Immunization programs against potentially immunosuppressive viral agents should be employed. There is no support for the concept that migrating larvae of *Parascaris equorum* might carry *R. equi* from the intestine to the lung, but this theory seems plausible and a good deworming program is recommended. The assurance of colostral intake by foals is essential. The organism's robust and ubiquitous nature precludes the usefulness of simple disinfection procedures.

CONCLUSIONS

Rhodococcus equi is an opportunistic, intracellular organism that has similar structure, resistance, and pathogenic mechanisms as some *Mycobacterium* species. Components of the humoral and cell-mediated immune systems are activated after exposure to *R. equi,* but these are not always sufficiently protective to ward off infection. The prognosis for foals with *R. equi* pneumonia has improved with the use of specific antibiotic combinations and with increased early diagnosis. Immunotherapy seems to be useful as well.

REFERENCES

1. Magnusson H: Spezifische infektiöse Pneumonie beim Fohlen. Ein neuer Eiterreger beim Pferd. *Arch Wiss Prakt Tierheilkd* 50:22, 1923.
2. Miessner H, Wetzel R: Beitrag zur schmiedhofferschen Streptokokkenpneumonie der Saugfohlen. *Wien Tierarztl Wochenschr* 31:449, 1923.
3. Bernheimer AW, Linder R, Avigad LS: Stepwise degradation of membrane sphingomyelin by corynebacterial phospholipases. *Infect Immun* 29:123, 1980.
4. Harrington BJ: A numerical taxonomical study of some corynebacteria and related organisms. *J Gen Microbiol* 45:31, 1966.
5. Goodfellow M, Alderson G: The actinomycete-genus *Rhodococcus:* A home for the "rhodochrous" complex. *J Gen Microbiol* 100:99, 1977.
6. Rowbotham TJ, Cross T: Ecology of *Rhodococcus coprophilus* and associated actinomycetes in fresh water and agricultural habitats. *J Gen Microbiol* 100:231, 1977.
7. Prescott JF: *Rhodococcus equi:* An animal and human pathogen. *Clin Microbiol Rev* 4:20, 1991.
8. Skerman VBD, McGowan V, Sneath PHA: Approved lists of bacterial names. *Int J Syst Bacteriol* 30:225, 1980.
9. Chaparas SD, Krichersky MI, Benedict FA: Analysis of antigens of *Rhodococcus* species by rocket immunoelectrophoresis. *Int J Syst Bacteriol* 32:288, 1982.
10. Mordarski M, Goodfellow M: Deoxyribonucleic acid reassociation in the classification of the genus *Rhodococcus* 1891 (approved list). *Int J Med Microbiol* 30:521, 1980.
11. Barton MD, Hughes KL: Ecology of *Rhodococcus equi*. *Vet Microbiol* 9:65, 1984.
12. Barton MD, Hughes KL: *Corynebacterium equi:* A review. *J Clin Microbiol* 50:65, 1980.
13. Keddie RM, Cure GL: The cell wall composition and distribution of free mycolic acids in named strains of coryneform bacteria and in isolates from natural sources. *J Appl Bacteriol* 42:220, 1977.
14. Magnusson H: Pyaemia in foals caused by *Corynebacterium equi*. *Vet Rec* 50:1459, 1938.
15. Magnusson H: Pyämie beim und tuberkuloseähnliche Herde

der Schweine, verursacht durch *Corynebacterium equi*. *Z Infektkr Haustiere* 56:199, 1940.
16. Nordmann P, Keller M, Espinasse F, et al: Correlation between antibiotic resistance, phage-like particle presence, and virulence in *Rhodococcus equi* human isolates. *J Clin Microbiol* 32:377, 1994.
17. Reddy R: Value of acid metabolic products in identification of certain corynebacteria. *J Clin Microbiol* 7:428, 1978.
18. Goodfellow M, Minnikin DE: Nocardioform bacteria. *Annu Rev Microbiol* 31:159, 1977.
19. Yamada K, Komagata K: Taxonomic studies on coryneform bacteria. IV. Morphological, cultural, biochemical and physiological characteristics. *J Appl Bacteriol* 18:399, 1972.
20. Ellenberger MA, Genetzky RM: *Rhodococcus equi* infections: Literature review. *Compendium Continuing Educ Pract Vet* 8:S414, 1986.
21. Bowles PM, Woolcock JB, Mutimer MD: Early events associated with experimental infection of the murine lung with *Rhodococcus equi*. *J Comp Pathol* 101:411, 1989.
22. Nakazawa M, Nemoto H: Synergistic hemolysis phenomenon of *Listeria monocytogenes* and *Corynebacterium equi*. *Jpn J Vet Sci* 42:603, 1994.
23. Carter GR, Hylton GA: An indirect hemagglutination test for antibodies to *Corynebacterium equi*. *Am J Vet Res* 35:1393, 1974.
24. Takai S, Kawazu S, Tsubaki S: Enzyme-linked immunosorbent assay for diagnosis of *Corynebacterium (Rhodococcus) equi* infection in foals. *Am J Vet Res* 46:2166, 1985.
25. Takai S, Koike K, Ohbushi S, et al: Identification of 15- to 17-kilodalton antigens associated with virulent *Rhodococcus equi*. *J Clin Microbiol* 29:439, 1991.
26. Barton MD: Antibiotic sensitivity of *Corynebacterium equi*. *Aust Vet J* 56:339, 1980.
27. Prescott JF, Markham RJF, Johnson JA: Cellular and humoral immune response of foals to vaccination with *Corynebacterium equi*. *Can J Comp Med* 43:356, 1979.
28. Sippel WL, Keahey EE, Bullard TL: *Corynebacterium* infection in foals: Etiology, pathogenesis, and laboratory diagnosis. *J Am Vet Med Assoc* 153:1610, 1968.
29. Wilson MM: A study of *Corynebacterium equi* infection in a study of thoroughbred horses in Victoria. *Aust Vet J* 31:175, 1955.
30. Hughes KL, Sulaiman I: The ecology of *Rhodococcus equi* and physicochemical influences on growth. *Vet Microbiol* 14:241, 1987.
31. Takai S, Fujimori T, Katsuzaki K, et al: Ecology of *Rhodococcus equi* in horses and their environment on horse-breeding farms. *Vet Microbiol* 14:233, 1987.
32. Woolcock JB, Mutimer MD, Farmer AMT: Epidemiology of *Corynebacterium equi* in horses. *Res Vet Sci* 28:87, 1980.
33. Takai S, Narita K, Ando K, et al: Ecology of *Rhodococcus (Corynebacterium) equi* in soil on a horse-breeding farm. *Vet Microbiol* 12:169, 1986.
34. Carman MG, Hodges RT: Distribution of *Rhodococcus equi* in animals, birds and from the environment. *N Z Vet J* 35:114, 1987.
35. Mutimer MD, Woolcock JB, Sturgess BR: *Corynebacterium equi* in human faeces. *Med J Aust* 2:422, 1979.
36. Barton MD, Hughes KL: Comparison of three techniques for isolation of *Rhodococcus (Corynebacterium) equi* from contaminated sources. *J Clin Microbiol* 13:219, 1981.
37. Takai S, Tsubaki S: The incidence of *Rhodococcus (Corynebacterium) equi* in domestic animals and soil. *Jpn J Vet Sci* 47:493, 1985.
38. Nakazawa M, Sugimoto C, Isayama Y: Quantitative culture of *Rhodococcus equi* from the feces of horse. *Natl Inst Anim Health Q* 23:67, 1983.
39. Takai S, Ohkura H, Watanabe Y, Tsubaki S: Quantitative

aspects of fecal *Rhodococcus (Corynebacterium) equi* in foals. *J Clin Microbiol* 23:794, 1986.

40. Skalka B: Dynamics of *equi*-factor antibodies in sera of foals kept on farms with differing histories of *Rhodococcus equi* pneumonia. *Vet Microbiol* 14:269, 1987.

41. Takai S, Ohbushi S, Koike K, et al: Prevalence of virulent *Rhodococcus equi* in isolates from soil and feces of horses from horse-breeding farms with and without endemic infection. *J Clin Microbiol* 29:2887, 1991.

42. Prescott JF, Hoffman AM: *Rhodococcus equi. Vet Clin North Am Equine Pract* 9:375, 1993.

43. Sweeney CR, Sweeney RW, Divers TJ: *Rhodococcus equi* pneumonia in 48 foals: response to antimicrobial therapy. *Vet Microbiol* 14:329, 1987.

44. Woolcock JB, Farmer AMT, Mutimer MD: Selective medium for *Corynebacterium equi* isolation. *J Clin Microbiol* 9:640, 1979.

45. Cotchin E: *Corynebacterium equi* in the submaxillary lymph nodes of swine. *J Comp Pathol* 53:298, 1943.

46. Zink MC, Yager JA: Experimental infection of piglets by aerosols of *Rhodococcus equi. Can J Vet Res* 51:290, 1987.

47. Rajagopalan VR: The occurrence of *Corynebacterium equi* in a she-buffalo. *Indian J Vet Sci Anim Husbandry* 7:38, 1938.

48. Carrigan MJ, Links IJ, Morton AG: *Rhodococcus equi* infection in goats. *Aust Vet J* 65:331, 1988.

49. Diteko T, Winnen GM, Manthe LM: Isolations of *Rhodococcus (Corynebacterium) equi* from goats in Botswana. *Zimbabwe Vet J* 19:11, 1988.

50. Fitzgerald SD, Walker RD, Parlor KW: Fatal *Rhodococcus equi* infection in an Angora goat. *J Vet Diagn Invest* 6:105, 1994.

51. Ojo MO, Njoku CO, Freitas J, et al: Isolation of *Rhodococcus equi* from the liver abscess of a goat in Trinidad. *Can Vet J* 34:504, 1993.

52. Roberts MC, Hodgson DR, Kelly WR: *Corynebacterium equi* infection in an adult horse. *Aust Vet J* 56:96, 1980.

53. Elliot G, Lawson GHK, Mackenzie CP: *Rhodococcus equi* infection in cats. *Vet Rec* 118:693, 1986.

54. Mutimer MD, Prescott JF, Woolcock JB: Capsular serotypes of *Rhodococcus equi. Aust Vet J* 58:67, 1982.

55. Rhaman A: The sensitivity of various bacteria to chemotherapeutic agents. *Br Vet J* 113:175, 1957.

56. Bauwens LE, Van Dyck E, De Meurichy W, et al: *Corynebacterium equi* pneumonia in three baikal seals (*Pusa sibirica*). *Aquatic Mammals* 13:17, 1987.

57. Stein FJ, Scott G: *Corynebacterium equi* in the cottontop marmoset (*Saguinus oedipus*): a case report. *Lab Anim Sci* 29:519, 1979.

58. Ishino S, Nakazawa M, Matsuda I: Pathological findings of guinea-pigs infected intratracheally with *Rhodococcus (Corynebacterium) equi. Jpn J Vet Sci* 49:395, 1987.

59. Jasmin AM, Carroll JM, Baucom JN: *Corynebacterium equi* infection in the American alligator (*Alligator missippiensis*) and the American crocodile (*Crocodilus acutus*). *J Comp Lab Med* 3:71, 1969.

60. Van Etta LL, Filice GA, Ferguson RM, et al: *Corynebacterium equi:* A review of 12 cases of human infection. *Rev Infect Dis* 5:1012, 1983.

61. Drancourt M, Bonnet E, Gallais H, et al: *Rhodococcus equi* infection in patients with AIDS. *J Infect* 24:123, 1992.

62. Emmons W, Reichwein B, Winslow DL: *Rhodococcus equi* infection in the patient with AIDS: Literature review and report of an unusual case. *Rev Infect Dis* 13:91, 1991.

63. Magnani G, Elia GF, McNeil MM, et al: *Rhodococcus equi* cavitary pneumonia in HIV-infected patients: An unsuspected opportunistic pathogen. *J Acquir Immune Defic Syndr* 5:1059, 1992.

64. Pialoux G, Fournier S, Dupont B, et al: Abcès pulmonaire à *Rhodococcus (Corynebacterium) equi* lors d'une infection a VIH. Deux observations. *Presse Med* 21:417, 1992.

65. Mastroianni CM, Lichtner M, Vullo V, et al: Humoral immune response to *Rhodococcus equi* in AIDS patients with *R. equi* pneumonia. *J Infect Dis* 169:1179, 1994.

66. Ebersole L, Paturzo JL: Endophthalmitis caused by *Rhodococcus equi* prescott serotype 4. *J Clin Microbiol* 26:1221, 1988.

67. Hillman D, Garretson B, Fiscella R: *Rhodococcus equi* endophthalmitis. *Arch Ophthalmol* 107:20, 1989.

68. Muller F, Schaal KP, Graevenitz A, et al: Characterization of *Rhodococcus equi*-like bacterium isolated from a wound infection in a noncompromised host. *J Clin Microbiol* 26:618, 1988.

69. Ellenburger MA, Kaeberle ML, Roth JA: Equine cell–mediated immune response to *Rhodococcus. Am J Vet Res* 45:2424, 1984.

70. Prescott JF, Johnson JA, Markham RJF: Experimental studies on the pathogenesis of *Corynebacterium equi* infection in foals. *Can J Comp Med* 44:280, 1980.

71. Johnson JA, Prescott JF, Markham RJF: The pathology of experimental *Corynebacterium equi* infection in foals following intrabronchial challenge. *Vet Pathol* 20:440, 1983.

72. Johnson JA, Prescott JF, Markham RJF: The pathology of experimental *Corynebacterium equi* infection in foals following intragastric challenge. *Vet Pathol* 20:450, 1983.

73. Martens RJ, Fiske RA, Renshaw HW: Experimental subacute foal pneumonia induced by aerosol administration of *Corynebacterium equi. Equine Vet J* 14:111, 1982.

74. Rooney JR: Corynebacterial infections in foals. *Mod Vet Pract* 47:43, 1966.

75. Elissalde GS, Waldberg JA, Renshaw HW: *Corynebacterium equi*: An interhost review with emphasis on the foal. *Comp Immunol Microbiol Infect Dis* 3:433, 1980.

76. McKenzie RA, Donald BA, Dimmock CK: Experimental *Corynebacterium equi* infections of cattle. *J Comp Pathol* 91:347, 1981.

77. McKenzie RA, Ward WH: *Rhodococcus (Corynebacterium) equi:* A possible cause of reactions to the complement fixation test for Johne's disease of cattle. *Aust Vet J* 57:200, 1981.

78. Ellenberger MA, Kaeberle ML, Roth JA: Effect of *Rhodococcus equi* on equine polymorphonuclear leukocyte function. *Vet Immunol Immunopathol* 7:315, 1984.

79. Ellenberger MA, Kaeberle ML, Roth JA: Equine cell-mediated immune response to *Rhodococcus. Am J Vet Res* 45:2424, 1984.

80. Ardans AA, Hietala SK, Spensley MS, et al: Studies of naturally occurring and experimental *Rhodococcus equi (Corynebacterium equi)* pneumonia in foals. *Proc Am Assoc Equine Pract* 32:129, 1986.

81. Hietala SK, Ardans AA, Sansome A: Detection of *Corynebacterium equi*–specific antibody in horses by enzyme-linked immunosorbent assay. *Am J Vet Res* 46:13, 1985.

82. Ainsworth DM, Weldon AD, Beck KA, et al: Recognition of *Pneumocystis carinii* in foals with respiratory distress. *Equine Vet J* 25:103, 1993.

83. Burrows GE: *Corynebacterium equi* infection in two foals. *J Am Vet Med Assoc* 152:1119, 1968.

84. Hietala SK, Ardans AA: Interaction of *Rhodococcus equi* with phagocytic cells from *R. equi*–exposed and non-exposed foals. *Vet Microbiol* 14:279, 1987.

85. Knight HD: Corynebacterial infections in the horse: Problems of prevention. *J Am Vet Med Assoc* 155:446, 1969.

86. Zink MC, Yager JA, Prescott JF, et al: In vitro phagocytosis and killing of *Corynebacterium equi* by alveolar macrophages of foals. *Am J Vet Res* 46:2171, 1985.

87. Martens JG, Martens RJ, Renshaw HW: *Rhodococcus (Cory-*

nebacterium) equi: Bactericidal capacity of neutrophils from neonatal and adult horses. *Am J Vet Res* 49:295, 1988.

88. Martens RJ, Martens JG, Fiske RA: *Rhodococcus equi* foal pneumonia: Pathogenesis and immunoprophylaxis. *Proc Am Assoc Equine Pract* 35:199, 1990.

89. Ellenberger MA, Kaeberle ML, Roth JA: Equine humoral immune response to *Rhodococcus (Corynebacterium) equi.* *Am J Vet Res* 45:2428, 1984.

90. Prescott JF, Ogilvie TH, Markham RJF: Lymphocyte immunostimulation in the diagnosis of *Corynebacterium equi* pneumonia of foals. *Am J Vet Res* 41:2073, 1980.

91. Takai S, Kawazu S, Tsubaki S: Immunoglobulin and specific antibody responses to *Rhodococcus (Corynebacterium) equi* infection in foals as measured by enzyme-linked immunosorbent assay. *J Clin Microbiol* 23:943, 1986.

92. Takai S, Kawazu S, Tsubaki S: Humoral immune response of foals to experimental infection with *Rhodococcus equi.* *Vet Microbiol* 14:321, 1987.

93. Martens RJ, Martens JG, Fiske RA, et al: *Rhodococcus equi* foal pneumonia: Protective effects of immune plasma in experimentally infected foals. *Equine Vet J* 21:249, 1989.

94. Martens RJ, Martens JG, Renshaw HW, et al: *Rhodococcus equi:* Equine neutrophil chemiluminescent and bactericidal responses to opsonizing antibody. *Vet Microbiol* 14:277, 1987.

95. Lederer E, Adam A, Ciobura R: Cell walls of mycobacteria and related organisms: Chemical and immunostimulant properties. *Mol Cell Biochem* 7:87, 1975.

96. Prescott JF, Machang'u R, Kwiecien J, et al: Prevention of foal mortality due to *Rhodococcus equi* pneumonia on an endemically affected farm. *Can Vet J* 30:871, 1989.

97. Nordmann P, Ronco E, Guenounou M: Involvement of interferon-gamma and tumor necrosis factor-alpha in host defense against *Rhodococcus equi.* *J Infect Dis* 167:1456, 1993.

98. Kanaly ST, Hines SA, Palmer GH: Failure of pulmonary clearance of *Rhodococcus equi* infection in CD4 + T-lymphocyte–deficient transgenic mice. *Infect Immun* 61:4929, 1993.

99. Nordmann P, Ronco E, Nauciel C: Role of T-lymphocyte subsets in *Rhodococcus equi* infection. *Infect Immun* 60:2748, 1992.

100. Bowles PM, Woolcock JB, Mutimer MD: Experimental infection of mice with *Rhodococcus equi:* Differences in virulence between strains. *Vet Microbiol* 14:259, 1987.

101. Nakazawa M, Haritani M, Sugimoto C, et al: Virulence of *Rhodococcus equi* for mice. *Jpn J Vet Sci* 45:679, 1983.

102. Takai S, Michizoe T, Matsumura K, et al: Correlation of *in vitro* properties of *Rhodococcus (Corynebacterium) equi* with virulence for mice. *Microbiol Immunol* 29:1175, 1985.

103. Kanno T, Asawa T, Ito H, et al: Restriction map of a virulence-associated plasmid of *Rhodococcus equi.* *Plasmid* 30:309, 1993.

104. Takai S, Iie M, Watanabe Y, et al: Virulence-associated 15- to 17-kilodalton antigens in *Rhodococcus equi:* Temperature-dependent expression and location of the antigens. *Infect Immun* 60:2995, 1992.

105. Takai S, Sasaki Y, Ikeda T, et al: Virulence of *Rhodococcus equi* isolates from patients with and without AIDS. *J Clin Microbiol* 32:457, 1994.

106. Takai S, Sekizaki T, Ozawa T, et al: Association between a large plasmid and 15- to 17-kilodalton antigen in virulent *Rhodococcus equi.* *Infect Immun* 59:4056, 1991.

107. Tkachuk-Saad O, Prescott J: *Rhodococcus equi* plasmids: Isolation and partial characterization. *J Clin Microbiol* 29:2696, 1991.

108. Gotoh K, Mitsuyama M, Imaizumi S, et al: Mycolic acid-containing glycolipid as a possible virulence factor of *Rhodococcus equi* for mice. *Microbiol Immunol* 35:175, 1991.

109. Leitch RA, Richards JC: Structural analysis of the specific capsular polysaccharide of *Rhodococcus equi* serotype 1. *Biochem Cell Biol* 68:778, 1990.

110. Machang'u RS, Prescott JF: Purification and properties of cholesterol oxidase and choline phosphohydrolase from *Rhodococcus equi.* *Can J Vet Res* 55:332, 1991.

111. Hondalus MK, Diamond MS, Rosenthal LA, et al. The intracellular bacterium *Rhodococcus equi* requires Mac-1 to bind to mammalian cells. *Infect Immun* 61:2919, 1993.

112. Ezoe H, Furuichi K, Katoh H, et al: Regulation of allergic reactions by aerobic *Corynebacterium equi* extract, CEF. II. Inhibition of heterologous PCA and antigen-induced histamine release in rats. *Int Arch Allergy Appl Immunol* 66:237, 1981.

113. Furuichi K, Ezoe H, Katoh H, et al: Regulation of allergic reactions by aerobic *Corynebacterium equi* extract, CEF. I. Antigen nonspecific suppression of reaginic antibody response in mice. *Int Arch Allergy Appl Immunol* 66:345, 1981.

114. Baldwin JL, Bertone JJ, Sommer MM, et al: *Rhodococcus equi* enteritis, colonic lymphadenitis, and peritonitis in three foals with nonresponsive *Rhodococcus equi* bronchopneumonia. *Equine Pract* 14:15, 1992.

115. Zink MC, Yager JA, Smart NL: *Corynebacterium equi* infections in horses, 1958–1984: A review of 131 cases. *Can J Vet Res* 27:213–219, 1986.

116. Bull LB: Corynebacterial pyaemia of foals. *J Comp Pathol Ther* 37:294, 1924.

117. Collatos C, Clark ES, Reef VB, et al: Septicemia, atrial fibrillation, cardiomegaly, left atrial mass, and *Rhodococcus equi* septic osteoarthritis in a foal. *J Am Vet Med Assoc* 197:1039, 1990.

118. Firth EC, Alley MR, Hodge H: *Rhodococcus equi*–associated osteomyelitis in foals. *Aust Vet J* 70:304, 1993.

119. Freestone JF, Shoemaker S, McClure JJ: Pulmonary abscessation, hepatoencephalopathy and IgM deficiency associated with *Rhodococcus equi* in a foal. *Aust Vet J* 66:343, 1989.

120. Giguere S, Lavoie JP: *Rhodococcus equi* vertebral osteomyelitis in 3 Quarter Horse colts. *Equine Vet J* 26:74, 1994.

121. Novak RM, Polisky EL, Janda WM, et al: Osteomyelitis caused by *Rhodococcus equi* in a renal transplant. *Infection* 16:186, 1988.

122. Olchowy TWJ: Vertebral body osteomyelitis due to *Rhodococcus equi* in two arabian foals. *Equine Vet J* 26:79, 1994.

123. Prescott JF: *Rhodococcus equi* vertebral osteomyelitis in foals. *Equine Vet J* 26:1, 1994.

124. Genetzky RM, Bettcher LH, White PL: *Corynebacterium equi* infection in a mare. *Mod Vet Pract* 63:876, 1982.

125. Simpson R: *Corynebacterium equi* in adult horses in Kenya. *Epizootiol Dis Afr* 12:303, 1964.

126. Smith BP, Robinson RC: Studies of an outbreak of *Corynebacterium equi* pneumonia in foals. *Equine Vet J* 13:223, 1981.

127. Falcon J: Clinical and radiographic findings in *Corynebacterium equi* pneumonia of foals. *J Am Vet Med Assoc* 186:593, 1985.

128. King GK: Equine thoracic radiography. Part I. *Compendium Continuing Educ Pract Vet* 3:S278, 1981.

129. King GK: Equine thoracic radiography. Part II. *Compendium Continuing Educ Pract Vet* 3:S283, 1981.

130. Nakazawa M, Isayama Y, Kashiwazaki M, et al: Diagnosis of *Rhodococcus equi* infection in foals by the agar gel diffusion test with protein antigen. *Vet Microbiol* 15:105, 1987.

131. Prescott JF, Coshan-Gauthier R, Barksdale L: Antibody to *equi* factor(s) in the diagnosis of *Corynebacterium equi* pneumonia of foals. *Can J Comp Med* 48:370, 1984.

132. Takai S, Kazama N, Tsubaki S: Radial immunodiffusion enzyme assay for detection of antibody to *Rhodococcus equi* in horse sera. *Jpn J Vet Sci* 52:653, 1990.

133. Takai S, Iie M, Kobayashi C, et al: Monoclonal antibody

specific to virulence-associated 15- to 17-kilodalton antigens of *Rhodococcus equi*. *J Clin Microbiol* 31:2780, 1993.

134. Burrows GE, MacAllister CG, Beckstrom DA, et al: Rifampin in the horse: comparison of intravenous, intramuscular, and oral administrations. *Am J Vet Res* 46:442, 1985.

135. Barton MD, Embury DH: Studies of the pathogenesis of *Rhodococcus equi* infection in foals. *Aust Vet J* 64:332, 1987.

136. Nordmann P, Ronco E: In-vitro antimicrobial susceptibility of *Rhodococcus equi*. *J Antimicrob Chemother* 29:383, 1992.

137. Prescott JF, Nicholson VM: The effects of combinations of selected antibiotics on the growth of *Corynebacterium equi*. *J Am Vet Med Assoc* 7:61, 1984.

138. Hillidge CJ: Review of *Corynebacterium (Rhodococcus) equi* lung abscesses in foals: Pathogenesis, diagnosis and treatment. *Vet Rec* 119:261, 1986.

139. Prescott JF, Sweeney CR: Treatment of *Corynebacterium equi* pneumonia of foals: A review. *J Am Vet Med Assoc* 187:725, 1985.

140. Burrows GE, MacAllister CG, Ewing P, et al: Rifampin disposition in the horse: Effects of age and method of oral. *J Vet Pharmacol Ther* 15:124, 1992.

141. Hillidge CJ: Use of erythromycin-rifampin combination in treatment of *Rhodococcus equi* pneumonia. *Vet Microbiol* 14:337, 1987.

142. Kohn CW, Sams R, Kowalski JJ, et al: Pharmacokinetics of single intravenous and single and multiple dose oral administration of rifampin in mares. *J Vet Pharmacol Ther* 16:119, 1993.

143. Wilson WD, Spensley MS, Baggot JD, et al: Pharmacokinetics, bioavailability, and in vitro antibacterial of rifampin in the horse. *Am J Vet Res* 49:2041, 1988.

144. Zertuche JML, Hillidge CJ: Therapeutic considerations for *Rhodococcus equi* pneumonia in foals. *Compendium Continuing Educ Pract Vet* 9:965, 1987.

145. Ewing PJ, Burrows G, MacAllister C, et al: Comparison of oral erythromycin formulations in the horse using pharmacokinetic profiles. *J Vet Pharmacol Ther* 17:17, 1994.

146. Knottenbelt DC: *Rhodococcus equi* infection in foals: A report of an outbreak on a thoroughbred stud in Zimbabwe. *Vet Rec* 132:79, 1993.

147. Prescott JF: The susceptibility of isolates of *Corynebacterium equi* to antimicrobial drugs. *J Vet Pharmacol Ther* 4:27, 1981.

148. Genetzky RM, McNeel SV, Loparco FV: *Rhodococcus equi* pneumonia in foals. *Mod Vet Pract* 65:787, 1984.

149. Nordmann P, Kerestedjian JJ, Ronco E: Therapy of *Rhodococcus equi* disseminated infections in nude mice. *Antimicrob Agents Chemother* 36:1244, 1992.

150. Nordmann P, Chavanet P, Caillon J, et al: Recurrent pneumonia due to rifampicin-resistant *Rhodococcus equi* in a patient infected with HIV (letter). *J Infect* 24:104, 1992.

151. Nordmann P, Rouveix E, Guenounou M, et al: Pulmonary abscess due to a rifampin and fluoroquinolone resistant *Rhodococcus equi* strain in an HIV infected patient (letter). *Eur J Clin Microbiol Infect Dis* 11:557, 1992.

152. Ainsworth DM, Beck KA, Boatwright CE, et al: Lack of residual lung damage in horses in which *Rhodococcus equi*–induced pneumonia had been diagnosed. *Am J Vet Res* 54:2115, 1993.

153. Vivrette S: The diagnosis, treatment, and prevention of *Rhodococcus equi* pneumonia in foals. *Vet Med* 87:144, 1992.

154. Madigan JE, Hietala S, Muller N: Protection against naturally acquired *Rhodococcus equi* pneumonia in foals by administration of hyperimmune plasma. *J Reprod Fertil Suppl* 44:571, 1991.

155. Muller NS, Madigan JE: Methods of implementation of an immunoprophylaxis program for the prevention of *Rhodococcus equi* pneumonia: Results of a 5-year field. *Proc Am Assoc Equine Pract* 39:193, 1993.

156. Chirino-Trejo JM, Prescott JF, Yager JA: Protection of foals against experimental *Rhodococcus equi* pneumonia by oral immunization. *Can J Vet Res* 51:444, 1987.

Chapter 19

Toxicologic Problems

David G. Schmitz, DVM, MS

In today's society, any list of substances that are toxic, or potentially toxic, is probably incomplete. Our industrial society is continuously producing new and different compounds that are potentially hazardous or fatal to humans and many species of animals. Our knowledge of toxic compounds and the mechanisms whereby they produce disease is also constantly changing, so certain substances that previously were thought to be inert are now known to affect the health of animals or humans.

It behooves the veterinary clinician to be as informed as possible concerning the potentially toxic substances found in the environment. Not all toxins are uniformly distributed in nature (this is particularly true of toxic plants), so it also seems reasonable to assume that in any given geographical area, certain toxicities will be much more common than others.

Many factors influence the toxicity of a given substance, and it is not within the scope of this chapter to expound on these in any great detail. Books have been written on specific aspects of toxicity and all the different mechanisms that come into play relating to a specific substance causing harm to a specific animal at a specific point in time. The reader is referred to other sources for information regarding general toxicologic principles and measurements and quantification. It should be noted that factors such as age, species of animal, reproductive status, nutritional status, management, diet, and numerous other factors relating to the animal itself can influence the toxicity of a given substance. Other factors related to the compound itself, such as its bioavailability, its chemical form or structure, its concentration, and so forth, can also influence the toxicity of a substance at any point in time.

Most toxins do not preferentially damage a solitary tissue, organ, or organ system, but frequently affect several organs or body systems at the same time. Although it is not unusual for clinical signs to be related predominately to a single organ system, multiple organ involvement is the rule rather than the exception. This necessitates a thorough examination and evaluation of any animal presented for diagnosis of possible toxicosis. All body systems should be adequately evaluated in the animal that is presented with suspected toxicity.

The clinical manifestations of many toxicologic problems occur some time following initial exposure to the toxin. This can make diagnosis and treatment difficult. For this reason, many cases of suspected toxicity are treated empirically. If a specific antidote is available or indicated, however, it should be employed in the treatment regimen. General rules of thumb regarding treatment of suspected toxicoses include (1) removal of the source from the environment, if possible; (2) removal of the toxin from the animal's body, if possible; (3) cleaning the skin or contact surface with suitable agents if the route of exposure is superficial; (4) evacuation of the gastrointestinal tract by appropriate means if contamination was oral; (5) maintenance of normal body functions and physiologic processes as much as possible by means of fluid administration and blood pH and electrolyte modification; (6) maintenance of body functions not affected by the toxin; (7) aiding elimination of the toxin source from the animal's system as expeditiously as possible; (8) not causing damage to a secondary organ or system while treating the primary toxicosis; and (9) preventing reexposure or recontamination of the animal by the toxic substance.

In this chapter, the toxins have been divided into broad categories of general clinical signs. A toxin is most completely discussed under the system to which the major clinical signs are referable. It must be remembered, however, that most toxins involve more than one organ system, so there will be a number of toxins that can be found in several categories. Specific antidotes are given where appropriate, and treatment aimed at symptomatic care is given at the end of each section.

TOXICOSES CAUSING SIGNS RELATING TO THE GASTROINTESTINAL SYSTEM

Plants

Oak (Quercus *species*)

Clinical Signs. Oak blossoms, buds, leaves, stems, and acorns can all be toxic to livestock. Most reports of toxicosis in livestock involve cattle and sheep, with rare occurrence in the horse. Clinical signs attributed to acorn toxicosis in horses are acute onset of severe abdominal pain, rectal straining, hemorrhagic diarrhea, and pronounced intestinal borborygmus. Acorn parts may be noted in feces. Occasionally horses are found dead, but other signs noted are hemoglobinuria and elevated heart and respiratory rates.

Pathophysiology. The toxicity of oak is attributed to tannins or their metabolites. Digallic acid is the major active metabolite produced by oak tannins. Following bacterial fermentation, digallic acid is converted to gallic acid and pyrogallol, both of which are considered toxic.[1] Pyrogallol and gallic acid are extremely toxic to renal tubules and result in acute tubular necrosis, anuria, electrolyte abnormalities, and uremia.[1, 2] Pyrogallol is also responsible for causing hemorrhagic gastroenteritis, subcutaneous hemorrhage, and hemolysis. Tannic acid itself is thought to result in increased vascular permeability, hemorrhage, and subsequent fluid loss into body spaces.[1]

Diagnosis. The diagnosis of oak toxicity is based on clinical signs and a history of exposure to the plant. Under adequate forage conditions, horses would seem to have a distaste for oak leaves and acorns, so most horses exposed to the plant will not develop toxicity. Toxicosis is more likely to result when abnormal conditions coupled with environmental factors result in large numbers of acorns being produced and becoming accessible to horses.

Laboratory findings compatible with oak toxicosis include dehydration or hemoconcentration to varying degrees, azotemia, hyperphosphatemia, hypocalcemia, and hypoproteinemia. Abnormal urine findings might include occult blood, proteinuria, and casts. An increase in gallic acid equivalent content in urine has also been used to support a diagnosis of oak toxicity.[1]

Necropsy findings suggestive of oak toxicosis include pericardial, thoracic, and peritoneal effusion; gastrointestinal and mesenteric edema; and pale and swollen kidneys that may bulge on cut surface. The intestinal tract may contain large quantities of acorn parts, and colonic ulceration has been reported.[1]

Specific Treatment and Management. No specific antidote for oak toxicity is available. Animals should be removed from further access to oak. Treatment of the acutely affected animal is aimed at maintaining fluid and acid-base balance, and correction of any electrolyte abnormalities. Balanced polyionic fluids given intravenously to promote diuresis are the basic therapy. This should be supplemented with calcium, bicarbonate, and other electrolytes as necessary. Anuric animals may gain additional benefit from furosemide 1 mg/kg IV or dimethyl sulfoxide (DMSO) 1 g/kg IV given as a 10% solution in addition to fluid therapy. Evacuation of the intestinal tract should be attempted by use of mineral oil or other suitable laxative.

The prognosis for affected horses is guarded. There is a paucity of information concerning mortality rates in affected horses, but death due to ingestion of acorns has been reported.[1]

Oleander (Nerium oleander)

Clinical Signs. Sudden death is the most common sign attributed to oleander poisoning in the literature. Other reports suggest that affected horses exhibit lethargy, inappetence, and occasional signs of abdominal pain.[3, 4] Profuse, watery, catarrhal, or bloody diarrhea may also occur within a few hours of ingestion.[5] Cardiac irregularities, including alternating bradycardia and tachycardia, may be accompanied by a variety of arrhythmias.[5, 6] The extremities may feel cold to the touch and mucous membranes can have a blanched appearance. Profuse sweating and muscle twitching

are followed by weakness and death. Death may occur less than 12 hours following ingestion.

The green plant apparently is unpalatable to horses. Most toxicities occur when leaves have been incorporated into lawn clippings and offered to horses. Drying does not affect the toxicity of the leaves; therefore, leaves incorporated into hay may also be toxic. Reportedly, 0.005% of body weight of green oleander is lethal to horses.[3]

Pathophysiology. Common oleander contains at least five cardiac glycosides that are found in all parts of the plant.[3, 5, 7] These glycosides (oleandrin, digitoxigenin, neriin, folinerin, rosagenin) inhibit the Na^+,K^+-ATPase (adenosine triphosphatase) system, resulting in hyperkalemia, conduction abnormalities, and ventricular arrhythmias. Which glycosides or metabolites cause specific symptoms is unclear because of undefined pharmacokinetics of the individual glycosides.[7]

Diagnosis and Treatment. Exposure to the plant along with the clinical signs described above should alert the clinician to the possibility of oleander toxicity. The rapidity of onset of clinical signs or the finding of dead animals may preclude any effective treatment. Symptomatic therapy should be initiated in those animals in which toxicosis is suspected. Evacuation of the intestinal tract by laxatives and enemas may be useful. Atropine and propranolol have been advocated, but they must be used with extreme caution.[5, 6] Fluids containing calcium should not be used, as they may augment the glycoside's effects on the myocardium.[3]

Castor Bean (Ricinus communis)

Clinical Signs. Castor beans contain ricin, a protein phytotoxin that acts as a potent proteolytic enzyme with significant antigenic qualities.[8] A latent period ranging from hours to several days usually occurs prior to the onset of clinical signs in affected horses. The bean is apparently very distasteful to horses, and intoxication is most likely to occur when the bean is inadvertently mixed into the feed source.

The most commonly reported clinical signs of castor bean toxicosis described in the literature are varying degrees of abdominal pain, diarrhea, depression, incoordination, profuse sweating, and increased body temperature.[8, 9] Muscle twitching, convulsions, and prominent cardiac contractions are occasionally observed. If enough ricin is absorbed, signs of shock and anaphylaxis predominate.[8, 9] Death may ensure as soon as 24 to 36 hours following ingestion.

Ricin is reported to be very toxic to horses. One reference cites a dosage of 0.1 μg/kg as a lethal dose,[8] and a second source indicates 25 g of castor beans is lethal.[9] No recent report of ricin or castor bean toxicosis could be found, but a published report in 1945 describes seven deaths attributed to castor bean toxicosis from a stable of 48 horses in London in 1931.[10] The exact number of affected horses was not reported. A recent review of the human literature suggests that castor bean (ricin) toxicosis in humans is not nearly as lethal as reported in the early twentieth-century literature.[11] Whether this holds for horses is open to speculation.

Pathophysiology. The oil extract of the bean contains ricinoleic acid. Within the small intestine, ricinoleate acts to reduce net absorption of fluid and electrolytes, and stimulates peristalsis.[12] The fibrous residue of the seed contains the water-soluble toxalbumin, ricin. Ricin is absorbed from the gastrointestinal tract and is a potent inhibitor of protein synthesis. Ricin contains two polypeptide chains. Chain B, a lectin, binds to the cell surface to facilitate toxin entry into the cell. Chain A disrupts protein synthesis by activating the 60S ribosomal subunit. The red blood cell (RBC) agglutinating properties of ricin are independent of these toxic effects.[13]

Diagnosis. The diagnosis is made by a combination of history of exposure to the plant, clinical signs, and the identification of seeds in feed material or feces. Radioimmunoassay for ricin content in urine is available from certain laboratories.[13]

Treatment. There is no specific antidote for ricin. Initial therapy is aimed at combating shock, abdominal pain, and evacuation of the bowel. Maintenance of fluid and electrolyte balance is important. Various sedatives and analgesics may be useful to control abdominal pain, if present. Oral administration of laxatives and protectants such as mineral oil and charcoal is indicated. Antihistamines have also been recommended.[8]

Pokeweed (Phytolacca americana)

Clinical Signs. No reports of pokeweed intoxication in horses could be found in the literature. However, one text reports that horses show signs of gastrointestinal irritation and abdominal discomfort as the primary clinical signs. The plant also produces a burning sensation of the oral mucous membranes and may cause a hemolytic crisis.[14] Fatalities due to pokeweed ingestion are said to result from respiratory failure and convulsions.[14]

Pathophysiology. The plant contains phytolaccine, a powerful gastrointestinal irritant, which in humans causes symptoms ranging from a burning sensation of the alimentary tract to severe hemorrhagic gastritis.[15] Five nonspecific mitogens that have hemagglutinating and mitotic activity have been isolated. These substances vary in concentration in the plant throughout the growing season. Noncardiac steroids and triterpenoid glycosides (saponins) are also present in significant quantities, but their role in pokeweed toxicity is not known.[15] Saponins may potentiate gastrointestinal toxicity, and produce vasodilation when given parenterally.

Diagnosis and Treatment. No specific diagnostic test is available. Horses with suspected toxicosis must be treated symptomatically. Evacuation of the gastrointestinal tract with the use of laxatives should be attempted. Adsorbents such as charcoal and protectants may be useful. If animals develop a hemolytic crisis, ancillary therapy such as whole-blood transfusions may be lifesaving. Fluid and electrolyte balance must be maintained in such animals to attempt to prevent or minimize hemoglobin nephrosis.[14]

Nightshade (Solanum species)

Clinical Signs. A number of species of *Solanum* have been incriminated in causing toxicity in horses. However, these plants are rarely a source of natural intoxication to horses. Reported clinical signs are referable to the gastrointestinal and central nervous systems. The primary gastrointestinal signs noted are salivation, abdominal pain, increased borborygmi, and diarrhea. Signs of central nervous system (CNS) dysfunction include mydriasis, dullness, depression, weakness, and progressive paralysis, which can lead to prostration and death.[16, 17]

Pathophysiology. Solanine is the toxic substance found in *Solanum* species. It is a water-soluble glycoalkaloid capable of producing local irritation.[16–18] It is poorly absorbed from the gastrointestinal tract.[18] Intravenous doses caused ventricular fibrillation in rabbits, and intraperitoneal doses caused mild-to-moderate inhibition of both specific and nonspecific cholinesterases.[18]

Diagnosis and Treatment. No specific diagnostic test is available. Animals with suspected toxicosis should be treated symptomatically. Evacuation of the gastrointestinal tract by the use of laxatives and protectants is indicated. Charcoal has also been recommended for treatment of human toxicosis.[18] Fluid, electrolyte, and acid-base status of affected animals should be monitored and corrections made as needed.

Blue-Green Algae

Clinical Signs. The occurrence of algal poisoning in livestock is sporadic, and reports of intoxication in horses are rare. Most cases of toxicity involve other grazing animals, principally cattle and sheep, but horses are reported to be affected.[19] Toxicity may occur during times that favor algal growth in surface water. The two most important factors that favor algal growth are a nutrient source (such as nitrogen or phosphate) and warm temperature. Therefore, toxicosis is most likely to occur during periods of warm weather (late spring through fall) when surface water may be contaminated with fertilizer runoff or organic waste high in nitrogen, such as that from feedlots.[19, 20]

At least eight genera of blue-green algae are known to be toxic. These are *Anabaena, Aphanizomenon, Microcystis, Coelosphaerium, Gloeotrichia, Lyngbya, Nodularia,* and *Nostoc,* but the first three are of most concern in veterinary medicine. Common signs of algal poisoning are rapid appearance of signs of abdominal pain, diarrhea, muscle tremors, dyspnea and cyanosis, prostration, and death. These signs frequently develop within a few minutes (< 1 hour) of ingestion. Some cases may show rapid onset of CNS dysfunction with seizures, prostration, and death. Animals surviving several days may exhibit hemorrhagic diarrhea, muscle tremors, signs of liver damage, and photosensitization.[19, 20]

Pathophysiology. *Anabaena flos-aquae* contains a low-molecular-weight alkaloid named anatoxin A, or very-fast-death factor. This toxin produces a potent postsynaptic depolarizing neuromuscular blocking agent that has a curarelike action. Death results from respiratory arrest.[19, 21] Blooms of *Aphanizomenon flos-aquae* produce a neurotoxin (saxitoxin) and at least three related toxic compounds of unknown structure.[19, 21] Saxitoxin blocks sodium conductance through excitable membranes, which subsequently stops nerve action potential. Death resulting from saxitoxin is due to respiratory neuromuscular paralysis.[19]

Microcystis aeruginosa produces at least two toxic substances. Microcystin (fast-death factor) is a lethal, low-molecular-weight cyclic peptide endotoxin that is released by *M. aeruginosa* upon cellular decomposition.[19, 21] This algal species also contains a cyclic peptide hepatotoxin that is potent, rapid-acting, and causes hepatocellular necrosis and collapse of the hepatic parenchyma. The immediate cause of death is hemorrhagic shock, secondary to the liver lesions.[22]

Diagnosis and Treatment. No practical means of isolating and identifying toxins from affected animals or suspect water is available. Because the concentration of algae and toxins can vary tremendously over a very short time period, recovery of the toxin from water may not be possible when clinical signs are noted. Likewise, no specific assay for toxin has been developed for use on animal tissues. A presumptive diagnosis at best can be made when conditions favoring algal overgrowth are present, coupled with exposure of animals to the algal source, and the development of rapid onset of clinical signs. Water samples can be analyzed for identification of specific blue-green algae, and their presence may support a diagnosis of algal toxicity.[19]

There is no specific antidote and animals are often found dead before treatment can be initiated.[19] Algal growth in surface water can be controlled by a variety of herbicides and copper sulfate. Care must be taken when treating water with these compounds, to ascertain they are being used in a safe manner for all susceptible livestock.

MEDICATIONS

Lincomycin and Clindamycin

Clinical Signs. Signs of illness in horses are generally not seen until 2 to 4 days following exposure. Subsequently, affected horses show signs of colitis and endotoxemia, with development of moderate-to-severe abdominal pain, tachycardia, congested mucous membranes, loose-to-watery feces that may contain blood, and elevated rectal temperature. Leukopenia may be present initially, and dehydration can develop rapidly. Some horses also develop laminitis during the episode or following acute illness.[23, 24]

Pathophysiology. Lincomycin is elaborated by an actinomycete, *Streptomyces lincolnensis,* and has largely been replaced in human medicine by its derivative, clindamycin.[25] Although no reports of equine toxicosis involving clindamycin were found, the antibiotic should be considered potentially toxic to horses because of its similarity to its parent compound, lincomycin. The oral minimal toxic dose of lincomycin in horses has not been established, but in one report, a dosage of less than 0.5 mg/kg body weight daily for 2 days caused clinical illness.[24]

Several mechanisms have been suggested to cause the necrotic and pseudomembranous lesions seen in the colon of affected horses. These have included bacterial overgrowth of certain pathogens, particularly *Salmonella, Clostridium*

perfringens, and *Clostridium difficile*; direct toxic action of the antibiotic; and a hypersensitivity reaction to the drug.[23, 24, 26] It is now thought that overgrowth of *C. difficile* is the primary reason for the toxic signs seen in humans.[25] Since these drugs have the potential to disrupt the normal cecal and colonic microflora, it has been suggested that their toxicity may involve colonization and invasion of the colon by pathogenic bacteria and release of bacterial toxins.[26]

Diagnosis and Treatment. A history of exposure to lincomycin, accompanied by a delayed onset of acute diarrhea and signs of endotoxic shock, suggest possible toxicosis.[23] Signs of colitis and endotoxemia from other causes are similar to those seen with lincomycin and clindamycin. Feed can be analyzed for lincomycin content.

Specific antidotes are not available. The suspect feed should be immediately removed, and affected horses should be treated symptomatically. Evacuation of the bowel by use of laxatives, and orally administered gastrointestinal protectants may be useful to prevent further colonization and invasion of pathogenic bacteria. Maintenance of fluid volume and normal electrolyte and acid-base concentrations should be accomplished by appropriate means. Other specific therapies for acute colitis, endotoxemia, and laminitis may be found elsewhere in this book.

Other Antibiotics

The oral administration of certain other antibiotics is also reported to induce colitis in horses. The use of trimethoprim-sulfa and erythromycin base has been associated with diarrhea in a small number of horses.[26] The mechanism whereby they induce colitis may also be related to their ability to alter normal intestinal microflora and allow overgrowth of pathogenic bacteria.

Imidocarb

Imidocarb diproprionate has been used for treatment of *Babesia* infections in horses. The recommended dose for *Babesia caballi* is 2 mg/kg IM for each of 2 consecutive days. *Babesia equi* is more difficult to eliminate from the horse and a dosage of 4 mg/kg IM at 72-hour intervals for a total of five injections is recommended. However, even this high dosage cannot be relied upon to eradicate *B. equi.* Higher doses than this are usually toxic to the animal.[27, 28]

Clinical Signs. The clinical signs of toxicity are dose-dependent. All horses given an intramuscular dose of 4 mg/kg exhibited signs of parasympathetic stimulation characterized by lacrimation, excessive sweating, and serous nasal discharge for 30 minutes after treatment.[27] Larger doses, including 16 mg/kg and 32 mg/kg, resulted in horses showing pronounced systemic signs of violent peristalsis and projectile diarrhea, colic, dyspnea, miosis, and depression leading to recumbency for 1 to 4 hours following treatment. Subsequently these horses became anorectic 1 to 2 days following injection. Local swelling at the injection site is almost always present. Fatal intoxications induced profound depression prior to coma and death. The median lethal dose

LD_{50} was determined to be approximately 16 mg/kg, with mortalities occurring within 6 days of the first injection.[27]

Pathophysiology. It has been proposed that imidocarb exerts its parasympathomimetic activity by inhibiting cholinesterase.[27] Imidocarb is rapidly absorbed from muscle, is disseminated widely in tissues, but selectively concentrates in the CNS, kidney, and liver. It causes diffuse, acute necrosis of the proximal convoluted tubules in the kidney and hepatocellular necrosis and biliary stasis in the liver. The degree of hepatic and renal damage is dose-dependent.[27] The toxic mechanism at the cellular level has not been elucidated.

Diagnosis and Treatment. Diagnosis of toxicity must be consistent with exposure to the drug. Certain clinicopathologic abnormalities are common in affected horses. Laboratory evidence of hepatic and renal damage is evidenced by increased serum concentrations of aspartate aminotransferase (AST), sorbitol dehydrogenase, and urea nitrogen. Elevated creatine kinase (CK) concentration in serum is probably a reflection of the myositis that develops at the injection site.[27]

There is no specific antidote for imidocarb toxicity. Therapy is largely symptomatic and must be aimed at supportive therapy for the liver and kidney. Since the toxicity is dose-dependent, no therapy is effective for horses receiving a lethal dose of greater than 16 mg/kg body weight.

Atropine

Atropine is a commonly used medication in equine practice, in both diagnosis and treatment of a variety of disorders. Toxicity from atropine administration is most likely to result from its physiologic effects on the different body organs and systems, rather than any toxic effect of atropine itself. Complications of excessive atropine administration principally involve abnormal function of the gastrointestinal system.

Clinical Signs. Clinical signs of atropine overdose in the horse essentially are those of colic.[29] Reduced gastrointestinal motility and ileus may lead to signs of severe abdominal pain characterized by sweating, pawing or kicking at the abdomen, attempts to lie down and roll, and so forth. The severity of signs is dependent upon the amount and degree of gaseous distention of the bowel, the tolerance of the horse to painful stimuli, and any complication associated with severely distended bowel impinging upon or affecting another organ or tissue. Reduced motility may be present for several hours. If secondary problems are avoided, the horse usually returns to normal within 12 to 24 hours.

Pathophysiology. Atropine interacts with muscarinic receptors of effector cells, and by competitive antagonism prevents acetylcholine from affixing to the receptor area. The net effect is that physiologic responses to parasympathetic nerve stimulation are attenuated or abolished. Although atropine acts immediately distal to all postganglionic cholinergic nerve endings, the net pharmacologic effect in a particular organ is influenced by the relative dominance of sympathetic or parasympathetic tone in that organ. Salivary and sweat glands are susceptible to small doses of atropine, and increasing dosages are required for a vagolytic effect on the heart and for relaxation of gastrointestinal and urinary tract smooth muscle.

Diagnosis and Treatment. Most cases of atropine toxicity occur when the drug is being used therapeutically. Therefore, the primary treatment should be withdrawal or reduced administration of the drug, and treatment of any secondary complications of sympathetic nervous stimulation, if necessary. Unless horses become violently painful because of gastrointestinal gas distention, withdrawal of the drug until symptoms subside is usually all that is necessary. Since atropine blockade of muscarinic sites of cardiac muscle, smooth muscle, and glands is due to competitive antagonism, large doses of acetylcholine or other cholinomimetic drugs may overcome the inhibitory effects of atropine at these sites.

Dioctyl Sodium Sulfosuccinate (DSS)

DSS is an anionic surface active agent that is commonly used for treatment of constipation and intestinal impaction in horses. The recommended dose of DSS is 17 to 66 mg/kg with a maximum dose of 200 mg/kg.[30, 31]

Clinical Signs. Signs of overdose commence within 60 to 120 minutes in affected horses. Initial signs are restlessness and increased intestinal sounds accompanied by steadily increasing heart and respiratory rates. Abdominal pain, watery diarrhea, and dehydration become apparent afterward, and horses gradually deteriorate to lateral recumbency and death within 14 to 72 hours.

Pathophysiology. Much information about the pharmacologic action of DSS remains uncertain.[32] The primary organ of involvement is the small intestine, where epithelial denudation, villous atrophy, and submucosal edema and congestion occur. It has been suggested that DSS could cause epithelial detachment by lowering the surface tension on the basement membranes of intestinal epithelial cells.[31] Once detachment occurs, there is extreme loss of fluid and electrolytes into the intestinal lumen. The absorptive capacity of the epithelium is lost and the osmotic effect of intestinal content causes further loss of fluid into the lumen. With extensive mucosal damage, the horse also becomes much more susceptible to endotoxemia. The rapid death in affected animals is due to hypovolemic shock, endotoxemia, and circulatory collapse as a consequence of the loss of fluids and electrolytes into the intestinal lumen.

Diagnosis and Treatment. Diagnosis of DSS toxicity is dependent upon observation of the above clinical signs in conjunction with oral DSS administration. There is no specific antidote for DSS, and once clinical signs commence, treatment is aimed at circulatory support and combating the effects of systemic endotoxin. Specific treatment for circulatory collapse and endotoxemia is covered elsewhere, but medications that might be useful include polyionic electrolyte solutions, electrolyte supplementation, corticosteroids, nonsteroidal anti-inflammatory agents (NSAIDs), bicarbonate, and orally administered gastrointestinal protectants.

Nonsteroidal Anti-inflammatory Agents

This group of drugs is used extensively in equine practice, and until recently were thought to be relatively nontoxic. However in recent years, excessive intake of these agents has been shown to produce signs of toxicity and death. Phenylbutazone has been most widely studied, but flunixin meglumine (Banamine, Schering Corp., Kenilworth, N.J.) has also been demonstrated to have toxic effects.

The toxic dose of phenylbutazone appears to be 8 to 10 mg/kg body weight, which must be administered for several days to cause signs of toxicosis.[33–36] Dosages of 15 mg/kg or greater, when given on multiple days, can be lethal to horses, with death occurring as early as day 4 of treatment.[34] Ponies may be at greater risk of developing toxicosis, as 10 mg/kg given once-daily to ponies resulted in death of several of the animals by day 7 of administration.[35] It has been suggested that foals may be more susceptible than adult horses to developing toxicosis when phenylbutazone is given in therapeutic dosages.[37]

Flunixin meglumine appears to be less toxic than phenylbutazone, but foals given 1.1 mg/kg for 30 days developed signs of toxicosis.[38] In another study, administration of flunixin meglumine at a dosage of 6.6 mg/kg/day IV for 5 days was necessary to produce signs of toxicosis in a group of foals.[39]

Excessive intake of NSAIDs has been associated with three syndromes: (1) gastrointestinal ulceration,[33–39] (2) renal medullary crest necrosis,[34–35, 40] and (3) ulceration of only the right dorsal colon.[37, 41, 42] Phenylbutazone toxicosis has caused all three syndromes, but flunixin meglumine has been associated only with gastrointestinal lesions. Ulceration and erosion of the digestive tract almost always affect the glandular stomach, large colon, and cecum. The small intestine can be affected, but the predominant lesions tend to involve the large colon.[33–39] Extensive edema of the colonic mucosa often occurs, and may precede the development of erosions and ulcers in the large bowel. In isolated cases, only the right dorsal colon has been affected. Renal medullary crest necrosis is seen along with renal tubular epithelial cell necrosis. Renal dysfunction occurs in horses with toxicosis, and may progress to acute or chronic renal failure. In clinical situations, renal dysfunction may also be a manifestation of more prolonged use of NSAIDs, or the concurrent use of these products in horses with already compromised renal function.

The NSAIDs should be used with caution in horses that are dehydrated, hypovolemic, or have preexisting renal disease, as these animals are at greater risk of developing toxicosis. Additional factors that may increase the risk of toxicosis include concomitant use of other NSAIDs or other medications with nephrotoxic potential, and administration of phenylbutazone in amounts greater than 8.8 mg/kg/day for periods longer than 4 days.

Clinical Signs. Signs of NSAID toxicosis include anorexia, depression, colic, diarrhea, melena, weight loss, ventral and peripheral edema, petechial hemorrhages and cyanosis of mucous membranes, and ulcerations of the oral cavity and digestive tract.[33–39, 41, 42] Oral ulcerations can be extensive and can involve the tongue, hard palate, and mucocutaneous junction at the commissure of the lips. Other signs of endo-toxemia, that is, fever, impaired cardiovascular function, hemoconcentration, and neutropenia, may be present in some horses. Renal medullary crest necrosis is rarely considered a primary cause of any clinical sign, but signs of renal dysfunction can accompany some horses with NSAID toxicity. Signs of toxicity can occur as early as the second to fourth day of treatment, when excessive quantities are given.[34]

Pathophysiology. The mechanisms whereby NSAIDs cause gastrointestinal damage and ulceration are still being elucidated. These agents may exert a local irritative effect on the oral and gastrointestinal tract mucosa.[33, 37] However, the major mechanism whereby damage occurs may be by inhibition of prostaglandin synthesis in the bowel, which is necessary for normal mucosal integrity and function.

Prostaglandins are formed in various body tissues by the action of cyclooxygenase on arachidonic acid. The intermediate endoperoxides formed are then converted by specific enzymes to metabolically active prostaglandins. Within the gastrointestinal tract, prostaglandins E_1 and E_2 (PGE_1, PGE_2) are of primary importance, and exert a number of beneficial effects. They enhance mucosal microcirculatory blood flow, promote reepithelialization following mucosal injury, stimulate bicarbonate and mucous secretion at the mucosal surface, and decrease hydrochloric acid and pepsin secretions in the stomach. They also appear to have other cytoprotective properties that are elucidated by unknown mechanisms.[36, 39]

NSAIDs inhibit prostaglandin synthesis by inhibition of cyclooxygenase. Within the gastrointestinal tract mucosa, depletion of endogenous PGE_1 and PGE_2 is suggested to result in vasoconstriction of the microvasculature, leading to mucosal ischemia and subsequent ulcer formation.[36, 37] Support for this theory stems from the ability of synthetic PGE_2 to prevent mucosal injury induced by phenylbutazone administration.[36]

Arachidonic acid metabolism may have other effects on gastrointestinal tract function. Several lipoxygenase enzymes act on arachidonic acid to form leukotrienes, which have a variety of effects upon the gastrointestinal tract. These substances influence inflammatory cell chemotaxis, fluid and electrolyte secretion, vasoconstriction, and vasodilation. Therefore, the use of NSAIDs may shunt arachidonic acid metabolism toward production of these endogenous eicosanoids, as well as modify the synthesis of prostaglandins within the gastrointestinal tract and other organ systems.

A recent study proposes that phenylbutazone-induced gastrointestinal ulceration results from direct toxic injury to the mucosal microvasculature.[43] This study suggests that the initial toxic injury induced by phenylbutazone in the intestinal tract is damage to the endothelial cells of the microvasculature. As a result, vascular swelling, stagnation and occlusion of blood flow, fibrin formation, and perivascular leakage occur, with subsequent formation of edema, thrombosis, and necrosis of the mucosa. Eventually the mucosal epithelium is sloughed. This study concluded that vasoconstriction was not the primary cause of the mucosal necrosis, and that once formed, erosions and ulcers may be perpetuated by other non-prostaglandin–mediated processes such as bacterial invasion.

The mechanisms involved in production of right dorsal colon ulceration are probably similar to those involved in ulcerogenesis in other regions of the digestive tract. Why the lesion is expressed only in the right dorsal colon in some horses is unknown.

Gastrointestinal edema and ulceration are responsible for most of the clinical signs noted with NSAID toxicity. Protein loss, diarrhea, melena, abdominal pain, and endotoxemia are all directly related to abnormal gastrointestinal function induced by toxic levels of NSAIDs.

Renal medullary crest necrosis is thought to be caused by inhibition of prostaglandin synthesis within the kidney by NSAIDs.[44] PGE_2, $PGF_{2\alpha}$, prostacyclin, and thromboxane are all produced in the kidney, with greater amounts being generated in the medulla than in the cortex. The renal prostaglandins are thought to function as local vasodilators to maintain renal blood flow and glomerular filtration rate under adverse conditions, but have little or no control over basal renal blood flow and glomerular filtration rate in healthy animals. As a consequence of prostaglandin inhibition, renal medullary ischemia can occur, leading to medullary crest necrosis.[44] Dehydration and hypovolemia may play a significant role in the development of this lesion, along with concurrent phenylbutazone administration.[40]

Diagnosis and Treatment. NSAID toxicity should be suspected when compatible clinical signs are evident and the animal has a history of inappropriate drug administration. In addition, certain clinicopathologic abnormalities are fairly characteristic of NSAID toxicosis, and aid in diagnosis. Hypoproteinemia and hypoalbuminemia are hallmarks of NSAID toxicity, and serum protein concentration can become dangerously low.[33–37, 39, 41, 42] Other abnormalities that are frequently present include increased concentrations of serum urea nitrogen, creatinine, and phosphorus. Serum bilirubin and AST concentrations are occasionally elevated. Serum calcium concentration is invariably decreased and is another consistent abnormal finding. Decreased serum chloride concentration is occasionally seen, and many horses are neutropenic.[33–37]

Treatment of NSAID toxicity is largely symptomatic and directed toward the specific disorders that are present. In all cases, use of NSAIDs should be critically evaluated, and withdrawn if possible. Plasma should be administered to severely hypoproteinemic horses, and broad-spectrum antibiotic therapy may be indicated if signs of sepsis or septicemia are present. Antimicrobials with minimal to no nephrotoxic potential should be chosen, if necessary. Fluid, electrolyte, and acid-base abnormalities should be corrected, but caution should be used when giving fluids to an already hypoproteinemic horse. Treatment of gastric ulceration, endotoxemia, and renal failure are discussed elsewhere.

Miscellaneous Agents

Arsenic

Arsenicals are found in a number of products, including insecticides, herbicides, defoliants, rodenticides, livestock dips, medications, wood preservatives, paint pigments, detergents, and certain insulation materials.[45, 46] Horses are most likely to be exposed to arsenic by eating contaminated forage.[46]

Clinical Signs. The clinical signs associated with arsenic toxicity are essentially those of a severe gastrointestinal irritant. Most toxicities are a result of inorganic forms of arsenic, and signs are similar in several animal species.

In peracute cases, the animals may be found dead with no premonitory signs. Acute signs of toxicity include severe colic, staggering, weakness, salivation, diarrhea that may contain blood or shreds of mucosa, and signs of shock that indicate cardiovascular collapse. Death usually occurs in 1 to 3 days.[45, 46] In subacute poisoning, animals may live for several days exhibiting signs of depression, anorexia, colic, diarrhea that may contain blood and mucus, polyuria followed by anuria, and subsequent shock and death. Horses that are poisoned by topical application of arsenic can show signs of blistering and edema of the skin.[45] Chronic arsenic poisoning is rarely seen in domestic animals.

Pathophysiology. Many factors play a role in the development of arsenic toxicosis in horses. In general, horses that are debilitated, weak, or dehydrated are more susceptible to toxicosis than normal animals. The formulation of the compound (trivalent arsenicals are more toxic than pentavalent forms), the solubility of the compound, the route of exposure, the rate of absorption from the gastrointestinal tract, and the rate of metabolism and excretion by the individual animal are all factors that can influence the toxicity of the various arsenic formulations.[45] The most hazardous preparations are products in which the arsenical is in a highly soluble trivalent form, usually trioxide or arsenite. Sodium arsenite is 3 to 10 times more toxic than arsenic trioxide. The average total oral lethal doses of these compounds for the horse are arsenic trioxide 10 to 45 g and sodium arsenite 1 to 3 g.[45, 46]

Soluble forms of arsenic are absorbed from all body surfaces. Less soluble arsenicals such as arsenic trioxide are poorly absorbed from the gastrointestinal tract and are essentially excreted unchanged in the feces. Following absorption, trivalent arsenic is readily excreted via the bile into the intestine, and pentavalent arsenic is excreted via the kidney.[45] Regardless of whether an introduced arsenical is in the trivalent or pentavalent form, all the major actions can be attributed to the trivalent form.[45]

All arsenicals are thought to exert their effects by reacting with sulfhydryl groups in cells. Trivalent arsenic acts primarily by combining with the two sulfhydryl groups of lipoic acid, thereby inactivating this essential cofactor necessary for the enzymatic decarboxylation of the keto acids pyruvate, ketoglutarate, and ketobutyrate. By inactivating lipoic acid, arsenic inhibits the formation of acetyl, succinyl, and propionyl coenzymes A (CoA). The net effect is the blocking of fat and carbohydrate metabolism and cellular respiration.[45, 46] Trivalent arsenic may also inactivate sulfhydryl groups of oxidative enzymes and the sulfhydryl group of glutathione and other essential monothiols and dithiols. Arsenic also causes a local corrosive action on the intestine.[46]

Arsenic seems to prefer tissues rich in oxidative enzymes such as the liver, kidney, and intestine. The capillary endothelial cells in these organs appear extremely sensitive to arsenic, because it causes a relaxation of capillaries and an increase in capillary permeability. Blood vessels with smooth muscle in their walls also dilate. In the intestinal tract, the mucosa easily sloughs away because of the accumulation of fluid in the submucosa.[46] In the kidney, renal tubular degeneration occurs.[46]

Diagnosis. The clinical signs described above should cause inorganic arsenic poisoning to be considered. Antemortem laboratory findings are consistent with gastrointestinal, hepatic, and renal damage. Feces may contain blood, mucus, and increased numbers of white blood cells (WBCs). The liver enzymes sorbitol dehydrogenase, lactate dehydrogenase (LDH), AST, and γ-glutamyltransferase (GGT) may be increased in serum, and urine might contain protein, RBCs, and casts. Urine arsenic concentration in affected animals often exceeds 2 ppm.[45]

Postmortem findings are fairly characteristic of a severe gastroenteritis and may include hepatic lipidosis and necrosis. In suspect horses, liver, kidney, stomach and intestinal contents, and urine should be evaluated for arsenic content. Blood and milk can also be tested. Levels above 10 ppm are confirmatory of arsenic toxicosis.[45]

Treatment. Specific therapy for arsenic toxicity is dimercaprol (BAL). This chelating agent forms a relatively nontoxic and easily excretable complex with arsenic. However, dimercaprol may mobilize stored arsenic in tissues and cause an initial exacerbation of clinical signs by allowing more arsenic to circulate to the intestine and liver. BAL can also be toxic if overdosed. Signs of overdosage include tremors, convulsions, coma, and death. In horses, the recommended dose is 3 mg/kg IM as a 5% solution in a 10% solution of benzyl benzoate in peanut oil. This dose is given every 4 hours for the first 2 days, every 6 hours on the third day, and twice-daily for the next 10 days until recovery.[46]

Sodium thiosulfate has also been advocated for treatment of arsenic toxicosis, but its efficacy is questionable. The recommended dose for horses is 20 to 30 g PO in 300 mL water, plus 8 to 10 g IV in a 10% to 20% solution.[46]

Symptomatic care of affected animals includes evacuation of the gastrointestinal tract with laxatives, and oral demulcents to coat the intestinal tract. Fluid, acid-base, and electrolyte indices should be evaluated and supported if necessary. Since endotoxemia may develop as a consequence of the intestinal and liver lesions, prophylactic use of flunixin meglumine at a dosage of 0.25 mg/kg t.i.d. may be beneficial. Other therapy to prevent shock and cardiovascular collapse may also be indicated.

Petroleum Distillates

Horses are exposed to excessive amounts of crude oil or petroleum distillates primarily by contamination of rangeland with byproducts of the oil industry; or by iatrogenic application, since petroleum distillates are commonly used as carrier agents for many insecticides.

Clinical Signs. The most noted signs associated with ingestion of petroleum products are essentially those of gastrointestinal and respiratory dysfunction. Petroleum products are very irritating to mucous membranes, hence, prominent signs of gastrointestinal dysfunction might include salivation and fluid feces. The feces may actually contain oil or oily substances. Chronically affected animals may also exhibit anorexia and weight loss over several days' to weeks' duration.

Signs of respiratory dysfunction are a common manifestation of petroleum toxicity. Aspiration of the oil or fumes is very irritating to pulmonary tissue, and aspiration pneumonia is probably the most serious consequence of petroleum toxicity.[47] Signs of toxicity include increased respirations, anorexia, depression, weight loss, a variable degree of fever, and possibly increased nasal discharge.

Products that are inadvertently applied to the skin might cause some degree of respiratory embarrassment, but they are more likely to cause signs related to the absorption of excessive lead or toxic hydrocarbons.[48] Topically applied agents may also cause signs associated with a contact irritant.

Pathophysiology. The toxicity of crude oil is correlated with the relative amounts of gasoline, naphtha, and kerosene content in the oil. Crude oil rich in these low-temperature distillates is more toxic than petroleum containing a lot of sulfur but less of the low-temperature distillates.[48] Petroleum products are very irritating to mucous membranes, and their oily nature makes them very difficult to remove from skin and mucous membranes, and virtually impossible to remove from the respiratory epithelium. Once aspirated, they serve as a focus for foreign body pneumonia that may progress to abscessing pneumonia, pleuritis and pleural effusion, and death.

Diagnosis. History of possible exposure, clinical signs, and pathophysiologic signs are very important in establishing a diagnosis.[47] Suspect contents, that is, gastrointestinal content, may be mixed with water, and if oil is present, it will float to the surface to be readily visible. Infrared spectrophotometry can sometimes be used to establish the identity of an oil.[47]

Treatment. Treatment is supportive. The gastrointestinal tract should be evacuated and protected by laxatives and demulcents. Products applied to the skin can be removed by soap and water. Aspiration pneumonia may be very frustrating to treat, and supportive care such as fluids and electrolytes, NSAIDs, and broad-spectrum antimicrobial therapy is potentially helpful.

Slaframine

Slaframine is an indole alkaloid produced by *Rhizoctonia leguminicola,* a mold that infects red clover and other legumes.[49–51] *Rhizoctonia leguminicola* is a ubiquitous soil fungus that infects certain legumes during conditions of high rainfall or humidity.[51] The toxin can survive and persist in dried and baled hay.[49]

Clinical Signs. The most consistently reported clinical sign is excessive salivation characterized by profuse, viscous, clear saliva.[51] Salivation may begin within 30 to 60 minutes after eating the affected plants, and response from one feeding may persist for up to 24 hours.[49] Other clinical signs are anorexia, polyuria, and sometimes watery diarrhea.[49] One case of abortion in an affected mare has been reported.[51] Clinical signs generally abate within 48 to 96 hours once infected hay is removed from the diet.[49]

Pathophysiology. Slaframine is apparently activated by liver microsomes following absorption. The active compound seems to have direct histaminergic effects or possibly a histamine-releasing effect. This is borne out in laboratory animal studies, in which clinical signs responded better to antihistamines than to atropine.[50]

Diagnosis. The combination of acute clinical signs of excessive salivation coupled with digestive disturbances and identification of *R. leguminicola* in forage is generally adequate to establish a diagnosis. Slaframine can be identified by chemical means, but usually such procedures are unnecessary.[49]

Treatment. No specific treatment is usually necessary. Animals generally recover uneventfully in 48 to 96 hours following withdrawal of the contaminated forage.[49] Atropine and antihistaminic therapies have both been suggested to help control clinical signs,[49, 50] but their efficacy is questionable.

Pentachlorophenol ("Penta")

Documented instances of horses becoming intoxicated with pentachlorophenol (PCP) are rare. However, since PCP is routinely used as a wood preservative, and since other domestic animals, including cattle and swine, are affected, some aspects of this toxin will be described.

The chlorophenols (which include PCP) are generally not very water-soluble, but are soluble in oils and organic solvents.[52, 53] PCP is volatile and can give off toxic vapors.[52] The chlorophenols are readily absorbed from the gastrointestinal tract, by inhalation, from intact skin, and are excreted fairly rapidly via the kidney.[52, 53]

Several factors affect the toxicity of chlorophenols. High ambient temperature, physical activity, poor body condition, oily or organic solvent vehicles, prior exposure, and hyperthyroid states all serve to enhance toxicity in humans and other animal species. Cold temperatures, antithyroid drugs, and increased amounts of body fat help to diminish their toxicity.[52]

The mechanism whereby the chlorophenols exert their toxicity involves the energy production sites of mitochondria, where they uncouple oxidative phosphorylation. The chlorophenols act at sites of adenosine triphosphate (ATP) production to decrease or block their production without blocking the electron transport chain. Free energy from the electron transport chain then is converted to body heat. As the body temperature is increased, the heat-dissipating mechanisms are overcome and metabolism is increased. The electron transport chain responds by utilizing more oxygen in an effort to produce ATP, but much of the free energy is liberated as more body heat. Eventually the oxygen demand overcomes the oxygen supply and energy reserves become depleted.[52]

Clinical signs, if observed, include fever, tachycardia, dyspnea, sweating, lethargy, incoordination, weakness, cyanosis, collapse, and death. Less severely affected animals may primarily manifest signs of hyperthermia and oxygen deficiency.[52] PCP in high doses to pregnant animals is also reported to cause embryonic and fetal deaths, but is not teratogenic.[54]

Diagnosis of PCP toxicity is associated with the combination of clinical signs and blood PCP levels above 40 ppm. There is no specific treatment, but saline diuresis has been suggested to be helpful in certain instances of human toxicosis.[54]

Chlorates

Chlorate salts (sodium or potassium chlorate) are commonly used as herbicides and defoliants. Horses become exposed by grazing areas that have been recently sprayed, or by the mistaken substitution of sodium chlorate for sodium chloride as a feed additive.

Clinical Signs. Initial signs are those of gastrointestinal irritation and include colic and diarrhea. Hematuria and hemoglobinuria are also present early in the disease course. Within hours, there are dyspnea, cyanosis, and increased respiratory effort. Death can occur suddenly without obvious symptoms.[55]

Pathophysiology. Chlorate is readily absorbed from the intestine, and once absorbed it continues to exert its damaging effects as long as it is present.[55, 56] A dose of 250 g is reported to be lethal to horses.[55]

Chlorate causes toxic changes by three different mechanisms of action. (1) it is directly irritating to the gastrointestinal tract; (2) it oxidizes hemoglobin to methemoglobin; and (3) it causes severe hemolysis by some undetermined action on erythrocyte membranes. The net effect of methemoglobinemia and hemolysis is a severe compromise in the oxygen-carrying capacity of blood, and animals may be affected severely enough to die from anoxia.[56]

Diagnosis. The prolonged, extensive methemoglobinemia found in affected animals should alert the veterinarian to the possibility of chlorate poisoning. These clinical signs should also be accompanied by a history of exposure to chlorate to form a presumptive diagnosis. Chlorate concentration in blood, urine, or tissues can be analytically determined, and since it is not normally found in animals, its presence in a suspect sample would be confirmatory of poisoning if clinical signs, history, lesions, and response to therapy also suggest this diagnosis.[56]

Treatment. Once the diagnosis is made, the chlorate source should be immediately sought and removed from the horse's environment. Methemoglobinemia is treated with methylene blue at a dose of 4.4 mg/kg given as a 1% solution by intravenous drip. This dose may be repeated in 15 to 30 minutes if clinical response is not obtained.[56, 57] Other recommended therapeutic measures include gastric lavage with 1% sodium thiosulfate, and the oral administration of intestinal protectants and demulcents.[55, 57] Blood transfusion and oxygen supplementation may be beneficial in certain instances.[56]

Pyriminil ("Vacor")

Pyriminil currently is not commercially available, but in previous years was marketed as a rodenticide. Reports of toxicosis in horses are rare,[58] and deaths due to pyriminil ingestion are not reported.[58, 59]

Clinical Signs. Reported signs in affected horses include severe muscular fasciculation, profuse sweating, dehydration, and mydriasis with a weak pupillary response.[58] Hindlimb weakness, ataxia, persistent inappetence, and abdominal pain have also been reported.[58] Hyperglycemia is a fairly consistent laboratory finding.[58, 60]

Pathophysiology. Pyriminil is absorbed from the gastrointestinal tract and excreted in the urine. It acts as a nicotinamide antagonist but its exact mechanism of action is unknown.[59–61] Pyriminil has also been shown to damage the pancreatic beta cells and to depress glucose uptake by erythrocytes.

Diagnosis. Presumptive diagnosis is based on compatible clinical signs and history of exposure to the rodenticide.

Treatment. Specific therapy for pyriminil toxicity is reported to be nicotinamide. However, its use in humans appears to be effective only when given within 1 hour of ingestion of pyriminil. The reported dosage is nicotinamide 50 to 100 mg IM every 4 hours for up to eight injections. This dosage is followed by 25 to 50 mg orally three to five times daily for 7 to 10 days.[60] Other symptomatic therapies that may be beneficial include gastric lavage and the oral administration of mineral oil and activated charcoal.[59, 60] Apparently, affected horses recover, as no deaths due to pyriminil toxicosis are recorded.

Tetrachlorodibenzodioxin (TCDD, "Dioxin")

The polychlorinated dibenzodioxins include a large number of isomers that differ chemically only in the number and location of chlorine atoms on the dioxin nucleus, but that vary greatly in their toxic potential to various animal species. Of the 75 possible isomers of polychlorinated dibenzodioxin, the specific isomer designated 2,3,7,8-tetrachlorodibenzodioxin (TCDD) is most toxic, and is generally considered the most toxic synthetic molecule known.[62] TCDD is a contaminant of certain herbicides, and is a byproduct of certain chemical manufacturing and combustion processes.[62] It is a highly stable contaminant in the environment, with a half-life in soil of about 1 year.[63]

Clinical Signs. In one reported outbreak, the initial signs began 4 days following exposure and included abdominal pain, polydipsia, anorexia, severe weight loss, alopecia, skin and oral ulcers, conjunctivitis, dependent edema, joint stiffness, and laminitis. A total of 85 horses were exposed, 58 became ill, and 43 subsequently died. The length of illness varied from 4 to 132 weeks in the terminally ill horses, with those having a heavier exposure exhibiting a shorter disease course (average of 32 weeks) than others (average of 74 weeks' duration). In addition, abortions occurred in pregnant mares, and many foals that were exposed only in utero died either at birth or shortly thereafter.[63] Other reported signs in animals include gastrointestinal hemorrhage with necrosis and ulceration of the gastrointestinal mucosa, cerebrovascular hemorrhage, hepatotoxicity, and thymic and peripheral lymph node atrophy.[62, 63]

Pathophysiology. TCDD is readily absorbed by oral and dermal routes, and following absorption appears to be retained primarily by liver and adipose tissue. The mechanism of action of TCDD in various organs in not well defined. TCDD is known to induce microsomal mixed function oxidases in liver and kidney, and hepatic δ-aminolevulinic acid synthetase and aryl hydrocarbon hydroxylase, but the role of these processes in the induction of toxicity of TCDD remains to be elucidated.[62] The mechanism whereby TCDD induces immunosuppression by causing thymic and peripheral lymph node atrophy is undetermined.

Diagnosis. A combination of the described clinical signs and possible exposure to industrial waste oil products should alert the veterinarian to the possibility of TCDD toxicity. Dioxin content in tissue can be confirmed by means of gas-liquid chromatography and mass spectroscopy, but few laboratories offer this service, and the analysis is generally expensive.[62]

A characteristic liver lesion seen at necropsy in a number of horses was microscopic evidence of bile stasis, hepatocyte necrosis, bile duct proliferation, and extensive fibrosis that was very pronounced around the central veins but minimal in the peripheral liver lobules. Other microscopic changes noted were thickened vascular walls and endothelial proliferation in the smaller blood vessels of several different organs.[63]

Treatment. No known antidote exists for TCDD toxicity once clinical signs develop. Following their onset, symptomatic and supportive care only can be offered, and every precaution should be employed to prevent laminitis. Soil and activated charcoal appear to bind strongly to TCDD and inhibit its absorption, so if known ingestion has occurred, immediate oral administration of activated charcoal may have beneficial effects by reducing the amount absorbed.[62]

Monensin

Monensin is one of several biologically active compounds categorized as ionophore antibiotics because they can form lipid-soluble complexes with specific alkali metal cations and transport them across biological membranes. Monensin is produced by the fungus *Streptomyces cinnamonensis* and is selective in transporting sodium and potassium ions between intracellular and extracellular spaces.[64–66] It is routinely used as a poultry coccidiostat and as a feed additive to improve feed efficiency in pasture and feedlot cattle. Horses are the most sensitive domestic animal to monensin toxicosis. The LD_{50} of monensin for the horse is 2 to 3 mg/kg.[64]

Clinical Signs. Several syndromes of toxicity occur and seem to be dose-related. Peracute toxicity may manifest as a progressive, severe hemoconcentration, hypovolemic shock, and death within a few hours of ingestion. The acute form of the disorder is characterized by partial-to-complete anorexia, abdominal pain, occasional watery diarrhea, intermittent profuse sweating, stiffness and progressive muscle weakness most prominent in the hindquarters, progressive ataxia, tachycardia, hypotension, dyspnea, and polyuria. Affected horses may show clinical signs for 1 to 4 days prior to death.[66] Horses surviving sublethal doses of monensin exhibit signs of reduced athletic performance, unthriftiness, and cardiac failure.[64] Cardiac arrhythmias, including atrial fibrillation and tachycardia, a prominent jugular pulse, and pleural and pericardial effusion can be seen.[64] Intravascular hemolysis may also occur to a limited degree.[65]

Pathophysiology. The primary action of monensin is selective transport of sodium and potassium ions between the intracellular and extracellular spaces. Two mechanisms have been suggested to explain the toxic action.

One theory suggests that monensin interacts with the mechanism regulating potassium entry into cell organelles, especially the mitochondria.[64] Low concentrations of monensin lead to a net accumulation of potassium within the cell, while higher doses cause a net loss of potassium from the cell.[65] Since potassium is required for ATP hydrolysis by the mitochondria, the effect of monensin might be to inhibit ATP hydrolysis in mitochondria. As a result, cell energy production is decreased and can result in loss of cell function and death.[64, 65]

The second hypothesis suggests that increased intracellular calcium concentration is the mechanism responsible for cell death. When the intracellular calcium concentration is increased, the mitochondria are forced to maintain calcium homeostasis by sequestering the excess calcium. This requires energy, which could take priority over ATP production. When the mitochondria become overloaded with calcium, oxidative phosphorylation is inhibited and less energy is produced to pump calcium out of the cell. When intracellular calcium levels reach a critical level, degradative enzymes are released, swelling of the mitochondria and sarcoplasmic reticulum occur, and cell necrosis and death follow.[64, 65]

The heart is the primary target organ of monensin toxicosis, and electron microscopic studies of acute monensin toxicosis in ponies have shown structural changes in myocardial cells consistent with severe mitochondrial damage.[67] In horses ingesting a sublethal dose of monensin, the myocardial sarcolemma is damaged, and is replaced by fibrous tissue in the healing process. Myocardial lesions are characterized microscopically by pale myofibers, loss of fiber striation, multifocal vacuolar degeneration, and scattered areas of necrosis. The end result is a structurally weakened heart that can succumb to stress and cause acute collapse of the horse.[64, 65] Other lesions that may be present in affected horses include pericardial, pleural, and peritoneal effusions; hemopericardium; and epicardial hemorrhage. Chronically affected horses may also have hepatic congestion with centrilobular necrosis and hydropic degeneration of the renal tubules.[64, 65]

Diagnosis. Monensin toxicosis should be suspected when horses show clinical signs of anorexia, muscle weakness, and heart failure, and when a possible exposure to contaminated feed has occurred. Suspect feeds can be evaluated for monensin content.

Clinicopathologic abnormalities are nonpathognomonic, but include early signs of severe hemoconcentration and dehydration in horses affected peracutely. Serum potassium and calcium may be moderately decreased in the first 12 to 16 hours, but then tend to come back to normal levels. Blood urea nitrogen (BUN) and creatinine concentrations are elevated in horses acutely affected, but return to normal in surviving animals. Other enzymes that show elevated serum activity include CK, AST, and LDH isoenzyme fractions 1 (cardiac muscle) and 2 (RBC origin). Total serum bilirubin may also be elevated.[64, 65]

Abnormal findings in urine can include a progressive decrease in urine osmolality during the initial few hours of the disease course.[64] Elevations in urinary activity of renal tubular enzymes such as GGT and N-acetylglucosaminidase might also be expected. Urinalysis abnormalities tend to correlate fairly well with the degree of renal insult, and are nonspecific indicators of renal damage.

Treatment. There is no specific antidote for monensin. Horses that have ingested a large amount should be treated early and aggressively with polyionic fluids to combat hemoconcentration and hypovolemic shock. Electrolyte and acid-base analysis should be performed, if possible, and deficiencies be corrected. Evacuation of the bowel should be attempted by use of oral laxatives such as mineral oil, and oral activated charcoal may help decrease the absorption of monensin. Affected horses should be kept as quiet and nonstressed as possible for weeks following exposure, to allow the damaged myocardium to heal.[64, 65]

Digitalis glycosides should never be used in acutely affected horses because they and monensin have been shown to be synergistic and immediately fatal to cardiac muscle cells.[65] The use of digitalis glycosides should only be used with great caution in the weeks following recovery from the toxic episode. Likewise, calcium should not be given to acutely affected horses for two reasons. Firstly, serum hypocalcemia is transitory, and serum calcium usually recovers to normal by 24 hours. Secondly, calcium can be dangerously irritating to an already injured myocardium.[65]

It must be noted that affected horses are extremely susceptible to cardiac damage, which is often permanent. It is therefore judicious to critically evaluate the cardiac function and integrity of any previously intoxicated horse that is destined to return to some form of athletic endeavor.

Lasalocid

Lasalocid is another carboxylic ionophore antibiotic. It is a fermentation product of the mold *Streptomyces lasaliensis,* and is commercially used as a poultry coccidiostat and as a feed additive to improve feed efficiency in ruminants.

Clinical Signs. The signs observed in horses given toxic amounts of lasalocid are similar to those of monensin toxicosis. Affected horses exhibited depression, ataxia, paresis, and paralysis with partial anorexia.[68] Once recumbent, some horses would rise when given assistance. Most horses that survived appeared normal 2 to 3 days following exposure. The lowest dose that caused fatality was 15 mg/kg body weight, but the LD_{50} for a single oral dose of lasalocid was estimated to be 21.5 mg/kg. Death occurred between 31 and 96 hours following oral dosing in the nonsurvivors.[68]

Results of a toxic feeding study indicated that poultry

rations containing approved concentrations of lasalocid (75–125 g/metric ton) are not toxic or lethal to horses. This study revealed that horses voluntarily reduced their feed intake with increasing amounts of lasalocid in the ration, and refused to eat the commercial premix when offered in place of their normal ration.[68]

Pathophysiology. The mechanism of action of lasalocid is thought to be similar to that of monensin. Lasalocid is the least toxic of the ionophores and differs from monensin in that it accepts both divalent and monovalent cations.[69]

Diagnosis. No signs or laboratory findings are pathognomonic for lasalocid toxicity. In suspect horses, feedstuffs can be analyzed for lasalocid content.

Abnormal laboratory findings in affected horses include hypocalcemia, hypophosphatemia, and hypokalemia early in the disease course (within 24 hours of exposure), but these values returned to normal ranges by 120 hours post ingestion. Serum activity of AST is frequently increased, as is total serum bilirubin and glucose concentrations. Occasionally BUN is increased.[68]

Treatment. Initial treatment should include removal of all suspected feed sources and the oral administration of laxatives to enhance evacuation of the gastrointestinal tract. Other nonspecific supportive care may be helpful, but horses receiving a sublethal dose will probably recover with minimal assistance. If a lethal dose is forced into an animal inadvertently, oral laxatives and adsorbents such as activated charcoal may help bind lasalocid and reduce the amount absorbed.

Salinomycin

Salinomycin is an ionophore, also marketed as a coccidiostat, that is more closely related to monensin than is lasalocid. The ionic affinity of salinomycin is predominantly to sodium and potassium, and its mode of action and cellular effects are similar to those of monensin.[70]

In one report of affected horses, the clinical signs were similar to those of the other ionophore toxicoses. The range of clinical signs included anorexia, depression, occasional sweating, colic, dyspnea, weakness, ataxia, and recumbency. Occasionally, horses showed reduced performance for several weeks following exposure, but many horses that became recumbent were humanely destroyed.[71] The clinicopathologic abnormalities exhibited by affected horses included elevated serum activities of CK, AST, and alkaline phosphatase (ALP).[71]

The diagnosis of salinomycin toxicity is hampered by the facts that none of the clinical signs are pathognomonic, and tissue samples do not reveal toxic levels. However, suspect feed and intestinal content can be assayed for the presence and quantity of salinomycin.

Treatment of affected horses is largely symptomatic, since no specific antidote is available. Evacuation of the bowel by laxatives may be helpful in reducing the amount of toxic material available for absorption. Fluid balance and electrolyte and acid-base indices should be maintained within normal ranges. Affected horses generally require an extended

convalescent period, and the possibility of a persistent cardiomyopathy should be considered.[71] Affected horses should undergo a rigorous cardiac examination prior to returning to performance events.

Cantharidin Toxicosis (Blister Beetle Toxicosis)

Cantharidin toxicosis results from ingestion of dead blister beetles that become entrapped in hay during harvesting. Essentially all reports are of horses being fed alfalfa hay or alfalfa products, but anecdotal reports of horses intoxicated by ingesting grass hay have been communicated to me. There are over 200 species of blister beetles in the continental United States, but toxicity results primarily from beetles of the genus *Epicauta*.[72]

Cantharidin is the sole toxic principle, and is contained in the hemolymph, genitalia, and possibly other tissues of the beetle. It is a highly irritating substance that causes acantholysis and vesicle formation when in contact with skin or mucous membranes. Cantharidin is absorbed from the gastrointestinal tract and rapidly excreted by the kidney. Storage of hay does not reduce the toxicity of cantharidin.[72]

Clinical Signs. The signs associated with toxicosis are many and varied, and are somewhat dose-dependent. Horses affected with a minimal dose may show only signs of depression, anorexia, and occasionally polyuria, whereas horses ingesting a lethal dose may show signs of profound shock, gastrointestinal and urinary tract irritation, myocardial dysfunction, and hypocalcemia.[72, 73] The onset and duration of clinical signs vary from hours to days, but horses that succumb to cantharidin generally die within 48 hours of onset of signs. Horses that live longer than 48 hours have a better prognosis for recovery if no complications arise.

The most commonly observed clinical signs include varying degrees of abdominal pain, anorexia, depression, and repeatedly submerging the muzzle in water or frequently drinking small amounts of water. The respiratory and cardiac rates are elevated, and cardiac contractions are occasionally forceful enough to be observed through the thoracic wall. Mucous membranes are very congested and cyanotic, and capillary refill time is prolonged. The feces may be watery in consistency but rarely contain blood or mucus. Profuse sweating is typical of horses more severely affected, and may be a sign of severe abdominal pain. Affected horses often make frequent attempts to void urine. The urine is grossly normal early in the disease course, but later may become blood-tinged or contain clots of blood. Gross hematuria, if it occurs, is usually in the later stages of the disease process. Less commonly observed signs include synchronous diaphragmatic flutter, erosions of the gingival and oral mucous membranes, and occasionally a stiff, short-strided gait similar to that seen in acute myositis. Sudden death has also been reported.[72]

Pathophysiology. The mechanism of action of cantharidin at the cellular level has not been fully elucidated. Acantholysis and vesicle formation occur as a result of disrupted cell membranes. Cantharidin does not have a direct effect on membranes, but is thought to interfere with oxidative enzymes bound to mitochondria. These enzyme systems are directly involved in active transport across the plasma membrane, and their failure results in cell death due to marked permeability changes in the cell membrane.[72]

Hypovolemic shock and pain develop rapidly in more severely affected horses. The normal transfer of fluid, nutrients, and electrolytes across the intestinal mucosa is disrupted because of the morphologic changes induced by cantharidin. Although renal tubular damage is not severe enough to cause death, changes in the renal tubular epithelium may also be related to the development of fluid, acid-base, and electrolyte abnormalities.[72, 73]

Hypoproteinemia develops later in the disease course, probably as a result of protein loss across the damaged intestinal mucosa. Protein is also lost into the peritoneal space, and a minor amount may be lost via the urine.[72]

The profound hypocalcemia and hypomagnesemia that occur in many horses have not been fully explained. Calcium loss or derangement of calcium homeostasis or a combination of both, is the most likely explanation, because the acute onset of the disease eliminates reduced intake as a possible cause. Calcium can be lost via urine, sweat, and as protein-bound calcium through the damaged intestinal wall. There may also be an influx of intracellular calcium in certain tissues. It is unknown if cantharidin has an effect on calcium binding sites on proteins or in cells.[72]

The low urine specific gravity seen in most horses may be due to decreased permeability of the collecting ducts to water. Other findings, however, point to a mild pathologic insult as a cause of the low urine specific gravity. These findings include the facts that a low specific gravity occurs suddenly within hours of toxin exposure; specific gravity returns to normal in 2 to 4 days in surviving horses; only mild to moderate changes are noted in other renal function tests; and the histologic renal lesions are mild and neither acute nor chronic renal failure is associated with cantharidin toxicosis in horses.[72]

Myocardial necrosis is a common finding in affected horses, and may be caused by the direct effect of cantharidin on cardiac muscle. Dose-related intracellular changes involving the mitochondria, cristae, nuclear chromatin, sarcoplasmic reticulum, and myofibrils have been observed in the cardiac muscle of rabbits that were given cantharidin. A proposed mechanism for these changes suggests that there is an excess transport of calcium into the myocardial cells, leading to an intracellular calcium overload. This may result in a high-energy phosphate deficiency within the cell, leading to necrosis and cell death.[72]

Diagnosis. Cantharidin toxicosis should be considered when horses exhibit signs of abdominal pain, depression, or polyuria, and their diet contains alfalfa hay or alfalfa products. The diagnosis can be made when horses have clinical signs and laboratory findings compatible with cantharidin toxicosis, and beetles are found in the hay. The beetles can be very difficult to identify in hay, so a thorough search should be made. Cantharidin can be assayed by use of high-pressure liquid chromatography and gas chromatography–mass spectrometry techniques.[72, 74] Samples to be tested are urine and stomach content from suspect horses.

Laboratory findings are nonpathognomonic, but several abnormalities are typically noted. Packed cell volume (PCV)

and serum protein concentrations are elevated early, but hypoproteinemia frequently develops after about 24 hours. Mild hypokalemia can occur, but is not a striking feature of this disease. BUN may be moderately elevated, and hyperglycemia is almost always present initially.[72]

Serum calcium and magnesium concentrations are significantly decreased in most horses, and remain low for longer than 48 hours if untreated. The urine generally contains RBCs and has a low specific gravity, even in the face of clinical dehydration. Abnormal peritoneal fluid findings include increased protein concentration, but relatively normal fibrinogen and WBC values. Feces are often positive for occult blood. Serum CK activity may be quite elevated in more severely affected horses, and augurs a poor prognosis.[72] Although not diagnostic, laboratory findings of prolonged hypocalcemia and hypomagnesemia, and elevated CK concentration may help differentiate cantharidin toxicosis from other causes of acute abdominal crisis.

Treatment. No specific antidote is available for cantharidin. Once the diagnosis is suspected, all suspect feed should be removed from the horse's environment, and hay subsequently fed to horses should be carefully examined for the presence of beetles.

Mineral oil should be given early to suspect horses. This helps in evacuation of the bowel and may also help reduce the amount of cantharidin available for absorption, since cantharidin is lipid-soluble. Activated charcoal given via nasogastric tube may also have beneficial effects.[72]

Intravenous polyionic fluids should be administered throughout the disease course, to correct dehydration and promote diuresis. Diuretics may also be given once the horse is volume-loaded. Analgesics are usually required because of the severity of the abdominal pain, and glucocorticoids may be necessary to aid in treatment of shock. Calcium gluconate should be given to elevate the serum calcium concentration, and calculated deficits of magnesium should be replaced by slow intravenous infusion.[72]

Phosphorus

Elemental phosphorus is available in red and white forms. Red phosphorus is used in manufacturing fertilizers and safety matches, and is considered inert and nontoxic.[75] White phosphorus is used as a rodenticide and is commercially available in pastes containing from 1.5% to 5.0% phosphorus. The reported toxic dose for horses is 0.5 to 2.0 g.[75]

Clinical Signs. The toxic manifestations of phosphorus poisoning are generally threefold. Initially, toxic signs commence within hours of ingestion. This is followed by a latent period of 48 hours to several days when the animal may appear recovered, and finally there is a recurrence of clinical signs, which are usually severe.

The initial signs are characterized by severe abdominal pain and gastrointestinal irritation, with occasional episodes of diarrhea. Blood may be present in feces. Cardiac arrhythmias may occur during this phase, and if the dose is sufficiently large, cyanosis, shock, incoordination, and coma can develop, and the animal may die before the second and third stages develop.[75]

The latent period may occur from 48 to 96 hours following the onset of clinical signs, and during this time period the animal may appear normal. The third stage presents as a recurrence of severe abdominal pain, and signs of liver dysfunction may become evident. Icterus and a tendency to bleed from the gingiva, stomach, intestine, or kidney may be noted.[75]

Pathophysiology. Phosphorus is absorbed from both the gastrointestinal and respiratory tracts. Although dermal exposure may cause skin irritation or burning, absorption does not occur via this route. The mechanism of action of phosphorus is unknown, but it is noted for causing irritation and necrosis of affected tissue. Phosphorus is also known to cause peripheral vasodilation.[75]

Diagnosis and Treatment. Clinicopathologic abnormalities reflect hepatic and renal damage. Hypoglycemia may be pronounced, and liver enzymes such as AST, LDH, and sorbitol dehydrogenase are elevated. Renal damage is reflected by increased BUN and creatinine. Albumin, blood, and increased concentrations of amino acids may be found in urine. The phosphorus concentration in blood is usually normal.[75] Although elemental phosphorus in tissues can be assayed, in time a large portion may be oxidized to phosphates, thereby making confirmation of poisoning difficult by chemical means.[75]

No specific antidote is available for phosphorus intoxication. Therapy is essentially symptomatic and supportive.

Thallium

Thallium is toxic to all animals, including humans, but no reports of clinical toxicosis in horses could be found in the literature. However, a dose of thallus acetate 27 mg/kg PO has been suggested as potentially lethal to horses.[76] Thallium has been used in recent years as a rodenticide, but its use is now restricted only to government agencies.

Clinical Signs. Thallium ingestion can result in acute, subacute, or chronic syndromes. In the acute form, clinical signs usually begin within 1 to 4 days of ingestion. Initial signs are those of severe gastrointestinal insult and include vomiting, severe hemorrhagic diarrhea, abdominal pain, and anorexia. Labored breathing can be seen early in the disease course, and motor paralysis and trembling may occur. Signs suggestive of renal dysfunction may also be seen.[77]

The subacute form generally manifests signs in 3 to 7 days post ingestion. Signs of gastric distress and motor disturbances are less marked than in the acute form, but they persist for a longer period of time. In this form, there is a reddening of the skin, and pustule formation. There is also a very pronounced reddening of the oral mucous membranes that seems to be unique to this particular toxicosis. Other clinical signs observed include conjunctivitis, hair loss, and crusty skin lesions. Secondary bacterial infections may also develop in affected animals.[77]

The chronic stage requires 7 to 10 days to appear. Signs of gastrointestinal and nervous system dysfunction are mild, but hair loss and dry, scaly skin become pronounced.[77]

Pathophysiology. Thallium is readily absorbed from the intestinal tract or through the skin. It is distributed in all body tissues but higher levels accumulate in the kidneys and liver. It is excreted principally in feces, and to a lesser extent in urine, and undergoes an enterohepatic cycle for resorption and excretion.[76]

Thallium is thought to combine with mitochondrial sulfhydryl enzymes at a specific, yet unknown, place in the scheme of sulfur metabolism. It therefore interferes with oxidative phosphorylation within cells. Recent evidence suggests that thallium exchanges for potassium in muscle and nerve cells primarily, and it also has a necrotizing effect on the intestinal tract, kidney, and occasionally, the brain.[76, 77]

Diagnosis. Thallium toxicosis can be suspected on the basis of clinical signs, and urine can be assayed for thallium content. The finding of thallium in tissue in any amount is diagnostic, but liver and kidney levels tend to be higher than in other tissues.

Treatment. Chelation therapy using diphenylthiocarbazone (dithizone) at a dosage of 70 mg/kg PO t.i.d. has been recommended for use in dogs.[77] However, cats react adversely to this agent. Its effect in horses is unknown.

Potassium chloride may aid in the elimination of thallium. It can be given intravenously or orally, but the oral route is contraindicated in animals that are also being treated with an ion exchange agent.

Trapping thallium in the intestine can be attempted by use of the ion exchange agent potassium ferric cyanoferrate-II (potassium-Prussian blue, PPB). Experimentally, PPB is not absorbed from the intestinal tract and acts to immobilize the thallus ion by exchanging with the potassium of PPB. Once trapped, thallium is not readily released from PPB, and fecal excretion of thallium is increased.[76, 77]

Other forms of symptomatic therapy include intestinal protectants and demulcents, fluid and electrolyte support, analgesics, oral activated charcoal, and general nursing care.[76]

TOXICOSES CAUSING SIGNS OF CENTRAL NERVOUS SYSTEM STIMULATION
Plants
Locoweed

A nervous syndrome in horses, cattle, and sheep has long been associated with eating plants of the genera *Astragalus* and *Oxytropis*. This group of plants is quite large. The *Astragalus* species that grow in North America number greater than 300. Not all species of *Astragalus* and *Oxytropis* are toxic, however, and some species make nutritious forage for livestock.[78] Some debate still exists over the taxonomy of these species, but their clinical signs are essentially the same, and they will be discussed together.

The toxic species of *Astragalus* produce three different syndromes in livestock. Some species contain nitroglycosides, which cause methemoglobinemia and competitive inhibition of certain cellular enzymes; others accumulate toxic levels of selenium; and a third group contains alkaloids that cause locoism.[78, 79] The first group of plants is of very minor importance to the horse and the selenium concentrators are discussed in the section on selenium toxicosis. Here I discuss the clinical syndrome called locoism.

The species of *Astragalus* and *Oxytropis* that induce locoism include *A. lentiginosus* (36 varieties); *A. mollissimus* (11 varieties); *A. wootonii* (2 varieties); *A. thurberi; A. nothoxys; O. sericea; O. lambertii;* and *A. soximontana.*[78] Additional *Astragalus* species incriminated in causing disease include *A. argillophilus, A. bisulcatus,* and *A. earlei.*[79] Geographically, locoweeds are found from western Canada southward, to include the western United States and northern Mexico.[78]

Clinical Signs. Locoweeds cause a number of problems in livestock, including neurologic and reproductive dysfunction, emaciation, and habituation.[78] Typical signs exhibited by affected horses include a slow staggering gait, depression, an unthrifty appearance, emaciation, muscular incoordination, and nervousness, especially when the animal is stressed. The affected horse may become solitary and hard to manage, and may have difficulty in eating and drinking. In some animals, sexual activity may become suppressed. Visual impairment also occurs in some horses, and mares ingesting locoweed during pregnancy have been known to abort or produce foals with various limb deformities.[79, 80] Horses that are chronically affected are generally useless for riding or draft purposes, because their behavior is so unpredictable.[78]

The onset of clinical signs varies from as short as 2 weeks to as long as 2 months after the horse starts to graze the plant. The plants are generally considered nonpalatable to horses, but once they start to ingest the plant, they seem to become addicted to it, and will search it out.[78] The addiction can extend to subsequent growing seasons, so clinical signs can progressively worsen in successive years if animals continue to graze the plant.[79] Affected horses can recover if feeding or grazing is discontinued before they become too emaciated, and if nutritious forage is given.[78] However, the syndrome may eventually lead to death in chronically affected horses.[79]

Pathophysiology. The indolizidine alkaloids swainsonine and swainsonine *N*-oxide have been suggested as the toxic principle in locoweeds.[79] These alkaloids were first recovered from *Swainsona* species in Australia.[78, 79] Swainsonine inhibits α-mannosidase, a lysosomal enzyme essential in the cellular metabolism of oligosaccharides. As a result, mannose-rich oligosaccharides accumulate in lysosomes and disrupt cellular function. These accumulations are seen microscopically as intracytoplasmic vacuoles.[79] Vacuolization of the renal cortical tubular cells can occur as early as 4 days after feeding of locoweed is started, and neurons of the CNS, including Purkinje cells, may show vacuolization by 8 days. The vacuoles disappear shortly after consumption ceases in the early stages of disease, but if grazing is prolonged, permanent cellular damage occurs. Continuous feeding of the plant for 30 days or longer results in vacuolization of almost all tissues of the body except skeletal and cardiac muscle.[79]

Neurologic signs are a result of vacuolization of the axons, glial cells, and Purkinje cells of the cerebellum and cerebral cortex. The weight loss and emaciation result from impairment of the liver, pancreas, thyroid, and parathyroid glands. Vacuolization of cells of the retina and decreased lacrimation are responsible for impaired vision in some animals. Vacuoles also occur in lymph nodes, placenta, testicles, and lymphocytes.[78, 79] The pathogenesis and lesions of locoism are very similar to mannosidosis, a heritable lysosomal storage disease of Angus and Murray Grey cattle.[79]

Diagnosis and Treatment. No pathognomonic test is available for diagnosis of locoism. The diagnosis should be suspected when horses show clinical signs compatible with locoism, and there is history of exposure to the plant. Laboratory testing is nonspecific and test results consistent with multiple organ dysfunction can be expected. Microscopic lesions of intracytoplasmic vacuolization in various organs, including the CNS, are compatible with a diagnosis of locoism.[78, 79] Peripheral lymphocytes that contain intracytoplasmic vacuoles are also considered indicative of locoism, if clinical signs are present.[79]

There is no effective cure for horses with chronic locoism that have had clinical signs for some time. Mild cases usually resolve in 1 to 2 weeks once ingestion ceases, so successful recovery from locoism is dependent upon early recognition of the disease syndrome, and preventing horses from further consumption of the plants. Reserpine has been suggested to be helpful in relieving some of the clinical signs of locoism in horses.[79]

"Nervous Ergotism"

There are two forms of ergotism observed in domestic animals, a nervous or convulsive form and a gangrenous form. Horses appear to be rarely affected with ergotism, but the nervous form is reported to occur much more frequently in horses than the gangrenous form.[81, 82] Ergotism is caused by a number of alkaloids contained in *Claviceps purpura,* a fungus infecting many grains, such as wheat, barley, rye, and oats, and wild grasses, such as quackgrass, smooth brome grass, wheat grass, bluegrasses, and wild rye.[81] The fungal mass, or sclerotium, replaces the seed or kernel of the plant, and may have the same general configuration of the seed, but is usually larger, dark-colored, and hard.[81] Ergotism is rarely of concern in dry seasons, but abundant fungal growth can occur during wet periods.[81] Although well-documented cases of ergotism due to *C. purpura* in horses are absent in the literature, a nervous syndrome typical of *Claviceps paspali* poisoning has been observed in horses in Australia. However, the cause of the clinical signs in these horses was suggested to have been due to the tremorogenic mycotoxins in *C. paspali* rather than the alkaloids found in ergot.[83]

Clinical Signs. Reportedly, the first sign of nervous ergotism is dizziness or an unsteady gait. This phase may be interrupted by convulsions and temporary posterior paralysis and drowsiness.[81] Other behavioral effects that have been described include incoordination, lameness, difficulty in breathing, excessive salivation, and diarrhea.[82]

Pathophysiology. Approximately 40 different alkaloids have been isolated from *C. purpura.* All of these alkaloids are derivatives of the tetracyclic compound 6-methylergoline, a lysergic acid base structurally similar to a number of biogenic amines such as dopamine, serotonin, and norepinephrine.[81, 84] The most pharmacologically potent alkaloids in ergot are ergonovine, ergotamine, ergotsine, ergocristine, ergocryptine, and ergocornine.[81] Additionally, tyrosine, tryptophan, tyramine, histamine, histidine, choline, and acetylcholine have been isolated from ergot sclerotia, but their clinical significance is uncertain.[84]

The mechanism whereby ergot alkaloids induce central nervous signs in horses has not been elucidated. Of the ergot alkaloids known to affect the nervous system in humans, bromocriptine is the prototype. Bromocriptine is a long-acting dopamine agonist that has central stimulating effects and may cause hypotension.[84] Another ergot alkaloid, isoergine (lysergic acid amide), has one-tenth the mind-altering potency of the structurally related compound lysergic acid diethylamide (LSD).[84] LSD is thought to produce hallucinations by a series of complex agonist and antagonist actions on several central monoamine neurotransmitters, particularly serotonin.[85]

Diagnosis and Treatment. The diagnosis of nervous ergotism in horses is based primarily upon clinical signs, and eliminating other causes of CNS stimulation. The ergot alkaloid content of feed can be assayed, but detailed analysis is required to determine the quantity of individual alkaloids present and their potency.[81]

No specific antidote exists for ergot alkaloid toxicity. Treatment of affected horses is largely symptomatic. Recommendations for control include the use of ergot-free feed, crop rotation, plowing deeply because shallow cultivation and seeding leave the sclerotia near the soil surface where they can germinate more readily, and mowing surrounding grasses to limit the spread of fungus into the cultivated crop.[82] Pasture grasses that may be infested with ergot should be mowed prior to the development of seed heads, since *Claviceps* replaces the seed or kernel of the plant.

Medications

Carbamates

The carbamate pesticides are composed of cyclic or aliphatic derivatives of carbamic acid, and numerous ones are commercially available.[86, 87] Carbamates are readily absorbed through the lungs, gastrointestinal tract, and skin. They do not accumulate in any particular tissue, but do cross the rat placenta, depress fetal acetylcholinesterase, and are not readily metabolized in the fetus.[87] In humans, the carbamates poorly penetrate the blood-brain barrier and therefore produce few CNS symptoms.[88] Carbamates do not require activation by liver enzymes to exert their effect. Toxicity data are not complete for several domestic animals, but lethal doses of the different compounds vary from less than 1 up to several hundred milligrams per kilogram of body weight.[87] Carbamates are not very stable in the environment and are fairly insoluble in water, but organic solvents and oils can carry the compounds across cell barriers.[87]

Clinical Signs. Clinical signs can commence within a few minutes to several hours following exposure, but are rela-

tively short-lived. The clinical episode frequently is less than 36 to 48 hours in length, with the animal either succumbing or recovering during this time period.[86, 87]

Signs of toxicity in horses are a reflection of muscarinic and nicotinic cholinergic overstimulation. The signs suggestive of muscarinic cholinergic overstimulation include profuse salivation, severe gastrointestinal disturbances characterized by hypermotility, severe pain, abdominal cramps and diarrhea, excessive lacrimation, miosis, sweating, dyspnea, cyanosis, and urinary and fecal incontinence. Affected animals may also cough frequently as a sign of excessive accumulation of respiratory tract secretions. The signs reflected by nicotinic overstimulation include excessive stimulation of the skeletal muscles. The muscles of the face, eyelids, tongue, and the general musculature may twitch. Some animals exhibit signs of generalized tetany whereby they walk in a stiff-legged fashion. This hyperactivity may be followed by weakness and paralysis of the skeletal muscles.[86]

Signs of CNS involvement in domestic food-producing animals may include hyperactivity reflective of excessive stimulation of the CNS, but domestic animals rarely exhibit convulsive seizures. CNS depression is reported to occur more commonly than CNS stimulation.[86]

Pathophysiology. Carbamates induce excessive stimulation of the parasympathetic nervous system by inhibiting both acetylcholinesterase and pseudocholinesterase. The carbamate pesticides occupy both the anionic and esteratic sites of acetylcholinesterase, with the esteratic site being carbamylated. Acetylcholinesterase can hydrolyze carbamate pesticides but at a slower rate than that for acetylcholine. Therefore, carbamates are reversible inhibitors of acetylcholinesterase but toxicosis occurs when the amount of pesticide is large enough that the rate of carbamylation of acetylcholinesterase exceeds the rate of hydrolysis of pesticide by the enzyme.[87] As a result, acetylcholine accumulates in neuroeffector and synaptic regions, resulting in the observed clinical signs of parasympathetic overstimulation.

The continuous stimulation of secretory glands leads to excessive salivation and accumulation of fluid within the respiratory tract and within the lumen of the bowel. Extensive pulmonary edema may occur and, along with bronchoconstriction, can lead to death in affected animals.[86]

Carbamates are removed from the circulation largely by spontaneous hydrolysis of the carbamate-cholinesterase complex. In addition, blood esterases can also inactivate a portion of the circulating carbamate, and certain liver microsomal enzymes break down the compounds within hours of exposure.[87, 88] The clinical signs associated with carbamate toxicity are generally rather short-lived, with recovery occurring in less than 36 to 48 hours in most animals.

Diagnosis and Treatment. Diagnosis is most likely made from a history of possible exposure, clinical signs, and response to atropine treatment. Chemical analyses of body tissue for carbamate residue are usually unrewarding, probably because of the rapid metabolism of the compound. However, finding the pesticide in stomach content or in feed samples in sufficient quantities to cause toxicosis could confirm the diagnosis.[86]

Cholinesterase activity in blood and tissue can also be used to confirm a diagnosis. However, discretion must be used when interpreting these results, as recommended therapeutic levels of carbamates applied to animals can result in some depression of blood cholinesterase activity.[86] In one author's opinion, clinical signs of acute carbamate toxicity are associated with blood cholinesterase activity of less than 20% of normal values.[86] Since the inactivation of cholinesterase by carbamates involves a much weaker and less stable binding than that by organophosphates, blood samples from suspect animals should not be diluted and they should be refrigerated and analyzed as soon as possible.[86]

Affected animals should be treated as quickly as possible. Initial therapy should consist of atropine sulfate 0.2 mg/kg body weight. This initial dose should be divided, with approximately one-fourth of the dose given intravenously and the remainder subcutaneously or intramuscularly. Repeated doses of atropine may be required, but should only be used to counteract the parasympathetic signs. The skeletal muscle tremors may not respond to atropine therapy.[86]

Oral adsorbents such as activated charcoal may be useful in binding ingested pesticide, and aqueous cathartics may further aid in evacuation of the intestinal tract. Oral mineral oil should probably not be used in suspect cases, as organic solvents and oils can carry the compound across cell barriers. Dermally exposed animals should be washed with soap and water to prevent further exposure. The oximes, such as pralidoxime (2-PAM), are of no benefit in treating carbamate toxicosis, and their use may or may not worsen the animals' condition.[86, 87]

Organophosphates

The organophosphates are increasingly being used in a variety of ways. Some of the typical uses for these compounds include animal insecticides and parasiticides; plant insecticides; soil nematocides, fungicides, herbicides, and defoliants; rodenticides; insect repellents; and chemosterilants.[89] Horses can become intoxicated in a variety of ways, since these products are so commonly used in our environment.

A wide variety of organophosphorous compounds have been developed, and their toxicity varies dramatically among compounds and among animal species. A good list of various organophosphorous compounds and their relative toxicities has been tabulated by Osweiler, et al.[86] In addition to variations in compound toxicity, a number of physicochemical factors can also affect the toxicity of organophosphorous compounds. The toxicity of these compounds decreases as they are degraded by sun, water, microbes, alkali, or metal ions such as iron or copper.[89] An increase in toxicity may occur by storage activation, a process in which highly toxic isomers of certain pesticides are formed spontaneously in polar solvents or water. This reaction is speeded by heat. Parathion, malathion, fenthion, chloropyrifos, diazinon, and coumaphos are some of the compounds that can undergo this type of storage activation.[89] The storage activation phenomena provide good reasons to use only freshly prepared preparations of organophosphate compounds on horses.

Other factors that can influence the toxicity of a particular organophosphorous compound are ambient temperature (higher temperatures may increase the toxicity of certain compounds); the vehicle in which the pesticide is dispersed; the age and sex of the animal; and the presence of other chemicals that may alter organophosphate toxicity. The combined effects of two organophosphates may be synergistic or antagonistic, and drugs that compete with organophosphates for target esterases, such as succinylcholine, phenothiazine, and procaine, may enhance organophosphate toxicity. In addition, drugs that have neuromuscular blocking properties (inhalant anesthetics, magnesium ion, certain aminoglycoside antibiotics, and the depolarizing and nondepolarizing neuromuscular blocking agents) may also enhance organophosphate toxicity.[89] The organophosphates are poorly soluble in water, but are soluble in organic solvents, fats, and oils. Oily vehicles or organic solvents can also facilitate passage of the organophosphates through the skin.[89]

Clinical Signs. Clinical signs of organophosphate toxicity are similar to those of carbamate toxicity, and essentially are those of overstimulation of the parasympathetic nervous system, skeletal muscles, and the CNS.

Overstimulation of muscarinic cholinergic sites results in profuse salivation and lacrimation; serous or seromucous nasal discharge; increased respiratory sounds resulting from bronchoconstriction and excessive bronchial secretions; profound gastrointestinal disturbances of increased motility, abdominal pain, and diarrhea; bradycardia; miosis; sweating; coughing; and frequent urination. Signs of nicotinic cholinergic overstimulation include muscle fasciculations, tremors, twitching, spasms, and a stiff or rigid gait. CNS signs frequently include anxiety, restlessness, and hyperactivity.[86, 89] If the exposure is not severe enough to result in death of the horse, several days or weeks may be required for complete recovery.[89]

Pathophysiology. Organophosphates can be absorbed from the gastrointestinal tract, lungs, or through the skin. Following absorption, they are distributed throughout the body, but do not accumulate in any particular tissue. Most of the organophosphates must be activated by hepatic microsomal oxidative enzymes before they become potent esterase inhibitors. Phosphorothiolate and the phosphate class of organophosphates do not require activation and can inhibit esterases immediately upon entry into the bloodstream.[89]

Organophosphates act as irreversible inhibitors of true cholinesterase and pseudocholinesterase in mammals. They irreversibly phosphorylate the esteratic site of cholinesterases throughout the body. As a result, endogenous acetylcholine is not inactivated. Therefore acetylcholine accumulates in neuromuscular junctions, parasympathetic postganglionic sites in smooth muscle, cardiac muscle and glands, in all autonomic ganglia, and in cholinergic synapses within the CNS. The result is overstimulation of these sites, leading to clinical signs of toxicosis.[86, 89]

Lethal amounts of organophosphates cause death by a combination of effects of nicotinic, muscarinic, and central cholinergic overstimulation or receptor paralysis. These effects include hypotension, bradycardia, bronchoconstriction and excessive bronchial secretion, inability of the respiratory muscles to work properly, cyanosis, and central respiratory depression. The animal actually dies of asphyxia.[89]

Detoxification of organophosphates is largely accomplished by serum and liver esterases. However, other enzymes in the liver and in other tissues may attack the pesticides at rates dependent upon the class of pesticide, the species, and the age of the animal. Water-soluble metabolites may be rapidly formed and the pesticide excreted quickly in the urine.[86, 89]

Diagnosis and Treatment. Diagnosis is suspected when there is a history of possible exposure within the past 48 hours, in conjunction with characteristic signs of parasympathetic overstimulation. Tests for organophosphate content in body tissues or specimens and in other suspect materials can be performed, but the process is tedious. Body specimens analyzed for organophosphate content often yield negative results because the compounds do not stay in tissues very long after the animal has been exposed.[86, 89]

A test for cholinesterase activity in blood or tissue is the most important aid in determining if an animal has been exposed to excessive amounts of a cholinesterase inhibitor. Blood cholinesterase activity values of less than 20% to 25% of normal are compatible with exposure of the animal to excess organophosphates or other cholinesterase inhibitors. It should be noted that some depression of blood cholinesterase activity occurs when therapeutic levels of organophosphates or carbamates are used, so these results need to be viewed with discretion.[86, 89]

Treatment should involve immediate use of atropine sulfate at 0.2 mg/kg body weight. Approximately one fourth of this dose should be given intravenously and the remainder subcutaneously or intramuscularly. It is usually necessary to repeat this dose at 3- to 6-hour intervals for a day or more. Since atropine does not block the nicotinic cholinergic effects, the horse may continue to show signs of muscle fasciculation or tremors.[86, 89] Atropine should be used with great discretion in the horse so as not to cause further complications such as gut stasis with atropine overdosage (see section on atropine toxicity).

The oximes, such as 2-PAM and pralidoxime chloride, act specifically on the organophosphorus-enzyme complex to free the enzyme. They also react directly with the organophosphate to form a relatively nontoxic complex that is excreted in urine. The use of these products in horses, though, may be economically unfeasible. The recommended dose varies between 20 mg/kg,[90] and 25 to 50 mg/kg given as a 20% solution intravenously over several minutes.[89] Oximes are reported to work best in the presence of atropine, so they should be given to the animal following atropine administration.[89] Treatment with the oximes can be repeated if signs reappear.[89]

Other treatment measures include removal of the source, if possible; use of orally administered activated charcoal; laxatives to aid in evacuation of the bowel; washing with soap and water if dermal exposure has occurred; and supportive therapy such as fluids and electrolyte administration, if necessary. *Drugs to be avoided in treating organophosphate toxicosis include phenothiazine tranquilizers, succinylcholine, and morphine.*[86, 89]

Chlorinated Hydrocarbons

The use of chlorinated hydrocarbon pesticides is being discontinued or severely restricted because of their persistence in the environment and their incorporation into the food chain. However, certain agents are still being used, primarily as contact insecticides and as ectoparasiticides.[90–92]

The chlorinated hydrocarbon insecticides are poorly soluble in water but soluble in organic solvents and oils. Also, oily vehicles or organic solvents can facilitate penetration of the insecticide through intact skin. This group of compounds is also characterized by volatility, so exposure to the pesticide can occur via inhalation of the vaporized compound.[92] Since these compounds accumulate in body tissues, primarily adipose tissue, signs of toxicosis can occur following repeated exposure to lesser amounts or subsequent to a single excessive dose.[90] Toxicity varies greatly among the different compounds, and Osweiler, et al.[91] have tabulated the toxicity of a number of these compounds for various animal species.

Clinical Signs. The chlorinated hydrocarbons act as diffuse stimulants or depressants of the CNS, with the onset of signs ranging from several minutes to several days following exposure. The signs displayed may be progressively severe or explosive and fulminating.[91] Initially, the animal may be hypersensitive, apprehensive, or belligerent. These behavioral aberrations may progress to abnormal posturing or frenzied or maniacal behavior. Nervous signs can begin with hypersensitivity and muscle fasciculations beginning around the head and facial area, and proceeding caudally to eventually include the hindquarters. These muscle spasms can occur intermittently or continuously. Clonic-tonic seizures often follow, which may result in death or be followed by intermittent periods of CNS depression. Autonomic manifestations of profuse salivation, mydriasis, diarrhea, urination, and bradycardia or tachycardia with arrhythmias may occur. Some animals may lose coordination and stumble while walking, walk aimlessly, or move in circles. Other signs noted may include increased rate and depth of respiration and fluid sounds in the lungs. Death may occur within minutes, hours, or days, or not at all.[90–92]

Pathophysiology. Chlorinated hydrocarbon pesticides gain entry into the body via the gastrointestinal and respiratory tracts and absorption through the skin. Once they gain entry into the bloodstream, they are thought to bind to serum lipoproteins and are distributed throughout the body. Eventually an equilibrium is reached in which the pesticide concentration varies among different body compartments. Most of the absorbed pesticide is stored in fat, but brain and fetus can also accumulate significant amounts.[91–92]

Adipose tissue is the main storage tissue for chlorinated hydrocarbons, and as such can retain some of these compounds for an extended period of time. The pesticide is also slowly mobilized from fat, which can account for the presence of the pesticide in blood and milk for weeks to months.[92]

The chlorinated hydrocarbons are broken down by liver microsomal enzymes and the pesticide and its metabolites are excreted in urine, bile, milk, and feces. This first stage of elimination is fairly rapid and may account for 40% to 50% of the compound being eliminated during the first 3 to 4 days after exposure.[92]

The exact mechanism of action of the chlorinated hydrocarbons is unknown, but they act as nonspecific stimulants of the CNS. A suggested mechanism is that the compounds easily enter neural membranes and prolong the time during which some of the sodium channels in the membrane are open during depolarization. In addition, potassium efflux from the cell is hindered. The net effect of these ion imbalances is a decreased transmembrane resting potential that causes a decreased firing threshold and an increased neuronal excitability.[92]

An increase in whole-brain free ammonia concentration and brain glutamine also occurs, but it is unknown if these changes are a cause or an effect of the sodium-potassium flux defect. However, the onset and disappearance of convulsions in animals is correlated with an increase and decrease of brain ammonia concentration.[92]

The depression produced by some chlorinated hydrocarbons may result from rapid depolarizing blockade of neurons of the reticular activating system. Excessive depolarization of the medullary neurons may be responsible for respiratory failure, which is the usual cause of death in chlorinated hydrocarbon pesticide toxicosis.[92] The muscle tremors seen in chlorinated hydrocarbon toxicosis are thought to be partly central in origin and partly caused by direct depolarizing effects on peripheral motor nerves.[92]

Diagnosis and Treatment. A tentative diagnosis can be made when animals are known to have been exposed to an insecticide and they are exhibiting signs of convulsive seizures and neuromuscular dysfunction. Tissue samples may be assayed for residues of the specific compound, but results must be interpreted with caution, as some of the compounds may be found in fat of normal animals as a result of exposure to small concentrations in the environment. However, parts per million concentrations may have diagnostic significance if history and clinical signs are consistent with chlorinated hydrocarbon poisoning. Brain concentrations of pesticide are reported to be better correlated with toxicosis than are concentrations in body fat.[92] Other suitable tissue specimens include blood, milk, liver, kidney, and gastrointestinal contents.[91]

No specific antidote is available for the chlorinated hydrocarbons, so treatment is symptomatic. Animals exhibiting convulsive seizures or neuromuscular hyperactivity can be given chloral hydrate or pentobarbital intravenously very carefully to effect. Sedative doses of these two agents should control most of the behavioral, nervous, and locomotor signs. Sedation can usually be discontinued after 24 to 48 hours.

Oral exposure should be treated with saline cathartics and an adsorbent such as activated charcoal. If exposure was via the dermal route, the animal should be thoroughly bathed with soap and water. As in all cases of pesticide toxicity, the source of contamination should be eliminated if possible.[91, 92]

Strychnine

The present-day use of strychnine is primarily as a rodenticide. Although it is available to the public through many retail outlets, instances of horses becoming intoxicated by strychnine are quite rare.[93–95] The approximate oral lethal dose for horses is 0.5 mg/kg.[93]

Clinical Signs. The clinical manifestation of strychnine toxicosis can appear as rapidly as 10 minutes to 2 hours following ingestion. Initial signs include apprehension, nervousness, and muscle stiffness. These signs are followed by violent tetanic seizures that may appear spontaneously or be initiated by stimuli such as sound, touch, or light. These tetanic spasms may vary from a few seconds to a minute or more in duration, and are characterized by extreme extensor muscle rigidity. Apnea frequently occurs during the seizure.[93, 94] Intermittent periods of relaxation occur between seizures, but become less frequent as the clinical episode progresses. In lethal cases, the convulsive seizures become more frequent until death eventually occurs during a seizure or from exhaustion and anoxia. The entire clinical episode may last less than 2 hours.[93, 94]

Additional signs that are reported in horses include sweating, incoordination, prostration, convulsions, and death within approximately 2 hours.[94]

Pathophysiology. Strychnine is rapidly absorbed from the intestinal tract, but not from the stomach. The alkaloid nature of the compound promotes its ionization within an acid medium, hence minimal absorption occurs from the stomach.[93] Once absorbed, it is readily distributed throughout the body. It does not accumulate in any given tissue, but significant concentrations occur in blood, liver, and kidney.[93, 94] Strychnine is metabolized in the liver by hepatic microsomal enzymes, and it and its metabolites are excreted in urine.[93] Excretion of strychnine is very rapid, with most of a lethal dose being eliminated within 24 hours.[94]

Glycine is an inhibitory neurotransmitter in the spinal cord and medulla which serves to "dampen" or modulate efferent motor neuron activity. The purpose of this modulating effect is to provide smooth, coordinated muscle contraction and activity that are appropriate and consistent with the requirements for locomotion and respiration. Strychnine acts to competitively antagonize glycine by blocking its uptake at postsynaptic sites on receptors in the spinal cord and brainstem. The result of this blockade is hyperexcitation of muscle groups from lack of normal inhibition. Muscle reflex activity is allowed to proceed in basically an uncontrolled manner. All striated muscles are affected, but the more powerful extensor muscles tend to predominate and produce generalized rigidity and tonic seizures.[93, 94]

Diagnosis and Treatment. Diagnosis of strychnine poisoning may be tentatively made based upon history of possible exposure, characteristic clinical signs, and a rapid recovery in animals treated in time. To confirm the diagnosis, tissue samples may be submitted for evaluation. Liver, kidney, and stomach contents are the most suitable specimens for analysis, but urine and CNS tissues may also be used.[93, 94]

Treatment of strychnine poisoning is symptomatic, since no specific antidote is available. The horse should be kept in a quiet environment with minimal stimulation. Of primary importance is maintenance of relaxation and prevention of asphyxia. Pentobarbital or chloral hydrate solutions should be given intravenously to effectively produce sedation. It is usually not required or desired to completely anesthetize the horse. Other medications have been recommended for use in dogs, and should be effective in horses as well. These include the centrally acting muscle relaxants methocarbamol 150 mg/kg IV and guaifenesin 110 mg/kg IV repeated as needed; diazepam and xylazine to control seizures; and inhalation anesthetics if necessary.[93] Oxygen therapy and assisted ventilation may be necessary in some animals.

Additional agents that may prove beneficial are activated charcoal given orally, followed by a laxative to evacuate the bowel. Acidification of urine with oral ammonium chloride 132 mg/kg may also enhance excretion of strychnine. Although toxic doses of strychnine may be depleted from the body in a very short time, relaxation and sedation may have to be maintained for 24 to 48 hours.[93]

Metaldehyde

Metaldehyde is used primarily as a molluscicide in snail and slug baits in coastal and low-lying areas. The baits are generally in the form of meal or pellets and are placed around crops or ornamental plants.[96, 97] Horses can become poisoned through inadvertent exposure to these baits. No specific toxicity studies could be found regarding horses, but it is reported that horses may be more susceptible to toxicosis than dogs, in which the acute oral LD_{50} may be as little as 60 to 100 mg/kg.[97] In two separate reports, horses died following ingestion of as little as 60 mg/kg[98] and 120 mg/kg.[99] Experimentally, a parasitized yearling colt died following exposure to 0.1 mg/kg.[99]

Clinical Signs. The clinical signs reported in horses include acute onset of signs within 1 hour following exposure, excessive sweating, profuse salivation and restlessness, hyperesthesia, incoordination, and tachycardia. Terminally, one horse exhibited violent muscle spasms just prior to death.[98] Other signs include muscle fasciculation, clonic spasms, and very rapid and deep respiratory movements.[99] Death occurs rapidly (3–5 hours) in horses exposed to a lethal amount of the substance[98, 99] and is thought to result from acute respiratory failure.[97] Reportedly, dogs also exhibit signs of convulsions and extremely elevated body temperature.[96, 97]

Pathophysiology. Metaldehyde is readily absorbed from the gastrointestinal tract. Gastric hydrochloric acid enhances its decomposition to acetaldehyde, and both metaldehyde and acetaldehyde are absorbed and readily cross the blood-brain barrier. The exact mechanism of action of metaldehyde is yet to be elucidated.[97]

Diagnosis and Treatment. A history of possible exposure to a molluscicide coupled with the appropriate clinical signs can lead to a tentative diagnosis of metaldehyde toxicity. Stomach content can be analyzed for acetaldehyde, and a formaldehyde-like odor may be present in the stomach content.[96, 97]

No antidote is available for metaldehyde. Treatment is symptomatic and aimed at sedation, removing the compound from the stomach, and supportive therapy such as maintaining proper fluid, electrolyte, and acid-base indices. Sedatives such as xylazine, acepromazine, and diazepam may be useful to control convulsive behavior. Methocarbamol may help control muscle spasms and fasciculations, and mineral oil can be given orally to aid in evacuation of the gastrointestinal tract.[96, 97]

Methiocarb

This molluscicide has been reported to cause toxicity in two horses: one died, and the other fully recovered.[100, 101] In each instance, the amount ingested was estimated to be from 100 to 125 g of a 4% w/v preparation.

Clinical Signs. The onset of signs was very rapid, beginning within a few minutes of ingestion. Muscle tremors, which became severe, and profuse sweating and salivation were noted.[101] Both horses had elevated heart and respiratory rates, and the surviving horse also exhibited signs of abdominal discomfort.[101] Clinical signs gradually lessened until they became absent approximately 12 hours following onset in the surviving horse.[101] The horse fatally intoxicated died about 12 hours after initially showing signs. Postmortem findings included severe generalized pulmonary congestion with froth accumulation in the airways, and a number of large hemorrhagic areas scattered throughout the intestinal tract.[100]

Treatment. The specific antidote for methiocarb is atropine sulfate.[100, 101] Repeated dosing may be necessary. Other suggested remedies include supportive therapy consisting of sedatives, calcium solutions, and mineral oil.[101]

4-Aminopyridine

This product is used commercially as a bird repellent that is often mixed with grain prior to its distribution. In the one reported instance of 4-aminopyridine toxicity, affected horses were exposed to corn that contained the substance.[102]

Clinical Signs. The two affected horses began showing signs of profuse sweating, severe convulsions, behavioral abnormalities, and rapid fluttering of the third eyelid. Both horses died within 2 hours of the onset of clinical signs, and about 8 hours after ingesting the contaminated corn.[102] No specific lesions were noted at necropsy. The estimated lethal dose of 4-aminopyridine for these two horses was 2 to 3 mg/kg body weight.[102]

Pathophysiology. The mechanism whereby 4-aminopyridine causes death has not been elucidated. However, this substance readily crosses the blood-brain barrier and may enhance the release of acetylcholine and other neurotransmitters from prejunctional nerve endings.[103, 104] The result is a stimulatory effect upon the CNS.

Diagnosis and Treatment. Diagnosis of suspected toxicity can be confirmed by testing the suspect material and stomach content of affected horses. High-performance liquid chromatography can be utilized to identify and quantitate 4-aminopyridine in these samples.[102] No specific antidote for 4-aminopyridine toxicity is suggested, but affected horses can be given supportive therapy and mineral oil orally to enhance evacuation of the intestinal tract. From the known mechanism of action of this compound, it would seem that CNS depressants such as phenobarbital may have some value in treating the CNS signs of affected horses. However, the efficacy of this treatment regimen has not been proved, and cannot be recommended at this time.

Levamasol

Levamasol has not gained widespread use as an equine anthelmintic, principally because of its limited efficacy in destroying strongyles, and because its toxic dose is extremely close to its therapeutic dose. Levamasol is effective, however, in eliminating lungworms, ascarids, and adult pinworms from horses. It has also been used in humans and other animal species in an attempt to enhance immune system function.

Clinical Signs. Clinical signs associated with levamasol toxicity occur within 1 hour of administration and include hyperexcitability, muscle tremors, hyperactivity, and excessive sweating and lacrimation. These signs may be followed by recumbency, but animals that recover generally appear normal by 12 hours' post exposure.[105–107] Adverse effects are more likely following subcutaneous injection than by oral drenching.[107] The toxic dose of 20 mg/kg is extremely close to the therapeutic dose of 15 mg/kg, and 20 mg/kg may cause death in some horses.[108]

Diagnosis and Treatment. The diagnosis is suspected when horses exhibit clinical signs suggestive of levamasole toxicosis, and exposure is known to have occurred. There is no specific antidote, so therapy is largely aimed at supportive care. Most animals recover uneventfully if a sublethal dose has been given.

Carbon Disulfide

Carbon disulfide is seldom used as an anthelmintic in present times, but has enjoyed widespread use in past years for treatment of infestation caused by *Parascaris equorum* and *Gastrophilus* species.[109] It is a manmade product used as a solvent for resins, pesticides, and waxes, and as an agent to remove greases. It is widely used as a fumigant to control insects in stored grain.[110] Carbon disulfide is an exceptional fat solvent, and in the pure state it is a clear, colorless volatile liquid with a sweet, aromatic odor resembling that of decaying cabbage.[110, 111] It is well absorbed through the skin and lungs and following ingestion.[110, 111]

Clinical Signs. Reported signs of acute toxicity in animals include dyspnea and cyanosis, spasmodic tremors, vascular collapse, prostration, convulsions, coma, and death.[110] Signs referable to local irritation following inhalation might include salivation and coughing. A combination product of piperazine–carbon disulfide and phenothiazine caused transitory signs of overtranquilization and unsteady gait when dosed 8 oz/45 kg body weight.[109] It was not determined if any of these effects were directly related to carbon disulfide.

Chronic exposure causes neuropsychiatric changes, peripheral neuropathies, and cranial nerve dysfunction in humans,[111] but chronic exposure in horses is unlikely.

Pathophysiology. Since carbon disulfide is a potent fat solvent, local skin contact results in erythema and pain, and prolonged contact produces chemical burns and vesiculation.[111] It is very irritating to mucous membranes when inhaled or ingested.[109, 111]

At the cellular level, carbon disulfide acts to block enzymatic processes by reacting with nucleophilic compounds including pyridoxamine, monoamine oxidase in the cerebrum, and dopamine decarboxylase. Carbon disulfide binds to microsomal enzymes, thereby reducing their activity, and produces a centrilobular hepatic necrosis. In addition, carbon disulfide chelates copper and zinc and therefore can produce disturbances in tract mineral balance.[111]

Diagnosis and Treatment. No specific diagnostic test is available for use on animals suspected of suffering from carbon disulfide toxicosis. In one report, affected animals had increased BUN and bilirubin concentrations, increased serum activities of AST and alanine aminotransferase (ALT), and increased serum cholesterol concentration. Affected horses also had depressed serum concentrations of protein-bound iodine and magnesium.[109]

In humans, the iodine-azide test is used to identify carbon disulfide metabolites in urine,[111] but the efficacy of this procedure for diagnostic use in horses is unknown.

Treatment of toxicosis primarily involves removal of the source and symptomatic care.

Miscellaneous Agents
Nicotine

Nicotine is an alkaloid contained in tobacco leaves. Although toxicosis might occur from ingestion of excessive amounts of tobacco leaves or cured tobacco in cigarettes or cigars, this route of toxicosis is probably rare in horses. Horses are more likely to be intoxicated by ingestion or exposure to the salt, nicotine sulfate.[112, 113] A concentrated solution of nicotine sulfate (Blackleaf 40) has been used to control leaf-eating insects and occasionally as a premises spray to control certain ectoparasites.[112, 114] Horses may ingest this substance from spills of the solution, from contaminated containers, or from foliage that has been sprayed with the product.[113] Topical exposure may result when horses are housed in stables where this product has been used for mite control.[114] The lethal dose of nicotine in the horse is 100 to 300 mg.[112]

Clinical Signs. The signs of nicotine toxicity are very rapid in onset, often occurring within a few minutes following exposure. Initially, the signs noted are those of cholinergic overstimulation, that is, excitement, increased respiration, and salivation. Increased peristalsis and diarrhea can also occur.[112, 114] These signs are transitory, and are rapidly followed by depression, muscle weakness and ataxia, slow and shallow respiration, and an increased heart rate. Convulsions can also occur. In fatal cases, these signs progress to collapse, coma, and death within minutes to hours following the onset of clinical signs.[112–114]

Pathophysiology. Nicotine is readily absorbed from the oral mucosa, respiratory tract, gastrointestinal tract (excluding the stomach), and through intact skin.[112, 115] If ingested, it can also exert a direct, rapid caustic action on the mucosa of the mouth and throat, esophagus, and stomach.[112] The substance is primarily metabolized in the liver, and nicotine and its metabolites are excreted in urine.[115] In humans, urinary acidification greatly enhances clearance of nicotine and its metabolites.[115]

Initially, and only for a short period of time, nicotine stimulates the autonomic nervous system ganglia, neuromuscular junctions, and some synapses in the CNS by depolarization of the postsynaptic membrane.[112, 115] With toxicosis, however, the stimulation is followed rapidly by a depolarizing-type blockade of all these nicotinic cholinergic receptors.[112, 113, 115] Large doses result in a descending paralysis of the CNS, and death is due to respiratory failure caused by paralysis of the diaphragm and chest muscles.[112, 113] The effects of a sublethal dose should diminish in a few hours.[112]

Diagnosis and Treatment. No diagnostic lesions are present at necropsy. However, the distinct odor of nicotine may be present in stomach content.[112, 113] Urine, blood, liver, kidney, and other tissues can be evaluated for nicotine content in suspect cases.[112]

Treatment often is ineffective because of the rapid course of the toxicosis. However, since no specific antidote exists for nicotine toxicity, affected horses should be treated symptomatically. If exposure has been via the dermal route, washing with soap and water is indicated.[112] Following oral exposure, affected horses can be treated with oral laxatives, tannic acid, or potassium permanganate in an attempt to reduce absorption of the toxin. Activated charcoal may also be beneficial in adsorbing residual nicotine in the intestinal tract.[112, 114] Atropine sulfate is reported to be without value in affected horses because it does not protect vital nicotinic receptors in the respiratory muscles and in the CNS from the effects of nicotine.[113] Artificial respiration becomes the only means of maintaining life once the respiratory depression reaches a critical level. This last-ditch effort usually fails.[113]

Ammonia

Ammonia toxicosis in the horse can occur in two ways: either by primary exposure to ammonia gas or by secondary metabolism of urea to ammonia within the body (see discussion of Urea Toxicity).[116, 117]

Primary exposure to toxic concentrations of ammonia gas is probably very rare in horses, even though ammonia is the air pollutant most frequently found in high concentrations in animal facilities.[116] The concentrations of ammonia found in stables may be irritating to horses, but will probably never reach lethal concentrations. Another source of ammonia toxicosis to horses might be compressed anhydrous ammonia, which is used as an agricultural fertilizer. An accidental spill or spray of anhydrous ammonia onto a horse could have disastrous results that might be lethal.[116] In humans, the odor of ammonia can be detected at a concentration of 30 ppm, eye and nasal irritation occurs near 50 ppm, and severe pulmonary dysfunction results from concentrations above 1,000 ppm. Immediate death occurs at concentrations nearing 1,500 ppm.[117]

Clinical Signs. Signs associated with low concentrations of aerial ammonia are those of irritation to the eyes and respiratory tract. Excessive tearing, shallow breathing, coughing, and nasal discharge are common findings. Higher concentra-

tions can induce laryngospasm and pulmonary edema.[117] Exposure to anhydrous ammonia can result in permanent or impaired loss of eyesight, respiratory disease, and skin burns.[116]

Pathophysiology. Ammonia is a highly water-soluble, irritating alkaline gas that causes liquefactive necrosis at high concentrations.[117] Because it is so highly water-soluble, it readily reacts with the mucous membranes of the eye and the respiratory tract.[116]

Diagnosis and Treatment. A diagnosis of aerial ammonia toxicosis is primarily based on history and physical examination findings.[116] Laboratory evaluation is of little value in establishing a diagnosis of inhalation exposure,[116] but laboratory evaluation can be useful to assess the degree of damage to the respiratory tract, and to evaluate the effectiveness of therapy.

Treatment involves removing the horse from the source of exposure. If exposure has been severe enough to result in ophthalmic or respiratory tract disease, these conditions should be treated accordingly.

Urea and Nonprotein Nitrogen Substances

Urea and other nonprotein nitrogen substances, including various ammonium salts, are added to ruminant rations as a source of nonprotein nitrogen, since ruminants can utilize these compounds to provide a large percentage of their protein nitrogen requirements. Urea has additional uses as a fertilizer and as a substitute for salt in melting snow and ice in metropolitan areas.[118, 119] Horses are only mildly susceptible to urea toxicosis and it is highly unlikely that horses would ingest sufficient urea or urea-containing feedstuffs to cause clinical signs.[118, 120] However, horses are more susceptible to toxicosis by ingestion of ammonium salts,[118] which may occur by accidental exposure to these substances. In horses, urea is lethal when ingested at a rate of 4 g/kg body weight, and ammonium salts are lethal at a dose of 1.5 g/kg body weight.[119] Urea and other nonprotein nitrogen formulations are toxic to animals simply because they are hydrolyzed to ammonia, which is responsible for causing the derangements associated with toxicosis. Therefore, urea and non-aerosol ammonia toxicosis will be considered together.

Clinical Signs. The spectrum and intensity of signs seen in ruminants with urea toxicosis are quite varied, and the same is probably true for horses. The clinical course is usually acute and very rapid, often occurring from a few minutes to a few hours following consumption.[118] Occasionally animals are found dead, or they may die quickly following signs of weakness, dyspnea, colic, and terminal tonic convulsions. Other varied signs can be present. Behavioral abnormalities such as restlessness and dullness may be present. These signs can be followed by excitement and even belligerency. Nervous signs, including hyperesthesia, tremors, and muscle twitching and spasms, can occur. Autonomic nervous system derangements can include salivation, bradycardia, hypertension, and severe colic.[119] More terminal signs can include increased and labored respirations, cardiac arrhythmias, frothing at the mouth, and cyanosis. Intermittent tonic-opisthotonic seizures can also be elicited near death.[119] The onset of signs may range from 10 minutes to 4 hours, and death may occur in a few hours to 3 to 4 days.[119]

Pathophysiology. Urea is hydrolyzed to ammonia by the action of the enzyme urease. This reaction is speeded by an alkaline pH, and in the horse these requirements are all found in the cecum. In horses, urea is absorbed from the small intestine and excreted via the urine.[120] The only urea that might contribute to toxicity in the horse would be that excessive amount that reaches the cecum and is available for hydrolysis.[120]

In normal animals, ammonia liberated from nonprotein nitrogen sources can be in the form of ammonium ion (NH_4^+). This ion is soluble but its charge prevents it from being absorbed across membranes.[119] Ammonia (NH_3), however, is also soluble, but since it lacks an ionic charge, it can readily be absorbed across membranes to enter the bloodstream.[119]

Ammonia is a normal byproduct of tissue metabolism, and in the hepatocytes it is converted to urea by the urea cycle or is incorporated into glutamic acid in the synthesis of glutamine.[119] Toxicosis occurs when the amount of ammonia absorbed into the bloodstream exceeds the horse's ability to detoxify it.[119]

The primary mechanism of ammonia toxicosis is thought to be inhibition of the citric acid cycle, but the exact mechanism by which this occurs is not known.[119] It is suggested that ammonia saturation of the glutamine-synthesizing system has an inhibitory effect on the citrate cycle, creating a decrease in its intermediates and a subsequent decrease in cellular energy production and respiration. As the citrate cycle fails, cells begin to malfunction. Cellular energy and respiration deficits may be the cause of ultrastructural damage leading to degenerative changes and eventual cell death. The role of ammonia in causing signs of encephalopathy is controversial and not well understood.[121]

Laboratory abnormalities associated with ammonia toxicosis include elevated serum potassium, phosphorus, lactic acid, glucose, and concentration of the liver enzyme AST. Urine output decreases and PCV increases as impending cardiac failure and shock ensue.[119]

The ultimate cause of death is inconsistent in urea toxicosis and poisoning by ammonium compounds. Cardiac failure may be induced by hyperkalemia, or ventricular fibrillation may result from the myocardial effects of ammonia itself.[119] Convulsions may be prolonged and responsible for fatal anoxia. Pulmonary edema may be a complicating factor in some cases. Death has also been postulated to result from asphyxiation.[119]

Diagnosis and Treatment. Animals that die of ammonia toxicosis exhibit no characteristic lesions. Generalized venous stasis and congestion of organs may be present, along with pulmonary edema and scattered petechiation and ecchymoses. A strong odor of ammonia may be present, but this is probably much more characteristic of ruminants than of monogastric animals.[119]

Clinical signs and history can be helpful in establishing a diagnosis. Laboratory evaluation for blood ammonia can be

performed, but the results must be interpreted with caution.[119] Storage of the sample, length of time between death and time of sampling, and length of time between sampling and analysis can all influence the blood ammonia concentration. Suspect tissue specimens should be frozen immediately if they are to be analyzed.[118] Suspect feeds can also be analyzed for urea or nonprotein nitrogen content.

Treatment is often unrewarding because of the rapidity of onset. There is no specific antidote for ammonia,[119] so therapy is largely symptomatic. Orally administered laxatives such as mineral oil may be beneficial. Any deficits in fluid volume or abnormalities in acid-base or electrolyte concentrations should be corrected. Horses that are convulsing should be controlled with pentobarbital. A patent airway should be maintained. Assisted ventilation, if necessary, is usually futile because of the extremely poor survival of animals affected so severely.[119]

TOXICOSES CAUSING SIGNS RELATING TO CENTRAL NERVOUS SYSTEM DEPRESSION

Plants

Black Locust (Robinia pseudoacacia)

No clinical reports of black locust toxicity were found in the literature. The tree has been described as being toxic to horses, however.[122, 123]

The toxic principle is classified as a lectin, which is present in seeds, sap, roots, wood, leaves, and bark of the plant. This lectin has been used in cytologic research because of its ability to stimulate glycoprotein biosynthesis and cell proliferation in lymphocytes of various animal species.[124] Horses may become intoxicated by ingesting the bark. Reportedly, only small amounts precipitate clinical disease.[123]

The clinical signs reported are mental depression, weakness, posterior paralysis, an irregular heart rate, pale mucous membranes, and anorexia. Abdominal discomfort and diarrhea of varying degrees may also be noted.[122, 123]

No definitive diagnostic test is available. Treatment of suspected toxicosis is largely symptomatic, and should include removal of the source, evacuation of the intestinal tract, and maintenance of normal fluid, electrolyte and acid-base indices.

Bracken Fern (Pteridium aquilinum)

Bracken fern is most commonly found in forested areas, burns, or in abandoned fields in the northern and western United States.[125] Toxicity can occur at any time of year, but horses are more likely to consume the plant in late summer and fall when other forage is scarce.[126] However, horses might also acquire a taste for the plant in pastures, or when it is incorporated in bedding. Horses can also become intoxicated from hay contaminated with large amounts of bracken fern. The entire plant is considered to be toxic.[126]

Clinical Signs. Signs of toxicosis occur after the horse has been consuming the plant for 30 to 60 days. Horses can also exhibit signs even if they have not ingested bracken fern for 2 to 3 weeks.[126] The signs most frequently reported are incoordination, which may progress to severe ataxia; postural abnormalities, including arching of the back, crouching, and a base-wide stance; muscle fasciculations, which can progress to severe tremors; and bradycardia with cardiac arrhythmias early in the disease course, but tachycardia is most prevalent terminally.[125, 126] Terminal stages of the disease are characterized by signs of opisthotonus and clonic convulsions.[125, 126] There is also one report of an affected horse showing signs of colic and acute hemolytic anemia.[127]

Pathophysiology. The agent in bracken fern that is toxic to horses is thiaminase.[125, 126] Bracken fern is also reported to contain a heat-stabile antithiamine factor,[128] a radiomimetic factor capable of inducing bone marrow suppression, and a β-glucopyranoside which may enhance the release of endogenous histamine.[125] The significance of these last two compounds in the development of toxicity in horses is unknown. Thiamine plays an integral role in carbohydrate, fat, and protein metabolism, where it acts as a cofactor in enzymatic pathways responsible for energy production. Thiamine is an important cofactor in the decarboxylation of pyruvate to acetyl CoA, which subsequently enters the tricarboxylic acid cycle.

Thiamine deficiency acts to interrupt these cellular energy processes, and also limits certain metabolic pathways available for pyruvate metabolism, resulting in the systemic accumulation of a variety of metabolites, including pyruvate and lactate.

Diagnosis and Treatment. History and clinical signs are helpful in arriving at a diagnosis. There are no pathognomonic lesions or laboratory abnormalities, but expected laboratory findings would include elevated blood pyruvate concentration and decreased plasma thiamine and RBC transketolase concentrations.[125]

Thiamine should be administered to affected horses at a dose of 0.25 to 0.5 mg/kg body weight daily either intravenously, subcutaneously, or intramuscularly for several days. Initially, thiamine can be given at a dose of 5 to 10 mg/kg IV, but this dose should be diluted in fluids and given slowly because of the frequency of adverse reactions when thiamine is given intravenously.[125] Prevention of thiamine deficiency can usually be accomplished by dietary supplementation of yeast or cereal grains.[125]

Equisetum (Equisetum arvense)

This plant, commonly called horsetail, mare's-tail, or scouring rush, has geographical distribution similar to that of bracken fern. Like bracken fern, equisetum is unpalatable to horses, and toxicosis usually results from hay contaminated with the plant.[129, 130]

Thiaminase is the toxic principle found in equisetum, and the clinical signs, pathogenesis, and treatment are virtually identical to those of bracken fern.[129, 130]

Milkweed (Asclepias species)

Several species of Asclepias have been reported to be toxic to large animals,[131, 132] but no specific reports of horses intoxicated by this plant were found. The plants are reported to be very distasteful to animals, and not commonly grazed, but the plant may become incorporated into hay.

Affected animals are reported to have a weak, rapid pulse; dyspnea; loss of muscular control; and muscular spasms. Salivation, bloating, and convulsions may also occur.[131, 132] Most animals that reach the convulsive stage die.[132]

Numerous compounds have been isolated from Asclepias species, including resinoids and cardioactive glycosides. One resinoid produces smooth muscle spasms of the gastrointestinal tract.[131] The mechanism of action of the other toxins has not been elucidated.

No specific antidote is available,[131] but supportive care, including evacuation of the gastrointestinal tract, is indicated.

White Snakeroot (Eupatorium rugosum) and Rayless Goldenrod (Isocoma wrightii)

Cases of white snakeroot intoxication have primarily been reported in the eastern half of the United States, from Michigan, south to Alabama, and eastward.[133] The toxic principle is trematol, which has been described as a fat-soluble, high-molecular-weight alcohol.[134, 135] Tremetol poisoning is reported to be most prevalent in dry years or in circumstances where animals are subjected to inadequate pasturage.[133] The toxin is slowly excreted and therefore tends to accumulate in animals grazing the plant. Because of this cumulative effect, repeated small doses can result in toxicosis, as well as a single, larger exposure to the plant. A total amount of green plant varying from 1% to 10% of body weight may be lethal to horses.[133] The toxic principle remains in the dried plant after freezing.[134] In the southwestern United States, Rayless goldenrod is the source of tremetol, and ingestion of this plant produces the same clinical syndrome as that of white snakeroot intoxication.

Clinical Signs. Depression, a stiff gait with frequent crossing of the rearlimbs, and patchy, profuse sweating seem to be the most profound signs noted with tremetol toxicity. Other, less frequently noted findings include muscle tremors, particularly of the shoulders and limbs; labored or shallow respirations; normal-to-subnormal body temperature; pupillary dilatation; cardiac arrhythmias; and darkly discolored urine.[133, 134]

The time of onset of signs can vary considerably, from less than 2 days to as long as 3 weeks after the last exposure to the plant. Most horses showing clinical signs die. Recovery is reported to be rare, and is usually prolonged and often incomplete. However, a recent report describes two horses that apparently fully recovered from suspected tremetol toxicity.[134] Death often follows the appearance of clinical signs within 1 to 3 days.[133]

Laboratory abnormalities routinely noted include hematuria, hemoglobinuria and proteinuria, mild elevations in serum ALP activity, elevated AST concentration, and marked elevation of serum CK activity. Acidosis, hyperglycemia, and glucosuria have also been documented.[133, 134]

Postmortem findings primarily consist of mild renal tubular degeneration and necrosis; nonsuppurative colitis; pulmonary congestion; increased amounts of pleural and peritoneal fluid; and moderate-to-severe centrolobular vacuolar changes in the liver. Other significant findings can include pericarditis, and extensive, patchy myocardial degeneration and necrosis. Extensive, minute epicardial hemorrhage has also been reported.[133, 134] One reported case also exhibited moderate, multifocal degeneration of skeletal muscle.[133]

Pathophysiology. The mechanism whereby tremetol causes the lesions and signs described above remains unknown.

Diagnosis and Treatment. Diagnosis of tremetol toxicity is based on observation of the described clinical signs and concurrent clinicopathologic abnormalities. Additionally, evidence that the affected horses have been exposed to white snakeroot should be present, and necropsy findings, when available, should be compatible with those described for tremetol toxicity. Isolation of tremetol from suspect samples has not been reported, and attempts at recovering the substance from blood, urine, liver, kidney, and stomach and cecal contents from affected horses have been unsuccessful.[133]

Treatment is symptomatic. The primary goal of therapy is promptly removing the horse from exposure to the plant, and providing supportive care. Evacuation of the gastrointestinal tract with laxatives such as mineral oil should be attempted. Activated charcoal has also been suggested as being beneficial in removal of the toxin.[134] Based upon observed histopathologic abnormalities, volume diuresis of affected animals seems appropriate, and maintenance of normal acid-base and serum electrolyte concentrations should be attempted. All affected horses and herdmates should be provided with adequate and suitable forage, and ample fresh water.

Yellow Star Thistle (Centauria solstitialis) and Russian Knapweed (Centauria repens)

Both yellow star thistle and Russian knapweed cause nigropallidal encephalomalacia in horses. These plants are found scattered over much of the western United States, and are most abundant in nonirrigated pastures during the dry seasons of summer and fall. Both plants have a minimal moisture requirement, and so may be the only green plants remaining in a dry season. Consequently, most poisonings occur during the summer or fall months.[136–138]

Horses apparently reject the plants when more suitable vegetation is available, as the disease does not occur in horses grazing improved pastures or grassland range.[138] However, it is reported that some horses develop a craving for the plant and selectively seek it out.[136] Horses may eat the weeds, either occasionally or frequently, without becoming ill,[138] and continuous and protracted exposure to the plants is necessary for toxicosis to develop under experimental conditions.[138] Feeding trials have shown that horses must consume an amount of weed equivalent to 59% to 200% of their body weight of yellow star thistle, and 59% to 63% of their body weight of Russian knapweed, for a period of 3 to 11 weeks of continuous feeding before clinical signs develop.[138] The plants retain their toxicity when dried and incorporated into hay.[138] All ages may be affected, but in general, younger horses seem more prone to the disease. One study reported a median age of about 2 years in affected horses.[138] Horses appear to be the only animals that develop nigropallidal encephalomalacia when exposed to these plants.

Clinical Signs. The onset of signs is always sudden, beginning with variable degrees of impairment of eating and drinking. Coordinated movements of prehension, mastication, and deglutition are often lacking. Affected horses are unable to adequately chew and propel the food to the back of the mouth. Some horses may show only faulty prehension, while others are unable to eat at all. Most horses, however, appear to be able to swallow if feed and/or water gains access to the posterior pharynx. More severely affected horses may attempt to drink by immersing their muzzle deeply into the water in an attempt to force water into the posterior pharynx.[136, 138–140]

Hypertonicity of the facial muscles is a characteristic sign, particularly when feed is offered.[136] The mouth is often held partially opened with the lips retracted, resulting in a fixed facial expression.[136, 140] The tongue may protrude from the mouth, and many horses display constant chewing movements.[136, 140]

Other characteristic signs include weight loss, mild-to-moderate depression, and yawning.[136, 140] Most horses can readily be roused from somnolence by mild stimulation. Few animals may show aimless, slow walking or circling early in the disease course. The gait is usually normal, but occasional deficits, including stiffness, slowness, ataxia, tetraparesis, and conscious proprioceptive deficits, are noted.[136, 140] In prolonged cases, a wobbly, shuffling gait may occur because of weakness.[140] Sensation and reflexes appear normal, and the animals are afebrile.[140]

Horses less severely affected may adopt unusual means of eating, by scooping feed into the mouth. These animals may survive for months, but complete recovery has not been observed in confirmed cases of the disease. In some instances, however, residual signs may become almost undetectable.[138] Death of affected horses is due to starvation and dehydration.

Pathophysiology. The pathogenesis of the lesions is unknown, but it has been postulated that these plants may either contain a specifically toxic substance, or they may lack some nutritional component necessary for the health and well-being of the horse.[139, 140] Several sesquiterpene lactones and polyacetylenes have been isolated from these plants, but their significance remains undetermined.[141]

Diagnosis and Treatment. The antemortem diagnosis of nigropallidal encephalomalacia is based largely upon observation of clinical signs, and prolonged exposure of the horse to the plants, either by grazing or by severely contaminated hay. Characteristic necropsy findings include bilaterally symmetric softening and necrosis in areas of the globus pallidus and substantia nigra. These areas are usually sharply defined and may be cavitary.[136, 140]

No known treatment exists for affected horses. Prevention is accomplished by avoiding exposure to the plant and by providing adequate, suitable forage.

Milkvetch, Timber Milkvetch (Astragalus species)

Most of the *miser* species of *Astragalus* are referred to as timber milkvetch or milkvetch. These plants are found primarily in the western United States, from northern Mexico to Canada, and are essentially a cause of toxicosis to ruminants. Horses are reported to be poisoned by this group of plants, but there are no reports of the lesions.[142]

The disease in ruminants is primarily characterized by general depression, mental dullness, incoordination, and eventual rearlimb paralysis. Respiratory distress, cyanosis, and acute collapse may also be noted. Both acute and chronic forms of the syndrome are reported.[142]

The toxic principle, referred to as miserotoxin, is a β-D-glycoside of 3-nitro-1-propanol. It is metabolized in the intestinal tract to the highly toxic compound 3-nitro-1-propanol. Miserotoxin is broken down into inorganic nitrite and a three-carbon side chain. The nitrite is responsible for producing methemoglobinemia in animals, but is not the primary cause of death.[142]

No specific antidote is recommended. Poisoning is prevented by controlling the plants with herbicides and preventing livestock from grazing the plant.

Medications

Piperazine

Piperazine has been widely used as an equine anthelmintic, particularly because of its efficacy against ascarids. Numerous derivatives, principally salts of piperazine, have been developed, and these compounds have a wide margin of safety in all animals. Chemically, piperazine is a diethylenediamine that is freely soluble in water and glycerol. It is a strong base and therefore readily absorbs water and carbon dioxide.[143]

Piperazine and its salts are readily absorbed from the anterior gastrointestinal tract. Following absorption, piperazine is partially metabolized in tissues, but approximately 30% to 40% is excreted in urine. Urinary excretion is usually complete within 24 hours. Piperazine is reported to be virtually nontoxic under ordinary circumstances for both adult horses and foals.[143]

Reports of toxicity in horses are rare, but the amount of compound necessary to produce clinical signs of toxicity apparently varies among the different piperazine salts. Foals treated with six times the normal dosage of piperazine adipate failed to show any ill effects.[144] However, foals and adult horses treated with six times the normal dosage of piperazine citrate[145] and piperazine monohydrochloride[146] showed clinical signs of toxicity. Toxicity apparently results from the inadvertent overdosage of certain of the piperazine salts.

Clinical Signs. The clinical signs of piperazine toxicity are primarily those of depression and incoordination. Horses given excessive amounts of piperazine citrate began to show clinical signs over a period of 12 to 48 hours following ingestion.[145] The horses were depressed and incoordinated. Walking produced a moderate incoordination in all legs and when standing, affected horses would sway, as if their sense of balance were adversely affected. Hyperesthesia to touch but not to sound was noted. Other findings included dilated pupils that responded slowly to light, gross muscle tremors, and constipation. All laboratory values measured were within normal limits. These included a hemogram and serum electrolyte and muscle enzyme concentrations. Appetite was initially depressed in affected horses, but returned to normal with recovery.[145]

The one horse experimentally intoxicated with piperazine monohydrochloride began showing signs of CNS depression 6 hours after treatment. By 24 hours post-treatment, the horse was very unsteady and reluctant to move. By 4 days post-treatment, the horse stood quietly in a normal stance. Anorexia was noted during the entire posttreatment period, and the horse died on the 11th day following treatment.[146]

Pathophysiology. The mechanism whereby piperazine produces its toxic effects in horses has not been elucidated. Piperazine and its derivatives have an anticholinergic action at the myoneural junction in ascarids. The resulting neuromuscular blockade produces a narcotizing or paralytic effect on the worm.[143] Whether this same mechanism is responsible for the toxic effects observed in horses remains to be proved.

Diagnosis and Treatment. Diagnosis of piperazine toxicity is dependent upon observation of clinical signs and a history of inadvertent overdosage. No laboratory values appear to be altered in affected horses, but since the drug is readily excreted in the urine, measurement of urinary piperazine concentrations would seem valuable. This procedure should be attempted early in the disease course, as urinary excretion is practically complete within 24 hours following ingestion.

No treatment other than supportive care is indicated. All horses intoxicated with piperazine citrate made a complete recovery within 2 to 3 days. The one horse that died following piperazine monohydrochloride administration was not treated, and necropsy abnormalities were only related to debilitation from prolonged anorexia.[146]

Reserpine

Reserpine is the most widely used and studied pure alkaloid prepared from the plant *Rauwolfia serpentina* and other *Rauwolfia* species.[147] The drug has found very little application in clinical veterinary medicine, but has been used in horses when a period of prolonged tranquilization lasting several days is desired.[148, 149] The therapeutic and toxic dosages of reserpine are extremely close in horses, which increases the likelihood of toxicosis even under the most judicious circumstances. An effective parenteral dose of 1 to 4 mg/450 kg body weight has been suggested, but 5 to 10 mg/450 kg has resulted in signs of toxicity.[149]

Reserpine is readily absorbed from the oral and intramuscular routes, and peak blood levels in humans are reached in 1 to 2 hours. The compound is widely distributed into a variety of tissues, including the brain, liver, spleen, kidneys, and adipose tissue. The alkaloid also localizes in the adrenergic neurons. It is metabolized in the liver and gastrointestinal tract, and approximately 6% of the dose is excreted in the urine within the first 24 hours. Up to 60% of a dose is excreted in the feces within 96 hours.[147]

Clinical signs. Signs of toxicosis in horses can occur rapidly, within 3 to 6 hours following intravenous administration.[149, 150] Initial signs include marked depression, generalized profuse sweating, and flatulence. Horses may exhibit sporadic episodes of violent colic-like behavior followed by abrupt recumbency and somnolence. Additional signs noted early in the disease course are increased gastrointestinal sounds and diarrhea, muscle trembling, sinus bradycardia, and second-degree atrioventricular (AV) blockade. Affected horses will also have miosis and ptosis of the upper eyelids, and males will develop paraphimosis.[149, 150] Signs of tranquilization will persist in affected horses until norepinephrine stores are replenished.[149] In horses experimentally intoxicated with reserpine, clinical signs had abated within 60 hours of exposure.[150]

Pathophysiology. Reserpine is a sympatholytic agent that acts at the presynaptic nerve terminal of postganglionic adrenergic neurons to cause a depletion of norepinephrine. It impairs the magnesium- and ATP-dependent uptake mechanism whereby norepinephrine is accumulated and stored in intraneuronal vesicles within the terminal sympathetic nerve endings. As a result, norepinephrine is released from granular storage sites into the neuronal cytoplasm, where it is metabolized by cytoplasmic monamine oxidase.[147, 148] Reserpine interferes with catecholamine synthesis by blocking dopamine uptake into storage vesicles, where it is enzymatically converted to norepinephrine. Reserpine also crosses the blood-brain barrier, where it causes the brain neurons to become depleted of serotonin, dopamine, and norepinephrine.[147, 148]

The end result is that norepinephrine is no longer available to cross the synaptic cleft and excite the postsynaptic membrane receptor. This transient deficiency of an adrenergic neurotransmitter allows a physiologic state to develop whereby profound parasympathetic tone predominates. Reserpine binding at the presynaptic neuron site is reversible. The prolonged effects are a result of the high lipid-solubility of the drug, which allows it to persist in the body.[147, 149]

Diagnosis and Treatment. Qualitative analysis for reserpine can be performed on serum and urine samples, but testing is not easily available at most commercial laboratories. Thin-layer or high-performance liquid chromatography is used to identify the drug, which can be detected in serum up to 5 days following a 2- to 4-mg intravenous dose.[149]

No specific antidote is available.[147] Treatment of affected horses is largely symptomatic, but pressor agents such as methamphetamine have been recommended.[149] The use of such agents should only be initiated in horses that are volume-loaded, so fluid, acid-base, and electrolyte indices should also be maintained in a normal range.

Iron

Iron toxicosis in horses usually results from iatrogenic overdose of injected or oral products given to foals, or from accidental consumption of iron-containing supplements.[151] Supplemental iron is available in injectable and oral formulations, and presently there are over 120 iron preparations on the market.[151] Iron dextrin, iron polysaccharide, iron sorbitol,

and ferric ammonium citrate are available injectable preparations. Oral formulations include such iron salts as ferris sulfate, citrate, or ammonium citrate; ferrous sulfate, chloride, glutamate, lactate, fumarate, or carbonate; or ferric phosphate with sodium citrate. Chelated iron compounds are about one-fourth as toxic as other compounds.

The toxicity of iron is least by the oral route, with intramuscular and intravenous routes being increasingly more toxic. Since most animals do not have a mechanism for iron excretion, the toxicity of iron is dependent upon the amount of iron already present in the body.

Clinical Signs. In animals, two syndromes of iron toxicosis are reported. A peracute syndrome is represented by sudden death within a few minutes to hours after injection. This syndrome may resemble an anaphylactic reaction, but the triggering mechanism is unknown. A subacute reaction characterized by progressive depression, icterus, and disorientation leading to coma and death seems to be the more typical syndrome seen in horses.[151–153]

Pathophysiology. Experimentally, 5% to 10% of oral iron is absorbed in the small intestine, primarily from the duodenum and jejunum, by a rate-limited mucosal transfer system. The ferrous forms are absorbed to a greater extent than the ferric forms, but both can be absorbed if they are in the ionized state. Phosphates will reduce the absorption of iron, and a high sugar diet will increase absorption. Once absorbed, iron is bound in serum by transferrin.[151]

Toxic doses of oral iron overwhelm the mechanism controlling absorption of iron from the intestine, resulting in massive iron absorption. Toxicity occurs when serum iron levels exceed the iron-binding capacity of transferrin. Free circulating iron then damages blood vessels, may cause erosion and ulceration of the stomach and intestine, causes hepatocellular necrosis and fatty degeneration of the myocardium, and can produce cerebral edema.[151, 154] In horses, hepatic failure appears to be the cause of death.[152]

At the cellular level, excessive iron causes extensive peroxidation of lipids in biological membranes. A resulting decline in the unsaturated:saturated fatty acid ratio leads to increased membrane rigidity, reduction of membrane potential, and increased permeability to various ions, leading to rupture of the membrane. The intracellular organelles adversely affected include the mitochondria and the lysosomal and sarcoplasmic membranes.[155] Elevated serum iron also inhibits the thrombin-induced conversion of fibrinogen to fibrin, thereby adversely affecting coagulation and enhancing any hemorrhagic process.[154] Histologically, affected livers are characterized by small size, have prominent bile duct proliferation, periportal fibrosis, and hepatocellular necrosis.[152]

Diagnosis

Measurement of serum iron concentration is the best method of confirming a diagnosis of iron toxicity.[151] In addition, a history of iron administration coupled with clinical signs and laboratory evidence of hepatocellular damage and cardiovascular collapse is highly suggestive of toxicity.

Abnormal laboratory findings include prolonged partial

thromboplastin time (PTT) and prothrombin time (PT), high concentrations of aromatic amino acids (tyrosine, phenylalanine, tryptophan, methionine), elevated plasma ammonia concentration, and increased activities of the liver-derived enzymes ALP and GGT. In addition, a high ratio of aromatic-to-branched-chain amino acids and an elevated total serum bilirubin content are often found.[152]

Treatment

Treatment of peracute iron toxicosis is usually unrewarding. Once clinical signs become evident, major organ damage is usually present. No specific treatment for horses affected with iron toxicity is known. Treatment of affected dogs has included supportive therapy with glucose and norepinephrine, and magnesium oxide given orally to help complex the ingested iron. Experimentally, a specific chelator of ferric iron, deferoxamine (Desferal, Ciba-Geigy Corp., Summit, N.J.) has been used at 0.75 mg/kg/min IV to chelate the circulating iron in dogs. This drug should be given slowly by intravenous drip because it can cause a sharp decline in blood pressure. Plasma extenders and intravenous fluids have also been used to counteract cardiovascular shock present in some dogs.[151]

In cases of human toxicosis, gastric lavage, chelating agents, and cathartics (sodium sulfate and magnesium sulfate) have all been employed. The use of oral bicarbonate solutions to decrease iron absorption is controversial, and activated charcoal is given orally to absorb the iron-deferoxamine complex, even though charcoal does not effectively bind free iron.[154]

The chelator of choice in human toxicosis is deferoxamine. It is produced by the bacteria *Streptomyces pilosis,* and is a specific chelator of ferric iron. It is given intravenously for maximum effect, and has a plasma half-life of about 1 hour. Deferoxamine is detoxified by the liver, but the iron-deferoxamine complex is excreted via the kidney.[154]

Carbon Tetrachloride

There is no current indication for carbon tetrachloride therapy in horses; therefore, toxicosis results from accidental exposure to the substance. This product is currently used in the industrial manufacture of aerosol propellants, solvents, and fluorocarbon refrigerants. It is a clear, colorless, highly volatile but nonflammable liquid that has an odor similar to that of ether. It is well absorbed by the lungs and gastrointestinal tract and is concentrated in fat stores in the body.[156]

Clinical signs. In animals, death following exposure to carbon tetrachloride occurs either peracutely, that is, within 24 hours, as a result of anesthetic depression and severe pulmonary edema, or 3 to 7 days later as a result of hepatic and renal failure.[157] The latter syndrome is most typical of farm animals exposed to carbon tetrachloride. The peracute syndrome is characterized by immediate onset of staggering and falling, with progressive narcosis, collapse, convulsions, and death following. The more typical syndrome is characterized by anorexia, depression, weakness, jaundice, and diarrhea of several days' duration. In sheep, death is usually preceded by coma. Affected animals occasionally exhibit other signs

of hepatic failure, such as photosensitization, and they are reported to be more sensitive to various environmental stressors.[157] Since carbon tetrachloride is also a potent renal tubular toxin, affected animals can exhibit signs suggestive of acute renal failure (see section on renal disease).

Pathophysiology. Carbon tetrachloride causes acute fatty degeneration of the liver by blocking the formation and release of low-density lipoproteins.[156] Carbon tetrachloride also induces hepatic necrosis, but the exact mechanism whereby this occurs has not been fully elucidated. Cleavage of the carbon-chloride bond, which is thought to proceed via the microsomal cytochrome P-450 reductase and NADPH-dependent reductive pathways, produces trichloromethyl and monoatomic chlorine-free radicals. These radicals lead to lipid peroxidation, and energy processes and protein synthesis within the endoplasmic reticulum are subsequently disrupted. Binding of these radicals to cell organelles, in addition to the lipid peroxidation, contributes to the hepatic damage.[156]

Carbon tetrachloride also produces acute tubular necrosis primarily of the proximal tubules and the loop of Henle in the kidney.[156] Inhalation of carbon tetrachloride causes immediate, acute CNS depression, and diffuse pulmonary edema.[156, 157]

Diagnosis. The diagnosis of carbon tetrachloride toxicity should be suspected when horses show clinical signs and laboratory evidence of acute hepatorenal disease, and exposure to the toxin is known to have occurred. Laboratory findings suggestive of acute hepatic dysfunction include elevations in serum activities of the liver enzymes sorbitol dehydrogenase, AST, and isoenzyme 5 of LDH.[158] Increases in plasma bile acid concentration and plasma bilirubin are also noted.[159]

Laboratory findings suggestive of renal tubular damage include elevated BUN and creatinine, and abnormal urine findings of proteinuria, casts, and occasionally blood cells. Affected horses may be expected to lose their urine concentrating ability, and urinary activity of renal tubular enzymes such as GGT and LDH should be increased early in the course. As a result of renal dysfunction, other homeostatic mechanisms are disturbed, which can lead to changes in fluid balance, acid-base disturbances, and serum electrolyte abnormalities.

Treatment. There is no specific antidote for carbon tetrachloride toxicity. Supportive therapy for acute hepatic and renal dysfunction should be initiated. (See sections on treatment of acute hepatic failure and acute renal failure.)

Propylene Glycol

Propylene glycol is used commercially as a diluent for injectable drugs, and as a glucose precursor in the treatment of hypoglycemia in ruminants. Horses may become intoxicated by the inadvertent use of propylene glycol, when it may be mistaken for a similar-appearing liquid paraffin preparation. Reports of toxicosis in horses are rare.[160, 161]

Propylene glycol has a low oral toxicity in humans. Approximately 45% of the absorbed dose is excreted unchanged via the kidney, while the remainder is metabolized by hepatic alcohol dehydrogenase to acetate, pyruvate, and lactate.[162]

Clinical Signs. Adverse signs occur within 10 to 30 minutes following a toxic dose of propylene glycol. Initial findings include salivation and profuse sweating, ataxia, depression, and tachypnea. Additional signs can include cyanosis, seizures, and coma.[160] Diarrhea has also been reported in one horse experimentally given a large dose of propylene glycol.[161] Death has occurred 1 to 3 days following ingestion of excessive amounts of the product.[160, 161]

Pathophysiology. Propylene glycol is metabolized by hepatic alcohol dehydrogenase to form acetate, lactate, and pyruvate. Following a large exposure, excessive amounts of these products accumulate, resulting in severe systemic lactic acidosis.[162] The clinical signs and toxicologic findings result from the effects of this severe acidemia on various body organs and tissues.

The acute oral LD_{50} for horses has not been established, but the doses for rats, rabbits, and dogs are 32, 18, and 9 mL/kg respectively.[160] One 450-kg horse died following intubation with 3.8 L (7.6 mL/kg) of propylene glycol,[160] but other horses have survived this dose.[161] Toxic signs were reported in horses receiving 1.9 to 7.6 L of propylene glycol, but the only death occurred in the horse getting 7.6 L.[161]

Diagnosis and Treatment

Exposure to propylene glycol can be confirmed by chemical analysis of serum and tissues, and by use of gas chromatography with flame ionization.[160] Necropsy findings associated with propylene glycol toxicosis may be minimal.[160] The horse given 7.6 L exhibited sloughing of the gastric mucosa, diffuse enterocolitis, renal congestion, and brain edema.[161] Histopathologic findings typically include hepatic necrosis, renal tubular necrosis and infarcts, myocardial perivascular edema, and pulmonary edema.[160, 161]

Since no specific antidote is available, treatment of propylene glycol toxicosis is aimed at the severe acidemia that develops, and at supportive care for the other organs and tissues that may become compromised. Sodium bicarbonate solutions should be given to treat the acidosis. Where possible, blood pH should be monitored, and bicarbonate administration adjusted according to need. Intravenous fluids should be given to aid diuresis as well as maintain normal fluid volume. Pulmonary and renal function should be thoroughly evaluated in affected horses, and precautions should be taken to prevent further pulmonary edema from developing. This may require the use of diuretics and careful monitoring of the fluid administration rate.

Serum electrolyte concentrations should be maintained in normal ranges, and oxygen therapy may be beneficial in horses exhibiting tachypnea and cyanosis. Activated charcoal has been recommended in treating human toxicosis.[162]

MISCELLANEOUS AGENTS
Triclopyr

Triclopyr is a herbicide used to control hardwood species on road rights of way, industrial sites, and forest planting sites.

Horses may become exposed to the herbicide by grazing areas that have been previously treated with the product. Spontaneously occurring instances of triclopyr toxicity were not found in the literature.

An experimental study has been conducted to determine the toxic level of triclopyr to ponies.[163] Ponies given 60 mg/kg/day for 4 days did not show any clinical sign of illness. Ponies given 300 mg/kg/day for 4 days did develop clinical signs. This study indicated that the toxic dosage in ponies was five times the estimated maximal intake for the highest recommended usage rate as a herbicide.[163] Therefore, poisoning from the proper use of this herbicide is unlikely.

Clinical Signs. Initial signs of depression and decreased gastrointestinal motility were first noticed on the fourth day of the trial. Additional signs that developed were ataxia, weakness, muscle tremors, increased respiratory rate, cyanotic mucous membranes, and normal-to-slightly elevated body temperature. Some ponies became recumbent as clinical signs progressed. Two ponies died on the fifth and sixth days of the trial and two other ponies were euthanized on the fifth day. The remaining two ponies were only mildly affected and recovered.

No significant changes were seen in clinical chemistry values. Gross necropsy lesions consisted of pale livers and pale swollen kidneys, and a few horses had excessive intestinal fluid contents. Microscopic changes were mild, and were those of nonspecific hepatosis and nephrosis.[163]

Pathophysiology. The mechanism whereby triclopyr produces clinical disease in horses has not been elucidated.

Diagnosis and Treatment. Toxicosis due to triclopyr appears highly unlikely under natural circumstances.[163, 164] Diagnosis of suspect cases is based on clinical signs and a history of exposure to the herbicide. No specific antidote is available. Supportive and symptomatic care should be given to affected individuals.

Aflatoxin

Aflatoxicosis is apparently a rarely documented disorder of horses, as evidenced by the paucity of clinical cases reported in the literature.[165–167] In reported instances, toxicosis developed in horses being fed contaminated feedstuffs, but horses have also been affected experimentally by forced feeding of aflatoxin-contaminated material.[168, 169]

Aflatoxins are toxic metabolites produced by the fungi *Aspergillus flavus* and *Aspergillus parasiticus*. These molds are ubiquitous in nature and can normally be found in stored feeds. The molds are not inherently toxigenic, but under environmental conditions of adequate temperature and humidity, the molds can grow rapidly and produce large amounts of aflatoxin. Many feedstuffs can support the growth of these molds, but cereal grains, cottonseed meal and cake, and peanuts seem to be most commonly affected.[170]

These molds produce five major aflatoxins: B1 and B2, which fluoresce blue under long-wave ultraviolet light; G1 and G2, which fluoresce green; and M1 aflatoxin, which is present in milk. Of these, B1 is the most important, because of its toxicity and because it occurs most abundantly under natural conditions.[170]

Aflatoxins are a group of polycyclic, unsaturated compounds that have a coumarin nucleus coupled to a reactive bifuran system and either a pentenone or lactone. These toxins are insoluble in water and are relatively heat-resistant. They are rapidly absorbed from the gastrointestinal tract and bound to serum albumin. Most of the toxins are removed from the bloodstream in the liver, where aflatoxins bind to macromolecules such as DNA, endoplasmic steroid-binding sites, and certain enzymes within the hepatocytes. Here, a variety of metabolites are produced at rates that vary among species. The metabolites may be either lipid-soluble or water-soluble conjugates, and are excreted in bile. At least some of the metabolites undergo an enterohepatic cycle of absorption-excretion. The aflatoxins and their metabolites are excreted in urine and feces, and complete elimination may take several days. The aflatoxins are not known to be stored in any particular tissue.[170]

Both acute and chronic aflatoxicosis are reported in a variety of animal species, including man. However, clinical reports of equine disease are primarily concerned with acute intoxication. The acute oral LD_{50} of aflatoxin B1 in horses is reported to be greater than 2 mg/kg, and for foals is 2.0 mg/kg.[170] One author reported signs of toxic hepatopathy and gastrointestinal upset in horses that consumed feed containing 2 to 50 parts per billion of aflatoxin B1.[170] Toxicity of aflatoxins is also reported to be enhanced by riboflavin, exposure to light, and a diet low in protein, choline, and vitamin B_{12}.[170]

Clinical Signs. Clinical signs associated with acute aflatoxicosis include anorexia, elevated temperature and heart and respiratory rates, ataxia, depression, lethargy, convulsions, icterus, colic and abdominal straining, bloody feces, and death. These signs were exhibited by horses experimentally intoxicated with aflatoxin at dosages of 2 to 5 mg/kg. Onset of signs began as early as 4 hours post dosing, and deaths occurred from 68 hours to 32 days' post intoxication.[166, 168, 169] An additional sign noted in a naturally occurring instance of toxicosis was subcutaneous hemorrhages.[166]

The feed concentration of aflatoxin B1 necessary to cause signs of chronic aflatoxicosis in horses has not been established,[170] and reports of chronic aflatoxicosis were not found in the literature. Signs of chronic aflatoxicosis in other species have included reduced feed efficiency, rough hair coats, anemia, anorexia, depression, mild jaundice, and occasionally abortion.[170] It should be noted that experimental trials have indicated that some horses will refuse mold-contaminated grain, and that well-fleshed animals may be at lesser risk of developing aflatoxicosis than unthrifty animals.[166, 168]

Pathophysiology. The hepatic cytotoxicity of aflatoxins is thought to be related to their binding to intracellular macromolecules. Aflatoxin B1 binds to nuclear DNA to inhibit RNA synthesis, which subsequently inhibits synthesis of intracellular enzymes and other proteins. Aflatoxin also binds to endoplasmic steroidal ribosome-binding sites, resulting in ribosomal disaggregation. Metabolites of aflatoxin B1 can also bind to cellular macromolecules, and most of the cytotoxicity of aflatoxin B1 appears to be the result of

binding of certain of these metabolites, rather than of aflatoxin B1 itself.[170] This impairment of protein synthesis and the related ability to mobilize fats is thought to cause the early lesions of hepatic necrosis and fatty degeneration of the liver seen in aflatoxicosis.[171]

It has been suggested that there may be other mechanisms responsible for the other signs and lesions noted with aflatoxicosis. Aflatoxins are known to be carcinogenic, they can be immunosuppressive, and they also can inhibit synthesis of clotting proteins. The mechanisms whereby these changes take place have not been well described.[170]

Diagnosis and Treatment. Definitive diagnosis of aflatoxicosis can be difficult because of the non-specificity of many clinical signs, and because the disease can mimic many other conditions. Experimentally intoxicated horses have elevations in serum concentrations of AST, ALT, GGT, iditol dehydrogenase, and arginase.[166, 168, 169] Other laboratory abnormalities have included hypoglycemia, hyperlipidemia, lymphopenia, and elevated PT.[165, 166, 169]

Gross necropsy lesions typically consist of variable degrees of hepatic degeneration and necrosis, visceral petechial hemorrhages, and hemorrhagic enteritis.[165, 166, 169] Other lesions noted at necropsy include encephalomalacia of the cerebral hemispheres, myocardial degeneration, fatty infiltration of the kidney, and subcutaneous and intramuscular hemorrhage.[165, 166] Histopathologic abnormalities may include fatty degeneration and necrosis of hepatocytes, bile duct hyperplasia, periportal fibrosis, and inflammatory cell infiltration into the liver. Renal lesions have included lipid accumulation in the tubular epithelial cells of the proximal tubules and protein precipitation in the tubular lumen.[165, 169]

Although metabolites of *Aspergillus* species fluoresce under ultraviolet light, the presence of fluorescence in suspect feed samples is not pathognomonic for aflatoxin. Aflatoxin can be definitively assayed in feed samples using a minicolumn technique utilizing thin-layer chromatography.[166] Aflatoxin can also be quantitated in animal tissues.[165, 169] Mold culture is nondiagnostic.[170]

Treatment is largely symptomatic and must include removal of the offending feed material, if it is still being fed. An easily digested, low fat diet containing appropriate protein has been recommended.[170] Multiple vitamin supplementation might be beneficial, and treatment of specific organ dysfunction should be initiated. In acutely intoxicated horses, charcoal administered orally has been recommended.[170] Prevention of the condition should be aimed at storing feeds in a suitable environment that discourages mold growth, and the feeding of noncontaminated feedstuffs.

Leukoencephalomalacia

Equine leukoencephalomalacia (ELEM), a sporadically occurring disease of horses, ponies, donkeys, and mules, has a worldwide distribution. The disease is usually seasonal, with most cases occurring from late fall through early spring, and most outbreaks have been associated with a dry growing period followed by a wet period.[172, 173]

This malady is caused by the mycotoxin fumonisin B1 (FB1), a metabolite of *Fusarium moniliforme*. Equidae become affected usually by ingesting *F. moniliforme*–infected corn, but the problem has also been associated with the consumption of commercially prepared diets.[172–175] Infected kernels often have a pink-to-reddish-brown discoloration, and damaged kernels and cob parts have a much greater concentration of FB1 than do undamaged kernels.[173, 175] Feeds containing less than 10 ppm FB1 have not been associated with disease, but concentrations of greater than 10 ppm can be lethal to horses.[176]

Clinical Signs. Two clinical syndromes are associated with FB1 intoxication. The more common is the classic neurotoxic syndrome, but hepatotoxicosis also occurs in some horses.[172, 173] Older animals may be more susceptible than younger animals, and clinical signs become evident approximately 3 to 4 weeks following daily ingestion of contaminated feed. Onset of signs is typically abrupt and death usually occurs within 2 to 3 days.[172, 173] Occasionally, horses are found dead with no premonitory signs.[172]

The neurologic syndrome is characterized initially by incoordination, aimless walking, intermittent anorexia, lethargy, depression, blindness, and head-pressing. These signs may be followed by hyperexcitability, belligerence, extreme agitation, profuse sweating, and delirium.[172, 173] Recumbency and clonic-tetanic convulsions may occur prior to death. Recovery from acute episodes has been reported, but some horses retain neurologic deficits.[173]

Clinical signs associated with the hepatotoxic syndrome are swelling of the lips and nose, somnolence, severe icterus and petechiae of mucous membranes, abdominal breathing, and cyanosis. Affected horses also had acute onset of clinical signs with death occurring within a few hours to days.[172, 173]

Pathophysiology. The gross lesions typical of ELEM include liquefactive necrosis and degeneration of the cerebral hemispheres, but degenerative changes also can occur in the brainstem, cerebellum, and spinal cord.[172–175] Necrotic areas can vary in size, and regions adjacent to the necrosis are often edematous and rarefied.[173, 174]

Gross hepatic lesions in affected horses are generally not pronounced. The liver may be slightly swollen, have a yellowish-brown discoloration, and contain irregular foci or nodules scattered throughout the parenchyma. Histologic abnormalities noted in the liver may include centrilobular necrosis and fibrosis, fatty infiltration of hepatocytes, portal fibrosis, biliary stasis, and bile duct proliferation.[172–174]

The mechanism(s) whereby these changes occur has not been elucidated. It has been suggested that the brain lesions are induced by smaller quantities of infected corn ingested during a long period, and that ingestion of higher quantities can produce fatal hepatotoxicosis in a shorter time.[173, 177] Several metabolites of *F. moniliforme* have been identified in feeds associated with outbreaks of ELEM. These include fusarin C, moniliformin, fusaric acid, 2-methoxy-4-ethylphenol, FB1, and fumonisin B2 (FB2).[174, 175] Toxicity information about FB2 is unknown, but moniliformin, fusaric acid, and 2-methoxy-4-ethylphenol do not produce leukoencephalomalacia when injected intravenously into donkeys.[174] Their role in the pathogenesis of the liver lesions seen in ELEM is likewise unknown. However, both the neurologic and hepatotoxic syndromes can be produced by oral and intravenous administration of FB1.[174]

Diagnosis and Treatment. The diagnosis of ELEM has largely been based on observation of clinical signs coupled with a history of exposure to moldy corn. Typical postmortem lesions, when available, confirm the diagnosis.

Clinicopathologic abnormalities are nonspecific and usually indicate some degree of liver dysfunction. Increased serum concentrations of bilirubin, AST, GGT, and LDH have been reported.[172, 174, 177] Cerebrospinal fluid (CSF) abnormalities can include increased protein and total nucleated cell counts, and an increased concentration of myelin basic protein.[173, 177]

With the recent identification of FB1 as the causative agent, however, analytic methods have been developed to assay this toxic metabolite in feed material. Suspect feed samples can be analyzed for FB1 by thin-layer chromatography, high-performance liquid chromatography or gas chromatography/mass spectroscopy. Feed containing greater than 10 ppm FB1 is not safe to feed to horses.[176] Since the disease requires a fairly prolonged exposure to infected corn, an appropriate feed sample should be submitted for analysis. Feed currently being ingested may not be contaminated with the mold.

Treatment of ELEM is largely supportive as there is no specific antidote to FB1. Horses that are hyperexcitable should be sedated to minimize injury to themselves and their handlers. Supportive therapy for hepatic dysfunction should be initiated if there is evidence of liver damage, and some horses may require forced feeding and watering if they become unable to eat and drink. Mannitol or DMSO may be given to aid resolution of cerebral edema. Laxatives and activated charcoal can be given to eliminate toxins already in the digestive tract, but their usefulness is probably minimal as this disease is not an acute intoxication. Contaminated feed should be immediately removed from all exposed horses, and pastured horses should be moved to pastures without access to corn. Prevention is aimed at providing suitable feed material to horses, and storing grains, particularly corn, under conditions that discourage mold growth.

Trichothecenes

The trichothecenes are a group of compounds elaborated primarily by *Fusarium tricinctum* and other *Fusarium* species. There are only four of approximately 40 trichothecene derivatives that have been found naturally occurring in feedstuffs. These four include T-2 toxin, deoxynivalenol, diacetoxyscirpenol, and nivalenol.[178, 179] Of these, only one reported episode of T-2 intoxication in horses was found in the literature.[179]

In the reported outbreak, horses showed clinical signs and laboratory abnormalities similar to those of ELEM caused by FB1. Gross lesions in necropsied horses were also similar to those of ELEM. *Fusarium tricinctum* was isolated from all suspect feed samples and T-2 toxin was detected in varying concentrations in all examined feed samples. Other *Fusarium* metabolites detected in this outbreak included HT-2, verrucarin A and J, and roridin A. The toxicity of these metabolites in farm animals is not yet determined.[179]

Lead

Lead is reported to be one of the more common toxicants found in veterinary practice. Materials that can serve as a source of lead toxicity to animals include lead-based paints, putty and caulking materials, used crankcase oil, greases, linoleum, leaded gasoline, solid lead solder, roofing materials, asphalt, and industrial effluents contaminating streams or forage. Discarded automobile batteries and water from lead plumbing might also serve as a source of toxicity.[180, 181]

Both acute and chronic forms of toxicosis can occur, depending upon the amount of lead ingested and the time frame in which ingestion occurs. Lead toxicosis in horses is usually chronic, and is associated with some type of forage contamination.[182, 183] Foliage near lead smelters often contains excessive lead, and grasses located near busy highways have been reported to contain high lead concentrations.[180, 183] Horses appear to be much more sensitive than cattle to prolonged, low-dose exposure to lead, yet they are much less sensitive than cattle to short-term exposure of large doses.[181, 182] The acute oral lethal dose of lead acetate in horses is 500 to 750 g total dose, but chronic toxicosis can arise when 1 to 7 mg/kg/day is ingested over a period of days, weeks, or months.[181]

Numerous factors can influence the toxicity of lead in horses. Young animals and malnourished animals are reportedly more susceptible than older animals; solid lead is not as toxic as the more soluble salts, which are more readily absorbed; and concurrent exposure to lead and cadmium results in increased severity of clinical signs of lead poisoning. In addition, lead may interact with other minerals to affect toxicity. High levels of dietary calcium cause decreased gastrointestinal absorption of lead.[180, 181, 183]

Clinical Signs. The clinical signs of lead toxicity in horses are primarily due to peripheral nerve dysfunction. The motor nerves are at greater risk, with minimal sensory perception loss in affected horses. Initially, affected horses may appear weak or have slight incoordination. Depression and weight loss become apparent and worsen over the disease course. Laryngeal and pharyngeal paralysis, dysphagia, dysphonia, and proprioceptive deficits occur. As the disease progresses, horses may exhibit flaccidity of the rectal sphincter, paresis of the lower lip, and difficulty in prehension, mastication, and deglutition. Aspiration pneumonia secondary to dysphagia and regurgitation of food is common and fine muscle tremors may occur intermittently. Terminally, horses may show severe incoordination, anorexia, emaciation, and almost complete pharyngeal and esophageal paralysis with inability to swallow food or water. Seizures may also occur terminally. Colic and diarrhea may be noted but they are not common signs.[180, 182, 183] Progression of these disease signs may require weeks.

Dietary lead crosses the placental barrier, and mares chronically exposed to lead in late pregnancy may deliver premature or small, weak foals. These foals are at greater risk of developing secondary disease complications.[182]

Pathophysiology. Lead enters the body primarily through ingestion. Inorganic lead cannot readily penetrate the skin, but organic forms such as tetraethyl lead and tetramethyl lead are absorbed through the skin. However, exposure of horses to organic lead compounds would seem to be a rare occurrence. Metallic lead shot or bullets lodged in tissues do not dissolve because tissue pH is too high.[181]

Metallic lead and lead sulfide are less absorbed than the acetate, carbonate, hydroxide, oxide, and phosphate salts. Only 1% to 2% of ingested lead is absorbed, but if sufficient quantities of soluble salts are ingested, a significant amount of lead can cross into blood. Even though intestinal absorption is relatively inefficient, increases in blood lead concentrations are seen within 3 hours of dosing.[180, 181]

Once absorbed, a large portion of lead is carried on erythrocyte membranes where it is irreversibly bound to erythrocyte proteins. Much of the remaining lead becomes bound to albumin, and only a very small proportion of the absorbed lead is actually free in serum. Unbound lead is in equilibrium with lead bound to erythrocytes and albumin, and distribution to various tissues takes place from the unbound fraction.

Much of the blood lead is removed in the liver. Within the liver, cellular trapping of lead is thought to occur by lead binding to cytoplasmic proteins called metallothioneins.[181] Lead also accumulates within the renal cortex, where it becomes trapped as intranuclear lead proteinate inclusions in tubular epithelial cells. Unbound lead is excreted into milk, and it readily passes membrane barriers such as the placenta and the blood-brain barrier to become distributed in many body tissues.[181]

Unbound lead becomes immobilized and bound to bone substance, particularly in the physeal region, by an unknown mechanism. However, bone is considered to be the "sink" for lead, and may eventually contain greater than 90% of the total body burden of lead. Deposition of lead into bone is a slow, gradual process, entailing redistribution of lead from other soft tissues. In this manner, bone serves as a detoxification mechanism under conditions of chronic exposure to small concentrations. Bone cannot hold an infinite amount of lead, however, and when saturation occurs, signs of toxicosis may appear suddenly because of rising blood and soft tissue concentrations following continued exposure.[181]

Bile and feces are thought to be the primary pathways of excretion of lead, and feces may contain unabsorbed lead as well as lead that has undergone enterohepatic circulation. Gastrointestinal secretions, including pancreatic secretions, might also be involved in elimination of lead from the body.[180, 181]

The mechanism(s) of action of lead at the cellular level is still under scrutiny. The known toxic effects of lead include inhibition of sulfhydryl groups of enzymes essential to cellular metabolism, and inhibition of heme synthesis. Lead is also known to cause a decrease in local concentrations of the essential trace metals copper, iron, and zinc. These metals have important functions in mitochondrial enzymes, and interference by lead of these may adversely affect cellular respiration, oxidative phosphorylation, and the ATP synthetase complex.[181]

The peripheral neuropathy associated with lead toxicosis in horses is thought to be due to peripheral nerve segmental demyelination. This impedes nerve impulse conduction and contributes to the clinical signs observed. The metabolic inhibitory effects of lead are speculated to cause the demyelination.[181, 182]

Lead is known to damage the blood-brain barrier and capillary endothelial cells, resulting in cerebral edema and hemorrhage. Additionally, the damaged blood-brain barrier may allow cytotoxic solutes normally excluded from the brain to enter the brain substance.[181] It is unknown if these mechanisms have any appreciable effect on the development of clinical signs observed in the horse.

Inhibition of heme synthesis is an important aspect of lead toxicosis in several animal species. This pathologic mechanism also occurs in the horse, but its significance to the overall disease course is somewhat limited. The result of heme metabolism interference and altered function of other erythrocyte proteins is a shortened erythrocyte half-life. This can produce a normochromic, normocytic anemia, which is generally marginal in affected horses (PCV of 25%–30%).[182, 183] The anemia may also be accompanied by nucleated RBCs and Howell-Jolly bodies in peripheral blood.[183]

Two enzymes in the heme synthesis pathway that are particularly susceptible to lead are δ-aminolevulinic acid dehydratase (ALA dehydratase) and ferrochelatase. Inhibition of ALA dehydratase results in reduced levels of porphobilinogen in erythrocytes, and an accumulation of ALA, which is excreted in urine. Interference with ALA dehydratase may also be partly responsible for brain damage associated with lead toxicity in some species.[180] Inhibition of ferrochelatase limits the formation of heme from protoporphyrin, resulting in an accumulation of unmetabolized porphyrins. These include protoporphyrin I, which is retained in the erythrocyte; uroporphyrins, which are excreted in urine; and coproporphyrins, which are excreted in feces. Lead also interferes with pyrimidine-specific 5′-nucleotidase activity, resulting in basophilic stippling of affected erythrocytes.[180]

Another important implication of lead toxicity is the suggestion that lead may be immunosuppressive via interference with cell-mediated immune responses.[180, 181] The mechanism of this effect is unknown, and its significance to equine lead toxicosis in unclear.

Diagnosis and Treatment. Confirmation of suspected lead poisoning is often based upon determination of blood or tissue lead concentrations. Blood levels of 0.35 ppm or greater are diagnostic if horses are showing clinical signs, but blood lead concentrations are not reflective of the severity of poisoning.[182, 183] Lead concentrations greater than 4 ppm in liver, 5 ppm in kidney, and 30 ppm in bone are considered diagnostic of lead intoxication in horses.[181]

In instances of chronic toxicity, however, blood lead values may be within a normal range. In such instances, diagnosis of toxicity may be aided by administration of calcium disodium ethylenediaminetetraacetic acid (EDTA), which chelates lead in bone stores and increases the lead concentration in plasma. The soluble lead complexes are then excreted in urine, with a resultant many-fold increase in urinary lead concentration within a few hours of EDTA administration.[180–182] The recommended dose of calcium disodium EDTA is 75 mg/kg IV.[180]

Clinicopathologic aberrations include increased concentrations of erythrocyte aminolevulinic acid and erythrocyte porphyrins, and decreased activity of erythrocyte ALA dehydratase. Increased amounts of coproporphyrins, uroporphyrins, and aminolevulinic acid are found in urine, but measurement of erythrocytic ALA is considered more diagnostic than measuring urinary ALA content.[180–182] Increased blood concentration of zinc protoporphyrin has also been documented in an affected horse.[184]

Hematologic abnormalities in affected horses can include a marginal anemia frequently accompanied by metarubricytes and Howell-Jolly bodies in peripheral blood.[180, 183] Anisocytosis, poikilocytosis, hypochromasia, polychromasia, and basophilic stippling can also occur. These changes are suggestive, but not pathognomonic, of lead toxicity in horses.[180] Concentration of lead in soil and in forages can also be measured. Poisoning in horses has been reported when grazed forage contained greater than 300 ppm lead.[180, 183]

Treatment of affected horses should include immediate elimination of the lead source if possible, and prompt initiation of chelation therapy. Calcium disodium EDTA is the chelator of choice. It chelates osseous lead but not tissue-bound lead. The chelated lead then becomes soluble and is excreted by the kidney. The unsaturated bone stores then reequilibrate with the lead in soft tissues.[180] Calcium disodium EDTA can be given by slow intravenous infusion at a dosage of 75 mg/kg body weight daily for 3 to 5 days. A 2-day non-treatment period to allow reequilibration of soft tissue and bone lead may be followed by an additional 5-day treatment regimen if needed. An alternative dosage schedule is 110 mg/kg IV twice-daily for 2 days. Following a 2-day non-treatment period, this same regimen may be repeated. The decision to continue therapy with EDTA should be based on post-treatment blood lead concentrations and renal function tests.[180]

Additional therapy should include fluid and nutritional support. Although thiamine administration has been advocated in conjunction with chelation therapy in ruminant lead toxicosis,[180] its efficacy in treating horses with lead poisoning has not been investigated. Dietary calcium supplementation may have some beneficial effect by helping to reduce further gastrointestinal absorption of lead.

Methods aimed at reducing exposure to lead and preventing intoxication include appropriate cutting and disposal of contaminated forage, tilling or burning the stubble, and addition of lime to the soil.[182] Use of alfalfa as a roughage might also be beneficial. This may be a result of the high calcium content in alfalfa, since intoxication is more difficult to produce experimentally in horses when alfalfa is being fed, and because increased dietary calcium decreases the gastrointestinal absorption of lead.[180, 182]

Toxicoses Causing Signs Relating to the Cardiovascular System

Plants

Red Maple (Acer rubrum)

Intoxication of the horse by leaves of the red maple tree is a seasonal disorder that occurs during the summer and fall months, primarily in the eastern United States.[185, 186] Fresh leaves present no problem to the horse, but wilted or dried leaves are toxic, and overnight freezing and storage of dried leaves for 30 days does not alter their toxicity.[187] Experimentally, dried leaves are toxic when administered at a dose of 1.5 mg/kg body weight.[186, 187] The toxin present in red maple leaves is unknown, but the clinical syndrome produced is one of acute hemolytic anemia with methemoglobinemia and

Heinz body production.[185-188] Red maple toxicity has only been recognized in horses,[188] and they will electively ingest the leaves when other suitable forage is available.

Clinical Signs. Signs of toxicity generally commence within 48 hours of ingestion. Affected horses show acute onset of lethargy, anorexia, weakness, and depression. Elevated heart and respiratory rates are typical, and the animals are afebrile. Two outstanding characteristics of most affected horses are the obvious presence of icterus or brown discoloration of mucous membranes, and a brownish discoloration of blood and urine. Many horses may appear cyanotic, and petechiation of mucous membranes has been reported. Signs of secondary acute renal failure have also been documented.[188] Death, when it occurs, generally happens 3 to 7 days following ingestion.[185-188]

The above signs are representative of naturally occurring instances of toxicity. In an experimental study, however, two patterns of toxicity were recognized.[187] One group of ponies given dried leaves accumulated prior to September 15 exhibited signs of the typical hemolytic syndrome and died 3 to 5 days later. Ponies given leaves collected after September 15 died within 18 hours of dosing, and exhibited clinical signs only of cyanosis and depression.[187] The reason(s) for this disparity of signs was not offered.

Pathophysiology. Although the toxin in wilted or dried red maple leaves has not been identified, it produces an acute hemolytic anemia with methemoglobinemia and Heinz body production in affected horses. The mechanism of erythrocyte damage has not been determined but these hematologic abnormalities are all characteristic of an oxidant.[186-188]

Heinz bodies are intracellular precipitates of oxidized hemoglobin that result from oxidant injury to erythrocytes. They damage the erythrocyte membrane and produce both intravascular and extravascular hemolysis. Intravascular hemolysis results when erythrocyte membrane functions involving active and passive ion transport become impaired. The hyperpermeability changes that then occur alter the osmotic gradient of the erythrocyte and cause rupture of the affected RBC. Extravascular hemolysis occurs when the RBC remains intact, but the damaged erythrocyte is removed from circulation by cells of the reticuloendothelial system.[185, 186, 188]

Methemoglobin is formed when hemoglobin is oxidized from the ferrous (Fe^{2+}) to the ferric (Fe^{3+}) form of iron. A certain amount of direct oxidation of hemoglobin to methemoglobin occurs naturally, but erythrocytes are able to reduce methemoglobin back to hemoglobin. Excessive production of methemoglobin occurs under conditions of excessive oxidative stress, or when methemoglobin reduction is impaired.[185, 187] Although methemoglobin itself does not produce hemolysis, it is incapable of transporting oxygen and therefore contributes to hypoxia. When present in sufficient quantities, it imparts a brown discoloration to peripheral blood and mucous membranes.

Diagnosis and Treatment. Red maple leaf toxicosis occurs under rather specific conditions, but is characterized by an acute onset of hemolytic anemia with methemoglobinemia and Heinz body production. The typical clinical signs and conditions supporting red maple leaf intoxication should be in evidence prior to making a diagnosis. Since the toxic principle is yet unidentified, no specific assay of feed or tissue specimens is available.

Hematologic abnormalities noted in affected horses include moderate to severe anemia (PCV often <10% in severely affected horses), hemoglobinemia, methemoglobinemia, Heinz bodies, anisocytosis, hyperbilirubinemia, and increased erythrocyte fragility.[185-188] Blood chemistry analysis may reveal depletion of erythrocyte reduced glutathione and increased serum concentrations of LDH, creatine phosphokinase, AST, and sorbitol dehydrogenase.[185-188] Transient hypercalcemia has been recorded in some horses,[185] and elevations in BUN and creatinine can be expected in horses undergoing significant renal insult secondary to hemolysis.[188] Urine analysis may indicate varying degrees of hemoglobinuria, hematuria, bilirubinuria, and proteinuria.[185-187]

Treatment of affected horses is primarily symptomatic. Exposure to red maple leaves should be eliminated immediately, and affected horses should be maintained in a quiet, calm environment. Oxygen therapy may be beneficial in selected cases, and blood transfusions can be administered to severely affected individuals.

Balanced, polyionic fluid administration is extremely important to maintain renal function and to aid in diuresis, since affected horses may be at great risk of developing hemoglobin nephrosis and acute renal failure. Blood electrolyte and acid-base parameters should be monitored, and abnormalities corrected as needed. Acute renal failure, if it develops, should be treated appropriately.

Prevention of the disease is accomplished by preventing exposure of horses to leaves from red maple trees.

Onion (Allium *species*)

Onion toxicosis in horses is a rare event, and occurs when horses are fed large amounts of cull onions (from commercial onion farms) or when forced to eat wild onions because of inadequate available forage. Horses appear to avoid these plants when suitable forage is available.[189, 190] The toxic principle in onions, n-propyl disulfide, only affects circulating erythrocytes, where it causes oxidant injury to the RBC with resultant Heinz body formation and subsequent hemolytic anemia. Severely affected horses can succumb to onion toxicosis because of severe anemia or secondary renal failure due to hemoglobin nephropathy.

The clinical signs, laboratory values, and pathogenesis of the anemia are all similar to those of red maple leaf toxicosis, with the exception that methemoglobin formation does not seem to be nearly as pronounced in onion toxicity as in the former. Horses dying from onion toxicosis may have an "onion odor" of the carcass noticeable at necropsy.[189]

Affected horses may recover from onion toxicity if they are removed from the onion source soon enough, and the anemia is not pronounced. Treatment is largely symptomatic and should include removal of the onion source and provision of adequate, suitable forage. Hematinics are of little value, but oxygen therapy and blood transfusions may be indicated in more severely affected animals.

Maintenance of renal function is of primary concern because affected horses are at risk of developing secondary hemoglobin nephropathy. Balanced, polyionic fluids should be given to promote diuresis, and electrolyte and acid-base abnormalities should be corrected. Diuretics should be used with caution, but they may be of value in the volume-loaded horse.

Medications

Heparin

Heparin is an anionic sulfated glycosaminoglycan polysaccharide found normally in mast cells. It is commercially available as a calcium or sodium salt, and is prepared from either bovine lung tissue or porcine intestinal mucosa.[191] Its use in humans and animals is primarily as an anticoagulant, and in horses it has been used as adjunct therapy in treatment of acute laminitis, septic peritonitis, DIC, and in horses at risk of developing thrombosis. It also has been used for prevention of peritoneal fibrin deposition following abdominal surgery, and in attempts to prevent DIC in horses suffering from various systemic diseases.[192–194]

Heparin is strongly acidic and is not absorbed from the gastrointestinal tract. Intramuscular injection often leads to painful, large hematomas at the injection site, so administration is limited to the intravenous and subcutaneous routes.[191, 195] Heparin is bound primarily to low-density lipoproteins, globulins, and fibrinogen, and is metabolized in the liver by heparinase.[191] In humans, the inactive metabolic products are excreted in urine along with a small fraction of unchanged drug. Heparin apparently is removed from the circulation primarily by the reticuloendothelial system, and localizes on arterial and venous endothelium.[191] The plasma half-life of heparin is approximately 1.5 hours.[195]

Clinical Signs. One adverse effect of heparin overdose is hemorrhage, as heparin acts as an anticoagulant, but the primary problem associated with heparin therapy in the horse is that of induced reduction of RBC mass.[192–194] In experimental studies, dosages of 160 units/kg body weight or greater, SC b.i.d., resulted in reduction of the measured circulating RBC mass, and an increase in measured mean corpuscular volume (MCV). The RBC mass was reduced as much as 57% in some horses. A dosage of 40 units/kg b.i.d. had no effect on measured blood parameters.[192] In reports of clinical cases, a dosage of 80 units/kg SC b.i.d. also resulted in reduced PCV and increased MCV.[193]

In affected horses, the PCV begins to decrease by 12 to 24 hours after initiation of a "toxic" dose, and appears to remain depressed while the horse remains on heparin therapy. The PCV begins to increase by 24 hours after cessation of heparin therapy, and approaches baseline values in 72 hours.[192, 196] One anecdotal report indicated that horses maintained on heparin therapy would also exhibit a rebound in PCV in several days, even though heparin administration was continued.[197] Other hematologic abnormalities that may be noted in affected horses include an increase in serum bilirubin concentration,[196] and decreased serum concentrations of hemoglobin and platelets.[192] These hematologic discrepancies have been induced in horses given heparin at a dosage that maintained the activated PTT (APTT) within a therapeutic range of 1.5 to 2.0 times the normal mean.[192]

Pathophysiology. Heparin by itself is inactive. It produces its anticoagulant action by combining with antithrombin III, an endogenous α_2-globulin, which must be present in adequate amounts for the process to proceed. The heparin–antithrombin III complex markedly accelerates the antagonistic action of antithrombin III on thrombin, thereby restricting the conversion of fibrinogen to fibrin. This complex is also inhibitory to kallikrein, and to the activated forms of clotting factors IX, X, XI, and XII.[195] In addition, heparin acts as an opsonin, and may augment certain phagocytic activities of the reticuloendothelial system.[192, 196]

The mechanism whereby heparin causes a reduction in circulating RBC mass is still under scrutiny. Initially, heparin was suggested to cause extravascular hemolysis by enhanced phagocytosis of RBCs by the reticuloendothelial system.[192, 196] More recent evidence, however, strongly suggests that the deleterious effects of heparin on formed blood elements are largely artifactual, and that the measured abnormalities are a result of erythrocyte agglutination.[193, 194] Further investigation is required to determine if this agglutination also occurs in vivo in heparinized horses.

Diagnosis and Treatment

The rapid onset of dramatic reduction in PCV in horses treated with heparin implies either acute hemorrhage or the above-described adverse reaction of heparin on the formed blood elements of the horse. The specific antidote for heparin is protamine sulfate, which can be given at a dose not to exceed 1 mg for every 90 to 100 units of heparin administered.[195, 198] Whole, fresh blood or plasma transfusions can also be given to reverse or antagonize the anticoagulant effect.[195]

It is unlikely that the above treatments would be required, except in instances of hemorrhage due to heparin overdose. Removal of heparin from the treatment regimen is usually all that is necessary to stop the decline in PCV. Normal numbers of circulating erythrocytes should reappear by approximately 72 hours after cessation of heparin therapy, if this adverse reaction to heparin is the cause of the lowered PCV.

Coumarin Derivatives

Coumarin is normally present in some species of sweet clover, and has no anticoagulant action. However, coumarin derivatives are widely used as anticoagulants, with bishydroxycoumarin (dicumarol) and 3-(α-acetonylbenzyl)-4-hydroxycoumarin (warfarin sodium) being the first oral anticoagulants developed from coumarin.[199] These compounds are used therapeutically as anticoagulants and as rodenticides. In horses, warfarin has been used therapeutically to treat thrombotic disorders such as thrombophlebitis, and more recently in the treatment of navicular disease.[200, 201] Horses may exhibit signs of toxicity while being medicated with warfarin, if a therapeutic concentration is exceeded. Rarely are horses exposed to warfarin or other coumarin derivatives used as rodenticides around buildings or feed storage areas.

Clinical Signs. The clinical signs of toxicity noted with warfarin or other coumarin derivatives are largely those of a hemorrhagic diathesis. Onset of signs is usually acute, and may include hematoma formation, epistaxis, anemia, weakness, pale mucous membranes or ecchymoses of mucous membranes. Hematuria and melena can occur, and hemorrhage into various body compartments may result in secondary signs caused by malfunction of the involved organ or tissue. Occasionally, affected animals may be found dead.[202] Multiple fractional doses given over several days may be more toxic to horses than a single, relatively larger dose.[200]

The onset of clinical signs is delayed somewhat from the time of ingestion. In an experimental model, the hypothrombogenic effect of warfarin anticoagulation was noticed 60 hours following an acute dose.[203] This effect persisted for approximately 30 hours.

Pathophysiology. Warfarin is readily absorbed from the gastrointestinal tract, but may also be administered intravenously for therapeutic purposes.[199, 200] Once absorbed, warfarin is highly bound (> 90%) to plasma proteins and some is stored in the liver.[199, 200, 203] Warfarin is hydroxylated by hepatic enzymes to inactive compounds that are eliminated by the kidney. The metabolites have no anticoagulant effect,[199] and the biological half-life of warfarin in the horse is approximately 13 hours.[203] Coumarins also cross the placenta and are secreted in milk.[199]

Protein binding of warfarin is reversible, and the protein-bound, pharmacologically inactive warfarin serves as a reservoir. The unbound portion remains fairly constant in plasma.[199, 200]

A number of factors can influence the amount of unbound free warfarin in serum. Drugs that are protein-bound, such as phenylbutazone, chloral hydrate, and sulfonamides, may enhance the toxicity of warfarin by displacing warfarin from protein-binding sites. This allows a greater proportion of the drug to be in the free form and thus able to exert its pharmacologic effect.[199, 202] Corticosteroids and thyroxine (T_4) may lower the therapeutic dose of warfarin by increasing both clotting factor catabolism and receptor site affinity.[200]

Certain physiologic factors may also enhance the toxicity of warfarin. Hypoalbuminemia may result in fewer binding sites available, thereby increasing the amount of free drug. Hepatic dysfunction may impede metabolism of warfarin, and reduced amounts of vitamin K in the diet may predispose to toxicity.[199]

Some drugs reduce the therapeutic response to a given dose of warfarin. Barbiturates, rifampin, and chloramphenicol induce hepatic microsomal enzyme activity, thereby accelerating metabolism of warfarin. If these drugs are withdrawn during warfarin therapy, toxicosis may result.[199, 200] Likewise, excessive dietary intake of vitamin K (such as alfalfa) or vitamin K administration can reduce or inhibit the anticoagulant effects of warfarin.[200]

Warfarin acts as an anticoagulant by inhibiting production of the vitamin K–dependent clotting factors II, VII, IX, and X. Vitamin K is a cofactor in the synthesis of clotting factors II, VII, IX, and X, and also acts on all clotting factor precursors to convert glutamyl residues to α-carboxyglutamyl residues. During this carboxylation process, vitamin K_1 is converted to vitamin K_1 2,3-epoxide, an inactive metabolite. This epoxide returns to active vitamin K_1 by action of the microsomal enzyme vitamin K_1 epoxide reductase. The coumarin anticoagulants inhibit vitamin K_1 epoxide reductase, thereby creating a vitamin K_1 "deficiency." The result is decreased production and subsequent deficiency of the vitamin K–dependent clotting factors.[204] The delayed onset of action of the coumarin derivative anticoagulants is a result of this impediment to clotting factor synthesis, rather than a direct effect on the clotting mechanism per se.

The various blood clotting factors have different plasma half-lives. Factor VII has a shorter half-life than the other clotting factors, so the earliest laboratory indication of warfarin toxicity is a prolongation of PT. As the other clotting factors become depleted, APTT also increases as toxicity continues.[200] Horses given warfarin therapeutically should be closely monitored for clotting abnormalities. Prolongation of PT by 1.5 to 2.0 times baseline has been suggested as the effective range of anticoagulation. However, some horses maintained in this range may show signs of hemorrhage.[201]

Diagnosis and Treatment. The diagnosis of warfarin or other coumarin derivative anticoagulant intoxication is based on evidence of exposure to the drug, presence of a bleeding diathesis, and prolongation of PT with or without prolonged APTT. Since warfarin only affects certain clotting factors, other elements of the clotting profile are not affected. The platelet count, fibrinogen concentration, fibrin degradation product concentration, and antithrombin III activity all remain within their respective normal range of activity.[200, 202]

Tissue concentration of warfarin can also be evaluated on postmortem specimens. Liver, kidney, spleen, stomach and intestinal content, feces, and unclotted blood can be submitted for evaluation. Specimens should be frozen for transportation to the laboratory.[202, 203]

In horses intoxicated by warfarin, discontinuance of warfarin therapy or removal of the product from the horse's environment is of primary importance. Vitamin K_1 is the specific antidote for coumarin derivatives, and should be given at a dosage of 300 to 500 mg SC every 4 to 6 hours until PT returns to the baseline value. Thereafter, PT should be monitored daily for 3 to 4 days to ensure stability. The subcutaneous route of vitamin K_1 administration is preferred because of the possibility of adverse reactions if the product is given intravenously or intramuscularly. Intravenous injection of vitamin K_1 may result in transient restlessness, tachypnea, tachycardia, and sweating. Intramuscular administration of vitamin K_1 results in erratic response times, and therefore may be inappropriate for a hemorrhaging patient.[205] Alternative doses for vitamin K_1 administration are 0.3 to 0.5 mg/kg IV, and a dosage of greater than 0.5 mg/kg IV has been suggested to inhibit coumarin activity for several days.[200] If the intravenous route is chosen, vitamin K_1 should be diluted in 5% dextrose or saline, and given slowly.[202]

If bleeding is serious, fresh blood or fresh plasma given intravenously may be necessary to control hemorrhage and to help correct hypovolemia. Other supportive measures, such as bandaging and keeping the animal in a quiet environment, may be helpful. Organ dysfunction induced by hemorrhage should be treated appropriately. The prognosis for affected horses is good if the disorder is recognized early and appropriate therapy is instituted.

Prevention of warfarin toxicosis is aimed at minimizing exposure of horses to the product and carefully monitoring the therapeutic use of the drug in the horse. Contraindications to its use include any clinical or laboratory suggestion of hepatic disease, hypoproteinemia, or other condition that might increase the risk of toxicity. The concurrent use of other medications should be evaluated, as they may affect the potential for toxicosis to develop, and the dosage of warfarin administered should be reevaluated if other concurrent medications are changed. Additionally, the potential for traumatic injury should be minimized in horses undergoing warfarin therapy.

Dimethyl Sulfoxide (DMSO)

This byproduct of the papermaking industry is a colorless liquid originally used as an industrial solvent. It is a polar compound that readily mixes with ethyl alcohol and many organic solvents. It is extremely hygroscopic and can absorb more than 70% of its weight of water from air.[206] DMSO possesses some antimicrobial and antifungal activity, but its primary medical use has been as an anti-inflammatory agent and as a transdermal transport agent.[206] More recently, it has found use as a diuretic and has shown very promising results when used in the treatment of acute cranial and spinal cord trauma.[206, 207]

The systemic toxicity of DMSO is considered to be very low, and its greatest toxic potential appears to result from its combination with other toxic agents.[208] However, in an experimental study, rapid infusion of DMSO in 20% and 40% concentrations caused hemolysis, hemoglobinuria, diarrhea, muscle tremors, and signs of colic in some horses.[209] The LD_{50} of DMSO has not been established for horses, but it ranges from 2.5 to 9.0 g/kg as a single intravenous dose in a number of animal species.[208] A dose of 1 g/kg intravenously has been suggested for use in horses. This dose should be diluted to a 10% to 20% solution and administered slowly when given intravenously.[207, 208]

DMSO produces hemolysis when given intravenously in concentrations of 20% to 50% or greater.[206–208] If hemolysis is severe, affected horses may be at increased risk of developing hemoglobin nephrosis. Concentrations of 10% or less are considered suitable for intravenous injection in horses.[206, 207, 209] Additionally, increased WBC adherence and fibrinogen precipitation have been reported when concentrations greater than 50% are administered.[206]

DMSO is a mild cholinesterase inhibitor, and its concurrent use with organophosphates or other cholinesterase inhibitors is not recommended.[206, 208] DMSO is also known to induce histamine release from mast cells, but the significance of this phenomenon is uncertain.[208]

Skin reactions to topical DMSO can occur. Varying degrees of erythema, pruritus, drying, hardening, and desquamation of normal skin may be noted. These reactions are usually self-limiting and typically diminish with repeated applications.[208]

The greatest risk of toxicity resulting from DMSO is probably a consequence of its concomitant use with other toxic or potentially toxic agents. DMSO may aid transport of a variety of toxic compounds across skin, thereby inducing toxicosis from the transported agent. For example, mercury toxicity has been reported in a horse that had a DMSO and mercury–containing blister applied topically to a leg.[210] In such instances, the specific toxic reaction(s) should be

treated appropriately. No specific antidote is recognized for DMSO, other than its judicious and conscientious use when being administered to horses. The above-described precautions should be heeded when administering the drug.

Phenothiazine

Phenothiazine is an anthelmintic that has a narrow spectrum of activity in horses. It is active only against strongyles. It is moderately effective in removing large strongyles but is more effective against small strongyles.[211] This drug is rarely used as an equine anthelmintic because of its side effects, and because safer and more efficacious anthelmintics with broader spectra of activity have been developed.

Clinical Signs. Phenothiazine administration has resulted in acute and unpredictable signs of toxicity in horses. Debilitated, weak, and anemic animals are reportedly more susceptible to toxicosis, yet toxic reactions have been seen at normal therapeutic doses.[211, 212] Fifteen grams may be toxic to horses and 30 g may be lethal.[213] The common signs of toxicity reported are hemolytic anemia with subsequent hemoglobinuria and icterus, anorexia, weakness, CNS disturbances, and photosensitization.[211, 212]

Pathophysiology. Phenothiazine is absorbed from the intestinal tract after it is converted to phenothiazine sulfoxide by cellular enzymes of the intestinal epithelium. Once absorbed, it is further oxidized in the liver to leukophenothiazone and leukothionol. These two substances are then excreted primarily in urine.[212]

Phenothiazine acts as an oxidant to RBCs, resulting in the production of Heinz body anemia. The pathogenesis of this condition is described in detail elsewhere (see discussion of red maple leaf toxicosis).

Photosensitization may not be a problem in horses intoxicated by phenothiazine.[212] However, in other species, photosensitization can occur because of abnormal accumulation of phenothiazine sulfoxide. Normally, this product is converted to phenothiazone by the liver. When high doses of phenothiazine are given, or if liver dysfunction impairs the conversion of phenothiazine sulfoxide to phenothiazone, the sulfoxide diffuses into the general circulation and ultimately into the aqueous humor of the eye. Upon exposure to ultraviolet light, the phenothiazine sulfoxide produces photosensitization in unpigmented skin and a photosensitive keratitis. The keratitis may be manifested by corneal ulceration and blindness.[212]

The mechanism whereby phenothiazine may induce CNS derangements has not been elucidated.

Diagnosis and Treatment. Diagnosis of phenothiazine toxicity is based primarily upon history of exposure to the drug, and compatible clinical signs. No specific antidote is available, so symptomatic therapy is indicated. Heinz body anemia should be treated as previously described. Photosensitization can be prevented by keeping treated animals out of direct sunlight for 2 to 3 days following therapy. Debilitated, weak animals, and those with evidence of liver disease should not be given phenothiazine.

Digoxin

Digoxin has been used to treat congestive heart failure in many species, including horses. However, reports of digoxin toxicity in horses are rare.[214] There is a narrow margin between therapeutic and toxic doses in many species, and wide variations in individual tolerance to the drug are seen. Therefore, signs of toxicity may develop in horses given a normal dose of digoxin.[214]

Clinical Signs. The clinical signs reported in one instance of digoxin intoxication were anorexia, depression that became more pronounced over time, muscle tremors, and colic. Cardiac abnormalities included a slower, somewhat irregular pulse rate, and electrocardiographic (ECG) findings of a prolonged PQ interval with increased duration (widening) of the P wave were seen. The horse was also hyponatremic and hypochloremic.[214]

Signs of toxicity reported in other species, including humans, are anorexia, vomiting, salivation, diarrhea, abdominal pain, depression, skin rashes, neurologic signs, nausea, and various cardiac arrhythmias.[214, 215] The most frequently encountered arrhythmias include incomplete or complete heart block, junctional escape rhythms and ventricular premature beats, ventricular bigeminy, and paroxysmal ventricular or atrial tachycardia with block. Death, when it occurs, is due to cardiac arrhythmias.[215]

Pathophysiology. Digoxin can be administered via the intravenous or oral route, but the latter is preferred in the horse. Intravenous administration of the drug results in an initial high serum concentration, and is an unsatisfactory means of providing long-term therapy. Absorption of digoxin is rapid and occurs largely in the small intestine, but the bioavailability of the drug is low (approximately 20%) and considerable variation in absorption occurs among horses.[215, 216] Following absorption, digoxin is bound primarily to serum albumin, but again, there is wide individual variation in the amount of protein binding in normal horses.[217] The biological half-life of digoxin in the horse is reported to range from 17 to 23 hours,[216, 218] and elimination is largely through urinary excretion of unchanged drug.[217]

The suggested therapeutic range for digoxin in the horse is a serum concentration of 0.5 to 2.0 ng/mL. This concentration has been achieved by administering an oral dose of 35 μg/kg/24 hr.[216] However, it must be remembered that no dosage regimen is absolute because of the extreme individual variation in absorption and protein binding of the drug. Repeated clinical monitoring of treated horses is imperative, with dosage adjustments based on clinical improvement, development of early signs of toxicosis, and assay of plasma digoxin concentration.[216]

Digoxin acts as a positive ionotrope and a negative chronotrope. The cellular mechanisms of inotropic action of digoxin are still being evaluated, but it is known that digoxin inhibits the Na^+K^+-ATPase–dependent transport system. This results in an intracellular loss of potassium and an intracellular elevation of sodium and calcium. The resting membrane potential is therefore reduced, making the cardiac cells more excitable. Another hypothesis is that the increased intracellular sodium concentration augments transmembrane exchange of intracellular sodium for extracellular calcium.

The increased calcium delivered to the contractile proteins may be partially responsible for the positive inotropic effect.[215]

Digoxin acts as a negative chronotrope by decreasing sinus rate and slowing conduction of the AV impulse. These effects are the result of increased vagal tone and secondary hemodynamic improvement in digitalized animals. The increased vagal tone has been attributed to at least three mechanisms: (1) direct stimulation of vagal centers in the brain, (2) sensitization of baroreceptors in the carotid sinus to blood pressure, and (3) enhanced pacemaker response to acetylcholine at the myocardial level.[215] The circulatory improvement following digitalization tends to remove the stimuli responsible for reflex sinus tachycardia, a compensatory effort seen in many instances of congestive heart failure. As a result, the sinus rate can return toward normal.[215]

Toxic effects of digoxin on cardiac muscle are seen when the above mechanisms proceed beyond a beneficial level. Increased cardiac automaticity and excitability, coupled with excessive refractoriness at the AV node and decreased refractoriness of the atria and ventricles, can lead to extrasystoles and tachyarrhythmias. These dysrhythmias can be severe enough to result in cardiac failure and death.[219]

Many factors may enhance digoxin toxicity in humans. Diseases such as renal failure, hypothyroidism, myocardial infarction, and myocarditis can have an additive effect on toxicity. Certain drugs, including quinidine, verapamil, amiodarone, spironolactone, and indomethacin, act to increase serum digoxin levels, and abnormal electrolyte concentrations can enhance digoxin toxicity. Hypokalemia, hyperkalemia, hypomagnesemia, hypernatremia, and alkalosis can contribute to digoxin toxicity.[219]

The mechanisms responsible for the noncardiac signs of digoxin toxicity have not been elucidated.

Diagnosis and Treatment. Diagnosis of digoxin toxicity may be difficult to differentiate from continuing cardiac compromise. If compatible clinical and ECG findings of toxicity are present, measurement of serum digoxin concentration should verify the diagnosis. However, some horses may exhibit signs of toxicity even though the serum concentration is within the suggested nontoxic range of 0.5 to 2.0 ng/mL.

Treatment of digoxin toxicosis should begin with drug withdrawal. Serum electrolyte concentrations and acid-base status should be evaluated, and abnormalities should be treated appropriately.[215, 219] Oral charcoal administration has been advocated in instances of human toxicosis,[219] but its efficacy in equine poisoning remains undetermined. Horses that require digoxin therapy should be started on a relatively low dose, with the dosage increased as needed over time.

Bicarbonate

Sodium bicarbonate is one of the most common alkalizing agents used in animals, including horses. It is specifically indicated in the treatment of acute, severe metabolic acidosis because of its rapid effect on blood pH when given intravenously.[220] Sodium bicarbonate has also been used in performance horses both in treatment of exertional myopathies and in attempts to prevent rhabdomyolysis. More recently, sodium bicarbonate administration in performance horses has been investigated because of its suggested role in limiting or preventing systemic lactic acidosis, thereby enhancing the performance level of the horse.[221, 222] The adverse effects of bicarbonate administration occur when it is given too rapidly, or in excessive quantities, or when it is given in the presence of certain other systemic abnormalities.

Clinical Signs. Animals, including horses, that suffer from an acute overdose of bicarbonate may exhibit signs of delirium, depression, and coma. Rapidly induced alkalosis has also been associated with cardiac dysrhythmias.[220]

Horses that are volume-depleted and have sustained excessive electrolyte loss through sweat, such as endurance horses or racehorses, often have clinicopathologic changes of hypokalemia, hypochloremia, hypocalcemia, and metabolic alkalosis. When such horses are given bicarbonate, dramatic deleterious effects are noted. These animals may exhibit signs of muscle fasciculation, synchronous diaphragmatic flutter, bruxism, and decreased respiratory rate. Clinical evidence of further dehydration may also be noted, such as increased capillary refill time, delayed jugular distensibility, diminished skin turgor, and decreased arterial pulse.[222]

Pathophysiology. The rapid administration or overdose of sodium bicarbonate has been associated with extracellular hyperosmolality, intracranial hemorrhage, and CSF acidosis. Hyperosmolality is the consequence of hypernatremia, since sodium bicarbonate dissociates into sodium ions and bicarbonate ions. An abrupt increase in serum osmolality can lead to intracranial hemorrhage, as intracellular water moves into the extracellular space. This extracellular fluid accumulation may result in engorgement of perivascular spaces, with subsequent tearing of bridge veins and resultant hemorrhage. The CSF acidosis is a consequence of the rapid diffusion of generated carbon dioxide into the CSF. Carbon dioxide enters the CSF almost instantaneously, establishing new steady-state levels within minutes. Bicarbonate ion, on the other hand, is very slow to enter the CSF, and requires hours to days to achieve new steady-state levels. With sodium bicarbonate administration, the increasing amount of carbon dioxide generated readily enters the CSF disproportionately more than does the bicarbonate ion. As a consequence, the CSF becomes acidic.[223] These mechanisms, either individually or collectively, are thought to be responsible for development of the clinical signs observed with rapid or excessive administration of sodium bicarbonate solution.

Another effect of alkalosis is a shift to the left of the oxyhemoglobin dissociation curve. This left shift indicates an increased affinity of hemoglobin for oxygen, with a resultant decrease in the amount of oxygen available for cellular use. This change in hemoglobin affinity for oxygen has been associated with cardiac dysrhythmias following rapidly induced alkalosis.[220]

Horses undergoing extensive exercise or horses that are treated with furosemide (primarily as prerace medication for exercise-induced pulmonary hemorrhage) are at risk of developing hypochloremic, hypokalemic metabolic alkalosis. When sodium bicarbonate is given to these volume-depleted horses with electrolyte loss and concurrent metabolic alkalosis, another deleterious series of events can result. Further reduction of the circulating fluid volume may occur, along with development of serum hyperosmolality, electrolyte abnormalities of hypernatremia, hypokalemia, hypochloremia, and hypocalcemia, and further development of metabolic alkalosis.[222]

Excess sodium bicarbonate produces hyperosmolality due to hypernatremia, since sodium bicarbonate dissociates into sodium and bicarbonate ions. The hypokalemia is partially explained by the intracellular shift of potassium in response to metabolic alkalosis, and the bicarbonate ion adds further to the alkalosis already present. Furosemide administration causes urinary loss of potassium, chloride, and calcium, and sweating can also result in significant loss of chloride and calcium. Additionally, rapid intravenous infusion of 5% sodium bicarbonate in normal horses results in hypochloremia.[224]

The muscle fasciculations and diaphragmatic flutter noted in some horses is likely a consequence of hypocalcemia.[222] The total serum calcium concentration may be within a normal range, but alkalosis causes a reduction in the amount of circulating ionized calcium. Since ionized calcium is responsible for neuromuscular function, reduction in this fraction can cause clinical signs of hypocalcemia.

Diagnosis and Treatment. Horses being treated with sodium bicarbonate solutions should be closely monitored for clinical signs of alkalosis. Blood pH is obviously elevated, but rapid infusion of sodium bicarbonate or excessive use in horses already sustaining fluid and electrolyte loss can result in a number of clinicopathologic alterations. Affected horses typically exhibit elevations in PCV, total serum protein, and serum bicarbonate and sodium concentrations. Additional findings of hypokalemia, hypochloremia, and hypocalcemia are usually present.

Treatment of affected horses involves cessation of bicarbonate administration and correction of the alkalosis and electrolyte abnormalities. Potassium chloride administration is indicated in horses with hypokalemic, hypochloremic metabolic alkalosis, and is much more effective in correcting these electrolyte abnormalities than is sodium chloride. Potassium chloride has also been shown to cause a prompt, significant decline in venous blood pH in these horses.[222]

It is apparent that hypertonic sodium bicarbonate solutions should not be used in dehydrated horses. The concurrent use of furosemide and sodium bicarbonate also appears to be contraindicated, or at best, used with extreme caution and close observation with laboratory assessment. Sodium bicarbonate should not be mixed with fluids containing calcium, as insoluble complexes may form. The use of sodium bicarbonate orally in horses subjected to short-term, intense exercise is still controversial.

Miscellaneous Agents

Nitrates and Nitrites

Nitrates are an important component in the naturally occurring nitrogen cycle, and as such, are present in soils, ground water, forages, row crops, weeds, animal tissues, and excreta. Nitrates are also widely used in fertilizers. Toxicity problems can arise when animals consume plants, feed, or water containing excessive amounts of nitrate or when they ingest nitrate fertilizers or residues. Nitrates naturally undergo microbial decomposition to nitrites, so nitrite toxicity can occur when animals ingest feed or water in which the nitrates have decomposed to yield large amounts of nitrites. This can occur in moist haystacks, water troughs, farm ponds, silages, and pig swills. Nitrite is also administered intravenously in treatment of cyanide poisoning, and overzealous use of this therapy can result in toxicity.[225]

The primary exposure to nitrate or nitrite for most animals is the plants they consume. Many plants and forages are known to be nitrate accumulators, and a number of factors influence the uptake of nitrates in plants. Nitrate concentration by plants is enhanced by low soil pH; low soil molybdenum, sulfur, or phosphorus content; low soil temperature; drought; soil aeration; decreased light; and use of phenoxyacetic acid herbicides such as 2,4-D. Nitrate and nitrite accumulation in ponds and ground water is due to water runoff from nitrate-rich soils, or by direct contamination with nitrates and nitrites.[225, 226] Both nitrates and nitrites are water-soluble, and are easily carried from feedlots, pigpens, and fertilized areas into the soil and subsequently into plants, wells, and ponds.

The most important aspect of nitrates is their ease of microbial conversion to nitrites. It is nitrite that is responsible for the primary signs associated with toxicity in nitrate poisoning.

Clinical Signs. Although apparently rare, horses are reported to be susceptible to nitrate intoxication. Experimentally, an oral dose of 1 g/kg potassium nitrate caused illness but not death in horses.[225] However, nitrates have been associated with death of horses under field conditions.[225]

In monogastric animals, nitrate ingestion is reported to produce gastrointestinal irritation with resulting emesis or enteritis. Salivation, diarrhea, colic, and frequent urination may be noted if the nitrate is concentrated enough. Since there is no mechanism whereby these animals can rapidly reduce nitrate to nitrite, they are generally much more tolerant of nitrate than are ruminants.[226]

Signs of acute poisoning with nitrites usually commence within one-half to 4 hours following ingestion of high nitrite feed or water. The most characteristic signs are those referable to respiratory insufficiency, and include dyspnea, cyanosis, rapid and weak pulse, and anxiety. Exertion may exacerbate these signs, and induce muscle tremors and collapse. There may be terminal clonic convulsions. The blood of affected animals is usually brown or chocolate-colored, and will impart a cyanotic appearance to mucous membranes. Death may occur within several hours or be delayed until 12 to 24 hours post ingestion.[225, 226]

Pathophysiology. Nitrites are rapidly absorbed from the gastrointestinal tract into the bloodstream. The nitrite ion acts directly on vascular smooth muscle to cause relaxation, and easily enters erythrocytes in exchange for chloride ion. Nitrite can also pass the placenta to enter fetal erythrocytes, which are especially sensitive to nitrite. The biological half-life of blood nitrate in horses is 4.8 hours. Only small amounts of nitrate or nitrite are bound to plasma proteins.[225, 227]

Nitrite causes acute poisoning by two mechanisms. The primary action of nitrite is to interact with hemoglobin to form methemoglobin. One molecule of nitrite interacts with two molecules of hemoglobin, causing the oxidation of normal ferrous (Fe^{2+}) hemoglobin to ferric (Fe^{3+}) hemoglobin, which is called methemoglobin. Methemoglobin is incapable of transporting oxygen to tissues, and if sufficient quantities are formed, severe oxygen deficiency can occur. Clinical signs become evident when methemoglobin levels approach 30% to 40%, and death occurs when 80% to 90% of hemoglobin is oxidized to methemoglobin.[225, 226] However, death can occur in active animals with only 50% to 60% methemoglobin.[225]

Normally, methemoglobin is converted back to ferrous hemoglobin by two reducing enzyme systems: NAD-dependent diaphorase I and NADP-dependent diaphorase II. This conversion occurs rather slowly, and in instances of nitrate toxicity, methemoglobin formation far exceeds the ability of these enzyme systems to regenerate hemoglobin.[225]

The second action of nitrite is to cause direct relaxation of smooth muscle, particularly vascular smooth muscle. The mechanism by which this occurs is unknown, but the physiologic changes brought about by the vasodilating action of nitrite include pulmonary arterial, central venous, and systemic arterial hypotension and decreased cardiac output. These changes may contribute to tissue anoxia, and act to enhance tissue oxygen starvation already initiated by methemoglobin.[225]

Diagnosis and Treatment. The diagnosis of nitrate or nitrite toxicity is based upon compatible clinical signs; methemoglobinemia; history of exposure to nitrate- or nitrite-containing plants, water, or fertilizers; and nitrate quantitation in blood. Serum nitrate and methemoglobin determinations should be performed quickly following collection, as they are not stable in refrigerated, heparinized blood for more than a few hours. However, blood mixed with a phosphate buffer will preserve the methemoglobin present, and allow shipment to a diagnostic laboratory. Forage, hay, and water samples can be analyzed for nitrate or nitrite content, as can other body fluids, such as urine, aqueous humor, and intestinal content.[226]

Treatment is directed toward reduction of methemoglobin back to hemoglobin. Mildly affected animals may recover spontaneously if the toxic source is removed and if they are given sufficient time for normal methemoglobin reduction processes to occur. Methylene blue may be used to treat more severely affected horses, at a suggested dose of 4.4 mg/kg IV given slowly as a 1% solution in isotonic saline. The dose can be repeated in 30 minutes if clinical response is unsatisfactory.[225] Caution should be exercised with this product, however, as excess methylene blue may directly oxidize hemoglobin to methemoglobin.[225] Methylene blue is converted to leukomethylene blue by an $NADPH_2$-dependent system. Leukomethylene then reduces methemoglobin to hemoglobin. In this reaction, leukomethylene blue is oxidized back to methylene blue, but can be reconverted to leukomethylene blue as long as sufficient $NADPH_2$ is available. If this $NADPH_2$ system becomes saturated with methylene blue, excess methylene blue may directly oxidize hemoglobin to more methemoglobin.[225]

Other nonspecific therapies that may be employed include blood transfusion, oxygen therapy, and laxatives such as mineral oil to aid evacuation of the gastrointestinal tract.[225]

Cyanide

Hydrogen cyanide, cyanide, hydrocyanic acid, and prussic acid are all terms relating to the same toxic substance. Horses become exposed primarily through ingestion of certain plants that contain cyanogenic glycosides, but compounds containing cyanide are also used as fumigants, rodenticides, and fertilizers.[228, 229]

A number of plants or plant parts may accumulate large quantities of cyanide or cyanogenic glycosides, and a more complete description of them can be found elsewhere.[230] When these cyanogenic glycosides undergo hydrolysis, free HCN is formed.[229] Plant cells contain degradative enzymes that can hydrolyze these glycosides, but under natural conditions, the enzymes are kept spatially separated from the glycosides in intact cells. Damage to the plant cells by wilting, freezing, or stunting allows enzymatic degradation of the glycoside.[229] Rapid hydrolysis and release of HCN occurs only when the plant cell structure is disrupted. When the glycoside is exposed to an acid medium, or when maceration of the plant occurs within the intestinal tract, hydrolysis and subsequent formation of HCN also occurs.

A number of factors can influence the toxic potential of cyanogenic plants. Since plant cyanogenic glycosides and degradative enzymes are both genetically controlled by a dominant gene, it is possible to selectively breed plants with low cyanogenic potential. Therefore, species and varieties of forage affect cyanogenic content. High nitrogen fertilization, nitrogen and phosphorus imbalance in soil, and drought conditions can also influence cyanide potential in plants.[229]

Most of the cyanogenic activity in the plant is located in the leaves and seeds, and immature and rapidly growing plants have the greatest potential for high glycoside levels. Conditions that damage the plant, such as drought, wilting, or freezing, may allow for more rapid combination of glycoside and enzyme, thereby enhancing plant toxicity.[229] Other factors that may affect toxicity are the size of the animal, speed of ingestion, the type of food ingested along with the cyanogen, and the presence of active degradative enzymes in the plant and in the horse's digestive tract.[229]

Clinical Signs. Since cyanide is such a potent, rapidly acting poison, affected animals are commonly found dead. When clinical signs are observed, they may range from mild tachypnea and anxiousness to severe panting, gasping, and behavioral excitement. Salivation, lacrimation, muscle tremors, defecation, urination, and mydriasis may be noted. These signs are followed by prostration, clonic convulsions, and death. The mucous membranes typically have a bright red appearance, and blood color is a bright cherry-red. Clinical signs may last from only several minutes to a few hours, but horses that survive longer than 90 to 120 minutes following exposure usually survive.[228, 229, 231]

Pathophysiology. HCN is rapidly absorbed from the gastrointestinal tract or from the lungs. Following absorption, endogenous thiosulfate combines with the cyanide ion to form thiocyanate, which is relatively harmless. This reaction occurs in the liver and other tissues, and the generated thiocyanate is excreted in urine. Another inherent detoxification mechanism involves inactivation of HCN in the bloodstream by combining with the ferric iron of methemoglobin.

However, since there is normally a very small amount of methemoglobin present in blood, and endogenous stores of thiosulfate can be rapidly depleted, these two endogenous mechanisms of detoxification are rapidly overcome in cases of clinical toxicity.[228, 229]

Excess cyanide ion reacts readily with the trivalent (ferric) iron of cytochrome oxidase to form a very stable cyanide–cytochrome oxidase complex. When iron is maintained in the ferric form, electron transport can no longer occur, and the chain of cellular respiration is brought to a halt. As a consequence, hemoglobin is unable to release its oxygen to the electron transport system, and cellular hypoxia results. This action occurs despite a large concentration of oxygen in the bloodstream. Cytochrome oxidase is most concentrated in tissues that have a high oxidative metabolic rate, such as the CNS and cardiac muscle. All tissues can be affected from this lack of usable oxygen, but death is primarily due to anoxia in the brain.[228, 229]

The acute oral LD_{50} of HCN is 2.0 to 2.3 mg/kg, and rapid intake of plant material equivalent to about 4 mg/kg is thought to be a lethal amount.[228]

Diagnosis and Treatment. Cyanide poisoning should be considered when animals consuming cyanogenic plants are affected with acute signs of oxygen starvation and bright-red blood. Chemical confirmation can be accomplished, and forage, blood, liver, muscle, brain, and heart may be submitted. All samples should be quick-frozen as soon as possible, and shipped in a frozen state.[228, 229] Plant materials containing greater than 200 ppm HCN, and concentrations in brain and ventricular myocardium greater than 100 μg/100 g wet tissue are considered significant.[229]

Treatment is aimed at splitting the cyanide–cytochrome oxidase complex, with subsequent removal of the cyanide complex, and to augment available thiosulfate in the bloodstream. Sodium nitrite is used to displace the cyanide molecule from the cytochrome enzyme. Sodium nitrite changes some of the hemoglobin to methemoglobin, which then competes with cytochrome oxidase for the cyanide ion. In this process, methemoglobin and the cyanide ion form cyanomethemoglobin, and cytochrome oxidase is subsequently regenerated. Sodium nitrite should be used cautiously because of the possible danger of producing nitrite toxicosis, but reportedly it can be administered intravenously at doses ranging from 6 mg/kg, given as a 20% solution,[231] to 15 to 25 mg/kg.[228]

Sodium thiosulfate reacts with the cyanide ion in the blood or liberated from cyanomethemoglobin, and forms thiocyanate. Thiocyanate is essentially harmless and is excreted in urine. Sodium thiosulfate is also given intravenously at doses ranging from 60 to 660 mg/kg, as a 20% solution,[231] to 1.25 g/kg.[228] Additional recommended therapies include large doses of hydroxycobalamin (vitamin B_{12}) and mineral oil. The cobalt in the vitamin B_{12} preparation may bind additional cyanide in the circulation, and mineral oil is used to aid evacuation of the gastrointestinal tract.[228] Animals that survive 24 hours usually do not require further treatment.[228]

Sodium Fluoroacetate (1080)

Sodium fluoroacetate and fluoroacetamide are both highly toxic to many animal species. They are used as rodenticides and in predator control, and because of their toxicity are available only from licensed exterminators. The compounds are odorless, tasteless, and water-soluble, and are typically incorporated into baits composed of carrot chunks, bread, bran, or meats. In the United States, these compounds are mixed with a black dye prior to being placed in baits. Horses may become intoxicated by inadvertent exposure to these baits.[223, 233]

Clinical Signs. Sodium fluoroacetate causes signs primarily related to cardiac dysfunction in herbivores. The onset of signs usually occurs from one-half to 2 hours following ingestion. When signs begin, their onset is usually acute and follow a rapid, usually violent course. Marked cardiac arrhythmias with rapid, weak pulse and eventual ventricular fibrillation are typical findings. Horses may exhibit staggering, trembling, restlessness, urination, and defecation. Moaning and bruxism may be noted along with profuse sweating and colicky signs. Terminal convulsions may also occur. Ventricular fibrillation is the cause of death, and some horses may be found dead with no outward signs of struggle.[232, 233]

Pathophysiology. Fluoroacetate is readily absorbed from the gastrointestinal tract, lungs, or open wounds, but not through intact skin. Following absorption, it is distributed throughout the body and does not accumulate in any specific tissue. The acute oral LD_{50} of fluoroacetate in horses is 0.35 to 0.55 mg/kg.[232]

Following entry into cells, fluoroacetate can replace acetyl CoA, combining with oxaloacetate to form fluorocitrate. Fluorocitrate then competes with citrate for the active site of aconitase, a Krebs cycle enzyme, and also inhibits succinate dehydrogenase, which catalyzes succinate metabolism. The inhibition of these two enzymes and the subsequent accumulation of citrate block the Krebs cycle, leading to decreased glucose metabolism, energy stores, and cellular respiration. These actions occur in all cells, but organs with high metabolic rates (such as brain and heart) are affected most severely.[232-234]

The short latent period between ingestion and onset of signs is because fluoroacetate must be converted to the more toxic fluorocitrate. The accumulation of toxic levels of fluorocitrate therefore requires some time.[233]

Diagnosis and Treatment. Diagnosis of fluoroacetate toxicity must rely heavily on history of exposure, compatible clinical signs, and absence of other pathologic findings. Laboratory detection of these compounds can be very difficult, but specimens can be subjected to analysis by both gas-liquid and high-performance liquid chromatography.[233, 234] Fluoride ion–specific electrodes are also used to detect the compound in suspect samples. Suspect baits, stomach content, liver, and kidney are the best samples to submit for evaluation.[232, 233] Marked elevation of kidney citrate levels is suggestive of 1080 toxicity.[232]

Laboratory abnormalities in affected animals might include hyperglycemia and lactic acidemia.[233] However, these findings are inconclusive, and accompany many disease states in the horse.

There is no specific antidote. Therapy is largely supportive

and apparently unrewarding in horses already showing signs of toxicity. Intestinal decontamination may be attempted by use of oral mineral oil and activated charcoal. If hypocalcemia develops, calcium gluconate or calcium chloride may be administered. Glycerol monoacetate 0.1 to 0.5 mg/kg IM with hourly repeat treatments has been suggested, but may not be effective after onset of clinical signs.[233, 235]

TOXICOSES CAUSING SIGNS RELATING TO THE EPITHELIUM, SKELETAL SYSTEM, AND GENERAL BODY CONDITION

Plants

Black Walnut (Juglans nigra)

Shavings and aqueous extracts from black walnut trees are responsible for a toxic syndrome in horses characterized by acute onset of laminitis and variable degrees of limb edema.[236-238]

Clinical Signs. Horses begin showing signs of toxicity within 10 to 12 hours of being bedded with black walnut shavings. The primary signs are those of laminitis, and include reluctance to move, shifting weight from limb to limb, increased digital pulse and temperature of the hoof, and positive response to hoof testers. The severity of the laminitis can vary from mild to severe.[236-238] Another very characteristic finding is that of limb edema, which can become fairly pronounced. Additional signs noted may include increased respiratory rate with flared nostrils, anorexia and lethargy, and abdominal pain.[237] Horses removed from the bedding after clinical signs have developed have a good prognosis for full recovery.[236, 237]

Pathophysiology. The toxic principle involved in toxicosis is yet unidentified. Earlier, juglone, a naphthoquinone found in roots, bark, and nuts of black walnut trees, was suggested to be the causative agent.[236-238] Further work has shown, however, that an aqueous soluble toxin other than juglone, and found in the heartwood, is more likely to be responsible for generation of clinical signs.[238] The mechanism of action of this soluble toxin has not been fully elucidated, but it has been shown to reversibly enhance vasoconstriction of isolated digital vessels in vitro induced by administration of epinephrine potentiated with hydrocortisone.[239]

Diagnosis and Treatment. Diagnosis of black walnut–induced laminitis is based primarily on known exposure to shavings containing the plant and subsequent development of clinical signs. The treatment of laminitis is covered elsewhere, but horses have a good prognosis for recovery if they are removed from the offending bedding. Black walnut shavings should not be used as bedding for horses.

Wild Jasmine (Cestrum diurnum)

Cestrum diurnum (wild jasmine, day cestrum, day-blooming jessamine, king-of-the-day, Chinese inkberry) is a tropical-to-subtropical plant native to the West Indies, but has been widely introduced and cultivated as an ornamental in southern parts of the United States, including Florida, Texas, and California. The plant grows rapidly from seeds, and birds may contribute to spread of the plant because of their appetite for ripe berries which contain seeds. The plant is naturalized in Hawaii and India also, and it tends to multiply along fence rows, roadsides, and in neglected pastures and fields. Horses show signs of disease following ingestion of the plant for several weeks to months.[240]

Clinical Signs. Affected horses show signs primarily of weight loss and lameness. Weight loss occurs over several weeks to months in spite of normal appetite. Lameness is usually of increasing severity, and may begin with signs of generalized stiffness. Eventually, the fetlock joints may become overextended and horses may exhibit kyphosis. The flexor tendons, and particularly the suspensory ligament become sensitive to palpation. The lameness can become so severe as to require euthanasia.[240] Signs of renal failure may also become evident in isolated cases.

Pathophysiology. *Cestrum diurnum* and certain other members of the Solanaceae family contain a potent steroid glycoside with vitamin D-like activity. The toxic agent is a 1,25-dihydroxycholecalciferol [1,25(OH)2D$_3$] glycoside found in the leaves of the plant.[241, 242] Normally, vitamin D$_3$ is acquired from the diet or is produced in the skin by a reaction dependent on ultraviolet light. Vitamin D$_3$ is hydroxylated in the liver to yield 25-hydroxycholecalciferol, which is subsequently hydroxylated in the kidney to 1,25(OH)2D$_3$. This compound is the most active form of the vitamin, and acts to increase calcium absorption and stimulate production of calcium-binding protein in the intestine.[241]

The normal rate of production 1,25(OH)2D$_3$ is regulated by a negative feedback mechanism. Calcium or phosphorus deprivation stimulates the production of 1,25(OH)2D$_3$, and a decreased rate of production occurs when calcium or phosphorus is present in adequate amounts.[241]

This natural feedback mechanism is bypassed when 1,25(OH)2D$_3$ is supplied exogenously, as in the case of ingestion of *C. diurnum*. As a consequence, excessive calcium-binding protein is synthesized in the intestine, and excessive amounts of calcium and phosphorus are absorbed. If the calcium load exceeds the kidneys' capacity to excrete it, soft tissue mineralization (dystrophic calcification) and osteopetrosis occur.[241] In horses ingesting toxic amounts of *C. diurnum*, calcification of the flexor tendons, suspensory ligament, and other elastic tissues appears to predominate over deposition of calcium into other soft tissues.[240] Osteopetrosis is thought to result from sustained hypercalcemia and secondary elevation of calcitonin.[240]

Diagnosis and Treatment

Diagnosis of the condition should be suspected when horses exhibit signs of weight loss and lameness, and they have known prolonged access to *C. diurnum*. Affected horses typically are hypercalcemic, but serum phosphorus concentration is usually within a normal range. Renal dysfunction, if present, may be characterized by elevations in BUN and creatinine. Urine analysis may indicate an increased frac-

tional excretion of sodium, potassium, and phosphorus, along with other laboratory findings associated with renal failure.

No treatment for vitamin D toxicosis in known. Horses should be denied access to *C. diurnum* plants.

Hairy Vetch (Vicia villosa)

One report of toxicosis suspected to be the result of ingestion of hairy vetch is described.[243] The affected horse was a 1-year-old crossbred female presented for euthanasia because of severe weight loss and bilateral corneal ulceration with perforation.

The clinical signs reported were weight loss despite good appetite, fluctuating body temperature, subcutaneous swelling that started around the lips and spread to involve the rest of the body, and bilateral corneal ulceration with eventual perforation.

The only recorded abnormal laboratory findings consisted of elevated serum concentrations of LDH and AST measured 2 weeks after onset of clinical signs. Histologic lesions consisted of multifocal to diffuse granulomatous inflammation of the heart, lungs, kidneys, skin, lymph nodes, ileum, colon, skeletal muscle, and choroid.

The toxic substance has not been identified, and no specific therapy has been recommended. A similar toxic condition is occasionally seen in cattle grazing hairy vetch, with most cases of toxicosis occurring between April and July.

Photosensitizing Plants

Many plants can cause photosensitive reactions in horses. Some plants contain photodynamic substances that are absorbed from the gastrointestinal tract, either intact or in a form metabolically altered into an active compound (primary photosensitizing plants). Other plants may cause photodermatitis secondary to liver dysfunction, in which the photodynamic toxin is a metabolite normally excreted in bile (secondary photosensitivity). Because of hepatic damage induced by the plant, these metabolites enter the circulation and subsequent interaction with light results in clinical manifestation of disease. A list of plants[244–246] known to induce photosensitization in herbivores is shown in Table 19–1.

Clinical Signs. Signs of photosensitization are similar, regardless of the cause, and vary in degree. Factors that influence the severity of signs include the amount of reactive pigment present in the skin at a given time, the degree of exposure to light of appropriate wavelength, and the severity of hepatic damage, if hepatogenous photosensitization is the cause.[245]

Restlessness and discomfort are usually the first signs noted. Erythema may be noted, followed by edema of affected areas. Blister formation and subsequent serum exudation and scab formation occur as the condition progresses. Affected sites are usually painful to touch, and animals often attempt to protect themselves from direct sunlight.[245, 246]

The light-colored or nonpigmented areas of skin are most severely affected, particularly those areas involving the face, nose, back, escutcheon, and coronary band. Severely affected animals may also have involvement of pigmented areas of skin, and secondary self-trauma and bacterial infection may

Table 19–1. Plants Inducing Photosensitization in Herbivores

Primary Photosensitizers

Hypericum perforatum (Saint Johnswort, Klamath weed)—contains the naphthodianthrone derivative hypericin
Fagopyrum sagittatum (buckwheat)—contains the naphthodianthrone derivative fagopyrin
Cymopterus watsoni (spring parsley)—contains furocoumarins
Ammi majus (bishop's weed)—contains furocoumarins
Avena fatua (oat grass)
Brassica (rape)
Cooperia pedunculata
Erodium (trefoil)
Perennial rye grass
Ricinus communis (castor bean)
Rutaceae
Trifolium (clover)
Umbelliferae

Secondary or Hepatogenous Photosensitizers

Tetradymia glabrata (spineless horsebrush)
Tetradymia canescens (gray horsebrush)
Agave lecheguilla (lechuguilla)
Nolina texana (sacahuiste)
Tribulus terrestris (puncture vine)
Lantana spp.
Panicum spp. (panic grass, kleingrass)
Brassica napus (cultivated rape)
Senecio spp. (ragwort, groundsels)
Blue-green algae
Brachiaria brizantha
Brassia hyssopifolia
Holocalyx glaziovii
Lippia rehmanni
Myoporum laetum (ngaio)
Narthecium ossifragum (bog asaphodel)
Pithomyces chartarum and *Pithomyces minutissima*

Other Photosensitizers

Avena (oats)
Medicago (alfalfa)
Trifolium (clover)
Sorghum vulgare (Sudan grass)
Polygonum spp. (smartweed)
Euphorbia maculata (milk purslane)
Kochia scoparia (summer cyprus, fireweed)
Vicia spp. (vetches)

---

arise from the animal's attempts at rubbing the affected areas. Horses may lose patches of skin that slough in large, leathery plaques.[245, 246]

Pathophysiology. Plants causing primary photosensitization contain a photodynamic agent that is absorbed from the gastrointestinal tract either intact, or that is metabolically altered later into an active compound. Secondary photosensitizing plants induce hepatic damage of sufficient magnitude to inhibit adequate clearance of photodynamic agents. Normally, these photodynamic toxins are metabolites excreted in bile. When the liver is damaged sufficiently or bile flow is hindered, these metabolites enter the circulation. Phylloerythrin, a normal chlorophyll breakdown product, is considered the only important photodynamic substance in instances of secondary photosensitization.[247] These photodynamic agents are then circulated throughout the body, eventually reaching the dermal capillaries.

Interaction of long-wave ultraviolet light with these photodynamic agents circulating in the skin capillaries results in chemical excitement of these substances. As a consequence, free radicals are formed that are highly inflammatory and cause degradation of cell phospholipid membranes, polypeptide proteins, and nucleic acids.[246, 247] These processes are disruptive to cells and ultimately result in the dermal lesions noted with this toxicity. It should be remembered that drugs and diseases that cause liver damage can potentially also cause photosensitivity.

Diagnosis and Treatment. Clinical signs of photosensitivity are fairly typical and seldom confused with other afflictions of skin. When clinical signs become evident, the horse should be thoroughly evaluated for evidence of hepatopathy, since both primary and secondary photosensitivity produce the same clinical signs. If hepatic disease is present, the cause should be ascertained and appropriate therapy instituted.

Primary photodynamic agents can be identified with several biological assay systems. A mouse assay system and a microbial assay involving the use of *Candida albicans* are both available for this purpose.[246]

Specific therapy for photodermatitis is not available. Horses should be removed from direct sunlight until skin lesions are healed and the offending plant is removed from the environment. Various topical agents may be employed to help skin healing. Superficial bacterial dermatitis should be treated with appropriate antibiotics, and nonsteroidal anti-inflammatory therapy may be beneficial during initial stages of the disease process.

Pyrrolizidine Alkaloids

Pyrrolizidine alkaloid toxicity results from consumption of plants that contain various pyrrolizidine alkaloids. Horses can become intoxicated by ingestion of both fresh plants and dried plants incorporated into hay. As with many toxic plants, though, these plants are frequently unpalatable to most horses, yet certain conditions may render them more appetizing. This toxicity is characterized by a chronic, progressive disorder manifested by signs of liver failure. The more common plants that cause toxicosis in horses include *Senecio jacobaea* (tansy ragwort), *Senecio vulgaris* and, *Senecio longilobus* (groundsel), *Amsinckia intermedia* (fiddleneck), *Crotalaria* species (rattlebox), *Eichium plantagineum* (viper's bugloss), *Heliotropium europaeum* (common heliotrope), and *Cynoglossum officinale* (hound's-tongue).[248, 249]

Clinical Signs. Signs of pyrrolizidine alkaloid intoxication in horses are essentially those of liver failure. The more frequent signs noted include weight loss of weeks' to months' duration, icterus, and behavioral abnormalities. The behavioral changes are indicative of hepatoencephalopathy, and may include aimless pacing or wandering, ataxia, licking inanimate objects, blindness, head-pressing, and uncharacteristic aggression. Convulsions and coma may precede death. Clinical signs of abnormal behavior usually are a terminal event in the disease process, and typically have an acute onset.[249, 250] Other signs less frequently reported include diarrhea, photosensitization of nonpigmented areas of skin, hemoglobinuria, and inspiratory dyspnea.[249, 251] Abortion and poor exercise tolerance (reduced athletic performance) have also been observed in horses following ingestion of sublethal amounts.[252] Because toxicity of these plants is related to liver dysfunction, clinical signs of disease may not become apparent for weeks to months following ingestion.

Pathophysiology. There are a number of pyrrolizidine alkaloids present in various plant species, and some plants may contain multiple alkaloids. These substances are absorbed from the gastrointestinal tract and carried to the liver where they are metabolized by hepatic microsomal enzymes to pyrroles. These pyrroles can then cross-link double-stranded DNA, and bind to proteins and nucleic acid within hepatocytes.[248, 249]

The cross-linking of DNA has an antimitotic effect on hepatocytes. The hepatocytes are unable to divide and subsequently become megalocytes. As these cells die, they are replaced by fibrous tissue rather than normal hepatocytes. Binding of protein and nucleic acid results in inhibition of cytoplasmic protein synthesis. These changes may lead to more rapid death of hepatocytes and cause centrilobular necrosis. Eventually, liver function begins to fail because of progressive hepatocellular death and subsequent fibrosis.[248, 249] As the disease progresses, generalized fibrosis develops. Once connective tissue bridges form between portal areas, the disease is fatal.[248]

Variation in the dosage and frequency of administration of alkaloids results in a wide spectrum of hepatic lesions. Acute toxicosis resulting from massive doses is more likely to produce centrilobular necrosis with hemorrhage. Chronic doses tend to produce hepatocellular death in the portal areas, along with megalocytosis, fibrosis, biliary hyperplasia, and occlusion of hepatic veins.[248, 249] Liver failure is thought to be ultimately responsible for the clinical signs observed in pyrrolizidine alkaloid toxicosis.

The toxic dose of dried *Senecio* is estimated to be 5% of the horse's body weight. This amount does not need to be ingested all at once, however, as the effects are cumulative. The total dose of alkaloids consumed determines the toxic effect, regardless of the amount of time in which they were consumed.[248, 249]

Diagnosis and Treatment. Most cases of pyrrolizidine alkaloid toxicosis are diagnosed based upon history, compatible clinical signs, serum liver enzyme activities, and liver biopsy findings. When active hepatocellular damage is occurring early in the disease process, sorbitol dehydrogenase and LDH are usually elevated, but they often decline to normal values by the time the horse is showing clinical signs. Serum GGT, ALP, and AST activities all tend to be elevated throughout the disease course. Serum concentration of bile acids is also reported to be elevated in affected horses. Serum bilirubin concentration tends to be elevated in later stages of disease and hypoglycemia and hypoalbuminemia are rarely seen except in cases of severe hepatic disease.[248, 249, 251, 252]

Other diagnostic aids that may be useful from both a diagnostic and prognostic standpoint include measurement of the ratio of branched-chain to aromatic amino acids in serum, and liver biopsy. The branched-chain amino acids isoleucine, leucine, and valine are catabolized primarily in muscle and the aromatic amino acids phenylalanine and tyrosine are catabolized mainly in the liver. The ratio of the sums of these amino acids (branched-chain to aromatic) has been shown to progressively decrease from normal in horses affected with pyrrolizidine alkaloid toxicosis.[253] If the ratio is below normal range and the horses are continually exposed to alkaloid-containing plants, they have a poor chance of survival. Some affected horses also showed a dramatic decrease in this ratio just prior to death.[253] Liver biopsy findings of a triad of fibrosis, bile duct proliferation, and megalocytosis are highly suggestive of pyrrolizidine alkaloid toxicosis. Liver biopsy samples can also help in establishing prognosis, as the presence of advanced or generalized hepatic fibrosis warrants a grave prognosis.[248, 249]

Feed samples may be analyzed for pyrrolizidine alkaloid content, but the process is often time-consuming and relatively expensive.[248]

No specific treatment for pyrrolizidine alkaloid toxicity exists. Affected horses may survive if they are denied further exposure to alkaloid-containing plants, and are fed a suitable diet. However, some horses may still show signs of liver disease even though they have not had exposure to the plant for some time. Specific treatment of acute and chronic liver failure is discussed elsewhere.

Prevention is accomplished by keeping horses away from pasture or feed contaminated with pyrrolizidine alkaloid–containing plants.

Tall Fescue (Festuca arundinacea)

Horses grazing or being fed tall fescue hay preparations may develop a condition termed "summer slump" or "summer syndrome."[254, 255] The disorder is characterized by anorexia, weight loss, poor hair coat quality, pyrexia, and hypersalivation. Additionally, mares may sustain a variety of pregnancy- and reproductive-related disorders. Typical findings include the presence of a thick, tough placenta, prolonged gestation, abortion, birth of dead or very weak foals, and high perinatal foal mortality. Mares are frequently affected also with agalactia, retained placenta, and rebreeding difficulties.[254–256]

The causative agent of this disorder is suggested to be *Acremonium coenophialum,* a fungal endophyte that grows within the grass blade of fescue.[256] This endophyte is highly indigenous to many areas of the United States, and may contaminate as much as 90% of fescue pastures in certain geographical areas.[256]

The toxic agent in *Acremonium* is yet unidentified. Pyrrolizidine alkaloids and ergopeptine alkaloid compounds are contained in the fungus, but their role in the pathogenesis of this disorder is unknown.[256]

Treatment is largely symptomatic, as no specific therapy is available. Prevention is accomplished by restricting access to *Acremonium*-infested fescue pastures, but this may be very difficult to accomplish in some instances. Pasture management and use of alternative forages may be required to limit the incidence of the disorder. Local or regional authorities should be consulted for current methods of management of infected pastures.

Medications
Iodine

Iodine toxicosis or iodism is a rarely reported cause of toxicosis in horses. When it occurs, it is most likely due to iatrogenic administration of iodine-containing substances. Many rations contain iodine in the form of various iodized salts, and sodium and potassium iodide, along with the organic iodide compound ethylenediamine dihydroiodide, are used in treatment of various medical conditions.[257, 258]

Clinical Signs. Nonpruritic generalized alopecia and diffuse scaliness of the skin were reported in a horse given 45 g of ethylenediamine dihydroiodide twice-daily for 14 days.[259] Other reported clinical signs include goiter secondary to excessive iodine intake, increased secretions of the respiratory tract, nasal discharge, intermittent nonproductive cough, and excessive lacrimation.[257, 259, 260] Pregnant mares receiving excessive amounts of iodine may produce weak foals with enlarged thyroid glands. Such foals have a high mortality rate.[257]

Pathophysiology. Both organic and inorganic forms of iodine are rapidly and almost completely absorbed from the gastrointestinal tract in the ionic form, and distributed throughout the body. Iodine is excreted primarily in the urine, but smaller amounts are present in feces, sweat, and milk.[258, 260] The only known metabolic role of iodine is involvement in synthesis of the thyroid hormones T_4 and triiodothyronine (T_3).[260]

Oral iodine salts, whether organic or inorganic, taken in higher doses stimulate nerve receptors in the stomach wall. Subsequently, the vagus nerve becomes stimulated and causes reflex secretion by cells in the upper respiratory tract.[260, 261] Excessive iodine intake causes thyroidal organic iodine formation to increase to a maximal amount, then a sharp decline in organic iodine formation occurs. Excessive iodine also inhibits release of organic iodine from the thyroid gland if the gland is stimulated by thyroid-stimulating hormone (TSH). The net results are clinical signs of increased amount and viscosity of respiratory tract secretions, and occasional goiter development.[261] The mechanism underlying the development of the dermal lesions associated with iodism is unknown.[259]

Diagnosis and Treatment. Diagnosis of iodism is based on a history of exposure to high levels of iodine for a prolonged period of time, coupled with compatible clinical signs of nasal discharge and excessive lacrimation, intermittent nonproductive cough, and nonpruritic generalized alopecia and scaling. Serum iodine concentrations can be measured and are elevated in cases of iodism, but blood levels decrease rapidly to near background levels within a few days if iodine exposure is discontinued.[260] Serum concentrations of T_4 and T_3 may be below normal values in affected horses.[259]

Treatment consists in removing the source of the iodine. Since iodine is rapidly mobilized and excreted from tissues,

clinical signs usually subside fairly rapidly when excessive iodine is removed.[258, 260]

Miscellaneous Agents
Snake Venom

The venomous snakes in North America belong to the families Crotalidae (pit vipers), Elapidae (cobra), and Viperidae (true vipers). The vast majority of poisonous snakebites reported in humans are inflicted by members of the Crotalidae family, and the same is probably true for horses as well. Of this family, *Crotalus* (rattlesnakes), *Agkistrodon* (copperhead, cottonmouth), and *Sistrurus* (pigmy rattlesnake, massasauga) are the three genera most commonly involved. The eastern coral snake *(Micrurus fulvius)* and the Arizona coral snake *(Micruroides euryxanthus)* are two members of the Elapidae family indigenous to the United States, but they account for only about 3% of poisonous bites reported in humans.[262, 263] No documentation of coral snakebite affecting horses could be found in the literature.

Venom injected into prey is an aid to digestion and greatly reduces the time for complete digestion to occur in the snake. The amount of venom injected at a given time is under voluntary control, and larger amounts are injected into larger prey or when the snake strikes for defensive purposes. Not all bites result in envenomation, and it is estimated that rattlesnakes fail to inject venom in up to 20% of bites.[262, 263]

Snake venom is a highly complex mixture of enzymes, lipids, biogenic amines, free amino acids, metal ions, proteins, and polypeptides. Most snake venoms contain up to 25 different fractions, yet many of them are not yet identified.[262] Venom composition and toxic properties vary among *Crotalus* species and between individuals within the same species. Factors influencing venom composition include age, time from last feeding, and seasonal influences related to changes in feeding patterns or physiologic responses such as hibernation.[262] The LD_{50} in mice exposed to venom of *Crotalus* species ranges from 0.23 mg/kg for the Mojave rattlesnake *(C. scutulatus)* to 3.77 mg/kg for the red diamond rattlesnake *(C. ruber ruber)*. The mouse LD_{50} for the copperhead *(Agkistrodon contortrix)* and cottonmouth *(Agkistrodon piscivorus)* is 10.92 mg/kg and 4.17 mg/kg, respectively.[262] This large variation in dose and chemical composition of venom accounts for the extreme amount of variation in the physiologic responses of animals to these substances.

Clinical Signs. The clinical signs associated with snakebite in horses are usually the result of the local effects of the venom. Death from snakebite is rare in horses, as are systemic manifestations of envenomation. The classic signs noted in most horses are very acute onset of swelling and edema at the bite site. Usually the head and muzzle are affected because of the inquisitive nature of horses, but bites can also occur on the limbs or other parts of the body. The muzzle and nasal passages may become swollen to the extent that respiration can become extremely labored, necessitating a tracheotomy. Initially, fang marks may be noted, but they soon disappear with the onset of extensive swelling. Skin discoloration at the injection site is a common occurrence with many rattlesnakes, but rarely occurs with copperhead and Mojave rattlesnake bites.[263] Varying degrees of necrosis of local tissue may occur as well as secondary bacterial infections at the wound site. In my opinion, bites involving the distal extremities of horses frequently have a prolonged convalescent period that may be accompanied by residual lameness.

Systemic manifestations of snake envenomation are rare in horses but may be seen when venom is injected intravascularly or perivascularly. Labored respiration may result from pulmonary edema caused by passive congestion secondary to vascular hypotension or precipitation of pulmonary emboli. Cardiac and neurologic dysfunction rarely occurs, but muscle fasciculation may be evident.[263] An exception to the above may be the venom of the Mojave rattlesnake, which produces respiratory paralysis that may result in death in humans.[262]

The venom of coral snakes produces neurologic signs in affected humans, with death occurring within 24 hours as a result of respiratory depression, hypotension, and cardiovascular collapse.[262] However, the coral snake requires prolonged contact (30 seconds or greater) to work the venom into the skin of its prey. It therefore seems improbable that horses would become exposed to coral snake venom except under extremely unusual circumstances.

Pathophysiology. The venoms of Crotalidae are rich in enzymes. Proteases cause severe tissue damage by digesting tissue proteins and peptides, and hyaluronidase allows rapid spread of venom through tissue by hydrolyzing connective tissue hyaluronic acid. L-amino acid oxidase, L-arginine ester hydrolases, and 5′-nucleotidase may also contribute to tissue destruction. Phospholipases A, B, C, and D hydrolyze lipids and cause hemolysis by destroying lecithin in the RBC membranes. They also disrupt neurotransmission at both the presynaptic and postsynaptic junctions. Other enzymes present in crotalid venom include ribonuclease, deoxyribonuclease, transaminase, phosphomonoesterase, phosphodiesterase, ATPase, DNAase, ALP, acid phosphatase, and endonuclease.[262]

Crotalid venom contains a number of polypeptides in addition to the enzymes. These polypeptides are low-molecular-weight proteins that are 5 to 20 times more lethal than crude venom in animal models, and they do not have enzymatic activity. They are present in higher concentrations in cobra venom than in rattlesnake venom, and are mainly responsible for blood dyscrasias and coagulopathies. Small peptides are partly responsible for the generation of DIC, and a venom fraction of the timber rattlesnake *(Crotalus horridus horridus)* causes platelet aggregation with resultant thrombocytopenia. Additionally, the venoms of the Mojave and Southern Pacific rattlesnakes contain a direct cardiotoxin.[262]

Rattlesnake venom contains substances with anticoagulant, procoagulant, and plasminogen-induced fibrinogenolytic properties. The coagulopathy that occurs in a given instance is variable, and is dependent upon the content of the various venom components, and upon the dose of venom injected. The anticoagulant activity of crotalid venom appears to result from reversible binding of venom to prothrombin. Thrombinlike enzymes produce hypofibrinogenemia and increased concentration of fibrin degradation products. They are also capable of directly converting fibrinogen to fibrin, which may result in excessive fibrin

formation and rapid DIC. The fibrinolytic characteristics of crotalid venom occur either directly or indirectly through the activation of endogenous plasminogen.[262, 263]

Diagnosis and Treatment. Diagnosis of snakebite is usually dependent upon clinical signs and accessibility to poisonous snakes. Laboratory abnormalities that may be present in affected horses include thrombocytopenia, hypofibrinogenemia, anemia, prolonged PT and PTT, hematuria, proteinuria, and myoglobinuria.[262, 263]

Affected horses should be kept calm and quiet. Incision over the fang marks and suction are rarely indicated and probably of minimal value except in the immediate time frame of the bite, since the venom is almost immediately absorbed into the surrounding tissues. Tracheotomy is indicated in those horses that develop excessive edema and swelling of the head and external nares to the point that respiration becomes impaired. Topical cold therapy may have some beneficial effect if applied early and for short time periods. Prolonged or excessive cold application, however, may enhance further tissue necrosis. Antivenom therapy is commonly used in instances of human snakebite, but is often considered unnecessary in horses because of the low mortality rate, financial considerations, and availability of other therapies. An exception may be the extremely valuable animal or foals.

Tetanus prophylaxis and systemic antibiotic therapy should be initiated. Broad-spectrum antimicrobials should be employed since both gram-positive and gram-negative organisms are found in the mouth of North American pit vipers. The most common organisms isolated include *Proteus vulgaris, Escherichia coli, Corynebacterium, Streptococcus,* and enterobacteria.[262]

NSAIDs should not be used during the very early stages, because they may enhance the thrombocytopenia frequently induced by snake venom. They may be used in the later stages of the disease to help reduce pain, swelling, and inflammation. Corticosteroids should be used with caution, since they may diminish the clearance of fibrin degradation products from the peripheral vasculature by the reticuloendothelial system, and they may increase susceptibility to wound infection at the site. Corticosteroids may be beneficial, however, in treating severe hypotensive shock in young animals or in patients with intravenous envenomation. Heparin therapy has also been suggested to be helpful in instances of thrombus formation.[263]

Animals affected with systemic hypotension and cardiac dysrhythmias should be treated appropriately. This may include the administration of intravenous fluids and plasma, and the use of specific antiarrhythmic medications.

Fluoride

Fluoride toxicosis in horses is apparently an extremely rare event.[264] Although acute and chronic fluoride toxicosis have been described in various animals, chronic fluorosis appears more common. Common sources of fluoride in chronic fluorosis include forages subjected to airborne contamination from nearby industrial plants such as aluminum smelters, steel mills, or fertilizer plants that heat fluorine-containing materials and discharge fluorides; drinking water containing excessive fluoride; feed supplements and vitamin and mineral additives with high fluoride concentration; and vegetation grown on soils containing high fluoride levels.[265]

Animals normally ingest small amounts of fluoride throughout their lives, and it accumulates in the body as long as constant or increasing amounts are ingested. Chronic toxicosis can result from prolonged ingestion of sufficiently high levels. The long-term dietary tolerance for fluoride in the horse is reported to be 40 to 60 ppm dietary fluoride.

Fluoride is almost totally absorbed from the gastrointestinal tract. Once absorbed, approximately half is rapidly excreted in urine with the remaining half being stored in bone and teeth. Fluoride accumulates in calcified tissues, but once exposure ceases, bone fluoride will be depleted slowly over a period of months to years.

Clinical Signs. Chronic fluorosis in the horse is a rare event. In one suspected case, the affected horse exhibited chronic weight loss of months' duration, poor growth, difficulty in mastication, and deformed, discolored, and absent deciduous incisors. The horse was also missing some deciduous premolars and molars.[264] Classic dental abnormalities reported in other species include mottled, hypoplastic enamel and brown discoloration with uneven wear of teeth.[265] Additional signs associated with chronic fluorosis in other animals include hyperostosis, enlargement and roughening of involved bones, intermittent lameness and generalized stiffness, dry and roughened hair coat, and decreased weight and milk production.[265] Because of the insidious nature of chronic fluorosis, it must be remembered that there may be a time lag between ingestion of excessive fluoride and the appearance of clinical signs.

Pathophysiology. Excessive fluoride produces dental abnormalities by affecting the teeth during development. The primary effect of fluorine is thought to be a delaying and alteration of normal mineralization of the pre-enamel, predentine, and precementum. High fluoride levels appear to cause specific ameloblastic and odontoblastic damage. The matrix laid down by these damaged cells fails to accept minerals normally, resulting in faulty mineralization of the tooth bud. Once the tooth is fully formed, the ameloblasts have lost their constructive ability and the enamel lesions cannot be repaired. However, odontoblasts can produce secondary dentine to compensate for deficiencies brought about by excessive fluoride.[265] The brown-to-black discoloration of affected teeth is the result of oxidation of organic material in the teeth.

The pathogenesis of bone lesions associated with fluoride toxicosis is still undecided. One theory is that high fluoride levels lead to inadequate matrix and defective, irregular mineralization of bone. Another theory is that hydroxyl radicals in the hydroxyapatite crystal structure are replaced by fluoride ions, resulting in a decrease in crystal lattice dimensions.[265] The pathologic results of skeletal fluorosis include dissociation of normal sequences of osteogenesis, production of abnormal bone, accelerated remodeling of bone, and occasional accelerated bone resorption.[265]

Diagnosis and Treatment. Diagnosis of chronic fluorosis is primarily based on clinical findings and history of possible exposure to fluorides. Confirmation of fluorosis is usually accomplished by analysis of skeletal or dental tissues for fluoride content, and evaluation of fluoride concentration in urine. Water and feed consumed by the animals should also be analyzed for fluoride content.

Treatment of chronic fluorosis is largely aimed at dietary restriction of fluoride-containing substances. Aluminum sulfate, aluminum chloride, calcium aluminate, calcium carbonate, and defluorinated phosphate have been used to reduce the toxic effects of fluoride, but no substance will completely prevent the toxic effects of ingesting excessive amounts of fluorides.

Zinc

Zinc intoxication is a problem of young growing horses. Sources of excessive zinc are usually soil and forage contamination from nearby smelters and following top-dressing of pastures with zinc oxide.[266, 267] Classic signs of zinc toxicity have also been produced by experimental feeding of excess zinc to young foals.[268, 269] Skeletally mature horses do not appear to be susceptible to the effects of zinc-contaminated pastures.[269]

Clinical Signs. Typical signs associated with zinc toxicity include swelling at the physeal region of long bones, gradual onset of lameness and stiffness that may become so severe that affected animals are reluctant to rise from lateral recumbency, swollen joints resulting from synovial effusion, unthriftiness, and weight loss despite normal appetite.[266–268] Anemia may also develop in more chronically affected individuals.[268] The joint swellings in affected horses are typical of those of osteochondrosis desiccans, and severe generalized osteochondrosis also develops in zinc-intoxicated horses.[266, 267, 269]

Pathophysiology. Zinc toxicity in horses actually appears to be a manifestation of copper deficiency and the subsequent development of hypocupremic-induced articular cartilage disease.[266, 269] Copper is an essential cofactor for lysyl oxidase, an enzyme involved in the formation of collagen cross-links. Copper deficiency interferes with collagen metabolism and results in production of weak connective tissue. This allows articular cartilage fractures and growth physeal fractures to occur in the zone of hypertrophic cells, producing the clinical syndrome of osteochondrosis desiccans.

The mechanism of zinc-induced copper deficiency is not totally understood. Experimentally intoxicated foals at necropsy had high hepatic copper content despite low serum copper concentration, suggesting that the hepatic copper was not readily available for production of ceruloplasmin or it could not be mobilized rapidly enough for use by other tissues.[269] Excess zinc stimulates production of metallothionein, an intestinal cell protein that binds to excess zinc, copper, and other divalent metal ions and facilitates their excretion in bile, feces, and saliva. Copper has a higher affinity for metallothionein than does zinc, and increased production of metallothionein, with subsequent binding to copper, may lead to copper deficiency via increased copper excretion.[270]

Diagnosis and Treatment. Once signs of osteochondrosis develop, the condition should be treated appropriately. Diagnosis of zinc toxicity may be somewhat difficult in that zinc is rapidly excreted following absorption, and blood and tissue zinc concentrations tend to quickly decline to normal levels with cessation of intake.[271] Liver, kidney, and serum zinc concentrations can be measured, but fecal samples collected from affected horses may be more suitable. Feed and water supplies can also be evaluated for zinc content.[271]

Treatment of affected horses is aimed at restoring proper copper concentration in the diet, and removing the source of excess zinc. Diets containing 7.7 mg of copper/kg and 250 mg of zinc/kg of dry weight were sufficient to maintain normal serum copper and zinc concentrations, and did not induce disease in treated foals. Diets containing 1,000 mg/kg or greater of zinc caused hypocupremia and subsequent osteochondrosis desiccans when fed to foals over a period of several weeks.[269] Osteochondrosis desiccans is treated surgically.

Selenium

Selenium toxicity in horses usually occurs as a result of prolonged ingestion of plants containing excessive amounts of selenium. Intoxication can result from horses foraging on soil with high levels of selenium, as well as from ingestion of selenium-accumulating plants growing on soils with minimal amounts of selenium.[272–275] Acute toxicosis can also occur through inadvertent overdose of selenium supplements added to rations or given by parenteral injection.[276] The acute single oral toxic dose of selenium given as sodium selenite lies between 3.3 and 6 mg/kg for the horse.[274, 277]

Clinical Signs. Three different syndromes are attributed to selenium intoxication—acute toxicity and two chronic forms described as "blind staggers" and "alkali disease." Signs of acute toxicity develop within 6 hours of ingestion, and include sweating, diarrhea, tachycardia, tachypnea, mild pyrexia, lethargy, and mild to severe colic. Death may occur within 24 hours, and some horses exhibit a dumb attitude prior to death. Head-pressing prior to death is suggested as a classic sign of acute selenosis.[274, 277]

Chronic selenium intoxication described as "blind staggers" results from frequent ingestion of plants over a period of weeks to months. Signs associated with this syndrome include aimless wandering or circling, muscle weakness, incoordination, respiratory difficulty, and decreased vision. In classic cases, blindness eventually develops and is followed by paralysis and death.[278]

Alkali disease also occurs from ingestion of plants and signs may develop within 3 weeks. Initially, lameness and swelling of the coronary band regions are noted, along with anorexia and mild depression. These signs progress to transverse cracking of the hoof wall distal to the coronary band with associated lameness. The hooves may eventually be sloughed. Loss of hair from the mane and tail occur because the hairs become brittle and are easily broken. Compromised reproductive function may also develop in affected horses.[272–276]

Pathophysiology. Selenium is absorbed readily from the gastrointestinal tract, but organic forms of selenium are generally retained in greater amounts than are inorganic forms.

Elimination occurs fairly rapidly through urine, sweat, feces, and exhaled air. Hoof and hair must also be recognized as routes of excretion, since excess selenium is deposited in these structures.[276] This latter fact has important diagnostic implications.

The mechanism whereby excess selenium produces these signs is not fully elucidated. Selenium functions in a number of enzymatic and physiologic processes. The toxic effects of selenium have been associated with its affinity for reacting with sulfur-containing amino acid residues, such as cystine, which are synthetically incorporated into biologically active glycoproteins and polypeptides. As a result, various selenosulfides are formed as a substitute for disulfide bonds.[279]

Diagnosis and Treatment. A presumptive diagnosis of selenium intoxication can be made based upon typical clinical signs and history of possible exposure to selenium—either iatrogenically in the form of selenium supplementation, or via ingestion of appropriate plants. A definitive diagnosis can be attempted by assaying serum, hair, and hoof material for selenium content. In acute fatal selenosis, serum selenium concentration may exceed 1 ppm.[274, 277] Selenium concentration greater than 5 ppm in hair and hoof wall can be considered diagnostic of selenosis.[272, 274, 275] Selenium concentration can also be measured in liver and kidney samples.

Treatment of affected horses involves removing the selenium source coupled with symptomatic treatment of lesions and good nursing care. Oral dosing of naphthalene 4.5 g/day for 5 days, waiting 5 days, then repeating the dose for an additional 5 days has been suggested for treatment of adult horses.[272, 274] Prevention of selenosis has been attempted by adding copper,[277] methionine,[280] or sodium arsenite[272, 274] to the diet of at-risk animals.

Gangrenous Ergotism (Clavaceps purpurea)

Clavaceps purpurea is a fungal parasite that invades the developing ovary of the grass flower and cereal grains. Rye, oats, wheat, and Kentucky bluegrass are commonly parasitized by this fungus, and are most often associated with outbreaks of gangrenous ergotism. The fungus replaces the seed ovary with a dark-brown-to-purple oblong body called a sclerotium. Sclerotia are slightly larger than the original whole grain seed, and their growth is promoted by warm, moist conditions. Horses are rarely affected with this condition, in part because of the distasteful nature of affected feedstuffs and because most fungal elements are removed during commercial grain processing procedures.[281, 282]

Clinical Signs. Signs may become apparent if infected feeds are ingested over a period of several days to weeks. Dry gangrene of the extremities is the classic sign associated with *C. purpurea* toxicosis. The limbs, nose, ears, and tail can be affected. Early signs of toxicosis are lameness and cool extremities. The hindlimbs are often affected first, with swelling and tenderness in the fetlock area. The involved tissues become dark and discolored and a transverse line of demarcation may occur between normal skin and the distal parts of the limb. Eventually, the hoof and associated bones and tissue may slough. This same sequence can involve the nose, ears, and tail. Gangrenous signs may be preceded by colic and constipation or diarrhea. Subacute effects can include depression, partial anorexia, general unthriftiness, and increased pulse and respiratory rates.[281, 282]

Pathophysiology. The major toxic alkaloids in ergot are divided into three groups: ergotamine, ergotoxine, and ergometrine. They are absorbed slowly and incompletely from the gastrointestinal tract, reaching peak plasma concentrations in approximately 2 hours. The liver is the primary site of metabolism and approximately 90% of metabolites are excreted in bile. Small amounts of unmetabolized alkaloids are excreted in urine. The total concentration and proportions of alkaloids present in ergot sclerotia may vary with species and environmental conditions.[281, 282]

Ergotamine and ergotoxine are polypeptide derivatives of lysergic acid. The varied physiologic effects of ergot are caused primarily by mixtures of levoisomers of ergotamine, coupled with smaller amounts of acetylcholine, histamine, and tyramine.[281]

Ergotamine is a vasoactive substance that causes both arterial and venous constriction. It may also damage capillary endothelium. The combined effects of vasoconstriction and endothelial damage produce increased blood pressure, decreased blood flow through the extremities, vascular stasis, thrombosis, and eventually gangrene.[281, 282]

The ergotoxine group of alkaloids produce α-adrenergic blockade and antagonize 5-hydroxytryptamine. This produces an increase in blood pressure as a result of peripheral vasoconstriction, particularly in postcapillary vessels.[281]

Diagnosis and Treatment. Tentative diagnosis of ergotism is based upon clinical signs and exclusion of other disease processes. Ergot sclerotia can be readily identified in grains by the experienced person. However, once grinding of feed has occurred, ergot can only be recognized by microscopic examination or chemical analysis for ergot alkaloids. Ergot alkaloids can be identified and quantitated by chromatographic methods, and a sample of the individual grain components should be obtained for analysis whenever possible.[281]

No specific treatment exists for gangrenous ergotism. The offending grain should be removed, and affected animals should be kept warm to avoid cold-induced further vasoconstriction in the extremities. Supportive therapy in the form of antibiotics and analgesics may be indicated. The use of anti-α-adrenergic pharmaceuticals to effect vasodilation may also be helpful. Such agents might include acepromazine, isoxsuprine, phenoxybenzamine, or similar products.[281, 282]

TOXICOSES CAUSING SIGNS RELATING TO THE URINARY SYSTEM

Plants

Oxalate Toxicosis

The most common source of oxalates to livestock is plants, particularly those of the Chenopodiaceae family. These plants contain varied amounts of soluble oxalates, usually in the form of sodium or potassium salts. However, since plants containing oxalates are generally unpalatable to horses,

plant-associated oxalate intoxication is rare. The following plants contain large amounts of soluble oxalates:

Amaranthus spp.	Pigweed
Beta vulgaris	Beet, mangold
Chenopodium album	Lamb's quarters
Halogeton glomeratus	Halogeton
Oxalis spp.	Wood sorrel, soursop
Portulaca oleracea	Purslane
Rheum rhaponticum	Rhubarb
Rumex spp.	Sorrel, dock
Salsola kali	Russian thistle
Sarcobatus vermiculatus	Black greasewood

Of these, *Halogeton* and *Sarcobatus* seem to be the primary offenders in range animals in the western United States.[283]

Since oxalates accumulate in the plants throughout the growing season, the incidence of toxicosis may be highest in the fall and winter months.[284] The oxalate content is highest in the leaves, with a lesser amount in seeds and a minimal amount present in the stems. The nonfatal toxic dosage of sodium oxalate for adult horses is approximately 200 g/day for 8 days.[283]

Clinical Signs. Affected horses may begin to show signs of depression, mild-to-moderate colic, muscular weakness, and irregular gait within 2 to 6 hours of ingestion. Weakness may proceed to lateral recumbency, unconsciousness, and death in 10 to 12 hours. Some animals may exhibit convulsions prior to succumbing.[283] The observed clinical signs of acute toxicity are typical of those of hypocalcemia.

Pathophysiology. Oxalates combine with serum calcium ions to form insoluble calcium oxalate. The result is a functional hypocalcemia in acute cases, with associated signs of altered behavior and neuromuscular abnormalities.

More chronic ingestion of oxalates can result in renal failure. Insoluble calcium oxalate crystals can lodge in the renal tubules, producing tubular blockage and necrosis. Oxalates may also crystallize in the vasculature and infiltrate blood vessel walls, producing necrosis and hemorrhage.[283]

Diagnosis and Treatment. In instances of acute toxicosis, consistent clinicopathologic abnormalities include moderate-to-marked hypocalcemia and varied electrolyte alterations. In chronic toxicity, urinalysis may reveal the presence of characteristic calcium oxalate crystals upon microscopic examination. Impending renal failure is also characterized by elevations in BUN and creatinine concentrations.[283]

Treatment is usually of little value once clinical signs have appeared. Calcium gluconate can be administered intravenously but usually provides only temporary relief of signs. Balanced electrolyte solutions are indicated to aid diuresis, and diuretics may also have benefit in the volume-loaded patient. Prevention is primarily aimed at avoidance of the plants by means of providing adequate suitable sources of feed.[283]

Rayless Goldenrod (Isocoma wrightii)

Ingestion of rayless goldenrod may produce renal tubular nephrosis and signs of renal failure, but tremetol is the most significant toxin present in the plant.[285, 286] For a detailed discussion of tremetol toxicity, see the discussion of white snakeroot toxicity.

Sorghum

Ingestion of *Sorghum* species and certain hybrid Sudan grasses has been associated with the development of an ataxia-cystitis syndrome.[287, 288] The toxicity occurs when horses graze the plants. More cases occur when the plant is young and rapidly growing, but mature and second-growth plants have also been incriminated. Horses being fed well-cured *Sorghum* species hay have not developed signs of toxicity. Occurrence of toxicity may increase during seasons of medium-to-high rainfall, but no cases have been recognized following the date of the first frost. Signs of toxicity may develop following a grazing period of 1 week to several months.[287]

Clinical Signs. The primary clinical signs noted are those of posterior ataxia and urinary incontinence or cystitis. The neurologic signs usually develop first and begin as posterior ataxia and incoordination. Affected horses may sway from side to side if forced to move, and signs tend to worsen upon backing the animal. Occasionally the rearquarters may drop almost to the ground, and flaccid paralysis of the tail and the rear legs may develop within 24 hours of the onset of neurologic signs. Affected horses remain alert and afebrile, and have a normal appetite and pulse and respiratory rates. Mares frequently exhibit continual opening and closing of the vulva, and relaxation of the perineal muscles. Males typically have a relaxed and extended penis.[287, 288]

Urinary incontinence exhibited by continual urine dribbling is prominent in both sexes and urine scalding on dependent skin becomes pronounced. The urinary bladder is typically distended and atonic, resulting in moderate-to-severe cystitis. Urethritis and ureteritis may also develop, and in horses that die from the disease, ascending pyelonephritis is usually the cause of death. Other clinical signs noted include abortion, and birth of foals with multiple arthrogryposis.[287, 288]

Pathophysiology. The clinical signs noted are a result of axonal degeneration and demyelination of nerve fibers in the spinal cord, particularly in the lumbar and sacral segments. The toxic substance in *Sorghum* species responsible for causing this change is unknown. Most *Sorghum* species are cyanogenic plants and contain various amounts of HCN. It has been suggested that exposure to multiple sublethal doses of HCN may induce axonal degeneration and demyelination.[287] Another hypothesis is that sorghum plants contain lathrogenic precursors and that this toxicosis may be caused by the ingestion of lathrogenic nitriles present in rapidly growing plants.[288, 289]

Diagnosis and Treatment. Diagnosis of sorghum ataxia-cystitis is primarily based upon appropriate clinical signs, history of grazing the plants, and exclusion of other known causes of posterior ataxia or paresis. No specific diagnostic tests are available. Cystitis and pyelonephritis are diagnosed by standard laboratory methods.

No specific treatment is available. Affected horses should be removed from the offending feed immediately. Once the feed is removed, affected horses usually show gradual improvement over several weeks to months, but complete recovery may not occur. Supportive and symptomatic therapy should include appropriate antibiotic treatment of bacterial urinary tract infections, and topical treatment of urine scald dermatitis. Periodic manual decompression of the urinary bladder may be helpful. Catheterization and frequent aspiration of bladder contents may be necessary to aid resolution of cystitis.

Medications
Aminoglycosides

The aminoglycoside antibiotics are commonly used because of their wide spectrum of bactericidal activity against gram-negative organisms. However, these drugs have significant toxic potential. Toxicity in horses is manifested almost exclusively by nephrotoxicosis, but eighth cranial nerve dysfunction, neuromuscular blockade, and direct myocardial depression have been described in other species, including humans.[290]

The development of toxicity is dependent upon a number of variables. Of the group, streptomycin is least nephrotoxic, neomycin is most nephrotoxic, and gentamicin, kanamycin, and amikacin are intermediate in their ability to cause renal damage. Since the aminglycosides are eliminated primarily by the kidney, any cause of reduced renal function can result in increased serum concentration of the drug and increased potential for nephrotoxicity. Other factors that enhance the toxic potential of these agents include acidosis, dehydration, hypovolemia, endotoxemia, increased dose or frequency of administration of the drug, and prolonged use of the drug. The concurrent use of other potentially nephrotoxic drugs, such as NSAIDs, may also predispose to aminoglycoside nephrotoxicity.[290-292] Although foals have not been shown to be more sensitive than adults to aminoglycoside nephrotoxicity, use of these products should be closely monitored in young animals that have potential for sepsis, hypotension, or dehydration.[293]

Clinical Signs. The clinical signs of aminoglycoside nephrotoxicity are those of acute renal failure. Anorexia and depression may be noted while the horse is being medicated or shortly after treatment has stopped. Most cases of acute renal failure due to aminoglycoside toxicity are nonoliguric, and polyuria is a frequently reported clinical finding. A discussion of the clinical signs of acute renal failure is found in Chapter 16.

Pathophysiology. The aminoglycosides are highly polar cations that are poorly lipid-soluble but highly water-soluble. They are minimally absorbed from the intestinal tract, but rapid absorption occurs from intramuscular and subcutaneous sites of injection.[294, 295] Distribution is essentially to the extracellular fluid space in the body and high concentrations of drug occur only in the renal cortex and the endolymph and perilymph of the inner ear.[295] Binding to plasma proteins is minimal, and excretion occurs almost entirely by glomerular filtration of unchanged drug.

A small portion of filtered aminoglycoside binds to phospholipid receptors on the brush border of cells of the proximal convoluted tubules and pars recta. Subsequently, the drug is reabsorbed, primarily by pinocytosis, and accumulates in lysosomes and other subcellular compartments of proximal tubular cells. This net reabsorption results in high concentrations of aminoglycoside within the renal cortex.[295, 296] Concentrated aminoglycoside within the renal cortex forms a poorly exchangeable drug pool, with a renal tissue half-life of several hundred hours. This contrasts to the serum half-life of aminoglycosides, which is several hours. Therefore, an aminoglycoside may be slowly excreted in urine for weeks after dosage is discontinued, even if serum levels are undetectable.

Eventually, proximal tubular cell damage and death occur. The mechanisms resulting in cell death are poorly understood, but several have been hypothesized: binding of aminoglycosides to plasma phospholipids, inducing alterations in plasma membrane structure and function; altered phospholipid accumulation and metabolism, resulting in impairment of lysosomal degradation and phagocytosis of cellular debris; activation of cellular phospholipases; damage to mitochondrial respiration, leading to reduced production of cellular ATP; and altered Na^+, K^+-ATPase activity. Although all of these actions may occur, it is still unclear which mechanism is primary. The ultimate step leading to cell death may involve changes in subcellular calcium homeostasis, but the precise mechanism is unknown.[296]

In addition to proximal tubular dysfunction, aminoglycoside toxicity also results in a decreased glomerular filtration rate. Proposed mechanisms for this phenomenon include release of vasoactive hormones causing alterations in renal blood flow; damage to proximal tubular cells leading to backleak of fluid and waste products across the damaged epithelium; and obstruction of individual nephrons causing increased hydrostatic pressure within the tubular lumen with subsequent reduction in the net ultrafiltration pressure within the glomerular capillaries.[296] With aminoglycoside nephrotoxicity, acute severe tubular necrosis rarely occurs, and impaired renal function is almost always reversible because of the capacity of the proximal tubular cells to regenerate.[295]

Diagnosis and Treatment. Aminoglycoside nephrotoxicity is initially manifested by evidence of proteinuria, hematuria, cylindruria, polyuria, and enzymuria. Under experimental conditions, a rise in the urinary GGT ratio was the earliest detectable laboratory change noted with gentamicin toxicity, and preceded increases in urinary protein and fractional excretion of phosphate by about 48 hours.[297] Proteinuria and cylindruria may be present 3 to 6 days after initiation of treatment, and may precede elevations in serum creatinine and urea nitrogen concentrations by several days.[290, 292] From a practical standpoint, monitoring urine for the presence of protein appears to be a sensitive means of detecting early drug toxicosis. If aminoglycoside toxicity results in acute renal failure, other clinicopathologic findings compatible with acute renal failure would be evident.

Therapeutic drug monitoring has been shown to be an effective means of decreasing the incidence of aminoglycoside nephrotoxicity in human patients. Measuring serum peak and trough concentrations of aminoglycosides allows for individual dosage regimens to be employed, particularly in the high-risk patient. In human patients and foals, elevated trough values have been associated with an increased incidence of nephrotoxicity,[298, 299] and are more predictable indicators of toxicity than are serum peak concentrations. In high-risk patients, frequent monitoring of serum peak and trough concentrations should be employed. In humans, trough concentrations less than 2 μg/mL for gentamicin and tobramycin, and less than 5 μg/mL for amikacin are desirable.[300] Optimal trough concentrations for the aminoglycosides in equine patients have not been established, but extrapolation from human values may provide useful guidelines. In my laboratory, trough concentrations of less than 1 μg/mL for gentamicin and tobramycin, and less than 2.5 μg/mL for amikacin are considered desired values.

Treatment of aminoglycoside nephrotoxicity is usually accomplished by drug dosage adjustment (with the aid of therapeutic drug monitoring) or drug withdrawal, fluid diuresis, and alkalinization of urine. In patients that require aminoglycoside therapy, increased dosage interval or reduced dosage may be necessary to minimize nephrotoxicity. Horses receiving moderate-to-large volumes of fluid therapy rarely develop nephrotoxicity, and, in fact, usually have less than the expected serum concentration of aminoglycoside when given at recommended dosages.

Diet may also influence the nephrotoxic potential of gentamicin, as oat-fed horses had a greater degree of gentamicin-induced nephrotoxicosis than did horses fed only alfalfa.[301] Low dietary calcium, sodium, and potassium have been shown to potentiate gentamicin-induced nephrotoxicosis in laboratory animals, and high dietary calcium provided a protective effect against gentamicin-induced nephrotoxicity in rats.[302] The effect of increased dietary calcium, sodium, and potassium on the nephrotoxic potential of the aminoglycosides in horses warrants further study. Additional treatments suggested for aminoglycoside-induced nephrotoxicity have included peritoneal dialysis, plasmapheresis, and hemodialysis to reduce the serum concentration of these drugs.[293]

Amphotericin B

Amphotericin B is a polyene antibiotic used in treatment of systemic fungal diseases, including blastomycosis, coccidioidomycosis, histoplasmosis, candidiasis, sporotrichosis, mucormycosis, chromoblastomycosis, aspergillosis, and pithiosis. Its use in the horse is rarely reported, but horses with histoplasmosis and subcutaneous pithiosis have been successfully treated with the drug.[303, 304] Amphotericin B is a known nephrotoxin and therapeutic and toxic levels of the drug overlap.[300]

Clinical signs of toxicity reported in horses include depression, anorexia, weight loss, anemia (ranging from mild to severe), and fever.[303, 304] One horse receiving treatment for an extended period of time also developed polyuria and polydipsia.[304] All clinical signs abated following cessation of therapy.

Amphotericin B causes distal tubular epithelial cell damage and renal ischemia. Tubular cell damage results from amphotericin B combining with sterols on the cholesterol-rich lysosomal membranes of the distal tubular cells. Direct injury to the cell membrane allows for increased cell permeability, leakage of cytosol, and cell death. Excessive potassium, bicarbonate, and water are lost into the urine, and hydrogen ions gain entrance back into the epithelial cells. Hypokalemia and metabolic acidosis can develop and lead to death, if renal disease is progressive.[305]

Renal vasoconstriction also plays a role in toxicity of amphotericin B. Significant afferent arteriolar vasoconstriction occurs by mechanisms not fully elucidated, but activation of the tubuloglomerular feedback system has been suggested as a possible cause.[300]

Diagnosis of toxicity is based largely upon increasing concentration of BUN and abnormal urine findings of cylindruria, hematuria, and proteinuria. In human patients, a rise in BUN above 40 to 50 mg/dL is cause for reduced dosage or temporary discontinuance of the drug.[306]

Treatment of toxicosis involves fluid diuresis and reduced dosage or temporary discontinuance of the drug until the BUN reaches a normal value. Because nephrotoxicity caused by this drug is reversible, cessation of treatment results in return of renal function to almost normal levels. Additional therapies that may be utilized include the concomitant use of mannitol, and oral sodium loading in an attempt to decrease the occurrence of azotemia.[300]

Sulfonamides

The sulfonamides are a group of antimicrobial agents widely used in equine practice for treatment of gram-positive and gram-negative bacterial infections. Historically, they have been incriminated as a cause of renal dysfunction, but currently are probably rarely involved in nephrotoxicity.

The sulfonamides are poorly soluble in water but highly soluble in alkaline solutions. They are excreted via the kidney. Their nephrotoxic potential results from their precipitation into crystals in renal tubules, leading to obstruction and anuria or tubular epithelial necrosis. Crystal formation increases with increasing urine acidity, and ultimately leads to acute renal failure.[300, 307] Animals that are hypovolemic or have reduced renal function from other causes may be at greater risk of developing nephrotoxicity than other animals.

Diagnosis is based largely on signs of acute renal failure in conjunction with a history of drug use and presence of sulfonamide crystalluria. Treatment is aimed at fluid diuresis and concurrent urine alkalinization.[300]

The potentiated sulfonamides (trimethoprim-sulfonamide combinations) have much greater urine solubility and have not been incriminated as a cause of nephrotoxicity in horses. There are no documented adverse effects of these products in horses, but anecdotal reports have associated their use with acute-onset diarrhea.[308] Drug withdrawal is usually sufficient therapy in such cases. In Great Britain, the concomitant use of intravenous trimethoprim-sulfadoxine with detomidine or halothane has been associated with severe cardiac dysrhythmias and sudden death in several horses.[309, 310] The simultaneous use of these products in horses should be avoided if possible.

Vitamins D₂ and D₃

Horses are capable of meeting their requirement for vitamin D if they are exposed to sunlight or have access to sun-cured forages. Although dietary requirements for the horse have not been established, a maximum safe level of 44 IU/kg body weight per day has been proposed for long-term feeding (>60 days).[311] Most cases of vitamin D intoxication are iatrogenic, resulting from overzealous use of vitamin supplements or from improperly formulated vitamin D–supplemented feeds. Ingestion of *Cestrum diurnum* (wild jasmine) can also result in vitamin D toxicosis, since this plant contains a metabolically active glycoside of 1,25-dihydroxycholecalciferol (see discussion of *Cestrum diurnum*).

Both vitamins D₂ (ergocalciferol) and D₃ (cholecalciferol) are potentially toxic, but vitamin D₃ is much more active and results in more severe lesions with wider tissue distribution than does an equivalent dose of vitamin D₂.[312, 313] Other variables that may affect toxicosis include duration of treatment and route of administration. High concentrations of dietary calcium might also enhance the effects of excessive amounts of vitamin D. The effect of vitamin D supplementation is cumulative, and signs of toxicity may occur weeks after supplementation has begun.

The clinical signs associated with vitamin D toxicosis are associated with impairment of the renal, cardiovascular, or musculoskeletal systems. Signs may include depression, anorexia, weakness, polyuria and polydipsia, cardiac murmurs and tachycardia, limb stiffness with impaired mobility, and recumbency. Calcification of tendons, ligaments, and other soft tissue structures may be palpable upon physical examination.[312, 313] Ultrasonographic examination of these structures may also demonstrate abnormal mineralization within the tissues.

The toxicity of excessive amounts of vitamin D₃ is a result of extensive dystrophic mineralization, rather than any inherent toxicity of vitamin D itself. Soft tissue sites most frequently affected include the kidneys, the endocardium and walls of large blood vessels, and tendons and ligaments.[312, 313]

Laboratory findings associated with toxicosis can vary with the organ system affected, but generally include pronounced and persistent hyperphosphatemia and hypercalcemia, although the latter can be somewhat variable on a daily basis. Serum calcium concentration may remain within a normal range in some horses. Other laboratory evidence of chronic renal failure may become evident with progression of toxicosis. Definitive diagnosis can be made by measuring serum concentrations of vitamins D₂ and D₃, and 1,25-dihydroxycholecalciferol.[313]

Treatment of vitamin D intoxication should include removal of all exogenous sources of vitamin D. A cation chelator such as sodium phytate may be helpful in reducing intestinal absorption of calcium, but the efficacy of this product has not been determined. Symptomatic therapy for renal insufficiency and failure should be employed, if necessary. Recovery may take months in less severely affected horses,[313] but treatment is usually unrewarding if excessive mineralization has occurred.

Menadione Sodium Bisulfite (Vitamin K₃)

Vitamin K₃ is a reported cause of acute renal failure in horses,[314] but the product has been withdrawn from the United States market. When the product was given at the manufacturer's recommended dosage of 2.2 to 11 mg/kg IV or IM, signs of toxicity became evident within 6 to 48 hours following injection in affected horses. Clinical signs included depression, anorexia, colic, hematuria, and stranguria. Azotemia, electrolyte abnormalities, proteinuria, and isosthenuria were also noted. Pathologic lesions noted at necropsy were those of acute tubular necrosis. Interstitial fibrosis and chronic renal failure were also present in one horse.[314] Treatment of affected horses is symptomatic for acute or chronic renal failure.

Miscellaneous Agents

Cadmium

Intoxication with cadmium is rarely reported in horses, but has been seen in animals raised near smelting operations.[315] Environmental contamination of soil and forage by cadmium and zinc was the cause of excessive intake.

Affected horses exhibited signs of unthriftiness, lameness, and swollen joints. Some of these signs were attributed to excess zinc in the diet, but the horses also had pronounced osteoporosis and nephrocalcinosis, which, along with proteinuria, are typical findings of cadmium toxicosis in humans.[315]

Serum concentrations of zinc and potassium were elevated in these horses, and the serum magnesium concentration was very low in one foal. Sodium, calcium, chloride, and bicarbonate concentrations were also decreased. Extensive nephrocalcinosis was characterized by multifocal loss of cortical tubules, which were replaced by dense deposits of calcium phosphate crystals.

Cadmium induces change in proximal renal tubular cells by an unknown mechanism. However, increased numbers of lysosomes and mitochondrial swelling in the proximal tubular cells are early changes noted. Proteinuria is usually the first abnormality noted in humans and laboratory animals. With continued chronic exposure, fibrosis and atrophy consequent to interstitial nephritis may ensue, leading to chronic renal failure.[316]

In humans, treatment is essentially supportive, with elimination of exposure to cadmium being imperative. Research data suggest a possible beneficial role of zinc, vitamin B complex, and nickel preparations, but their clinical efficacy is unproven.[316]

Hemoglobin and Myoglobin

These two endogenous substances can be a cause of acute renal failure in horses when they are present in serum in excessive amounts. Myoglobin nephrosis may occur following severe muscle damage such as extensive crushing or bruising injuries, large burns, heatstroke, or exertional rhabdomyolysis (tying-up). Excessive hemoglobinemia usually results from extensive intravascular hemolysis caused by acute hemolytic anemia, incompatible blood transfusions, or intravenous administration of certain medications, that is, hypotonic fluids and concentrated DMSO solutions. Possible causes of acute hemolytic anemia include *Babesia caballi* or *Babesia equi* infection, neonatal isoerythrolysis, phenothiazine toxicosis, onion (*Allium* species) toxicosis, and ingestion of withered red maple (*Acer rubrum*) leaves. Severe intravascular hemolysis may also occur with fulminant hepatic failure and with immune-mediated hemolytic anemia

caused by anti-erythrocyte antibodies. Equine infectious anemia may cause intravascular hemolysis, but hemoglobinuria and pigment nephrosis are rarely associated with this disease.[291]

Clinical Signs. Clinical signs of pigment nephropathy are those of acute renal failure in conjunction with grossly discolored urine. Urine of affected horses is usually red to brown-tinged in color, which can vary in intensity. Additionally, horses with myoglobinuria would be expected to exhibit some degree of muscle soreness or inflammation, or have a history of muscle trauma.

Pathophysiology. Excessive amounts of hemoglobin or myoglobin presented to the kidney result in tubular nephrosis by yet undetermined mechanisms. Hemoglobin casts are usually present within the renal tubules of affected horses, and may induce ischemic injury to the tubular cells. Hemoglobin nephropathy has also been suggested to be caused by RBC stromal elements rather than by hemoglobin itself.[317] More recent studies in rats suggest that iron may play a significant role in the development of pigment nephropathy caused by hemoglobin or myoglobin. Iron liberated from the hemoglobin or myoglobin molecule can promote formation of oxygen free radicals, which then initiate lipid peroxidation and other reactions, leading to renal injury.[318] In these studies, hemoglobin-induced renal injury was markedly attenuated by deferoxamine, an iron chelator that binds ferric iron (Fe^{3+}). Additional factors that may contribute to the development of pigment nephropathy include hypovolemia or dehydration, circulatory failure, endotoxemia, acidosis, and hypoxia.

Diagnosis and Treatment. The appearance of blood or hemoglobin in urine is not specific for pigment nephropathy, so other signs and laboratory findings are important for diagnosis. Hematuria, hemoglobinuria, and myoglobinuria all result in a positive orthotoluidine reaction for occult blood on multitest dipsticks. However, hematuria is evidenced by the presence of intact RBCs seen on microscopic examination of urine sediment, and anemia may be present if hematuria is of sufficient magnitude. With hemolysis, the serum is usually discolored pink, and hemoglobinemia can be verified by routine laboratory methods. Anemia may also be present if hemolysis is severe. Elevated serum CK concentration is characteristic of rhabdomyolysis, and affected horses usually exhibit some degree of muscle soreness or have a history of muscle trauma. Myoglobin is poorly bound to plasma proteins and is rapidly filtered through the glomerulus. As a result, the serum remains a normal color. Definitive tests for myoglobin in urine include electrophoresis or immunoassay techniques.[291, 319]

Treatment of pigment nephropathy is essentially supportive and consistent with that of acute renal failure due to other causes. Any predisposing cause of excessive myoglobin or hemoglobin should be identified and removed if possible. Compatible blood transfusions may be necessary in horses with severe hemolytic anemia, and horses with exertional rhabdomyolysis or other muscle injury should be treated accordingly.

Mercury

Mercury exists in a variety of organic and inorganic forms. Both forms can be toxic to horses but more recently reported cases involve acute toxicity resulting from inorganic mercury-containing blistering agents topically applied to skin.[320, 321] Ingestion of feed or seed grain contaminated with organic mercurial seed preservatives has been a source of contamination in previous years.

Acute and chronic forms of toxicosis can occur in horses. The acute toxic dose of inorganic mercury in adults is 5 to 10 g.[322] Experimentally, chronic toxicity from inorganic mercury has been produced by ingestion of mercuric chloride 0.8 mg/kg/day over a 14-week period.[323] Chronic organic mercury toxicosis has also been produced experimentally by feeding methyl mercury 0.4 mg/kg/day for a 10-week period.[324]

Clinical Signs. Signs associated with toxicity of the various mercurial compounds can differ, but they all include some degree of renal dysfunction. Acute toxicity resulting from inorganic mercury can cause signs of acute renal failure, including oliguria and depression, and signs of gastrointestinal irritation. Ulcerative stomatitis, excessive salivation, colic, and diarrhea are common findings associated with gastrointestinal tract disturbances.[320, 321] Chronic intoxication with inorganic mercury can result in signs of oral ulceration, reduced appetite and weight loss, alopecia, progressive respiratory difficulty, gradually increasing urine production, and terminal azotemia.[323] Signs reported with chronic organic mercury toxicity include development of neurologic dysfunction characterized by proprioceptive deficits, exudative dermatitis, reluctance to move, reduced appetite and weight loss, dullness, and renal changes exhibited by a steadily increasing BUN concentration and glucosuria.[324]

Pathophysiology. Inorganic mercury compounds are absorbed from the lungs and gastrointestinal tract, but poorly through the skin. Following ingestion and absorption, accumulation in the liver and particularly the kidney occur. Organic mercury is absorbed from the lung, gastrointestinal tract, and also through the skin. Some forms of organic mercury are degraded in the body to inorganic forms, which then also accumulate in the kidney prior to excretion.[322]

Inorganic mercury is concentrated to high levels within the proximal renal tubular cells. Metallothionein, a low-molecular-weight metal-binding protein is synthesized within 48 hours following exposure to heavy metals. This protein binds mercuric ions within the endoplasmic reticulum of the tubular epithelial cells and then slowly releases mercury. This slow release of sequestered mercury can cause continuing damage to tubular cells after the source of mercury is removed.[325] Hence, the development of mercury nephropathy appears to be a function of the amount of protein-bound mercury concentrated in the renal tubules. Bound mercury can persist in the kidneys for several weeks following exposure.[323] Acute toxicity results in massive tubular necrosis and acute renal failure, and chronic exposure may cause renal interstitial fibrosis leading to chronic renal failure.

Methylmercury can be biotransformed in the body to inorganic mercury, but methylmercury also accumulates in the brain to a much greater extent than do other forms of mercury.[322] The exact mechanism whereby methyl- and other alkylmercurials damage the nervous system is not understood.[324]

At the cellular level, mercury combines with sulfhydryl groups within cells. As a result, sulfhydryl enzyme systems essential to cellular metabolism and respiration are inhibited, resulting in cell death.

Diagnosis and Treatment. Mercury intoxication should be suspected when horses show compatible clinical signs and have a history of exposure. Laboratory abnormalities are similar to those of other causes of acute or chronic renal failure and irritative gastrointestinal diseases. Definitive diagnosis is usually based on measurement of mercury concentrations in kidney and liver.[322] Stomach and intestine may also be submitted for analysis in more acute cases.

Treatment of mercury intoxication initially involves removal of the source. In acute toxicity, evacuation of the bowel with a mild laxative may be helpful. The oral administration of 500 g of activated charcoal might help block absorption of mercury, but its efficacy has not been demonstrated. Dimercaprol (used to inactivate circulating mercury) can be given at a dosage of 3 mg/kg IM every 4 hours for the first 2 days, four times on the third day, and twice-daily for the next 10 days until recovery is complete.[322] Other principles of therapy for acute or chronic renal failure should also be employed. Treatment of chronic mercury intoxication is usually unrewarding.

REFERENCES

1. Anderson GA, Mount ME, Vrins AA, et al: Fatal acorn poisoning in a horse: Pathologic findings and diagnostic considerations. *J Am Vet Med Assoc* 182:1105, 1983.
2. Smith BP: Diseases of the alimentary system. In Smith BP, ed: *Large Animal Internal Medicine.* St Louis, Mosby–Year Book, 1990, p 814.
3. Knight AP: Oleander poisoning. *Compendium Continuing Educ Pract Vet* 10:262, 1988.
4. Oleander poisoning in equines. *J R Army Vet Corps* 42:8, 1971.
5. Oehme FW: Plant toxicities. In Robinson NE, ed: *Current Therapy in Equine Medicine,* ed 2. Philadelphia, WB Saunders, 1987, p 674.
6. Coyne CP, Oehme FW: Disorders caused by toxins. In Smith BP, ed: *Large Animal Internal Medicine.* St Louis, Mosby–Year Book, 1990, p 1649.
7. Ellenhorn MJ, Barceloux DG: *Medical Toxicology.* New York, Elsevier Science, 1988, p 1252.
8. Coyne CP, Oehme FW: Disorders caused by toxins. In Smith BP, ed: *Large Animal Internal Medicine.* St Louis, Mosby–Year Book, 1990, p 1653.
9. Oehme FW: Plant toxicities. In Robinson NE, ed: *Current Therapy in Equine Medicine,* ed 2. Philadelphia, WB Saunders, 1987, p 673.
10. McCunn J: Castor bean poisoning in horses. *Vet J* 101:136, 1945.
11. Rauber A, Heard J: Castor bean toxicity re-examined: A new perspective. *Vet Hum Toxicol* 27:498, 1985.
12. Brunton LL: Agents affecting gastrointestinal water flux and motility, digestants, and bile acids. In Gilman AG, Rall TW, Nies AS, et al, eds: Goodman and Gilman's The *Pharmaco-*

logical Basis of Therapeutics, ed 8. Elmsford, NY, Pergamon Press, 1990, p 922.

13. Ellenhorn MJ, Barceloux DG: *Medical Toxicology.* New York, Elsevier Science, 1988, p 1223.

14. Coyne CP, Oehme FW: Disorders caused by toxins. In Smith BP, ed: *Large Animal Internal Medicine.* St Louis, Mosby–Year Book, 1990, p 1657.

15. Ellenhorn MJ, Barceloux DG: *Medical Toxicology.* New York, Elsevier Science, 1988, p 1272.

16. Coyne CP, Oehme FW: Disorders caused by toxins. In Smith BP, ed: *Large Animal Internal Medicine.* St Louis, Mosby–Year Book, 1990, p 1646.

17. Oehme FW: Plant toxicities. In Robinson NE, ed: *Current Therapy in Equine Medicine,* ed 2. Philadelphia, WB Saunders, 1987, p 677.

18. Ellenhorn MJ, Barceloux DG: *Medical Toxicology.* New York, Elsevier Science, 1988, p 1229.

19. Osweiler GD, Carson TL, Buck WB, et al: *Clinical and Diagnostic Veterinary Toxicology,* ed 3. Dubuque, Iowa, Kendall/Hunt, 1985, p 451.

20. Zin LL, Edwards WC: Toxicity of blue-green algae in livestock. *Bovine Pract* 14:151, 1979.

21. Ellenhorn MJ, Barceloux DG: *Medical Toxicology.* New York, Elsevier Science, 1988, p 1199.

22. Theiss WW, Carmichael WW: Physiological effect of a peptide toxin produced by the freshwater cyanobacteria (blue-green algae) *Microcystis aeruginosa* strain 7820. In Steyn PS, Vleggaar R, eds: *Mycotoxins and Phycotoxins—A Collection of Invited Papers Presented at the Sixth International IUPAC Symposium on Mycotoxins and Phycotoxins.* Amsterdam, Elsevier Science, 1986, p 353.

23. Osweiler GD, Carson TL, Buck WB, et al: *Clinical and Diagnostic Veterinary Toxicology,* ed 3. Dubuque, Iowa, Kendall/Hunt, 1985, p 207.

24. Raisbeck MF, Holt GR, Osweiler GD: Lincomycin-associated colitis in horses. *J Am Vet Med Assoc* 179:362, 1981.

25. Sande MA, Mandell GL: Antimicrobial agents [continued]: Tetracyclines, chloramphenicol, erythromycin, and miscellaneous antibacterial agents. In Gilman AG, Rall TW, Nies AS, et al, eds: *Goodman and Gilman's The Pharmacological Basis of Therapeutics,* ed 8. Elmsford, NY, Pergamon Press, 1990, p 1134.

26. Murray MJ: Diseases of the alimentary system. In Smith BP, ed: *Large Animal Internal Medicine.* St Louis, Mosby–Year Book, 1990, p 661.

27. Adams LG: Clinicopathological aspects of imidocarb dipropionate toxicity in horses. *Res Vet Sci* 31:54, 1981.

28. Roberson EL: Antiprotozoan drugs. In Booth NH, McDonald LE, eds: *Veterinary Pharmacology and Therapeutics,* ed 5. Ames, Iowa State University Press, 1982, p 888.

29. Ducharme NG, Fubini SL: Gastrointestinal complications associated with the use of atropine in horses. *J Am Vet Med Assoc* 182:229, 1983.

30. Cox JH, Oehme FW: Disorders caused by toxins. In Smith BP, ed: *Large Animal Internal Medicine.* St Louis, Mosby–Year Book, 1990, p 1628.

31. Moffatt RE, Kramer LL, Lerner D, et al: Studies on dioctyl sodium sulfosuccinate toxicity: Clinical, gross and microscopic pathology in the horse and guinea pig. *Can J Comp Med* 39:434, 1975.

32. Brunton LL: Agents affecting gastrointestinal water flux and motility, digestants, and bile acids. In Gilman AG, Rall TW, Nies AS, et al, eds: *Goodman and Gilman's The Pharmacological Basis of Therapeutics,* ed 8. Elmsford, NY, Pergamon Press, 1990, p 922.

33. Snow DH, Douglas TA, Thompson H, et al: Phenylbutazone toxicosis in equidae: A biochemical and pathophysiologic study. *Am J Vet Res* 42:1754, 1981.

34. MacKay RJ, French TW, Nguyen HT, et al: Effects of large doses of phenylbutazone administration to horses. *Am J Vet Res* 44:774, 1983.

35. MacAllister CG: Effects of toxic doses of phenylbutazone in ponies. *Am J Vet Res* 44:2277, 1983.

36. Collins LG, Tyler DE: Experimentally induced phenylbutazone toxicosis in ponies: description of the syndrome and its prevention with synthetic prostaglandin E$_2$. *Am J Vet Res* 46:1605, 1985.

37. Traub JL, Gallina AM, Grant BD, et al: Phenylbutazone toxicosis in the foal. *Am J Vet Res* 44:1410, 1983.

38. Traub-Dargatz JL, Bertone JJ, Gould DH, et al: Chronic flunixin meglumine therapy in foals. *Am J Vet Res* 49:7, 1988.

39. Carrick JB, Papich MG, Middleton DM, et al: Clinical and pathological effects of flunixin meglumine administration to neonatal foals. *Can J Vet Res* 53:195, 1989.

40. Gunson DE: Renal papillary necrosis in horses. *J Am Vet Med Assoc* 182:263, 1983.

41. Simmons TR, Gaughan EM, Ducharme NG, et al: Treatment of right dorsal ulcerative colitis in a horse. *J Am Vet Med Assoc* 196:455, 1990.

42. Karcher LF, Dill SG, Anderson WI, et al: Right dorsal colitis. *J Vet Intern Med* 4:247, 1990.

43. Meschter CL, Gilbert M, Krook L, et al: The effects of phenylbutazone on the intestinal mucosa of the horse: A morphological, ultrastructural and biochemical study. *Equine Vet J* 22:255, 1990.

44. Rubin SI: Nonsteroidal antiinflammatory drugs, prostaglandins, and the kidney. *J Am Vet Med Assoc* 188:1065, 1986.

45. Osweiler GD, Carson TL, Buck WB, et al: *Clinical and Diagnostic Veterinary Toxicology,* ed 3. Dubuque, Iowa, Kendall/Hunt, 1985, p 72.

46. Hatch RC: Poisons causing abdominal distress or liver or kidney damage. In Booth NH, McDonald LE, eds: *Veterinary Pharmacology and Therapeutics,* ed 5. Ames, Iowa State University Press, 1982, p 1023.

47. Osweiler GD, Carson TL, Buck WB, et al: *Clinical and Diagnostic Veterinary Toxicology,* ed 3. Dubuque, Iowa, Kendall/Hunt, 1985, p 177.

48. Hatch RC: Poisons causing respiratory insufficiency. In Booth NH, McDonald LE, eds: *Veterinary Pharmacology and Therapeutics,* ed 5. Ames, Iowa State University Press, 1982, p 941.

49. Osweiler GD, Carson TL, Buck WB, et al: *Clinical and Diagnostic Veterinary Toxicology,* ed 3. Dubuque, Iowa, Kendall/Hunt, 1985, p 436.

50. Hatch RC: Poisons having unique effects. In Booth NH, McDonald LE, eds: *Veterinary Pharmacology and Therapeutics,* ed 5. Ames, Iowa State University Press, 1982, p 1055.

51. Sockett DC, Baker JC, Stowe CM: Slaframine (*Rhizoctonia leguminicola*) intoxication in horses. *J Am Vet Med Assoc* 181:606, 1982.

52. Hatch RC: Poisons causing respiratory insufficiency. In Booth NH, McDonald LE, eds: *Veterinary Pharmacology and Therapeutics,* ed 5. Ames, Iowa State University Press, 1982, p 962.

53. Exon JH: A review of chlorinated phenols. *Vet Hum Toxicol* 26:508, 1984.

54. Osweiler GD, Carson TL, Buck WB, et al: *Clinical and Diagnostic Veterinary Toxicology,* ed 3. Dubuque, Iowa, Kendall/Hunt, 1985, p 239.

55. Osweiler GD, Carson TL, Buck WB, et al: *Clinical and Diagnostic Veterinary Toxicology,* ed 3. Dubuque, Iowa, Kendall/Hunt, 1985, p 251.

56. Hatch RC: Poisons causing respiratory insufficiency. In Booth NH, McDonald LE, eds: *Veterinary Pharmacology and Therapeutics,* ed 5. Ames, Iowa State University Press, 1982, p 947.

57. Cox JH, Oehme FW: Disorders caused by toxins. In Smith BP, ed: *Large Animal Internal Medicine.* St Louis, Mosby–Year Book, 1990, p 1634.

58. Russel SH, Monin T, Edwards WC: Rodenticide toxicosis in a horse. *J Am Vet Med Assoc* 172:270, 1978.

59. Peoples SA, Maddy KT: Poisoning of man and animals due to ingestion of the rodent poison, vacor. *Vet Hum Toxicol* 21:266, 1979.

60. Osweiler GD, Carson TL, Buck WB, et al: *Clinical and Diagnostic Veterinary Toxicology,* ed 3. Dubuque, Iowa, Kendall/Hunt, 1985, p 357.

61. Cox JH, Oehme FW: Disorders caused by toxins. In Smith BP, ed: *Large Animal Internal Medicine.* St. Louis, Mosby–Year Book, 1990, p 1637.

62. Osweiler GD, Carson TL, Buck WB, et al: *Clinical and Diagnostic Veterinary Toxicology,* ed 3. Dubuque, Iowa, Kendall/Hunt, 1985, p 179.

63. Kimbrough RD, Carter CD, Liddle JA, et al: Epidemiology and pathology of a tetrachlorodibenzodioxin poisoning episode. *Arch Environ Health* 32:77, 1977.

64. Osweiler GD, Carson TL, Buck WB, et al: *Clinical and Diagnostic Veterinary Toxicology,* ed 3. Dubuque, Iowa, Kendall/Hunt, 1985, p 152.

65. Amend JF, Mallon FM, Wren WB, Kamos AS: Equine monensin toxicosis: Some experimental clinicopathologic observations. *Compendium Continuing Educ Pract Vet* 11:S173, 1980.

66. Matsuoka T: Evaluation of monensin toxicity in the horse. *J Am Vet Med Assoc* 169:1098, 1976.

67. Mollenhauer HH, Rowe LD, Cysewski SJ, Witzel DA: Ultrastructural observations in ponies after treatment with monensin. *Am J Vet Res* 42:35, 1981.

68. Hanson LJ, Eisenbeis HG, Givens SV: Toxic effects of lasalocid in horses. *Am J Vet Res* 42:456, 1981.

69. Roberson EL: Antiprotozoan drugs. In Booth NH, McDonald LE, eds: *Veterinary Pharmacology and Therapeutics,* ed 5. Ames, Iowa State University Press, 1982, p 878.

70. Roberson EL: Antiprotozoan drugs. In Booth NH, McDonald LE, eds: *Veterinary Pharmacology and Therapeutics,* ed 5. Ames, Iowa State University Press, 1982, p 878.

71. Rollinson J, Taylor FGR, Chesney J: Salinomycin poisoning in horses. *Vet Rec* 121:126, 1987.

72. Schmitz DG: Cantharidin toxicosis in horses. *J Vet Intern Med* 3:208, 1989.

73. Schoeb TR, Panciera RJ: Blister beetle poisoning in horses. *J Am Vet Med Assoc* 173:75, 1978.

74. Ray AC, Kyle ALG, Murphy MJ, et al: Etiologic agents, incidence, and improved diagnostic methods of cantharidin toxicosis in horses. *Am J Vet Res* 50:187, 1989.

75. Osweiler GD, Carson TL, Buck WB, et al: *Clinical and Diagnostic Veterinary Toxicology,* ed 3. Dubuque, Iowa, Kendall/Hunt, 1985, p 358.

76. Hatch RC: Poisons causing abdominal distress or liver or kidney damage. In Booth NH, McDonald LE, eds: *Veterinary Pharmacology and Therapeutics,* ed 5. Ames, Iowa State University Press, 1982, p 1027.

77. Osweiler GD, Carson TL, Buck WB, et al: *Clinical and Diagnostic Veterinary Toxicology,* ed 3. Dubuque, Iowa, Kendall/Hunt, 1985, p 349.

78. James LF, Hartley WJ, Van Kampen KR: Syndromes of *Astragalus* poisoning in livestock. *J Am Vet Med Assoc* 178:146, 1981.

79. Knight AP: Locoweed poisoning. *Compendium Continuing Educ Pract Vet* 9:F418, 1987.

80. McIlwraith CW, James LF: Limb deformities in foals associated with ingestion of locoweed by mares. *J Am Vet Med Assoc* 181:255, 1982.

81. Burfening PJ: Ergotism. *J Am Vet Med Assoc* 163:1288, 1973.

82. Hintz HF: Ergotism. *Equine Pract* 10:6, 1988.

83. Mantle PG: Ergotism in horses. In Wyllie TD, ed: *Mycotoxic Fungi, Mycotoxins, Mycotoxicoses,* New York, LG Moorehouse, 1978, p 185.

84. Ellenhorn MJ, Barceloux DG: *Medical Toxicology.* New York, Elsevier Science, 1988, p 1317.

85. Ellenhorn MJ, Barceloux DG: *Medical Toxicology.* New York, Elsevier Science, 1988, p 664.

86. Osweiler GD, Carson TL, Buck WB, et al: *Clinical and Diagnostic Veterinary Toxicology,* ed 3. Dubuque, Iowa, Kendall/Hunt, 1985, p 298.

87. Hatch RC: Poisons causing nervous stimulation or depression. In Booth NH, McDonald LE, eds: *Veterinary Pharmacology and Therapeutics,* ed 5. Ames, Iowa State University Press, 1982, p 992.

88. Ellenhorn MJ, Barceloux DG: *Medical Toxicology.* New York, Elsevier Science, 1988, p 1077.

89. Hatch RC: Poisons causing nervous stimulation or depression. In Booth NH, McDonald LE, eds: *Veterinary Pharmacology and Therapeutics,* ed 5. Ames, Iowa State University Press, 1982, p 984.

90. Cox JH, Oehme FW: Disorders caused by toxins. In Smith BP, ed: *Large Animal Internal Medicine.* St. Louis, Mosby–Year Book, 1990, p 1630.

91. Osweiler GD, Carson TL, Buck WB, et al: *Clinical and Diagnostic Veterinary Toxicology,* ed 3. Dubuque, Iowa, Kendall/Hunt, 1985, p 286.

92. Hatch RC: Poisons causing nervous stimulation or depression. In Booth NH, McDonald LE, eds: *Veterinary Pharmacology and Therapeutics,* ed 5. Ames, Iowa State University Press, 1982, p 999.

93. Osweiler GD, Carson TL, Buck WB, et al: *Clinical and Diagnostic Veterinary Toxicology,* ed 3. Dubuque, Iowa, Kendall/Hunt, 1985, p 345.

94. Hatch RC: Poisons causing nervous stimulation or depression. In Booth NH, McDonald LE, eds: *Veterinary Pharmacology and Therapeutics,* ed 5. Ames, Iowa State University Press, 1982, p 994.

95. Lilley CW: Strychnine poisoning in a horse. *Equine Pract* 7:7, 1985.

96. Osweiler GD, Carson TL, Buck WB, et al: *Clinical and Diagnostic Veterinary Toxicology,* ed 3. Dubuque, Iowa, Kendall/Hunt, 1985, p 325.

97. Hatch RC: Poisons causing nervous stimulation or depression. In Booth NH, McDonald LE, eds: *Veterinary Pharmacology and Therapeutics,* Ed 5. Ames, Iowa State University Press, 1982, p 1012.

98. Sutherland C: Metaldehyde poisoning in horses. *Vet Rec* 112:64, 1983.

99. Harris WF: Metaldehyde poisoning in three horses. *Mod Vet Pract* 56:336, 1975.

100. Edwards HG: Methiocarb poisoning in a horse. *Vet Rec* 119:556, 1986.

101. Alexander KA: Methiocarb poisoning in a horse. *Vet Rec* 120:47, 1987.

102. Ray AC, Dwyer JN, Fambro GW, et al: Clinical signs and chemical confirmation of 4-aminopyridine poisoning in horses. *Am J Vet Res* 39:329, 1978.

103. Booth NH: Stimulants. In Booth NH, McDonald LE, eds: *Veterinary Pharmacology and Therapeutics,* ed 5. Ames, Iowa State University Press, 1982, p 350.

104. Kitzman JV, Wilson RC, Hatch RC, et al: Antagonism of xylazine and ketamine anesthesia by 4-aminopyridine and yohimbine in geldings. *Am J Vet Res* 45:875, 1984.

105. Drudge JH, Lyons ET, Swerczek TW: Critical tests and safety studies on a levamisole-piperazine mixture as an anthelmintic in the horse. *Am J Vet Res* 35:67, 1974.

106. DiPietro JA, Todd KS: Anthelmintics used in treatment of

parasitic infections of horses. *Vet Clin North Am Equine Pract* 3:1, 1987.

107. Marriner S: Anthelmintic drugs. *Vet Rec* 118:181, 1986.

108. Roberson EL: Antinematodal Drugs. In Booth NH, McDonald LE, eds: *Veterinary Pharmacology and Therapeutics,* ed 5. Ames, Iowa State University Press, 1982, p 819.

109. Glenn MW, Burr WM: Toxicity of a piperazine-carbon disulfide-phenothiazine preparation in the horse. *J Am Vet Med Assoc* 160:988, 1972.

110. Osweiler GD, Carson TL, Buck WB, et al: *Clinical and Diagnostic Veterinary Toxicology,* ed 3. Dubuque, Iowa, Kendall/Hunt, 1985, p 201.

111. Ellenhorn MJ, Barceloux DG: *Medical Toxicology.* New York, Elsevier Science, 1988, p 818.

112. Osweiler GD, Carson TL, Buck WB, et al: *Clinical and Diagnostic Veterinary Toxicology,* ed 3. Dubuque, Iowa, Kendall/Hunt, 1985, p 273.

113. Hatch RC: Poisons causing nervous stimulation or depression. In Booth NH, McDonald LE, eds: *Veterinary Pharmacology and Therapeutics,* ed 5. Ames, Iowa State University Press, 1982, p 999.

114. Cox JH, Oehme FW: Disorders caused by toxins. In Smith BP, ed: *Large Animal Internal Medicine.* St Louis, Mosby–Year Book, 1990, p 1631.

115. Ellenhorn MJ, Barceloux DG: *Medical Toxicology.* New York, Elsevier Science, 1988, p 912.

116. Osweiler GD, Carson TL, Buck WB, et al: *Clinical and Diagnostic Veterinary Toxicology,* ed 3. Dubuque, Iowa, Kendall/Hunt, 1985, p 369.

117. Ellenhorn MJ, Barceloux DG: *Medical Toxicology.* New York, Elsevier Science, 1988, p 871.

118. Osweiler GD, Carson TL, Buck WB, et al: *Clinical and Diagnostic Veterinary Toxicology,* ed 3. Dubuque, Iowa, Kendall/Hunt, 1985, p 160.

119. Hatch RC: Poisons causing abdominal distress or liver or kidney damage. In Booth NH, McDonald LE, eds: *Veterinary Pharmacology and Therapeutics,* ed 5. Ames, Iowa State University Press, 1982, p 1029.

120. Cox JH, Oehme FW: Disorders caused by toxins. In Smith BP, ed: *Large Animal Internal Medicine.* St Louis, Mosby–Year Book, 1990, p 1641.

121. Morris DD, Henry MM: Hepatic encephalopathy. *Compendium Continuing Educ Pract Vet* 13:1153, 1991.

122. Oehme FW: Plant toxicities. In Robinson NE, ed: *Current Therapy in Equine Medicine,* ed 2. Philadelphia, WB Saunders, 1987, p 678.

123. Coyne CP, Oehme FW: Disorders caused by toxins. In Smith BP, ed: *Large Animal Internal Medicine.* St Louis, Mosby–Year Book, 1990, p 1657.

124. Fleischmann G, Rudiger H: Isolation, resolution and partial characterization of two *Robinia pseudoacacia* seed lectins. *Biol Chem Hoppe Seyler* 367:27, 1986.

125. Coyne CP, Oehme FW: Disorders caused by toxins. In Smith BP, ed: *Large Animal Internal Medicine.* St Louis, Mosby–Year Book, 1990, p 1648.

126. Oehme FW: Plant toxicities. In Robinson NE, ed: *Current Therapy in Equine Medicine,* ed 2. Philadelphia, WB Saunders, 1987, p 676.

127. Kelleway RA, Geovjian L: Acute bracken fern poisoning in a 14-month-old horse. *Vet Med/Small Anim Clin* 73:295, 1978.

128. Hintz HF: Bracken fern. *Equine Pract* 12:6, 1990.

129. Coyne CP, Oehme FW: Disorders caused by toxins. In Smith BP, ed: *Large Animal Internal Medicine.* St Louis, Mosby–Year Book, 1990, p 1648.

130. Oehme FW: Plant toxicities. In Robinson NE, ed: *Current Therapy in Equine Medicine,* ed 2. Philadelphia, WB Saunders, 1987, p 677.

131. Coyne CP, Oehme FW: Disorders caused by toxins. In Smith

BP, ed: *Large Animal Internal Medicine.* St Louis, Mosby–Year Book, 1990, p 1656.

132. Sperry OE, Dollahite JW, Hoffman GO, et al: *Texas Plants Poisonous to Livestock.* College Station, Tex, Texas Agricultural Extension Service, Texas Agricultural Experiment Station publication no. B-1028, p 10.

133. Olson CT, Keller WC, Gerken DF, et al: Suspected tremetol poisoning in horses. *J Am Vet Med Assoc* 185:1001, 1984.

134. Smetzer DL, Coppock RW, Ely RW, et al: Cardiac effects of white snakeroot intoxication in horses. *Equine Pract* 5:26, 1983.

135. Hatch RC: Poisons having unique effects. In Booth NH, McDonald LE, eds: *Veterinary Pharmacology and Therapeutics,* ed 5. Ames, Iowa State University Press, 1982, p 1055.

136. George LW: Diseases of the nervous system. In Smith BP, ed: *Large Animal Internal Medicine.* St Louis, Mosby–Year Book, 1990, p 978.

137. Farrell RK, Sande RD, Lincoln SD: Nigropallidal encephalomalacia in a horse. *J Am Vet Med Assoc* 158:1201, 1971.

138. Young S, Brown WW, Klinger B: Nigropallidal encephalomalacia in horses caused by ingestion of weeds of the genus *Centaurea. J Am Vet Med Assoc* 157:1602, 1970.

139. Mettler FA, Stern GM: Observations on the toxic effects of yellow star thistle. *J Neuropathol Exp Neurol* 22:164, 1963.

140. Cordy DR: Nigropallidal encephalomalacia in horses associated with ingestion of yellow star thistle. *J Neuropathol Exp Neurol* 13:330, 1954.

141. Stevens KL, Wong RY: Structure of chlororepdiolide, a new sesquiterpene lactone from *Centaurea repens.* J Nat Prod 49:833, 1986.

142. James LF, Hartley WJ, Van Kampen KR: Syndromes of *Astragalus* poisoning in livestock. *J Am Vet Med Assoc* 178:146, 1981.

143. Roberson EL: Antinematodal drugs. In Booth NH, McDonald LE, eds: *Veterinary Pharmacology and Therapeutics,* ed 5. Ames, Iowa State University Press, 1982, p 806.

144. Proctor DL, Singer RH, Sutton HH: Clinical evaluation of piperazine adipate as an anthelmintic in horses. *Vet Med* 50:575, 1955.

145. McNeil PH, Smyth GB: Piperazine toxicity in horses. *J Equine Med Surg* 2:321, 1978.

146. Drudge JH, Lyons ET, Swerczek TW: Critical tests and safety studies on a levamisole-piperazine mixture as an anthelmintic in the horse. *Am J Vet Res* 35:67, 1974.

147. Ellenhorn MJ, Barceloux DG: *Medical Toxicology.* New York, Elsevier Science, 1988, p 295.

148. Adams HR: Adrenergic and antiandrenergic drugs. In Booth NH, McDonald LE, eds: *Veterinary Pharmacology and Therapeutics,* ed 5. Ames, Iowa State University Press, 1982, p 110.

149. Lloyd KCK, Harrison I, Tulleners E: Reserpine toxicosis in a horse. *J Am Vet Med Assoc* 186:980, 1985.

150. Tobin T: Pharmacology review: A review of the pharmacology of reserpine in the horse. *J Equine Med Surg* 2:433, 1978.

151. Osweiler GD, Carson TL, Buck WB, et al.: *Clinical and Diagnostic Veterinary Toxicology,* ed 3. Dubuque, Iowa, Kendall/Hunt, 1985, p 104.

152. Divers TJ, Warner A, Vaala WE, et al: Toxic hepatic failure in newborn foals. *J Am Vet Med Assoc* 183:1407, 1983.

153. Arnbjerg J: Poisoning in animals due to oral application of iron with description of a case in a horse. *Nord Vet Med* 33:71, 1981.

154. Ellenhorn MJ, Barceloux DG: *Medical Toxicology.* New York, Elsevier Science, 1988, p 1023.

155. Hershko C: Mechanism of iron toxicity and its possible role in red cell membrane damage. *Semin Hematol* 26:277, 1989.

156. Ellenhorn MJ, Barceloux DG: *Medical Toxicology.* New York, Elsevier Science, 1988, p 969.

157. Blood DC, Radostits OM, Henderson JA: *Veterinary Medicine,* ed 6. London, Bailliere Tindall, 1983, p 1131.

158. Bernard WV, Divers TJ: Variations in serum sorbitol dehydrogenase, aspartate transaminase, and isoenzyme 5 of lactate dehydrogenase activities in horses given carbon tetrachloride. *Am J Vet Res* 50:622, 1989.

159. Anwer MS, Engelking LR, Gronwall R, et al: Plasma bile acid elevation following CC14 induced liver damage in dogs, sheep, calves and ponies. *Res Vet Sci* 20:127, 1976.

160. Dorman DC, Haschek WM: Fatal propylene glycol toxicosis in a horse. *J Am Vet Med Assoc* 198:1643, 1991.

161. Myers VS, Usenik EA: Propylene glycol intoxication of horses. *J Am Vet Med Assoc* 155:1841, 1969.

162. Ellenhorn MJ, Barceloux DG: *Medical Toxicology.* New York, Elsevier Science, 1988, p 809.

163. Osweiler GD: Toxicology of triclopyr herbicide in the equine. *Proc Am Assoc Vet Lab Diagn* 26:193, 1983.

164. Whisenant SG, McArthur ED: Triclopyr persistence in northern Idaho forest vegetation. *Bull Environ Contam Toxicol* 42:660, 1989.

165. Angsubhakorn S, Poomvises P, Romruen K, et al: Aflatoxicosis in horses. *J Am Vet Med Assoc* 178:274, 1981.

166. Asquith RL, Edds GT: Investigations in equine aflatoxicosis. *Proc Annu Meet Am Assoc Equine Pract* 26:193, 1980.

167. Greene HJ, Oehme FW: A possible case of equine aflatoxicosis. *Vet Toxicol* 17:76, 1975.

168. Aller WW, Edds GT, Asquith RL: Effects of aflatoxins in young ponies. *Am J Vet Res* 42:2162, 1981.

169. Bortell R, Asquith RL, Edds GT, et al: Acute experimentally induced aflatoxicosis in the weanling pony. *Am J Vet Res* 44:2110, 1983.

170. Hatch RC: Poisons causing abdominal distress or liver or kidney damage. In Booth NH, McDonald LE, eds: *Veterinary Pharmacology and Therapeutics,* ed 5. Ames, Iowa State University Press, 1982, p 1034.

171. Osweiler GD, Carson TL, Buck WB, et al: *Clinical and Diagnostic Veterinary Toxicology,* ed 3. Dubuque, Iowa, Kendall/Hunt, 1985, p 415.

172. Buck WB, Haliburton JC, Thilsted JP, et al: Equine encephalomalacia: comparative pathology of naturally occurring and experimental cases. *Proc Annu Meet Am Assoc Vet Lab Diagn* 22:239, 1979.

173. McCue PM: Equine leukoencephalomalacia. *Compendium Continuing Educ Pract Vet* 11:646, 1989.

174. Marasas WFO, Kellerman TS, Gelderblom WCA, et al: Leukoencephalomalacia in a horse induced by fumonisin B1 isolated from *Fusarium moniliforme. Onderstepoort J Vet Res* 55:197, 1988.

175. Wilson TM, Ross PF, Rice LG, et al: Fumonisin B1 levels associated with an epizootic of equine leukoencephalomalacia. *J Vet Diagn Invest* 2:213, 1990.

176. Ross PF, Rice LG, Reagor JC, et al: Fumonisin B1 concentrations in feeds from 45 confirmed equine leukoencephalomalacia cases. *J Vet Diagn Invest* 3:238, 1991.

177. Brownie CF, Cullen J: Characterization of experimentally induced equine leukoencephalomalacia (ELEM) in ponies *(Equus caballus)*: Preliminary report. *Vet Hum Toxicol* 29:34, 1987.

178. Booth NH: Drug and chemical residues in the edible tissues of animals. In Booth NH, McDonald LE, eds: *Veterinary Pharmacology and Therapeutics,* ed 5. Ames, Iowa State University Press, 1982, p 1096.

179. Gabal MA, Awad YL, Morcos MB, et al: Fusariotoxicoses of farm animals and mycotoxic leucoencephalomalacia of the equine associated with the finding of trichothecenes in feedstuffs. *Vet Hum Toxicol* 28:207, 1986.

180. George LW: Diseases of the nervous system. In Smith BP, ed: *Large Animal Internal Medicine.* St Louis, Mosby–Year Book, 1990, p 956.

181. Hatch RC: Poisons causing nervous stimulation or depression. In Booth NH, McDonald LE, eds: *Veterinary Pharmacology and Therapeutics,* ed 5. Ames, Iowa State University Press, 1982, p 1005.

182. Burrows GE: Lead poisoning in the horse. *Equine Pract* 4:30, 1982.

183. Burrows GE, Borchard RE: Experimental lead toxicosis in ponies: Comparison of the effects of smelter effluent–contaminated hay and lead acetate. *Am J Vet Res* 43:2129, 1982.

184. Kowalczyk DF, Naylor JM, Gunson D: The value of zinc protoporphyrin in equine lead poisoning: A case report. *Vet Hum Toxicol* 23:12, 1981.

185. Tennant B, Dill SG, Glickman LT, et al: Acute hemolytic anemia, methemoglobinemia, and Heinz body formation associated with ingestion of red maple leaves by horses. *J Am Vet Med Assoc* 179:143, 1981.

186. Divers TJ, George LW, George JW: Hemolytic anemia in horses after the ingestion of red maple leaves. *J Am Vet Med Assoc* 180:300, 1982.

187. George LW, Divers TJ, Mahaffey EA, et al: Heinz body anemia and methemoglobinemia in ponies given red maple *(Acer rubrum* L.) leaves. *Vet Pathol* 19:521, 1982.

188. Plumlee KH: Red maple toxicity in a horse. *Vet Hum Toxicol* 33:66, 1991.

189. Pierce KR, Joyce JR, England RB, et al: Acute hemolytic anemia caused by wild onion poisoning in horses. *J Am Vet Med Assoc* 160:323, 1972.

190. Hutchison TWS: Onion toxicosis. *J Am Vet Med Assoc* 172:1440, 1978.

191. Ellenhorn MJ, Barceloux DG: *Medical Toxicology.* New York, Elsevier Science, 1988, p 221.

192. Duncan SG, Meyers KM, Reed SM: Reduction of the red blood cell mass of horses: Toxic effect of heparin anticoagulant therapy. *Am J Vet Res* 44:2271, 1983.

193. Mahaffey EA, Moore JN: Erythrocyte agglutination associated with heparin treatment in three horses. *J Am Vet Med Assoc* 189:1478, 1986.

194. Moore JN, Mahaffey EA, Zboran M: Heparin-induced agglutination of erythrocytes in horses. *Am J Vet Res* 48:68, 1987.

195. Adams HR: Hemostatic and anticoagulant drugs. In Booth NH, McDonald LE, eds: *Veterinary Pharmacology and Therapeutics,* ed 5. Ames, Iowa State University Press, 1982, p 430.

196. Engelking LR, Mariner JC: Enhanced biliary bilirubin excretion after heparin-induced erythrocyte mass depletion. *Am J Vet Res* 46:2175, 1985.

197. Meyers KM, Duncan SG, Reed S: Research in anticoagulation in equine gastrointestinal disease. In *Proceedings Equine Colic Research Symposium,* Athens, GA, University of Georgia, September 1982, p 129.

198. Byars TD, Wilson RC: Clinical pharmacology of heparin. *J Am Vet Med Assoc* 178:739, 1981.

199. Adams HR: Hemostatic and anticoagulant drugs. In Booth NH, McDonald LE, eds: *Veterinary Pharmacology and Therapeutics,* ed 5. Ames, Iowa State University Press, 1982, p 431.

200. Vrins A, Carlson G, Feldman B: Warfarin: A review with emphasis on its use in the horse. *Can Vet J* 24:211, 1983.

201. Scott EA, Byars TD, Lamar AM: Warfarin anticoagulation in the horse. *J Am Vet Med Assoc* 177:1146, 1980.

202. Osweiler GD, Carson TL, Buck WB, et al: *Clinical and Diagnostic Veterinary Toxicology,* ed 3. Dubuque, Iowa, Kendall/Hunt, 1985, p 334.

203. Thijssen HHW, van den Bogaard AEJM, Wetzel JM, et al:

Warfarin pharmacokinetics in the horse. *Am J Vet Res* 44:1192, 1983.

204. Ellenhorn MJ, Barceloux DG: *Medical Toxicology*. New York, Elsevier Science, 1988, p 217.

205. Byars TD, Greene CE, Kemp DT: Antidotal effect of vitamin K_1 against warfarin-induced anticoagulation in horses. *Am J Vet Res* 47:2309, 1986.

206. Alsup EM, DeBowes RM: Dimethyl sulfoxide. *J Am Vet Med Assoc* 185:1011, 1984.

207. Blythe LL, Craig AM, Appell LH, Lassen ED: Intravenous use of dimethyl sulfoxide (DMSO) in horses: Clinical and physiologic effects. *Proc Am Assoc Equine Practn* 32:441, 1986.

208. Brayton CF: Dimethyl sulfoxide (DMSO): A review. *Cornell Vet* 76:61, 1986.

209. Blythe LL, Craig AM, Christensen JM, et al: Pharmacokinetic disposition of dimethyl sulfoxide administered intravenously to horses. *Am J Vet Res* 47:1739, 1986.

210. Schuh JCL, Ross C, Meschter C: Concurrent mercuric blister and dimethyl sulfoxide (DMSO) application as a cause of mercury toxicity in two horses. *Equine Vet J* 20:68, 1988.

211. DiPietro JA, Todd KSJ: Anthelmintics used in treatment of parasitic infections of horses. *Vet Clin North Am: Equine Pract* 3:1, 1987.

212. Roberson EL: Antinematodal drugs. In Booth NH, McDonald LE, eds: *Veterinary Pharmacology and Therapeutics*, ed 5. Ames, Iowa State University Press, 1982, p 803.

213. Osweiler GD, Carson TL, Buck WB, et al: *Clinical and Diagnostic Veterinary Toxicology*, ed 3. Dubuque, Iowa, Kendall/Hunt, 1985, p 227.

214. Pearson EG, Ayres JW, Wood GL, Watrous BJ: Digoxin toxicity in a horse. *Compendium Continuing Educ Pract Vet* 9:958, 1987.

215. Adams HR: Digitalis and other inotropic agents. In Booth NH, McDonald LE, eds: *Veterinary Pharmacology and Therapeutics*, ed 5. Ames, Iowa State University Press, 1982, p 447.

216. Button C, Gross DR, Johnston JT, et al: Digoxin pharmacokinetics, bioavailability, efficacy, and dosage regimens in the horse. *Am J Vet Res* 41:1388, 1980.

217. Baggot JD, Davis LE: Plasma protein binding of digitoxin and digoxin in several mammalian species. *Res Vet Sci* 15:81, 1973.

218. Brumbaugh GW, Thomas WP, Enos LR, et al: A pharmacokinetic study of digoxin in the horse. *J Vet Pharmacol Ther* 6:163, 1983.

219. Ellenhorn MJ, Barceloux DG: *Medical Toxicology*. New York, Elsevier Science, 1988, p 200.

220. Hartsfield SM, Thurmon JC, Benson GJ: Sodium bicarbonate and bicarbonate precursors for treatment of metabolic acidosis. *J Am Vet Med Assoc* 179:914, 1981.

221. Lawrence L, Kline K, Miller-Graber P, et al: Effect of sodium bicarbonate on racing standardbreds. *J Anim Sci* 68:673, 1990.

222. Freestone JF, Carlson GP, Harrold DR, et al: Furosemide and sodium bicarbonate–induced alkalosis in the horse and response to oral KCl or NaCl therapy. *Am J Vet Res* 50:1334, 1989.

223. Posner JB, Swanson AG, Plum F: Acid-base balance in cerebrospinal fluid. *Arch Neurol* 12:479, 1965.

224. Rumbaugh GE, Carlson GP, Harrold D: Clinicopathologic effects of rapid infusion of 5% sodium bicarbonate in 5% dextrose in the horse. *J Am Vet Med Assoc* 178:267, 1981.

225. Hatch RC: Poisons causing respiratory insufficiency. In Booth NH, McDonald LE, eds: *Veterinary Pharmacology and Therapeutics*, ed 5. Ames, Iowa State University Press, 1982, p 943.

226. Osweiler GD, Carson TL, Buck WB, et al: *Clinical and Diagnostic Veterinary Toxicology*, ed 3. Dubuque, Iowa, Kendall/Hunt, 1985, p 460.

227. Schneider NR, Yeary RA: Nitrite and nitrate pharmacokinetics in the dog, sheep, and pony. *Am J Vet Res* 36:941, 1975.

228. Hatch RC: Poisons causing respiratory insufficiency. In Booth NH, McDonald LE, eds: *Veterinary Pharmacology and Therapeutics*, ed 5. Ames, Iowa State University Press, 1982, p 960.

229. Osweiler GD, Carson TL, Buck WB, et al: *Clinical and Diagnostic Veterinary Toxicology*, ed 3. Dubuque, Iowa, Kendall/Hunt, 1985, p 455.

230. Kingsbury JM: *Poisonous Plants of the United States and Canada*. Englewood Cliffs, NJ, Prentice-Hall, 1964, p 26.

231. Coyne CP, Oehme FW: Disorders caused by toxins. In Smith BP, ed: *Large Animal Internal Medicine*. St Louis, Mosby–Year Book, 1990, p 1649.

232. Hatch RC: Poisons causing nervous stimulation or depression. In Booth NH, McDonald LE, eds: *Veterinary Pharmacology and Therapeutics*, ed 5. Ames, Iowa State University Press, 1982, p 997.

233. Osweiler GD, Carson TL, Buck WB, et al: *Clinical and Diagnostic Veterinary Toxicology*, ed 3. Dubuque, Iowa, Kendall/Hunt, 1985, p 340.

234. Ellenhorn MJ, Barceloux DG: *Medical Toxicology*. New York, Elsevier Science, 1988, p 1085.

235. Cox JH, Oehme FW: Disorders caused by toxins. In Smith BP, ed: *Large Animal Internal Medicine*. St Louis, Mosby–Year Book, 1990, p 1635.

236. Ralston SL, Rich VA: Black walnut toxicosis in horses. *J Am Vet Med Assoc* 183:1095, 1983.

237. Uhlinger C: Black walnut toxicosis in ten horses. *J Am Vet Med Assoc* 195:343, 1989.

238. Minnick PD, Brown CM, Braselton WE, et al: The induction of equine laminitis with an aqueous extract of the heartwood of black walnut (*Juglans nigra*). *Vet Hum Toxicol* 29:230, 1987.

239. Galey FD, Beasley VR, Schaeffer D, et al: Effect of an aqueous extract of black walnut (*Juglans nigra*) on isolated equine digital vessels. *Am J Vet Res* 51:83, 1990.

240. Krook L, Wasserman RH, Shively JN, et al: Hypercalcemia and calcinosis in Florida horses: Implication of the shrub, *Cestrum diurnum*, as the causative agent. *Cornell Vet* 65:26, 1975.

241. Wasserman RH: The nature and mechanism of action of the calcinogenic principle of *Solanum malacoxylon* and *Cestrum diurnum*, and a comment on *Trisetum flavescens*. In Keeler RF, Van Kampen KR, James LF, eds: *Effects of Poisonous Plants on Livestock*. New York, Academic Press, 1978, p 545.

242. Hughes MR, McCain TA, Chang SY, et al: Presence of 1,25-dihydroxy-vitamin D_3-glycoside in the calcinogenic plant *Cestrum diurnum*. *Nature* 268:347, 1977.

243. Anderson CA, Divers TJ: Systemic granulomatous inflammation in a horse grazing hairy vetch. *J Am Vet Med Assoc* 183:569, 1983.

244. Kingsbury JM: *Poisonous Plants of the United States and Canada*. Englewood Cliffs, NJ, Prentice-Hall, 1964, p 56.

245. Johnson AE: Toxicologic aspects of photosensitization in livestock. *J Natl Cancer Inst* 69:253, 1982.

246. Coyne CP, Oehme FW: Disorders caused by toxins. In Smith BP, ed: *Large Animal Internal Medicine*. St Louis, Mosby–Year Book, 1990, p 1652.

247. Hatch RC: Poisons causing lameness or visible disfigurement. In Booth NH, McDonald LE, eds: *Veterinary Pharmacology and Therapeutics*, ed 5. Ames, Iowa State University Press, 1982, p 1049.

248. Pearson EG: Diseases of the hepatobiliary system. In Smith BP, ed: *Large Animal Internal Medicine*. St Louis, Mosby–Year Book, 1990, p 850.

249. Knight AP, Kimberling CV, Stermitz FR, et al: *Cynoglossum officinale* (hound's-tongue)—a cause of pyrrolizidine alkaloid poisoning in horses. *J Am Vet Med Assoc* 185:647, 1984.

250. Giles CJ: Outbreak of ragwort (*Senecio jacobea*) poisoning in horses. *Equine Vet J* 15:248, 1983.

251. Pearson EG: Liver failure attributable to pyrrolizidine alkaloid toxicosis and associated with inspiratory dyspnea in ponies: Three cases (1982–1988). *J Am Vet Med Assoc* 198:1651, 1991.

252. Lessard P, Wilson WD, Olander HJ, et al: Clinicopathologic study of horses surviving pyrrolizidine alkaloid (*Senecio vulgaris*) toxicosis. *Am J Vet Res* 47:1776, 1986.

253. Gulick BA, Liu IKM, Qualls CW, et al: Effect of pyrrolizidine alkaloid-induced hepatic disease on plasma amino acid patterns in the horse. *Am J Vet Res* 41:1894, 1980.

254. Hatch RC: Poisons causing lameness or visible disfigurement. In Booth NH, McDonald LE, eds: *Veterinary Pharmacology and Therapeutics,* ed 5. Ames, Iowa State University Press, 1982, p 1048.

255. Coyne CP, Oehme FW: Disorders caused by toxins. In Smith BP, ed: *Large Animal Internal Medicine.* St Louis, Mosby–Year Book, 1990, p 1660.

256. Putnam MR, Bransby DI, Schumacher J, et al: Effects of the fungal endophyte *Acremonium coenophialum* in fescue on pregnant mares and foal viability. *Am J Vet Res* 52:2071, 1991.

257. Cox JH, Oehme FW: Disorders caused by toxins. In Smith BP, cd: *Large Animal Internal Medicine.* St Louis, Mosby–Year Book, 1990, p 1629.

258. Stowe CM: Iodine, iodides, and iodism. *J Am Vet Med Assoc* 179:334, 1981.

259. Fadok VA, Wild S: Suspected cutaneous iodism in a horse. *J Am Vet Med Assoc* 183:1104, 1983.

260. Osweiler GD, Carson TL, Buck WB, et al: *Clinical and Diagnostic Veterinary Toxicology,* ed 3. Dubuque, Iowa, Kendall/Hunt, 1985, p 145.

261. Schwink AL: Toxicology of ethylenediamine dihydriodide. *J Am Vet Med Assoc* 178:996, 1981.

262. Ellenhorn MJ, Barceloux DG: *Medical Toxicology.* New York, Elsevier Science, 1988, p 1112.

263. Coyne CP, Oehme FW: Disorders caused by toxins. In Smith BP, ed: *Large Animal Internal Medicine.* St Louis, Mosby–Year Book, 1990, p 1662.

264. Stewart KA, Genetzky RM: Odontodysplasia in a horse. *Mod Vet Pract* 65:87, 1984.

265. Osweiler GD, Carson TL, Buck WB, et al: *Clinical and Diagnostic Veterinary Toxicology,* ed 3. Dubuque, Iowa, Kendall/Hunt, 1985, p 183.

266. Gunson DE, Kowalczyk DF, Shoop CR, et al: Environmental zinc and cadmium pollution associated with generalized osteochondrosis, osteoporosis, and nephrocalcinosis in horses. *J Am Vet Med Assoc* 180:295, 1982.

267. Messer NT: Tibiotarsal effusioin associated with chronic zinc intoxication in three horses. *J Am Vet Med Assoc* 178:294, 1981.

268. Willoughby RA, MacDonald E, McSherry BJ, et al: Lead and zinc poisoning and the interaction between Pb and Zn poisoning in the foal. *Can J Comp Med* 36:348, 1972.

269. Bridges CH, Moffitt PG: Influence of variable content of dietary zinc on copper metabolism of weanling foals. *Am J Vet Res* 51:275, 1990.

270. Ringenberg QS, Doll DC, Patterson WP, et al: Hematologic effects of heavy metal poisoning. *South Med J* 81:1132, 1988.

271. Seawright AA, Hrdlicka J, Ng JC: Heavy Metal Intoxications in Horses. In Ruckebusch Y, Toutain PL, Koritz GD, eds: *Veterinary Pharmacology and Toxicology.* Lancaster, England, MTP Press, 1983, p 700.

272. Hultine JD, Mount ME, Easley KJ, et al: Selenium toxicosis in the horse. *Equine Pract* 1:57, 1979.

273. Crinion RAP, O'Connor JP: Selenium intoxication in horses. *Ir Vet J* 32:81, 1978.

274. Seawright AA, Hrdlicka J, Ng JC: Heavy metal intoxications in horses. In Ruckebusch Y, Toutain PL, Koritz GD, eds: *Veterinary Pharmacology and Toxicology.* Lancaster, England, MTP Press, 1983, p 703.

275. Traub-Dargatz JL, Knight AP, Hamar DW: Selenium toxicity in horses. *Compendium Continuing Educ Pract Vet* 8:771, 1986.

276. Dewes HF, Lowe MD: Suspected selenium poisoning in a horse. *N Z Vet J* 35:53, 1987.

277. Stowe HD: Effects of copper pretreatment upon the toxicity of selenium in ponies. *Am J Vet Res* 41:1925, 1980.

278. James LF, Van Kampen KV, Hartley WJ: *Astragalus fisulcatus:* A cause of selenium or locoweed poisoning. *Vet Hum Toxicol* 25:86, 1983.

279. Painter EP: The chemistry and toxicity of selenium compounds with special reference to the selenium problem. *Chem Ref* 28:179, 1941.

280. Sellers EA, Vou RW, Lucas CC: Lipotropic agents in liver damage produced by selenium or carbon tetrachloride. *Proc Soc Exp Biol Med* 75:118, 1950.

281. Osweiler GD, Carson TL, Buck WB, et al: *Clinical and Diagnostic Veterinary Toxicology,* ed 3. Dubuque, Iowa, Kendall/Hunt, 1985, p 428.

282. Hatch RC: Poisons causing lameness or visible disfigurement. In Booth NH, McDonald LE, eds: *Veterinary Pharmacology and Therapeutics,* ed 5. Ames, Iowa State University Press, 1982, p 1048.

283. Osweiler GD, Carson TL, Buck WB, et al: *Clinical and Diagnostic Veterinary Toxicology,* ed 3. Dubuque, Iowa, Kendall/Hunt, 1985, p 471.

284. Hulbert LC, Oehme FW: *Plants Poisonous to Livestock,* ed 3. Manhattan, Kansas State University, 1968, p 35.

285. Sperry OE, Dollahite JW, Hoffman GO, et al: *Texas Plants Poisonous to Livestock.* College Station, Tex, Texas A&M University, Texas Agricultural Extension Service, Texas Agricultural Experiment Station, B-1028, 1974, p 27.

286. Marsh CD, Roe GC, Clawson AB: *Rayless Goldenrod (Aplopappus heterophyllus) as a Poisonous Plant, Bulletin 1391.* Washington, DC, US Department of Agriculture, 1926, p 1.

287. Adams LG, Dollahite JW, Romane WM, et al: Cystitis and ataxia associated with sorghum ingestion by horses. *J Am Vet Med Assoc* 155:518, 1969.

288. Van Kampen KR: Sudan grass and sorghum poisoning of horses: A possible lathyrogenic disease. *J Am Vet Med Assoc* 156:629, 1970.

289. Osweiler GD, Carson TL, Buck WB, et al: *Clinical and Diagnostic Veterinary Toxicology,* ed 3. Dubuque, Iowa, Kendall/Hunt, 1985, p 455.

290. Riviere JE, Coppoc GL: Selected aspects of aminoglycoside antibiotic nephrotoxicosis. *J Am Vet Med Assoc* 178:508, 1981.

291. Schmitz DG: Toxic nephropathy in horses. *Compendium Continuing Educ Pract Vet* 10:104, 1988.

292. Riviere JE, Traver DS, Coppoc GL: Gentamicin toxic nephropathy in horses with disseminated bacterial infection. *J Am Vet Med Assoc* 180:648, 1982.

293. Divers TJ: Diseases of the Renal System. In Smith BP, ed: *Large Animal Internal Medicine.* St Louis, Mosby–Year Bauler, 1990, p 872.

294. Burrows GE: Aminocyclitol antibiotics. *J Am Vet Med Assoc* 176:1280, 1980.

295. Sande MA, Mandell GL: Antimicrobial agents [continued]: aminoglycosides. In Gilman AG, Goodman LS, Rall TW, et

al F, eds: *Goodman and Gilman's The Pharmacological Basis of Therapeutics,* ed 7. New York, Macmillan, 1985, p 1154.

296. Appel GB: Aminoglycoside nephrotoxicity. *Am J Med* 88(suppl 3C):3C–16S, 1990.

297. Hinchcliff KW, McGuirk SM, MacWilliams PS: Gentamicin toxicity in pony mares. In *Proceedings of the Fifth Annual Veterinary Medical Forum (ACVIM),* San Diego, May 1987, p 896.

298. Taketomo RT, McGhan WF, Fushiki MR, et al: Gentamicin nephrotoxicity: Application of multivariate analysis. *Clin Pharmacol* 1:544, 1982.

299. Riviere JE, Coppoc GL, Hinsman EJ, et al: Species dependent gentamicin pharmacokinetics and nephrotoxicity in the young horse. *Fundam Appl Toxicol* 3:448, 1983.

300. Engelhardt JA, Brown SA: Drug-related nephropathies part II. Commonly used drugs. *Compendium Continuing Educ Pract Vet* 9:281, 1987.

301. Schumacher J, Wilson RC, Spano JS, et al: Effect of diet on gentamicin-induced nephrotoxicosis in horses. *Am J Vet Res* 52:1274, 1991.

302. Quarum ML, Houghton DC, Gilbert DN, et al: Increasing dietary calcium moderates experimental gentamicin nephrotoxicity. *J Lab Clin Med* 103:104, 1984.

303. McMullan WC, Joyce JR, Hanselka DV, et al: Amphotericin B for the treatment of localized subcutaneous phycomycosis in the horse. *J Am Vet Med Assoc* 170:1293, 1977.

304. Cornick JL: Diagnosis and treatment of pulmonary histoplasmosis in a horse. *Cornell Vet* 80:97, 1990.

305. Cheville NF: *Cell Pathology,* ed 2. Ames, Iowa State University Press, 1983, p 575.

306. Pyle RL: Clinical pharmacology of amphotericin B. *J Am Vet Med Assoc* 179:83, 1981.

307. Osweiler GD, Carson TL, Buck WB, et al: *Clinical and Diagnostic Veterinary Toxicology,* ed 3. Dubuque, Iowa, Kendall/Hunt, 1985, p 221.

308. Divers TJ, Sweeney RW, Perkons S: Miscellaneous groups of antimicrobial agents. Sulfonamides, trimethoprim, rifampin, metronidazole, spectinomycin, vancomycin and polymixin. *Proc Am Assoc Equine Pract* 32:195, 1986.

309. Dick IGC, White SK: Possible potentiated sulphonamide-associated fatality in an anaesthetised horse. *Vet Rec* 121:288, 1987.

310. Taylor PM, Rest RJ, Duckham TN, et al: Possible potentiated sulphonamide and detomidine interactions. *Vet Rec* 122:143, 1988.

311. *Nutrient Requirements of Horses.* Washington, DC, National Academy of Sciences, 1989, p 21.

312. Harrington DD: Acute vitamin D_2 (ergocalciferol) toxicosis in horses: Case report and experimental studies. *J Am Vet Med Assoc* 180:867, 1982.

313. Harrington DD, Page EH: Acute vitamin D_3 toxicosis in horses: Case reports and experimental studies of the comparative toxicity of vitamins D_2 and D_3. *J Am Vet Med Assoc* 182:1358, 1983.

314. Rebhun WC, Tennant BC, Dill SG, et al: Vitamin K_3–induced renal toxicosis in the horse. *J Am Vet Med Assoc* 184:1237, 1984.

315. Gunson DE, Kowalczyk DF, Shoop CR, et al: Environmental zinc and cadmium pollution associated with generalized osteochondrosis, osteoporosis, and nephrocalcinosis in horses. *J Am Vet Med Assoc* 180:295, 1982.

316. Roxe DM, Krumlovsky FA: Toxic interstitial nephropathy from metals, metabolites, and radiation. *Semin Nephrol* 8:72, 1988.

317. Friedman H, De Venuto F, Lollini L, et al: Morphologic effects following massive exchange transfusions with a stroma-free hemoglobin solution. *Lab Invest* 40:655, 1979.

318. Paller MS: Hemoglobin- and myoglobin-induced acute renal failure in rats: Role of iron in nephrotoxicity. *Am J Physiol* 255:F539, 1988.

319. Kent JE, Harris P: Myoglobinuria: Methods for diagnosis. In Blackmore DJ, ed: *Animal Clinical Biochemistry.* Cambridge, England, Cambridge University Press, 1988, p 191.

320. Markel MD, Dyer RM, Hattel AL: Acute renal failure associated with application of a mercuric blister in a horse. *J Am Vet Med Assoc* 185:92, 1984.

321. Schuh JCL, Ross C, Meschter C: Concurrent mercuric blister and dimethyl sulfoxide (DMSO) application as a cause of mercury toxicity in two horses. *Equine Vet J* 20:68, 1988.

322. Osweiler GD, Carson TL, Buck WB, et al: *Clinical and Diagnostic Veterinary Toxicology,* ed 3. Dubuque, Iowa, Kendall/Hunt, 1985, p 121.

323. Roberts MC, Seawright AA, Ng JC, et al: Some effects of chronic mercuric chloride intoxication on renal function in a horse. *Vet Hum Toxicol* 24:415, 1982.

324. Seawright AA, Roberts MC, Costigan P: Chronic methylmercurialism in a horse. *Vet Hum Toxicol* 20:6, 1978.

325. Gonick HC: Nephropathies of heavy metal intoxication. In Massry SG, Glassock RJ, eds: *Textbook of Nephrology,* ed 1, vol 1. Baltimore, Williams & Wilkins, 1983, p 6.184.

Index

Note: Page numbers in *italics* refer to illustrations; page numbers followed by t refer to tables.

ISBN   0-7216-3524-5

90038